Skeletal Imaging

ATLAS OF THE SPINE AND EXTREMITIES

John A. M. Taylor, D.C., D.A.C.B.R.
Associate Professor
New York Chiropractic College
Seneca Falls, New York

Formerly:
Associate Professor of Radiology
Western States Chiropractic College
Portland, Oregon

Donald Resnick, M.D.
Chief, Osteoradiology Section
Department of Radiology
Veterans Affairs Medical Center
University of California San Diego
San Diego, California

W.B. SAUNDERS COMPANY
A Harcourt Health Sciences Company
Philadelphia London New York St. Louis Sydney Toronto

W.B. SAUNDERS COMPANY
A Harcourt Health Sciences Company

The Curtis Center
Independence Square West
Philadelphia, Pennsylvania 19106

Library of Congress Cataloging-in-Publication Data

Taylor, John A. M.

Skeletal imaging: atlas of the spine and extremities / John A. M. Taylor, Donald Resnick.—1st ed.

p. cm.

ISBN 0–7216–7510–7

1. Skeleton—Imaging—Atlases. I. Resnick, Donald. II. Title. [DNLM: 1. Spine—radiography—Atlases. 2. Bone and Bones—radiography—Atlases. 3. Diagnostic Imaging—Atlases. 4. Extremities—radiography—Atlases. WE 17 T243s 2000]
RC930.5.T39 2000 616.7′10754—dc21

DNLM/DLC 99–059402

Editorial Manager: Lisette Bralow
Developmental Editor: Catherine Fix
Manuscript Editor: Mary Reinwald
Production Manager: Frank Polizzano
Illustration Specialist: Walt Verbitski
Book Designer: Nicholas Rook

SKELETAL IMAGING: Atlas of the Spine and Extremities ISBN 0–7216–7510–7

Printed in the United States of America.

Last digit is the print number: 9 8 7 6 5 4 3 2 1

To the memory of my parents,
Ronald and Marion Taylor,
and to the memory of my brothers,
Ronnie and Kenny;

And to my teachers, friends, and mentors,
Douglas G. Brandvold, Peter H. Broomhall,
Alan Dawe, Ray A. Sherman, Felix G. Bauer,
Joseph W. Howe, and Donald Resnick.

J.A.M.T.

To my coauthor, John,
whose energy, enthusiasm, and dedication
were, in reality, the driving force
during the preparation of this text.

D.R.

Preface

Four years ago, the authors identified the need for a text of skeletal imaging organized according to anatomic region, a single-volume atlas designed for radiologists and other clinicians who routinely interpret images of the musculoskeletal system. Both authors believed that such a text would serve as a useful study guide for radiology residents and other clinicians-in-training who were preparing for certification examinations.

This atlas emphasizes the everyday appearance of skeletal disorders in routine radiographs but also includes computed tomographic (CT) scans, radionuclide studies, and magnetic resonance (MR) images. It includes a description of the appearance of normal developmental anatomy and major anomalies and anatomic variants, and it demonstrates the full range of the most frequently encountered conditions including dysplasias, physical injuries, internal derangements of joints, articular disorders, and bone tumors, as well as metabolic, hematologic, and infectious diseases.

With regard to organization of this text, Chapter 1, "Introduction to Skeletal Disorders: General Concepts," consists of 17 tables summarizing the general characteristics of the most common disorders discussed and illustrated throughout the text. These tables offer an overview of information such as age of onset, sites of involvement, clinical features, and general imaging features. This chapter was developed to avoid repetition of background material about disorders that affect several anatomic regions. Chapters 2 to 17 represent stand-alone monographs, each dealing with a specific anatomic site. The tables in these chapters emphasize only the site-specific manifestations of each entity, and they provide a sense of the range of disorders that characteristically affect that site. Furthermore, in each of these regional chapters, most of the important conditions are illustrated with routine radiographs, some of which are supplemented with conventional tomograms, CT or bone scans, or MR images, or combinations of these. In addition, the chapters dealing with spinal regions and joints contain tables and illustrations of the normal developmental anatomy of that region through infancy, childhood, and adolescence. When reading these chapters, it may be useful, or even necessary, to refer to Chapter 1 for a more detailed discussion of the general features of a particular disorder.

The major emphasis of this work, however, is on the illustrations that the authors believe represent the most characteristic or typical presentations of disease entities. For the most part, the cases include commonly encountered disorders, although some disorders that are seen less commonly also are included because they are important to consider with regard to differential diagnosis. Purposely, the illustrations are as large as possible in order to best display the imaging findings. Each is accompanied by a detailed legend beginning with the primary diagnosis and followed by a discussion of the imaging findings and any available and important clinical data. When MR imaging is displayed, detailed imaging parameters are included in the legend.

At least one useful reference for each condition has been included. The references are indicated not only in the tables but also in the figure legends. These reference citations indicate the major sources of material and serve to direct the reader to further discussion. In Chapter 1, a bibliography of recommended readings includes many textbooks dealing with various aspects of skeletal radiology that served as sources for information.

It is hoped that the regional format, along with the inclusion of numerous tables, large, crystal-clear illustrations, and comprehensive figure legends, significantly increases the utility of this atlas as an everyday reference source. Further, it is both authors' hope that this book serves to increase the likelihood of accurate diagnosis when imaging studies of the musculoskeletal system are interpreted.

John A. M. Taylor
Donald Resnick

Acknowledgments

The authors wish to acknowledge their appreciation of several persons who have generously contributed their time, effort, and case material during the production of this text. First, as is indicated in the legends associated with the illustrations, approximately 140 colleagues contributed one or more cases for inclusion in this atlas. Their willingness to share case material with us is very much appreciated. Of these persons, many deserve special mention for their donation of several cases: Drs. John Amberg, Appa Anderson, Richard Arkless, Felix Bauer, Gabrielle Bergman, Eve Bonic, Enrique Bosch, Sevil Kursunoglu Brahme, Thomas Broderick, Ann Brower, Clement Chen, Armando D'Abreu, Larry Danzig, Steven Eilenberg, Douglas Goodwin, Guerdon Greenway, Jorg Haller, Al Nemcek, Beverly Harger, Brian Howard, Roger Kerr, Phillipe Kindynis, Michael Mitchell, Arthur Newberg, Mini Pathria, Carlos Pineda, Jean Schils, Jack Slivka, Gary Smith, Richard Stiles, Phillip VanderStoep, Christopher Van Lom, and Vinton Vint. Numerous radiographs illustrating normal developmental anatomy were donated by Dr. David Sartoris from the University of California, San Diego; Dr. Jeffrey Cooley from Los Angeles College of Chiropractic; and Dr. Beverly Harger from Western States Chiropractic College. The authors also wish to acknowledge a number of persons who have willingly proofread portions of the manuscript at various stages of completion: Bill Adams, Eve Bonic, Todd Knudsen, Chad Warshel, Peter Broomhall, and especially Gary Smith, who was kind enough to carefully read and reread every chapter.

The atlas would not have been possible without the input of a team of professionals at W.B. Saunders: Lisette Bralow, Frank Polizzano, Mary Reinwald, Walt Verbitski, Nicholas Rook, and Nancy Matthews. Their expertise and advice were crucial to the production of the atlas.

Finally, two members of our team who from the outset were absolutely essential to the completion of the text deserve recognition for their extraordinary efforts. Debra Trudell, our technical assistant, produced the photographic reproductions. Catherine Fix, our copy editor, meticulously edited every table, caption, and reference throughout the text. Their expertise, attention to detail, and demand for excellence are evident throughout the atlas. The authors are deeply indebted to Debra and Catherine and, indeed, to all of the persons cited here.

Contents

CHAPTER 1

Introduction to Skeletal Disorders: General Concepts

Many bone and joint disorders affect multiple regions of the skeleton. The tables in this chapter list anomalies and anatomic variants (Table 1–1), skeletal dysplasias (Table 1–2), fractures (Tables 1–3 and 1–4), articular injuries (Table 1–5), articular disorders (Tables 1–6 to 1–9), bone tumors (Tables 1–10 and 1–11), tumor-like lesions of bone (Table 1–12), metabolic, nutritional, and endocrine disorders (Table 1–13), hematologic disorders (Table 1–14), osteonecrosis (Table 1–15), osteochondroses (Table 1–16), and infectious disorders of bones and joints (Table 1–17). These tables are intended to provide the reader with an overview of the common clinical, laboratory, and radiographic features of the more common disorders that typically appear in more than one skeletal location. Site-specific findings and features unique to each anatomic region are discussed further in subsequent chapters.

TABLE 1–1. Developmental Anomalies, Anatomic Variants, and Sources of Diagnostic Error: Concepts and Terminology*

Entity	Characteristics	Terminology	Examples	
			Spine	*Extremities*
Developmental anomaly	Marked deviation from normal standards as a result of a congenital or hereditary defect; such malformations usually represent a primary problem in the morphogenesis of a tissue May be asymptomatic or associated with significant clinical manifestations Spinal anomalies—general concepts: 1. Most spinal anomalies occur at transitional areas such as the craniocervical, cervicothoracic, and thoracolumbar regions 2. When one anomaly is identified, always search for more because anomalies may be multiple 3. Anomalies may be isolated or associated with a syndrome 4. Osseous anomalies may be associated with underlying neurologic or visceral anomalies	Nonsegmentation or synostosis Aplasia or agenesis Hypoplasia Hyperplasia Supernumerary bones	Block vertebrae Odontoid agenesis Hypoplastic C1 posterior arch Transverse process hyperplasia Transitional segments	Tarsal coalition Radial aplasia Glenoid hypoplasia Focal gigantism Polydactyly
Anatomic variant	A modification of some anatomic characteristic that is considered normal Usually not associated with clinical manifestations; often encountered as an incidental finding	Areas of normal trabecular diminution or prominence	Prominent Hahn's venous channels	Humeral pseudocyst Ward's triangle of femur Pseudocystic region of calcaneus
		Normal sites of osseous irregularity	Cupid's bow configuration of vertebral body simulating end-plate fracture or Schmorl's nodes	Avulsive cortical irregularity of the femur
Sources of diagnostic error	Misdiagnosis may occur under various conditions: Normal structures may be interpreted as abnormal owing to overlying shadows created by gas, soft tissue, or malpositioned structures	Overlying normal anatomy	Mach effect overlying odontoid, simulating fracture	Quadriceps muscle plane overlying femur, simulating fracture
	Rarefactions, irregularities, depressions, or proliferations of bone may be mistaken for evidence of disease	Anatomic irregularities	Normal notch in superior articulating process, simulating cervical pillar fracture	Normal sclerosis and fragmentation of calcaneal apophysis, simulating osteochondrosis
	Slight modifications in osseous anatomy may be judged to be significant	Anatomic variants	Osteosclerotic anterior arch of atlas, simulating an osteoblastic lesion	Rhomboid fossa in clavicle, simulating a destructive lesion

*The differentiation of anomalies, anatomic variants, and sources of error often is indistinct, owing to considerable overlap in the definitions.
Data from Smith DW: Recognizable Patterns of Human Deformation. Identification and Management of Mechanical Effects of Morphogenesis. Philadelphia, WB Saunders, 1981.

TABLE 1–2. Skeletal Dysplasias and Other Congenital Disorders

Entity	General Characteristics	General Radiographic Findings
Achondroplasia	Relatively common rhizomelic dwarfism Accentuated lumbar lordosis, waddling gait, prominent forehead, depressed nasal bridge, trident hand Short proximal extremities, normal length of spine ***Complications:*** Spinal stenosis Brain stem compression from narrow foramen magnum	Spinal stenosis with posterior scalloping of vertebral bodies and decreased spinal canal diameter Vertebral bodies may be flattened or wedge-shaped Diaphyseal widening of long bones Narrow thorax, champagne glass pelvis Splayed and cupped metaphyses of long bones
Diastrophic dysplasia	Rare autosomal recessive dwarfing dysplasia	Short stature, progressive scoliosis, kyphosis
Spondyloepiphyseal dysplasia	***Congenita form:*** Autosomal recessive, rhizomelic dwarfism Short trunk, respiratory and visual complications ***Tarda form:*** Milder, X-linked recessive form seen only in males ***Rare lethal form:*** Also termed hypochondrogenesis	***Congenita form:*** Scoliosis, accentuated kyphosis and lordosis, pectus carinatum, delayed ossification, platyspondyly, hypoplasia of the odontoid with atlantoaxial instability ***Tarda form:*** Heaped-up vertebrae, platyspondyly, disc space narrowing
Dysplasia epiphysealis hemimelica	Trevor's disease Uncommon developmental disorder Asymmetric cartilaginous overgrowth in one or more epiphyses May be localized or generalized Joint dysfunction, pain, limitation of motion, and a mass may accompany the disease	Resembles large eccentric osteochondroma arising from epiphyses particularly about the knee and ankle Bulky irregular ossification extending into soft tissues Computed tomographic (CT) or magnetic resonance (MR) imaging may be useful to show the exact location and extent of the lesion as well as the presence of joint involvement
Mucopolysaccharidosis (MPS)	Enzyme deficiencies result in radiographic changes termed dysostosis multiplex Two types most commonly encountered: Hurler's and Morquio's syndromes	***MPS I-H (Hurler's syndrome):*** Atlantoaxial instability may be present Rounded anterior vertebral margins with inferior beaking Posterior scalloping of vertebral bodies Paddle ribs, flared ilia, coxa valga and coxa vara deformities ***MPS IV (Morquio's syndrome):*** Hypoplastic or absent odontoid process with atlantoaxial instability Flattened vertebral bodies (platyspondyly) Posterior scalloping of vertebral bodies Short, thick tubular bones
Fibrodysplasia ossificans progressiva	Rare autosomal dominant disease Progressive ossification of skeletal muscle Results in limitation of motion, weakness, and eventual respiratory failure	Sheet-like ossification within soft tissues of neck, trunk, and extremities Hypoplastic vertebral bodies and intervertebral discs Apophyseal joint ankylosis Shortening of thumbs and great toes
Cleidocranial dysplasia	Rare autosomal dominant disorder characterized by incomplete ossification Widened cranial vault Drooping shoulders Abnormal gait, scoliosis, hypermobility, and dislocations of shoulders and hips Deafness, severe dental caries, and, infrequently, basilar impression	Absent or hypoplastic clavicles Spine: multiple midline defects of the neural arch (spina bifida) Pelvis: widened symphysis pubis, coxa valga, coxa vara, underdeveloped bones with small pelvic bowl Skull: wormian bones, persistent metopic suture

Table continued on following page

TABLE 1–2. Skeletal Dysplasias and Other Congenital Disorders *Continued*

Entity	General Characteristics	General Radiographic Findings
Osteopetrosis	Sclerosing dysplasia Benign, intermediate, and lethal forms Complications: anemia, osteomyelitis, blindness, deafness, hemorrhage; brittle bones predispose to bone fragility and pathologic fracture	Patterns of osteosclerosis: diffuse osteosclerosis, bone-within-bone appearance, sandwich vertebrae
Osteopoikilosis	Asymptomatic sclerosing dysplasia No associated complications	Multiple 2- to 3-mm circular foci of osteosclerosis Symmetric periarticular lesions resembling bone islands predominate about the hip, shoulder, and knee
Osteopathia striata	Extremely rare asymptomatic sclerosing dysplasia No associated complications	Regular, linear, vertically oriented bands of osteosclerosis extending from the metaphysis for variable distances into the diaphysis Metaphyseal flaring also may be seen May be related to cranial sclerosis and focal dermal hypoplasia (Goltz's syndrome)
Melorheostosis	Rare sclerosing dysplasia *Clinical findings:* May be associated with intermittent joint swelling, pain and limitation of motion, muscle contractures, tendon and ligament shortening, growth disturbances in affected limbs, and other musculoskeletal abnormalities	Usual pattern: hemimelic involvement of a single limb Peripherally located cortical hyperostosis resembling flowing candle wax on the surface of bones Para-articular soft tissue calcification and ossification may occur and may even lead to joint ankylosis May be positive on bone scans
Mixed sclerosing bone dystrophy	Rare condition in which patients have radiologic findings characteristic of more than one, and occasionally all, of the sclerosing dysplasias	Combinations of osteopetrosis, osteopoikilosis, osteopathia striata, and melorheostosis
Chondrodysplasia punctata	Conradi-Hünermann syndrome or stippled epiphyses Several different types of this rare multiple epiphyseal dysplasia have been identified, including mild and lethal forms Mild dwarfism, mental retardation, and joint contractures	Stippled calcification of vertebral bodies and epiphyses of the extremities In the rhizomelic form, coronal clefts are present within the vertebral bodies
Osteogenesis imperfecta	Inherited connective tissue syndrome Type II, congenital lethal form, has a high infant mortality rate Type I, the more common form, exhibits milder changes and is associated with a normal life expectancy Associated with osteoporosis and bone fragility, various degrees of dwarfism, blue sclera, ligament laxity, dentinogenesis imperfecta, and premature otosclerosis Complicated by multiple fractures, deafness, and pneumonia	Severe osteoporosis Pencil-thin cortices Multiple fractures of vertebrae and long bones Bowing deformities of long bones, especially lower extremity Rare cystic form—ballooning of bone, metaphyseal flaring, and honeycombed appearance of thick trabeculae
Progressive diaphyseal dysplasia	Rare autosomal dominant disorder also termed Camurati-Engelmann disease Typically bilateral and confined to the diaphyseal region of bone Progressive diaphyseal dysplasia affects predominantly the lower extremity Usually self-limited, resolving by 30 to 35 years of age	Bilateral fusiform thickening of the diaphysis of the long bones Cortical thickening and hyperostosis result in increased diaphyseal radiodensity
Hereditary osteo-onychodysostosis syndrome	Also termed Fong's syndrome, HOOD syndrome, and nail-patella syndrome Associated with abnormalities of the fingernails and toenails	Absent or hypoplastic patellae Patellar dislocation, iliac horns, and radial head dislocation

TABLE 1–2. Skeletal Dysplasias and Other Congenital Disorders *Continued*

Entity	General Characteristics	General Radiographic Findings
Marfan syndrome	Autosomal dominant connective tissue disorder Muscular hypoplasia, joint laxity, dislocations, cataracts Complications: aortic aneurysm, lens dislocation	Long slender bones, arachnodactyly, thin cortices Kyphoscoliosis in 40 to 60 per cent of persons Posterior vertebral body scalloping from dural ectasia
Ehlers-Danlos syndrome	Rare connective tissue disorder characterized by joint hypermobility, blood vessel fragility, and skin elasticity; many forms identified Complications: valvular insufficiency, aortic aneurysm and dissection	Posterior scalloping of vertebral bodies Platyspondyly and kyphoscoliosis Genu recurvatum and other joint subluxations Heterotopic myositis ossificans Subcutaneous hemangiomas (calcified phleboliths)

For more detailed discussion, refer to:

Murray RO: The Radiology of Skeletal Disorders. 3rd Ed. New York, Churchill Livingstone, 1989.
Taybi H, Lachman RS: Radiology of Syndromes, Metabolic Disorders and Skeletal Dysplasias. 4th Ed. St. Louis, Mosby–Year Book, 1996.
Yochum TR, Rowe LJ: Essentials of Skeletal Radiology. 2nd Ed. Baltimore, Williams & Wilkins, 1996.

TABLE 1–3. Fractures in Adults: Concepts and Terminology

Entity	Classification	Typical Sites of Involvement	Characteristics
Acute fractures	Orientation	Any tubular bone	*Transverse:* bending or angular forces in long bones; tensile or traction forces in short bones; also pathologic fracture such as occurs with tumors *Oblique:* compression, bending, and torsion forces *Oblique-transverse:* combination of axial compression and bending forces *Spiral:* torsion forces
	Alignment	Any tubular bone, particularly lower extremity	Varus angulation: angulation of the distal fragment toward the midline of the body Valgus angulation: angulation of the distal fragment away from the midline of the body Anterior or posterior angulation: anterior or posterior angulation of the distal fragment
	Position	Any tubular bone	Relationship of fracture fragments, exclusive of angulation: displaced or undisplaced fractures *Displacement:* abnormalities of apposition and rotation *Apposition:* degree of bone contact at the fracture site: undisplaced fractures have 100 per cent apposition; fracture surfaces may be separated and are termed distracted fractures; overlapping of fracture surfaces with consequent shortening is termed a bayonet deformity *Rotation:* rotation about the longitudinal axis; difficult to assess from routine radiographs
	Open fracture	Any site, particularly femur, tibia, and humerus	Communication between fracture and outside environment because of disruption of the skin Radiographic findings: soft tissue defect, bone protruding beyond soft tissues, subcutaneous or intra-articular gas, foreign material beneath skin, absent pieces of bone Associated with high-impact trauma; high rate of infection
	Closed fracture	Any bone Most fractures are closed	Simple fracture in which the bone does not break through the skin

Table continued on following page

TABLE 1–3. Fractures in Adults: Concepts and Terminology *Continued*

Entity	Classification	Typical Sites of Involvement	Characteristics
	Comminuted fracture	Any bone, especially long, tubular bones	Fracture with more than two fracture fragments Associated with high-impact injuries and crush injuries
	Butterfly fragment	Femoral and humeral diaphyses	Wedge-shaped fragment arising from the shaft of a tubular bone at the apex of the force input
	Segmental fracture	Femur, rib (flail chest)	Fracture lines isolate a segment of the shaft of a tubular bone
Impaction fractures	Depression fracture	Tibial plateau	One hard bone surface is driven into an apposing softer bone surface
	Compression fracture	Vertebral body	Forceful flexion of the spine resulting in a wedge fracture of the vertebral body with depression of the end plate within the spongiosa bone of the vertebral body
Pathologic fractures		Sites of skeletal metastasis, simple bone cyst, enchondroma, giant cell tumor, plasma cell myeloma, lymphoma, Ewing's sarcoma, and other large osteolytic or osteosclerotic lesions	Fracture through a bone weakened by a disease process (such as osteoporosis, neoplasm, infection, or metabolic disease) with forces insufficient to fracture a normal bone *Insufficiency fracture* is a term commonly applied to pathologic fractures occurring at sites of nontumorous lesions (see stress fractures)
Stress fractures	Fatigue fracture	Pars interarticularis of lumbar vertebrae (spondylolysis), metatarsal bones in military recruits (march fracture), and the lower extremity in athletes, joggers, and dancers	Fracture resulting from repeated cyclic loading applied to normal bones, with the load being less than that which causes acute fracture of bone Athletic, recreational, and occupational injuries are most common causes Tibial or femoral fatigue fractures may be longitudinal, involving a major portion of the diaphysis
	Insufficiency fracture	Sacrum, pubic rami, and lower extremity about the ankle, foot, knee, and hip	Pathologic fracture through a bone weakened by a disease process, initiated with forces insufficient to fracture a normal bone Disease processes include rheumatoid arthritis, osteoporosis, Paget's disease, osteomalacia or rickets, hyperparathyroidism, renal osteodystrophy, osteogenesis imperfecta, osteopetrosis, fibrous dyplasia, and irradiation High signal intensity on T2-weighted and low signal intensity on T1-weighted spin echo magnetic resonance (MR) sequences; scintigraphy also positive
Acute chondral and osteochondral fractures		Distal portion of femur, patella, humeral head, glenoid rim, elbow, or hip	Fracture of cartilage alone: chondral fracture Fracture of bone and cartilage: osteochondral fracture Shearing, rotational, or tangentially aligned impaction forces generated by abnormal joint motion may result in fractures of two apposing joint surfaces Momentary, persistent, or recurrent dislocations and subluxations may result in these injuries Associated with painful joint effusion, joint locking, clicking, and limitation of motion; intra-articular bodies common; bodies may attach to synovium and eventually resorb

Table continued on following page

TABLE 1–3. Fractures in Adults: Concepts and Terminology *Continued*

Entity	Classification	Typical Sites of Involvement	Characteristics
Osteochondritis dissecans		Femoral condyles and talus most typical sites Less common sites: other tarsal bones, tibia, humeral head, glenoid cavity, acetabulum, and elbow (capitulum) Patellar involvement is rare	Fragmentation and possible separation of a portion of the articular surface Adolescent onset most frequent, but occurs from childhood to middle age Male>female Symptoms and signs usually begin in patients between ages 15 and 20 years; painful or painless joint effusion, joint locking, clicking, and limitation of motion Significant history of trauma in 50 per cent of cases MR arthrography and computed tomographic arthrography are the most useful imaging techniques
Avulsion injuries	Avulsion fracture	Tibial tubercle, olecranon, pelvis, hip, tibial eminence, spinous process	Osseous fragment is pulled from the parent bone by a tendon, ligament, or portion of the joint capsule
Improper fracture healing	Delayed union	Scaphoid and improperly immobilized fracture sites	Conversion of fibrocartilage to bone is delayed or temporarily stopped
	Nonunion	Scaphoid, femoral neck, tibia, clavicle, odontoid process (os odontoideum), or any site improperly immobilized Also occurs in neurofibromatosis and fibrous dysplasia	Fracture site fails to heal completely during a period of 6 to 9 months after the injury Characterized by a pseudarthrosis consisting of a synovium-lined cavity and fluid typically related to persistent motion at the nonunion site
	Malunion	Any bone, especially long bones such as the tibia and clavicle	Fracture that heals in an improper position Excessive angular or rotational deformity Adults: leads to deformity that may require surgical correction Children: often temporary phenomenon that may disappear spontaneously with further skeletal growth

TABLE 1–4. Fractures in Children: Concepts and Terminology

Entity	Classification	Typical Sites of Involvement	Characteristics
Incomplete fractures	Greenstick fracture	Proximal metaphysis of the tibia and the middle third of the radius and ulna	Incomplete fracture that perforates one cortex, extends into the medullary bone, and does not involve the opposite cortex
	Torus fracture	Distal end of radius and ulna and, less commonly, the tibia	Incomplete fracture resulting in buckling of the cortex Usually involves a longitudinal compression force insufficient to create a complete discontinuity of the bone Most frequent in children and osteoporotic persons
	Lead pipe fracture	Radius	Combined compressive and angular forces result in a combination of greenstick and torus fractures Most frequent in children
	Bowing fracture	Radius and ulna; less commonly, the clavicle, ribs, tibia, humerus, fibula, and femur	Plastic response of a long tubular bone to longitudinal stress Bowing occurs in the absence of cortical discontinuity; in the case of neighboring bones (radius and ulna or tibia and fibula), one bone typically fractures or dislocates, whereas bowing is identified in the adjacent bone Seen almost exclusively in children

Table continued on following page

TABLE 1–4. Fractures in Children: Concepts and Terminology *Continued*

Entity	Classification	Typical Sites of Involvement	Characteristics
Toddler's fractures		Distal tibial diaphysis, fibula, femur, metatarsal bones, and, less commonly, the calcaneus, cuboid bone, pubic rami, or patella	Acute onset of fracture in children between the ages of 1 and 3 years Radiographs may initially be negative; scintigraphy useful in detecting such occult fractures Classic toddler's fracture: nondisplaced, oblique fracture of the distal tibial diaphysis
Trauma to synchondroses (growth plate injuries)		Distal end of radius (50 per cent) Distal end of humerus (17 per cent) Distal end of tibia (11 per cent) Distal end of fibula (9 per cent) Distal end of ulna (6 per cent) Proximal end of humerus (3 per cent)	Up to 15 per cent of all fractures to the tubular bones in children younger than 16 years of age involve the growth plate and neighboring bone 25 to 30 per cent of patients develop some degree of growth deformity
	Salter-Harris classification:		
	Type I (6 per cent)		Pure epiphyseal separation; fracture of cartilaginous growth plate; no fracture of adjacent bones Slipped capital femoral epiphysis
	Type II (75 per cent)		Growth plate fracture with associated metaphyseal fracture; metaphyseal fragment termed Thurston-Holland fragment or "corner sign"
	Type III (8 per cent)		Growth plate fracture with associated vertically oriented epiphyseal fracture
	Type IV (10 per cent)		Vertical fracture through the epiphysis, growth plate, and metaphysis
	Type V (1 per cent)		Crushing or compressive injury of the growth plate with no associated osseous fracture Frequently overlooked
	Chronic stress injury	Growth centers of the distal end of the radius and ulna in competitive gymnasts; also proximal portion of the humerus, distal ends of the femur and tibia in other young athletes	Chronic application of stress to the developing growth center in vigorous or repetitious physical activity Part of the physis appears widened and irregular with accompanying sclerosis of the adjacent metaphysis; often unilateral or asymmetric distribution
Child abuse	Traumatic abuse of children	Fractures: Ribs Humerus Femur Tibia Small bones of hands and feet Skull Spine (rare) Sternum (rare) Lateral portion of clavicle (rare) Scapula (rare)	An estimated 200,000 reports of child abuse and 2500 deaths are attributed to child abuse in the United States annually About 10 per cent of children younger than the age of 5 years seen for trauma by emergency room physicians have inflicted injuries that are detectable radiographically in 50 to 70 per cent of cases Typical age range is between 1 and 4 years; after this age, children generally are able to escape the abuser or at least verbalize what has occurred Humeral fractures in infants and femoral fractures in crawling children should raise suspicion of abuse *Radiographic findings:* Fractures in different phases of healing, subperiosteal hemorrhage with periostitis, metaphyseal corner fractures, physeal injuries, and transverse diaphyseal or metaphyseal fractures *Differential diagnosis:* Accidental fractures such as torus fractures of the distal end of radius, toddler's fractures of the tibia, clavicular and skull fractures; normal periostitis of infancy, metaphyseal changes of normal growth, congenital insensitivity to pain, rickets, osteogenesis imperfecta, metaphyseal and spondylometaphyseal dysplasia, Menkes' kinky hair syndrome, congenital syphilis, and infantile cortical hyperostosis (Caffey's disease)

TABLE 1–5. Articular Injuries: Concepts and Terminology

Entity	Typical Sites of Involvement	Characteristics
Joint effusion	Knee Elbow Tibiotalar joint Hip Glenohumeral joint	Accumulation of excessive synovial fluid within joint Bland effusion associated with acute injury or internal joint derangement Nonbloody effusions usually appear 12 to 24 hours after injury Absence of effusion with severe trauma may indicate capsular rupture of such a degree that fluid extravasates into the soft tissues surrounding the joint (especially the knee) Proliferative effusion associated with synovial proliferation as in inflammatory arthropathy and villonodular synovitis Pyarthrosis: purulent material in joint from pyogenic septic arthritis
Hemarthrosis	Any injured joint	Accumulation of blood within joint Hemarthroses usually result in joint effusion within the first few hours after injury May result from acute ligament injury, villonodular synovitis, hemophilia, synovial hemangioma, or other articular diseases
Lipohemarthrosis	Knee Glenohumeral joint Hip	Accumulation of blood and lipid material within synovial joint Fat-blood interface seen on cross-table horizontal beam lateral radiographs as well as on transaxial and sagittal magnetic resonance (MR) images Double fluid-fluid levels on MR images are more specific for lipohemarthrosis than a single fluid-fluid level Usually related to acute intra-articular fracture
Pneumolipohemarthrosis	Hip	Accumulation of gas, blood, and lipid material within synovial joint Typically seen after fracture-dislocation Most evident on computed tomography (CT) scans
Sprain	Acromioclavicular joint Tibiotalar joint Knee Elbow	Grade I: Mild sprain—stretching of the ligament but no tear Grade II: Moderate sprain—partial ligamentous disruption Grade III: Complete ligamentous rupture (with or without dislocation)
Subluxation	Glenohumeral joint, patellofemoral joint, and many other sites	Partial loss of contact between two osseous surfaces that normally articulate
Dislocation	Glenohumeral joint, acromioclavicular joint, patellofemoral joint, hip joint, apophyseal joints, and many other sites	Complete loss of contact between two osseous surfaces that normally articulate
Trauma to symphyses	Symphysis pubis, discovertebral joint, and manubriosternal joint	Abnormal separation of a joint containing fibrocartilage that normally is only slightly movable Cartilaginous nodes, posttraumatic annular vacuum cleft, limbus vertebrae, and apophyseal ring avulsion fractures resulting from discovertebral trauma
Heterotopic ossification	Large muscle groups in thigh, leg, upper arm	Self-limiting posttraumatic myositis ossificans Usually results from ossification of a chronic muscle hematoma *Radiographic findings:* Faint calcific intermuscular or intramuscular shadow may appear within 2 to 6 weeks of injury Well-defined region of ossification aligned parallel to the long axis of the tibia and fibula may be evident within 6 to 8 weeks Zonal phenomenon—ossific periphery with radiolucent center Cleavage plane may be evident between ossification and adjacent bone, helping to differentiate it from parosteal osteosarcoma Associated periostitis may relate to subperiosteal hemorrhage May be surrounded by edema seen on MR images *Differential diagnosis:* Aggressive neoplasms such as parosteal, periosteal, and soft tissue osteosarcoma, as well as Ewing's sarcoma, liposarcoma, and synovial sarcoma

TABLE 1–6. Degenerative Joint Disease and Related Disorders

Entity	Typical Age of Onset (Years)	Sex	Target Sites of Involvement	Clinical Characteristics	General Radiographic Findings
Primary osteoarthrosis	>40	Female : male, 10 : 1	Knee Hip Hand Foot Acromioclavicular joint Sacroiliac joint	Articular degeneration in the absence of any obvious underlying abnormality Accompanies aging *Clinical findings:* Variable, depending on site of involvement Periarticular bony enlargement; e.g., Heberden's nodes Pain and tenderness variable Joint stiffness and decreased mobility Joint crepitus Occasional instability Subluxation and deformity	Nonuniform or, less commonly, uniform joint space narrowing Osteophytes Subchondral sclerosis Subchondral cysts Subluxation, deformity, malalignment Buttressing Intra-articular osseous bodies; rarely, secondary synovial osteochondromatosis Absence of soft tissue swelling Absence of osteoporosis Fibrous ankylosis (rare) Unilateral or bilateral asymmetric distribution
Secondary osteoarthrosis	>25	Male = female	Glenohumeral joint Elbow Knee Hip Hand Foot Sacroiliac joint Acromioclavicular joint	Articular degeneration that is produced by alterations from a preexisting affliction; some of these are as follows: Previous septic arthritis or inflammatory arthritis, slipped capital epiphysis, developmental dysplasia of the hip, fracture or dislocation, obesity, Legg-Calvé-Perthes disease, osteonecrosis, acromegaly, ochronosis, and occupational or athletic injury Also occurs with crystal deposition diseases, synovial inflammatory processes, and other articular diseases *Clinical findings:* Same as those of primary osteoarthrosis; findings may coexist with, or be obscured by, those of the primary disorder	(See Primary osteoarthrosis) Appearance of osteoarthrosis may obscure (or be obscured by) that of the primary articular process
Erosive (inflammatory) osteoarthritis	>40	Female	Hand	Unique form of inflammatory interphalangeal osteoarthritis *Clinical findings:* Acute, inflammatory painful episodes of swelling and erythema overlying the interphalangeal joints of the fingers Prominent subluxation and osseous nodules (Heberden's nodes) May clinically resemble synovial inflammatory diseases	Central erosions Nonuniform joint space narrowing Subchondral sclerosis Osteophytes Subluxation

TABLE 1–6. Degenerative Joint Disease and Related Disorders *Continued*

Entity	Typical Age of Onset (Years)	Sex	Target Sites of Involvement	Clinical Characteristics	General Radiographic Findings
Degenerative spine disease	>30	Male = female	C5-C7 T2-T5 T10-T12 L4-S1 Discovertebral junction Uncovertebral joint Apophyseal joint Costovertebral joint	Degenerative spine disease includes: Intervertebral osteochondrosis Spondylosis deformans Uncovertebral osteoarthrosis Apophyseal joint osteoarthrosis Costovertebral joint osteoarthrosis *Clinical findings:* Variable, depending on anatomic site and severity Symptoms range from absent to severe and include acute or chronic pain, stiffness, radiculopathy (rare), and associated muscle spasm Poor correlation between symptoms and radiographic findings; patients with severe degenerative changes may have minimal or no symptoms, whereas those with minimal degenerative changes may have considerable symptoms	Spondylosis deformans: Osteophytes and osseous ridging Intervertebral osteochondrosis: Disc space narrowing Intradiscal vacuum phenomenon Disc calcification (rare) Subchondral bone sclerosis Schmorl's (cartilaginous) nodes Uncovertebral joint osteoarthrosis: Sclerosis, hypertrophy, and joint space narrowing Apophyseal (facet) joint osteoarthrosis: Sclerosis, hypertrophy, joint space narrowing, subluxation, capsular laxity, and synovial cysts Frequently contributes to foraminal stenosis
Diffuse idiopathic skeletal hyperostosis (DISH)	>50	Male>female	Thoracic spine Cervical spine Lumbar spine T7-T11 most common segments	DISH affects 25 per cent of men and 15 per cent of women older than 50 years of age *Clinical findings:* Symptoms are mild in comparison with the often dramatic radiographic signs Middle to lower back pain and stiffness Restricted motion Recurrent Achilles tendinosis Recurrent "tennis elbow" Cervical dysphagia Palpable calcaneal, patellar, and olecranon enthesophytes	Axial skeleton: Flowing hyperostosis: thick (1 to 20 mm) linear shield of ossification along the anterolateral aspect of the spine (see Diagnostic criteria) Appendicular skeleton: Enthesopathy and ligament ossification about the pelvis, hip, knee, foot, heel, and other extra-axial sites *Diagnostic criteria:* 1. Flowing calcification and ossification along the anterolateral aspect of at least four contiguous vertebral body segments with or without associated localized pointed excrescences at the intervening vertebral body–intervertebral disc junctions 2. Relative preservation of intervertebral disc height in the involved vertebral segment and absence of extensive degenerative disc disease 3. Absence of apophyseal joint bony ankylosis and sacroiliac joint erosion, sclerosis, or intra-articular osseous fusion

TABLE 1–7. Inflammatory Articular Disorders

Entity	Typical Age of Onset (Years)	Sex	Target Sites of Involvement	Clinical Characteristics	Laboratory and Radiographic Findings
Rheumatoid arthritis	25–55	Female : male, 2 or 3 : 1	Hand Foot Wrist Knee Elbow Glenohumeral joint Acromioclavicular joint Cervical spine	Bilateral symmetric polyarticular synovial inflammatory process Five to 15 times as common as ankylosing spondylitis *Clinical findings:* Acute or chronic episodes of painful joint swelling Prodromal symptoms: fatigue, anorexia, weight loss, malaise, muscular pain and stiffness Capsular and ligamentous laxity Muscular contraction and spasm Bursitis, tendinitis, and tenosynovitis *Diagnostic criteria*:* 1. Morning stiffness in and around joints lasting at least 1 hour before maximal improvement 2. Soft tissue swelling (arthritis) of three or more joint areas observed by a physician 3. Swelling (arthritis) of the proximal interphalangeal, metacarpophalangeal, or wrist joints 4. Symmetric swelling (arthritis) 5. Rheumatoid nodules 6. The presence of rheumatoid factor 7. Radiographic erosions or periarticular osteopenia, or both, in hand or wrist joints, or in both Rheumatoid arthritis is defined by the presence of four or more criteria; criteria 1 through 4 must have been present for at least 6 weeks	*Laboratory findings:* Normochromic or hypochromic normocytic anemia (common) Leukocytes: normal, elevated, or, infrequently, decreased Erythrocyte sedimentation rate: markedly elevated Rheumatoid factor: present in high titers Positive LE phenomenon (8 to 27 per cent of patients) *Radiographic findings:* Fusiform soft tissue swelling (early finding) Concentric joint space narrowing (early finding) Marginal and central subchondral erosions Subchondral cysts Cortical atrophy and osteolysis Absent or mild sclerosis Periarticular osteoporosis Synovial cysts Joint instability, particularly atlantoaxial joint Fibrous ankylosis and, infrequently, bony ankylosis Deformity, subluxation, dislocation Pathologic fractures
Juvenile chronic arthritis	5–10	Variable, depending on disorder	Hand Wrist Knee Cervical spine Foot Ankle Elbow Heel Hip	Several arthropathies have been identified in children *Disorders:* 1. Juvenile-onset adult type (seropositive) rheumatoid arthritis 2. Still's disease Systemic disease Polyarticular disease Pauciarticular or monoarticular disease 3. Juvenile-onset ankylosing spondylitis and other seronegative spondyloarthropathies *Clinical findings:* Variable, depending on disorder Subcutaneous nodules Acute joint swelling, pain, and erythema Systemic manifestations: Vasculitis Hepatosplenomegaly Iridocyclitis	Soft tissue swelling Periarticular osteoporosis with metaphyseal lucent bands Diffuse joint space loss (late finding) Erosions (late finding) Periostitis Growth disturbances Apophyseal joint ankylosis Extra-axial joint ankylosis Atlantoaxial instability Bony proliferation and periostitis Epiphyseal compression fractures

Ankylosing spondylitis	15–35	Male : female, 4 : 1 to 10 : 1	Sacroiliac joint Thoracolumbar spine Cervical spine Symphysis pubis Hip Shoulder Heel	Most common seronegative spondyloarthropathy ***Clinical findings:*** Axial skeleton: Middle and low back pain and stiffness Limited lumbar and thoracic spine motion Limited chest expansion (1 inch or less) Sacroiliac joint pain Radiating pain to lower extremity (50 per cent) Muscle spasm Increased thoracic kyphosis Extra-axial skeleton: As many as 50 per cent of patients affected Mild symmetric involvement is typical Pain, tenderness, and swelling Extraskeletal findings: Iritis (20 per cent of cases) Aortic insufficiency and aneurysms Pulmonary fibrosis (upper lobes) Pleuritis Inflammatory bowel disease Amyloidosis (especially kidney)	***Laboratory findings:*** Elevated erythroctye sedimentation rate Negative rheumatoid and LE factors HLA-B27 histocompatibility antigen present in 90 per cent of patients (6 to 8 per cent of general population) ***Radiographic findings:*** Spine: marginal syndesmophytes, erosions, ligament ossification (see Tables 3–9 and 3–10) Sacroiliac joints: bilateral symmetric involvement; joint erosion initially with eventual ankylosis Extra-axial skeleton: joint erosions; partial or complete osseous ankylosis
Psoriatic arthropathy	20–50	Male = female	Hand Foot Sacroiliac joint Thoracolumbar spine Cervical spine	Seronegative spondyloarthropathy Less common than ankylosing spondylitis Two to 6 per cent of patients with psoriatic skin lesions have associated psoriatic arthropathy ***Clinical patterns:*** 1. Polyarthritis with distal and proximal interphalangeal joint involvement 2. Deforming arthritis characterized by ankylosis and arthritis mutilans 3. Symmetric rheumatoid–like arthritis (rare) 4. Asymmetric oligoarthritis or monoarthritis 5. Combination of spondyloarthropathy and sacroiliitis ***Signs and symptoms:*** Long history of psoriatic skin lesions: patchy, scaly macular lesions Nail changes: pitting, discoloration, splintering, erosion, thickening, and detachment Low back pain, fever, fatigue, stiffness, conjunctivitis, iritis, and scleritis Sternocostoclavicular hyperostosis; pustular lesions of the skin in the hand and foot (pustulosis palmaris et plantaris) are observed in some patients with hyperostosis of the clavicles, ribs, and sternum and may be related to psoriasis, chronic recurrent multifocal osteomyelitis, and the synovitis-acne-pustulosis-hyperostosis-osteomyelitis (SAPHO) syndrome	***Laboratory findings:*** HLA-B27 antigen present in as many as 60 per cent of patients with psoriatic arthropathy Mild anemia Elevated erythrocyte sedimentation rate Elevated serum uric acid levels (occasionally) Negative for rheumatoid factor ***Radiographic findings:*** Axial skeleton: Paravertebral ossification (nonmarginal parasyndesmophytes) Unilateral or bilateral asymmetric sacroiliitis Atlantoaxial instability Extra-axial skeleton: Soft tissue swelling: periarticular or involving entire digit (sausage digit) Absence of osteoporosis Severe joint space destruction with marginal erosions New bone formation: whiskering, enthesopathy Ray pattern: involvement of all joints in one digit, frequently associated with sausage digit Tuft resorption and proliferation (ivory phalanx)

Table continued on following page

TABLE 1–7. Inflammatory Articular Disorders *Continued*

Entity	Typical Age of Onset (Years)	Sex	Target Sites of Involvement	Clinical Characteristics	Laboratory and Radiographic Findings
Reiter's syndrome	15–35	Male : female, 5 : 1 to 50 : 1	Foot Heel Ankle Knee Hip Sacroiliac joint Spine Hand (rare) Shoulder (rare) Elbow (rare)	*Clinical findings:* Urethritis (often first symptom) Ocular abnormalities Early: transient conjunctivitis (common) Later: episcleritis, keratitis, uveitis Circinate balanitis Keratoderma blenorrhagicum Keratosis of the nails Other findings: fever, weight loss, thrombophlebitis, amyloidosis, arthritis	*Laboratory findings:* HLA-B27 antigen present in as many as 75 per cent of patients Leukocytosis Anemia Elevated erythrocyte sedimentation rate *Radiographic findings:* Axial skeleton: Paravertebral ossification (nonmarginal parasyndesmophytes) Unilateral or bilateral asymmetric sacroiliitis Atlantoaxial instability Extra-axial skeleton: Soft tissue swelling: periarticular or involving entire digit (sausage digit) Absence of osteoporosis Diffuse joint space loss New bone formation: whiskering, enthesopathy
Enteropathic arthropathy	Variable, depending on underlying condition	Variable, depending on underlying condition	Sacroiliac joint Spine	Seronegative spondyloarthropathy resembling ankylosing spondylitis radiographically Associated with many inflammatory enteropathic diseases, as follows: ulcerative colitis, Crohn's disease, Whipple's disease, *Salmonella*, *Shigella*, and *Yersinia* infections, and intestinal bypass surgery Frequency of chronic inflammatory bowel disease in ankylosing spondylitis varies from 2 to 18 per cent	*Laboratory findings:* HLA-B27 antigen present in 90 per cent of patients with ulcerative colitis and Crohn's disease who develop spondylitis or sacroiliitis *Radiographic findings:* Spondylitis and sacroiliitis identical to those of ankylosing spondylitis Occasional peripheral joint abnormalities
Dermatomyositis and polymyositis	5–10 and 30–50	Female : male, 2 : 1	Soft tissues of the thigh, leg, and arm	Diseases characterized by diffuse inflammation and degeneration of striated muscle with widespread sheet-like calcification in soft tissues Unknown cause; affects patients of all ages Dermatomyositis affects skin and muscle, and polymyositis affects only muscle *Clinical findings:* Progressive, symmetric, proximal weakness, Raynaud's phenomenon (33 per cent of cases) and arthralgia (50 per cent of cases)	*Laboratory findings:* Elevated serum muscle enzyme or urinary creatinine excretion levels Abnormal electromyogram results Abnormal muscle biopsy *Radiographic findings:* Initial soft tissue edema Soft tissue atropy Sheet-like soft tissue calcification and infrequently, ossification Phalangeal tuft resorption
Scleroderma (progressive systemic sclerosis)	20–50	Female > male	Hand Wrist Foot Ribs Spine (rare)	Uncommon collagen vascular disease that affects skin, lungs, gastrointestinal tract, heart, kidneys, and musculoskeletal system Two types: Localized scleroderma: scleroderma without systemic involvement Progressive systemic sclerosis: scleroderma with systemic involvement	*Laboratory findings:* Elevated erythrocyte sedimentation rate (60 to 70 per cent of patients) Positive rheumatoid factor (30 to 40 per cent of patients) Presence of antinuclear antibodies (35 to 96 per cent of cases) High levels of protein in aspirated synovial fluid

				Clinical findings: Raynaud's phenomenon or syndrome Muscle weakness Dysphagia (smooth muscle weakness) Edema, rigidity, thickening, and tightening of the skin of the hands, feet, and face Melanotic hyperpigmentation, vitiligo, and telangiectasis Secondary infection Pulmonary or renal involvement	*Radiographic findings:* Globular accumulations of periarticular and subcutaneous soft tissue calcinosis Phalangeal tuft erosion Conical appearance of fingertips resulting from soft tissue resorption Erosions of superior aspect of ribs Paraspinal calcification
Systemic lupus erythematosus (SLE)	20–45	Female > male	Hand Osteonecrosis in femoral head, femoral condyles, and humeral head	Relatively common connective tissue disorder characterized by significant immunologic abnormalities, involvement of numerous organ systems, and musculoskeletal involvement *Clinical findings:* Variable depending on organ system involvement; most common manifestations include malaise, weakness, fever, anorexia, weight loss, polyarthritis, skin rashes (erythema nodosum and butterfly rash on face), neurologic findings, and several visceral inflammatory processes	*Laboratory findings:* Anemia (70 to 80 per cent of patients) Leukopenia Plasma protein abnormalities False-positive serologic test for syphilis Formation of LE cells and other antinuclear factors Autoagglutination of red blood cells *Radiographic findings:* Symmetric, deforming nonerosive arthropathy Acrosclerosis Erosions and subchondral cysts (rare) Phalangeal tuft resorption Osteonecrosis: occurs in patients regardless of whether they received corticosteroid therapy; possibly caused by vasculitis; hip most common site Tendon weakening and rupture Insufficiency fracture Osteomyelitis and septic arthritis
Mixed connective tissue disease	20–50	Female > male	Hand Wrist Foot	Overlap syndromes and mixed connective tissue diseases include combinations of rheumatoid arthritis, dermatomyositis, scleroderma, and systemic lupus erythematosus *Clinical findings:* Variable, depending on predominant connective tissue diseases involved	*Laboratory findings:* Presence of ribonuclease-sensitive extractable nuclear antigen *Radiographic findings:* Radiographic features variable; may result in diffuse joint space narrowing, erosions, soft tissue calcinosis, deforming nonerosive arthropathy, osteonecrosis, phalangeal tuft resorption, marginal erosions

*Arnett FC, Edworthy SM, Bloch DA, et al: The American Rheumatism Association 1987 revised criteria for the classification of rheumatoid arthritis. Arthritis Rheum 31:315, 1988.

TABLE 1–8. Articular Disorders: Crystal Deposition Diseases and Metabolic Disorders

Entity	Typical Age of Onset (Years)	Sex	Target Sites of Involvement	Clinical Characteristics	Laboratory and Radiographic Findings
Calcium pyrophosphate dihydrate (CPPD) crystal deposition disease	>50	Male = female	Knee Symphysis pubis Hand Wrist Hip Shoulder Elbow Spine	Common disorder characterized by CPPD crystal deposition within soft tissues May be precipitated by local damage *Clinical patterns:* Most persons are asymptomatic; several types of symptomatic disease include the following: 1. Pseudodegenerative joint disease 2. Pseudogout 3. Pseudorheumatoid arthritis 4. Pseudoneuropathic osteoarthropathy 5. Miscellaneous patterns *Clinical findings:* Asymptomatic, or may be characterized by acute, subacute, or chronic self-limited attacks of joint pain, swelling, and erythema Flexion contractures, morning stiffness, fatigue, restricted joint motion Many associated diseases and disorders have been reported	*Laboratory findings:* Pyrophosphate crystals in synovial fluid aspirate Elevated erythrocyte sedimentation rate *Radiographic findings:* Bilateral asymmetric involvement Local soft tissue swelling Calcification of intra-articular hyaline cartilage and fibrocartilage as well as synovium, capsules, tendons, and ligaments Pyrophosphate arthropathy: articular space narrowing, prominent subchondral sclerosis, cyst formation, and osteophytes Advanced disease: articular destruction and fragmentation resembling neuropathic osteoarthropathy Features characteristic of CPPD crystal deposition disease allowing differentiation from degenerative joint disease include prominent calcification, involvement of unusual joints and compartments, and the presence of extensive sclerosis, cysts, fragmentation, osseous debris, and variable osteophyte formation
Calcific bursitis and tendinitis	40–70	Male = female	Shoulder Rare sites: Wrist Hand Elbow Hip Neck	Calcium hydroxyapatite crystal deposition in tendons and bursae about the joints Calcific tendinitis of the rotator cuff is the most common clinical condition *Clinical findings:* Solitary or multiple periarticular calcific deposits can be asymptomatic or may be associated with painful episodes Acute symptoms: pain, tenderness on pressure, local edema or swelling, restricted active or passive motion and, infrequently, mild fever Chronic symptoms: mild, nonincapacitating pain and tenderness More common in manual workers than sedentary workers Often associated with acute or chronic trauma	*Laboratory findings:* Elevated erythrocyte sedimentation rate Identification of calcium hydroxyapatite crystals by electron microscopy, radioisotope techniques, or x-ray diffraction analysis (tests that are performed only infrequently) *Radiographic findings:* Single or multiple cloud-like, linear, triangular, or circular soft tissue calcifications at tendon insertion sites and within bursae Occasionally, large tumor-like accumulations of calcification are seen about joints in patients with chronic renal disease or collagen vascular disorders

Gouty arthropathy	>40	Male : female, 20 : 1	Common: Foot Hand Wrist Elbow Knee Uncommon or rare: Hip Shoulder Spine	Hyperuricemia develops from overproduction of uric acid, decreased renal excretion of uric acid, or a combination of both Primary gout results from an inborn error of uric acid metabolism; secondary gout arises as a consequence of other disorders *Clinical findings:* Four phases 1. Asymptomatic hyperuricemia: prolonged hyperuricemia without signs or symptoms; 20 per cent of patients develop acute arthritis or renal calculi, marking the end of this phase 2. Acute gouty arthritis: often dramatic acute inflammatory episode; monoarticular, oligoarticular, or, occasionally, polyarticular; severe pain, tenderness, swelling, erythema overlying affected joints 3. Interval phase of gout (intercritical gout): asymptomatic period between gouty attacks 4. Chronic tophaceous gout: visible tophaceous deposits with repeated episodes of pain	*Laboratory findings:* Hyperuricemia Monosodium urate crystals in synovial fluid aspirate *Radiographic findings:* Most commonly present with chronic gouty arthropathy Extra-articular erosions with overhanging edges of cortex Intra-articular erosions Tophi (soft tissue deposition of urate crystals) Absence of osteoporosis Relative absence of joint space narrowing Subperiosteal bone apposition Intraosseous calcification Predilection for first metatarsophalangeal joint
Hemochromatosis	40–60	Male : female, 10 : 1 to 20 : 1	Hand Wrist Knee Hip Shoulder	Rare progressive disorder involving articular damage from excessive iron deposition Classified into primary and secondary forms *Clinical findings:* Classic triad: bronze skin pigmentation, liver cirrhosis, and diabetes mellitus Joint pain, stiffness, and swelling; usually bilateral	*Laboratory findings:* Elevated eryrthrocyte sedimentation rate Elevated serum iron concentration Increased saturation of the plasma iron-binding protein tranferrin Characteristic findings on liver biopsy *Radiographic findings:* Bilateral symmetric involvement Osteoporosis Chondrocalcinosis related to CPPD crystal deposition Signs of secondary osteoarthrosis Predilection for metacarpophalangeal joints
Alkaptonuria	Present at birth, but asymptomatic until 30 or 40 years of age	Male = female	Spine Hip Knee	Rare hereditary metabolic disorder characterized by absence of homogentisic acid oxidase *Clinical findings:* Usually asymptomatic until adulthood Ochronosis: brown-black pigmentation in connective tissues (rare in patients younger than age 20 years) Discoloration of urine Ochronotic arthropathy: acute excerbations of arthriits, joint effusions, stiffness and restriction of motion, low back pain, thoracic kyphosis, lumbar hypolordosis, or disc prolapse Ochronotic deposition in other organs may lead to various systemic abnormalities	*Laboratory findings:* When urine is allowed to stand, homogentisic acid oxidizes to a melanin-like product, causing the urine to turn black Presence of homogentisic acid in urine and plasma *Radiographic findings:* Ochronotic arthropathy: accelerated degenerative disc and joint disease, disc calcification and peripheral joint chondrocalcinosis, diffuse joint space narrowing, sclerosis, fragmentation, osteophytosis, and eventual bamboo spine from syndesmophyte formation

TABLE 1–9. Miscellaneous Articular Disorders

Disorder	Typical Age of Onset (Years)	Sex	Target Sites of Involvement	Clinical Characteristics	General Radiographic Findings
Hemophilic arthropathy	2–3	Male	Common sites: Knee Elbow Rare sites: Ankle Hip Shoulder Hand Foot	Group of disorders characterized by deficiency in specific plasma clotting factors and defective blood coagulation Results in easy bruising and prolonged and excessive bleeding Manifested in men and carried by women Two main X-linked recessive types result in musculoskeletal manifestations: Hemophilia A: Classic form; deficiency of factor VIII (antihemophilic factor) Hemophilia B: Christmas disease; deficiency of factor IX (plasma thromboplastin component) *Clinical findings:* Three phases: 1. Acute hemarthrosis. Rapid onset of bleeding; tense, stiff, red joint; pain, tenderness, muscle spasm; fever and leukocytosis; symptoms decrease with administration of clotting factor 2. Subacute hemarthrosis. After two or more acute hemarthroses; periarticular swelling, contractures, muscle spasm, and mild pain 3. Chronic hemarthrosis. Six months to 1 year after subacute phase; more severe and persistent fibrosis, joint destruction, and contractures	Radiodense joint effusions Osteoporosis Epiphyseal overgrowth Accelerated localized skeletal maturation Osseous erosions and cysts Joint space narrowing Sclerosis and osteophytes Osteonecrosis Radiographic appearance of joints closely resembles that of juvenile chronic arthritis Hemophilic pseudotumors (<2 per cent of patients); intraosseous hemorrhage with multiloculated osteolytic lesions
Neuropathic osteoarthropathy	Variable, depending on cause	Variable, depending on cause	Knee Hip Ankle Spine Shoulder Elbow Wrist Foot	Central (upper motor neuron) and peripheral (lower motor neuron) lesions can lead to neuropathic osteoarthropathy *Underlying disorders:* Syringomyelia, diabetes mellitus, tabes dorsalis, meningomyelocele, trauma, multiple sclerosis, leprosy, alcoholism, amyloidosis, infection, and congenital insensitivity to pain	Hypertrophic and atrophic forms *Axial skeleton:* widespread discovertebral and zygapophyseal joint destruction May resemble infectious spondylodiscitis Joint collapse, bone fragmentation, pseudarthrosis, and kyphosis *Appendicular skeleton:* joint disorganization, osseous debris, distention, dislocation, fragmentation, increased density, deformity, and subluxation

Neurologic injury: heterotopic ossification	Any age	Male > female	Hip Knee Shoulder Elbow	Extensive periarticular soft tissue ossification occurs in as many as 53 per cent of paraplegic and quadriplegic patients after brain and spinal cord injury—as in burns, mechanical trauma, and venous stasis ***Clinical findings:*** Some patients have no symptoms other than those of their primary neurologic disorder itself Others have pain, swelling, restricted joint motion, or synovitis	Periarticular osseous deposits begin to appear 2 to 6 months after injury Begin as poorly defined opaque areas, typically progress to large accumulations possessing trabeculae Often result in complete osseous ankylosis
Pigmented villonodular synovitis	20–40	Slight male predominance	Knee Hip Elbow Ankle	Monoarticular synovial proliferative disorder of unknown cause 50 per cent of patients have history of trauma Extra-articular form is termed giant cell tumor of the tendon sheath and is seen most commonly in the hand and foot ***Clinical findings:*** Monoarticular distribution is typical May have symptoms of internal joint derangement Slowly progressive joint pain, swelling, warmth, tenderness, and stiffness Aspiration: acute or chronic hemorrhage	Soft tissue swelling Cystic erosions on both sides of the joint Hemorrhagic joint effusion Eventual osteoporosis Well-preserved joint space until late in the disease Radiographs may be normal Magnetic resonance (MR) imaging is useful in evaluation
Idiopathic synovial osteochondromatosis	20–50	Male : female, 2 : 1	Knee Hip Elbow	Monoarticular metaplastic or neoplastic proliferation of cartilaginous and osteocartilaginous bodies by the synovial membrane Idiopathic form: unknown cause Secondary form: secondary to degenerative disease or trauma ***Clinical findings:*** Several years of joint pain with limitation of motion; pain may resemble that of an internal joint derangement Joint locking and instability may occur Focal recurrence after surgery Malignant degeneration (rare)	Multiple intra-articular or periarticular collections of calcification of variable size and density Erosion of adjacent bone Secondary osteoarthrosis Noncalcified bodies are best demonstrated with arthrography or MR imaging Secondary synovial osteochondromatosis may occur as a result of degenerative joint disease

TABLE 1–10. Malignant Bone Tumors and Myeloproliferative Disorders

Entity	Typical Age of Onset (Years)	Sex (Male : Female)	Most Frequent Skeletal Locations* (Per Cent)	General Characteristics	General Radiographic Findings
Secondary malignant tumors of bone					
Skeletal metastasis	50–75	Variable: depends on source	Spine (40) Pelvis (15) Ribs, sternum (30) Skull (10) Femur (<10) Humerus (<10) Hand and foot (rare)	Most common malignant tumor of bone Most frequent primary sources in adults: carcinoma of the breast, prostate, lung, kidney, bladder, and thyroid gland Most frequent primary sources in children: neuroblastoma, Ewing's sarcoma, and osteosarcoma *Clinical findings:* Bone pain, bone tenderness, soft tissue mass, osseous deformity, unexplained weight loss *Laboratory findings:* Elevated serum calcium, serum alkaline phosphatase, and urinary hydroxyproline levels; anemia; elevated prostate-specific antigen level in prostate carcinoma	Multiple skeletal sites typically involved Permeative or moth-eaten osteolysis (75 per cent of patients) Diffuse or patchy osteosclerosis or mixed pattern of osteolysis and osteosclerosis (25 per cent of patients) Pathologic fracture Soft tissue mass (rare) Periosteal reaction (rare) Bone expansion (rare) *Cortical metastasis:* Prevalent in the long bones, especially in patients with metastasis resulting from bronchogenic carcinoma Small radiolucent, eccentric, saucer-shaped, scalloped erosions, which sometimes occur near the entrance of nutrient arteries into the bone (cookie-bite lesions)
Primary malignant tumors of bone					
Osteosarcoma (conventional)	10–25	2 : 1	Femur (46) Tibia (21) Humerus (11) Pelvis (7)	Readily metastasizes to other bones and lung and may result from malignant transformation of benign neoplasms *Clinical findings:* Pain, swelling, restriction of motion, warmth, and pyrexia	Osteolytic, osteosclerotic, or mixed patterns of medullary and cortical destruction Prominent aggressive periosteal reaction common Preferential involvement of the metaphysis
Osteosarcoma (parosteal)	20–45	1 : 1	Femur (64) Humerus (15) Tibia (11)	*Clinical findings:* Insidious onset of pain, swelling, and palpable mass (often about the knee)	Osteosclerotic surface lesion of bone Large radiodense, oval sessile mass with smooth or irregular margins Lesion may have cleavage plane separating it from the parent bone Ossification begins centrally and progresses outwardly, opposite that of benign heterotopic bone formation (myositis ossificans)
Osteoblastoma (aggressive)	10–30	2 : 1	Spine (23) Tibia (13) Pelvis (13) Femur (11) Foot (11)	Aggressive (malignant) osteoblastomas recur in 50 per cent of cases, whereas only 10 per cent of conventional (benign) osteoblastomas recur Aggressive osteoblastomas have histologic and radiographic characteristics of malignancy and can be difficult to differentiate from osteosarcoma May lead to patient's death in some cases	Variable appearance that may resemble osteosarcoma or conventional osteoblastoma Expansile osteolytic lesion that may be partially ossified or contain calcium Metaphyseal location; may extend into epiphysis Soft tissue involvement

Chondrosarcoma (conventional)	30–60	3:2	Femur (24) Pelvis (24) Humerus (10) Ribs (8) Tibia (7) Spine (6)	Several forms: conventional, juxtacortical, clear cell, mesenchymal, and dedifferentiated types Further classified as peripheral or central Patients with peripheral chondrosarcoma tend to be slightly younger than those with central chondrosarcoma *Clinical findings:* Pain, tender soft tissue mass, pathologic fracture, warmth, and erythema	*Central chondrosarcoma:* Elongated poorly defined lesions May have soft tissue mass Multilobulated, osteolysis, cortical destruction, cortical thickening, periostitis, endosteal scalloping, and calcification *Peripheral chondrosarcoma:* Arise from preexisting osteochondroma or, infrequently, from the periosteal membrane in the form of juxtacortical chondrosarcoma *Calcification characteristics:* Present in more than 60 per cent of cases Well-organized calcific rings in low-grade chondrosarcomas Amorphous, punctate, scattered, or irregular calcification in high-grade chondrosarcomas
Giant cell tumor (aggressive)	30–50	3:2	Femur Tibia Radius Spine Humerus	Locally aggressive or malignant form of giant cell tumor is more common in men than in women Five to 10 per cent of giant cell tumors are malignant; radiographic appearance is an inaccurate guide to determining malignancy of lesion; biopsy is necessary Vast majority of malignant giant cell tumors develop after irradiation of benign giant cell tumors Forty to 60 per cent recurrence rate for all giant cell tumors Tumor implantation may occur at distant sites, typically the lung, 2 to 5 years after surgical resection of tumor; more prevalent with lesions of the distal end of the radius *Clinical findings:* Pain, local swelling, pathologic fracture, and limitation of motion in adjacent joint Pain usually mild and of several months' duration, relieved by bed rest, aggravated by activity	Eccentrically located, subarticular osteolytic lesion extending into the metaphysis of long bones Cortical destruction and soft tissue mass are variable findings Spinal lesions predominate in the vertebral body and may result in vertebral collapse
Fibrosarcoma	25–55	1:1	Femur (39) Tibia (16) Humerus (11) Pelvis (10)	Rare malignant neoplasm of bone Fibrosarcomas of bone have a poorer prognosis than fibrosarcomas of soft tissue Two main types: 1. De novo form 2. Secondary form: in areas of Paget's disease, osteonecrosis, chronic osteomyelitis, or previously irradiated bone *Clinical findings:* Local pain, swelling, limitation of motion Pathologic fracture present at initial evaluation in 33 per cent of patients	Purely osteolytic destruction with wide zone of transition Large solitary metaphyseal lesion: 1.5 to 20 cm in size Usually moth-eaten or permeative destruction; may exhibit geographic destruction Sequestrum may be seen Minimal sclerotic reaction or periostitis Central or eccentric location in tubular bones Soft tissue masses are common

Table continued on following page

TABLE 1–10. Malignant Bone Tumors and Myeloproliferative Disorders *Continued*

Entity	Typical Age of Onset (Years)	Sex (Male : Female)	Most Frequent Skeletal Locations* (Per Cent)	General Characteristics	General Radiographic Findings
Chordoma	30–60	2 : 1	Spine (75) Skull (25)	Rare locally aggressive lesion of notochordal origin Predominate in the sacrum and clivus and, less commonly, the axis or thoracolumbar vertebral bodies *Clinical findings:* Vary according to location; symptoms may be mild initially and result from pressure on adjacent structures (rectum, bladder, nerve roots, and spinal cord)	Central vertebral body lesion; osteolytic destruction with expansion is the most common pattern; rarely osteosclerotic or mixed; soft tissue mass frequently encountered
Adamantinoma (angioblastoma)	Women, 10–30; men, 30–50	5 : 4	Tibia (85) Humerus (6) Ulna (4) Femur (3)	Rare locally aggressive or malignant lesion of bone May be related to ossifying fibroma in the immature skeleton	Central or eccentric, multilocular, slightly expansile, sharply or poorly delineated osteolytic lesion Reactive bone sclerosis Periostitis rare
Ewing's sarcoma	10–25	3 : 2	Femur (22) Pelvis (18) Tibia (11) Humerus (10) Fibula (9) Ribs (8) Scapula (5)	Rare in African Americans (fewer than 2 per cent of patients) Pain most common presenting symptom	Permeative or moth-eaten osteolysis, aggressive cortical erosion or violation, laminated (i.e., onionskin appearance) or spiculated periostitis, and soft tissue involvement Occasional bone sclerosis Pathologic fracture (15 per cent of patients) Most lesions central and diametaphyseal in location
Myeloproliferative disorders					
Plasma cell (multiple) myeloma	60–70	2 : 1	Spine (75) Pelvis (27) Ribs (26) Humerus (15)	Plasma cell (multiple) myeloma is a malignant disease of plasma cells and represents the most common primary malignancy of bone 75 per cent of cases of plasma cell myeloma are multiple myeloma Particularly common in African Americans *Clinical findings:* Bone pain, particularly in the back and chest, weakness, fatigue, fever, weight loss, bleeding, neurologic signs, and many other signs and symptoms Rare osteoblastic form may be associated with peripheral neuropathy *Laboratory findings:* Serum immunoelectrophoresis is positive in 80 to 90 per cent of cases, and Bence Jones proteinuria is present in 40 to 60 per cent of patients Normocytic normochromic anemia, rouleau formation, thrombocytopenia, leukopenia, hypercalcemia, hyperuricemia, elevated erythrocyte sedimentation rate	Early: Normal radiographs or diffuse osteopenia Later: Widespread well-circumscribed osteolytic lesions with discrete margins, which appear uniform in size Vertebral collapse common Pathologic fracture 97 per cent osteolytic; 3 per cent osteoblastic False-negative bone scans common

Solitary plasmacytoma	45–55	2 : 1	Spine (50) Pelvis (13) Femur (16) Sternum (15)	Localized form of plasma cell myeloma 25 per cent of cases of plasma cell myeloma are solitary plasmacytoma, but 70 per cent of these eventually develop into multiple myeloma *Clinical findings:* Bone pain is a common finding *Laboratory findings:* Serologic test results may be negative or similar to those of multiple myeloma	Solitary, geographic, expansile, multicystic osteolytic lesion with thickened trabeculae Frequently results in pathologic vertebral collapse If calcified, may relate to secondary amyloidosis
Hodgkin's disease	15–35	1 : 1	Spine (43) Ribs (16) Pelvis (11) Femur (10)	Skeletal abnormalities occur in 10 to 25 per cent of patients; more common in adults than in children Over 60 per cent of patients have multiple sites of skeletal involvement *Clinical findings:* Lymphadenopathy, masses, hepatomegaly, splenomegaly, fever, night sweats, weight loss	75 per cent of lesions are osteolytic; 25 per cent are osteosclerotic (ivory vertebra) Permeative or moth-eaten osteolysis Anterior vertebral body scalloping may occur secondary to direct invasion of lymph nodes
Primary lymphoma (non-Hodgkin's)	20–40	1 : 1	Femur (24) Pelvis (18) Spine (13) Tibia (9)	No race predilection *Clinical findings:* Localized pain and swelling, lymphadenopathy and splenomegaly Systemic signs and symptoms characteristically are absent Skeletal involvement in up to 30 per cent of patients with non-Hodgkin's lymphoma	May result in multiple moth-eaten or permeative osteolytic metaphyseal lesions Common cause of pathologic fracture Diffuse or localized sclerotic lesions are rare
Leukemia	Acute childhood type: 2–5; chronic adult type: 35–55	1 : 1	Long bones Spine	Poor correlation between the extent of bone lesions and the progress of leukemia *Clinical findings:* Vary according to type Lymphadenopathy, splenomegaly, bone pain, arthralgia, tenderness, swelling, bleeding episodes, recurrent infections *Laboratory findings:* Anemia, leukocytosis, neutropenia, and thrombocytopenia	Radiographic abnormalities more prevalent in childhood form (up to 70 per cent of cases) than adult form (less than 20 per cent of cases) Findings in acute childhood leukemia: Diffuse osteopenia (15 to 100 per cent of cases) Radiolucent or radiodense transverse metaphyseal bands (10 to 55 per cent of cases) Osteolytic lesions (30 to 50 per cent of cases) Periostitis (10 to 35 per cent of cases) Osteosclerosis (5 to 10 per cent of cases) Radiodense metaphyses more frequent in patients undergoing chemotherapy for leukemia; may resemble appearance of lead poisoning

*Numbers in parentheses indicate approximate percentages of the neoplasms that affect each skeletal site based on analysis of major reports containing the greatest number of cases. In cases in which no numbers are provided, the relative frequency at each site is unknown.

TABLE 1–11. Benign Bone Tumors

Entity	Typical Age of Onset (Years)	Sex (Male : Female)	Most Frequent Skeletal Locations* (Per Cent)	General Characteristics	General Radiographic Findings
Enostosis (bone island)	Any age	1 : 1	Femur (25) Pelvis (25) Ribs (12) Humerus (9) Wrist, hand (9)	Not a true neoplasm; painless, circular zone of osteosclerosis *Clinical findings:* Usually encountered as an incidental finding on radiographs obtained for unrelated reasons *Differential diagnosis:* Other osteosclerotic processes, such as osteoblastic metastases, osteomas, osteoid osteomas, enchondromas, bone infarcts, fibrous dysplasia, and osteopoikilosis	Solitary or multiple, discrete foci of osteosclerosis within the spongiosa of bone Round, ovoid, or oblong with brush border composed of radiating osseous spicules that intermingle with the surrounding trabeculae of the spongiosa Lesions may grow in size and, when large, exhibit activity on a bone scan even though they are benign Giant bone islands have been reported to reach proportions of up to 4 × 4 cm in diameter
Osteoid osteoma	7–25	3 : 1	Femur (32) Tibia (24) Wrist, hand (9) Humerus (7) Spine (6)	*Clinical findings:* Often results in severe dull or aching pain, classically worse at night and relieved by salicylates Spinal lesions: torticollis, scoliosis, spinal stiffness Intracapsular lesions: joint tenderness, swelling, synovitis, limitation of motion Laboratory studies usually are unremarkable	Cortical or subperiosteal lesion with reactive sclerosis surrounding central radiolucent nidus: nidus usually less than 1 cm in diameter and may not be visible on routine radiographs Computed tomography probably best technique to show nidus Intracapsular lesions provoke less reactive sclerosis and are more likely to cause joint pain
Osteoblastoma (conventional)	10–30	2 : 1	Spine (30) Femur (14) Tibia (10) Foot (7)	Approximately 95 per cent of osteoblastomas are benign *Clinical findings:* Mild local pain; usually not relieved by rest or salicylates Spinal lesions may be accompanied by muscle spasm, scoliosis, and neurologic manifestations	Osteolytic, osteosclerotic, or both Partially calcified matrix in many cases Often resembles large osteoid osteoma Spine: expansile, multiloculated lesion of the neural arch Tubular and flat bones: Cortical thinning Diaphyseal (75 per cent of cases) or metaphyseal location May be subperiosteal in location
Ossifying fibroma (osteofibrous dysplasia)	<1–20	1 : 1	Facial bones Tibia	Rare fibro-osseous lesion of tubular bones occurring almost exclusively in the tibia (and, infrequently, the ipsilateral fibula) Closely related to fibrous dysplasia and may resemble adamantinoma or a large nonossifying fibroma	Long diaphyseal lesion with intracortical osteolysis clearly marginated by a band of osteosclerosis Hazy or ground-glass appearance reminiscent of fibrous dysplasia Occasionally purely osteosclerotic Osseous expansion Bowing, deformity, and pathologic fracture
Enchondroma (solitary)	15–35	1 : 1	Wrist, hand (57) Femur (11) Foot (7) Humerus (7) Ribs (5)	Lesions usually are asymptomatic or associated with painless swelling Onset of pain should arouse suspicion of malignant transformation to chondrosarcoma (fewer than 1 per cent of cases) or pathologic fracture	Solitary, central or eccentric, medullary osteolytic lesion Metaphyseal location; may extend to include entire diaphyseal and subarticular regions of bone Lobulated endosteal scalloping Stippled calcification (50 per cent of lesions)

Enchondromatosis (Ollier's disease)	<10	1:1	Tibia Fibula Femur Hand, wrist	Rare nonhereditary disease ***Clinical findings:*** Palpable masses, asymmetric limb shortening, osseous deformities related to pathologic fracture Malignant transformation rate: 5 to 30 per cent	Multiple enchondromas Tubular radiolucent areas extending into the metaphysis from the physis Shortening and deformity of affected bones Frequent calcification of matrix
Maffucci's syndrome	<10	1:1	Tibia (50) Fibula (50) Hand, wrist Foot	Rare, congenital, nonhereditary mesodermal dysplasia Multiple enchondromas and soft tissue hemangiomas Unilateral distribution in 50 per cent of cases Malignant transformation rate: 20 to 40 per cent of cases (occurs in both bone and soft tissue)	Soft tissue hemangiomas: multiple phleboliths in the soft tissues Multiple central or eccentric radiolucent lesions containing variable amounts of calcification Shortening and deformity of affected bones
Chondroblastoma	10–25	2:1	Femur (33) Humerus (22) Tibia (18) Hands and feet (10)	Benign epiphyseal tumor of cartilage origin Frequently results in joint pain	Circular osteolytic lesion 5 or 6 cm in diameter Arise from epiphyses and apophyses of long bones; metaphyseal extension in 25 to 50 per cent of cases Thin sclerotic margin Calcification in matrix (30 to 50 per cent of cases) Soft tissue mass and pathologic fracture rare Occasionally periosteal reaction may be seen on routine radiographs and edema may be seen on magnetic resonance images
Chondromyxoid fibroma	10–25	Slight male predominance	Tibia (38) Femur (17) Fibula (8) Foot (6) Pelvis (6)	Least common benign tumor of cartilage Slowly progressive pain, tenderness, swelling, and restriction of motion; may infrequently be asymptomatic Pathologic fracture (rare)	Eccentric, elongated metaphyseal lesion 2 to 10 cm in length Cortical expansion, coarse trabeculation, endosteal sclerosis Calcification is rare (5–27 per cent of cases) May appear aggressive with large "bite" lesion penetrating cortex
Osteochondroma (solitary)	10–30	2:1	Femur (31) Humerus (19) Tibia (18) Foot (6) Hand, wrist (5) Fibula (4)	Represents either a true primary benign bone tumor, a developmental physeal growth defect, or a cartilaginous metaplasia within the periosteal membrane May occur spontaneously or secondary to injury or irradiation ***Clinical findings:*** Nontender, painless, slow-growing mass ***Complications:*** Fracture, osseous deformity, bursa formation, vascular injury, neurologic compromise, and malignant transformation (fewer than 1 per cent of solitary lesions)	Pedunculated or sessile cartilage-covered osseous excrescence arising from the surface of the metaphyses of long bones or, infrequently, flat bones Composed of cortex and medulla, which are continuous with the host bone Cartilage cap frequently contains calcification visible on radiographs Grows in a direction away from the adjacent joint Spinal lesions arise from the posterior arch ***Signs suggesting malignant transformation:*** Pain, soft tissue swelling, and soft tissue mass; growth of a previously stable lesion, bone erosion, irregular or scattered calcification, thick cartilage cap (>1 cm) These signs are not always reliable; a normal bone scan virtually excludes presence of malignancy; microscopic biopsy findings are most definitive

Table continued on following page

TABLE 1–11. Benign Bone Tumors *Continued*

Entity	Typical Age of Onset (Years)	Sex (Male : Female)	Most Frequent Skeletal Locations* (Per Cent)	General Characteristics	General Radiographic Findings
Hereditary multiple exostoses	10–30	1 : 1	Femur Tibia Fibula Humerus	Autosomal dominant disorder of metaphyseal overgrowth Also referred to as diaphyseal aclasis and multiple osteochondromatosis Characterized by multiple osteochondromas Malignant transformation rate: 3 to 25 per cent of cases	Multiple sessile and pedunculated osteochondromas numbering from a few to more than 100 Osseous deformities and abnormalities of modeling
Nonossifying fibroma and fibrous cortical defect	10–20	2 : 1	Tibia (43) Femur (38) Fibula (8) Humerus (5)	The terms nonossifying fibroma and fibrous cortical defect often are used interchangeably Common benign lesions consisting of whorled bundles of connective tissue cells Present in about 2 per cent of persons younger than 20 years of age, according to some estimates *Clinical findings:* Clinically silent; usually discovered incidentally or after fracture	Eccentric, multiloculated osteolytic lesion arising from metaphyseal cortex Resembles a well-circumscribed, blister-like shell of bone arising from the cortex Cortical thinning often is present Most lesions are replaced by normal bone, gradually disappearing over time; others grow large and may result in pathologic fracture Often bilateral and symmetric On serial radiographs, the lesion may appear to migrate away from the physis owing to normal longitudinal metaphyseal growth between the physis and the lesion
Giant cell tumor (benign)	20–40	Benign, 2 : 3; aggressive, 3 : 2	Femur (31) Tibia (27) Radius (10) Spine, especially sacrum (7) Humerus (6)	90 to 95 per cent are benign; 5 to 10 per cent are locally aggressive or malignant 40 to 60 per cent recurrence rate *Clinical findings:* Pain, local swelling, limitation of motion Pathologic fracture (10 per cent) Neurologic symptoms may accompany spinal or sacral lesions	Elongated, eccentric osteolytic neoplasm with a predilection for the subarticular region and metaphyses of the long bones Multiloculated, expansile, with delicate trabecular pattern Spinal and sacral lesions affect the vertebral body in an eccentric fashion and may extend into the posterior elements or cross the sacroiliac joint Radiographs are inaccurate in distinguishing benign from aggressive giant cell tumors
Intraosseous lipoma	30–50	1 : 1	Fibula (20) Calcaneus (15) Femur (15) Tibia (14) Humerus (9) Ribs (8)	Uncommon tumor or tumor-like osseous lesion that may be related to osteonecrosis or fat necrosis *Clinical findings:* Symptoms (in 66 per cent of patients) include localized pain and variable amounts of soft tissue swelling and tenderness to palpation Infrequent compression of adjacent neurovascular structures	Solitary osteolytic lesion surrounded by a thin, well-defined sclerotic border Central calcified or ossified focus is common Occasional lobulation or internal osseous ridges Osseous expansion (rare) Cortical destruction and periostitis absent

Hemangioma (solitary)	25–50	1:2	Skull (40) Spine (25) Ribs (9) Foot (5)	Vascular channels within bone: cavernous, capillary, or venous types Single lesions predominate, but multiple lesions occasionally are encountered ***Clinical findings:*** Usually discovered as an incidental finding Occasional soft tissue swelling or pain, particularly in presence of pathologic fracture Spinal lesions infrequently may be complicated by spinal cord compression from bone expansion, epidural tumor extension, epidural hemorrhage, or compression fracture	Radiolucent, slightly expansile intraosseous lesion Radiating, lattice-like or web-like trabecular pattern Spinal lesions exhibit characteristic corduroy cloth appearance: prominent vertical trabecular ridges within radiolucent spongiosa bone of vertebral body; may extend into neural arch Occasional cortical thinning Rarely, periostitis, soft tissue mass, or osteosclerosis Intracortical and periosteal hemangiomas (extremely rare) predominate in the tibia and fibula
Simple bone cyst	5–25	2:1	Humerus (56) Femur (27) Tibia (6) Fibula (5)	Fluid-filled solitary cyst of unknown cause and pathogenesis; not a true neoplasm Also termed solitary or unicameral bone cyst Flat bones (pelvic bones and calcaneus) more frequently involved in persons older than 20 years of age ***Clinical findings:*** Asymptomatic unless pathologic fracture occurs	Mildly expansile, solitary osteolytic lesion within metaphyseal medullary cavity of long bones May be multiloculated On serial radiographs, the lesion may appear to migrate away from the physis owing to normal longitudinal metaphyseal growth between the physis and the lesion May observe fallen-fragment sign in patients with pathologic fracture
Aneurysmal bone cyst	10–30	2:3	Tibia (15) Spine (14) Femur (13) Pelvis (9) Foot (8) Fibula (7) Hand, wrist (5)	Benign non-neoplastic lesion containing blood-filled cavities May develop after trauma or may accompany other benign processes, such as giant cell tumor, fibrous dysplasia, and chondroblastoma ***Clinical findings:*** Pain and swelling Spinal lesions may lead to neurologic compromise	Eccentric, thin-walled, expansile osteolytic lesion of the metaphysis of long bones Spinal lesions arise from the neural arch but often extend into the vertebral body Thin trabeculation with multiloculated appearance Buttressing at edge of lesion Typically more expansile than osteoblastoma

*Numbers in parentheses indicate approximate percentages of the neoplasms that affect each skeletal site based on analysis of major reports containing the greatest number of cases. In cases in which no numbers are provided, the relative frequency at each site is unknown.

TABLE 1–12. Tumor-Like Lesions of Bone

Entity	Typical Age of Onset (Years)	Sex (Male : Female)	Most Frequent Skeletal Locations* (Per Cent)	General Characteristics	General Radiographic Findings
Paget's disease	>55	2 : 1	Pelvis Femur Skull Tibia Spine Humerus	Unknown cause Results in deformity of bone *Clinical findings:* Asymptomatic in 90 per cent of patients Mild bone pain, worse with bowing deformities, pathologic fractures, and malignant transformation *Laboratory findings:* Elevated alkaline phosphatase, urinary hydroxyproline, and serum calcium levels; vary according to stage of involvement *Malignant transformation:* Malignant transformation rate: fewer than 2 per cent of cases; osteosarcoma, chondrosarcoma, and fibrosarcoma; femur is the most frequent site of malignant transformation Ominous signs for malignant transformation include increased pain, enlarging soft tissue mass, enlarging osteolytic lesion, further elevation of serum alkaline phosphatase levels	Usually polyostotic and may have unilateral involvement Coarsened trabeculae, cortical thickening, and bone enlargement Pathologic fracture Bowing deformities of bones Pseudofractures (i.e., insufficiency fractures) on convex surface of bowed bones Blade of grass (flame-shaped advancing edge of osteolysis) appearance seen in tubular bones Stages of involvement: I: osteolytic (50 per cent) II: osteosclerotic (25 per cent) III: mixed (25 per cent) IV: malignant transformation (fewer than 2 per cent)
Neurofibromatosis Type I (von Recklinghausen's disease)	Birth	1 : 1	Cranium Spine Ribs Tibia Femur	Inherited, autosomal dominant mesodermal dysplasia 50 per cent of patients develop skeletal lesions Approximately 5 per cent rate of malignant transformation to neurofibrosarcoma *Clinical findings:* Café-au-lait macules, neurofibromas, inguinal or axillary freckling, optic glioma, Lisch nodules, osseous lesions	Dysplastic bones with overconstriction, bowing deformities, pathologic fractures, and remodeling *Circumscribed cyst-like intraosseous lesions:* may result from subperiosteal hemorrhage with subsequent periosteal proliferation and repair or from the incorporation or overgrowth of periosteum around a previously external soft tissue lesion, such as a neurofibroma *Pseudarthroses:* when deformed bones fracture; precise cause of pseudarthrosis and defective fracture healing is not clear *Spinal involvement:* 60 per cent of patients; scoliosis or kyphoscoliosis, pedicle erosion, foraminal enlargement, penciling and spindling of transverse processes and ribs

Fibrous dysplasia				Nonhereditary, idiopathic, developmental anomaly of bone-forming mesenchyme in which osteoblasts fail to undergo normal morphologic differentiation and maturation	
Monostotic (70–80 per cent)	10–20	1 : 1	Rib (28) Femur (15) Tibia (10) Skull (common) Humerus (4)	***Clinical findings:*** Monostotic lesions tend to be asymptomatic unless pathologic fracture or stress fracture occurs ***Laboratory findings:*** Elevated serum alkaline phosphatase levels in one third of patients; poor correlation with extent of skeletal involvement	Thick rim of sclerosis surrounding a central or eccentric radiolucent lesion; hazy ground-glass appearance of matrix Lesions in long bones usually are intramedullary and diaphyseal in location Focal bone expansion and minimal bowing may occur
Polyostotic (20–30 per cent)	5–20	Slight female predominance	Femur (92)† Tibia (81) Pelvis (78) Foot (75) Fibula (62) Ribs (55) Hand, wrist (55) Humerus (50)	***Clinical findings:*** Initial symptoms may include osseous deformity or pathologic fracture May be associated with McCune-Albright syndrome: precocious female sexual development and cutaneous pigmentation	Polyostotic lesions are bilateral and asymmetric, or occasionally unilateral; tend to be larger, more expansile, and more multiloculated than monostotic lesions Bowing deformities more prominent
Langerhans' cell histiocytosis	5–10	Slight male predominance	Skull (>50) Pelvis (20) Femur (15) Ribs (7) Spine (6)	Histiocytic infiltration of tissue; unknown cause Three major conditions: 1. Eosinophilic granuloma: 80 per cent of patients; mildest, benign form characterized by single or multiple lesions of bone; usually asymptomatic 2. Hand-Schüller-Christian disease: 10 per cent of patients; most varied form with chronic dissemination of osseous lesions; associated with diabetes insipidus, exophthalmos, and severe visceral involvement 3. Letterer-Siwe disease: 10 per cent of patients; acute form with rapid dissemination, severe visceral involvement, and poor clinical prognosis; usually affects children younger than 3 years of age	*Long bones and flat bones:* osteolytic lesions may be multiloculated and expansile *Spine:* vertebra plana: with healing, the height of the pathologically collapsed vertebral body may be reconstituted, a finding more common in younger persons; bubbly, osteolytic, or expansile spinal lesions without collapse also may occur

*Numbers in parentheses indicate approximate percentages of lesions that affect each skeletal site based on analysis of major reports containing the greatest number of cases. The relative frequency of involvement in each location for Paget's disease and neurofibromatosis Type I is unknown.
†Numbers add up to more than 100% because several sites are involved simultaneously.

TABLE 1–13. Metabolic, Nutritional, and Endocrine Disorders of Bones and Joints

Entity	Typical Sites of Involvement	General Characteristics	General Radiographic Findings
Generalized osteoporosis	Predominates in the axial skeleton Osteoporotic fractures: Thoracolumbar spine Hip Distal end of radius Proximal end of humerus	*Causes:* Senile and postmenopausal states (most common) Medication Corticosteroids Heparin Endocrine states Hyperthyroidism Hyperparathyroidism Cushing's disease Acromegaly Pregnancy Diabetes mellitus Hypogonadism Deficiency states Scurvy Malnutrition Calcium deficiency Alcoholism and chronic liver disease Anemic states Osteogenesis imperfecta Idiopathic conditions	Uniform decrease in radiodensity, thinning of vertebral end plates, accentuation of vertical trabeculae Insufficiency fractures of the spine and hip common Wedge-shaped vertebral deformities caused by compression fractures are most common in thoracic spine; biconcave deformities are more common in the lumbar spine; vertebra plana deformities are more likely to be related to pathologic fracture caused by plasma cell myeloma, skeletal metastasis, or other destructive process Quantitative bone mineral analysis (densitometry) is necessary for accurate assessment of the presence and extent of diminished bone mineral content Dual energy x-ray absorptiometry is the most widely used method to assess bone mineral density because of its ease of use, high precision, and low radiation exposure to patients
Regional osteoporosis	Hip Knee Foot Hand Immobilized extremity	*Causes:* Transient regional osteoporosis Transient osteoporosis of the hip Regional migratory osteoporosis Reflex sympathetic dystrophy Immobilization and disuse Usually self-limited	Patchy, spotty, linear, or diffuse patterns of osteopenia in a regional distribution Regional involvement Magnetic resonance imaging findings of marrow edema
Osteomalacia	Diffuse skeletal involvement	Inadequate or delayed mineralization of osteoid in mature cortical and spongiosa bone *Causes:* Vitamin D deficiency Inadequate exposure to ultraviolet radiation Gastrointestinal malabsorption Abnormal vitamin D metabolism Liver disease Kidney disease Phosphate loss Associated tumors Anticonvulsant drugs	Diminished radiodensity and prominent coarsened trabeculae Bilateral and symmetric transverse insufficiency fractures: pseudofractures or Looser's zones, which, when seen in tubular bones, occur on the concave aspect of the bone Thickening of tubular bones from excessive osteoid deposition
Rickets	Findings are more prominent in the appendicular skeleton	Interruption in orderly development and mineralization of the growth plate *Causes:* Similar to those in osteomalacia *Clinical findings:* Muscle tetany, weakness, delayed skeletal maturation, small stature, irritability, osseous bowing deformities, rachitic rosary	General retardation in body growth Osteopenia Rachitic rosary (masses on anterior chest wall) at costochondral junctions *Deformities:* Bowing deformities of long tubular bones Scoliosis may develop with overall decrease in height Concave vertebral body deformities Basilar impression and acetabular protrusion *Growth plate changes:* Widening, cupping, and fraying of the metaphyses Decreased density at the metaphyseal zone of provisional calcification Irregularity of the metaphyseal zone of provisional calcification

TABLE 1–13. Metabolic, Nutritional, and Endocrine Disorders of Bones and Joints *Continued*

Entity	Typical Sites of Involvement	General Characteristics	General Radiographic Findings
Hyperparathyroidism	Resorption: phalangeal tufts, sacroiliac joint, symphysis pubis, periarticular regions, discovertebral joints, patellofemoral joints, medial tibial metaphysis, skull Brown tumors: tubular and flat bones	Three forms: primary, secondary, and tertiary *Primary form:* elevated parathyroid hormone secretion as a result of parathyroid gland hyperplasia or adenomas *Secondary form:* excessive parathyroid hormone secretion secondary to sustained hypocalcemic states such as those encountered in chronic renal failure, malabsorption syndromes, sprue, and gluten enteropathy *Tertiary form:* occurs in patients with chronic renal failure or malabsorption and long-standing secondary hyperparathyroidism who develop relatively autonomous parathyroid function and hypercalcemia *Clinical findings:* Widely variable owing to the many organ systems that can be involved; some findings include urinary tract calculi, peptic ulcer disease, pancreatitis, symptomatic bone disease (10 to 25 per cent of patients), and abnormalities of the skin, central nervous system, and cardiovascular system	Bone resorption: subperiosteal, subchondral, subligamentous, subtendinous, intracortical, endosteal Urate and calcium pyrophosphate dihydrate (CPPD) crystal deposition Osteosclerosis Rugger-jersey spine: horizontal bands of osteosclerosis adjacent to the superior and inferior surfaces of the vertebral body Brown tumor (osteoclastoma): solitary or multiple expansile osteolytic lesions containing fibrous tissue and giant cells; may disappear after treatment for hyperparathyroidism Tendon rupture Soft tissue and vascular calcification
Renal osteodystrophy		Uremic osteopathy in patients with chronic renal insufficiency Combination of osteomalacia or rickets and secondary hyperparathyroidism *Clinical findings:* Most patients have chronic renal disease and may be undergoing dialysis treatment	Findings of osteomalacia, rickets (in children), and hyperparathyroidism Osteosclerosis may be prominent
Dialysis spondyloarthropathy	Cervical and lumbar spine	Seen in as many as 25 per cent of patients who receive long-standing hemodialysis Middle-aged or elderly men or women May be related to amyloid deposition or, less commonly, calcium hydroxyapatite or calcium oxalate crystal deposition in disc Additional sites of amyloid deposition include shoulder with large masses (shoulder-pad sign), wrist with carpal tunnel syndrome, and hip (which may lead to fracture of the femoral neck)	Discovertebral joint erosions at one or more levels resembling those of infectious spondylodiscitis, neuropathic osteoarthropathy, and CPPD crystal deposition disease Rapidly progressive disc space narrowing, erosion, and sclerosis of vertebral end plates
Hypervitaminosis D	Tubular bones	Acute or chronic vitamin D poisoning occurs particularly in patients with preexisting renal or gastrointestinal dysfunction *Clinical findings:* Acute: vomiting, fever, dehydration, abdominal cramps, bone pain, convulsions, coma Chronic: lassitude, thirst, anorexia, polyuria, vomiting	*Infants and children:* Metaphyseal bands of increased density alternating with areas of increased radiolucency Cortical thickening or osteoporosis Widespread osteosclerosis and soft tissue calcification *Adults:* Focal or generalized osteoporosis Massive intra-articular and para-articular metastatic soft tissue calcification

Table continued on following page

TABLE 1–13. Metabolic, Nutritional, and Endocrine Disorders of Bones and Joints *Continued*

Entity	Typical Sites of Involvement	General Characteristics	General Radiographic Findings
Scurvy (hypovitaminosis C)	Long tubular bones	Ascorbic acid (vitamin C) deficiency Radiographic evidence of skeletal changes in scurvy is seen only in advanced disease of long duration Infantile scurvy: occurs in babies who are fed pasteurized or boiled milk; heating the milk disrupts vitamin C Adult scurvy: rarely encountered, only in severely malnourished persons, especially the elderly *Clinical findings:* Pale skin, petechial hemorrhage, bleeding gums, anorexia, weight loss	*Infantile scurvy:* Periostitis secondary to subperiosteal hemorrhage Transverse radiodense zone of provisional calcification (white line of Frankel) Transverse radiolucent metaphyseal line (scurvy line, Trümmerfeldzone) Beaklike metaphyseal excrescences (corner or angle sign) Radiodense shell surrounding epiphyses (Wimberger's sign of scurvy) Healing scurvy may result in increased radiodensity of the metaphyses and epiphyses
Hypervitaminosis A	Hyperostosis: ulnae, metatarsal bones, clavicles, tibiae, fibulae, metacarpal bones, other tubular bones, ribs Metaphyseal and epiphyseal changes: most prominent at distal end of femur	Acute or chronic vitamin A poisoning occurs in both children and adults *Clinical findings:* Acute form: nausea, vomiting, headache, drowsiness, irritabilty, and, in children, bulging of the fontanelles, drowsiness, and vomiting Chronic form: anorexia, itching, dry scaly skin, hair loss, digital clubbing, soft tissue swelling of the extremities, and osseous abnormalities on radiographs Similar findings may be seen with medications (e.g., *cis*-retinoic acid) used to treat skin disorders	Radiographic findings usually confined to children at the end of the first year of life Soft tissue nodules Hyperostosis and periostitis: cortical thickening of tubular bones involving the diaphysis Cupping, splaying, and shortening of the metaphysis; irregularity and narrowing of the growth plates; hypertrophy and premature fusion of the epiphyseal ossification centers
Fluorosis	Axial skeleton involvement is characteristic Infrequently may affect bones of the extremities	Endemic or industrial exposure to high concentrations of fluorine in water or air; also occurs in osteoporotic patients treated with sodium fluoride *Clinical findings:* Acute exposure: nausea, vomiting, constipation, anorexia, toxic nephritis Prolonged exposure: joint pain, restriction of motion, back stiffness, restriction of respiratory movements, dyspnea, paraplegia, and palpable thickening of superficial tubular bones *Differential diagnosis:* Osteopetrosis, Paget's disease, skeletal metastasis, other causes of diffuse osteosclerosis, and diffuse idiopathic skeletal hyperostosis (DISH)	*Spine:* osteosclerosis and ossification of the posterior longitudinal ligament, prominent osteophytosis, and periostitis *Tubular bones (rare):* osteosclerosis, periostitis, or osteoporosis (early in the disease) *Flat bones:* osteosclerosis, ligament calcification, and enthesopathy
Hypothyroidism	Entire skeleton, particularly long bones and spine	Thyroxine and triiodothyronine deficiency Primary and secondary forms *Clinical findings:* Dry, coarse skin and hair, fatigue, lethargy, edema, pallor, cold intolerance, decreased sweating, hoarseness, constipation, weight gain, hair loss, paresthesias	*General findings:* osteopenia, delayed skeletal development, epiphyseal dysgenesis and deformity, dystrophic calcification, slipped capital femoral epiphysis, CPPD crystal deposition, erosive osteoarthritis *Spine findings:* bullet vertebrae, thoracolumbar gibbus deformity, and widened disc spaces

TABLE 1–13. Metabolic, Nutritional, and Endocrine Disorders of Bones and Joints *Continued*

Entity	Typical Sites of Involvement	General Characteristics	General Radiographic Findings
Hyperthyroidism	Entire skeleton	Thyrotoxicosis from overproduction of thyroid hormone by the thyroid gland; common causes are Graves' disease and thyroid adenomas *Clinical findings:* Nervousness, hypersensitivity to heat, palpitation, fatigue, weight loss, tachychardia, dyspnea, weakness, hyperorexia, goiter, tremor, thyroid bruit, and eye signs and symptoms	Hyperthyroid osteopathy Osteoporosis Accelerated skeletal maturation
Thyroid acropachy	Metacarpals, metatarsals, middle and proximal phalanges, and, occasionally, long tubular bones	Occurs in patients after treatment for hyperthyroidism Unknown cause Present in less than 1 per cent of patients with thyrotoxicosis *Clinical findings:* Exophthalmos Soft tissue swelling Pretibial myxedema	Digital clubbing Asymmetric diaphyseal periostitis of tubular bones Periostitis is irregular or spiculated and is more prominent on the radial or tibial side of the bones
Acromegaly and gigantism	Acromegalic changes most prominent in acral parts, skull, mandible, and soft tissues Gigantism affects entire skeleton proportionately	Hypersecretion of growth hormone (somatotropin) results in acromegaly in adults and gigantism in children Often associated with acidophilic or chromophobic adenomas of the anterior lobe of the pituitary gland *Clinical findings:* Enlarged acral parts, menstrual disturbances, headaches, amenorrhea, increased basal metabolic rate, hyperhydrosis, cutaneous pigmentation, weight gain, hypertrichosis, back ache, limb arthropathy, compression neuropathy, neuromuscular symptoms, Raynaud's phenomenon	*Acromegaly:* Widening or enlargement of costochondral junctions, mandible, phalangeal tufts, heel pad, sella turcica, articular spaces, and disc spaces Enthesopathy, thickening of cranial vault, cortical thickening of tubular bones, osteophytosis, and premature degenerative disease *Spine:* elongation and widening of the vertebral bodies; ossification of the anterior portion of the disc; posterior scalloping of vertebral bodies occurs infrequently; increased disc height; premature degenerative disease, exuberant osteophytosis *Gigantism:* Symmetric and proportionate overgrowth of all tissues within the body
Growth recovery lines	Tubular bones, including femur, tibia, humerus	Transverse radiodense lines representing a sign of new or increased growth, presumably after a period of inhibited bone growth In children, growth recovery lines may be related to a previous episode of trauma, infection, malnutrition, or other chronic disease states Also seen in normal children without episodes of trauma or disease	Transverse radiodense lines across the metaphyseal region of tubular bones In adults, transverse bone bars or reinforcement lines may be present in persons with chronic osteoporosis and do not appear to be related to growth recovery or arrest

TABLE 1–14. Hematologic Disorders of Bone

Entity	Typical Sites of Involvement	General Characteristics	General Radiographic Findings
Mastocytosis	Axial skeleton: diffuse or focal lesions Appendicular skeleton: focal lesions predominate	Systemic mastocytosis is characterized by mast cell proliferation and histamine release *Clinical findings:* Resembles lymphoma and leukemia and typically results in edema, flushing, shock-like episodes, diarrhea, vomiting, anaphylaxis, bronchoconstriction, hepatosplenomegaly, weakness, and malaise	Skeletal changes include combinations of the following: Diffuse or focal osteosclerosis Diffuse osteopenia Focal osteolysis Pathologic fracture
Myelofibrosis	Axial skeleton and proximal long bones Spine, pelvis, skull, ribs	Rare disease of unknown cause characterized by fibrotic or sclerotic bone marrow and extramedullary hematopoiesis Middle-aged and elderly men and women Malignant or acute form: patients may die within a few months of initial diagnosis *Clinical findings:* Weakness, fatigue, weight loss, abdominal pain, anorexia, nausea, vomiting, and dyspnea; abdominal swelling, purpura, and hepatosplenomegaly Diagnosis established by bone marrow biopsy Elevated serum or urinary uric acid levels (50 to 80 per cent of patients) lead to secondary gout in as many as 20 per cent of patients	Osteosclerois is a predominant pattern (40 to 50 per cent of patients) Occasional sandwich vertebra appearance Normal or osteopenic bones or osteolytic lesions may be present Cortical thickening and endosteal sclerosis lead to obliteration of the normal demarcation between cortical and medullary bone
Gaucher's disease	Spine Long tubular bones Pelvis	Rare familial lipid storage disease characterized by marrow infiltration with Gaucher cells Caused by a deficiency of a specific enzyme (glucocerebroside hydrolase or beta glucosidase) that leads to abnormal accumulation of lipid material in reticuloendothelial cells *Type I:* chronic or adult form; most frequent form; Ashkenazic Jews; bone involvement common *Type II:* acute form: rare fatal neurodegenerative disorder; survival usually is 1 year or less *Type III:* subacute form: juvenile onset; convulsions and other neurologic signs *Clinical findings:* Hepatosplenomegaly, mental retardation (variable), spasticity, seizures, anemia, leukopenia, bleeding diathesis	Vertebral changes include diffuse vertebral body collapse and, infrequently, H-shaped step-like defects in the vertebral bodies Marrow infiltration results in osteopenia, osteolytic lesions, cortical diminution, and medullary widening Osseous weakening results in pathologic fractures Modeling deformities: Erlenmeyer flask deformity is the term applied to widening of the distal diametaphysis of the femur and other tubular bones Osteonecrosis
Sickle cell anemia	Can involve any skeletal site	Common disease among North-American and African blacks characterized by the presence of HbS, sickle-shaped erythrocytes *Clinical findings:* Symptomatic painful crises begin during second or third year of life and include anemia, fever, icterus, nausea, vomiting, abdominal pain, and prostration Other findings include hepatosplenomegaly, cardiac enlargement, chronic leg ulcers, infection, pulmonary infarction and pneumonia, abdominal pain, cholelithiasis, peptic ulcer disease, hematuria, priapism, neurologic findings, and lymphadenopathy Death may result from infection, cardiac decompensation related to severe anemia, or thrombosis and infarction of various organs	Diffuse osteopenia Vascular occlusion leading to osteonecrosis Growth disturbances Osteomyelitis and septic arthritis Uric acid and calcium pyrophosphate dihydrate (CPPD) crystal deposition Marrow hyperplasia Joint effusion and hemarthroses H-shaped vertebral body indentations occur as a result of vascular occlusion to the vertebral body growth centers; commonly encountered in severe cases of sickle cell anemia and other hemoglobinopathies; may simulate Schmorl's nodes or biconcave (fish) vertebrae associated with osteoporotic vertebral body fractures; compensatory vertical growth of adjacent vertebral bodies results in "tower vertebrae"

TABLE 1–14. Hematologic Disorders of Bone *Continued*

Entity	Typical Sites of Involvement	General Characteristics	General Radiographic Findings
β-thalassemia[128]	Skull, spine, ribs, and appendicular skeleton	Severe form of anemia associated with hepatosplenomegaly and bone abnormalities Typically encountered in patients of Mediterranean ancestry *Clinical features:* Homozygous β-thalassemia (thalassemia major): severe anemia, prominent hepatosplenomegaly, and early death, often in childhood Anemia leads to pallor, fatigability, jaundice, icterus, deficient growth, and significant osseous deformities, especially in the face Heterozygous β-thalassemia (thalassemia minor): milder signs and symptoms, including slight to moderate anemia, splenomegaly, and jaundice; most common in Mediterranean populations and affects 1 per cent of American blacks, most of whom are asymptomatic	Findings similar to those of sickle cell anemia Severe osteopenia—lace-like trabecular pattern H-shaped vertebral bodies (rare) Modeling deformities: Erlenmeyer flask appearance Multiple and recurrent fractures secondary to osteoporosis Uric acid and CPPD crystal deposition as well as hemochromatosis secondary to repeated transfusions

TABLE 1–15. Osteonecrosis

Entity	Typical Sites of Involvement	Causes and Associations	General Radiographic Findings
Epiphyseal osteonecrosis and osteonecrosis of the small or irregular bones	Femoral head Talus Distal femoral condyle Carpal lunate Humeral head	Trauma Hip dislocation Intracapsular hip fracture Hemoglobinopathies Sickle cell anemia Corticosteroid compounds Exogenous corticosteroid therapy Cushing's disease Inflammatory articular disorders Systemic lupus erythematosus Dysbaric disorders Divers Astronauts Pregnancy Irradiation Pancreatitis (alcoholism) Gout Renal transplantation Lymphoproliferative disorders Idiopathic	Routine radiographs may be negative Bone sclerosis Cysts Subchondral collapse (crescent sign) May be focal or segmental area of involvement Joint space narrowing in advanced cases Intravertebral vacuum phenomenon with pathologic vertebral body collapse Scintigraphy, computed tomography, and magnetic resonance imaging are important in assessing osteonecrosis
Medullary osteonecrosis	Long tubular bones, especially lower extremity	Same associations as epiphyseal osteonecrosis (above)	Metadiaphyseal involvement: also termed bone infarct Patchy intramedullary sclerosis with areas of radiolucency Irregular calcific deposits Closely resembles appearance of enchondroma Occurs within areas of fatty marrow Malignant transformation extremely rare
Vertebral body osteonecrosis	Vertebral body: lumbar and thoracolumbar segments	Frequently associated with corticosteroid use	Vertebral body collapse with linear zone of intraosseous gas (intravertebral vacuum)

TABLE 1–16. Osteochondroses and Other Epiphyseal Alterations

Entity	Site of Involvement	Age (yr)	Probable Mechanism
Legg-Calvé-Perthes disease	Femoral capital epiphysis	4–8	Osteonecrosis, perhaps caused by trauma
Freiberg's infraction	Metatarsal head	13–18	Osteonecrosis caused by trauma
Kienböck's disease	Carpal lunate	20–40	Osteonecrosis caused by trauma
Thiemann's disease	Phalanges of hand	11–19	Osteonecrosis, perhaps caused by trauma
Osgood-Schlatter disease	Tibial tubercle	11–15	Trauma or abnormal stress
Blount disease	Proximal tibial epiphysis	1–3 (infantile) 8–15 (adolescent)	Trauma or abnormal stress
Scheuermann's disease	Discovertebral junction	13–17	Trauma or abnormal stress
Sinding-Larsen-Johansson disease	Patella	10–14	Trauma or abnormal stress
Köhler's bone disease	Tarsal navicular	3–7	Osteonecrosis or altered sequence of ossification
Panner's disease	Capitulum of humerus	5–10	Osteonecrosis or abnormal ossification
Sever's disease	Calcaneal apophysis	4–10	Variation of normal ossification (no clinical significance)
Van Neck's disease	Ischiopubic synchondrosis	4–8	Normal bulbous appearance of ossification center (no clinical significance)

TABLE 1–17. Infectious Disorders of Bones and Joints

Entity	General Characteristics	General Radiographic Findings
Acute pyogenic osteomyelitis	Intravenous drug abusers, diabetics, and immunocompromised patients have a predisposition to osteomyelitis and septic arthritis of adjacent joints Routes of contamination: hematogenous, contiguous source, direct implantation, and postoperative Organisms: *Staphylococcus, Actinomyces, Pseudomonas, Brucella,* and many others	Metaphyses in children Spine and pelvis in adults Poorly defined permeative bone destruction
Pyogenic septic arthritis	Predisposing factors: intravenous drug abuse, joint surgery, immunocompromised states Routes of contamination: hematogenous, contiguous source, direct implantation, and postoperative Common organisms: *Staphylococcus aureus, Streptococcus, Haemophilus, Pseudomas,* gonococcus, and *Escherichia coli* Mycobacterial and fungal agents also may be implicated Neonatal septic arthritis is more common than childhood septic arthritis Infectious spondylodiscitis occurs most frequently after spine surgery	*Adult septic arthritis:* Rapid concentric joint space narrowing Periarticular osteoporosis Capsular distention from joint effusion Loss of definition and destruction of subchondral bone Marginal and central osseous erosions Bony ankylosis (rare) *Neonatal and childhood septic arthritis:* Soft tissue swelling or capsular distention Pathologic subluxation or dislocation: lateral displacement of ossification center Slipped capital femoral epiphysis Metaphyseal osteomyelitis Concentric joint space narrowing
Chronic osteomyelitis	*Signs of reactivation:* Change from a previous radiograph Poorly defined areas of osteolysis Thin linear periostitis Sequestration *Complication:* Marjolin's ulcer—squamous cell carcinoma at site of cloaca	Osteosclerosis and cortical thickening Thick, single layer of periosteal bone proliferation Areas of osteolysis and poorly defined areas of sclerosis Sequestrum and involucrum
Brodie's abscess	Subacute pyogenic osteomyelitis Most frequently found in children Predilection for the distal tibial metaphysis Rarely crosses into the epiphysis Tibia is the most common site of such infections Usually staphylococcal organisms	Circular, geographic zone of osteolysis Sharply circumscribed sclerotic margin Metaphyseal location Radiolucent channel may communicate with growth plate May resemble osteoid osteoma or stress fracture
Chronic recurrent multifocal osteomyelitis (CRMO)*	Unknown cause Occurs mainly in children and adolescents Diagnosis of exclusion: 1. Lack of causative organism 2. No abscess formation 3. Atypical location compared with infectious osteomyelitis 4. Often multifocal lesions 5. Radiographic findings suggesting acute or subacute osteomyelitis 6. Laboratory and histologic findings suggesting acute or subacute osteomyelitis	Initial osteolytic destruction of metaphysis adjacent to growth plate with no periosteal bone formation or sequestration Magnetic resonance imaging also useful in the diagnosis

TABLE 1–17. Infectious Disorders of Bones and Joints *Continued*

Entity	General Characteristics	General Radiographic Findings
	7. Prolonged, fluctuating course with recurrent episodes of pain occurring over several years, usually without systemic manifestations 8. May accompany pustulosis palmoplantaris or other skin lesions and may be closely related to synovitis, acne, pustulosis, hyperostosis, and osteitis (SAPHO) syndrome	
Tuberculous osteomyelitis: extraspinal sites	Tuberculosis confined to extraspinal bone is infrequent; bone involvement usually is associated with tuberculous arthritis of adjacent joints Affects persons of any age, especially those with underlying disorders, corticosteroid users, intravenous drug abusers, immigrants, and immunosuppressed persons Most common organism: *Mycobacterium tuberculosis* Can affect any bone: pelvis, phalanges and metacarpals (tuberculous dactylitis), long bones, ribs, sternum, scapula, skull, patella, and the carpal and tarsal regions	Osteolytic lesions Surrounding sclerosis and periostitis may occur Intracortical lesions are rare Cystic tuberculosis: disseminated lesions throughout the skeleton rarely occur Often begins in epiphysis and spreads to adjacent joint Metaphyseal lesions in children may violate the growth plate (helping to differentiate tuberculous osteomyelitis from pyogenic osteomyelitis)
Tuberculous arthritis: extraspinal sites	Affects persons of any age, especially those with underlying disorders, corticosteroid users, intravenous drug abusers, immigrants, and immunosuppressed persons Most common organism: *Mycobacterium tuberculosis* Other sites include the hip, knee, wrist, and elbow	Various degrees of soft tissue swelling Gradual joint space narrowing Juxta-articular osteoporosis Peripherally located erosions Subchondral erosions Periarticular abscess
Tuberculous spondylitis	Tuberculous spondylitis: spine is involved in 25 to 50 per cent of all cases of skeletal tuberculosis Thoracolumbar region most frequent site of involvement May affect solitary vertebra, but most cases affect two or more vertebrae In more than 80 per cent of patients, tuberculous infection begins in the vertebral body; less commonly affects posterior elements Most common organism: *Mycobacterium tuberculosis* Men > women; occurs in adults and children	Discovertebral lesions: osteolytic destruction of vertebral body margins and usual extension into the intervening intervertebral disc; eventual obliteration of the disc space and adjacent subchondral end plates; vertebral collapse and consequent kyphosis (gibbus) deformity may occur Paraspinal extension: frequent spread of infection from vertebral bodies and discs to adjacent ligaments and soft tissues; usual extension is anterolateral; rare epidural extension; subligamentous extension underneath the anterior and posterior longitudinal ligaments; abscesses (i.e., psoas abscesses) may extend for great distances and may penetrate adjacent viscera Other infrequent radiographic findings include bony ankylosis, ivory vertebrae, atlantoaxial instability (fewer than 2 per cent of tuberculous spondylitis patients), and spinal canal involvement
Congenital syphilis	Affects babies born to mothers who have been infected during pregnancy with the spirochete *Treponema pallidum*	Symmetric, transverse, radiolucent, metaphyseal bands or linear, longitudinal, alternating lucent and sclerotic bands (the "celery stalk" appearance) Other osseous abnormalities include osteochondritis, diaphyseal osteomyelitis, and gumma formation
Poliomyelitis	Paralysis results in muscle and bone atrophy May result in scoliosis and mechanical disorders of the spine and lower extremities	Asymmetric hypoplasia and osteopenia of the pelvic bones and femur Prominent scoliosis
Leprous osteomyelitis	Leprosy is an infectious disease caused by *Mycobacterium leprae,* rarely encountered in the United States; most common in Africa, South America, and Asia Patients also may contract neuropathic osteoarthropathy, secondary infection, and leprous arthritis	Periostitis Osteitis Osteomyelitis Neuropathic osteoarthropathy
Unusual bacterial and fungal forms of osteomyelitis	Disorders include the following: Actinomycosis Nocardiosis Cryptococcosis (torulosis) North American blastomycosis Coccidioidomycosis Histoplasmosis Sporotrichosis Candidiasis Maduromycosis (mycetoma)	Findings variable depending on causative organisms

*Data from Rosenberg ZS, Shankman S, Klein M, et al: Chronic recurrent multifocal osteomyelitis, AJR 151:142, 1988; Jurik AG, Egund N: MRI in chronic recurrent multifocal osteomyelitis, Skeletal Radiol 26:230, 1997.

RECOMMENDED READING*

Chapman S, Nakielny R: Aids to Radiological Differential Diagnosis. 3rd Ed. Philadelphia, WB Saunders, 1995.

Dorfman HD, Czerniak B: Bone Tumors. St. Louis, Mosby, 1998.

Edeiken J, Dalinka M, Karasick D: Edeiken's Roentgen Diagnosis of Diseases of Bone. 4th Ed. Baltimore, Williams & Wilkins, 1990.

Forrester DM, Kricun ME, Kerr R: Imaging of the Foot and Ankle. Rockville, MD, Aspen, 1988.

Frymoyer JW, Ducker TB, Hadler NM, et al (eds): The Adult Spine: Principles and Practice. 2nd Ed. New York, Raven Press, 1997.

Gehweiler JA Jr, Osborne RL Jr, Becker RF: The Radiology of Vertebral Trauma. Philadelphia, WB Saunders, 1980.

Gilula LA, Yin Y: Imaging of the Wrist and Hand. Philadelphia, WB Saunders, 1996.

Greenfield GB: Radiology of Bone Diseases. 2nd Ed. Philadelphia, JB Lippincott, 1975.

Greenspan A: Orthopedic Radiology: A Practical Approach. 3rd Ed. Philadelphia, JB Lippincott, 1999.

Harris JH Jr, Mirvis SE: The Radiology of Acute Cervical Spine Trauma. 2nd Ed. Baltimore, Williams & Wilkins, 1995.

Hilton SVW, Edwards DK: Practical Pediatric Radiology. 2nd Ed. Philadelphia, WB Saunders, 1994.

Huvos AG: Bone Tumors: Diagnosis, Treatment and Prognosis. 2nd Ed. Philadelphia, WB Saunders, 1991.

Keats TE, Smith TH: An Atlas of Normal Developmental Roentgen Anatomy. 2nd Ed. Chicago, Year Book Medical Publishers, 1988.

Keats TE: Atlas of Normal Roentgen Variants That May Simulate Disease. 6th Ed. Chicago, Year Book Medical Publishers, 1996.

Kleinman PK: Diagnostic Imaging of Child Abuse. 2nd Ed. Philadelphia, Mosby–Year Book, 1998.

Köhler A, Zimmer EA: Borderlands of Normal and Early Pathologic Findings in Skeletal Radiography. 4th Ed. New York, Thieme Medical Publishers, 1993.

Lovell WW, Winter RB: Pediatric Orthopedics. 4th Ed. Philadelphia, JB Lippincott, 1996.

Marchiori, D: Clinical Imaging: With Skeletal, Chest, and Abdomen Pattern Differentials. Philadelphia, Mosby–Year Book, 1998.

Mirra JM, Picci P, Gold RH: Bone Tumors: Clinical, Radiologic, and Pathologic Considerations. Philadelphia, Lea & Febiger, 1989.

Murray RO, Jacobson HG, Stoker DJ: The Radiology of Skeletal Disorders. 3rd Ed. New York, Churchill Livingstone, 1990.

Rockwood CA, Green DP, Bucholz RW: Rockwood and Green's Fractures in Adults. 4th Ed. Philadelphia, JB Lippincott, 1996.

Rockwood CA, Wilkins KE, Beaty JH: Fractures in Children. 4th Ed. Philadelphia, JB Lippincott, 1996.

Resnick D, Kang HS: Internal Derangements of Joints: Emphasis on MR Imaging. Philadelphia, WB Saunders, 1997.

Resnick D: Diagnosis of Bone and Joint Disorders. 3rd Ed. Philadelphia, WB Saunders, 1995.

Silverman FN, Kuhn JP (eds): Essentials of Caffey's Pediatric X-ray Diagnosis. Chicago, Year Book Medical Publishers, 1990.

Taybi H, Lachman RS: Radiology of Syndromes, Metabolic Disorders, and Skeletal Dysplasias. 4th Ed. St. Louis, Mosby–Year Book, 1996.

Unni KK, David C: Dahlin's Bone Tumors: General Aspects and Data on 11,087 Cases. 5th Ed. Baltimore, Williams & Wilkins, 1996.

Yochum TR, Rowe LJ: Essentials of Skeletal Radiology. 2nd Ed. Baltimore, Williams & Wilkins, 1996.

---

*Only major reference sources, primarily textbooks, are listed here. More specific references pertaining to individual disorders are cited in subsequent chapters.

CHAPTER 2

Cervical Spine

- ◆ Normal Developmental Anatomy
- ◆ Developmental Anomalies, Anatomic Variants, and Sources of Diagnostic Error
- ◆ Skeletal Dysplasias and Other Congenital Diseases
- ◆ Physical Injury
- ◆ Articular Disorders
- ◆ Bone Tumors
- ◆ Metabolic Diseases
- ◆ Intervertebral Disc Abnormalities
- ◆ Cervical Spine Surgery
- ◆ Vascular Disorders

Normal Developmental Anatomy

Accurate interpretation of pediatric cervical spine radiographs requires a thorough understanding of normal developmental anatomy. Table 2–1 outlines the age of appearance and fusion of the primary and secondary ossification centers. Figures 2–1 to 2–3 demonstrate the radiographic appearance of many important developmental landmarks at selected ages from birth to skeletal maturity.

Developmental Anomalies, Anatomic Variants, and Sources of Diagnostic Error

Radiographic interpretation of disease processes in the cervical spine may be difficult owing to many anomalies, variations, and other sources of diagnostic error that are frequently encountered in this region of the spine (Table 2–2). Although most of these processes are of no clinical significance, some anomalies may result in atlantoaxial instability and are of vital concern to the clinician and the patient (Table 2–3).

Skeletal Dysplasias and Other Congenital Diseases

Table 2–6 outlines a number of dysplastic and congenital disorders that affect the cervical spine; Figures 2–39 and 2–40 illustrate some of these disorders.

Physical Injury

Fractures, dislocations, and soft tissue injuries involving the spine are frequent, and often these lesions are associated with serious clinical manifestations. Tables 2–7 and 2–8 outline some of the more important injuries of the upper and lower portions of the cervical spine, respectively. The injuries are classified according to their anatomic locations, presumed mechanism of injury, and presence or absence of spinal instability. In addition, Figures 2–41 to 2–58 and Tables 2–9 and 2–10 demonstrate the most characteristic imaging manifestations of some of the more common examples of physical injury.

Articular Disorders

The cervical spine is a frequent and characteristic site of involvement for many forms of spondyloarthropathy. Tables 2–11 and 2–12 outline the degenerative, inflammatory, crystal-induced, infectious, and other articular diseases that commonly afflict the cervical spine, and Figures 2–59 to 2–83 reveal some of their radiographic manifestations.

Bone Tumors

A wide variety of malignant tumors, benign tumors, and tumor-like lesions affect the cervical spine. Table

2–13 reveals the spectrum of neoplasms that may affect the entire vertebral column (including the thoracic, lumbar, sacral, and coccygeal segments). The table also indicates some of the typical characteristics of each lesion as it is manifested in the cervical spine. Table 2–14 and Figures 2–84 to 2–96 illustrate some of the more common examples.

Metabolic Diseases

The skeletal manifestations of many metabolic disorders are frequently exhibited in the cervical spine. Some of the more common conditions are outlined in Table 2–15 and illustrated in Figures 2–97 to 2–99.

Intervertebral Disc Abnormalities

Herniation of one or more intervertebral discs in the cervical spine is a common cause of signs and symptoms in the cervical spine and upper extremity. Table 2–16 describes acute disc herniations and chronic degenerative spondylosis. Figure 2–100 illustrates the imaging of this common problem. Degenerative spine disease also is discussed under the heading of articular disorders earlier in this chapter.

Cervical Spine Surgery

Numerous surgical procedures are performed for pathologic conditions of the intervertebral disc, spinal stenosis, or other disorders. Table 2–17 lists a few of these procedures and some of their complications; Figures 2–101 to 2–103 show some of their imaging manifestations.

Vascular Disorders

Vascular disease may be encountered in the evaluation of cervical spine radiographs. Table 2–18 contains a description of three of these conditions, and Figure 2–104 illustrates a vertebral artery aneurysm.

TABLE 2–1. Approximate Age of Appearance and Fusion of Cervical Spine Ossification Centers[1–3] (Figs. 2–1 to 2–3)

Ossification Center	Primary or Secondary	No. of Centers	Age of Appearance* (Years)	Age of Fusion* (Years)	Comments
C1 posterior arch	P	2	Birth	3	
C1 anterior arch	P	1	Birth–1	6–7	
C1 tip of transverse process	S	2	18	21–25	
C2 odontoid	P	2	Birth	4	Fuses to body
C2 tip of odontoid	S	1	3–6	8–12	Fuses to odontoid
C2 body	P	1 or 2	Birth	4	Fuses to laminae
C2 neural arches (laminae)	P	2	Birth	2	Fuse together
C2 end-plate ring apophysis	S	1	Puberty	22–25	Fuses to body
C3-C7 body	P	1	Birth	3	Fuses to laminae
C3-C7 neural arches (laminae)	P	2	Birth	1	Fuse together in order from C7-C3
C3-C7 end-plate ring apophyses	S	2	11–12	17–18	Fuse to body

*Ages of appearance and fusion of ossification centers in girls typically precede those of boys. Ethnic differences also exist.
P, Primary; S, secondary.

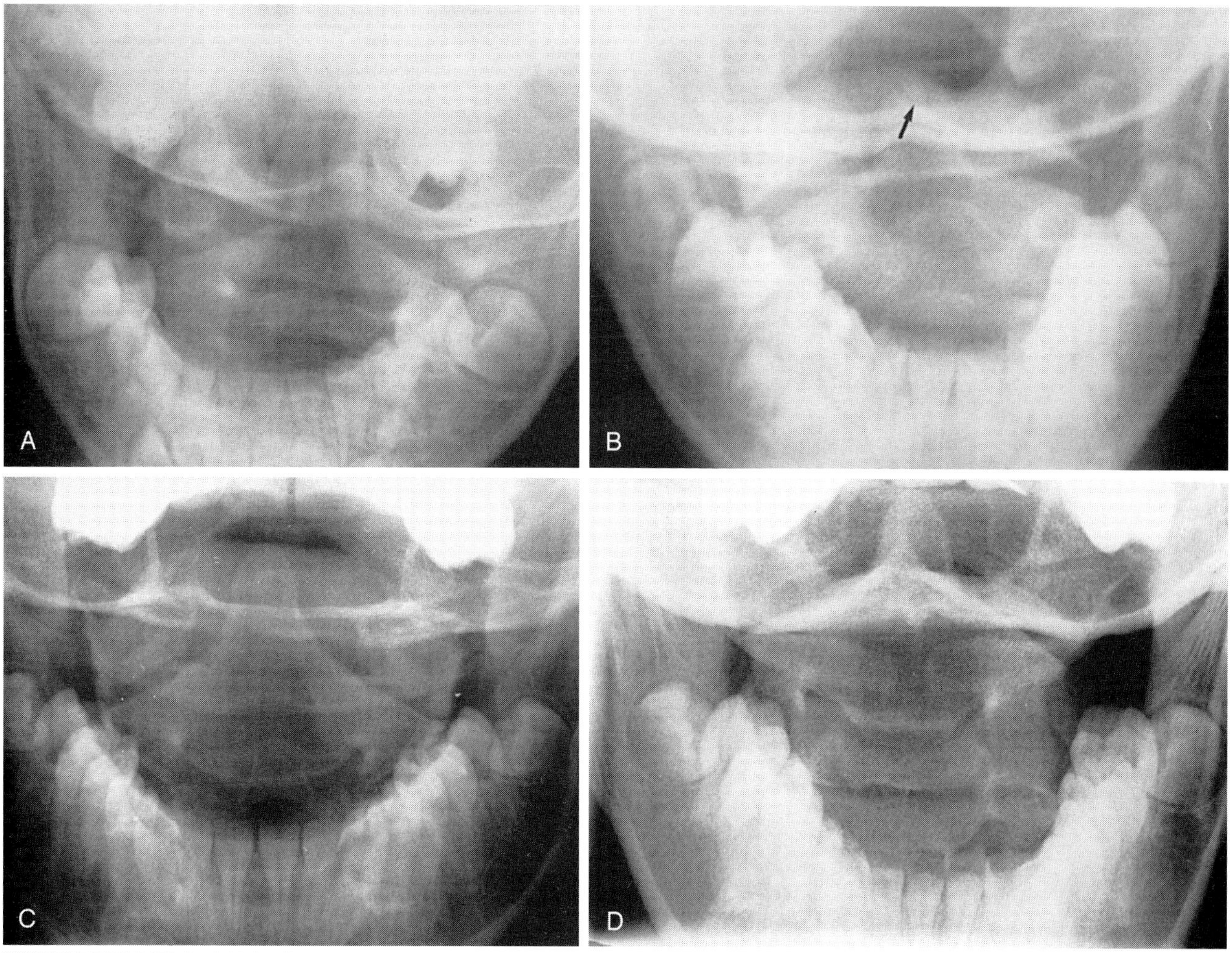

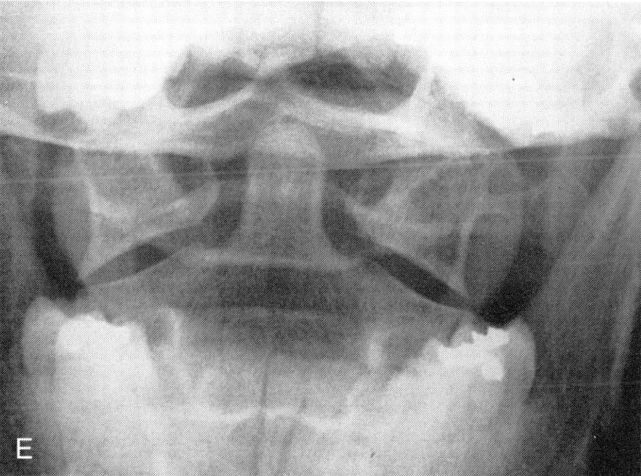

FIGURE 2–1. Skeletal maturation and normal development: Anteroposterior open mouth upper cervical spine radiographs.[1–3] A 3-year-old girl. The odontoid and lateral masses of the atlas are obscured by the occipital and dental structures. The atlas often appears wider than the axis until about the age of 5 years. B 5-year-old boy. The ossification center at the tip of the odontoid (arrow) typically appears at the age of 2 years and fuses to the odontoid by the age of 12 years. If it persists into adulthood, it is termed an os terminale of Bergmann and is considered a normal variant. C 11-year-old girl. The odontoid process usually is completely developed by this age. D 14-year-old girl. The posterior arch of the atlas, which usually fuses at about the age of 3 years, remains ununited in this child. Such incomplete fusion (spondyloschisis) at this level is a frequent occurrence. E Adult: 28-year-old man. The secondary ossification centers of the transverse processes typically are the last centers to fuse, usually by age 25 years, and such fusion signals complete development.

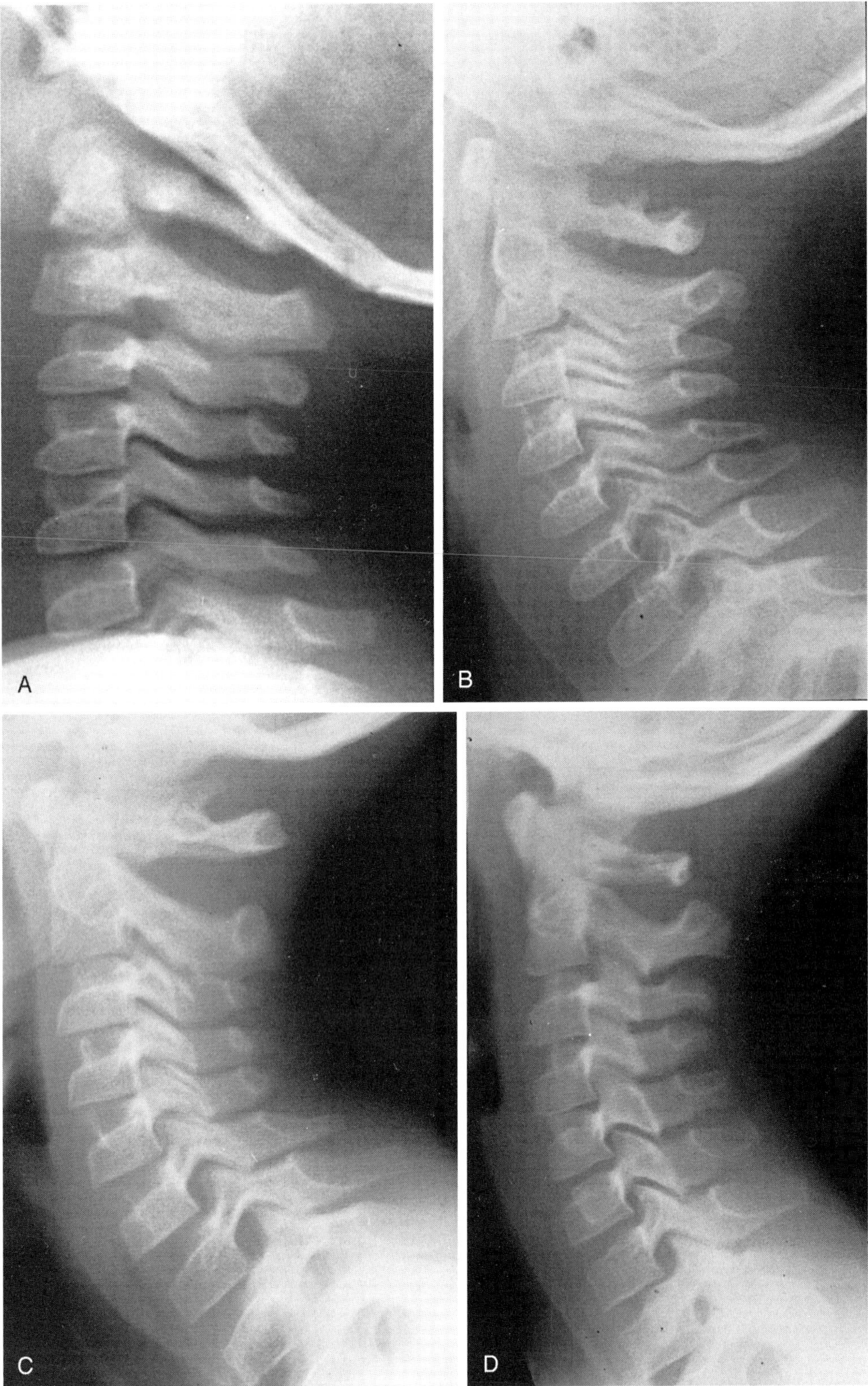

FIGURE 2–2. Skeletal maturation and normal development: Lateral cervical spine radiographs.[1–3] **A** 11-month-old girl. The odontoid is not yet fused with the body of C2. The vertebral bodies appear flattened, and the sagittal spinal canal diameter is disproportionately wide. **B** 3-year-old girl. The odontoid typically fuses to the body of C2 about the age of 3 years, and it is almost completely fused in this child. The superior aspects of the vertebral bodies are rounded, the spinal canal remains proportionately wide, and the posterior margins of the vertebral bodies are scalloped. The anterior arch of the atlas appears to be displaced superiorly in relation to the tip of the odontoid. This normal finding is the result of incomplete ossification of the odontoid and should not be mistaken for subluxation of the atlas. **C** 5-year-old boy. The vertebral bodies are wedge-shaped and their anterosuperior margins remain rounded. **D** 8-year-old boy. The superior margins of the vertebral bodies are beginning to appear less wedge-shaped.

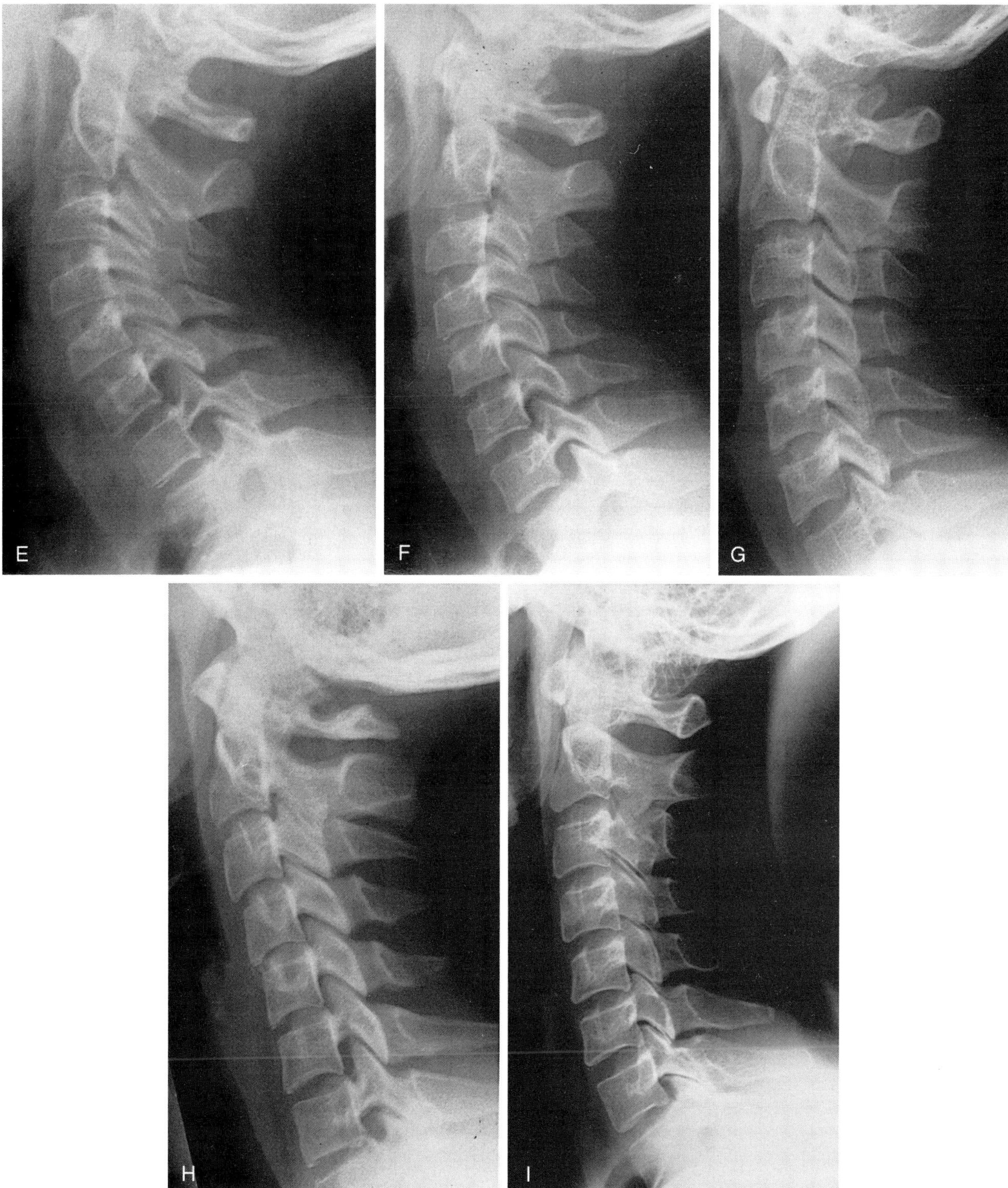

FIGURE 2–2 *Continued.* **E** 11-year-old girl. The secondary ring apophyses adjacent to the superior and inferior vertebral end plates begin to appear at puberty but may appear as early as age 7 years. The odontoid process usually is fully developed at this age. **F** 12-year-old boy. The midcervical vertebral bodies maintain a somewhat wedged appearance. Observe the ring apophyses and scalloped posterior body margins. **G** 15-year-old boy. The vertebral bodies have a more adult shape. Note the V-shaped predens space, a normal variant. **H** 16-year-old girl. The ring apophyses usually fuse with the vertebral bodies by the age of 17 years in girls and 18 years in boys. C3 often is the last cervical vertebra to retain its wedge-shaped configuration. The cervical lordosis is flattened in this girl. **I** Adult: 43-year-old woman. The vertebral bodies are squared, but their anterosuperior margins remain slightly rounded. The C2-C3 facet joints are not well visualized owing to their normal orientation. The superior articulating surface of the C7 articular process is notched, a normal variant frequently encountered in this region. The normal mastoid air cells overlying the atlanto-occipital region should not be confused with an expansile mass.

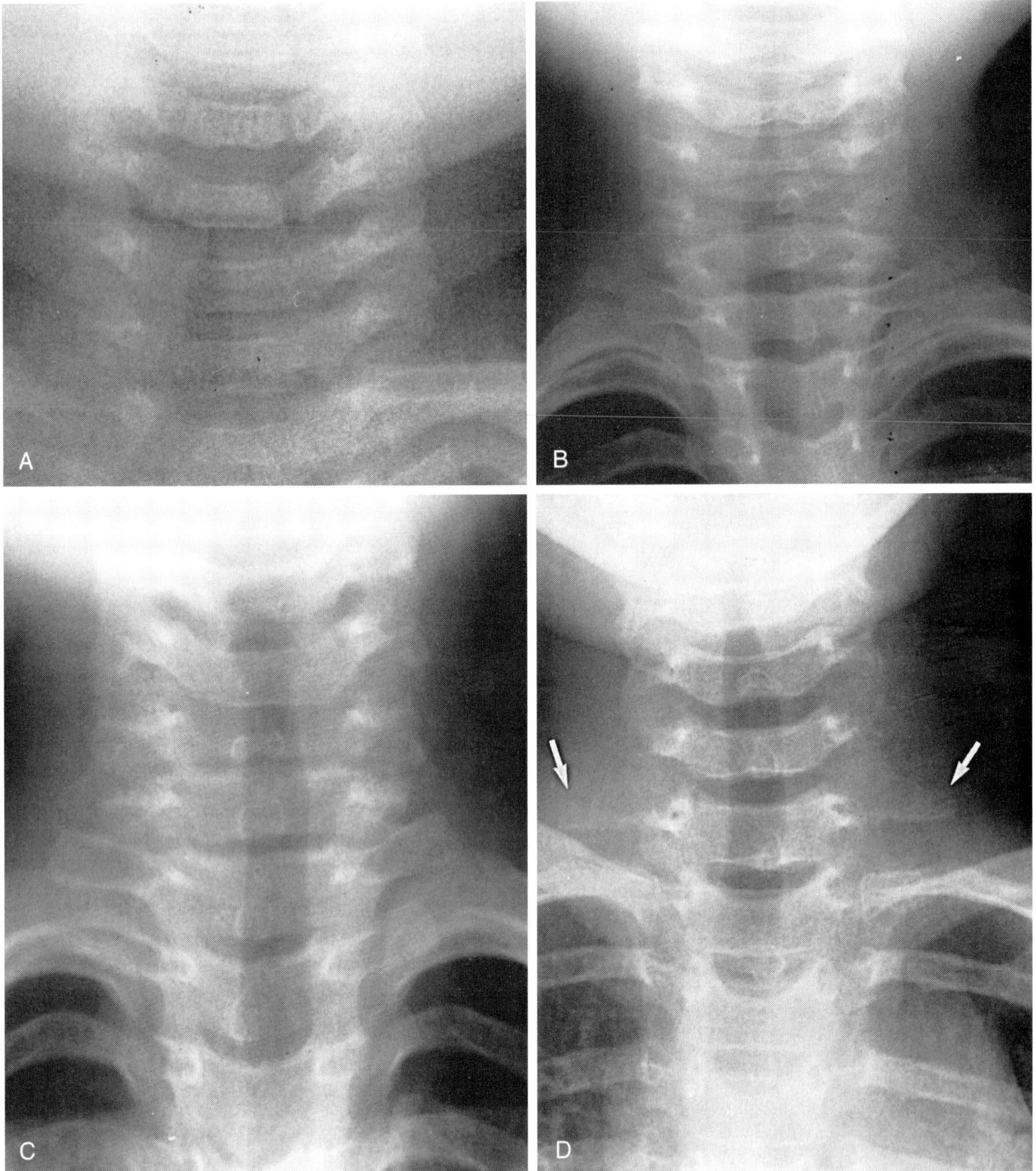

FIGURE 2–3. Skeletal maturation and normal development: Anteroposterior cervical spine radiographs.[1–3] A 11-month-old girl. Bilateral neural arch ossification centers, which usually fuse between 1 and 7 years of age, are evident in this infant. Incomplete development of the osseous structures results in a proportionately wide appearance of the spinal canal. Patient rotation has resulted in tracheal deviation. B 3-year-old girl. C 5-year-old boy. D 8-year-old girl. The C7 transverse processes are somewhat elongated (arrows), a common developmental anomaly. The obliquely oriented clavicles result from elevation of the patient's arms during exposure.

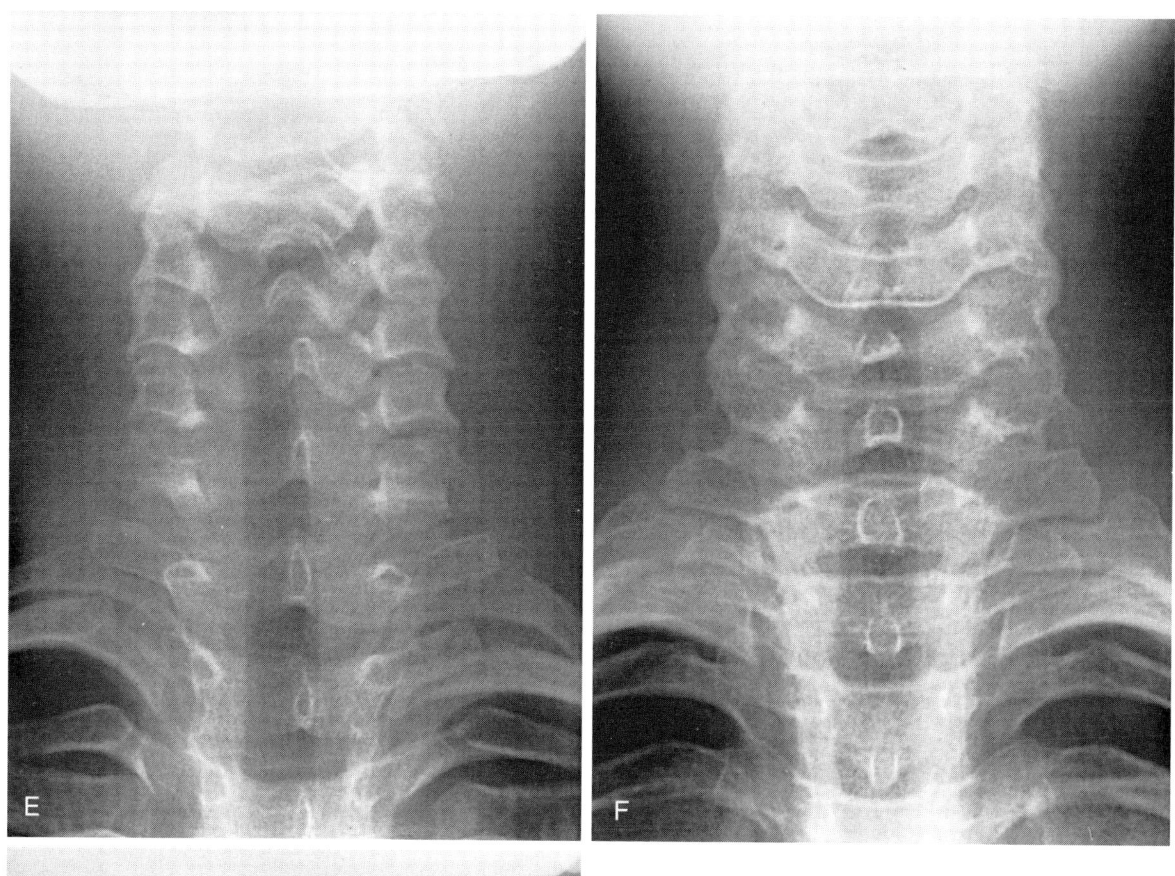

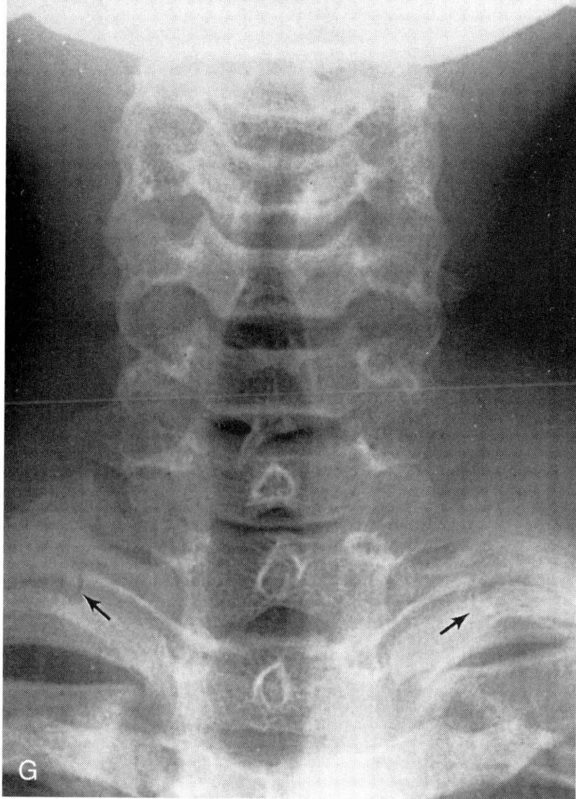

FIGURE 2–3 *Continued.* E 10-year-old boy. Inferior angulation of the x-ray beam allows visualization of the facet joint spaces. F 13-year-old boy. The cervical spine approaches adult proportions. G 15-year-old boy. The secondary ossification centers of the transverse processes usually appear about the age of 16 years. They are obvious at T2 (arrows) but indistinct at T1 in this person.

TABLE 2–2. Some Developmental Anomalies, Anatomic Variants, and Sources of Diagnostic Error Affecting the Upper Cervical Spine*

Entity	Figure(s)	Characteristics
Atlas (C1)		
Atlas assimilation[4] (occipitalization)	2–4	Failure of segmentation of the most caudal occipital sclerotome; atlas is fused to base of occiput Usually asymptomatic, but may be associated with pain, limitation of cervical motion, and neurologic signs May be associated with platybasia, basilar invagination, Chiari type I malformation, Sturge-Weber syndrome, and Klippel-Feil syndrome Atlantoaxial instability present in 50 per cent of persons with associated C2-C3 synostosis: flexion and extension radiographs should be considered to evaluate for such instability Premature degenerative disease at subjacent levels, especially C1-C2, observed in some patients with this anomaly
Posterior arch agenesis[4–8]	2–5, 2–6	Complete agenesis of posterior arch of atlas (a rare, usually asymptomatic anomaly characterized by incomplete ossification of the secondary growth center of the posterior arch) Partial agenesis, usually manifest as a midline cleft (spondyloschisis); a much more common anomaly than complete agenesis, present in 4 per cent of adults Often accompanied by compensatory hypertrophy and sclerosis of the anterior arch of C1 and hypertrophy of the spinous process of C2 (megaspinous process)—reliable signs that this is a long-standing condition rather than a rapid destructive process A cartilaginous or fibrous posterior arch is usually present, typically not resulting in instability; flexion and extension radiographs are useful in evaluating the integrity of the transverse ligament.
Anterior arch agenesis[4, 7]		Midline radiolucency on anterior arch from incomplete fusion of the ossification centers is extremely rare (0.1 per cent of persons); best seen on axial radiographs and computed tomographic (CT) scans
Accessory ossicles[9]	2–7	A variety of small ossicles may be present in the region of the atlas Usually of no clinical significance
Posterior ponticulus[6]	2–8	Ossification of posterior atlanto-occipital membrane present in 15 per cent of normal persons Arcuate foramen allows passage of the vertebral artery and C1 nerve Usually stable and benign; rarely related to vertebral artery compression, posttraumatic basal subarachnoid hemorrhage, and the Barré-Lieou syndrome
Sclerotic anterior tubercle[6]	2–9	Normal variant, not associated with osteosclerotic disorders Sclerosis and hypertrophy may be associated with chronic altered stresses related to posterior arch agenesis, os odontoideum, and other atlantoaxial anomalies
Asymmetry of atlas[7]	2–10	Lateral masses of atlas often develop asymmetrically and should not be mistaken for evidence of a compression injury of the lateral mass
Axis (C2) and C1-C2 articulations		
Normal transverse foramen[5, 7]	2–8	Normal anatomy: transverse foramen is seen on lateral radiograph as a circular radiolucency
Rotation simulating fracture[5, 7]	2–11	Rotation of lateral radiograph results in overlap of apophyseal joints, simulating fracture
Mach band effect[10]	2–12	Transverse zone of relative radiolucency overlying the base of the odontoid adjacent to the edge of the overlapping posterior arch of the atlas, simulating an odontoid fracture
Paraodontoid notch[5, 7]	2–13A	Normal bilateral notches adjacent to the base of the odontoid may simulate fractures
Incisors overlying odontoid[5]	2–13B	Normal space between incisors overlapping the odontoid may simulate a vertical fracture on anteroposterior open mouth radiograph
Os terminale of Bergmann[5, 7]	2–14	Unfused ossification center at the tip of the odontoid persisting past the age of 12 years, which may simulate a fracture

TABLE 2–2. Some Developmental Anomalies, Anatomic Variants, and Sources of Diagnostic Error Affecting the Upper Cervical Spine* *Continued*

Entity	Figure(s)	Characteristics
Os odontoideum[4, 7, 11]	2–15	Incomplete fusion of odontoid to C2 body Most likely represents a nonunion of a type II odontoid fracture rather than an anomaly Frequently results in multidirectional atlantoaxial instability that may lead to transient or progressive neurologic deficit and even death with trivial trauma
Odontoid agenesis and hypoplasia[7]		Incomplete development or absence of the odontoid Frequently results in atlantoaxial instability
Posterior inclination of odontoid[12]	2–16	Normal variation in the inclination of the odontoid that may simulate posterior displacement from an odontoid fracture or os odontoideum
V-shaped predens space[13]	2–2G, 2–17	Normal variation in which the predens space (atlantodental interspace) is V-shaped rather than parallel Accentuated on flexion radiographs Present in about 9 per cent of persons In some cases, may be due to increased flexion mobility with elongated or lax transverse ligament
Absence of transverse ligament[14]	2–18	Up to 20 per cent of children with Down syndrome (trisomy 21) are born with this anomaly, and many have hypoplasia or agenesis of the odontoid resulting in atlantoaxial instability and possible cord compression; these children should be screened with flexion and extension radiographs before participating in Special Olympics and other sporting events
Anomalous articulations[5, 7]	2–19	C1-C2 junction is a common site for several anomalies
C2 congenital spondylolysis[15]	2–20	Incomplete fusion of the C2 neural arches to the vertebral body results in a radiolucent defect and potential instability
Pseudosubluxation of C2[16, 17, 135]	2–21	Normal variant present in up to 24 per cent of infants and children up to age 8 years May be confused with an unstable fracture or ligament injury Excessive sagittal plane motion of the C2-C3 and C3-C4 segments, seen on flexion and extension radiographs in infants; is also a common finding attributed to normal ligamentous laxity
C2-C3 articulations		
Ball-and-socket articulation[5, 7]	2–22	Anomalous pronglike projection of the C3 articular process articulates with a concavity within the C2 articular process
Pseudofusion of C2-C3 apophyseal joints[18]	2–23	Normal orientation of the C2-C3 apophyseal joint surfaces often results in the appearance of joint ankylosis on lateral radiographs
Synostosis and other anomalies[5–7]	2–24; see Fig. 2–30	Developmental segmentation defects, frequently resulting in block vertebrae at the C2-C3 level; these synostoses are often accompanied by other anomalies

*See also Table 1–1.

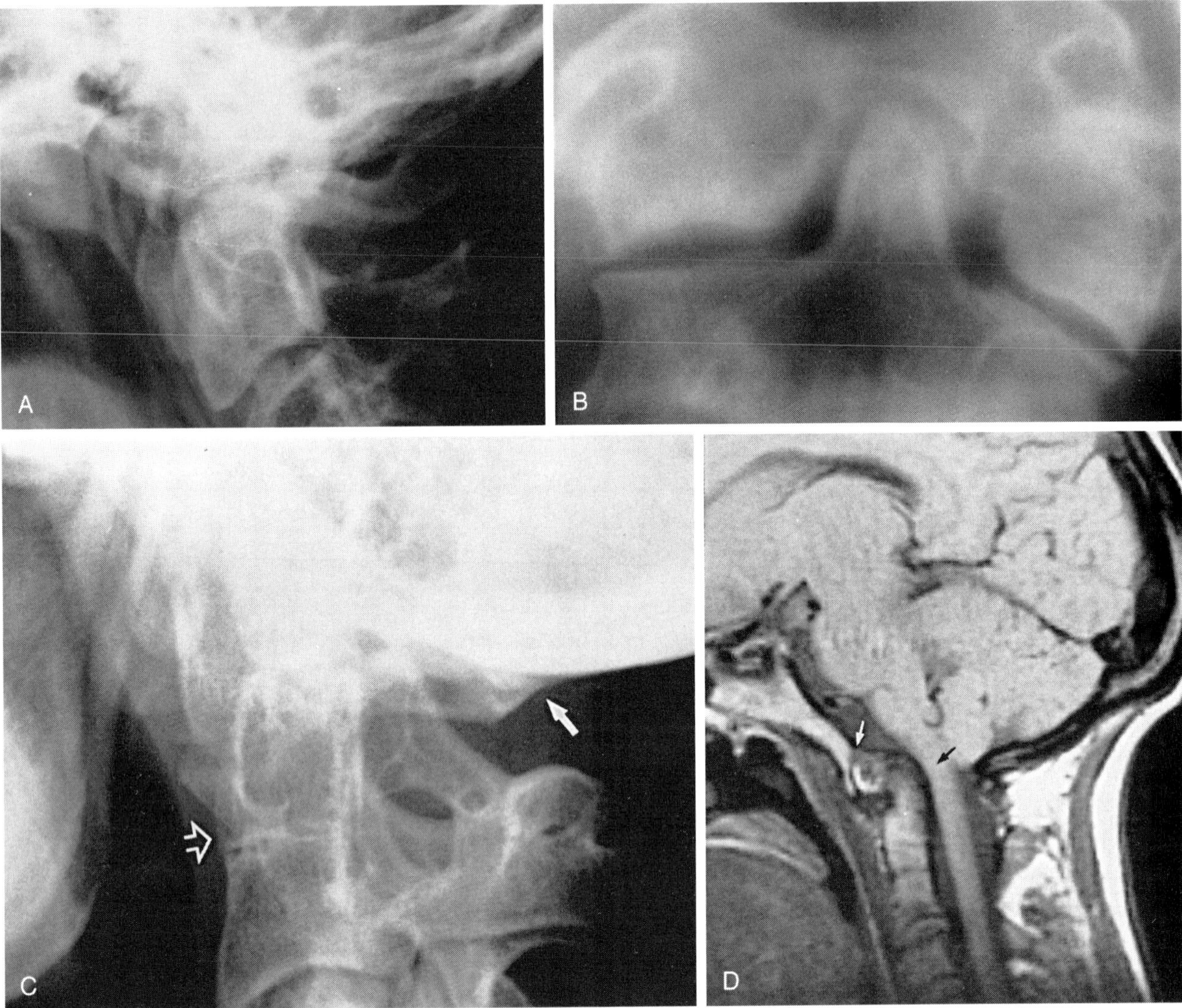

FIGURE 2–4. Atlanto-occipital assimilation (occipitalization).[4] A, B Lateral radiograph (A) and frontal conventional tomogram (B) demonstrate fusion of the occipital condyle with the lateral mass of C1 on the right side and, to a lesser extent, on the left. C, D Another patient: 27-year-old woman with stuttering and loss of memory after a motor vehicle accident. Lateral radiograph (C) shows assimilation of the atlas with the base of the occiput (arrow), synostosis (block vertebrae) of C2-C3 (open arrow), and mild basilar impression. Sagittal T1-weighted (TR/TE, 800/25) spin echo magnetic resonance (MR) image (D) reveals slight kinking of the spinomedullary junction (black arrow) and an unusually high position of the odontoid process within the foramen magnum. The anterior arch of atlas abuts on the clivus (white arrow). (C, D, *Courtesy of T. Wei, D.C., Portland, Oregon.*)

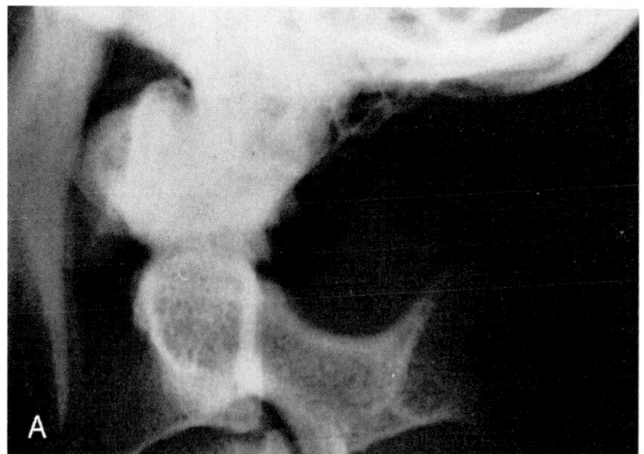

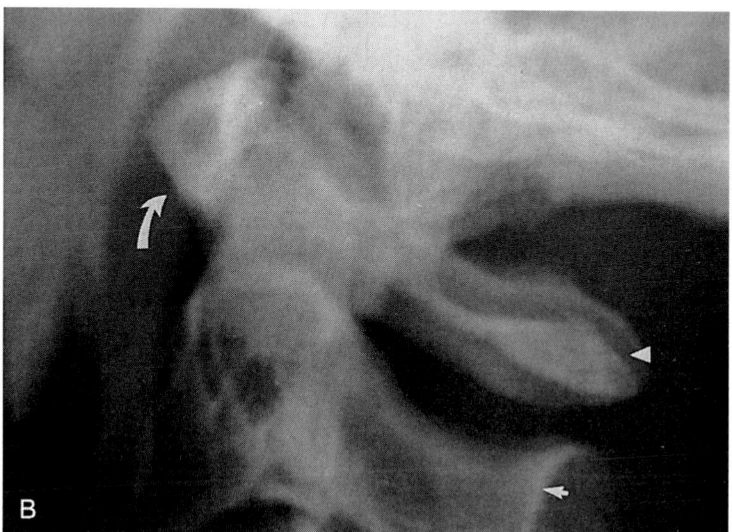

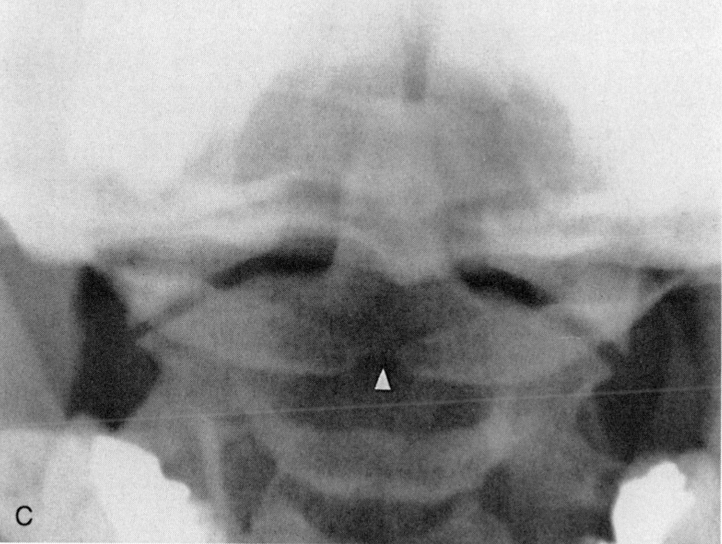

FIGURE 2–5. Agenesis of the posterior arch of C1.[4–8] A Complete agenesis. The posterior arch of the atlas remains unossified. B, C Partial agenesis (spondyloschisis). Lateral radiograph (B) shows a radiolucent cleft (arrowhead) and absence of the spinolaminar junction line. (Note the spinolaminar junction line identified at C2 by a straight arrow.) The anterior arch is hypertrophied and sclerotic (curved arrow). Frontal radiograph (C) demonstrates a median cleft in the posterior arch (arrowhead).

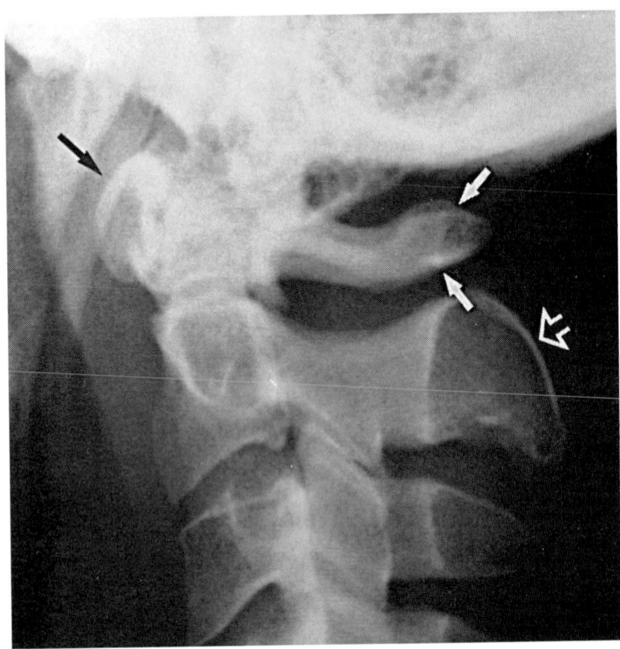

FIGURE 2–6. Anomalous atlantoaxial region.[4–8] The spinolaminar junction line at the posterior arch of atlas is incomplete (white arrows), indicating partial agenesis or spondyloschisis of the posterior arch of C1. The anterior arch of the atlas is hypertrophic and sclerotic (black arrow), and the C2 spinous process is enlarged and unusually shaped (open arrow). Hypertrophy and sclerosis of the anterior arch are commonly seen in patients with upper cervical spine anomalies, especially C1 spondyloschisis, agenesis of the posterior arch, and os odontoideum.

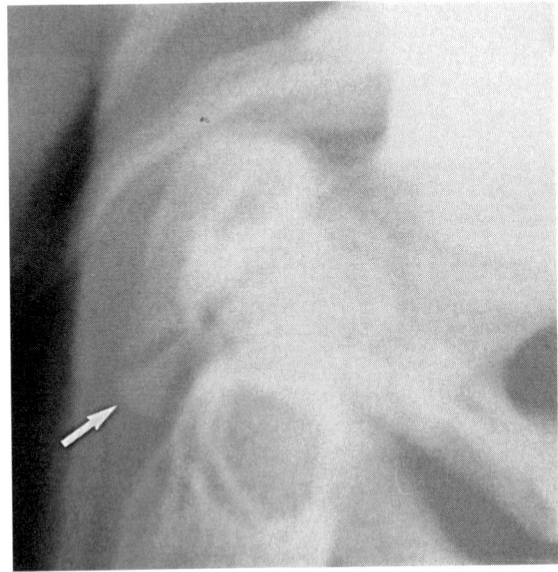

FIGURE 2–7. Accessory ossicle.[9] Observe the tiny ossicle of bone situated at the inferior aspect of the anterior arch of C1 (arrow). This painless normal variant should not be confused with an anterior arch fracture, hydroxyapatite crystal deposition within the longus colli tendon, or a degenerative osteophyte or enthesophyte.

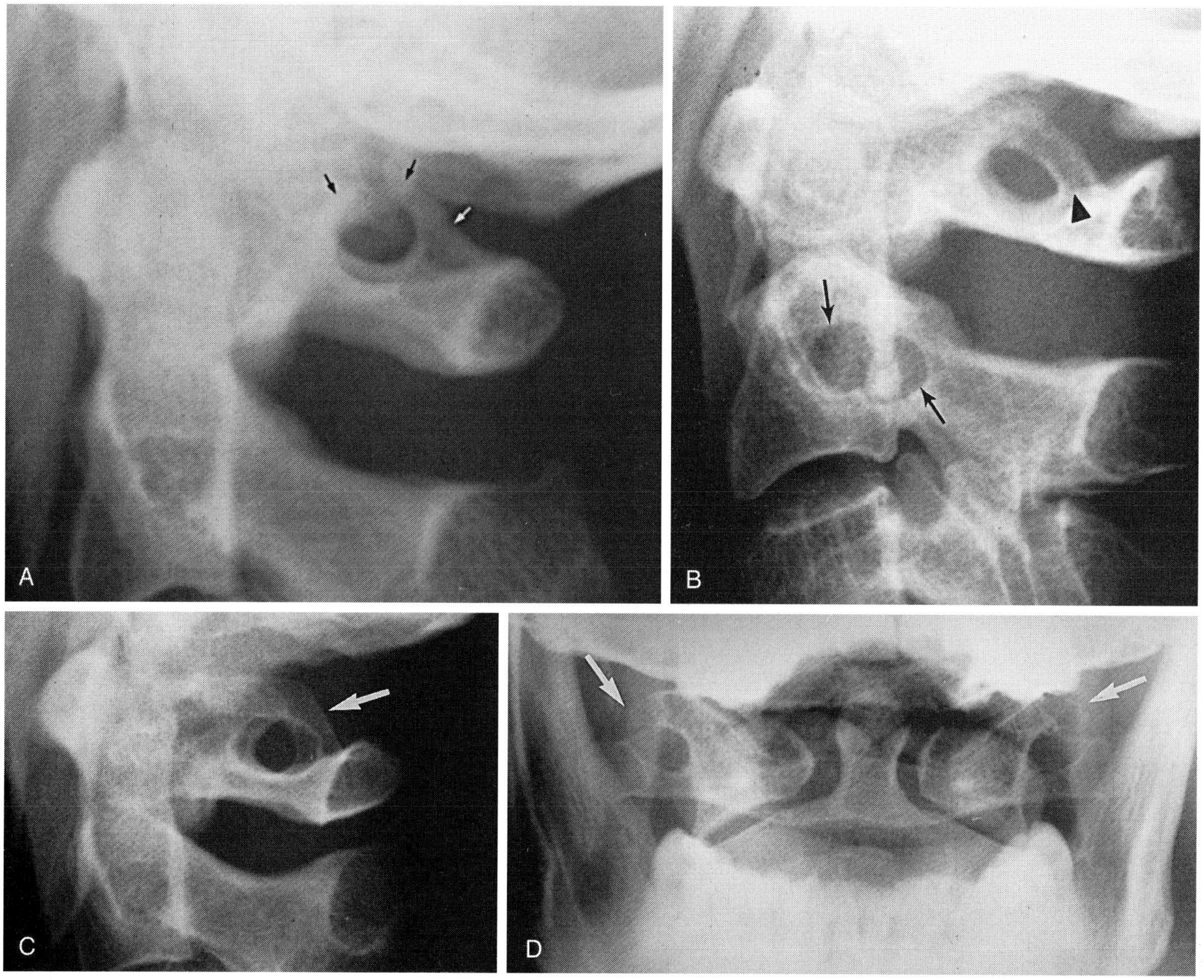

FIGURE 2–8. Posterior ponticulus (arcuate foramen).[5–7] **A** This curvilinear osseous bridge is best visualized on the lateral radiograph (arrows). The osseous bridge joins the posterior arch with the lateral mass of C1 and forms a circular opening (arcuate foramen) for the passage of the vertebral artery and the C1 nerve. **B** In this slightly rotated lateral radiograph from another patient with a posterior ponticulus anomaly (arrowhead), two circular radiolucent shadows overlying the C2 vertebral body also are present (arrows). These represent the normal foramina transversaria within the transverse processes of the axis. **C, D** Another patient. In **C,** curvilinear osseous bridges extending from the superior aspect of the lateral masses of the atlas to the posterior arches of the atlas are evident on the lateral radiograph (arrow). In **D,** the open mouth radiograph reveals that the osseous arches are continuous with the lateral masses (arrows).

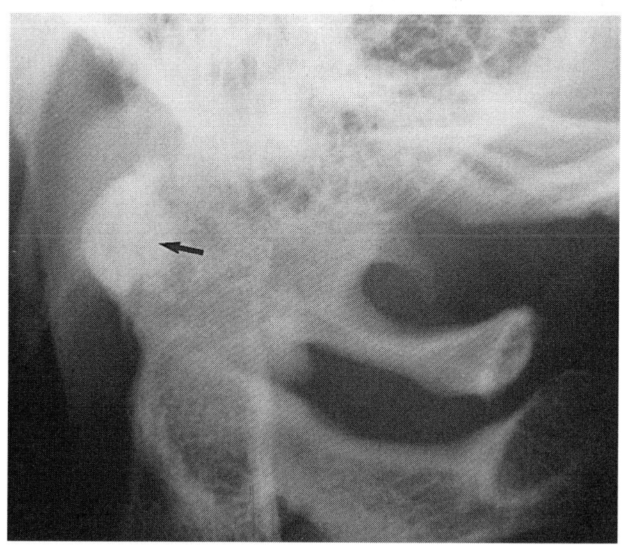

FIGURE 2–9. Sclerotic anterior tubercle.[6] The anterior arch of the atlas appears sclerotic (arrow). A partial posterior ponticulus also is present. Sclerosis, with or without hypertrophy, often occurs in conjunction with posterior arch agenesis, os odontoideum, and other anomalies of the atlantoaxial region.

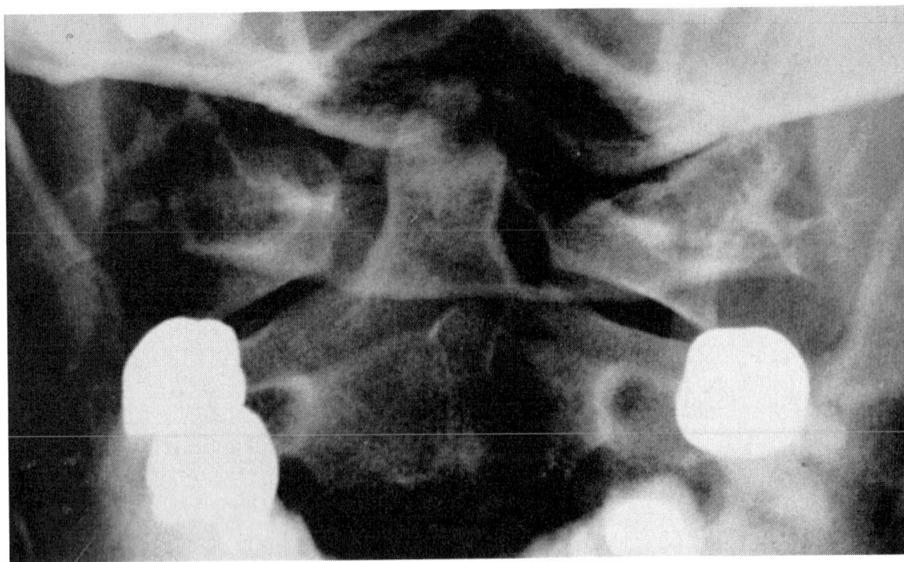

FIGURE 2–10. Asymmetric atlas.[7] The atlas has developed asymmetrically, simulating a compression fracture of the left lateral mass. Vertebral asymmetry is a common finding, especially at the transitional regions of the spine. *(Courtesy of A.L. Anderson, D.C., Portland, Oregon.)*

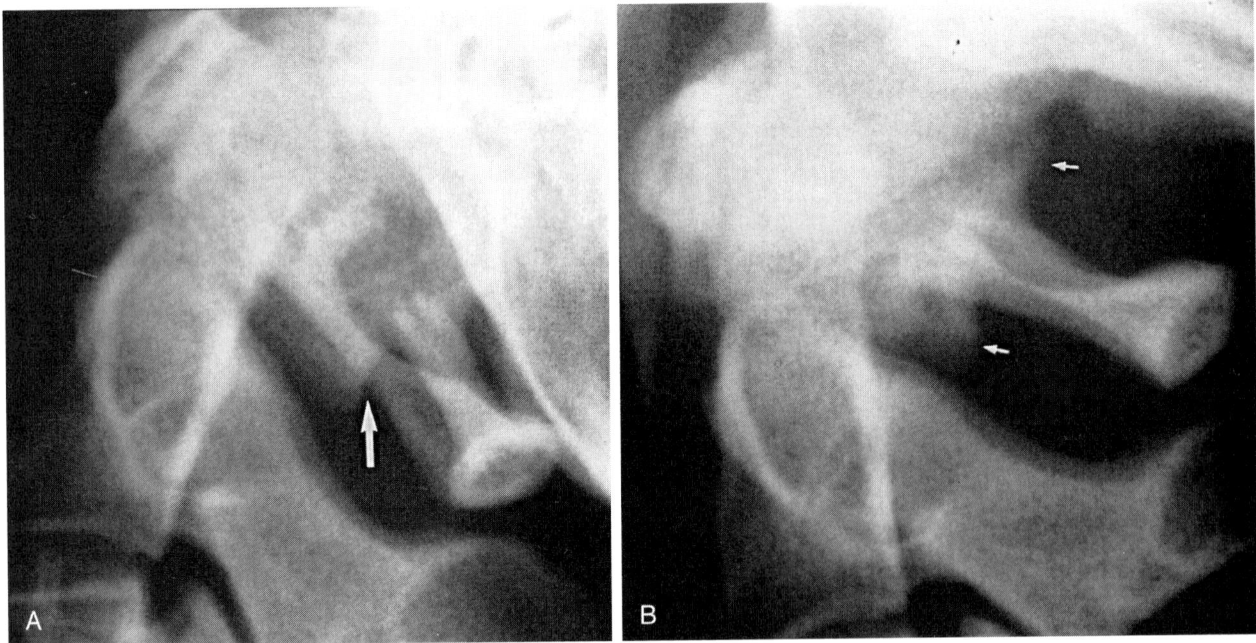

FIGURE 2–11. Simulated fracture produced by rotation.[5, 7] A Lateral radiograph taken in extension shows an apparent fracture of the posterior arch of atlas with offset of the fragments (arrow). B Neutral lateral film with normal alignment demonstrates that it is the overlying lateral masses of the atlas (arrows) that create the false appearance of a fracture.

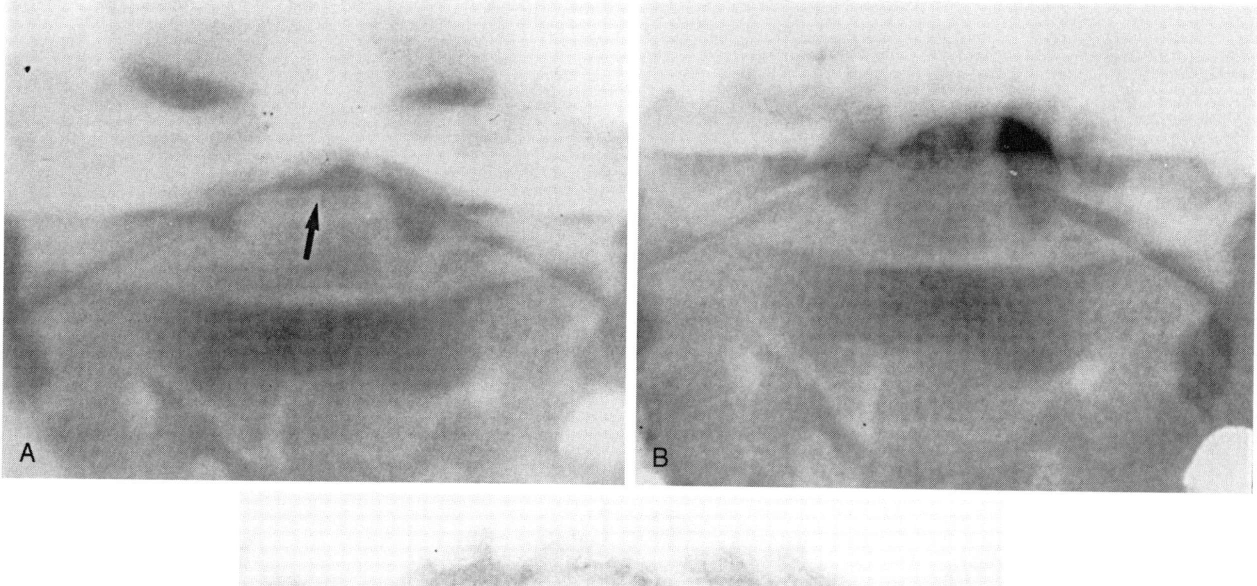

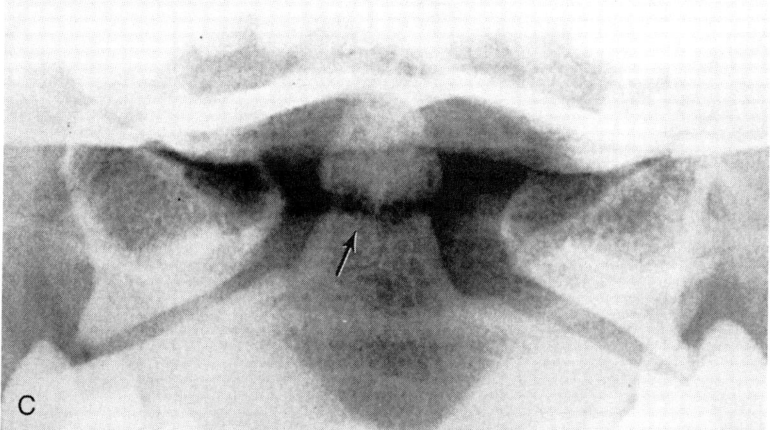

FIGURE 2–12. Mach band effect.[10] A, B This 37-year-old woman complained of pain and stiffness after a motor vehicle collision. Initial radiograph (A) shows a transverse radiolucent defect across the base of the odontoid process (arrow) resembling a type II odontoid fracture. A second radiograph (B) taken moments later with slightly different head position reveals that the base of the odontoid is intact. In this case, on the initial radiograph, the base of the occiput overlies the top of the odontoid, and the posterior arch of C1 overlies the lower odontoid and C2 vertebral body. The intervening portion of the odontoid has no overlying density, and, therefore, appears remarkably radiolucent—the Mach band effect. C In a second patient, a transverse radiolucent line across the odontoid process (arrow) is created by the space between the anterior and posterior arches of atlas, and this space should not be misinterpreted as an odontoid fracture.

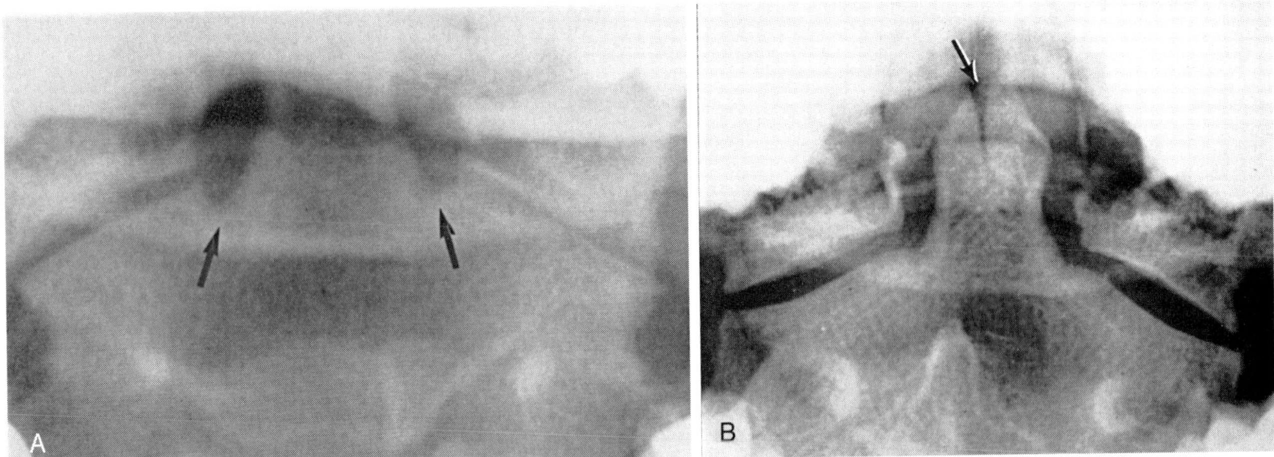

FIGURE 2–13. Normal anatomy simulating fractures.[5, 7] A Paraodontoid notches. Bilaterally symmetric notches adjacent to the base of the odontoid (arrows) are normal variants of no clinical consequence that may simulate fractures. B Overlying incisors. A vertical radiolucent shadow overlying the odontoid process (arrow) results from the space between the two overlying central incisors and should not be mistaken for a split odontoid or a fracture.

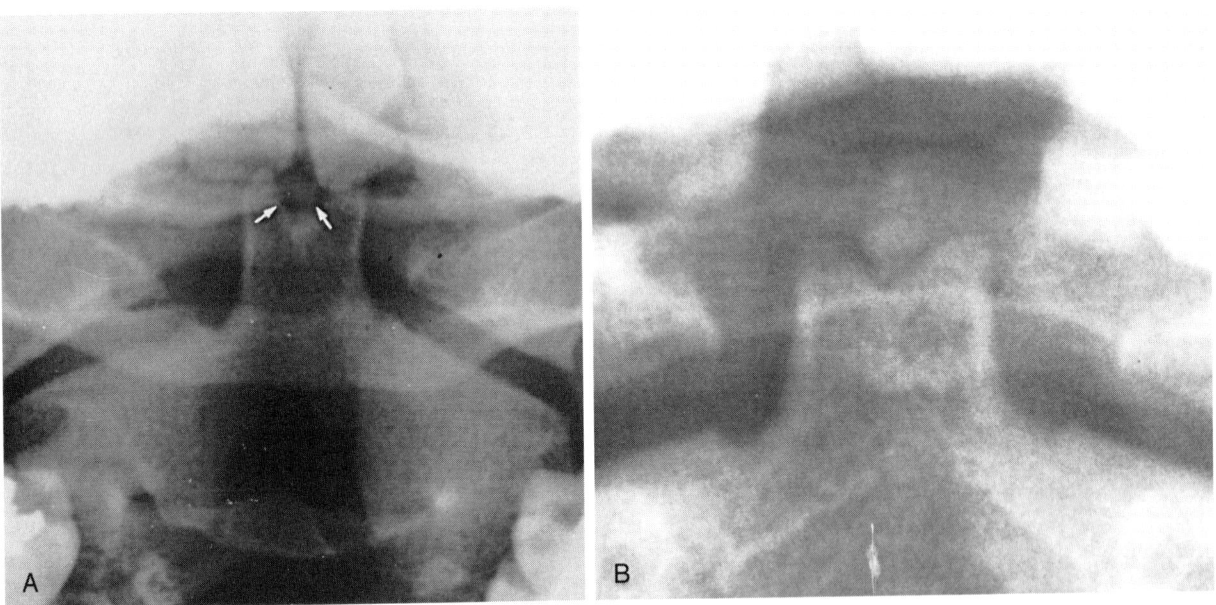

FIGURE 2–14. Os terminale of Bergmann.[5, 7] A Observe the small circular ossification center within the triangular or V-shaped radiolucent indentation (arrows). B In another patient, a more clearly defined diamond-shaped ossification center is present. The os terminale of Bergmann represents a persistent, ununited secondary growth center at the tip of the odontoid in a patient older than 12 years of age. This is of no clinical significance but must be differentiated from a fracture or an os odontoideum.

TABLE 2–3. Some Causes of Atlantoaxial Instability and Subluxation*[6, 19]

Common	Uncommon
Developmental anomalies and dysplasias	
Atlanto-occipital assimilation	Morquio's syndrome
Down syndrome (trisomy 21)	Hurler's syndrome
Os odontoideum	Spondyloepiphyseal dysplasia
Odontoid agenesis	Marfan syndrome
Odontoid hypoplasia	Metaphyseal dysplasia
Inflammatory arthropathies and connective tissue diseases	
Rheumatoid arthritis	Systemic lupus erythematosus
Ankylosing spondylitis	Behçet's syndrome
Psoriatic arthritis	Dialysis spondyloarthropathy
Reiter's syndrome	Rheumatic fever
Juvenile chronic arthritis	Multicentric reticulohistiocytosis
	Calcium pyrophosphate dihydrate crystal deposition disease
Physical injury	
Odontoid fracture	Some Jefferson fractures
	Rotatory atlantoaxial subluxation
	Transverse ligament rupture
Infection	
Retropharyngeal abscess (Grisel's syndrome)	

*Atlantoaxial instability and subluxation are present or should be questioned when the atlantodental interspace exceeds 5 mm in children and 3 mm in adults on neutral lateral or flexion radiographs, or when the interspace distance changes between flexion and extension.

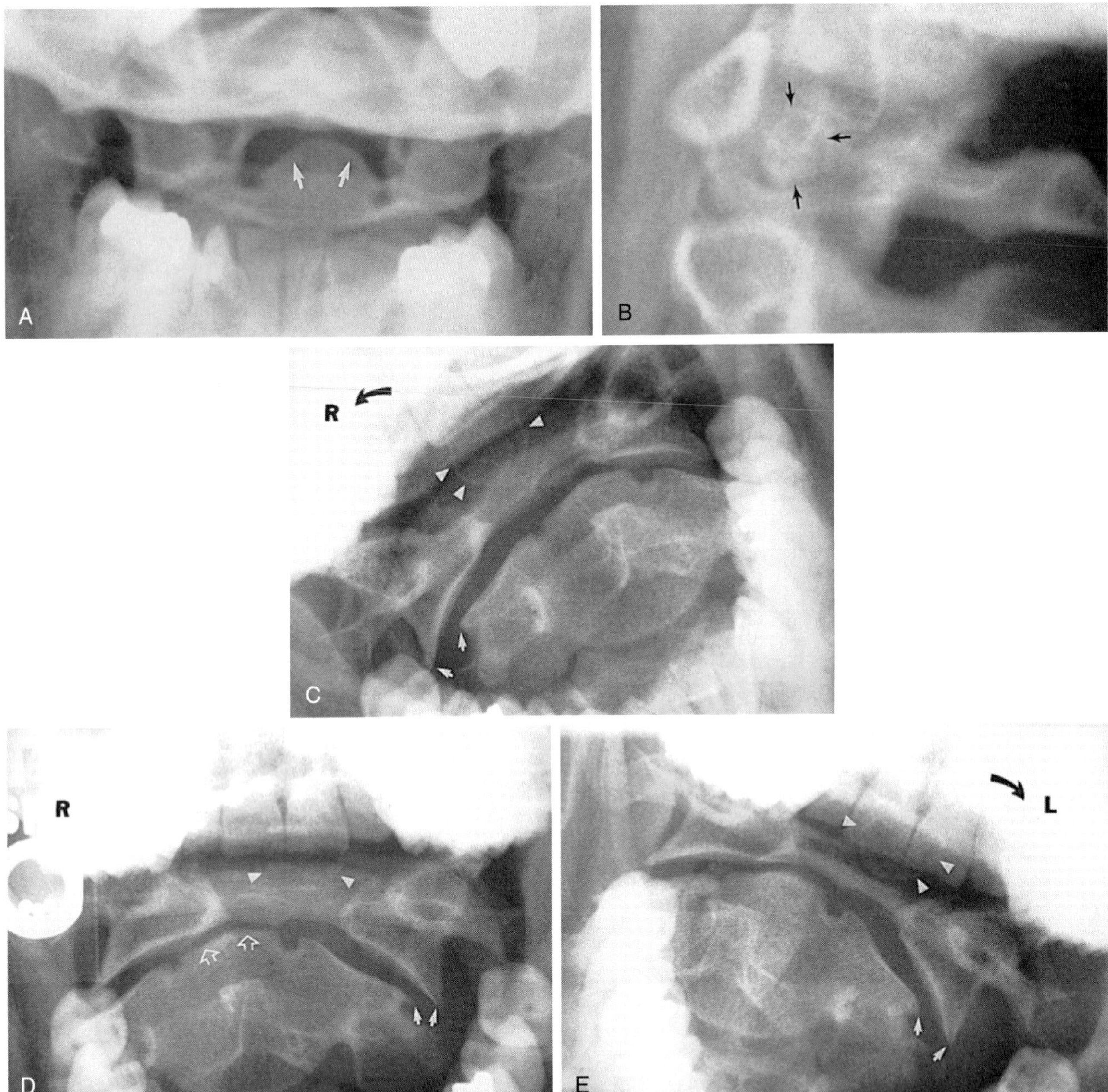

FIGURE 2–15. Os odontoideum.[4, 7, 11] A Anteroposterior open mouth view reveals an amputated appearance of the odontoid (arrows), and the ossicle is not visible. B Lateral radiograph reveals an incompletely developed ossicle (arrows) that is not fused to the C2 vertebral body. The anterior arch of atlas is sclerotic and hypertrophic, and the atlas is displaced posteriorly, indicating sagittal plane instability. C–E Coronal plane instability in another patient. Frontal open mouth radiographs obtained in active right lateral flexion (C), neutral posture (D), and active left lateral flexion (E) reveal a smooth cortical margin along the upper surface of the short odontoid (open arrows) and a separate, barely perceptible, dysplastic ossicle of bone above (arrowheads). Lateral translation of the lateral masses of the atlas in relation to C2 measured 16 mm, indicating coronal plane instability. (C–E, *From Ramos LS, Taylor JAM, Lackey G, et al: Top Diagn Radiol Adv Imaging 3:5, 1996.*)

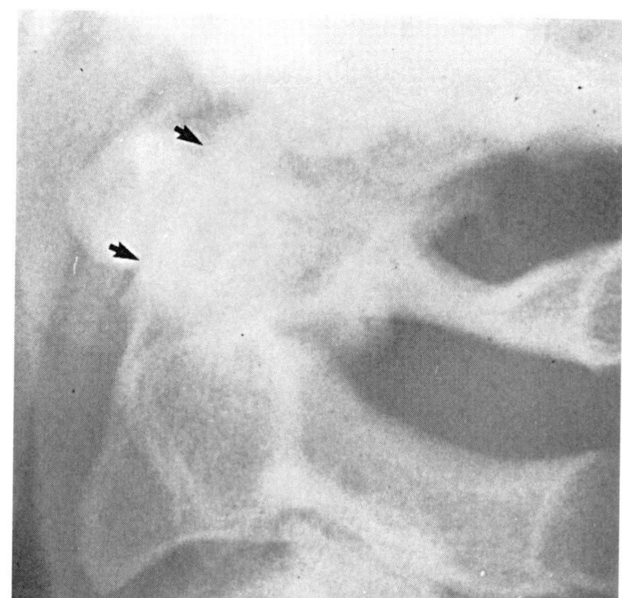

FIGURE 2–16. Posterior inclination of the odontoid.[12] The odontoid is tilted posteriorly (arrows) in this patient with no history of trauma. This peculiar posterior inclination is a variation of normal that may simulate a fracture. In cases of trauma, such a finding should lead to a careful search for an associated odontoid fracture. *(Courtesy of E.E. Bonic, D.C., Portland, Oregon.)*

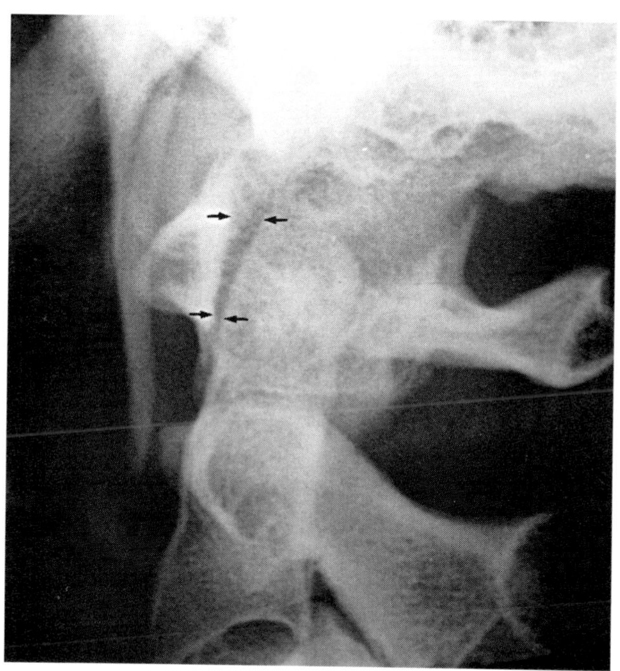

FIGURE 2–17. V-shaped predens space.[13] Observe the triangular atlantodental interspace in this patient (arrows). Such a V-shaped configuration is a variant of normal, and it should not automatically be considered an example of atlantoaxial instability. Bohrer and associates[13] postulate that this appearance may be due to increased flexion mobility at the atlantoaxial articulation, with developmental elongation or laxity of the cranial fibers of the transverse ligament or the posterior ligamentous complex, or both. In cases of suspected instability, flexion and extension radiographs should be obtained. The atlantodental interspace measured in the neutral, flexion, or extension position should be no more than 3 mm in adults or 5 mm in children. The measurement should be obtained at the central portion of this articulation.

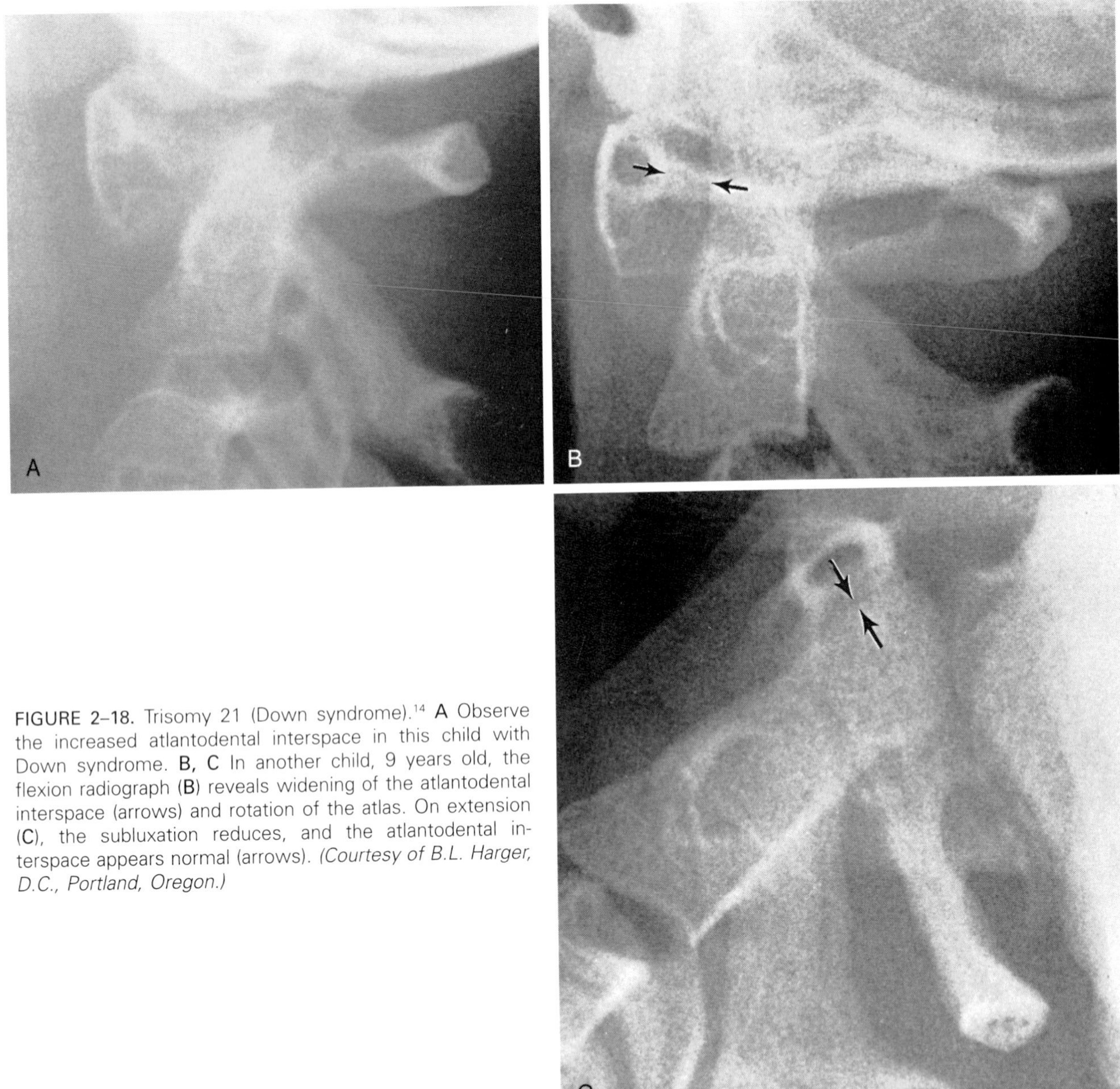

FIGURE 2–18. Trisomy 21 (Down syndrome).[14] **A** Observe the increased atlantodental interspace in this child with Down syndrome. **B, C** In another child, 9 years old, the flexion radiograph (**B**) reveals widening of the atlantodental interspace (arrows) and rotation of the atlas. On extension (**C**), the subluxation reduces, and the atlantodental interspace appears normal (arrows). *(Courtesy of B.L. Harger, D.C., Portland, Oregon.)*

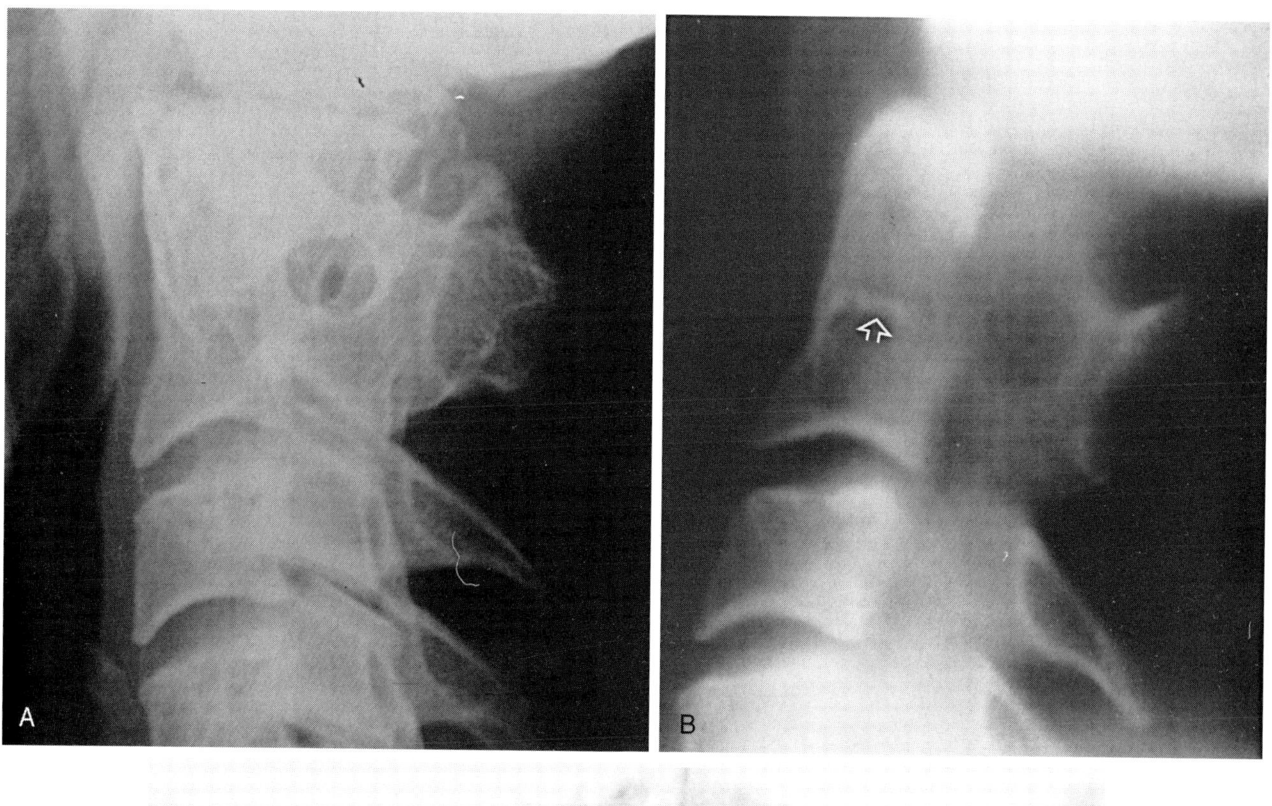

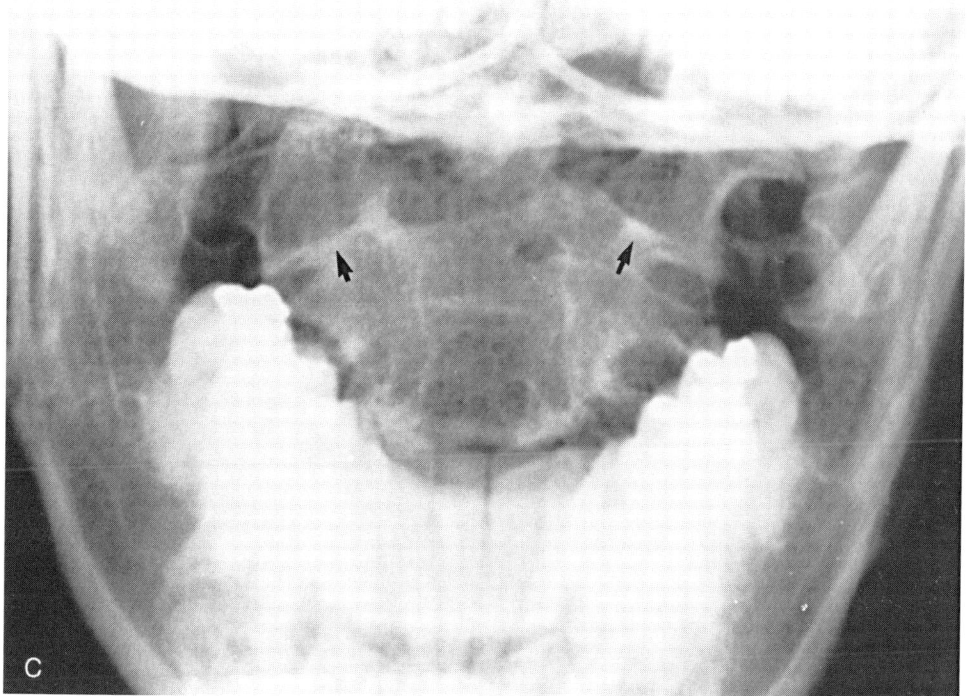

FIGURE 2–19. C1-C2 anomalies.[5, 7] A–C Synostosis. A Lateral radiograph reveals that the articulation between the atlas and axis is not visualized. The posterior arch of C1 is fused to the C2 spinous process and lamina, and an anomalous foramen is present between the C1 and C2 segments, resembling an intervertebral foramen. B Lateral conventional tomogram illustrates a partially calcified synchondrosis between the C2 vertebral body and odontoid process (open arrow) with a waist-like narrowing at this junction. C Anteroposterior open mouth radiograph reveals fusion of the C1-C2 apophyseal joints (arrows).

Illustration continued on following page

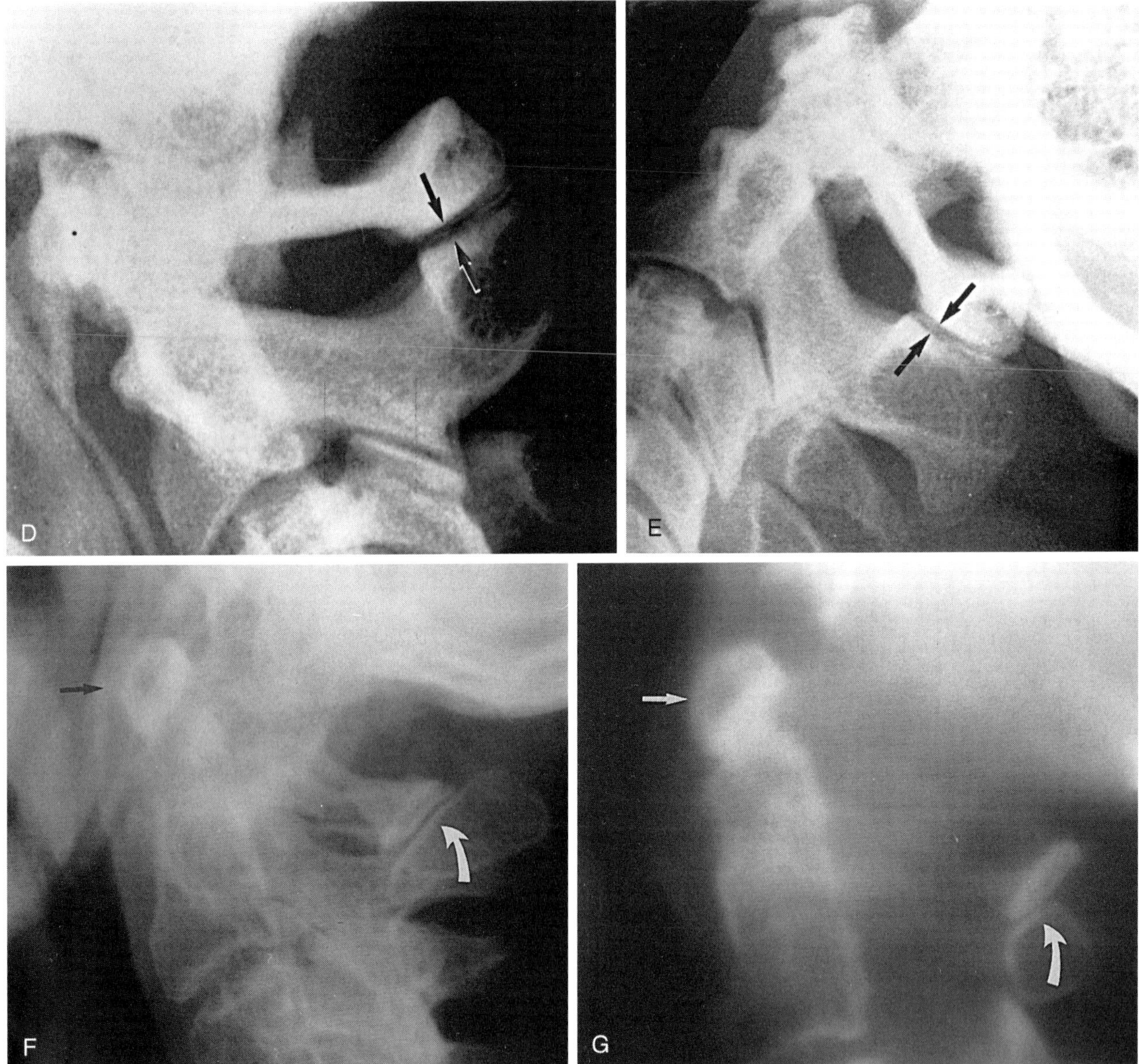

FIGURE 2–19 *Continued.* D, E Anomalous articulation. In another patient, observe the unusual articulation between the posterior arch of the atlas and the spinous process of the axis. Only minimal separation of the posterior elements (arrows) is evident in flexion (D) and extension (E) radiographs. F, G Complex atlantoaxial anomalies in an 87-year-old man with restriction of cervical flexion, extension, and rotation. Lateral radiograph (F) and conventional tomogram (G) reveal an anomalous tapered odontoid, high riding anterior arch of C1 (arrows), and an apparent pseudoarticulation between the posterior arch of C1 and the spinous process of C2 (curved arrows).

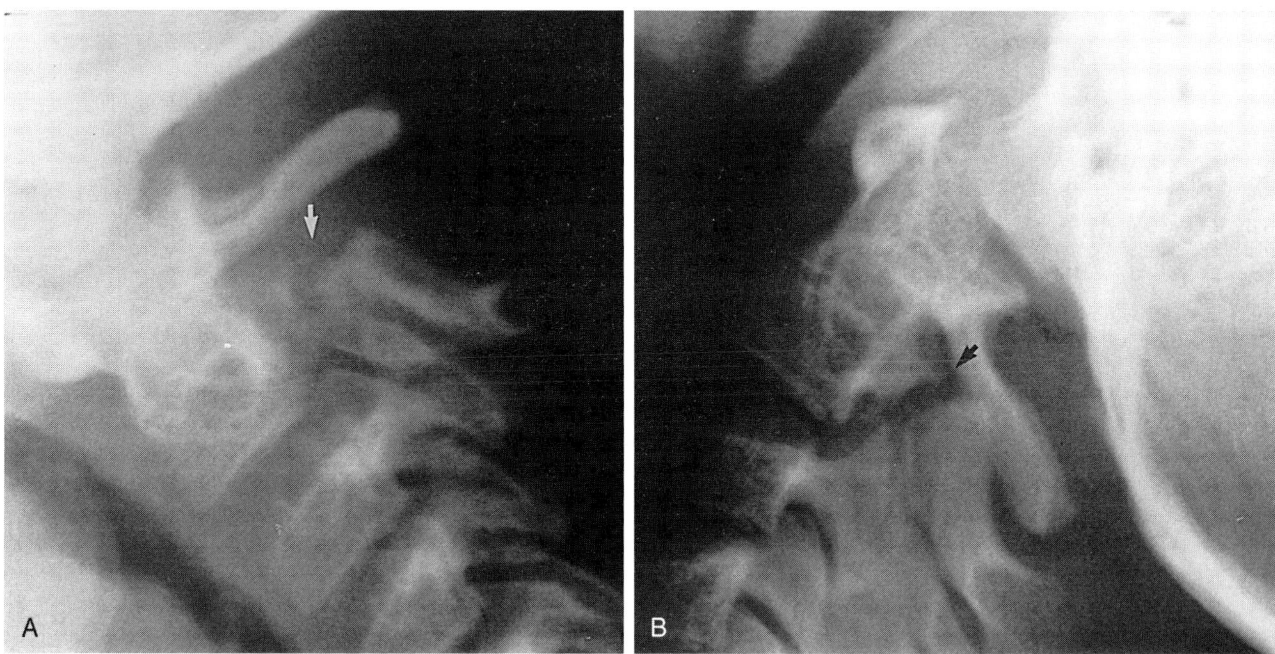

FIGURE 2–20. C2 spondylolysis.[15] This 9-year-old boy sustained mild head trauma. Flexion (A) and extension (B) films taken 1 week after the injury, when the patient was asymptomatic, show a radiolucent cleft in the neural arch of C2 (arrows) simulating a hangman's fracture. The flexion and extension films reveal no evidence of instability. Spondyloschisis and hypertrophy of the anterior arch also are present at C1. The diagnosis of fracture was excluded on the basis of absence of both symptoms and instability. This entity represents congenital spondylolysis of C2. Cervical spondylolysis and spondylolisthesis occur most commonly at C6 but also have been described at C2, as in this patient.

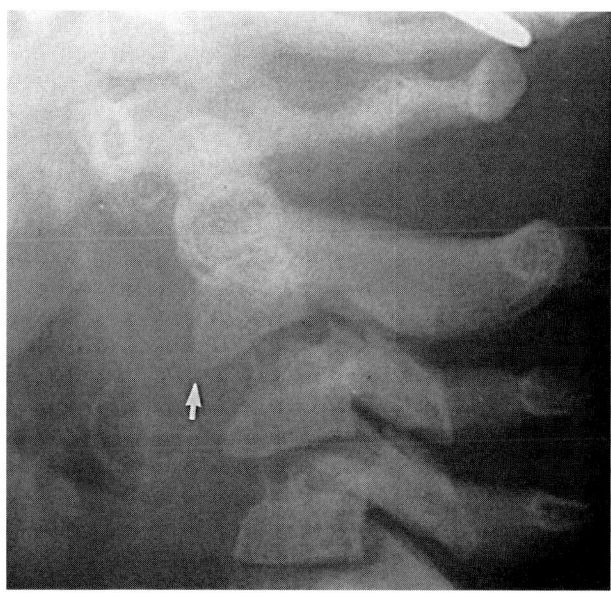

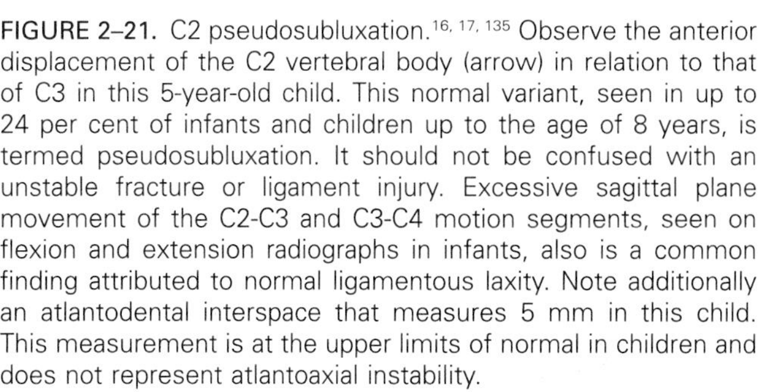

FIGURE 2–21. C2 pseudosubluxation.[16, 17, 135] Observe the anterior displacement of the C2 vertebral body (arrow) in relation to that of C3 in this 5-year-old child. This normal variant, seen in up to 24 per cent of infants and children up to the age of 8 years, is termed pseudosubluxation. It should not be confused with an unstable fracture or ligament injury. Excessive sagittal plane movement of the C2-C3 and C3-C4 motion segments, seen on flexion and extension radiographs in infants, also is a common finding attributed to normal ligamentous laxity. Note additionally an atlantodental interspace that measures 5 mm in this child. This measurement is at the upper limits of normal in children and does not represent atlantoaxial instability.

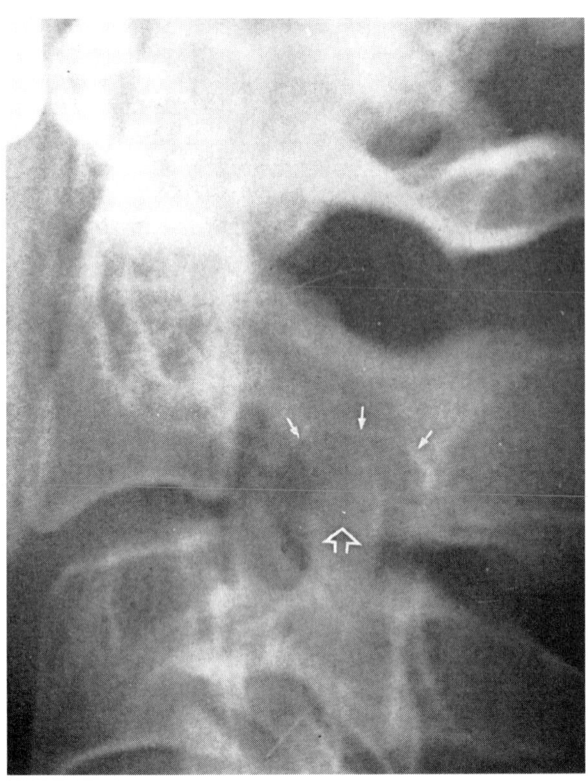

FIGURE 2–22. Anomalous C2-C3 facet articulation.[5, 7] An unusually bulbous superior articular process of C3 (open arrow) articulates with a concave inferior articular process of C2 (arrows) in a ball-and-socket fashion. This anomaly has no known clinical significance. Note also the posterior ponticulus of the atlas. *(Courtesy of D. McCallum, D.C., Vancouver, British Columbia, Canada.)*

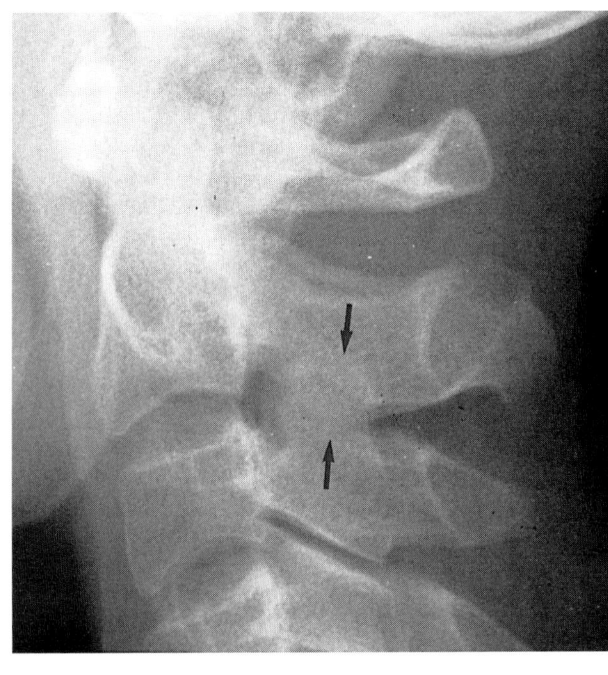

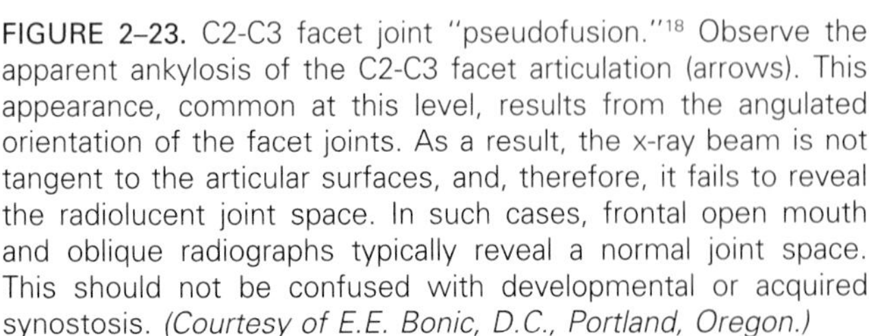

FIGURE 2–23. C2-C3 facet joint "pseudofusion."[18] Observe the apparent ankylosis of the C2-C3 facet articulation (arrows). This appearance, common at this level, results from the angulated orientation of the facet joints. As a result, the x-ray beam is not tangent to the articular surfaces, and, therefore, it fails to reveal the radiolucent joint space. In such cases, frontal open mouth and oblique radiographs typically reveal a normal joint space. This should not be confused with developmental or acquired synostosis. *(Courtesy of E.E. Bonic, D.C., Portland, Oregon.)*

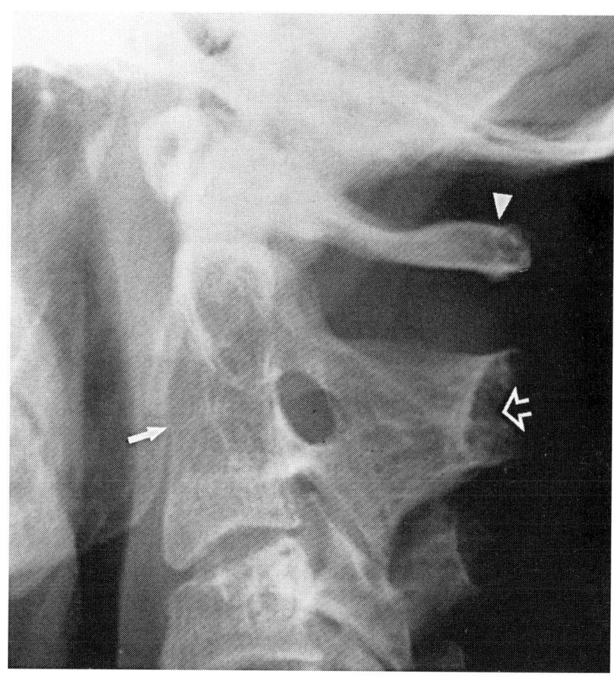

FIGURE 2–24. Upper cervical spine anomalies.[5–8] Lateral radiograph reveals absence of the spinolaminar junction line at C1, signifying spondyloschisis (nonunion of the posterior arch) (arrowhead). Congenital synostosis (block vertebra) of the C2-C3 level also is present with absence of the intervertebral disc space (arrow) and nonsegmentation of the lamina, articular processes, and spinous processes (open arrow). Observe the prominent intervertebral foramen at this level. Approximately 50 per cent of congenital block vertebrae also include nonsegmentation of the posterior elements.

TABLE 2–4. Some Developmental Anomalies, Anatomic Variants, and Sources of Diagnostic Error Affecting the Lower Cervical Spine (C3-C7)*

Entity	Figure(s), Table(s)	Characteristics
Normal ring apophyses[2]	2–25	Normal vertebral body ring apophyses may resemble tiny fractures
Nuclear impressions[2, 7]	2–26	Normal curvilinear concave depressions on the undersurface of vertebral bodies are believed to be notochordal remnants; developmental variant unrelated to osteopenia or mechanical stress on the spine Differential diagnosis: Schmorl's cartilaginous nodes, compression fractures, biconcave (fish vertebrae) deformities in osteoporosis, and H vertebrae characteristic of sickle cell anemia
Vertebra plana[7]	2–27	A change occurring in midcervical to lower cervical vertebral bodies in which the vertical height is diminished, resembling acute or pathologic collapse; characteristic of eosinophilic granuloma or normal variant
Elongated transverse processes[20, 21]	2–28	Developmental overgrowth and anomalous articulation of the anterior tubercles of two adjacent transverse processes May cause anterolateral neck pain and decreased range of motion
Notching of the articular processes[22]	2–29	Normal variant characterized by a smooth, well-corticated, curvilinear depression of the superior aspect of the articular facet that may resemble a pillar fracture or erosion Most common at C5-C7
Synostosis (block vertebra)[5–7, 23]	2–30	Developmental failure of segmentation of vertebral segments, most frequently present at C5-C6 and C2-C3 Often results in premature degenerative disease at adjacent vertebral levels owing to excessive intervertebral motion above and below the synostosis *Radiographic findings:* Waist-like constriction at the level of the intervertebral disc Disc space completely absent, or may be represented by a rudimentary, irregularly calcified structure Total height of the block vertebra less than expected from the number of segments involved Fusion of the posterior elements (50 per cent of cases) *Differential diagnosis:* Fusion from surgery or inflammatory arthropathy

Table continued on following page

TABLE 2–4. Some Developmental Anomalies, Anatomic Variants, and Sources of Diagnostic Error Affecting the Lower Cervical Spine (C3-C7)* *Continued*

Entity	Figure(s), Table(s)	Characteristics
Congenital spinal stenosis[6]		Developmental narrowing of the spinal canal is uncommon and may be seen as an isolated phenomenon or associated with achondroplasia Sagittal diameter of the cervical canal should never measure less than 12 mm Acquired (degenerative) stenosis is much more common than the congenital form and results from osteophyte proliferation into the spinal canal or nerve root canals
Klippel-Feil syndrome[24]	2–31 Table 2–5	Multiple segmentation defects and other anomalies
Pedicle agenesis[6]		Developmental absence of a pedicle Often results in sclerosis and hypertrophy of contralateral or adjacent pedicles May be associated with congenital spondylolisthesis and other anomalies
Spina bifida occulta[5, 7]	2–32	Midline defect within the neural arch in which the two laminae fail to fuse centrally at the spinolaminar junction, resulting in a radiolucent cleft or absent spinous process Seen as an isolated anomaly or in conjunction with other entities, such as congenital spondylolisthesis, cleidocranial dysplasia, or Klippel-Feil syndrome Osseous spina bifida rarely is associated with meningomyelocele (spina bifida vera), which represents protrusion of the meninges or spinal cord with consequent severe neurologic abnormalities
Congenital spondylolisthesis[25]	2–32	Most common at C6 Combination of anomalies, including spina bifida occulta, neural arch defect (such as pedicle agenesis), and anterolisthesis of the vertebral body
Persistent unfused ossification centers[7]	2–1E, 2–33	Any vertebral secondary ossification center may fail to fuse and may persist into adulthood, usually with no clinical consequences May simulate fractures At the corner of a vertebral body, they often are called limbus vertebrae, and may be associated with displacement of disc material underneath the ring apophysis
Cervical ribs and elongated C7 transverse processes[26]	2–34	Transverse processes of C7 typically are shorter than those of T1 Both elongated transverse processes and cervical ribs may contribute to neurovascular compression of the thoracic outlet Cervical ribs are present in 10 to 15 per cent of patients with the Klippel-Feil syndrome
Tracheal cartilage calcification[6]	2–35	Normal physiologic calcification of cartilaginous tracheal rings
Hair artifact[5]	2–36	Streaklike artifacts from unusual hairstyles
Lymph node calcification[6, 27]	2–37	Lobulated calcific collections in prevertebral and paravertebral locations Cervical lymph node calcification may be evidence of previous tuberculosis or other granulomatous disease, or, less likely, lymphoma or metastatic disease
Ossification of the stylohyoid ligaments[28]	2–38	Diffuse elongation and ossification or calcification of the stylohyoid ligaments May possess one or more articulations Usually an incidental finding, but fracture may occur and, in a condition termed "Eagle's syndrome," there may be symptoms of pain, dysphagia, and a sensation of a lump in the throat More common in patients with mucopolysaccharidoses and diffuse idiopathic skeletal hyperostosis (DISH)

*See also Table 1–1.

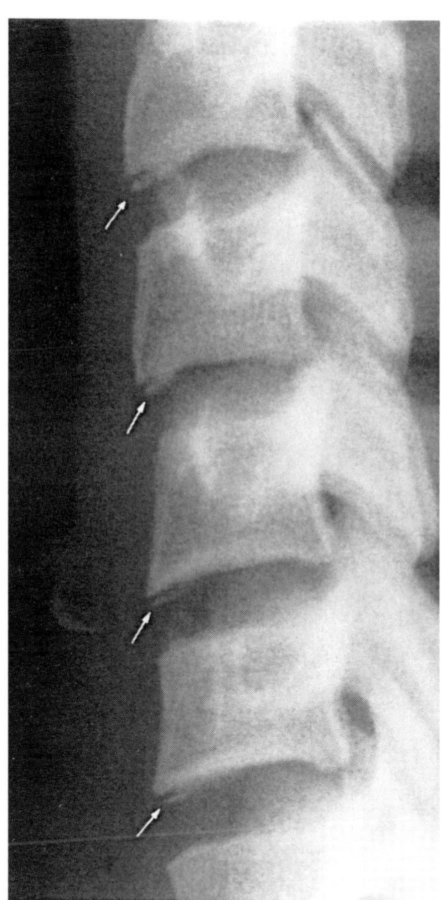

FIGURE 2–25. Normal ring apophyses.[2] Observe the tiny, linear, partially ossified secondary ossification centers (arrows) adjacent to the inferior vertebral end plates of C2-C6 on this radiograph of a 16-year-old boy.

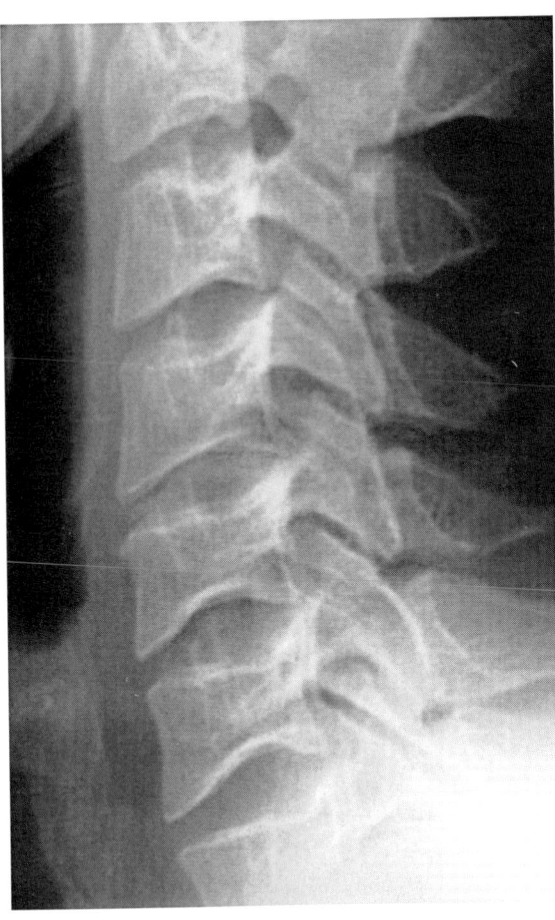

FIGURE 2–26. Nuclear impressions.[2, 7] Lateral radiograph reveals prominent, broad-based, curvilinear depressions of the superior and inferior vertebral end plates. These indentations, which are believed to be related to notochordal remnants, represent a developmental variant and are unrelated to osteopenia or mechanical stress on the spine.

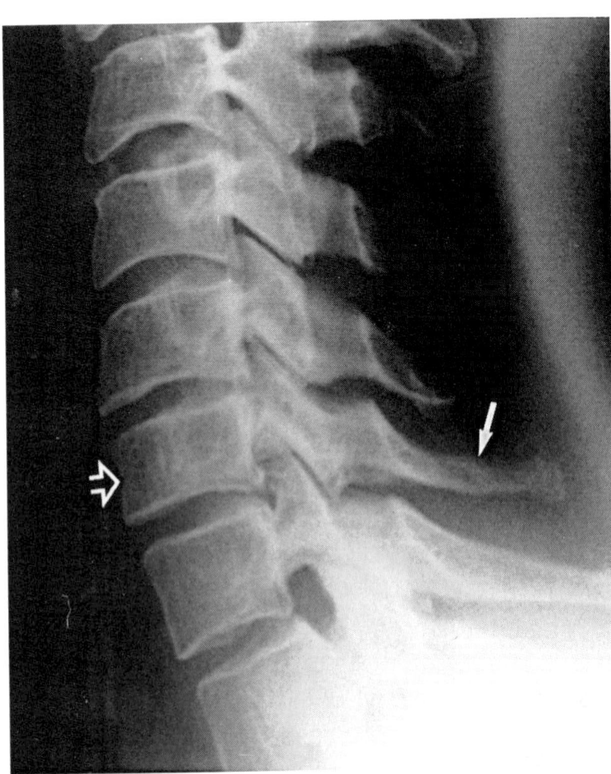

FIGURE 2–27. Anomalous development of C6.[7] The C6 vertebral body appears flattened (open arrow), and the spinous process is thin and attenuated (arrow). A radionuclide bone scan was normal, favoring the diagnosis of an isolated anomaly.

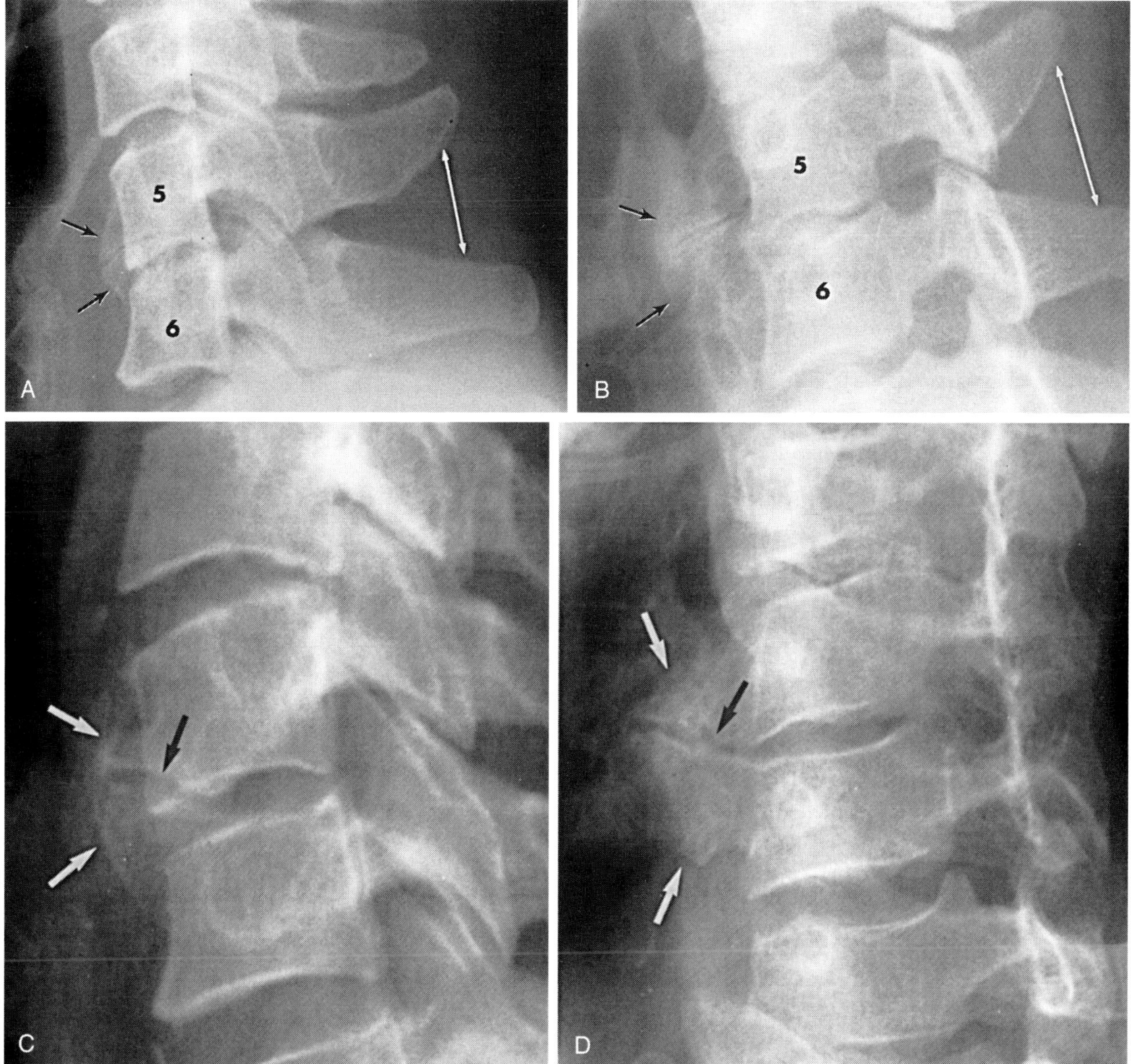

FIGURE 2–28. Elongated anterior tubercles of the transverse processes.[20, 21] A Lateral radiograph shows hypoplastic C5 and C6 vertebral bodies, narrowed disc space, and flaring of the spinous processes (double-headed white arrow). A thin projection of bone (black arrows) with a horizontal radiolucency is seen anterior to the disc space. B Oblique radiograph reveals that the bone projection (black arrows) represents elongated anterior tubercles of the C5 and C6 transverse processes that form an anomalous articulation. These elongated transverse processes with accompanying pseudarthrosis may be a source of anterolateral neck pain and limitation of motion. C, D In another patient, lateral (C) and oblique (D) radiographs show elongation of the anterior tubercles of the C5-C6 transverse processes (white arrows) with an anomalous articulation (black arrows).

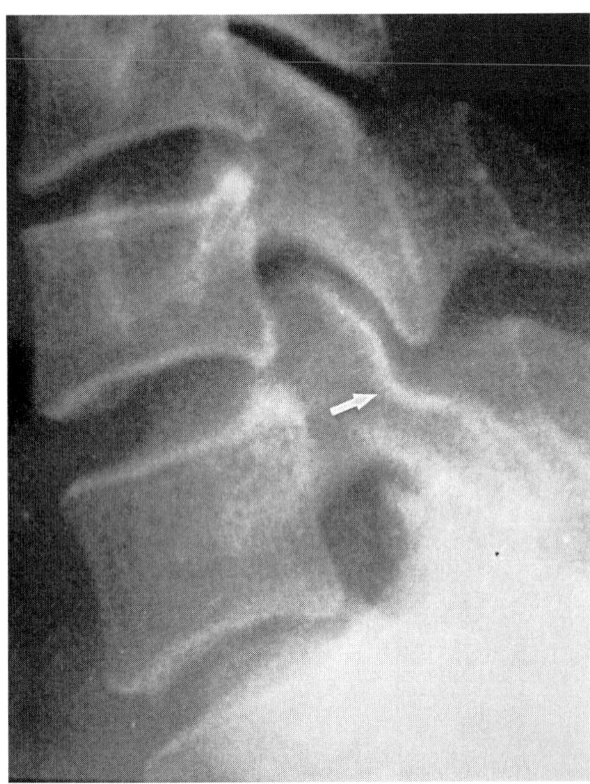

FIGURE 2–29. Articular process notching.[22] Notching of the superior apophyseal joint surface of C7 (arrow) represents a normal variation that may simulate an erosion or a fracture. Observe the well-corticated margin of the notch, characteristic of this normal variant.

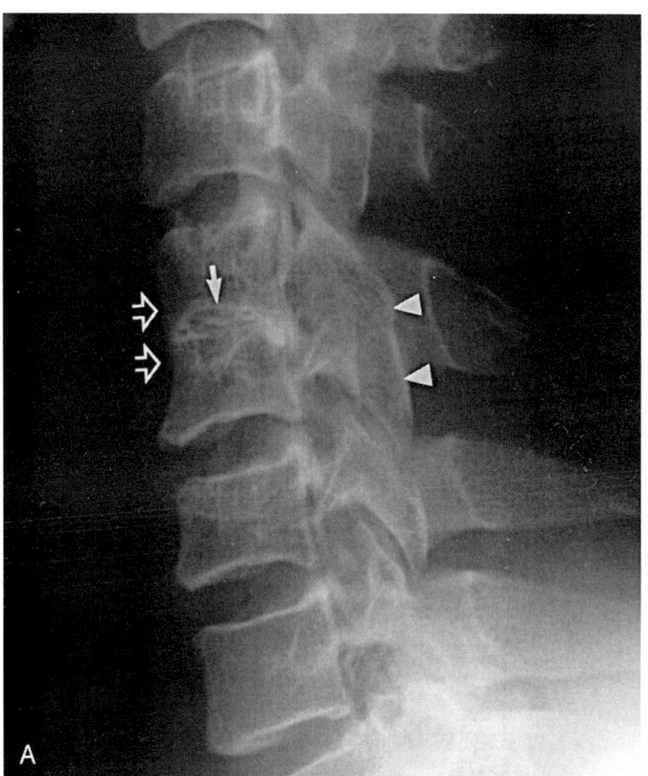

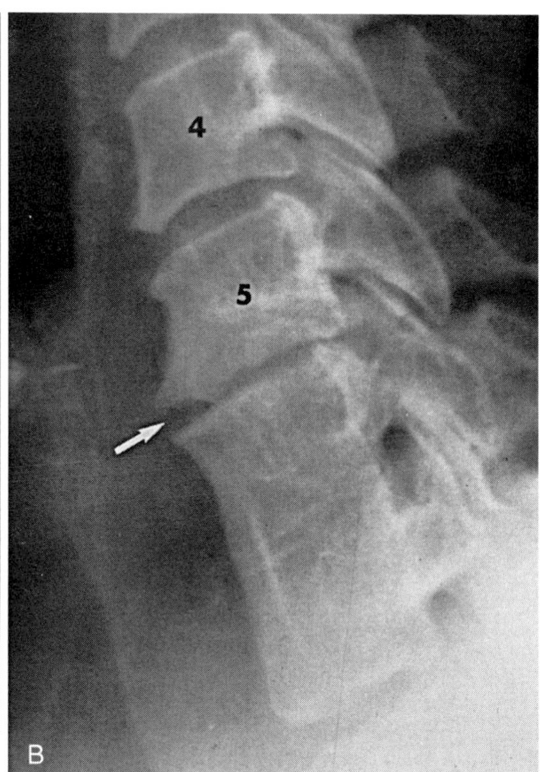

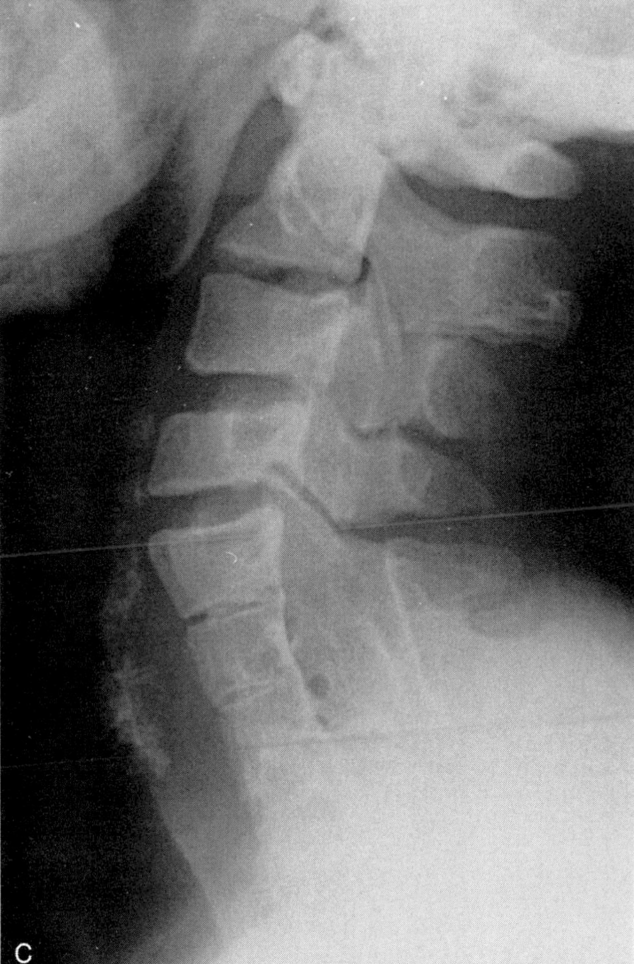

FIGURE 2–30. Block vertebrae (developmental synostosis).[5–7, 23] A In this patient, nonsegmentation of the bone is seen at C4-C5 with a hypoplastic intervertebral disc (arrow), hypoplasia of the two vertebral bodies (open arrows), and osseous fusion of the apophyseal joints (arrowheads). B In this 61-year-old woman, synostosis of C6-C7 with concomitant degenerative disease of the C5-C6 level (arrow) is seen. C Multiple block vertebrae. In another patient, observe the dramatic hypoplasia of the C5-T1 vertebral bodies and intervening intervertebral discs. The apophyseal joints and spinous processes also are fused. The C2-C4 vertebral bodies appear excessively elongated in their anterior to posterior dimension.

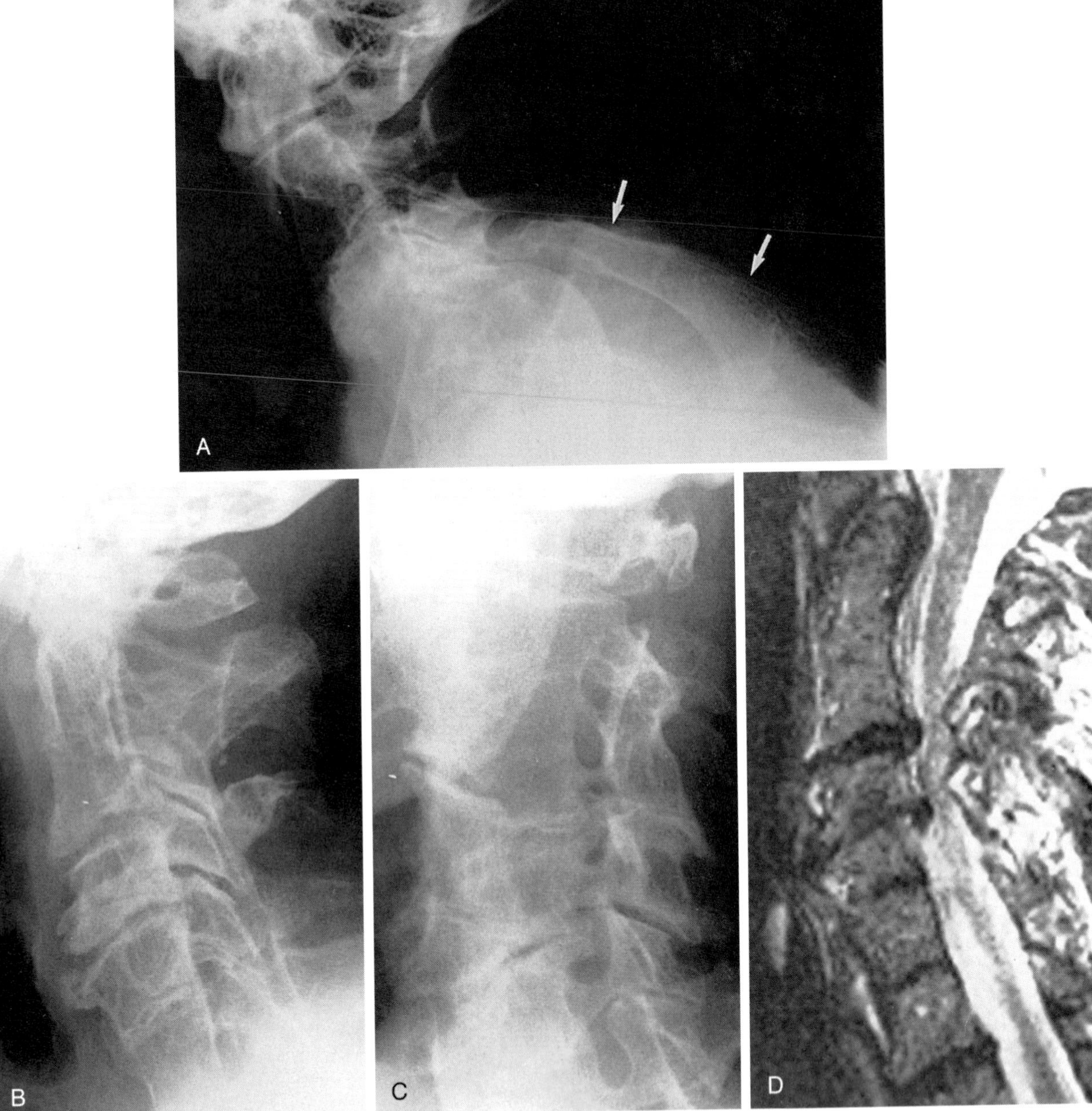

FIGURE 2–31. Klippel-Feil syndrome.[24] A Congenital synostosis (block vertebrae) at multiple levels is evident in this 88-year-old man. An omovertebral bone also is seen (arrows). B–D 58-year-old man with radiculopathy after an injury. Lateral radiograph (B) reveals synostosis of C2-C3 and C5-C7 with extensive associated degenerative disease. Oblique radiograph (C) reveals extensive foraminal encroachment from uncovertebral and facet joint osteophytes. A parasagittal T2-weighted (TR/TE, 4000/100) spin echo magnetic resonance (MR) image (D) shows disc protrusions and hypertrophic bone proliferation arising from the apophyseal joints and resulting in severe spinal canal stenosis at the C3-C4 and C4-C5 levels. Table 2–5 lists some of the malformations and complications commonly associated with Klippel-Feil syndrome. (B–D, *Courtesy of S. Maskall, D.C., Grand Forks, British Columbia, Canada.*)

TABLE 2–5 Klippel-Feil Syndrome[24]

Entity	Characteristics and Prevalence
Malformations	
Clinical appearance: short neck, low posterior hairline, limitation of cervical spine motion	Classic clinical triad present in about 50 per cent of cases
Multiple congenital synostoses (fusions) of cervical vertebrae	Most consistent osseous finding May involve any level, including upper thoracic vertebrae Fusions may be continuous or interrupted May result in extensive degenerative changes at adjacent spinal levels
Sprengel's deformity	20 to 25 per cent of cases Unilateral or bilateral elevation of scapula
Omovertebral bone	Found in 30 to 40 per cent of fixed elevated scapulae
Cervical ribs	10 to 15 per cent of cases Women > men
Hemivertebrae	15 to 20 per cent of cases Usually contributes to congenital scoliosis
Spina bifida occulta	May be present at one or more levels in patients with cervical fusions
Other anomalies	Kyphosis, scoliosis, spinal stenosis, and rib, cranial, brain, and visceral anomalies
Complications	
Spinal cord compression Nerve root compression Cord transection Central stenosis Foraminal stenosis Fractures	These neurologic sequelae may develop spontaneously or with minor or major trauma as a result of instability, degenerative changes, or osseous abnormalities

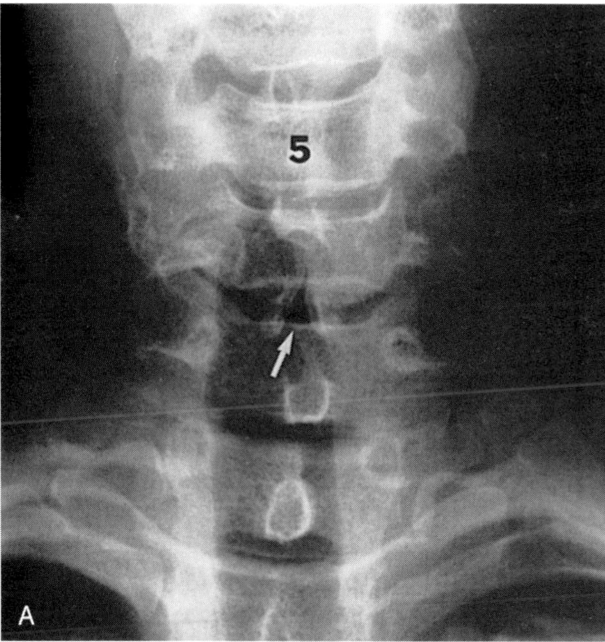

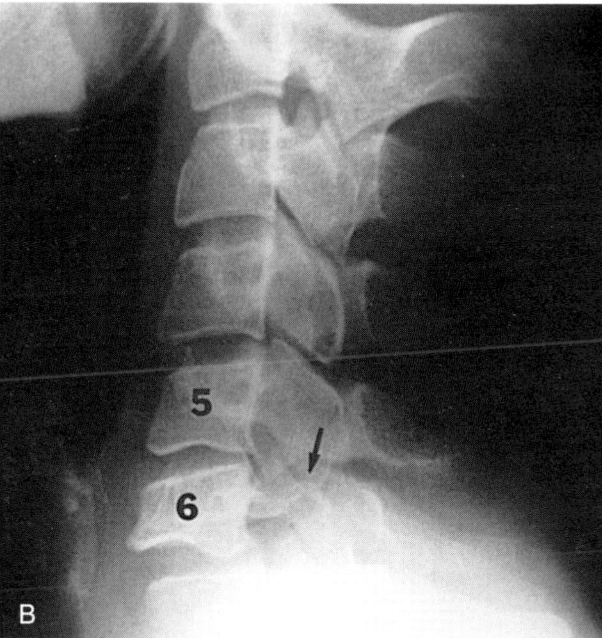

FIGURE 2–32. Congenital spondylolisthesis.[25] **A** An anteroposterior radiograph reveals spina bifida occulta at C6 (arrow). **B** Lateral radiograph shows minimal anterior displacement of C6 in relation to C7 and a neural arch defect consisting of incomplete ossification of the pedicles and articular processes of C6 (arrow). In addition, the C6 vertebral body is hypoplastic. *(Courtesy of E.E. Bonic, D.C., Portland, Oregon.)*

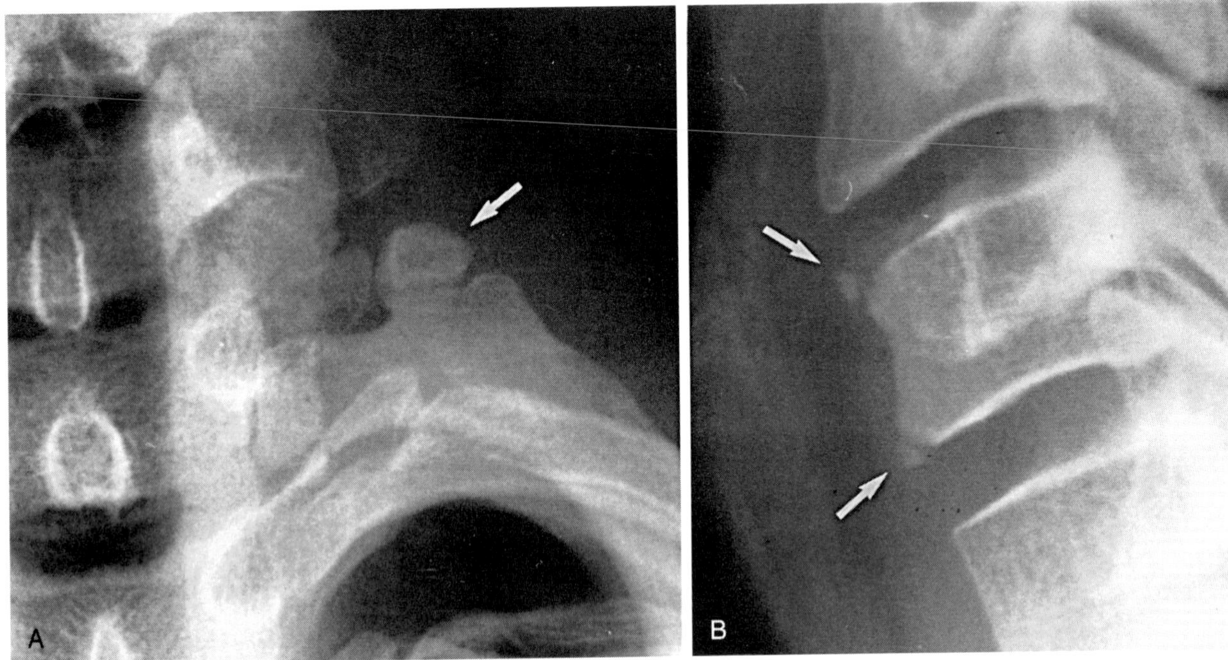

FIGURE 2–33. Persistent (ununited) secondary ossification centers.[7] A An anomalous ossicle is present adjacent to the tip of the T1 transverse process and first rib (arrow). This probably represents failure of fusion of the secondary ossification center at the tip of the transverse process, a structure that usually fuses by the age of 25 years. B In this 40-year-old man, two small triangular opacities are evident adjacent to the anterior corners of the C6 vertebral body (arrows). These ossification centers, which usually fuse to the vertebral body by the age of 17 or 18 years, may fail to fuse and persist into adulthood. These "limbus vertebrae" are variations of normal that may simulate a fracture.

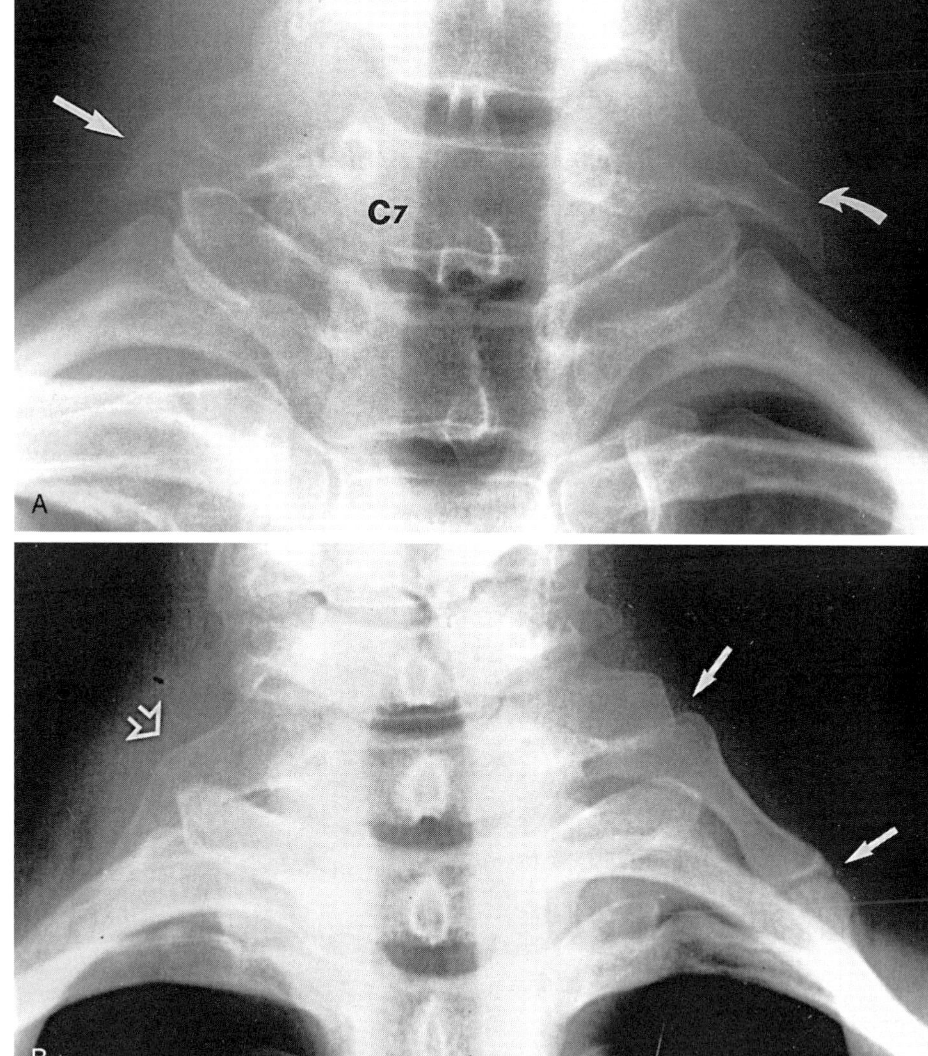

FIGURE 2–34. Cervical rib and elongated C7 transverse process.[26] A The left C7 transverse process is elongated and has a tapered, sharpened appearance (curved arrow). A small, articulating cervical rib is evident on the right (arrow). B In another patient, the right C7 transverse process is elongated and tapered (open arrow), and a cervical rib with two articulations (arrows) is present on the left.

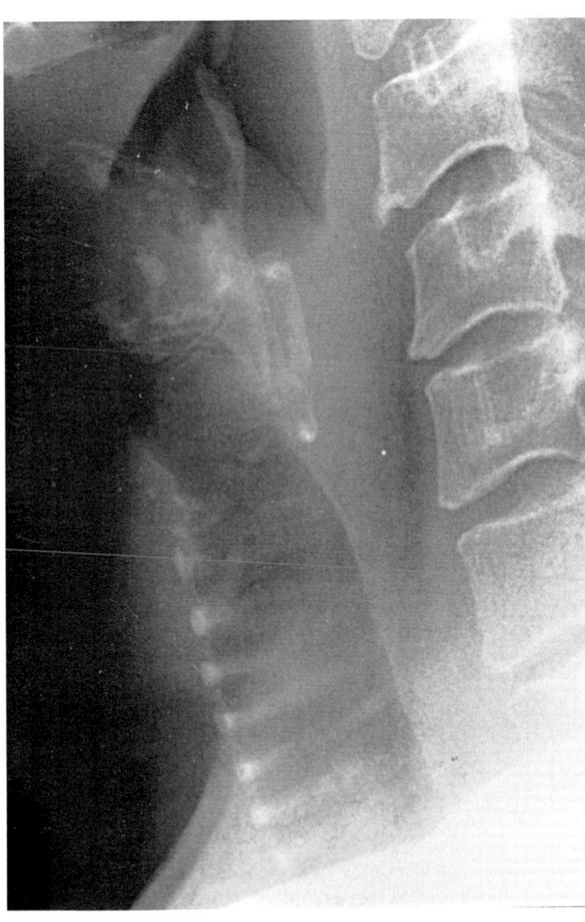

FIGURE 2–35. Tracheal ring calcification.[6] Prominent ringlike calcification of the tracheal cartilage is evident on a lateral radiograph of this 50-year-old woman. Such calcification is common in the elderly, is clinically asymptomatic, and is of no significance. *(Courtesy of E.E. Bonic, D.C., Portland, Oregon.)*

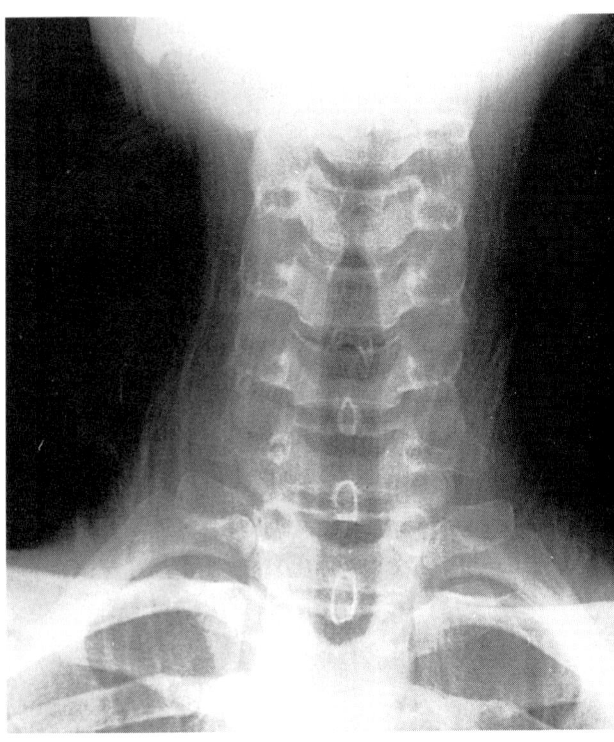

FIGURE 2–36. Hair artifact.[5] Streaky, vertically oriented opacities are seen over the cervical spine and soft tissues of the neck. This commonly encountered artifact results from overlying strands of hair. *(Courtesy of E.E. Bonic, D.C., Portland, Oregon.)*

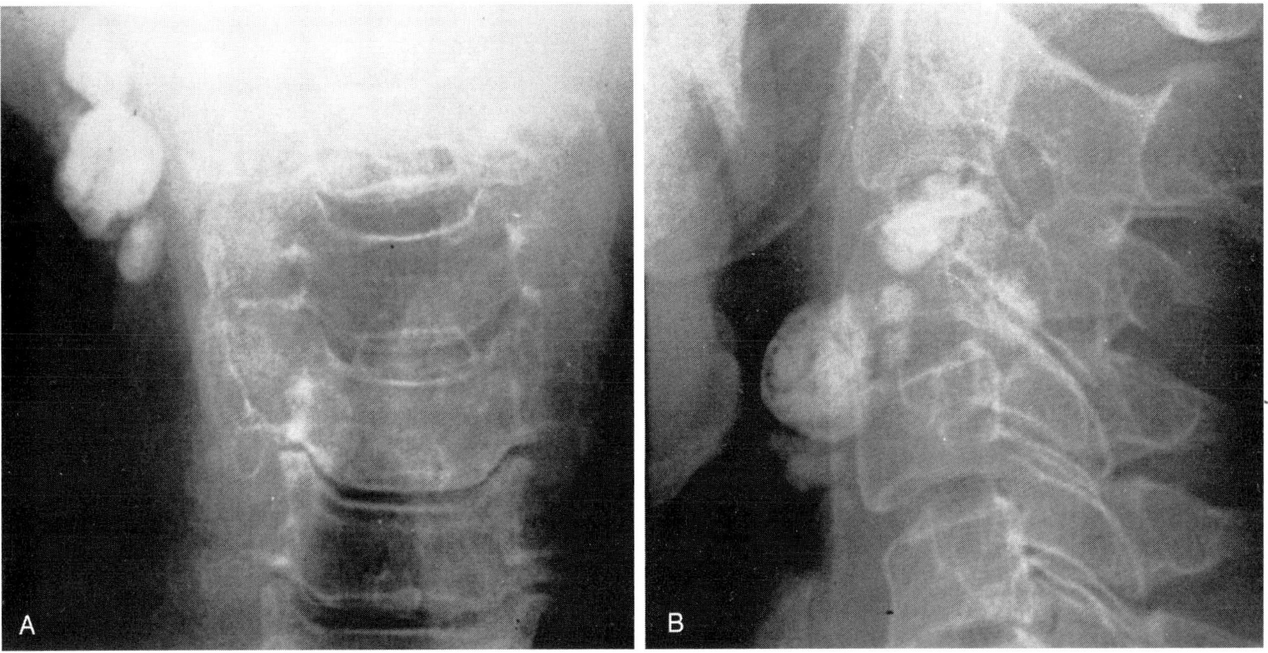

FIGURE 2–37. Cervical lymph node calcification.[6, 27] Lobulated accumulations of calcification (A, B) are evident within the paraspinal soft tissues of the neck. These calcifications are consistent with lymph node calcification and should not be confused with the periarticular calcifications seen in connective tissue and crystal deposition diseases. *(Courtesy of S. Maskall, D.C., Grand Forks, British Columbia, Canada.)*

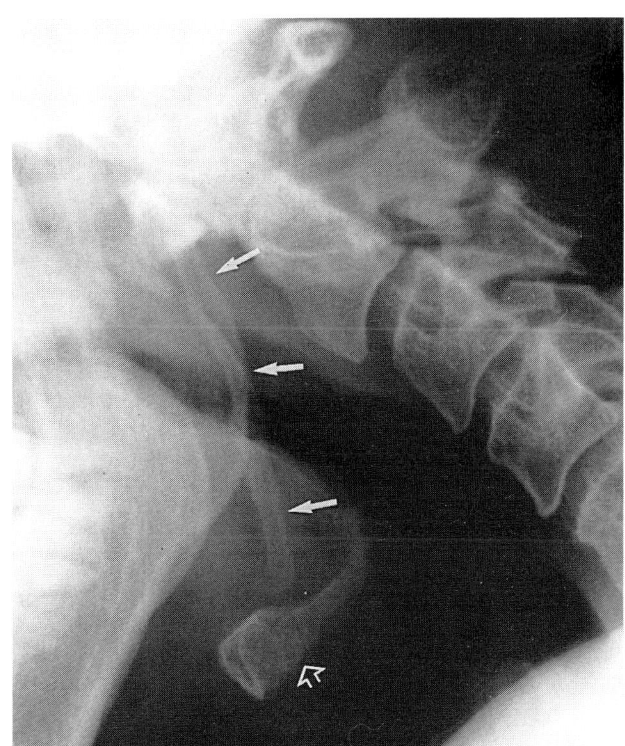

FIGURE 2–38. Ossification of the stylohyoid ligament.[28] In this lateral radiograph obtained in flexion, observe the vertical, linear ossified structure (arrows) overlying the prevertebral structures superior to the hyoid bone (open arrow). This represents ossification and elongation of the stylohyoid ligament, which usually is an incidental finding. This structure may possess one or more articulations, it may fracture, and, in a condition termed Eagle's syndrome, it may cause symptoms of pain, dysphagia, and a sensation of a lump in the throat. The prevalence of ossified stylohyoid ligaments is higher in patients with mucopolysaccharidoses and diffuse idiopathic skeletal hyperostosis (DISH).

TABLE 2–6. Skeletal Dysplasias and Other Congenital Diseases Affecting the Cervical Spine*

Entity	Figure(s)	Characteristics in the Cervical Spine
Achondroplasia[29]		Brain stem compression by narrow foramen magnum Spinal stenosis with posterior scalloping of vertebral bodies Vertebral bodies may be flattened
Spondyloepiphyseal dysplasia congenita[30]	2–39	Hypoplasia of the odontoid with atlantoaxial instability Platyspondyly
Mucopolysaccharidoses (MPS)[31, 32]		*MPS I-H (Hurler's syndrome):* Atlantoaxial instability may be present Rounded anterior vertebral margins with inferior beaking Posterior scalloping of vertebral bodies *MPS IV (Morquio's syndrome):* Hypoplastic or absent odontoid with atlantoaxial instability Platyspondyly Posterior scalloping of vertebral bodies
Fibrodysplasia ossificans progressiva[33]		Sheet-like ossification within soft tissues of neck Hypoplastic vertebral bodies and intervertebral discs Apophyseal joint ankylosis
Osteopetrosis[34, 35]	2–40	Patterns of osteosclerosis: diffuse osteosclerosis, bone-within-bone appearance, sandwich vertebrae
Osteopoikilosis[36]		Infrequently affects the spine Multiple punctate circular foci of osteosclerosis
Marfan syndrome[37]		Scoliosis in 40 to 60 per cent of persons Posterior vertebral body scalloping from dural ectasia

*See also Table 1–2.

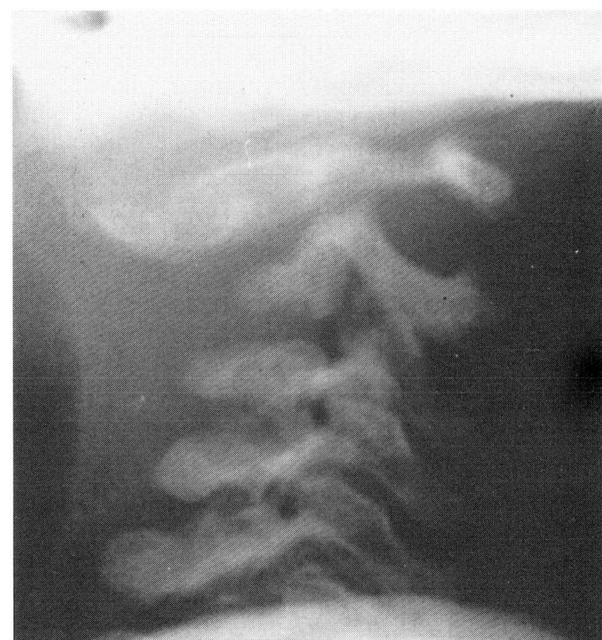

FIGURE 2–39. Spondyloepiphyseal dysplasia congenita.[30] This 5-year-old boy has platyspondyly, a hypoplastic odontoid process with atlantoaxial subluxation, instability, and craniocervical canal stenosis. Respiratory and visual complications may be severe, and a rare lethal form exists termed hypochondrogenesis.

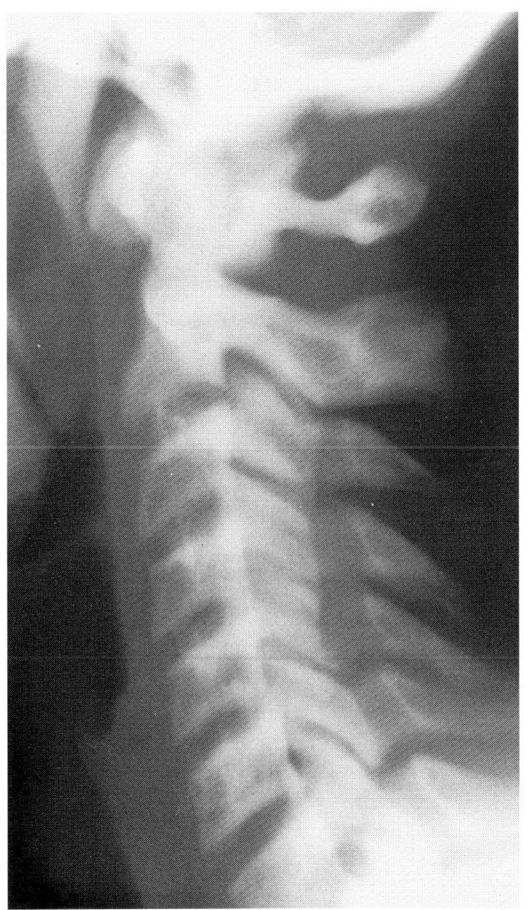

FIGURE 2–40. Osteopetrosis.[34, 35] Diffuse sclerosis predominates at the vertebral end plates of the cervical spine in this 15-year-old boy with osteopetrosis. The radiographic pattern in the spine may be diffusely sclerotic, or osteopetrosis may be manifest as "sandwich vertebrae" or as a "bone-within-bone" appearance. Generalized osteosclerosis in osteopetrosis results from an increased amount of bone, not from an increase in the percentage of mineralized bone per unit volume of tissue.

TABLE 2–7. Upper Cervical Spine Injuries[46, 50, 51]

Entity	Figure(s), Table(s)	Stability*	Mechanism	Characteristics
Atlas injuries				
Atlanto-occipital dislocation[38, 39]		Unstable	Hyperextension-shearing and distraction	Rare injury; almost always fatal Occurs with or without associated fracture Cranium usually is displaced anteriorly relative to the cervical spine Distance between the odontoid and basion is increased
Traumatic transverse ligament disruption[40]		Unstable	Poorly understood mechanism	Rupture of the transverse ligament with or without associated fractures Atlantoaxial instability invariable: atlantodental interspace more than 3 mm in adults and 5 mm in children Rare: only 1 per cent of all cervical injuries Nontraumatic causes of transverse ligament rupture much more frequent and include inflammatory arthritis, Down syndrome, anomalies, and infection
Rotatory atlantoaxial fixation[41–43]	2–41 Table 2–8	Variable	Hyper-rotation	Persistent pathologic fixation of the atlantoaxial joints in a rotated position such that the atlas and axis move as a unit rather than independently Patient typically has a persistent painful torticollis Occurs after rotational trauma, but also may occur after an inflammatory condition of the pharynx or upper respiratory tract, such as in Grisel's syndrome Dynamic or functional computed tomography (CT) is useful in identifying the presence and precise type of atlantoaxial rotatory fixation
Burst (Jefferson) fracture[44]	2–42	Variable Deemed unstable when the transverse ligament is ruptured or avulsed	Axial compression	May be unilateral or bilateral Axial compressive loading causes compression of the lateral masses of C1 between the occipital condyles and the C2 articular processes, resulting in two, three, or four fracture fragments of the atlas ring (classic Jefferson fracture is four-part) Unilateral or bilateral displacement of lateral masses on open mouth view Normal lateral offset (pseudospread) of the atlas is common in normal children and may measure 4 to 6 mm

TABLE 2–7. Upper Cervical Spine Injuries[46, 50, 51] *Continued*

Entity	Figure(s), Table(s)	Stability*	Mechanism	Characteristics
Atlas injuries *Continued*				
				Jefferson fracture should be suspected in patients with 3 mm or more of total lateral displacement, and transverse ligament damage should be suspected in patients with more than 7 mm of total lateral displacement seen on the anteroposterior view Permanent neurologic injury is uncommon with classic four-part Jefferson fractures
Posterior arch fracture[45]	2–43	Stable	Compressive hyperextension	Most common fracture of the atlas Results from compression of the atlas between the basiocciput and the posterior arch of C2 during hyperextension injury 90 per cent are bilateral; 10 per cent are unilateral Heals slowly, pseudarthroses are common
Anterior arch fracture[46]		Usually stable	Disruptive hyperextension	Horizontal fracture seen on lateral radiograph produced by avulsion of the tubercle of the anterior arch by the superior oblique portion of the longus colli muscle and the anterior longitudinal ligament Often associated with fractures of C1 posterior arch and odontoid
Isolated lateral mass fracture[46]		Usually stable	Axial compression or lateral hyperflexion	Extremely rare injury Fracture of the medial aspect of the lateral mass may result from avulsion by the transverse ligament
Isolated transverse process fracture[46]		Usually stable	Lateral hyperflexion	Extremely rare injury at C1 level Potential vertebral artery injury
Axis injuries				
Odontoid fracture[47, 48]			Complex and poorly understood mechanism including combinations of extreme flexion, extension, rotation, and shearing	Most common axis fracture: 55 per cent of C2 fractures; 7–13 per cent of all cervical spine injuries Up to 90 per cent of affected patients are intact neurologically at time of injury but may develop late-onset neurologic deficit Fracture-dislocation may complicate odontoid fractures Anterior odontoid displacement from flexion forces Posterior odontoid displacement from extension forces Lateral odontoid displacement from lateral flexion or rotational forces Three types of odontoid fracture based on fracture location

Table continued on following page

TABLE 2–7. Upper Cervical Spine Injuries[46, 50, 51] *Continued*

Entity	Figure(s), Table(s)	Stability*	Mechanism	Characteristics
Axis injuries *Continued*				
Type I		Stable		Least common type: believed to be caused by alar ligament avulsion Unilateral oblique fracture through the tip of the odontoid above the transverse ligament Nonunion and displacement rare
Type II	2–44	Unstable		Most common type Fracture occurs through the base of the odontoid at its junction with the C2 body; frequently disrupts the blood supply Nonunion occurs in more than 25 per cent of cases Displacement (more than 60 per cent of cases) and angulation (more than 25 per cent) increase likelihood of nonunion Popular theory holds that os odontoideum actually represents a chronic nonunion type II odontoid fracture rather than a developmental anomaly
Type III		Stable		Horizontal or oblique fracture line extends from the base of the odontoid into the cancellous bone of the vertebral body, typically exiting through the articular process of C2 into the C1-C2 articulation Anterior displacement occurs in 58 per cent of cases and lateral tilting of the odontoid greater than 5 degrees is present in about 66 per cent of cases Nonunion occurs in less than 13 per cent of cases
Odontoid fracture with distraction	2–45	Highly unstable	Distraction	Rare fracture of odontoid (usually type II) with wide separation at fracture site
Hangman's fracture[47–49]	2–46	Varies according to type	Varies according to type	Four to 23 per cent of all cervical spine fractures Sometimes termed traumatic spondylolisthesis of C2 Bilateral avulsion fractures of the neural arches from the C2 vertebral body Fractures occur through the pars interarticularis or adjacent portion of the articular processes Extension into the vertebral body occurs in as many as 18 per cent of cases Neurologic damage occurs in less than 13 per cent of cases but infrequently is permanent

TABLE 2–7. **Upper Cervical Spine Injuries**[46, 50, 51] *Continued*

Entity	Figure(s), Table(s)	Stability*	Mechanism	Characteristics
Axis injuries *Continued*				
Three types:				
Type I		Stable	Hyperextension	Nonangulated, nondisplaced (< 2 mm), and normal C2-C3 disc
Type II		Unstable	Hyperextension or flexion-distraction	Anterior displacement or angulation with C2-C3 disc injury
Type III		Unstable	Hyperflexion	Anterior displacement or angulation with bilateral facet dislocation
Extension teardrop fracture[46]		Unstable	Disruptive hyperextension	Avulsion fracture of a triangular fragment of the anteroinferior margin of the body by the anterior longitudinal ligament Most common at C2, but may occur at any level Fragment may be displaced, distracted, or rotated More common in elderly persons with osteoporosis and spondylosis Usually not associated with neurologic deficit
Avulsion fracture of C2 body from hyperextension dislocation[46]		Unstable	Disruptive hyperextension	Severe injury: avulsion fracture of anteroinferior corner of vertebral body mediated through Sharpey's fibers Usually occurs in lower cervical spine, but also seen at C2-C3 Frequently associated with acute cervical central cord syndrome
Oblique fracture of body[46]		Variable	Combinations of axial compression and rotation	Oblique fracture through the C2 vertebral body below the odontoid and articular processes Results in widened anteroposterior diameter of the C2 vertebral body: "fat C2 sign"
Isolated process fracture[46]		Usually stable	Hyperextension, rotation, hyperflexion, or direct trauma	Unilateral pedicle, lateral mass, or lamina Spinous process

*Clinical instability here is defined as the inability to maintain vertebral relationships in such a way that spinal cord and nerve root damage are avoided and subsequent deformity and excessive pain do not develop. From White AA, Southwick WO, Panjabi MM: Clinical instability in the lower cervical spine. Clin Orthop 109:85, 1975.

TABLE 2–8. **Some Causes of Asymmetric Lateral Atlantodental Space**[43]

Two- to 5-mm discrepancy in this space has been documented in normal persons
Correlation with other radiographic evidence is necessary to determine the significance of this measurement
Normal range of cervical motion and no fixed deformity
Congenital variation of odontoid shape
Slanting of odontoid process
Contour variations of C1 lateral articular masses
Restriction of cervical motion or fixed deformity
Rotatory atlantoaxial fixation (see Fig. 2–41)
Jefferson's fracture (see Fig. 2–42)

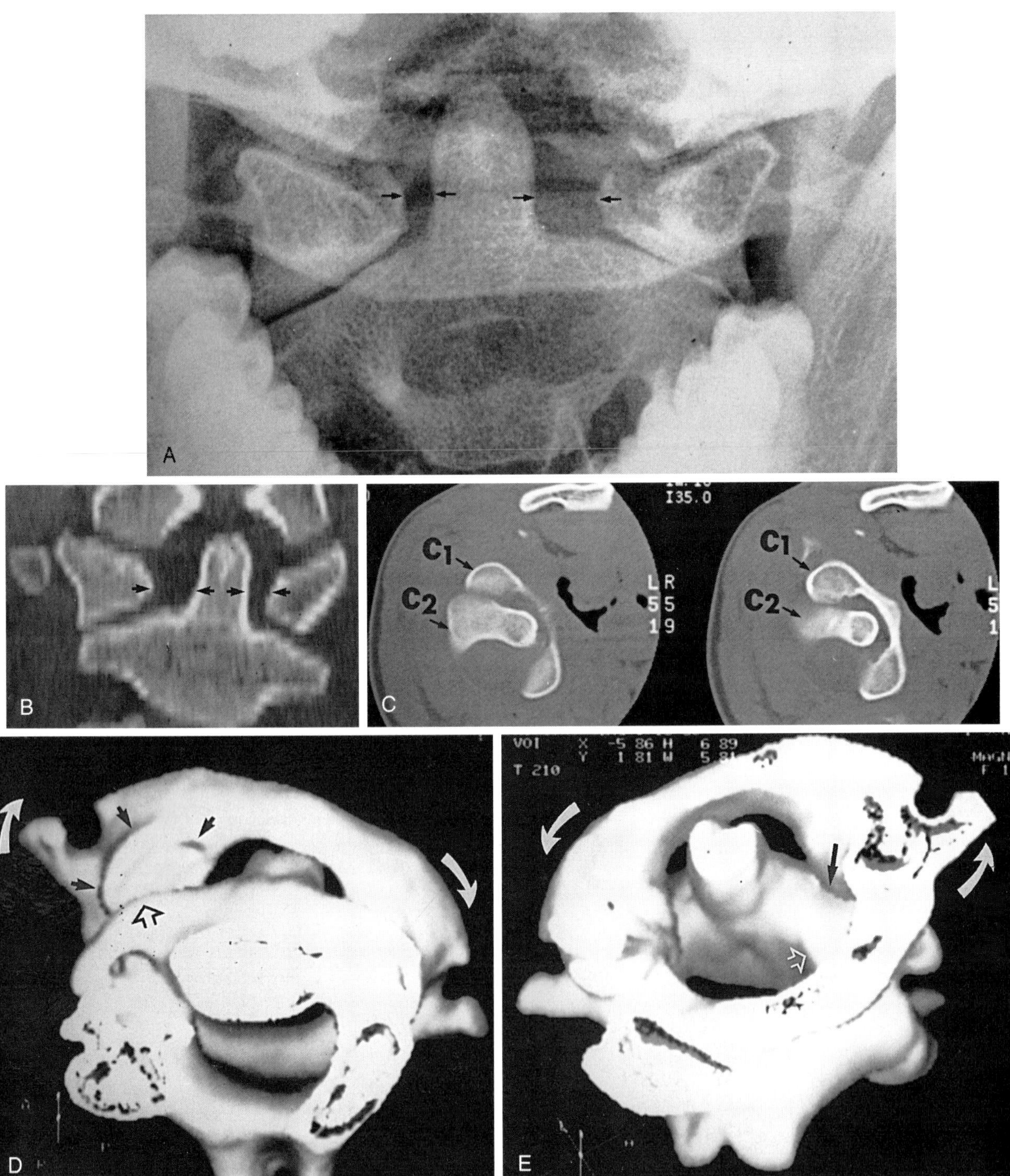

FIGURE 2–41. Rotatory atlantoaxial fixation.[41–43] A Plain film radiographic findings. Observe the asymmetric space between the odontoid process and the medial aspect of the lateral masses of the atlas (arrows). B–E CT findings. B Coronal reformation. In another patient, asymmetric alignment of atlas and axis (arrows) is evident on this coronal computed tomographic (CT) image. C, Transaxial images obtained with the patient's head and neck in full left rotation show the anterior displacement of the right lateral mass of atlas (C1) relative to the articulating facet of axis (C2). D, E Three-dimensional CT reconstruction in a third patient shows the direction of rotation of the atlas (curved arrows). In the first image, viewed from below (D), the right lateral mass of the atlas (arrows) is clearly situated anterior to the articulating surface of the C2 facet (open arrow). Viewed from above (E), the articulating surface of the right lateral mass of the atlas (arrow) is displaced anteriorly in relation to the axis articular surface (open arrow), and the facet joints are locked in this position. *(B–E, Courtesy of B.A. Howard, M.D., Charlotte, North Carolina.)*

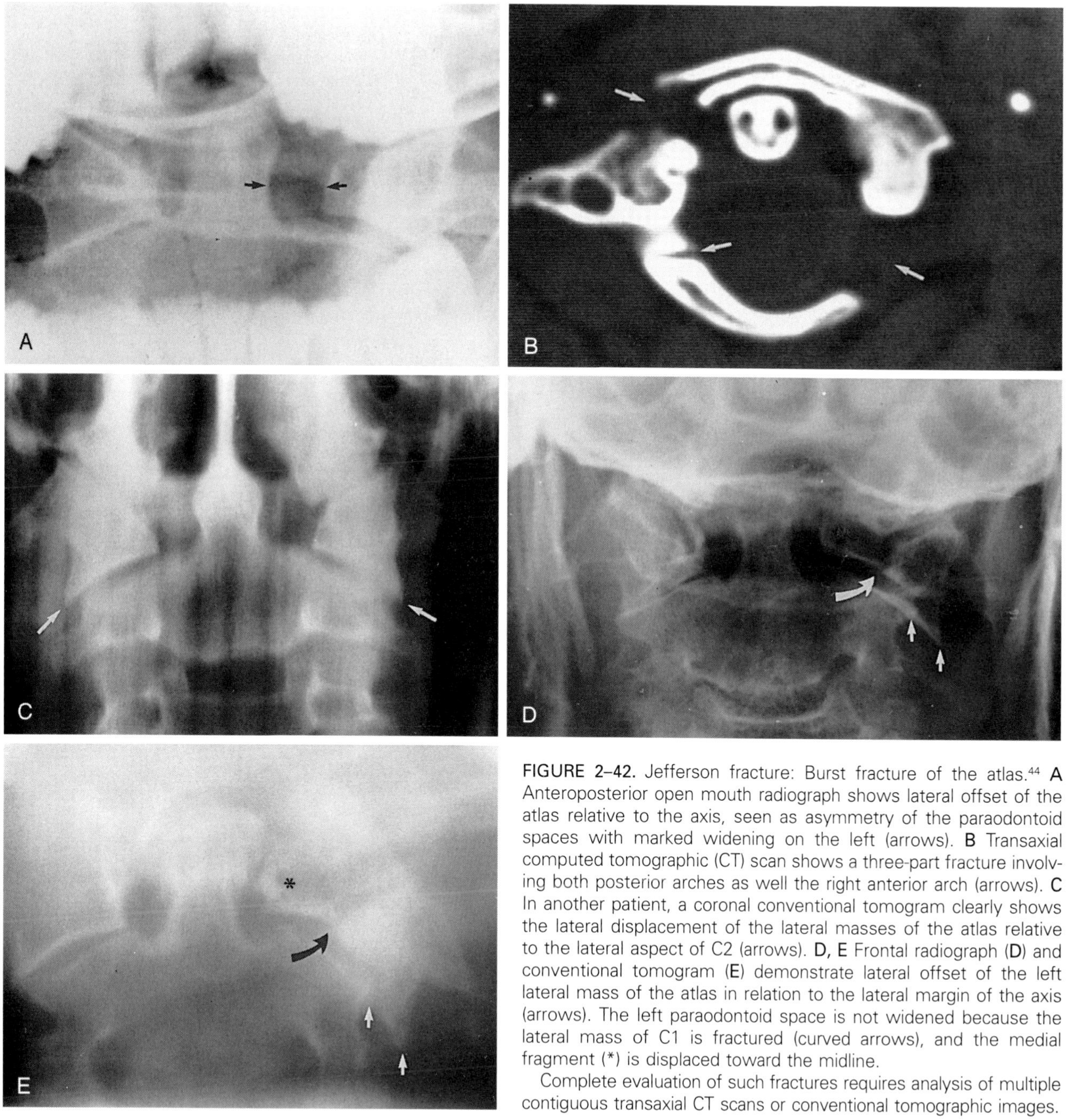

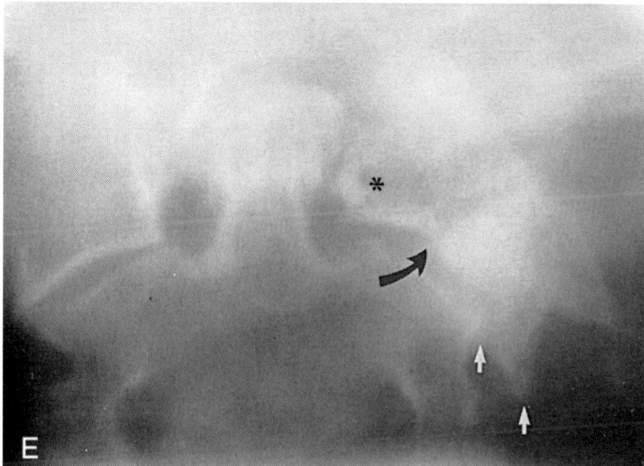

FIGURE 2–42. Jefferson fracture: Burst fracture of the atlas.[44] **A** Anteroposterior open mouth radiograph shows lateral offset of the atlas relative to the axis, seen as asymmetry of the paraodontoid spaces with marked widening on the left (arrows). **B** Transaxial computed tomographic (CT) scan shows a three-part fracture involving both posterior arches as well the right anterior arch (arrows). **C** In another patient, a coronal conventional tomogram clearly shows the lateral displacement of the lateral masses of the atlas relative to the lateral aspect of C2 (arrows). **D, E** Frontal radiograph (**D**) and conventional tomogram (**E**) demonstrate lateral offset of the left lateral mass of the atlas in relation to the lateral margin of the axis (arrows). The left paraodontoid space is not widened because the lateral mass of C1 is fractured (curved arrows), and the medial fragment (*) is displaced toward the midline.

Complete evaluation of such fractures requires analysis of multiple contiguous transaxial CT scans or conventional tomographic images.

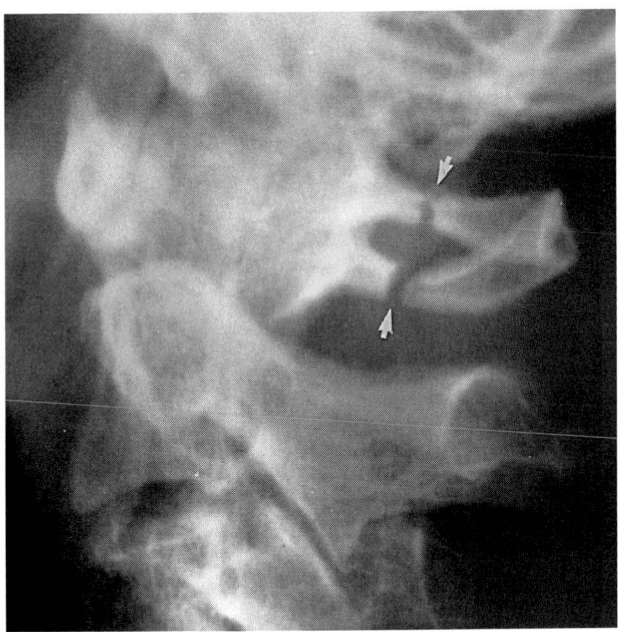

FIGURE 2–43. Posterior arch fracture.[45] Lateral radiograph shows bilateral fractures of the posterior arch of C1 that occurred after a hyperextension injury.

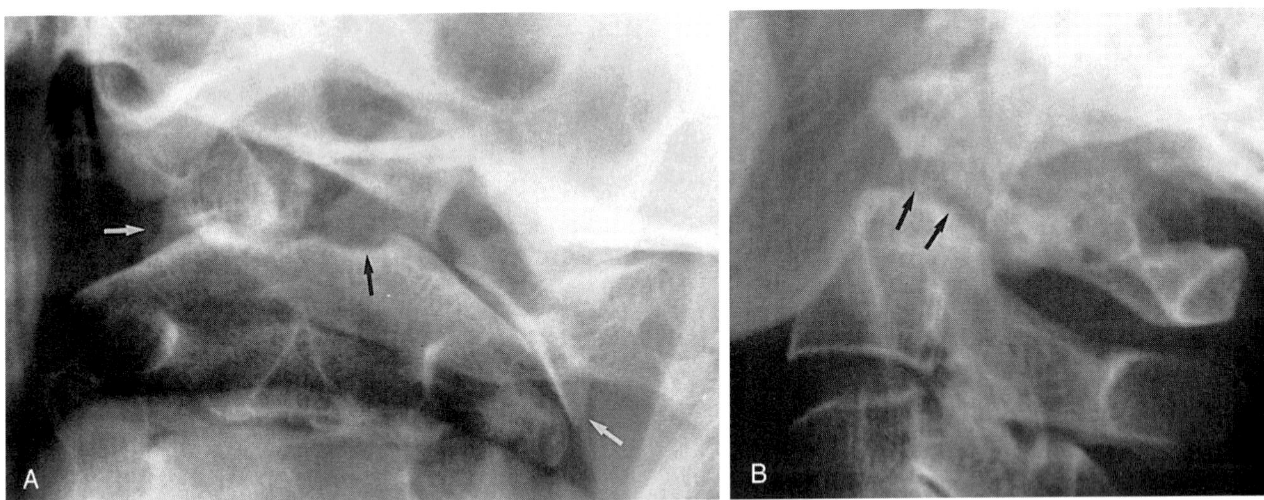

FIGURE 2–44. Odontoid fracture: Type II.[47, 48] This 84-year-old man fell on his face, injuring his cervical spine. A Anteroposterior open mouth radiograph demonstrates a radiolucent fracture cleft at the base of the laterally displaced odontoid process (black arrow). In addition, the lateral masses of the atlas are significantly displaced to the left (white arrows). B Lateral radiograph also shows the fracture line (arrows) and posterior displacement of the odontoid and the atlas in relation to the body of axis.

The type II odontoid fracture, occurring at the junction of the C2 body and the dens, is the most common type of odontoid fracture, is considered unstable, and frequently results in nonunion.

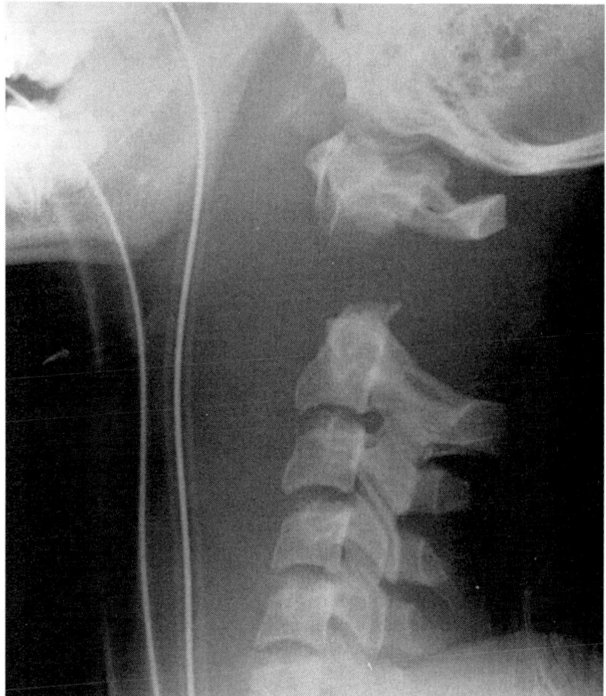

FIGURE 2–45. Odontoid fracture with severe distraction dislocation.[46] Observe the fracture through the base of the odontoid process. Dramatic prevertebral soft tissue swelling and hemorrhage also are evident. This rare type of odontoid fracture with severe distractive dislocation is secondary to massive trauma with predominantly distractive forces. Such injuries usually result in death. *(Courtesy of W. Pogue, M.D., San Diego, California.)*

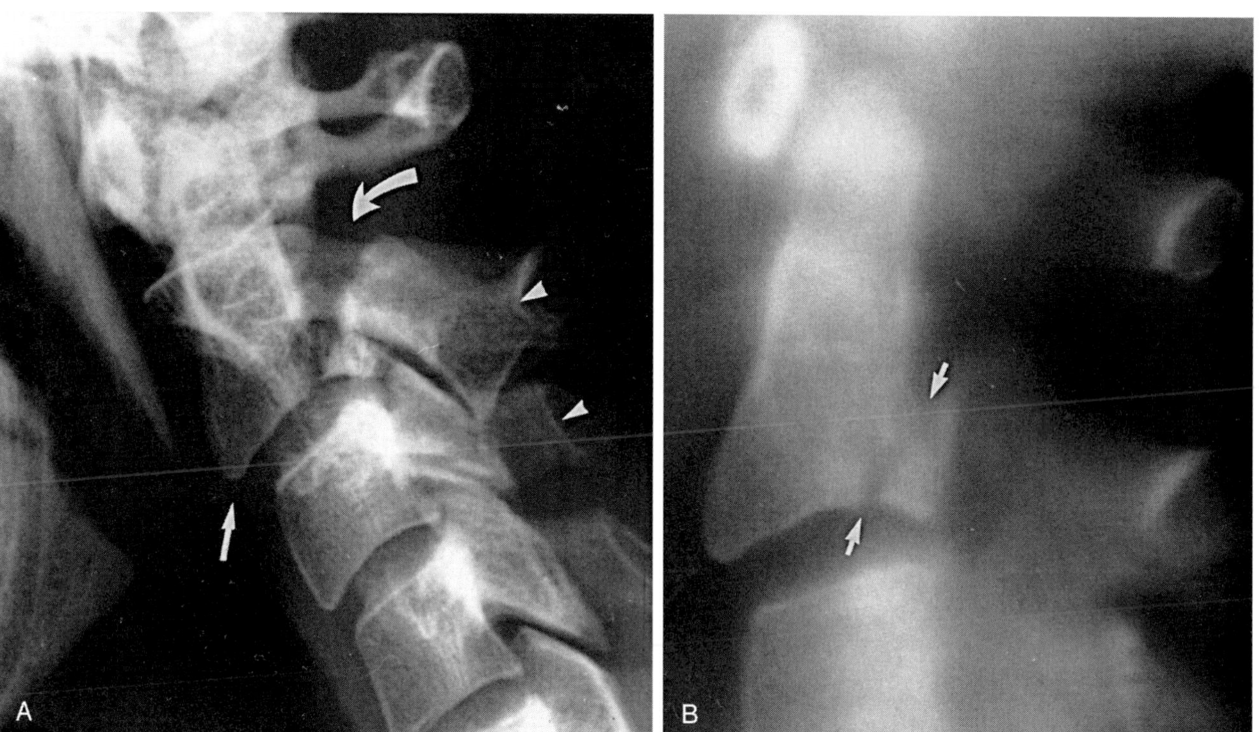

FIGURE 2–46. Hangman's fracture.[47–49] This 28-year-old man was involved in a high-speed motor vehicle accident in which his face struck the windshield and his neck was forced into hyperextension. **A** Lateral radiograph shows fractures through both pedicles of the axis (curved arrow) with anterior displacement of the C2 vertebral body (arrow). In this injury, the spinolaminar junction line remains in normal alignment (arrowheads). **B** Lateral conventional tomogram reveals more clearly the triangular fracture fragment of the posterior portion of the vertebral body (arrows).

TABLE 2–9. Lower Cervical Spine Injuries[46, 60, 61]

Entity	Figure(s), Table(s)	Stability*	Mechanism	Characteristics
Hyperflexion sprain[52]	2–47 Table 2–10	Unstable	Hyperflexion	Acute disruption of ligaments in the following order of injury: supraspinous, interspinous, ligamentum flavum, facet joint capsule; in severe cases, the posterior longitudinal ligament and posterior aspect of the annulus fibrosus also are disrupted C2-C3 and C3-C4 levels most frequent in children; lower cervical levels most frequent in adults Neurologic deficit usually mild and reversible Progressive kyphosis and delayed spinal instability develop in up to 33 per cent of patients treated conservatively Partial ligament disruptions respond well to conservative care, but complete ligament ruptures typically require anterior or posterior cervical fusion Operative fixation should be performed early with kyphosis exceeding 20 degrees in children and 10 degrees in adults Initial radiographs frequently appear normal despite clinically evident cord injury
Bilateral apophyseal joint dislocation[53]	2–48	Unstable	Hyperflexion	Bilateral facet dislocation: highly unstable injury associated with neurologic deficit (75 per cent of cases), disc herniations (as many as 50 per cent of cases), and fractures Rupture of the posterior portion of the annulus fibrosus, posterior longitudinal ligament, and the capsular, interspinous, and supraspinous ligaments Inferior articular processes of the vertebra above dislocate and become perched (locked) in front of the superior articular processes of the vertebra below, resulting in spinal canal and foraminal stenosis Anterior vertebral body displacement typically is more than half the width of the vertebral body; this displacement increases during flexion but fails to reduce during extension Computed tomography (CT) and magnetic resonance (MR) imaging are useful in assessing such injuries Flexion and extension radiographs in patients with severe cervical spine trauma should be obtained only under careful observation by a clinician and only in alert, cooperative patients who are able to actively perform these movements

TABLE 2–9. Lower Cervical Spine Injuries[46, 60, 61] *Continued*

Entity	Figure(s), Table(s)	Stability*	Mechanism	Characteristics
Unilateral facet dislocation[54–56]	2–49	Stable unless associated with facet fractures and neurologic deficit	Hyperflexion with rotation	In unilateral facet lock (dislocation), rupture of the interspinous ligament and capsule of the apophyseal joint allows the ipsilateral inferior facet of one vertebra to pivot, dislocate, and come to rest in the neural foramen anterior to the superior facet of the vertebra below Frequently accompanied by articular process fractures and bilateral damage of the rotated vertebra These injuries contribute to rotational instability and require specific internal fixation based on a precise delineation of all injuries Neurologic deficits, including radiculopathy, are relatively uncommon CT with parasagittal reformation is valuable in evaluating injuries in these patients
Spinous process fractures	2–50	Stable		Spinous process fractures generally are stable and do not result in neurologic injury Careful observation for evidence of other fractures or dislocations is essential
Two major types:				
Clay-shoveler's fracture[57]			Hyperflexion	Most common type: avulsion fracture of spinous process of C6-T2 levels Avulsed fragment typically is displaced inferiorly
Hyperextension type[46]			Hyperextension	Less common type: impaction injury of spinous processes Fracture from direct contact with adjacent spinous processes
Vertebral body compression fracture[46, 51]		Usually stable	Compressive hyperflexion	Wedgelike compression of vertebral body Usually spares the posterior ligaments and results in simple compression fractures of the anterior vertebral column Considered benign because these fractures do not compromise the spinal canal, and they result in uncomplicated healing
Flexion teardrop fracture[58]	2–51	Unstable	Compressive hyperflexion	Highly unstable comminuted fracture of the vertebral body that results in severe neurologic injury in almost 90 per cent of patients Injury occurs most frequently in diving and motor vehicle collisions Owing to the risk of neurologic injury related to instability, the lateral radiograph should be evaluated fully before flexion radiographs are obtained
Avulsion of the ring apophysis[46]		Stable	Hyperextension or, rarely, hyperflexion	Occurs in the vertebral body of the immature spine Usually not associated with neurologic damage, prevertebral soft tissue swelling, or other osseous injury Heals with an osseous excrescence at the inferior vertebral margin related to fusion of the avulsed apophysis with the vertebral body

Table continued on following page

TABLE 2–9. Lower Cervical Spine Injuries[46, 60, 61] *Continued*

Entity	Figure(s), Table(s)	Stability*	Mechanism	Characteristics
Extension teardrop fracture[59]		Variable	Hyperextension	Avulsion fracture of a triangular fragment of the anteroinferior margin of the body by the anterior longitudinal ligament Most common at C2 but may occur at any level Fragment may be displaced, distracted, or rotated More common in elderly persons with osteoporosis and spondylosis Usually not associated with any neurologic deficit
Posttraumatic discovertebral injury: lucent annular cleft sign[60]	2–52	May represent instability	Hyperextension most common, but also seen with hyperflexion	Lucent cleft sign, often seen after hyperextension injuries, is believed to represent nitrogen gas accumulating within a traumatic avulsion of the annulus fibrosus from its attachment to the anterior cartilaginous end plate Gas-filled cleft often is accentuated on radiographs taken in extension, can be associated with disc space widening, and may persist for as long as 5 years after trauma Posttraumatic vacuum cleft should not be confused with the more common intradiscal vacuum associated with degenerative disc disease, a condition that usually is accompanied by disc space narrowing, osteophyte formation, and a more extensive and irregular collection of gas
Hyperextension fracture-dislocation[46]		Unstable	Hyperextension	Injury usually ruptures the anterior longitudinal ligament or intervertebral disc, or, in as many as 65 per cent of patients, may result in avulsion of the anteroinferior corner of the vertebral body Severe hyperextension dislocation produces minimal radiographic findings but profound neurologic deficits In as many as 30 per cent of cases, the only radiographic finding is prevertebral hematoma; in some cases, retrolisthesis is evident Disc space widening can occur, but may be evident only during traction or extension Extension radiographs also may reveal radiolucent annular clefts C5-C6 and C4-C5 most common levels of involvement
Hyperextension sprain[61, 62]	2–53, 2–54	Generally considered stable	Hyperextension	Momentary dislocation that does not result in significant disruption of the spinal ligaments, osseous structures, or discs Neurologic damage is sustained, but stability usually is maintained May be impossible to differentiate sprain from reduced dislocation on radiographs Risk of neurologic injury is greater in patients with cervical spondylosis (because of acquired stenosis from osteophytes) and in patients with congenital spinal stenosis Typical neurologic injury is the central cord syndrome caused by hemorrhage in the central gray matter of the cervical cord

TABLE 2–9. Lower Cervical Spine Injuries[46, 60, 61] *Continued*

Entity	Figure(s), Table(s)	Stability*	Mechanism	Characteristics
Pillar fractures[63, 64]	2–55	Stable	Hyperextension and rotation	Unilateral (or, infrequently, bilateral) vertical, oblique, or crushing fracture of the articular process, most common at the C6 and C7 levels Represent 3 to 11 per cent of all cervical spine fractures and result in radiculopathy in 6 to 39 per cent of patients Special oblique or pillar views often are helpful, but CT or conventional tomography is definitive Normal bilateral asymmetry in the height of the articular pillars may be as great as 3 mm in about 40 per cent of normal persons, and this asymmetric configuration may simulate a fracture
Other vertebral arch fractures[46]		Variable	Compressive hyperextension	Fractures of the pedicles or laminae
C3-C7 burst fracture[65]	2–56	Variable	Axial compression combined with flexion	Comminuted fracture of the vertebral body, usually sustained in motor vehicle accidents and diving injuries Most common at C5, C6, and C7 Vertebral body usually is comminuted; injury often is not associated with cervical kyphosis, interspinous fanning, or facet joint dislocation or subluxation Sagittal fracture line, seen on the anteroposterior view, may be difficult to detect Ligaments usually remain intact Neurologic deficits present in as many as 85 per cent of patients owing to stretching of the cord across the posterior aspect of the vertebral body or compression of the cord by retropulsed fragments
Isolated sagittal fracture of the vertebral body[66]	2–57	Unstable	Axial compression	In this rare type of injury, routine radiography may be unreliable, failing to reveal the vertical fracture even though the patient may be quadriplegic CT is essential in such cases, reliably demonstrating fractures of the vertebral body, and, in most patients, associated posterior element fractures MR imaging is more useful for demonstrating spinal cord injury in these patients
Transverse process fracture[67]	2–58	Stable	Lateral hyperflexion	Uncommon
Uncinate process fracture[67]		Stable	Lateral hyperflexion	Uncommon
Nerve root or brachial plexus avulsion[67]		Variable	Lateral hyperflexion	Uncommon injury, most likely caused by motorcycle accidents and birth trauma Often associated with cervical fracture, dislocation, or both Myelography and CT myelography currently are superior to MR imaging for identifying nerve root avulsions
Lateral wedgelike compression of vertebral body[67]		Stable	Lateral hyperflexion	Uncommon Lateral wedging of vertebral body and its associated lateral mass

*Clinical instability here is defined as the inability to maintain vertebral relationships in such a way that spinal cord and nerve root damage are avoided and subsequent deformity and excessive pain do not develop. From White AA, Southwick WO, Panjabi MM: Clinical instability in the lower cervical spine. Clin Orthop 109:85, 1975.

TABLE 2–10. Radiographic Findings in Hyperflexion Sprain With Posterior Ligament Disruption and Instability[46] (Fig. 2–47)

Finding	Characteristics
Interspinous widening	Widening that is more than 2 mm greater than the interspinous width at both adjacent levels is indicative of instability; definite anterior cervical dislocation is present when the interspinous distance is more than 1.5 times that of both adjacent levels
Localized kyphosis	Focally exaggerated kyphosis is required to make the diagnosis of hyperflexion sprain Kyphosis at a single level measuring more than 11 degrees with persistent lordosis at adjacent levels is indicative of hyperflexion sprain and indicates posterior ligament damage
Posterior disc space widening	Widening of the posterior aspect of the disc space suggests annular disruption
Anterior vertebral displacement	Anterior rotation, or 1 to 3 mm anterior displacement of the superior vertebra, may be present with posterior ligament disruption
Abnormal movement or alignment on flexion and extension views	If this injury is suspected, clinician-supervised flexion and extension radiographs should be obtained only in alert, cooperative patients who are able to perform these motions actively Abnormal alignment is exaggerated with neck flexion and corrected with neck extension

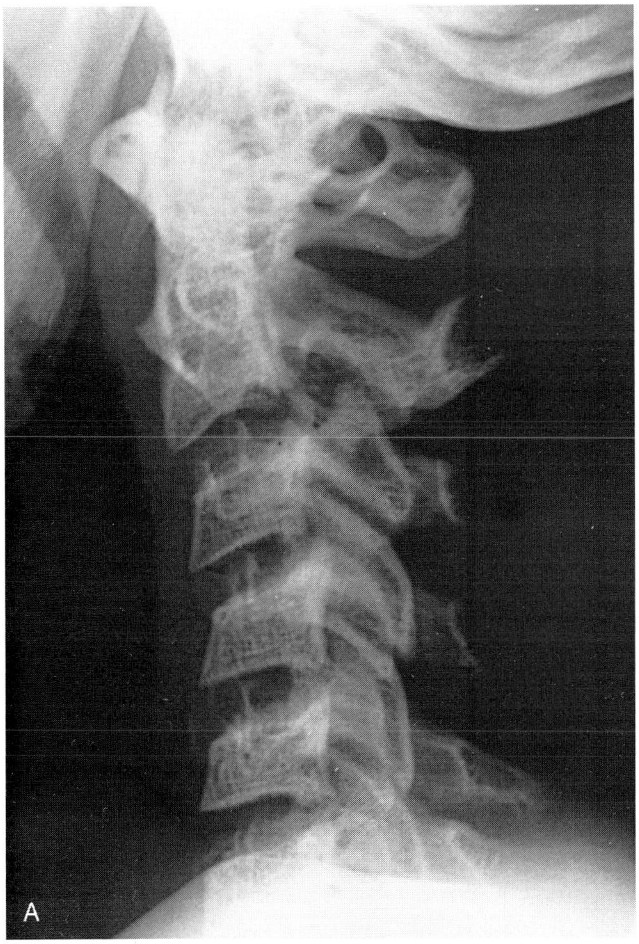

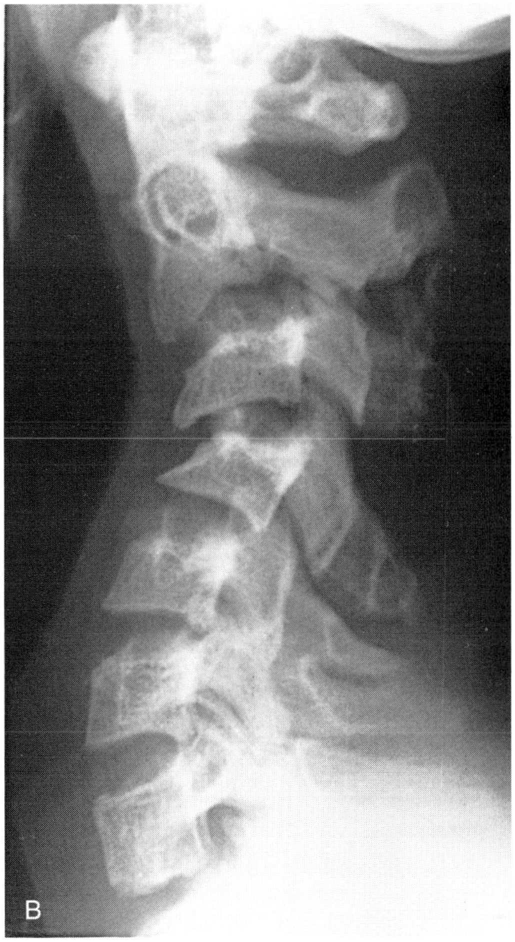

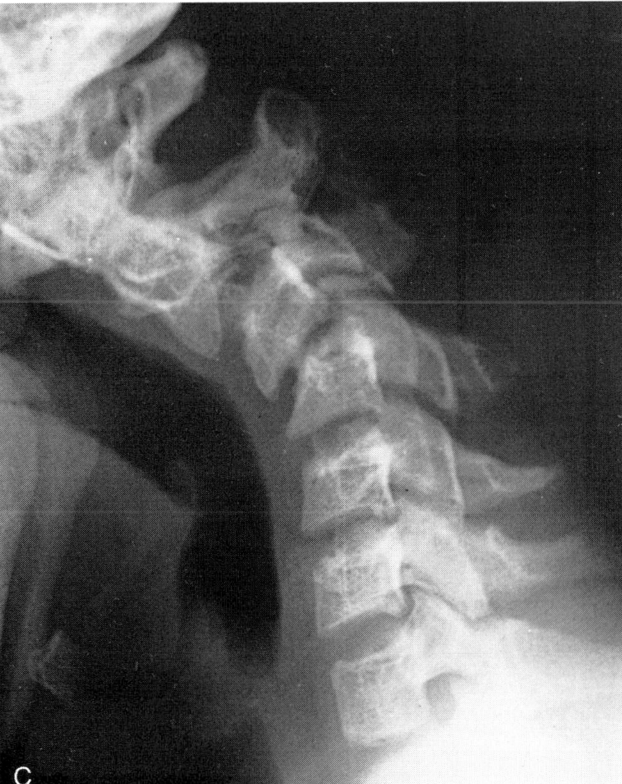

FIGURE 2–47. Acute unstable hyperflexion sprain: Progressive instability.[52] **A** Initial radiograph obtained at the time of a hyperflexion injury sustained in a motor vehicle accident reveals minimal reversal of the cervical lordosis and minimal anterolisthesis of C2 on C3. **B** Subsequent radiograph taken 10 months later shows progressive focal kyphosis, widening of the facet joints and interspinous space at C3-C4, and ossification of the interspinous ligaments at C2-C3, illustrating the consequences of an initially unrecognized hyperflexion injury. **C** Flexion radiograph obtained at the same time as **B** reveals excessive motion, acute angular kyphosis, and excessive translation of C3 on C4, indicative of marked instability. *(**A–C,** Courtesy of M.N. Pathria, M.D., San Diego, California.)*

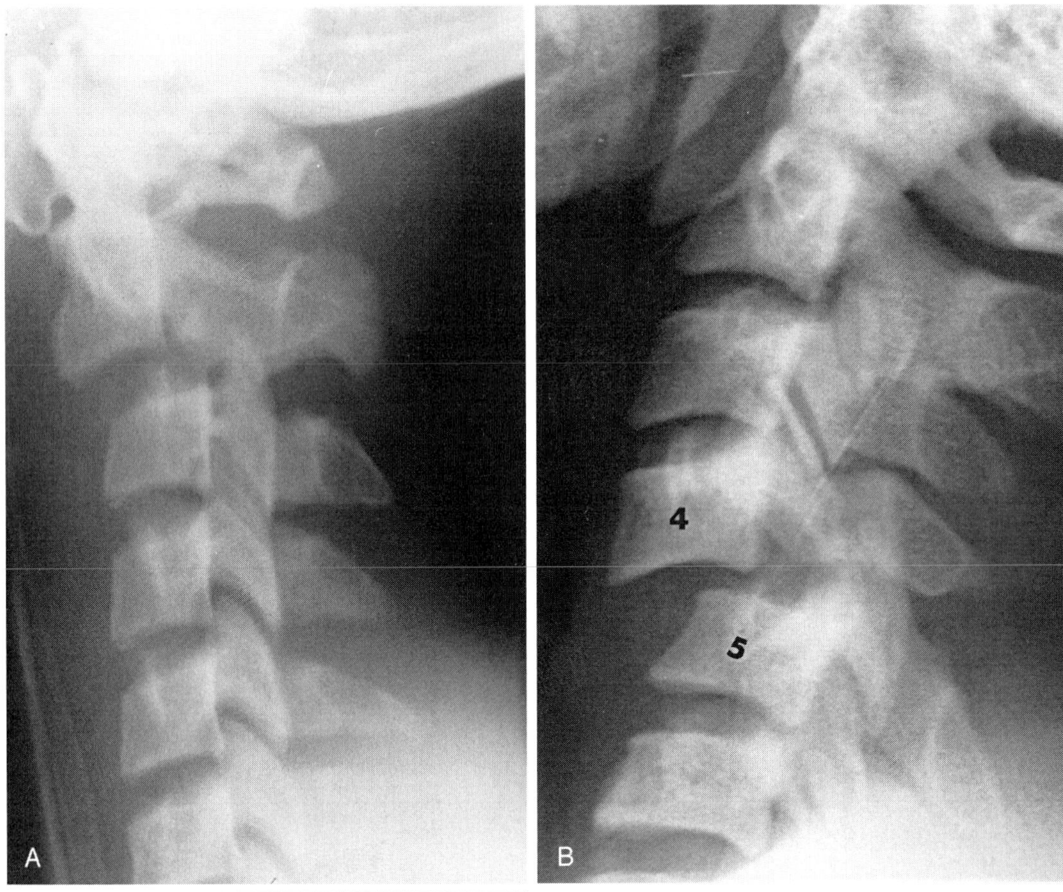

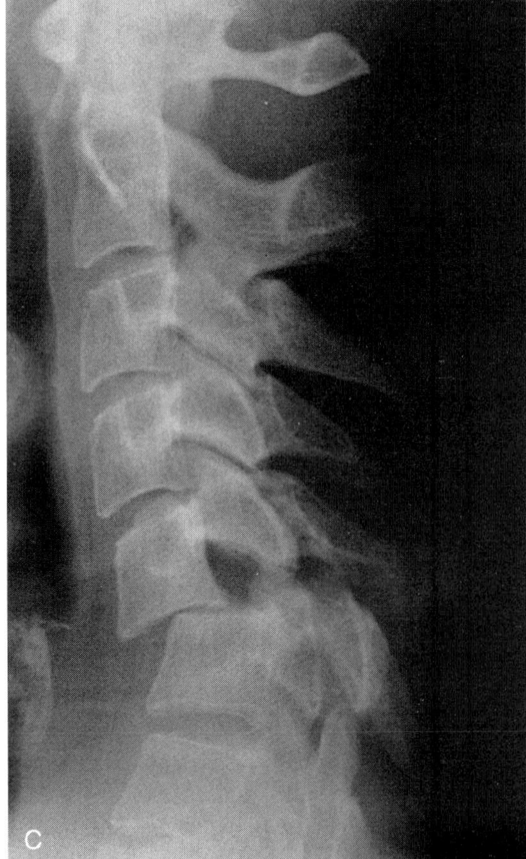

FIGURE 2–48. Bilateral apophyseal joint dislocation (facet lock).[53] **A** Acute bilateral apophyseal joint dislocation: C2-C3. This 16-year-old boy was paralyzed after a hyperflexion injury. Lateral radiograph demonstrates bilateral facet locks at the C2-C3 level. Note the anterior displacement of C2 on C3 measuring almost 50 per cent of the diameter of the vertebral body. Prevertebral soft tissue swelling also is present. **B** Acute bilateral apophyseal joint dislocation: C4-C5. This 27-year-old man was involved in a motor vehicle accident in which he sustained a hyperflexion injury. Observe the dislocation of C4 on C5 with a fracture of the inferior articular process of C4. **C** Chronic unreduced bilateral facet dislocation: C5-C6. This patient sustained a hyperflexion injury with bilateral facet dislocation. She did not seek treatment until several months after the injury. Lateral radiograph obtained at that time reveals persistent perching of the C5-C6 facet articulations with an associated focal kyphosis. *(**C**, Courtesy of G. Smith, D.C., Vancouver, Washington.)*

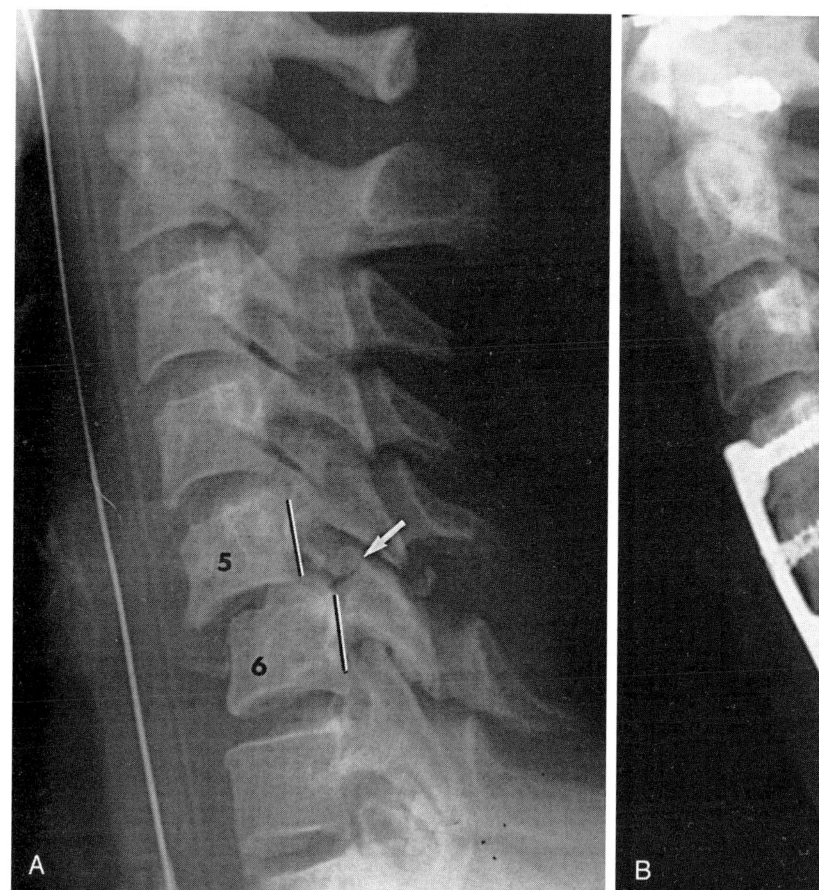

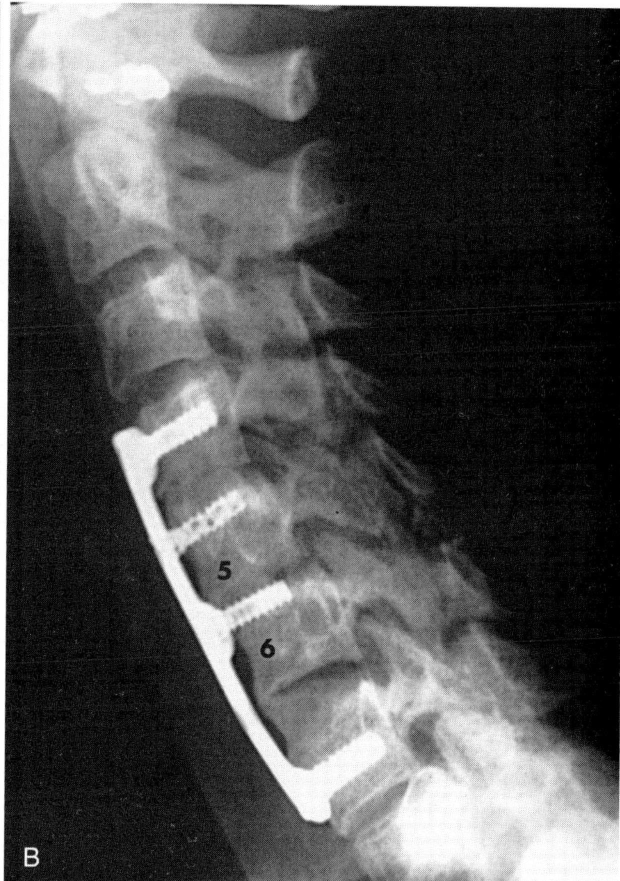

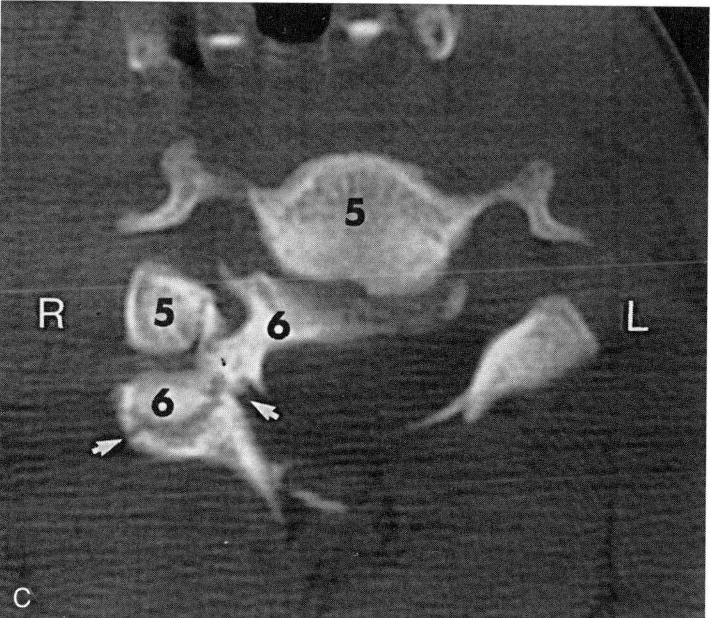

FIGURE 2–49. Unilateral facet joint dislocation with articular process fracture.[54–56] A Lateral radiograph obtained immediately after injury shows 7-mm anterior displacement of C5 on C6, malalignment of the C5-C6 facet joints, and a fracture (arrow) of the C6 superior articular process. B Lateral radiograph obtained after surgery demonstrates improved alignment and anterior cervical fusion with a fixation plate and cannulated screws. C Transaxial preoperative CT image shows the abnormal anatomic relationship of C5 and C6. The right C6 facet is seen dislocated in a position posterior to the C5 facet, which is perched (locked) anterior to its C6 counterpart. The body of C5 is rotated anteriorly on the right relative to the body of C6. A complex fracture of the C6 articular process (arrows) also is evident. *(Courtesy of M.N. Pathria, M.D., San Diego, California.)*

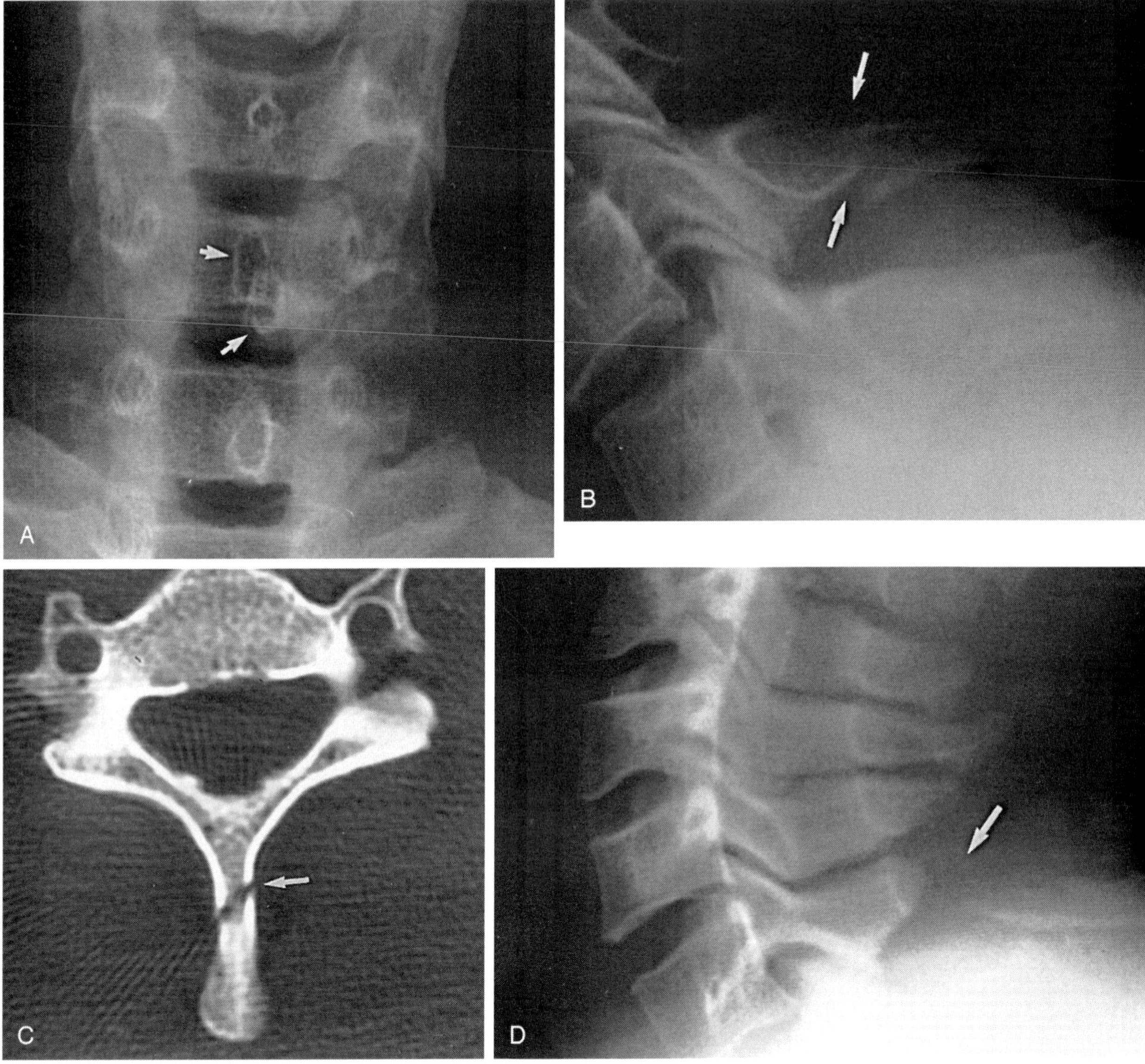

FIGURE 2–50. Spinous process fractures.[46, 57] A–C This 24-year-old man had a hyperflexion injury (clay-shoveler's fracture). A Anteroposterior radiograph shows a double spinous process sign, which relates to simultaneous visualization of the fractured base and the caudally displaced tip of the spinous process (arrows). B Lateral radiograph shows an oblique fracture of the tip of the C7 spinous process (arrows) with characteristic inferior displacement of the fracture fragment. C Transaxial CT image shows the fracture confined to the spinous process (arrow), with minimal displacement and an otherwise intact neural arch. D Hyperextension injury. This 22-year-old man suffered a hyperextension injury. Observe the fracture of the C7 spinous process (arrow) caused by forceful impaction of the posterior elements.

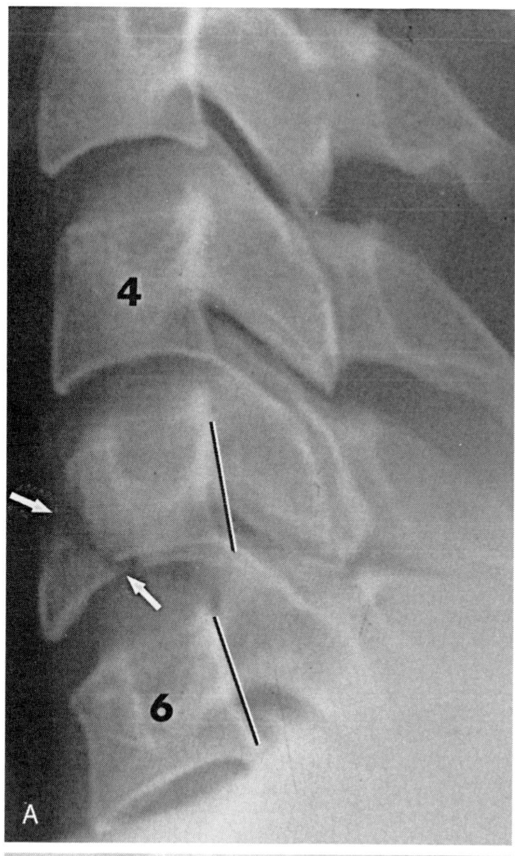

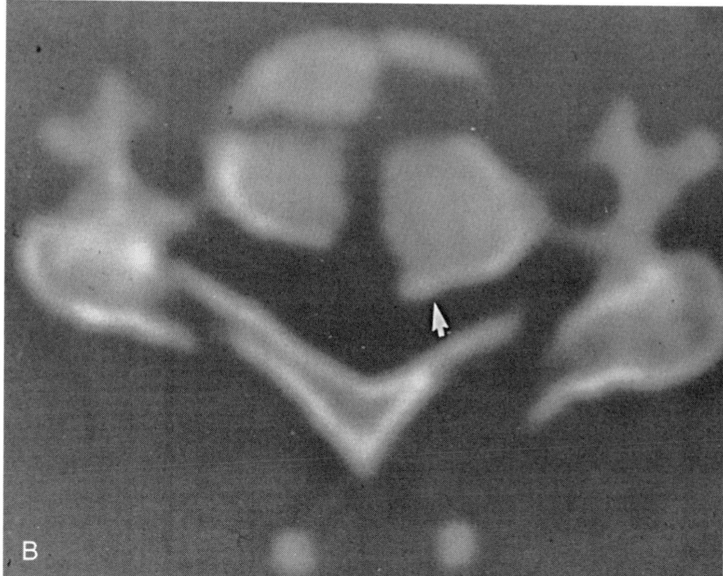

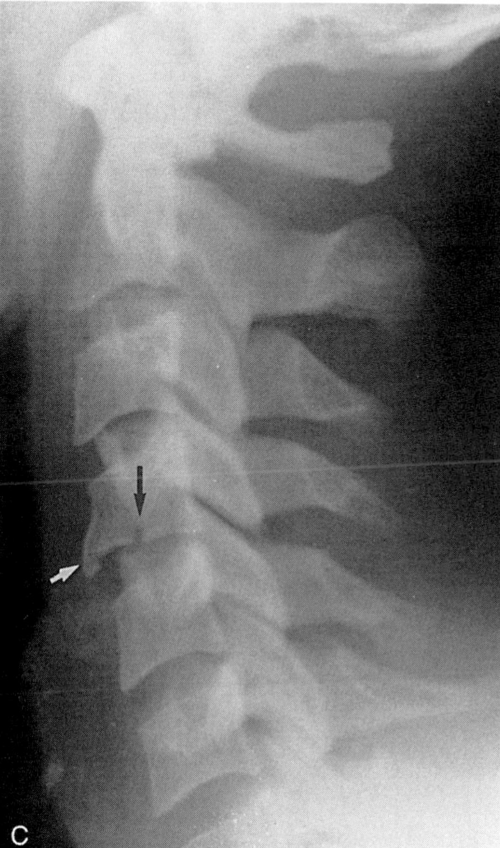

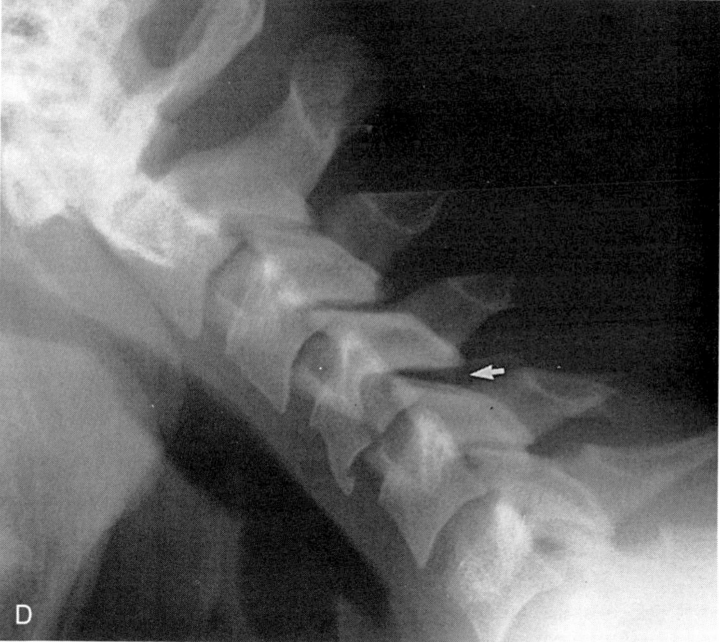

FIGURE 2–51. Flexion teardrop fractures.[58] A, B Lateral cervical radiograph (A) shows a triangular fracture of the anteroinferior margin of the C5 vertebral body (arrows). Slight retrolisthesis of C5 also is seen (note the posterior body lines of C5 and C6). Transaxial CT image (B) reveals comminution of the C5 vertebral body. The principal injury seen on the CT scan is a stellate, vertical fracture with coronal and sagittal components. Retropulsion of one of the osseous fragments (arrow) resulting in central stenosis is evident on the CT image but is imperceptible on the radiograph. C, D In another patient, the routine lateral cervical radiograph (C) shows a triangular fracture of the anteroinferior margin of the C5 vertebral body (white arrow) and a vertical fracture of the vertebral body (black arrow). A flexion radiograph (D) obtained prior to full evaluation of the neutral lateral radiograph shows excessive facet gapping (white arrow) and an increase in the interspinous space, both of which indicate ligamentous instability. *(A–D, Courtesy of M.N. Pathria, M.D., San Diego, California.)*

Illustration continued on following page

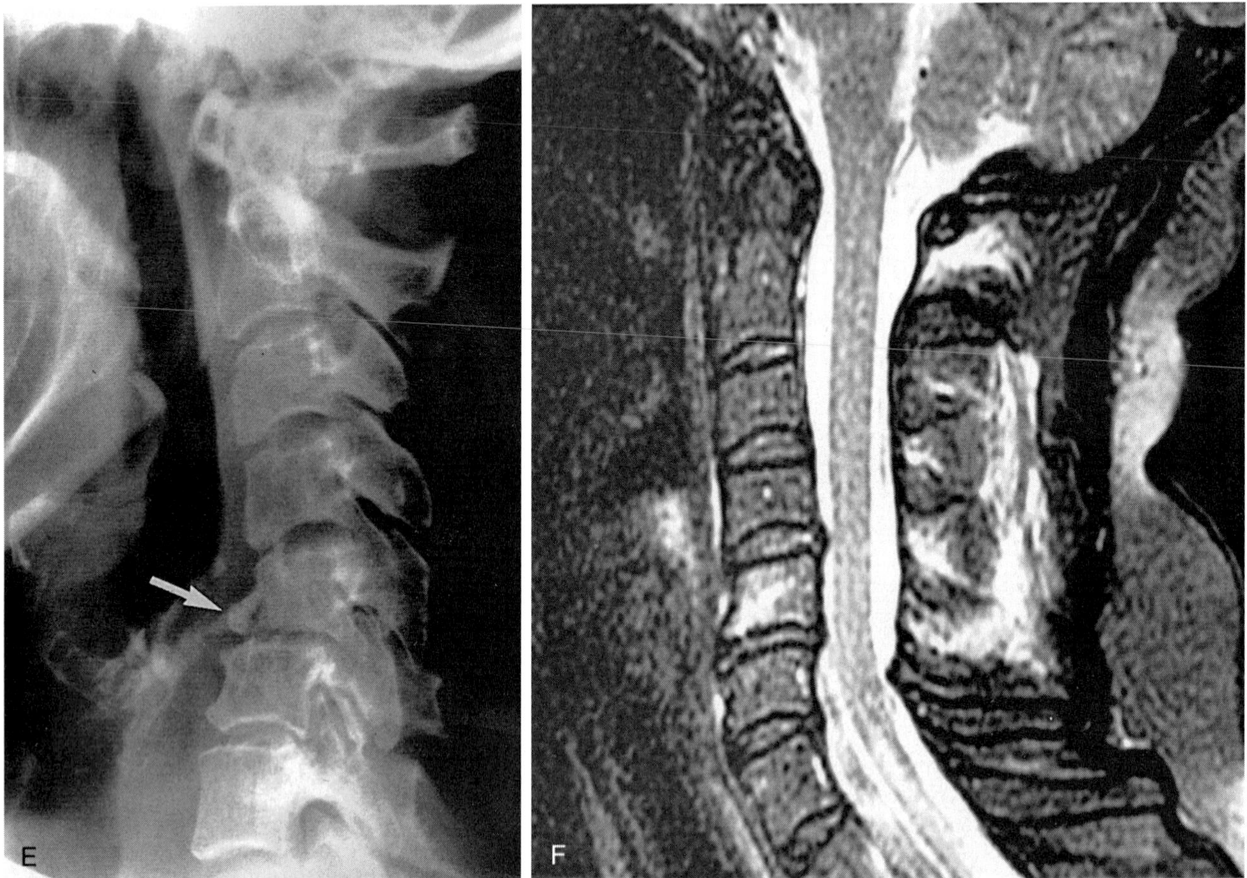

FIGURE 2–51 *Continued.* E, F This 57-year-old woman was involved in a motor vehicle accident. In E, a lateral radiograph shows a triangular fracture of the anteroinferior corner of the C5 vertebral body (arrow). Acute angular kyphosis, posterior body displacement, and a suggestion of widened facet joints are evident. In F, a sagittal T2-weighted (TR/TE, 2857/96 Ef) fast spin echo magnetic resonance (MR) image demonstrates high-signal intensity within the vertebral body and the spinal ligaments posteriorly, consistent with edema or hemorrhage, or both. *(*E, F, *Courtesy of D. Goodwin, M.D., Hanover, New Hampshire.)*

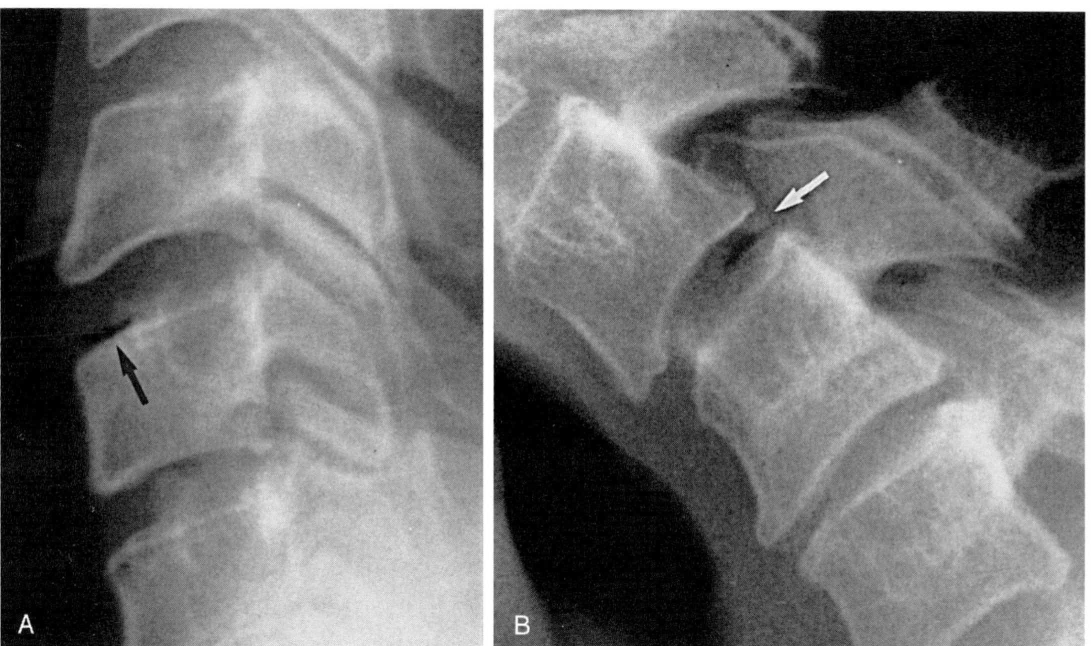

FIGURE 2–52. Posttraumatic discovertebral injury: Lucent annular cleft sign.[60] A Hyperextension injury. Lateral radiograph shows a linear collection of gas within the annular fibers of the intervertebral disc adjacent to the vertebral end plate. The lucent cleft sign (arrow), often seen after hyperextension injuries, is believed to represent traumatic avulsion of the annulus fibrosus from its attachment to the anterior cartilaginous end plate. B Hyperflexion injury. Observe the gas density within the posterior portion of the C4-C5 disc (arrow) on this lateral radiograph obtained in flexion. This patient was recently involved in a rear-end impact motor vehicle collision and had severe neck pain. *(Courtesy of M.N. Pathria, M.D., San Diego, California.)*

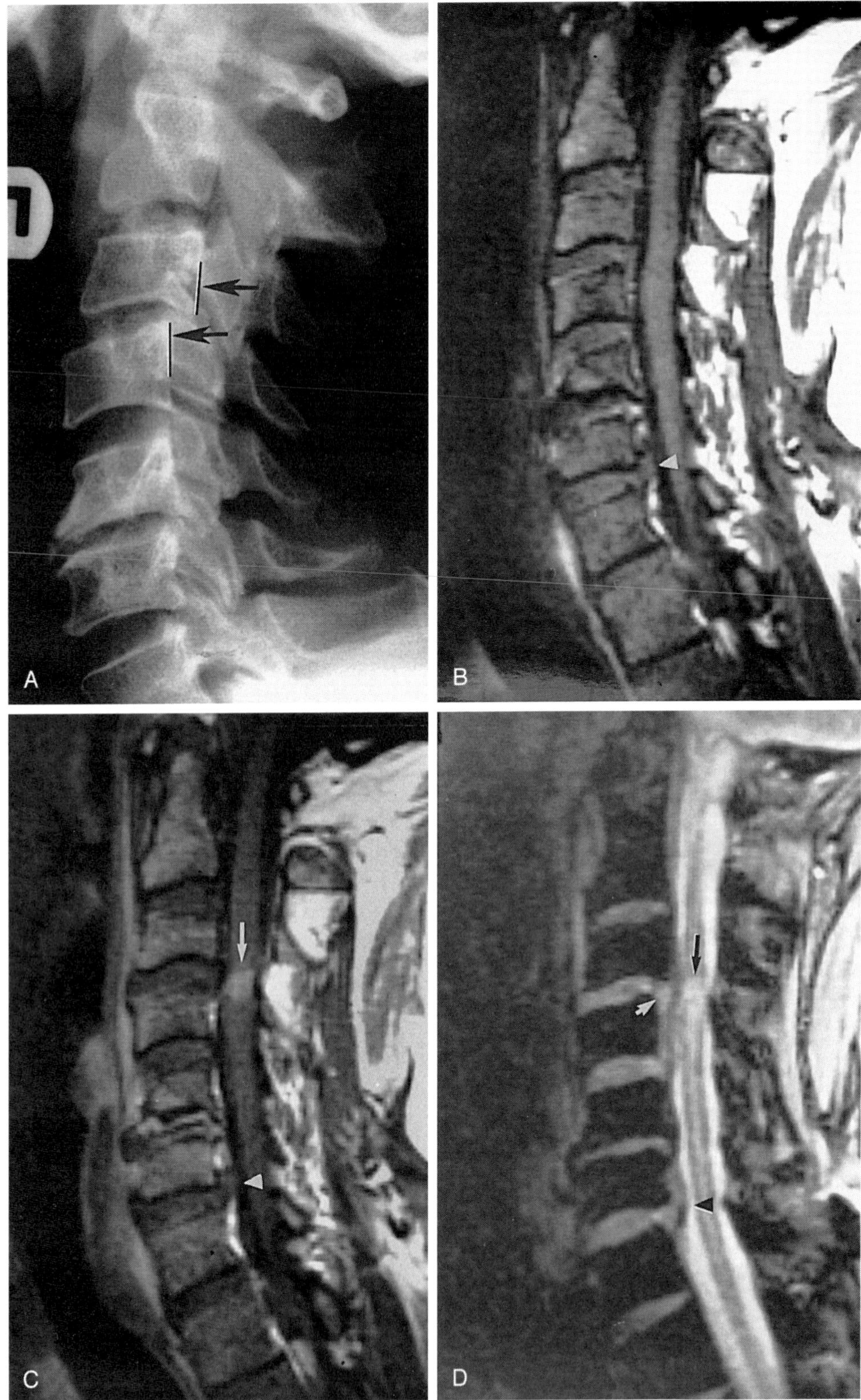

FIGURE 2–53. Acute hyperextension sprain.[61, 62] This 51-year-old man sustained a hyperextension injury in a motor vehicle collision. He developed persistent neurologic signs and symptoms. **A** Lateral radiograph. Observe the 5 mm of retrolisthesis of the C3 vertebral body relative to that of C4 (arrows). C5-C6 degenerative spondylosis also is seen. **B, C** Sagittal T1-weighted (TR/TE, 600/20) fat-suppressed spin echo magnetic resonance (MR) images before (**B**) and after (**C**) intravenous gadolinium administration. The postgadolinium image shows enhancement (high-signal intensity) of the injured spinal cord at the C3-C4 level (white arrow) not seen on the pregadolinium image. **D** Sagittal (TR/TE, 600/17) gradient echo MR image also demonstrates a high signal intensity focus representing spinal cord contusion (black arrow).

Disc herniations are seen at C6-C7 (arrowheads) on all MR imaging sequences and at C3-C4 on the gradient echo image (**D**) (small white arrow). *(Courtesy of M.N. Pathria, M.D., San Diego, California.)*

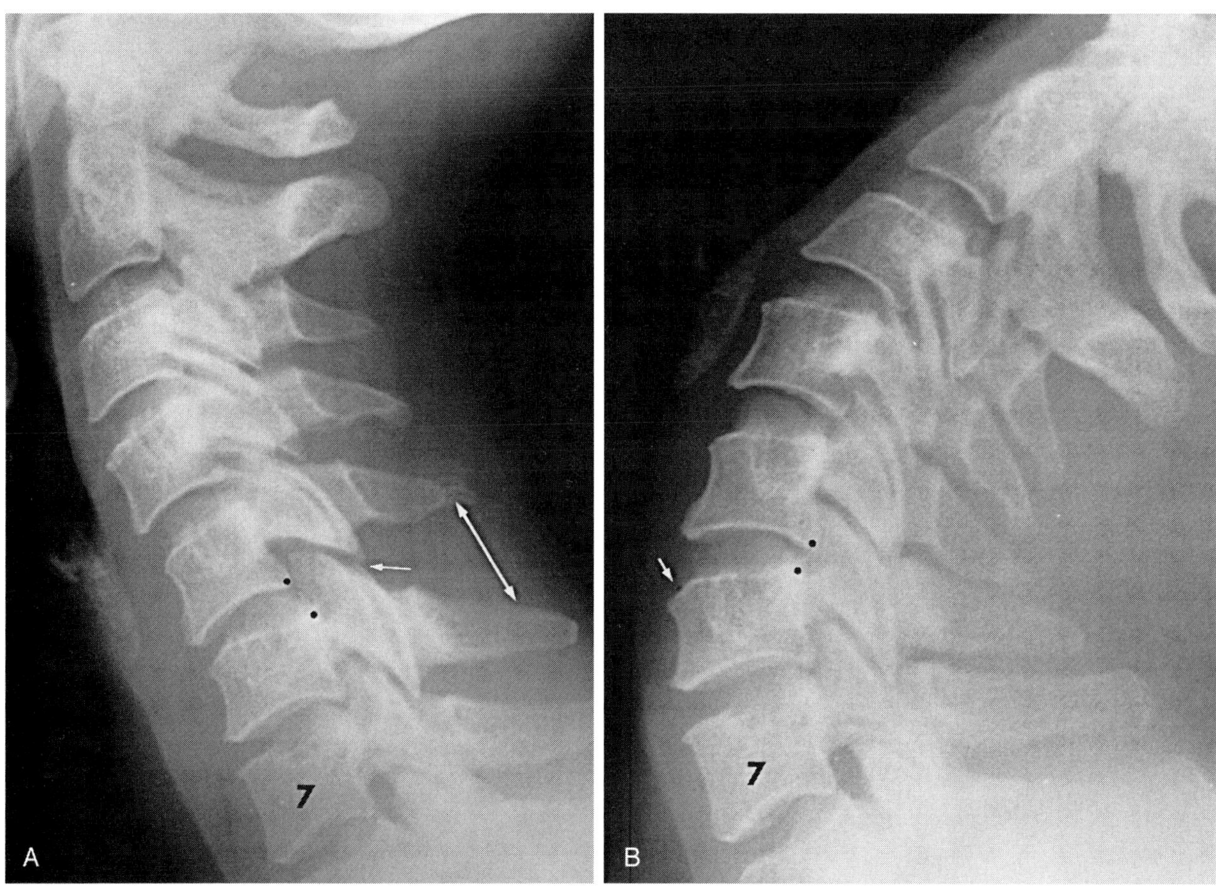

FIGURE 2–54. Hyperflexion-hyperextension sprain: Segmental instability.[61, 62] This 26-year-old woman had severe neck and radiating arm pain after a rear-end automobile collision. A Neutral lateral radiograph shows a reversal of the normal cervical lordosis, separation of the spinous processes (double-headed arrow) and facet joints (small arrow), and widening of the posterior C5-C6 intervertebral disc space (black dots). B Lateral radiograph obtained during neck extension reveals 5 mm of posterior translation of the C5 vertebral body in relation to the C6 vertebral body (black dots). A small radiolucent vacuum cleft (white arrow), not well visualized on this reproduction, is present within the anterior fibers of the C5-C6 intervertebral disc. Excessive intersegmental motion and intradiscal vacuum cleft are indicative of segmental instability.

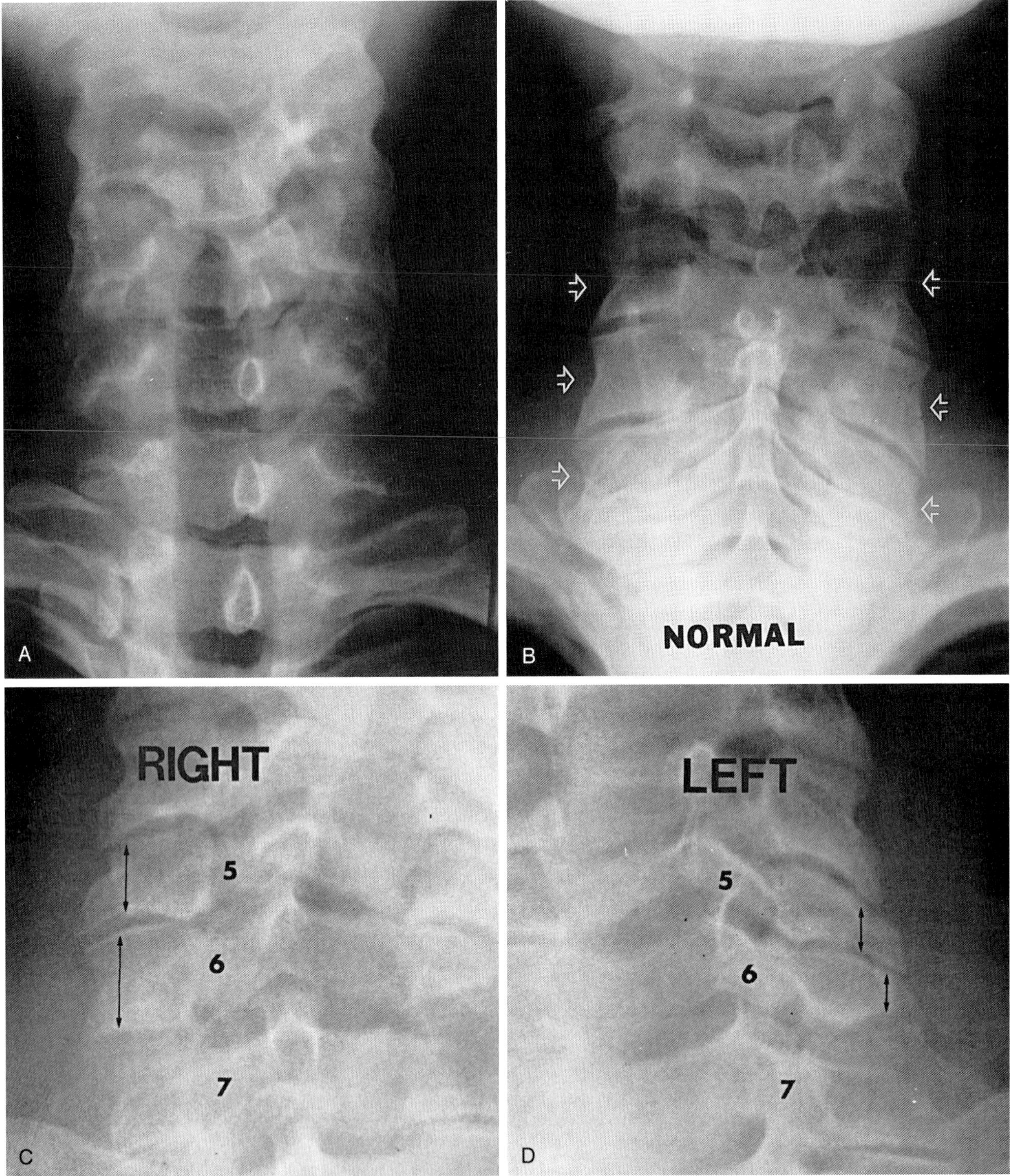

FIGURE 2–55. Pillar fracture: Value of pillar views.[63, 64] A Normal anteroposterior projection. The articular processes are not well visualized. B Normal anteroposterior pillar projection. The pillar radiograph is obtained using caudal tube angulation such that the beam is oriented along the plane of the facet joint, usually about 35 degrees caudally. Observe the symmetric and aligned articular processes, one on top of the other (open arrows). C, D This patient sustained a hyperextension-rotation injury compressing the left articular pillars. In C, the frontal pillar radiograph taken with left rotation. In D, the frontal pillar radiograph taken with right rotation. These radiographs reveal vertical compression of the left C5 and C6 articular processes (double-headed arrows).

The majority of pillar fractures occur at C4 through C7, with C6 involved in approximately 40 per cent of cases. It should be noted that 2 to 3 mm of asymmetry in height of the articular processes is present in over 45 per cent of normal persons and may lead to false-positive diagnoses. (C, D, *Courtesy of T. Hall, D.C., Long Beach, California.*)

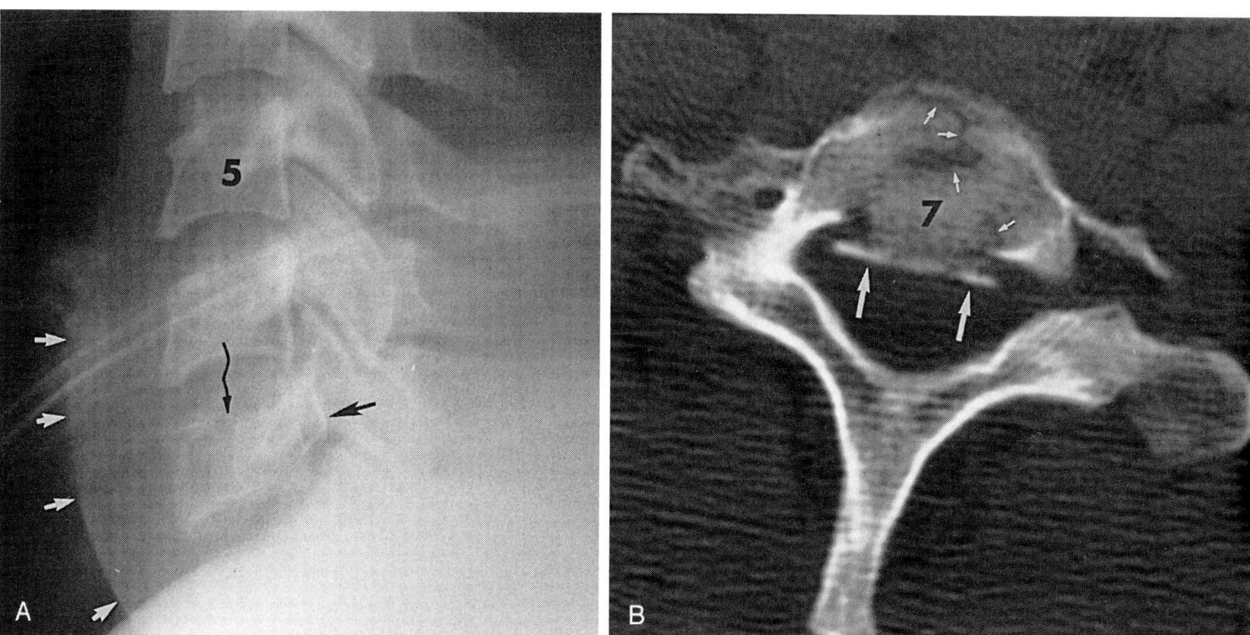

FIGURE 2–56. Burst fracture.[65] This 22-year-old man dove into a shallow pool. **A** Lateral radiograph shows loss of height of the C7 vertebral body, retropulsion of the posterior body margin into the spinal canal (black arrow), a vertical fracture through the end plate (wavy arrow), and prevertebral soft tissue swelling (white arrows). **B** Transaxial computed tomographic (CT) image through the C7 vertebral body shows the retropulsed bone fragment (large white arrows) resulting in canal stenosis. Comminution of the vertebral body also is noted (small white arrows).

Burst fractures of the cervical spine typically are sustained in motor vehicle collisions and diving injuries and result in neurologic deficits in about 85 per cent of patients. *(Courtesy of M.N. Pathria, M.D., San Diego, California.)*

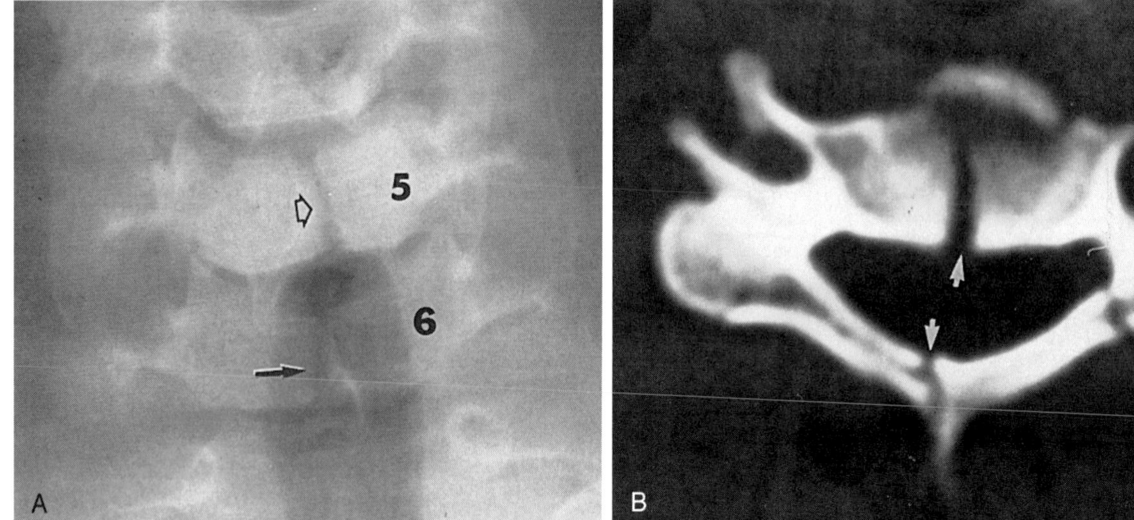

FIGURE 2–57. Axial compression injury: Sagittal fracture of C6 vertebral body.[66] This 23-year-old man dove into shallow water. Although he was quadriplegic immediately after the injury, he regained motor function of his arms and left leg, but pain and temperature sensation deficit persisted on his left side. Vibration and position sense remained intact. **A** Routine anteroposterior radiograph shows minimal compression and a vertical split in the vertebral body of C6 (arrow). The radiolucent vertical line (open arrow) through the C5 vertebral body represents the normal contracted larynx. **B** Transaxial computed tomographic (CT) scan shows the vertical fracture extending through the vertebral body as well as the neural arch (arrows).

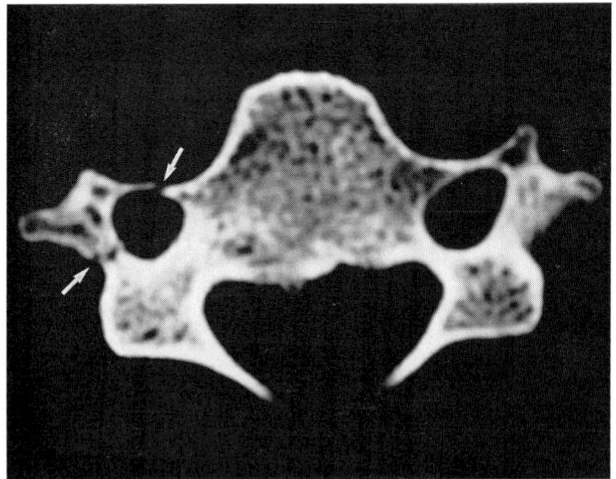

FIGURE 2–58. Isolated transverse process fracture.[67] This 34-year-old man was involved in a side-impact motor vehicle collision. He experienced anterolateral neck pain that failed to respond to conservative care. Routine radiographs (not shown) were normal. Transaxial computed tomographic (CT) image reveals a nondisplaced fracture across the transverse foramen and through both the anterior and posterior tubercles of the right transverse process of C4 (arrows). The patient experienced no signs or symptoms related to vertebral artery injury, and he had an uneventful recovery. *(Courtesy of M.A. Hubka, D.C., San Diego, California.)*

TABLE 2–11. Cervical Spine: Articular Disorders*

Entity	Figure(s) Table(s)	Characteristics	Target Sites of Involvement: Occiput, C1, C2	C2-C7 Disco-vertebral Joints	C2-C7 Apophyseal Joints	C3-C7 Unco-vertebral Joints
Degenerative and related disorders						
Degenerative disc disease[6, 68–70]	2–59, 2–60	*Spondylosis deformans:* Osteophytes and osseous ridging; Subchondral bone sclerosis		+ +		
		Intervertebral osteochondrosis: Disc space narrowing; Intradiscal vacuum phenomenon; Disc calcification (rare); Frequently contributes to foraminal stenosis		+ +		
Osteoarthrosis or arthrosis[71–73]	2–60, 2–61	*Uncovertebral joint arthrosis:* Sclerosis, hypertrophy and joint space narrowing				+ +
	2–62, 2–63	*Apophyseal (facet) joint osteoarthrosis:* Sclerosis, hypertrophy and joint space narrowing; Subluxation, capsular laxity, and synovial cysts may be present	+ +		+ +	
	2–64	*Degenerative spondylolisthesis:* Nonspondylolytic spondylolisthesis complicating degenerative disease; Involves midcervical to lower cervical segments		+	+	
Idiopathic childhood disc calcification[74]	2–65	Cause unknown; Boys = girls; 6 to 10 years of age; Disc calcification may be associated with disc displacement; C4-C7 levels involved most frequently; multiple discs affected in about 33 per cent of cases; Symptoms (including pain, stiffness, limitation of motion, dysphagia, torticollis) present in 75 per cent of affected children and resolve within a few days to weeks; Calcification usually disappears within months; May lead to neurologic findings		+ +		
Diffuse idiopathic skeletal hyperostosis diffuse idiopathic skeletal hyperostosis (DISH)[75]	2–66	Flowing anterior hyperostosis: prominent sheet of ossification on anterior aspect of spine; High rate of occurrence of ossification of the posterior longitudinal ligament		+ +		

Table continued on following page

TABLE 2–11. Cervical Spine: Articular Disorders* *Continued*

Entity	Figure(s) Table(s)	Characteristics	Target Sites of Involvement: *Occiput, C1, C2*	*C2-C7 Disco-vertebral Joints*	*C2-C7 Apophyseal Joints*	*C3-C7 Unco-vertebral Joints*
Degenerative and related disorders *Continued*						
Ossification of the posterior longitudinal ligament (OPLL)[76]	2–67	Occurs with increased frequency in patients with DISH Male:female, 2:1; most common in persons older than 50 years of age *Clinical findings:* May be asymptomatic or may exhibit paresthesias, weakness, incoordination, incontinence, or loss of libido Cord signs (56 per cent of symptomatic patients) Segmental signs (16 per cent of cases) Neck, arm, shoulder pain (28 per cent of cases) Symptoms vary according to thickness of ossification *Radiographic findings:* Segmental or continuous vertical sheet of ossification, as much as 1 to 5 mm thick, extending along the posterior margins of the vertebral bodies and discs within the spinal canal				
Inflammatory disorders						
Rheumatoid arthritis (adult)[78, 79]	2–68	*Upper cervical spine findings:* Atlantoaxial instability and subluxation Odontoid erosion and fracture Apophyseal joint erosion, sclerosis, and fusion	+ + Instability	+ +	+ +	+ +
	2–69	*Lower cervical spine findings:* Subaxial subluxation Apophyseal joint erosion, sclerosis, and fusion Intervertebral disc space narrowing Erosion and sclerosis of vertebral body margins Spinous process erosion Osteoporosis Absence of osteophytes and other osseous outgrowths				
Juvenile chronic arthritis[80, 81]	2–70, 2–71	Widespread discovertebral erosions and disc space narrowing Joint laxity with subluxation Odontoid erosions Diffuse apophyseal joint ankylosis Hypoplastic vertebral bodies at levels of apophyseal joint ankylosis Discs may be hypoplastic and calcified	+ + Instability	+ +	+ +	+ +

TABLE 2–11. Cervical Spine: Articular Disorders* *Continued*

Entity	Figure(s) Table(s)	Characteristics	Target Sites of Involvement: Occiput, C1, C2	C2-C7 Disco-vertebral Joints	C2-C7 Apophyseal Joints	C3-C7 Unco-vertebral Joints
Inflammatory disorders *Continued*						
Ankylosing spondylitis and enteropathic arthropathy[82, 83]	2–72, 2–73	Widespread marginal syndesmophytes, osteitis, disc calcification, osteoporosis, squaring of vertebral bodies, and disc ballooning Discovertebral and apophyseal joint erosion and eventual ankylosis Ossification of ligaments, joint capsules, and outer annular fibers Odontoid erosions and atlantoaxial instability Cervical spine in ankylosing spondylitis is especially susceptible to fractures that may result in neurologic injury and even death; these typically affect the lower cervical spine and occur chiefly as a result of hyperextension injuries Ulcerative colitis and regional ileitis are the most common inflammatory bowel diseases to result in enteropathic arthropathy: identical skeletal findings as those in ankylosing spondylitis	+ + Instability in 1 to 2 per cent of patients	+ +	+ +	+ +
Psoriatic arthropathy and Reiter's syndrome[84, 85]	2–74, 2–75, 2–76	Nonmarginal paravertebral ossification Apophyseal joint narrowing, sclerosis, bony ankylosis, atlantoaxial subluxation Cervical spine changes more common in psoriasis than in Reiter's syndrome	+ + Instability	+ +	+ +	
Crystal deposition disorders						
Calcium pyrophosphate dihydrate crystal deposition disease[86, 87]	2–77	Widespread secondary degenerative disease Disc space narrowing and chondrocalcinosis of the annulus fibrosus, joint capsules, apophyseal joints, and articular cartilage	+ + Instability	+ +	+	
Calcium hydroxyapatite crystal deposition[28]	2–78	Calcific tendinitis: amorphous collection of calcification within the longus coli muscle and tendon seen anterior to the C2 vertebral body May be asymptomatic or result in painful swallowing, fever, occipital pain, and neck rigidity Symptoms are self-limited, usually resolving within 2 weeks Infrequently, such crystals are deposited in ligamentum flavum in older patients				

Table continued on following page

TABLE 2–11. Cervical Spine: Articular Disorders* *Continued*

Entity	Figure(s) Table(s)	Characteristics	Target Sites of Involvement: *Occiput, C1, C2*	*C2-C7 Disco-vertebral Joints*	*C2-C7 Apophyseal Joints*	*C3-C7 Unco-vertebral Joints*
Crystal deposition disorders *Continued*						
Gout[89]		Rare involvement of spine Prominent disc space narrowing and erosion of subchondral end plate	+	+		
Alkaptonuria[90]	2–79	Widespread and severe disc space narrowing and diffuse annulus fibrosus calcification Intradiscal vacuum phenomenon Osseous bridging may resemble marginal syndesmophytes Eventual progression to bamboo spine	+ +			
Miscellaneous disorders						
Neuropathic osteoarthropathy[77]		Widespread discovertebral and zygapophyseal joint destruction May resemble infectious spondylodiscitis Joint collapse, bone fragmentation, and kyphosis Syringomyelia, diabetes mellitus, and tabes dorsalis often affect the spine; most frequently affects the thoracolumbar region		+ +	+	
Pyogenic spondylodiscitis[91–93]	2–80, 2–81 Table 2–12	Up to 21-day latent period before radiographic changes appear Initially involves disc and adjacent vertebral body Severe monoarticular disc space narrowing that eventually may spread to adjacent levels Obliteration of vertebral end plate and vertebral collapse in late stages Paravertebral soft tissue mass or abscess	+ Instability	+ +	+ (late)	+
Tuberculous spondylodiscitis[94]	2–82	Usually involves thoracolumbar region Typically begins in the anterior vertebral body and spreads to the disc Rare involvement of neural arch Slower process than pyogenic infection	+ + Instability	+ +	+	+
Dialysis spondyloarthropathy[95]	2–83	Seen in patients on long-standing hemodialysis May be related to amyloid deposition or, less commonly, calcium hydroxyapatite or calcium oxalate crystal deposition in disc Discovertebral joint erosions resembling those of infectious spondylodiscitis, neuropathic osteoarthropathy, and calcium pyrophosphate dihydrate crystal deposition disease Disc space narrowing, erosion, and sclerosis of vertebral end plates		+ +		

*See also Tables 1–6 to 1–9 and Table 1–17.

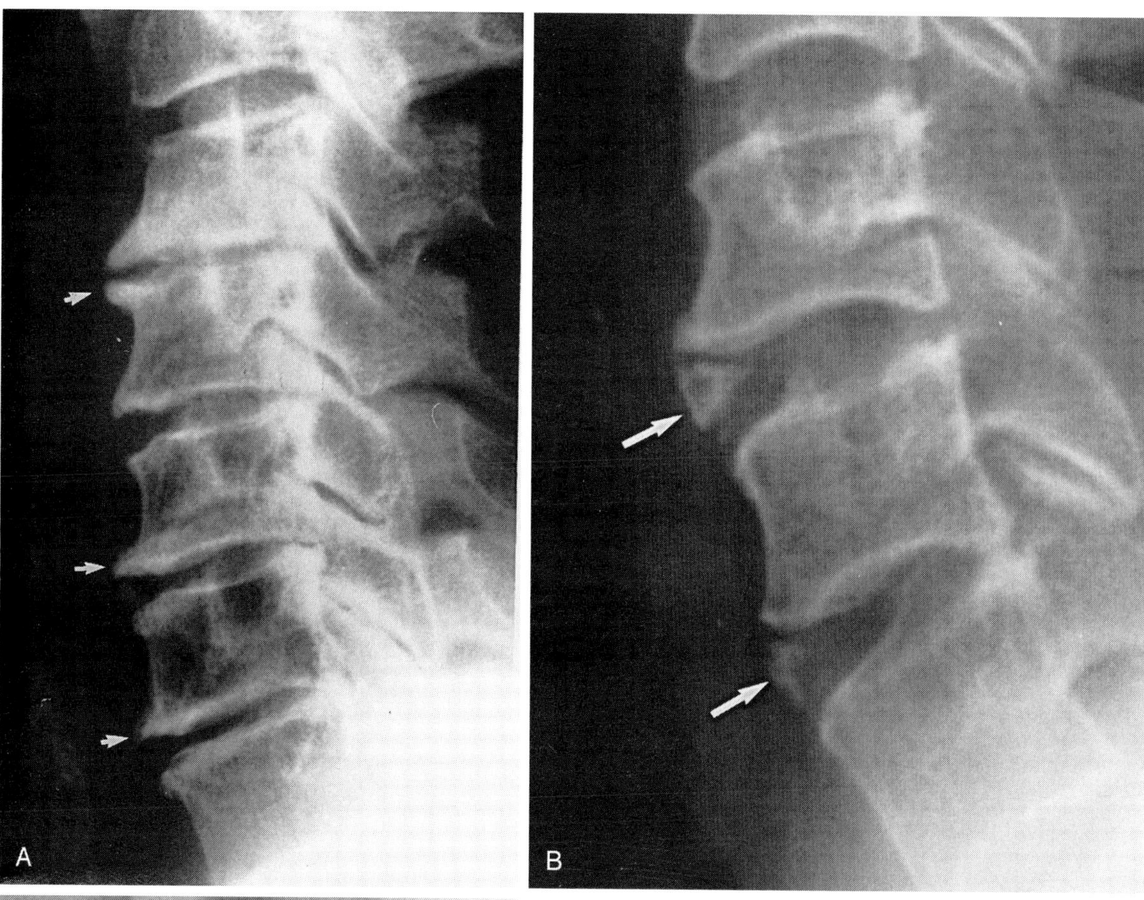

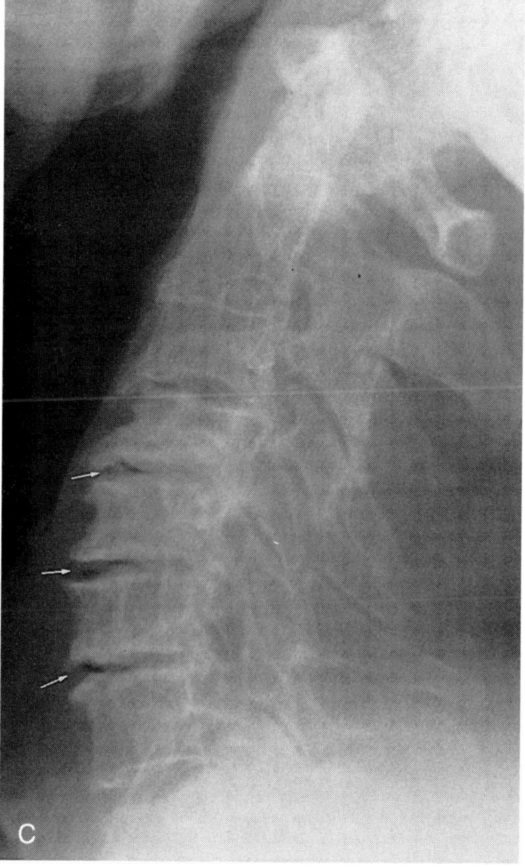

FIGURE 2–59. Degenerative spine disease.[6, 68–70] A Widespread disc space narrowing is associated with prominent osteophytes (arrows) and vertebral end-plate sclerosis. Observe also the narrowing of the apophyseal joints and sclerosis of the articular facet surfaces. B In another patient, small, triangular, well-corticated osseous densities are present within the anterior annular fibers (arrows). These ossicles have been termed intercalary bones and are a manifestation of degenerative disc disease. Intercalary bones differ from unossified secondary growth centers (limbus vertebrae) in that there is no corresponding wedge-shaped defect of the adjacent vertebral body corner. C Advanced changes. Diffuse disc space narrowing, vacuum phenomena (arrows), well-defined sclerotic vertebral margins, osteophyte formation, facet joint arthrosis, and uncovertebral arthrosis are all present in this 75-year-old man. Congenital synostosis of C2-C3 with facet joint ankylosis and a rudimentary disc space also is evident.

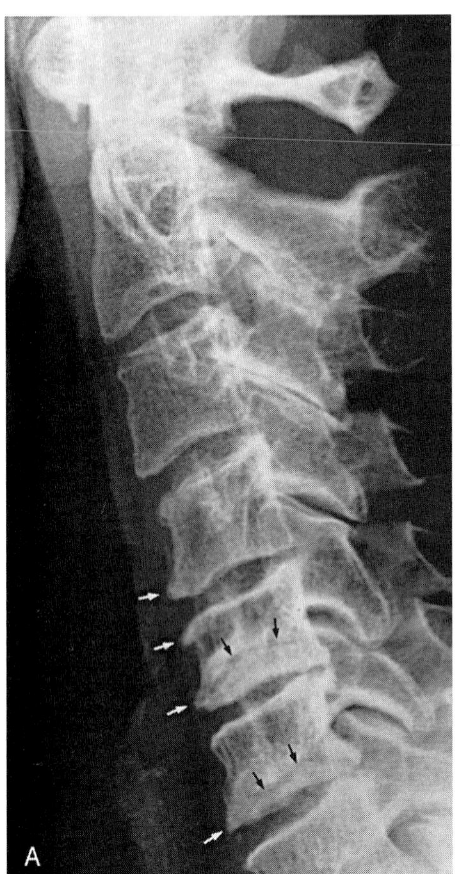

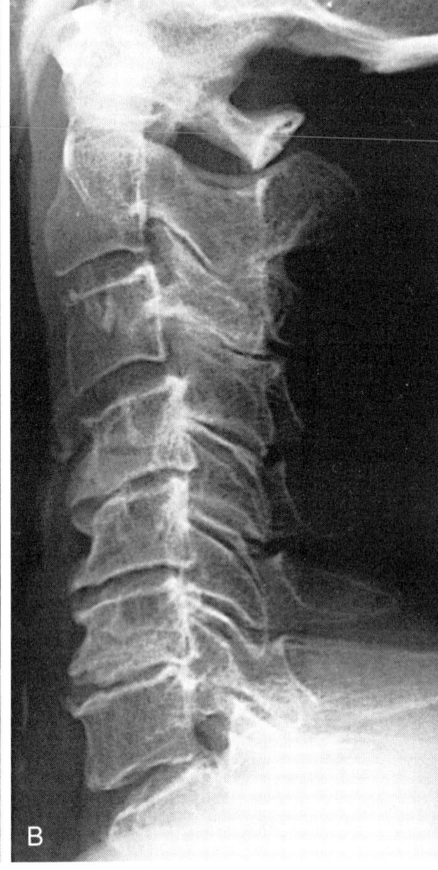

FIGURE 2–60. Degenerative spine disease.[71–73] A Lateral cervical radiograph of a 71-year-old man shows extensive osteoarthrosis of the apophyseal joints characterized by joint space narrowing and subchondral sclerosis. Narrowing of the C5-C6 and C6-C7 intervertebral disc spaces and osteophytes (white arrows) arising from the vertebral body margins are evidence of degeneration. Uncovertebral joint arthrosis appears as hypertrophy of the uncinate processes with horizontal clefts across the C5 and C6 vertebral bodies (black arrows), a phenomenon termed pseudofracture. B In another patient, similar findings are seen. The lordosis is reversed, and alignment abnormalities are seen involving C3 (anterolisthesis) and C4 (retrolisthesis). *(Courtesy of F.G. Bauer, D.C., Sydney, Australia.)*

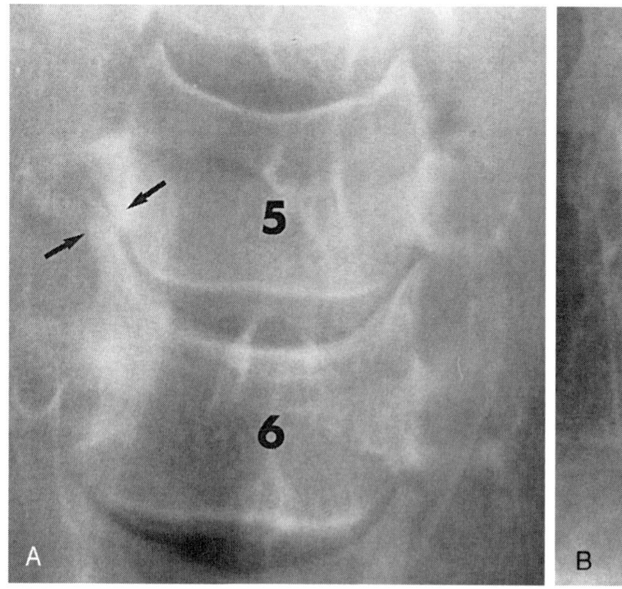

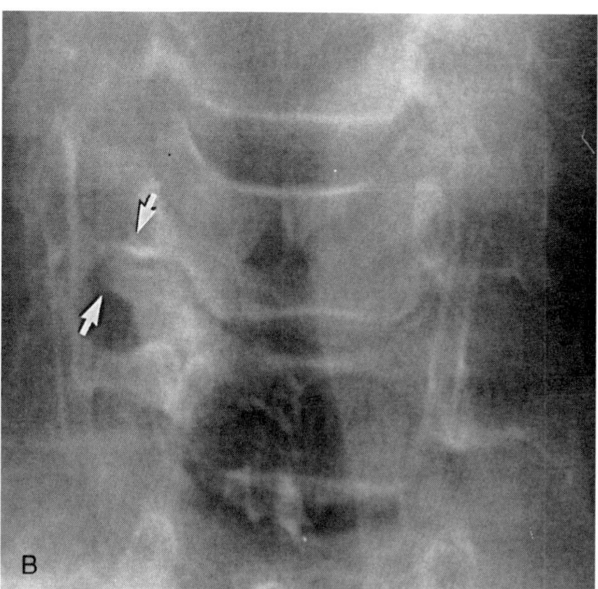

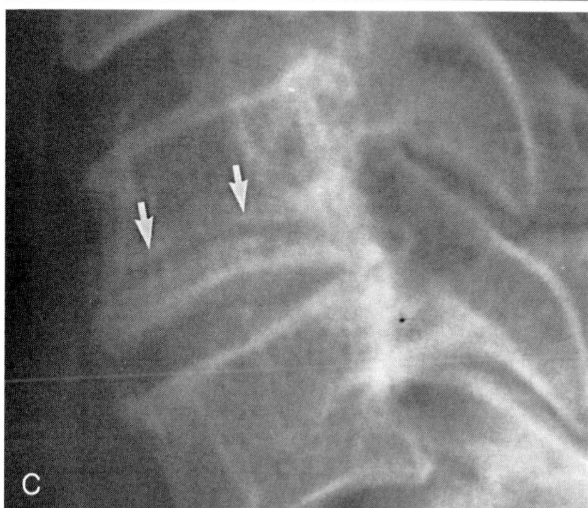

FIGURE 2–61. Uncovertebral joint arthrosis.[71–73] **A** Frontal radiograph of the cervical spine reveals the presence of hypertrophy and sclerosis of the C6 uncinate processes and corresponding narrowing of the uncovertebral articulation (arrows). **B, C** In another patient a frontal radiograph (**B**) shows prominent hypertrophy and osteophyte formation of the C6 uncinate processes and narrowing of the C5-C6 uncovertebral joint (arrows). Lateral radiograph (**C**) shows a horizontal radiolucent region (arrows) through the inferior aspect of the C5 vertebral body, which represents the joint line of the degenerated uncovertebral joint (pseudofracture effect).

Illustration continued on following page

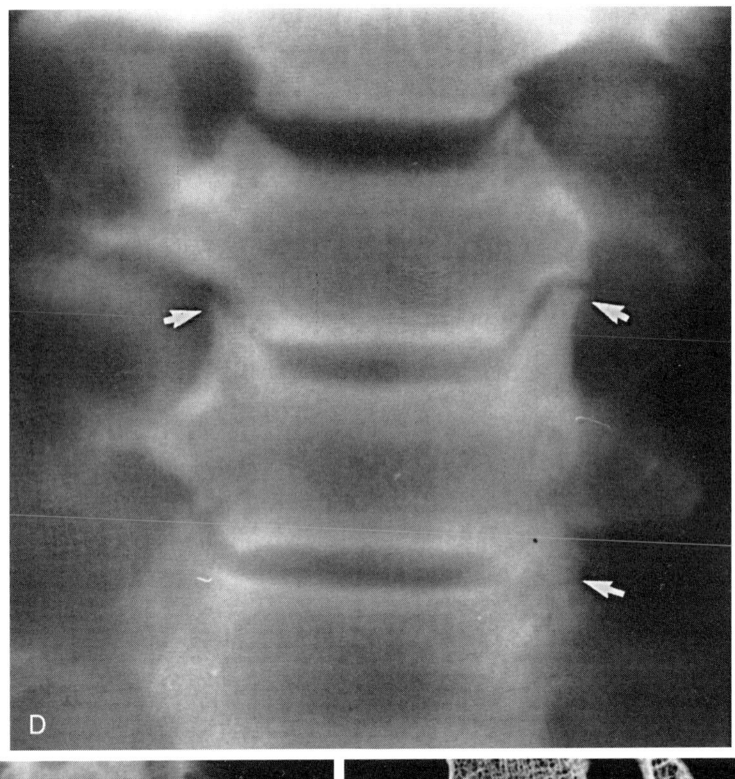

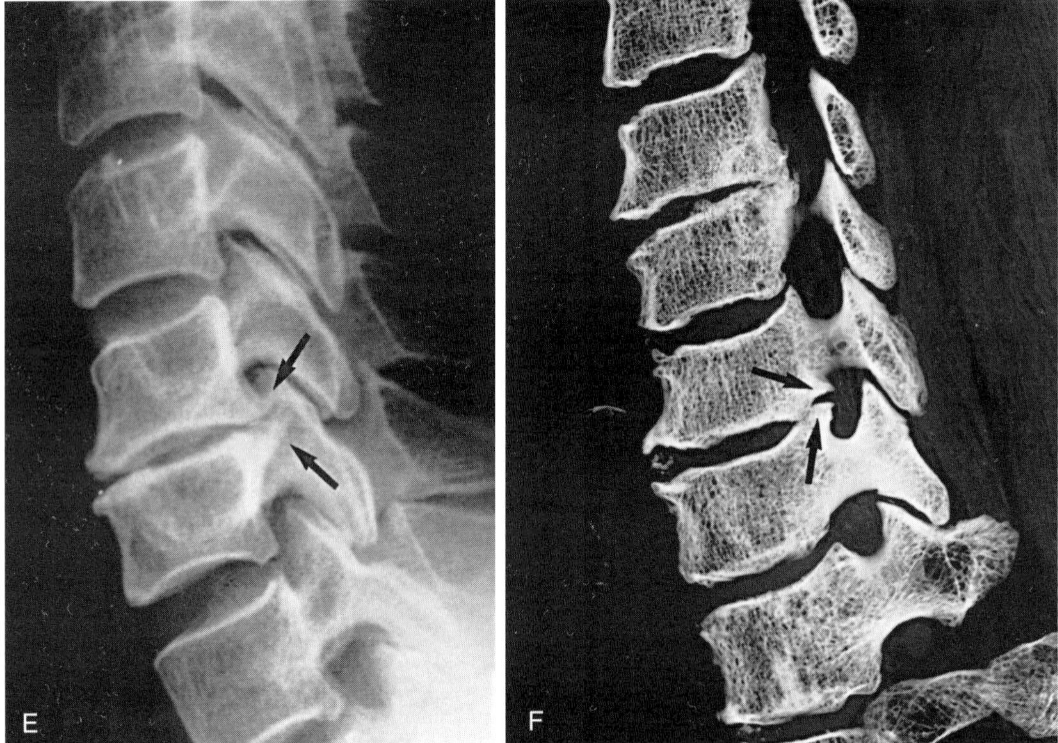

FIGURE 2–61 *Continued.* **D** Frontal conventional tomogram clearly illustrates the sclerosis, hypertrophy, and osteophytes arising from the uncinate processes (arrows), and the associated narrowing of the uncovertebral articulations. **E** Lateral cervical radiograph reveals disc space narrowing and marginal osteophytes arising from the discovertebral and uncovertebral margins. Large posterior osteophytes are evident (arrows). **F** Oblique radiograph of a cadaveric specimen demonstrates the stenotic effect of posterolateral uncovertebral osteophytes (arrows) on the neural foramen. Such osteophytes represent a significant factor in foraminal stenosis and may be a source of nerve root compression and radiculopathy.

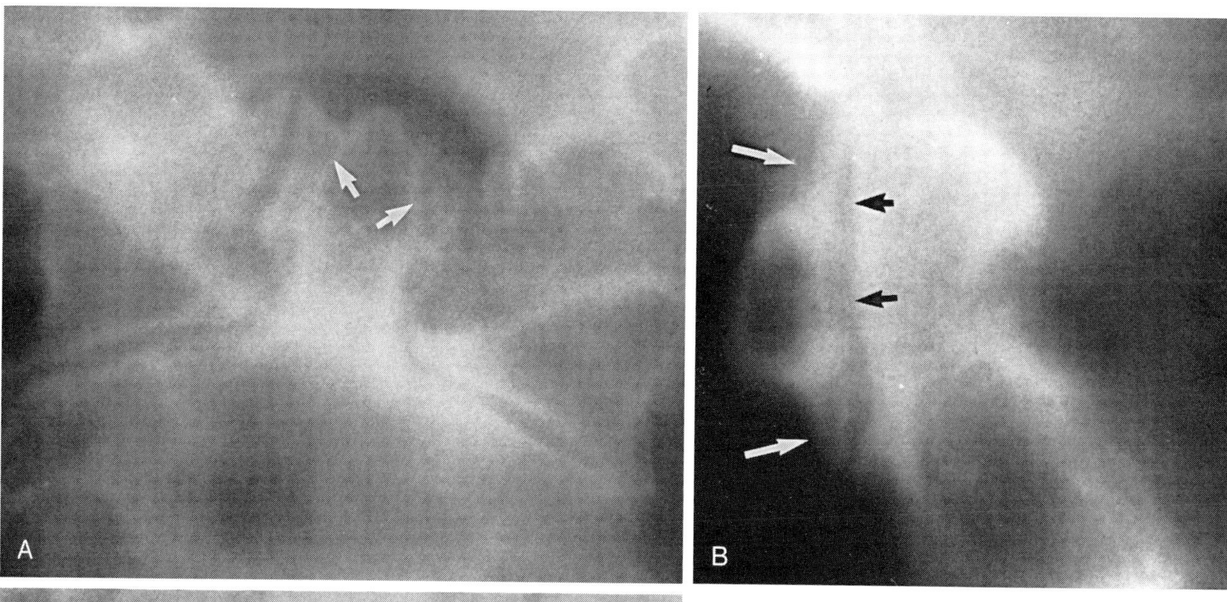

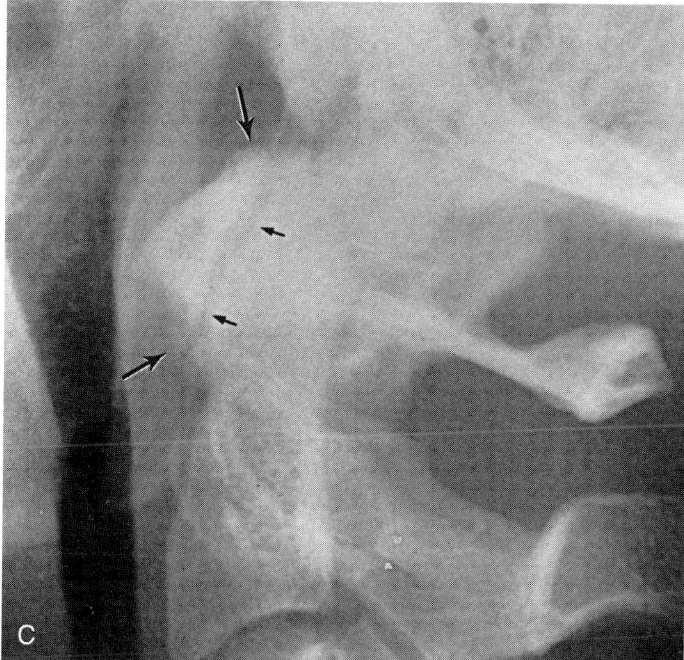

FIGURE 2–62. Osteoarthrosis: C1-C2 articulations.[71–73] A, B Conventional tomogram in the frontal plane (A) shows narrowing of the lateral atlantoaxial synovial articulations as well as considerable bone proliferation about the odontoid process (arrows). Lateral conventional tomogram (B) demonstrates marked narrowing of the anterior median atlantoaxial articulation (black arrows). Prominent osteophytes also are seen arising from the inferior and superior margins of the anterior arch of the atlas (white arrows). C Another case reveals narrowing of the atlantodental interspace (small arrows), sclerosis, and osteophytes (large arrows).

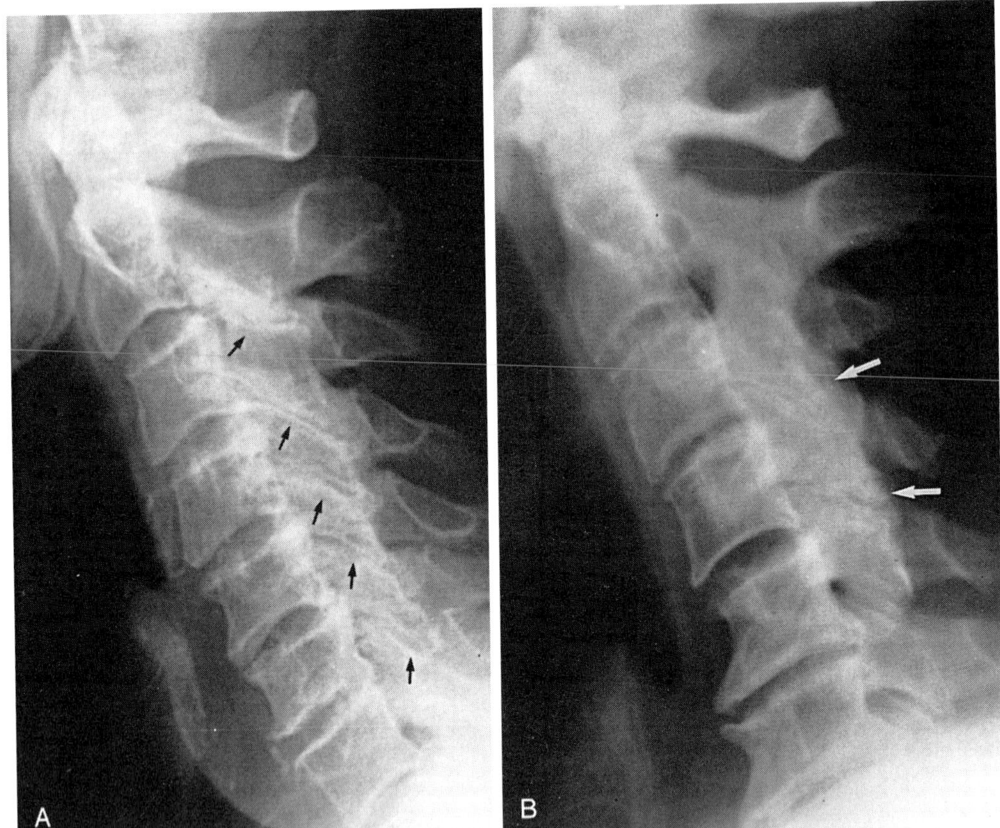

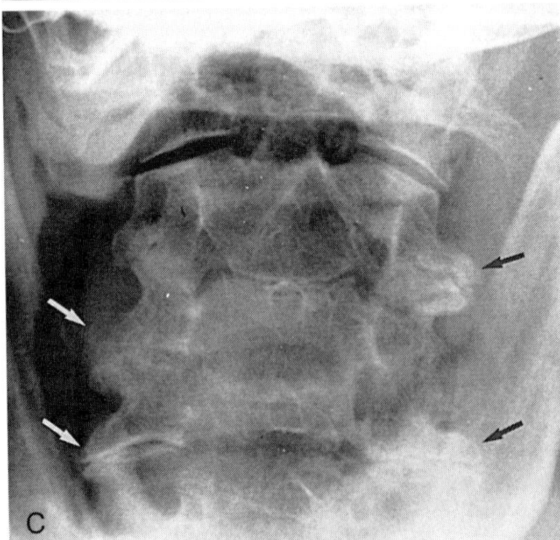

FIGURE 2–63. Osteoarthrosis (degenerative joint disease): Apophyseal joints.[71–73] A In this 77-year-old man, apophyseal joint space narrowing, osteophyte formation, and sclerosis are noted throughout the cervical spine (arrows). B This 79-year-old man complained of progressive cervical spine stiffness and pain. Lateral radiograph reveals extensive sclerosis of the articular processes of C2 to C5 combined with dramatic joint space narrowing of the apophyseal joints (arrows). Marked degenerative disc disease also is present at the C5-C6 and C6-C7 levels. C Frontal open mouth radiograph from this elderly patient reveals dramatic osteophyte formation arising from the facet articulations throughout the cervical spine (arrows). (C, *Courtesy of L. Hoffman, D.C., Portland, Oregon.*)

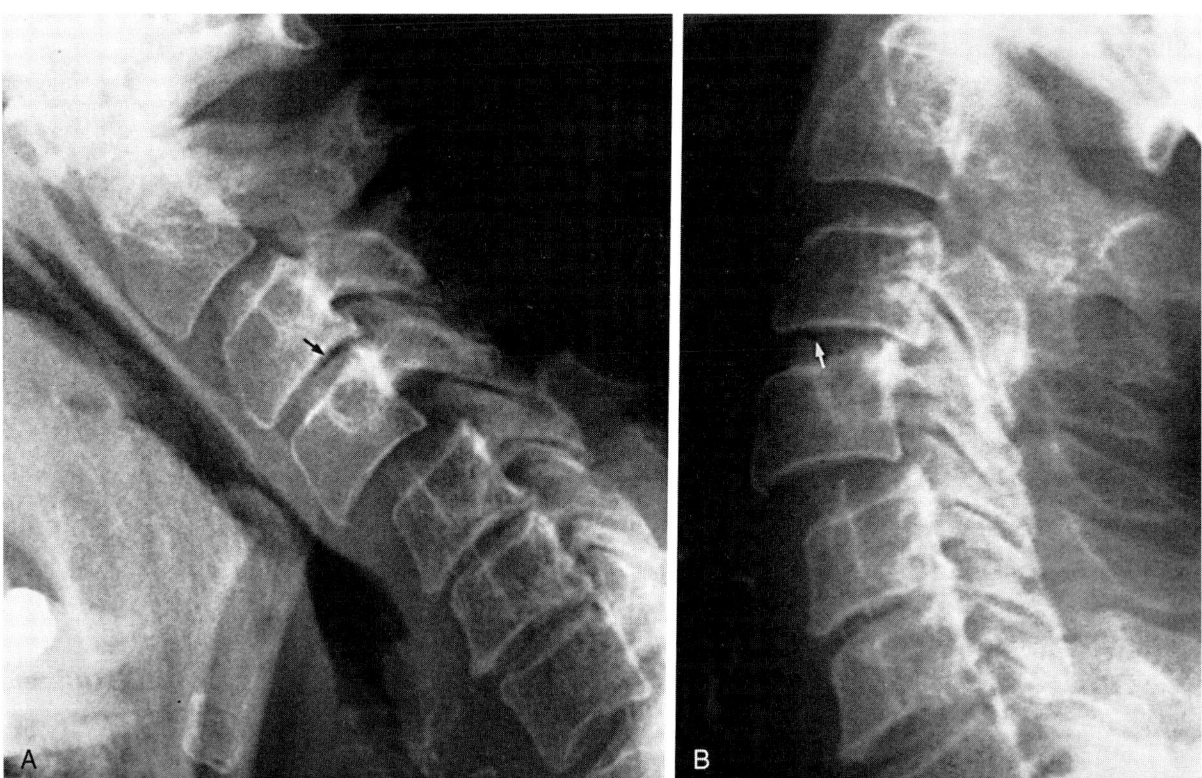

FIGURE 2–64. Degenerative spondylolisthesis.[71–73] This 73-year-old woman had neck pain and stiffness. Lateral radiographs taken in flexion (A) and extension (B) reveal extensive apophyseal joint space narrowing and sclerosis with anterolisthesis of C4 on C5. Minimal translation is present at C4-C5 between flexion and extension. At the C3-C4 level, however, disc space narrowing and a vacuum phenomenon (arrows) are present, and approximately 4 mm of translation is evident, suggesting instability. *(Courtesy of W. Longstaffe, D.C., Vancouver, British Columbia, Canada.)*

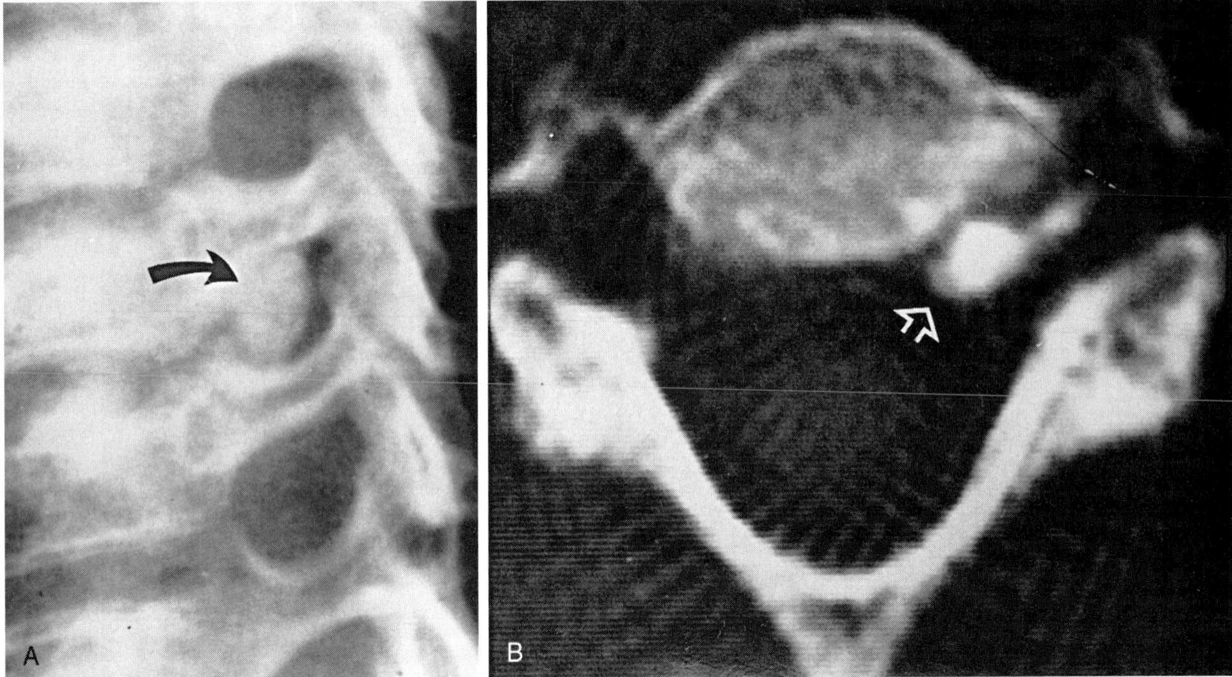

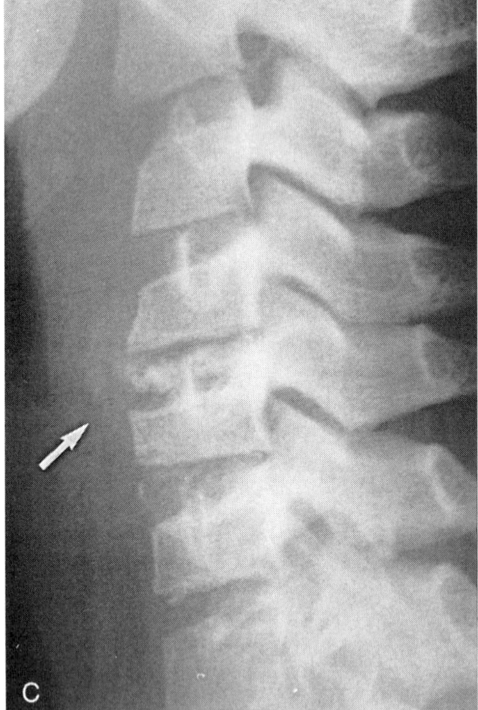

FIGURE 2–65. Idiopathic intervertebral disc calcification.[74] A In this child, a calcified mass is seen in the neural foramen on the oblique radiograph (curved arrow). B Transaxial computed tomography (CT) scan reveals a calcified extruded intervertebral disc extending into the neural foramen (open arrow). *(A, B, Courtesy of M. Alcaraz, M.D., Madrid, Spain.)* C In another child, anterior extrusion and extensive calcification of the C4-C5 intervertebral disc are seen (arrow). *(C, Courtesy of P. Wilson, M.D., Eugene, Oregon.)*

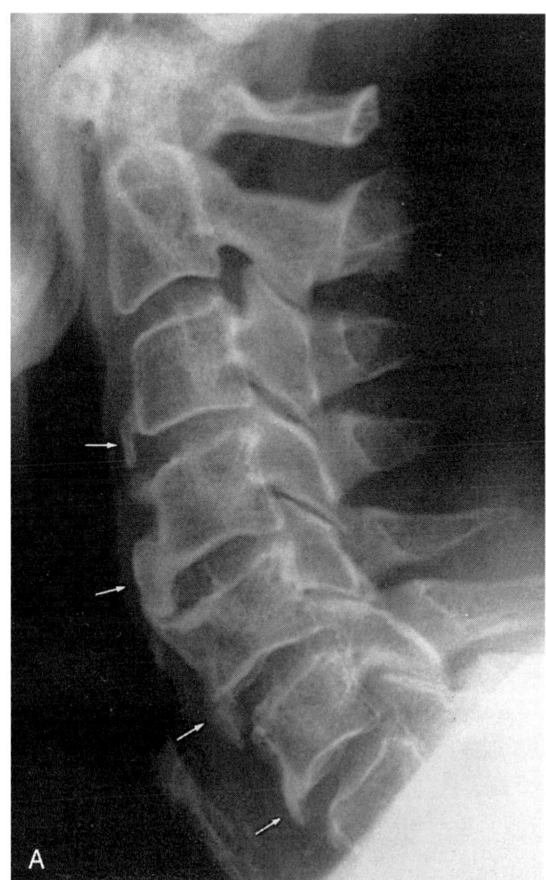

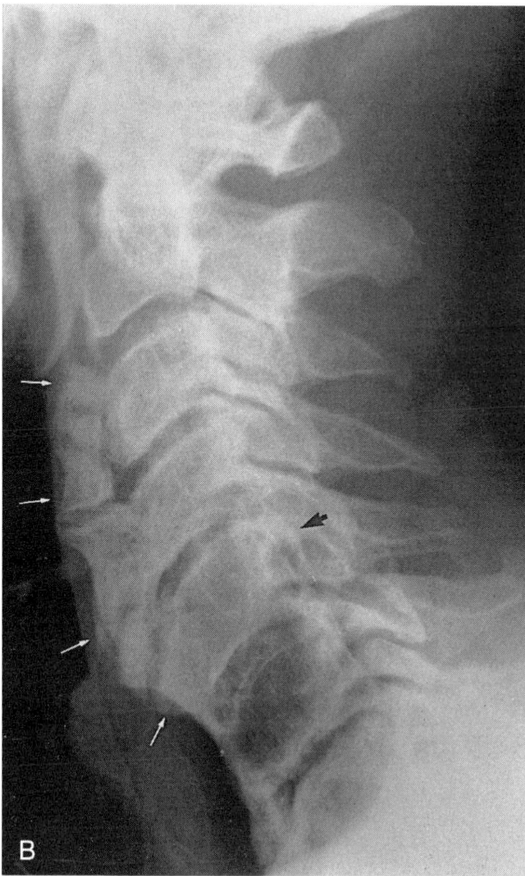

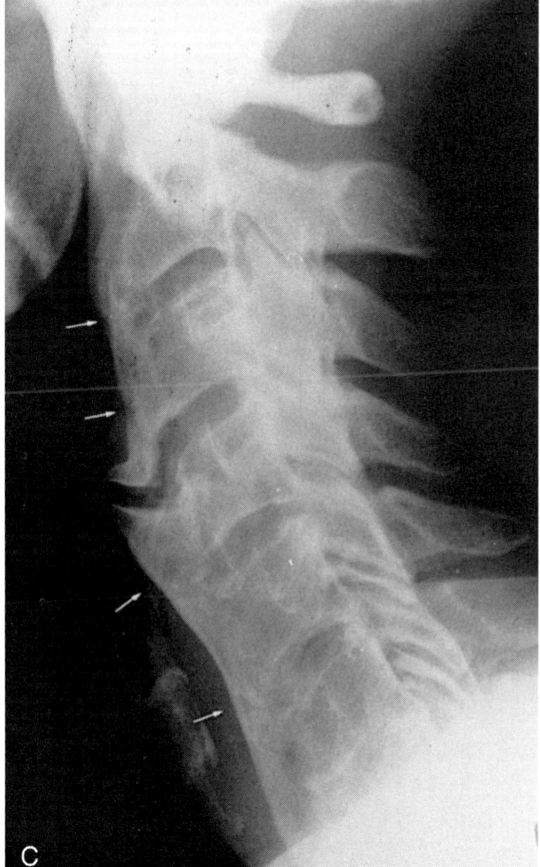

FIGURE 2–66. Diffuse idiopathic skeletal hyperostosis (DISH): Spectrum of abnormalities.[75] **A** Early changes. Intermittent segments of ossification (arrows) are seen along the anterior aspect of several vertebral bodies. The disc spaces are well preserved. **B** Advanced changes. A thick layer of ossified bone is present along the anterior aspect of the cervical spine (white arrows). The ossification is not continuous at all levels, but is more continuous than in **A.** This patient also has ossification of the posterior longitudinal ligament (black arrow), resulting in spinal stenosis. **C** Severe changes. In a third patient, continuous thick ossification bridges the anterior aspects of several lower cervical vertebrae (arrows). Interruption of the osseous segment is seen at the C3-C4 disc level. The disc spaces are preserved. (**C,** *Cour[illegible]of L. Bogle, M.D., San Diego, California.*)

Illustration continued on following page

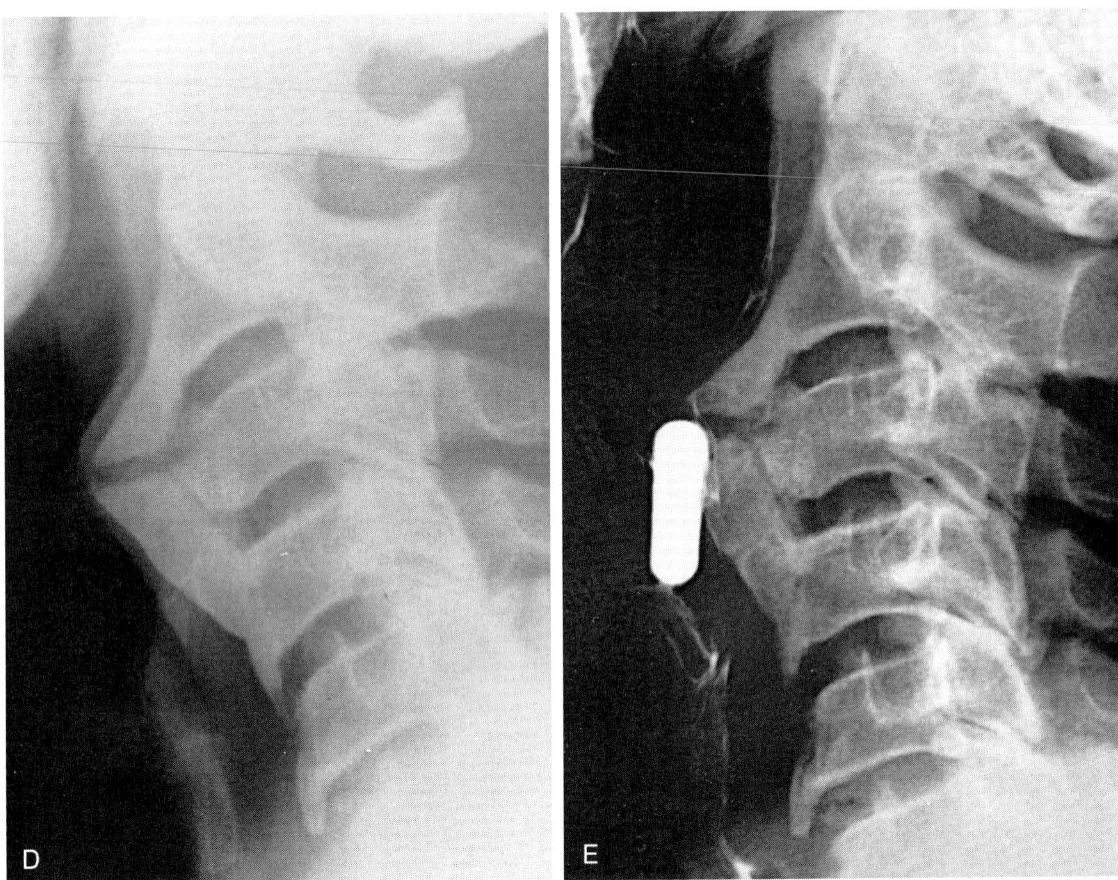

FIGURE 2–66 *Continued.* **D, E** Severe changes. This patient had dysphagia. Routine radiograph (**D**) shows dramatic protuberant ossification. Radiograph obtained while the patient was swallowing a barium contrast tablet (**E**) documents esophageal obstruction at the site of osseous protrusion. *(**D, E,** Courtesy of C. Cortes, M.D., Santiago, Chile.)*

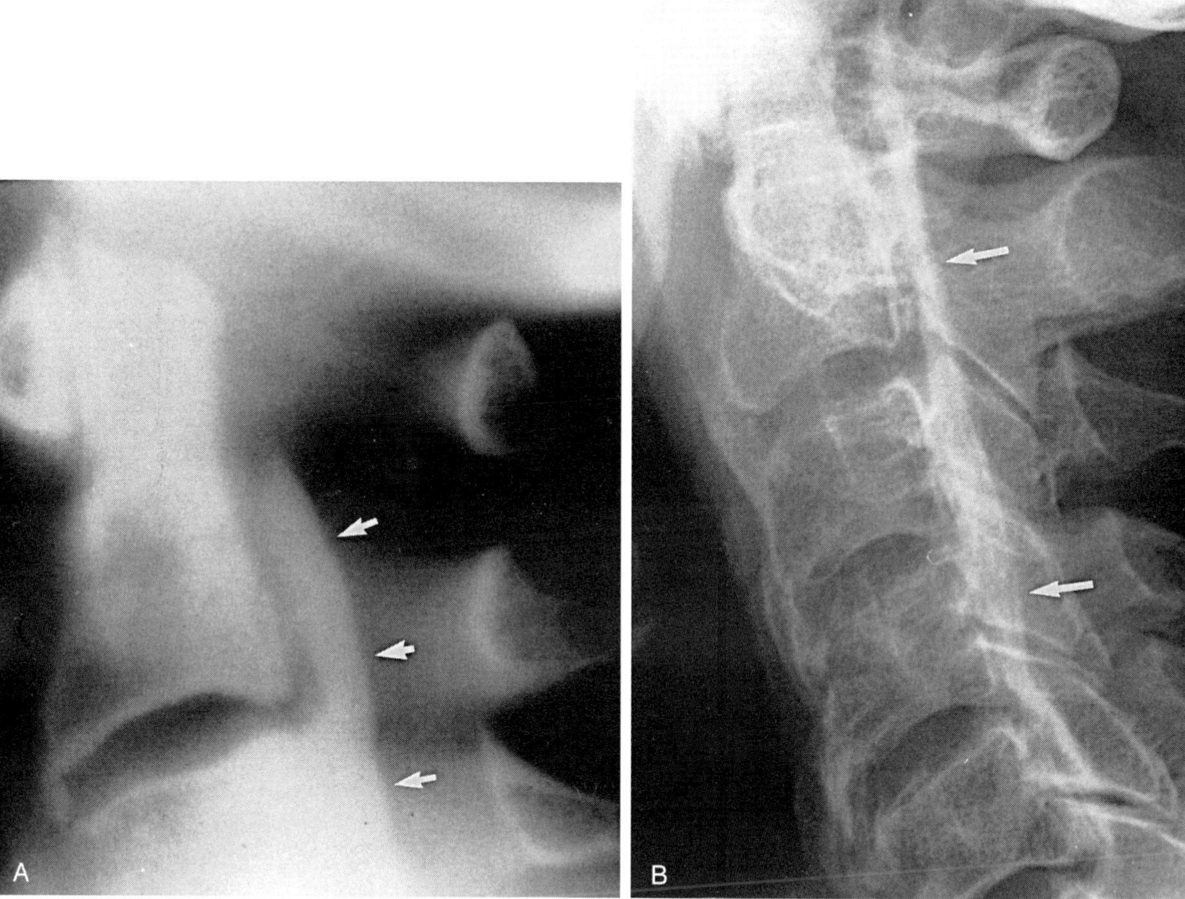

FIGURE 2–67. Ossification of the posterior longitudinal ligament in diffuse idiopathic skeletal hyperostosis (DISH).[76] **A** A thick, vertical, linear band of ossification (arrows) is seen in the spinal canal of the upper cervical spine in this conventional tomogram of a patient with DISH. *(A, Courtesy of J. Mink, M.D., Los Angeles, California.)* **B, C** A 57-year-old man with neck pain. In **B,** a linear sheet of ossification within the spinal canal extending from C1 to C5 (arrows) is evident in this patient with DISH.

Illustration continued on following page

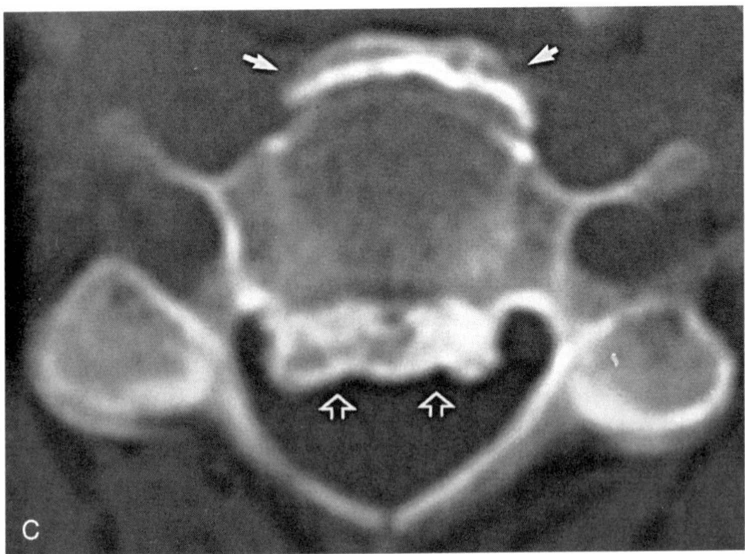

FIGURE 2–67 *Continued.* In C, a transaxial CT scan at the C3 level reveals a thick layer of ossification (open arrows) occupying approximately 30 per cent of the sagittal canal diameter. Observe also the ossification anterior to the vertebral bodies (arrows). *(B, C, Courtesy of E. Bosch, M.D., Santiago, Chile.)*

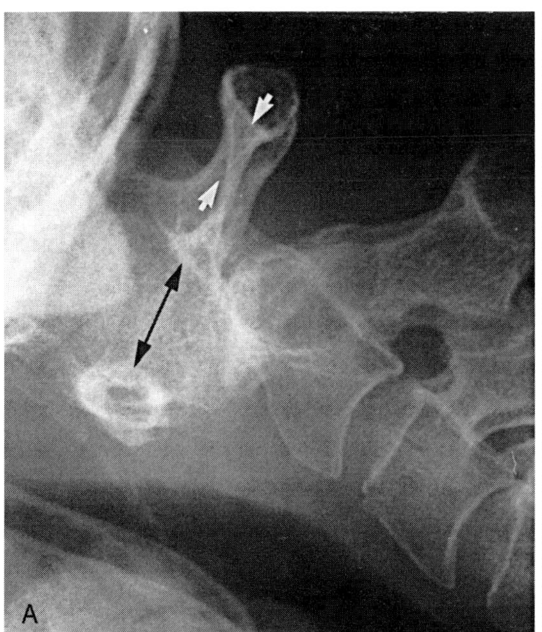

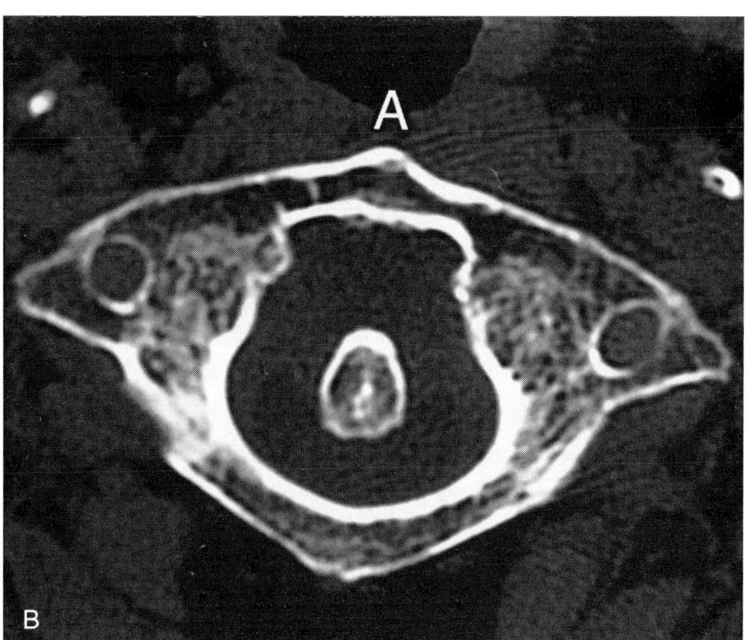

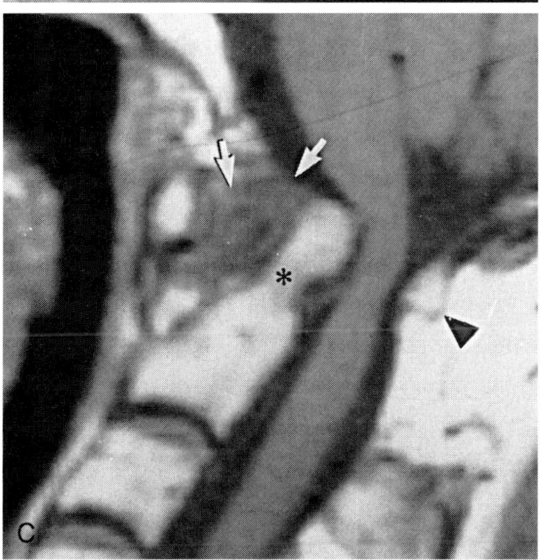

FIGURE 2–68. Rheumatoid arthritis: Atlantoaxial abnormalities.[78, 79] **A–C** Atlantoaxial instability in a 55-year-old woman with no neurologic deficit. In **A**, a lateral radiograph obtained in flexion shows dramatic anterior displacement of the atlas in relation to the axis. The atlantodental interspace (predens space) measures 15 mm (black double-headed arrow). The sagittal canal diameter, measured between the posterior aspect of the odontoid and the spinolaminar junction line (white arrows), measures only 8 mm. In **B**, a transaxial computed tomography (CT) scan confirms the atlantoaxial instability revealing that the odontoid process is situated posterior to the midline of the spinal canal rather than anteriorly adjacent to the anterior arch. The spinal cord is being compressed between the odontoid and the posterior arch. (A = anterior.) In **C**, compression of the spinomedullary junction by the odontoid process anteriorly and the posterior arch of the atlas posteriorly (arrowhead) is clearly evident on this sagittal T1-weighted (TR/TE, 600/12) spin echo magnetic resonance (MR) image. The atlantodental interspace is widened and contains low-signal intensity pannus (arrows). It is the inflammatory synovial pannus that results in disruption of the transverse ligament and consequent erosion of the base of the odontoid (*). *(***A–C***, Courtesy of M.N. Pathria, M.D., San Diego, California.)*

Illustration continued on following page

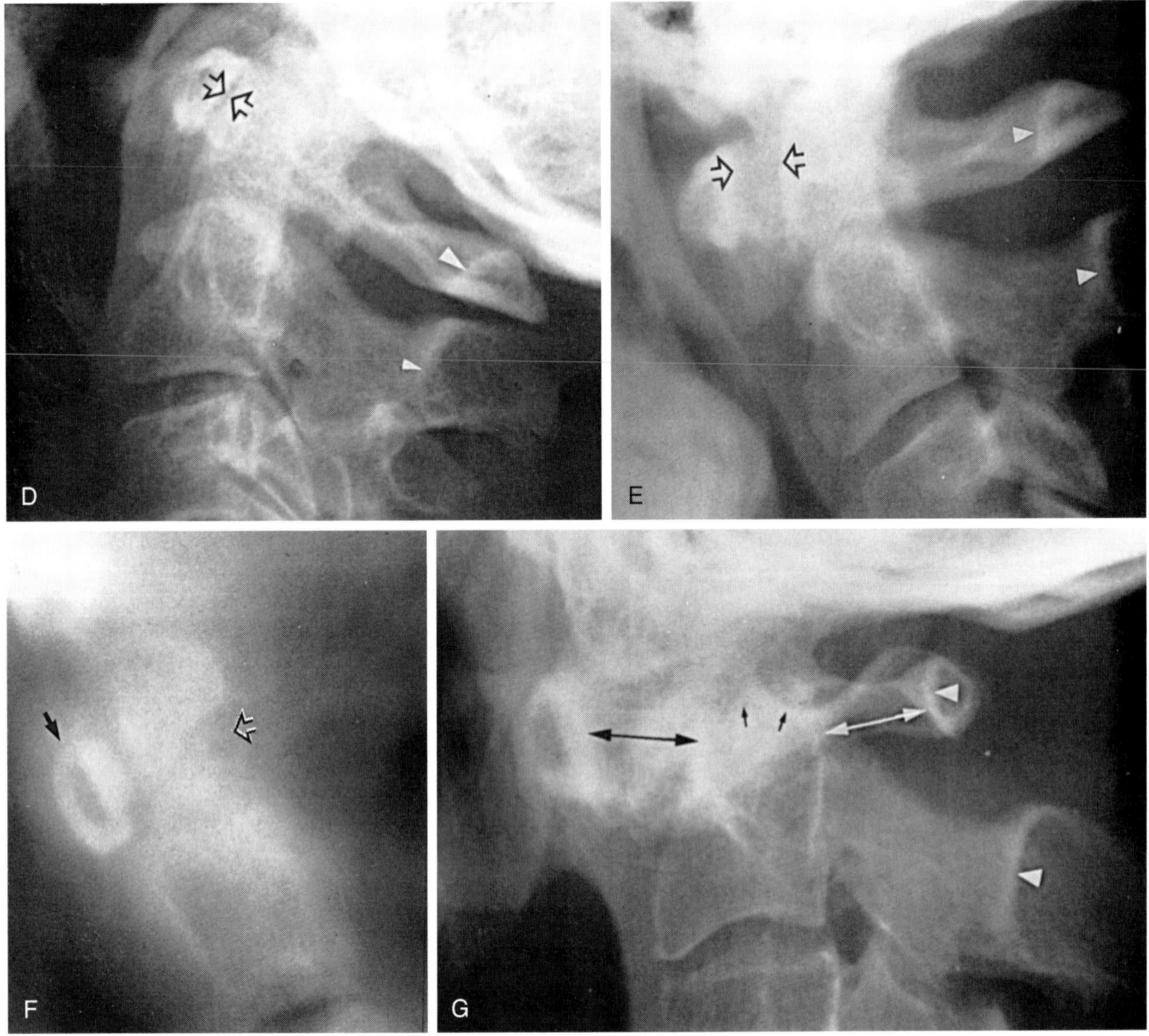

FIGURE 2–68 *Continued.* D, E Atlantoaxial instability: Value of functional radiographs. In D, a lateral radiograph obtained in extension shows a normal atlantodental interspace (open arrows) and normal alignment of the C1 and C2 spinolaminar junctions (arrowheads). In E, a lateral radiograph obtained in flexion reveals widening of the atlantodental interspace (open arrows) and anterior displacement of the C1 spinolaminar junction line in relation to that of C2 (arrowheads), documenting atlantoaxial instability. Atlantoaxial instability exists when the atlantodental interspace exceeds 3 mm in adults and 5 mm in children. F In another patient, a lateral conventional tomogram shows erosion of the posterior aspect of the odontoid at the point of contact with the synovial compartment of the transverse ligament (open arrow). Also evident is inferior subluxation of the atlas relative to the odontoid (arrow), a condition termed cranial settling. G Cranial settling, anterior subluxation, and extensive odontoid erosions resulting in an amputated appearance (arrows) are observed in a male patient with chronic rheumatoid arthritis. Observe the displacement of the spinolaminar junction line between C1 and C2 (arrowheads), widening of the atlantodental interspace (double-headed black arrow), and the severely compromised sagittal canal diameter and space available for the cord (double-headed white arrow).

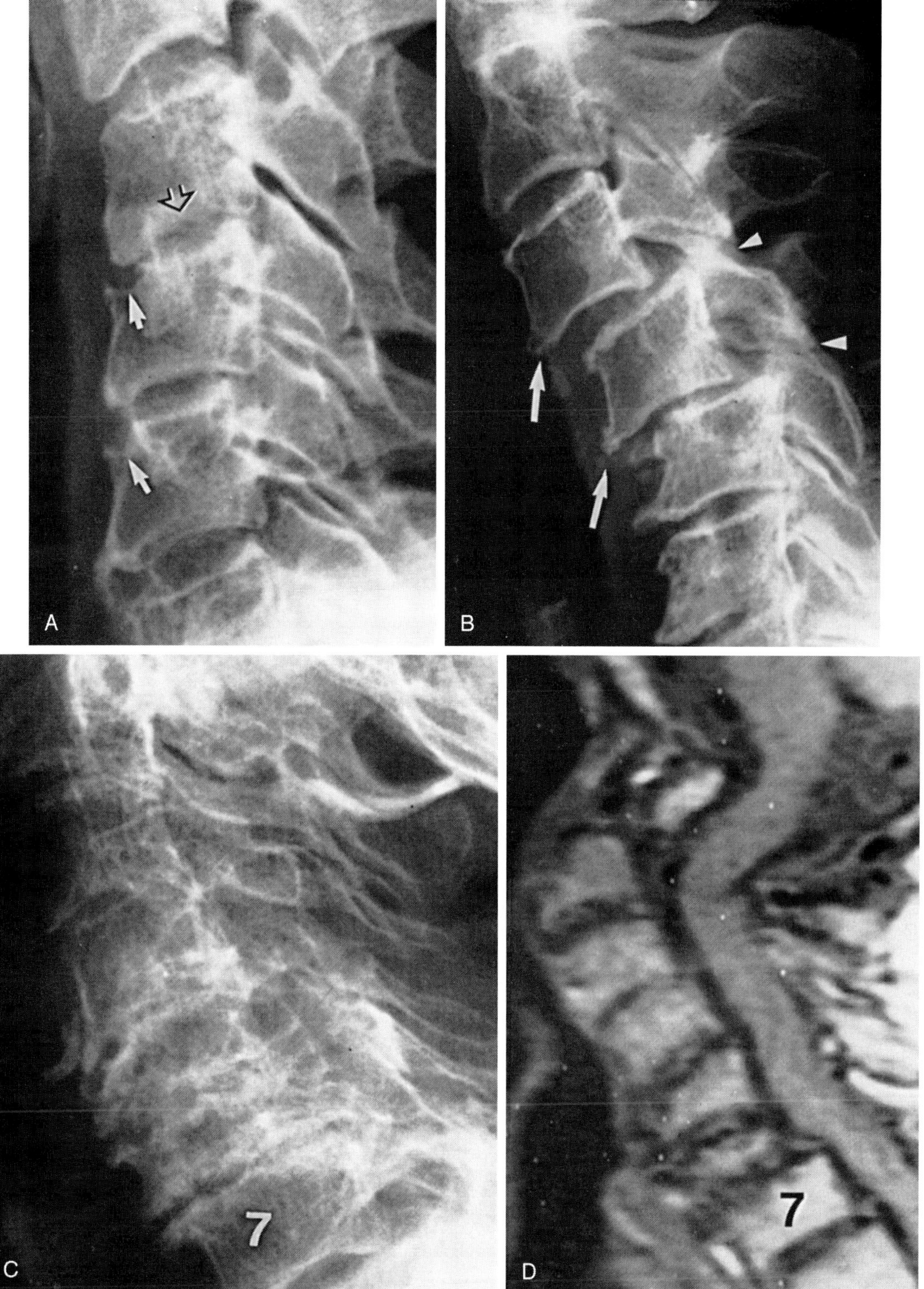

FIGURE 2–69. Rheumatoid arthritis: Midcervical and lower cervical spine abnormalities.[78, 79] **A** Discovertebral joint changes. In this patient with early erosive changes, multiple intervertebral discs are narrowed and the vertebral end plates at C3-C4 are indistinct (open arrow). Discovertebral erosions are evident at the anterosuperior vertebral body margins (arrows). In the absence of osteophytes and subchondral sclerosis, such findings are highly suggestive of an inflammatory arthropathy. **B** Subaxial joint subluxation: Advanced changes. In this patient with advanced rheumatoid arthritis, dramatic anterior subluxation of C3 on C4 and C4 on C5 is seen (arrow). Several disc spaces are narrowed, and osteophytes are small and poorly developed. Apophyseal joint narrowing, sclerosis, and subluxation also are present (arrowheads). **C, D** Advanced changes in a 66-year-old man. In **C,** severe disc space narrowing, indistinct and irregular end plates and apophyseal joint erosion, narrowing, and subluxation are evident. Atlantoaxial instability with posterior dislocation of the atlas is also present. In **D,** a sagittal proton density–weighted (TR/TE, 1200/20) spin echo magnetic resonance (MR) image reveals dramatic subluxation at C1-C2 and at C6-C7. Discovertebral junction erosions are prominent. The odontoid process appears to be eroded or fractured, and the spinal cord at C2-C3 appears kinked.

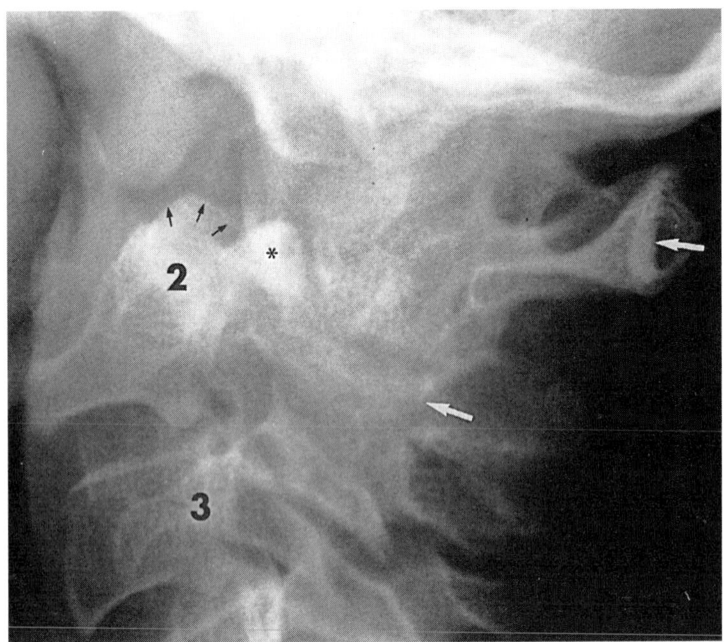

FIGURE 2–70. Juvenile chronic arthritis: Upper cervical spine.[80, 81] Severe atlantoaxial instability with posterior dislocation of the atlas is seen in this 27-year-old woman with long-standing juvenile rheumatoid arthritis. The anterior arch of the atlas (*) is dislocated in a posterior position with respect to the eroded odontoid process (black arrows) of C2 (2). Posterior dislocation of the atlas also is indicated by the malalignment of the spinolaminar junction lines of C1 and C2 (white arrows). The vertebral bodies of C2 (2) and C3 (3) reveal abnormal translation. *(Courtesy of J. Bramble, M.D., Kansas City, Missouri, and M. Murphy, M.D., Washington, D.C.)*

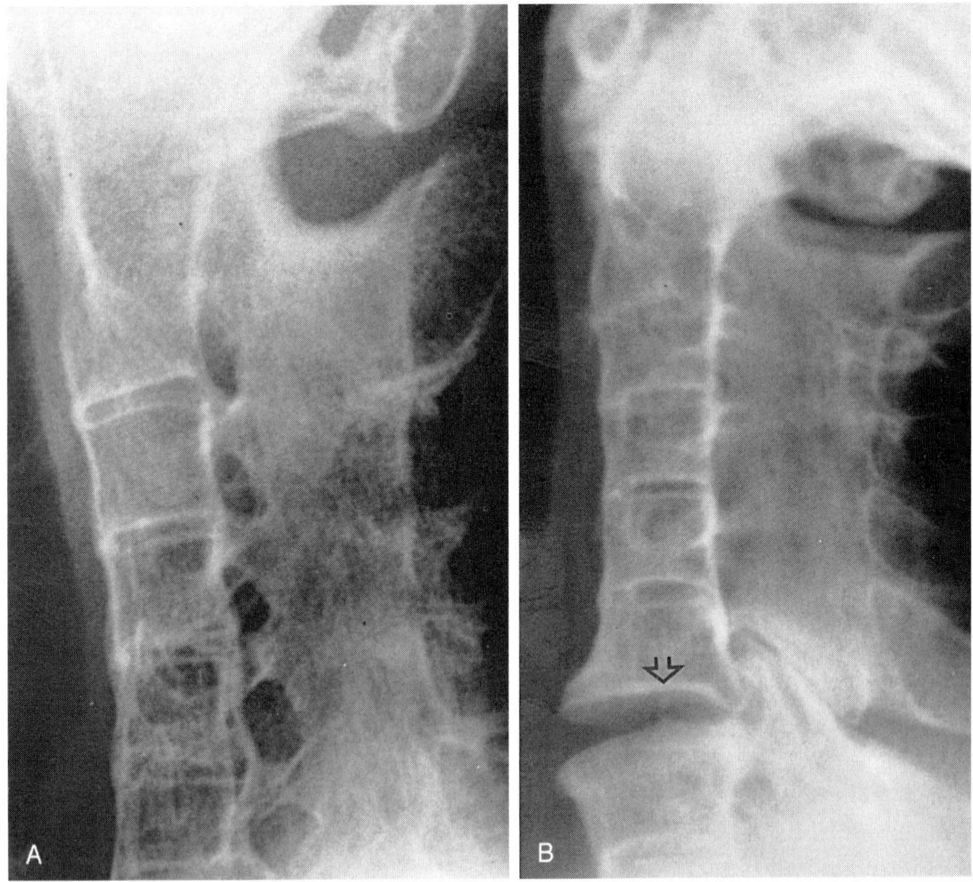

FIGURE 2–71. Juvenile chronic arthritis: Cervical spine.[80, 81] A Observe the widespread apophyseal joint ankylosis, disc space narrowing, and hypoplasia of the vertebral bodies in this 6-year-old girl with severe juvenile rheumatoid arthritis. *(A, Courtesy of V. Vint, M.D., San Diego, California.)* B Widespread ankylosis, disc space narrowing, and hypoplasia of the vertebral bodies are seen in a 25-year-old woman. Atlantoaxial instability also is present. The C6-C7 interspace is not ankylosed (open arrow), and in the presence of such widespread ankylosis of the adjacent segments, it may be a source of excessive motion and potential instability.

The differential diagnosis in such cases includes juvenile-onset ankylosing spondylitis and Klippel-Feil syndrome. *(***B***, Courtesy of C. Pineda, M.D., Mexico City, Mexico.)*

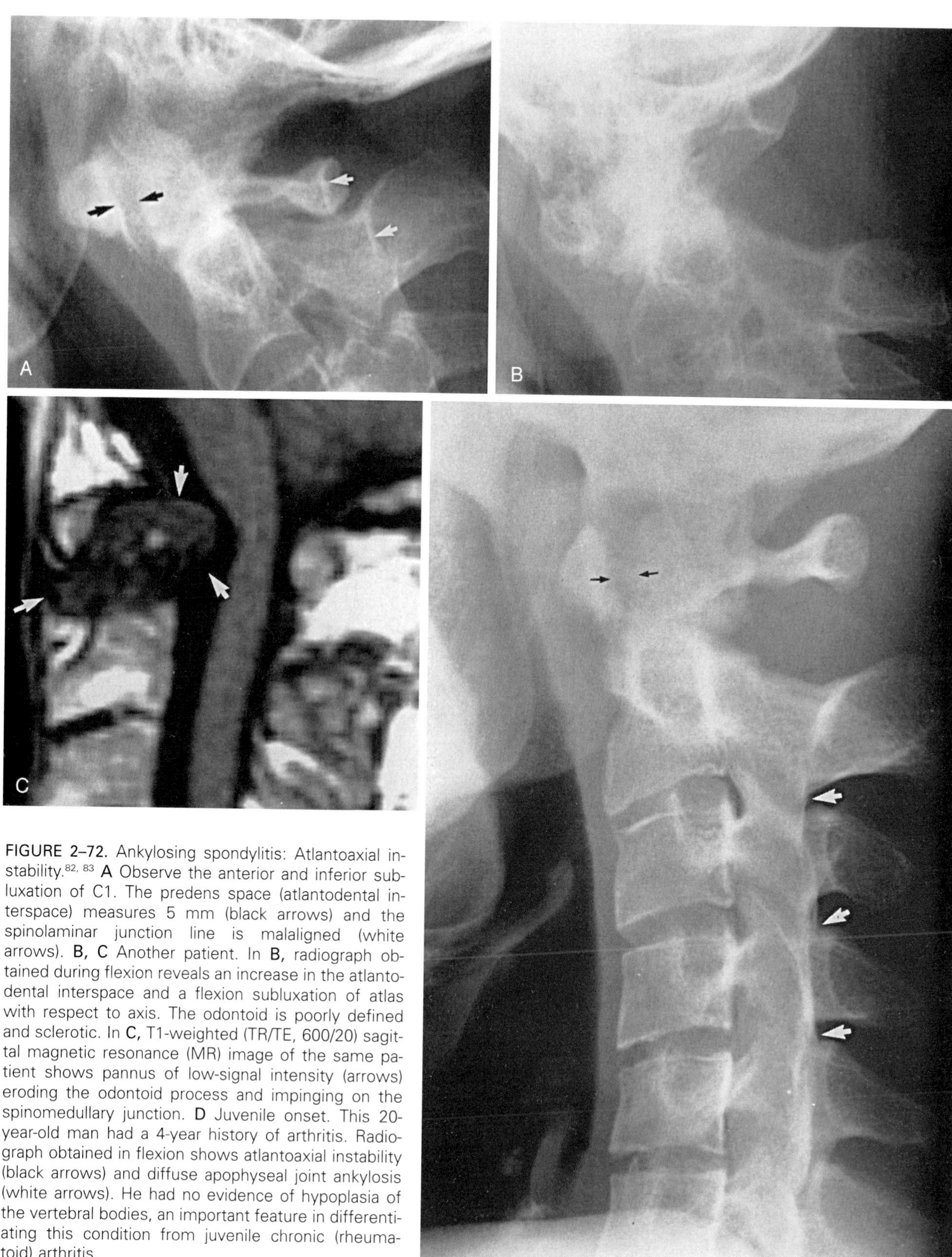

FIGURE 2–72. Ankylosing spondylitis: Atlantoaxial instability.[82, 83] A Observe the anterior and inferior subluxation of C1. The predens space (atlantodental interspace) measures 5 mm (black arrows) and the spinolaminar junction line is malaligned (white arrows). B, C Another patient. In B, radiograph obtained during flexion reveals an increase in the atlantodental interspace and a flexion subluxation of atlas with respect to axis. The odontoid is poorly defined and sclerotic. In C, T1-weighted (TR/TE, 600/20) sagittal magnetic resonance (MR) image of the same patient shows pannus of low-signal intensity (arrows) eroding the odontoid process and impinging on the spinomedullary junction. D Juvenile onset. This 20-year-old man had a 4-year history of arthritis. Radiograph obtained in flexion shows atlantoaxial instability (black arrows) and diffuse apophyseal joint ankylosis (white arrows). He had no evidence of hypoplasia of the vertebral bodies, an important feature in differentiating this condition from juvenile chronic (rheumatoid) arthritis.

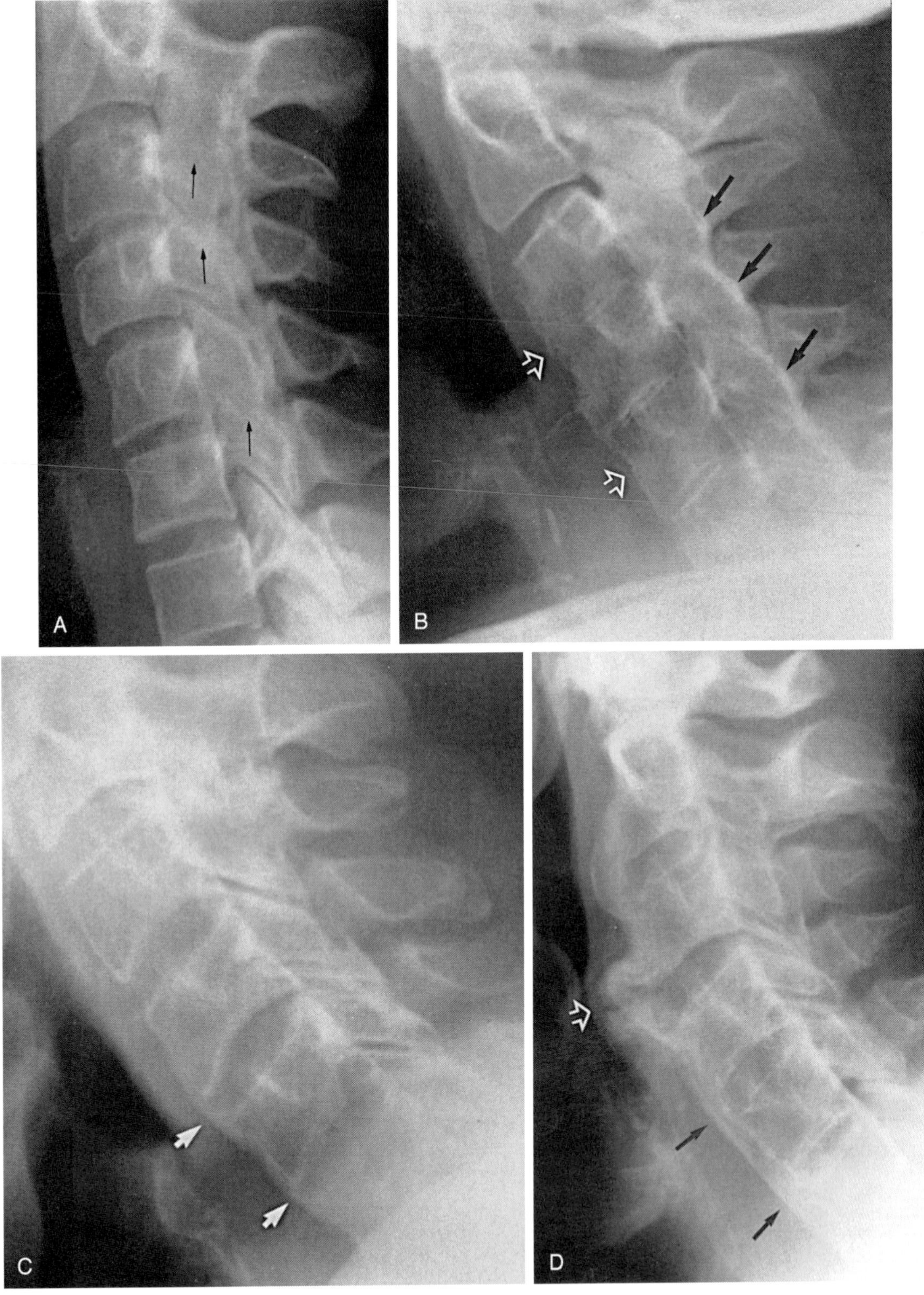

FIGURE 2–73. Ankylosing spondylitis: Spectrum of radiographic abnormalities.[82, 83] A Lateral radiograph of this 38-year-old woman reveals extensive ankylosis of the apophyseal joints (arrows) with no evidence of syndesmophyte formation. B In another patient, diffuse apophyseal joint ankylosis (arrows), disc space narrowing, and anterior vertebral body ankylosis (open arrows) are noted. An abnormal posture, in which the head is thrust forward, is also a frequent finding in ankylosing spondylitis. C In a third patient, marginal syndesmophytes predominate in the lower cervical spine (arrows). The apophyseal joints appear somewhat irregular, but no ankylosis is evident. D This patient has diffuse syndesmophyte formation at several levels and more prominent osteophyte formation at the C3-C4 level (arrows), perhaps secondary to excessive motion (open arrow).

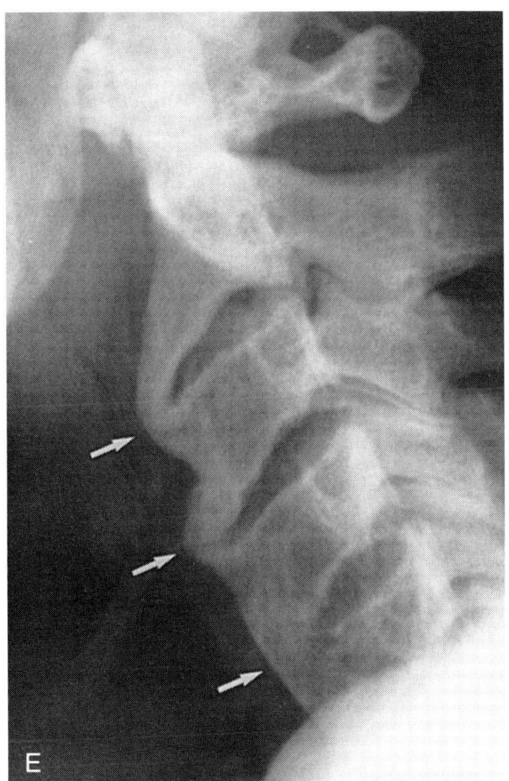

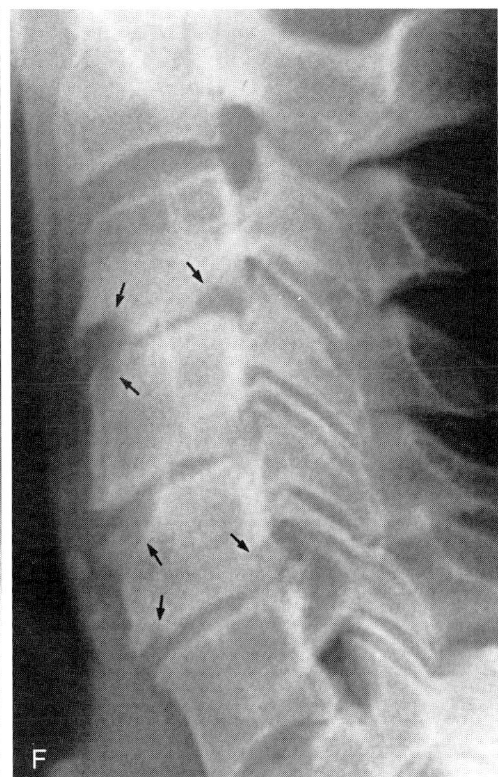

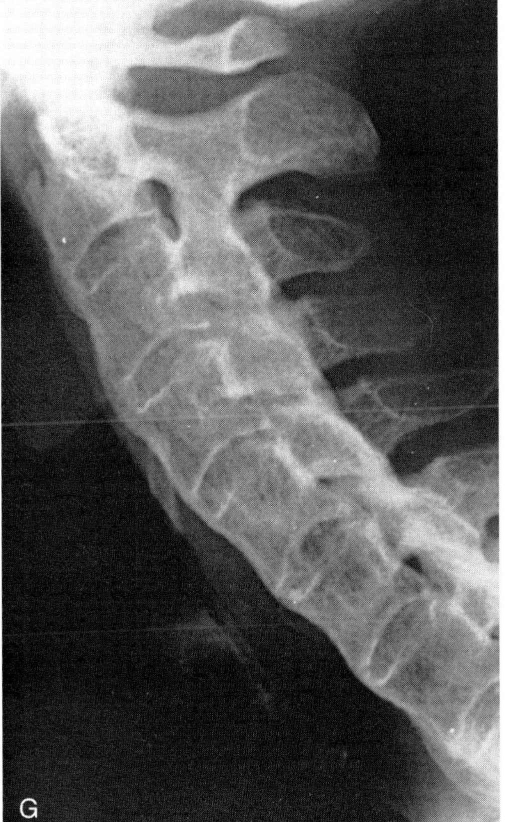

FIGURE 2–73 *Continued.* E An atypical presentation of thick DISH-like flowing hyperostosis (arrows) is evident in this 49-year-old man with positive HLA-B27 and classic lumbar spine and sacroiliac changes of ankylosing spondylitis. F Prominent disc space narrowing, peripheral endplate erosions (arrows), and osteitis of the vertebral bodies predominate in another patient with early ankylosing spondylitis. G Advanced disease is characterized by diffuse ankylosis of the apophyseal joints, diffuse syndesmophyte formation, and ballooning of the discs.

Illustration continued on following page

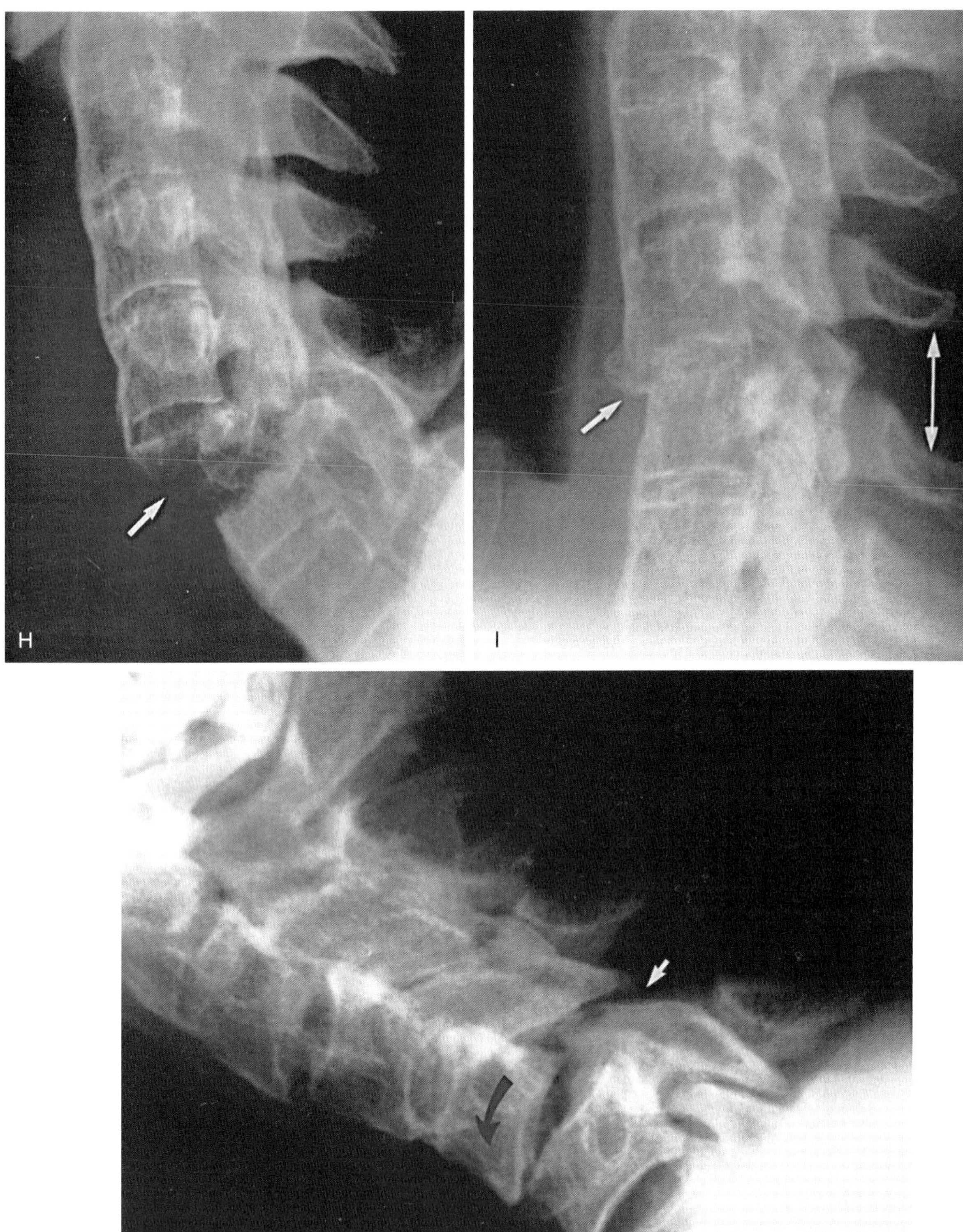

FIGURE 2–73 *Continued.* Fractures. In **H**, the patient had had a fall that resulted in a fracture of his ankylosed C6 vertebral body (arrow) and apophyseal joints. In **I**, another patient, a lateral radiograph reveals a fracture of the ankylosed cervical spine at C4-C5. The fracture extends through the apophyseal joints and results in anterior displacement of C4 (arrow) and divergence of the C4-C5 spinous processes (double-headed arrow) with instability. **J** Hyperflexion sprain. This 42-year-old man with ankylosing spondylitis sustained a cervical spine hyperflexion injury in a motor vehicle collision. A flexion radiograph reveals facet gapping (arrow), anterior C5 vertebral body subluxation (curved arrow), and disc space wedging at the C5-C6 level. *(**J**, Courtesy of D. Goodwin, M.D., Lebanon, New Hampshire.)*

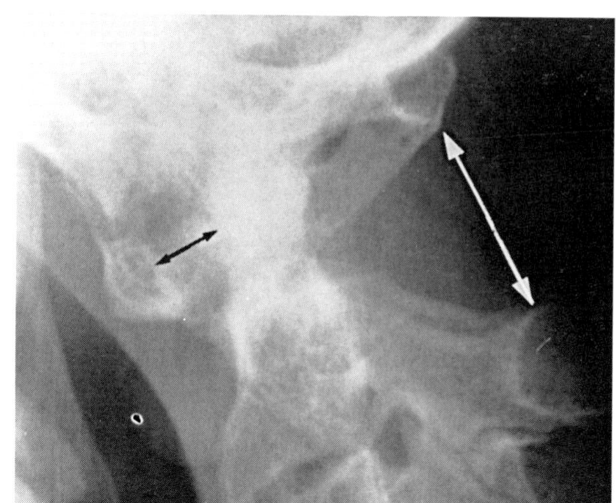

FIGURE 2–74. Psoriatic arthropathy: Atlantoaxial instability.[84] Lateral radiograph obtained during flexion shows dramatic atlantoaxial subluxation in which the anterior arch of atlas has translated anteriorly (black double-headed arrow) and inferiorly in relation to the odontoid process. The space between the posterior arch of atlas and the C2 spinous process is widened (white double-headed arrow).

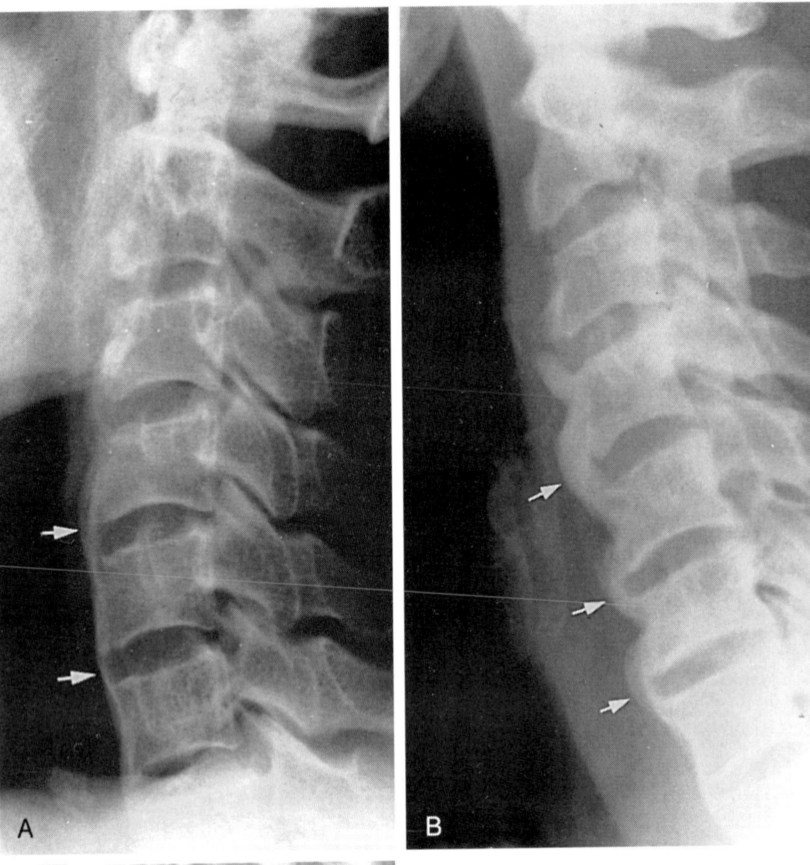

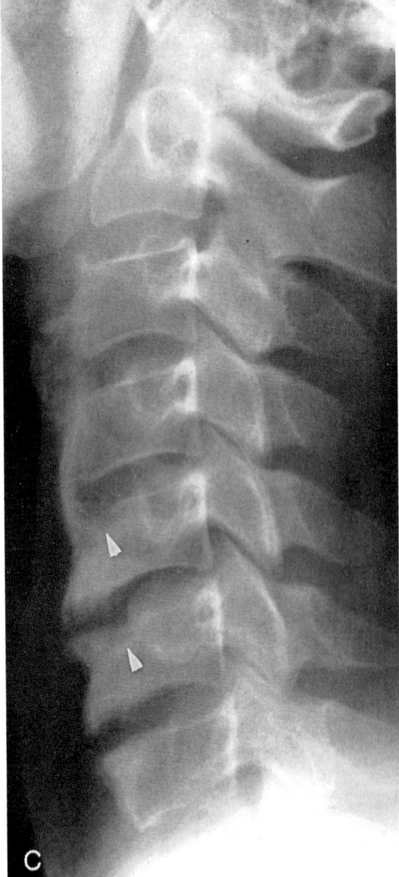

FIGURE 2–75. Psoriatic arthropathy.[84] A A thin sheet of paravertebral ossification is seen spanning the anterior aspect of the lower cervical spine (arrows). The disc spaces and apophyseal joints are well preserved. B In another patient, a thicker, more prominent pattern of ossification is present (arrows). The spinal outgrowths are nonmarginal, arising from the central portion of the anterior aspect of the vertebral body. The disc spaces are preserved. C Acne congoblata. In a patient with this rare skin disease, the osseous outgrowths are seen as hyperostosis and sheet-like proliferation similar to findings seen in classic psoriatic arthritis. The disc and apophyseal joint spaces are intact, but erosions of the C5 and C6 vertebral end plates are evident (arrowheads). *(C, Courtesy of N. Kinnis, M.D., Chicago, Illinois.)*

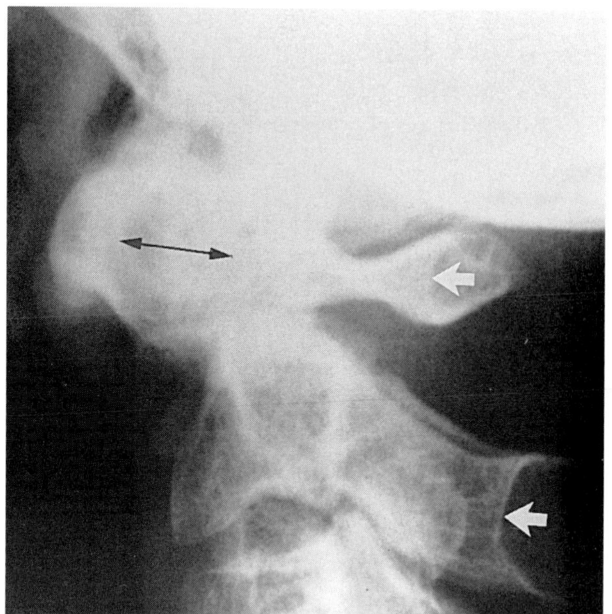

FIGURE 2–76. Reiter's syndrome: Atlantoaxial instability.[85] Observe the anterior translation of C1 in relation to C2. The atlantodental interspace measures 14 mm (black double-headed arrow), and the C1 spinolaminar junction line is significantly displaced in relation to that of C2 (white arrows).

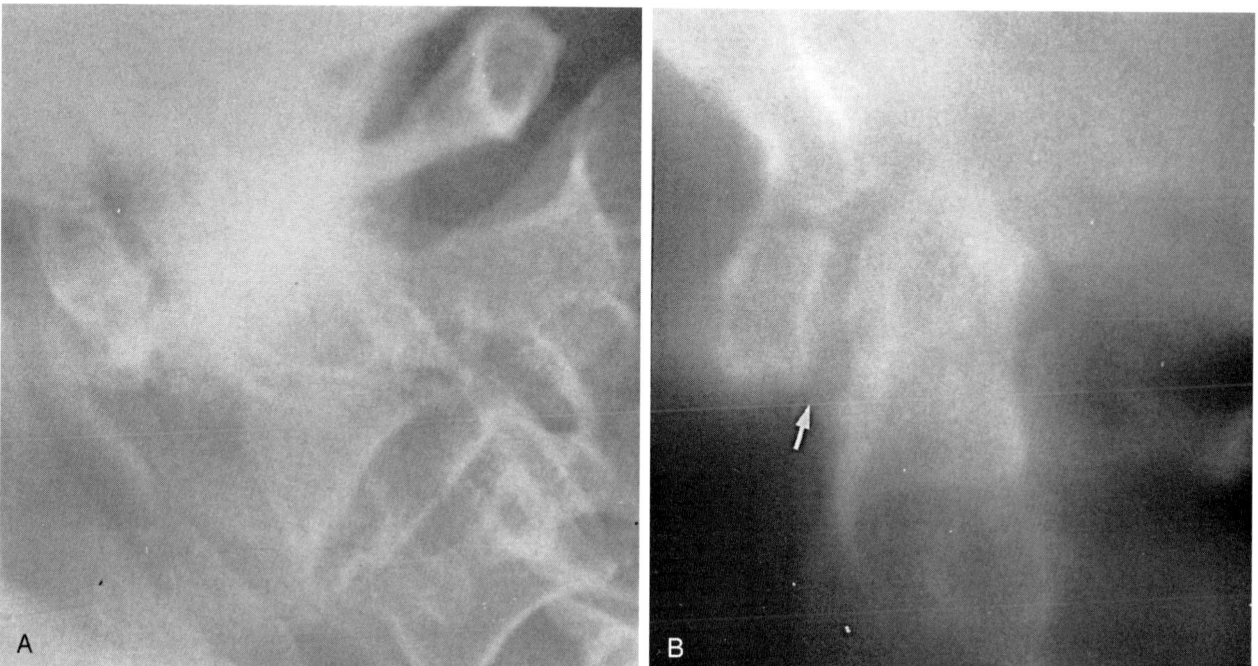

FIGURE 2–77. Calcium pyrophosphate dihydrate (CPPD) crystal deposition disease.[86, 87] A In a 76-year-old man, a lateral radiograph obtained in flexion reveals erosion and sclerosis of the atlantoaxial articulation. B Lateral conventional tomogram reveals atlantoaxial instability (arrow) and irregularity of the articular surfaces.

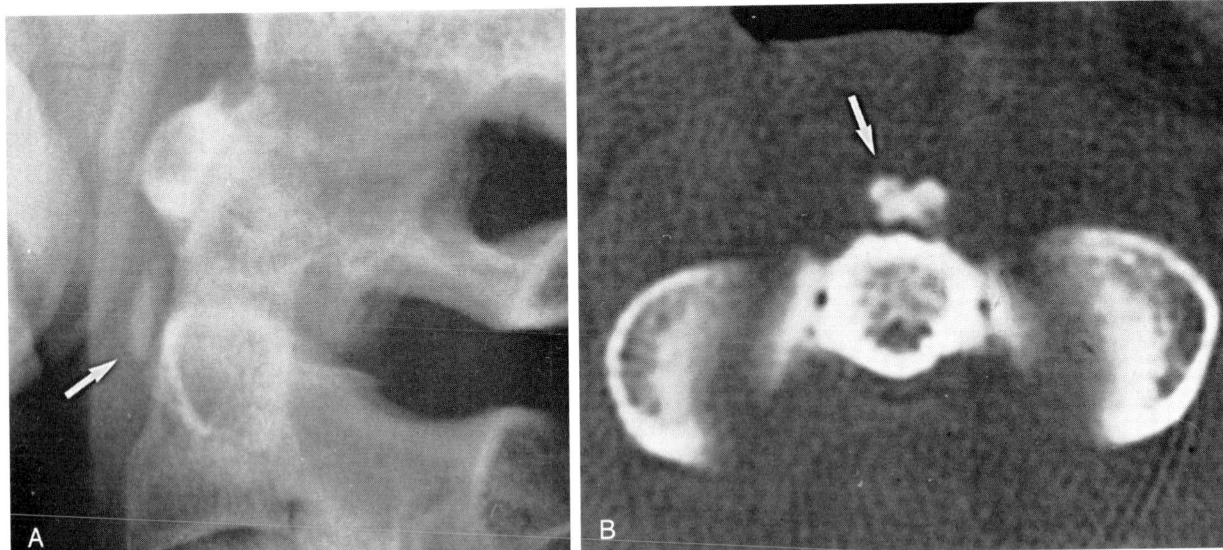

FIGURE 2–78. Calcium hydroxyapatite crystal deposition disease (HADD): Longus colli muscle and tendon.[88] **A** In this 46-year-old woman with neck pain, fever, and limitation of motion, a globular collection of calcification is seen within the soft tissues adjacent to the anterior aspect of the C2 vertebral body (arrow). **B** In a 28-year-old man, a transaxial CT scan reveals that the calcification is located within the longus colli muscle and tendon (arrow) anterior to the base of the odontoid and posterior to the pharynx.

Calcific tendinitis at this site is a self-limited condition that typically affects middle-aged persons. It may be asymptomatic or result in acute neck pain, torticollis, occipital pain, nuchal rigidity, and dysphagia. *(**A, B,** Courtesy of G. Greenway, M.D., Dallas, Texas.)*

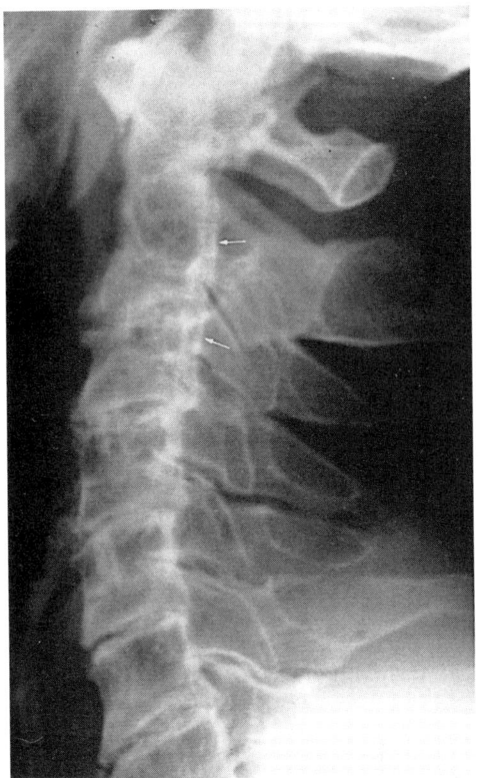

FIGURE 2–79. Alkaptonuria.[90] Prominent intervertebral disc narrowing, calcification, and ossification are evident in this patient with long-standing ochronosis. Note also the presence of vertebral end-plate sclerosis. A vertical linear radiodense band within the spinal canal at the C2-C3 level (arrows) represents ossification of the posterior longitudinal ligament, a complication that may result in spinal stenosis.

TABLE 2–12. MR Imaging Findings in Vertebral Osteomyelitis*[92]

Loss of end-plate definition (95 per cent)
Contrast enhancement of both disc and vertebral body (94 per cent)
Signal intensity changes of both the vertebral body on T1-weighted images and of the disc on T1-weighted and T2-weighted images (85 per cent)
Signal intensity changes of both vertebral body and disc on T1-weighted and T2-weighted images (46 per cent)
Ring enhancement correlated at surgery with abscess
Homogeneous enhancement correlated at surgery with phlegmon

Signal Change	Imaging Protocol	Site	Per Cent
Decreased	T1-weighted	Vertebral body	91
Increased	T2-weighted	Vertebral body	56
Increased	T2-weighted	Disc	95

*N = 37 patients, 41 vertebral levels; modified from ref. 92.

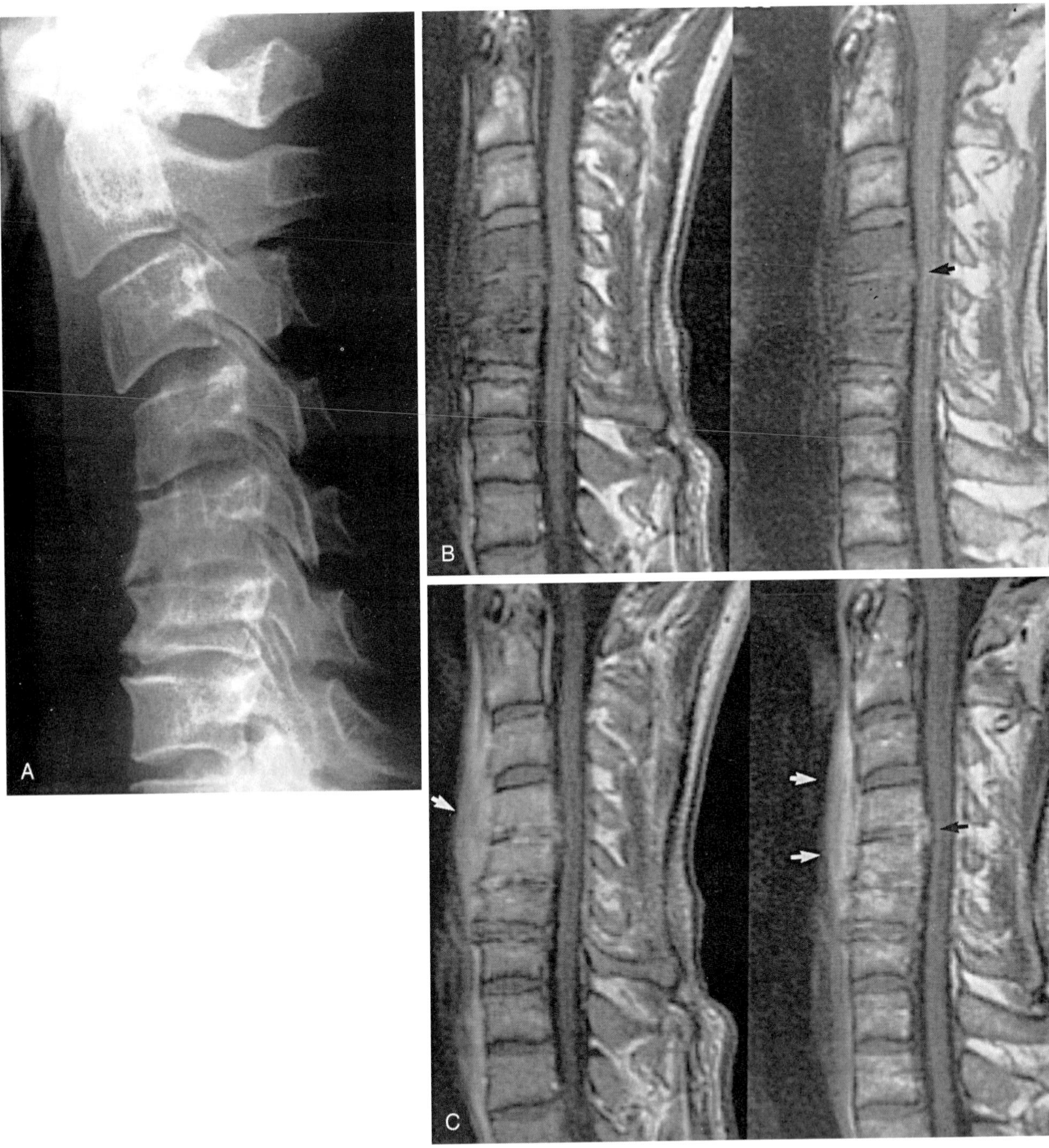

FIGURE 2–80. Infectious (pyogenic) spondylodiscitis: Direct implantation.[91–93] This 40-year-old man had persistent neck pain after a discogram. **A** Lateral radiograph reveals a kyphotic posture and marked disc space narrowing at C4-C5 and C5-C6. Osteophytes and other degenerative changes are absent. **B** The routine sagittal T1-weighted (TR/TE, 450/20) spin echo magnetic resonance (MR) images demonstrate low signal intensity in the marrow of the C4, C5, and C6 vertebral bodies. The intervertebral disc spaces are narrowed and erosions of the vertebral end plates are evident. **C** Sagittal T1-weighted (TR/TE, 450/20) spin echo magnetic resonance (MR) images obtained after intravenous gadolinium administration demonstrate marked enhancement within the vertebral bodies, prevertebral soft tissues (white arrows), and a small epidural abscess that extends into the spinal canal at the C4-C5 level (black arrow). *Staphylococcus aureus* was cultured, and the patient was treated with antibiotics.

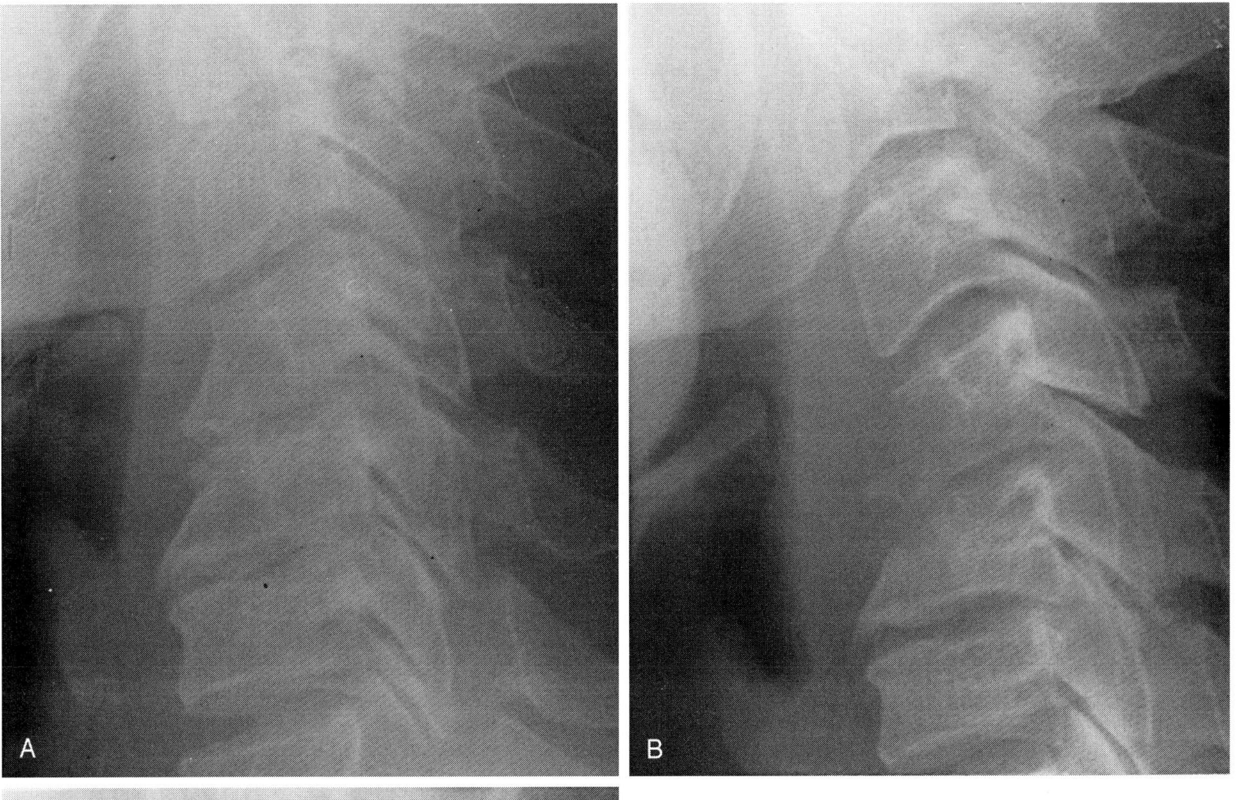

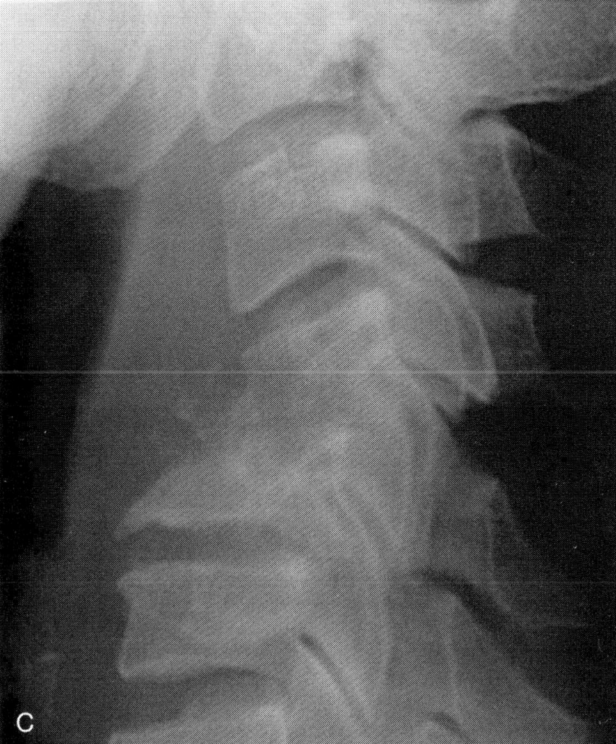

FIGURE 2–81. Infectious (pyogenic) spondylodiscitis.[91–93] Serial radiographs from this 40-year-old male heroin addict taken initially (**A**) and 3 weeks (**B**) and 6 weeks (**C**) later reveal rapid destruction of the C4-C5 discovertebral junctions. Observe the progressive obliteration of the cortical margins of the vertebral end plates and eventual pathologic vertebral collapse, resulting in dramatic subluxation. The organism cultured was *Klebsiella pneumoniae,* an extremely rare cause of musculoskeletal infection, usually found only in patients with diminished resistance.

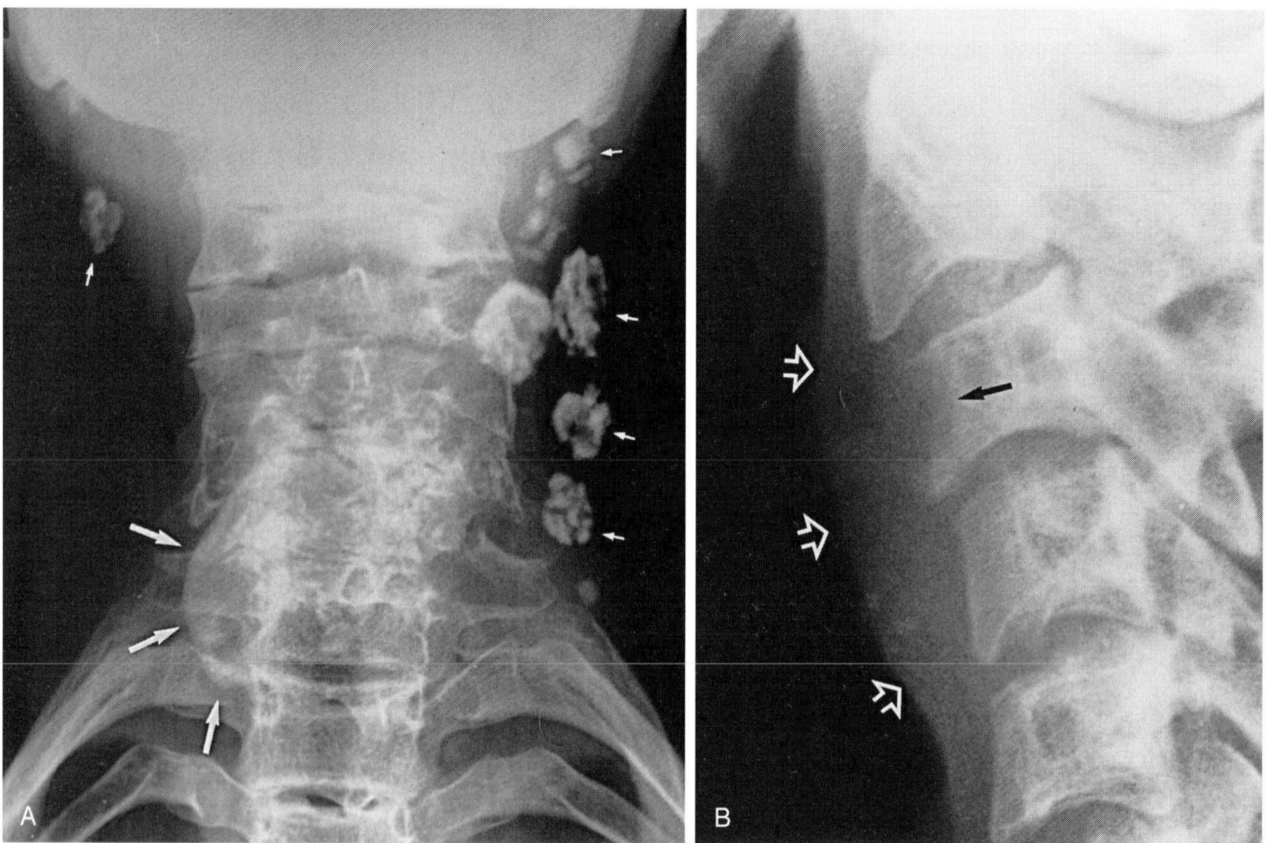

FIGURE 2–82. Tuberculous spondylodiscitis.[94] A Calcified paravertebral abscess. Observe a diffuse curvilinear zone of calcification overlying the cervicothoracic region, representing a tuberculous abscess (large arrows). Extensive popcorn-like calcifications also are noted in the paravertebral lymph nodes (small arrows). Extension of tuberculosis from vertebral and discal sites to the adjacent ligaments and soft tissues is frequent. Extension usually is anterolateral, but it may occur posteriorly into the peridural space. B Prevertebral abscess. Prevertebral soft tissue swelling (open arrows) indicates extraspinal extension of an abscess in this patient. Note also the erosion of the third cervical vertebral body (black arrow). *(A, B, Courtesy of A. D'Abreu, M.D., Porto Alegre, Brazil)*

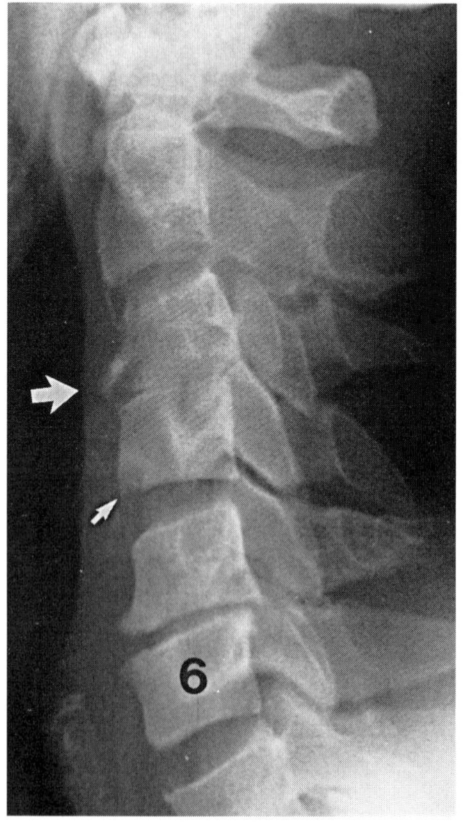

FIGURE 2–83. Dialysis spondyloarthropathy.[95] A radiograph from this hemodialysis patient demonstrates disc space destruction, vertebral end-plate erosion, and vertebral body collapse at the C3-C4 level (large arrow). A small erosion is seen at the inferior aspect of the C4 vertebral body (small arrow), and early C5-C6 disc space narrowing also is evident. This peculiar type of destructive spondyloarthropathy, well recognized in patients undergoing hemodialysis for a period of years, must be differentiated from spinal infection, neuropathic osteoarthropathy, and calcium pyrophosphate dihydrate or calcium hydroxyapatite crystal deposition disease.

TABLE 2–13. Tumors and Tumor-like Lesions Affecting the Cervical Spine*

Entity	Figure(s), Table(s)	Characteristics
Malignant		
Skeletal metastasis[96]	2–84	75 per cent osteolytic; 25 per cent osteoblastic or mixed pattern Usually multiple sites of involvement Pathologic vertebral collapse, pedicle destruction, or ivory vertebra
Primary malignant neoplasms of bone		
Osteosarcoma (conventional)[97]		Very rare occurrence in the spine Vertebral body involvement often leads to vertebral collapse Readily metastasizes to other bones and lung
Osteoblastoma (aggressive)[98]	2–85	23 per cent of aggressive osteoblastomas affect the spine Expansile osteolytic lesion of the neural arch that may be partially ossified or contain calcium
Chondrosarcoma (conventional)[99]		Extremely rare: only 6 per cent affect the spine Often contain calcification
Giant cell tumor (aggressive)[100]		Eccentric osteolytic lesion, rare in the spine
Fibrosarcoma[101]		Extremely rare in the spine
Ewing's sarcoma[102]		Extremely rare in the cervical spine
Chordoma[103]	2–86	75 per cent of all chordomas affect the spine; some of these involve the axis Most common pattern: central osteolytic, expansile destruction of the vertebral body; infrequently, osteosclerotic or mixed; soft tissue mass
Myeloproliferative disorders		
Plasma cell myeloma[104]		Common malignancy of the spine
Multiple myeloma (75 per cent of all plasma cell myeloma)	2–87	75 per cent of patients have spinal lesions Early: Normal radiographs or diffuse osteopenia Later: Multiple well-circumscribed osteolytic lesions Pathologic vertebral collapse False-negative bone scans common
Solitary plasmacytoma (25 per cent of all plasma cell myeloma)		50 per cent of plasmacytomas affect the spine Solitary, geographic, expansile, osteolytic lesion that frequently results in pathologic collapse 70 per cent eventually develop into multiple myeloma
Hodgkin's disease[105]		43 per cent of all skeletal lesions in Hodgkin's disease affect the spine More than 60 per cent of patients have multiple sites of involvement 75 per cent of lesions are osteolytic; 25 per cent are osteosclerotic
Primary lymphoma (non-Hodgkin's)[106, 107]	2–88	Spinal involvement in 13 per cent of patients with non-Hodgkin's lymphoma May result in multiple moth-eaten or permeative osteolytic lesions, with pathologic vertebral collapse Common cause of pathologic fracture Diffuse or localized sclerotic lesions are rare
Leukemia[108]		Osteoporosis, compression fractures, and radiolucent bands adjacent to the end plates
Benign		
Primary benign neoplasms of bone		
Enostosis[109]		Only 2 per cent affect the spine Painless, circular zone of osteosclerosis May be normal or warm on bone scan
Osteoid osteoma[110]	2–89	6 per cent of osteoid osteomas affect the spine Reactive sclerosis of the pedicle or other part of the neural arch Central radiolucent nidus usually is less than 1 cm in diameter and often is not visible on routine radiographs
Osteoblastoma (conventional)		30 per cent of osteoblastomas affect the spine Approximately 95 per cent of osteoblastomas are benign Expansile lesion of neural arch, usually purely osteolytic with a predilection for C4, C5, and C6
Osteochondroma (solitary)[111, 112]	2–90	Only 2 per cent occur in the spine Pedunculated or sessile cartilage-covered osseous excrescence arising from the surface of a lamina, transverse process, or spinous process
Hereditary multiple exostosis[113]		Infrequently involves spine: multiple lesions, each with same appearance as solitary osteochondroma

Table continued on following page

TABLE 2–13. Tumors and Tumor-like Lesions Affecting the Cervical Spine* *Continued*

Entity	Figure(s), Table(s)	Characteristics
Benign *Continued*		
Giant cell tumor (benign)[114]		Only 7 per cent affect the cervical spine Eccentric osteolytic neoplasm 90 to 95 per cent of all giant cell tumors are benign
Hemangioma (solitary)[115]	2–91	25 per cent affect the spine Corduroy cloth appearance of vertebral body related to accentuated vertical striations
Aneurysmal bone cyst[116, 117]	2–92	14 per cent of all lesions affect the spine Eccentric, expansile osteolytic lesion arising from the neural arch; isolated involvement of the vertebral body is uncommon and usually is associated with simultaneous involvement of the posterior elements Typically more expansile than osteoblastoma
Tumor-like lesions		
Paget's disease[118, 119]	2–93	Predilection for upper cervical segments, but may affect any level Usually polyostotic and expansile and is one cause of ivory vertebrae Coarsened trabeculae and end plates may create picture-frame vertebrae Vertebral enlargement common Spinal involvement may be osteolytic, osteosclerotic, or mixed Contiguous vertebrae may be involved, obliterating the disc spaces and resembling developmental synostosis
Neurofibromatosis Type I (von Recklinghausen's disease)[120, 121]	2–94 Table 2–14	50 per cent of patients develop skeletal lesions Posterior vertebral scalloping and enlargement of the neural foramina Associated with short, angular kyphoscoliosis (50 per cent of cases) and dramatic cervical kyphosis
Fibrous dysplasia[122] Monostotic (70–80 per cent) Polyostotic (20–30 per cent)	2–95	Monostotic and polyostotic forms Monostotic spinal involvement extremely rare (less than 1 per cent of lesions) 21 per cent of patients with polyostotic fibrous dysplasia have spine involvement Thick rim of sclerosis surrounding a radiolucent lesion within multiple vertebral bodies with or without pathologic collapse
Langerhans' cell histiocytosis[123, 124]	2–96	6 per cent of all lesions affect the spine Flattened vertebral bodies or, less commonly, bubbly, lytic, or expansile lesions without vertebral body collapse With healing, the height of the pathologically collapsed vertebral body may be reconstituted, a finding more common in younger persons Thoracic and lumbar lesions are more common than cervical spine lesions

*See also Tables 1–10 to 1–12.

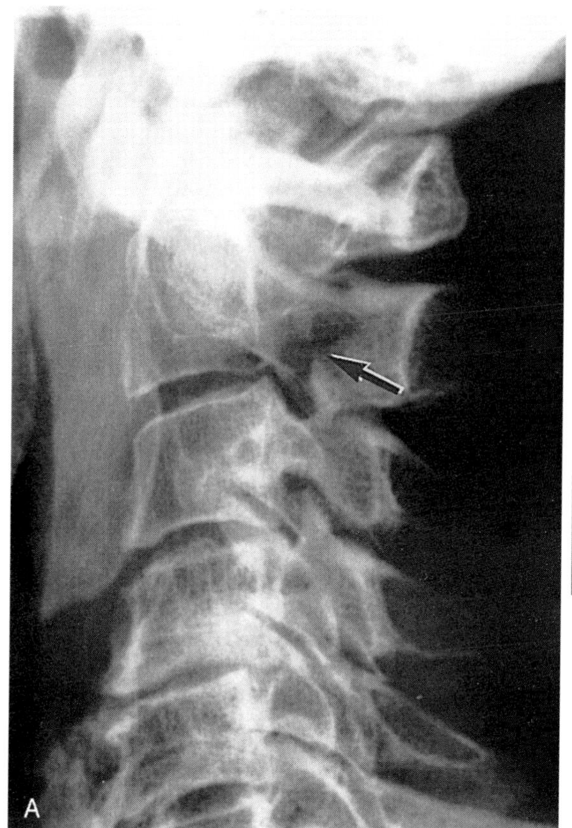

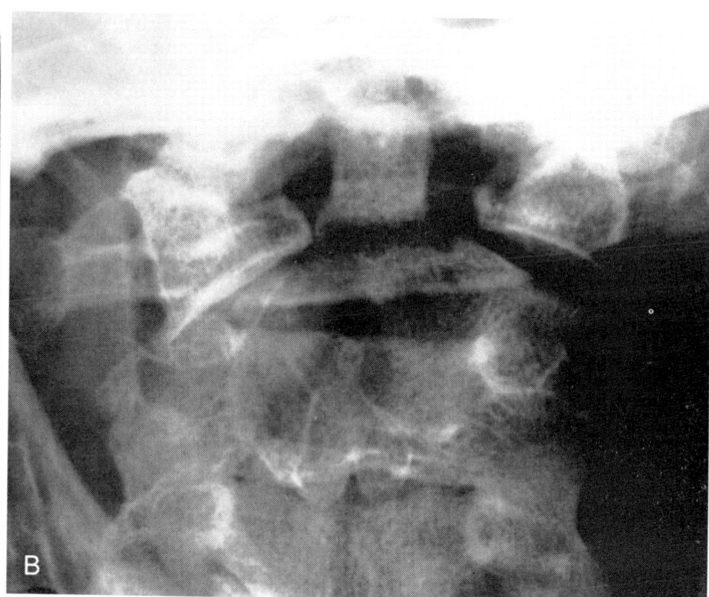

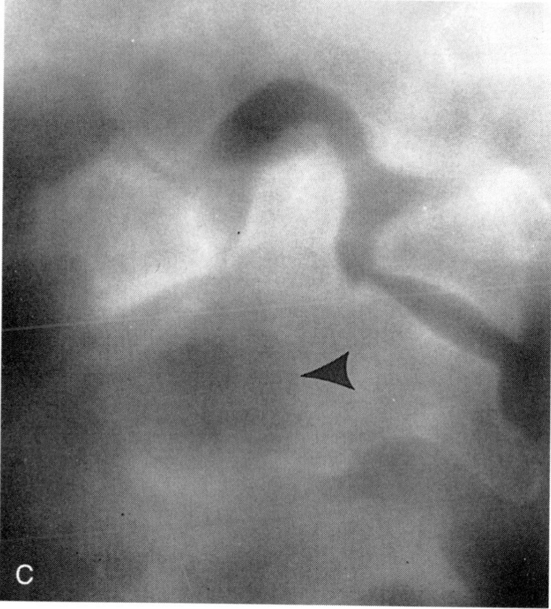

FIGURE 2–84. Skeletal metastasis.[96] Bronchogenic carcinoma: Osteolytic pattern. This 67-year-old man with lung cancer developed neck pain. A, B Lateral cervical spine (A) and anteroposterior open mouth upper cervical (B) radiographs reveal barely perceptible osteolytic destruction and collapse of the second cervical vertebral body. In A, a fracture is seen through the neural arch (arrow), and severe lateral offset of the atlas in relation to the axis is present. C Conventional tomogram more clearly defines the size and location of osteolytic destruction (arrowhead).

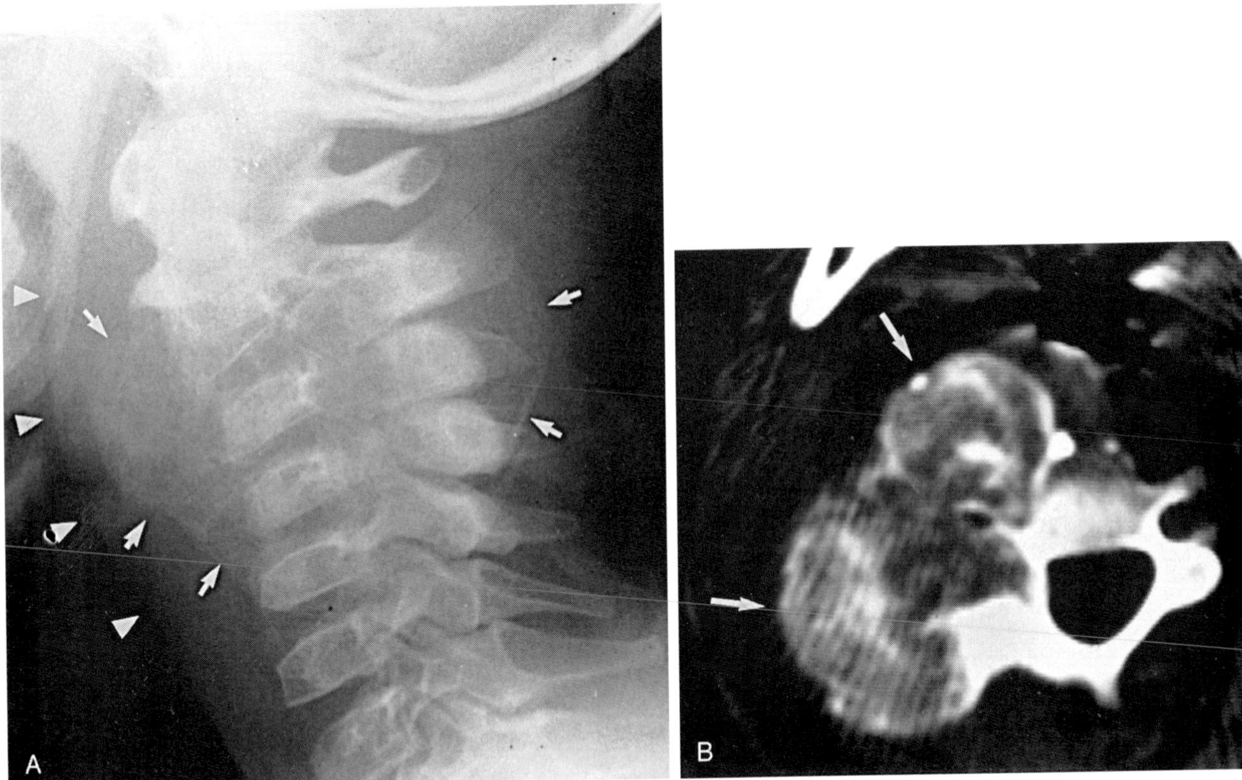

FIGURE 2–85. Aggressive osteoblastoma.[98] A Lateral cervical spine radiograph of this 6-year-old boy shows a large, expansile lesion overlying the C2 to C5 cervical vertebrae (arrows). The articular processes of C2 and C3 appear radiolucent. Observe the prominent prevertebral soft tissues caused by swelling and extraosseous tumor extension (arrowheads). B Transaxial CT scan through the C3 vertebral body documents the location, extent of osseous expansion, and partially calcified osteolytic matrix of the tumor.

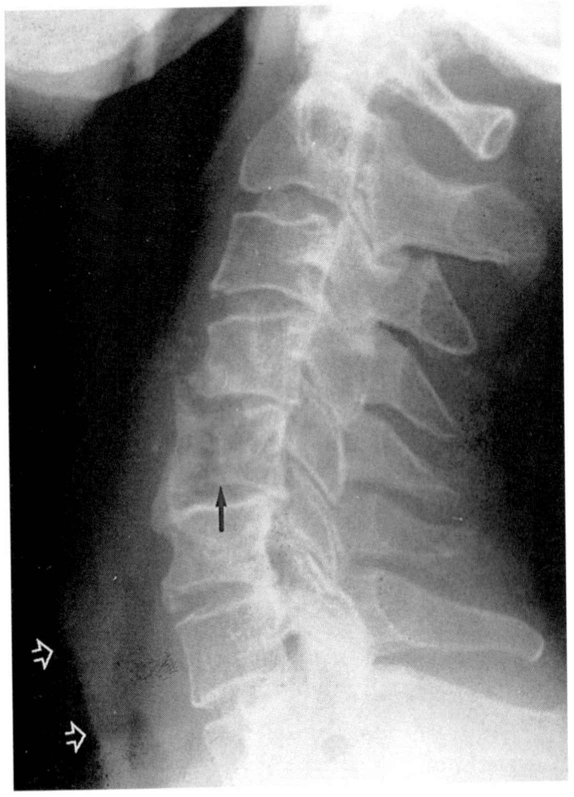

FIGURE 2–86. Chordoma.[103] A large, permeative, osteolytic lesion of the C5 vertebral body is seen (arrow). Note the osteolysis of the C5 vertebral end plates. Observe also the prominent prevertebral soft tissues, indicating swelling or neoplastic extension (open arrows).

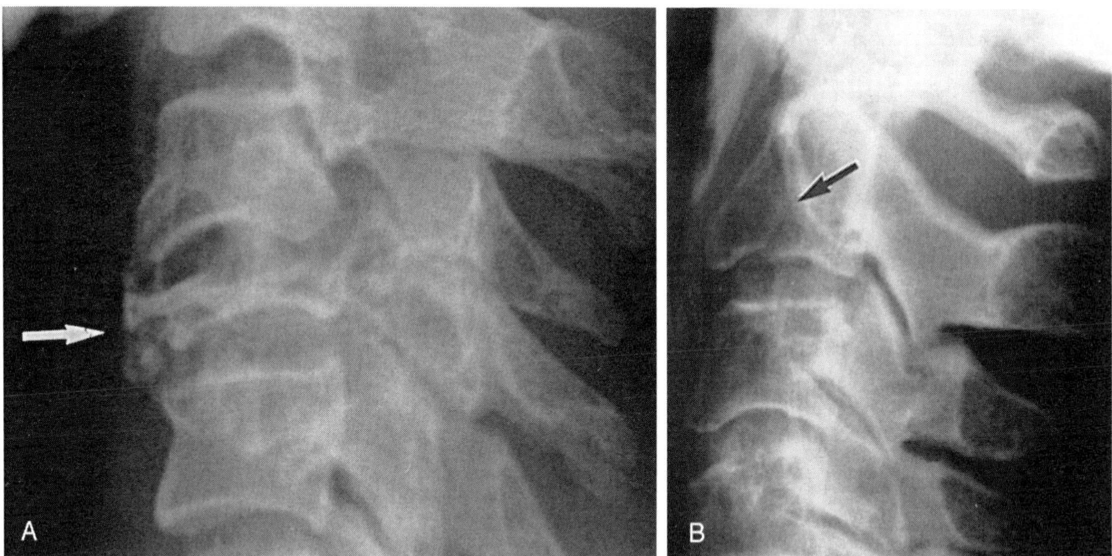

FIGURE 2–87. Plasma cell myeloma.[104] A Complete collapse of the fourth cervical vertebral body (arrow) is seen in this 40-year-old man. B In another patient, an osteolytic lesion within the vertebral body of C2 is seen (arrow). Diffuse osteopenia of the entire cervical spine is also present.

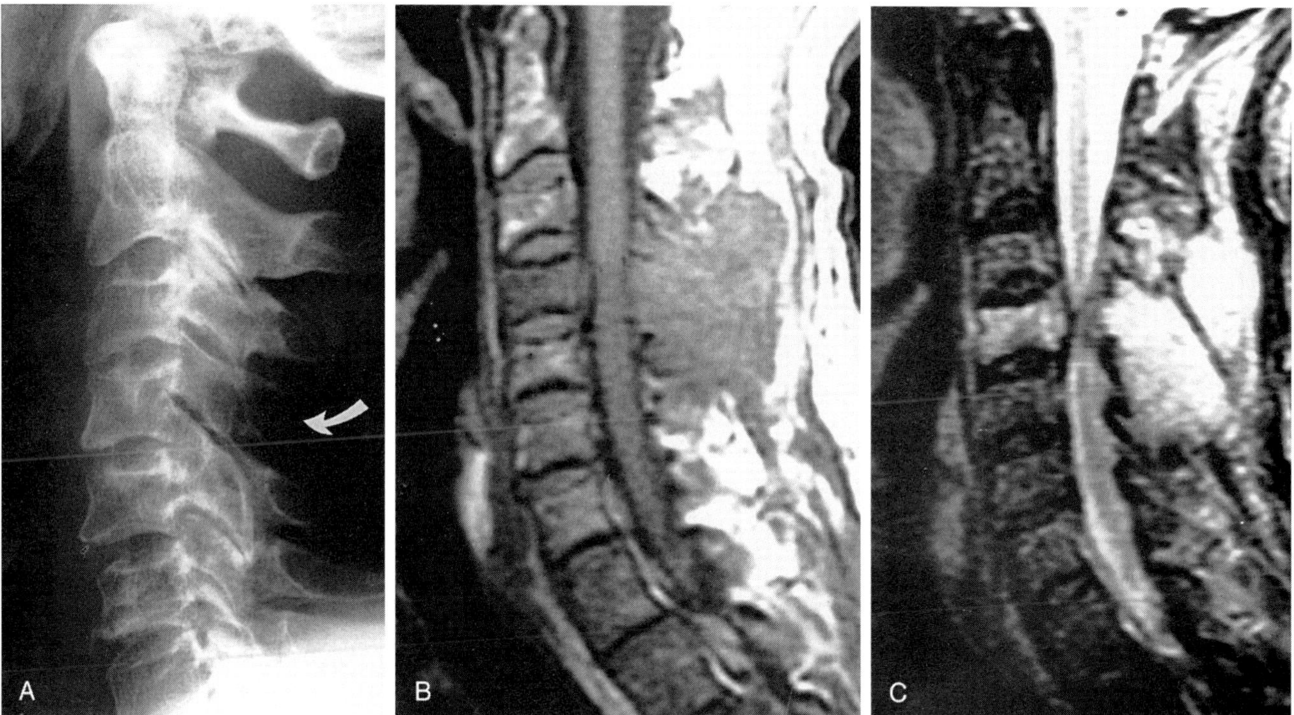

FIGURE 2–88. Non-Hodgkin's lymphoma: Large cell type.[106, 107] Spinal involvement in a 65-year-old man. A Routine radiograph reveals diffuse osteopenia and focal osteolysis of the fourth cervical spinous process (curved arrow). B, C Sagittal T1-weighted (TR/TE, 600/11) (B) and T2-weighted (TR/TE, 2000/70) (C) spin echo magnetic resonance (MR) images reveal destruction of this spinous process and a soft tissue mass that results in spinal canal stenosis. The high signal intensity in the C4 vertebral body on the T2-weighted image represents bone marrow edema or tumor infiltration.

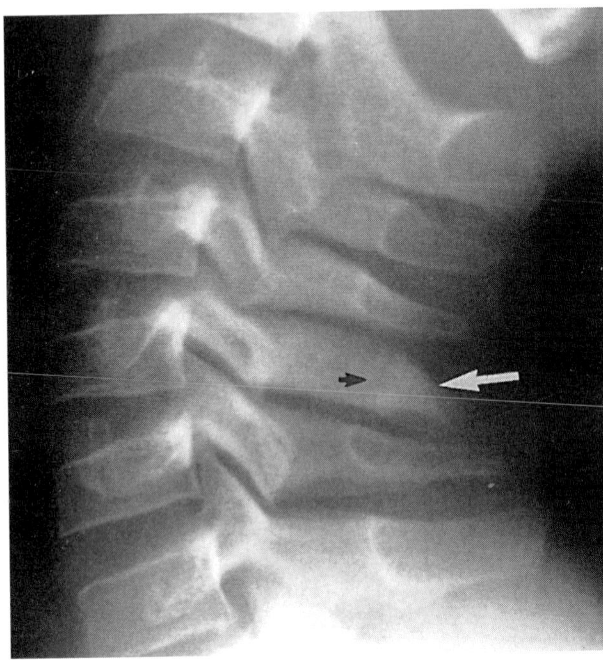

FIGURE 2–89. Osteoid osteoma.[110] In this 12-year-old boy with severe neck pain and rigidity, the spinous process of C5 appears sclerotic (large arrow). The spinolaminar junction line is obliterated, and a tiny circular radiolucent nidus is seen (small arrow). A biopsy revealed osteoid osteoma, and the lesion was surgically resected.

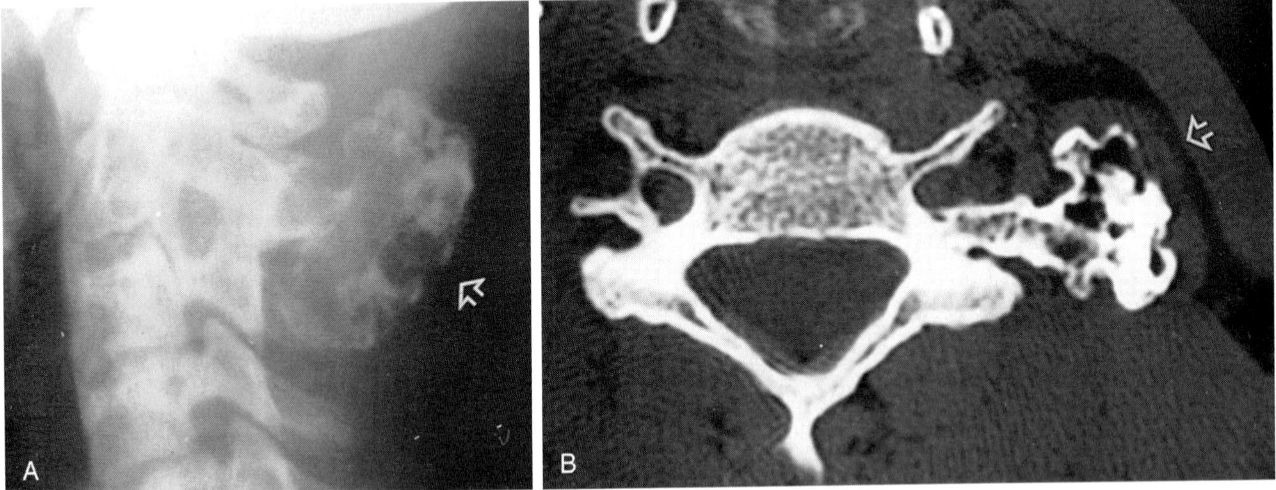

FIGURE 2–90. Solitary osteochondroma.[111, 112] A Oblique cervical spine radiograph from this 7-year-old child reveals an irregular, pedunculated osseous exostosis arising from the spinous process of C2 (open arrow). B In another patient, a transaxial computed tomography (CT) image reveals a large osteocartilaginous lesion. Observe that the cortex and medulla of the tumor are continuous with those of the posterior tubercle of the transverse process. The cartilaginous cap displaces the soft tissues of the anterolateral neck (open arrow). (*B, Courtesy of G.D. Schultz, D.C., Costa Mesa, California.*)

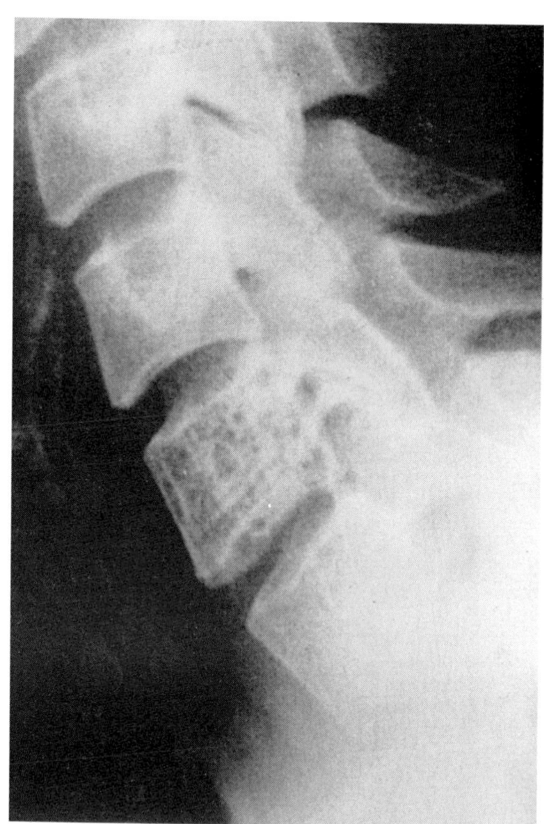

FIGURE 2–91. Hemangioma.[115] Observe the striated, lace-like trabeculae within the C6 vertebral body. The cortex and vertebral end plates are intact, and there is no evidence of vertebral body expansion. Hemangiomas may occasionally extend from the vertebral body into the neural arch but not in this case. *(Courtesy of A.L. Anderson, D.C., Portland, Oregon.)*

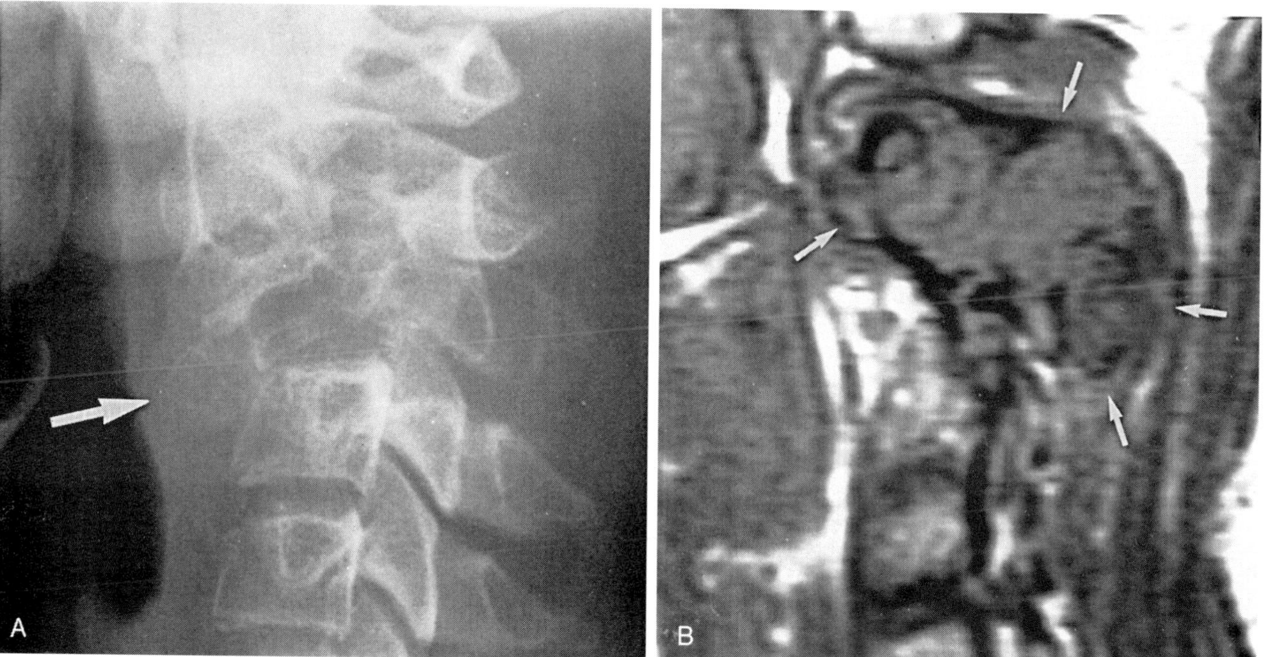

FIGURE 2–92. Aneurysmal bone cyst.[116, 117] In this 10-year-old child, a routine lateral cervical radiograph (**A**) reveals an expansile osteolytic lesion of the C3 vertebral body and neural arch (arrow). Sagittal T1-weighted (TR/TE, 700/20) spin echo magnetic resonance (MR) image (**B**) more clearly defines the extent (arrows) and nature of the tumor and its widespread destruction and soft tissue infiltration. The lesion was biopsied and the histologic diagnosis was aneurysmal bone cyst. *(Courtesy of L. Pinckney, M.D., San Diego, California.)*

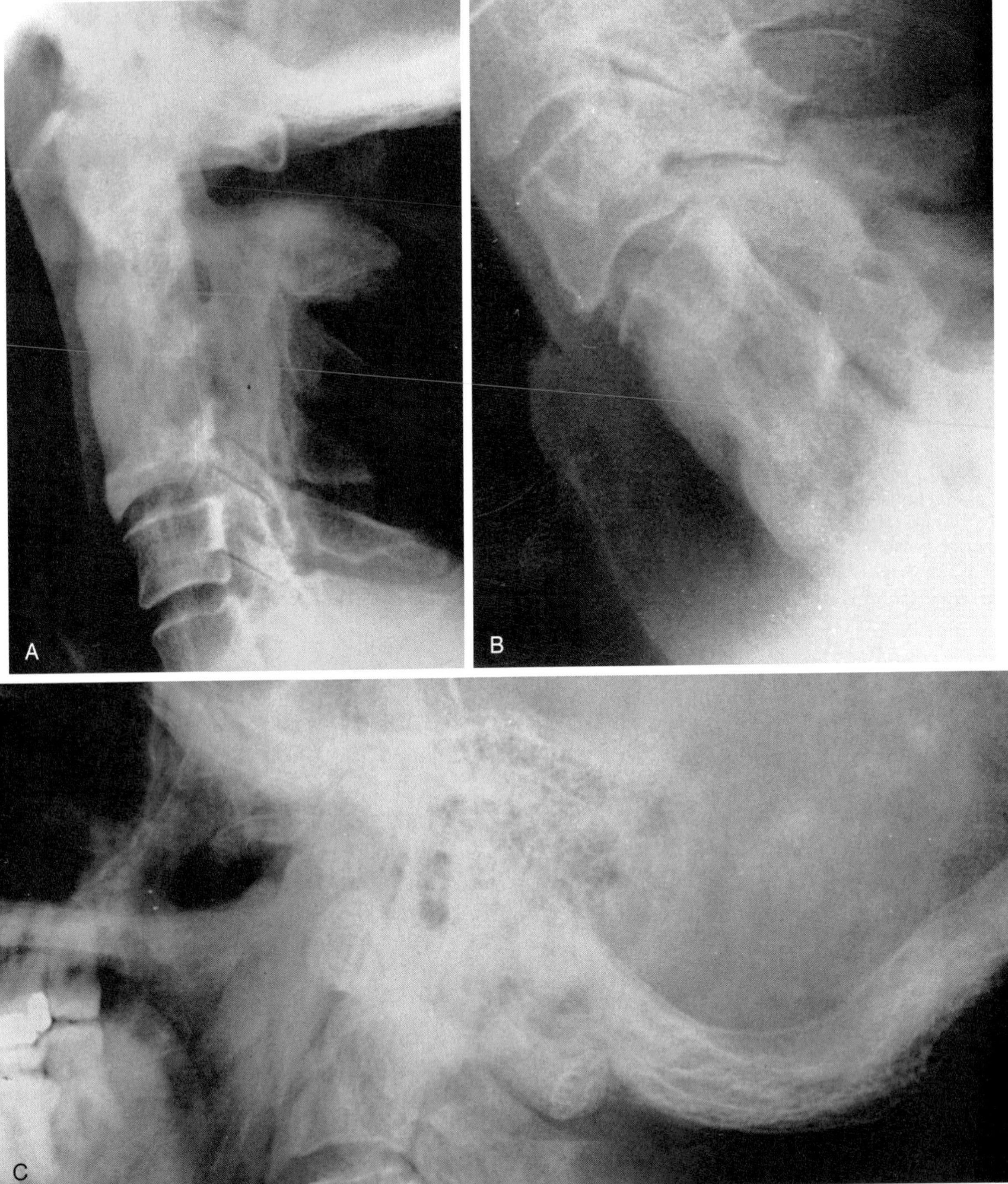

FIGURE 2–93. Paget's disease.[118, 119] A Observe the expansion, fusion, and trabecular thickening involving the C2-C4 vertebrae in this patient with polyostotic Paget's disease. B In another patient, observe a similar pattern of osseous fusion affecting the C5-C7 levels. C In a third patient, extensive upper cervical spine changes typical of Paget's disease are evident. The base of the skull exhibits characteristic calvarial thickening and basilar invagination, complicating features of this bone-softening disease.

TABLE 2–14. Some Causes of Enlarged Cervical Intervertebral Foramen[6, 19]

Neural causes	Vertebral artery abnormalities
Neurofibroma* (Fig. 2–94)	Vertebral artery tortuosity
Meningioma	Vertebral artery aneurysm (see Fig. 2–104)
Meningocele	Arteriovenous malformation
Bone neoplasms	Pseudoaneurysm
Aneurysmal bone cyst	Aortic coarctation
Skeletal metastasis	Subclavian steal syndrome
Osteoblastoma	Carotid artery obstruction
	Anomalous arterial loop
	Congenital
	Pedicle agenesis

*Most common cause.

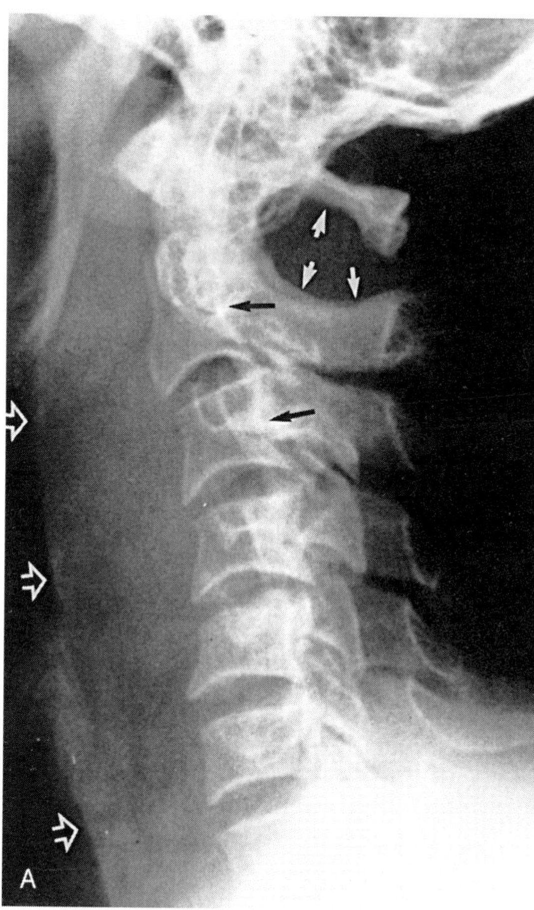

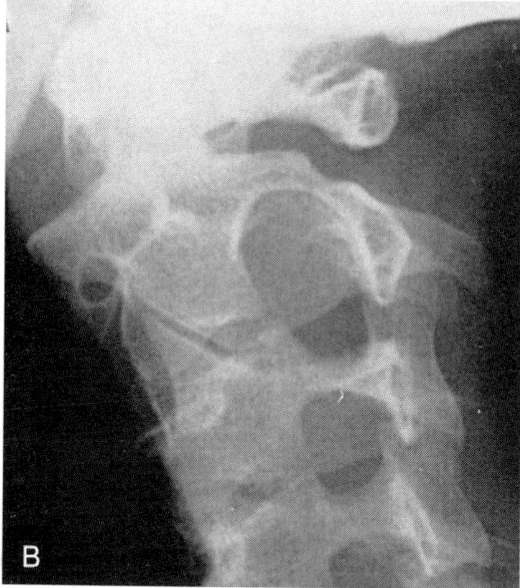

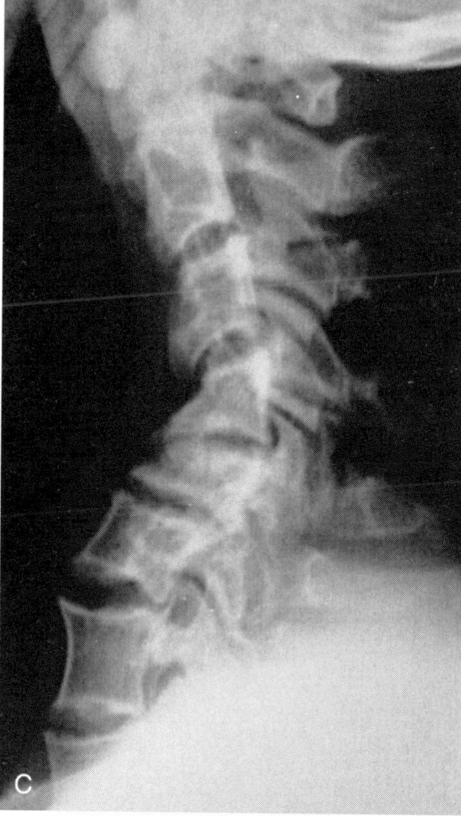

FIGURE 2–94. Neurofibromatosis Type I (von Recklinghausen's disease).[120, 121] A Note the posterior scalloping of the C2 and C3 vertebral bodies (black arrows), erosion of the C1 and C2 neural arches (white arrows), and dramatic prevertebral soft tissue widening (open arrows) caused by neurofibromas in the soft tissues. B In another patient, an oblique cervical spine radiograph reveals characteristic enlargement of the neural foramina of C2-C3 owing to gradual scalloped erosion of the posterior vertebral bodies and adjacent pedicles. C In a third patient, a severe kyphotic deformity with vertebral wedging is noted.

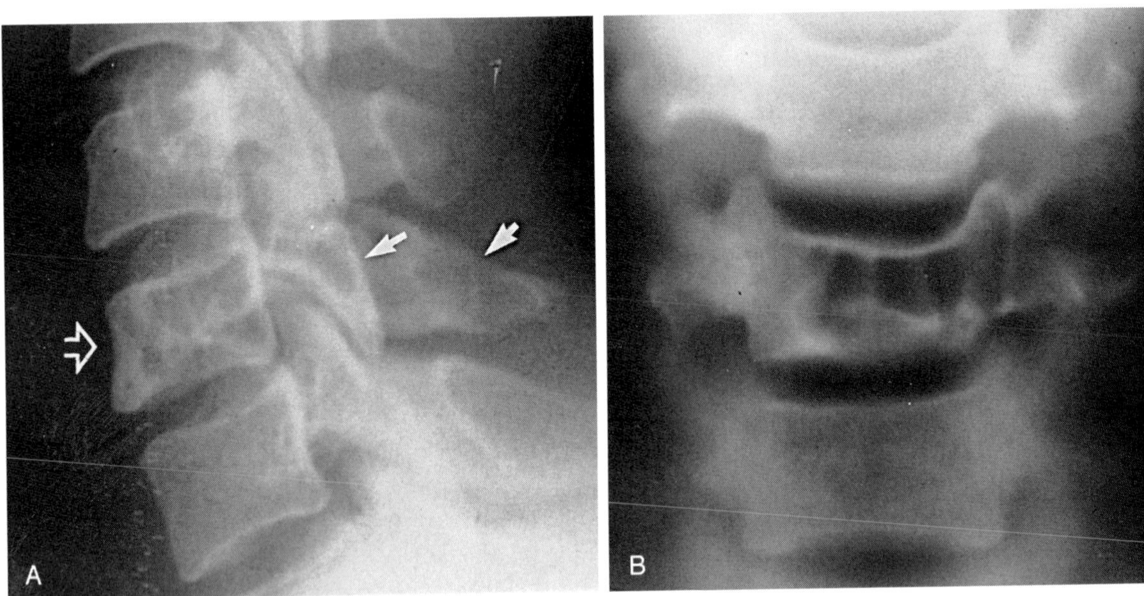

FIGURE 2–95. Fibrous dysplasia.[122] A Lateral radiograph demonstrates trabecular alterations of the C6 vertebral body (open arrow) and neural arch (arrows), with areas of osteolysis and osteosclerosis. B Frontal conventional tomogram more clearly delineates the osteolytic, multilocular appearance of the lesion. Pathologic collapse has occurred.

Spinal involvement is infrequent in polyostotic fibrous dysplasia, and it is even more rare in monostotic disease.

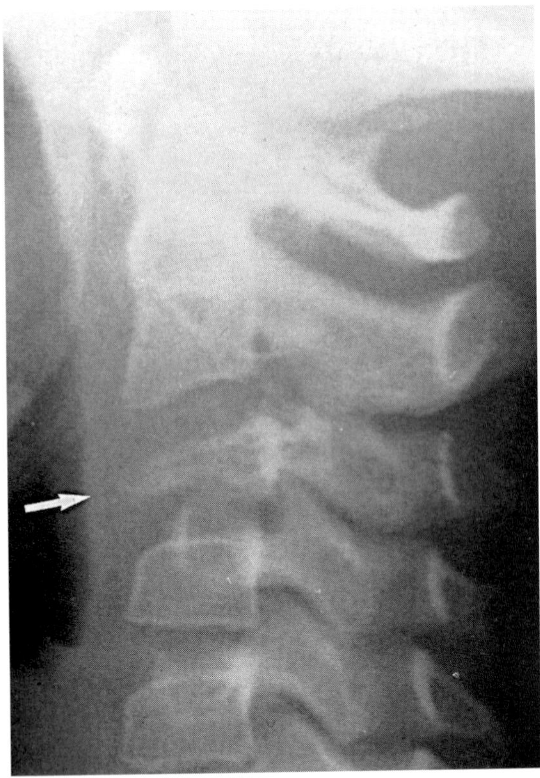

FIGURE 2–96. Langerhans' cell histiocytosis: Eosinophilic granuloma.[123, 124] In this 6-year-old girl, a characteristic flattened C3 vertebral body (vertebra plana) is observed (arrow). *(Courtesy of L. Danzig, M.D., Santa Ana, California.)*

TABLE 2–15. Metabolic Disorders Affecting the Cervical Spine*

Entity	Figure(s)	Characteristics
Generalized osteoporosis[125, 126]	2–97	Uniform decrease in radiodensity, thinning of vertebral end plates, accentuation of vertical trabeculae, and fish vertebrae Most vertebral fractures occur in the thoracolumbar spine Routine radiographs may suggest the presence of osteoporosis, but bone densitometry is necessary for accurate assessment of the presence and extent of diminished bone mineral content See Chapters 1, 4, and 7 for more extensive discussions of osteoporosis
Osteomalacia[127]		Diminished radiodensity and prominent coarsened trabeculae Vertebral body fractures
Hyperparathyroidism and renal osteodystrophy[127]		Subchondral resorption at discovertebral junctions Rugger-jersey spine: bandlike sclerosis adjacent to superior and inferior surfaces of the vertebral body Vertebral fracture with biconcave deformities (more prominent in thoracolumbar spine)
Acromegaly[128]	2–98	Elongation and widening of the vertebral bodies, less common in the cervical than in the thoracic and lumbar regions Ossification of the anterior portion of the disc and posterior scalloping of vertebral bodies occur infrequently
Fluorosis[129]	2–99	Diffuse osteosclerosis and ossification of the posterior longitudinal ligament are the predominant spinal findings Prominent osteophytosis and periostitis also may be encountered Differential diagnosis includes DISH, osteopetrosis, skeletal metastasis, and other causes of diffuse osteosclerosis

*See also Table 1–13.

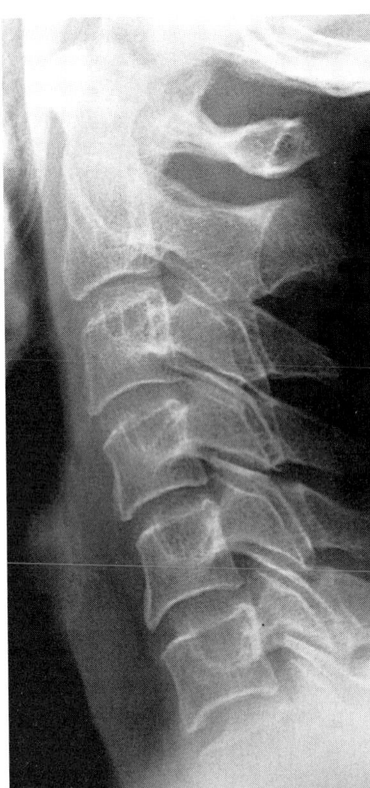

FIGURE 2–97. Generalized osteoporosis.[125, 126] Marked thinning of the cortical margins and increased radiolucency of the vertebral bodies and posterior elements are seen in this 55-year-old postmenopausal woman. Although radiographs are relatively insensitive to changes in bone density, they may suggest the presence of osteopenia.

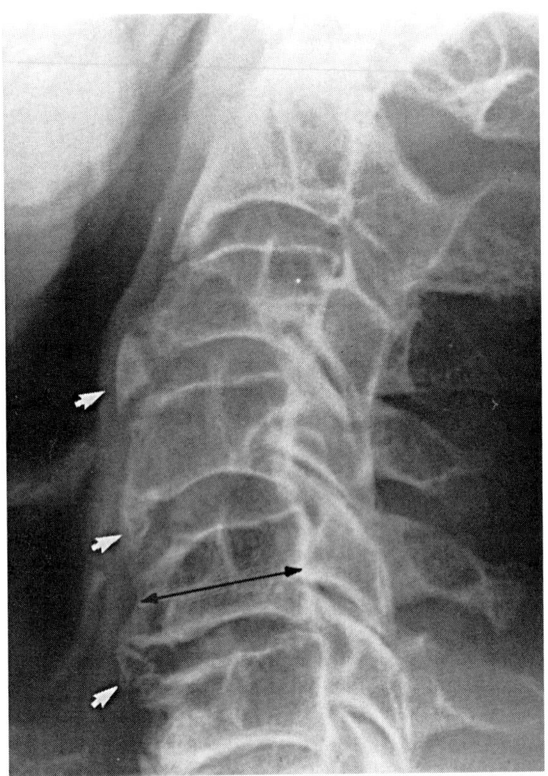

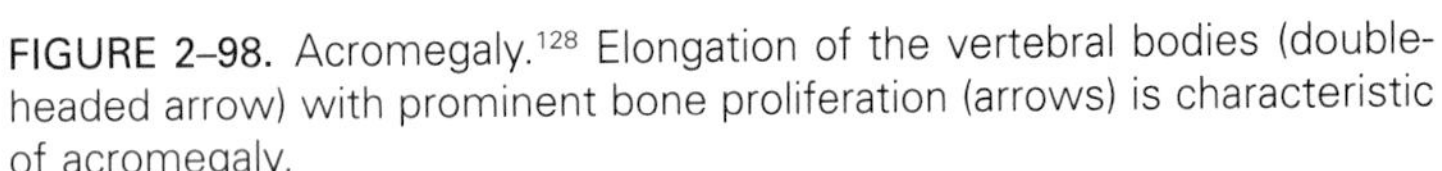

FIGURE 2–98. Acromegaly.[128] Elongation of the vertebral bodies (double-headed arrow) with prominent bone proliferation (arrows) is characteristic of acromegaly.

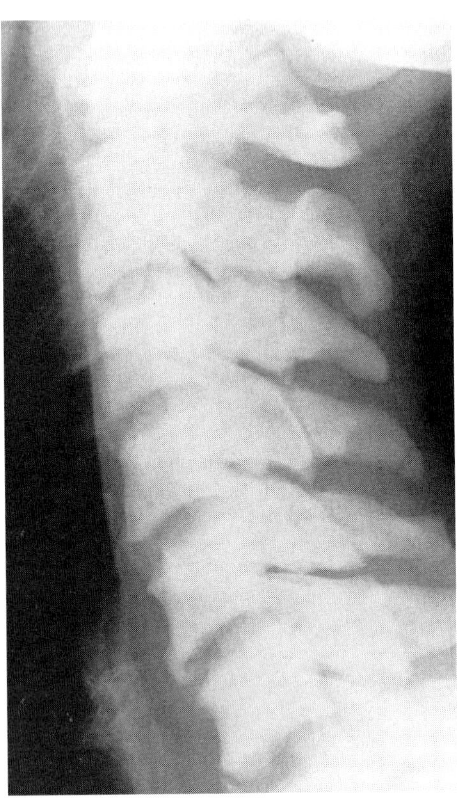

FIGURE 2–99. Fluorosis.[129] Observe the extensive ossification of the paraspinal ligaments and the generalized increased radiodensity of the spine in this patient with fluoride poisoning. *(Courtesy of G. Beauregard, Montreal, Quebec, Canada.)*

TABLE 2–16. Cervical Intervertebral Disc Abnormalities

Entity	Figure(s), Table(s)	Characteristics
Acute disc herniation[130]	2–100	Peak prevalence is in the third and fourth decades of life Patients may have radiculopathy, neck pain, or myelopathy Most frequent sites are C6-C7 (60 to 75 per cent) and C5-C6 (20 to 30 per cent) Uncalcified (soft) disc herniations are not visible on plain radiographs; best imaged using magnetic resonance (MR) imaging, computed tomography (CT), or CT myelography Two major types identified: Central (median) and foraminal (paramedian) *Central disc herniation:* Central disc herniations may be compressive or noncompressive. Often those that compress the thecal sac may be as large as 3 to 5 mm without causing significant symptoms, such as radiculopathy Larger central herniations may compress the thecal sac and nerve roots, contributing to significant stenosis and resulting in radiculopathy or even myelopathy *Foraminal disc herniation:* Lateral protrusions of disc material Owing to limited space within the nerve root canal, these herniations more frequently result in nerve root compression and radiculopathy than do central lesions Foraminal herniations may be more difficult to visualize than central lesions on MR images because of volume averaging and decreased conspicuousness within the nerve root canal Differentiation of disc herniations from degenerative osteophytes arising from the posterior discovertebral margins and uncovertebral joints may be difficult on MR imaging and myelography
Chronic cervical spondylosis[68–73]	2–61	See also earlier discussion (degenerative diseases) Degenerative disc disease (spondylosis) is very common in elderly patients and usually is asymptomatic Chronic degeneration leading to posterior discovertebral, apophyseal, and uncovertebral marginal osteophytes may result in spinal stenosis, foraminal encroachment, and compression of cervical nerve roots (radiculopathy) or cord (myelopathy) Patients with degenerative (or congenital) stenosis are much more likely to develop myelopathy and are more susceptible to cord or nerve root damage from minor trauma MR imaging interpretation tends to overestimate the degree of foraminal stenosis

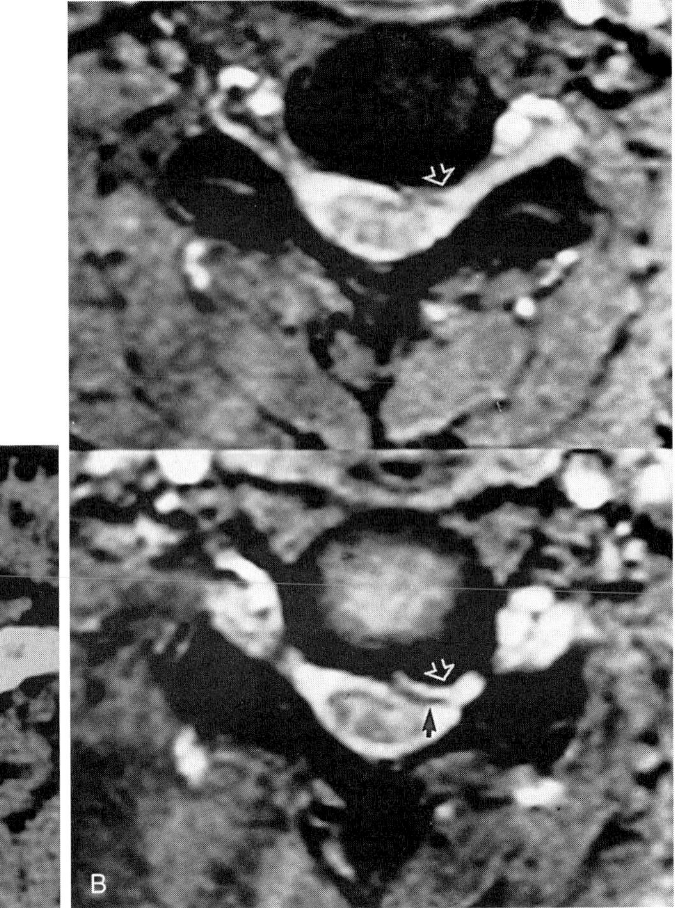

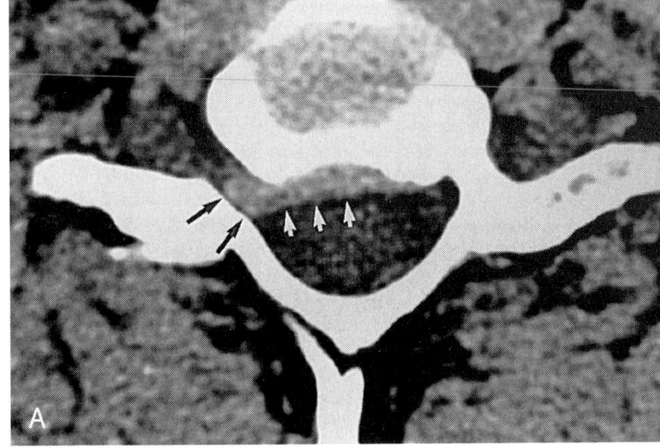

FIGURE 2–100. Intervertebral disc herniation.[130] A Computed tomographic (CT) abnormalities: Transaxial soft tissue window computed tomographic (CT) image shows a right paramedian foraminal disc protrusion (white arrows) with herniation of disc material into the right nerve root canal (black arrows). With the advent of magnetic resonance (MR) imaging, CT scanning has taken on a secondary role in the evaluation of disc protrusions. *(A, Courtesy of J. Haller, M.D., Vienna, Austria.)* B Magnetic resonance (MR) imaging abnormalities: This 40-year-old man developed left upper extremity weakness and radiculopathy. Transaxial gradient echo T2-weighted (TR/TE/flip angle, 500/20/30 degrees) MR images reveal a left C5-C6 posterolateral disc herniation. This lesion displaces the posterior longitudinal ligament (arrow), compresses and displaces the thecal sac, and obliterates the nerve root canal. Uncovertebral joint osteophytes are evident (open arrows) and contributed, with the disc herniation, to foraminal stenosis. Subsequent discectomy and fusion resulted in complete recovery. *(B, Courtesy of B. Carson, D.C., Kamloops, British Columbia, Canada.)*

TABLE 2–17. Cervical Spine Surgery

Entity	Figure(s)	Indications	Complications
Spinal fusion[131, 132]	2–101, 2–102	Disc pathology Fracture with instability Atlantoaxial instability Unstable developmental anomalies	Spinal cord compression Thecal sac encroachment Screw malpositioning Fracture or displacement of screw, plate, or wire Graft dislodgment Osteomyelitis Postoperative kyphosis Failed interbody plug fusion Pseudarthrosis Postoperative prevertebral swelling Epidural hematoma Cerebrospinal fluid leak
Laminectomy[133]	2–103	Decompression for spinal stenosis	Postlaminectomy instability Postlaminectomy kyphosis

Adapted from Pathria MN, Garfin SR: Imaging after spine surgery. *In* Resnick D (Ed): Diagnosis of Bone and Joint Disorders. 3rd Ed. Philadelphia, WB Saunders, 1995; Karasick D, Schweitzer ME, Vaccaro AR: Complications of cervical spine fusion: Imaging features. AJR 169:869, 1997.

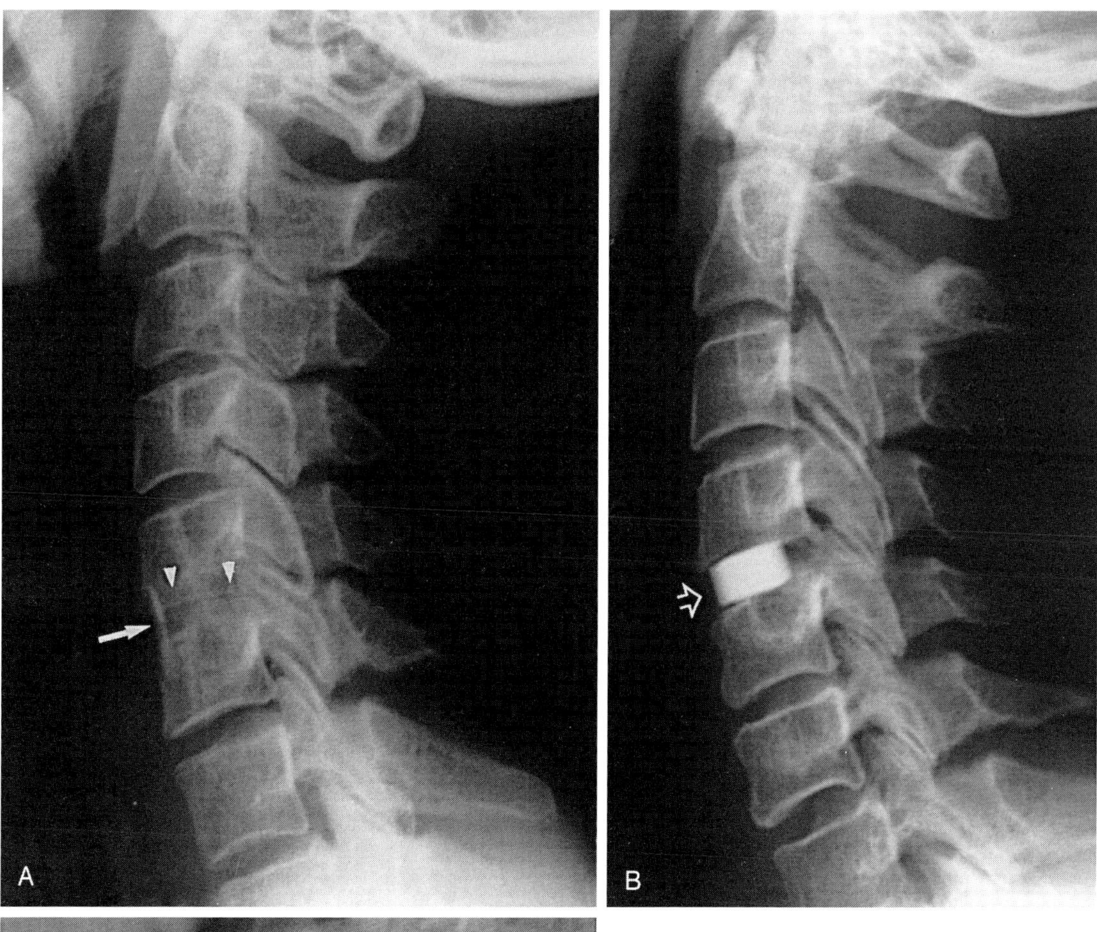

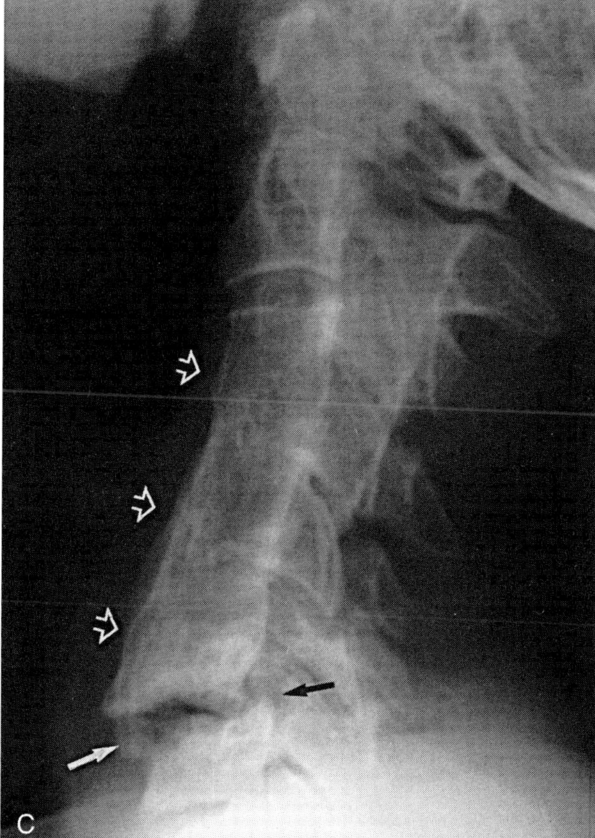

FIGURE 2–101. Spine surgery: Spinal fusion.[131, 132] A Anterior surgical fusion. Observe the thin linear zone of ossification representing successful bone graft between the C5 and C6 vertebral bodies (arrow). Cortical or cancellous bone graft material typically is harvested from the iliac bone. Note the relative preservation of the disc space and the obliteration of the vertebral end plates at the fusion site (arrowheads). B Hydroxyapatite (sea coral) graft. This patient had a C4-C5 discectomy followed by placement of a radiopaque interbody coraline-based hydroxyapatite graft (open arrow). Once incorporated into host bone, these constructs are structurally stronger than bone and function to maintain separation of the adjacent vertebral bodies after discectomy. C Multilevel anterior fusion. This patient had surgical arthrodesis of the C3-C6 levels (open arrows). Observe the degenerative disc disease with an intradiscal vacuum phenomenon and spondylolisthesis at C6-C7 (arrows). Accelerated degenerative changes are a common complication at spinal levels adjacent to levels of surgical or congenital spinal fusion.

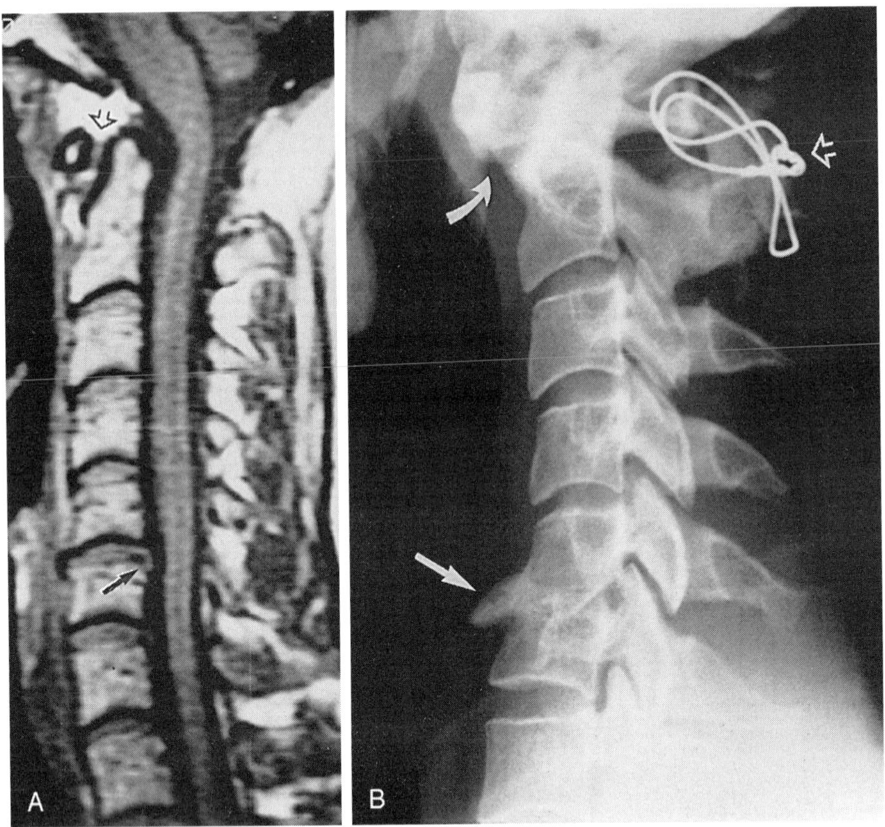

FIGURE 2–102. Spine surgery: Atlantoaxial fusion and C5-C6 discectomy.[131] **A, B** This 39-year-old man injured his neck while launching his boat, and he immediately developed upper extremity radiculopathy. Initial radiographs (not shown) revealed atlantoaxial subluxation and C5-C6 disc space narrowing secondary to disc degeneration. The atlantoaxial subluxation was determined to be related to a chronic tear of the transverse ligament that occurred many years earlier. In **A**, a sagittal T1-weighted (TR/TE, 600/20) spin echo magnetic resonance (MR) image reveals wide separation of the atlantodental interspace (open arrow) and a C5-C6 disc herniation (arrow). This patient subsequently underwent two separate surgeries: C5-C6 discectomy and atlantoaxial stabilization. In **B**, a postoperative radiograph shows the bone graft and wires from a Gallie procedure used to stabilize the atlantoaxial articulation (open arrow). The atlantodental interspace remains widened (curved arrow). In addition, graft material in the C5-C6 disc space has become dislodged anteriorly (arrow), which necessitated another surgical procedure to repair this complication. *(Courtesy of J. Upton, D.C., Victoria, British Columbia, Canada.)*

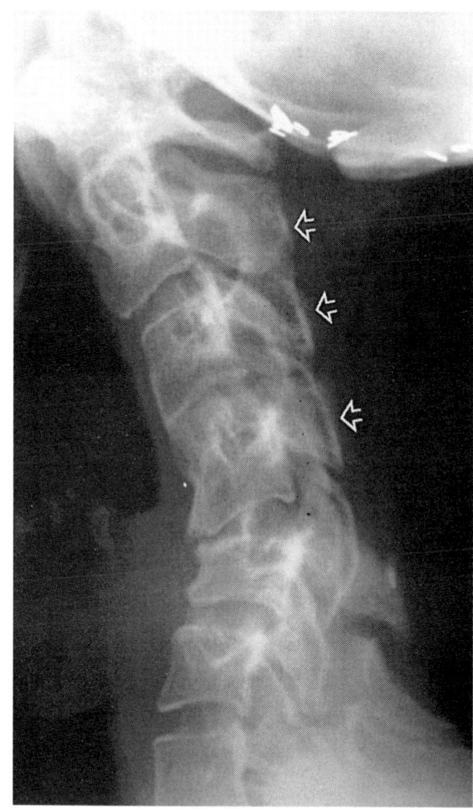

FIGURE 2–103. Postlaminectomy kyphosis: Swan-neck deformity.[133] This 28-year-old woman developed a severe kyphosis after multiple-level cervical spine laminectomies. The operation was performed to remove a benign intraspinal tumor that extended from the brain stem into the lower cervical spinal canal. The spinous processes and laminae of C2-C5 have been excised (open arrows), and an acute angular kyphosis is present at the C4-C5 level. This swan-neck deformity, which is seen in patients with multilevel laminectomies, presumably results from loss of posterior ligamentous and osseous stability and muscle weakness. *(Courtesy of B.F. Dickson, D.C., Vancouver, British Columbia, Canada.)*

TABLE 2–18. Vascular Disorders Affecting the Cervical Spine

Entity	Figure(s)	Characteristics
Carotid artery atherosclerosis[6]		Mottled calcification of the carotid arteries visible on frontal radiographs lateral to the spine Most common site is at the bifurcation of the carotid artery
Tortuous vertebral artery[134]		Tortuosity of the vertebral artery can occur in elderly persons as a result of aging and may result in erosion of the posterior arch of atlas, pedicles, intervertebral foramina, or foramen transversarium of axis May result in vertebrobasilar insufficiency MR angiography is helpful in the evaluation of the vertebral arteries
Vertebral artery aneurysm[6]	2–104	Rare occurrence in the vertebral artery: vessel dilatation and possible dissection May be congenital or occur secondary to atherosclerosis, infection (mycotic aneurysm), poststenotic dilatation, syphilis, or arteritis May result in vertebrobasilar insufficiency MR angiography is helpful in the evaluation of the vertebral arteries

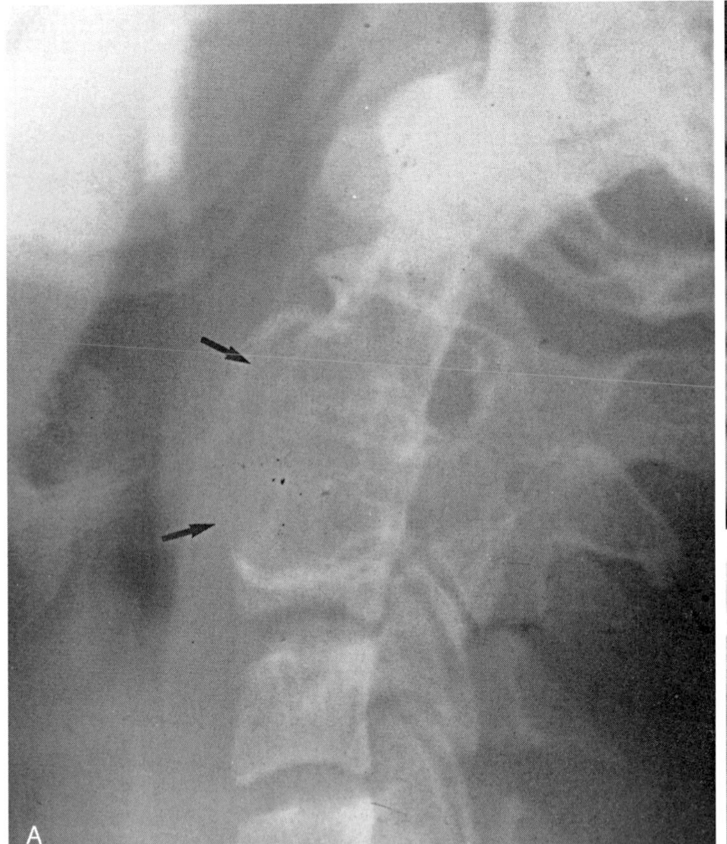

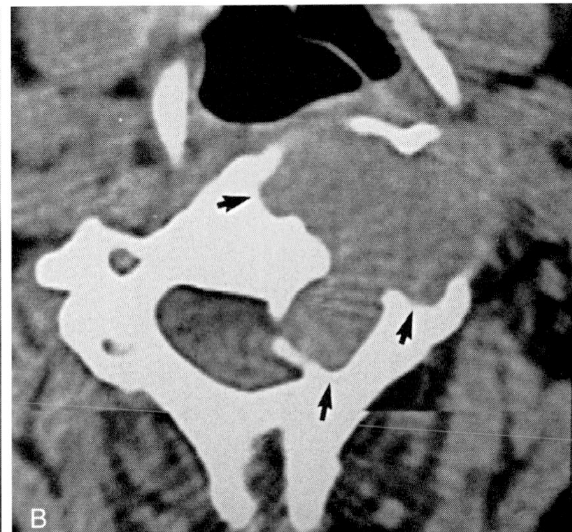

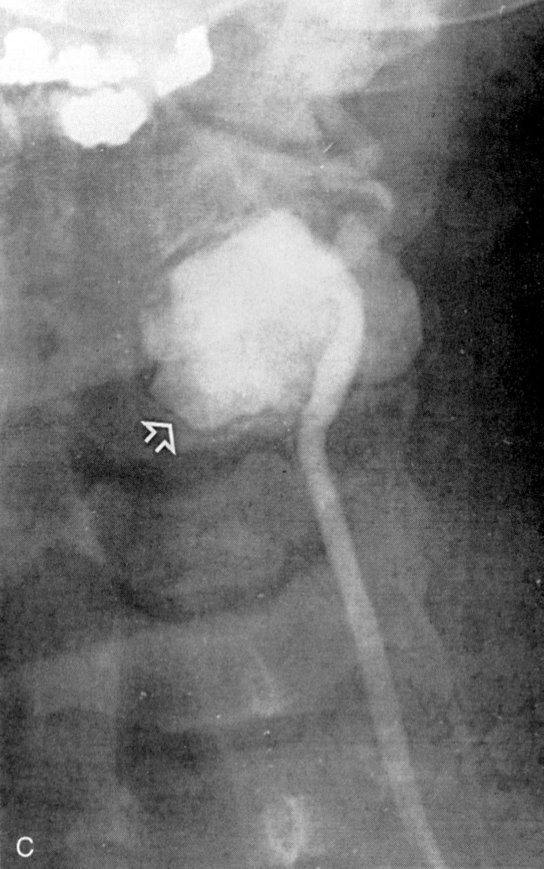

FIGURE 2–104. Vertebral artery aneurysm.[6] 17-year-old woman with a mycotic vertebral artery aneurysm. **A** A large, expansile, destructive lesion involving the C2 and C3 vertebral bodies is evident on this lateral radiograph (arrows). **B** A transaxial computed tomographic (CT) image reveals destruction of approximately one half of the vertebral body (arrows) with extension into the spinal canal. **C** A vertebral artery angiogram demonstrates a large lobulated collection of contrast material in the aneurysm (open arrow) that erodes the C2 and C3 vertebrae.

This rare condition occurs most frequently at the C1-C2 region. It often results in erosion of adjacent osseous structures, including the pedicle, transverse process, and vertebral body. Other causes of vertebral erosion are listed in Table 2–13.

REFERENCES

1. Edeiken J, Dalinka M, Karasick D: Edeiken's Roentgen Diagnosis of Diseases of Bone. 4th Ed. Baltimore, Williams & Wilkins, 1990.
2. Keats TE, Smith TH: An Atlas of Normal Developmental Roentgen Anatomy. 2nd Ed. Chicago, Year Book, 1988.
3. Greenfield GB: Radiology of Bone Diseases. 2nd Ed. Philadelphia, JB Lippincott, 1975.
4. Smoker WRK: Craniovertebral junction: Normal anatomy, craniometry, and congenital anomalies. RadioGraphics 14:255, 1994.
5. Keats TE: Atlas of Normal Roentgen Variants That May Simulate Disease. 6th Ed. Chicago, Year Book Medical Publishers, 1996.
6. Yochum TR, Rowe LJ: Essentials of Skeletal Radiology. 2nd Ed. Baltimore, Williams & Wilkins, 1996.
7. Köhler A, Zimmer EA: Borderlands of Normal and Early Pathologic Findings in Skeletal Radiography. 4th Ed. New York, Thieme Medical Publishers, 1993.
8. Gehweiler JA, Daffner RH, Roberts L: Malformations of the atlas simulating the Jefferson's fracture. AJR 140:1083, 1983.
9. Keats TE: Inferior accessory ossicle of the anterior arch of the atlas. AJR 101:834, 1967.
10. Daffner RH: Pseudofracture of the dens: Mach bands. AJR 128:607, 1977.
11. Ramos LS, Taylor JAM, Lackey G, et al: Os odontoideum with sagittal and coronal plane instability: A report of three cases. Top Diagn Radiol Adv Imaging 3:5, 1996.
12. Swischuk LE, Hayden CK Jr, Sarwar M: The posteriorly tilted dens: A normal variation mimicking a fractured dens. Pediatr Radiol 8:27, 1979.
13. Bohrer P, Klein A, Martin W III: "V" shaped predens space. Skeletal Radiol 14:111, 1985.
14. Tredwell SJ, Newman DE, Lockitch G: Instability of the cervical spine in Down syndrome. J Pediatr Orthop 10:602, 1990.
15. Riebel GD, Bayley JC: A congenital defect resembling the hangman's fracture. Spine 16:1240, 1991.
16. Swischuk LE: Anterior dislocation of C2 in children: Physiologic or pathologic? Radiology 122:759, 1977.
17. Cattell ES, Filtzer DL: Pseudosubluxation and other normal variations in the cervical spine in children. J Bone Joint Surg [Am] 47:1295, 1965.
18. Massengill AD, Huynh SL, Harris JH Jr: C2-3 facet joint "pseudo-fusion": Anatomic basis of a normal variant. Skeletal Radiol 26:27, 1997.
19. Chapman S, Nakielny R: Aids to Radiological Differential Diagnosis. 3rd Ed. Philadelphia, WB Saunders, 1995.
20. Applebaum Y, Gerald P, Bryk D: Elongation of the anterior tubercle of a cervical vertebral transverse process: An unusual variant. Skeletal Radiol 10:265, 1983.
21. Lapayowker MS: An unusual variant of the cervical spine. AJR 83:656, 1960.
22. Keats TE, Johnstone WH: Notching of the lamina of C7: A proposed mechanism. Skeletal Radiol 7:273, 1982.
23. Lovell WW, Winter RB: Pediatric Orthopedics. Philadelphia, JB Lippincott, 1978.
24. Karasick D, Schweitzer ME, Vaccaro AR: The traumatized cervical spine in Klippel-Feil syndrome: Imaging features. AJR 170:85, 1998.
25. Black KS, Gorey MT, Seidman B, et al: Congenital spondylolisthesis of the 6th cervical vertebra: CT findings. J Comput Assist Tomogr 15:335, 1991.
26. Adson AW: Surgical treatment for symptoms produced by cervical ribs and the scalenus anticus syndrome. Clin Orthop 207:3, 1986.
27. Som PM, Bergeron RT: Head and Neck Imaging. St. Louis, Mosby-Year Book, 1991, p 574.
28. Langlais R, Miles DA, Van Dis ML: Elongated and mineralized stylohyoid ligament complex: A proposed classification and report of a case of Eagle's syndrome. Oral Surg 61:527, 1986.
29. Kao SCS, Wazin MH, Smith WL, et al: MR imaging of the craniovertebral junction, cranium, and brain in children with achondroplasia. AJR 153:565, 1989.
30. Harding CO, Green CG, Perloff WH, et al: Respiratory complications in children with spondyloepiphyseal dysplasia congenita. Pediatr Pulmonol 9:49, 1990.
31. Thomas SL, Childress MH, Quinton B: Hypoplasia of the odontoid with atlantoaxial subluxation in Hurler's syndrome. Pediatr Radiol 15:353, 1985.
32. Holzgrave W, Grobe H, von Figura K, et al: Morquio syndrome: Clinical findings of 11 patients with MPS IV-A and 2 patients with MPS IV-B. Hum Genet 57:360, 1981.
33. Bridges AL, Kou-Ching H, Singh A, et al: Fibrodysplasia (myositis) ossificans progressiva. Semin Arthritis Rheum 24:155, 1994.
34. Kovanlikaya A, Luiza Loro M, Gilsanz V: Pathogenesis of osteosclerosis in autosomal dominant osteopetrosis. AJR 168:929, 1997.
35. Kahler SG, Burns JA, Aylsworth AS: A mild autosomal recessive form of osteopetrosis. Am J Genet 17:451, 1984.
36. Benli IT, Akalin S, Boysan E, et al: Epidemiological, clinical, and radiological aspects of osteopoikilosis. J Bone Joint Surg [Br] 74:504, 1992.
37. Joseph KN, Kane HA, Milner RS, et al: Orthopedic aspects of the Marfan phenotype. Clin Orthop 277:251, 1992.
38. Harris JH, Carson GC, Wagner LK: Radiologic diagnosis of traumatic occipitovertebral dissociation: 1. Normal occipitovertebral relationships on lateral radiographs of supine subjects. AJR 162:881, 1994.
39. Harris JH, Carson GC, Wagner LK, et al: Radiologic diagnosis of traumatic occipitovertebral dissociation: 2. Comparison of three methods of detecting occipitovertebral relationships on lateral radiographs of supine subjects. AJR 162:887, 1994.
40. Shapiro R, Youngberg AS, Rothman SLG: The differential diagnosis of traumatic lesions of the occipito-atlanto-axial segment. Radiol Clin North Am 11:505, 1973.
41. Fielding JW, Stillwell WT, Chynn KY, et al: Use of computed tomography for the diagnosis of atlantoaxial rotatory fixation. J Bone Joint Surg [Am] 60:1102, 1978.
42. Kowalski HM, Cohen WA, Cooper P, et al: Pitfalls in the CT diagnosis of atlantoaxial rotary subluxation. AJNR 8:697, 1987.
43. Mirvis SE: Atlantoaxial relationships: Questions and answers. AJR 170:1106, 1998.
44. Lee C, Woodring JH: Unstable Jefferson variant atlas fractures: An unrecognized cervical injury. AJR 158:113, 1992.
45. Suss RA, Bundy KJ: Unilateral posterior arch fracture of the atlas. AJNR 5:783, 1984.
46. Pathria M: Physical injury: Spine. *In* Resnick D: Diagnosis of Bone and Joint Disorders. 3rd ed. Philadelphia, WB Saunders, 1995, p 2825.
47. Hadley MN, Browner C, Sonntag VKH: Axis fractures:

A comprehensive review of management and treatment in 107 cases. Neurosurgery 17:281, 1985.
48. Effendi B, Roy D, Cornish B, et al: Fractures of the ring of the axis: A classification based on the analysis of 131 cases. J Bone Joint Surg [Br] 63:319, 1981.
49. Pech P, Kilgore DP, Pojunas KW, et al: Cervical spine fractures: CT detection. Radiology 157:117, 1985.
50. Gehweiler JA Jr, Osborne RL Jr, Becker RF: The Radiology of Vertebral Trauma. Philadelphia, WB Saunders, 1980.
51. Harris JH Jr, Mirvis SE: The Radiology of Acute Cervical Spine Trauma. 2nd Ed. Baltimore, Williams & Wilkins, 1995.
52. Fazl M, LaFebvre J, Willinsky RA, et al: Posttraumatic ligamentous disruption of the cervical spine, an easily overlooked diagnosis: Presentation of three cases. Neurosurgery 26:674, 1990.
53. Salamone JA, Steele MT: An unusual presentation of bilateral facet dislocation of the cervical spine. Ann Emerg Med 16:1390, 1987.
54. Scher AT: Unilateral locked facet in cervical spine injuries. AJR 129:45, 1977.
55. Shanmuganathan K, Mirvis SE, Levine AM: Rotational injury of cervical facets: CT analysis of fracture patterns with implications for management and neurologic outcome. AJR 163:1165, 1994.
56. Andreshak JL, Dekutoski MB: Management of unilateral facet dislocations: A review of the literature. Orthopedics 20:917, 1997.
57. Cancelmo JJ Jr: Clay shoveler's fracture: A helpful diagnostic sign. AJR 115:540, 1972.
58. Kim KS, Chen HH, Russell HJ, et al: Flexion teardrop fracture of the cervical spine: Radiographic characteristics. AJR 152:319, 1989.
59. Edeiken-Monroe B, Wagner LK, Harris JH Jr: Hyperextension dislocation of the cervical spine. AJR 146:803, 1986.
60. Bohrer SP, Chen YM: Cervical spine annulus vacuum. Skeletal Radiol 17:324, 1988.
61. Davis SJ, Teresi LM, Bradley WG Jr, et al: Cervical spine hyperextension injuries: MR findings. Radiology 180:245, 1991.
62. Cintron E, Gilula LA, Murphy WA, et al: The widened disc space: A sign of cervical hyperextension injury. Radiology 141:639, 1981.
63. Lee C, Woodring JH: Sagittally oriented fractures of the lateral masses of the cervical vertebrae. J Trauma 31:1638, 1991.
64. Miller MD, Gehweiler JA, Martinez S, et al: Significant new observations on cervical spine trauma. AJR 130:659, 1978.
65. Harris JH Jr: Acute injuries of the spine. Semin Roentgenol 13:53, 1978.
66. Lee C, Kwang SK, Rogers LR: Sagittal fracture of the cervical vertebral body. AJR 139:55, 1982.
67. Schaaf RE, Gehweiler JA, Miller MD, et al: Lateral hyperflexion injuries of the cervical spine. Skeletal Radiol 3:73, 1978.
68. MacNab I: Cervical spondylosis. Clin Orthop 109:69, 1975.
69. Wilkinson HA, LeMay ML, Ferris EJ: Roentgenographic correlations in cervical spondylosis. AJR 105:370, 1969.
70. Lestini WF, Wiesel SW: The pathogenesis of cervical spondylosis. Clin Orthop 239:69, 1989.
71. Goldberg RP, Vine HS, Sacks BA, et al: The cervical split: A pseudofracture. Skeletal Radiol 7:267, 1982.
72. Halla JT, Hardin JG Jr: Atlantoaxial (C1-C2) facet joint osteoarthritis: A distinctive clinical syndrome. Arthritis Rheum 30:577, 1987.
73. Fletcher G, Haughton VM, Ho K-C, et al: Age-related changes in the cervical facet joints: Studies with cryomicrotomy, MR, and CT. AJNR 11:27, 1990.
74. Wong CC, Pereira B, Pho RWH: Cervical disc calcification in children: A long-term review. Spine 17:139, 1992.
75. Suzuki K, Ishida Y, Ohmori K: Long term follow-up of diffuse idiopathic skeletal hyperostosis in the cervical spine: Analysis of progression of ossification. Neuroradiology 33:427, 1991.
76. Widder DJ: MR imaging of ossification of the posterior longitudinal ligament. AJR 153:194, 1989.
77. Kapila A, Lines M: Neuropathic spinal arthropathy: CT and MR findings. J Comput Assist Tomogr 11:736, 1987.
78. Boden SD, Dodge LD, Bohlman HH, et al: Rheumatoid arthritis of the cervical spine: A long-term analysis with predictors of paralysis and recovery. J Bone Joint Surg [Am] 75:1282, 1993.
79. Aisen AM, Martel W, Ellis JH, et al: Cervical spine involvement in rheumatoid arthritis: MR imaging. Radiology 165:159, 1987.
80. Espada G, Babini JC, Maldonado-Cocca JA, et al: Radiologic review: The cervical spine in juvenile rheumatoid arthritis. Semin Arthritis Rheum 17:185, 1988.
81. Azouz EM, Duffy CM: Juvenile spondyloarthropathies: Clinical manifestations and medical imaging. Skeletal Radiol 24:399, 1995.
82. Suarez-Almazor ME, Russell AS: Anterior atlantoaxial subluxation in patients with spondyloarthropathies: Association with peripheral disease. J Rheumatol 15:973, 1988.
83. Amamilo SC: Fractures of the cervical spine in patients with ankylosing spondylitis. Orthop Rev 18:339, 1989.
84. Killebrew K, Gold RH, Sholkoff SD: Psoriatic spondylitis. Radiology 108:9, 1973.
85. Halla JT, Bliznak J, Hardin JG: Involvement of the craniocervical junction in Reiter's syndrome. J Rheumatol 15:1722, 1988.
86. Resnick D, Pineda C: Vertebral involvement in calcium pyrophosphate dihydrate crystal deposition disease: Radiographic-pathologic correlation. Radiology 153:55, 1984.
87. Steinbach LS, Resnick D: Calcium pyrophosphate dihydrate crystal deposition disease revisited. Radiology 200:1, 1996.
88. Hall FM, Docken WP, Curtis HW: Calcific tendinitis of the longus colli: Diagnosis by CT. AJR 147:742, 1986.
89. Alarcón GS, Reveille JD: Gouty arthritis of the axial skeleton including the sacroiliac joints. Arch Intern Med 147:2018, 1987.
90. Justesen P, Andersen PE Jr: Radiologic manifestations in alkaptonuria. Skeletal Radiol 11:204:1984.
91. Osti OL, Fraser RD, Vernon-Roberts B: Discitis after discography: The role of prophylactic antibiotics. J Bone Joint Surg [Br] 72:271, 1990.
92. Dagirmanjian A, Schils J, McHenry M, et al: MR imaging of vertebral osteomyelitis revisited. AJR 167:1539, 1996.
93. Broom MJ, Beebe RD: Emphysematous septic arthritis due to *Klebsiella pneumoniae*. Clin Orthop 226:219, 1988.
94. Hsu LCS, Leong JCY: Tuberculosis of the lower cervical spine (C2 to C7): A report on 40 cases. J Bone Joint Surg [Br] 66:1, 1984.
95. Naito M, Ogata K, Nakamoto M, et al: Destructive spondyloarthropathy during long-term haemodialysis. J Bone Joint Surg [Br] 74:686, 1992.

96. Wong DA, Fornasier VL, MacNab I: Spinal metastases: The obvious, the occult, and the impostors. Spine 15:1, 1990.
97. Barwick KW, Huvos AG, Smith J: Primary osteogenic sarcoma of the vertebral column: A clinicopathologic correlation of ten patients. Cancer 46:595, 1980.
98. Mitchell M, Ackerman LV: Metastatic and pseudomalignant osteoblastoma: A report of two unusual cases. Skeletal Radiol 15:213, 1986.
99. Brien EW, Mirra JM, Kerr R: Benign and malignant cartilage tumors of bone and joint: Their anatomic and theoretical basis with an emphasis on radiology, pathology and clinical biology. 1. The intramedullary cartilage tumors. Skeletal Radiol 26:325, 1997.
100. Dahlin DC: Giant cell tumor of bone: Highlights of 407 cases. AJR 144:955, 1985.
101. Huvos AG, Higinbotham NL: Primary fibrosarcoma of bone: A clinicopathologic study of 130 patients. Cancer 35:837, 1975.
102. Dahlin DC, Coventry MB, Scanlon PW: Ewing's sarcoma: A critical analysis of 165 cases. J Bone Joint Surg [Am] 43:185, 1961.
103. Sudaresan N: Chordomas. Clin Orthop 204:135, 1986.
104. Kyle RA: Multiple myeloma: Review of 869 cases. Mayo Clin Proc 50:29, 1975.
105. Franczyk J, Samuels T, Rubenstein J, et al: Skeletal lymphoma. J Can Assoc Radiol 40:75, 1989.
106. Hermann G, Klein MJ, Fikry Abedlewahab I, et al: MRI appearance of primary non-Hodgkin's lymphoma of bone. Skeletal Radiol 26:629, 1997.
107. Clayton F, Butler JJ, Ayala AG, et al: Non-Hodgkin's lymphoma in bone: Pathologic and radiologic features with clinical correlates. Cancer 60:2494, 1987.
108. Epstein BS: Vertebral changes in childhood leukemia. Radiology 68:65, 1957.
109. Greenspan A: Bone island (enostosis): Current concept—a review. Skeletal Radiol 24:111, 1995.
110. Zwimpfer TJ, Tucker WS, Faulkner JF: Osteoid osteoma of the cervical spine: Case reports and literature review. Can J Surg 25:637, 1982.
111. Fielding JW, Ratzan S: Osteochondroma of the cervical spine. J Bone Joint Surg [Am] 55:640, 1973.
112. Karasick D, Schweitzer ME, Eschelman DJ: Symptomatic osteochondromas: Imaging features. AJR 168:1507, 1997.
113. Schmale GA, Conrad EV, Raskind WH. The natural history of hereditary multiple exostosis. J Bone Joint Surg [Am] 76:986, 1994.
114. Dahlin DC: Giant cell tumor of bone: Highlights of 407 cases. AJR 144:955, 1985.
115. Laredo J-D, Reizine D, Bard M, et al: Vertebral hemangiomas: Radiologic evaluation. Radiology 161:183, 1986.
116. De Dios AMV, Bond JR, Shives TC, et al: Aneurysmal bone cyst: A clinico-pathologic study of 238 cases. Cancer 69:2921, 1992.
117. Papagelopoulos PJ, Currier BJ, Shaughnessy WJ, et al: Aneurysmal bone cyst of the spine: Management and outcome. Spine 23:621, 1998.
118. Hadjipavlou A, Lander P: Paget disease of the spine. J Bone Joint Surg [Am] 73:1376, 1991.
119. Mirra JM, Brien EW, Tehranzadeh J: Paget's disease of bone: Review with emphasis on radiologic features. II. Skeletal Radiol 24:173, 1995.
120. Leeds NE, Jacobson HG: Spinal neurofibromatosis. AJR 126:617, 1976.
121. Mitchell GE, Lourie H, Berne AS: The various causes of scalloped vertebrae with notes on their pathogenesis. Radiology 89:67, 1967.
122. Resnik CS, Liniger JR: Monostotic fibrous dyplasia of the cervical spine: Case report. Radiology 151:49, 1984.
123. Stull MA, Kransdorf MJ, Devaney KO: Langerhans' cell histiocytosis of bone. RadioGraphics 12:801, 1992.
124. Kilpatrick SE, Wenger DE, Gilchrist GS, et al: Langerhans' cell histiocytosis (histiocytosis X) of bone: A clinicopathologic analysis of 263 pediatric and adult cases. Cancer 76:2471, 1995.
125. Michel BA, Bjorkengren AG, Lambert E, et al: Estimating lumbar bone mineral density from routine radiographs of the lumbar spine. Clin Rheumatol 12:49, 1993.
126. Genant HK, Engelke K, Fuerst T, et al: Noninvasive assessment of bone mineral and structure: State of the art. J Bone Miner Res 11:707, 1996.
127. Resnick D, Niwayama G: Parathyroid disorders and renal osteodystrophy. *In* Resnick D: Diagnosis of Bone and Joint Disorders. 3rd Ed. Philadelphia, WB Saunders, 1995, p 2036.
128. Mikawa Y, Watanabe R, Nishishita Y: Cervical myelopathy in acromegaly: Report of a case. Spine 17:1542, 1992.
129. Wang Y, Yin Y, Gilula LA, et al: Endemic fluorosis of the skeleton: Radiographic features in 127 cases. AJR 162:93, 1994.
130. Willing SJ: Atlas of Neuroradiology. Philadelphia, WB Saunders, 1995.
131. Karasick D: Anterior cervical spine fusion: Struts, plugs and plates. Skeletal Radiol 22:85, 1993.
132. Karasick D, Schweitzer ME, Vaccaro AR: Complications of cervical spine fusion: Imaging features. AJR 169:869, 1997.
133. Sim FH, Svien HJ, Bickel WH, et al: Swan-neck deformity following extensive cervical laminectomy. J Bone Joint Surg [Am] 56:564, 1974.
134. Kricun R, Levitt LP, Winn HR: Tortuous vertebral artery shown by MR and CT. AJR 159:613, 1992.
135. Shaw M, Burnett H, Wilson A, et al: Pseudosubluxation of C_2 on C_3 in polytraumatized children—Prevalence and significance. Clin Radiol 54:377, 1999.

CHAPTER 3

Thoracic Spine

- Normal Developmental Anatomy
- Developmental Anomalies, Anatomic Variants, and Sources of Diagnostic Error
- Skeletal Dysplasias and Other Congenital Diseases
- Alignment Abnormalities
- Physical Injury
- Articular Disorders
- Bone Tumors
- Metabolic and Hematologic Disorders

Normal Developmental Anatomy

Accurate interpretation of pediatric thoracic spine radiographs requires a thorough understanding of normal developmental anatomy. Table 3–1 outlines the age of appearance and fusion of the primary and secondary ossification centers. Figures 3–1 and 3–2 demonstrate the radiographic appearance of many important developmental landmarks at selected ages from birth to skeletal maturity.

Developmental Anomalies, Anatomic Variants, and Sources of Diagnostic Error

Many anomalies, normal variations, and other sources of diagnostic error encountered in the thoracic spine may simulate disease processes (Table 3–2) and result in misdiagnosis. This chapter describes most of the more common processes, which are shown in Figures 3–3 to 3–8.

Skeletal Dysplasias and Other Congenital Diseases

Table 3–3 lists a number of dysplastic and congenital disorders that affect the thoracic spine, and Figures 3–9 to 3–13 illustrate some of these manifestations.

Alignment Abnormalities

A wide spectrum of alignment abnormalities may be encountered in the thoracic spine. These include alterations of the normal kyphotic curve (Table 3–4) and several types of scoliosis (Table 3–5). Many of these conditions are illustrated in Figures 3–14 to 3–22.

Physical Injury

Fractures, dislocations, and soft tissue injuries involving the thoracic spine are frequent, and often they are are associated with serious clinical manifestations. Table 3–6 outlines the more important injuries of the upper, middle, and lower portions of the thoracic spine. The injuries are classified according to their most typical anatomic location and their presumed mechanisms of injury. The differential diagnosis of acute versus chronic compression fractures is detailed in Table 3–7. In addition, Figures 3–23 to 3–30 demonstrate the most characteristic imaging manifestations of common thoracic spine injuries.

Articular Disorders

The thoracic spine is a frequent target site of involvement for many forms of degenerative, inflammatory, crystal-induced, and infectious spondyloarthropathies and other articular disorders. Table 3–8 lists these diseases, and Figures 3–31 to 3–47 illustrate the characteristic radiographic manifestations. Tables 3–9 and 3–10 describe osseous outgrowths of the spine and terminology applied to ankylosing spondylitis.

Bone Tumors

A wide variety of malignant, benign, and tumor-like lesions affect the spine. Table 3–11 lists the neoplasms illustrated in this chapter in Figures 3–48 to 3–63. A more complete description of bone neoplasms is found in Table 1–10.

Metabolic and Hematologic Disorders

A number of metabolic disorders are manifest in the thoracic spine and are outlined in Table 3–12 and illustrated in Figures 3–64 to 3–70.

TABLE 3–1. Thoracic Spine: Approximate Age of Appearance and Fusion of Ossification Centers*[1–3] (Figs. 3–1 and 3–2)

Ossification	Primary or Secondary	No. of Centers	Age of Appearance (Years)	Age of Fusion (Years)	Comments
Neural arches (laminae)	P	2	Birth	1–1.5	Fuse together in midline in ascending order from T12 to T1
Vertebral body	P	1	Birth	4–5	Fuse to laminae
Spinous process	S	1	11–16	17–25	
Transverse processes	S	2	11–16	17–25	
Articular processes	S	4	11–16	17–25	
End-plate ring apophyses	S	2	11–16	17–25	Fuse to body

*Ages of appearance and fusion of ossification centers in girls typically precede those of boys. Ethnic differences also exist.
P, Primary; S, secondary.

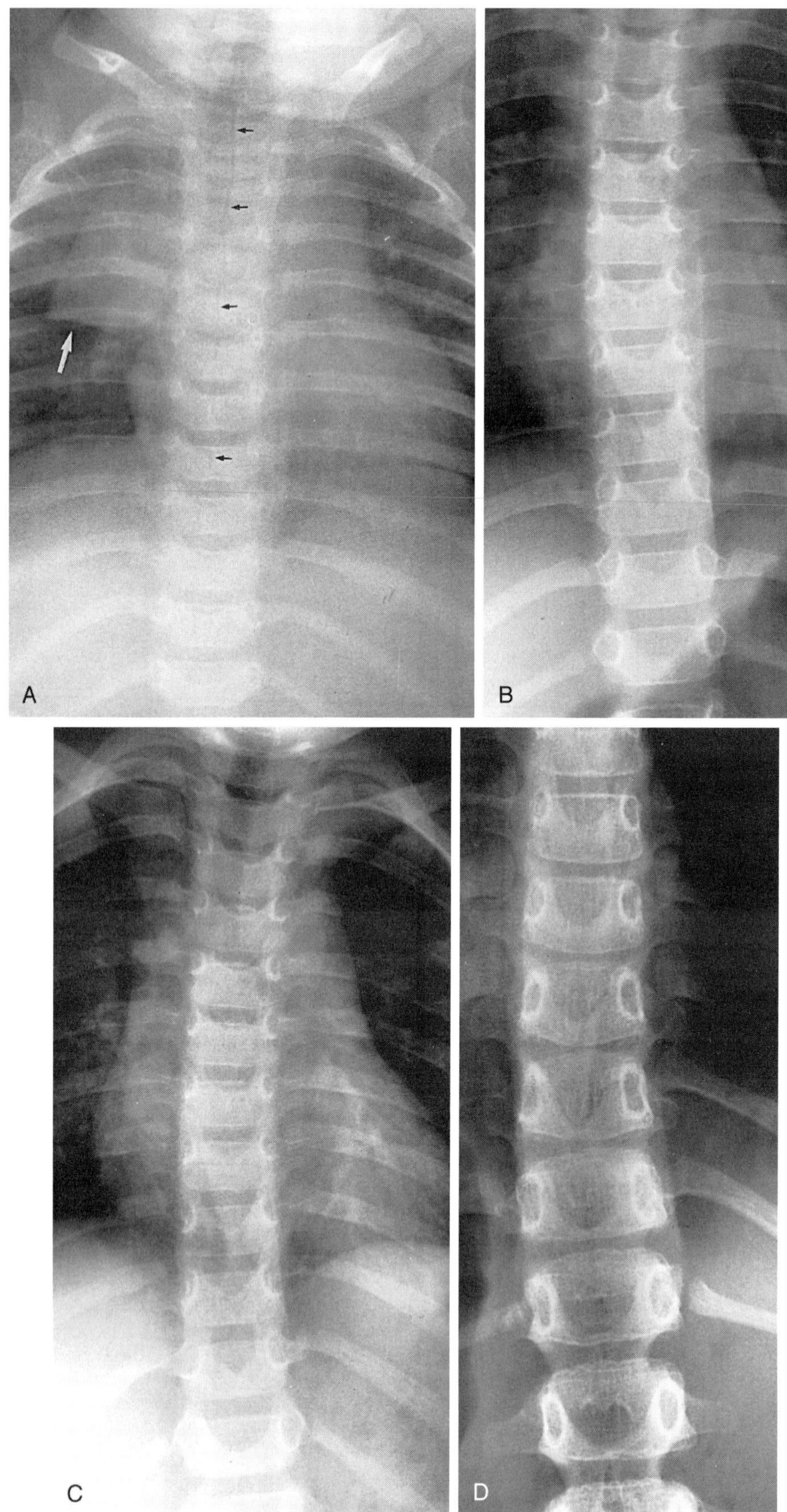

FIGURE 3–1. Skeletal maturation and normal development: Anteroposterior thoracic spine radiographs.[1–3] A 5-month-old boy. Observe the multiple midline radiolucent areas (black arrows) representing the unfused primary ossification centers of the neural arches. The neural arches usually start to fuse within the first year, beginning with T12 and progressing to T1 within the next 6 months. In this child, the lower thoracic centers have fused somewhat prematurely. The spinal canal appears proportionately wide, and a prominent thymus (sail sign) is evident (white arrow). B 3-year-old girl. The ossification centers of the neural arches typically fuse to the vertebral bodies about the age of 3 years. C 5-year-old boy. D 6-year-old girl. Irregularity of the superior and inferior vertebral body margins is common just prior to appearance of the secondary ring apophyses. The vertebral bodies are somewhat oval.

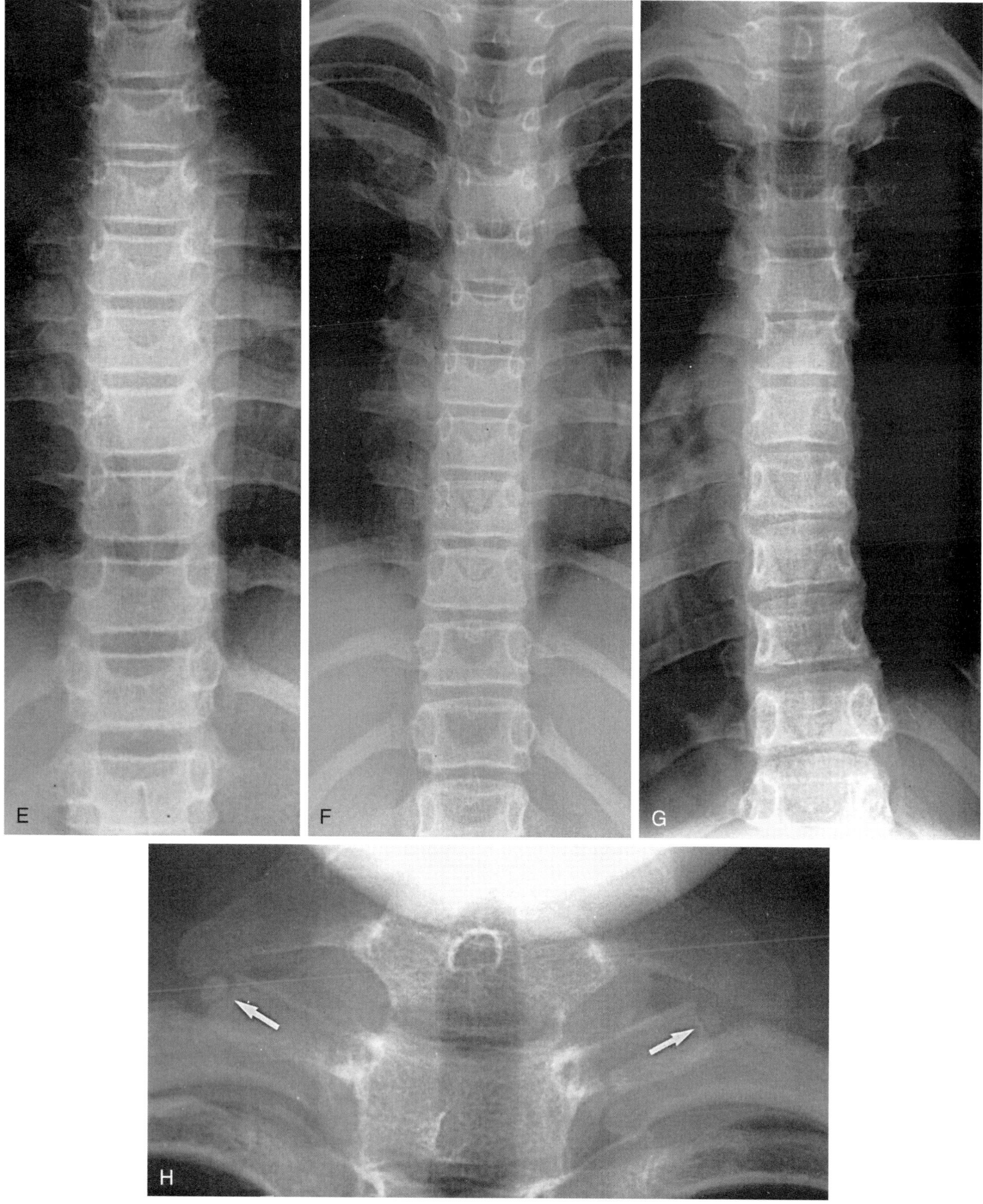

FIGURE 3–1 *Continued.* E 10-year-old boy. F 11-year-old girl. The vertebrae exhibit an adult configuration. G 13-year-old boy. The spine has an adult appearance. H 13-year-old girl. Observe the circular secondary ossification centers at the tips of the transverse processes of T1 (arrows). These centers usually appear at about the age of 16 years and fuse to the parent bone by the age of 25 years. The transverse processes of C7 are markedly elongated, a common developmental anomaly.

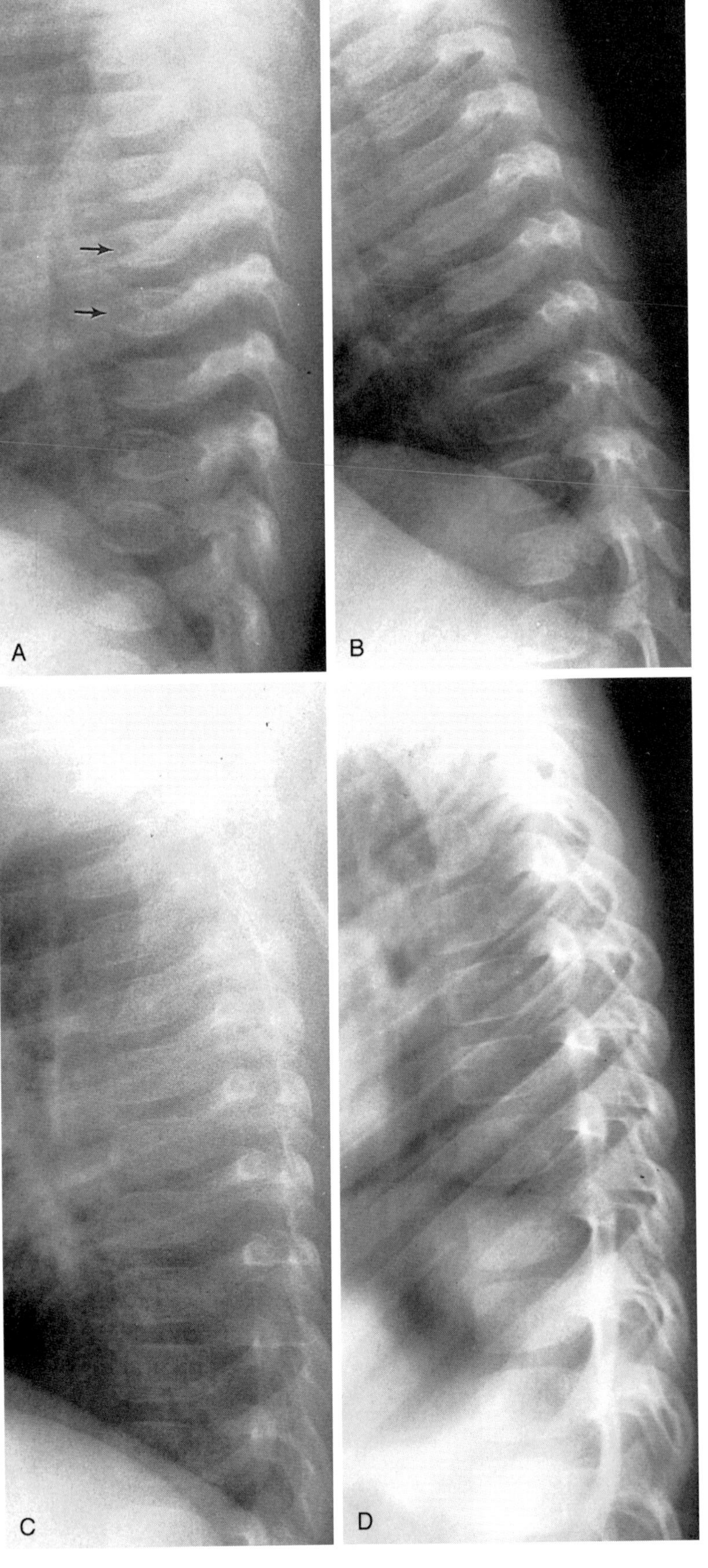

FIGURE 3–2. Skeletal maturation and normal development: Lateral thoracic spine and chest radiographs.[1–3] A 2-month-old boy. The vertebral bodies are oval, and prominent vascular notches (Hahn's venous channels) are present within the anterior margins (arrows). The neural arches have not fused to the vertebral bodies, and the spinal canal appears proportionately wide. B 5-month-old boy. The neural arches have not yet completely fused to the vertebral bodies. C 13-month-old girl. D 3-year-old girl.

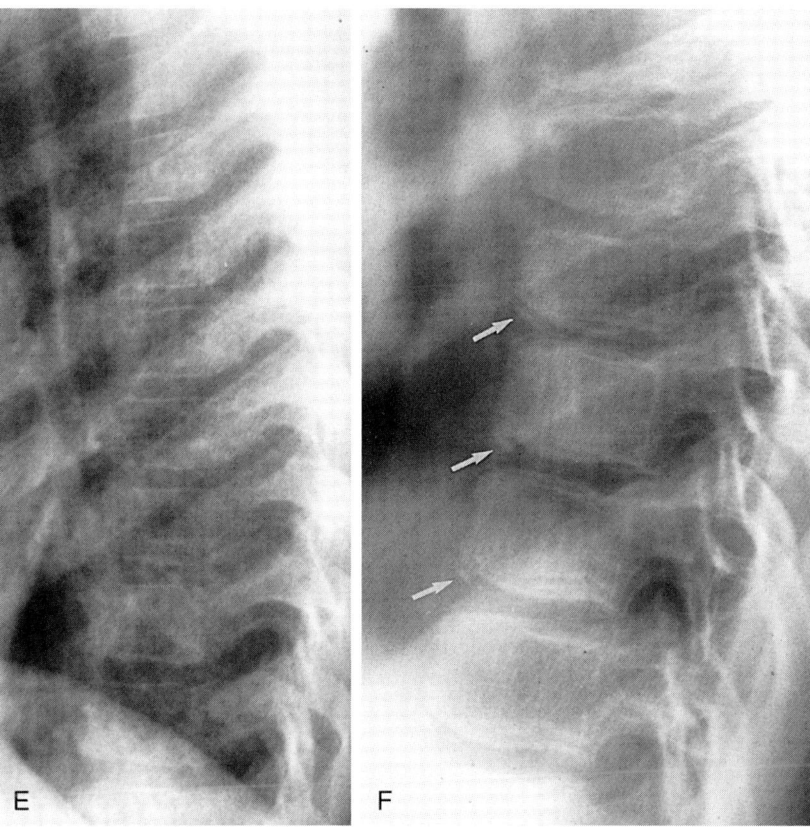

FIGURE 3–2 *Continued.* E 5-year-old boy. The vertebral body margins appear more square. The neural arches have fused to the vertebral bodies, a process that normally occurs between the ages of 4 and 6 years. F 13-year-old boy. The vertebral bodies are more rectangular. The secondary ring apophyses of the vertebral bodies have begun to appear (arrows). These typically begin to ossify at puberty, although such ossification may be apparent as early as 7 years of age. These secondary ring apophyses usually fuse to the vertebral bodies between the ages of 17 and 25 years.

TABLE 3–2. Developmental Anomalies, Anatomic Variants, and Sources of Diagnostic Error Affecting the Thoracic Spine*

Entity	Figure(s)	Characteristics
Normal ring apophyses[4]	3–1 to 3–3	Normal vertebral body ring apophyses may resemble fractures or limbus vertebrae
Hahn's venous channels[5]	3–4	Normal anatomy: a central horizontal vascular groove or channel that traverses the vertebral body These channels are quite prominent beginning with the first year of life but tend to disappear with age; even when they persist into adulthood, they are of no clinical significance
Spina bifida occulta[6]	3–5	Extremely common developmental anomaly consisting of a midline defect within the neural arch in which the two laminae fail to fuse centrally at the spinolaminar junction Spina bifida occulta results in a radiolucent cleft or an absent spinous process, or both; it occurs most frequently at the L5-S1 and T11-T12 levels Seen as an isolated anomaly or in conjunction with other entities, such as congenital spondylolisthesis, cleidocranial dysplasia, or Klippel-Feil syndrome Cleft usually is occupied by strong cartilage and fibrous tissue and generally is of no clinical consequence Spina bifida may infrequently be associated with meningomyelocele, which represents protrusion of the meninges or spinal cord, or both; meningomyelocele may result in severe neurologic abnormalities
Hemivertebra[7, 8]	3–6; see 3–17	Vertebral body originally develops from paired chondral centers, which at a later stage form a single ossification focus that is separated transiently by the notochordal remnant into anterior and posterior centers *Lateral hemivertebra* results from failure of development of one of the paired chondral centers Lateral hemivertebra might involve a normally occurring vertebra or it might be supernumerary; one pedicle may be normal or enlarged and its counterpart at the same level may be absent or hypoplastic; the incomplete segment may articulate with or be fused to the adjacent vertebra Frequently results in congenital scoliosis and may be associated with segmentation anomalies *Dorsal and ventral hemivertebrae* result from agenesis of either the anterior of posterior portion of the growth center, respectively; these occur much less frequently than lateral hemivertebrae
Butterfly vertebra[8]	3–7	Incomplete fusion of the two lateral chondral centers of the vertebral body results in a central sagittal constriction of the vertebral body, which is seen on a frontal radiograph and is considered a variant of enchondral ossification Interpedicle distance of the butterfly vertebra may be widened, and the adjacent vertebrae usually remodel to conform to the shape of the butterfly vertebra
Synostosis (block vertebra)[8]	2–30, 4–6	Developmental failure of segmentation of vertebral somites with subsequent fusion of adjacent vertebrae Often results in premature degenerative disease at adjacent vertebral levels owing to excessive intervertebral motion above and below the synostosis Findings include waist-like constriction at the level of the intervertebral disc; complete absence of disc space or a disc represented by a rudimentary, irregularly calcified structure; total height of the block vertebra is less than expected from the number of segments involved; fusion of the posterior elements (50 per cent of cases) Differential diagnosis: surgical fusion or ankylosis from inflammatory arthropathy or previous infection
Tracheal cartilage calcification[7]	3–8	Normal physiologic calcification of cartilaginous tracheal rings; no clinical significance

*See also Table 1–1.

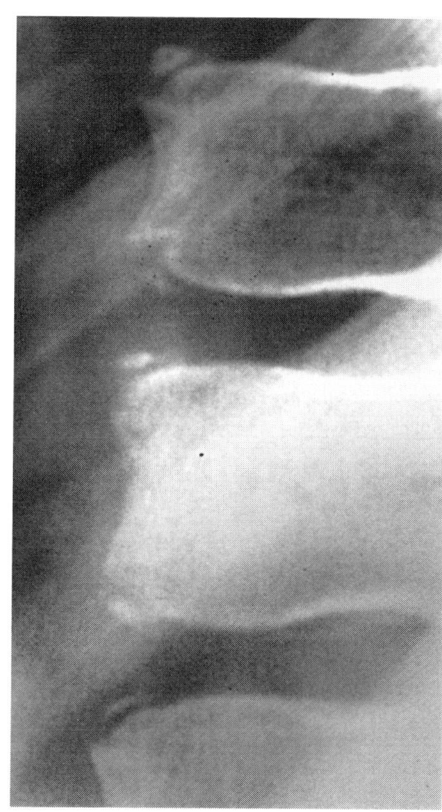

FIGURE 3–3. Normal ring apophyses.[4] Small triangular ossification centers are present at the anterosuperior and anteroinferior corners of the vertebral bodies in this 15-year-old boy. Notching and rounding of the adjacent corners of the vertebral bodies also are evident. This appearance of the normal vertebral body ossification centers should not be confused with fractures or limbus vertebrae.

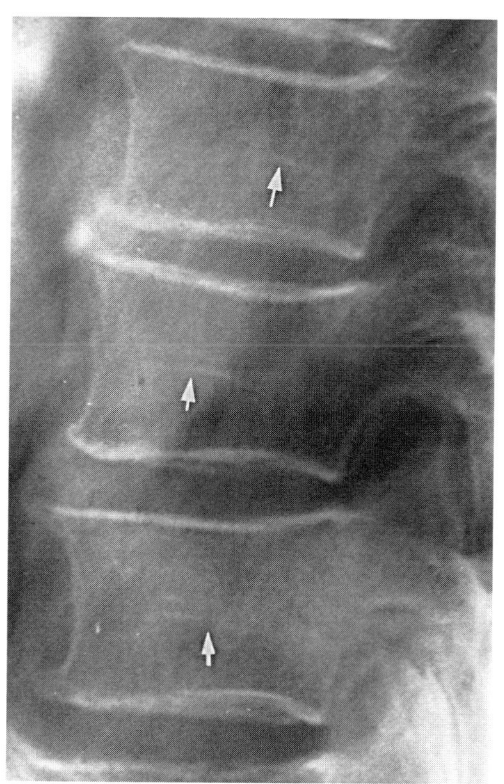

FIGURE 3–4. Hahn's venous channels.[5] Horizontal radiolucent grooves through the central portion of the vertebral bodies (arrows) are seen most frequently in the lower thoracic spine and represent residual venous sinus channels that accommodate vertebral veins.

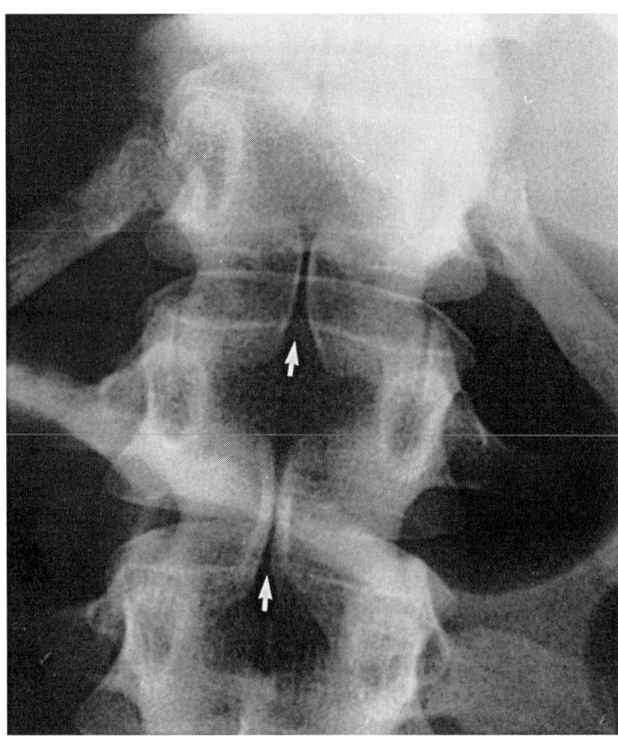

FIGURE 3–5. Spina bifida occulta.[6] Midline vertical radiolucent clefts in the thoracolumbar region (arrows) represent failure of union of the paired ossification centers of the neural arches.

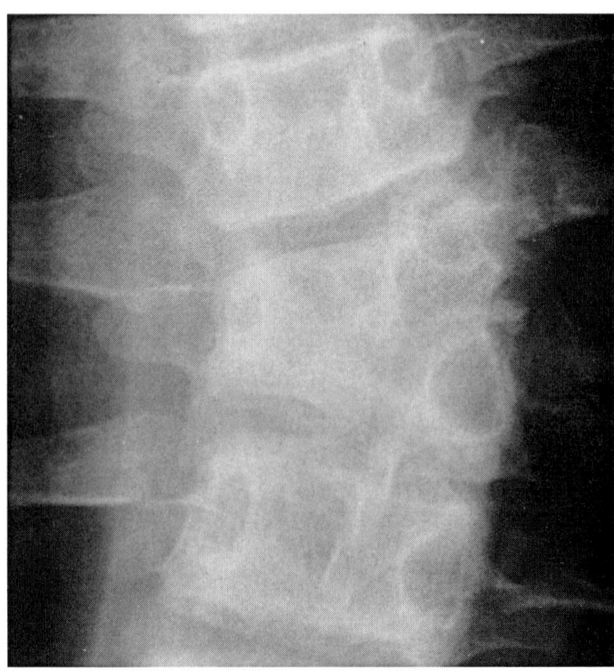

FIGURE 3–6. Lateral hemivertebra.[7, 8] Observe the triangular appearance of the vertebral body in the lower thoracic spine. The anomalous vertebra possesses two pedicles and costovertebral articulations on the left and one pedicle and costovertebral articulation on the right, resulting in a congenital scoliosis. *(Courtesy of A. Manne, D.C., Minneapolis, Minnesota.)*

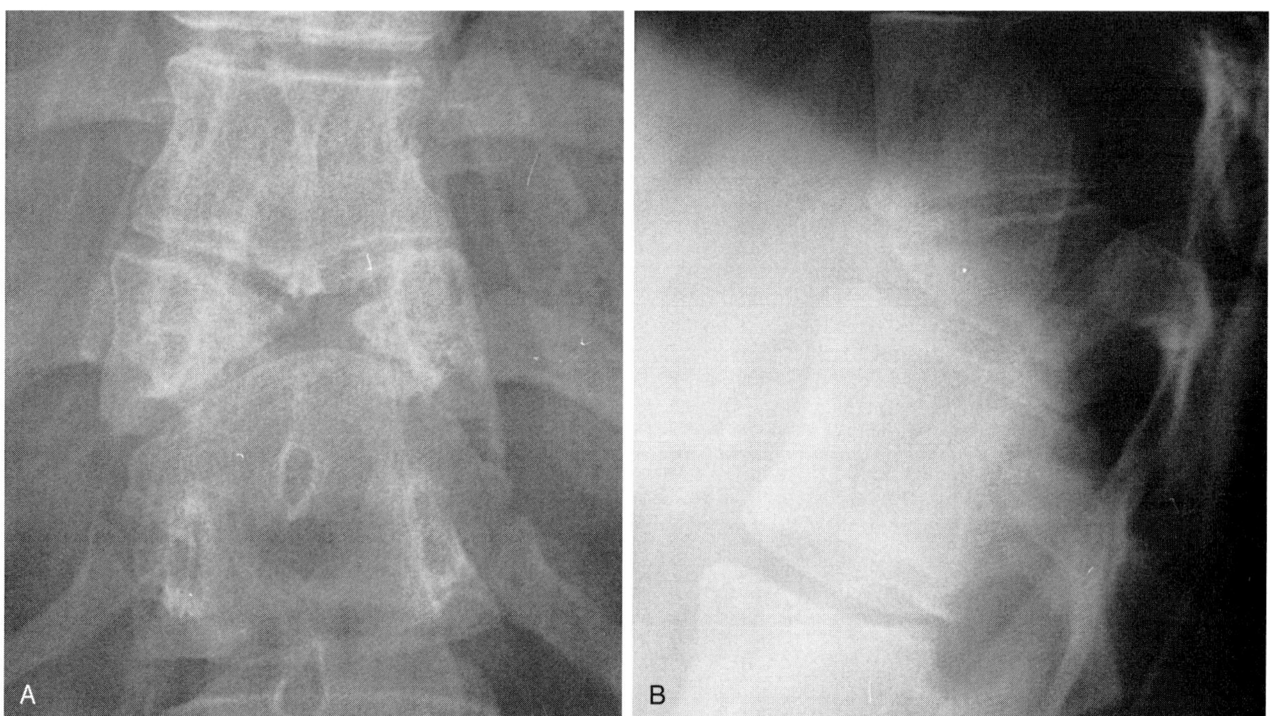

FIGURE 3–7. Butterfly vertebra.[8] Frontal (A) radiograph demonstrates a classic butterfly vertebra. The interpedicle distance is widened. A midline, vertically oriented sagittal defect in the vertebral body appears to divide the vertebra into two triangular segments, resembling a butterfly. The adjacent vertebral bodies have remodeled such that they appear to fit into the sagittal cleft defect much like the pieces of a jigsaw puzzle. This feature helps to distinguish butterfly vertebrae from vertebral body fractures. Lateral radiograph (B) reveals a tapered appearance of the vertebral body anteriorly.

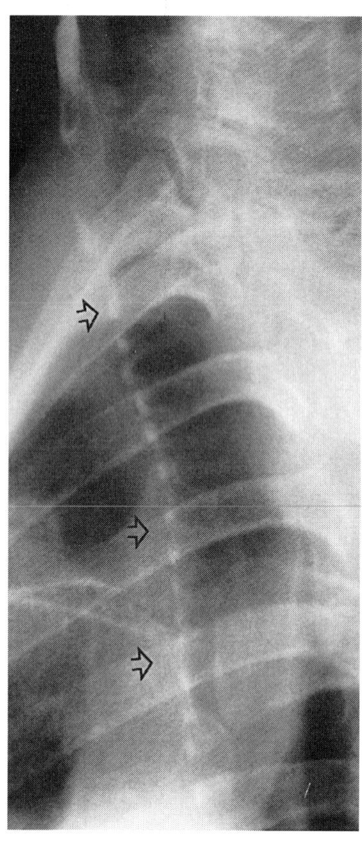

FIGURE 3–8. Tracheal cartilage calcification.[7] Extensive ringlike calcification of the tracheal cartilage (open arrows) is evident on an oblique radiograph from this 58-year-old woman. Such calcification is common in the elderly, is asymptomatic, and is of no clinical significance.

TABLE 3–3. Skeletal Dysplasias and Other Congenital Diseases*

Entity	Figure(s)	Characteristics
Achondroplasia[9]		Spinal stenosis Vertebral bodies may be flattened and may demonstrate posterior scalloping
Spondyloepiphyseal dysplasia congenita[10]	3–9	Platyspondyly and the "heaped-up" vertebral appearance in which the posterior aspect of the vertebral body is taller than the anterior aspect
Mucopolysaccharidoses (MPS)[11, 12]	3–10	Two types most frequently affect the thoracic spine: *MPS I-H (Hurler's syndrome):* Thoracolumbar gibbus deformity and posterior scalloping of vertebral bodies Rounded anterior vertebral body margins with inferior beaking *MPS IV (Morquio's syndrome):* Platyspondyly Posterior vertebral body scalloping and kyphoscoliosis
Osteopetrosis[13, 14]	3–11	Patterns of osteosclerosis: diffuse osteosclerosis; bone-within-bone appearance; sandwich vertebrae Bones are brittle and fracture easily
Osteopoikilosis[15]		Infrequently affects the spine Multiple punctate circular foci of osteosclerosis
Marfan syndrome[16]		Kyphoscoliosis in 40 to 60 per cent of persons Posterior vertebral body scalloping from dural ectasia
Osteogenesis imperfecta[17]	3–12	Osteoporosis and bone fragility Multiple compression fractures and severe kyphoscoliosis common
Chondrodysplasia punctata[18]	3–13	Stippled calcification of vertebral bodies Coronal clefts are present within the vertebral bodies of patients with the rhizomelic form

*See also Table 1–2.

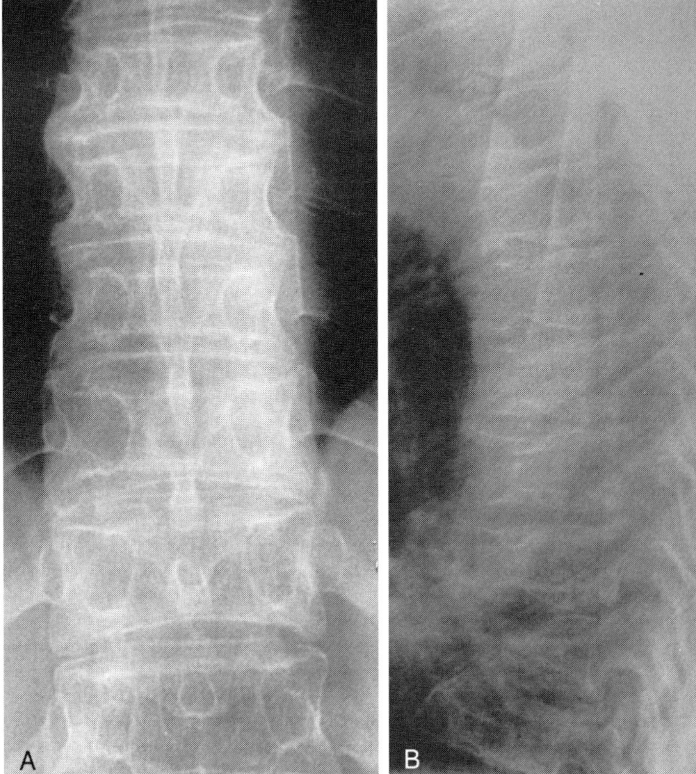

FIGURE 3–9. Spondyloepiphyseal dysplasia congenita.[10] Frontal (A) and lateral (B) routine radiographs reveal intervertebral disc spaces that appear narrow posteriorly and wide anteriorly owing to osseous humps that arise from the central and posterior portions of the vertebral end plates. This vertebral body shape is sometimes referred to as the heaped-up appearance. On the frontal view (A), the vertebral bodies appear flattened. These patients often have associated thoracic disc herniations.

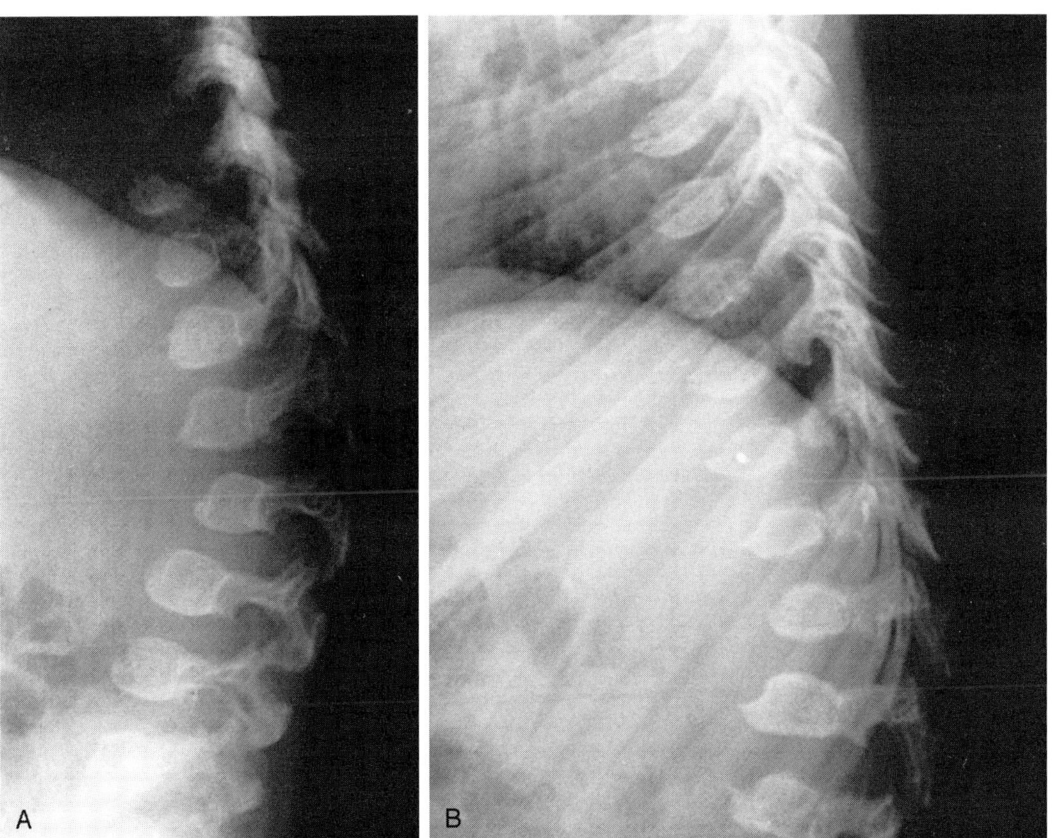

FIGURE 3–10. Mucopolysaccharidoses (MPS).[11, 12] A Hurler's syndrome (MPS 1-H). In this 3-year-old child, beaklike projections are noted arising from the anteroinferior vertebral bodies. A thoracolumbar gibbus deformity also is present. These two findings are characteristic of this rare autosomal recessive mucopolysaccharidosis. B Morquio's syndrome (MPS IV). This child is of short stature and has a thoracolumbar kyphoscoliosis. Characteristic central tonguelike anterior beaking and rounding of the vertebral bodies are observed. In adults, the vertebrae typically appear flat and rectangular, with irregular margins.

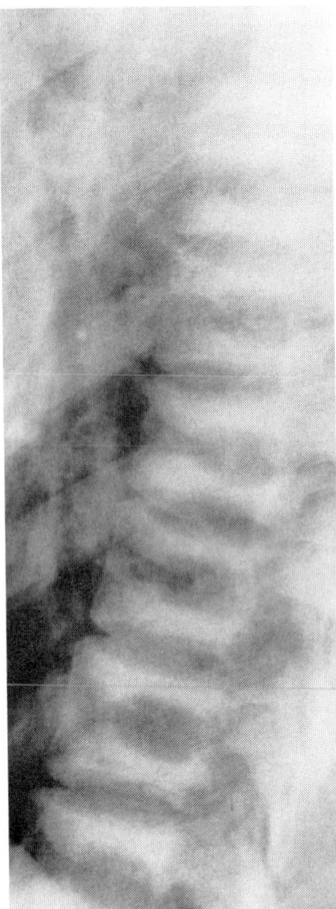

FIGURE 3–11. Osteopetrosis.[13, 14] Dense sclerosis is noted adjacent to the superior and inferior vertebral end plates of the thoracic spine in this patient. This pattern of vertebral sclerosis is described as "sandwich" vertebrae; however, diffuse sclerosis and the "bone-within-bone" appearance also may be encountered.

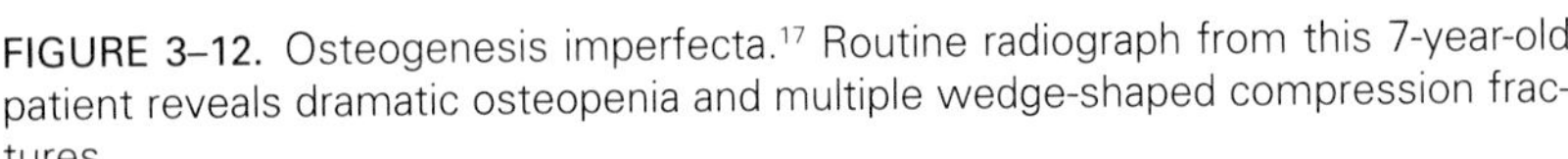

FIGURE 3–12. Osteogenesis imperfecta.[17] Routine radiograph from this 7-year-old patient reveals dramatic osteopenia and multiple wedge-shaped compression fractures.

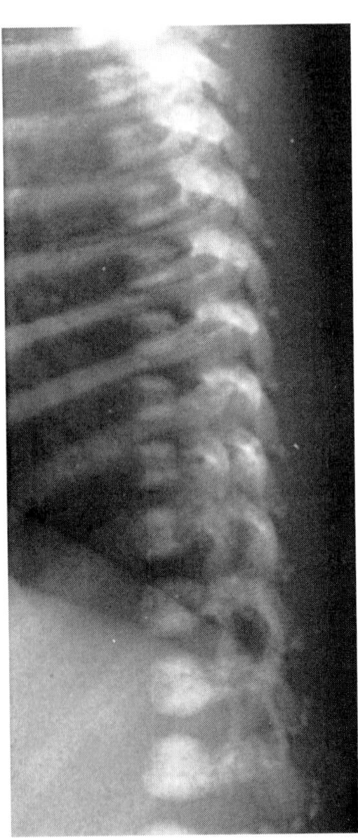

FIGURE 3–13. Chondrodysplasia punctata.[18] Radiograph from this 2-day-old infant shows the characteristic finding of stippled calcification of the thoracic vertebral bodies and neural arches. Several different forms of this rare multiple epiphyseal dysplasia have been identified.

TABLE 3–4. Alterations of Kyphosis

Entity	Figure(s)	Characteristics
Normal kyphosis[7, 19]	3–14 A, B	Modified Cobb method is used to measure the thoracic kyphosis Normal maximum kyphosis ranges from 36 to 56 degrees in women and 40 to 66 degrees in men; measurements tend to increase with age
Congenital kyphosis[8]		Agenesis or underdevelopment of the anterior portion of the vertebral body ossification center results in a dorsal hemivertebra and subsequent kyphotic deformity; less likely to be caused by failure of segmentation of the anterior portion of two adjacent vertebral bodies, forming a congenital bar
Senile kyphosis[19]	3–14 C	Kyphosis secondary to severe degeneration of the anulus fibrosus Occurs mostly in nonosteoporotic persons who are in their seventh and eighth decades Men > women
Osteoporotic kyphosis[19]	3–14 D; see 3–64	In older person, generalized osteoporosis results in wedging or collapse of the anterior aspect of the vertebral bodies, especially the T6 and T7 levels Women > men May also occur in Cushing's disease and other secondary causes of osteoporosis
Tuberculous spondylodiscitis[20]	See Figs. 3–46, 3–47	Thoracolumbar vertebral body collapse results in accentuated gibbus deformity and is seen in advanced tuberculous spondylodiscitis (Pott's disease)
Ankylosing spondylitis[19]		Advanced ankylosis and syndesmophyte formation result in exaggerated kyphosis and flattening of the lumbar lordosis
Thoracolumbar injury[21]	See Fig. 3–25	Thoracolumbar compression fractures, burst fractures, or other hyperflexion-distraction or hyperflexion-shearing injuries may result in accentuation of the thoracic kyphosis
Straight back syndrome[7, 22]	3–14 E	Flattening or reversal of the thoracic curve, which may alter intracardiac blood flow dynamics and be manifested as a functional cardiac murmur
Scheuermann's disease[23]	3–15; see 3–14B	Common form of osteochondrosis that usually begins between the ages of 13 and 17 years, and affects 4 to 8 per cent of the adolescent population, with a slight predilection for male patients Diagnostic criteria include involvement of at least three contiguous vertebrae, each with wedging of 5 degrees or more, multiple Schmorl's nodes, and undulating surfaces of the vertebral end plates Increased thoracic kyphosis is present in 75 per cent of patients; kyphosis may initially be correctable but may become progressively more fixed in position with age; other postural findings include increased lumbar lordosis or thoracolumbar kyphosis Many patients are asymptomatic; others may experience fatigue, aching back pain, stiffness, and discomfort usually occurring around the time of puberty; an increasd prevalence of scoliosis and disc displacement also has been noted Multiple Schmorl's nodes frequently are seen in patients with Scheuermann's disease, although the precise cause is unclear; factors that appear to play a role in some cases of Scheuermann's disease include: 1. stress-induced intraosseous disc, displacements through congenitally or traumatically weakened portions of cartilaginous end plate 2. osteoporosis during growth spurts 3. genetic factors 4. athletic activity
Gibbus deformity	See Figs. 3–10, 3–27, 3–28, 3–46, 3–47, 3–65	Acute angular kyphosis, typically affecting the thoracolumbar region, found in tuberculous spondylitis, hypothyroidism, achondroplasia, mucopolysaccharidoses, various other bone dysplasias, and some severe thoracolumbar flexion injuries

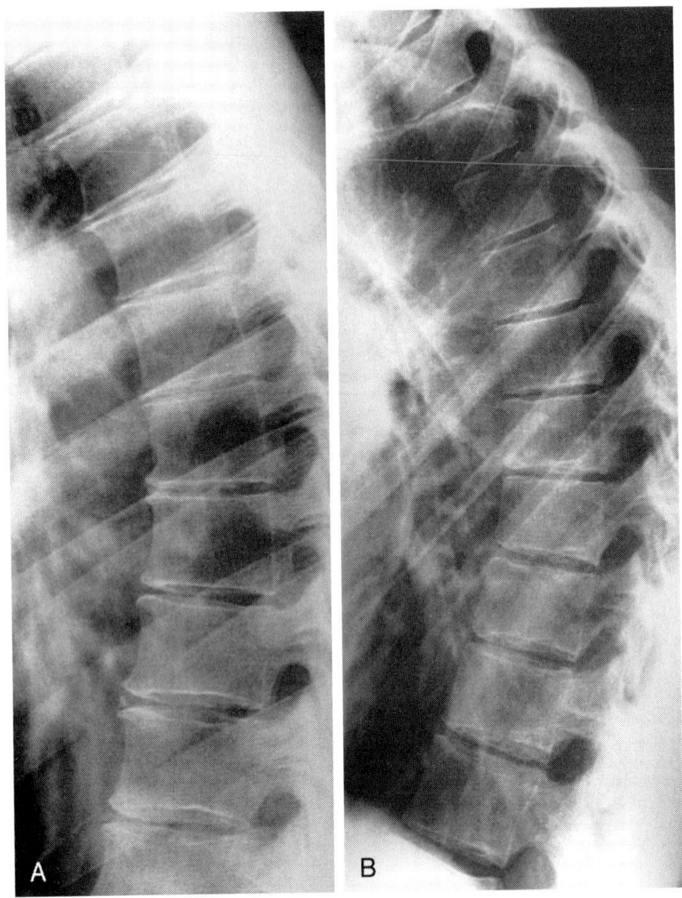

FIGURE 3–14. Thoracic kyphosis: Normal and abnormal appearance. A Normal kyphosis.[23] In a 37-year-old man, observe the normal thoracic kyphosis. In addition, early degenerative disc disease is noted, characterized by disc space narrowing, osteophytes, and calcification of the anterior annular fibers. B Scheuermann's kyphosis.[7, 19] In another patient, observe a slightly exaggerated thoracic kyphosis. Mild irregularity of the vertebral end plates represents Schmorl's cartilaginous nodes, and the findings are compatible with Scheuermann's disease.

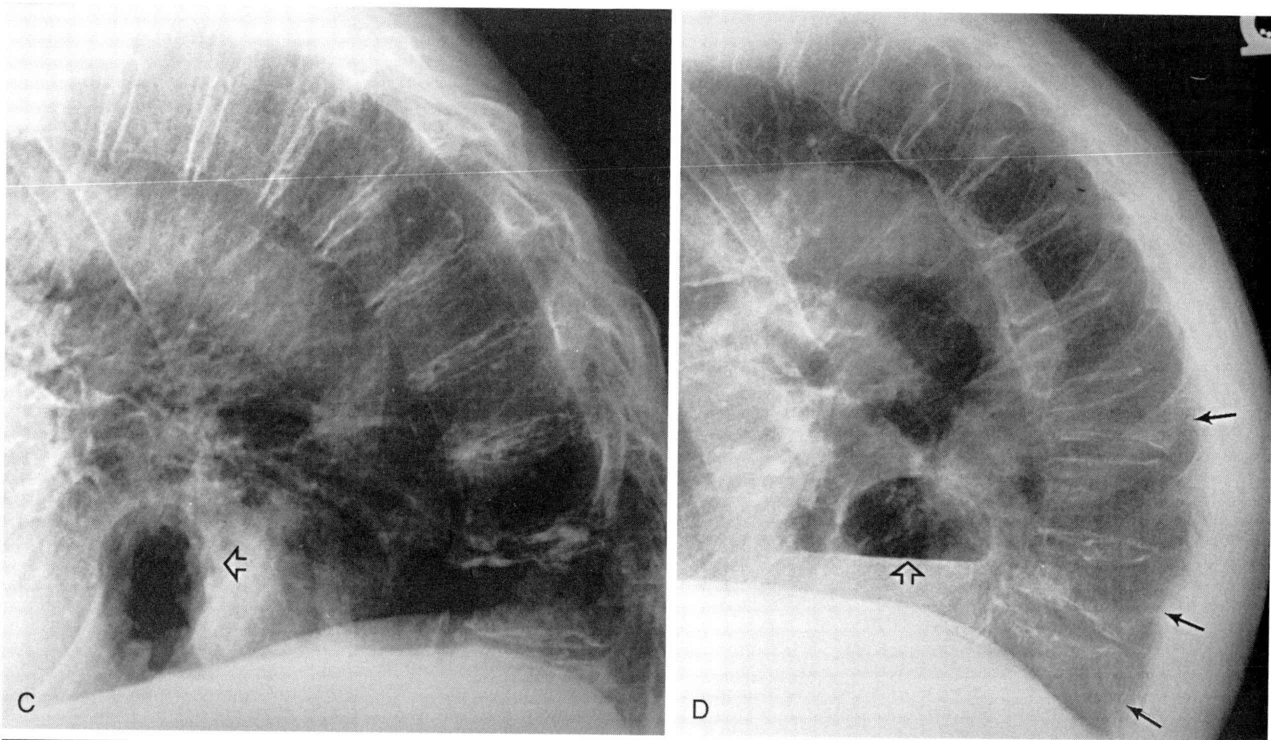

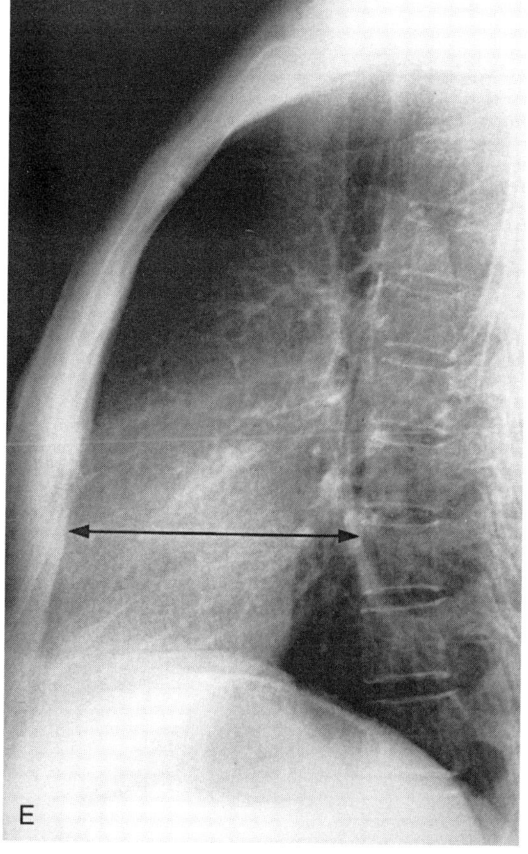

FIGURE 3–14 *Continued.* C Senile kyphosis.[19] This 73-year-old woman with advanced postmenopausal osteoporosis and concomitant degenerative disc disease with intervertebral disc calcification has dramatic kyphosis measuring 102 degrees. Although mild anterior vertebral body wedging is noted at several levels, no frank compression fractures are present. The air density in the mediastinum (open arrow) represents a hiatal hernia. D Osteoporotic kyphosis.[19] Severe kyphosis, anterior vertebral body ossification and multiple compression fractures (arrows) are evident in this 82-year-old woman. She also has osteoporosis and a hiatal hernia (open arrow). E Reversed kyphosis or lordosis.[7, 22] The thoracic spine of this 36-year-old woman has a lordotic, reversed kyphotic curve. This flattening of the thoracic kyphosis and the anteroposterior diameter of the chest may lead to a condition termed the straight back syndrome. In this syndrome, the sagittal dimension of the thoracic cage (double-headed arrow) measures less than 13 cm in men and 11 cm in women (on a 72-inch source-image receptor distance (SID) chest radiograph). Cardiac compression and a functional cardiac murmur have been identified in patients with this syndrome.

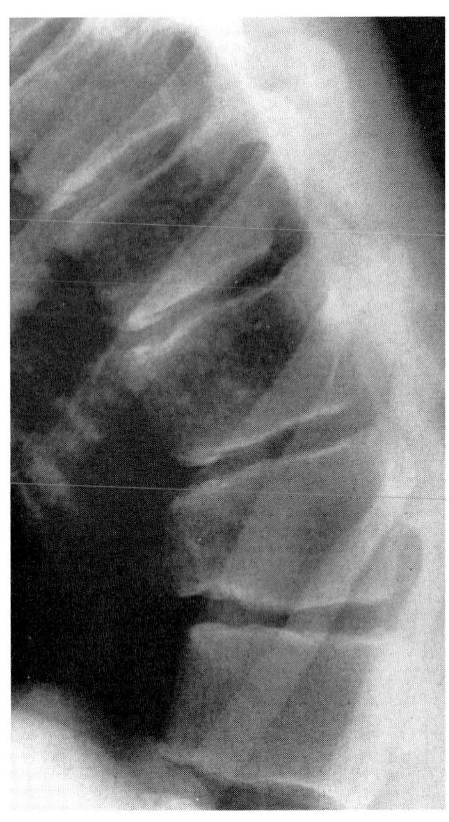

FIGURE 3–15. Scheuermann's disease.[23] In a 22-year-old man with back pain, abnormalities include kyphosis, multiple end plate irregularities, disc space narrowing, and wedge-shaped vertebral bodies, which are characteristic of this disease. Schmorl's nodes and limbus vertebrae, not prominent in this case, also occur in Scheuermann' s disease.

TABLE 3–5. Scoliosis

Entity	Figure(s)	Characteristics
Idiopathic scoliosis		
Infantile[8]		Onset: children younger than 4 years of age; not present at birth, but develops within first 6 months of life Rare in the United States; more common in the United Kingdom Resolution occurs in 74 per cent of patients; progression mainly occurs with curves > 50 degrees
Juvenile[8]		Onset: 4 to 9 years of age 13 per cent of all cases of scoliosis are detected in this age range Boys > girls before age of 6 years; girls > boys from ages 7 to 9 years Almost invariably progresses with growth
Adolescent[4, 24]	3–16	Onset: 10 years of age to skeletal maturity Most common type of idiopathic scoliosis Girls: boys, 4:1 to 8:1
Congenital scoliosis		
Secondary to developmental anomalies[25]	3–17; see 3–6	Failure of segmentation (unilateral block vertebra, pedicle bar, or neural arch fusion), partial duplication (supernumerary hemivertebra), or failure of formation (hemivertebra) results in structural lateral curvatures of the spine Progression is seen in 75 per cent of cases Associated findings: rib, genitourinary tract, and thumb anomalies, congenital heart disease, and undescended scapula
Neurofibromatosis Type I (von Recklinghausen's disease)[26]	3–18; see 3–61	Often appears initially as an acute scoliotic angulation and associated kyphosis; it also may resemble a smooth idiopathic curve May be associated with posterior scalloping of vertebral bodies and enlarged neural foramina

TABLE 3–5. Scoliosis *Continued*

Entity	Figure(s)	Characteristics
Congenital scoliosis *Continued*		
Marfan syndrome[16]		Scoliosis occurs in 40 to 60 per cent of patients Male = female Smooth, long sweeping curve resembles that of idiopathic scoliosis In young people, the curve progresses more rapidly than in idiopathic scoliosis Thoracic scoliosis often is associated with posterior scalloping of vertebral bodies from dural ectasia
Diastematomyelia[8]		Two thirds of patients have scoliosis; diastematomyelia occurs in 15 per cent of all patients with congenital scoliosis; often associated with other vertebral anomalies and short angular kyphosis Girls: boys, 2:1 Congenital longitudinal diastasis of the spinal canal and spinal cord with increased interpedicle distance Septum (ossified or unossified) divides the cord in 50 to 75 per cent of affected persons
Neuromuscular scoliosis		In general, scoliotic curves in neuromuscular diseases tend to be long, sweeping, and C-shaped
Neuropathic[8]		Cerebral palsy: most common cause of neuromuscular scoliosis Syringomyelia: up to 70 per cent of patients have scoliosis Traumatic paraplegia and quadriplegia: result in neuromuscular scoliosis, especially when injury occurs before skeletal maturation Poliomyelitis: no longer a common cause of neuropathic scoliosis
Myopathic[27]	3–19	Duchenne's muscular dystrophy frequently results in proximal muscle weakness and incapacitation by adolescence Spinal deformity, including kyphosis and scoliosis, occurs in 60 to 95 per cent of children older than age 10 years who are confined to a wheelchair; may be complicated by respiratory failure, pneumonia, and eventual cardiac failure, which may be fatal, commonly by the third decade of life Asymmetric hip contractures, muscle weakness, and pelvic obliquity contribute to the scoliosis
Trauma		
Fracture[8]		Fractures may result in an antalgic curve convex to the side of injury
Back pain[8]		Muscle splinting often results from low back pain due to disc displacements and other causes of mechanical pain; may result in self-limited lumbar and thoracic scoliosis
Radiation[28]		Radiation therapy for tumors of the kidney, thorax, or retroperitoneum causes asymmetric growth of vertebral structures within the radiation field; frequently results in scoliosis Scoliosis complicating radiation treatment is seen in 70 per cent of patients with Wilms' tumor and 76 per cent of 5-year survivors of neuroblastoma
Neoplasms		
Bone tumors[29]	3–20; 3–57	Osteoid osteoma and osteoblastoma often result in painful scoliosis These tumors generally are seen on the concave side of the scoliosis at or near the apex of the curve
Spinal cord tumors[30]		10 per cent of intraspinal tumors are associated with scoliosis May be associated with pedicle erosion, spinal canal widening, or paravertebral masses
Other disorders		
Ossified disc fragment[31]	3–21	Thoracic disc herniations may calcify or ossify and result in a compensatory antalgic scoliosis
Secondary to leg length inequality[32]		Functional lumbar curve convex to the side of the shorter leg; compensatory thoracic curve in the opposite direction
Treatment for scoliosis		
Spinal instrumentation[33]	3–22	Many different surgical methods used to treat severe scoliosis

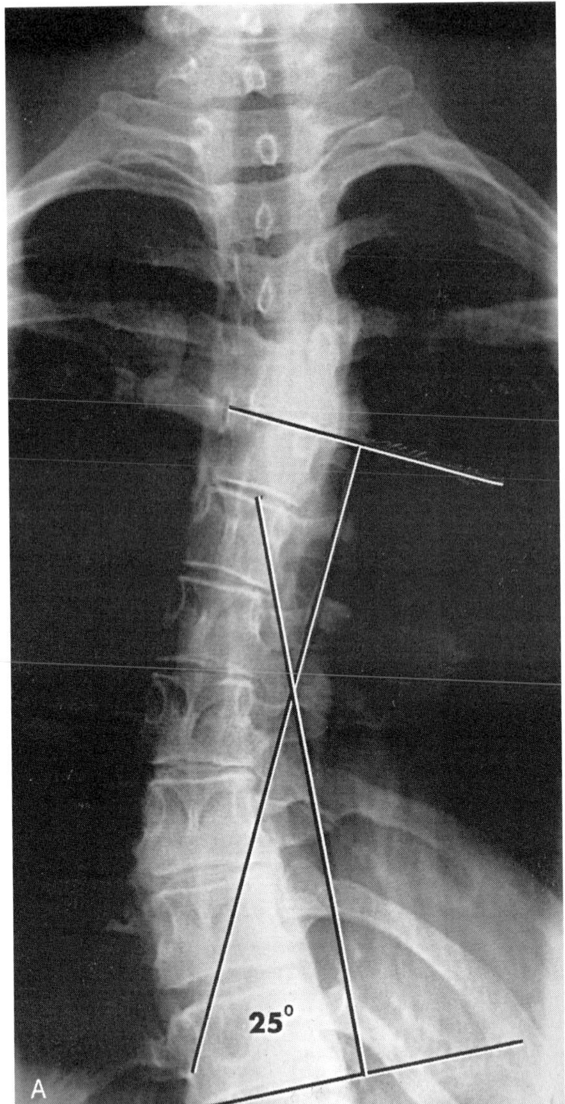

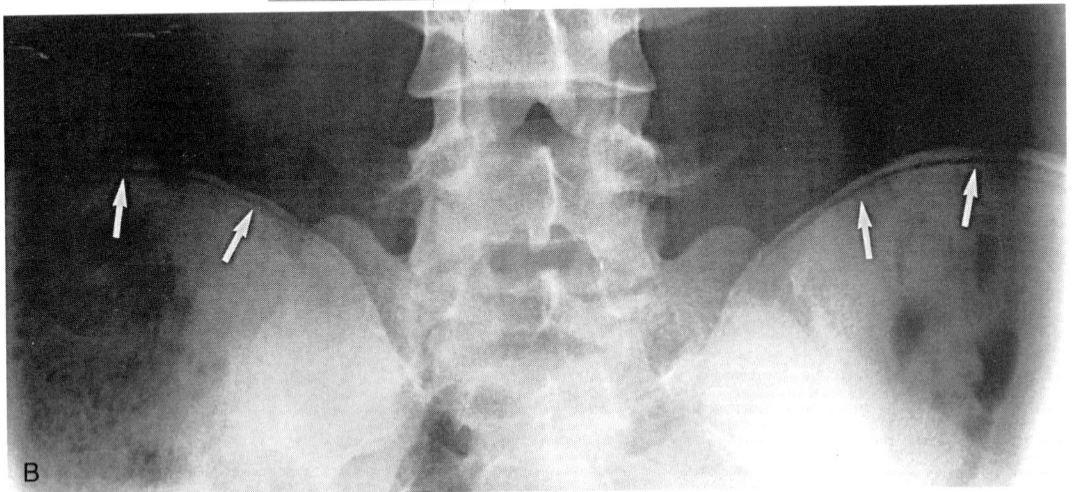

FIGURE 3–16. Adolescent idiopathic scoliosis.[4, 24] A This 26-year-old woman was diagnosed as having idiopathic adolescent scoliosis at the age of 13 years. A right convex curve extending from T5 to T12 measures 25 degrees using the Cobb method. A smaller left convex curve extends from T1 to T5. B Determination of skeletal maturity: Risser sign. The normal iliac apophysis just prior to fusion in this 19-year-old man appears as a curvilinear ossified rim along each iliac crest (arrows). The iliac apophyses begin to appear between the ages of 12 and 15 years, typically at the time of menarche in women. They may ossify multicentrically and appear rippled. Fusion of the apophysis to the iliac crest takes place between the ages of 21 and 25 years, a feature helpful in the determination of skeletal maturity in scoliotic patients (Risser sign).

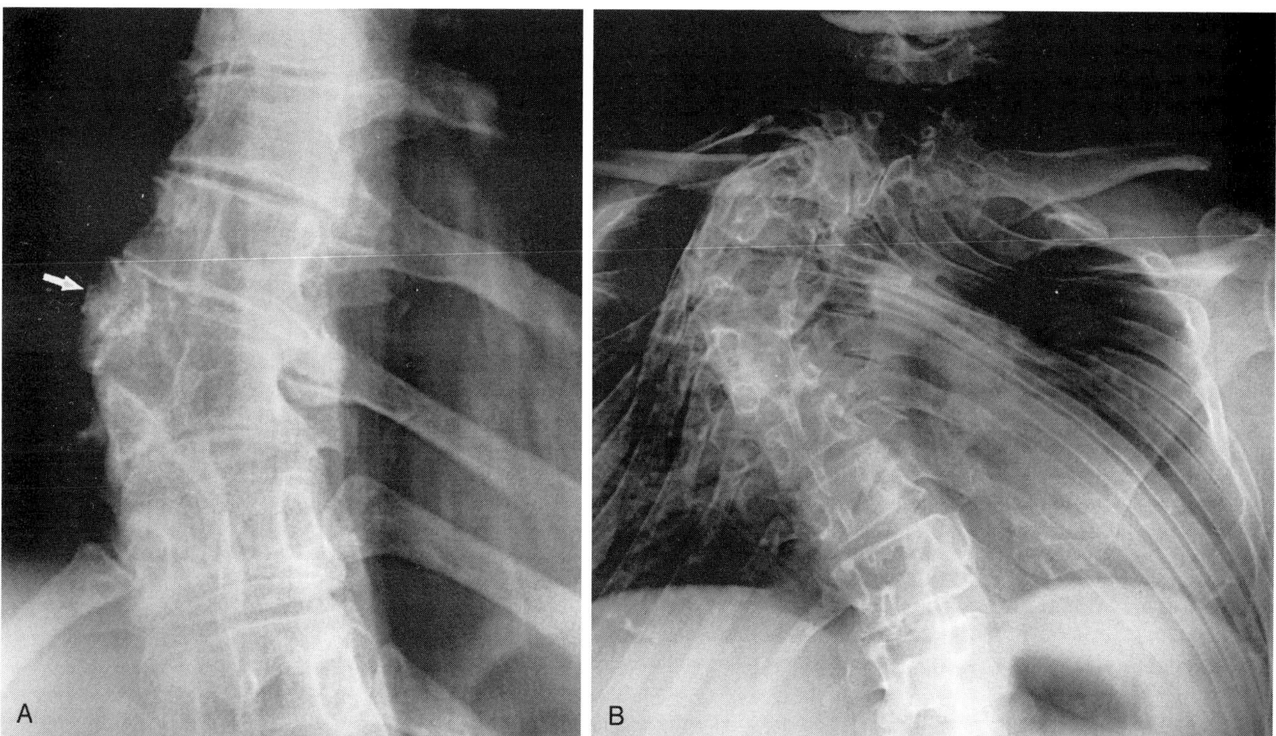

FIGURE 3–17. Congenital scoliosis.[25] A Lateral hemivertebra. A frontal radiograph from this 25-year-old woman demonstrates short, angular lower thoracic scoliosis. A small incomplete triangular vertebral body and its associated pedicle (arrow) are interposed between two relatively normal vertebrae on the right side. *(A, Courtesy of S. O'Connor, D.C., Toronto, Ontario, Canada.)* B Severe thoracic scoliosis with crowding of the ribs, thoracic cage deformity, and numerous cervicothoracic anomalies is seen in another patient. *(B, Courtesy of R.D. Stonebrink, D.C., Portland, Oregon.)*

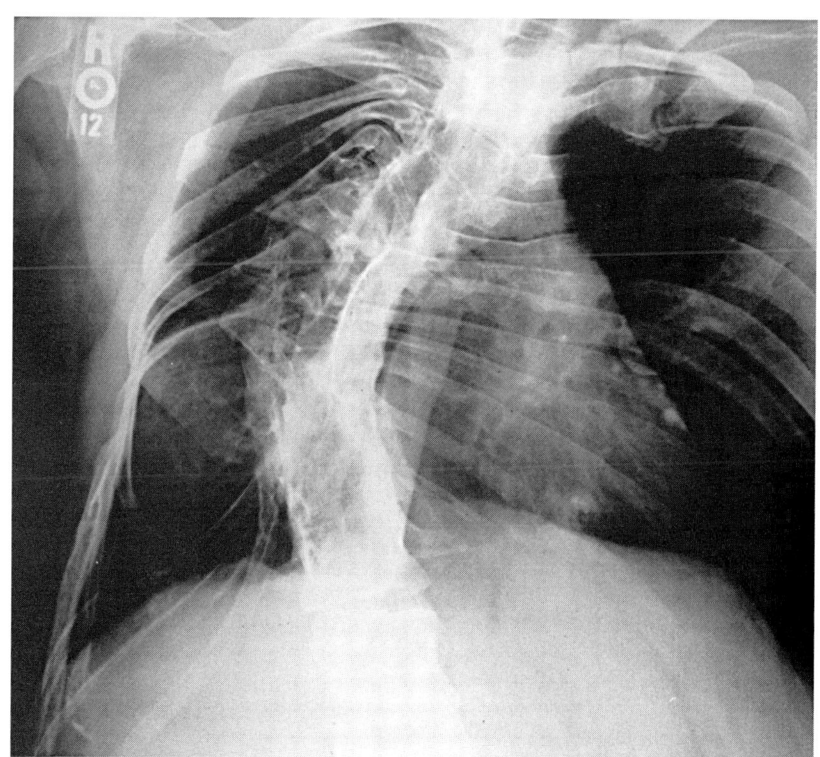

FIGURE 3–18. Scoliosis: Neurofibromatosis Type I (von Recklinghausen's disease).[26] A severe S-shaped scoliosis with multiple rib deformities and ribbon-like ribs are seen. Scoliosis (with or without kyphosis) is the most common spinal manifestation of neurofibromatosis. The scoliosis associated with this disease can take one of two forms: The first resembles an ordinary idiopathic scoliosis with a long sweeping curve; the second is dysplastic, may be rapidly progressive, and is a sharply angulated, short-segment kyphoscoliosis. This latter type commonly involves fewer than six middle or lower thoracic vertebral segments. *(Courtesy of S.K. Brahme, M.D., San Diego, California.)*

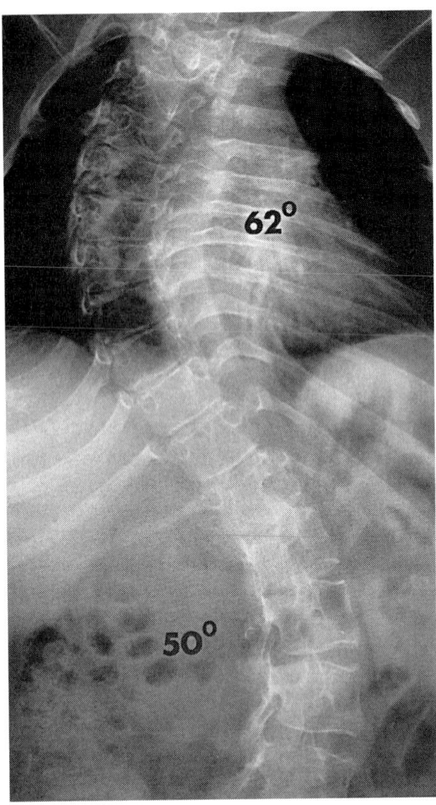

FIGURE 3–19. Scoliosis: Neuromuscular disease—myopathic.[27] Frontal radiograph from this 15-year-old boy with Duchenne muscular dystrophy reveals severe scoliosis. The thoracic curve measures 62 degrees, and the lumbar curve measures 50 degrees.

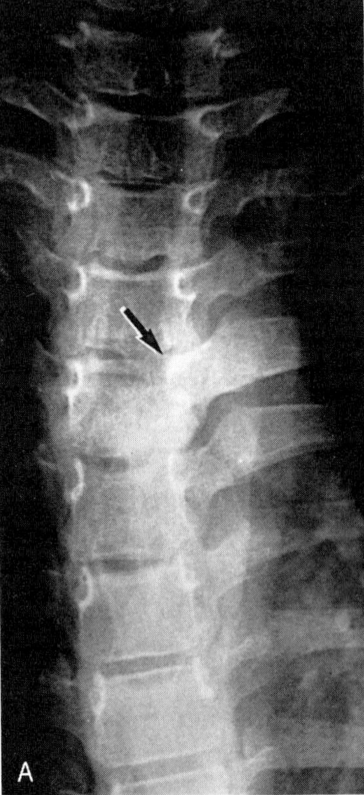

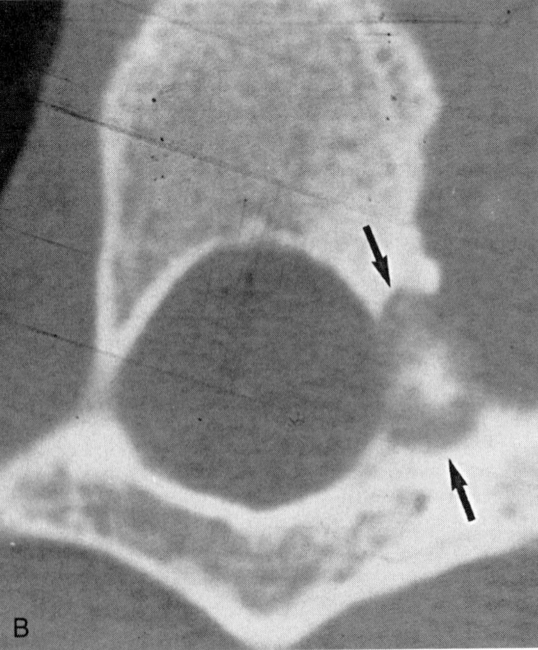

FIGURE 3–20. Scoliosis: Osteoid osteoma.[29] This 9-year-old girl has painful scoliosis. Routine radiograph (A) shows scoliosis and sclerosis within the left T5 pedicle (arrow). Transaxial CT image (B) demonstrates the radiolucent nidus (arrows) and central calcification surrounded by reactive sclerosis within the left pedicle and lamina.

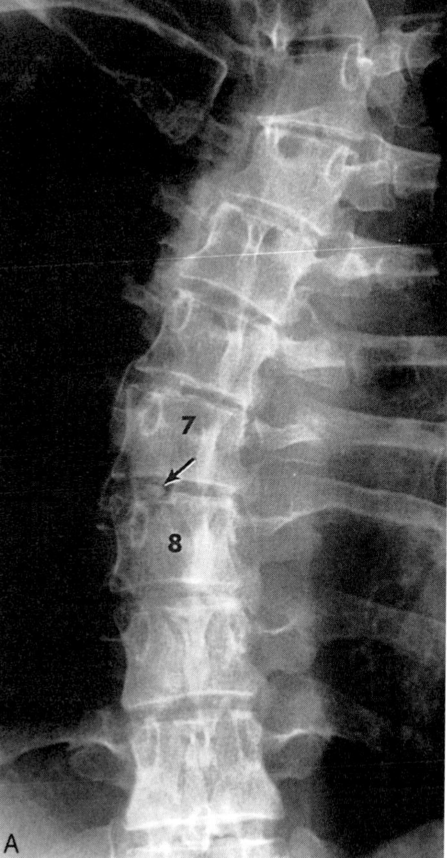

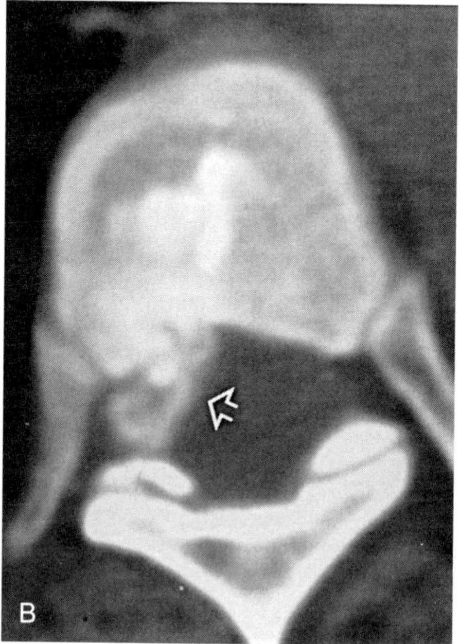

FIGURE 3–21. Scoliosis: Extradural mass from ossified disc herniation.[31] This 40-year-old woman has persistent thoracic spine pain and an antalgic scoliosis. A Frontal radiograph reveals a left cervicothoracic and right thoracic scoliosis. A small focus of calcification (arrow) is seen within the right T7-T8 disc space. B Transaxial CT scan shows extensive calcification within both the T7-T8 disc and herniated disc fragment (open arrow), the latter displacing the thecal sac. Thoracic disc herniations frequently calcify or ossify. *(Courtesy of M. Gallagher, M.D., Billings, Montana.)*

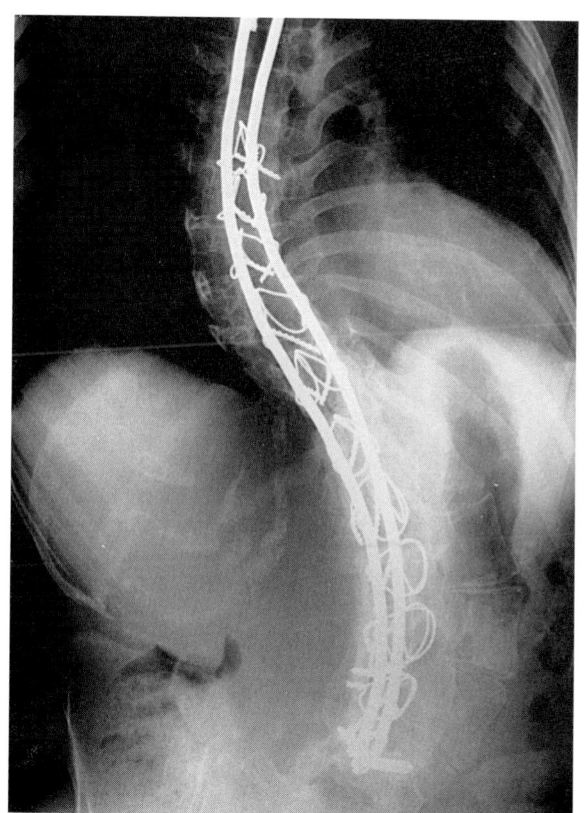

FIGURE 3–22. Scoliosis: Management with spinal instrumentation.[33] This patient with severe scoliosis has Luque L-shaped rods implanted to help correct the deformity and stop progression of the scoliosis. This is only one of many surgical procedures used for the management of scoliosis.

TABLE 3–6. Fractures and Dislocations of the Thoracic Spine

Entity	Figure(s)	Characteristics
Upper thoracic spine (T1-T4)		
Vertebral body compression fractures[34]		Rare site for this injury; high likelihood of associated neurologic deficit More frequent in younger people Mechanisms: electric shock, seizures, motor vehicle accidents, motorcycle accidents, direct trauma, athletic injuries When compression fractures occur in the upper thoracic spine, the possibility of pathologic fracture secondary to tumor should be considered
Midthoracic spine (T5-T9)		
Vertebral body compression fracture[35]	3–23	Frequent occurrence in osteoporotic persons Low prevalence of neurologic deficit Mechanism: single incident of trivial trauma, repeated minor trauma, or slow bone remodeling resulting from ongoing chronic microfractures
Schmorl's cartilaginous nodes[36]	3–24	Displacement of intervertebral disc material through the cartilaginous end plate and subchondral bone plate Isolated Schmorl's nodes may occur with acute trauma, degenerative disc disease, osteoporosis, osteomalacia, Paget's disease, hyperparathyroidism, infection, and neoplasm May be painful, but usually have no neurologic complication Gadolinium-enhanced MR images reveal that larger Schmorl's nodes often are vascularized, frequently are associated with bone marrow edema, and are more common in symptomatic patients than in asymptomatic patients Presence of multiple Schmorl's nodes in an adolescent thoracic spine suggests the diagnosis of Scheuermann's disease
Thoracolumbar spine (T10-L2)*		
Vertebral body compression fracture[35, 37–39]	3–23, 3–26	Most common thoracolumbar spine injury Very common in elderly persons Low prevalence of neurologic deficit Affects only the anterior column Mechanism: trivial trauma, repeated minor trauma, or slow bone remodeling resulting from ongoing chronic microfractures, or hyperflexion-compression injury
Burst fracture[40]		14 per cent of all thoracolumbar spine injuries Discussed in depth in Chapter 4
Thoracolumbar flexion injury: seat belt fracture[41–44]	3–27, 3–28	Most common in younger persons Affects middle and posterior (and occasionally anterior) columns and often results in thoracolumbar facet instability Approximately 15 per cent of patients have neurologic deficits; visceral injuries are common Mechanism: flexion-distraction over a fulcrum, such as that occurring in motor vehicle accidents in persons wearing a lap belt Occurs frequently in children restrained by lap belts in motor vehicle accidents *Injury patterns:* 1. Disruption of posterior and middle column ligaments, compression fracture of anterior body, intact anterior ligaments (Fig. 3–28) 2. Disruption of anterior, middle, and posterior ligaments 3. Classic osseous Chance-type fracture: horizontal fracture through the body, pedicles, pars interarticularis, and spinous and transverse processes (Fig. 3–27)
Fracture-dislocation[34]	3–29	10 to 20 per cent of all thoracolumbar spine injuries; may also occur at the T3 to T8 region Complete disruption of three columns 53 to 93 per cent of patients develop permanent neurologic deficit Mechanisms: compression (anterior column); rotation, shear, and distraction (middle and anterior columns) Often severe injuries, usually with polytrauma
Any region of thoracic spine		
Abused child syndrome[45]	3–30	Spine trauma is rare in child abuse Injuries include compression fractures of the vertebral body, acute disc displacement, avulsion of the posterior elements, and thoracolumbar fracture-dislocation

*From Denis F: The three column spine and its significance in the classification of acute thoracolumbar spinal injuries. Spine 8:817, 1983.

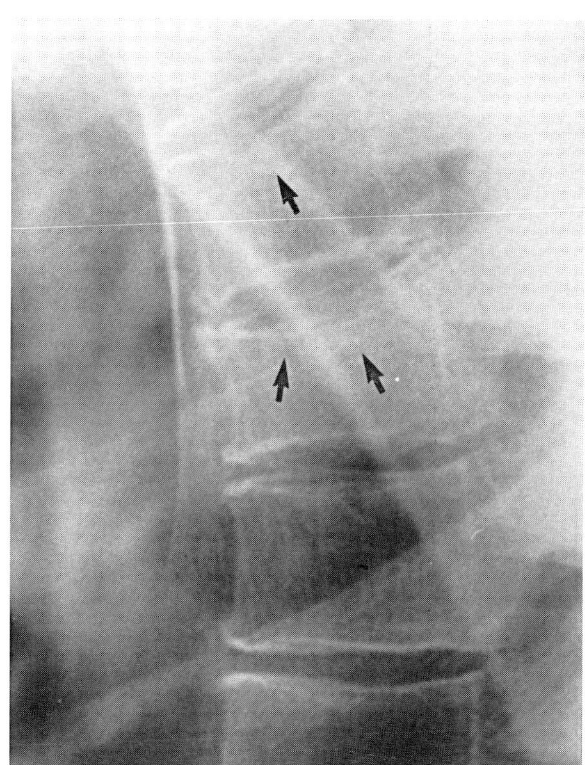

FIGURE 3–23. Compression fractures.[34, 35] Routine radiograph from this 73-year-old man demonstrates anterior wedge-shaped compression fractures of the fourth and fifth thoracic vertebral bodies. Observe the anterior and central end-plate depressions (arrows).

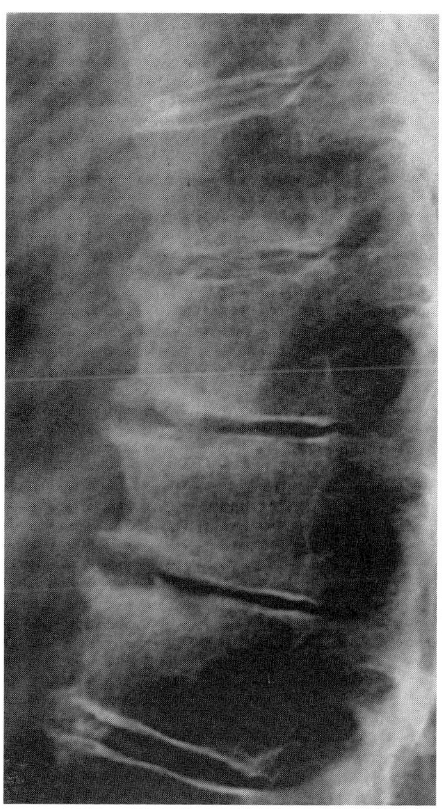

FIGURE 3–24. Schmorl's (cartilaginous) nodes.[36] Irregularity of the vertebral end plates, lucent areas, and adjacent sclerosis typical of cartilaginous nodes throughout the thoracic spine is seen in this elderly patient.

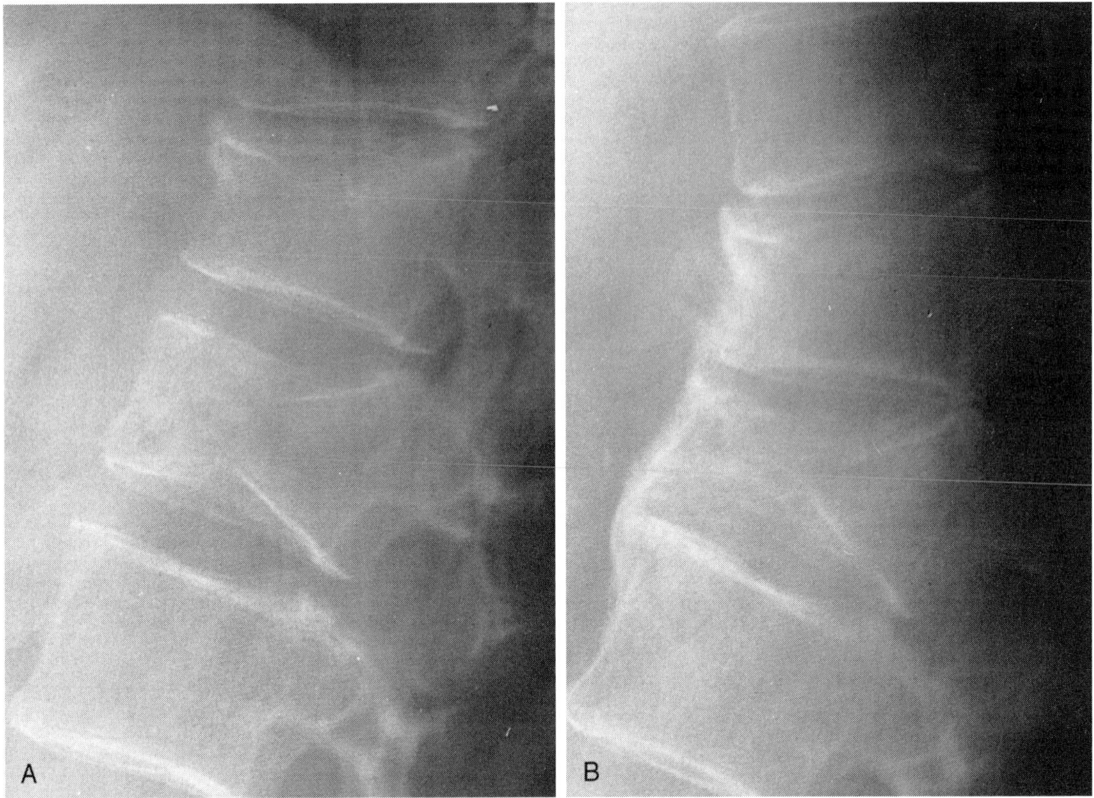

FIGURE 3–25. Compression fractures: natural history.[35, 37–39] A Initial radiograph taken at the time of injury shows generalized osteopenia and central end-plate depressions of the T12 and L1 vertebral bodies. B Radiograph obtained 2 years later reveals extensive osseous bridging of the anterior aspects of the compressed vertebrae and more advanced collapse of the L1 vertebral body. The presence of secondary degenerative ossification, as seen in this patient, is a reliable sign that the fracture occurred at least 18 months earlier (Table 3–7).

TABLE 3–7. Differential Diagnosis: Acute Versus Chronic Compression Fractures[7]

Features	Acute (Recent) Fracture (Within Last 2 Months)	Chronic (Remote) Fracture (Before Last 2 Months)
Vertebral body wedging	Present	Present; may progress with time
Step defect	Present	Absent
Sclerotic zone of impaction	Present	Absent
Disc space narrowing	Absent	Often present owing to degenerative disc disease
Paravertebral soft tissue hemorrhage	Present (variable)	Absent
Scintigraphy	Positive	Positive up to 18 to 24 months after fracture
MR imaging characteristics:		
T1-weighted	Low signal intensity	Isointense to normal vertebral bodies
T1-weighted with gadolinium	High signal intensity	Isointense to normal vertebral bodies
T2-weighted	High signal intensity	Isointense to normal vertebral bodies

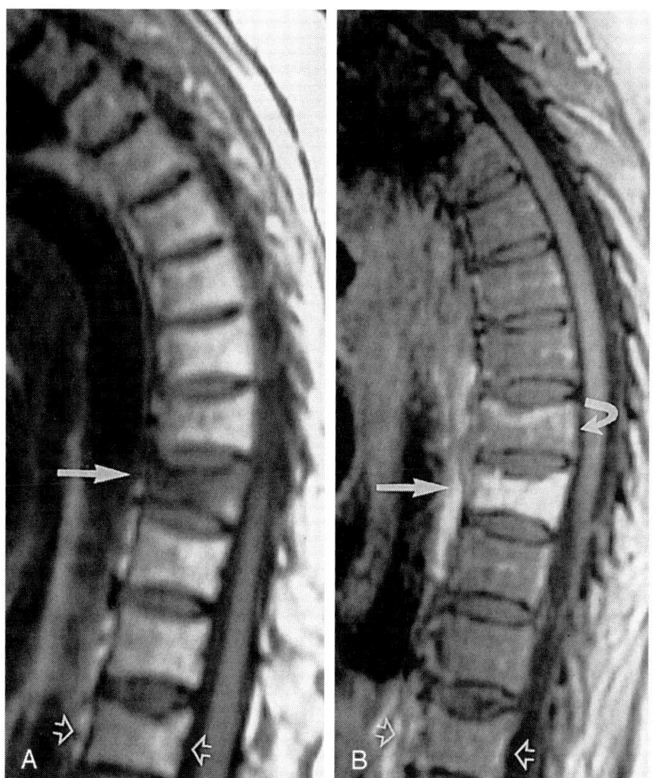

FIGURE 3–26. Acute compression fracture: Magnetic resonance (MR) imaging abnormalities.[35, 37–39] **A, B** 63-year-old woman with severe kyphosis and acute thoracic spinal pain. Sagittal T1-weighted spin echo MR images obtained before (TR/TE, 500/12) **(A)** and after (TR/TE, 800/12) **(B)** intravenous administration of gadolinium contrast agent reveal a wedge-shaped compression deformity of T10 vertebral body (arrow). Low signal intensity is seen in the pregadolinium image **(A)** and high signal intensity in the postgadolinium image **(B)**, characteristic of a recently fractured vertebra. Compare the findings of the acute fracture in T10 to those of a remote, healed fracture of L1 (open arrows). In the remote fracture, the signal intensity of the L1 vertebral body is the same as that of the adjacent vertebral bodies before **(A)** and after **(B)** contrast agent administration. A subacute fracture of T9 also is evident (curved arrow) in which the signal is less intense than that of the acute fracture on the postgadolinium image **(B)**. Note high signal intensity in the prevertebral soft tissues in **B**. Compression fractures are common, especially in older women. MR imaging can be useful in differentiating between recent (acute) and long-standing (chronic) spine fractures and is well suited for assessing spinal cord and soft tissue injury (Table 3–7). However, differentiating between benign compression fractures and neoplastic, pathologic fractures can be difficult. The finding on MR images of a fluid collection within a collapsed vertebral body may represent osteonecrosis secondary to vertebral collapse. *(Courtesy of M.N. Pathria, M.D., San Diego, California.)*

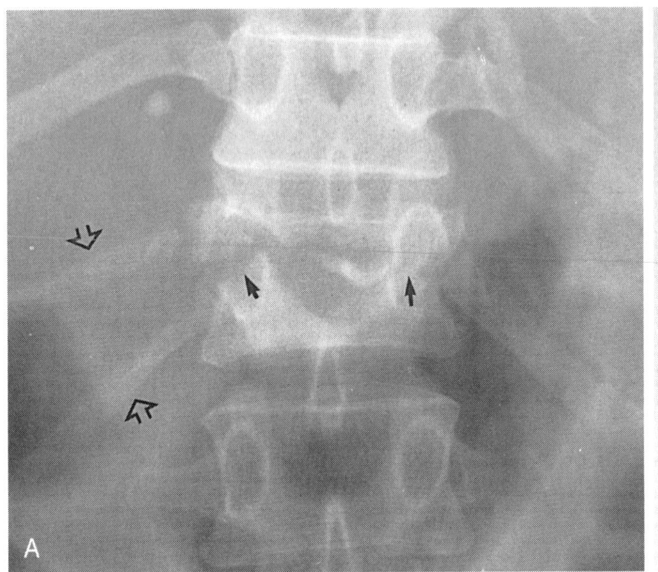

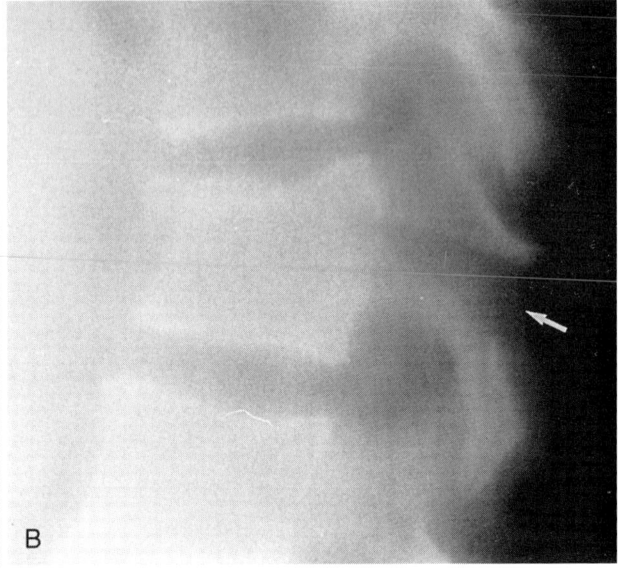

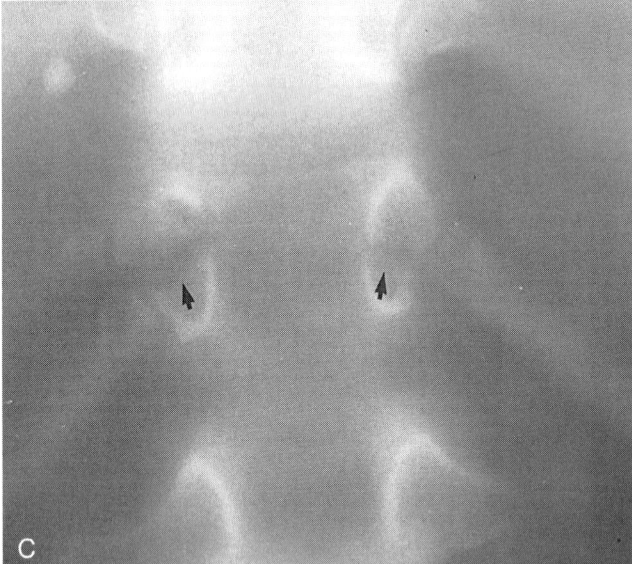

FIGURE 3–27. Thoracolumbar flexion instability: Seat belt fracture.[41–44] A, B Anteroposterior radiograph (A) and lateral (B) conventional tomogram reveal anterior vertebral body wedging and a horizontal fracture through the vertebral body and neural arch (arrows). The twelfth rib also is split horizontally (open arrows), although it remains unclear whether this represents a horizontal fracture of the rib or a preexisting anomaly. C Frontal conventional tomogram confirms the horizontal split through the pedicles (arrows).

The seat belt (or lap belt) injury of the thoracolumbar spine is caused by tensile failure of the spine, which results from a combination of forced hyperflexion and distraction over a fulcrum. This is the most common type of flexion-distraction injury (sometimes referred to as a Chance fracture) and results in a horizontal splitting of the posterior osseous elements from distraction and minimal compression of the anterior portion of the vertebral body.

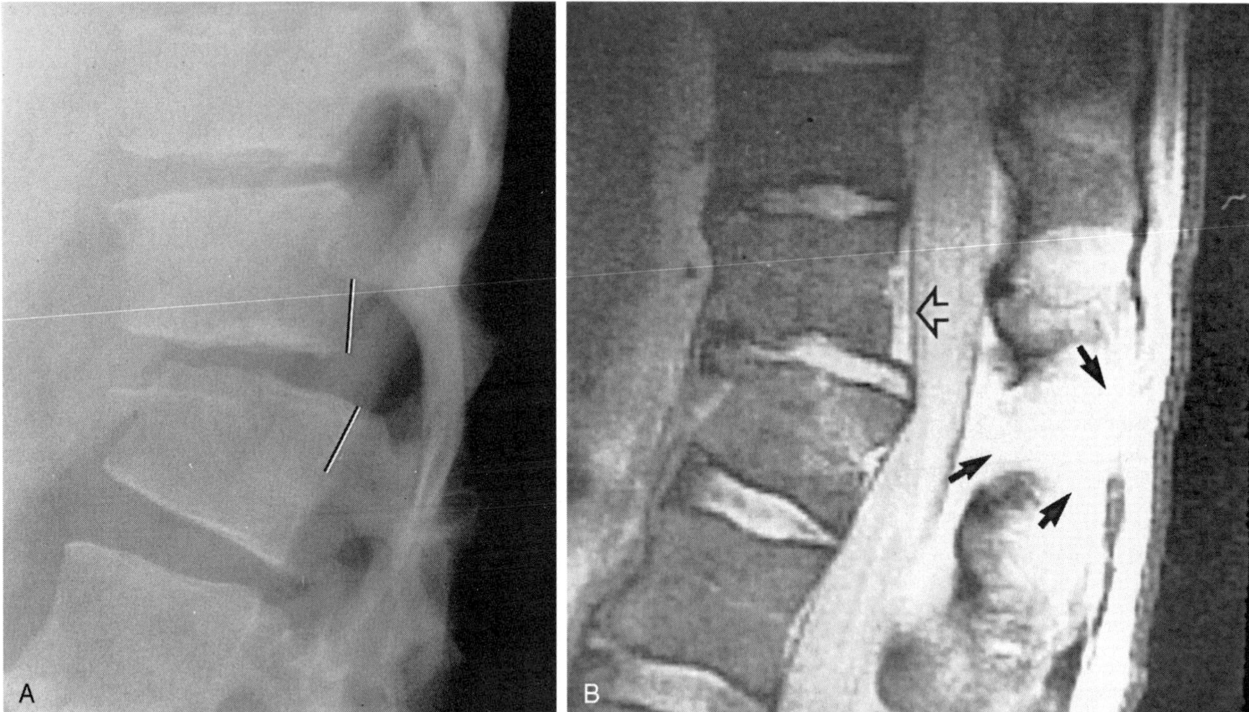

FIGURE 3–28. Thoracolumbar flexion instability: Ligament disruption.[41–44] A Lateral radiograph shows compression of the anterior aspect of the L1 vertebral body, anterior translation of the T12 vertebral body (vertical lines show displacement), and separation of the posterior elements, suggesting the possibility of an acute facet lock. B Sagittal T2-weighted (TR/TE, 2700/60) spin echo magnetic resonance (MR) image demonstrates disruption of the supraspinous and interspinous ligaments (arrows). High signal intensity within these ligaments and the L1 vertebral body is characteristic of hemorrhage or edema. In addition, the posterior longitudinal ligament is stripped from the displaced T12 vertebral body (open arrow), and the thecal sac is kinked and compressed. *(Courtesy of M.N. Pathria, M.D., San Diego, California.)*

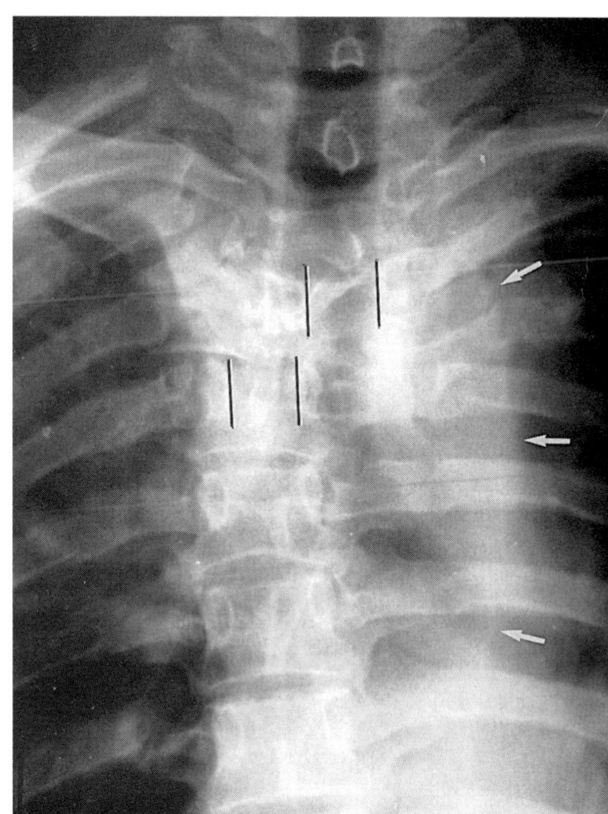

FIGURE 3–29. Fracture-dislocation.[34] Frontal radiograph shows widening of the mediastinum (arrows) consistent with the presence of hematoma or aortic arch injury in this patient with a T3-T4 fracture-dislocation. The vertical lines demarcate the inner margins of the pedicles of T3 and T4 and illustrate the extent of lateral dislocation. These severe, unstable injuries are associated with an extremely high rate of neurologic injury, most commonly complete paraplegia. They occur most frequently at the T3 to T8 levels. Widening of the mediastinum should raise suspicion also of aortic arch injury.

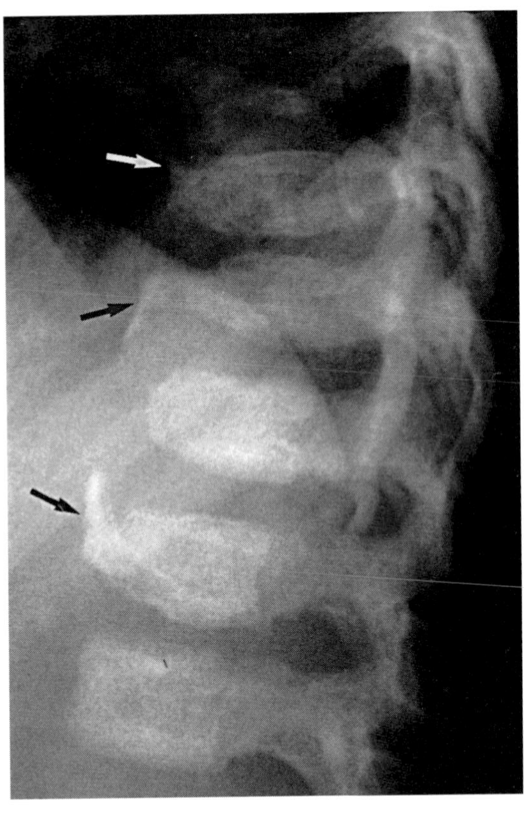

FIGURE 3–30. Abused child syndrome.[45] This 3-year-old girl was repeatedly subjected to physical abuse. Observe the multiple thoracolumbar spine fractures at different stages of healing. Flattening of several vertebral bodies and associated anterior tongue-like projections of bone proliferation are evident (arrows).

TABLE 3–8. Thoracic Spine: Articular Disorders*

Entity	Figure(s), Table(s)	Characteristics
Degenerative and related disorders		
Degenerative disc disease[46]	3–31 Table 3–9	*Spondylosis deformans:* Osteophytes and osseous ridging Subchondral bone sclerosis *Intervertebral osteochondrosis:* Disc space narrowing Intradiscal vacuum phenomenon Disc calcification (rare)
Costovertebral osteoarthrosis[46]	3–32	Sclerosis and hypertrophy of costotransverse and costovertebral articulations secondary to degeneration Osteophytes may be prominent Ipsilateral rib hypertrophy may be present May be painful and result in limitation of motion CT is the best imaging technique, but it is seldom used because of its expense and the benign nature of costovertebral osteoarthrosis
Degenerative disc calcification[47]	3–33A	Chronic degenerative calcific deposits occur primarily in the anulus fibrosus; affects older persons and may be asymptomatic Men > women It is unclear what proportion of these patients is symptomatic Calcification predominates in the midthoracic and upper lumbar intervertebral discs
Idiopathic childhood disc calcification[96]	3–33 B–D	Disc calcification in children, often associated with disc displacements, is symptomatic in 75 per cent of cases Symptoms and signs include pain, stiffness, limitation of motion, and torticollis; fever, leukocytosis, and elevated erythrocyte sedimentation rate Symptoms generally resolve within a few days to weeks; calcification typically disappears within a few weeks to months Boys = girls
Ossified disc displacement[31]	3–34	Ossification of a disc herniation or fragment Calcification or ossification of thoracic discs in adults May be asymptomatic or may cause chronic or acute symptoms secondary to compression of the thecal sac

TABLE 3–8. Thoracic Spine: Articular Disorders* *Continued*

Entity	Figure(s), Table(s)	Characteristics
Degenerative and related disorders *Continued*		
Diffuse idiopathic skeletal hyperostosis (DISH)[48–51]	3–35, 3–36	Flowing anterior hyperostosis: prominent vertical sheet of ossification along the anterior vertebral bodies and anulus fibrosus (Table 3–8) Relative absence of degenerative changes and preservation of disc height Involvement of at least four contiguous segments Relatively normal apophyseal and sacroiliac joints T7-T11 most frequent sites of involvement
Ossification of the posterior longitudinal ligament (OPLL)[52]	3–37	Segmental or continuous vertical sheet of ossification of the posterior longitudinal ligament, up to 5 mm thick; extends along the posterior margins of the vertebral bodies and discs within the spinal canal Often accompanies DISH and may contribute to central stenosis with or without symptoms
Neuropathic osteoarthropathy[53]		Infrequently involves the upper and middle thoracic spine, but syringomyelia, diabetes mellitus, and tabes dorsalis may affect the thoracolumbar region Widespread discovertebral and zygapophyseal joint destruction, collapse, bone fragmentation, and kyphosis May resemble infectious spondylodiscitis
Inflammatory disorders		
Ankylosing spondylitis and enteropathic arthropathy[54, 55]	3–38, 3–39 Table 3–9, 3–10	Widespread marginal syndesmophytes, osteitis, disc calcification, osteoporosis, squaring of vertebral bodies, and disc ballooning Erosion and eventual ankylosing of discovertebral junctions and apophyseal joints Ossification of ligaments, joint capsules, and outer annular fibers Ulcerative colitis and regional ileitis may result in identical radiographic findings to those of ankylosing spondylitis Thoracic spine in ankylosing spondylitis is susceptible to fractures and pseudarthrosis, both of which can result in neurologic injury
Psoriatic spondyloarthropathy and Reiter's syndrome[56, 57]	3–40, 3–41 Table 3–9	Unilateral or bilateral, asymmetric, nonmarginal, comma-shaped paravertebral ossification about the lower thoracic and upper lumbar spine in 10 to 15 per cent of patients with psoriasis Apophyseal joint narrowing, sclerosis, and bony ankylosis
Progressive systemic sclerosis (scleroderma)[58]	3–42	Paraspinal calcific deposits are composed predominantly of calcium hydroxyapatite crystals
Dermatomyositis and polymyositis[59]	3–43	Subcutaneous and intermuscular calcification frequently involves the chest wall; may be evident on thoracic spine radiographs
Crystal deposition disorders		
Calcium pyrophosphate dihydrate crystal deposition disease[60, 61]	3–44	May result in widespread secondary degenerative disease with disc space narrowing and chondrocalcinosis of the anulus fibrosus, joint capsules, apophyseal joints, and articular cartilage
Alkaptonuria[62]	3–45 Table 3–9	Widespread, severe disc space narrowing, diffuse anulus fibrosus calcification, and intradiscal vacuum phenomena Osteoporosis and loss of lumbar lordosis Osseous bridging may resemble marginal syndesmophytes Eventual progression to bamboo spine
Infection		
Pyogenic spondylodiscitis[63]		Up to 21-day latent period before radiographic changes appear Infection initially involves disc and adjacent vertebral body Severe one-level disc space narrowing that eventually may spread to adjacent levels, obliterating vertebral end plates and resulting in vertebral collapse in later stages Paravertebral soft tissue mass or abscess
Tuberculous spondylodiscitis[64, 65]	3–46, 3–47	25 to 60 per cent of cases of skeletal tuberculosis affect the spine, principally the thoracolumbar region Anterior vertebral destruction and collapse often results in an acute, angular gibbus deformity Classically, vertebral bodies and disc are involved; posterior elements are affected infrequently Slower progression compared with that of pyogenic spondylodiscitis Paravertebral abscess is common

*See also Tables 1–6 to 1–9 and Table 1–17.

TABLE 3–9. Osseous Outgrowths of the Spine

Entity	Figure(s)	Definition	Representative Disorders	Appearance
Osteophyte	3–31	Hypertrophic proliferation of bone at the attachment of the annular fibers to the vertebral body	Degenerative disc disease (spondylosis deformans)	Triangular outgrowth located several millimeters from edge of the vertebral body; may be claw-shaped and may bridge the discovertebral joint in advanced disease
Marginal syndesmophyte	3–38, 3–39	Ossification of the anulus fibrosus	Ankylosing spondylitis Alkaptonuria	Thin, symmetric, vertical outgrowth extending from the corner of one vertebral body margin to the next; results in the bamboo spine appearance
Flowing anterior hyperostosis	3–35, 3–36	Ossification of the intervertebral disc, anterior longitudinal ligament, and paravertebral connective tissue	Diffuse idiopathic skeletal hyperostosis (DISH)	Thick undulating outgrowth along the anterior aspect of the spine; may be intermittently separated from vertebral bodies by a radiolucent cleft
Nonmarginal paravertebral ossification	3–40, 3–41	Ossification of paravertebral connective tissue	Psoriatic arthropathy Reiter's syndrome	Poorly defined or well-defined, asymmetric outgrowth that may be comma-shaped; separated from the edge of the vertebral body and intervertebral disc

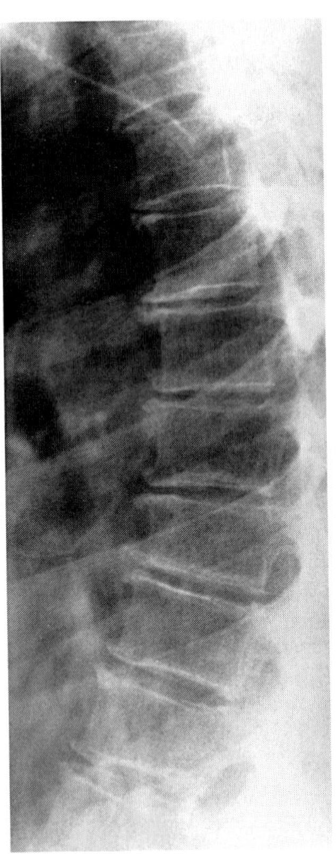

FIGURE 3–31. Degenerative disc disease.[46] Disc space narrowing, vertebral end-plate sclerosis, and osteophyte formation are evident in this 41-year-old woman.

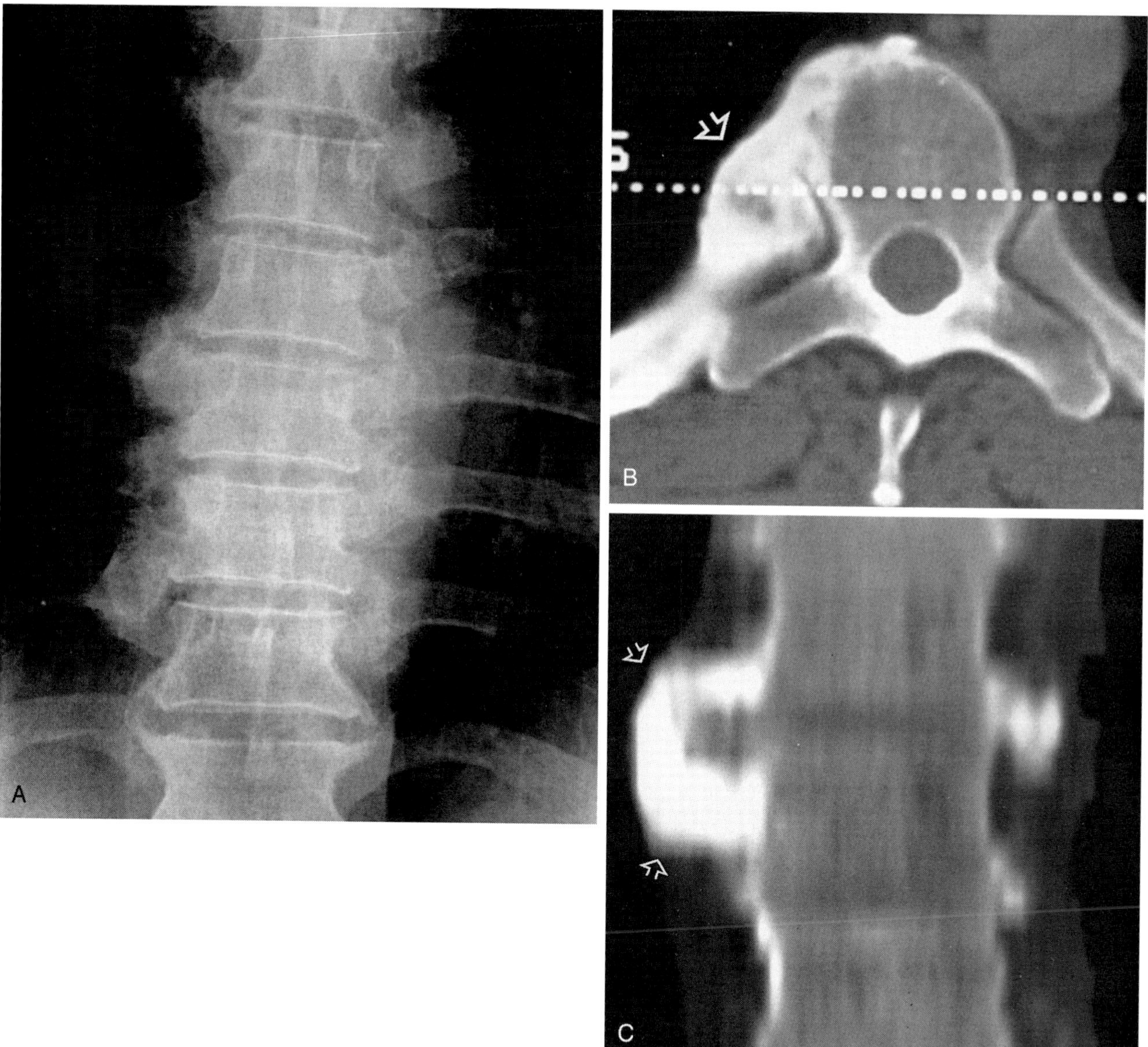

FIGURE 3–32. Costovertebral osteoarthrosis.[46] A Frontal radiograph of the thoracic spine in this 52-year-old man shows extensive hyperostosis of the costovertebral articulations, resulting in a bulbous appearance. B, C Transaxial (B) and coronal reformatted (C) computed tomographic (CT) images from another patient show marked hypertrophic bone arising from the costovertebral and costotransverse articulations (open arrows). Note the enlarged, dense rib in B, consistent with stress hypertrophy. *(B, C Courtesy of J. Haller, M.D., Vienna, Austria.)*

Illustration continued on following page

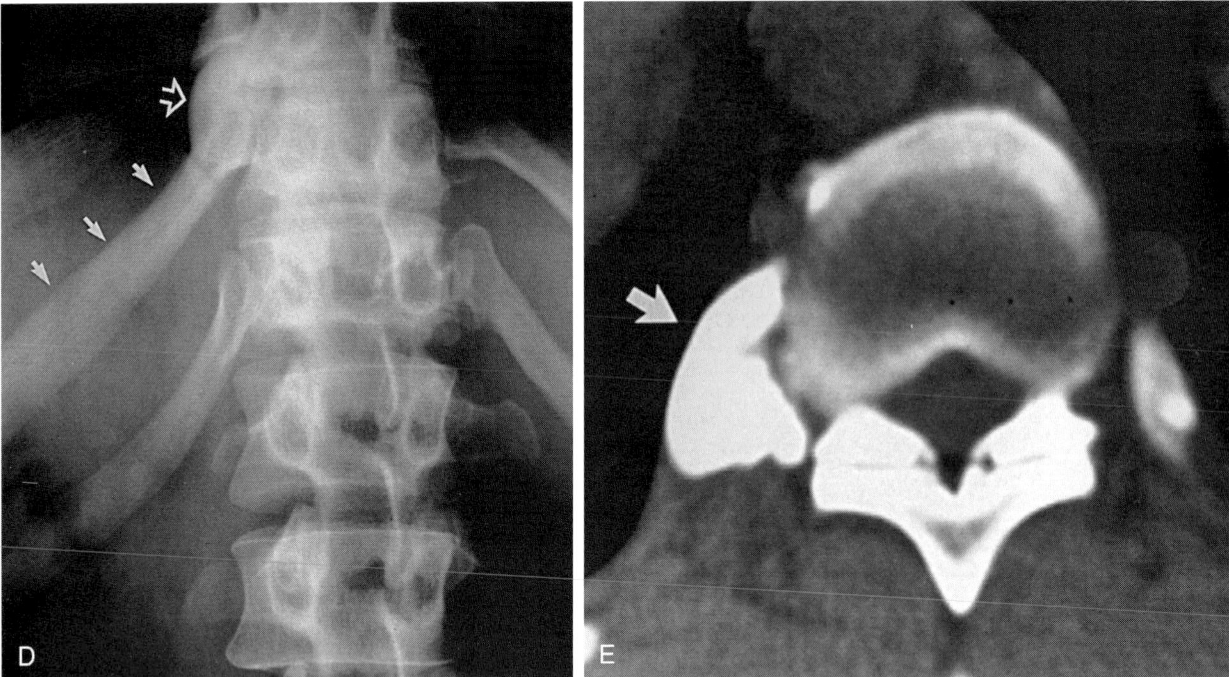

FIGURE 3–32 *Continued.* D, E In another patient, a thoracolumbar radiograph (D) reveals extensive rib hyperostosis (arrows) and enlargement and sclerosis of the costovertebral joint (open arrow). These findings are demonstrated (arrow) on the transaxial CT scan (E). Costovertebral joint degenerative disease tends to predominate on the right side of the spine. Cortical thickening and hyperostosis of the posterior portion of the ribs simulating Paget's disease (D, E) also may occur in ankylosing spondylitis, diffuse idiopathic skeletal hyperostosis, and psoriatic spondyloarthropathy.

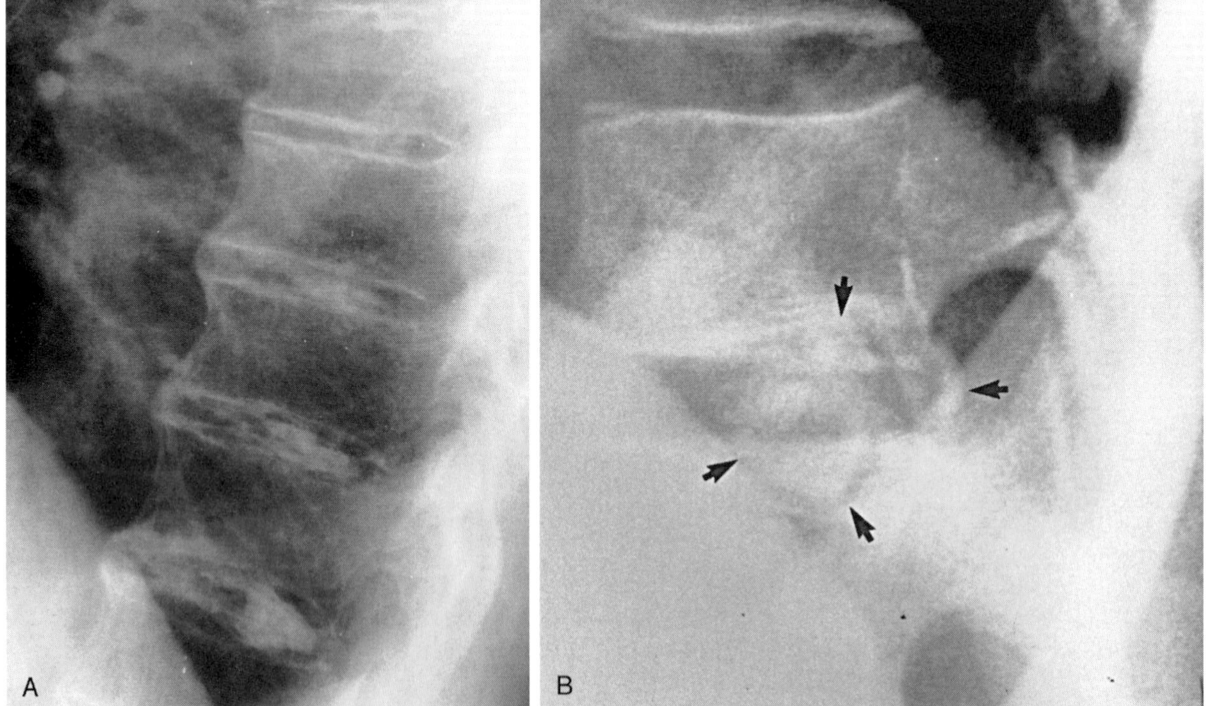

FIGURE 3–33. Disc calcification. A Degenerative disc calcification: Adult.[47] A 60-year-old woman had lower thoracic spine pain. Lateral radiograph shows calcification of multiple thoracic intervertebral discs. B–D Idiopathic childhood disc calcification.[96] This 11-year-old girl with back pain had a bone scan that was normal. In B, a lateral radiograph shows cloudy calcification overlying the T11-T12 disc space (arrows) with associated erosion of the inferior vertebral end plate of T11.

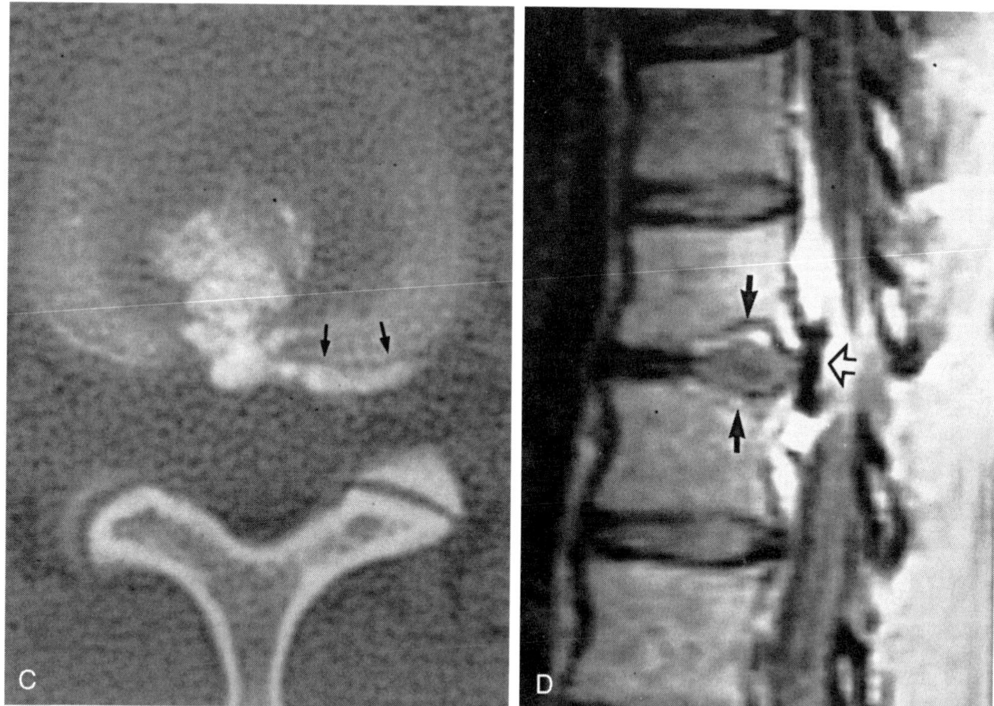

FIGURE 3–33 *Continued.* In **C**, a transaxial CT scan shows extensive circumferential calcification of the nucleus pulposus with posterior extension of calcified disc material extending posterolaterally into the left neural foramen (arrows). In **D**, a sagittal T1-weighted (TR/TE, 700/15) spin echo magnetic resonance (MR) image obtained after administration of intravenous gadolinium contrast agent reveals a large mass of intermediate signal intensity within the posterior aspect of the disc that erodes the adjacent vertebral bodies. The zone of high signal enhancement (arrows) probably represents edema. An additional low signal intensity mass corresponding to the posteriorly displaced calcified disc material and surrounding high signal intensity edema indent and displace the thecal sac (open arrow). *(**B–D,** Courtesy of K. Koeller, M.D., Washington, D.C.)*

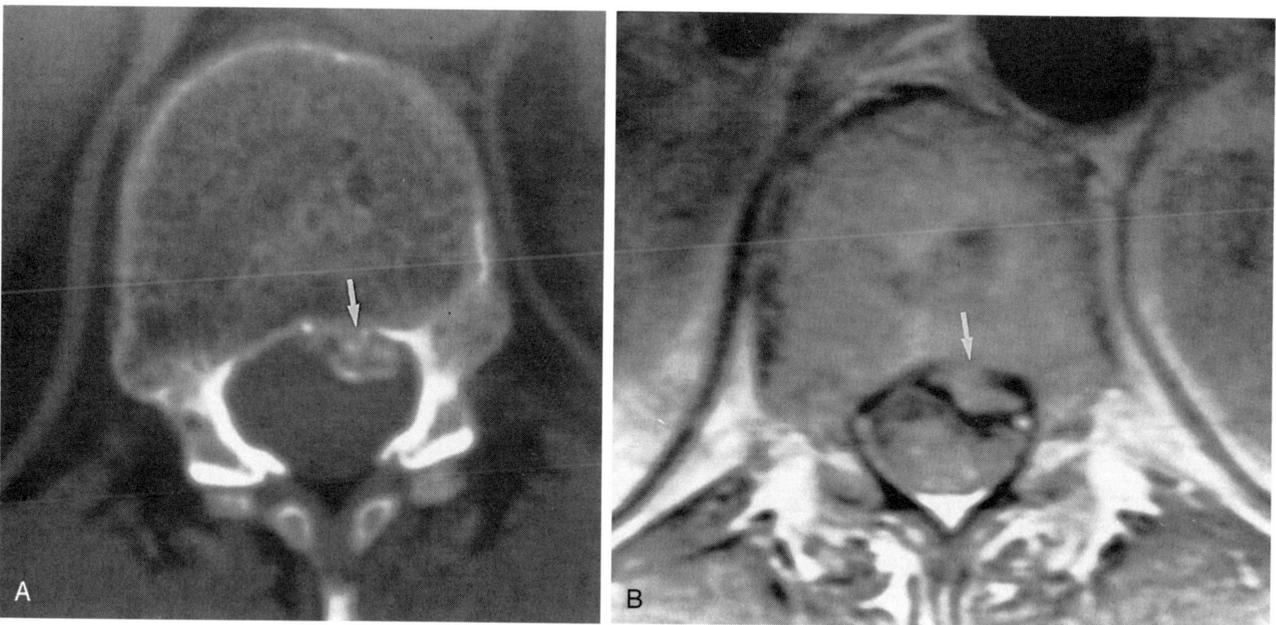

FIGURE 3–34. Ossification of a displaced disc fragment.[31] **A, B** 75-year-old woman. In **A**, a transaxial CT image shows an area of high attenuation within the displaced T11-T12 intervertebral disc fragment (arrow). In **B**, a corresponding transaxial fast spin echo (TR/TE, 2200/20) magnetic resonance (MR) image shows the mass (arrow) to be composed of cortical and medullary bone that is displacing and compressing the thecal sac. *(**A, B,** Courtesy of S. Eilenberg, M.D., San Diego, California.)*

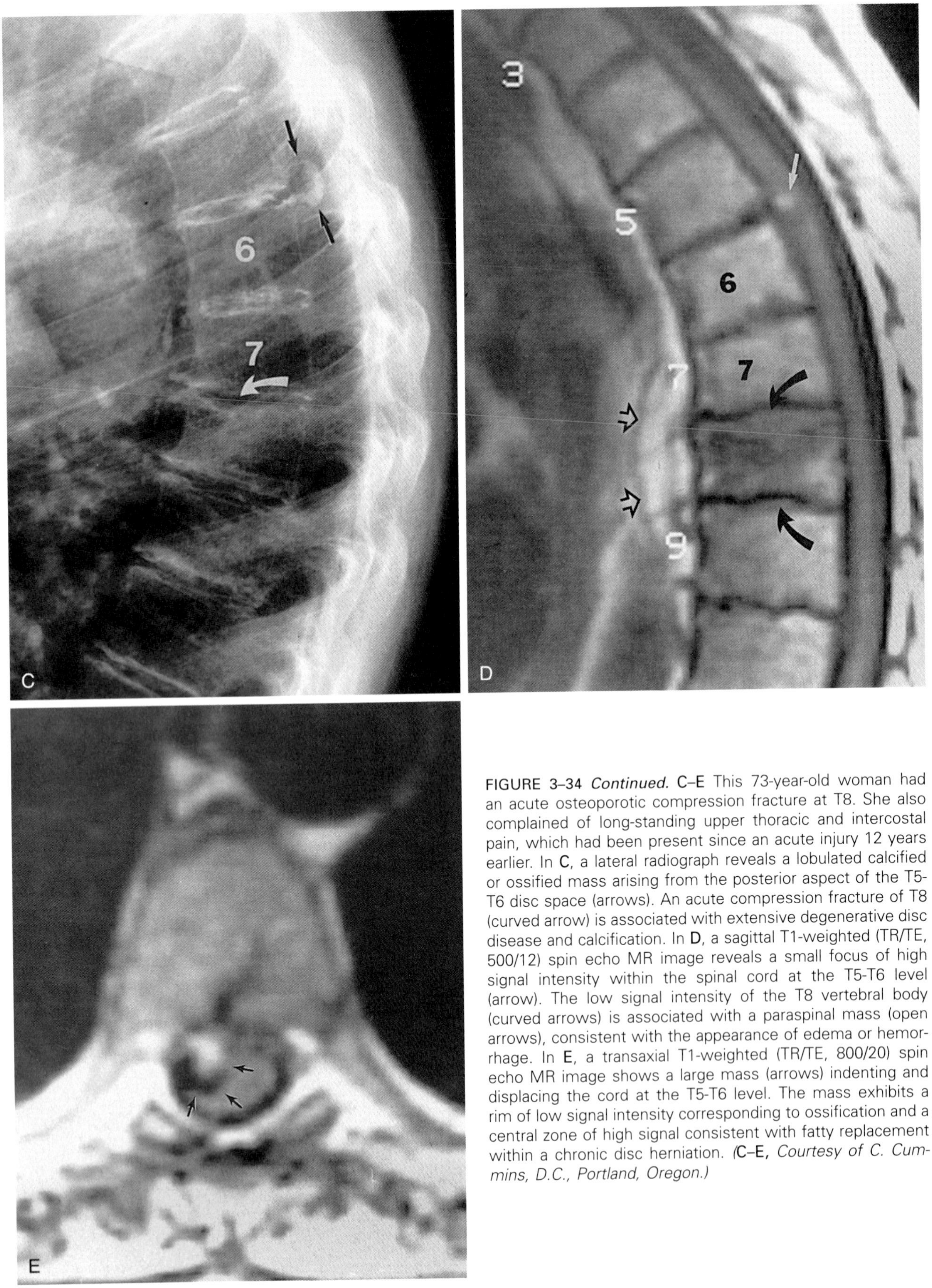

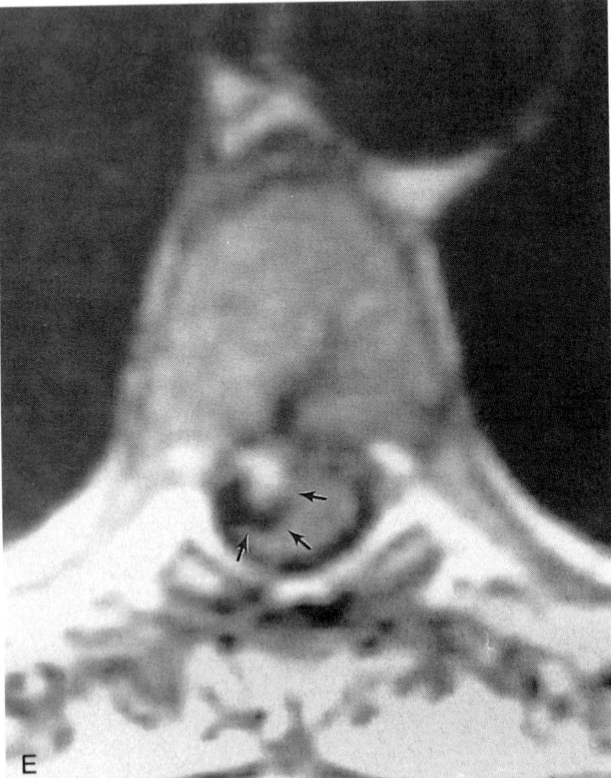

FIGURE 3–34 *Continued.* C–E This 73-year-old woman had an acute osteoporotic compression fracture at T8. She also complained of long-standing upper thoracic and intercostal pain, which had been present since an acute injury 12 years earlier. In C, a lateral radiograph reveals a lobulated calcified or ossified mass arising from the posterior aspect of the T5-T6 disc space (arrows). An acute compression fracture of T8 (curved arrow) is associated with extensive degenerative disc disease and calcification. In D, a sagittal T1-weighted (TR/TE, 500/12) spin echo MR image reveals a small focus of high signal intensity within the spinal cord at the T5-T6 level (arrow). The low signal intensity of the T8 vertebral body (curved arrows) is associated with a paraspinal mass (open arrows), consistent with the appearance of edema or hemorrhage. In E, a transaxial T1-weighted (TR/TE, 800/20) spin echo MR image shows a large mass (arrows) indenting and displacing the cord at the T5-T6 level. The mass exhibits a rim of low signal intensity corresponding to ossification and a central zone of high signal consistent with fatty replacement within a chronic disc herniation. (C–E, *Courtesy of C. Cummins, D.C., Portland, Oregon.)*

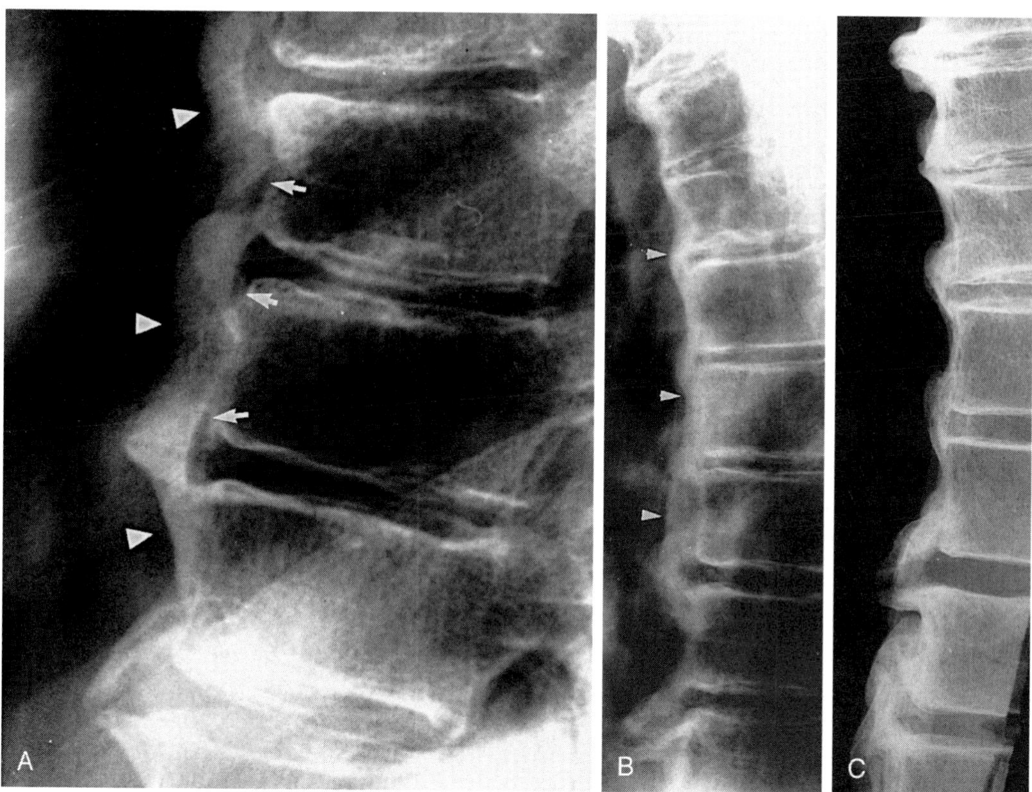

FIGURE 3–35. Diffuse idiopathic skeletal hyperostosis (DISH).[48–51] A Lateral radiograph demonstrates the characteristic flowing hyperostosis of DISH anterior to several contiguous vertebral bodies (arrowheads). Relative preservation of the disc spaces and the intermittent radiolucent zone between the ossification and the vertebral bodies (arrows) are well-recognized findings in this disease. B In another patient, undulating ossification anterior to the thoracic spine (arrowheads) is evident. C A specimen radiograph clearly reveals the flowing ossification typical of DISH. Observe the thick, bulky, undulating excrescences and normal disc spaces.

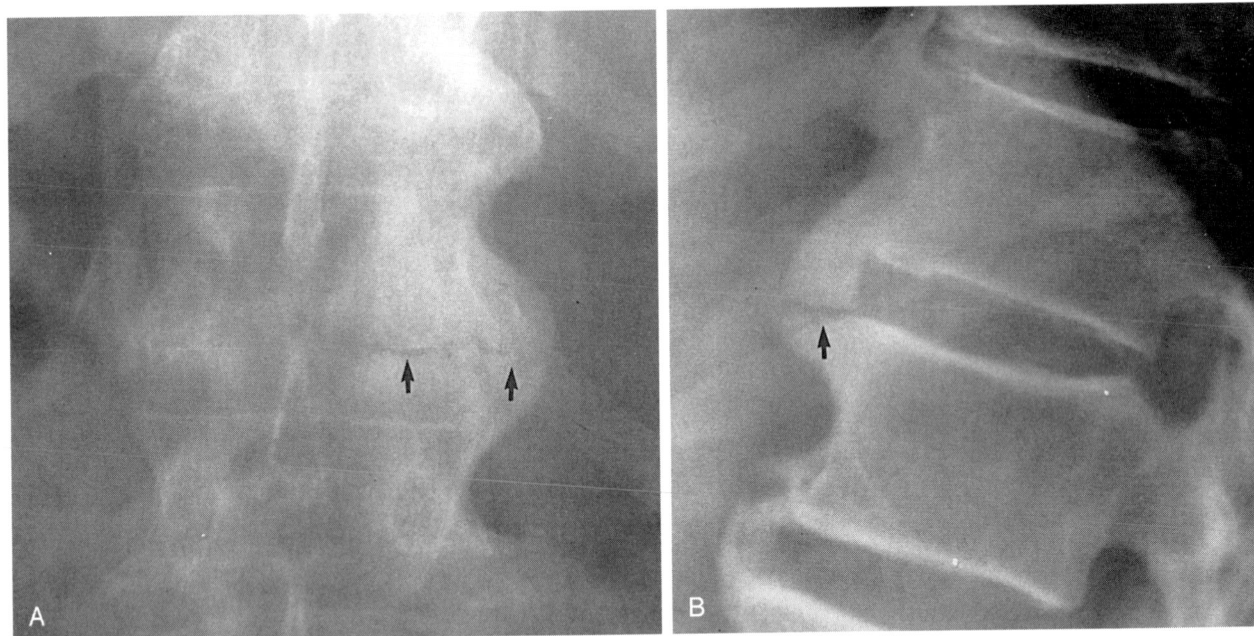

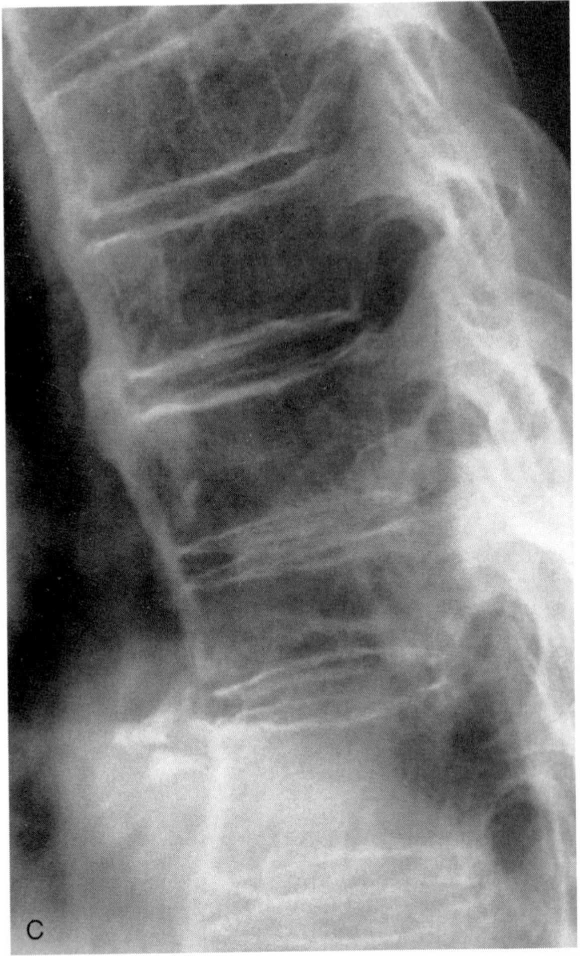

FIGURE 3–36. Diffuse idiopathic skeletal hyperostosis (DISH): Fracture through the region of hyperostosis.[50, 51] A, B This man with long-standing DISH had a 6-month history of thoracolumbar pain. He could not recall any specific injury to his back during the past year. A radiolucent cleft (arrows) traverses the bone outgrowth at T12-L1. Continued motion at such fracture sites frequently results in a pseudarthrosis. C In another patient with advanced DISH, a fracture has occurred through the region of hyperostosis, and the adjacent vertebral body is slightly diminished in height.

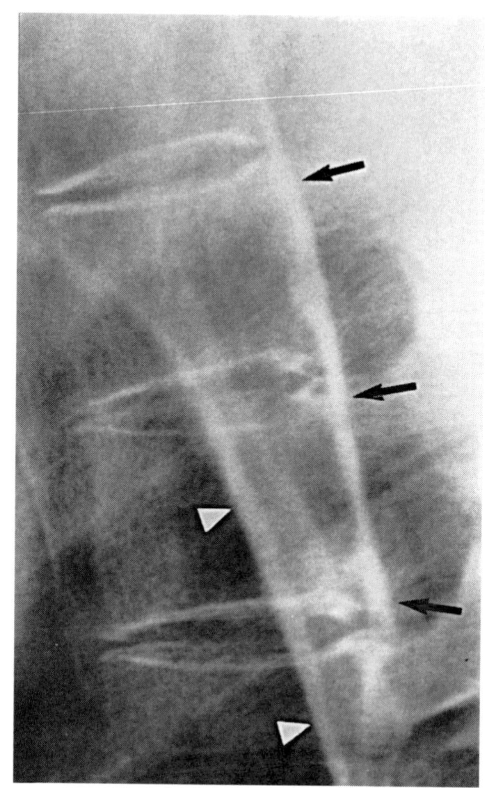

FIGURE 3–37. Ossification of the posterior longitudinal ligament (OPLL).[52] A thin linear sheet of ossification is observed within the spinal canal immediately posterior to the upper thoracic vertebral bodies (arrows). The overlying scapular margin (arrowheads) should not be confused with abnormal ossification. *(Courtesy of M. Mitchell, M.D., Halifax, Nova Scotia, Canada.)*

TABLE 3–10. Terminology Commonly Applied to Spinal Abnormalities in Ankylosing Spondylitis

Term	Definition
Osteitis	Enthesopathy occurring at discovertebral junction and associated with erosion, sclerosis, and syndesmophytes
"Shiny corner" sign	Increased radiodensity of the corners of the vertebral body related to "osteitis"
Squaring	Loss of normal anterior vertebral body concavity related to erosion and resulting in a flattened or convex anterior margin of the vertebral body
Syndesmophyte	Ossification of the outer fibers of the anulus fibrosus leading to thin, vertical spinal outgrowths
Bamboo spine	Undulating vertebral contour due to extensive syndesmophytosis
Discitis	"Erosive" abnormalities of the discovertebral junction
Disc ballooning	Biconcave shape of the intervertebral disc space related to osteoporotic deformity and central flattening or collapse of the vertebral body
"Trolley track" sign	Three vertical radiodense lines on frontal radiographs related to ossification of the supraspinous and interspinous ligaments and the apophyseal joint capsules
Dagger sign	Single central radiodense line on frontal radiographs related to ossification of the supraspinous and interspinous ligaments

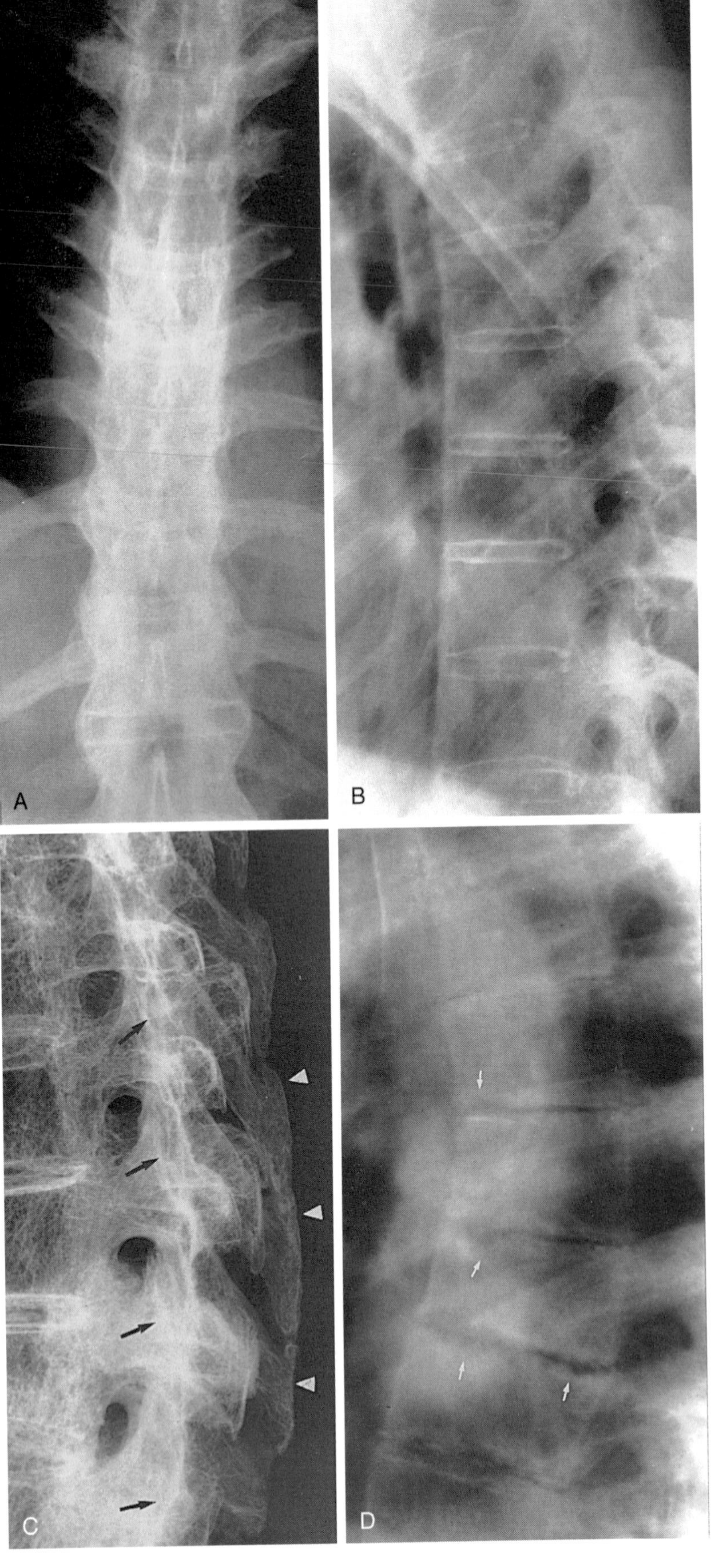

FIGURE 3–38. Ankylosing spondylitis: Spectrum of abnormalities.[54, 55] A, B A 75-year-old man with long-standing ankylosing spondylitis. In A, a frontal radiograph reveals extensive ankylosis of the apophyseal joints, marginal syndesmophytes, and hyperostosis of the costovertebral joints. In B, a lateral radiograph clearly demonstrates continuous syndesmophyte formation and ankylosis of the apophyseal joints. *(A, B, Courtesy of D. Goodwin, M.D., Lebanon, New Hampshire.)* C Ossification of the supraspinous ligament (arrowheads) and widespread apophyseal joint ankylosis (arrows) are seen throughout the thoracic spine in this specimen radiograph. D Erosive changes. In another patient, observe the diffuse disc space narrowing and vertebral end-plate erosions (arrows).

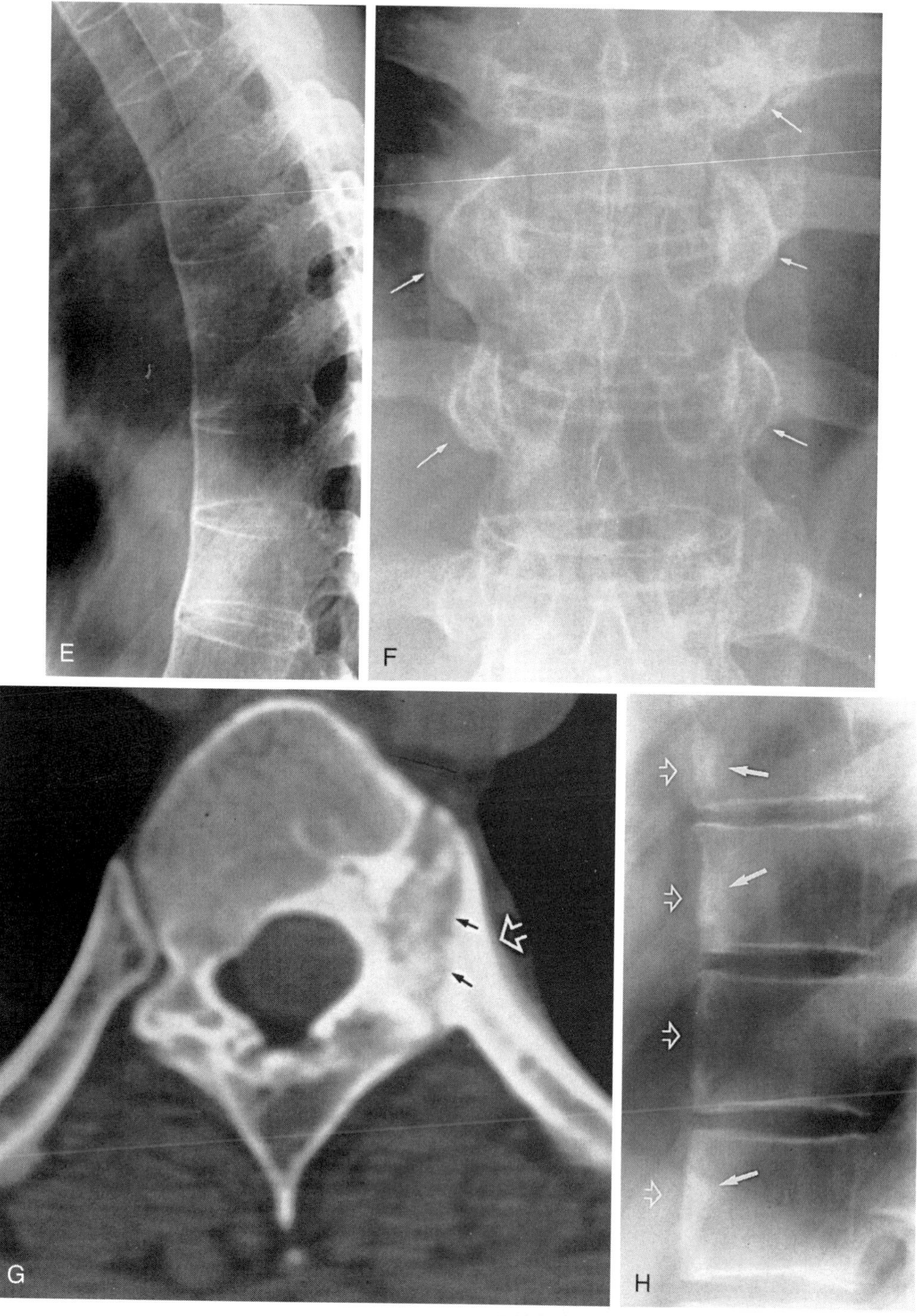

FIGURE 3–38 *Continued.* E In a 57-year-old man with advanced disease, observe the extensive syndesmophyte production, osteopenia, ballooning of the disc spaces, and marked kyphosis. F, G Costovertebral involvement. In F, a frontal radiograph shows prominent, bulbous enlargement of several costovertebral articulations (arrows). In G, a transaxial CT scan in another patient demonstrates costovertebral joint space obliteration, subchondral bone erosion (arrows), and cortical thickening of the adjacent rib (open arrow) and vertebral body. H Osteitis. Squaring (open arrows) and sclerosis (arrows) of the anterior margins of vertebral bodies ("shiny corner" sign) are characteristic signs of osteitis typically seen in early ankylosing spondylitis.

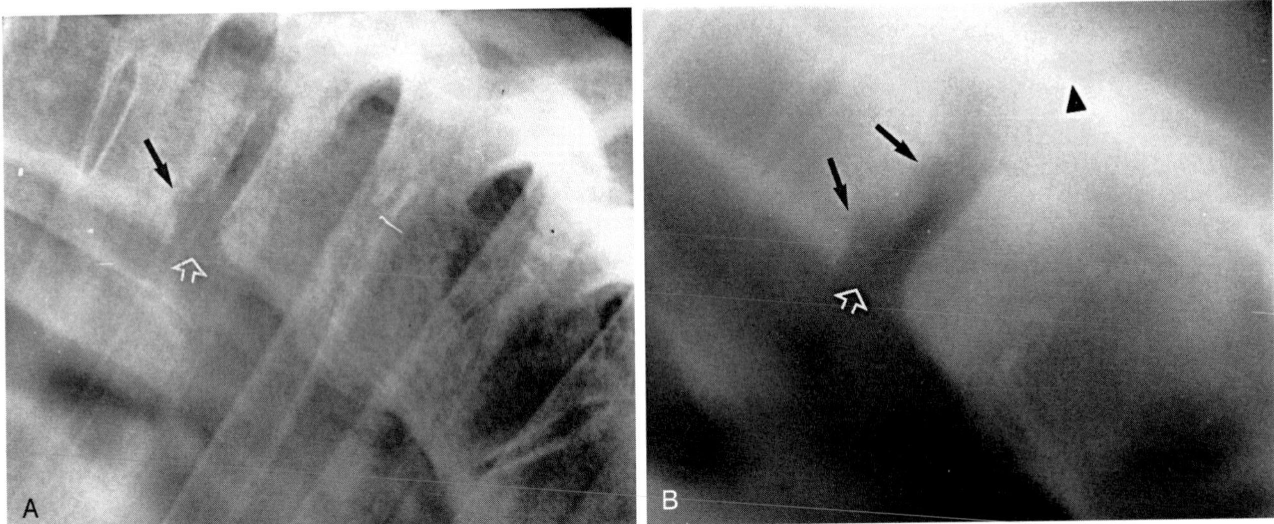

FIGURE 3–39. Ankylosing spondylitis: Pseudarthrosis.[55] Lateral radiograph (A) and sagittal conventional tomogram (B) from a 59-year-old man with advanced ankylosing spondylitis who gradually developed signs and symptoms of cord compression. Observe the absence of ankylosis at one level (open arrows) and extensive osseous resorption, sclerosis, and erosions (arrows) of the discovertebral junctions characteristic of a pseudarthrosis. The tomogram confirms presence of a fracture through the posterior elements (arrowhead). Pseudarthrosis may simulate spinal infection. Note also the widespread syndesmophyte formation, ankylosis, and kyphosis throughout the remainder of the spine.

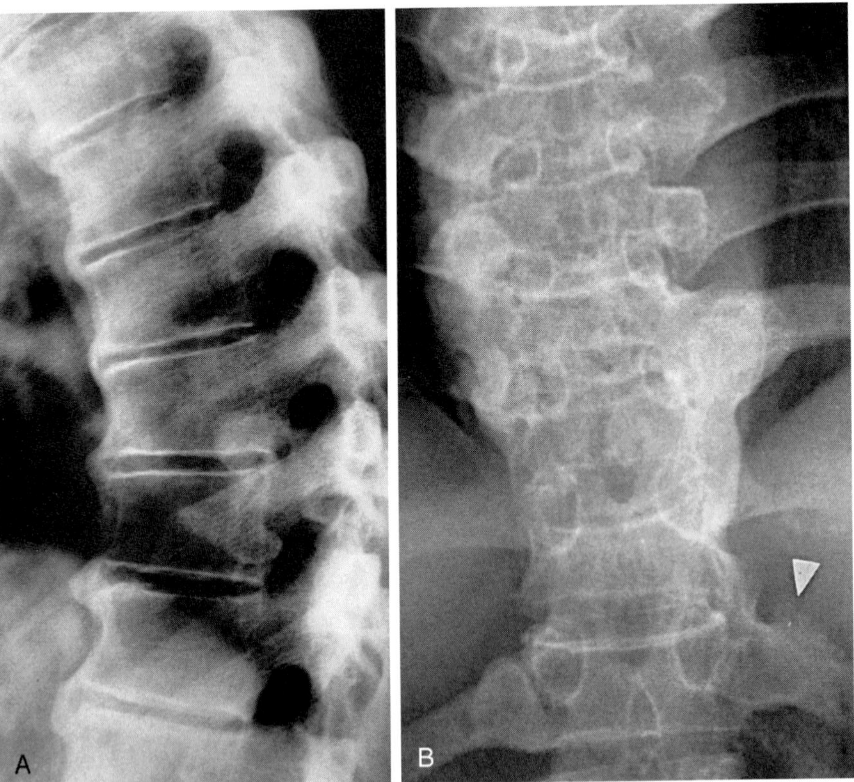

FIGURE 3–40. Psoriatic spondyloarthropathy.[56] A The paravertebral ossification in this patient with polyarticular psoriatic spondyloarthropathy and dermopathy resembles the flowing hyperostosis of diffuse idiopathic skeletal hyperostosis (DISH). B Prominent bulky paravertebral ossification is seen throughout the thoracic spine in this 28-year-old patient with long-standing psoriatic skin lesions and polyarticular arthropathy. Fluffy periostitis involving the twelfth rib (arrowhead), a finding characteristic of the seronegative spondyloarthropathies, also is evident.

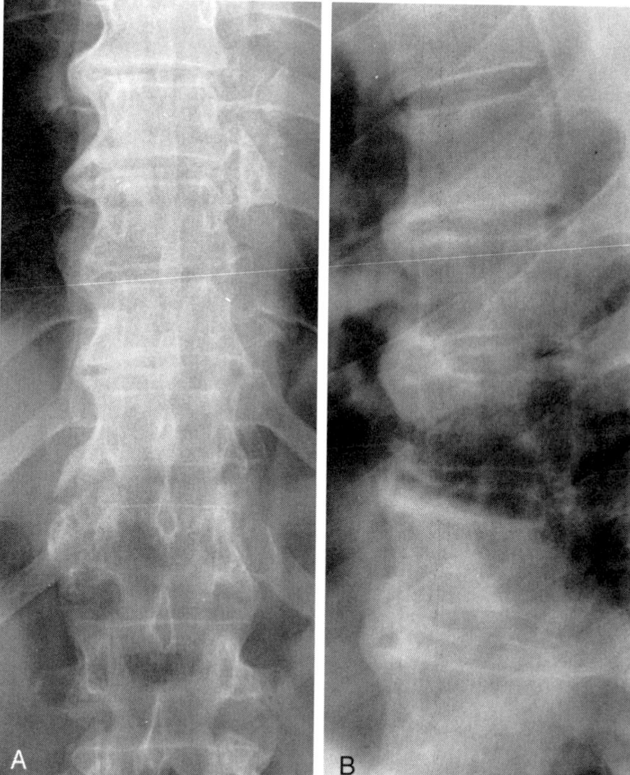

FIGURE 3–41. Reiter's syndrome.[57] Frontal (A) and lateral (B) radiographs of the thoracic spine in this 62-year-old man reveal paravertebral ossification in an asymmetric distribution. The characteristic pattern of ossification is that of comma-shaped, nonmarginal outgrowths. In this patient, some of the excrescences resemble the bridging osteophytes of degenerative disc disease and the flowing hyperostosis characteristic of diffuse idiopathic skeletal hyperostosis (DISH).

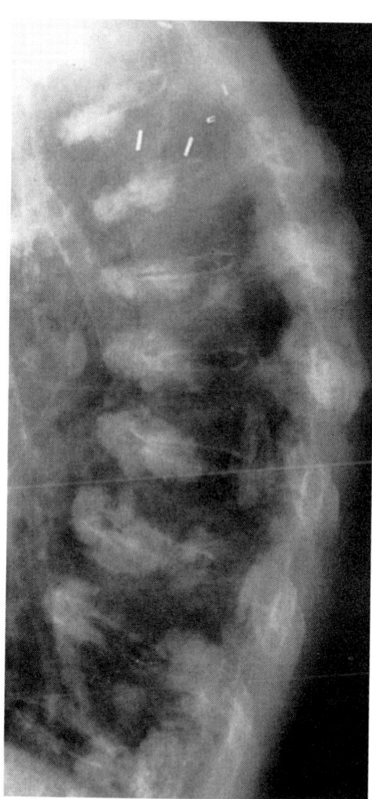

FIGURE 3–42. Progressive systemic sclerosis (scleroderma).[58] Extensive globular soft tissue calcification is seen adjacent to the intervertebral disc spaces and costovertebral joints. *(Courtesy of A. Nemcek, M.D., Chicago, Illinois, and L. Rogers, Winston-Salem, North Carolina.)*

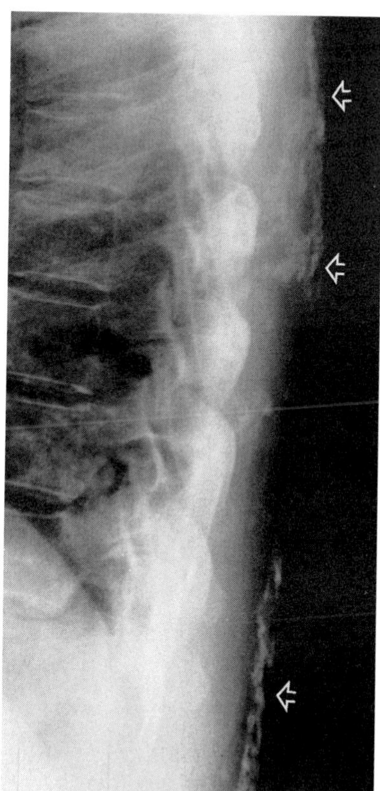

FIGURE 3–43. Dermatomyositis-polymyositis.[59] Diffuse subcutaneous calcification is seen in the paraspinal region posterior to the spine (open arrows). *(Courtesy of C. Pineda, M.D., Mexico City, Mexico.)*

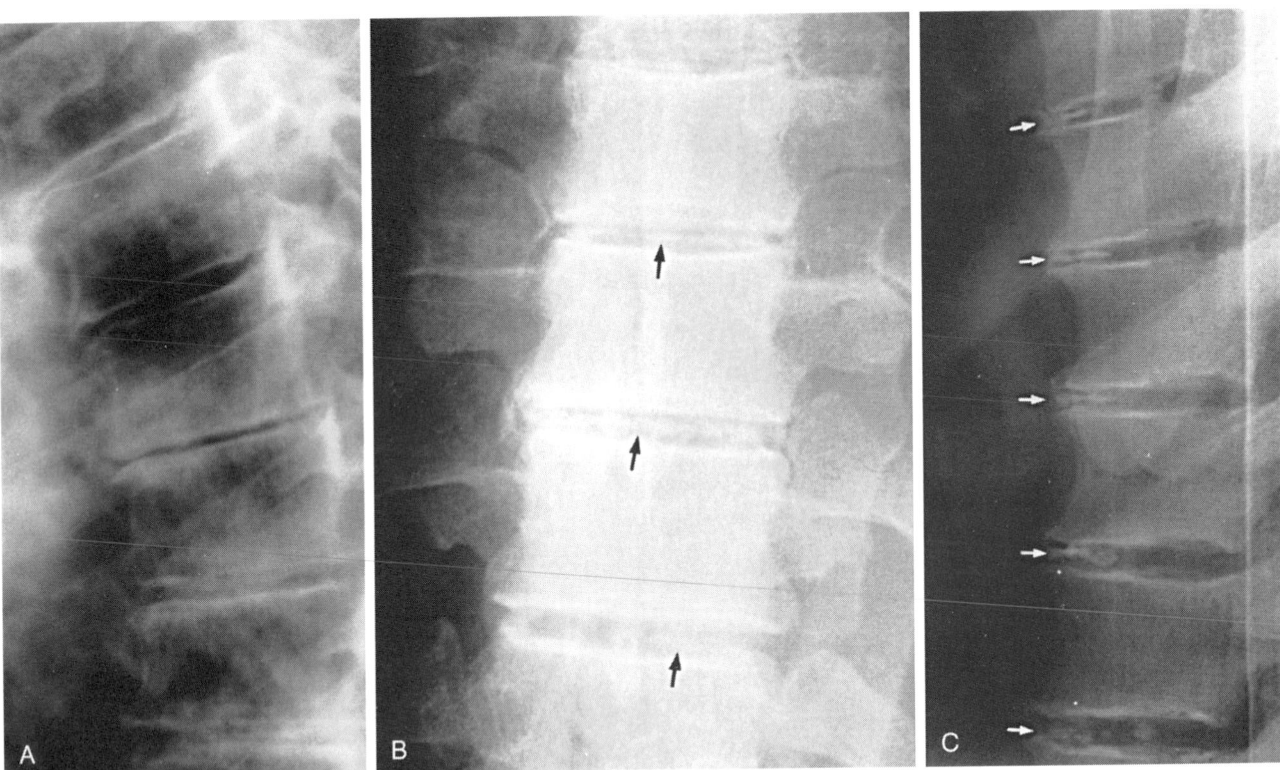

FIGURE 3–44. Calcium pyrophosphate dihydrate (CPPD) crystal deposition disease.[60, 61] A Severe disc space narrowing, calcification, and vacuum phenomena are accompanied by sclerosis of the vertebral end plates in this 77-year-old man. B, C Frontal (B) and lateral (C) radiographs from this 46-year-old man show extensive intervertebral disc calcification (arrows) and narrowing throughout the thoracic spine.

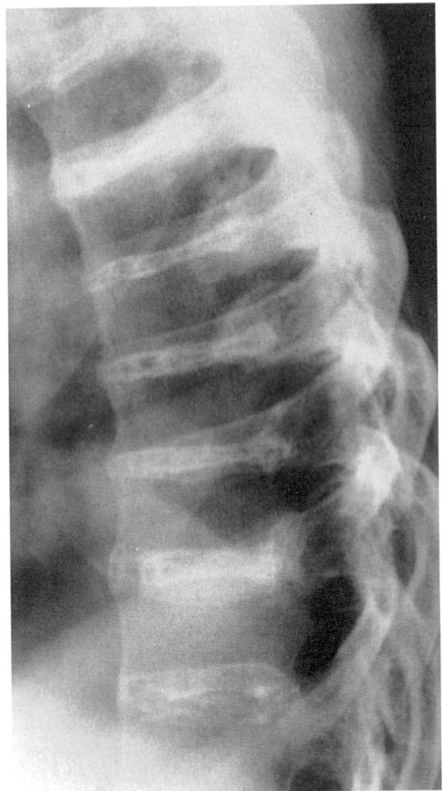

FIGURE 3–45. Alkaptonuria.[62] Diffuse disc space narrowing, calcification, and ossification, vertebral body osteoporosis, and small osteophytes are present in this patient.

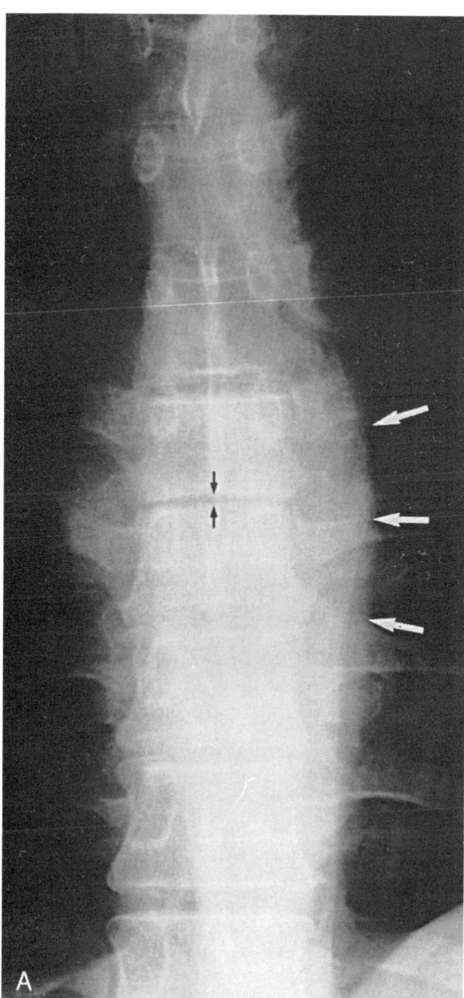

FIGURE 3–46. Tuberculous spondylitis: Paraspinal and epidural abscess.[64, 65] A Routine radiography. On this anteroposterior thoracic radiograph, the paraspinal tissues are distended, displacing the paraspinal line (white arrows). Narrowing of the intervertebral disc space also is demonstrated (black arrows). B, C MR imaging. Midsagittal (B) and parasagittal (C) T2-weighted (TR/TE 3500/112) fast-spin echo magnetic resonance (MR) images reveal pathologic collapse of the T2 vertebral body and a large paraspinal and epidural abscess of high signal intensity. The inhomogeneous abscess (white open arrows) extends anteriorly throughout the prevertebral soft tissues into the cervical region. The epidural extension of the abscess displaces and compresses the thoracic spinal cord (black arrow). Paraspinal subligamentous extension of tuberculous abscesses from vertebral and discal sites to the adjacent ligaments and soft tissues is frequent. Extension usually is anterolateral but may occur posteriorly into the peridural space, as in this case. *(B, C, Courtesy of T. Broderick, M.D., Orange, California.)*

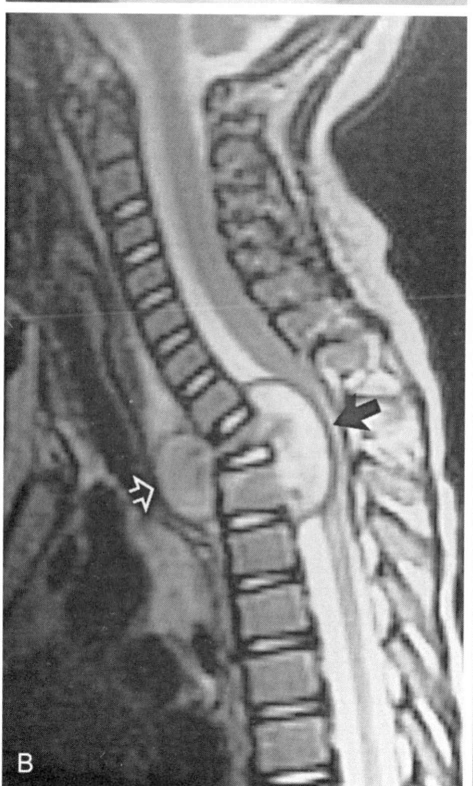

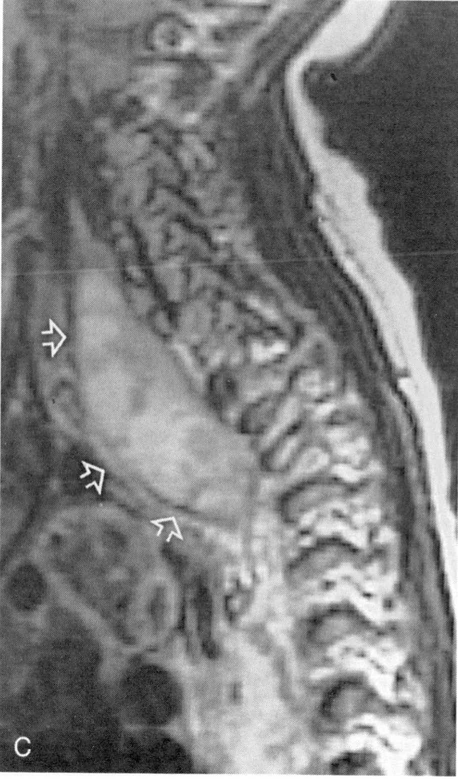

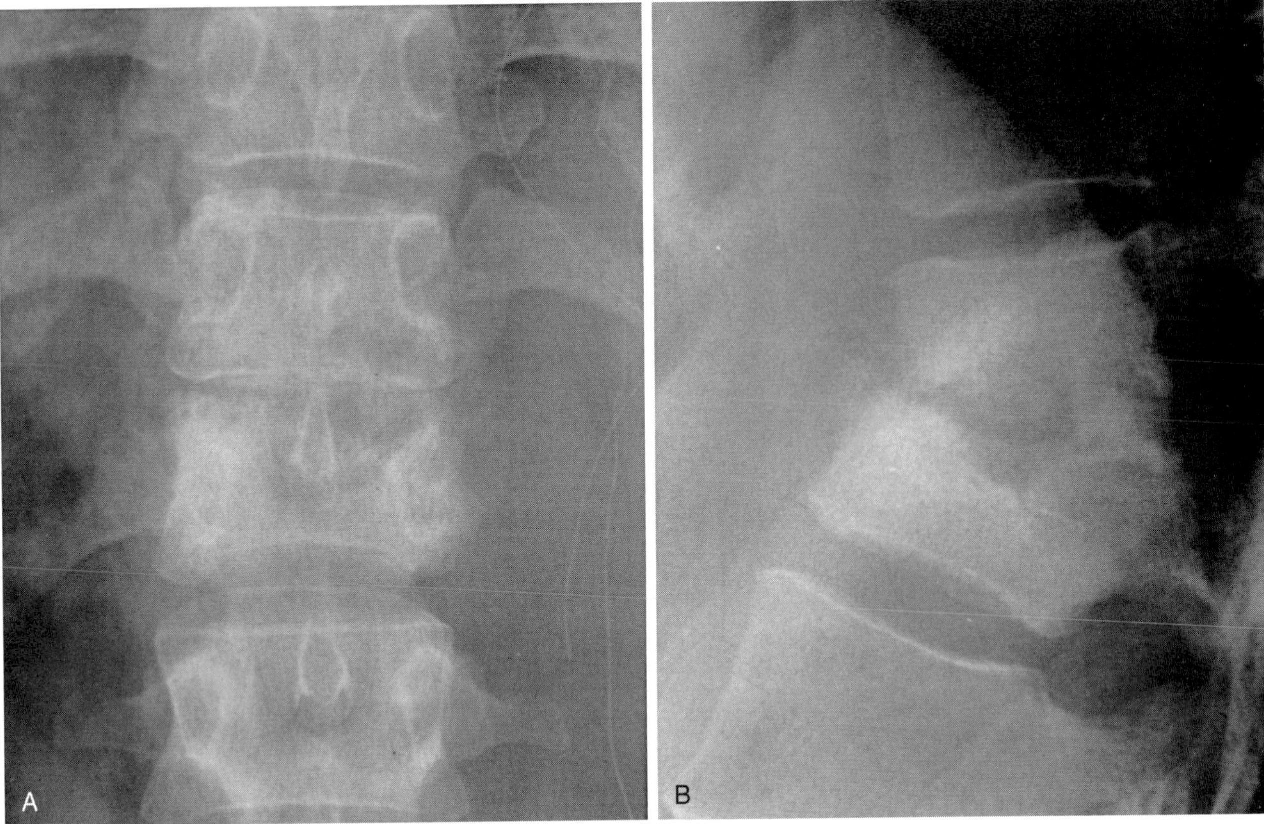

FIGURE 3–47. Tuberculous spondylodiscitis.[64, 65] Observe the marked erosion and destruction of the vertebral end plates with adjacent reactive sclerosis, obliteration of the intervening disc space, and pathologic collapse of the vertebral bodies of T11 and T12 in this 33-year-old woman with known pulmonary tuberculosis. The left twelfth rib had been removed surgically.

TABLE 3–11. **Thoracic Spine Neoplasms***

Entity	Figure(s)
Malignant neoplasms	
Skeletal metastasis[66–68]	3–48 to 3–50
Primary malignant neoplasms of bone	
Osteosarcoma (conventional)[69]	3–51
Myeloproliferative disorders	
Plasma cell myeloma[70, 71]	3–52
Myelofibrosis[72]	3–53
Hodgkin's disease[73]	3–54
Leukemia[74]	3–55
Benign neoplasms	
Enostosis[75]	3–56
Osteoid osteoma[76]	3–20, 3–57
Giant cell tumor (benign)[77]	3–58
Hemangioma (solitary)[78]	3–59
Tumor-like lesions	
Paget's disease[79, 80]	3–60
Neurofibromatosis Type I (von Recklinghausen's disease)[81, 82]	3–61
Fibrous dysplasia[83, 84]	3–62
Langerhans' cell histiocytosis[85, 86]	3–63

*This table lists only the neoplasms illustrated in this chapter; for a more complete discussion of neoplasms, see Tables 1–10 to 1–12 and Table 2–13.

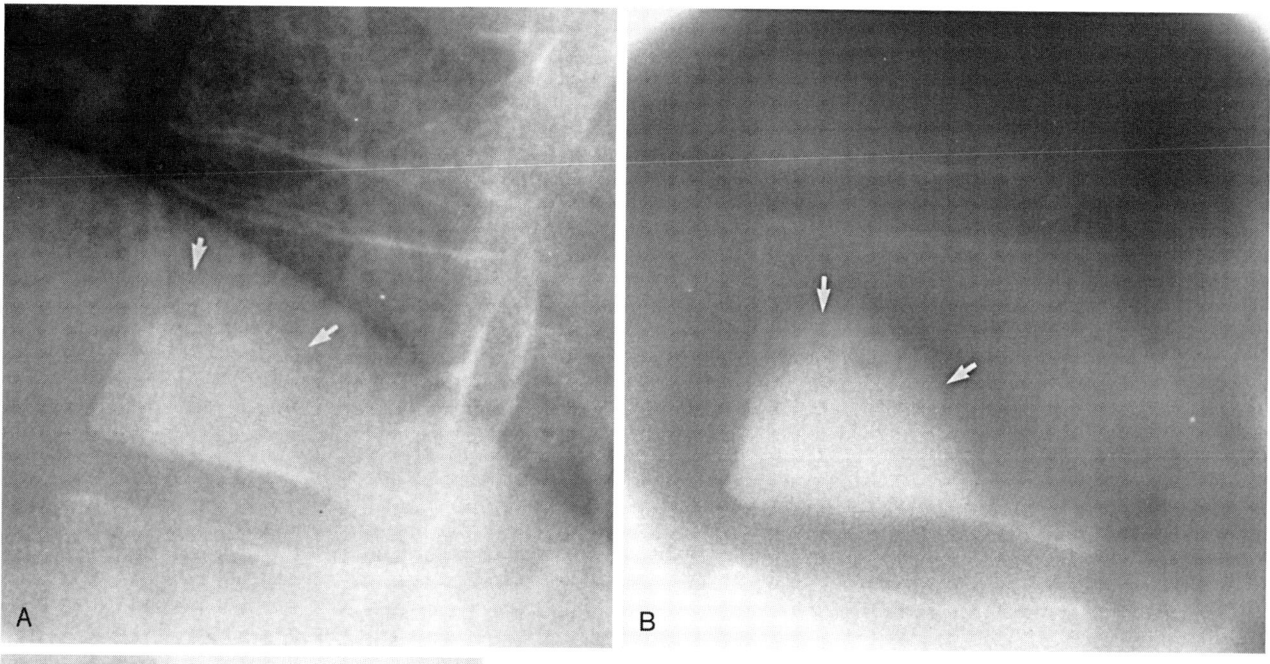

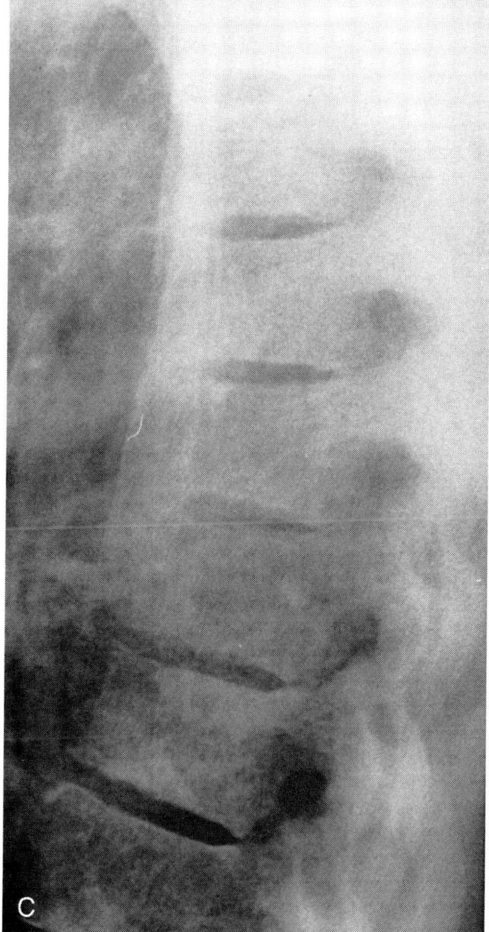

FIGURE 3–48. Skeletal metastasis: Carcinoma of the prostate—osteoblastic pattern.[66, 67] A, B This 54-year-old man had been diagnosed as having carcinoma of the prostate several years prior to this radiographic examination. Lateral thoracic radiograph (A) shows osteosclerosis of the T11 vertebral body (arrows). Conventional tomogram (B) clearly shows the osteosclerotic reaction of bone provoked by tumor infiltration (arrows). This appearance resembles that of idiopathic hemispherical segmental sclerosis of the vertebral body. C In another patient, a lateral thoracic radiograph shows a diffuse osteosclerotic pattern of metastatic disease uniformly involving all vertebrae. No evidence is seen of bone expansion, scalloping, or coarsened trabeculae, features that are helpful in differentiating osteoblastic metastatic disease from Hodgkin's disease or Paget's disease.

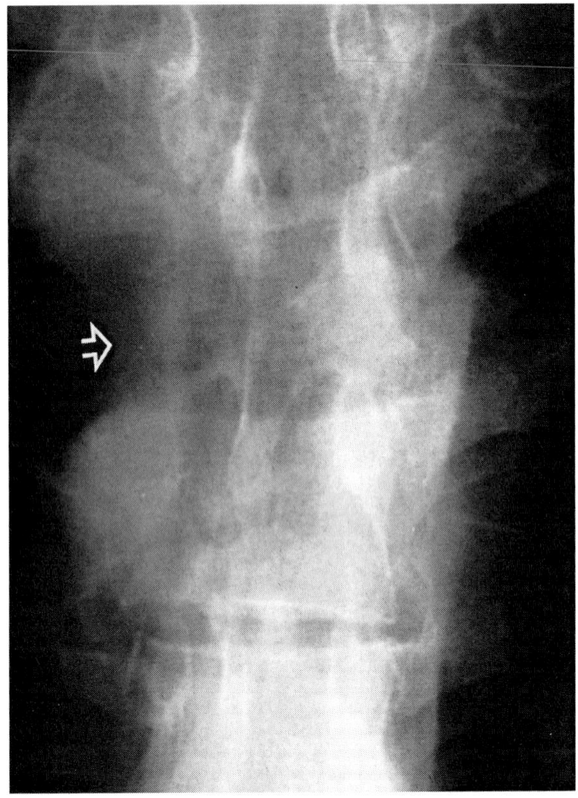

FIGURE 3–49. Skeletal metastasis: Missing pedicle sign.[66–68] In this patient with lung carcinoma, destruction of the pedicle and lateral portion of the vertebral body is seen on the frontal radiograph (open arrow). Osteolytic skeletal metastasis is the most common cause of a missing pedicle.

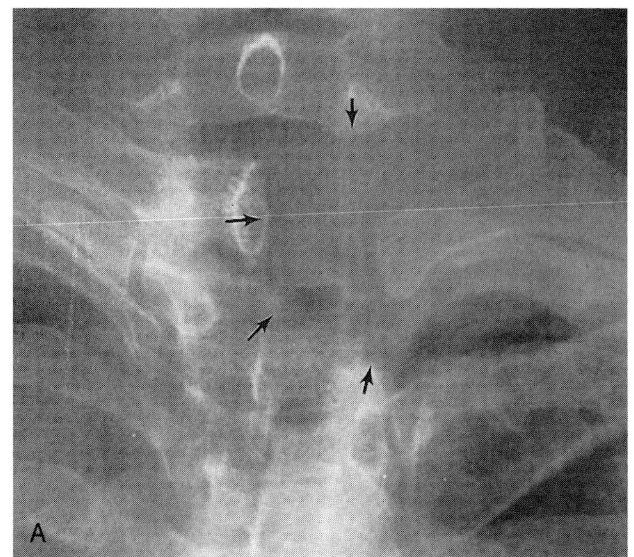

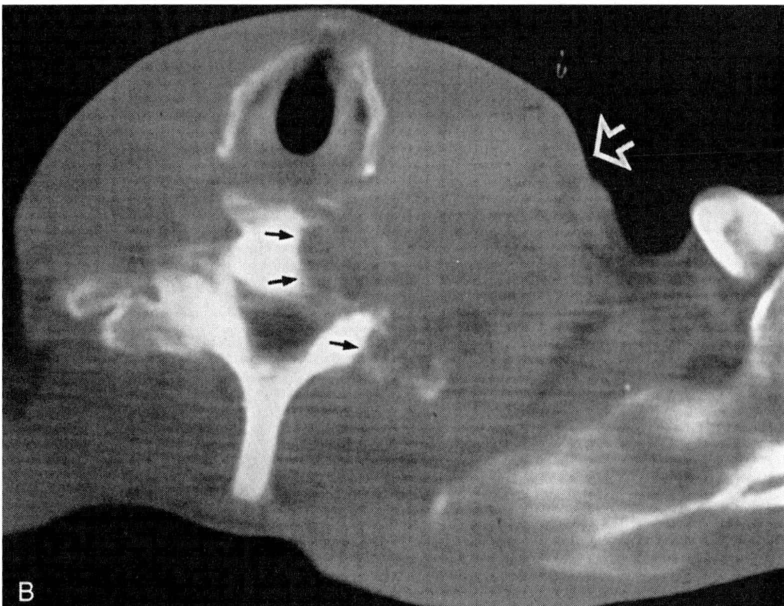

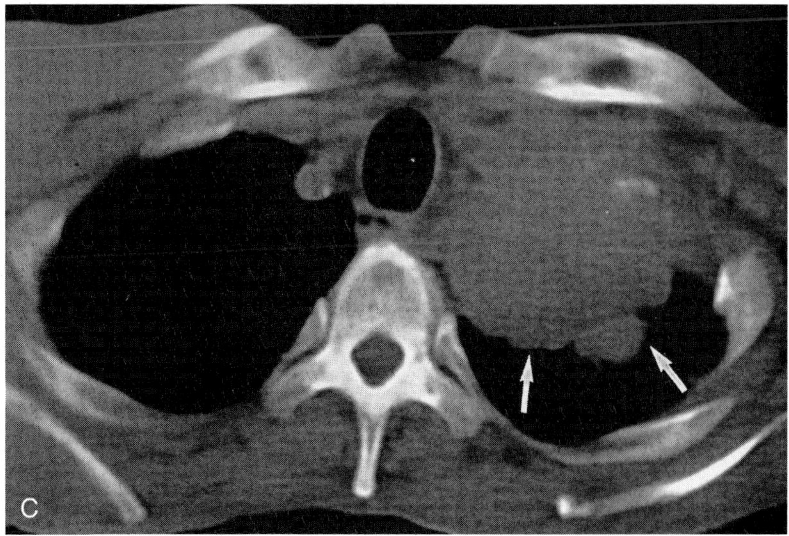

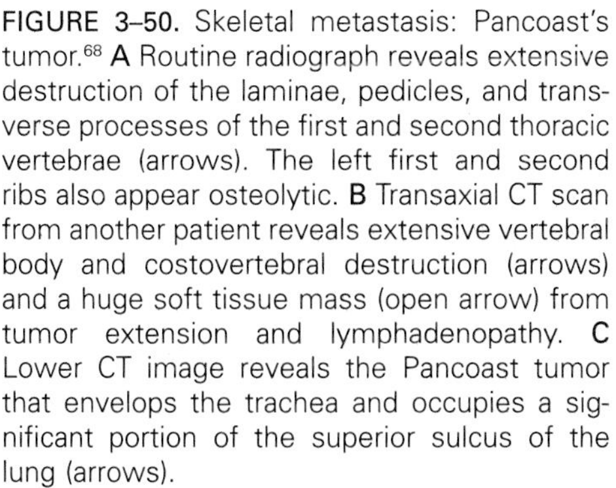

FIGURE 3–50. Skeletal metastasis: Pancoast's tumor.[68] **A** Routine radiograph reveals extensive destruction of the laminae, pedicles, and transverse processes of the first and second thoracic vertebrae (arrows). The left first and second ribs also appear osteolytic. **B** Transaxial CT scan from another patient reveals extensive vertebral body and costovertebral destruction (arrows) and a huge soft tissue mass (open arrow) from tumor extension and lymphadenopathy. **C** Lower CT image reveals the Pancoast tumor that envelops the trachea and occupies a significant portion of the superior sulcus of the lung (arrows).

In Pancoast's tumor, carcinoma of the apex of the lung most often invades adjacent ribs or cervicothoracic vertebrae via direct extension; or, less frequently, it spreads via hematogenous or lymphatic dissemination. *(Courtesy of B.A. Howard, M.D., Charlotte, North Carolina.)*

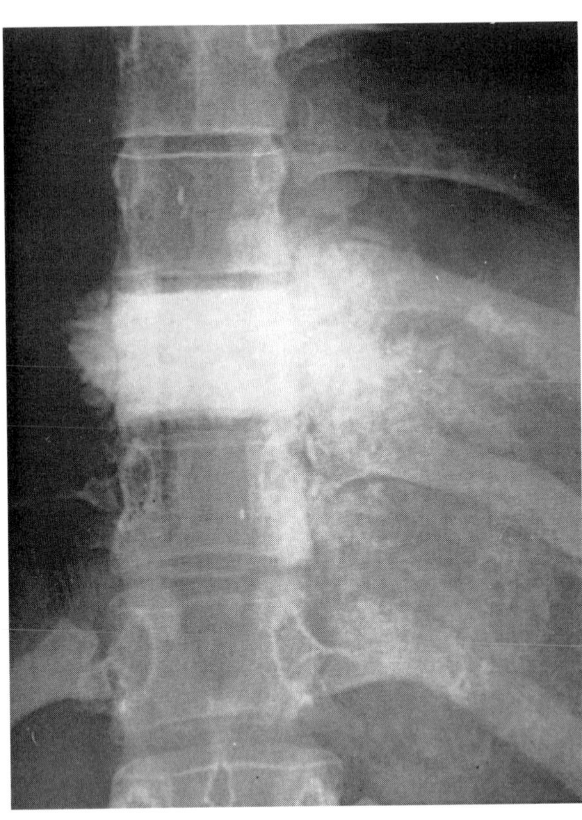

FIGURE 3–51. Osteosarcoma: Ivory vertebra.[69] Frontal radiograph of the spine in this 21-year-old woman demonstrates an osteosclerotic (ivory) vertebra with extraordinary proliferative ossification of the paraspinal soft tissues. Note the laminectomy defects from previous decompression surgery.

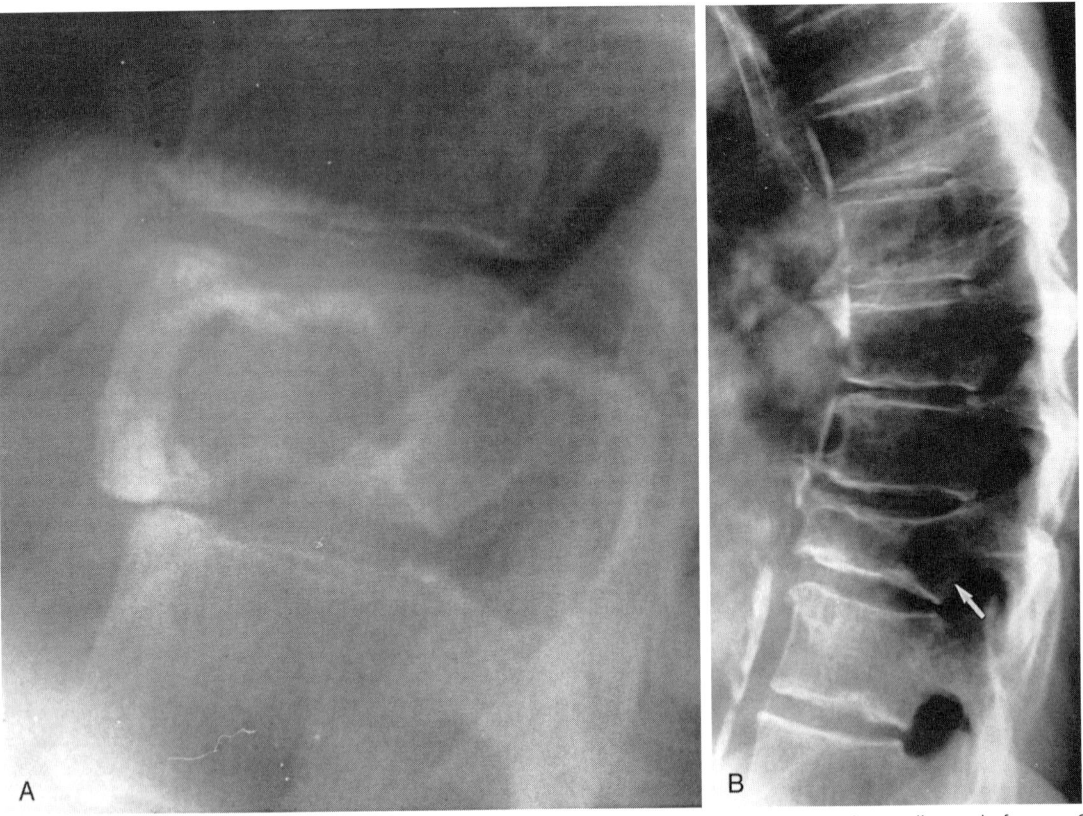

FIGURE 3–52. Plasma cell myeloma: Solitary plasmacytoma and multiple myeloma.[70, 71] **A** Routine radiograph from a 39-year-old woman with plasmacytoma shows a central radiolucent lesion within a partially collapsed lower thoracic vertebral body. A thick rim of sclerosis, a finding that resembles fibrous dysplasia, surrounds the radiolucent region. Plasmacytoma refers generally to solitary lesions of plasma cell myeloma. **B** Multiple myeloma. The prominent radiographic finding in this patient is diffuse osteopenia of the vertebral bodies. A pathologic vertebral compression fracture of T11 has occurred (arrow). Extensive vascular calcification within the posterior wall of the thoracic aorta also can be seen.

Plasma cell (multiple) myeloma is the most common primary malignant disease of bone. Infiltration of plasma cells occurs in patients 60 to 70 years of age and is particularly common in black persons.

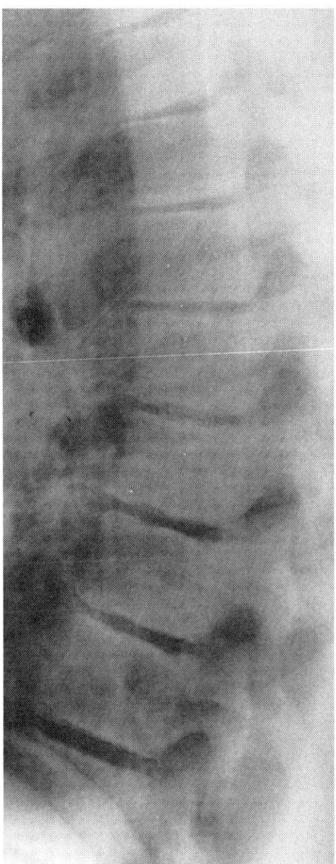

FIGURE 3–53. Myelofibrosis.[72] Diffuse osteosclerosis of the thoracic vertebrae is present in this patient. Myelofibrosis is an uncommon disease of middle-aged and elderly men and women. It is characterized by fibrotic or sclerotic bone marrow and extramedullary hematopoiesis. The main radiographic finding is osteosclerosis, but osteolysis or osteopenia also may occur occasionally. Patients usually have splenomegaly. *(Courtesy of M.N. Pathria, M.D., San Diego, California.)*

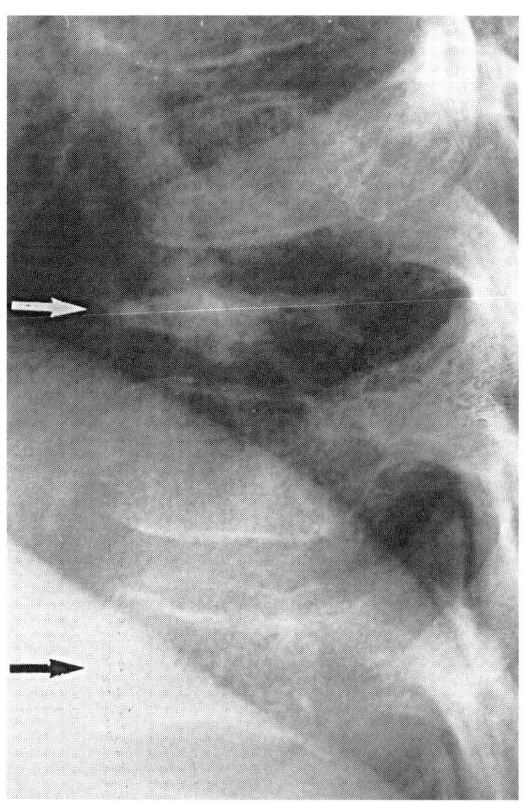

FIGURE 3–54. Hodgkin's disease.[73] Lateral radiograph of the spine in this child with Hodgkin's disease shows diffuse osteopenia. In addition, multiple collapsed vertebrae characterized by biconcave end-plate deformities (black arrow) and vertebra plana (white arrow) are evident. Hodgkin's disease may result in osteosclerosis, osteolysis, or a combination of the two.

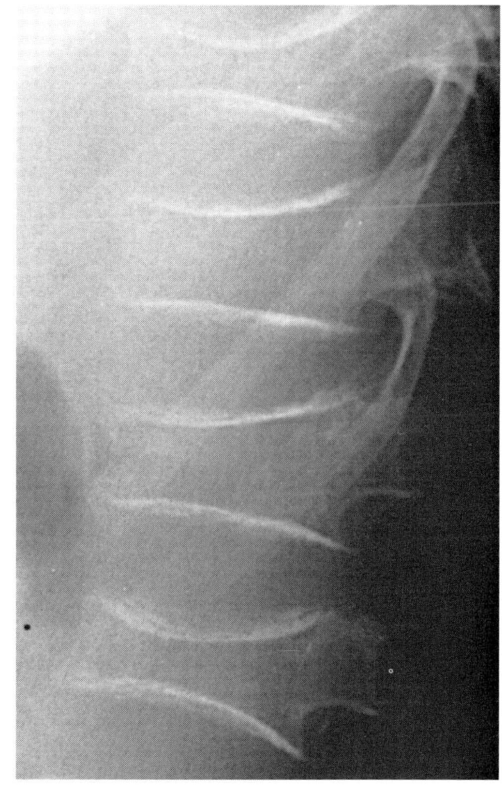

FIGURE 3–55. Acute childhood leukemia.[74] Multiple wedge-shaped and biconcave compression fractures are evident in this child.

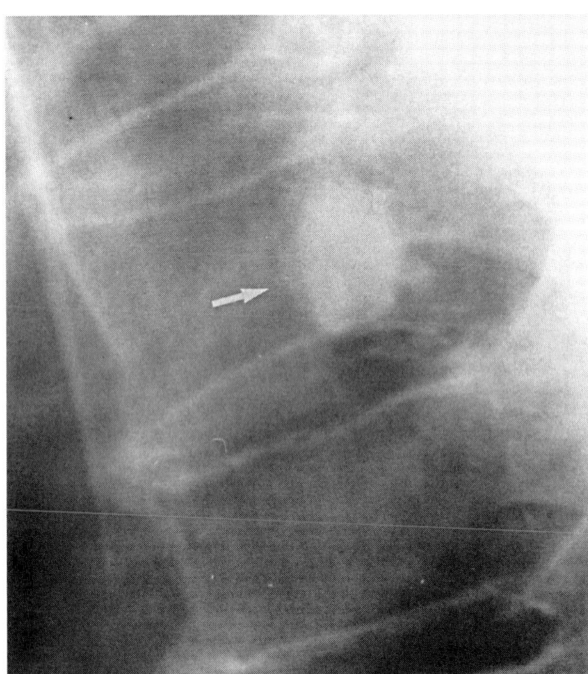

FIGURE 3–56. Bone island (enostosis).[75] A solitary, osteosclerotic lesion is seen in the vertebral body (arrow). Enostoses are solitary (or infrequently multiple) discrete foci of osteosclerosis within the spongiosa of bone. They may be round, ovoid, or oblong, may possess a brush border, and tend to be aligned with the long axis of trabecular architecture. Giant bone islands have been reported to reach proportions of 4 × 4 cm in diameter. Additionally, enostoses may increase or decrease in size and may even be positive on bone scans, particularly in large and growing lesions. Enostoses should be differentiated from other osteosclerotic processes, such as osteoblastic metastasis, osteomas, osteoid osteomas, enchondromas, bone infarcts, fibrous dysplasia, and osteopoikilosis.

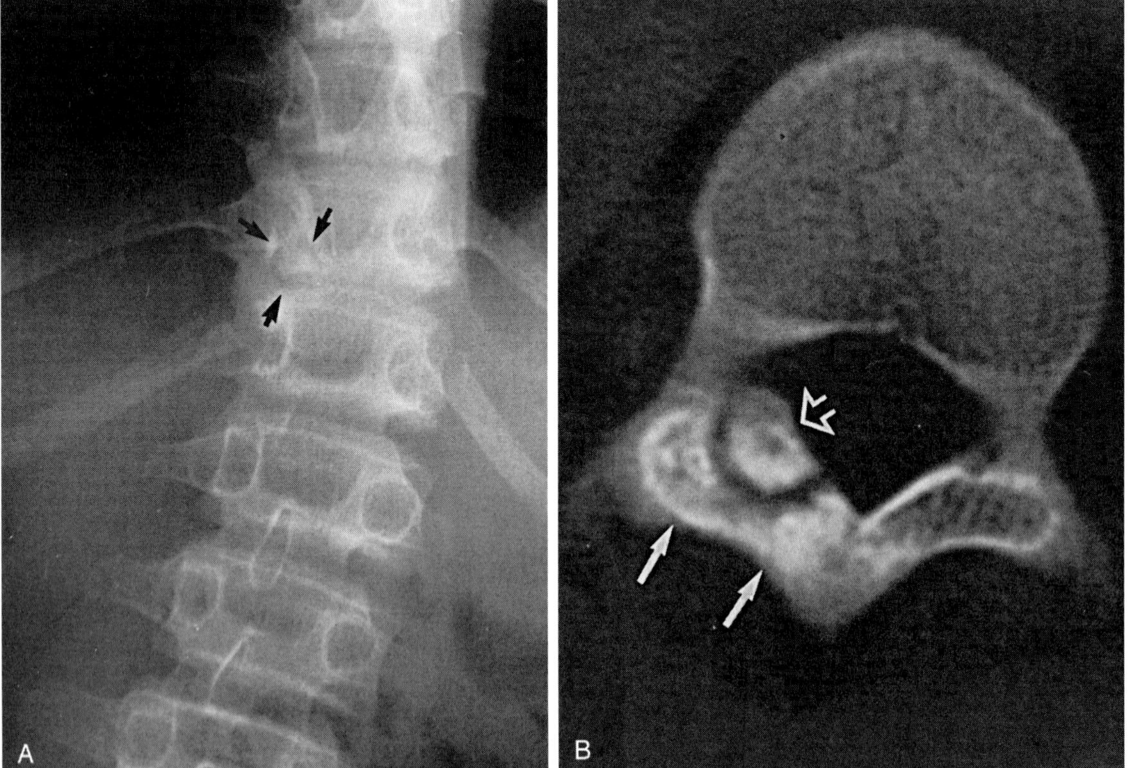

FIGURE 3–57. Osteoid osteoma.[76] 13-year-old boy with painful scoliosis. A Routine radiograph demonstrates an antalgic left thoracolumbar scoliosis. A circular radiolucent area with a central zone of calcification (nidus) is faintly visible within the right neural arch of T11 (arrows). B Transaxial CT image clearly shows the lesion localized to the right lamina of T11. A central zone of sclerosis representing the partially calcified nidus (open arrow) and reactive sclerosis of the adjacent bone (arrows) are evident.

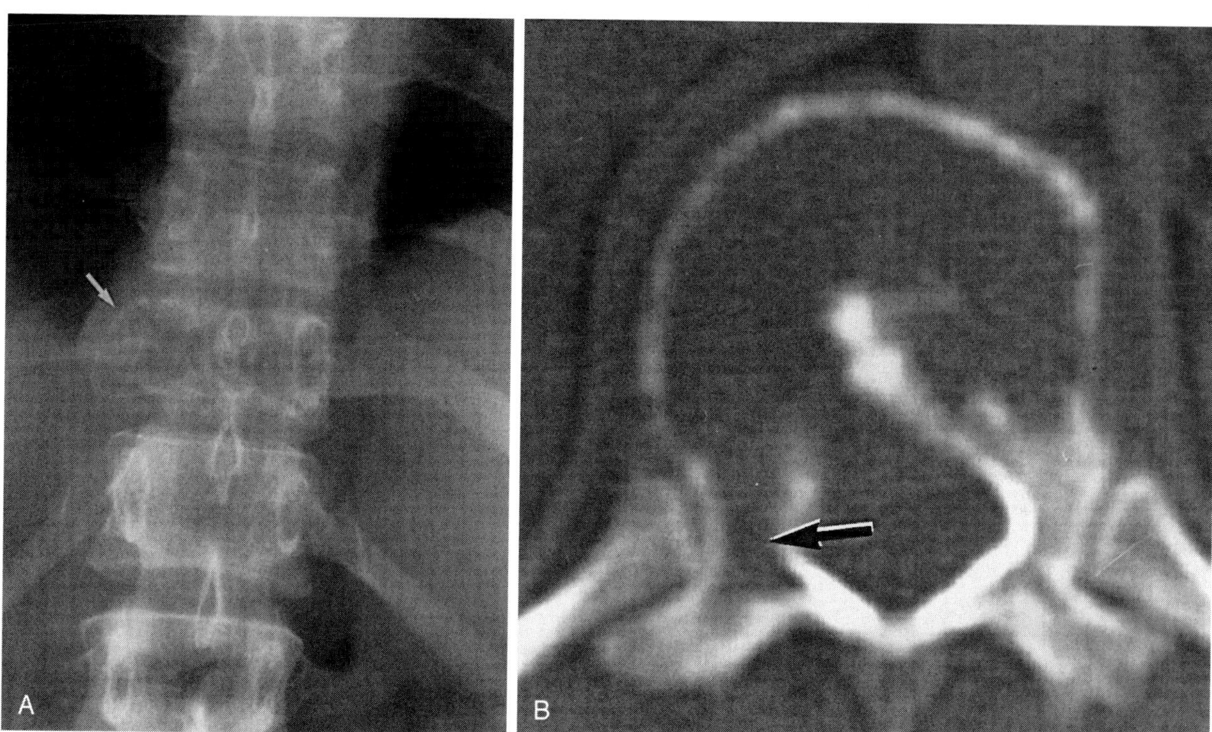

FIGURE 3–58. Giant cell tumor.[77] Radiographic investigation of back pain in this 29-year-old woman revealed an eccentric, expansile osteolytic lesion of the neural arch and partially collapsed vertebral body of T11. This is seen on the routine anteroposterior radiograph (A) (arrow) and is illustrated much more clearly on the transaxial CT image (B). The CT scan reveals that the lesion has destroyed the majority of the vertebral body and extends into the right pedicle and neural arch (arrow). Fewer than 10 per cent of all giant cell tumors affect the spine, and about 5 to 10 per cent of all giant cell tumors are malignant. *(Courtesy of C. Kusnick, M.D., Irvine, California.)*

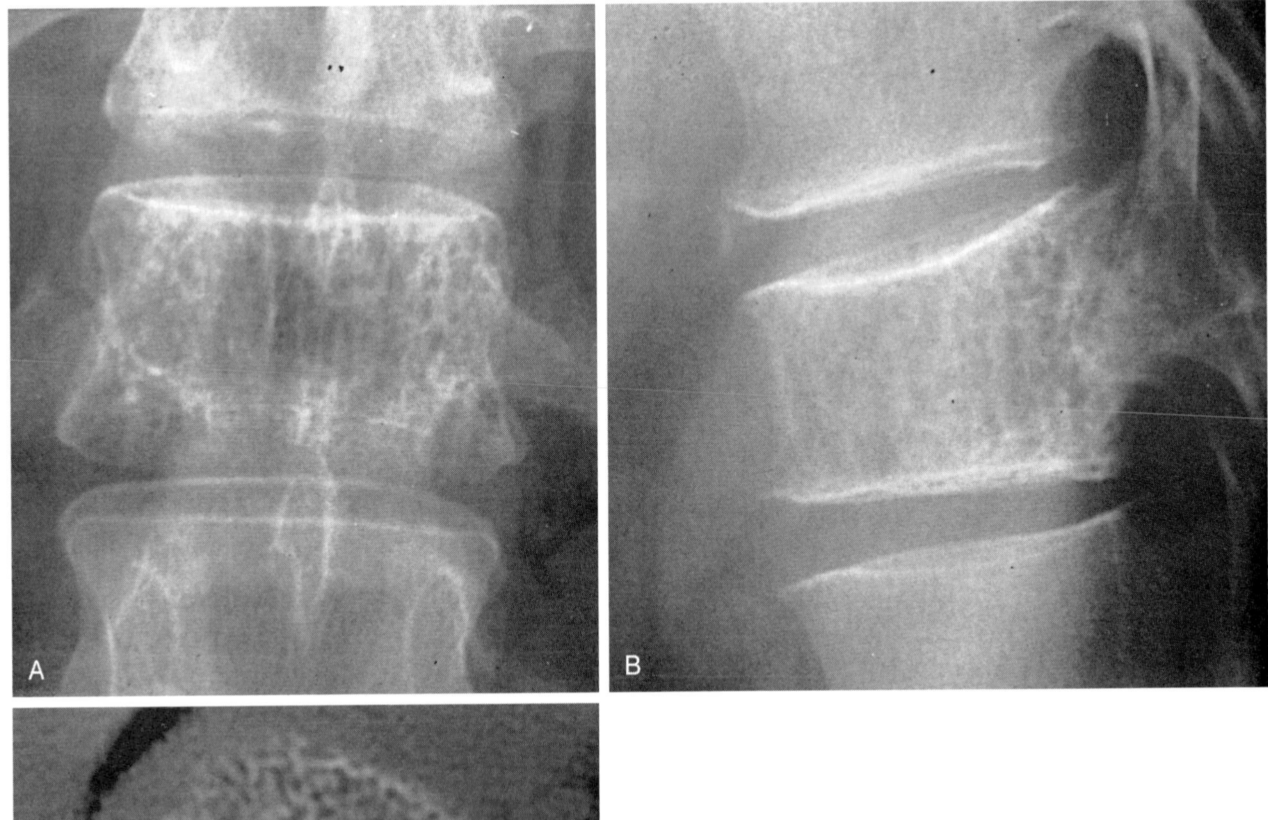

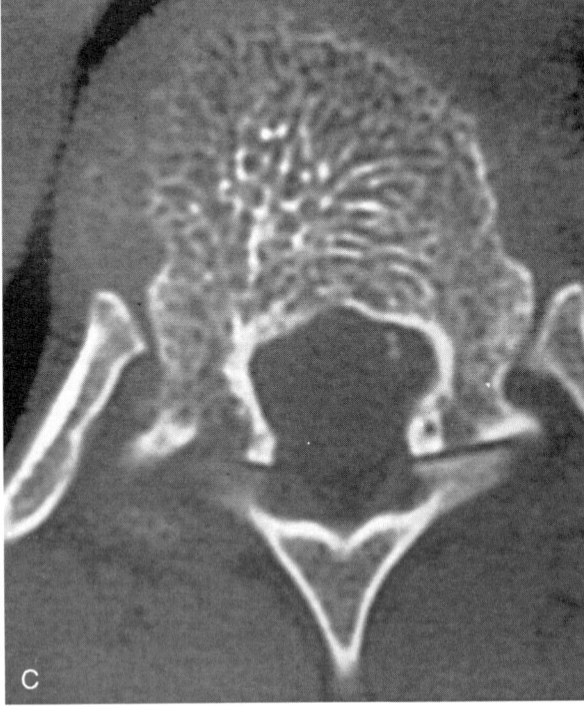

FIGURE 3–59. Hemangioma.[78] A, B A man in his late 30s had thoracolumbar pain. Frontal (A) and lateral (B) radiographs show a radiolucent vertebral body, accentuated vertical trabeculae, and a wedge-shaped compression fracture of the T12 vertebral body. This is an infrequent complication of benign hemangiomas. Pathologic fractures may cause spinal cord compression as a result of epidural extension of tumor, osseous displacement, or epidural hemorrhage. *(A, B, Courtesy of P.H. VanderStoep, M.D., St. Cloud, Minnesota.)* C In another patient, without a compression fracture, a transaxial computed tomographic (CT) scan of a thoracic vertebral hemangioma shows discrete columns of radiodense bone interspersed among the relatively osteopenic spongiosa of the vertebral body (the "corduroy cloth" appearance). Hemangiomas are considered the most common benign neoplasm of the spine.

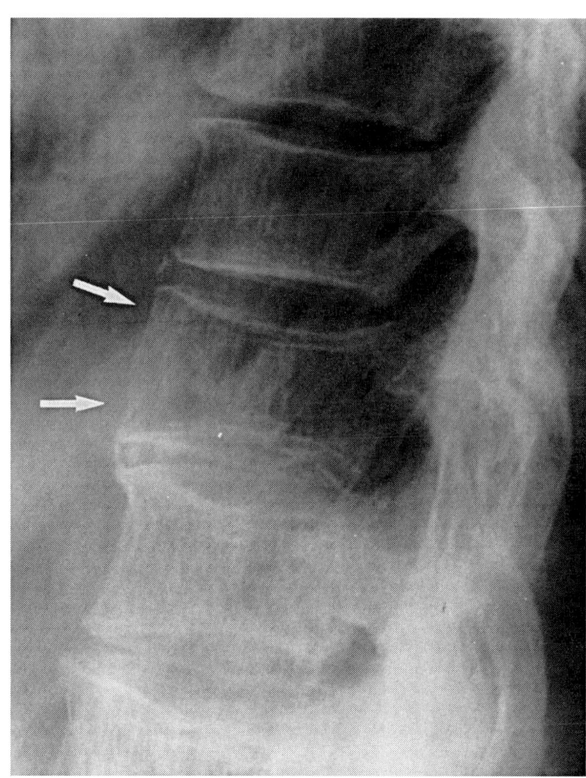

FIGURE 3–60. Paget's disease.[79, 80] Pagetic involvement of the thoracic spine is characterized by osseous enlargement and coarsening of trabeculae involving several vertebral bodies. Minimal collapse of the T11 vertebral body (arrows) also is present.

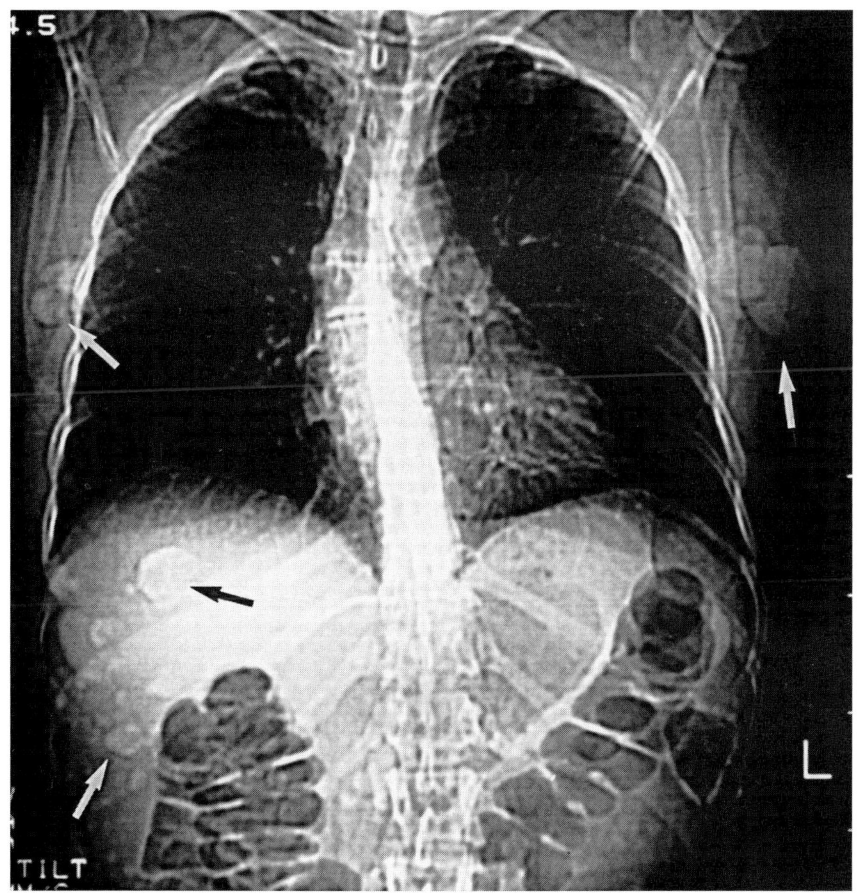

FIGURE 3–61. Neurofibromatosis Type I (von Recklinghausen's disease).[81, 82] Coronal CT localizer image from this 31-year-old man shows characteristic scoliosis and elevated skin lesions (fibroma molluscum) (arrows).

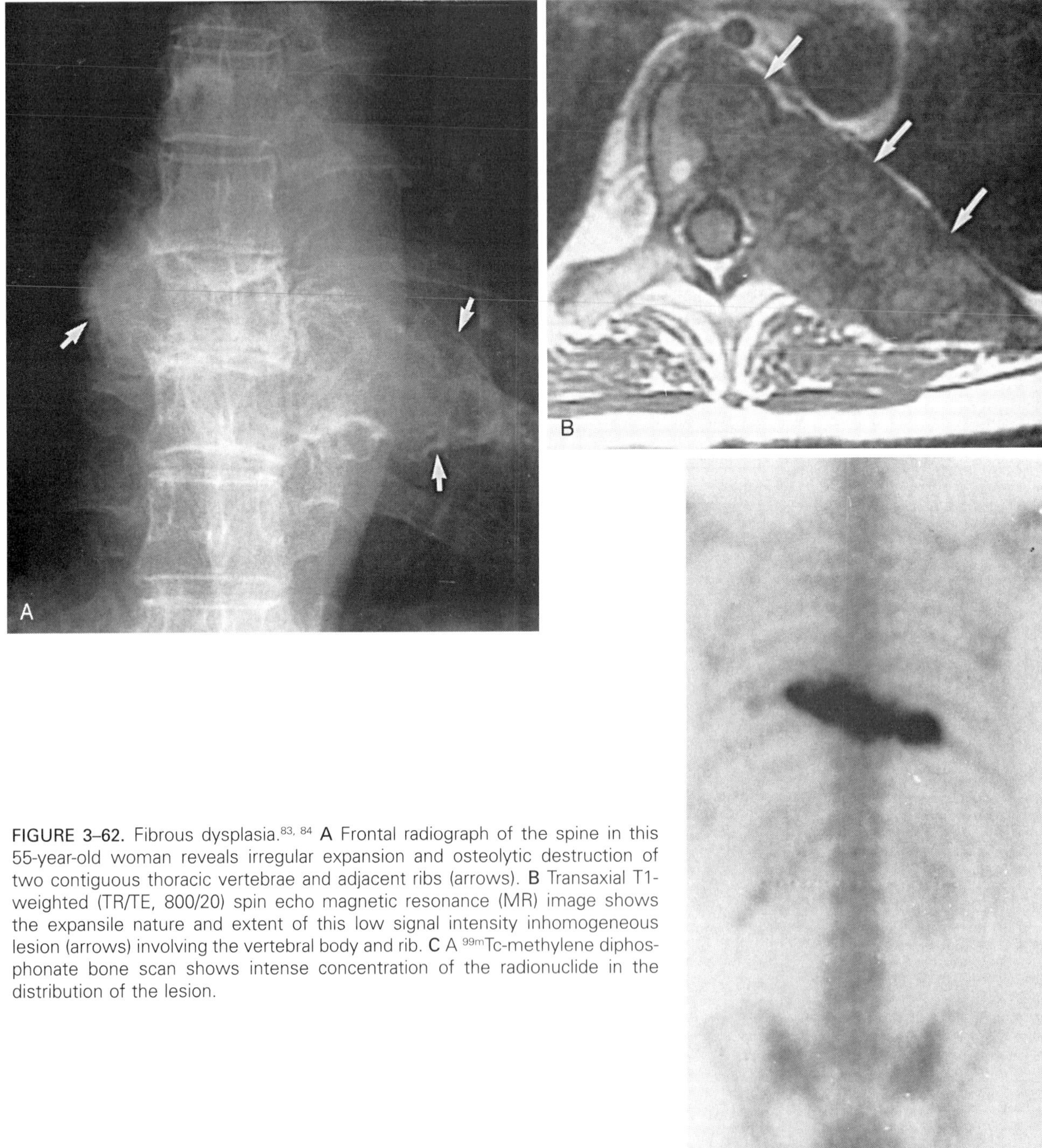

FIGURE 3–62. Fibrous dysplasia.[83, 84] A Frontal radiograph of the spine in this 55-year-old woman reveals irregular expansion and osteolytic destruction of two contiguous thoracic vertebrae and adjacent ribs (arrows). B Transaxial T1-weighted (TR/TE, 800/20) spin echo magnetic resonance (MR) image shows the expansile nature and extent of this low signal intensity inhomogeneous lesion (arrows) involving the vertebral body and rib. C A ^{99m}Tc-methylene diphosphonate bone scan shows intense concentration of the radionuclide in the distribution of the lesion.

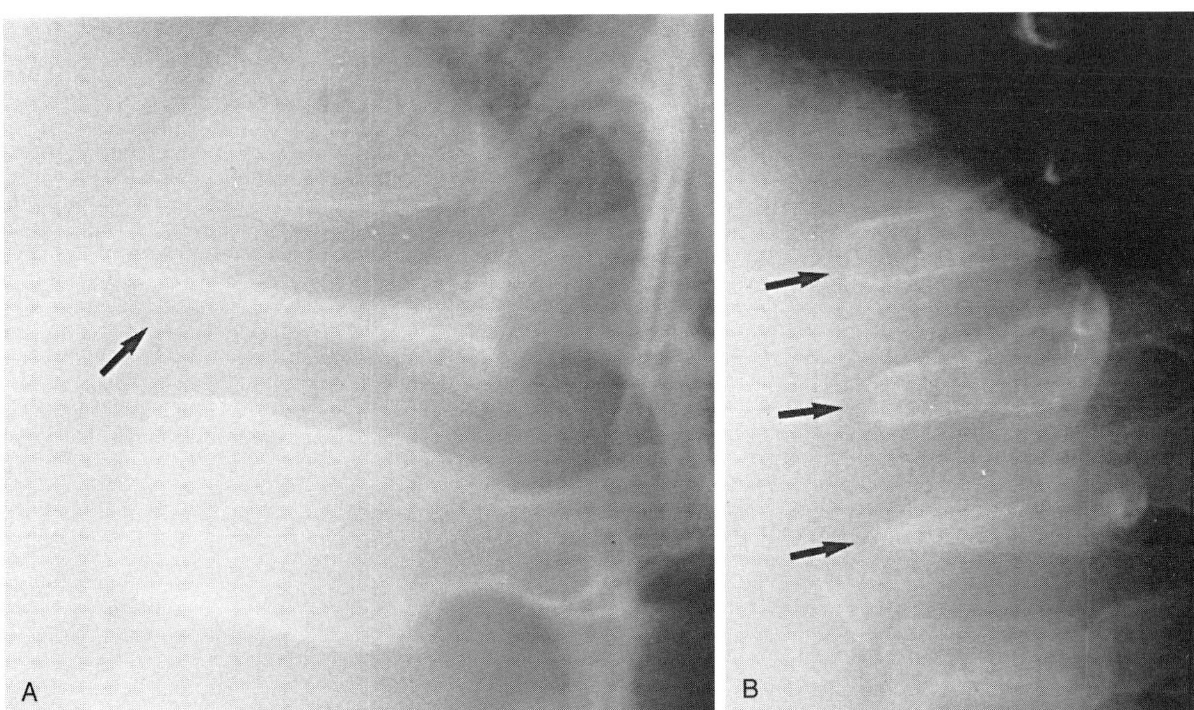

FIGURE 3–63. Langerhans' cell histiocytosis.[85, 86] A Eosinophilic granuloma. Observe vertebra plana involving a single vertebral body (arrow). B Letterer-Siwe disease. Vertebra plana involving multiple thoracic vertebral bodies (arrows) is seen in a patient with extensive bone involvement. Eosinophilic granuloma of bone is the most frequently encountered form of Langerhans' cell histiocytosis, a disease characterized by histiocytic infiltration of tissues. In addition to flattened vertebral bodies, bubbly, lytic, or expansile lesions without collapse may occur. With healing, the height of the vertebral body may be reconstituted, a finding more common in younger persons. Letterer-Siwe disease is the least common and most acute form of Langerhans' cell histiocytosis, usually affects children under the age of 3 years, and has the poorest clinical prognosis. It is characterized by histiocytic infiltration in multiple visceral organs. The intermediate form of histiocytosis—Hand-Schüller-Christian disease—is not illustrated.

TABLE 3–12. Metabolic and Hematologic Disorders Affecting the Thoracic Spine*

Entity	Figure(s)	Characteristics
Generalized osteoporosis[87]	3–64	Uniform decrease in radiodensity, thinning of vertebral end plates, accentuation of vertical trabeculae Thoracolumbar region of the spine is the most frequent site of osteoporotic compression fractures Wedge-shaped vertebral deformities are most common in thoracic spine compression fractures; vertebra plana deformities are more likely to be related to pathologic fracture caused by plasma cell myeloma or skeletal metastasis Bone densitometry is necessary for accurate assessment of the presence and extent of diminished bone mineral content See Chapters 1, 4, and 7 for more extensive discussions of osteoporosis
Osteomalacia[88]		Diminished radiodensity and prominent coarsened trabeculae Compression deformities of vertebral bodies
Hypothyroidism[89]	3–65	Bullet vertebrae, thoracolumbar gibbus deformity, osteoporosis, delayed development, ossification of the apophyses, and widened disc spaces
Hyperparathyroidism[90]		Findings are most prominent in the thoracolumbar spine Subchondral resorption at discovertebral junctions Rugger-jersey spine: band-like osteosclerosis on the superior and inferior surfaces of the vertebral body in secondary form
Renal osteodystrophy[90, 91]	3–66	Rugger-jersey spine Vertebral fracture results in bioconcave end-plate deformities, more prominent in thoracolumbar spine
Acromegaly[92]	3–67	Elongation and widening of the vertebral bodies Ossification of the anterior portion of the disc; posterior scalloping of vertebral bodies occurs infrequently
Fluorosis[93]	3–68	Predominant spinal findings include diffuse osteosclerosis and ossification of the posterior longitudinal ligament (OPLL), prominent osteophytosis, and periostitis Differential diagnosis includes diffuse idiopathic skeletal hyperostosis (DISH), osteopetrosis, skeletal metastasis, and other causes of diffuse osteosclerosis
Sickle cell anemia[94]	3–69	Diffuse osteopenia and H-shaped vertebra H-shaped vertebral body indentations may simulate Schmorl's nodes or bioconcave (fish) vertebrae associated with osteoporosis
Osteonecrosis of the vertebral body[95]	3–70	Intravertebral vacuum phenomenon with pathologic vertebral body collapse Frequently associated with corticosteroid use

*See also Tables 1–13 to 1–16.

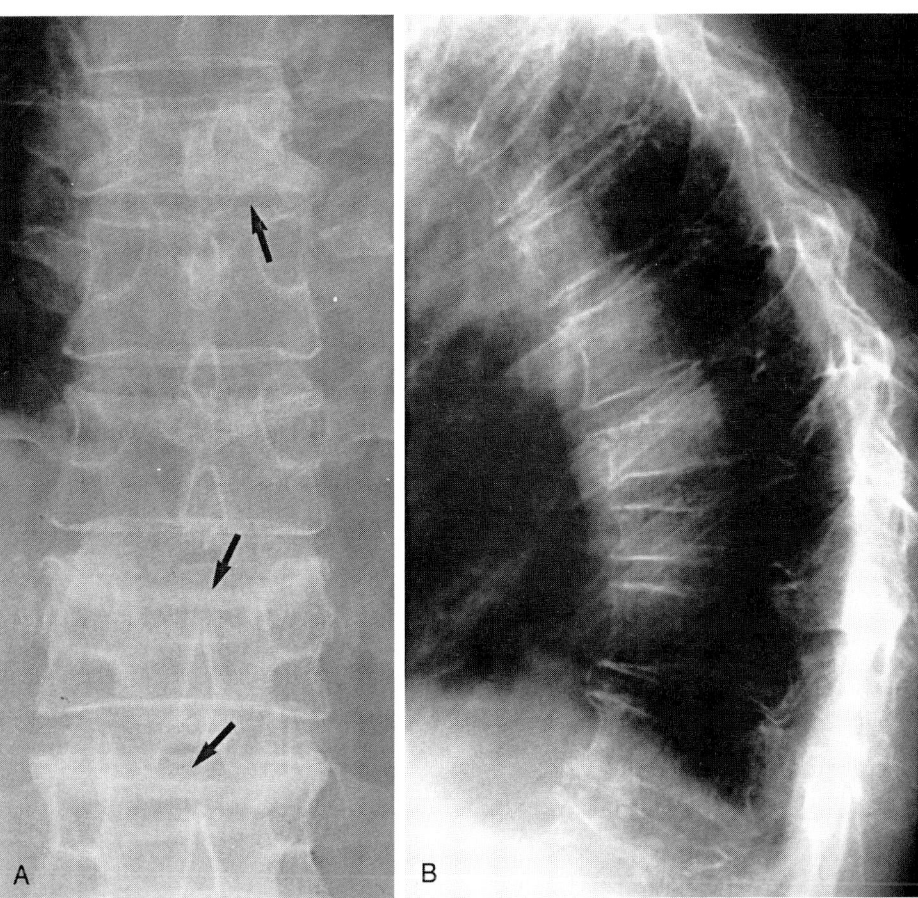

FIGURE 3–64. Osteoporosis. Spinal fractures.[87] A Frontal radiograph of the spine in this 59-year-old man with severe senile osteoporosis reveals fractures of several thoracolumbar vertebral bodies (arrows). B In a 61-year-old man with severe osteoporosis and multiple wedge-shaped vertebral body compression fractures, a dramatic kyphosis that measures greater than 100 degrees is observed. This kyphosis resulted in an insufficiency fracture of the sternum (not shown).

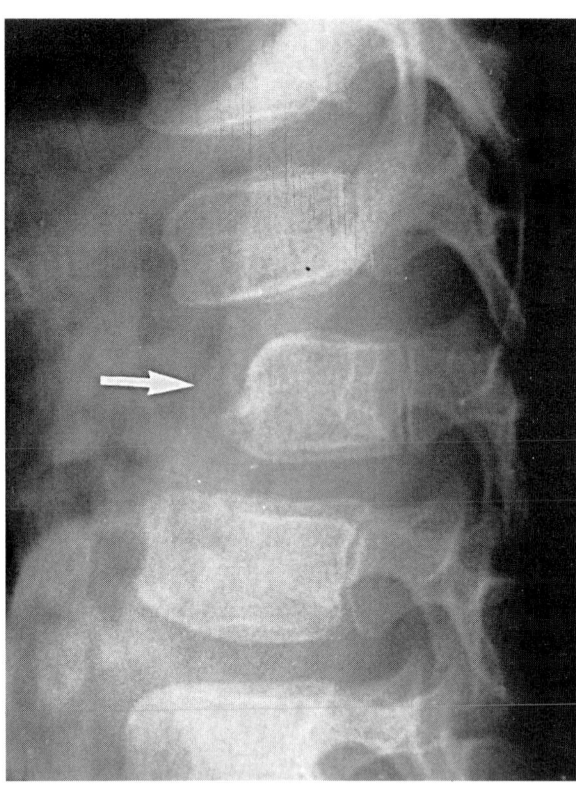

FIGURE 3–65. Hypothyroidism: Bullet vertebra.[89] A characteristic finding in cretinism is thoracolumbar bullet-shaped vertebrae (arrow).

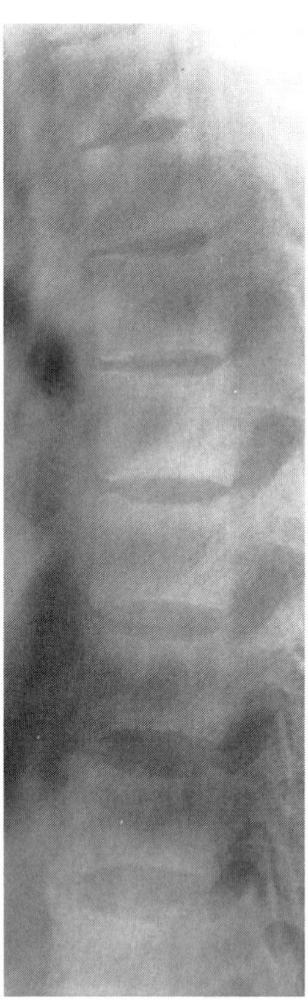

FIGURE 3–66. Renal osteodystrophy: Rugger-jersey spine.[90, 91] Horizontal linear bands of osteosclerosis within the superior and inferior aspects of the vertebral bodies are characteristic of the rugger-jersey spine appearance of renal osteodystrophy. This vertebral sclerosis may be accompanied by osteopenia of the intervening central portion of the vertebral body and may be associated with varying degrees of osseous collapse. The vertebral sclerosis may disappear after successful treatment.

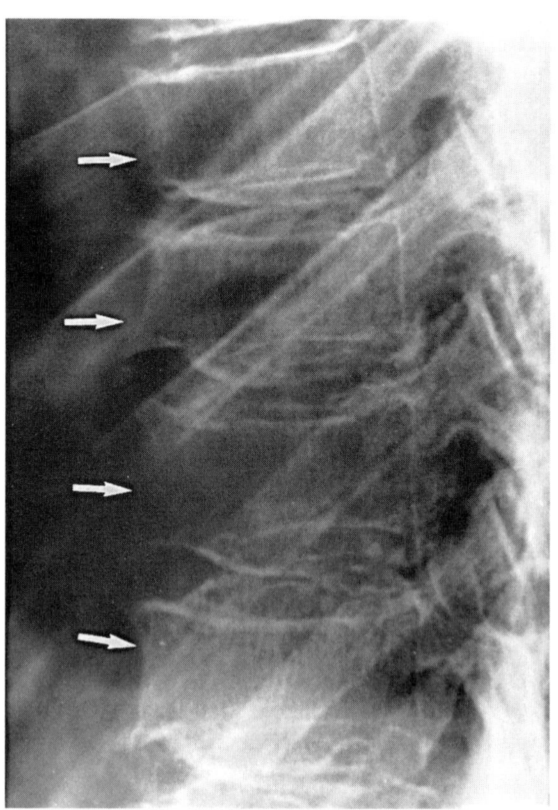

FIGURE 3–67. Acromegaly.[92] Observe the prominent flange-like bone formation and elongation of the vertebral bodies (arrows) in this 53-year-old man with long-standing acromegaly secondary to a pituitary adenoma.

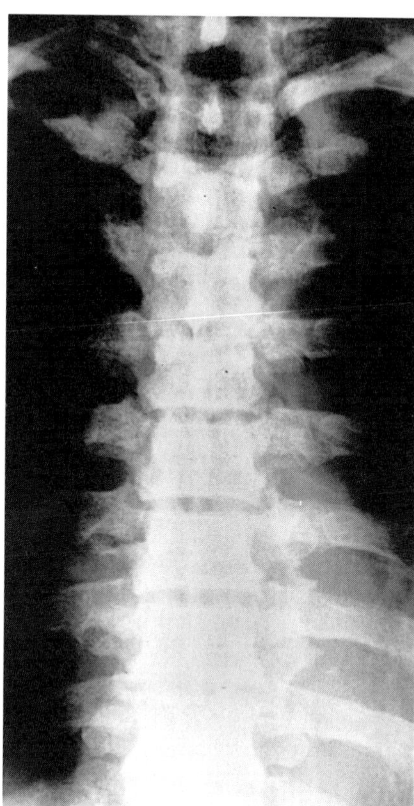

FIGURE 3–68. Fluorosis.[93] Observe the extensive ossification of the paraspinal ligaments and the generalized increased radiodensity of the spine in this patient with fluoride poisoning. *(Courtesy of G. Beauregard, Montreal, Quebec, Canada.)*

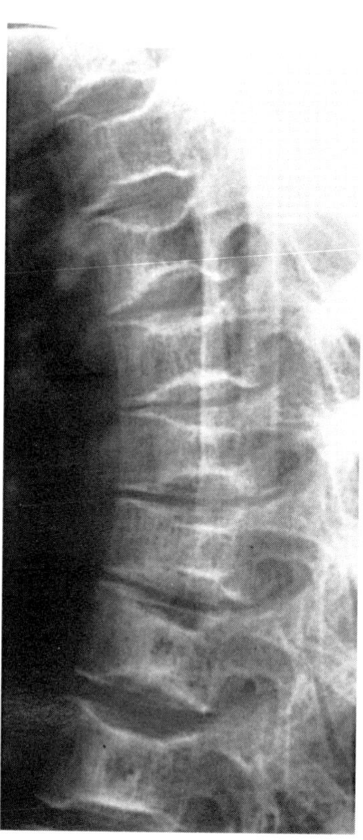

FIGURE 3–69. Sickle cell anemia.[94] H-shaped central end-plate depressions are evident throughout the vertebral bodies of the thoracic spine. Such indentations are characteristic of sickle cell anemia and other hemoglobinopathies.

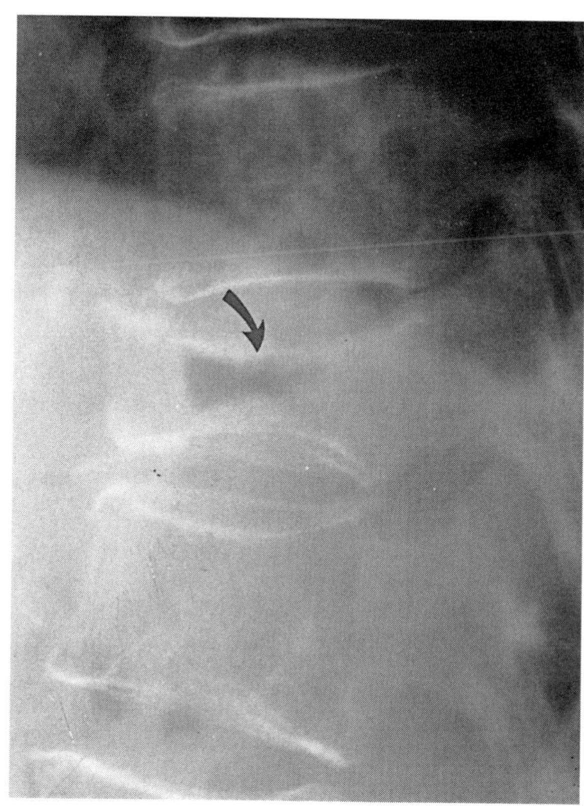

FIGURE 3–70. Steroid-induced osteonecrosis: Vertebral collapse.[95] This 90-year-old woman on long-term corticosteroid medication had acute back pain. Lateral radiograph reveals diffuse osteopenia. A radiolucent collection of gas is present within the collapsed lower thoracic vertebral body (curved arrow). This is termed the intravertebral vacuum cleft, and often it is a sign of vertebral osteonecrosis, frequently associated with the use of corticosteroid medication. *(Courtesy of P. Kindynis, M.D., Geneva, Switzerland.)*

REFERENCES

1. Edeiken J, Dalinka M, Karasick D: Edeiken's Roentgen Diagnosis of Diseases of Bone. 4th Ed. Baltimore, Williams & Wilkins, 1990.
2. Keats TE, Smith TH: An Atlas of Normal Developmental Roentgen Anatomy. 2nd Ed. Chicago, Year Book, 1988.
3. Greenfield GB: Radiology of Bone Diseases. 2nd Ed. Philadelphia, JB Lippincott, 1975.
4. Köhler A, Zimmer EA: Borderlands of Normal and Early Pathologic Findings in Skeletal Radiography. 4th Ed. New York, Thieme Medical Publishers, 1993.
5. Keats TE: Atlas of Normal Roentgen Variants That May Simulate Disease. 6th Ed. Chicago, Year Book Medical Publishers, 1996.
6. Magora A, Schwartz A: Relation between the low back pain syndrome and x-ray findings. 3. Spina bifida occulta. Scand J Rehabil Med 12:9, 1980.
7. Yochum TR, Rowe LJ: Essentials of Skeletal Radiology. 2nd Ed. Baltimore, Williams & Wilkins, 1996.
8. Ozonoff MB: Spinal anomalies and curvatures. *In* Resnick D: Diagnosis of Bone and Joint Disorders. 3rd Ed. Philadelphia, WB Saunders, 1995, p 4245.
9. Langer LO, Baumann PA, Gorlin RJ: Achondroplasia. AJR 100:12, 1967.
10. Langer LO: Spondyloepiphyseal dysplasia tarda, hereditary chondrodysplasia with characteristic vertebral configuration in the adult. Radiology 82:833, 1964.
11. Watts RWE, Spellacy E, Kendall BE, et al: Computed tomography studies on patients with mucopolysaccharidosis. Neuroradiology 21:9, 1981.
12. Holzgrave W, Grobe H, von Figura K, et al: Morquio syndrome: Clinical findings of 11 patients with MPS IV-A and 2 patients with MPS IV-B. Hum Genet 57:360, 1981.
13. Kovanlikaya A, Loro ML, Gilsanz V: Pathogenesis of osteosclerosis in autosomal dominant osteopetrosis. AJR 168:929, 1997.
14. Kahler SG, Burns JA, Aylsworth AS: A mild autosomal recessive form of osteopetrosis. Am J Genet 17:451, 1984.
15. Benli IT, Akalin S, Boysan E, et al: Epidemiological, clinical, and radiological aspects of osteopoikilosis. J Bone Joint Surg [Br] 74:504, 1992.
16. Magid D, Pyeritz RE, Fishman EK: Musculoskeletal manifestations of the Marfan syndrome: Radiologic features. AJR 155:99, 1990.
17. Root L: The treatment of osteogenesis imperfecta. Orthop Clin North Am 15:775, 1984.
18. Wardinski TD, Pagon RA, Powell BR, et al: Rhizomelic chondrodysplasia punctata and survival beyond one year: A review of the literature and five case reports. Clin Genet 38:84, 1990.
19. Fon GT, Pitt MJ, Thies AC Jr: Thoracic kyphosis: Range in normal subjects. AJR 134:979, 1980.
20. Rajasekaran S, Shanmugasundaram TK: Prediction of the angle of gibbus deformity in tuberculosis of the spine. J Bone Joint Surg [Am] 69:503, 1987.
21. Lund PJ, Ruth JT, Dzioba R, et al: Traumatic thoracolumbar facet instability: Characteristic imaging findings. Skeletal Radiol 26:360, 1997.
22. Kumar UK, Sahsasranam KV: Mitral valve prolapse syndrome and associated thoracic skeletal abnormalities. J Assoc Physicians India 39:536, 1991.
23. Lowe TG: Scheuermann disease. J Bone Joint Surg [Am] 72:940, 1990.
24. Perdriolle R, Vidal J: Thoracic idiopathic scoliosis curve: Evolution and prognosis. Spine 10:785, 1985.
25. McMaster MJ, Ohtsuka K: The natural history of congenital scoliosis: A study of two hundred and fifty-one patients. J Bone Joint Surg [Am]64:1128, 1982.
26. Hsu LCS, Lee PC, Leong JCY: Dystrophic spinal deformities in neurofibromatosis. J Bone Joint Surg [Br] 66:495, 1984.
27. Robin GC, Brief LP: Scoliosis in childhood muscular dystrophy. J Bone Joint Surg [Am] 53:466, 1971.
28. Mayfield JK, Riseborough EJ, Jaffe N, et al: Spinal deformity in children treated for neuroblastoma. The effect of radiation and other forms of treatment. J Bone Joint Surg [Am] 63:183, 1981.
29. Cohen MD, Harrington TM, Ginsbury WW: Osteoid osteoma: 95 cases and a review of the literature. Semin Arthritis Rheum 12:265, 1983.
30. DeSousa AL, Kalsbeck JE, Mealey J Jr, et al: Intraspinal tumors in children: A review of 81 cases. J Neurosurg 51:437, 1979.
31. Ryan RW, Lally JF, Kozic Z: Asymptomatic calcified herniated thoracic discs: CT recognition. AJNR 9:363, 1988.
32. Giles LGF, Taylor JR: Lumbar spine structural changes associated with leg length inequality. Spine 7:159, 1982.
33. Thometz JG, An HS: Luque instrumentation with sublaminar wiring. *In* An HS, Cotler JM (eds): Spinal Instrumentation. Baltimore, Williams & Wilkins, 1992, p 93.
34. El-Khoury G, Whitten CG: Trauma to the upper thoracic spine: Anatomy, biomechanics, and unique imaging features. AJR 160:95, 1993.
35. Kaplan PA, Orton DF, Asleson RJ: Osteoporosis with vertebral compression fractures, retropulsed fragments, and neurologic compromise. Radiology 165:533, 1987.
36. Stabler A, Bellan M, Weiss M, et al: MR imaging of enhancing intraosseous disk herniation (Schmorl's nodes). AJR 168:933, 1997.
37. Gehweiler JA, Osborne RL Jr, Becker RF: The Radiology of Vertebral Trauma. Philadelphia, WB Saunders, 1980.
38. Baker LL, Goodman SB, Perkash I, et al: Benign versus pathologic compression fractures of vertebral bodies: Assessment with conventional spin-echo, chemical-shift, and STIR MR imaging. Radiology 174:495, 1990.
39. Dupuy DE, Palmer WE, Rosenthal DI: Vertebral fluid collection associated with vertebral collapse. AJR 167:1535, 1996.
40. Saifuddin A, Noordeen J, Taylor BA, et al: The role of imaging in the diagnosis of thoracolumbar burst fractures: Current concepts and a review of the literature. Skeletal Radiol 25:603, 1996.
41. Lund PJ, Ruth JT, Dzioba R, et al: Traumatic thoracolumbar facet instability: Characteristic imaging findings. Skeletal Radiol 26:360, 1997.
42. Smith KS, Kaufer H: Patterns and mechanisms of lumbar injuries associated with lap seat belts. J Bone Joint Surg [Am] 51:239, 1988.
43. Terk MR, Hume-Neal M, Fraipont M, et al: Injury of the posterior ligament complex in patients with acute spinal trauma: Evaluation by MR imaging. AJR 168:1481, 1997.
44. Emery SE, Pathria MN, Wilber RG, et al: Magnetic resonance imaging of posttraumatic spinal ligament injury. J Spinal Disord 2:229, 1989.
45. Kleinman PK, Marks SC: Vertebral body fractures in child abuse: Radiologic-histopathologic correlates. Invest Radiol 27:715, 1992.
46. Resnick D: Degenerative disease of the spine. *In* Resnick D: Diagnosis of Bone and Joint Disorders. 3rd Ed. Philadelphia, WB Saunders, 1995, p 1372.
47. Weinberger A, Myers AR: Intervertebral disc calcification in adults: A review. Semin Arthritis Rheum 8:69, 1978.
48. Resnick D, Shaul SR, Robins JM: Diffuse idiopathic skeletal hyperostosis (DISH): Forestier's disease with extraspinal manifestations. Radiology 115:513, 1975.

49. Weinfeld RM, Olson PN, Maki DD, et al: The prevalence of diffuse idiopathic skeletal hyperostosis (DISH) in two large American Midwest metropolitan hospital populations. Skeletal Radiol 26:222, 1997.
50. Hendrix RW, Melany M, Miller F, et al: Fracture of the spine in patients with ankylosis due to diffuse idiopathic skeletal hyperostosis: Clinical and imaging findings. AJR 162:899, 1994.
51. Quagliano PV, Hayes CW, Palmer WE: Vertebral pseudoarthrosis associated with diffuse idiopathic skeletal hyperostosis. Skeletal Radiol 23:353, 1994.
52. Widder DJ: MR imaging of ossification of the posterior longitudinal ligament. AJR 153:194, 1989.
53. Kapila A, Lines M: Neuropathic spinal arthropathy: CT and MR findings. J Comput Assist Tomogr 11:736, 1987.
54. Pascual E, Castellano JA, Lopez E: Costovertebral joint changes in ankylosing spondylitis with thoracic pain. Br J Rheumatol 31:413, 1992.
55. Peh WCG, Ho TK, Chan FL: Case report: Pseudoarthrosis complicating ankylosing spondylitis—appearances on magnetic resonance imaging. Clin Radiol 47:359, 1993.
56. Sundaram M, Patton JT: Paravertebral ossification in psoriasis and Reiter's disease. Br J Radiol 48:628, 1975.
57. Martel W, Braunstein EM, Borlaza G, et al: Radiologic features of Reiter's disease. Radiology 132:1, 1979.
58. Czirjak L, Nagy Z, Szegedi G: Systemic sclerosis in the elderly. Clin Rheumatol 11:483, 1992.
59. Resnick D: Dermatomyositis and polymyositis. *In* Resnick D: Diagnosis of Bone and Joint Disorders. 3rd Ed. Philadelphia, WB Saunders, 1995, p 1218.
60. Resnick D, Pineda C: Vertebral involvement in calcium pyrophosphate dihydrate crystal deposition disease: Radiographic-pathologic correlation. Radiology 153:55, 1984.
61. Steinbach LS, Resnick D: Calcium pyrophosphate dihydrate crystal deposition disease revisited. Radiology 200:1, 1996.
62. Justesen P, Andersen PE Jr: Radiologic manifestations in alkaptonuria. Skeletal Radiol 11:204, 1984.
63. Dagirmanjian A, Schils J, McHenry M, et al: MR imaging of vertebral osteomyelitis revisited. AJR 167:1539, 1996.
64. Hoffman EB, Crosier JH, Cremin B: Imaging in children with spinal tuberculosis: A comparison of radiography, computed tomography and magnetic resonance imaging. J Bone Joint Surg [Br] 75:233, 1993.
65. Travlos J, Du Toit G: Spinal tuberculosis: Beware the posterior elements. J Bone Joint Surg [Br] 72:722, 1990.
66. Wong DA, Fornasier VL, MacNab I: Spinal metastases: The obvious, the occult, and the impostors. Spine 15:1, 1990.
67. Algra PR, Heimans JJ, Valk J, et al: Do metastases in vertebrae begin in the body or the pedicles? Imaging study in 45 patients. AJR 158:1275, 1992.
68. Garrett IR: Bone destruction in cancer. Semin Oncol 20:4, 1993.
69. Barwick KW, Huvos AG, Smith J: Primary osteogenic sarcoma of the vertebral column: A clinicopathologic correlation of ten patients. Cancer 46:595, 1980.
70. Kyle RA: Multiple myeloma: Review of 869 cases. Mayo Clin Proc 50:29, 1975.
71. Lecouvet FE, Vande Berg BC, Maldague BE, et al: Vertebral compression fractures in multiple myeloma. Part I: Distribution and appearance at MR imaging. Radiology 204:195, 1997.
72. Bouroncle BA, Doan CA: Myelofibrosis: Clinical, hematologic and pathologic study of 110 patients. Am J Med Sci 243:697, 1962.
73. Franczyk J, Samuels T, Rubenstein J, et al: Skeletal lymphoma. J Can Assoc Radiol 40:75, 1989.
74. Epstein BS: Vertebral changes in childhood leukemia. Radiology 68:65, 1957.
75. Greenspan A: Bone island (enostosis): Current concept—a review. Skeletal Radiol 24:111, 1995.
76. Gamba JL, Martinez S, Apple J, et al: Computed tomography of axial skeletal osteoid osteomas. AJR 142:769, 1984.
77. Dahlin DC: Giant cell tumor of bone: Highlights of 407 cases. AJR 144:955, 1985.
78. Graham JJ, Yang WC: Vertebral hemangioma with compression fracture and paraparesis treated with preoperative embolization and vertebral resection. Spine 9:97, 1984.
79. Hadjipavlou A, Lander P: Paget disease of the spine. J Bone Joint Surg [Am] 73:1376, 1991.
80. Mirra JM, Brien EW, Tehranzadeh J: Paget's disease of bone: Review with emphasis on radiologic features, part II. Skeletal Radiol 24:173, 1995.
81. Leeds NE, Jacobson HG: Spinal neurofibromatosis. AJR 126:617, 1976.
82. Mitchell GE, Lourie H, Berne AS: The various causes of scalloped vertebrae with notes on their pathogenesis. Radiology 89:67, 1967.
83. Gibson MJ, Middlemiss JH: Fibrous dysplasia of bone. Br J Radiol 44:1, 1971.
84. Jee W-H, Choi K-Y, Choe B-Y, et al: Fibrous dysplasia: MR imaging characteristics with radiopathologic correlation. AJR 167:1523, 1996.
85. Stull MA, Kransdorf MJ, Devaney KO: Langerhans' cell histiocytosis of bone. Radiographics 12:801, 1992.
86. Kilpatrick SE, Wenger DE, Gilchrist GS, et al: Langerhans' cell histiocytosis (histiocytosis X) of bone: A clinicopathologic analysis of 263 pediatric and adult cases. Cancer 76:2471, 1995.
87. Ryan PJ, Fogelman I: Osteoporotic vertebral fractures: Diagnosis with radiography and bone scintigraphy. Radiology 190:669, 1994.
88. Mankin HJ: Rickets, osteomalacia, and renal osteodystrophy. Orthop Clin North Am 21:81, 1990.
89. Resnick D: Thyroid disorders. *In* Resnick D: Diagnosis of Bone and Joint Disorders. 3rd Ed. Philadelphia, WB Saunders, 1995.
90. Resnick D, Niwayama G: Parathyroid disorders and renal osteodystrophy. *In* Resnick D (ed): Diagnosis of Bone and Joint Disorders. 3rd Ed. Philadelphia, WB Saunders, 1995.
91. Tigges S, Nance EP, Carpenter WA, et al: Renal osteodystrophy: Imaging findings that mimic those of other diseases. AJR 165:143, 1995.
92. Lang EK, Bessler WT: The roentgenologic features of acromegaly. AJR 86:321, 1961.
93. Wang Y, Yin Y, Gilula LA, et al: Endemic fluorosis of the skeleton: Radiographic features in 127 cases. AJR 162:93, 1994.
94. Rohlfing BM: Vertebral end-plate depression: Report of two patients with hemoglobinopathy. AJR 128:599, 1977.
95. Malghem J, Maldague B, Labaisse M-A, et al: Intravertebral vacuum cleft: Changes in content after supine positioning. Radiology 187:483, 1993.
96. Wong CC, Pereira B, Pho RWH: Cervical disc calcification in children: A long-term review. Spine 17:139, 1992.

CHAPTER 4

Lumbar Spine

- Normal Developmental Anatomy
- Developmental Anomalies, Anatomic Variants, and Sources of Diagnostic Error
- Skeletal Dysplasias and Other Congenital Disorders
- Spondylolysis and Spondylolisthesis
- Lumbar Scoliosis
- Physical Injury
- Intervertebral Disc Disorders
- Articular Disorders
- Bone Tumors
- Metabolic and Hematologic Disorders
- Lumbar Spine Surgery
- Vascular Disorders

Normal Developmental Anatomy

Accurate interpretation of pediatric lumbar spine radiographs requires a thorough understanding of normal developmental anatomy. Table 4–1 lists the age of appearance and fusion of the primary and secondary ossification centers. Figures 4–1 and 4–2 demonstrate the radiographic appearance of many important ossification centers and other developmental landmarks at selected ages from birth to skeletal maturity.

Developmental Anomalies, Anatomic Variants, and Sources of Diagnostic Error

The lumbar spine is a frequent site of anomalies, normal variations, and other sources of diagnostic error, many of which may simulate disease and result in misdiagnosis. Table 4–2 and Figures 4–3 to 4–16 are designed to familiarize the reader with the more common processes.

Skeletal Dysplasias and Other Congenital Disorders

Table 4–3 outlines a number of dysplastic and congenital disorders that affect the lumbar spine, and Table 4–4 lists some of the leading causes of vertebral scalloping. Figures 4–17 to 4–24 illustrate the radiographic manifestations of some of these disorders.

Spondylolysis and Spondylolisthesis

Spondylolysis (defects of the pars interarticularis) and spondylolisthesis (vertebral slippage) are encountered frequently on imaging studies of the lumbar spine. Table 4–5 lists the types of such disorders, Table 4–6 describes a measurement technique used in evaluation, and Figures 4–25 to 4–34 show radiographic examples.

Lumbar Scoliosis

The topic of scoliosis is discussed in more detail in Chapter 3 (see Table 3–5 and Figures 3–16 to 3–22). Scoliosis also exhibits important manifestations in the lumbar spine. Table 4–7 lists some types of scoliosis that affect the lumbar spine in addition to those listed in Chapter 3. Figures 4–35 to 4–38 illustrate the radiographic findings.

Physical Injury

Fractures, dislocations, and soft tissue injuries involving the lumbar spine are common, many of which are associated with serious clinical manifestations. Table 4–8 lists the important injuries of the lumbar spine and their characteristics. Table 4–9 addresses instability in burst fractures. In addition, Figures 4–39 to 4–45 represent examples of the most characteristic imaging manifestations of common lumbar spine injuries.

Intervertebral Disc Disorders

Table 4–10 lists several conditions involving lumbar intervertebral discs. Tables 4–11 to 4–15 deal with specific manifestations of disc disease. Figures 4–46 to 4–61 represent examples of imaging of intervertebral disc disorders.

Articular Disorders

The lumbar spine is a frequent target site of involvement for many forms of degenerative, inflammatory, crystal-induced, and infectious spondyloarthropathies and other articular disorders. Table 4–16 outlines these diseases and their characteristics, and Figures 4–62 to 4–76 illustrate the characteristic radiographic manifestations. Additionally, Chapter 3 provides discussions of osseous outgrowths of the spine (see Table 3–9) and terminology applied to ankylosing spondylitis (see Table 3–10).

Bone Tumors

A wide variety of malignant and benign tumors and tumor-like lesions affect the spine. Those neoplasms illustrated in this chapter are described in Table 4–17; examples are illustrated in Figures 4–77 to 4–92. A more complete list of neoplasms is found in Chapter 1 (Table 1–10). Table 4–18 lists the characteristics of several disorders that cause vertebral osteosclerosis.

Metabolic and Hematologic Disorders

A number of metabolic disorders involve the lumbar spine. These are outlined in Table 4–19 and illustrated in Figures 4–93 to 4–106.

Lumbar Spine Surgery

Surgical procedures for pathologic disc conditions, spinal stenosis, and other disorders are numerous. Table 4–20 lists a few of these procedures and their associated complications. Figures 4–107 and 4–111 illustrate the characteristic imaging findings of some surgical procedures.

Vascular Disorders

Aneurysms of the abdominal aorta and iliac arteries may be manifested clinically as low back pain, often simulating bone and joint disorders of the spine. A brief description of these aneurysms is provided in Table 4–21, and representative examples are shown in Figures 4–112 and 4–113.

TABLE 4–1. Lumbar Spine: Approximate Age of Appearance and Fusion of Ossification Centers*[1-3] (Figs. 4–1, 4–2)

Ossification Center	Primary Secondary	No. of Centers	Age of Appearance (Years)	Age of Fusion (Years)	Comments
L1-L4					
Neural arches (laminae)	P	2	Birth	1	Fuse together in order from L4 to L1
Vertebral body	P	1	Birth	5–6	Fuse to laminae
Spinous process	S	1	11–16	17–25	
Transverse processes	S	2	11–16	17–25	
Articular processes	S	4	11–16	17–25	
Mamillary processes	S	2	11–16	17–25	
Ring apophyses	S	2	11–16	17–25	Fuse to body
L5					
Neural arches (laminae)	P	2	Birth	5	Fuse together
Vertebral body	P	1	Birth	6	Fuse to laminae
Spinous process	S	1	11–16	17–25	
Transverse processes	S	2	11–16	17–25	
Articular processes	S	4	11–16	17–25	
Mamillary processes	S	2	11–16	17–25	
Ring apophyses	S	2	11–16	17–25	Fuse to body

*Ages of appearance and fusion of ossification centers in girls typically precede those of boys. Ethnic differences also exist.
P, Primary; S, Secondary.

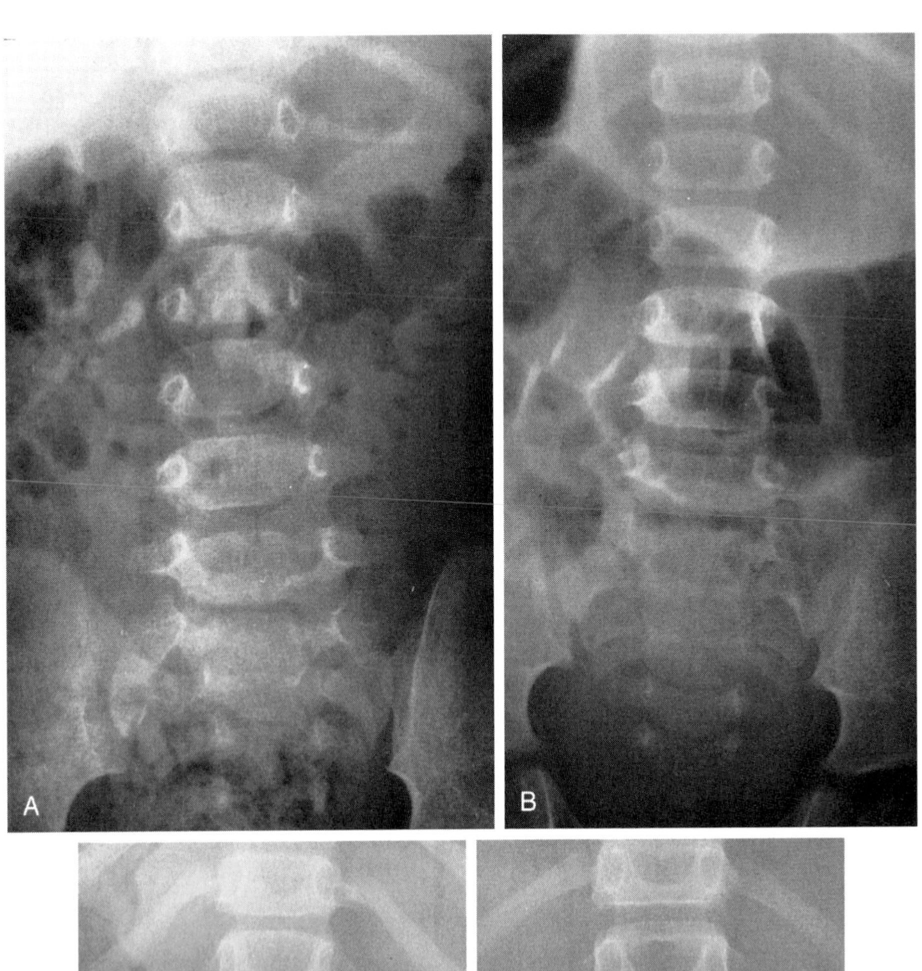

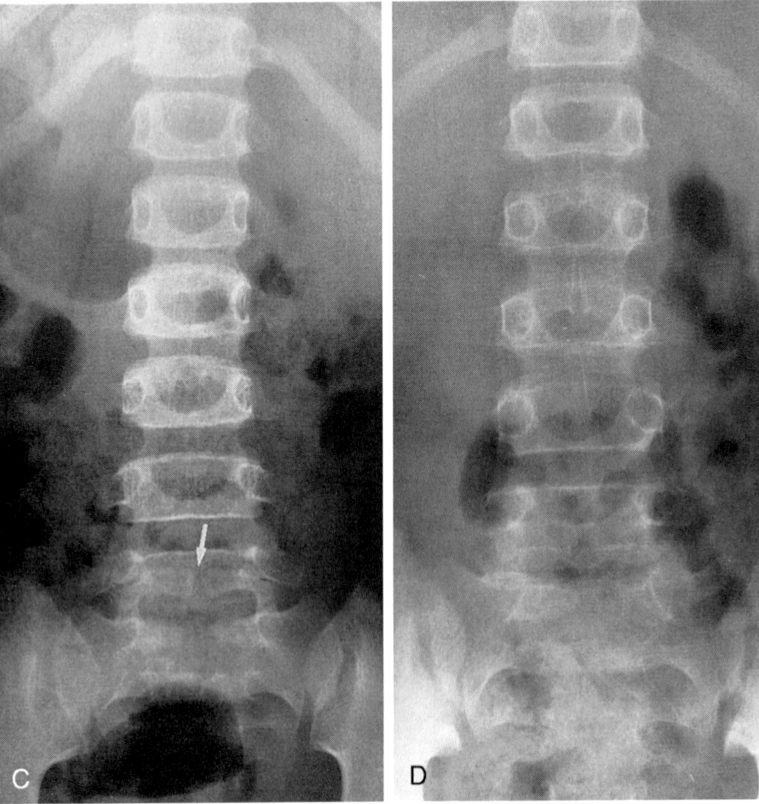

FIGURE 4–1. Skeletal maturation and normal development: Anteroposterior lumbar spine radiographs.[1–3] **A** 14-month-old girl. The spinal canal appears proportionately wide in relation to the vertebral bodies. The laminae are thin and the interlaminar spaces are wide. **B** 2-year-old boy. **C** 8-year-old boy. The neural arch of L5 usually fuses between the ages of 5 and 6 years, but it has not yet fused in this patient (arrow). Failure of fusion in adults (spina bifida occulta) at this level is a common developmental anomaly. Some of the vertebral end plates are jagged or serrated, a finding that often persists until complete fusion of the secondary ring apophysis to the vertebral body has occurred. **D** 10-year-old boy. The spinal canal remains disproportionately wide, and the superior vertebral end plates have a serrated appearance.

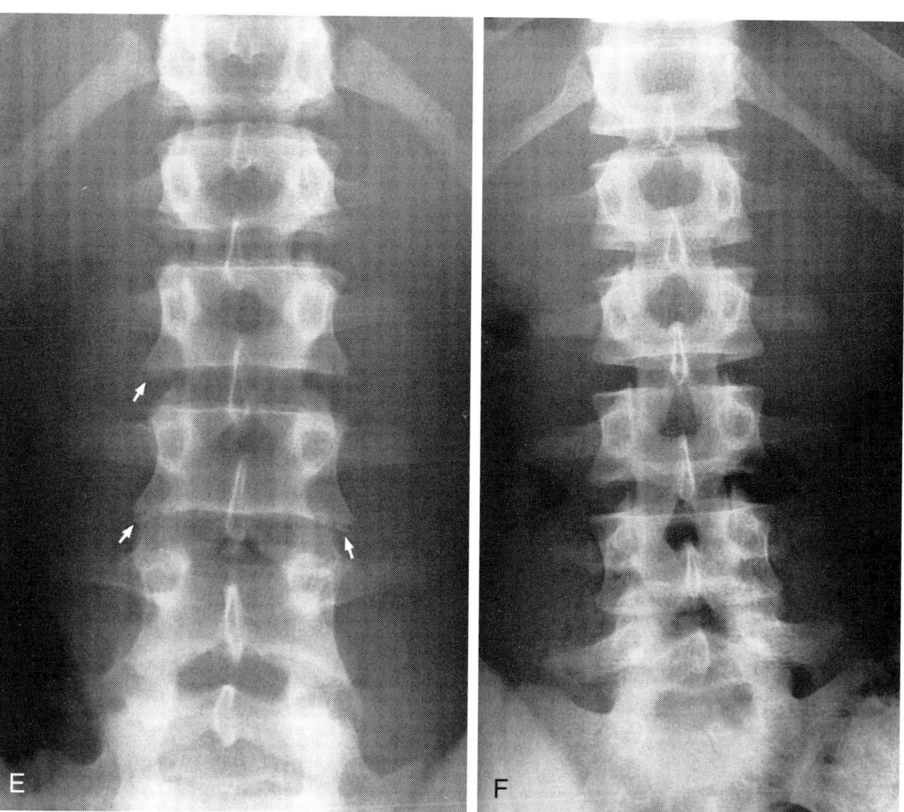

FIGURE 4–1 *Continued.* **E** 13-year-old boy. The secondary ring apophyses have begun to ossify and are readily visible, especially adjacent to the inferior end plates (arrows). Note also the serrated margins of the superior vertebral end plates. **F** 16-year-old boy. The vertebral bodies are more rectangular and the size of the spinal canal has begun to resemble that of the adult.

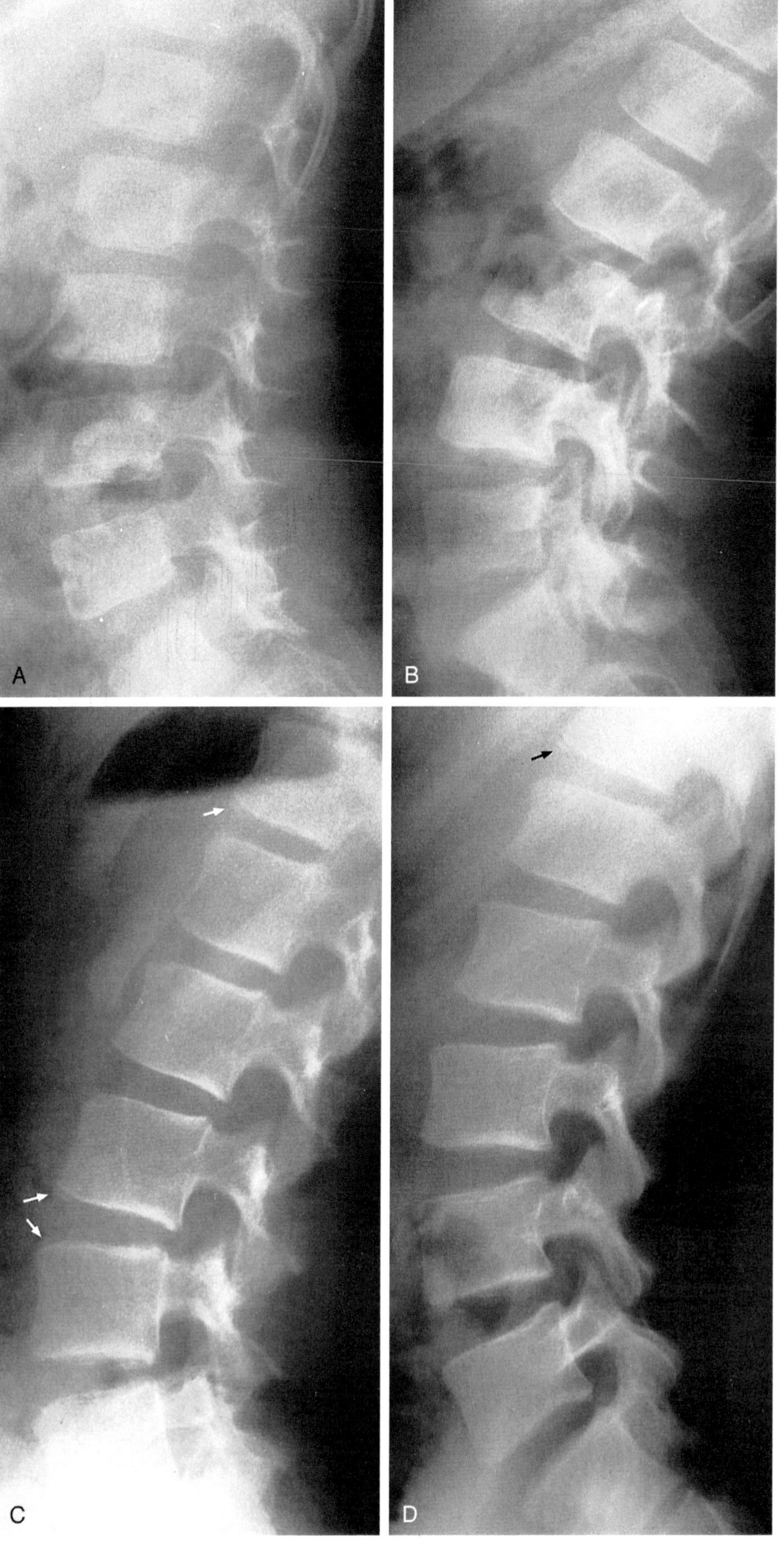

FIGURE 4–2. Skeletal maturation and normal development: Lateral lumbar spine radiographs.[1–3] A 30-month-old girl. The vertebral body contours are rounded and the spinal canal appears disproportionately wide in relation to the vertebral body width. In some children at this age, the anterior vascular notches may be prominent and the vertebral bodies may show anterior beaking (neither of which are present in this child). B 9-year-old girl. The posterior vertebral bodies exhibit normal physiologic scalloping, an appearance that may begin as early as the age of 2 years. The overall shape of the vertebral body is rectangular, but the corners remain rounded because the ring apophyses are not yet ossified. C 11-year-old girl. The secondary ring apophyses are seen adjacent to the notched anterior vertebral body margins (arrows). These ossification centers typically appear near the age of puberty but may appear as early as the age of 7 years. They fuse to the vertebral body between 17 and 25 years of age. D 13-year-old boy. The ring apophyses are visible at the thoracolumbar region (arrow). The posterior vertebral body contours remain scalloped.

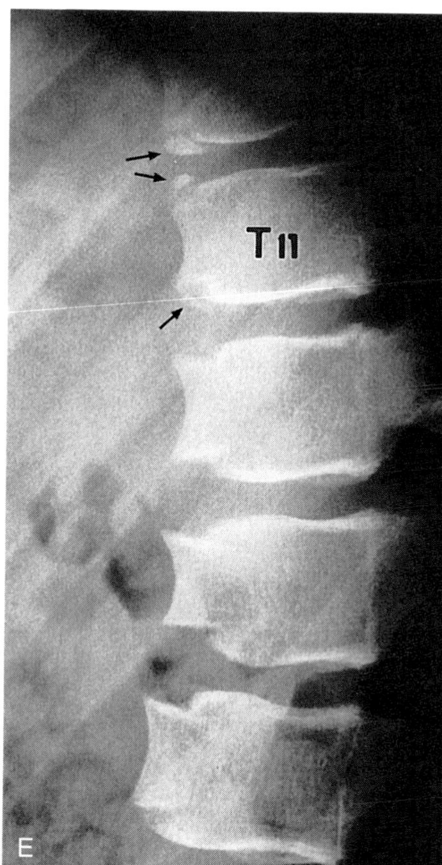

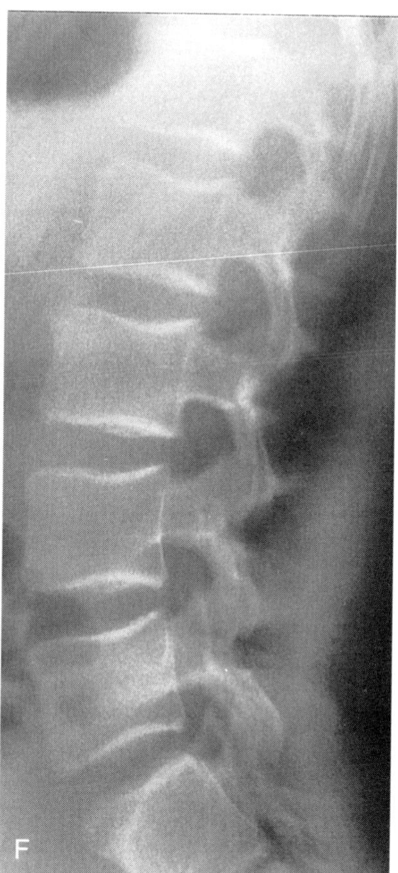

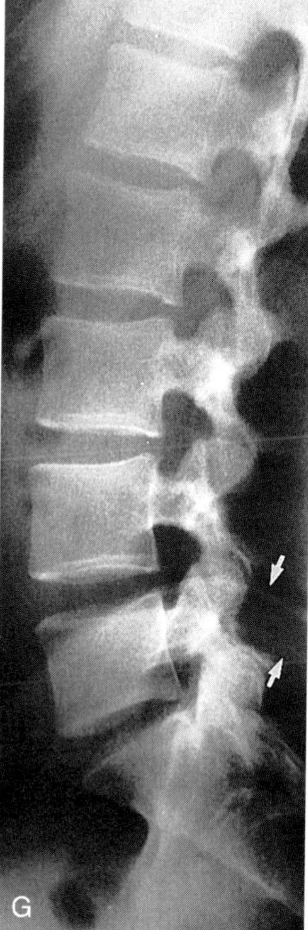

FIGURE 4–2 *Continued.* **E** 15-year-old boy. Observe the prominent notch-like defects of the vertebral bodies of T12, L1, and L2. These notches are normal in the juvenile spine and represent the space occupied by the unossified secondary ossification centers. Ossification of the ring apophyses is evident at the T10 and T11 levels (arrows). **F** 15-year-old boy. In another patient, the notches are less prominent and the ring apophyses are ossified. Note the normal curvilinear appearance of the inferior vertebral body surfaces. The ring apophyses typically fuse to the vertebral end plates at about the age of 19 years in male adolescents and 16 years in female adolescents. Fusion may occur as late as the age of 25 years. **G** Adult: 22-year-old man. All secondary ossification centers have fused to the vertebral bodies. The vertebral bodies are more rectangular, the posterior margin of each vertebral body is not scalloped, and the vertebral end plates have a less exaggerated curvilinear appearance. The secondary ossification centers of the iliac crests have yet to fuse to the ilium (arrows). *(E, Courtesy of G. Schultz, D.C., Costa Mesa, California.)*

TABLE 4–2. Developmental Anomalies, Anatomic Variants, and Sources of Diagnostic Error Affecting the Lumbar Spine*

Entity	Figure(s)	Characteristics
Normal ring apophyses[4]	4–2 C–F	Normal vertebral body ring apophyses may resemble fractures or limbus vertebrae
Hahn's venous channels[5]	4–3	Normal anatomy: a central horizontal vascular groove or channel that traverses the vertebral body; evident on radiographs, computed tomography (CT) scans, and magnetic resonance (MR) images These channels are quite prominent beginning with the first year of life, but they tend to disappear with age; they are of no clinical significance even when they persist into adulthood
Nuclear impressions[5, 10]	4–4	Broad-based curvilinear indentations of the lower lumbar vertebral end plates seen on lateral radiographs; represent a variation of normal May be related to notochordal remnants or the Cupid's bow contour seen on frontal radiographs Differential diagnosis: Schmorl's cartilaginous nodes, compression fractures with bioconcave deformities (fish vertebrae), and H vertebrae characteristic of hemoglobinopathy
Cupid's bow contour[10]	4–5	Paramedian curvilinear indentations, generally of the inferior vertebral end plates, seen on frontal radiographs, which represent a normal variation closely related to nuclear impressions Most common at L4 and L5 Unrelated to osteopenia, fracture, or mechanical stress on the spine
Synostosis (block vertebrae)[11]	4–6	Developmental failure of segmentation of vertebral somites with subsequent fusion of adjacent vertebral bodies Most common lumbar sites are T12-L1 and L4-L5 Often results in premature degenerative disease at adjacent vertebral levels owing to excessive intervertebral motion above and below the synostosis *Radiographic findings:* 1. Waist-like constriction at the level of the intervetebral disc 2. Completely absent or rudimentary disc space, with or without irregular calcification 3. Total height of the block vertebra is less than expected from the number of segments that are involved 4. Fusion (nonsegmentation) of the posterior elements (50 per cent of cases) Differential diagnosis: surgical fusion or ankylosis from inflammatory arthropathy or infectious discitis
Lumbar ribs[4]	4–7	Anomalous supernumerary ribs articulating with the transverse processes of the first lumbar vertebra Normal variant or developmental anomaly of no clinical significance
Spina bifida occulta[6, 12]	4–8	Extremely common developmental anomaly consisting of a midline defect within the neural arch resulting from failure of the two laminae to fuse centrally at the spinolaminar junction Radiolucent cleft, absent spinous process, or failure of fusion at the spinolaminar junction; most frequent at L5 and S1 Isolated anomaly, or occurring in conjunction with other entities, such as cleidocranial dysplasia or clasp-knife syndrome Strong cartilage and fibrous tissues fill the cleft; the anomaly generally is of no clinical consequence Spina bifida may infrequently be associated with meningomyelocele, which represents protrusion of the meninges or spinal cord, or both; meningomyelocele may result in severe neurologic abnormalities Higher prevalence of spondylolysis and spondylolisthesis is associated with L5 spina bifida occulta
Clasp-knife syndrome[13]	4–9	Spina bifida occulta of S1 and elongation of the L5 spinous process During trunk extension, the L5 spinous process may impinge on the spinal canal, irritating pain-sensitive structures
Developmental spinal stenosis[2, 4, 7]	4–10; see Fig. 4–17	Congenital narrowing or hypoplasia of the spinal canal Common finding in achondroplasia Developmental stenosis may be complicated in later life by other diseases, such as degenerative stenosis ***Lumbar spine radiographic measurements:*** 1. Eisenstein's method for sagittal canal measurement: Lower limits of normal 15 mm: suggests stenosis 12 mm: unequivocal evidence of stenosis 2. Interpedicle method for coronal canal measurement: Lower limits of normal 20 mm at any lumbar level: suggests stenosis Measurements of stenosis on routine radiographs may be misleading; cross-sectional CT or MR imaging and clinical correlation are necessary to fully evaluate patients with suspected stenosis
Hemivertebra[7, 8]	4–11	Vertebral body originally develops from paired chondral centers; at a later stage, a single ossification focus forms; this focus then separates transiently by the notochordal remnant into anterior and posterior centers *Lateral hemivertebra* results from failure of development of one of the paired chondral centers

Entity	Figure(s)	Characteristics
		Hemivertebra might involve a normally occurring vertebra or it might be supernumerary; one pedicle may be normal or enlarged and its counterpart at the same level may be absent or hypoplastic; the incomplete segment may articulate with or be fused to the adjacent vertebrae Frequently results in congenital scoliosis and may be associated with segmentation anomalies *Dorsal and ventral hemivertebrae* are much less frequent than lateral hemivertebrae and result from agenesis of either the anterior or posterior portion of the growth center, respectively
Butterfly vertebra[8, 9]		Incomplete fusion of the two lateral chondral centers of the vertebral body results in a central sagittal constriction of the vertebral body, which is seen on a frontal radiograph and is considered a variant of enchondral ossification Interpedicle distance of the butterfly vertebra may be widened, and the adjacent vertebrae usually remodel to conform to the shape of the butterfly vertebra
Facet tropism[2, 4, 7]	4–12	Asymmetric orientation of left and right lumbosacral facet joint of the same level Most common at L4-L5 and L5-S1 L1-L2 to L4-L5 facet joints usually are oriented predominantly in the sagittal plane; L5-S1 facet joints usually are oriented in the coronal plane; tropism is a variation in this orientation, usually visualized on frontal radiographs; cross-sectional imaging (CT or MR) best demonstrates exact orientation of the articular surfaces Clinical significance is controversial: Preponderance of evidence does not support a relationship between facet tropism and degenerative disc disease May result in pedicle sclerosis
Ununited ossification center of the articular process[2]	4–13	Failure of fusion of the secondary ossification center of the inferior articular process, also termed "Oppenheimer's ossicle" Most common sites: L3 and L4 inferior articular processes Smooth, nondisplaced, well-corticated fragment involving lower aspect of articular process Usually asymptomatic and of no clinical significance Differential diagnosis: fracture
Articular process agenesis[14]	4–14	Rare, stable anomaly that usually is asymptomatic and an incidental finding Most common site: L5 inferior articular process Nonossified, cartilaginous or fibrous analogue is present Differential diagnosis: pathologic destruction
Transitional lumbosacral segment[15–17]	4–15	Several different patterns of anomalous lumbosacral segmentation are referred to as "transitional vertebrae" and often are associated with other anomalies, such as spina bifida and neural arch defects; present in 5 to 8 per cent of the population Three typical patterns: 1. Bilateral symmetric assimilation of the fifth lumbar and first sacral segments (sacralization) resulting in four mobile lumbar-type vertebrae and elongation of the vertical height of the sacrum; assimilation can include complete osseous synostosis or incomplete synostosis in which a hyperplastic (spatulated) L5 transverse process forms an articulation with the sacral ala and may articulate with the ilium, forming the superior portion of the sacroiliac joint; lumbosacral disc space is decreased in height or absent 2. Bilateral symmetric segmentation of the first and second sacral segments (lumbarization) resulting in six mobile lumbar-type vertebrae and a decreased vertical height of the sacrum; the lowest mobile vertebra may resemble a normally formed lumbar vertebra with either a completely formed or rudimentary disc articulating with the sacrum 3. Unilateral or bilateral asymmetric variations of assimilation or nonsegmentation; a spatulated transverse process of the lowest lumbar vertebra may articulate with the sacral ala; this tendency toward assimilation may eventually lead to complete synostosis with the sacrum; sclerosis of the articulating surfaces might reflect uneven distribution of mechanical stress Literature on the relationship of transitional vertebrae to signs and symptoms is confusing and sometimes contradictory: Disproportionate degenerative changes often are encountered at articulations of transitional segments Patients with six lumbar-type vertebrae appear to be predisposed to disc protrusions[4] Sclerosis of articulating surfaces may be associated with pain and tenderness over the anomaly[4] Weight gain, trauma, and even pregnancy may exacerbate symptoms[4] Patients with spondylolisthesis and four lumbar-type vertebrae have greater slippage of their spondylolisthesis than patients with five lumbar-type vertebrae[16] Other reviews have found no relationship between transitional vertebrae and back pain[17]
Diastematomyelia[18]	4–16	Congenital longitudinal diastasis of the thoracic or lumbar spinal canal and spinal cord with increased interpedicle distance Present in 15 per cent of all patients with congenital scoliosis; two thirds of patients with diastematomyelia have scoliosis Often associated with other vertebral anomalies, short angular kyphosis, and tethering of the spinal cord Female:male, 2:1 50 to 75 per cent of persons have a septum (ossified or unossified) dividing the cord Plain film radiography often is inadequate to recognize a septum even when it is present, and MR imaging or CT with or without myelographic contrast is indicated when this condition is suspected

*See also Table 1–1.

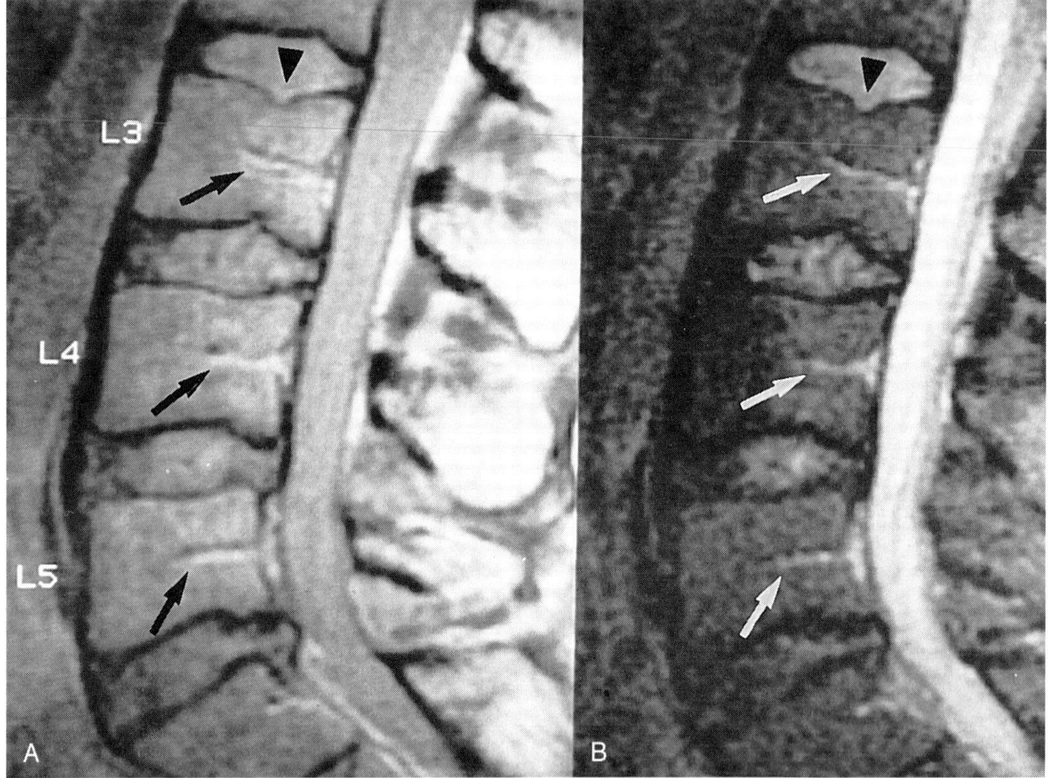

FIGURE 4–3. Hahn's venous channels: Magnetic resonance (MR) imaging.[4] Normal high signal intensity horizontal fissures (arrows) are seen within several vertebral bodies on proton density–weighted (A) and T2-weighted (B) sagittal spin echo MR images. These channels represent perforations for the vertebral veins and communicate posteriorly with the epidural venous plexus; therefore, they should not be misinterpreted as fractures. A Schmorl's node is present in the L3 superior end plate (arrowheads).

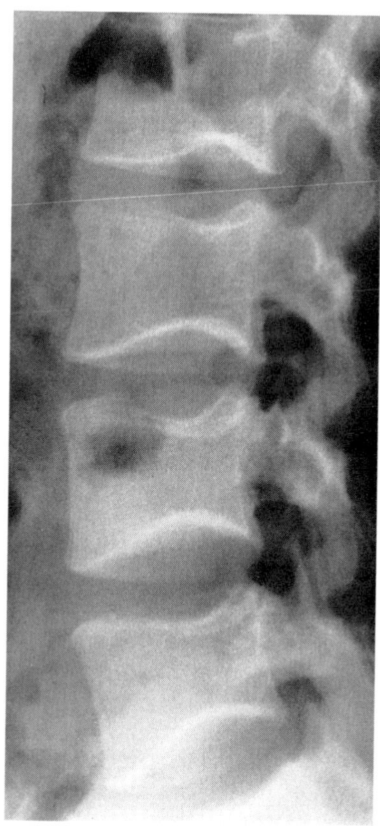

FIGURE 4–4. Nuclear impressions.[5, 10] Lateral lumbar radiograph from this 26-year-old man demonstrates prominent, broad-based, curvilinear depressions of the vertebral end plates. These nuclear impressions, usually more prominent at the inferior end plate, represent a normal variation of vertebral contour and should not be confused with fracture, Schmorl's nodes, or pathologic destruction.

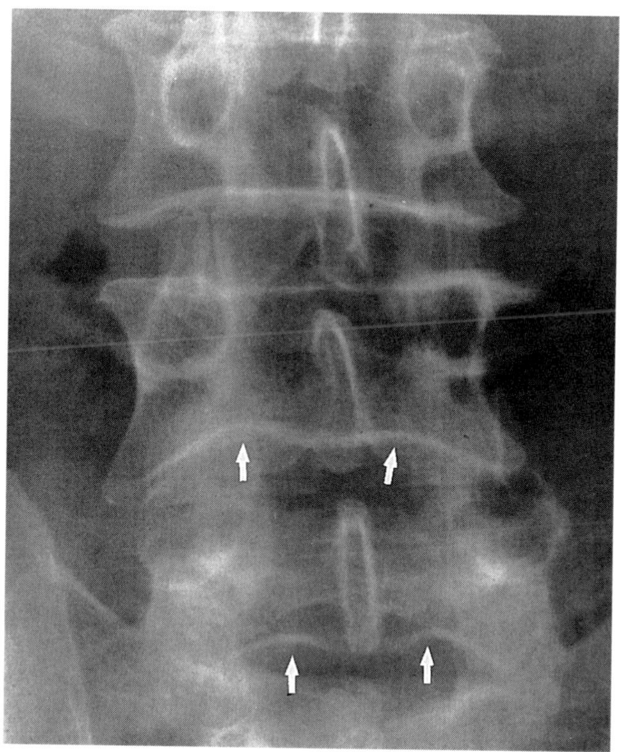

FIGURE 4–5. Cupid's bow contour.[10] Frontal radiograph reveals normal paramedian curvilinear impressions of the inferior end plates of the L4 and L5 vertebral bodies (arrows).

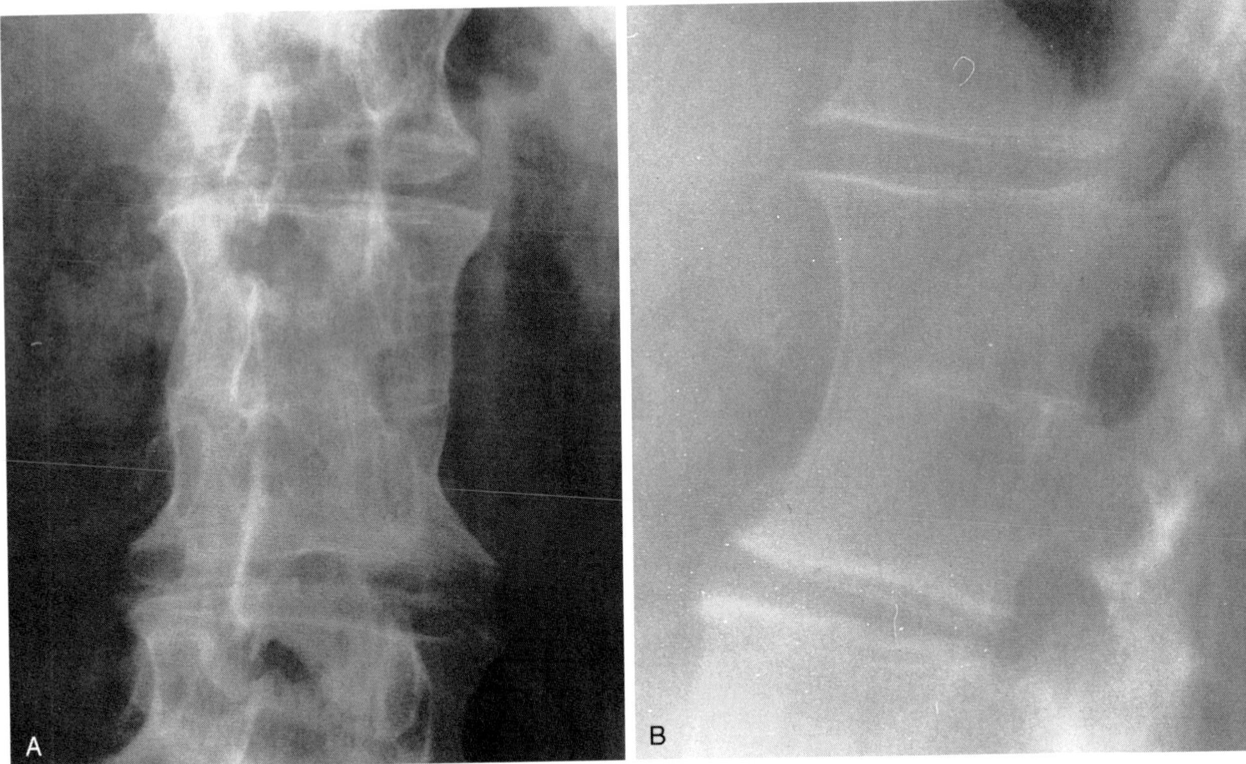

FIGURE 4–6. Developmental synostosis (block vertebrae).[11] Frontal (A) and lateral (B) radiographs demonstrate failure of segmentation of two contiguous vertebral segments. The intervening rudimentary intervertebral disc is calcified. The central portion of the vertebrae are hypoplastic (wasp-waist constriction). The degenerative intervertebral disc space narrowing and osteophyte formation, seen at adjacent levels, are frequent complications of block vertebrae. This degeneration occurs secondary to compensatory excessive motion at segments adjacent to block vertebrae.

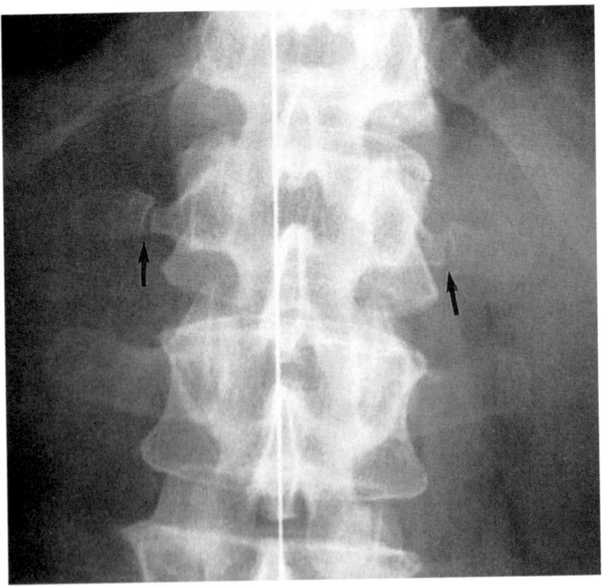

FIGURE 4–7. Lumbar ribs.[4] Small, hypoplastic transverse processes of L1 articulate with rudimentary anomalous ribs (arrows). This anomaly usually is an incidental finding of no clinical significance.

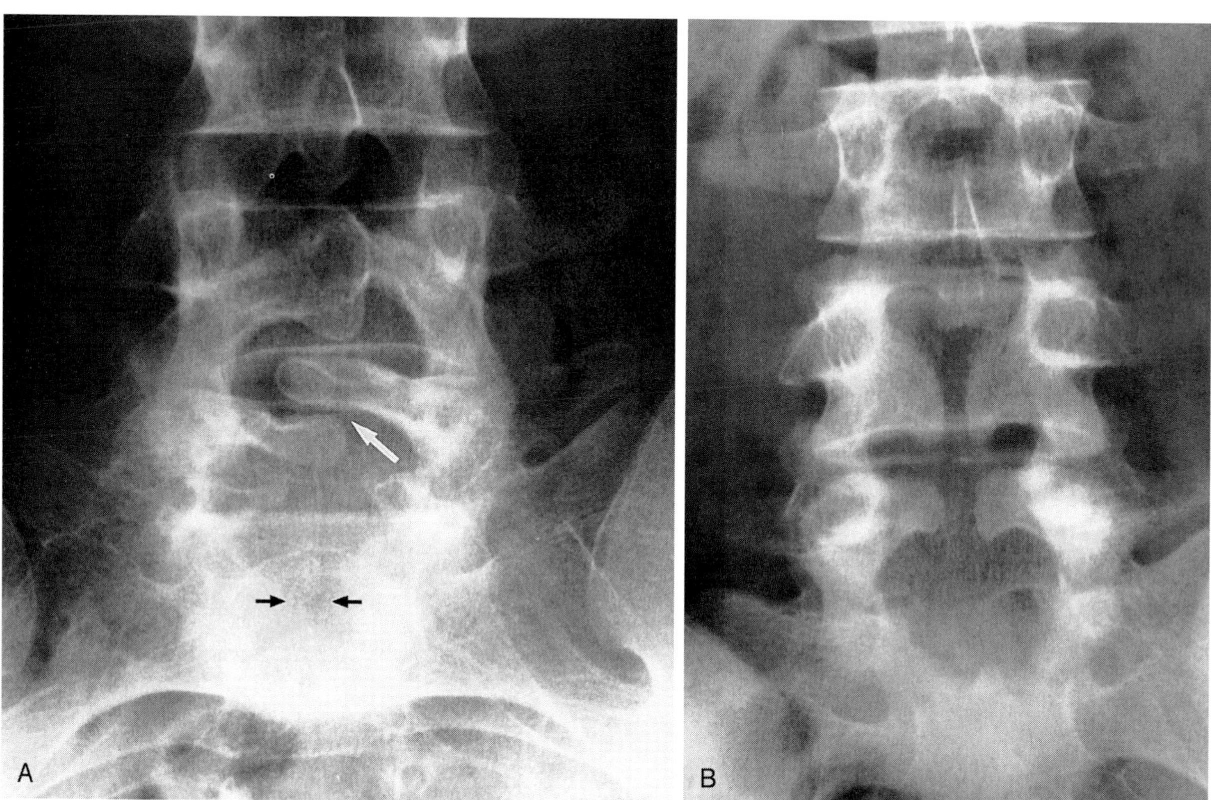

FIGURE 4–8. Spina bifida occulta.[6, 12] A In this 26-year-old man with a grade 1 spondylolytic spondylolisthesis, nonunion of the anomalous L5 laminae, seen as a radiolucent defect (white arrow), results in incomplete development of the spinous process. A small midline defect also is present at S1 (black arrows), representing another site of spina bifida occulta. B In another patient, midline radiolucent defects represent incomplete formation of the spinous processes of L4 and L5 and the first sacral tubercle.

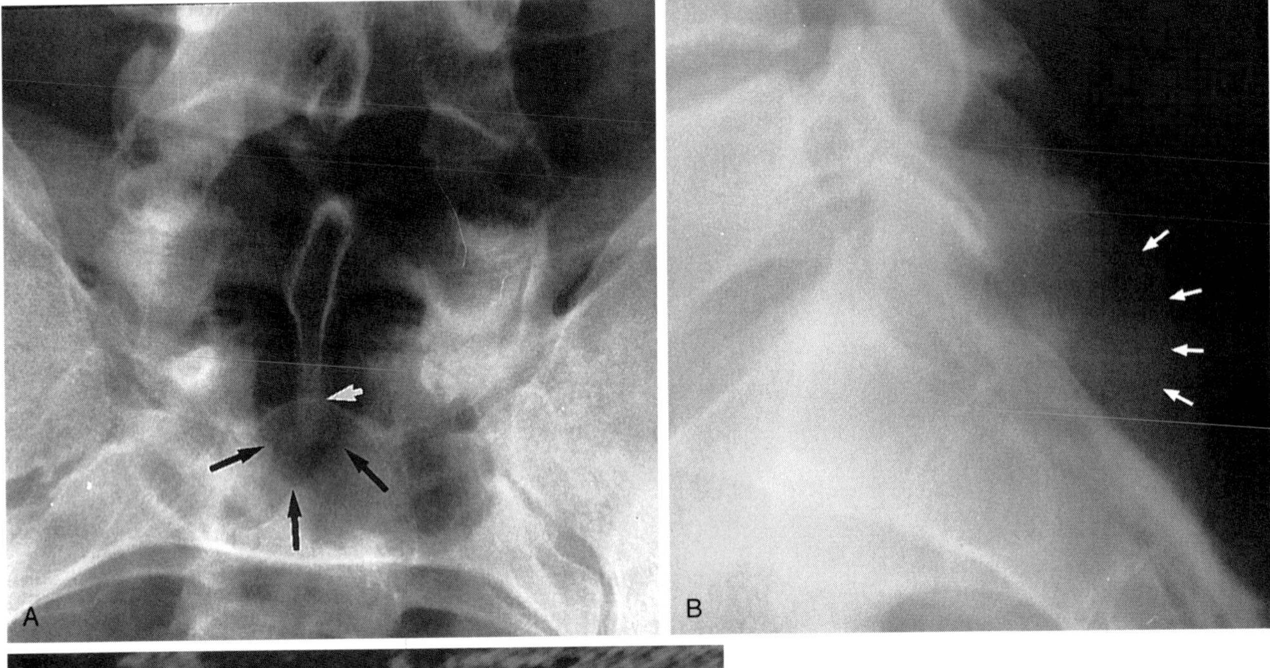

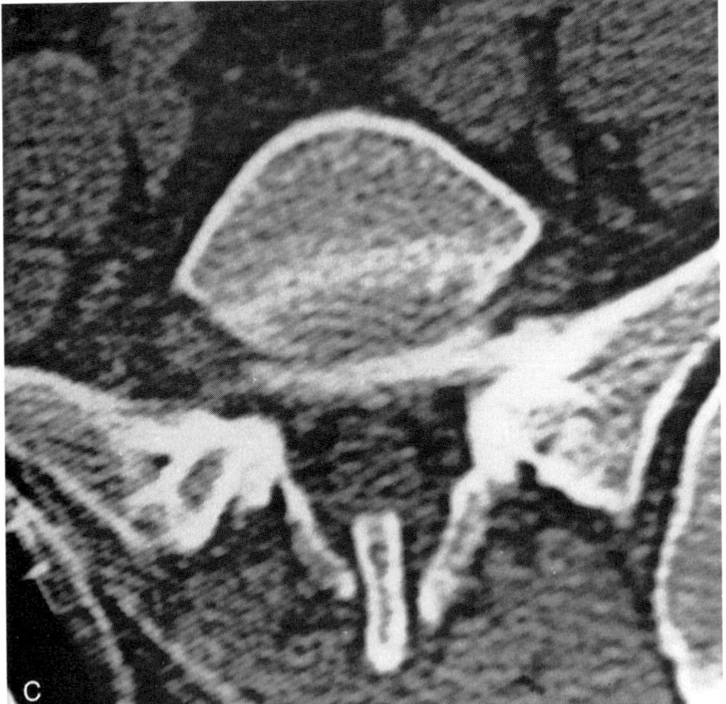

FIGURE 4–9. Clasp-knife deformity.[13] Frontal (A) and lateral (B) radiographs of the lumbar spine in a manual laborer with back pain exacerbated by trunk extension. Clasp-knife deformity involves inferior sloping and elongation of the L5 spinous process (white arrows) in conjunction with spina bifida occulta of S1 (black arrows). A transaxial CT scan (C) obtained during trunk extension in another patient shows the L5 spinous process penetrating the S1 spina bifida and contacting the thecal sac. During extension, the L5 spinous process may impinge on the spinal canal, irritating pain-sensitive structures.

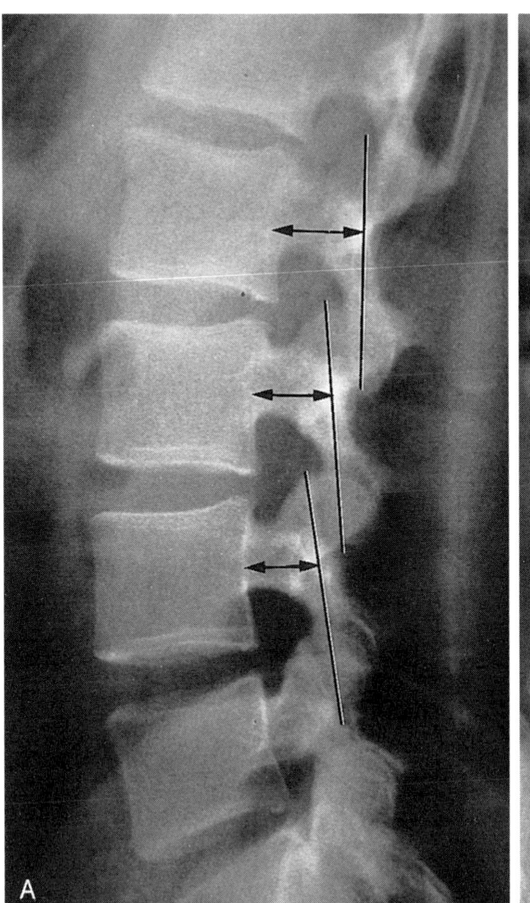

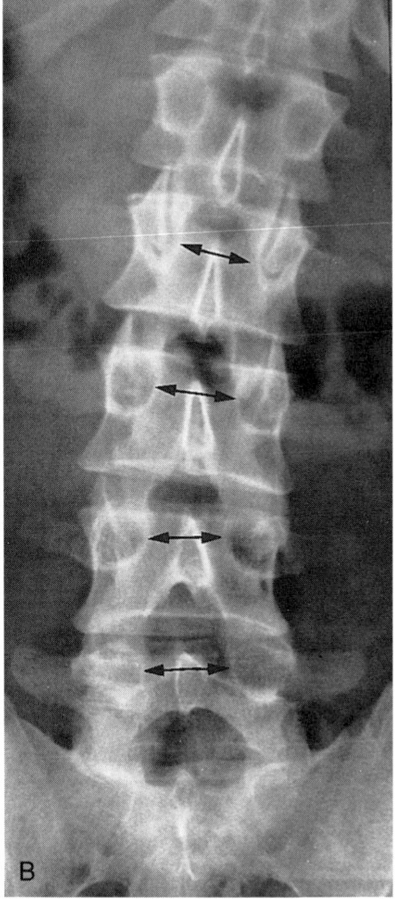

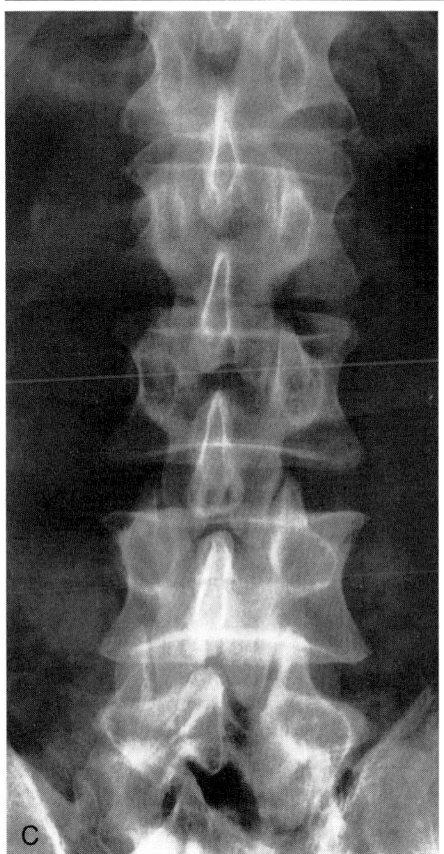

FIGURE 4–10. Developmental (congenital) spinal stenosis.[2, 4, 7] A, B Techniques of radiographic measurement.[7] In A, Eisenstein's method for measuring the sagittal diameter of the spinal canal is demonstrated. On a lateral radiograph, the first step is to construct the articular process line connecting the tips of the superior and inferior articular processes (straight lines). The next step is to identify the midpoint of the posterior body margin, midway between the superior and inferior end plates. The sagittal canal diameter is measured (in millimeters) between the articular process line and the posterior body margin (double-headed arrows). This measurement is obtained from L1 through L4. At the L5 segment, the measurement is obtained by measuring the distance between the spinolaminar junction line and the posterior body margin. Single measurements less than 15 mm at any lumbar level suggest stenosis, and those less than 12 mm represent unequivocal evidence of stenosis. In B, interpedicle distances for measuring the coronal diameter of the spinal canal are described. On a frontal radiograph, the shortest distance between the inner surfaces of the two pedicles is measured in millimeters (double-headed arrows). Normal measurements vary according to the spinal level. At the L1 to L4 levels, the measurement should be no less than 21 mm, and at L5, it should be no less than 23 mm. The interpedicle distance is narrowed in spinal stenosis and widened in patients with expanding spinal cord tumors. C This 59-year-old man had long-standing low back pain and bilateral leg pain. Frontal radiograph reveals that the interpedicle distances become progressively narrower in the lower lumbar spine in comparison with the upper lumbar spine. The measurement at L5 was 17 mm. Radiographic measurements of stenosis can be misleading, and cross-sectional methods employing computed tomographic (CT) or magnetic resonance (MR) imaging should be used to fully evaluate patients with suspected stenosis.

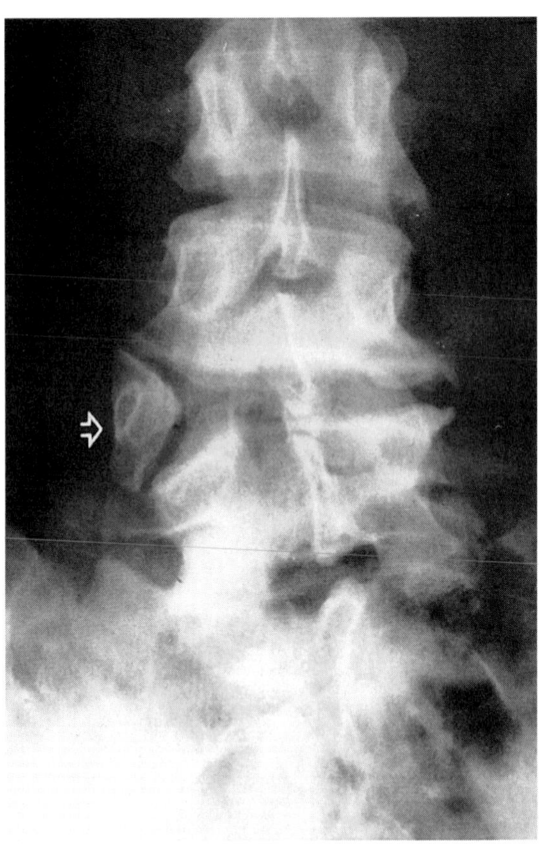

FIGURE 4–11. Lateral hemivertebra.[7, 8] An incomplete, triangular vertebral body and corresponding pedicle is incorporated (open arrow) within the L4-L5 intervertebral disc space. Compensatory remodeling of the adjacent vertebral bodies and asymmetric degenerative disc disease also are seen at this level. Hemivertebrae frequently result in congenital scoliosis.

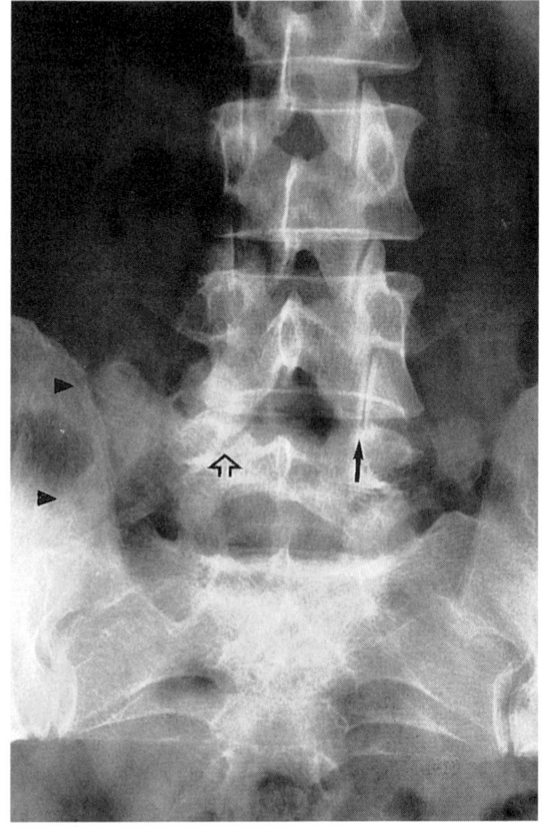

FIGURE 4–12. Facet tropism.[2, 4, 7] Observe the asymmetry of the lumbosacral apophyseal joint orientation: The left apophyseal joint is oriented in the sagittal plane (solid arrow), and the right apophyseal joint is oriented predominantly in the coronal plane (open arrow). Computed tomographic (CT) or magnetic resonance (MR) imaging is necessary to determine the precise facet joint orientation, but such sophisticated techniques usually are not warranted. Note also that the right transverse process of the lowest lumbar-type vertebra is spatulated (arrowheads) and appears to articulate with the sacral ala. The lumbosacral region is a common site for multiple developmental anomalies. *(Courtesy of F.G. Bauer, D.C., Sydney, New South Wales, Australia.)*

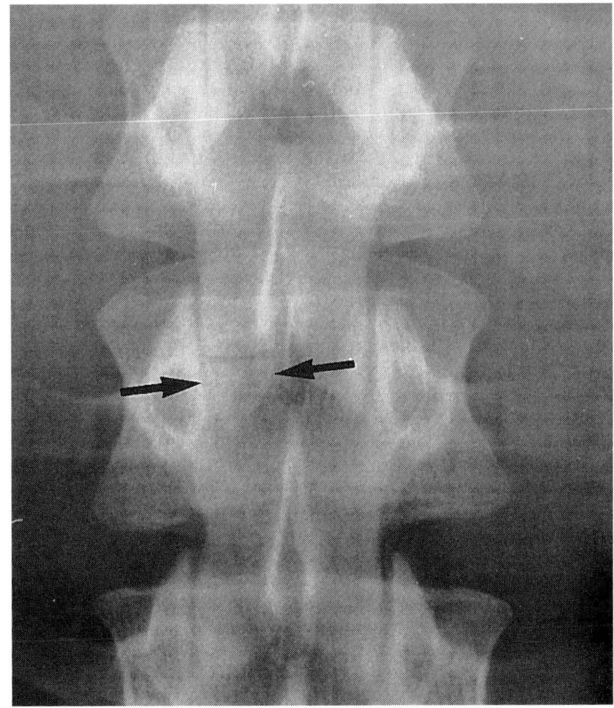

FIGURE 4–13. Ununited secondary ossification center of the articular process.[2] Failure of union of the secondary ossification center of the inferior articular process (arrows) is seen most frequently at L3 and L4 and has been referred to as "Oppenheimer's ossicle." This anomaly must be differentiated from a fracture.

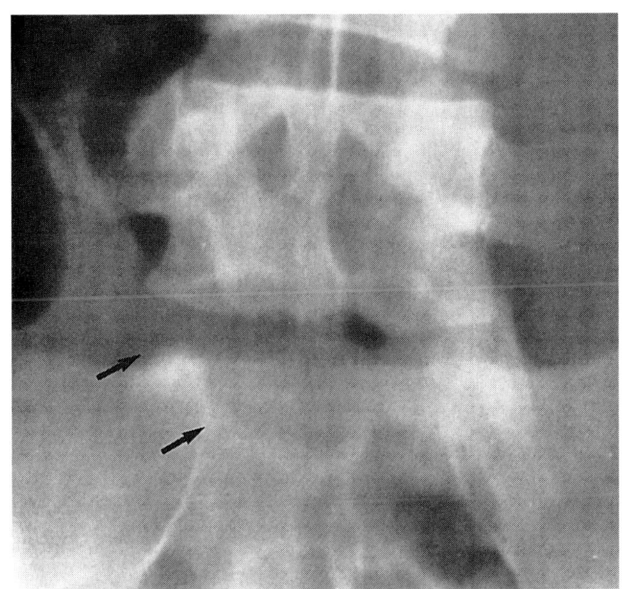

FIGURE 4–14. Agenesis of lumbosacral articular process.[14] Observe the absence of the right inferior articular process of L5 (arrows). In this rare, stable, and often asymptomatic anomaly, a nonossified, cartilaginous, or fibrous analogue is present. This anomaly frequently is identified as an incidental finding, but it may resemble pathologic destruction such as that seen in skeletal metastasis. *(From Mitchell R: Congenital absence of a lumbosacral facet. Top Diagn Radiol Adv Imaging 1:3, 1993.)*

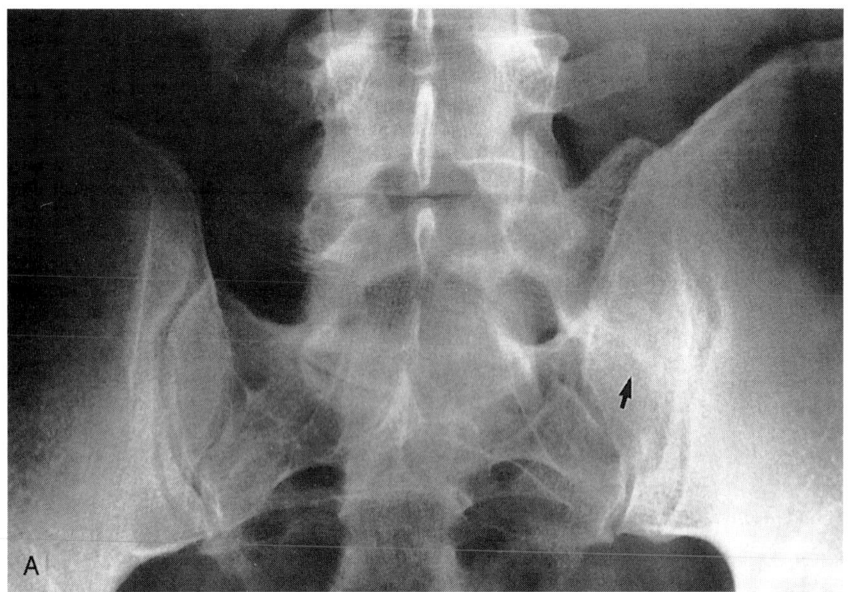

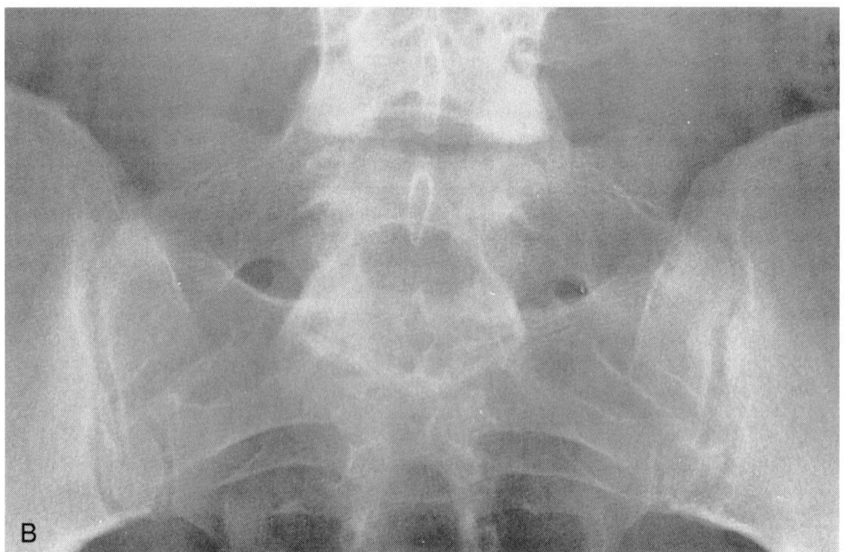

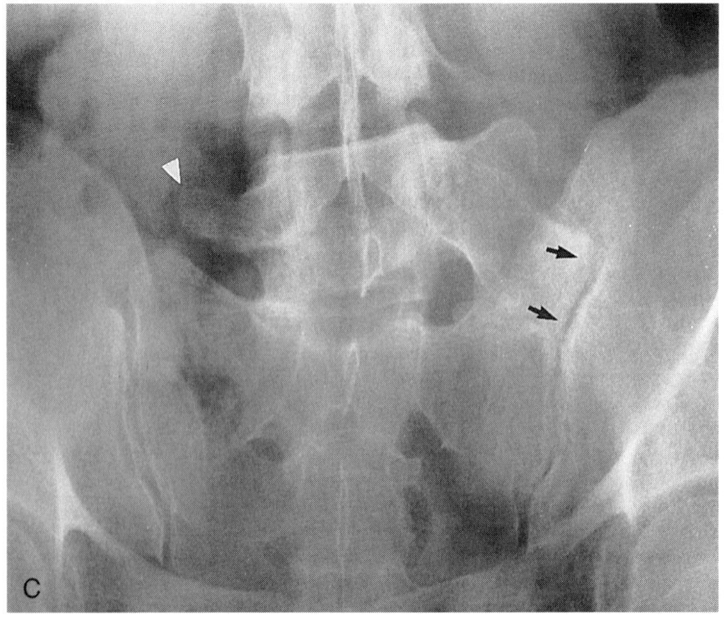

FIGURE 4–15. Transitional lumbosacral segment.[15–17] A Frontal radiograph demonstrates a large, spatulated left L5 transverse process that articulates with the sacral ala (arrow). B In a second patient, both L5 transverse processes are enlarged and spatulated and articulate with the sacral alae. On the lateral lumbar spine radiograph (not shown), only four movable lumbar-type vertebrae were present, a condition termed sacralization. C Observe the asymmetric growth of the transitional segment on this angulated radiograph. The left transverse process of the fifth lumbar vertebra is spatulated and forms an anomalous articulation with the first sacral segment and ilium, creating a portion of the sacroiliac joint (arrows). The right L5 transverse process is of normal size (arrowhead) and does not articulate with the sacrum or ilium.

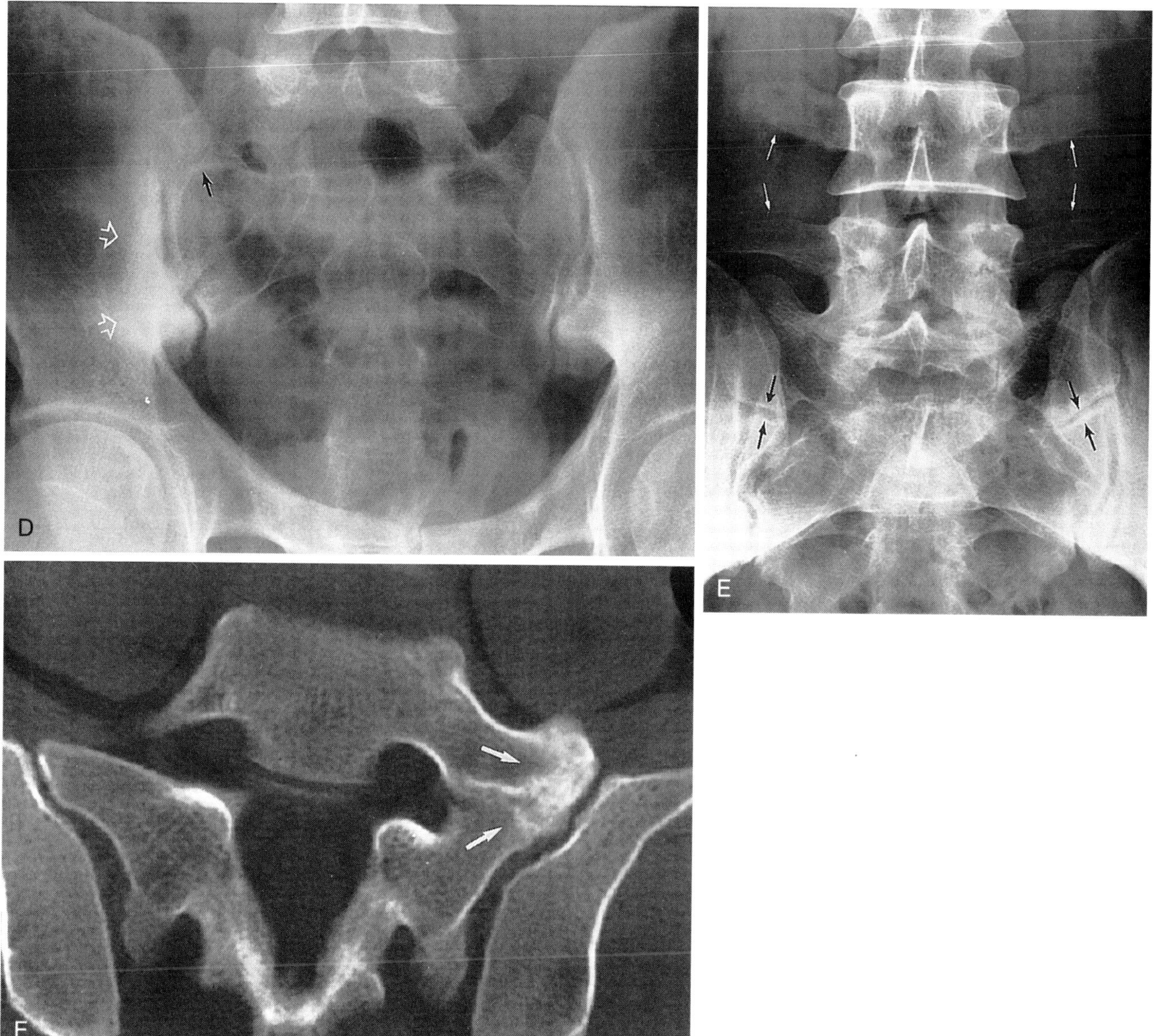

FIGURE 4–15 *Continued.* **D** In this 26-year-old man, note that the right transverse process of L5 appears to articulate with the sacral ala but not the ilium (arrow). Severe reactive sclerosis of the iliac side of the right sacroiliac joint is evident (open arrows). Serologic tests failed to reveal evidence of a seronegative spondyloarthropathy or other articular disease. The sclerosis, therefore, was presumed to be the result of mechanical stress. **E** In a third example, observe the elongated lower lumbar transverse processes (white arrows) and the large, spatulated transverse processes of the lowest lumbar-type vertebra. These spatulated transverse processes appear to articulate bilaterally with the sacrum (black arrows). **F** In another patient, a transaxial CT scan clearly demonstrates reactive degenerative sclerosis adjacent to the apposing surfaces of these partially fused anomalous segments (arrows). *(F, Courtesy of T. Learch, M.D., Los Angeles, California.)*

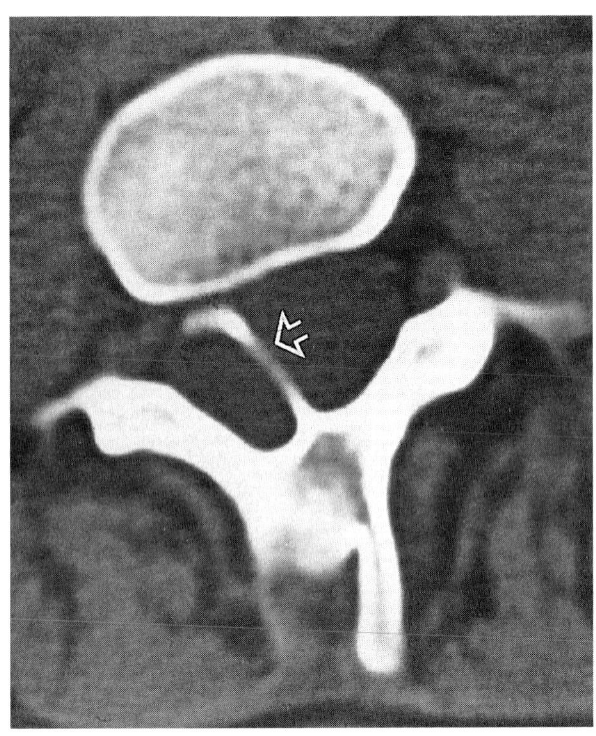

FIGURE 4–16. Diastematomyelia: CT scan.[18] A sagittally oriented vertical osseous bar (open arrow) divides the L3 thecal sac in this 22-year-old woman. Plain film radiography often is inadequate in the demonstration of this osseous or fibrous septum even when it is present. MR imaging or CT with or without myelographic contrast is indicated when this condition is suspected. *(Courtesy of B.L. Harger, D.C., Portland, Oregon.)*

TABLE 4–3. Skeletal Dysplasias and Other Congenital Disorders Affecting the Lumbar Spine*

Entity	Figure(s), Table(s)	Characteristics
Achondroplasia[19]	4–17	*Radiographic findings:* Spinal stenosis Thoracolumbar bullet vertebrae Posterior scalloping and flattening of vertebral bodies
Spondyloepiphyseal dysplasia congenita[20]		Platyspondyly and the "heaped-up" vertebra appearance
Mucopolysaccharidoses (MPS)[21, 22]	4–18	Two types most frequently affect the lumbar spine: *MPS I-H (Hurler's syndrome):* Thoracolumbar gibbous deformity and posterior scalloping of vertebral bodies Rounded anterior vertebral body margins with inferior breaking *MPS IV (Morquio's syndrome):* Platyspondyly Posterior vertebral body scalloping and kyphoscoliosis
Osteopetrosis[23, 24]	4–19; see Fig. 4–31	Patterns of osteosclerosis: diffuse osteosclerosis; "bone-within-bone" appearance, "sandwich vertebrae" Bones are brittle and fracture easily
Osteopoikilosis[25, 26]	4–20	Asymptomatic sclerosing dysplasia Multiple 2- to 3-mm circular foci of osteosclerosis Infrequently affects the spine; lumbar spinal stenosis has been reported as a rare complication of this dysplasia
Marfan syndrome[27, 28]	4–21; see Fig. 4–38 Table 4–4	Kyphoscoliosis in as many as 65 per cent of persons Posterior vertebral body scalloping secondary to dural ectasia Tall, elongated vertebral bodies with exaggerated biconcavity; long transverse processes; 18 per cent of patients have a lumbosacral transitional vertebra
Ehlers-Danlos syndrome[29]	4–22 Table 4–4	Posterior scalloping of vertebral bodies Platyspondyly and kyphoscoliosis
Osteogenesis imperfecta[30]		Osteoporosis and bone fragility Multiple compression fractures and severe kyphoscoliosis common
Chondrodysplasia punctata[31]	4–23	Stippled calcification of vertebral bodies Coronal clefts may be present within the vertebral bodies in the rhizomelic form
Diastrophic dysplasia[32]	4–24	Short stature, progressive scoliosis, kyphosis, and other abnormalities

*See also Table 1–2.

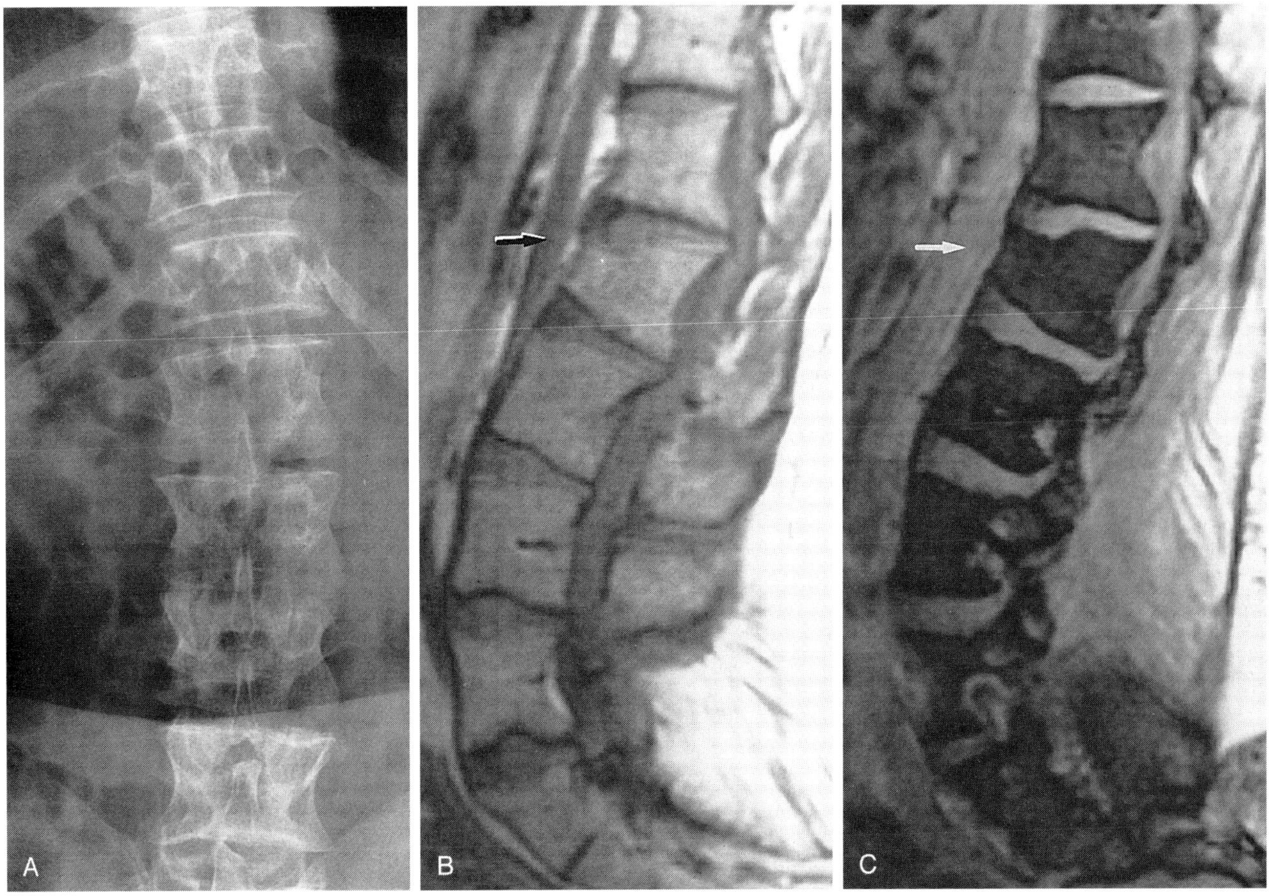

FIGURE 4–17. Achondroplasia.[19] Routine frontal radiograph (A) from this patient with heterozygous achondroplasia shows progressive narrowing of the lower lumbar interpedicle distances. Parasagittal T1-weighted (TR/TE, 600/20) spin echo (B) and multiplanar gradient recalled (MPGR) (TR/TE, 400/15; flip angle, 20 degrees) (C) magnetic resonance (MR) images reveal severe central stenosis, scalloping of the posterior vertebral body margins, and a bullet-shaped thoracolumbar vertebra (arrow).

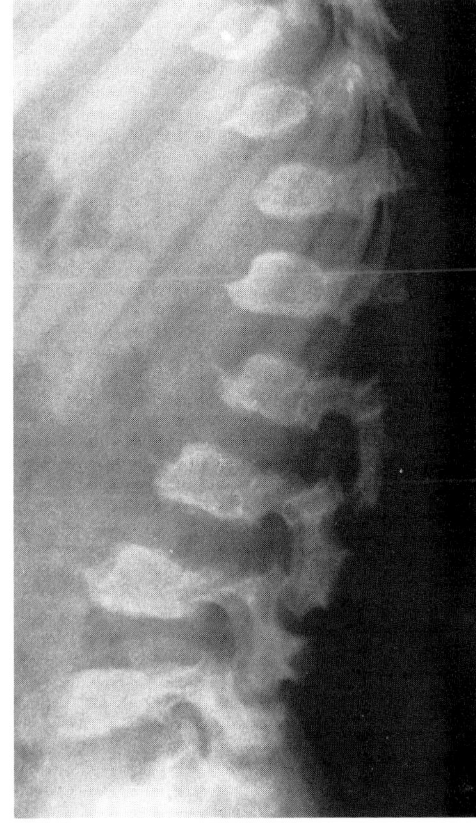

FIGURE 4–18. Morquio's syndrome (mucopolysaccharidosis [MPS] IV).[21, 22] This child with MPS IV has short stature and a thoracolumbar kyphoscoliosis. The central, tongue-like, anterior beaking and rounding of the vertebral bodies are typically seen in young patients with this syndrome. In adults, the vertebrae usually appear flat and rectangular, with irregular margins.

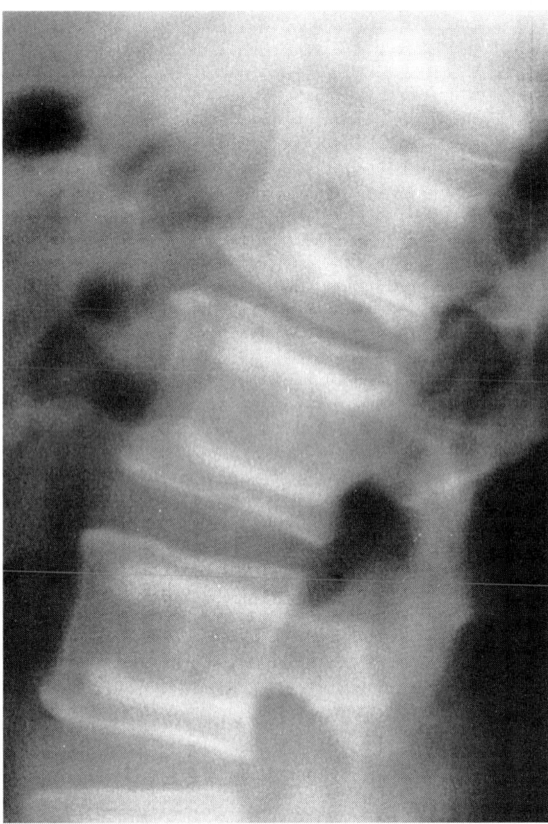

FIGURE 4–19. Osteopetrosis tarda.[23, 24] The peculiar pattern of sclerosis observed in this patient is termed the "bone-within-bone" appearance because it resembles smaller vertebral bodies within normal vertebral bodies. The radiographic pattern of osteopetrosis in the spine may also be that of diffuse sclerosis, or it may be manifest as horizontal bands of sclerosis adjacent to the vertebral end plates ("sandwich vertebrae"). *(Courtesy of R.B. Phillips, D.C., Ph.D., Los Angeles, California.)*

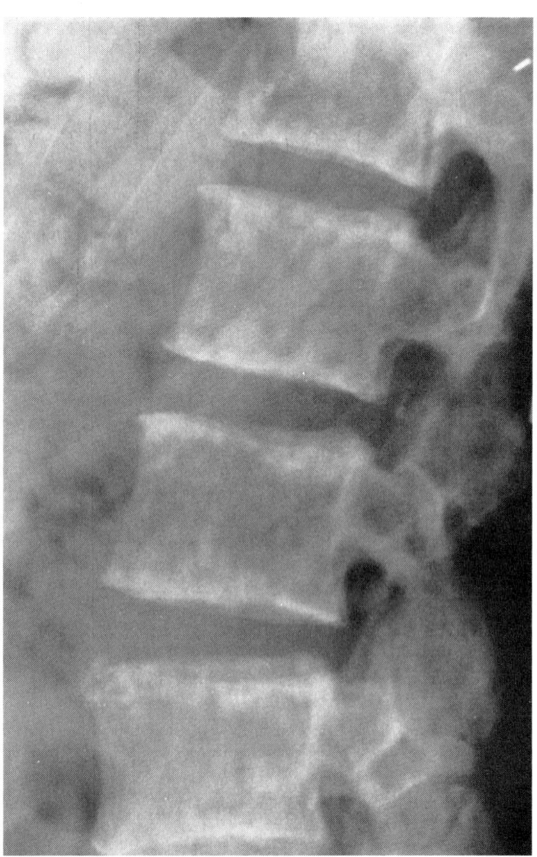

FIGURE 4–20. Osteopoikilosis.[25, 26] Note the symmetric, circular, and ovoid osteosclerotic foci within the vertebral bodies and posterior elements. This sclerosing dysplasia is asymptomatic and of no clinical significance.

TABLE 4–4. Some Causes of Scalloped Vertebrae*

Posterior vertebral body scalloping
- Increased intraspinal pressure
  - Intradural neoplasms
  - Intraspinal cysts
  - Syringomyelia and hydromelia
  - Communicating hydrocephalus
- Dural ectasia
  - Marfan syndrome (Fig. 4–21)
  - Ehlers-Danlos syndrome (Fig. 4–22)
  - Neurofibromatosis (Fig. 4–91)
- Bone resorption
  - Acromegaly
- Congenital disorders
  - Achondroplasia (Fig. 4–17)
  - Morquio's disease (Fig. 4–18)
  - Hurler's syndrome
- Physiologic scalloping (Figs. 4–2B to D)

Anterior vertebral body scalloping
- Lymphoma (Fig. 4–84C)
- Abdominal aortic aneurysm
- Lymphadenopathy
- Tuberculosis

*Adapted from Mitchell GE, Lourie H, Berne AS: The various causes of scalloped vertebrae with notes on their pathogenesis. Radiology 89:67, 1967.

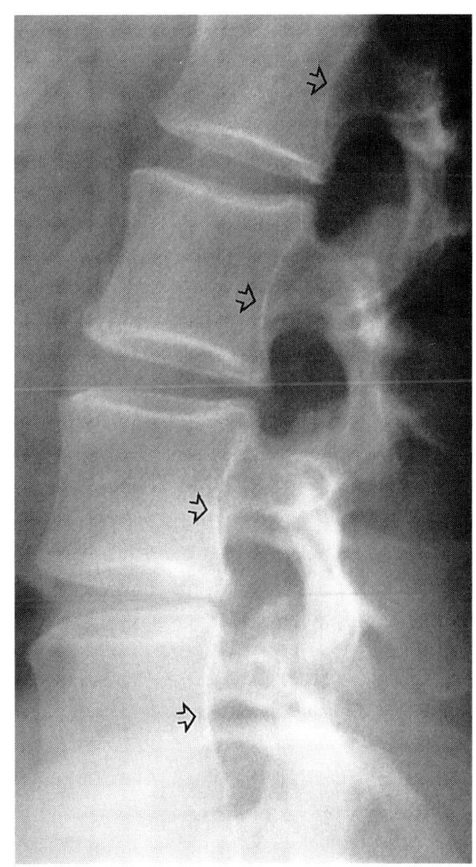

FIGURE 4–21. Marfan syndrome.[27, 28] In this 39-year-old man with Marfan syndrome, posterior scalloping secondary to dural ectasia (open arrows) is evident in the tall and slender vertebral bodies.

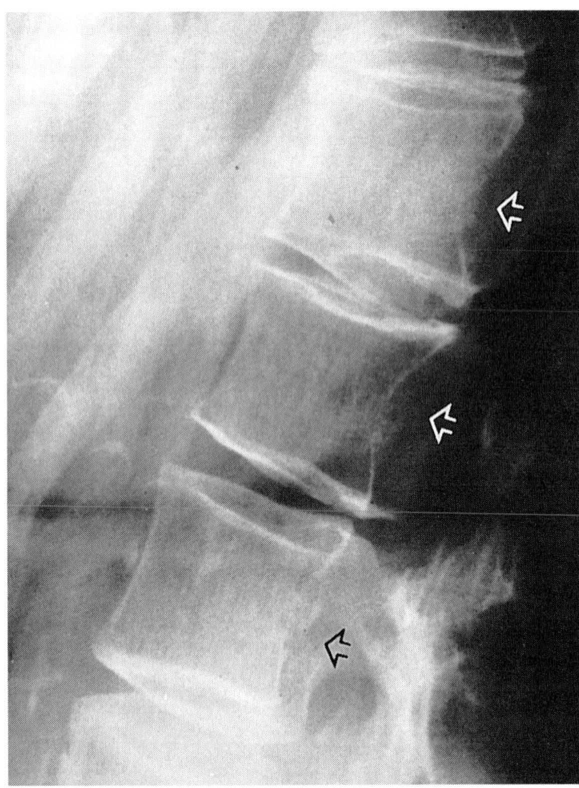

FIGURE 4–22. Ehlers-Danlos syndrome.[29] Lateral view of the lumbar spine reveals prominent scalloping of the posterior vertebral bodies (open arrows). Platyspondyly and thoracolumbar scoliosis (not evident in this patient) also may be seen in patients with Ehlers-Danlos syndrome.

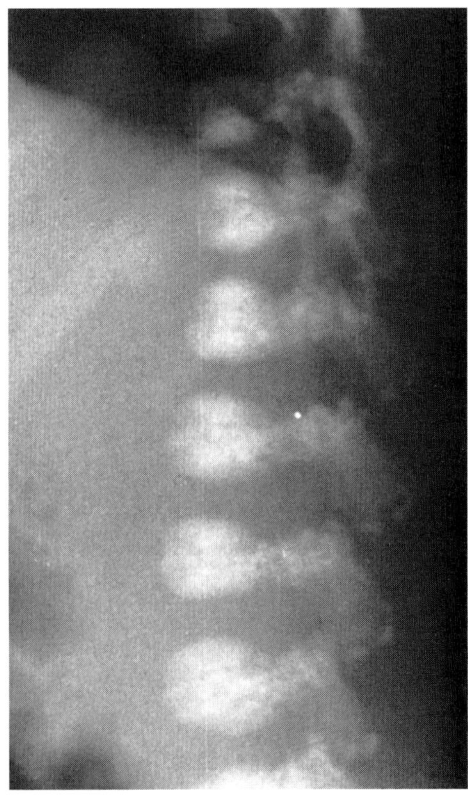

FIGURE 4–23. Chondrodysplasia punctata.[31] In this 2-day-old infant, the radiograph shows the characteristic stippled calcification of the lumbar vertebral bodies and neural arches.

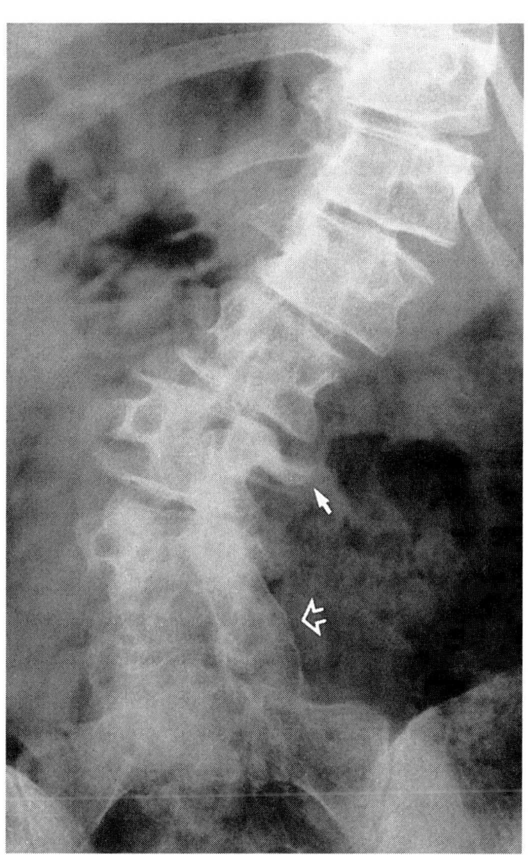

FIGURE 4–24. Diastrophic dysplasia.[32] A lumbar scoliosis is seen in this adult patient with diastrophic dysplasia. Observe the large degenerative osteophyte at the L2-L3 level (solid arrow). A lumbar laminectomy and spinal fusion also have been performed (open arrow).

TABLE 4–5. Spondylolysis and Spondylolisthesis

Entity	Type*	Figure(s)	Characteristics
Dysplastic spondylolisthesis[7, 33]	I	4–25	Developmental anomaly of the neural arch of L4 or L5 or of the sacrum, resulting in anterior displacement of the L4 or L5 segment Rare cause of spondylolisthesis
Spondylolytic (isthmic) spondylolisthesis[7, 34–36]	IIA	4–26, 4–27, 4–28	Fatigue (stress) fracture of the pars interarticularis (spondylolysis) with anterior vertebral body displacement (spondylolisthesis) Most common form of spondylolisthesis in persons under the age of 50 years 90 per cent of spondylolyses occur at L5, followed in frequency by L4 and L3 Spondylolysis present in approximately 7 per cent of Caucasians and as many as 16 per cent of athletes Most progression of displacement usually occurs by age 10 years, with progression almost never occurring after age 18 years Instability uncommon: measured by functional radiography—flexion-extension and compression-traction radiographs As many as 50 per cent of patients with spondylolysis or spondylolisthesis remain asymptomatic; patients with translation (instability) on functional radiographs have a higher prevalence of associated pain than those without translation; in patients without translation on functional radiographs, no relationship exists between pain and the amount of slippage Differentiation from acute isthmic fracture (type II C) requires clinical history, single photon emission computed tomographic (SPECT) imaging, or magnetic resonance (MR) imaging
Spondylolisthesis from elongated intact pars interarticularis[7, 33]	II B		Elongation of an intact pars interarticularis is extremely rare Believed to result from repetitive minor trabecular stress fractures of the pars interarticularis with consequent healing, sclerosis, hypertrophy, and elongation of this structure With progressive displacement, the pars interarticularis may fracture and separate becoming a type II A spondylolytic spondylolisthesis
Acute spondylolysis[37, 38]	II C	4–29	Acute fracture of the pars interarticularis is an extremely rare cause of spondylolysis and spondylolisthesis Hyperextension injuries are believed to be the most common cause of acute pars interarticularis fracture in young athletes Associated with disabling low back pain Acute fractures are seldom bilateral and symmetric, the fracture margins are not well corticated, and progression of spondylolisthesis is rare Diagnosed by identifying increased radiopharmaceutical uptake on SPECT imaging or bone marrow edema on MR imaging; such positive SPECT and MR imaging findings correlate well with acute pain Most authorities recommend immobilization in a back brace for the management of this acute form of fracture
Degenerative spondylolisthesis[39, 70]	III	4–30	Anterior vertebral displacement of one segment on another secondary to apophyseal joint degeneration without defects of the pars interarticularis Synonyms: pseudospondylolisthesis, nonspondylolytic spondylolisthesis, articular spondylolisthesis Most common at L4 in women who are older than 50 years of age; more common in black persons and in patients with transitional lumbosacral segments (synostosis of L5-S1); a higher prevalence is noted in patients with diabetes mellitus *Clinical findings:* Patients may be asymptomatic or may have back pain, sciatica, nerve root compression, intermittent claudication of the cauda equina; symptoms may be related to stenosis, disc herniation, or both; patients with progressive slippage are more likely to have pain; generally not associated with disability or long-term symptoms

TABLE 4–5. Spondylolysis and Spondylolisthesis *Continued*

Entity	Type*	Figure(s)	Characteristics
			Prevalence: 28 per cent in women who have borne children 16.7 per cent in nulliparous women 7.5 per cent in men *Radiographic findings:* Anterior vertebral displacement, apophyseal joint space narrowing, sclerosis, and osteophytes, remodeling of the neural arch, disc space narrowing, vacuum phenomenon, and hyperlordosis (variable) Flexion and extension radiographs are used to identify excessive translation and angulation indicative of segmental instability Forward slippage of the L4 vertebral body usually is less than 20 per cent of the anteroposterior diameter of the L5 vertebral body (grade I)
Traumatic spondylolysis[7, 33]	IV		Acute, severe injury resulting in fracture of the neural arch at a site other than the pars interarticularis Example: C2 hangman's fracture; rare in thoracic and lumbar spine
Pathologic spondylolysis[33, 40]	V	4–31	Spondylolysis through pathologic bone, with or without spondylolisthesis Some disorders include skeletal metastasis, osteopetrosis, and Paget's disease
Unilateral spondylolysis[7, 41]		4–32	Unilateral pars interarticularis defect may occur as a result of a fatigue fracture (type II A) or an acute fracture (type II C) Sclerosis of the opposite pedicle is believed to be secondary to redistribution of weight-bearing forces through the contralateral pedicle and neural arch
Unstable spondylolisthesis[42–44]		4–33	Instability is a rare complication of most types of spondylolisthesis Clinical utility of functional lateral radiographs—compression-traction and flexion-extension radiographs—is controversial, and the evidence is somewhat contradictory Compression-traction radiographs may be useful in revealing instability of motion segments in patients with spondylolytic spondylolisthesis[44] In patients with clinically suspected lumbar instability of all causes, flexion-extension radiographs obtained with the patient standing more frequently reveal signs of instability than traction-compression radiographs[43] Flexion-extension radiographs obtained in the lateral decubitus position reveal even more motion than those obtained in the standing position[42] Translational instability: total anterior to posterior intersegmental motion in excess of 4 mm or 8% of the sagittal diameter of the vertebral body Angular instability: total intersegmental angular motion in excess of 12 degrees[42] or 20 degrees[43]
Progressive spondylolisthesis[45]		4–34	Progression occurs before 18 years of age in most cases of progressive spondylolytic spondylolisthesis Infrequently, new vertebral displacement or progression of an existing displacement may occur in adult spondylolysis and isthmic spondylolisthesis of L5 without evidence of trauma Thick L5 transverse processes and iliolumbar ligaments protect against further slippage of L5

*Classification After Wiltse LL, Newman PH, MacNab I: Classification of spondylosis and spondylolysis. Clin Orthop 117:13, 1976.

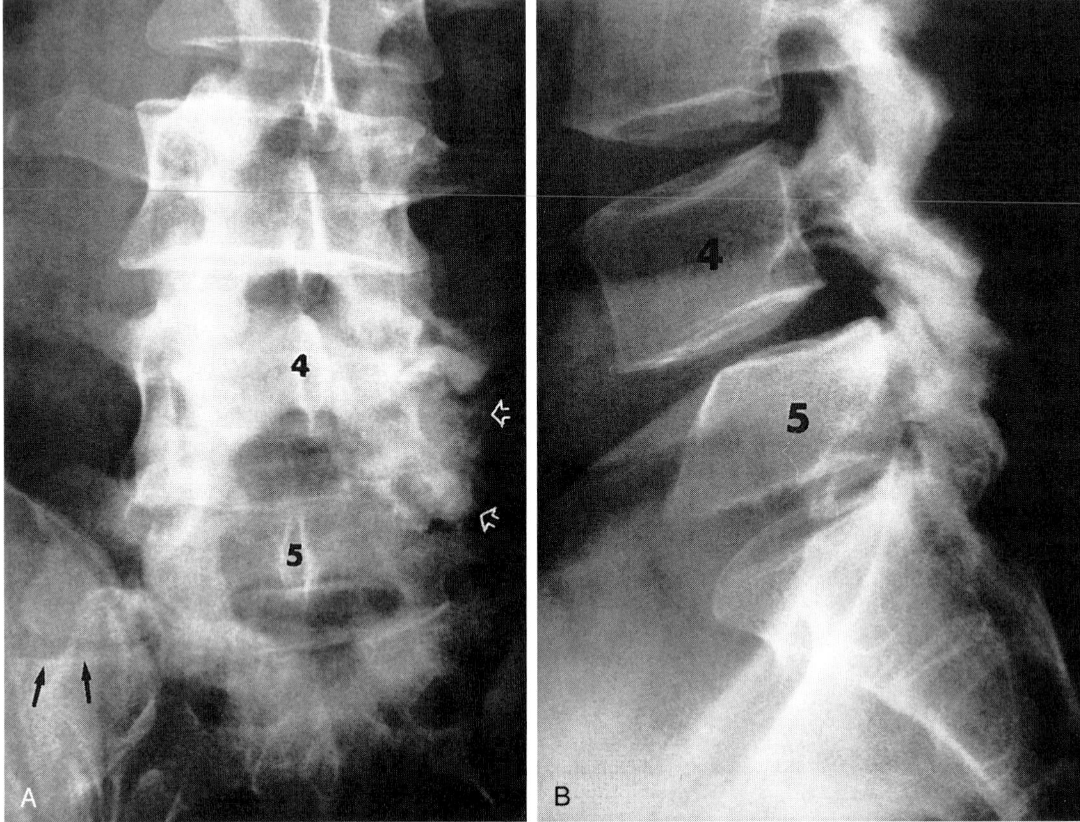

FIGURE 4–25. Dysplastic spondylolisthesis.[7, 33] This 29-year-old manual laborer had chronic low back pain. A Frontal radiograph reveals a transitional lumbosacral segment with a spatulated transverse process on the right that articulates with the sacrum (solid arrows). Extensive osteophyte formation and bone proliferation of the contralateral L4-L5 apophyseal articulation also are seen (open arrows). B Lateral radiograph shows a wedge-shaped, dysplastic appearance of the anterosuperior margin of the L5 vertebral body as well as short L5 pedicles. The L4 vertebral body exhibits marked anterior translation and angulation in relation to L5, and the neural arch is elongated and sclerotic. Dramatic apophyseal joint degeneration also is evident, especially at the L4-L5 level. This patient has a combination of dysplastic (type I) and degenerative (type III) spondylolisthesis. *(Courtesy of G. Murdoch, D.C., Smithers, B.C., Canada.)*

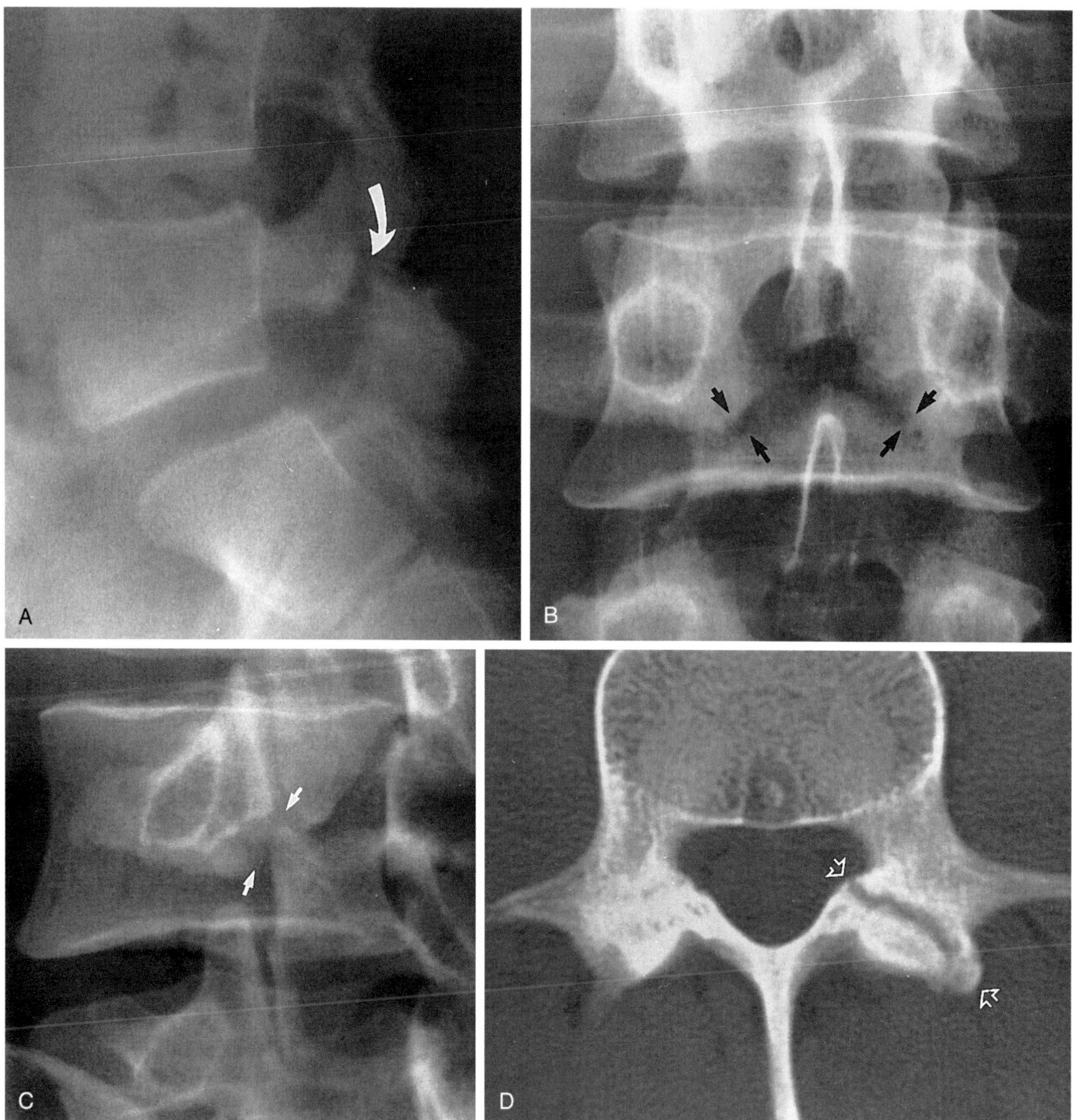

FIGURE 4–26. Spondylolysis.[7, 33] A Spondylolysis at L5. This 10-year-old girl complained of back pain after gymnastics. A radiolucent pars interarticularis defect (spondylolysis) is apparent at L5 (curved arrow). Spondylolisthesis is minimal and the vertebral body morphology is normal. *(A, Courtesy of M.N. Pathria, M.D., San Diego, California.)* B, C Spondylolysis. Frontal radiograph (B) shows the pars interarticularis defects (arrows). These defects are best demonstrated on lateral and oblique (C) radiographs (arrows). D Spondylolysis at L4: CT abnormalities. Transaxial CT bone window shows a unilateral radiolucent defect through the pars interarticularis of L4 (open arrows). Sclerosis and hypertrophic bone formation (callus) suggest that the fracture is healing. *(D, Courtesy of J. Amberg, M.D., San Diego, California.)*

TABLE 4–6. Myerding's Method of Measuring Spondylolisthesis[34]

Grade	Degree of Displacement
I	<25 per cent
II	26–50 per cent
III	51–75 per cent
IV	76–100 per cent
V	> 100 per cent (spondyloptosis)

*Myerding's method measures the amount of displacement of the posterior margin of the L5 vertebral body in relation to S1 on lateral radiographs (Fig. 4–27).

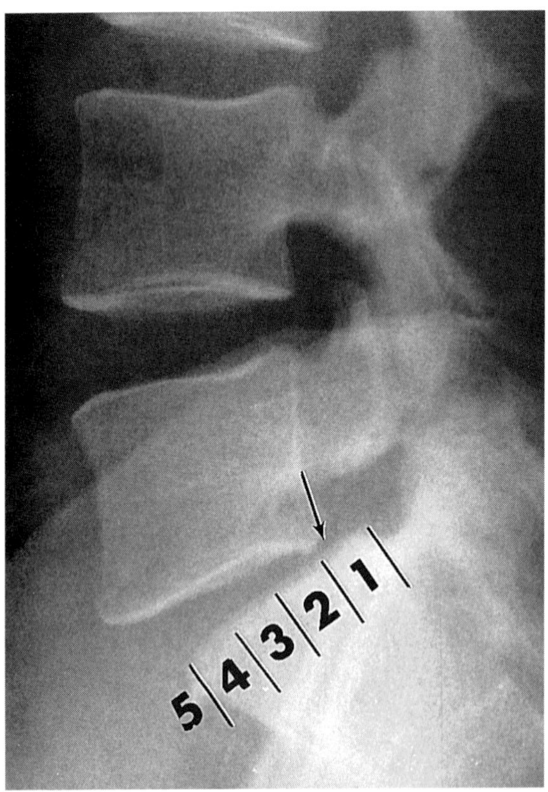

FIGURE 4–27. Measurement of spondylolisthesis: Myerding's method.[34] On the lateral radiograph, a line constructed along the sacral base divides the sacrum into four equal parts. Another line drawn along the posterior vertebral body of L5 (arrow) is extended inferiorly to intersect one of these quadrants. The extent of L5 vertebral body displacement is graded (into grades 1 through 4) according to the quadrant intersected. In cases in which the L5 body translates beyond the sacral promontory, the spondylolisthesis is termed grade 5 and is called spondyloptosis. In this case, the spondylolisthesis is grade 1 (Table 4–6).

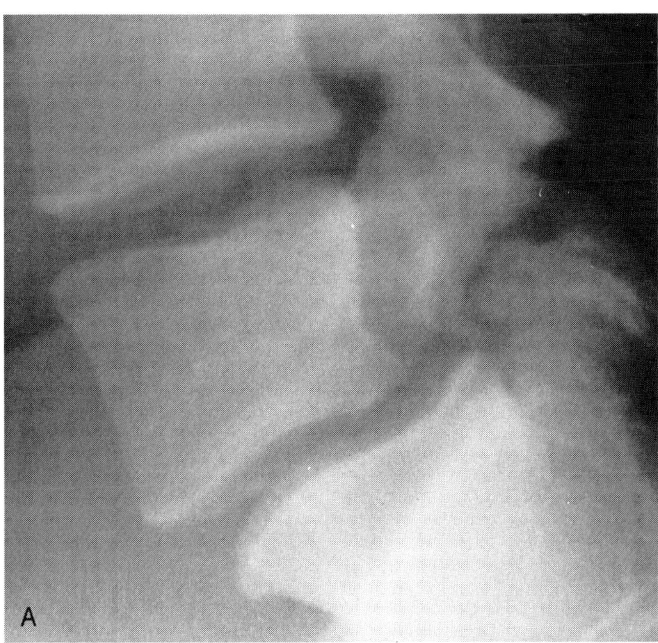

FIGURE 4–28. Spondylolytic (isthmic) spondylolisthesis.[35, 36] A Spondylolisthesis at L5. Lateral radiograph shows a grade 1 anterolisthesis of L5 and a pars interarticularis defect. Note the trapezoidal shape of the L5 vertebral body, a finding that may represent a normal contour and may also be exaggerated by bone remodeling in long-standing spondylolisthesis. B The "inverted Napoleon hat" sign. Frontal radiograph demonstrates the "inverted Napoleon hat" sign or "bowline of Brailsford" sign characteristic of grades 3 to 5 spondylolisthesis. In these cases, the L5 vertebral body is translated anteriorly, such that on the frontal radiograph, it is seen in the axial plane rather than in the conventional coronal plane. The arrows indicate the anterior aspect of the L5 vertebral body. C Degenerative sclerosis. Extensive sclerosis is observed in the lumbosacral vertebral bodies (open arrows) in this 50-year-old man with a long-standing grade II spondylolytic spondylolisthesis. Observe also the presence of buttressing at the anterior aspect of the sacrum (curved arrow). Sclerosis and buttressing are believed to be compensatory responses to mechanical stress from abnormal motion.

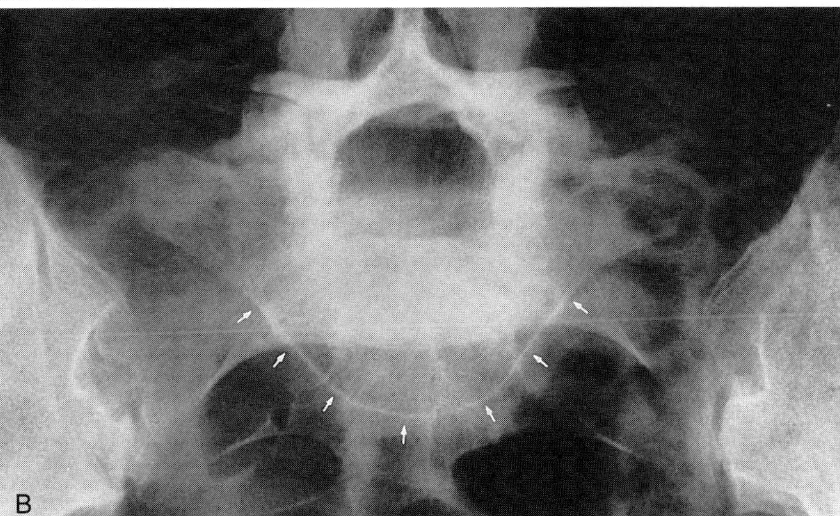

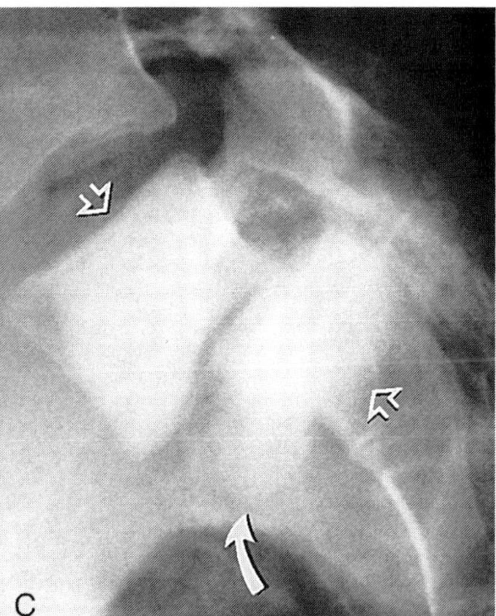

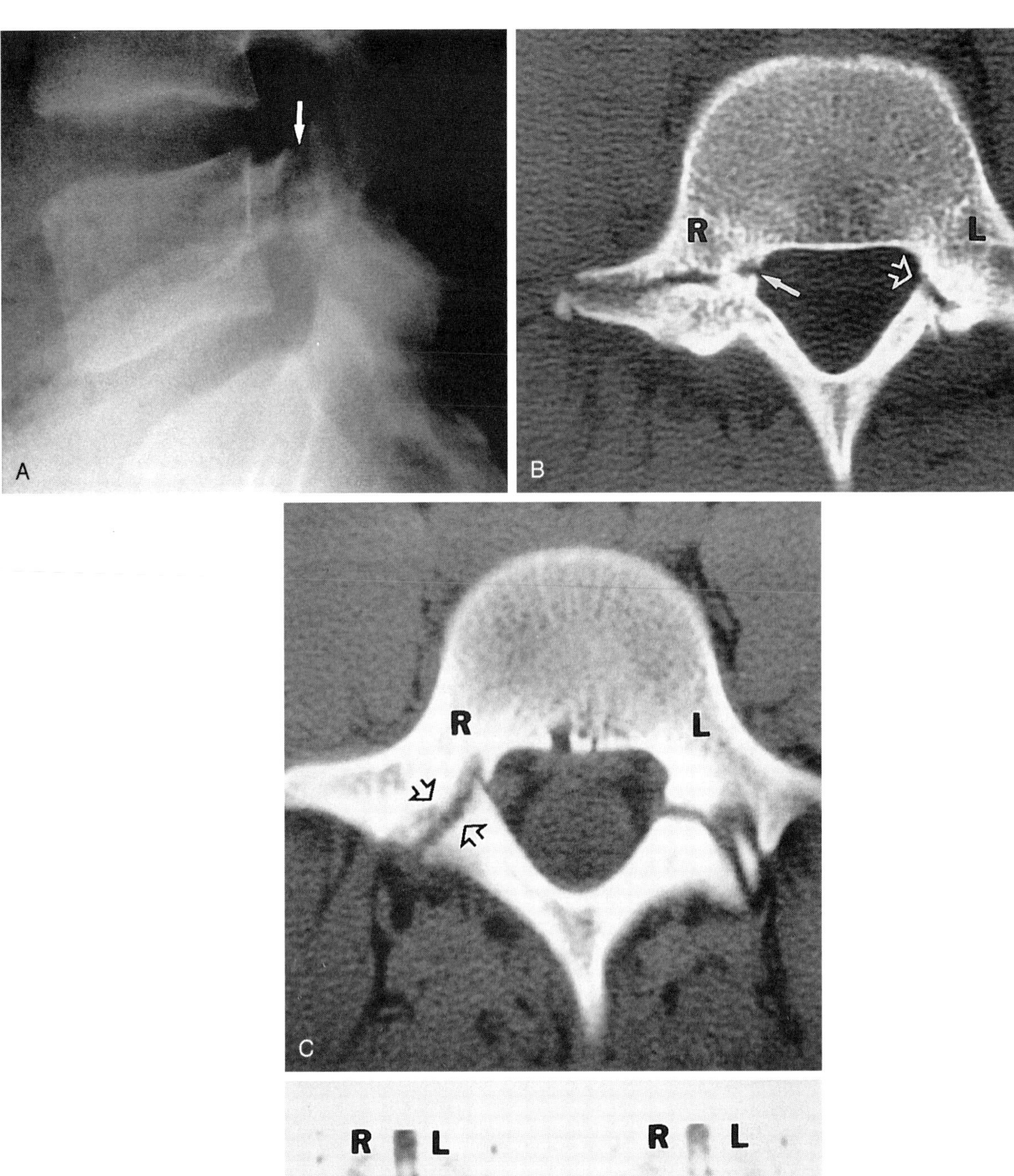

FIGURE 4–29. Acute spondylolysis.[37, 38] **A, B** Acute neural arch fracture in a 17-year-old boy who sustained a fall of 15 feet. Lateral radiograph **(A)** and transaxial computed tomographic (CT) image **(B)** demonstrate a coronally oriented vertical fracture line through the right transverse process (solid arrows) and an oblique fracture line through the left pedicle-lamina junction of L5 (open arrow). No anterior displacement of the vertebral body is seen. **C, D** Acute pars interarticularis fracture in a 16-year-old high school football player. Routine radiographs (not shown) revealed bilateral spondylolysis but no evidence of spondylolisthesis. In **C,** a transaxial CT scan obtained 9 months after the initial onset of pain shows bilateral defects of the pars interarticularis. The fracture margins on the left are sclerotic and well-defined; the fracture margins on the right (open arrows) are less sclerotic and more poorly defined with significant resorption of the apposing bone surfaces. These findings suggest that the fracture on the right is more acute than the fracture on the left. In **D,** images from a coronal single photon emission computed tomographic (SPECT) bone scan obtained at the same time as the CT scan **(C)** reveal intense uptake of the radiopharmaceutical agent in the right pars interarticularis (arrows) and only moderate uptake on the left side. These findings confirm the acute nature of the right pars fracture and the long-standing nature of the left pars defect. Acute traumatic fractures of the neural arch are rare, painful lesions that are best imaged with SPECT imaging. CT and magnetic resonance (MR) imaging also may be helpful in such cases. *(***C, D,** *Courtesy of S. Thorpe, D.C., Chicago, Illinois.)*

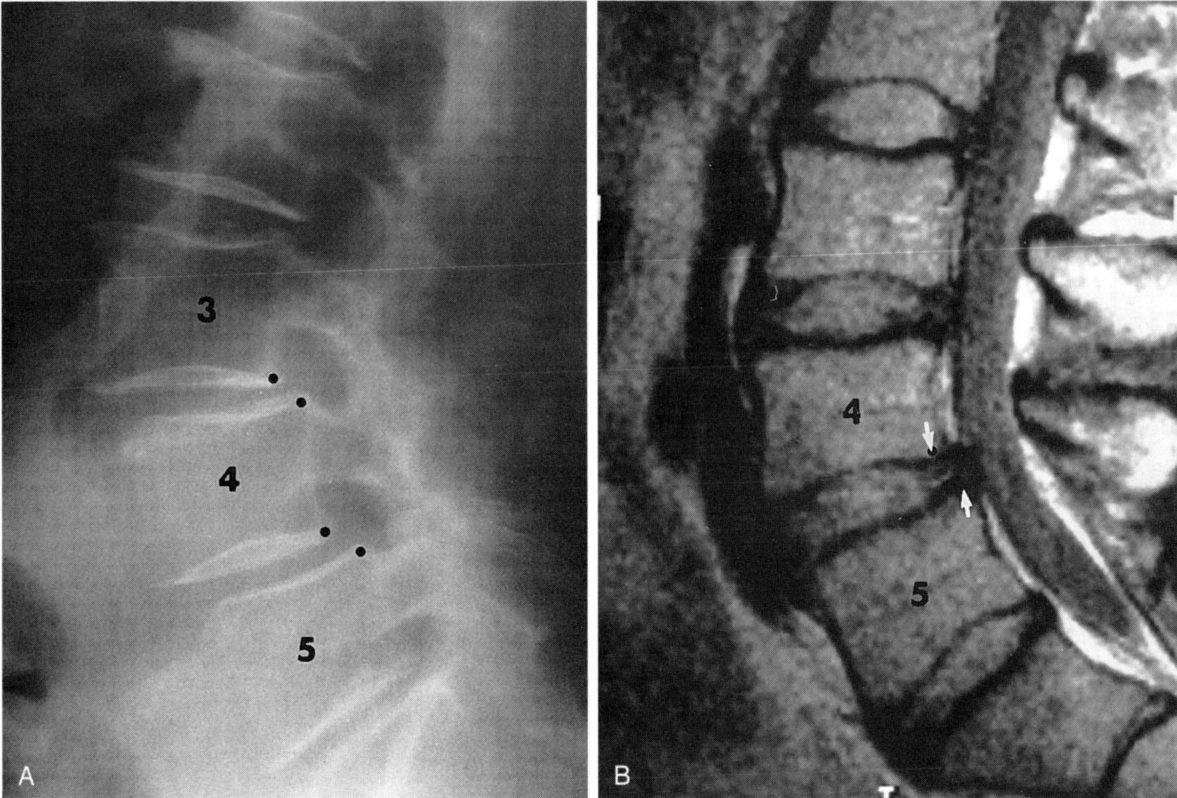

FIGURE 4–30. Degenerative spondylolisthesis.[39, 70] A Lateral radiograph from a 74-year-old woman with chronic low back pain reveals severe apophyseal joint osteoarthrosis and anterior displacement of both L3 and L4 (dots). B Midsagittal T1-weighted (TR/TE, 400/17) spin echo magnetic resonance (MR) image from another patient shows degenerative spondylolisthesis of L4 (arrows) and consequent spinal stenosis and thecal sac compression.

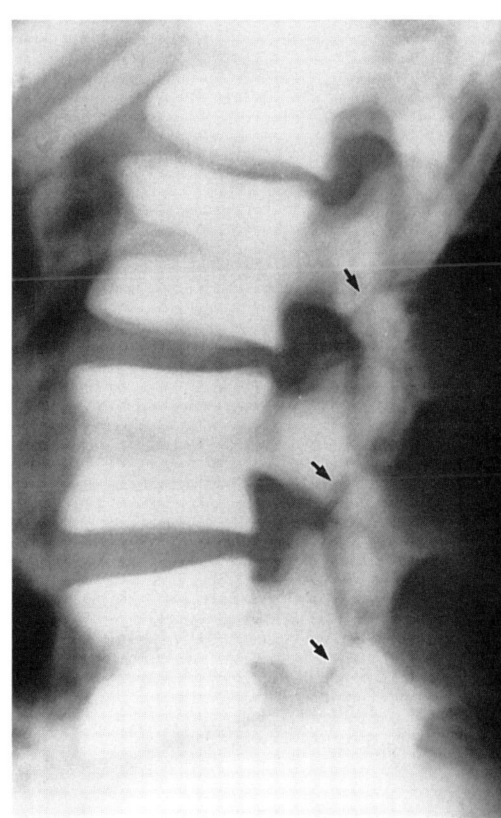

FIGURE 4–31. Pathologic spondylolysis: Osteopetrosis.[33, 40] In this 26-year-old man with episodic low back pain, the vertebral bodies appear diffusely sclerotic with an intervening central band of normal bone density ("sandwich vertebra"). The neural arches also are diffusely sclerotic, and pars interarticularis fractures are evident at three vertebral levels (arrows). These pathologic fractures of the pars interarticularis presumably occur as a result of brittle bones. *(From Khanchandani BA: Albers-Schonberg disease with multiple-level lumbar spondylolysis: A case report. Eur J Chiropr 37:5, 1989.)*

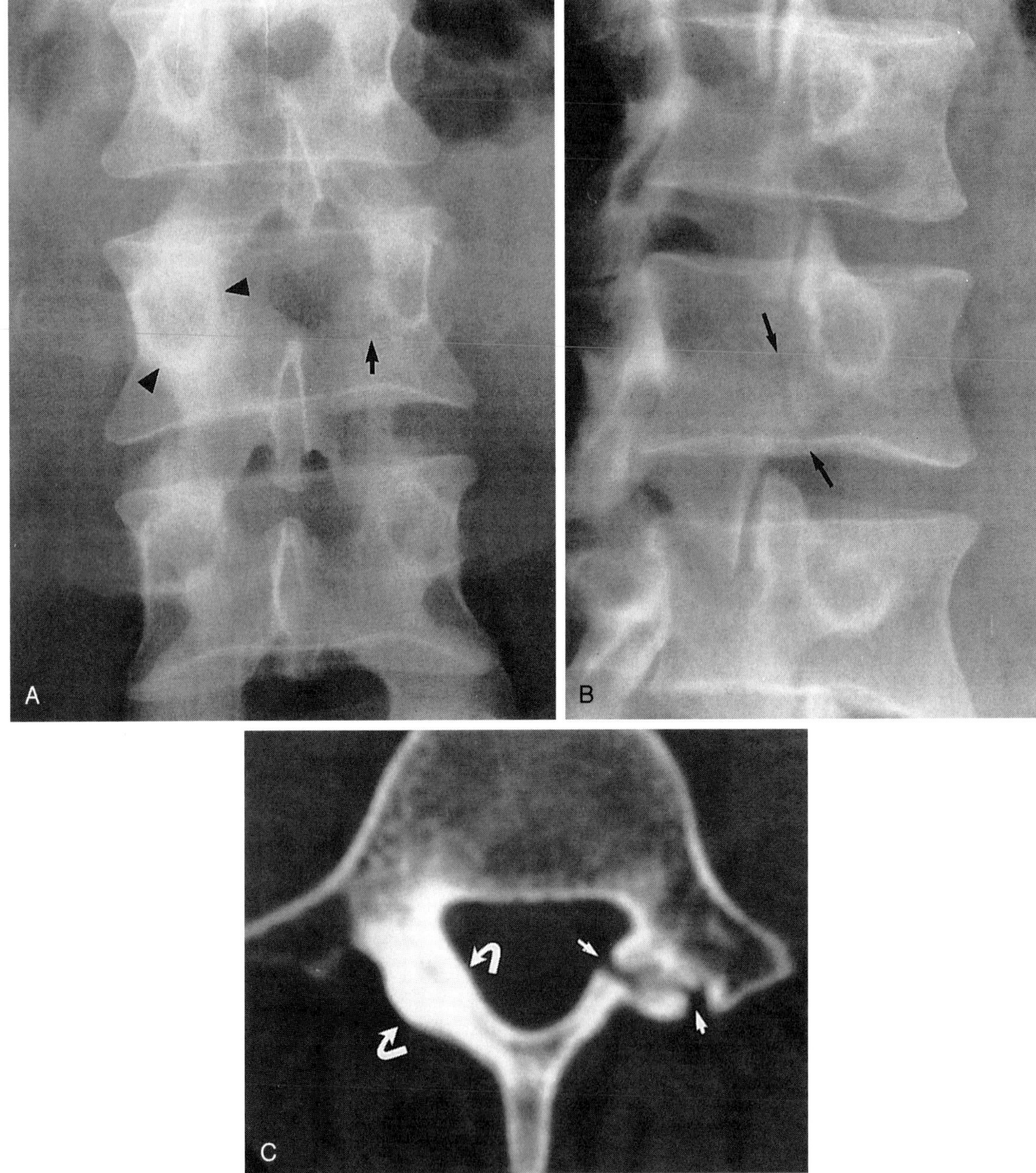

FIGURE 4–32. Unilateral spondylolysis.[7, 41] A Frontal radiograph shows a hypertrophic and sclerotic pedicle (arrowheads) and a poorly visualized pars interarticularis defect on the contralateral side (arrows). B Oblique radiograph shows a unilateral pars interarticularis defect (arrows). *(A, B, Courtesy of J. Grilliot, D.C., Toledo, Ohio.)* C Transaxial computed tomographic (CT) image from another patient illustrates a unilateral pars defect (arrows) with a contralateral sclerotic pedicle (curved arrows).

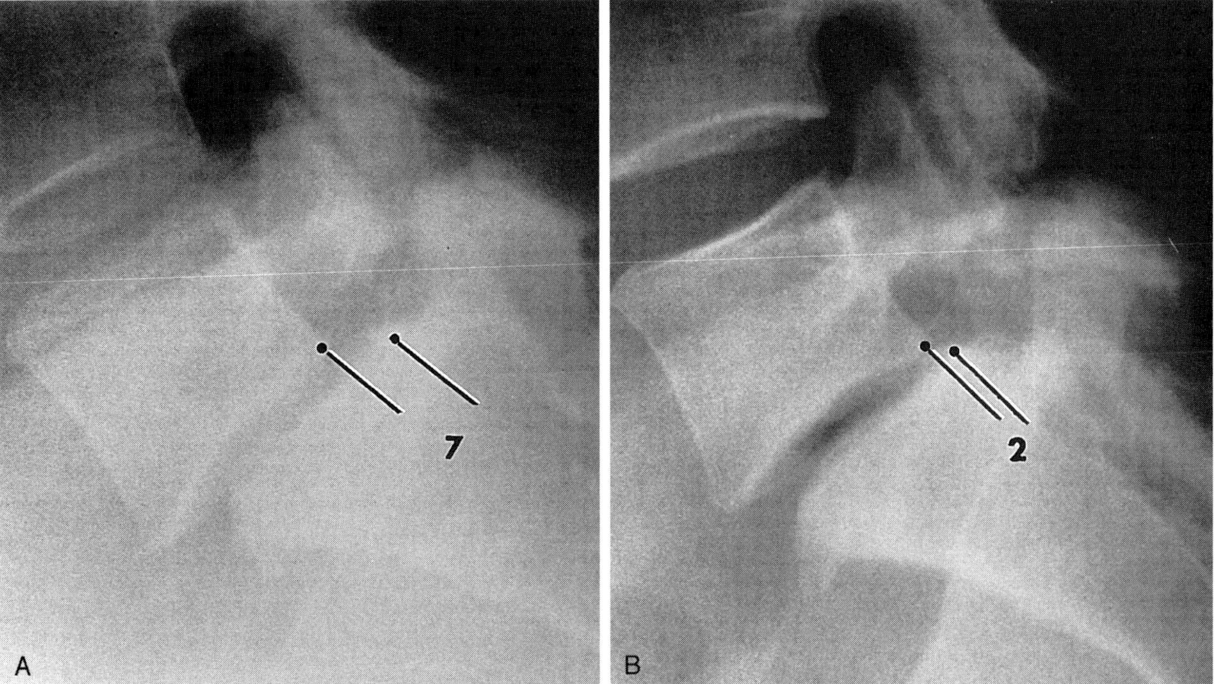

FIGURE 4–33. Spondylolisthesis: Instability evaluation with functional radiography.[42–44] A Radiograph obtained with compression shows 7 mm of anterior translation of L5 on S1 (vertical lines with dots). B Film obtained with traction reveals a reduction of the anterolisthesis to 2 mm (vertical lines with dots). In addition, the disc space has widened, and intradiscal gas (vacuum phenomenon) is evident. Sagittal translation on functional radiographs in excess of 4 mm indicates instability and implies a higher probability of progression of the spondylolisthesis.

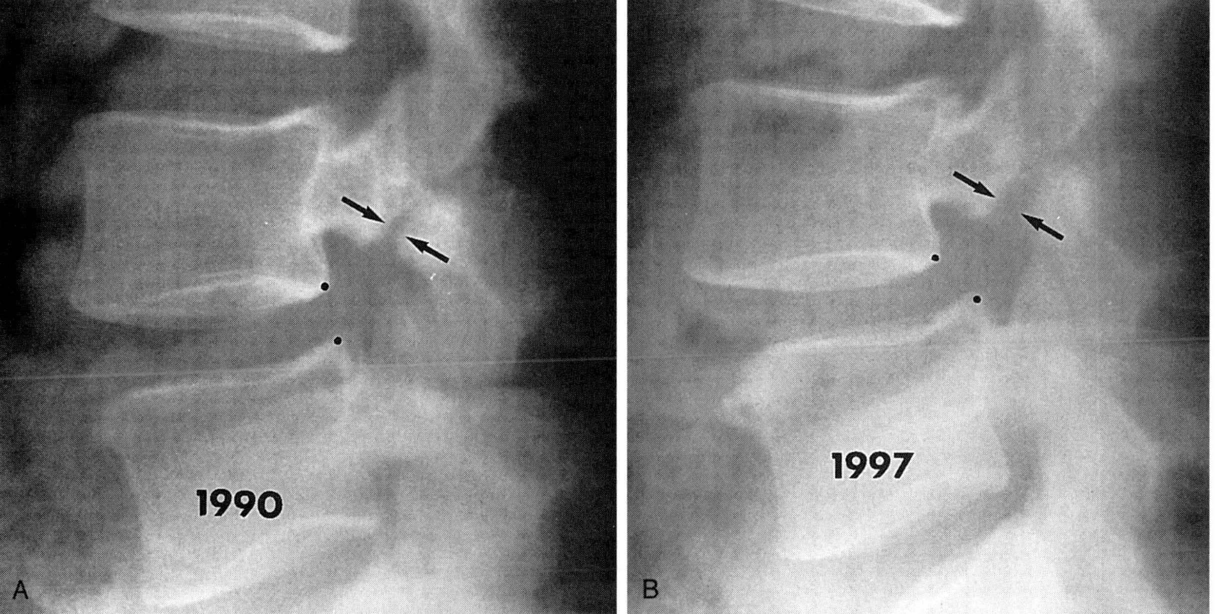

FIGURE 4–34. Spondylolytic spondylolisthesis: Serial progression in an adult.[45] A Upright (standing) spinal radiograph of a 42-year-old man obtained in 1990 reveals a spondylolysis of L4 with only minimal anterior displacement of L4 on L5. The pars interarticularis defects (arrows) are well visualized and the apposing margins appear sclerotic. B Another upright spinal radiograph of the same patient obtained 7 years later, after a motor vehicle collision, reveals separation of the pars interarticularis defects (arrows) and a 5-mm progression of anterior translation of L4. The apposing margins of the pars defect appear less sclerotic and distinct and suggest the presence of resorption at this site. In this case, it is impossible to determine if there is a causal relationship between the motor vehicle collision and progression of the spondylolisthesis. With spondylolytic spondylolisthesis, progression usually occurs before 16 to 18 years of age. In adults, however, new vertebral displacement or progression of an existing displacement of an L5 isthmic spondylolisthesis may rarely occur with no history of trauma. *(Courtesy of G.C. Stirling, D.C., Kelowna, British Columbia, Canada.)*

TABLE 4–7. Lumbar Scoliosis*

Entity	Figure(s), Table(s)	Characteristics
Idiopathic adolescent scoliosis[46]	4–35	Most common type of idiopathic scoliosis Typical pattern: right thoracic, left lumbar Onset: 10 years of age to skeletal maturity Girls: boys, 4:1 to 8:1
Degenerative scoliosis[47]	4–36 Table 4–15	Scoliosis in elderly persons is associated with advanced degenerative disease
Scoliosis secondary to leg length inequality[48]	4–37	Functional lumbar curve convex to the side of the shorter leg Compensatory thoracic curve in the opposite direction Functional curves typically are flexible in younger persons, but become more rigid and structural with advancing age through long-term changes from contracture or growth Sacral tilt also may result from pelvic asymmetry rather than leg length discrepancy
Marfan syndrome[27, 49]	4–38	Scoliosis occurs in as many as 65 per cent of patients No female predominance Smooth, long sweeping curve resembles that of idiopathic scoliosis In young people, the curve progresses more rapidly than in idiopathic scoliosis Thoracic scoliosis often is associated with posterior scalloping from dural ectasia

*Only the types of scoliosis illustrated in this chapter are listed; for a more complete discussion of scoliosis, see Table 3–5.

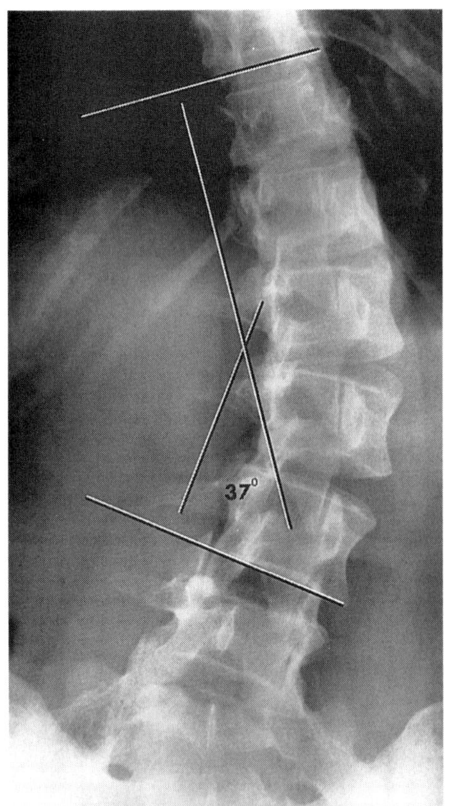

FIGURE 4–35. Idiopathic scoliosis.[46] This 26-year-old woman has idiopathic adolescent scoliosis that was diagnosed at 13 years of age. Using the Cobb measurement method, this left lumbar scoliosis measures 37 degrees. Marked vertebral body rotation also is noted.

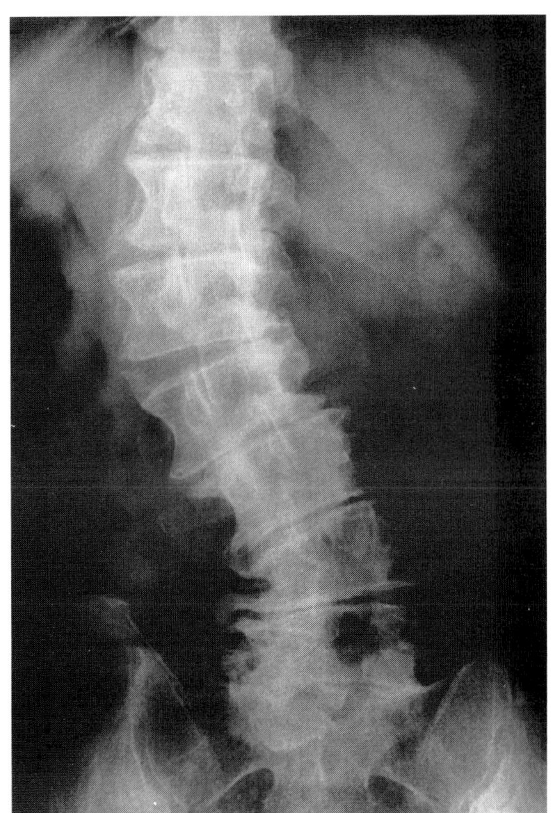

FIGURE 4–36. Degenerative scoliosis.[47] Right thoracolumbar and left lumbar idiopathic scoliosis in this 78-year-old man have been present since adolescence. Severe degenerative changes of both the discs and apophyseal joints are evident on the concave aspects of the curves. Despite these severe degenerative changes, this patient had only occasional back pain and aching. *(Reprinted with permission from Taylor JAM, Hoffman LE: The geriatric patient: Diagnostic imaging of common musculoskeletal disorders. Top Clin Chiropr 3:23, © 1996, Aspen Publishers, Inc.)*

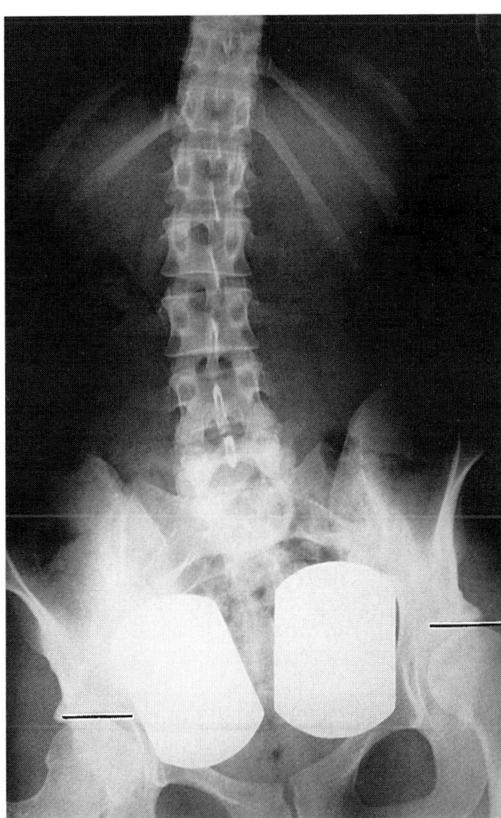

FIGURE 4–37. Scoliosis secondary to leg length discrepancy.[48] This patient sustained fractures of both the femur and the tibia during a motorcycle accident. After reduction and fixation, the right leg remained 8 cm short, resulting in prominent pelvic distortion and scoliosis seen on this upright radiograph. (Horizontal lines demonstrate the variation in height of the femoral heads.)

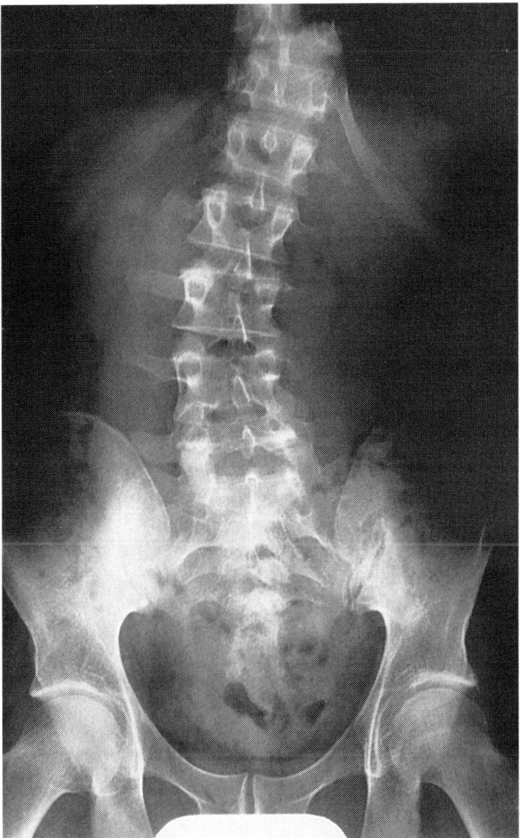

FIGURE 4–38. Scoliosis: Marfan syndrome.[27, 49] A lumbar scoliosis is seen in this 29-year-old man with Marfan syndrome. Scoliosis is evident in up to 65 per cent of patients with Marfan syndrome and exhibits a pattern similar to that of idiopathic scoliosis. In Marfan syndrome patients, however, the scoliosis typically begins earlier in life and progresses more rapidly.

TABLE 4–8. Fractures and Dislocations of the Lumbar Spine*

Entity	Figure(s), Table(s)	Characteristics
Vertebral body compression fracture[50]	4–39	Usually upper lumbar region Frequent occurrence in osteoporotic persons *Mechanisms:* Acute fracture from accidental, athletic, or occupational hyperflexion-compression injury; alternatively, trivial trauma, repeated minor trauma, or slow bone remodeling resulting from ongoing chronic microfractures Biconcave end-plate deformities are common in the lumbar spine May be quite painful, but the middle column (posterior vertebral body) generally remains intact, and, therefore, these fractures are considered stable, infrequently resulting in neurologic deficit Unstable fractures or ligament injuries may be misinterpreted as stable compression fractures; all radiographs should be examined closely for evidence of retropulsion of the posterior margin of the vertebral body, as seen in burst fractures, or disruption of the posterior elements, as seen in seat belt fractures, both of which are unstable injuries
Burst fracture[51, 52]	4–40 Table 4–9	More common in younger persons Most common in the thoracolumbar spine *Mechanisms:* Predominantly axial compression during motor vehicle accident Comminution of vertebral body, widened interpedicle distance, retropulsion of vertebral body fragments Fractures of anterior and middle columns Up to 50 per cent of patients have neurologic deficit May be unstable (Table 4–9)
Transverse process fracture[53, 54]	4–41, 4–42	*Mechanisms:* Direct blow or lateral flexion 13.6 per cent of all thoracolumbar spine injuries Often multiple transverse process fractures occur Abdominal visceral injury, including that to ureter and kidney in as many as 20 per cent of patients Heterotopic ossification related to associated hematoma may result in a vertical osseous bridge spanning adjacent transverse processes
Fracture-dislocation[55, 56]	4–43, 4–44	Rare injury of thoracolumbar or, less commonly, lumbosacral regions Highly unstable injury; results in complete disruption of all three columns Permanent neurologic deficit, usually complete paraplegia, in more than 90 per cent of cases *Mechanisms:* Compression (anterior column), rotation, shear, and distraction (middle and posterior columns) Often severe injuries associated with polytrauma
Thoracolumbar flexion injury (seat belt fracture)[55]	2–27, 2–28 Table 3–6	See Table 3–6
Acute pars interarticularis fracture[37, 38]	4–29 Table 4–5	Very uncommon form of spondylolisthesis
Apophyseal ring fracture (posterior limbus fracture)[57, 58]	4–45	Avulsion of the posterior vertebral ring apophysis; usually associated with disc protrusion L4 and L5 most common sites CT best for delineating osseous fragment; MR imaging best for evaluating disc, thecal sac, and surrounding soft tissues Frequent radiculopathy and other neurologic signs
Abused child syndrome[137]	3–30	Spine trauma is rare in child abuse Injuries include compression fractures of the vertebral body, acute disc displacement, avulsion of the posterior elements, and thoracolumbar fracture dislocation

*See also Tables 1–3 and 1–4.

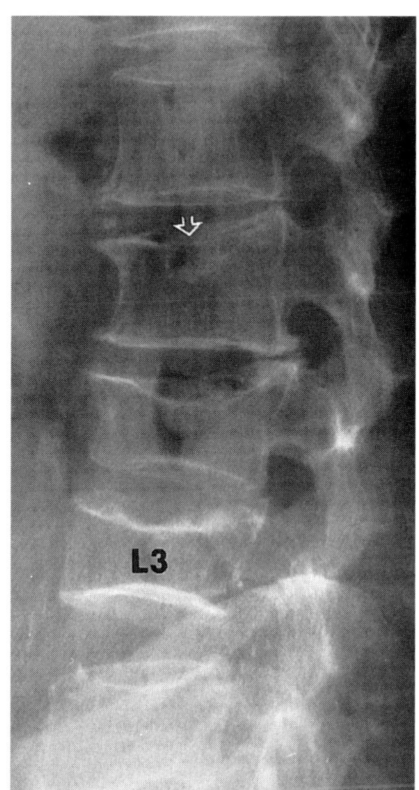

FIGURE 4–39. Acute vertebral body compression fractures.[50] Routine lateral radiograph from a 51-year-old man shows an anterior wedge-shaped deformity of the L2 vertebral body as well as a superior end-plate depression of L1 (open arrow) and biconcave end-plate deformities of L3.

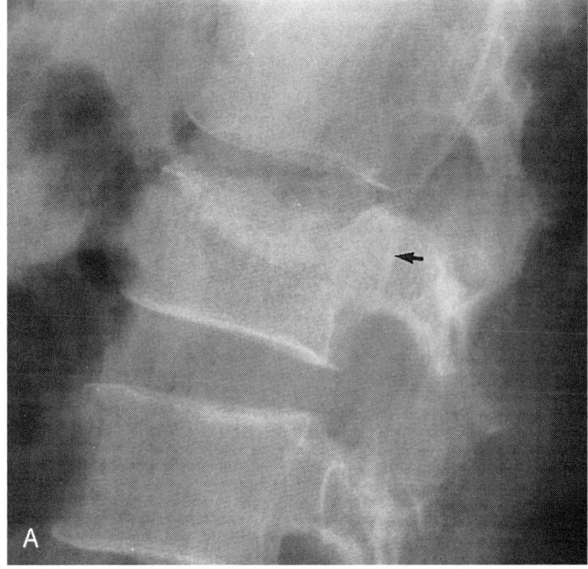

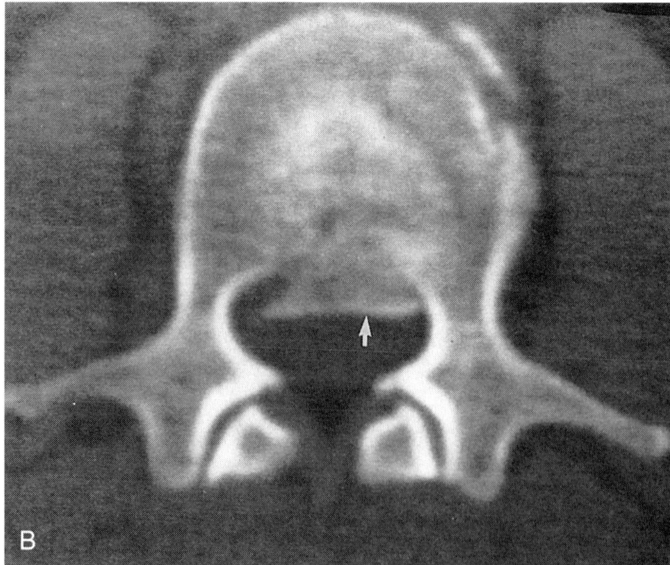

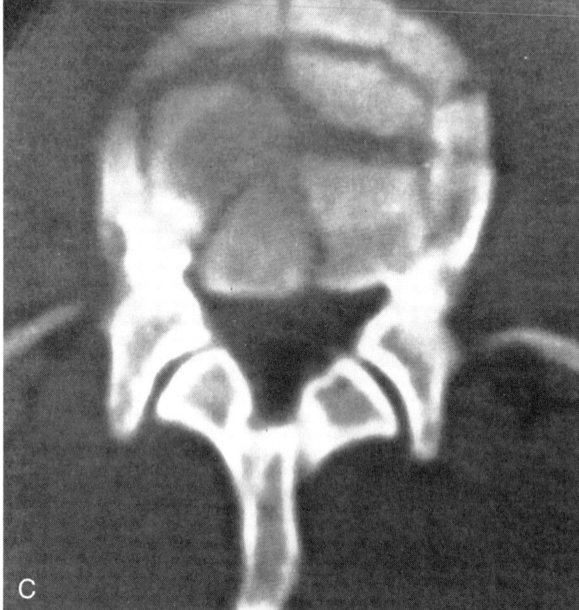

FIGURE 4–40. Burst fracture.[51, 52] **A, B** Lateral radiograph (**A**) and transaxial computed tomographic (CT) scan (**B**) of a 38-year-old man, which were taken after he had jumped from a 20-foot bridge, demonstrate a burst fracture of L2 with superior end-plate disruption, vertebral-body comminution, and retropulsion of bone fragments into the spinal canal (arrows). **C** In another patient with a burst fracture of L3, a transaxial CT image shows severe comminution and retropulsion of the vertebral body.

TABLE 4–9. Instability in Thoracolumbar Burst Fractures*

General features of unstable burst fractures
1. As many as 50 per cent of burst fractures are unstable
2. 40 per cent of cases involve disruption of the posterior ligament complex:
   Supraspinous ligament
   Interspinous ligament
   Ligamenta flava
   Facet joint capsule

Findings indicating instability in burst fractures
1. Progressive neurologic deficit
2. Posterior element disruption
3. Kyphosis that progresses 20 degrees or more in the presence of a neurologic deficit
4. Loss of height of the vertebral body of more than 50 per cent, with associated facet joint subluxation
5. Retropulsed bone fragments detectable on CT scans in the presence of an incomplete neurologic injury

*Adapted from McAfee PC, Hansen AY, Lasda NA: The unstable burst fracture. Spine 7:365, 1982.

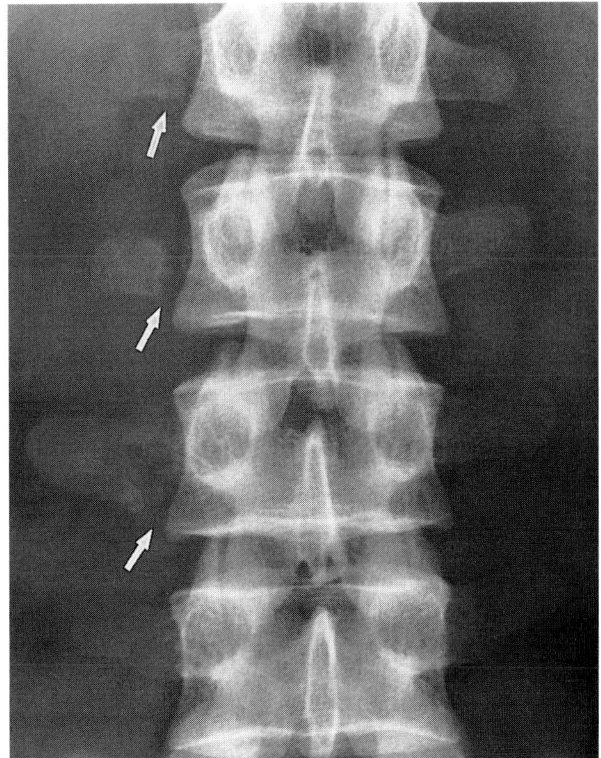

FIGURE 4–41. Transverse process fractures.[53, 54] This 18-year-old man was in a motor vehicle accident in which he suffered a direct blow from a door handle to the paraspinal region. Minimally displaced fractures of the L1, L2, and L3 transverse processes are seen (arrows). A scoliosis, convex to the side of the fractures, frequently accompanies this injury. Transverse process fractures are complicated by injury to the abdominal viscera, especially the kidney and ureter, in up to 20 per cent of cases. The patient should be questioned about the presence of hematuria, and intravenous urography or computed tomographic (CT) scanning may be indicated if abdominal injuries are suspected.

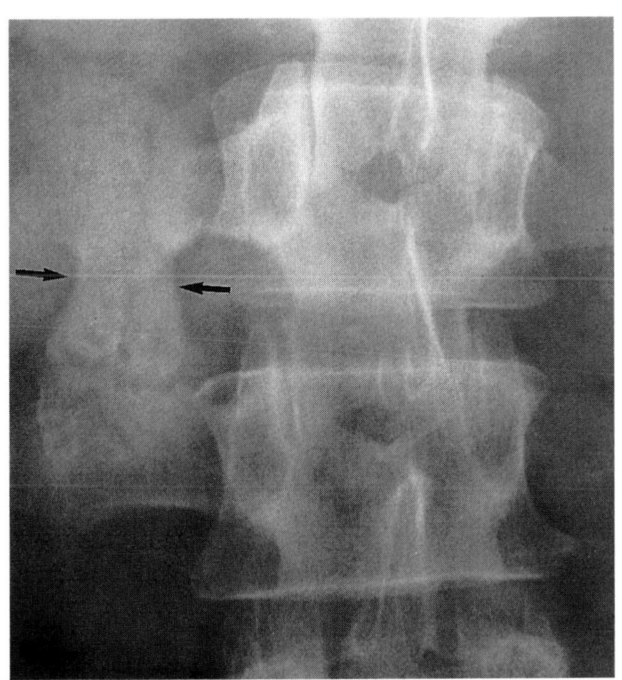

FIGURE 4–42. Osseous bridging of the transverse processes.[54] A unilateral, vertically oriented sheet of ossification is seen spanning the transverse processes of the lumbar spine (arrows). This finding usually is the result of ossification of a hematoma resulting from a previous injury. Osseous bars, which are developmental in nature, also may span the transverse processes. Although similar in appearance, these anomalies are rare.

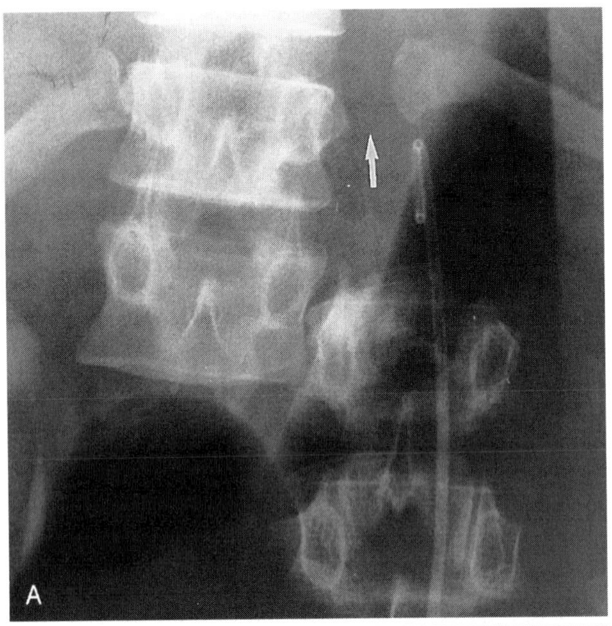

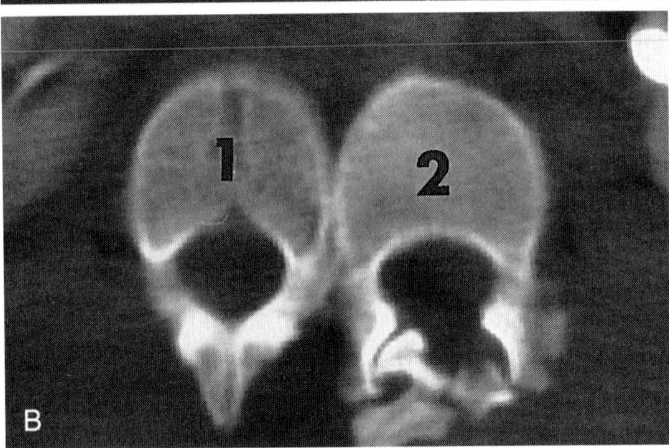

FIGURE 4–43. Fracture-dislocation.[55] A 28-year-old hearing-impaired man was struck by a train while walking on train tracks. **A,** Routine radiograph demonstrates a complete fracture-dislocation at the L1-L2 vertebral level. The left twelfth costovertebral joint is dislocated (arrow). **B,** In a computed tomographic (CT) scan, the dislocated first (1) and second (2) lumbar vertebral bodies are seen side-by-side on one transaxial slice. *(Courtesy of A. Nemcek, M.D., Chicago, Illinois.)*

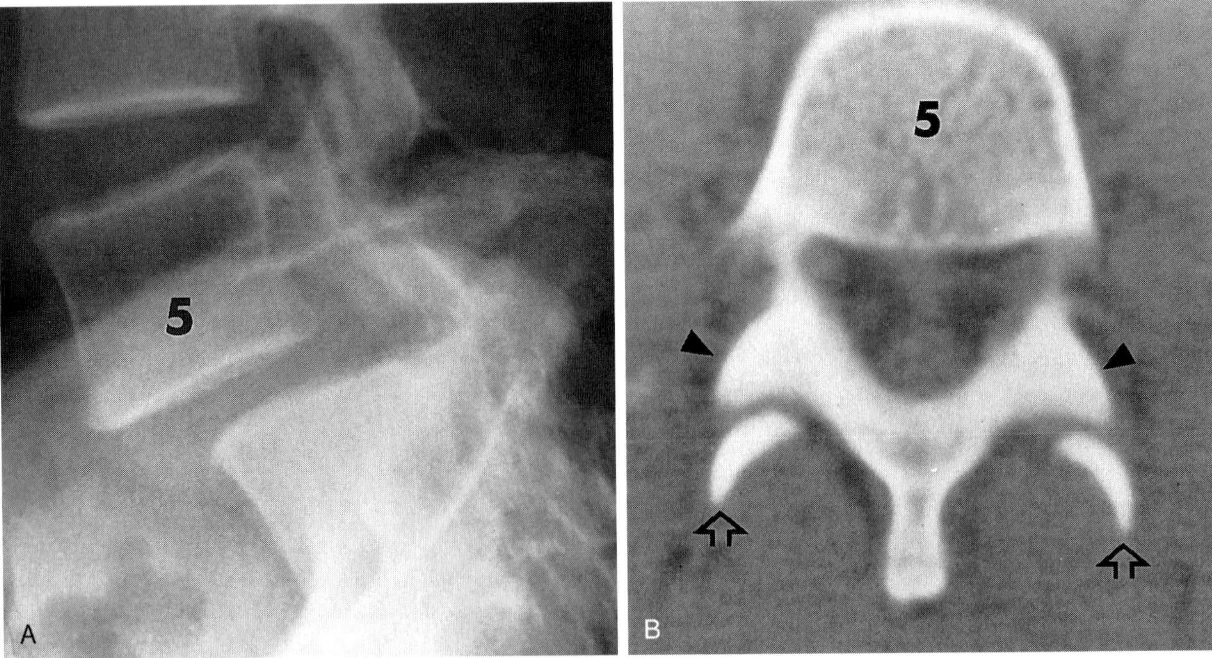

FIGURE 4–44. Lumbosacral apophyseal joint dislocation and facet lock.[56] **A** Routine radiograph shows abnormal alignment of the L5-S1 facet articulations. **B** The interlocked and dislocated position of the lumbosacral articular processes is better defined on a transaxial computed tomographic (CT) image. The L5 inferior articular processes (arrowheads) are situated anterior to the S1 superior articular processes (open arrows). This rare injury usually results from severe trauma involving a complex mechanism that includes compressive hyperflexion as well as rotational or shear forces. It often is associated with fractures of the sacrum and lower lumbar spine.

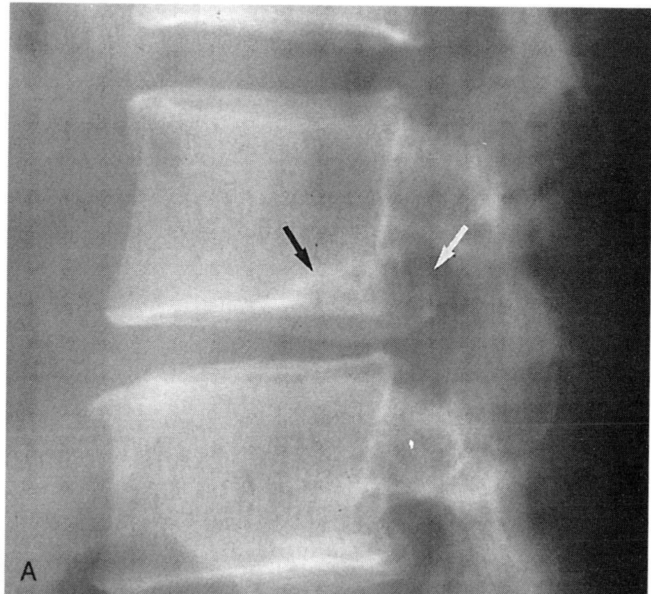

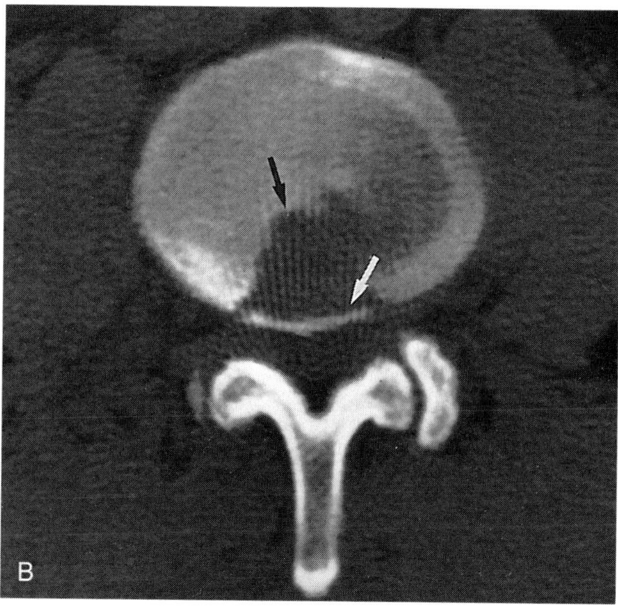

FIGURE 4–45. Posterior apophyseal ring avulsion fracture.[57, 58] A Lateral radiograph of this 35-year-old man shows a posterior fragment of bone projecting from the vertebral body into the spinal canal (white arrow). Observe also the triangular radiolucent defect in the vertebral body (black arrow). B Transaxial computed tomographic (CT) image shows a curvilinear rim of avulsed bone projecting into the spinal canal (white arrow) and a radiolucent Schmorl's node in the posterior vertebral body (black arrow). These bony injuries often are secondary to trauma that results in disc herniation and associated avulsion of the adjacent unfused ring apophysis. CT is excellent for assessing the osseous components, and magnetic resonance (MR) imaging is best suited to the evaluation of the soft tissue abnormalities.

TABLE 4–10. Lumbar Intervertebral Disc Disorders

Entity	Figure(s), Table(s)	Characteristics
Degenerative disc disease[47, 59–62]	4–46, 4–47, 4–48	*Spondylosis deformans:* Osteophytes and osseous ridging (Table 3–9) Subchondral bone sclerosis (Table 4–12) *Intervertebral osteochondrosis:* Disc space narrowing (Table 4–12) Intradiscal vacuum phenomenon (Table 4–11) Disc calcification is rare MR imaging signal changes in vertebral body bone marrow (Table 4–13) Degenerative diseases of the lumbar spine may result in several complications (Table 4–15)
Annular bulge[60]	4–48	Broad-based circumferential bulging of discal material beyond the margins of the vertebral body Present in 81 per cent of asymptomatic persons Degenerative disc bulges: very common in older persons; often are associated with extensive osteophyte formation, disc space narrowing, and loss of magnetic resonance (MR) imaging signal intensity in the disc secondary to degeneration
Disc herniation		Displaced nucleus pulposus extends through some or all of the fibers of the annulus fibrosus; associated with annular tears Annular tears present in 56 per cent of asymptomatic persons Three types of herniation relate to increasing stages of severity: prolapse, extrusion, and sequestration
1. Prolapse or protrusion[60, 63]	4–49	Displaced nucleus pulposus extends through some annular fibers but still is confined by the intact outermost annular fibers: contained herniation Infrequently results in direct nerve root compression Present in 33 per cent of asymptomatic persons
2. Extrusion[63–65]		Displaced nucleus pulposus penetrates all of the annular fibers and lies under the posterior longitudinal ligament: noncontained subligamentous herniation Usually associated with symptoms but infrequently results in cauda equina compression or permanent neurologic deficit

Table continued on following page

TABLE 4–10. Lumbar Intervertebral Disc Disorders *Continued*

Entity	Figure(s), Table(s)	Characteristics
3. Sequestration[64, 65]	4–50	Displaced nucleus pulposus penetrates or extends around the posterior longitudinal ligament and lies within the epidural space; alternatively, the displaced nucleus, although not extending through this ligament, migrates for a considerable distance cephalad or caudad as a fragment that is separate from the remaining portion of the intervertebral disc: noncontained herniation Usually associated with symptoms and commonly results in cauda equina compression or permanent neurologic deficit
Internal disc derangement[138]		Internal disruption and alteration in the internal structure and metabolic functions of one or more discs, usually after significant trauma Controversial condition diagnosed by discography; radial extension of dye associated with an overfilled nucleus May be associated with loss of MR imaging signal intensity of disc, normal disc height, and absence of extension of nuclear material into the annulus fibrosus May result clinically in back pain, referred leg pain, fatigue, weight loss, and accompanying psychologic disturbances
Schmorl's cartilaginous nodes[66]	4–51	Intravertebral disc herniation superiorly or inferiorly through the cartilaginous and osseous vertebral end plates, penetrating the spongiosa of the vertebral body Well-defined or poorly defined, punctate contour defect in vertebral end plate, often associated with surrounding osteosclerosis Occasionally painful, but these nodes usually are not associated with neurologic complications Isolated Schmorl's nodes may occur with acute trauma, degenerative disc disease, osteoporosis, osteomalacia, Paget's disease, hyperparathyroidism, infection, and neoplasm Gadolinium-enhanced MR images reveal that larger Schmorl's nodes are often vascularized, are frequently associated with bone marrow edema, and are more common in symptomatic than in nonsymptomatic patients Presence of multiple Schmorl's nodes in an adolescent thoracic spine suggests the diagnosis of juvenile lumbar osteochondrosis (Scheuermann's disease)
Limbus vertebra[67]	4–52	Intravertebral herniation of disc material extending beneath the vertebral ring apophyseal ossification center, separating it from the vertebral body Disc material also may dissect underneath the anterior longitudinal ligament, causing pressure erosions of the body or displacing the ligament anteriorly along with the attached apophyseal ring fragment Often the limbus fragment fails to fuse to the vertebral body and persists into older age, frequently resulting in extensive degenerative change, especially osteophyte formation Most limbus vertebrae occur anteriorly, but posterior limbus vertebrae also may occur, often resulting in severe nerve root compression with neurologic deficit
Apophyseal ring fracture (posterior limbus vertebra)[57, 58]	4–45 Table 4–8	Avulsion fracture of the posterior aspect of the ring apophysis associated with disc protrusion
Juvenile lumbar osteochondrosis[68]	4–53	Usually begins in adolescents and young adults and is more common in competitive athletes and in persons from rural communities Men > women Closely resembles Scheuermann's disease but usually is localized to the thoracolumbar and lower lumbar regions and may not be associated with thoracic kyphosis Multiple Schmorl's nodes, limbus vertebrae, undulating vertebral end-plate surfaces, and posterior disc displacements Many cases are asymptomatic but others are associated with low back pain, sciatica, and intermittent nonvascular claudication in the lower extremities Possible pathogenesis: repeated axial compression of the spine with injury to the cartilaginous end plates

TABLE 4–11. Vertebral Gas Collections: Vacuum Phenomena

Location	Causes
Intervertebral disc	Degenerative disc disease Extrusion of a disc fragment Vertebral collapse Trauma
Vertebral body	Steroid-induced ischemia: osteonecrosis Posttraumatic vertebral collapse of Kümmel Intraosseous cyst Intraosseous disc displacement: Schmorl's node
Apophyseal joints	Degenerative joint disease Synovial cyst
Spinal canal	Idiopathic Synovial cyst
Soft tissues	Surgery

TABLE 4–12. Intervertebral Disc Space Narrowing and Adjacent Sclerosis

Entity	Figure(s)	Mechanism	Radiographic Appearance	Vacuum Phenomena
Degenerative disc disease	4–46, 4–47, 4–48	Degeneration of disc and cartilaginous end plate Schmorl's nodes	Disc space narrowing Well-defined sclerotic vertebral margins	Present
Trauma	4–46, 4–47, 4–48	Disc injury and degeneration Schmorl's nodes	Disc space narrowing Well-defined sclerotic vertebral margins Fracture Soft tissue mass	Variable
Neuropathic osteoarthropathy	See Fig. 4–65	Loss of sensation and proprioception with repetitive trauma	Disc space narrowing Extensive vertebral body sclerosis Osteophytosis Fragmentation Malalignment	Prominent
Rheumatoid arthritis	See Fig. 4–66	Apophyseal joint instability with recurrent discovertebral trauma or Inflammatory tissue extending from neighboring articulations	Disc space narrowing Poorly defined or well-defined sclerotic vertebral margins Subluxation Apophyseal joint abnormalities (Usually confined to the cervical spine)	Absent
Calcium pyrophosphate dihydrate crystal deposition disease	See Fig. 4–72	Crystal deposition in cartilaginous end plate and intervertebral disc with degeneration	Disc space narrowing Calcification Poorly defined or well-defined sclerotic vertebral margins Fragmentation Subluxation	Variable
Alkaptonuria	See Fig. 4–73	Crystal deposition in cartilaginous end plate and intervertebral disc with degeneration	Disc space narrowing Well-defined sclerotic vertebral margins Extensive disc calcification	Prominent
Infectious spondylodiscitis	See Figs. 4–75, 4–76	Pyogenic or tuberculous osteomyelitis and spondylodiscitis	Disc space narrowing Poorly defined sclerotic vertebral margins Soft tissue abscess	Absent

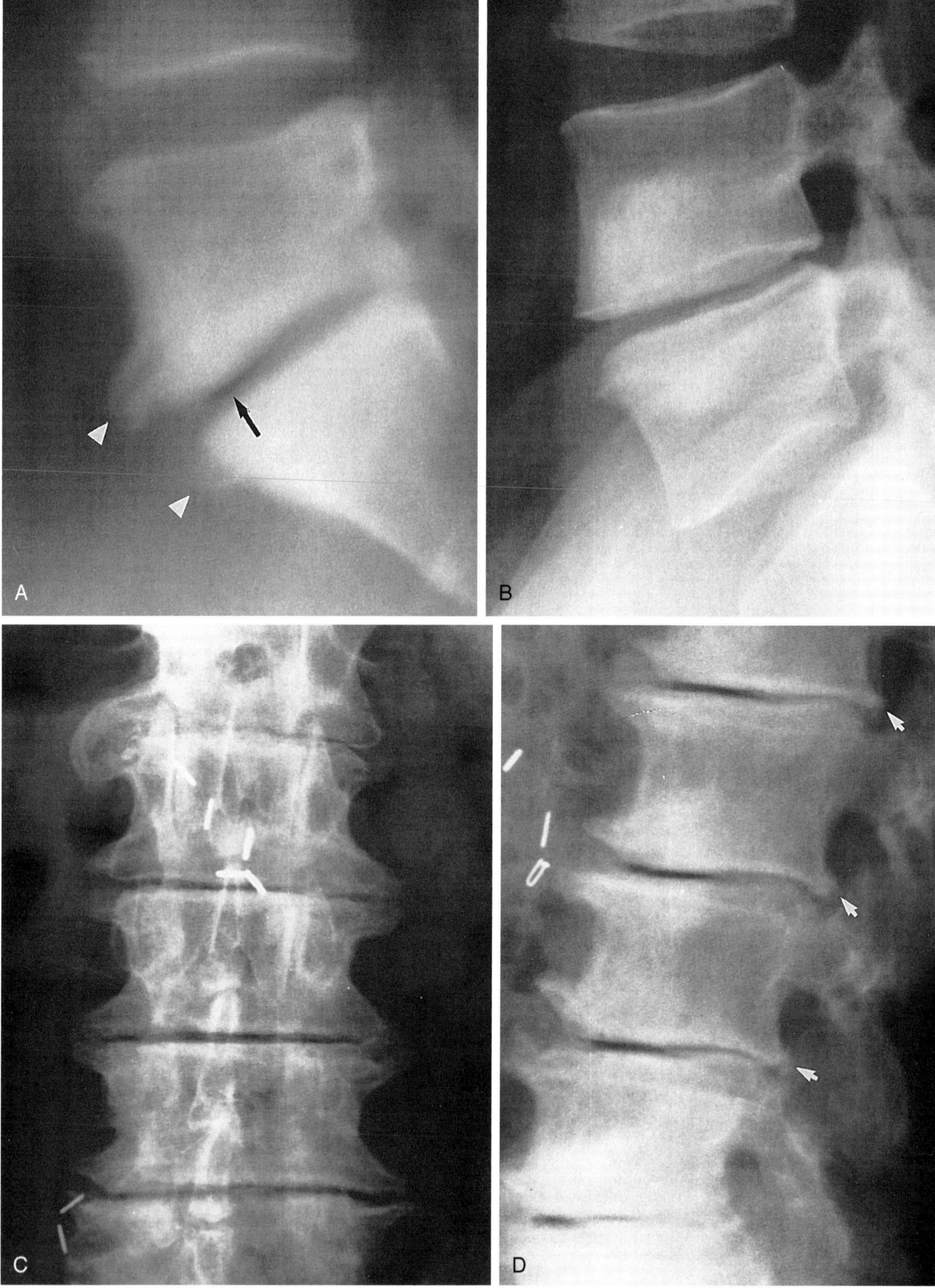

FIGURE 4–46. Degenerative disc disease.[47, 59–61] A Lateral conventional tomogram demonstrates disc space narrowing, intradiscal gas (vacuum phenomenon) (arrow), osteophytes (arrowheads), and sclerosis of the adjacent vertebral bodies. B Observe the disc space narrowing, and vertebral body sclerosis at the L4-L5 level in this 47-year-old woman. This pattern of vertebral body sclerosis, especially when it is an isolated finding, is termed idiopathic segmental sclerosis or hemispheric spondylosclerosis and may simulate osteoblastic skeletal metastasis. C, D In this 68-year-old man, extensive disc space narrowing, osteophytes, vacuum phenomena, and vertebral body sclerosis are evident. Observe also the posterior osteophytes (arrows) that may contribute to foraminal and central canal stenosis.

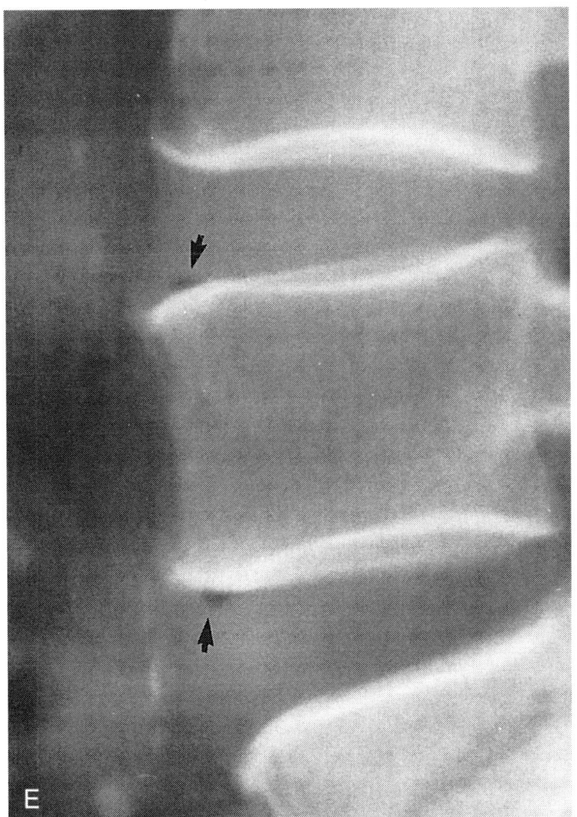

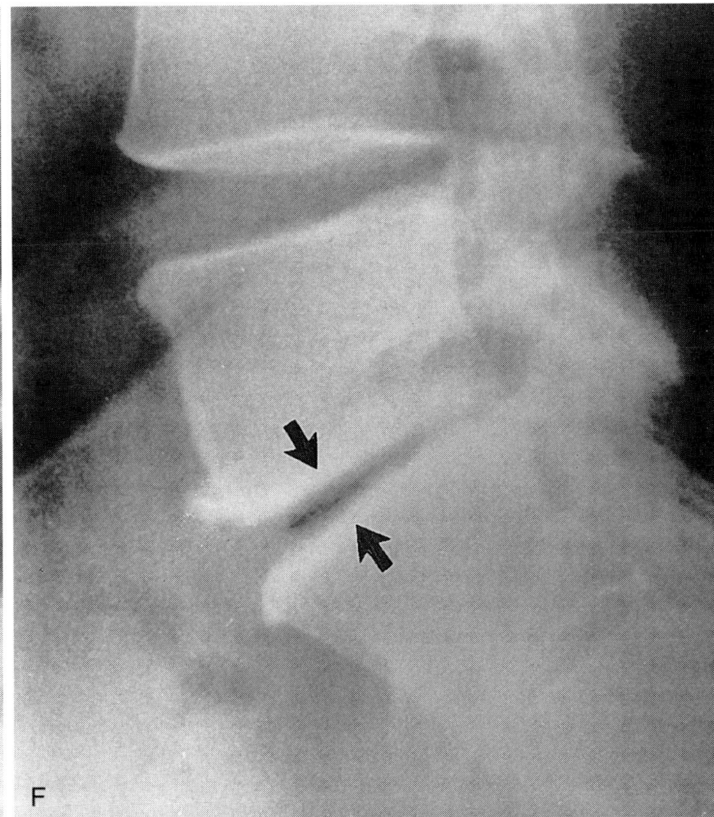

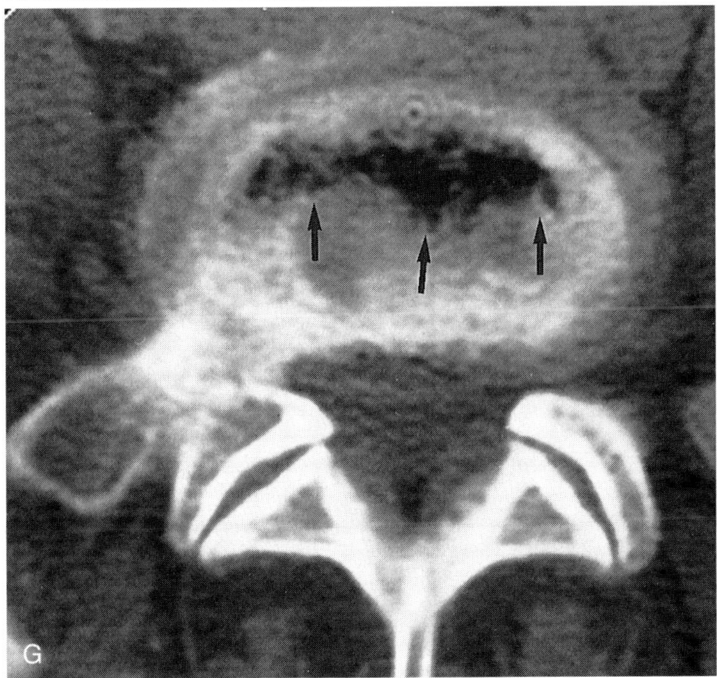

FIGURE 4–46 *Continued.* E In another patient, small collections of gas within the disc are localized to the discovertebral junctions adjacent to the L4 vertebral body (arrows). These focal vacuum phenomena probably are the result of annular degeneration. In the presence of acute trauma, especially in the cervical spine, these tiny "annular vacuum clefts" represent acute injuries of the annular fibers. F Lumbosacral degenerative disc disease is evident in a 58-year-old man with severe disc space narrowing, vacuum phenomenon (arrows), traction osteophytes, and subchondral sclerosis. G Vacuum phenomenon: Computed tomographic (CT) findings. Transaxial CT scan shows a collection of gas (arrows) within the degenerated L5-S1 intervertebral disc.

On routine lateral radiographs, a posterior disc height of the lumbosacral junction measuring less than 5.4 mm reliably indicates degenerative disc disease. Conversely, L5 posterior disc height measurements of more than 7.7 mm indicate the absence of degenerative disc disease. *(F, Reprinted with permission from Taylor JAM, Hoffman LE: The geriatric patient: Diagnostic imaging of common musculoskeletal disorders. Top Clin Chiropr 3:23, © 1996, Aspen Publishers, Inc.)*

TABLE 4–13. Magnetic Resonance (MR) Imaging of Vertebral Body Bone Marrow in Degenerative Disc Disease*

Type	Figure(s)	MR Imaging Signal Changes		Characteristics
		T1-Weighted	*T2-Weighted*	
I	4–47 A, B	Decreased	Increased	Fibrovascular marrow changes 4 per cent† May enhance with gadolinium contrast agent administration
II	4–47 C, D	Increased	Isointense or increased	Fatty marrow changes: conversion of hematopoietic to fatty marrow 16 per cent†
III		Decreased	Decreased	Sclerotic marrow changes: absence of bone marrow in regions of osteosclerosis Associated with considerable sclerosis on radiographs

*Adapted from Modic MT, Steinberg PM, Ross JS, et al: Degenerative disc disease: Assessment of changes in vertebral body marrow with MR imaging. Radiology 166:193, 1988.

†Percentage of patients undergoing MR imaging examination for lumbar disc disease who exhibit these findings.

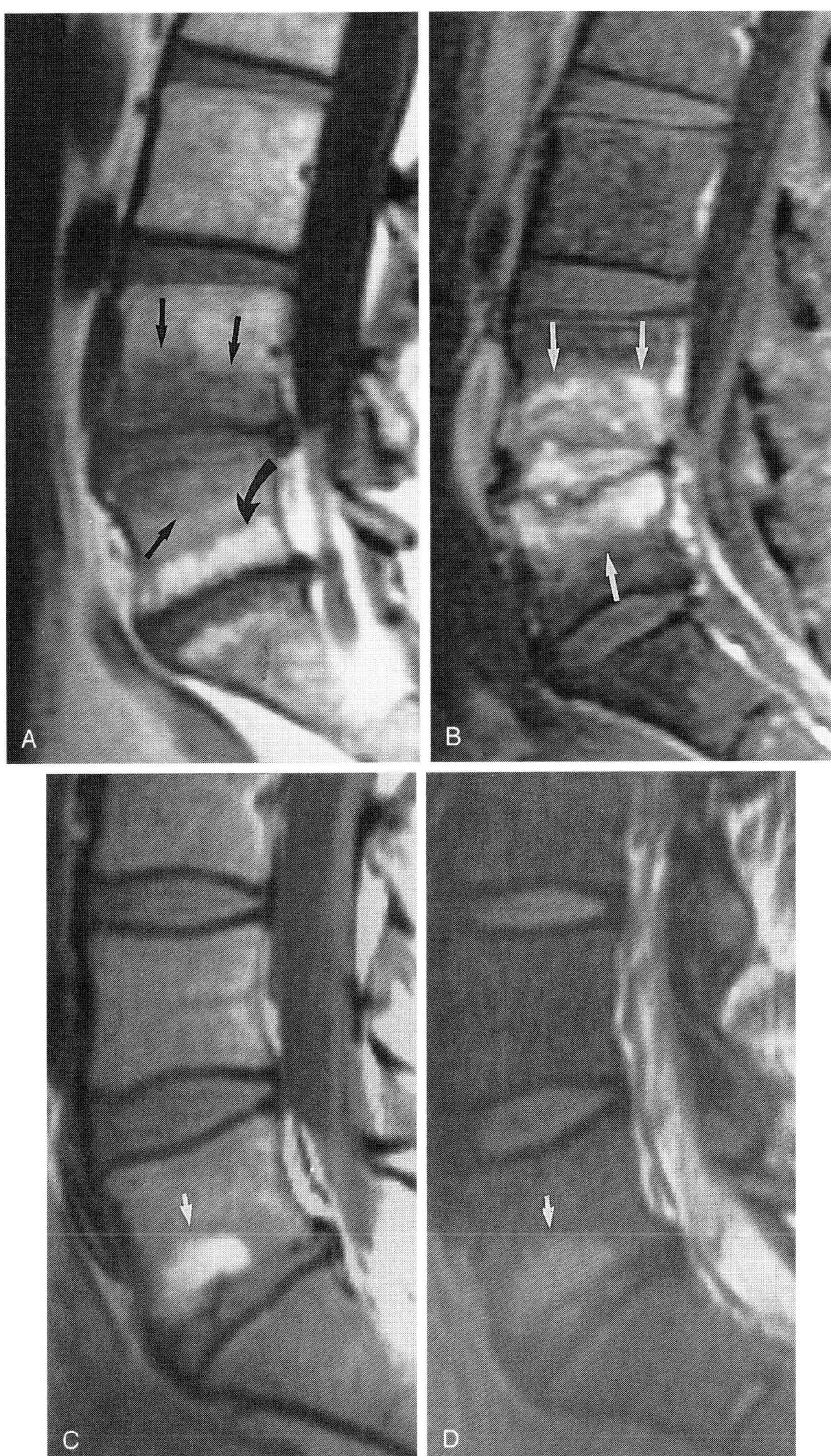

FIGURE 4–47. Degenerative disc disease: Magnetic resonance (MR) imaging of marrow changes within the vertebral body.[62] **A, B** Type I changes. In **A**, a sagittal T1-weighted (TR/TE, 600/20) spin echo MR image demonstrates degenerative disc narrowing at the L4-L5 level with decreased signal intensity (straight arrows) of the adjacent subchondral bone. Fat is seen within the subchondral marrow adjacent to the L5-S1 disc (curved arrow). In **B**, another sagittal T1-weighted spin echo MR image obtained with fat suppression after administration of gadolinium contrast agent demonstrates increased signal intensity of the adjacent subchondral bone (arrows). **C, D** Type II changes in a 34-year-old woman with low back pain. In **C**, a sagittal proton density–weighted (TR/TE, 1000/20) spin echo MR image demonstrates degenerative disc narrowing at the L5-S1 level with a focus of increased signal intensity within the adjacent subchondral bone of the L5 vertebral body (arrow). In **D**, a T2-weighted (TR/TE, 1000/90) spin echo MR image also exhibits increased signal intensity within the vertebral body (arrow) (Table 4–13).

TABLE 4–14. Lumbar Magnetic Resonance (MR) Imaging Findings in an Asymptomatic Population*

Finding	Prevalence (*n* = 36)
	Percentage of all subjects
Disc bulges	81
Mild or moderate disc degeneration	72
Annular tears	56
Severe disc degeneration	55
High-intensity zones within disc	47
Disc protrusions	33
Disc extrusions	0
Direct nerve root compression by disc protrusions	0
	Percentage of annular tears or protrusions
Gadolinium enhancement of annular tears	96
Gadolinium enhancement of disc protrusions	85
Interruption of annuloligamentous complex by annular tears	0

*Adapted from Stadnik TW, Lee RR, Coen HL, et al: Annular tears and disc herniation: Prevalence and contrast enhancement on MR images in the absence of low back pain or sciatica. Radiology 206:49, 1998.

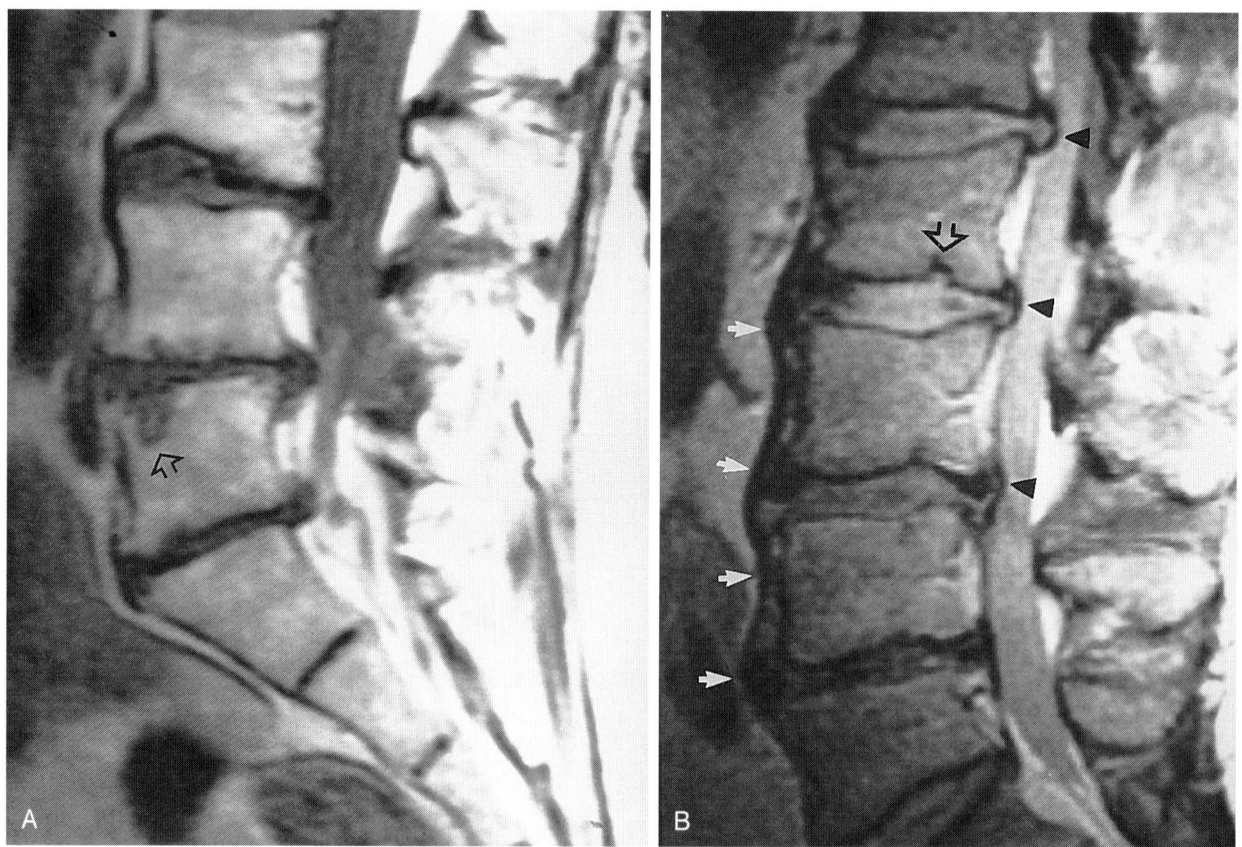

FIGURE 4–48. Degenerative disc disease and annular bulges: Magnetic resonance (MR) imaging abnormalities.[60] A Sagittal T1-weighted (TR/TE, 733/16) fast spin echo MR image of this 75-year-old woman shows extensive disc space narrowing and degenerative disc bulges at several levels. A Schmorl's (cartilaginous) node representing intravertebral disc displacement also is present (open arrow). B Midsagittal proton density–weighted (TR/TE, 2500/30) spin echo MR image reveals decreased signal intensity of the L3-L4, L4-L5, and L5-S1 lumbar discs and posterior degenerative disc bulges at the L1-L2, L2-L3, and L3-L4 levels (arrowheads). A Schmorl's node is evident in the L2 inferior end plate (open arrow). In addition, the anterior longitudinal ligament is stripped away from the vertebral bodies by anterior disc bulges and osteophytes (white arrows).

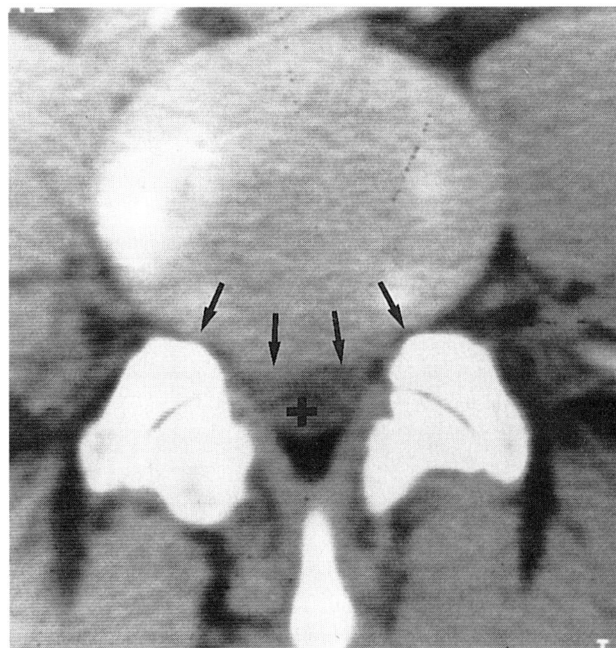

FIGURE 4–49. Intervertebral disc protrusion: Computed tomographic (CT) abnormalities.[60, 63] Transaxial CT image shows a broad-based central disc protrusion (black arrows) that displaces the thecal sac (+) and virtually obliterates the nerve root canals.

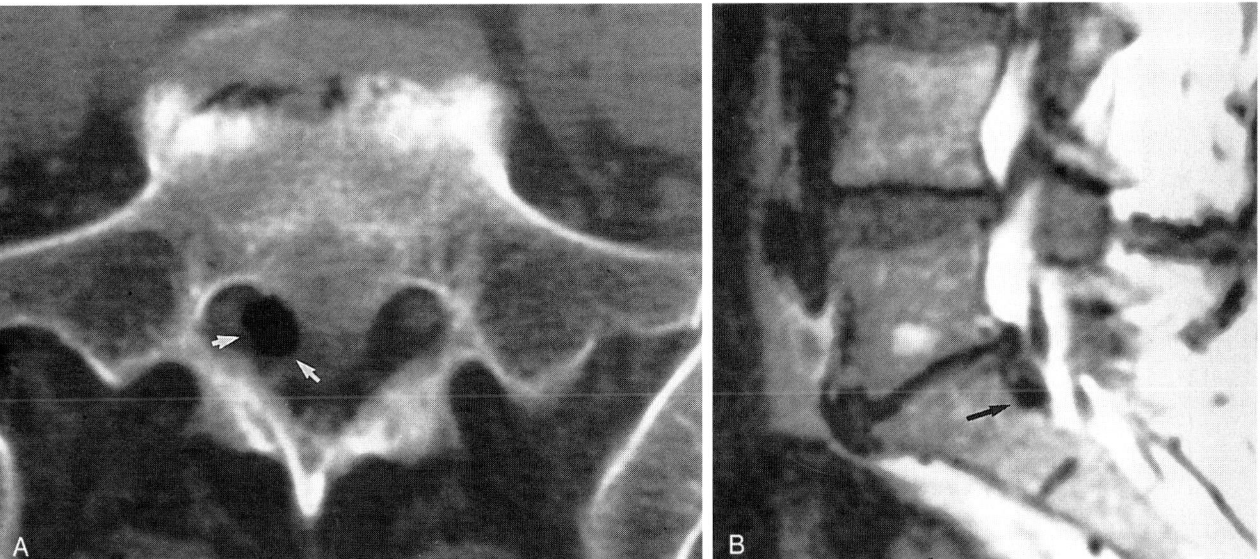

FIGURE 4–50. Intervertebral disc sequestration.[64, 65] **A, B** Sequestrated fragment with intradiscal vacuum phenomenon. In **A,** a transaxial computed tomographic (CT) image at the S1 level reveals an intradiscal vacuum phenomenon seen as a radiolucent collection of gas (arrows) within a large noncontained L5-S1 disc sequestration. In **B,** a sagittal T1-weighted (TR/TE, 400/17) spin echo magnetic resonance (MR) image of the same patient shows a focal area of signal void corresponding to the gas collection within the disc fragment (arrow). The L5-S1 disc is narrowed and the L4-L5 disc bulges posteriorly. A focal collection of fat is evident in the fifth lumbar vertebral body. *(A, B, Courtesy of S. Eilenberg, San Diego, California.)*

Illustration continued on following page

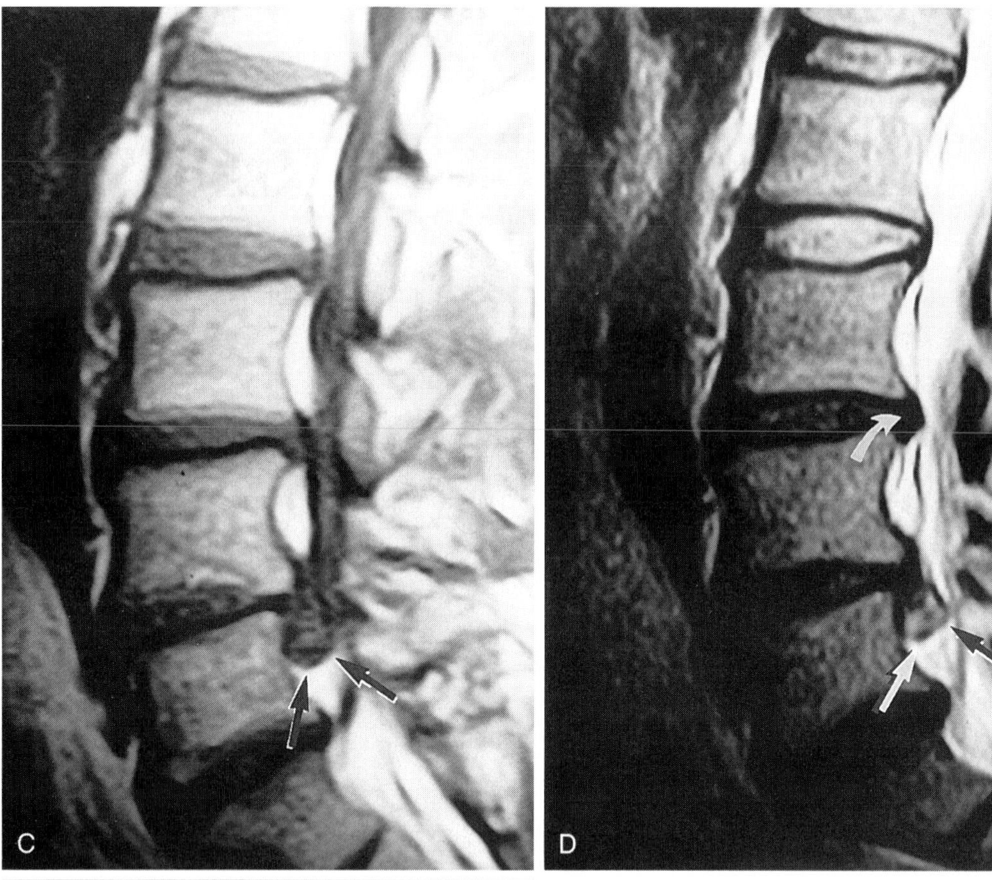

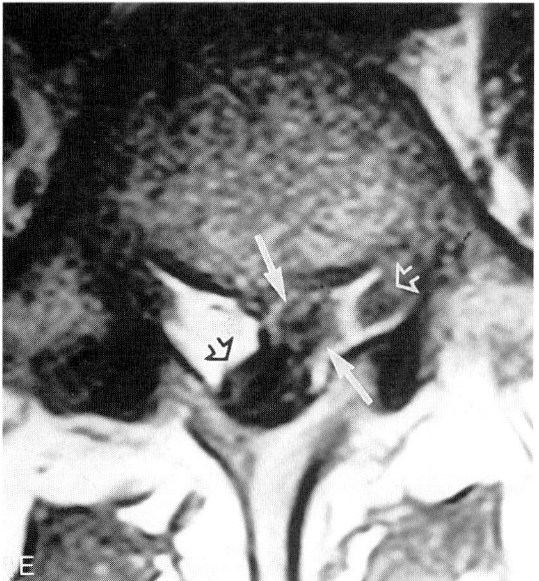

FIGURE 4–50 *Continued.* C–E MR images from another patient with severe low back pain and radiculopathy. In C, a sagittal T1-weighted (TR/TE, 457/20) spin echo MR image reveals a lobulated mass of intermediate to low signal intensity (arrows) within the spinal canal posterior to the L5 vertebral body and adjacent to a severely degenerated L4-L5 disc. In D, the sagittal T2-weighted (TR/TE, 3000/96) fast spin echo MR image reveals heterogeneous signal intensity within the noncontained mass (arrows). A contained L3-L4 disc protrusion also is present (curved arrow). In E, a transaxial T1-weighted (TR/TE, 744/20) spin echo MR image through the lesion at the level of the L5 lateral recess shows the sequestrated fragment (arrows) displacing the thecal sac posteriorly (black open arrow) and abutting on the nerve root (white open arrow). *(C–E, Courtesy of L. Ramos, D.C., Berlin, New Hampshire.)*

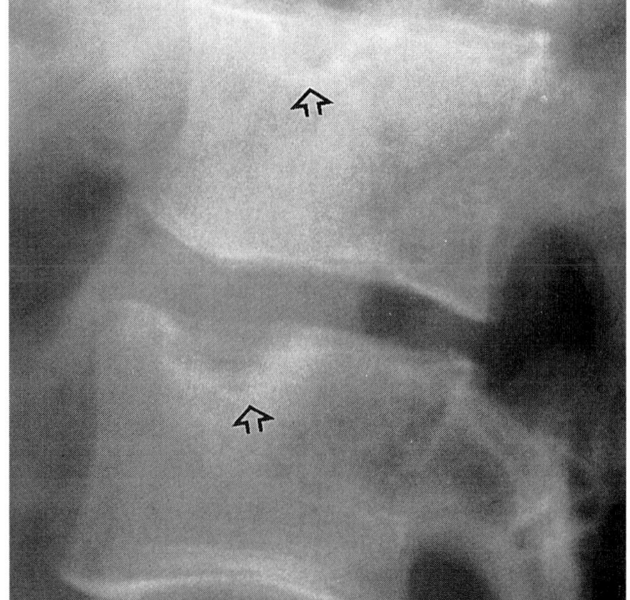

FIGURE 4–51. Schmorl's (cartilaginous) nodes.[66] Schmorl's nodes are evident in two adjacent vertebral bodies in this patient with Scheuermann's disease. Observe both the irregularity of the vertebral end-plate surfaces and focal radiolucent depressions with adjacent sclerotic margins (open arrows). Both of these findings are typical of Schmorl's nodes.

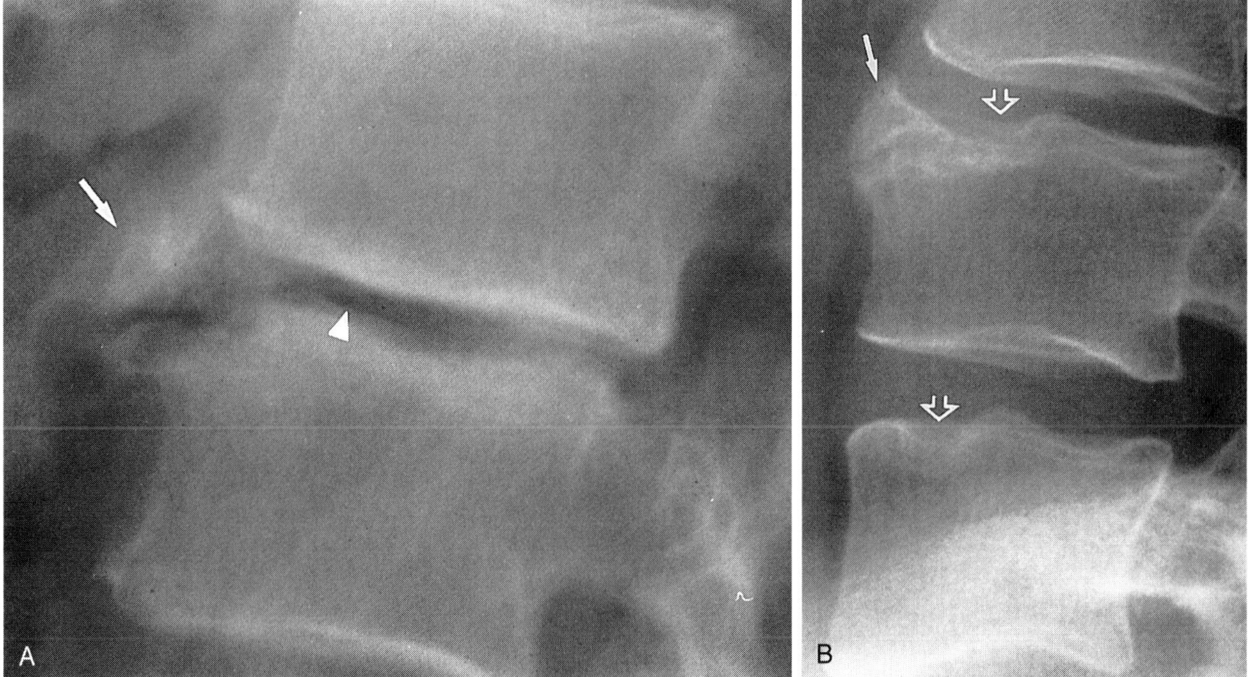

FIGURE 4–52. Limbus vertebra.[67] A A triangular, sclerotic bone fragment (arrow) is seen adjacent to the anterosuperior margin of the vertebral body. Note the radiolucent cleft separating the fragment from the vertebral body. Significant degenerative disease with a vacuum disc phenomenon also is present (arrowhead). B Lateral radiograph of a 38-year-old man demonstrates anterior Schmorl's nodes (open arrows) within the superior vertebral end plates of L4 and L5. At L4, the triangular osseous fragment, or limbus vertebra (arrow), represents the residual apophyseal ring that was separated from the vertebral body during adolescence. Associated degenerative changes also are apparent.

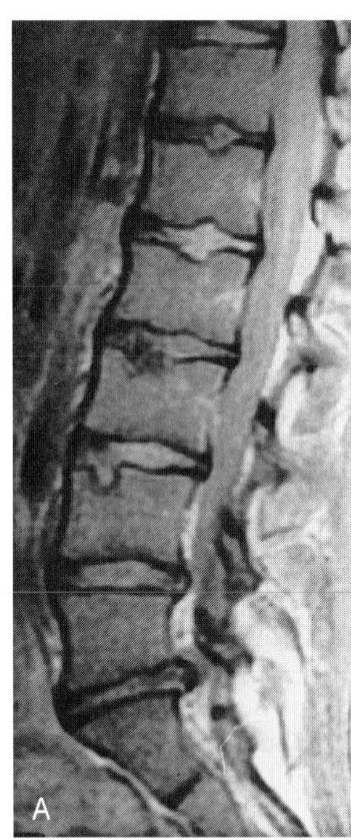

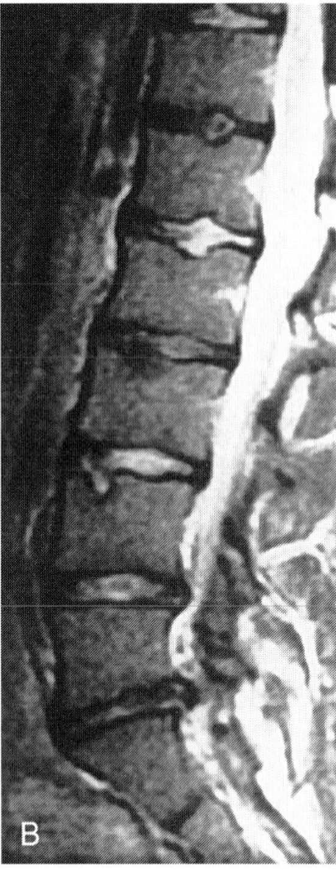

FIGURE 4–53. Juvenile lumbar osteochondrosis (lumbar Scheuermann's disease).[68] **A, B** Sagittal proton density–weighted (TR/TE, 2500/30) **(A)** and T2-weighted (TR/TE, 2500/70) **(B)** spin echo MR images from this 15-year-old boy demonstrate Schmorl's nodes, end-plate irregularities, and intervertebral disc calcification. Low signal intensity of the L2-L3 and L5-S1 discs and posterior disc displacement at the L4-L5 and L5-S1 levels also are evident. *(Courtesy of C. Gundry, M.D., Minneapolis, Minnesota.)*

TABLE 4–15. Complications of Degenerative Disease of the Lumbar Spine

Entity	Figure(s)	Characteristics
Alignment abnormalities		
Segmental instability[43, 44, 69]	4–54	Excessive or abnormal motion associated with degenerative disease of the lumbar spine *Findings suggestive of lumbar instability:* Static radiographic findings Gas within disc Traction osteophytes Radial fissure in disc during discography Functional radiographic findings on flexion-extension radiographs Forward or backward displacement of one vertebra on another in excess of 3 to 4 mm Narrowing of intervertebral foramina Loss of disc height Disc wedging in excess of 12 to 20 degrees Possible causes: trauma, spondylolisthesis, other pathologic processes, and spine surgery
Degenerative spondylolisthesis[39, 70–72]	4–55	See Table 4–4
Degenerative retrolisthesis[39]	4–56	Posterior vertebral displacement of one segment on another secondary to degenerative disc disease Decreased height of intervertebral disc, closer approximation of vertebral bodies, and gliding or telescoping of the corresponding articular processes *Radiographic findings:* Vacuum phenomenon, disc space narrowing, vertebral body marginal sclerosis, osteophytes, apophyseal joint instability and subluxation with posteroinferior displacement of the inferior articular processes of the upper vertebra in relation to the subjacent level L2 on L3 affected most commonly, but also occurs above and below this level Clinical findings are variable and include the following: pain, difficulty with trunk flexion or extension, spinal rigidity, and neurologic abnormalities related to stenosis and cord compression

TABLE 4–15. Complications of Degenerative Disease of the Lumbar Spine *Continued*

Entity	Figure(s)	Characteristics
Alignment abnormalities *Continued*		
Degenerative lumbar scoliosis[47, 71, 72]	4–57	Scoliosis in elderly persons that is associated with extensive degenerative changes; the scoliosis often precedes the degenerative changes, and the curve may progress slowly with continued degeneration *Radiographic findings:* Eccentric disc space narrowing, vertebral body sclerosis, osteophytes, vacuum phenomena, and apophyseal joint degeneration predominating on the concave side of the curve Clinical findings vary from asymptomatic cases to disabling low back and lower extremity pain, weakness, and neurogenic claudication Far-out syndrome: impingement of the fifth lumbar spinal nerve between the L5 transverse process and the sacrum; complication of degenerative lumbar scoliosis
Degenerative lumbar kyphosis[47]		Marked loss or even reversal of the lumbar lordosis in patients with extensive degenerative spine disease *Radiographic findings:* Loss of sacral base inclination, narrowing of disc spaces, decreased height of anterior portion of lumbar vertebral bodies
Baastrup's disease[47]	4–58	Enlarged spinous processes with flattened, sclerotic superior and inferior margins that approximate each other with trunk extension May be painful on extension
Intervertebral disc displacement		
Anterior, posterior, superior, or inferior disc displacement		See Table 4–10
Vertebral body sclerosis		
Segmental sclerosis of vertebral bodies[73]	4–59	Osteosclerosis of the vertebral body, which may occur alone or adjacent to a degenerative disc, associated with loss of disc height and vacuum phenomena Predilection for L3 and L4 anteroinferior vertebral bodies; may affect two adjacent vertebral bodies Magnetic resonance (MR) imaging: decreased signal on T1-weighted images; increased signal on T2-weighted images (resembling type I changes and infectious spondylodiscitis) Synonyms: hemispherical spondylosclerosis, pseudoinfection of the disc, nonneoplastic sclerosis of the vertebral body, idiopathic segmental sclerosis of the vertebral body, traumatic lesion of the discovertebral junction Also prominent in association with Schmorl's cartilaginous nodes Differential diagnosis of vertebral sclerosis includes infection, neoplasm, Paget's disease, osteopetrosis, and renal osteodystrophy (Tables 4–12 and 4–18)
Intervertebral disc calcification and ossification		
Calcification[47]		Chronic degenerative calcific deposits in older persons occur primarily in the annulus fibrosus Men > women Unclear what proportion of these patients have symptoms Calcification predominates in the midthoracic and upper lumbar intervertebral discs and may be associated with disc displacement
Ossification[47]		Disc degeneration or trauma may lead to proliferation of both fibrous tissue and blood vessels through clefts in the cartilaginous end plate; hypervascularity stimulates ossification within the intervertebral discs Ossified tissue possesses trabeculae, may simulate osteophytes, and may lead to decreased mobility
Spinal stenosis		
General concepts		Three types based on anatomic site of involvement: central, lateral recess, and foraminal stenosis Degenerative stenosis predominates in the lower lumbar segments and further complicates existing developmental stenosis Osteophytes, posterior or posterolateral disc displacements, apophyseal joint hypertrophy and subluxation, enlarged laminae, and buckling or hypertrophy of the ligamenta flava all may contribute to spinal canal narrowing Measurements of stenosis on routine radiographs may be misleading; cross-sectional computed tomographic (CT) or MR imaging and clinical correlation are necessary to fully evaluate patients with suspected stenosis

Table continued on following page

TABLE 4–15. Complications of Degenerative Disease of the Lumbar Spine *Continued*

Entity	Figure(s)	Characteristics
Intervertebral disc displacement *Continued*		
Central stenosis[74]	4–60	*Imaging findings:* Distortion of normal canal configuration by hypertrophic changes Compression of thecal sac in an anteroposterior direction Obliteration of adjacent epidural fat *Lumbar spine radiographic measurements:* 1. Eisenstein's method for sagittal canal measurement Lower limits of normal 15 mm: suggests stenosis 12 mm: unequivocal evidence of stenosis 2. Interpedicle method coronal canal measurement: Lower limits of normal 20 mm at any lumbar level: suggests stenosis *CT and MR imaging measurements:* Lower limits of normal: 11.5-mm midsagittal diameter 16-mm coronal diameter (interpedicle distance)
Lateral (subarticular) recess stenosis[47, 74]	4–60, 4–61	Bone hypertrophy about the superior articular process may result in lateral recess stenosis with compression or displacement of the nerve root and epidural and perineural fat *Borders of the lateral recess:* Anterior: posterior surface of vertebral body Posterior: superior articular process and pars interarticularis Lateral: medial margin of pedicle *CT and MR imaging measurements:* Anteroposterior dimension is measured at the superior aspect of the pedicle 4–5 mm: highly suggestive of lateral recess stenosis Less than 3 mm: definite lateral recess stenosis
Foraminal stenosis[47, 74]	4–60, 4–61	Nerve root occupies the uppermost region of the foramen directly beneath the pedicle of the upper vertebra; stenosis of this region is more significant than stenosis of the lower portion of the foramen *Borders of the intervertebral foramen:* Anterior: posterior aspect of vertebral bodies and disc Superior: pedicle of upper vertebra Inferior: pedicle of lower vertebra Posterior: superior articular process and pars interarticularis Foraminal stenosis may be caused by posterolateral disc displacements, osseous ridges or osteophytes arising from the posterior aspect of the vertebral body, synovial cysts, or postoperative fibrosis Radiography may show foraminal stenosis from osteophytes, but it is insensitive to soft tissue findings and correlates poorly with clinical findings CT and MR imaging reveal displacement or distortion of the exiting nerve root and the surrounding epidural or perineural fat

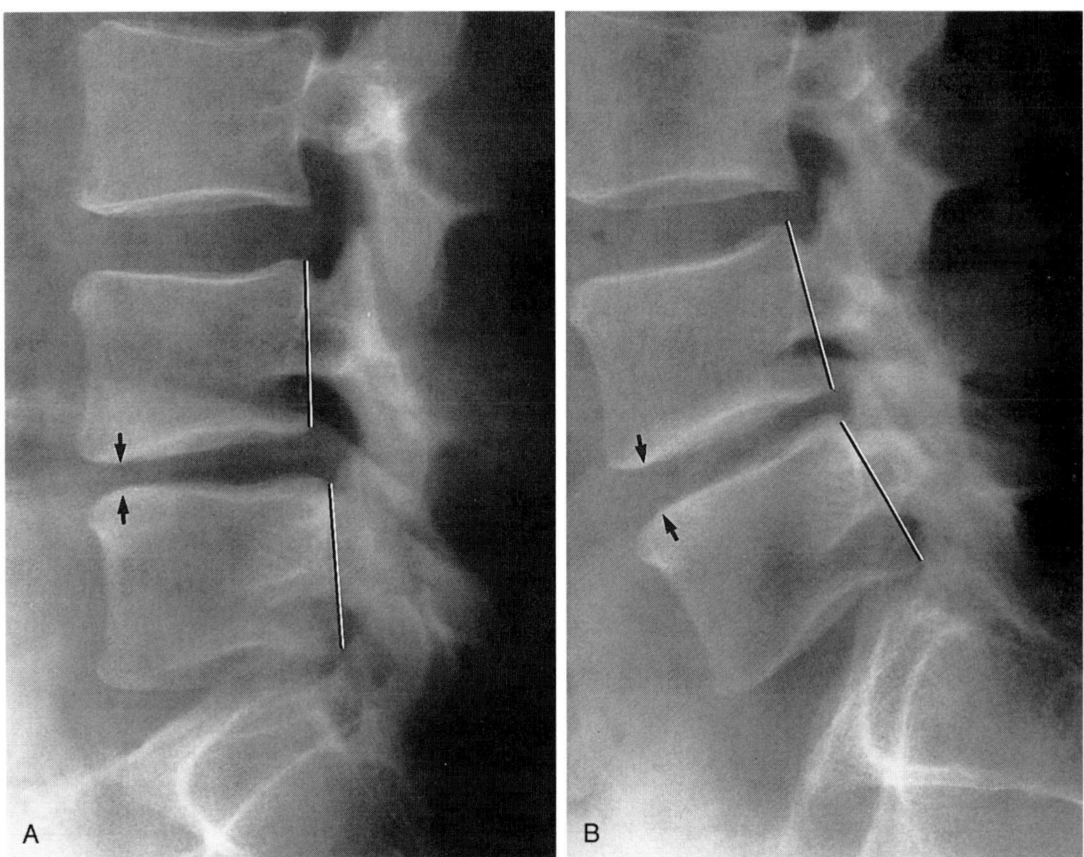

FIGURE 4–54. Segmental instability: Abnormal intersegmental motion.[43, 44, 69] Lateral lumbar radiographs obtained in flexion (A) and extension (B) reveal narrowing of the L4-L5 disc. The disc angle changes dramatically between flexion and extension (arrows), and the L4 vertebral body translates anteriorly with respect to L5 during flexion. This translation is illustrated by the change in position of the vertical lines along the posterior vertebral body margins. Segmental instability may be a complication of trauma, spondylolisthesis, spinal surgery, degenerative disease, and other causes.

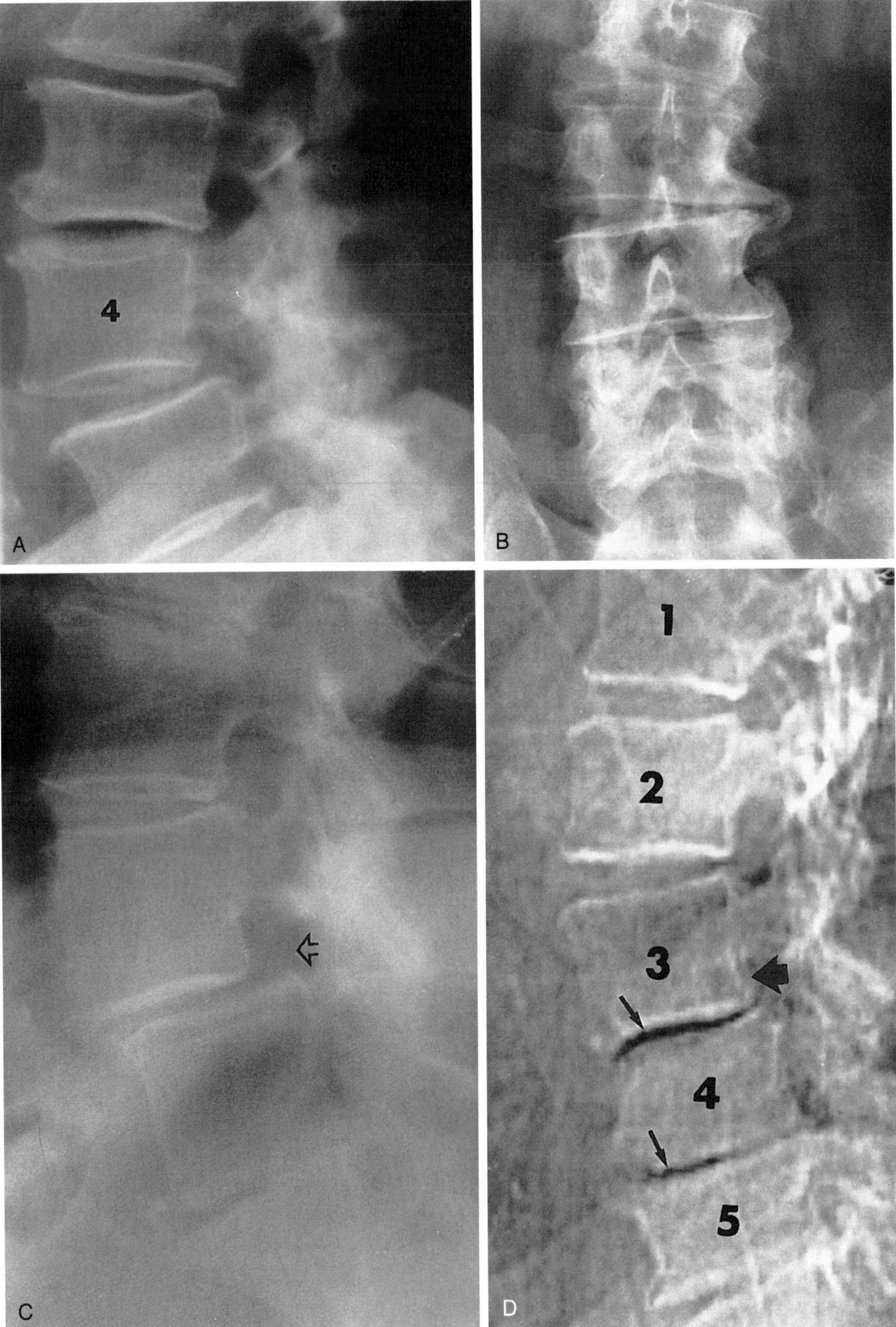

FIGURE 4–55. Degenerative disease—alignment abnormalities.[39, 70–72] A, B 79-year-old man. Lateral (A) and frontal (B) radiographs demonstrate extensive degenerative disc disease, vacuum disc phenomenon, apophyseal joint osteoarthrosis, and degenerative scoliosis. Degenerative spondylolisthesis is seen at L4 with anterior displacement relative to L5. Degenerative retrolistheses are evident at the L2-L3 and L3-L4 levels. C Degenerative spondylolisthesis of L4 (open arrow) is evident in another patient with severe apophyseal joint osteoarthrosis. D In a third patient, sagittal CT reconstruction reveals advanced L3-L4, L4-L5, and L5-S1 disc degeneration with intradiscal gas (small arrows) as well as L3 degenerative spondylolisthesis (large arrow).

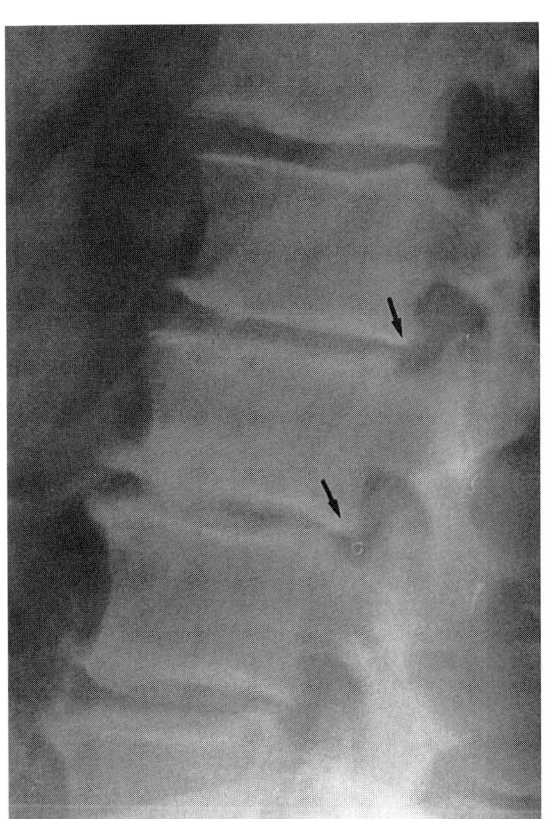

FIGURE 4–56. Degenerative retrolisthesis.[39] Degenerative retrolistheses at L2-L3 and L3-L4 (arrows) are associated with marked disc degeneration, apophyseal joint osteoarthrosis, and foraminal narrowing in this elderly patient.

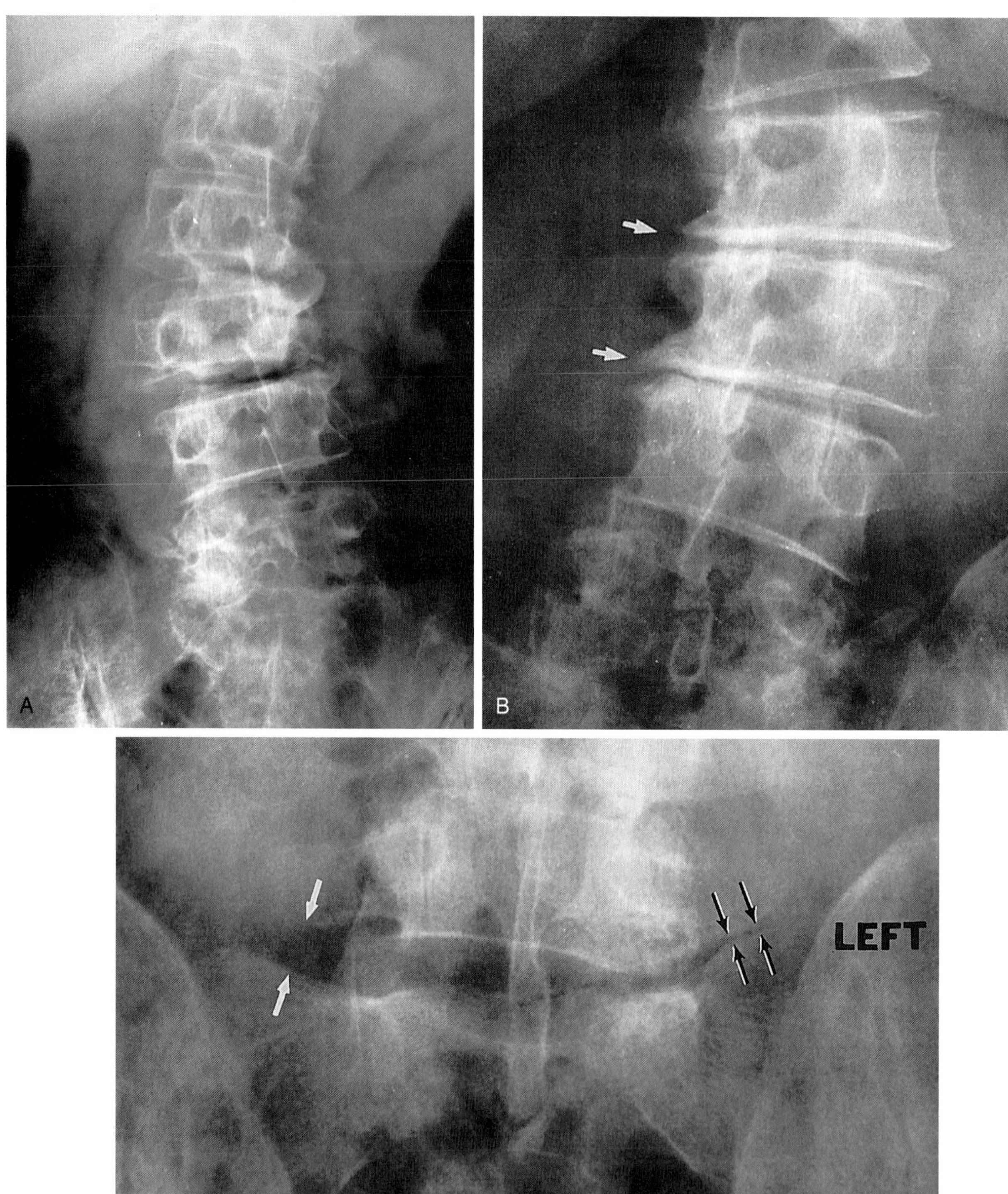

FIGURE 4–57. Degenerative scoliosis.[47, 71, 72] A This lumbar scoliosis is associated with asymmetric disc degeneration and extensive osteophytosis on the concave side of the curve. A prominent vacuum phenomenon is seen in the L3-L4 intervertebral disc. B, C The "far-out" syndrome in an 81-year-old woman with persistent back pain and left buttock pain. In B, a routine frontal radiograph shows severe scoliosis, asymmetric disc space narrowing, prominent osteophytosis, and bone sclerosis predominating on the concave side of the curve (white arrows). In C, an angulated frontal radiograph shows lateral flexion of the L5 vertebra with asymmetric disc space narrowing. The right L5 transverse process and sacral ala are normally spaced (white arrows), but impaction of the left L5 transverse process on the ipsilateral sacral ala is evident (black arrows). This abnormal alignment and impaction may result in entrapment of the L5 spinal nerve as it passes through this anatomic space, a condition termed the "far-out" syndrome. Surgery may be necessary to decompress the L5 nerve. *(B, C, Reprinted with permission from Taylor JAM, Hoffman LE: The geriatric patient: Diagnostic imaging of common musculoskeletal disorders. Top Clin Chiropr 3:23, © 1996, Aspen Publishers, Inc.)*

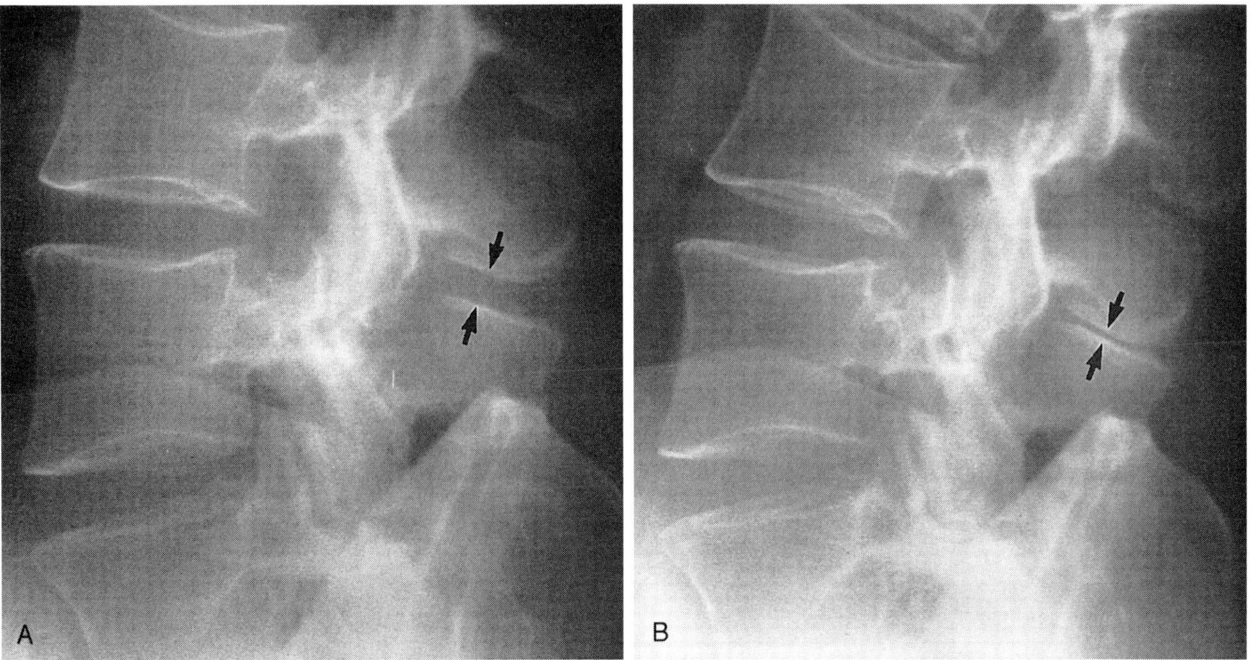

FIGURE 4–58. Baastrup's disease.[47] Lateral radiographs obtained in the neutral position (A) and in extension (B) reveal enlarged spinous processes with flattened, sclerotic superior and inferior margins (arrows). The spinous processes abnormally approximate on extension, often causing pain.

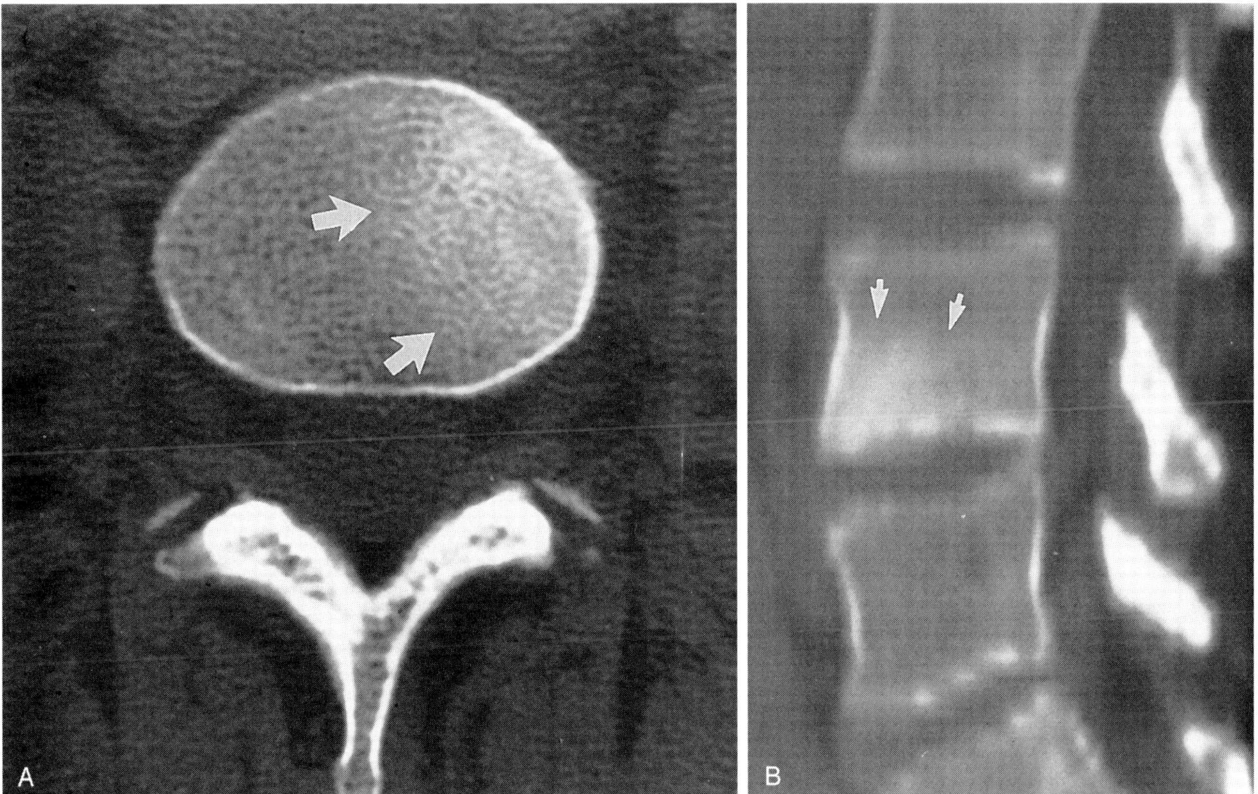

FIGURE 4–59. Segmental sclerosis of the vertebral body: Hemispheric spondylosclerosis.[73] Transaxial (A) and reconstructed sagittal (B) computed tomographic (CT) images show eccentric osteosclerosis of the L4 vertebral body (arrows) adjacent to the intervertebral disc. The differential diagnosis includes osteoblastic skeletal metastasis and other osteosclerotic lesions of bone. *(Courtesy of M.N. Pathria, M.D., San Diego, California.)*

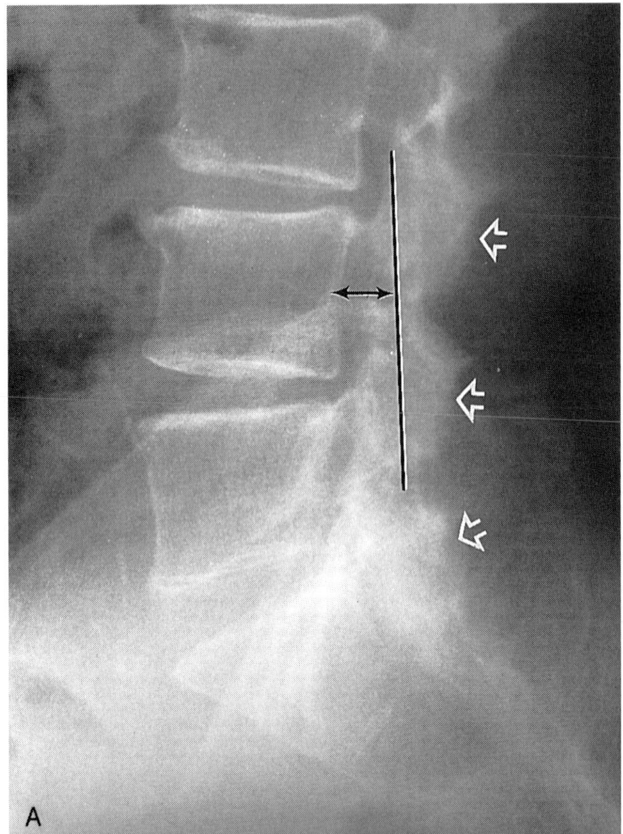

FIGURE 4–60. Degenerative disease—spinal stenosis.[74] A Lateral radiograph shows extensive sclerosis and osteophyte proliferation of the posterior facet articulations in the lower lumbar region (open arrows). The sagittal diameter of the spinal canal is narrowed (double-headed arrow). Measurements of spinal canal diameter obtained on routine radiographs may suggest the possibility of spinal stenosis, but they tend to be inaccurate and have poor correlation with signs and symptoms. B In another patient, transaxial computed tomographic (CT) images reveal hypertrophic osteophytes arising from the articular processes (white arrows) and discovertebral junctions (arrowheads), vacuum disc phenomenon (curved arrows), and ossification of the posterior longitudinal ligament (open arrow). The neural foramina are narrowed (small black arrows), and the thecal sac is compressed and displaced.

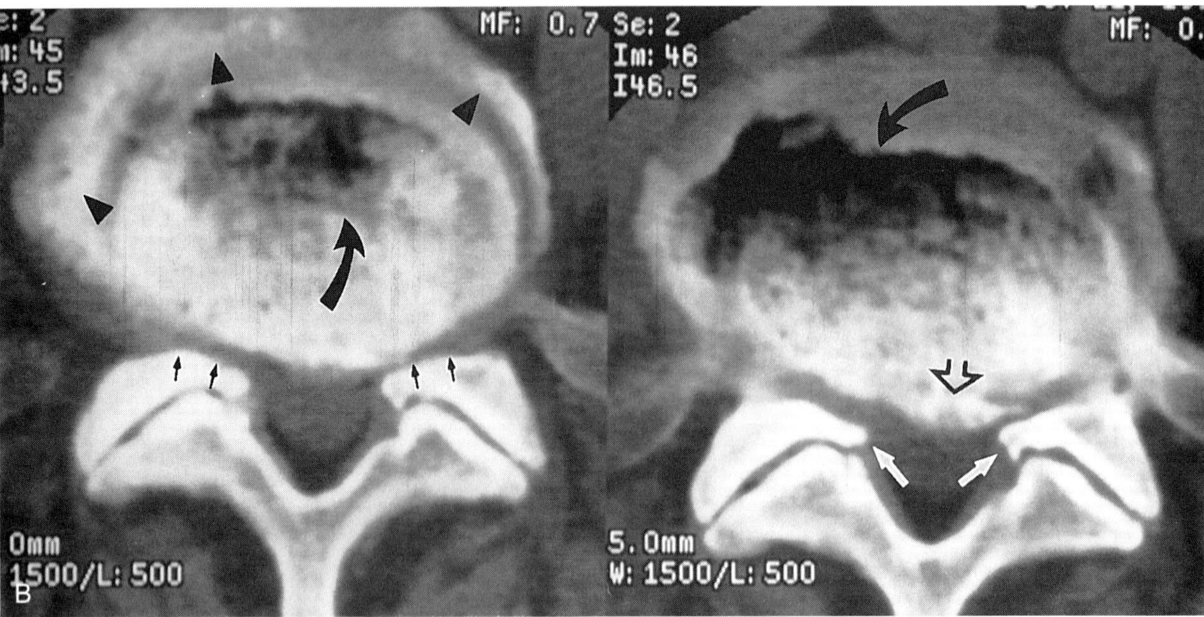

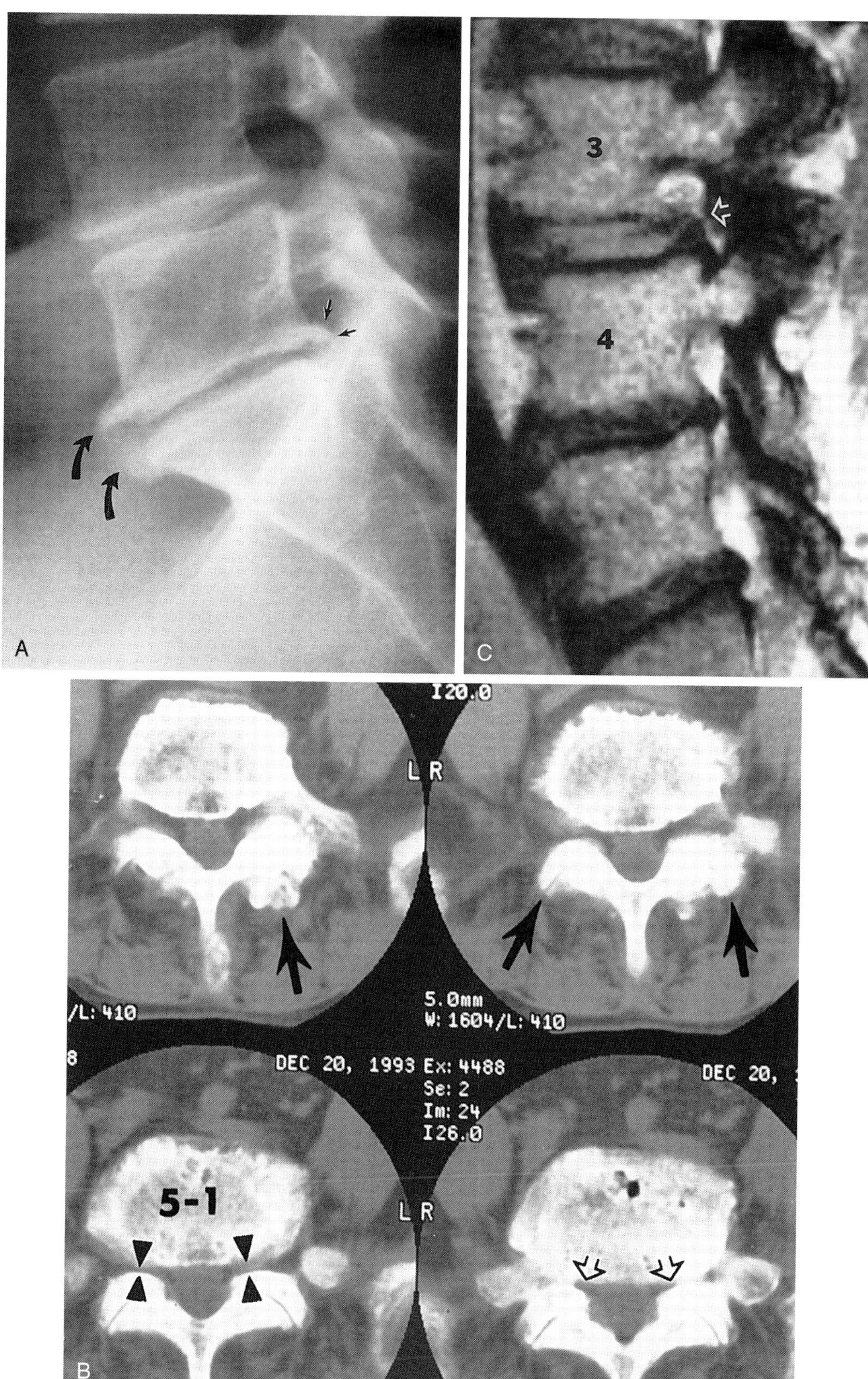

FIGURE 4–61. Degenerative disease: foraminal and lateral recess stenosis.[47, 74] A Anterior (curved arrows) and posterior (arrows) osteophytes are prominent in this patient with severe L4-L5 and L5-S1 degenerative disc space narrowing. The posterior osteophytes contribute to foraminal stenosis. (A, *Reprinted with permisson from Taylor JAM, Hoffman LE: The geriatric patient: Diagnostic imaging of common musculoskeletal disorders. Top Clin Chiropr 3:23, © 1996, Aspen Publishers, Inc.)* B Transaxial CT images from a 71-year-old woman with bilateral neurogenic claudication and a clinical diagnosis of degenerative spinal stenosis demonstrate severe hypertrophy of the articular processes (large arrows) and osseous encroachment of the intervertebral foramina (arrowheads), and lateral recesses (open arrows). (B, *Courtesy of D. Peterson, D.C., Portland, Oregon.)* C Parasagittal T2-weighted MR image of a patient with L3 degenerative spondylolisthesis shows narrowing and distortion of the L3-L4 intervertebral foramen by the hypertrophic and anteriorly subluxated apophyseal joints (open arrow).

TABLE 4–16. Lumbar Spine: Articular Disorder*

Entity	Figure(s), Table(s)	Characteristics
Degenerative and related disorders		
Degenerative spine disease[47, 58–62, 75]	4–46 to 4–48, 4–62	*Spondylosis deformans:* Osteophytes and osseous ridging (Table 3–9) Subchondral bone sclerosis *Intervertebral osteochondrosis:* Disc space narrowing Intradiscal vacuum phenomenon Disc calcification is rare *Apophyseal joint osteoarthrosis:* Subchondral bone sclerosis Articular process hypertrophy Joint space narrowing Synovial cysts in some cases Degenerative diseases of the lumbar spine may result in several complications (Table 4–15)
Diffuse idiopathic skeletal hyperostosis (DISH)[76]	4–63	*Radiographic findings:* 1. Flowing anterior hyperostosis: prominent vertical sheet of ossification along the anterior vertebral bodies and annulus fibrosus (Table 3–9) 2. Relative absence of degenerative changes and preservation of disc height 3. Involvement of at least four contiguous segments 4. Relatively normal apophyseal joints Fifty per cent of patients with DISH have associated ossification of the posterior longitudinal ligament (OPLL)
Ossification of the posterior longitudinal ligament (OPLL)[76]		Segmental or continuous vertical sheet of ossification of the posterior longitudinal ligament, up to 5 mm thick; extends along the posterior margins of the vertebral bodies and discs within the spinal canal Often accompanies DISH (more than 40 per cent of OPLL patients have DISH) L1 and L2 are the most common lumbar levels of involvement Frequently contributes to central stenosis with or without symptoms
Ossification and calcification of other spinal ligaments[77]	4–64	Ossification of the following spinal ligaments has been described in association with degenerative disease and DISH: Iliolumbar ligament Ligamenta flava Supraspinous ligament
Neuropathic osteoarthropathy[78]	4–65	Syringomyelia, tabes dorsalis, and diabetes mellitus may result in neuropathic osteoarthropathy affecting the thoracolumbar region Widespread discovertebral and zygapophyseal joint destruction, collapse, bone fragmentation, and kyphosis
Inflammatory disorders		
Rheumatoid arthritis[79]	4–66	Lumbar spine involvement rare Apophyseal joint erosion, sclerosis, and subluxation Intervertebral disc space narrowing Spinous process erosion Osteoporosis Absence of osteophytes and other osseous outgrowths
Ankylosing spondylitis and enteropathic arthropathy[80, 81]	4–67, 4–68 Tables 3–9, 3–10	Widespread marginal syndesmophytes, osteitis, disc calcification, osteoporosis, squaring of vertebral bodies, and disc ballooning Erosion and eventual ankylosis of discovertebral junctions and apophyseal joints Ossification of ligaments, joint capsules, and outer annular fibers (syndesmophytes) Ulcerative colitis and regional ileitis are the most common inflammatory bowel diseases to result in radiographic findings identical to those of ankylosing spondylitis Arachnoid diverticula also may complicate long-standing ankylosing spondylitis; can be associated with the cauda equina syndrome

TABLE 4–16. Lumbar Spine: Articular Disorder* *Continued*

Entity	Figure(s), Table(s)	Characteristics
Inflammatory disorders *Continued*		
Psoriatic spondyloarthropathy and Reiter's syndrome[82]	4–69, 4–70	Unilateral or bilateral, asymmetric, nonmarginal, comma-shaped paravertebral ossification about the thoracolumbar spine in 10 to 15 per cent of patients with psoriasis Paravertebral ossification—found in both psoriasis and Reiter's syndrome—may resemble the osseus outgrowths seen in other diseases (Table 3–9) Apophyseal joint narrowing, sclerosis, and bony ankylosis
Neurologic injury[83]	4–71	Patients with paraplegia and quadriplegia may develop spine changes identical to those of neuropathic osteoarthropathy, DISH, ankylosing spondylitis, psoriatic spondyloarthropathy, Reiter's syndrome, and degenerative disease Pseudarthrosis may occur as a result of improper fracture healing and may be accompanied by dramatic hypertrophic bone formation
Crystal deposition disorders		
Calcium pyrophosphate dihydrate crystal deposition disease[84, 85]	4–72	May result in widespread secondary degenerative disease (pyrophosphate arthropathy) with disc space narrowing and chondrocalcinosis of the annulus fibrosus, joint capsules, apophyseal joints, and articular cartilage
Alkaptonuria[86, 87]	4–73	Widespread, severe disc space narrowing, diffuse annulus fibrosus calcification, intradiscal vacuum phenomenon Osteoporosis and loss of lumbar lordosis Osseous bridging may resemble marginal syndesmophytes (Table 3–9) Eventual progression to complete ankylosis
Gouty arthropathy[88]	4–74	Spine involvement is extremely uncommon Osteophytosis and tophaceous erosive abnormalities of the apophyseal joints; discovertebral erosions may resemble those seen in infection and degenerative disc disease Paraspinal calcification may be seen
Infection		
Pyogenic spondylodiscitis[89, 90]	4–75 Table 2–12	Latent period of as long as 21 days before radiographic changes appear Infection initially involves disc and adjacent vertebral body Severe disc space narrowing at one level that eventually may spread to adjacent levels, obliterating vertebral end plates and resulting in vertebral collapse in later stages Paravertebral soft tissue mass or abscess
Tuberculous spondylodiscitis[91, 92]	4–76	Spine involvement in 25 to 60 per cent of cases of skeletal tuberculosis Thoracolumbar region is the most frequent site of infection Anterior vertebral destruction and collapse often result in an acute, angular gibbous deformity Classically, the vertebral bodies and disc are involved; the posterior elements are affected infrequently Paravertebral abscesses are common

*See also Tables 1–6 to 1–9 and Table 1–17.

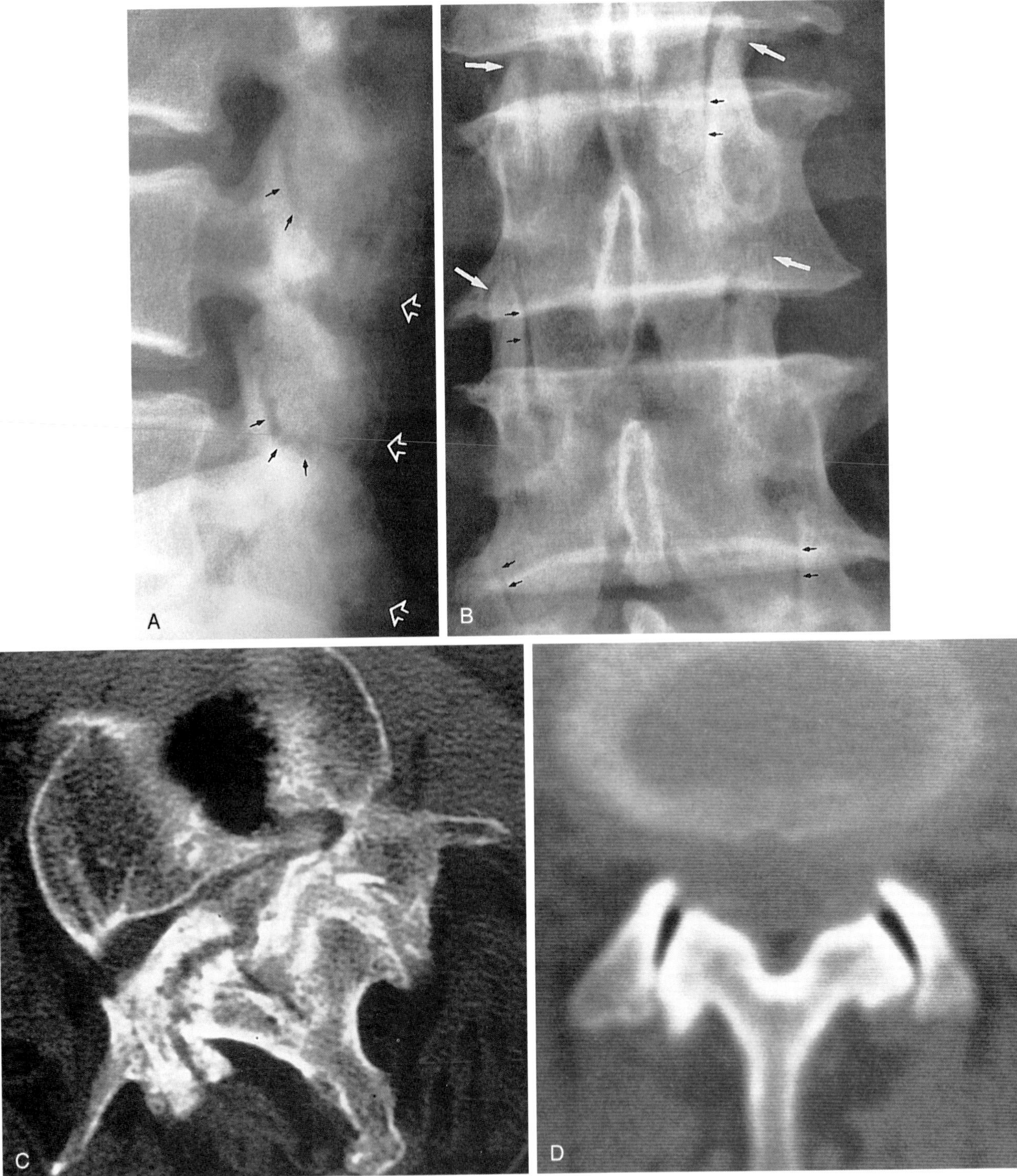

FIGURE 4–62. Apophyseal joint osteoarthrosis.[75] A Lateral radiograph reveals extensive bone proliferation, sclerosis (open arrows), and irregularity (arrows) of the apophyseal joints. B Anteroposterior radiograph shows joint space narrowing (black arrows), sclerosis, and hypertrophy of the superior articular processes (white arrows). (A, B, *Courtesy of E.E. Bonic, D.C., Portland, Oregon.*) C computed tomographic (CT) abnormalities in a patient with severe, long-standing idiopathic scoliosis. Transaxial CT image obtained after administration of myelographic contrast material shows extensive degeneration of the L3-L4 apophyseal joints. The findings include hypertrophy and sclerosis of the articular processes, osteophyte formation, apophyseal joint space narrowing with intra-articular gas (vacuum phenomenon), and dramatic central canal stenosis. (C, *Courtesy of W. Peck, M.D., Orange, California.*) D In another patient, a transaxial CT image reveals extensive intra-articular gas and subchondral sclerosis of the articular processes.

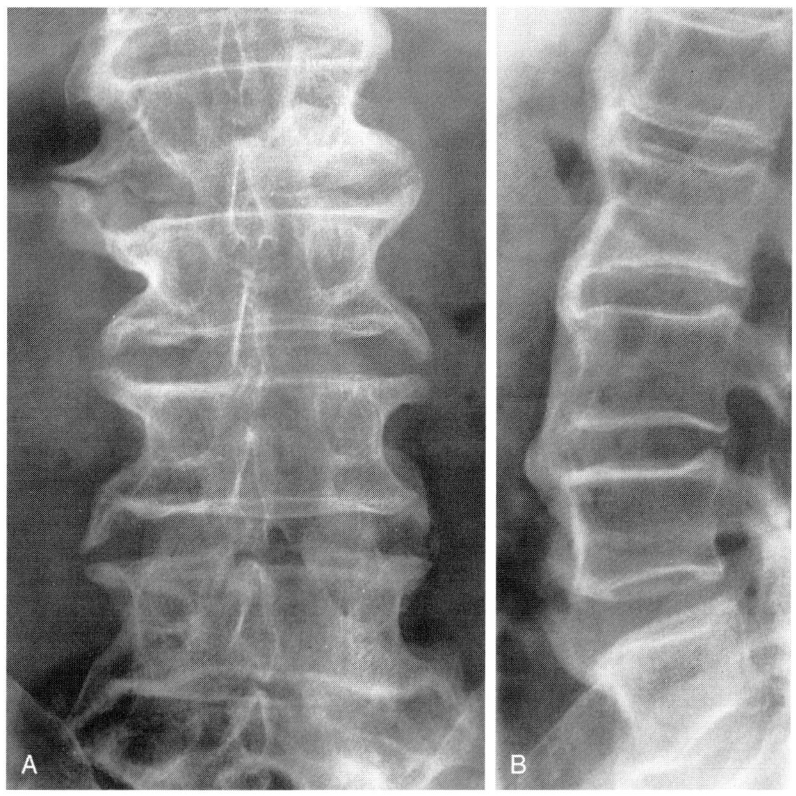

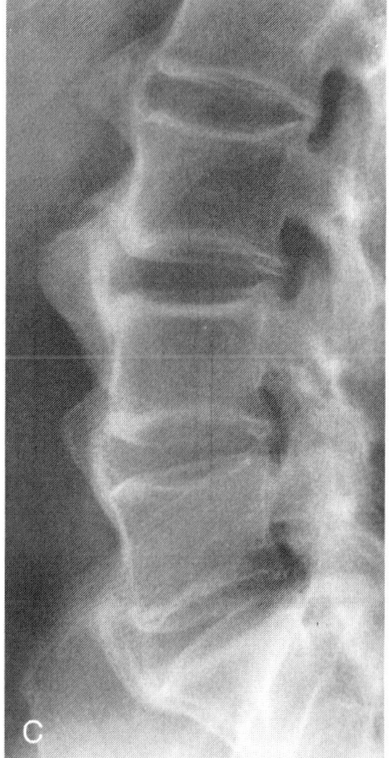

FIGURE 4–63. Diffuse idiopathic skeletal hyperostosis (DISH).[76] A Prominent flowing hyperostosis is seen arising from the central portion of the vertebral bodies on this anteroposterior radiograph. The disc spaces are preserved. B In another patient, the thick layer of ossification spans several vertebral levels, and the widths of the disc spaces are relatively well maintained. C Similar findings are evident in a third patient.

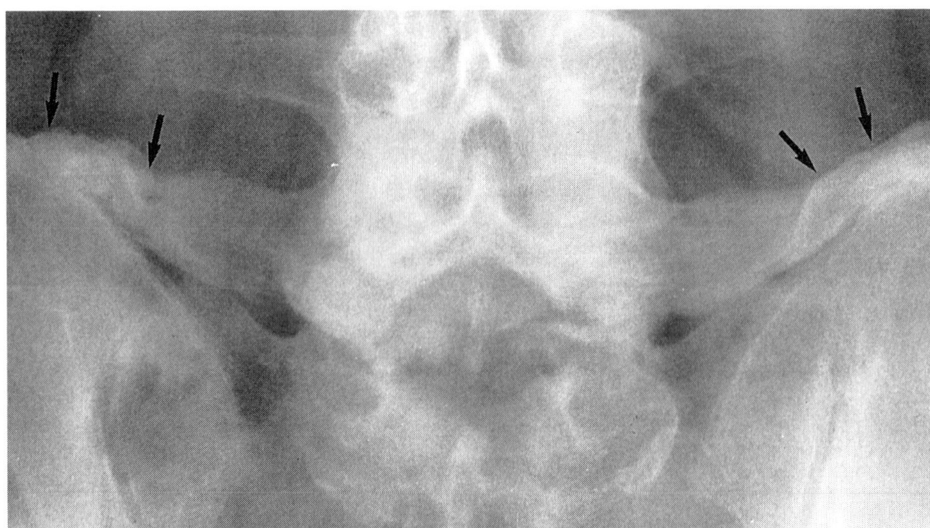

FIGURE 4–64. Iliolumbar ligament ossification.[77] Diffuse ossification of the iliolumbar ligaments (arrows) is a finding common to both degenerative disease and diffuse idiopathic skeletal hyperostosis (DISH). Deep palpation of the ossified iliolumbar ligaments may elicit pain.

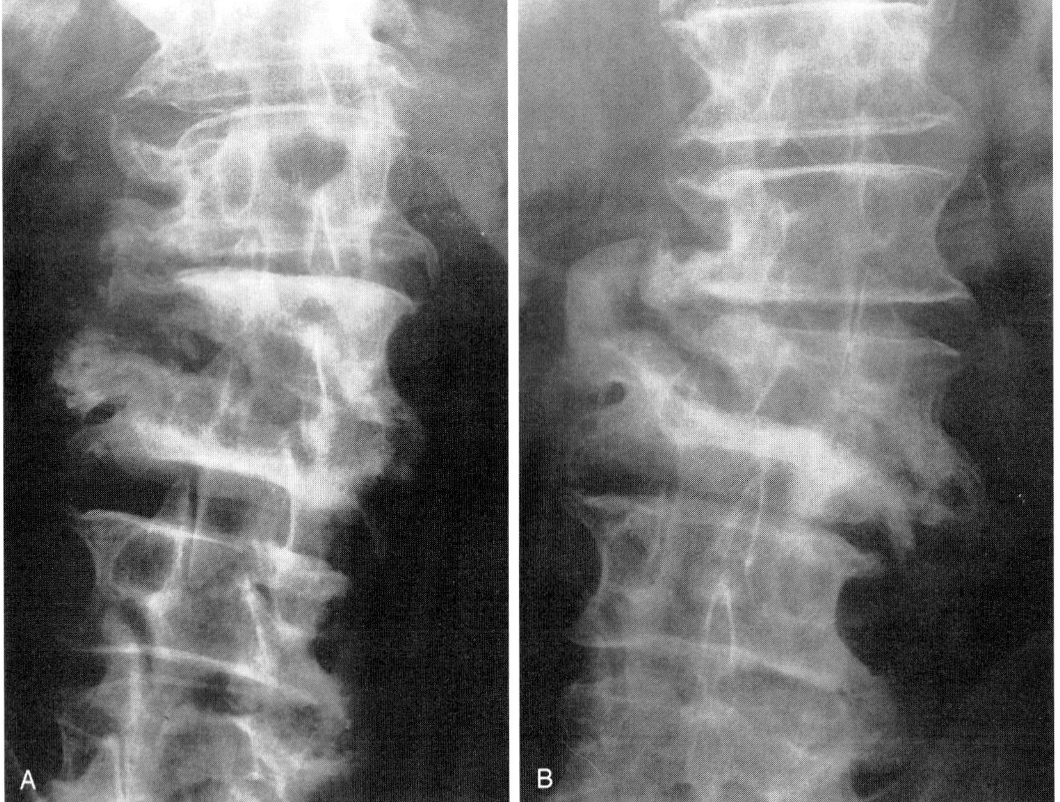

FIGURE 4–65. Neuropathic osteoarthropathy (Charcot's spine): Neurosyphilis.[78] This patient is a 65-year-old man with long-standing syphilis. **A** Initial radiograph shows extensive destruction and disorganization of the L2 and L3 vertebral bodies. Osteophyte formation and sclerosis also are apparent. **B** Radiograph obtained 2 years later shows progression of the destructive changes, marked sclerosis, and bulky osteophyte formation. This appearance resembles the improper fracture healing or pseudarthrosis seen in paralyzed patients.

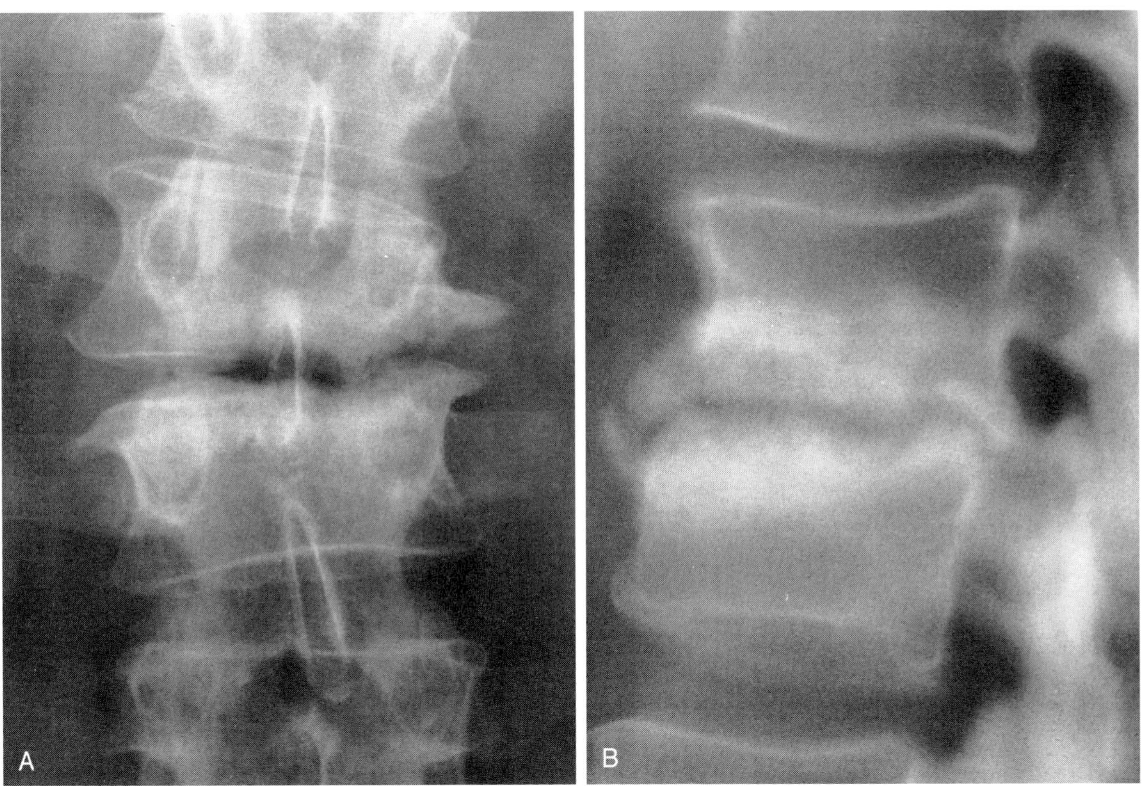

FIGURE 4–66. Rheumatoid arthritis.[79] In this 53-year-old patient with rheumatoid arthritis, a routine frontal radiograph (A) and a lateral conventional tomogram (B) reveal disc space narrowing, poorly defined osseous erosions, and sclerosis. These findings resemble those of infection, degenerative disc disease, and neuropathic joint disease. The presence of intradiscal gas and osteophytes is characteristic of degenerative disc disease. The indistinct vertebral end plates, however, are more typical of an inflammatory process. Although these joint changes may occasionally be found in patients with rheumatoid arthritis, their pathogenesis is debated.

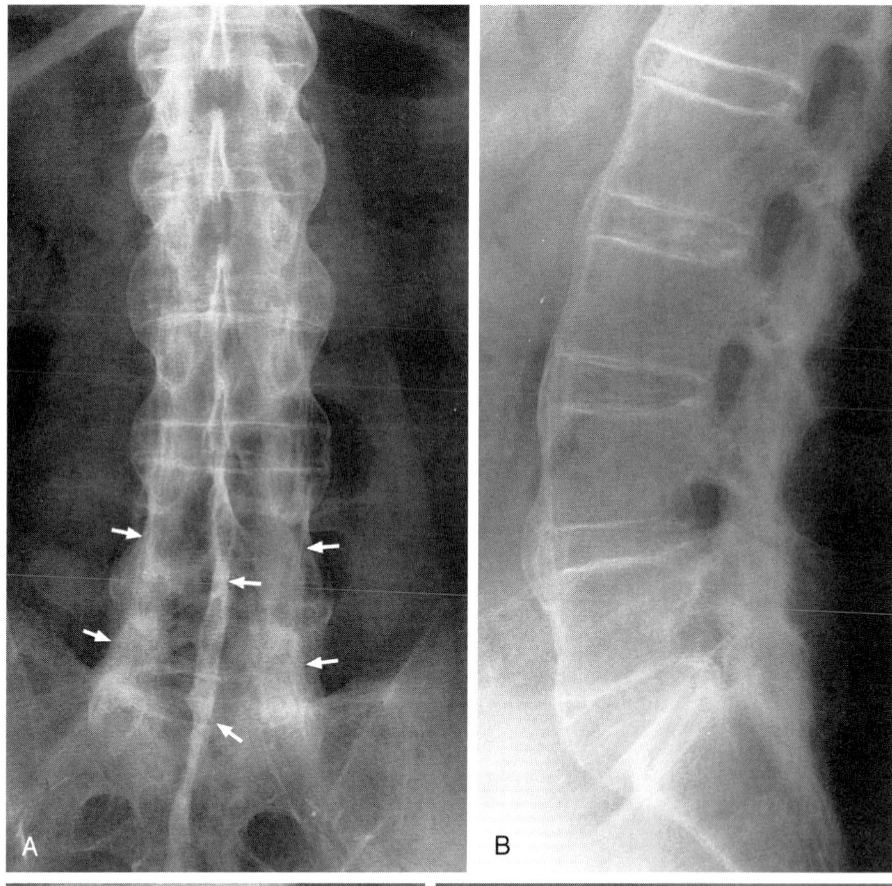

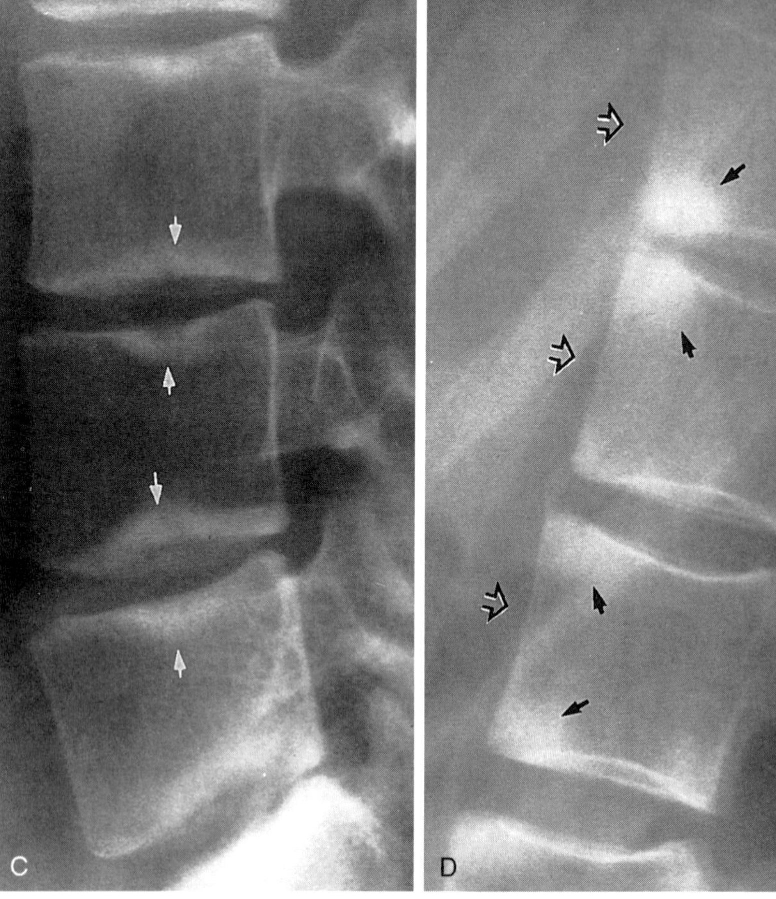

FIGURE 4–67. Ankylosing spondylitis: Spectrum of abnormalities.[80] **A, B** A 75-year-old man with long-standing ankylosing spondylitis. In **A,** a frontal radiograph reveals undulating syndesmophytes (bamboo spine). The presence of ossification and ankylosis of the apophyseal joints and supraspinous ligaments (arrows) is termed the "trolley track" sign. In **B,** a lateral radiograph demonstrates the continuous marginal syndesmophyte formation, ankylosis of the apophyseal joints, and discal calcification. *(***A, B,** *Courtesy of D. Goodwin, M.D., Lebanon New Hampshire.)* **C** Central discovertebral erosions. Observe the presence of multiple central discovertebral erosions throughout the lumbar spine (arrows). The erosions have an associated sclerotic margin and somewhat resemble Schmorl's nodes. This patient shows no evidence of syndesmophyte formation. *(***C,** *Courtesy of J. Amberg, M.D., San Diego, California.)* **D** "Shiny corner" sign. Osseous erosion and osteitis at the anterior aspects of the vertebral bodies adjacent to the discovertebral margin have resulted in sclerosis, which is referred to as the "shiny corner" sign (arrows). The loss of the normal anterior concavity of the vertebral bodies is a frequent finding termed "squaring" (open arrows). *(***D,** *Courtesy of A. Brower, M.D., Norfolk, Virginia.)*

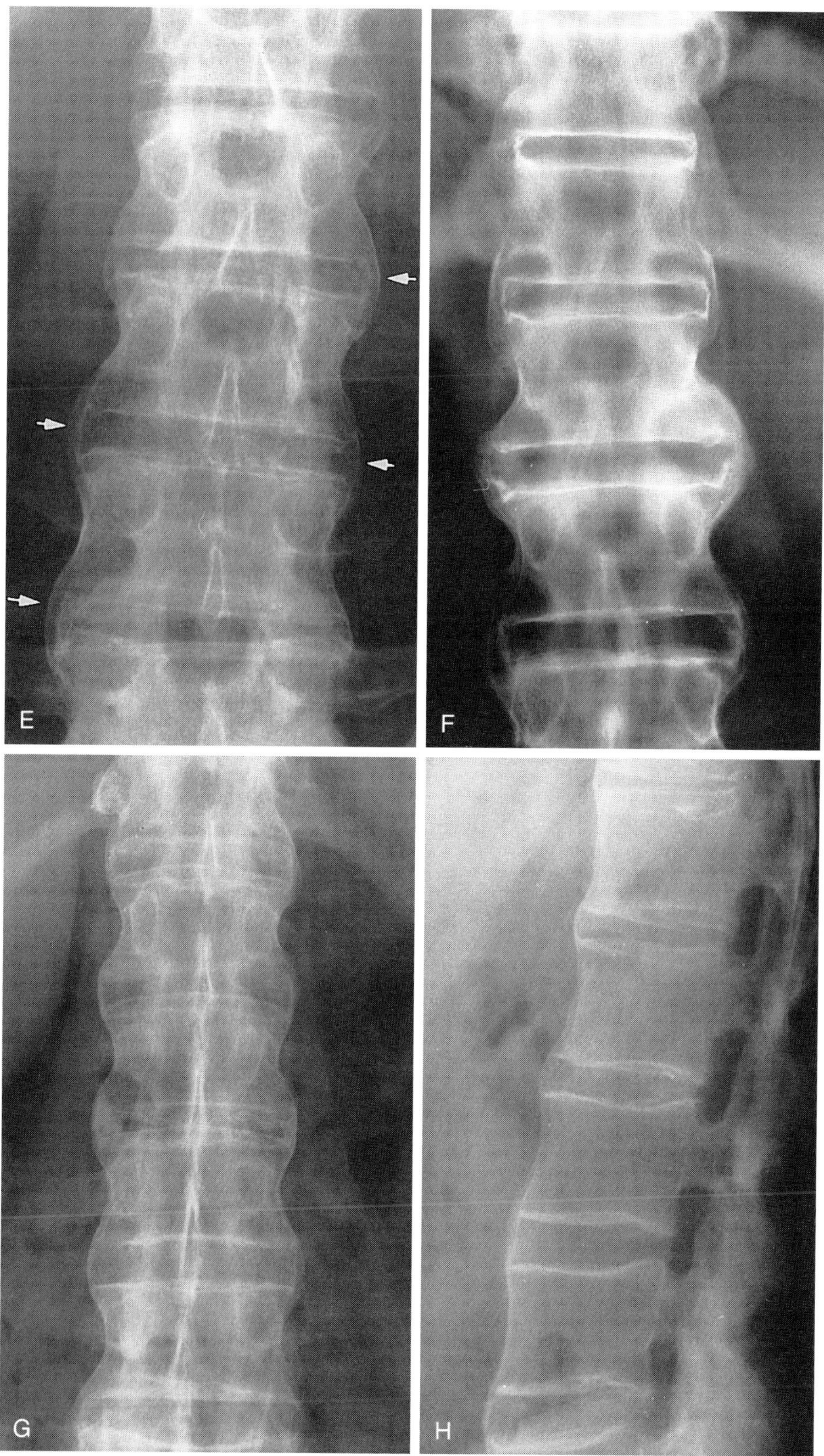

FIGURE 4–67 *Continued.* E Syndesmophytes. A routine radiograph demonstrates the characteristic thin, curvilinear, marginal syndesmophytes arising from the corners of the vertebral bodies throughout the lumbar spine (arrows). This appearance is sometimes referred to as the "bamboo spine" appearance. F In another patient, conventional tomography more clearly shows the slender marginal syndesmophytes. *(F, Courtesy of T. Broderick, M.D., Orange, California.)* G, H In another patient with ankylosing spondylitis, radiographs show extensive syndesmophyte formation. See also Table 3–10 for terminology applied to ankylosing spondylitis.

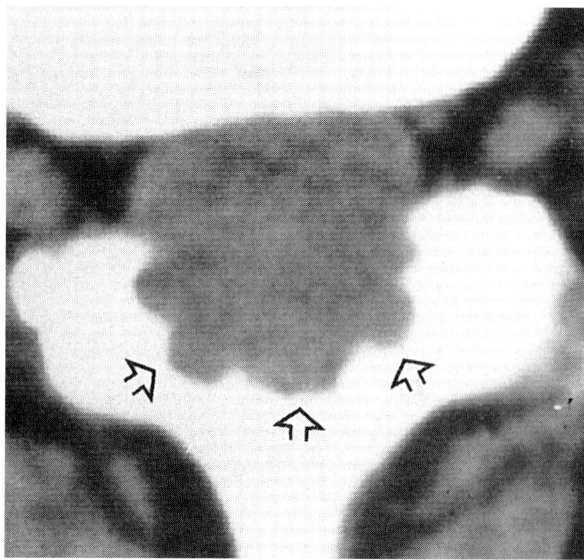

FIGURE 4–68. Ankylosing spondylitis: Arachnoid diverticula.[81] Observe the scalloped erosions of the neural arch (open arrows) on this computed tomographic (CT) scan from a patient with long-standing ankylosing spondylitis. Arachnoid diverticula are a rare complication of ankylosing spondylitis.

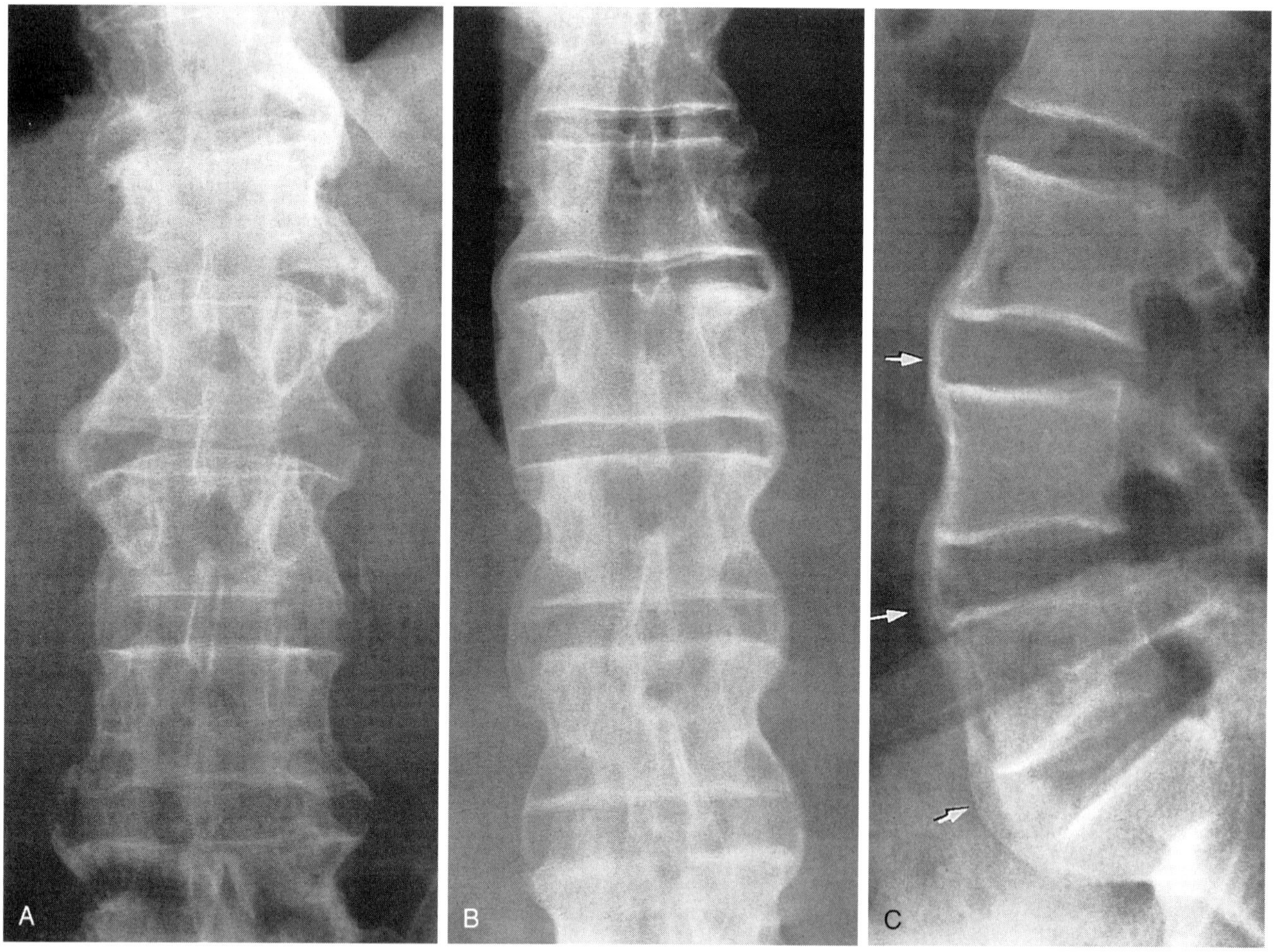

FIGURE 4–69. Psoriatic spondyloarthropathy.[82] **A** Asymmetric bulky osseous projections are seen arising several millimeters from the corners of the vertebral bodies and bridging several intervertebral discs. This asymmetric paravertebral ossification is characteristic of the spondyloarthropathy of psoriasis and Reiter's syndrome. **B, C** A 69-year-old man with long-standing psoriatic skin lesions and polyarticular joint disease. In **B**, an anteroposterior radiograph reveals prominent undulating paravertebral ossification throughout the lumbar spine. The continuous symmetric pattern of ossification in this patient is somewhat atypical of psoriatic spondyloarthropathy, resembling instead the more classic syndesmophytes of ankylosing spondylitis. In **C**, a lateral radiograph shows the characteristic undulating osseous outgrowths that span the anterior aspect of the lumbar vertebrae and disc spaces (arrows). The disc spaces are well preserved.

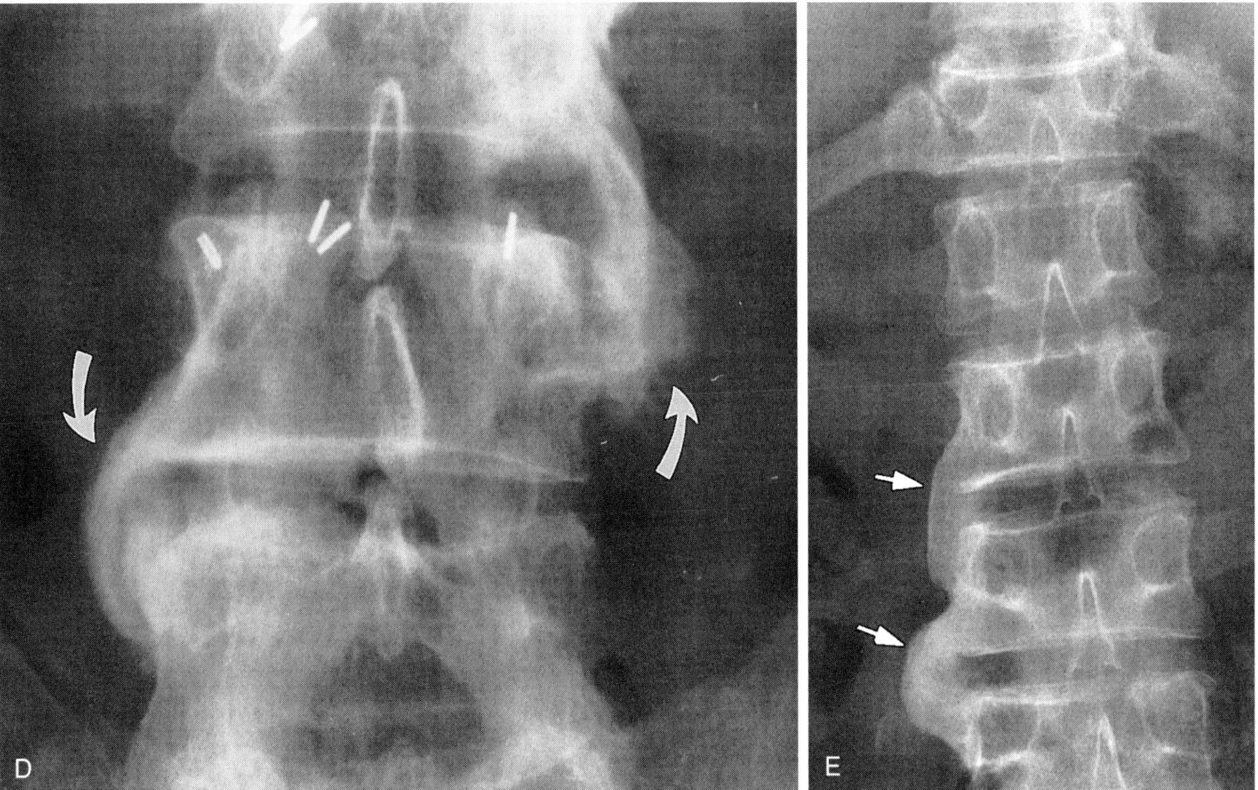

FIGURE 4–69 *Continued.* D In another patient, bulky asymmetric paravertebral ossification of the lumbosacral region is seen (curved arrows). E In a fourth patient, unilateral ossification spans the L2-L3 and L3-L4 intervertebral disc spaces (arrows). Unilateral or bilateral asymmetric paravertebral ossification of the lower thoracic and upper lumbar spine is evident radiographically in 10 to 15 per cent of patients with psoriasis. The paravertebral ossification, characteristic of both psoriatic spondyloarthropathy and Reiter's syndrome, may resemble the marginal syndesmophytes seen in ankylosing spondylitis, the flowing hyperostosis of diffuse idiopathic skeletal hyperostosis (DISH), or the osteophytes of degenerative disc disease. In psoriatic spondyloarthropathy and Reiter's syndrome, however, the excrescences may be large, bulky, or fluffy and often parallel the lateral surfaces of the vertebral bodies and intervertebral discs. The characteristic radiographic and clinical features usually allow differentiation of psoriatic spondyloarthropathy and Reiter's syndrome from these other conditions.

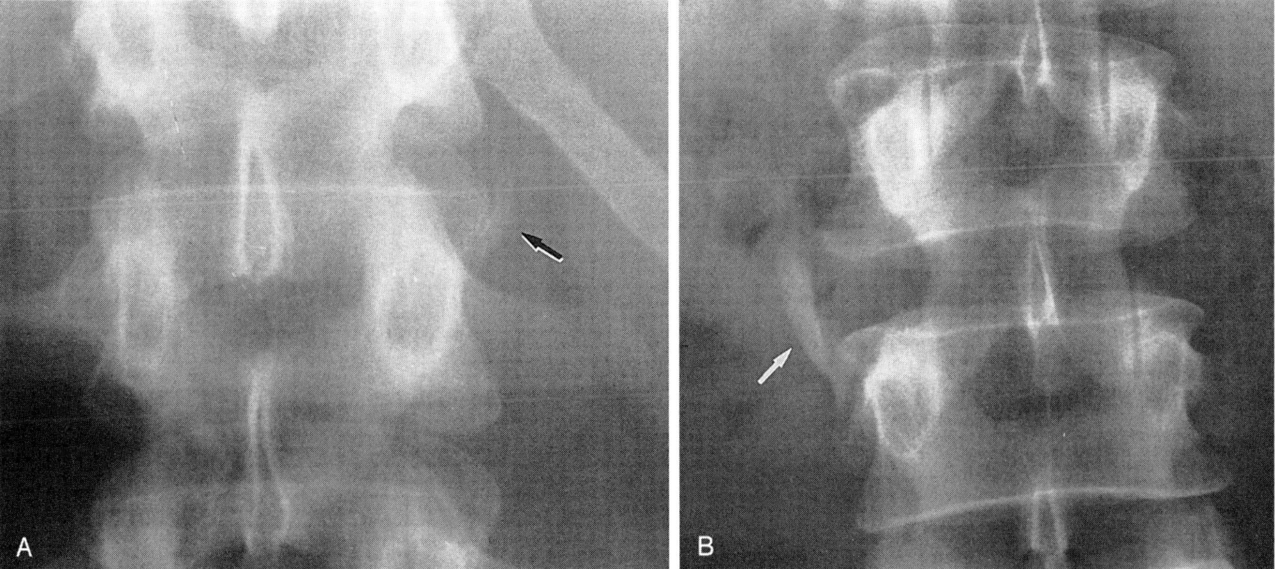

FIGURE 4–70. Reiter's syndrome: Paravertebral ossification.[82] A Observe the comma-shaped osseous excrescence arising from the lateral aspect of the vertebral body of L1 (arrow). This pattern is characteristic of seronegative spondyloarthropathies, such as Reiter's syndrome and psoriatic spondyloarthropathy. B In another patient, a characteristic nonmarginal paravertebral excrescence is seen spanning two adjacent lumbar vertebrae (arrow).

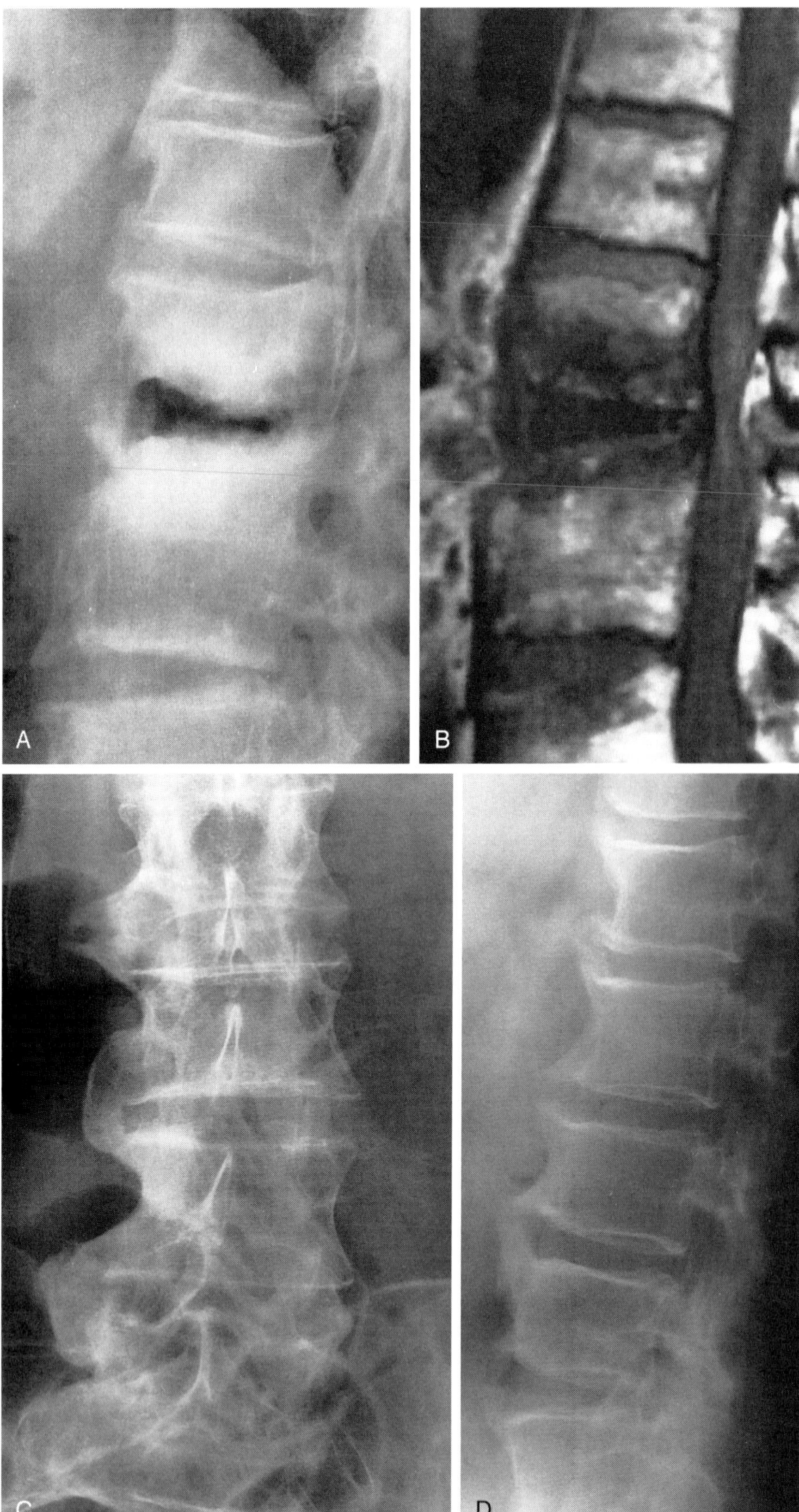

FIGURE 4–71. Neurologic injury: Spinal abnormalities.[83] **A, B** Neuropathic osteoarthropathy: Spine changes in a paraplegic man (Charcot's spine). In **A,** a routine radiograph shows intradiscal gas (vacuum phenomena) and vertebral body sclerosis. In **B,** a sagittal T1-weighted (TR/TE, 600/20) spin echo magnetic resonance (MR) image reveals low signal intensity within both the disc and the sclerotic portions of the adjacent vertebral bodies. **C, D** In a different patient with paralysis, frontal **(C)** and lateral **(D)** radiographs demonstrate thick, flowing hyperostosis and relative preservation of disc spaces, a pattern resembling the changes of diffuse idiopathic skeletal hyperostosis (DISH).

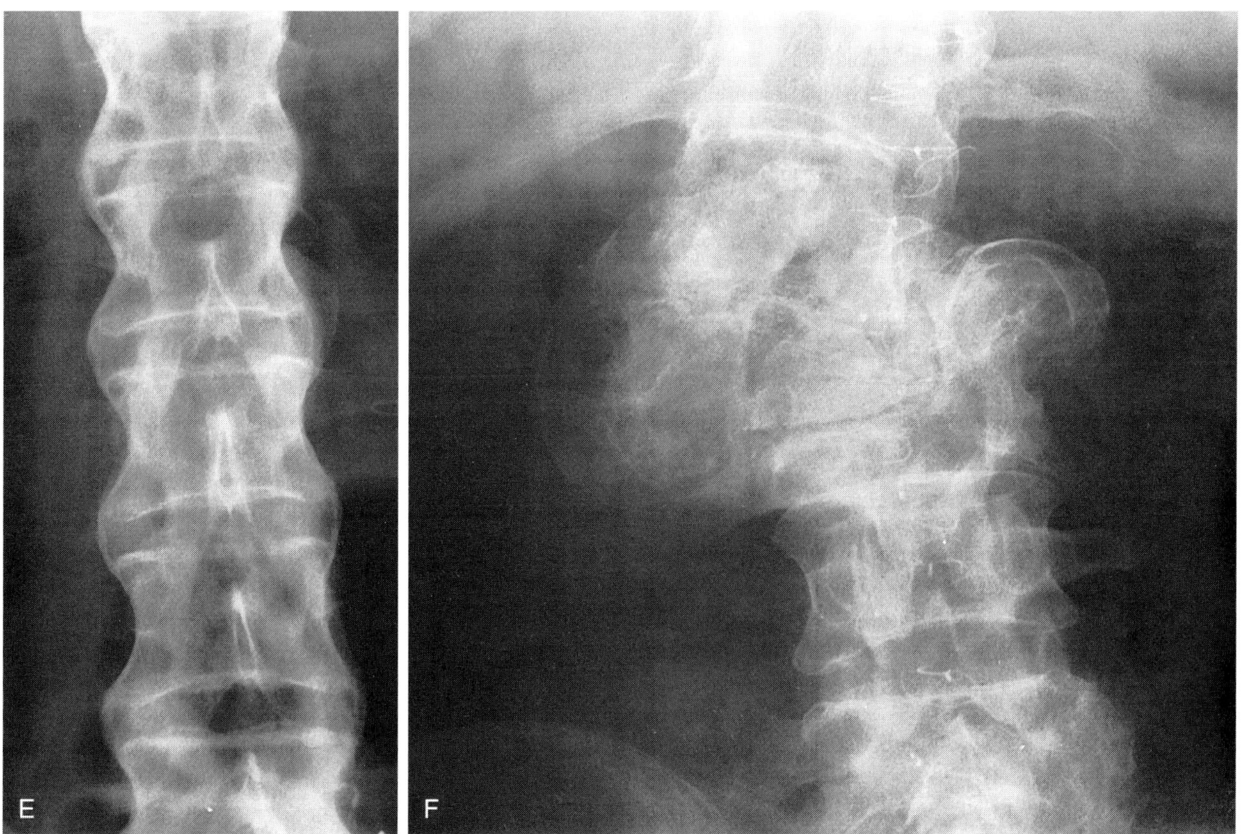

FIGURE 4–71 *Continued.* E In this quadriplegic man, the diffuse syndesmophyte formation is more typical of ankylosing spondylitis. F In another patient, a pseudarthrosis with bizarre hypertrophic bone formation is characteristic of improper fracture healing, a pattern occasionally seen in paralyzed patients. *(From Park Y-H, Huang G-S, Taylor JAM, et al: Patterns of vertebral ossification and pelvic abnormalities in paralysis: A study of 200 patients. Radiology 188:561, 1993.)*

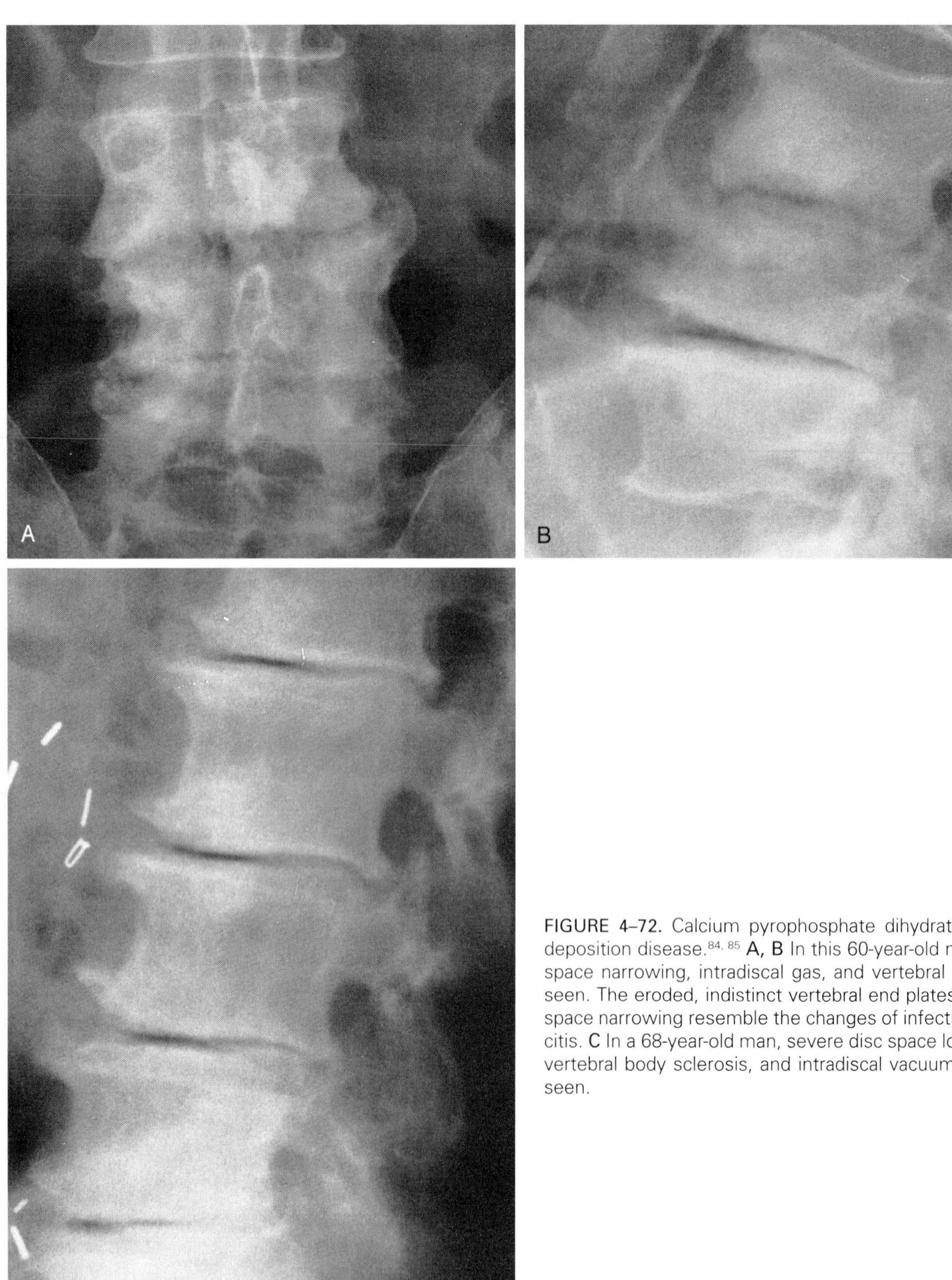

FIGURE 4–72. Calcium pyrophosphate dihydrate (CPPD) crystal deposition disease.[84, 85] A, B In this 60-year-old man, marked disc space narrowing, intradiscal gas, and vertebral body sclerosis is seen. The eroded, indistinct vertebral end plates and severe disc space narrowing resemble the changes of infectious spondylodiscitis. C In a 68-year-old man, severe disc space loss, osteophytes, vertebral body sclerosis, and intradiscal vacuum phenomena are seen.

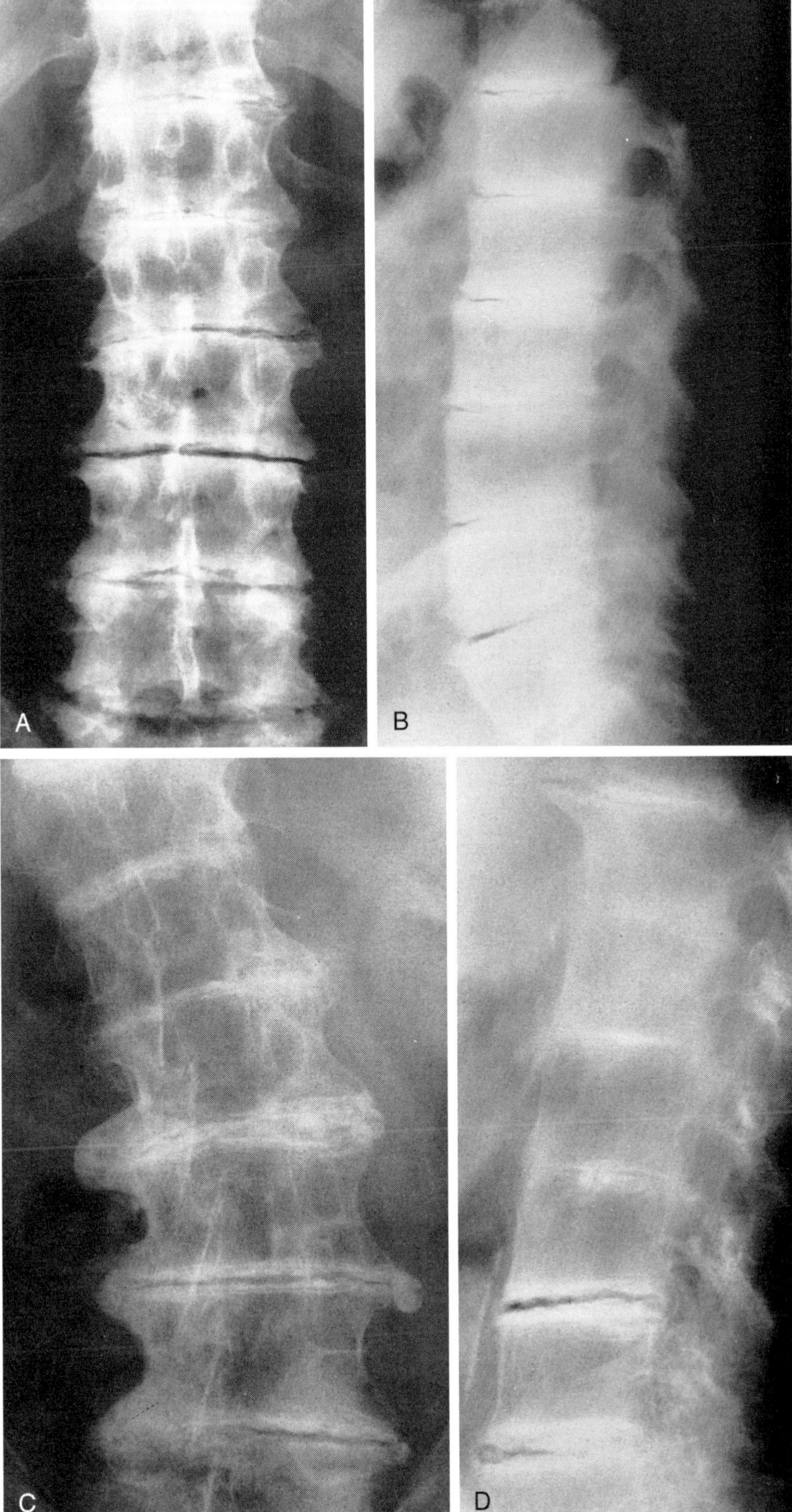

FIGURE 4–73. Alkaptonuria (ochronotic arthropathy).[86, 87] A, B Radiographs of this 42-year-old man exhibit severe, diffuse disc space narrowing, vacuum phenomena, and adjacent subchondral sclerosis. Disc calcification is not prominent in this patient. *(A, B, Courtesy of P. Katzenstein, M.D., Houston, Texas.)* C In another patient, observe the widespread disc space narrowing and calcification, vertebral end-plate sclerosis, and prominent osteophytosis. This patient also has scoliosis. *(C, Courtesy of G. Marques, M.D., São Paulo, Brazil.)* D In a third patient, widespread ossification of spinal ligaments and intervertebral discs results in ankylosis of several lumbar segments. Intradiscal gas is present within two lower lumbar intervertebral discs.

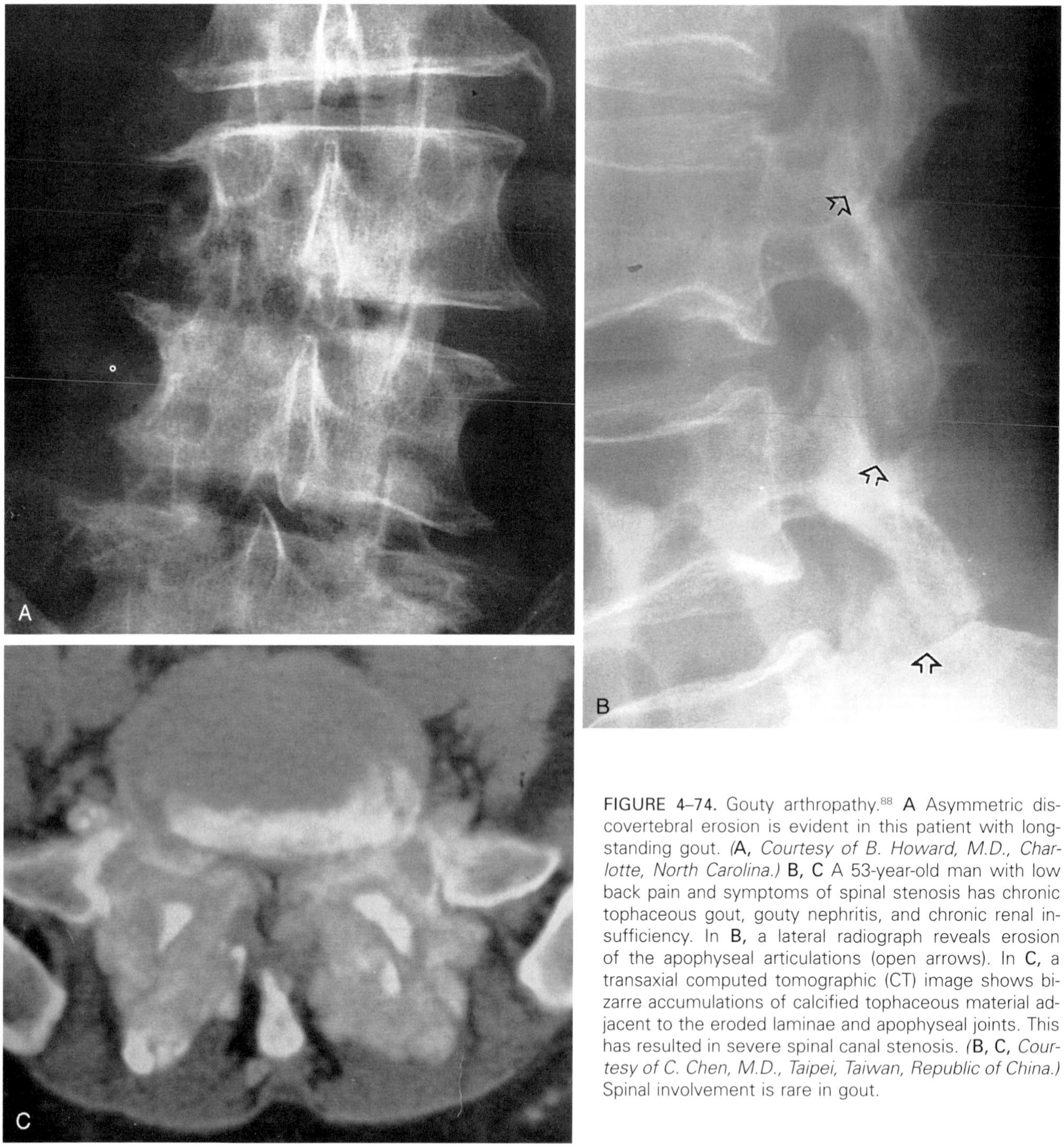

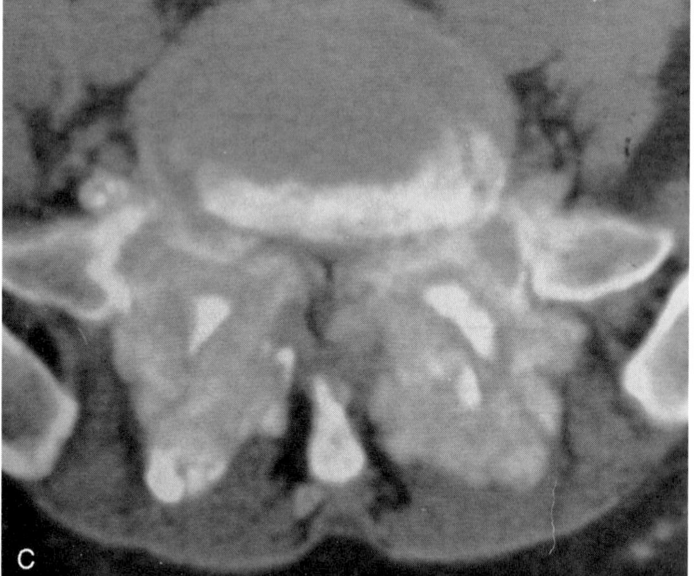

FIGURE 4–74. Gouty arthropathy.[88] **A** Asymmetric discovertebral erosion is evident in this patient with long-standing gout. *(**A**, Courtesy of B. Howard, M.D., Charlotte, North Carolina.)* **B, C** A 53-year-old man with low back pain and symptoms of spinal stenosis has chronic tophaceous gout, gouty nephritis, and chronic renal insufficiency. In **B**, a lateral radiograph reveals erosion of the apophyseal articulations (open arrows). In **C**, a transaxial computed tomographic (CT) image shows bizarre accumulations of calcified tophaceous material adjacent to the eroded laminae and apophyseal joints. This has resulted in severe spinal canal stenosis. *(**B, C**, Courtesy of C. Chen, M.D., Taipei, Taiwan, Republic of China.)* Spinal involvement is rare in gout.

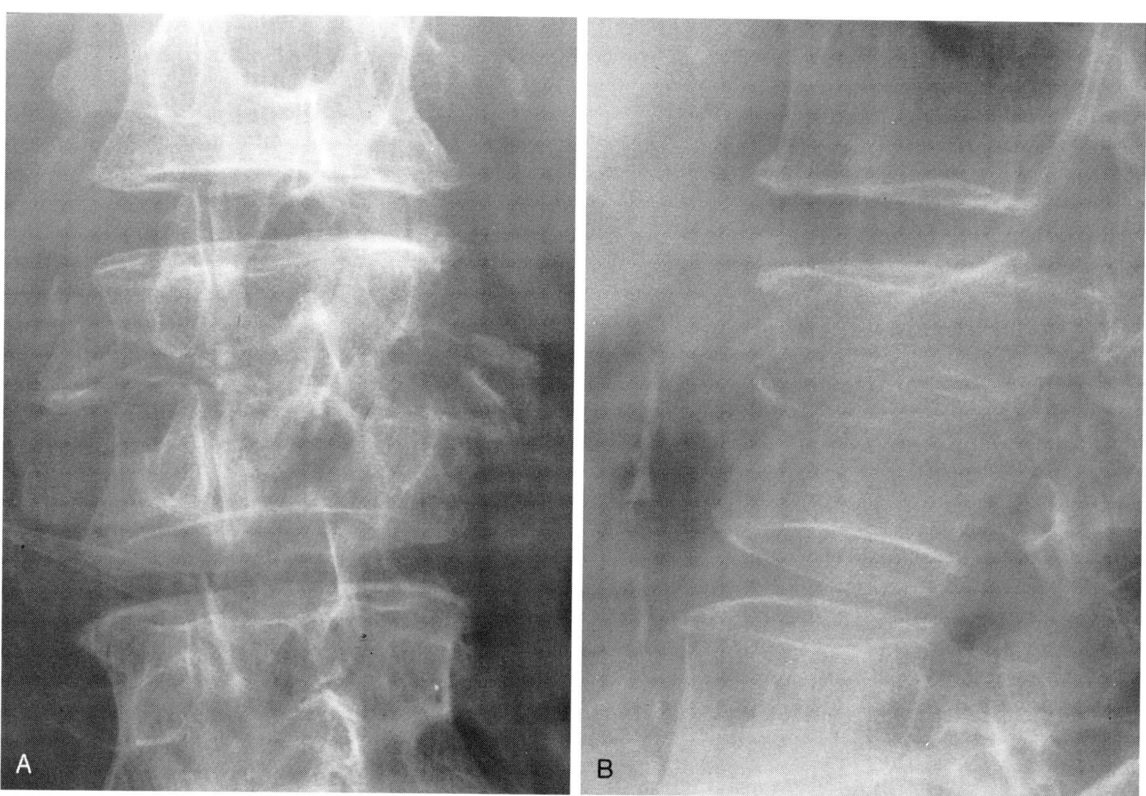

FIGURE 4–75. Pyogenic spondylodiscitis.[89, 90] A, B, Obliteration of the L2-L3 intervertebral disc space and destruction of the adjacent vertebral end plates and bodies are evident. Osseous debris is noted in the paraspinal region. Complete vertebral body collapse is imminent. Infectious spondylodiscitis occurs in up to 3.7 per cent of patients undergoing lumbar discectomy. Prophylactic antibiotic therapy is effective in preventing such postoperative infection. Refer also to Table 2–12 for MR imaging findings in spinal osteomyelitis.

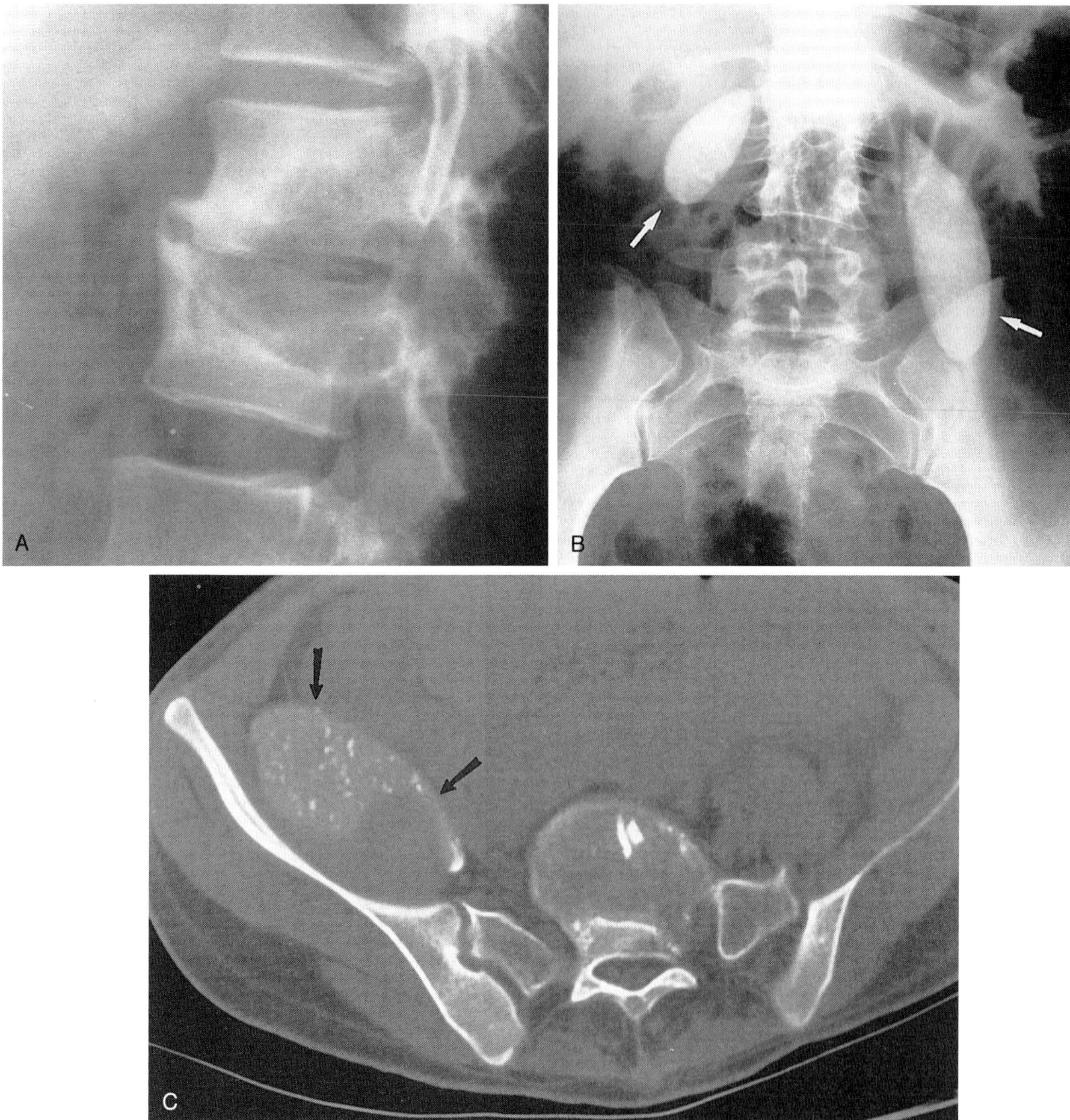

FIGURE 4–76. Tuberculous spondylitis.[91, 92] A Observe the loss of definition of the vertebral end plate, marked narrowing of the intervening disc space, and large scalloped erosions of the two adjacent vertebral bodies. B, C Psoas abscess. In B, a routine radiograph of a patient with spinal tuberculosis shows extensive calcification within bilateral psoas abscesses (arrows). In C, a transaxial computed tomographic (CT) image of a 13-year-old girl with long-standing tuberculosis shows a soft tissue mass in the vicinity of the iliopsoas muscle (arrows). Observe the punctate calcification within this tuberculous abscess about the L5-S1 disc. The spine is affected in 25 to 60 per cent of patients with skeletal tuberculosis. The vertebral bodies and disc typically are involved, although the posterior elements also may be affected. (C, *Courtesy of M.N. Pathria, M.D., San Diego, California.)*

TABLE 4–17. Lumbar Spine Neoplasms*

Entity	Figure(s)
Malignant neoplasms	
Skeletal metastasis[93–96]	4–77, 4–78, 4–79
Primary malignant neoplasms of bone:	
Chordoma[97]	4–80
Osteosarcoma (conventional)[98]	4–81
Myeloproliferative disorders:	
Plasma cell myeloma[99, 100]	4–82
Plasmacytoma[99]	4–83
Hodgkin's disease[95, 101]	4–84
Leukemia[102]	4–85
Benign neoplasms	
Primary benign neoplasms:	
Enostosis[103]	4–86
Osteochondroma[104, 105]	4–87
Aneurysmal bone cyst[106, 107]	4–88
Hemangioma[108]	4–89
Tumor-like lesions:	
Paget's disease[109, 110]	4–90
Neurofibromatosis Type I (von Recklinghausen's disease)[111]	4–91
Langerhans' cell histiocytosis[112, 113]	4–92

*This table lists only the neoplasms illustrated in this chapter; for a more complete discussion of neoplasms see Tables 1–10 to 1–12 and Table 2–13.

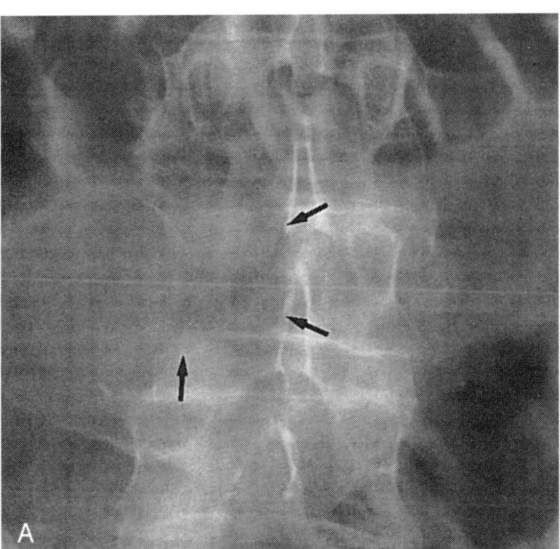

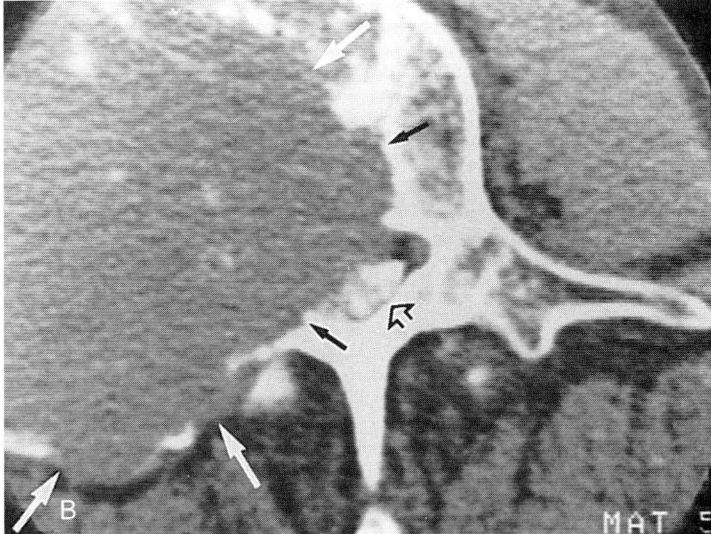

FIGURE 4–77. Skeletal metastasis: Vertebral destruction.[93] This 60-year-old man with known renal cell carcinoma developed back pain. A Frontal radiograph shows osteolytic destruction of the right L3 pedicle and vertebral body (arrows). B Transaxial CT-myelographic image shows widespread destruction of the vertebral body, pedicle, and lamina (black arrows). A huge soft tissue mass (white arrows) displaces the thecal sac, compressing it against the left lamina (open arrow). Unilateral pedicle destruction is termed the "winking owl" sign, and bilateral pedicle destruction has been referred to as the "blind vertebra" sign. Skeletal metastasis is the most common cause of a missing pedicle. CT, MR imaging, and scintigraphy play an essential role in the evaluation of patients with skeletal metastasis.

TABLE 4–18. Vertebral Osteosclerosis

Representative Disorders or Causes	Characteristics
Ivory vertebra and other sclerotic lesions of vertebral bodies	
Paget's disease[109, 110]	Older patient, expansion, coarse trabeculae, picture frame vertebrae
Hodgkin's disease[95, 101]	Younger patient, occasional anterior vertebral body scalloping
Osteoblastic metastasis[94–96]	Solitary, patchy, or diffuse sclerosis, history of primary carcinoma
Enostosis[103]	Giant bone island
Chordoma[97]	Solitary, rare cause of sclerotic vertebra
Infection[89, 90]	Rare cause of sclerotic vertebra, associated disc destruction
Hemangioma[108]	Striated corduroy cloth vertebra, usually solitary, rarely expansile
Osteopetrosis[23, 24]	Diffuse sclerosis, "sandwich vertebrae," or "bone-within-bone" appearance
Osteopoikilosis[15]	Rare in spine, multiple circular sclerotic lesions of uniform size
Fluorosis[122]	Diffuse osteosclerosis and osteophytosis
Sclerotic pedicle[41]	
Osteoblastic metastasis	Solitary lesions rare; bone scan usually reveals more lesions
Osteoid osteoma	Sclerosis, hypertrophy, small radiolucent nidus, severe pain
Osteoblastoma	Expansile lesions
Enostosis	Bone island within or overlying pedicle
Unilateral spondylolysis	Stress hypertrophy from contralateral pars interarticularis defect
Spina bifida occulta	Variable appearance, stress hypertrophy
Facet tropism	Stress hypertrophy
Laminectomy	Contralateral stress hypertrophy
Spinal fusion	Reactive sclerosis or graft bone
Agenesis or hypoplasia of contralateral pedicle or neural arch	Stress hypertrophy from absence of contralateral pedicle, lamina, or articular process

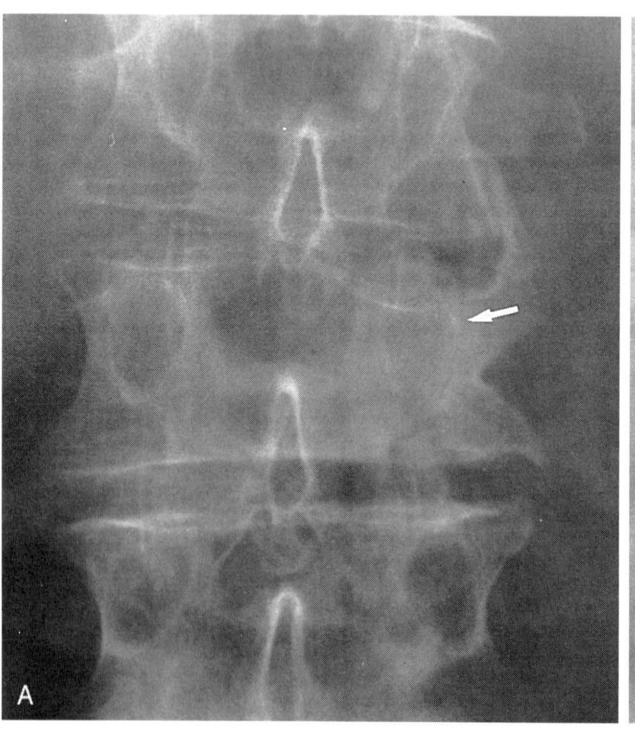

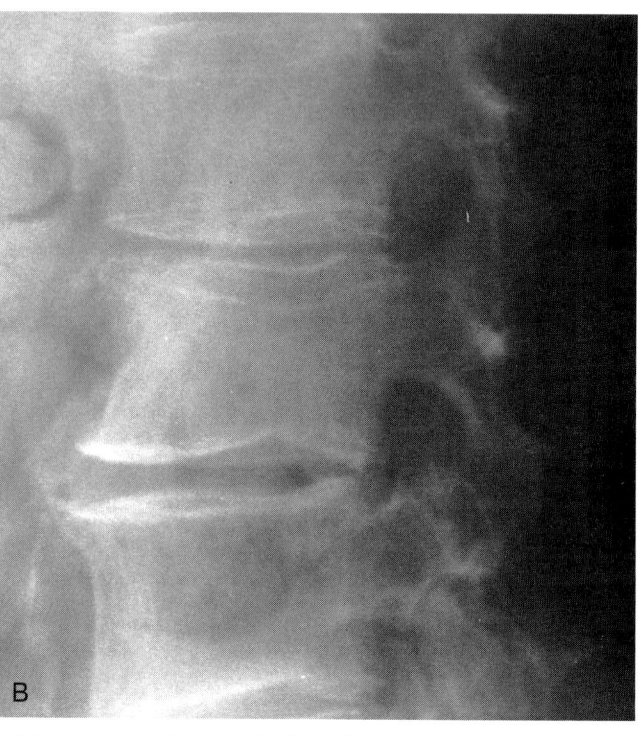

FIGURE 4–78. Skeletal metastasis[94, 95]: Prostate carcinoma—variable presentations. **A, B** An 83-year-old man with prostate carcinoma. Routine frontal (**A**) and lateral (**B**) radiographs of the lumbar spine show extensive osteolytic destruction of the L2 vertebral body. Collapse of the vertebral end plate and osteolysis of the left pedicle also are evident (arrow).

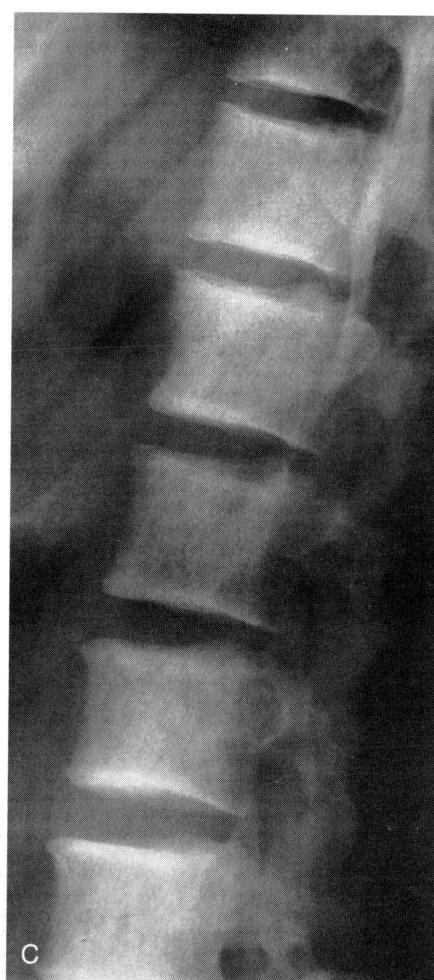

FIGURE 4–78 *Continued.* C Osteoblastic pattern. Lateral radiograph shows a diffuse osteosclerotic pattern of metastatic disease. No evidence is present of bone expansion, scalloping, or coarsened trabeculae. D, E In another man with prostate carcinoma, the radiographic appearance (D) of the L1 vertebral body is osteoblastic. The involved vertebral body has undergone pathologic collapse. A bone scan from this patient (E) reveals increased accumulation of the radiopharmaceutical agent localized to the L1 vertebra (arrows). In skeletal metastasis secondary to prostate carcinoma, the osteoblastic pattern is seen in approximately 80 per cent of cases, and the osteolytic or mixed patterns constitute the remaining 20 per cent of cases.

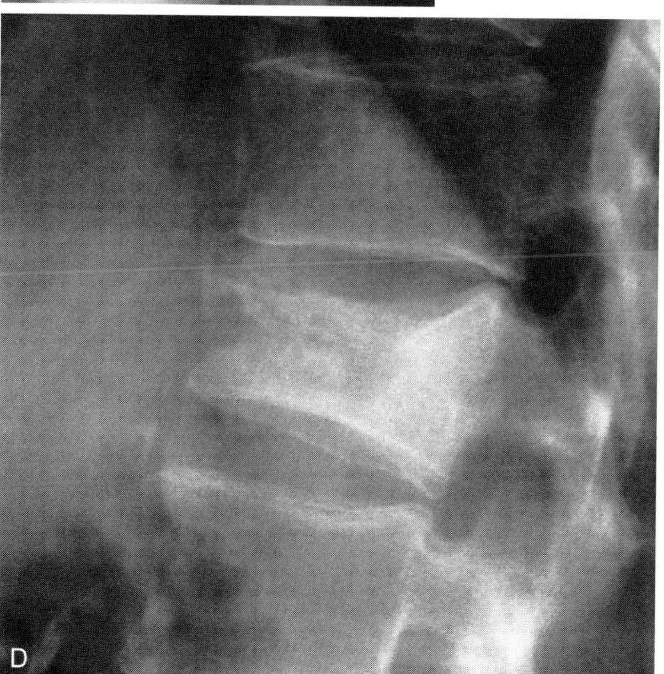

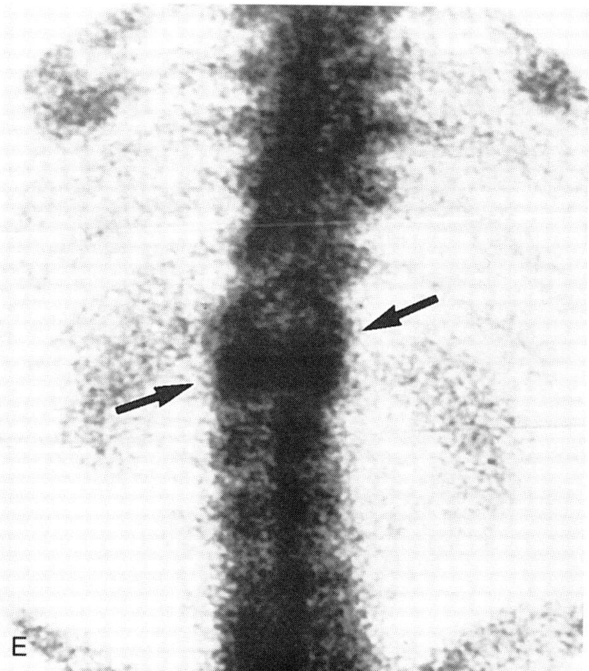

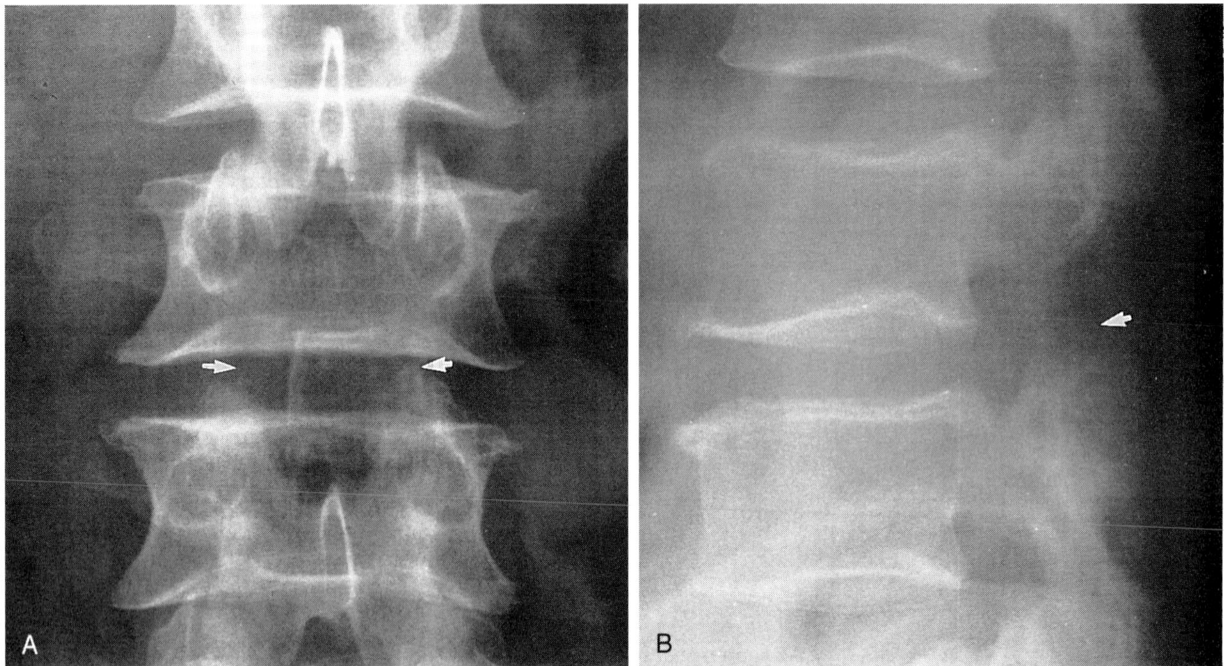

FIGURE 4–79. Skeletal metastasis: Osteolytic pattern.[96] In this patient, frontal (A) and lateral (B) radiographs demonstrate osseous destruction of the inferior articular processes (arrows), portions of the pedicles, the entire laminae, and the spinous process of the L3 vertebra.

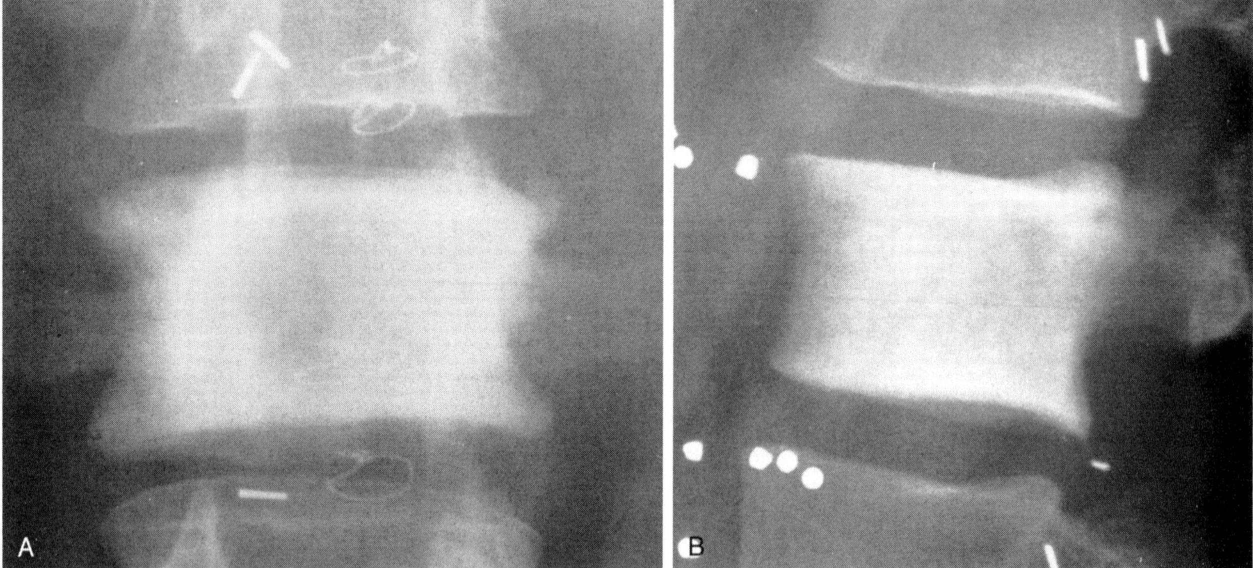

FIGURE 4–80. Chordoma: Ivory vertebra.[97] Frontal (A) and lateral (B) radiographs show osteosclerosis of the L2 vertebra of this 38-year-old man with chordoma. He developed neurologic signs and symptoms secondary to an epidural soft tissue mass and subsequently underwent a three-level laminectomy to decompress the spinal canal. Of incidental note are metal buckshot artifacts from an old hunting accident. Approximately 75 per cent of all reported chordomas occur in the vertebral column, sacrum, and coccyx.

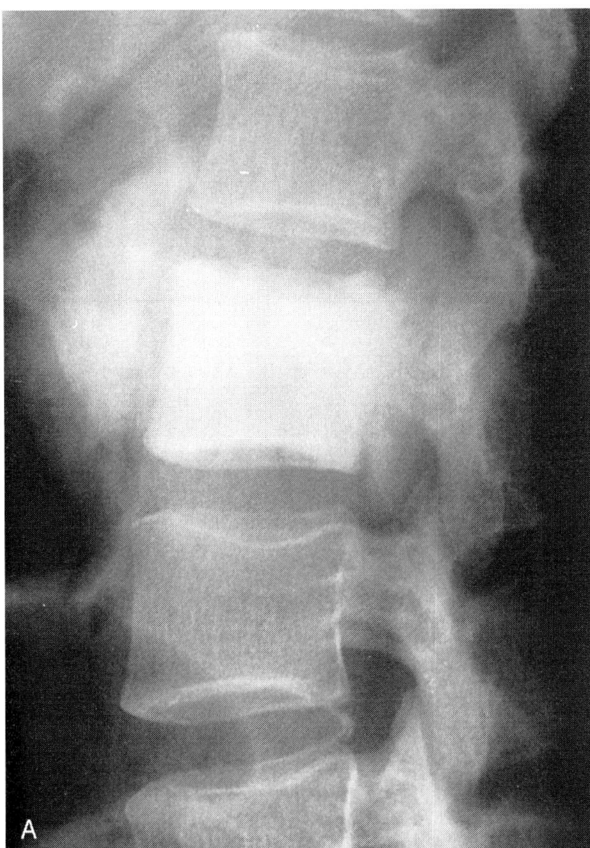

FIGURE 4–81. Osteosarcoma.[98] A 44-year-old woman had low back and leg pain. A Lateral radiograph reveals an osteosclerotic (ivory) vertebra and an associated radiodense mass in the soft tissues. B Transaxial CT scan shows the increased radiodensity of the vertebral body as well as paraspinal (open arrows) and epidural (arrows) extension of the neoplasm. C Sagittal T1-weighted (TR/TE, 700/20) spin echo magnetic resonance (MR) image demonstrates low signal intensity of the involved vertebral body. The histologic diagnosis was osteosarcoma. Osteosarcoma is a common primary malignant tumor of bone, but spinal osteosarcomas occur infrequently. Conventional osteosarcoma occurs most frequently in persons between the ages of 10 and 25 years, although it also affects older and younger patients. It is twice as common in men. The tumor may be osteoblastic, osteolytic, or more frequently a mixed appearance with both osteoblastic and osteolytic components. *(Courtesy of A. Deutsch, M.D., Los Angeles, California.)*

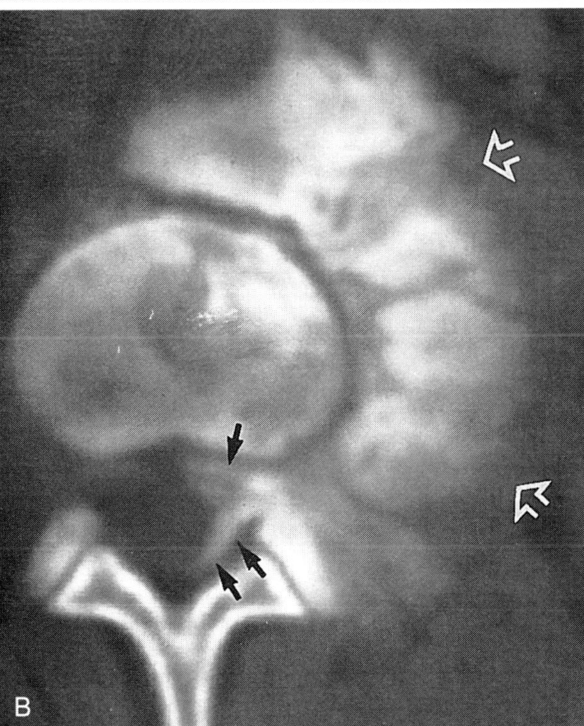

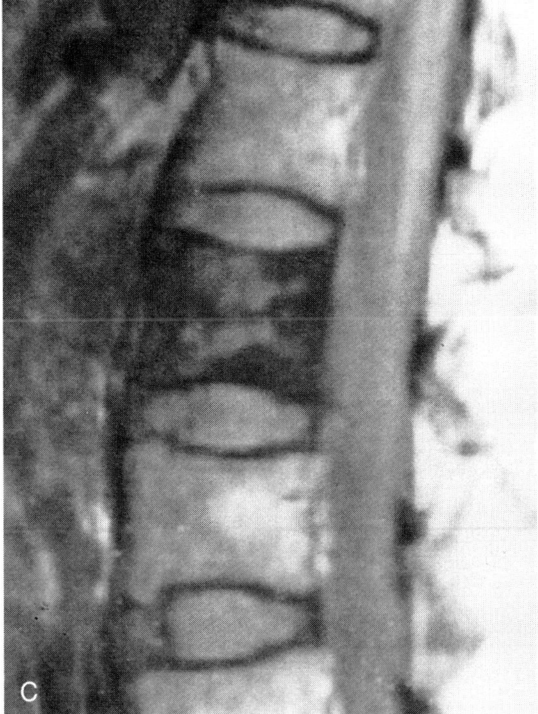

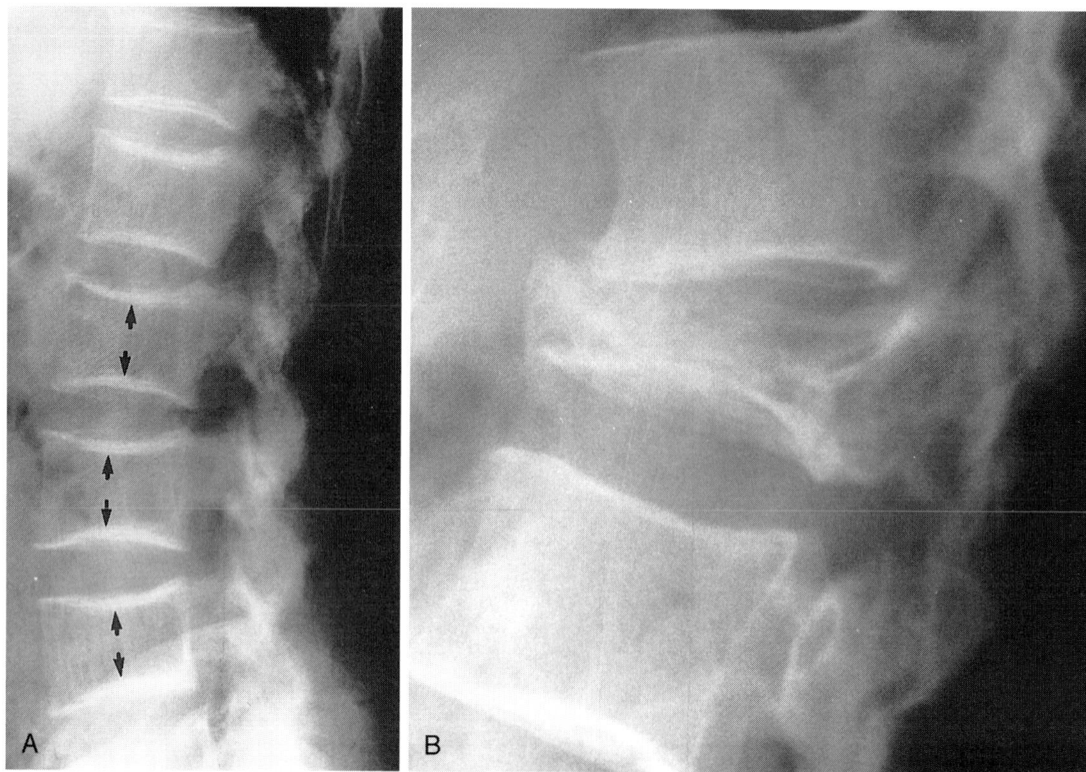

FIGURE 4–82. Plasma cell myeloma.[99, 100] A Diffuse osteopenia with increased radiolucency of the medullary portion of the vertebral bodies and early biconcave (fish) deformities (arrows) are seen in this patient with diffuse myeloma throughout the spine. The early changes of myeloma, as in this patient, are radiographically indistinguishable from the generalized osteoporosis of aging. B In this 40-year-old man, the L2 vertebra has undergone pathologic collapse. Plasma cell (multiple) myeloma is a common malignant disease of plasma cells that typically affects patients who are 60 to 70 years of age. It is particularly common in black persons. Clinically, these patients have bone pain, particularly in the back and chest, weakness, fatigue, fever, weight loss, bleeding, neurologic signs, and many other signs and symptoms. Serum electrophoresis is positive in 80 to 90 per cent of patients, and Bence Jones proteinuria is apparent in 40 to 60 per cent of patients with this disease. Classically, myeloma is first manifested as widespread osteolytic lesions with discrete margins, which appear uniform in size. Alternatively, diffuse osteopenia may be the only radiographic finding.

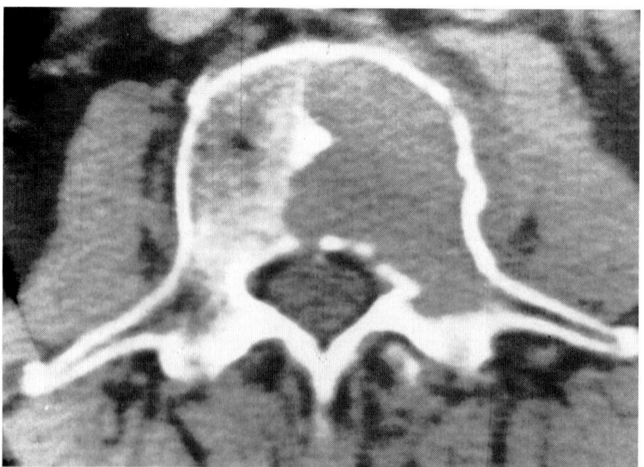

FIGURE 4–83. Plasmacytoma.[99] Transaxial CT scan of the lumbar spine in a patient with plasmacytoma shows medullary osteolysis of the left side of the lumbar vertebral body and a portion of the pedicle. Solitary plasmacytoma (solitary plasma cell myeloma), in comparison with multiple myeloma, is rare, affects younger patients (average age 50 years), can simulate giant cell tumor, and often results in neurologic manifestations. The lesion may be expansile and multicystic with thickened trabeculae, or it may be purely osteolytic. The spine is the most common site of involvement. Serum electrophoresis and Bence Jones proteinuria tests are not as reliable as they are in multiple myeloma.

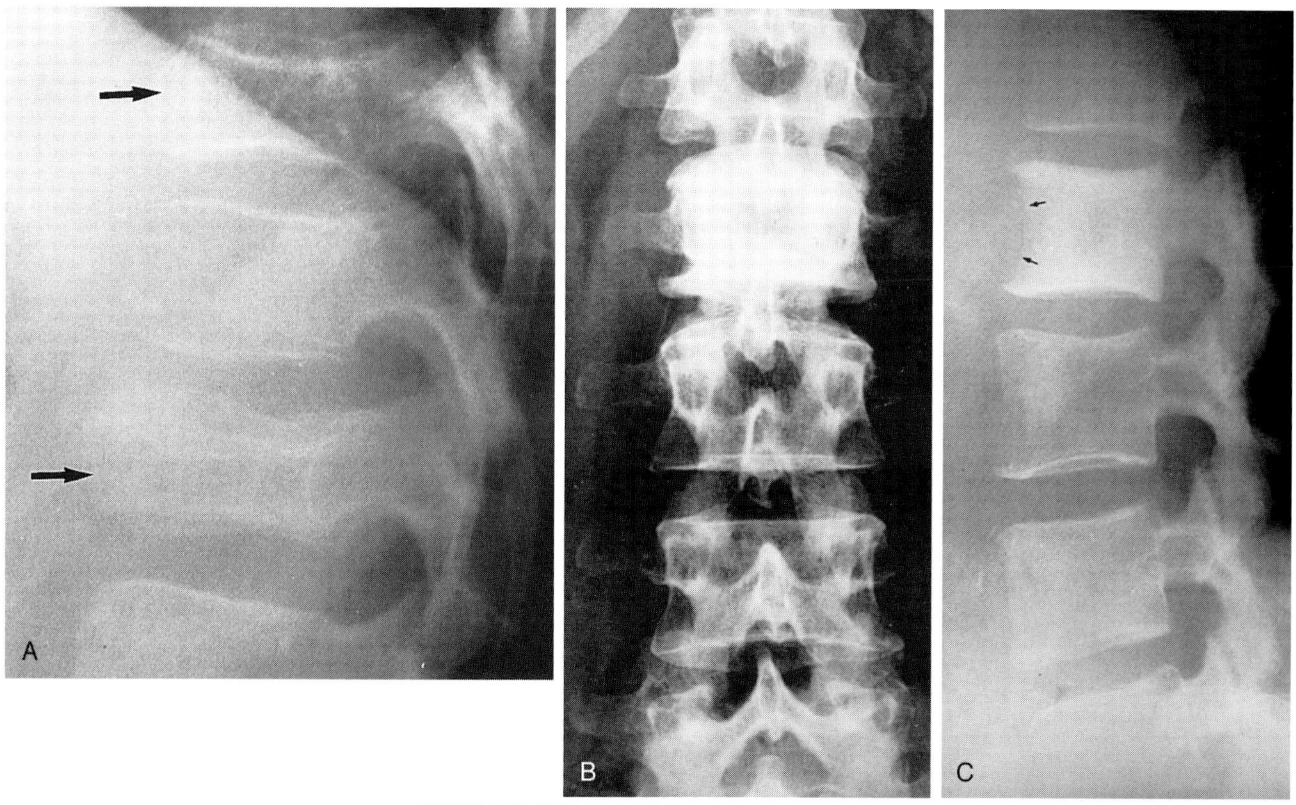

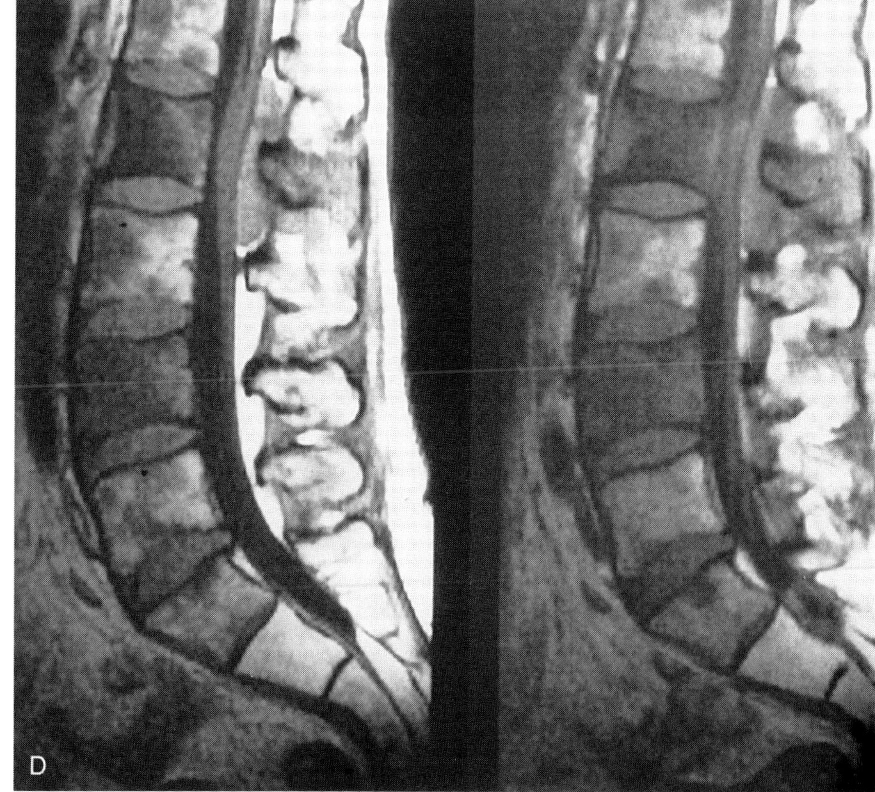

FIGURE 4–84. Hodgkin's disease.[95, 101] A Osteolytic pattern. Lateral radiograph of this child with Hodgkin's disease shows diffuse osteopenia and multiple biconcave collapsed vertebrae (arrows). B–D Osteosclerotic pattern—ivory vertebra. In a 38-year-old man, frontal (B) and lateral (C) radiographs reveal a diffusely sclerotic L2 vertebral body (ivory vertebra) (arrows). Mild anterior scalloping of the L2 vertebral body is evident on the lateral radiograph (arrows). Sagittal T1-weighted (TR/TE, 560/19) spin echo MR images (D) reveal inhomogeneous signal intensity of the bone marrow throughout the lumbar spine, indicating disseminated marrow infiltration with neoplastic lymphomatous cells. *(B–D, Courtesy of T. Hughes, M.D., Christchurch, New Zealand.)*

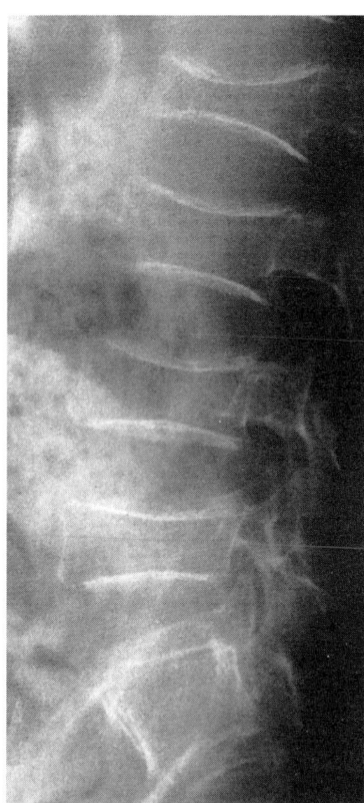

FIGURE 4–85. Acute childhood leukemia.[102] Multiple wedge-shaped and biconcave (fish vertebrae) compression fractures are apparent in this child with acute leukemia. Radiographic skeletal changes occur in up to 70 per cent of persons with acute childhood leukemia. These findings include diffuse osteopenia, osteolytic lesions, and, rarely, osteosclerosis.

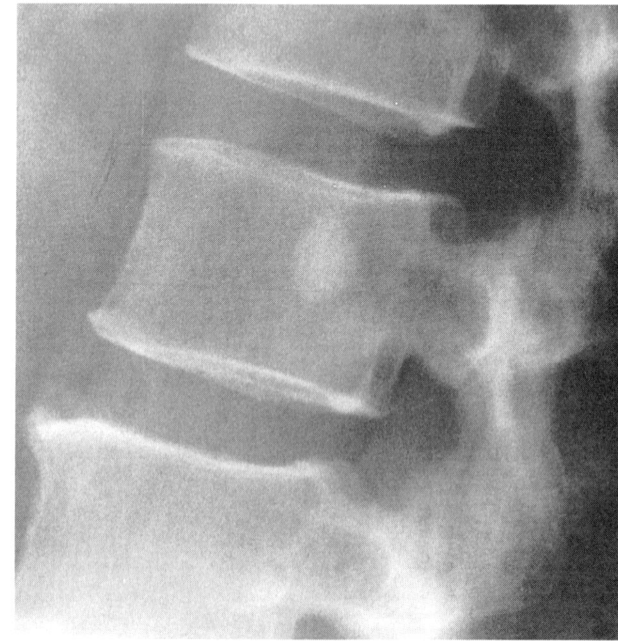

FIGURE 4–86. Enostosis (bone island).[103] Conventional radiograph shows a solitary, circular, osteosclerotic lesion in the L3 vertebral body of this 58-year-old man. A bone scan (not shown) revealed a slight increase in uptake of the bone-seeking radiopharmaceutical agent at the site of the lesion. Enostoses are solitary (or rarely multiple) discrete foci of osteosclerosis within the spongiosa of bone. They may be round, ovoid, or oblong and tend to be aligned with the long axis of the trabecular architecture. They often have a brush border composed of radiating osseous spicules that intermingle with the surrounding trabeculae of the spongiosa.

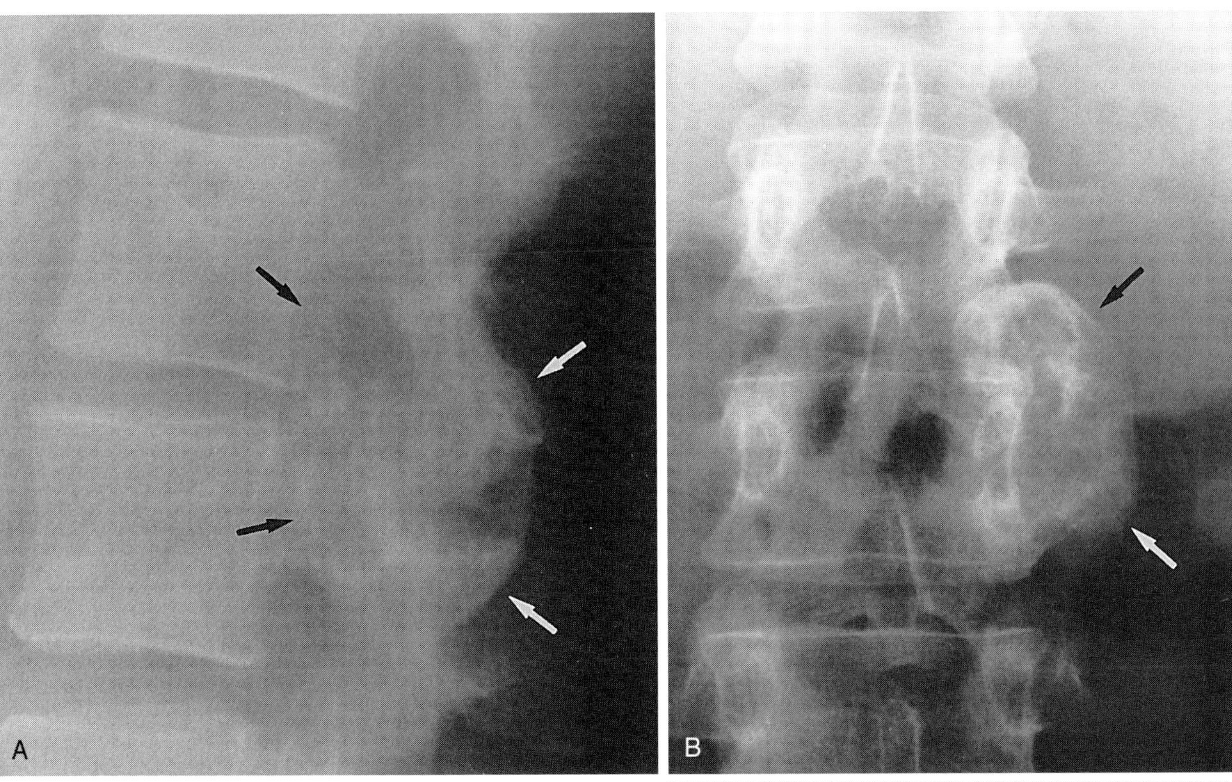

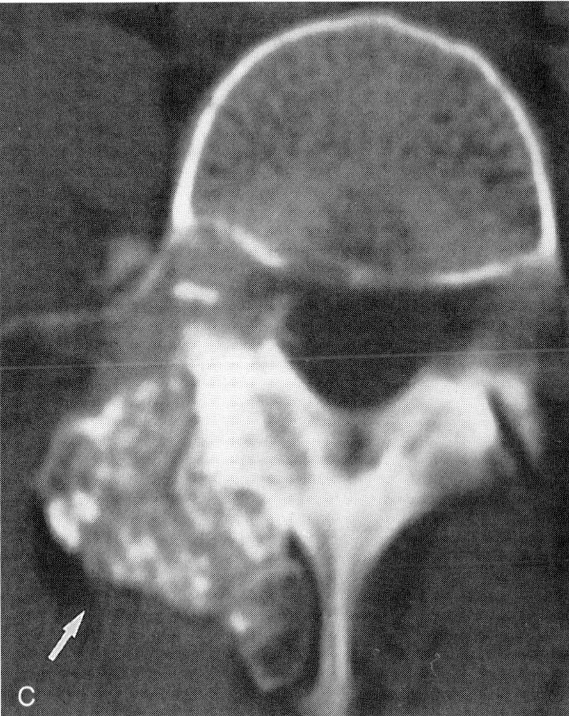

FIGURE 4–87. Spinal osteochondroma.[104, 105] A, B Anteroposterior (A) and lateral (B) radiographs reveal a large ovoid osteochondroma arising from the L3 neural arch (arrows). *(A, B, Courtesy of R. Kerr, M.D., Los Angeles, California.)* C In another patient, a transaxial CT bone window reveals a large broad-based osteocartilaginous mass arising from the right lamina and transverse process of the third lumbar vertebra (arrow). Spinal osteochondromas arise predominantly from the posterior elements and account for only about 2 per cent of all osteochondromas. These benign neoplasms are cartilage-covered osseous excrescences that arise from the surface of bones. They may be solitary or multiple (hereditary multiple exostoses). They may occur spontaneously or after accidental or iatrogenic injury or irradiation. Over 70 per cent of these painless, slow-growing masses occur in patients younger than 20 years of age. Symptoms and signs may occur after fracture, compression of adjacent neurovascular structures, or malignant transformation, a complication occurring in less than 1 per cent of solitary lesions and in up to 25 per cent of hereditary multiple exostoses. Rapid growth of an osteochondroma, although not pathognomonic of malignant transformation, is an ominous sign necessitating surgical removal of the lesion. *(C, Courtesy of L. White, M.D., Toronto, Ontario, Canada.)*

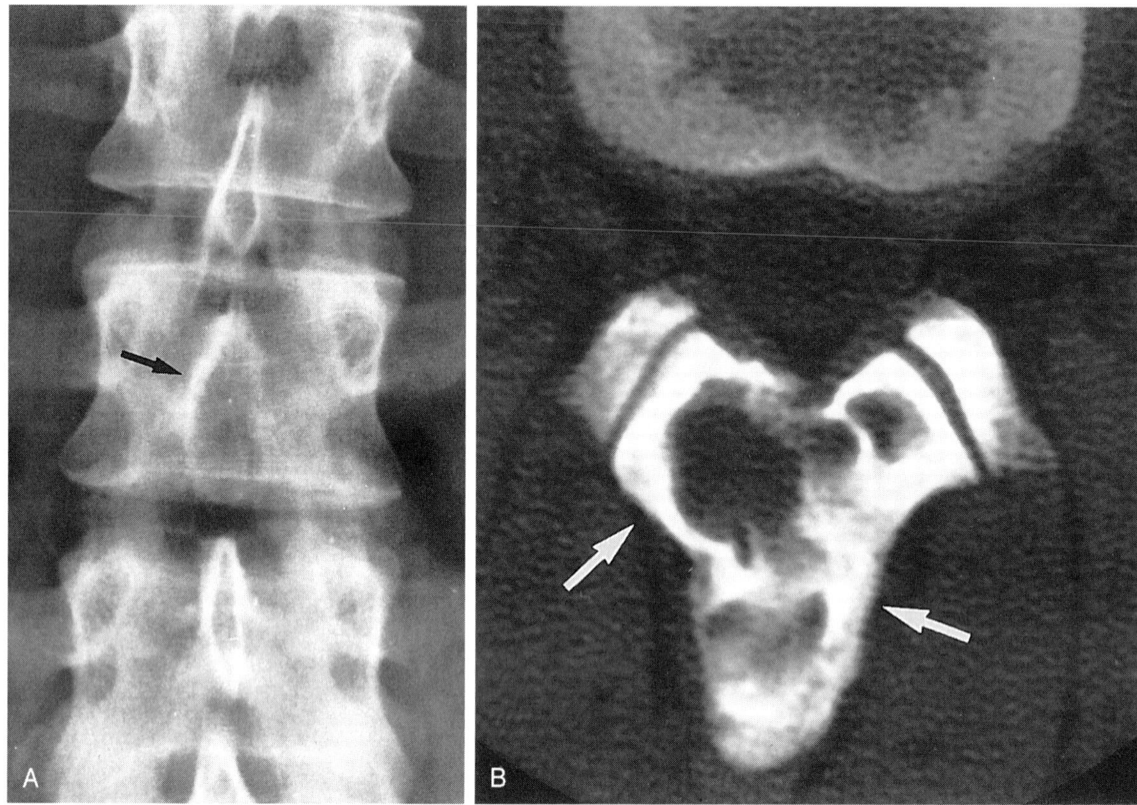

FIGURE 4–88. Aneurysmal bone cyst.[106, 107] An 18-year-old man had back pain. An anteroposterior radiograph **(A)** reveals subtle expansion and radiolucency of the L3 spinous process (arrow). A transaxial CT bone window image **(B)** more accurately shows the osseous expansion, osteosclerosis, and multiseptate osteolytic foci (arrows). Approximately 14 per cent of aneurysmal bone cysts occur in the spine, primarily in the posterior elements. This benign tumor is a thin-walled, expansile lesion containing blood-filled cystic cavities. Most aneurysmal bone cysts are discovered in patients younger than 20 years of age (age range, 3 to 70 years). Clinical findings include local pain and tenderness and, occasionally, neurologic symptoms. Acute, severe pain may accompany pathologic fracture of aneurysmal bone cysts. Ten per cent of spinal aneurysmal bone cysts recur within 6 months of surgery. *(Courtesy of P. Kindynis, M.D., Geneva, Switzerland.)*

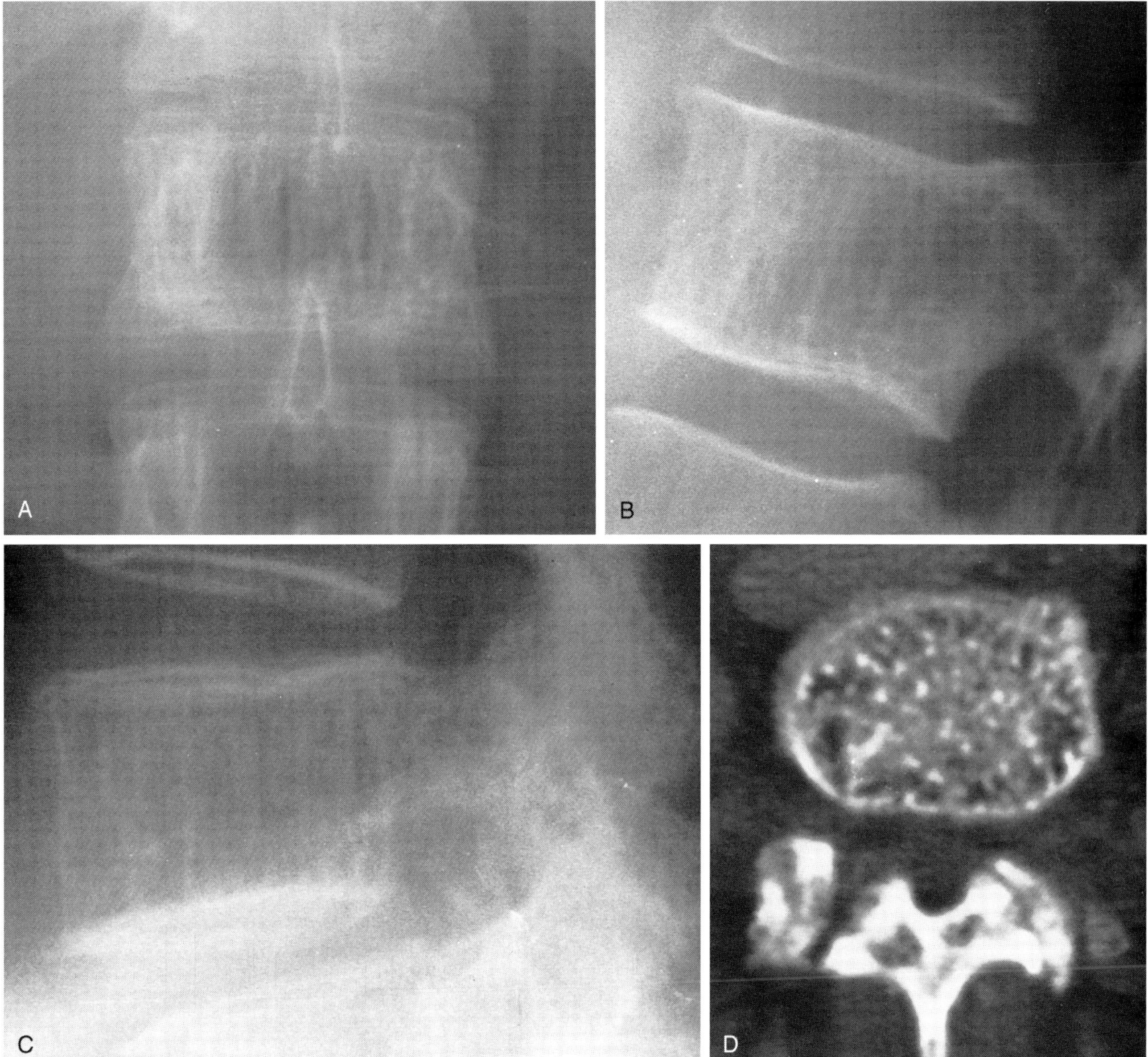

FIGURE 4–89. Hemangioma.[108] A, B 53-year-old man. Anteroposterior (A) and lateral (B) radiographs show the characteristic "corduroy cloth" appearance of a hemangioma affecting the L1 vertebral body. This appearance is produced by the coarse vertical radiodense striations that are interspersed among the relatively osteopenic spongiosa of the vertebral body. C, D This 77-year-old woman had multiple spinal hemangiomas. Lateral radiograph (C) demonstrates coarse vertical trabeculae within the osteopenic vertebral body and pedicle of L4. Transaxial CT image through L4 (D) demonstrates the radiodense vertical trabeculae within the osteopenic spongiosa of the vertebral body and posterior elements. Approximately 25 per cent of hemangiomas occur in the spine, and as such, are considered the most common benign neoplasm of the spine. (*C, D, Courtesy of V. Vint, M.D., San Diego, California.*)

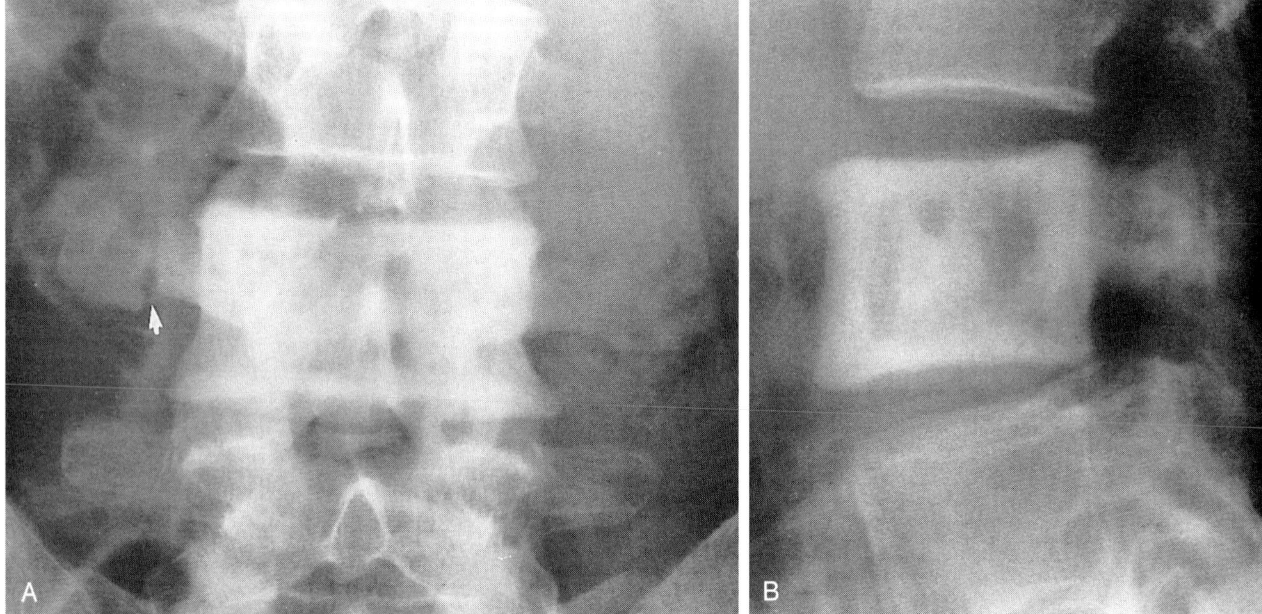

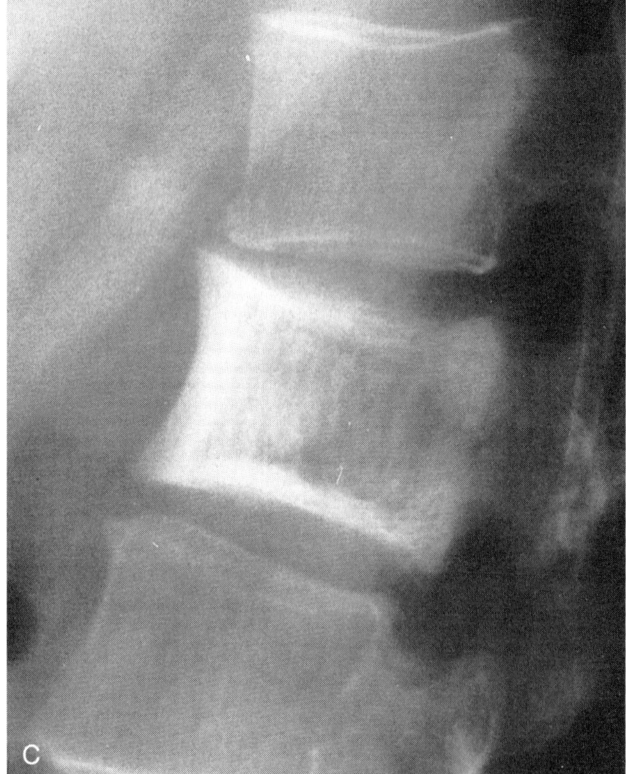

FIGURE 4–90. Paget's disease: Radiographic appearance.[109, 110] A, B Picture-frame vertebra. Frontal (A) and lateral (B) radiographs show sclerosis of the vertebral body and cortical thickening of its periphery. This pattern is best seen on the lateral film and is referred to as the picture frame vertebral body. A pathologic fracture of the transverse process also is seen (arrow). C In another patient, observe the characteristic picture-frame appearance with significant osseous enlargement of the vertebral body.

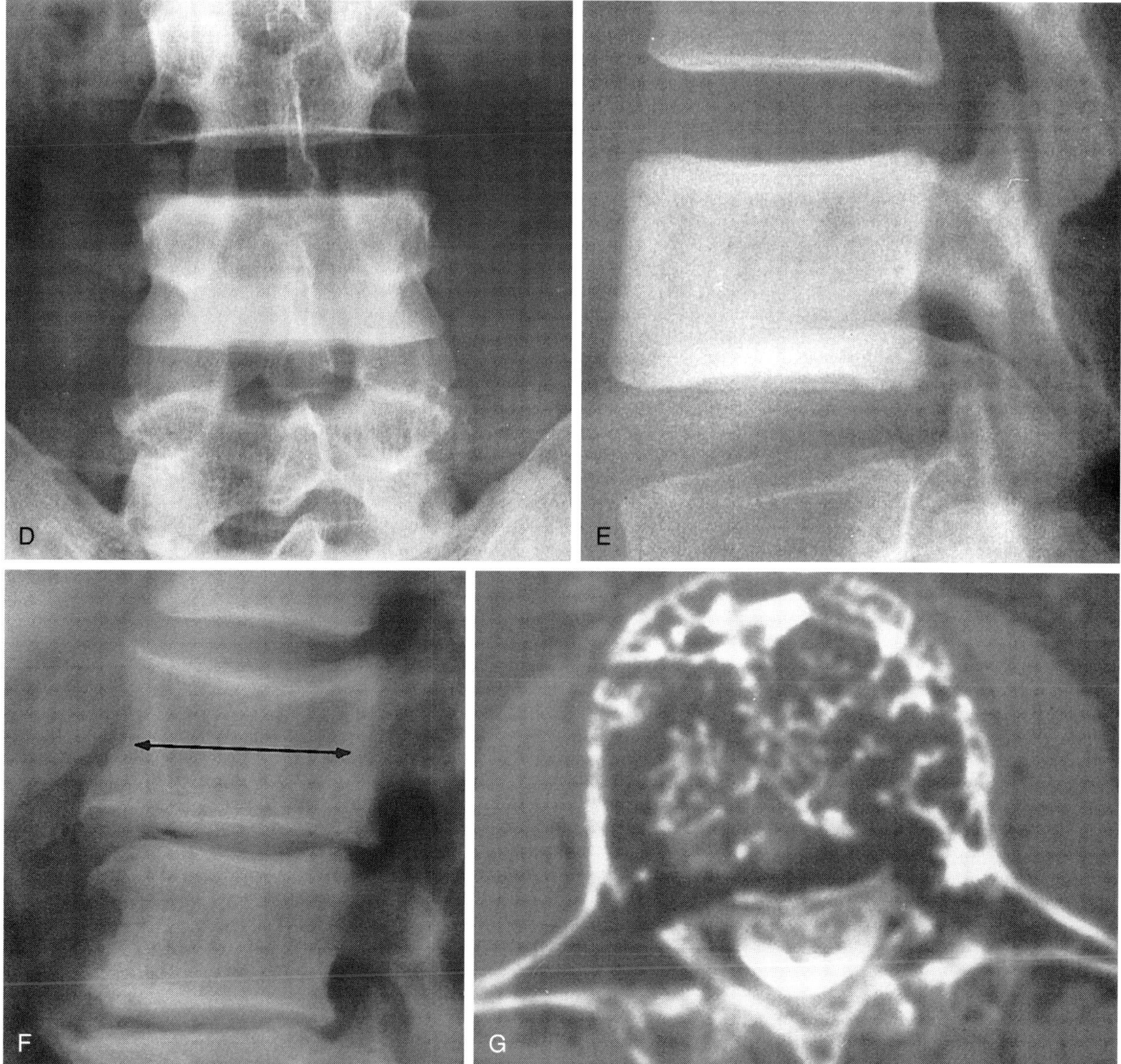

FIGURE 4–90 *Continued.* D, E Ivory vertebra. In a third patient, observe the diffuse sclerosis of the L4 vertebral body. The sclerosis dominates at the periphery of the vertebral body. Paget's disease is one cause of an ivory vertebra. F Vertebral enlargement. Observe the localized osseous expansion of the L2 vertebral body (double-headed arrow). G Computed tomographic (CT) findings. Transaxial CT–myelographic image shows the typical coarsened trabecular pattern, intervening radiolucency of medullary bone, and enlarged osseous contour typical of Paget's disease.

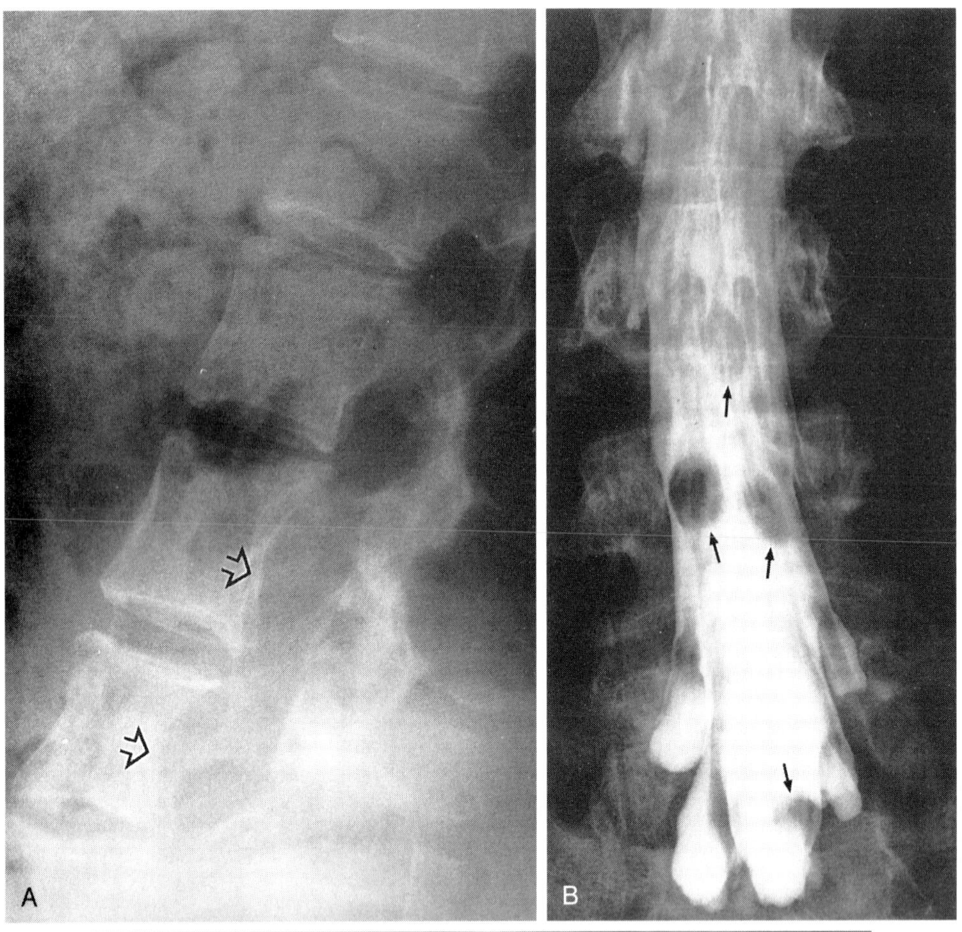

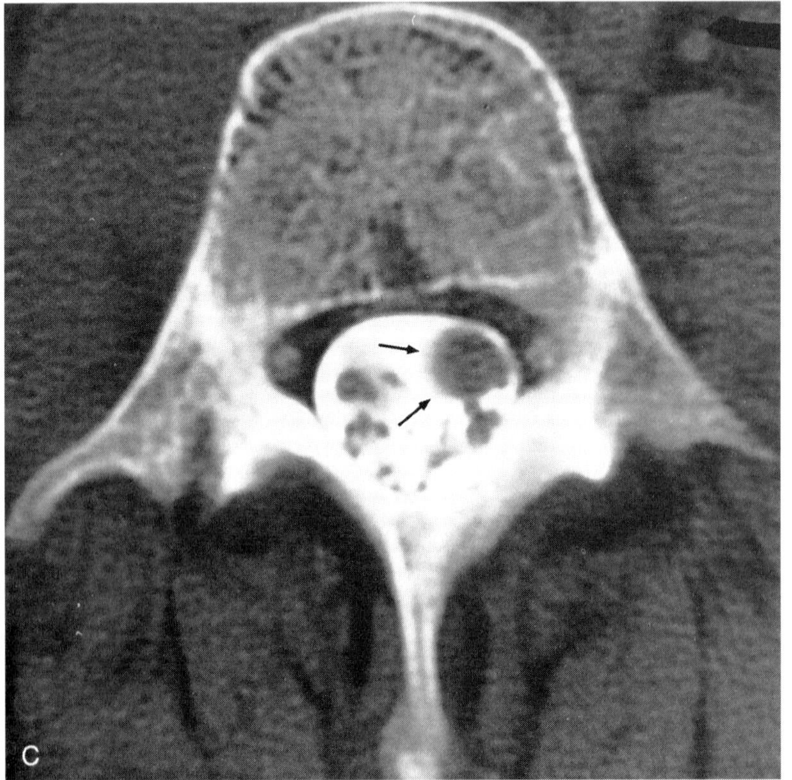

FIGURE 4–91. Neurofibromatosis Type I (von Recklinghausen's disease).[111] A Lateral radiograph shows posterior vertebral body scalloping and expansion primarily of the L3 and L4 neural foramina (open arrows). Scalloping results from intrinsic dysplastic changes in the bone or from neighboring dural ectasia rather than from mechanical pressure exerted by a local neurofibroma. *(A, Courtesy of G. Koors, D.C., Eugene, Oregon, and G. Smith, D.C., Portland, Oregon.)* B, C 23-year-old woman. Routine radiograph (B) and transaxial CT scan (C) after metrizamide myelography show lobulated intrathecal neurofibromas of varying size (arrows).

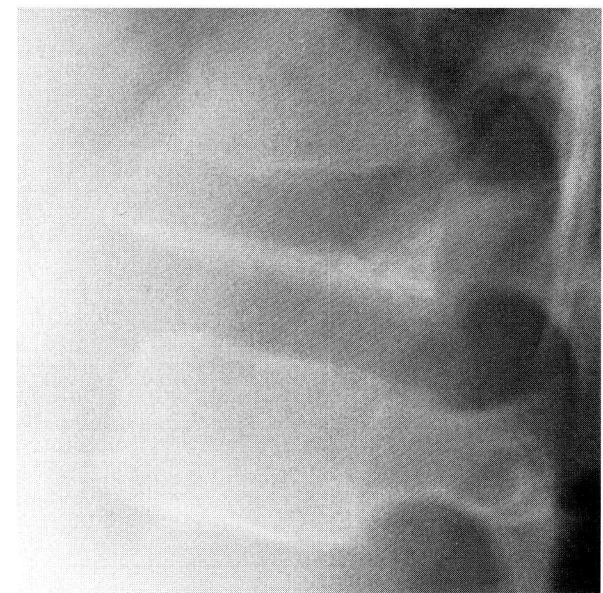

FIGURE 4–92. Langerhans' cell histiocytosis: Eosinophilic granuloma.[112, 113] Observe vertebra plana involving a thoracolumbar vertebral body. Eosinophilic granuloma of bone is the most frequent and mildest form of Langerhans' cell histiocytosis, a disease characterized by histiocytic infiltration of tissues. In addition to flattened vertebral bodies, eosinophilic granuloma may appear as bubbly, lytic, or expansile lesions without collapse. With healing, the height of the vertebral body may be reconstituted, a finding more common in younger persons.

TABLE 4–19. Metabolic and Hematologic Disorders Affecting the Lumbar Spine*

Entity	Figure(s)	Characteristics
Generalized osteoporosis[114–117]	4–93, 4–94, 4–95, 4–96	Uniform decrease in radiodensity, thinning of vertebral end plates, accentuation of vertical trabeculae Thoracolumbar region of the spine is the most frequent site of osteoporotic compression fractures Wedge-shaped vertebral deformities due to compression fractures are most common in thoracic spine; biconcave deformities are more common in the lumbar spine; vertebra plana deformities are more likely to be related to pathologic fracture due to plasma cell myeloma, skeletal metastasis, or other destructive process Quantitative bone mineral analysis (densitometry) is necessary for accurate assessment of the presence and extent of diminished bone mineral content Dual energy x-ray absorptiometry is the most widely used method to assess bone mineral density owing to its ease of use, high precision, and low radiation exposure to patients
Osteomalacia[118]	4–97	Diminished radiodensity and prominent coarsened trabeculae Vertebral compression fractures
Hypothyroidism[119]	4–98	Bullet vertebra, thoracolumbar gibbous deformity, osteopenia, delayed development, and widened disc spaces
Hyperparathyroidism[120]	4–99	Findings are most prominent in the thoracolumbar spine and include subchondral resorption at discovertebral junctions and the rugger-jersey spine—band-like osteosclerosis adjacent to the superior and inferior surfaces of the vertebral body
Renal osteodystrophy[120]		Rugger-jersey spine Vertebral fracture typically results in bioconcave thoracolumbar end-plate deformities
Acromegaly[121]	4–100	Elongation and widening of the vertebral bodies; ossification of the anterior portion of the disc; posterior scalloping of vertebral bodies occurs infrequently; increased disc height; premature degenerative disease, exuberant osteophytosis
Fluorosis[122]	4–101	Diffuse osteosclerosis and ossification of the posterior longitudinal ligament, prominent osteophytosis, and periostitis Differential diagnosis includes osteopetrosis, skeletal metastasis, other causes of diffuse osteosclerosis, and diffuse idiopathic skeletal hyperostosis (DISH) (Table 4–18)
Mastocytosis[123]	4–102	Spinal skeletal changes include combinations of diffuse or focal osteosclerosis, osteopenia, or osteolysis
Gaucher's disease[124]	4–103	Vertebral changes include diffuse vertebral body collapse and, infrequently, H-shaped, step-like defects in the vertebral bodies
Sickle cell anemia[125–127]	4–104	Diffuse osteopenia and H-shaped vertebra Compensatory vertical growth of adjacent vertebral bodies results in "tower vertebrae"
β-thalassemia[128]	4–105	Findings similar to those of sickle cell anemia with osteopenia, lace-like trabecular pattern, and, infrequently, H-shaped vertebral bodies
Osteonecrosis of the vertebral body[129]	4–106	Intravertebral vacuum phenomenon with pathologic vertebral body collapse Frequently associated with corticosteroid use

*See also Tables 1–13 to 1–16.

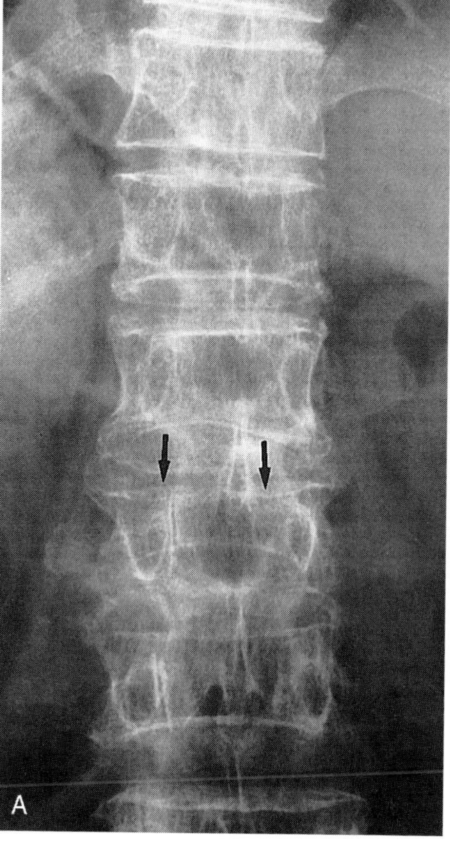

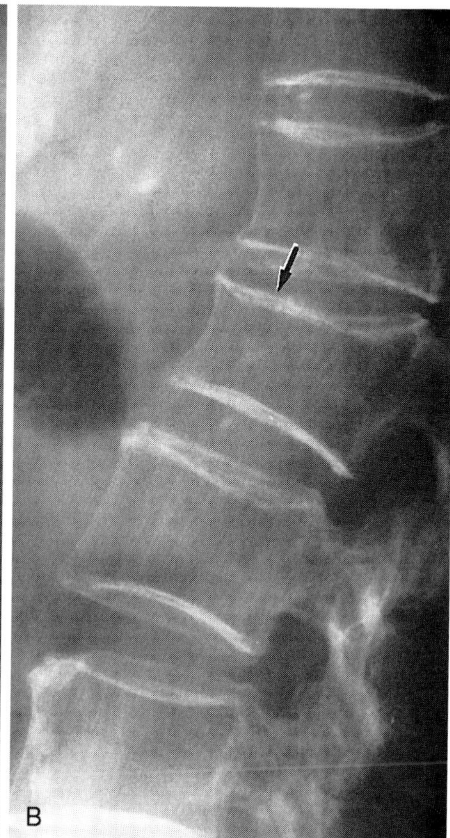

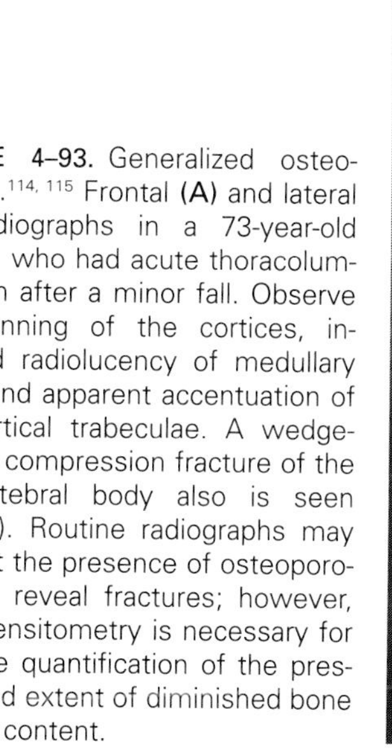

FIGURE 4–93. Generalized osteoporosis.[114, 115] Frontal (A) and lateral (B) radiographs in a 73-year-old woman who had acute thoracolumbar pain after a minor fall. Observe the thinning of the cortices, increased radiolucency of medullary bone, and apparent accentuation of the vertical trabeculae. A wedge-shaped compression fracture of the L2 vertebral body also is seen (arrows). Routine radiographs may suggest the presence of osteoporosis and reveal fractures; however, bone densitometry is necessary for accurate quantification of the presence and extent of diminished bone mineral content.

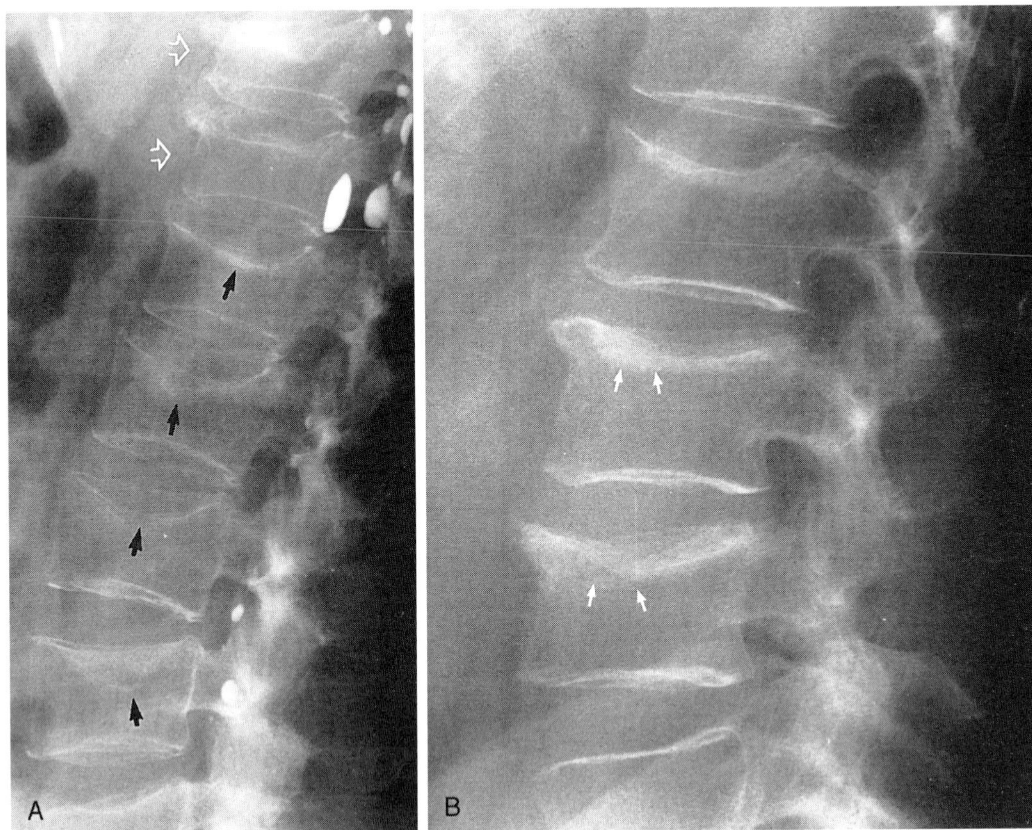

FIGURE 4–94. Osteoporosis: Spinal fractures.[114] **A** Senile osteoporosis. In this 68-year-old patient, observe the central end-plate deformities of all lumbar vertebral bodies (arrows) as well as wedge-shaped deformities of T11 and T12 (open arrows). Residual myelographic contrast material is incidentally seen within the spinal canal. **B** Corticosteroid-induced osteoporosis. This 67-year-old asthmatic man on long-term corticosteroid medication developed back pain but could not recall injuring his back. A radiograph shows diffuse, severe osteopenia, multiple biconcave vertebral body deformities, and a distinct zone of sclerosis along the superior end plates of L3 and L4 (arrows). This band of increased density is commonly encountered in steroid-induced vertebral fractures and may relate to abundant callus formation.

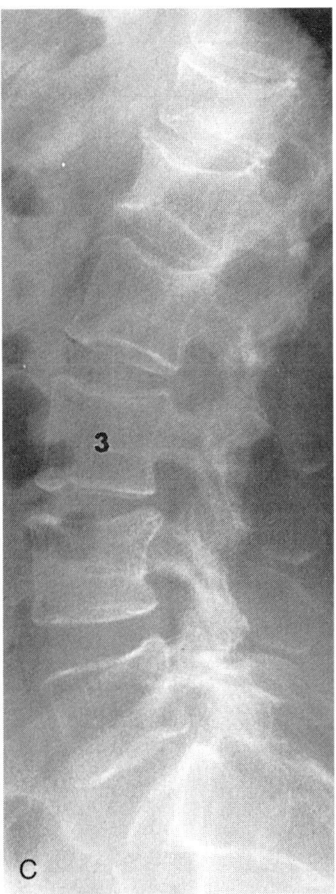

FIGURE 4–94 *Continued.* C–E Magnetic resonance (MR) imaging evaluation. A 49-year-old woman with acute back pain. In **C,** a routine radiograph shows diffuse osteopenia and vertebral end-plate fractures at T12, L1, and to a lesser extent, L4. In **D,** a sagittal T1-weighted (TR/TE, 800/16) fast spin echo MR image shows low signal intensity of the L4 marrow (arrow) and intermediate signal intensity of the T12 and L1 vertebral bodies (arrowheads). **E** A sagittal T2-weighted (TR/TE, 3800/102) fast spin echo MR image reveals high signal intensity in the L1 and L4 bodies (arrows), indicating that these two fractures are probably acute. The T12 vertebral body shows no hyperintensity, indicating that it most likely occurred at an earlier time. Of incidental note is a focus of high signal intensity in the L5 vertebral body on both T1- and T2-weighted images, characteristic of a hemangioma.

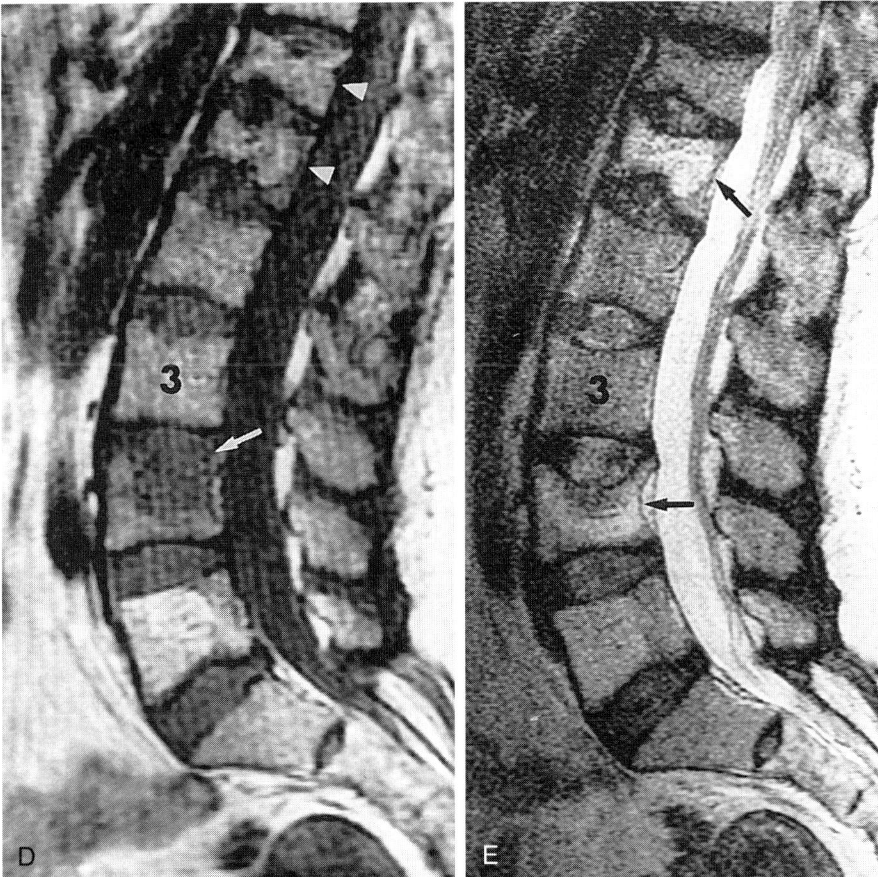

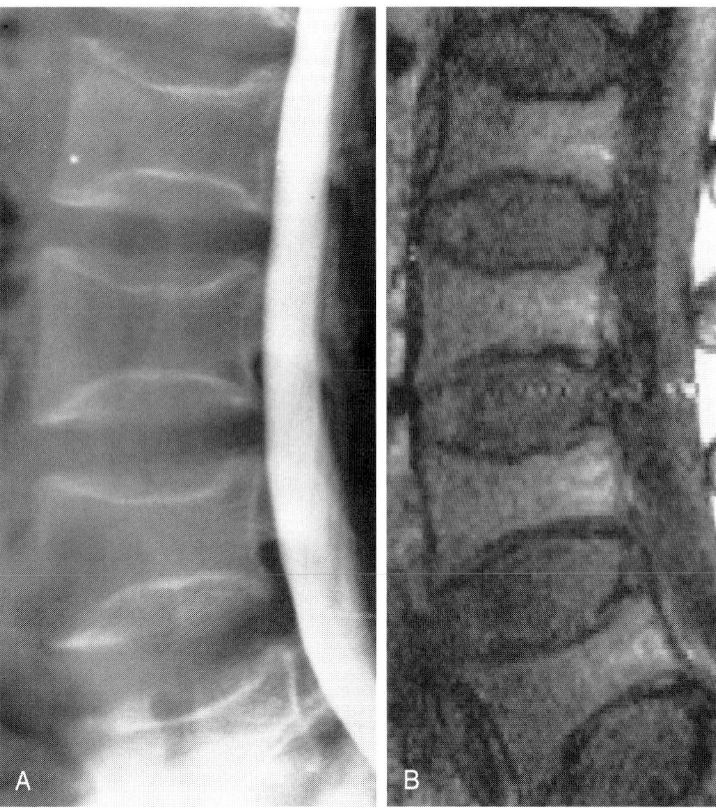

FIGURE 4–95. Corticosteroid-induced osteoporosis: Vertebral collapse.[116] This 22-year-old woman had received long-term corticosteroid medication as a child. A Lateral radiograph obtained during a myelographic examination shows diffuse osteopenia and widespread biconcave vertebral end-plate deformities. B Sagittal T1-weighted (TR/TE, 200/26) spin echo magnetic resonance (MR) image reveals the compressed vertebral bodies. Biconcave vertebral fractures often are termed "fish vertebrae" because they resemble the shape of normal vertebrae in fish. Osteoporosis and fractures may occur as a result of excessive exogenous corticosteroid administration or endogenous corticosteroid secretion, such as in Cushing's disease. *(Courtesy of G. Greenway, M.D., Dallas, Texas.)*

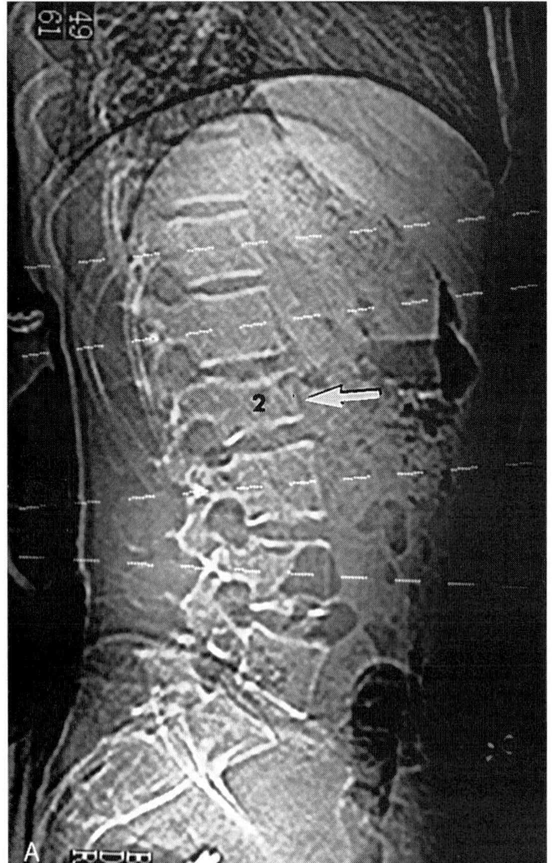

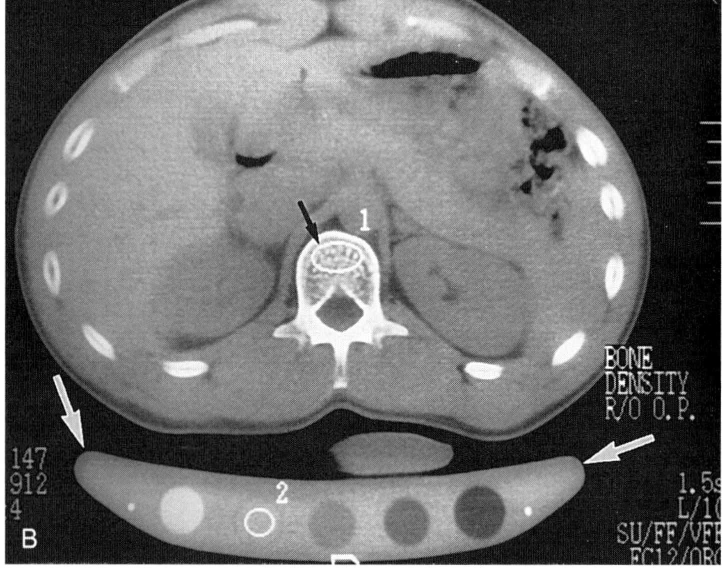

FIGURE 4–96. Quantitative bone mineral analysis (densitometry).[115, 117] A, B Quantitative computed tomography (QCT). In A, a lateral scout view localizes the midplane of four vertebral bodies to be sampled. A compression fracture of the L2 vertebral body is seen (arrow). In B, an 8- to 10-mm thick transaxial section is obtained at each level to be sampled. An oval cursor (black arrow) is positioned anteriorly within the spongiosa portion of the vertebral body that contains purely trabecular bone. During acquisition of the sections, the patient lies supine on a calibration phantom device with compartments containing solutions of K_2HPO_4 of predetermined densities (white arrows). The precise bone mineral density within the trabecular bone of the vertebral body is then computed by comparing it with these calibrated densities.

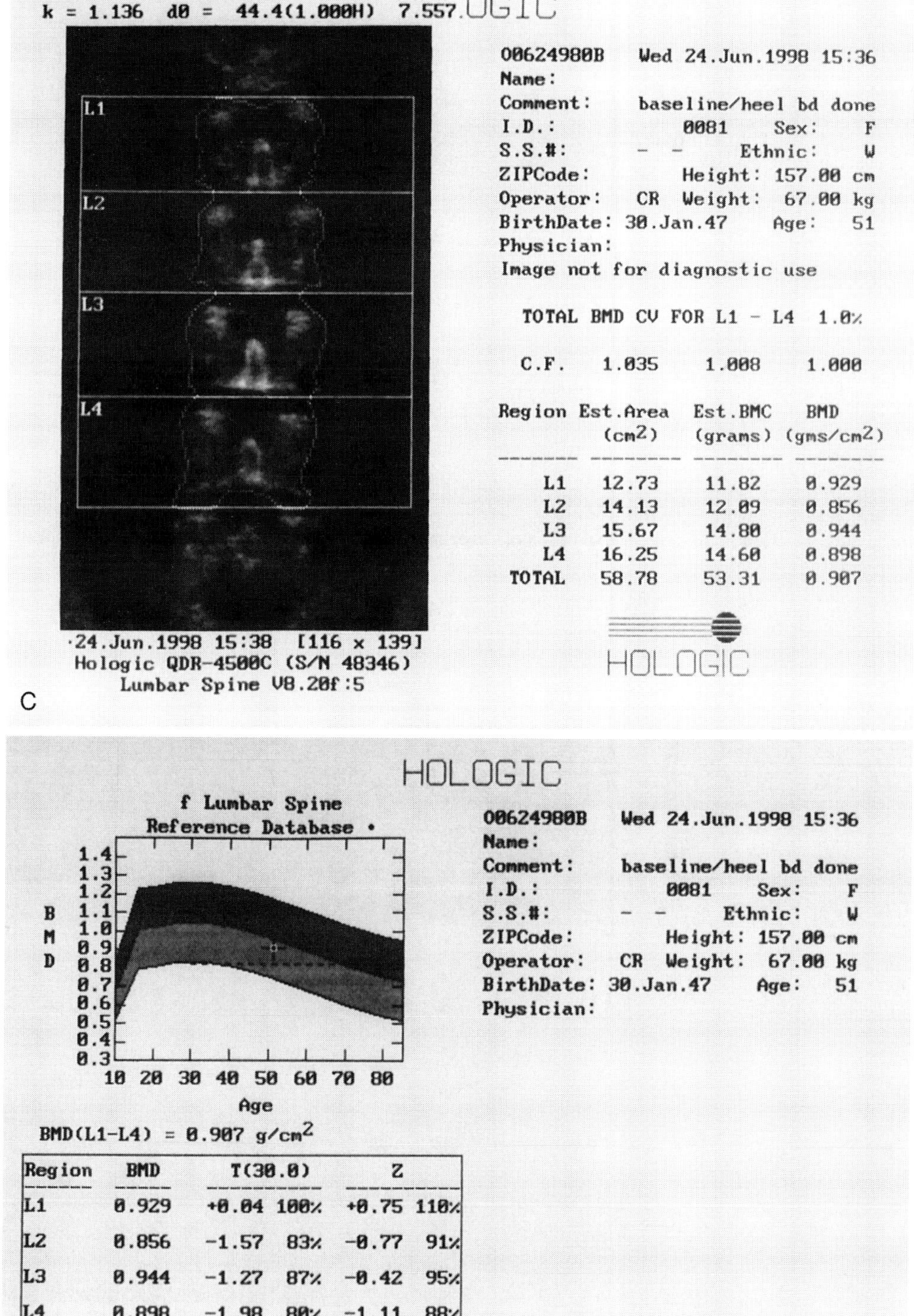

FIGURE 4–96 *Continued.* C, D Dual energy x-ray absorptiometry (DXA). C shows the lumbar spine as depicted on a DXA display and printout. Measured sites include the L1 to L4 vertebral bodies. For each region of interest, the area (cm²), bone mineral content (g), and bone mineral density (g/cm²) are computed. In D, further evaluation includes comparing the patient's bone mineral density with normal peak bone mass (T-score) and an age-matched (Z-score) control population, both of which are predetermined in a reference database. With both QCT and DXA, the patient's bone mineral density is expressed in terms of standard deviations from the normal, information that can be applied to management, prognosis, and estimation of fracture risk.

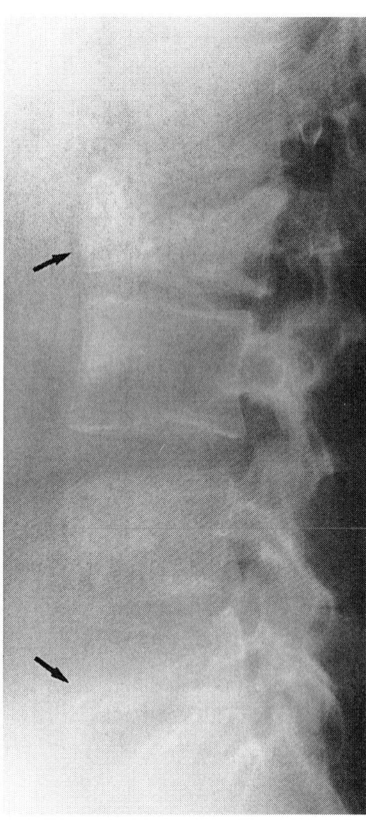

FIGURE 4–97. Osteomalacia: Spine fractures.[118] This young man with epilepsy had been on long-term phenytoin (Dilantin) therapy. He sustained compression fractures of the L2 and L5 vertebral bodies (arrows). Observe the diffuse osteopenia and abundant sclerosis associated with the L2 vertebral body. *(Courtesy of P. Fenton, M.D., Kingston, Ontario, Canada.)*

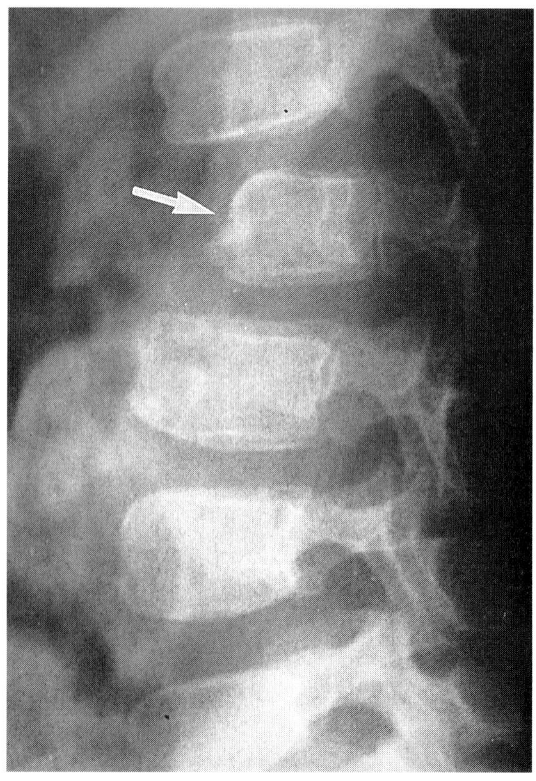

FIGURE 4–98. Hypothyroidism: Bullet vertebra.[119] A characteristic finding in cretinism is the thoracolumbar bullet-shaped vertebra (arrow). Additional spinal changes observed in hypothyroidism include gibbous deformity, osteoporosis, delayed epiphyseal development and ossification, and widened disc spaces.

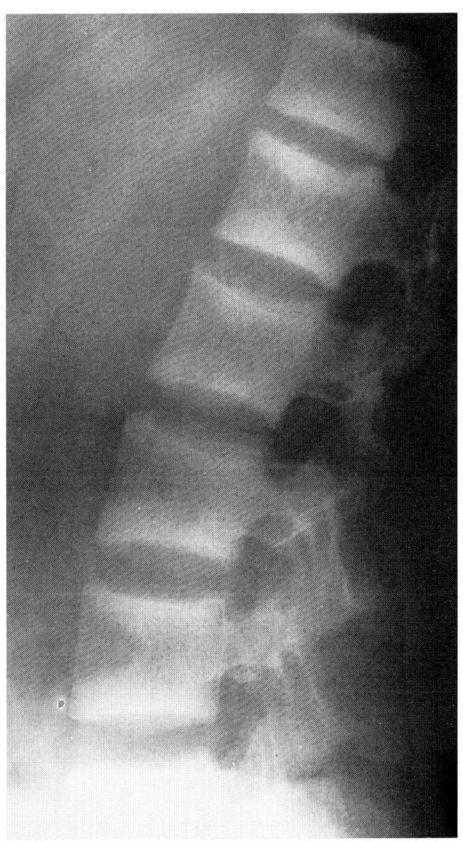

FIGURE 4–99. Hyperparathyroidism: Rugger-jersey spine.[120] Observe the horizontal bands of osteosclerosis affecting the superior and inferior aspects of the lumbar vertebral bodies. This sclerosis may disappear after treatment. Additional vertebral manifestations of hyperparathyroidism include diffuse osteopenia or osteosclerosis.

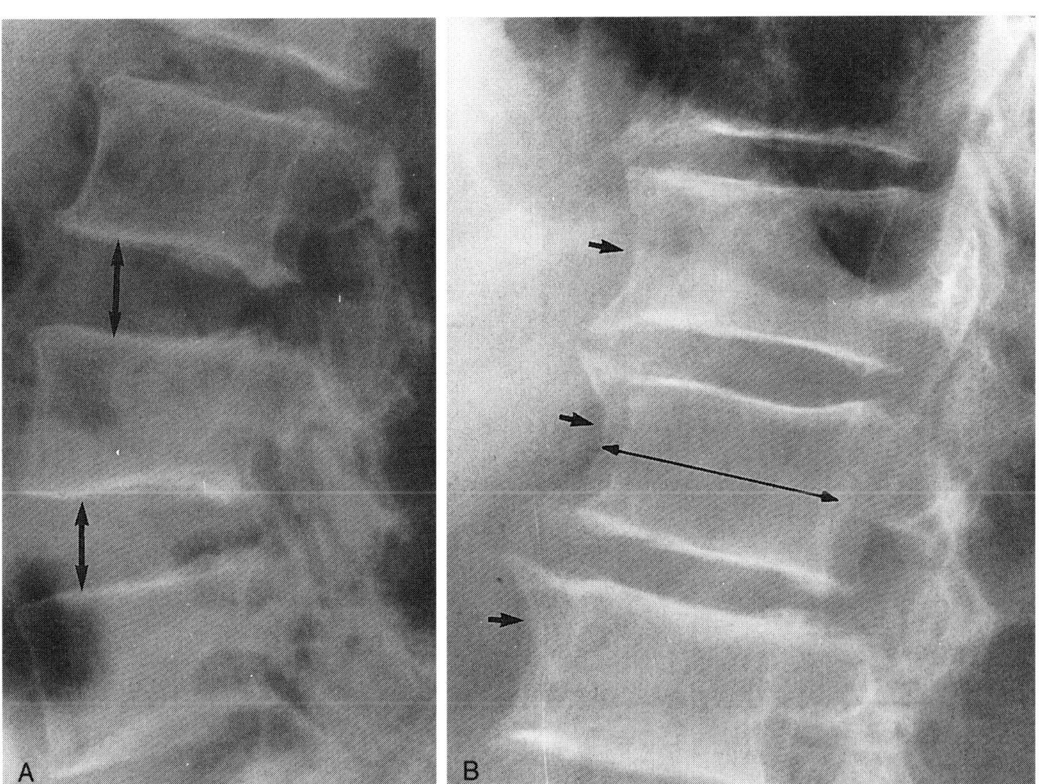

FIGURE 4–100. Acromegaly.[121] A Prominent disc space widening (double-headed arrows) is seen throughout the lumbar spine in this 53-year-old man with long-standing acromegaly. B In another patient, a 72-year-old man, thick flange-like bone proliferation at the anterior aspects of the vertebral bodies (arrows) contributes to an increased sagittal diameter of each vertebral body (double-headed arrow). Hypersecretion of growth hormone (somatotropin) from pituitary adenomas or hyperplasia in adults results in radiographic changes that relate to overgrowth of bone and soft tissues.

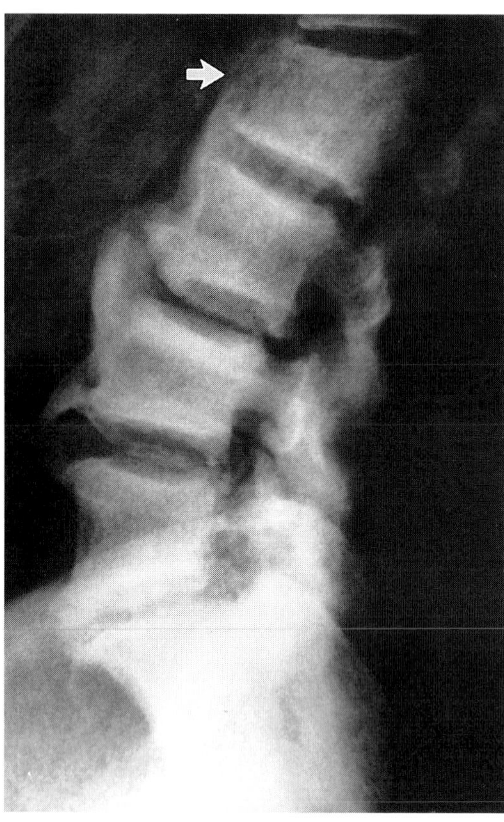

FIGURE 4–101. Iatrogenic fluorosis.[122] Long-term sodium fluoride was administered to this 80-year-old woman for treatment of osteoporosis. Extensive ossification of the paraspinal ligaments and generalized increased radiodensity of the spine are seen. A compression fracture of the L2 vertebral body (arrow) occurred prior to the fluoride treatment.

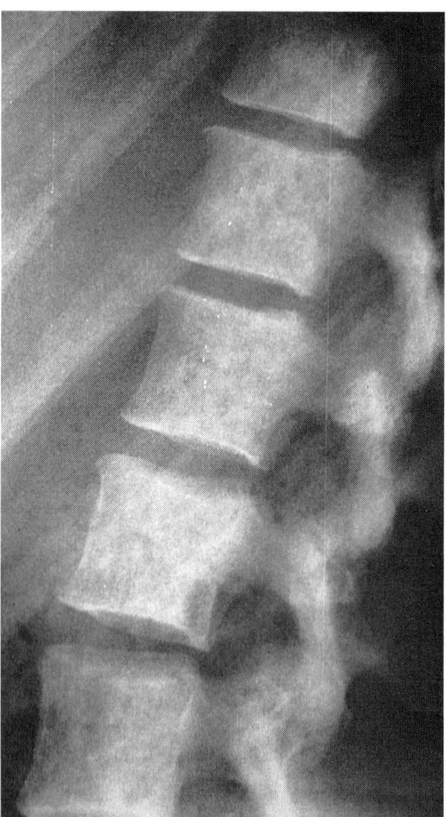

FIGURE 4–102. Mastocytosis.[123] Widespread, patchy osteosclerosis throughout the lumbar spine is evident in this 38-year-old woman with systemic mastocytosis. *(Courtesy of B. Holtan, M.D., Rock Springs, Wyoming.)*

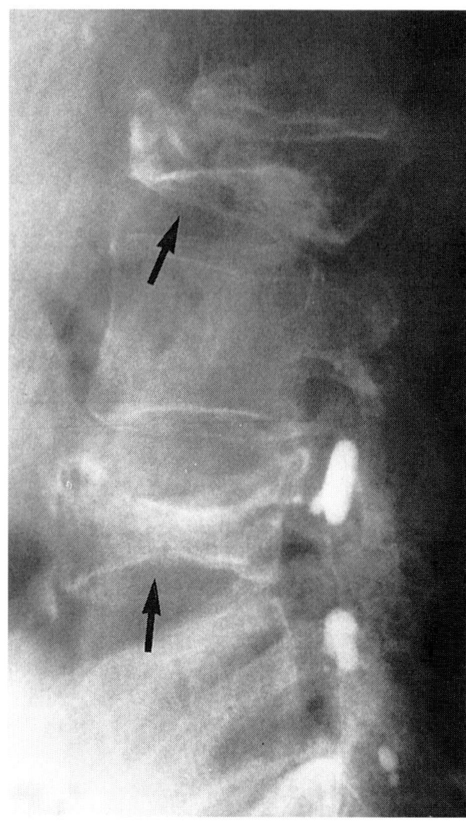

FIGURE 4–103. Gaucher's disease.[124] Observe the multiple collapsed vertebrae (arrows) in this patient with Gaucher's disease. *(Courtesy of A. Brower, M.D., Norfolk, Virginia.)*

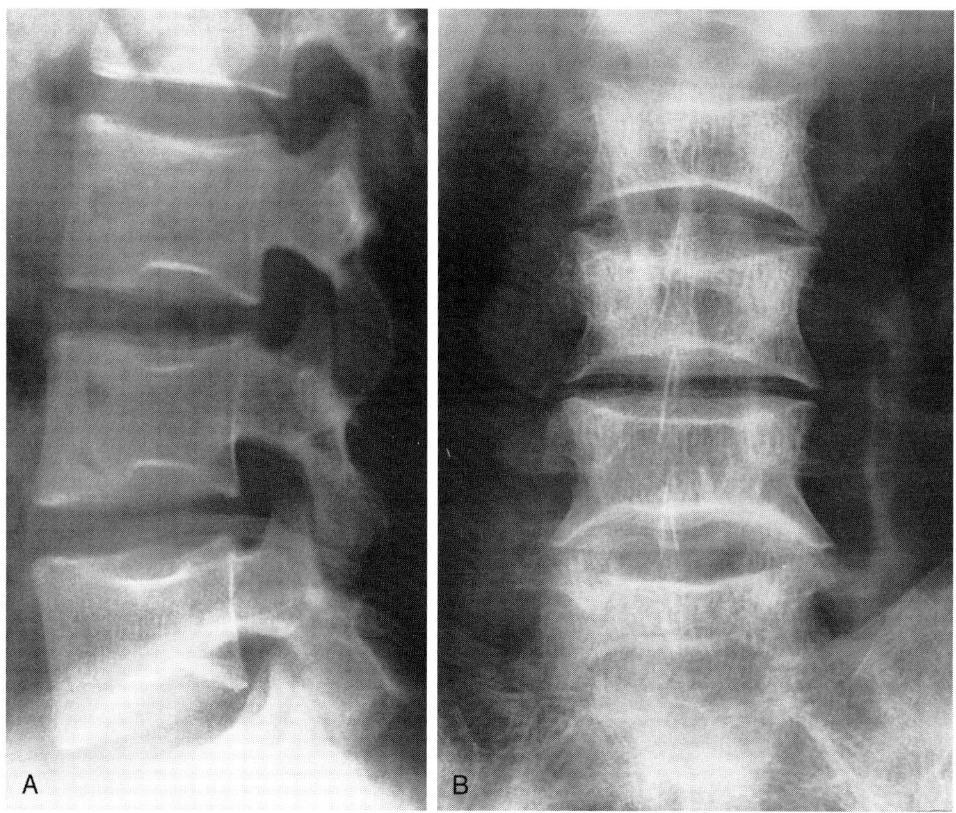

FIGURE 4–104. Sickle cell anemia.[125–127] A Radiograph from this 21-year-old man with anemia reveals several central indentations of osteopenic vertebral bodies. B Sickle cell hemoglobin C disease. In this 24-year-old man, the lumbar spine is osteosclerotic, the trabeculae are prominent, and the vertebral bodies exhibit H-shaped central end-plate depressions.

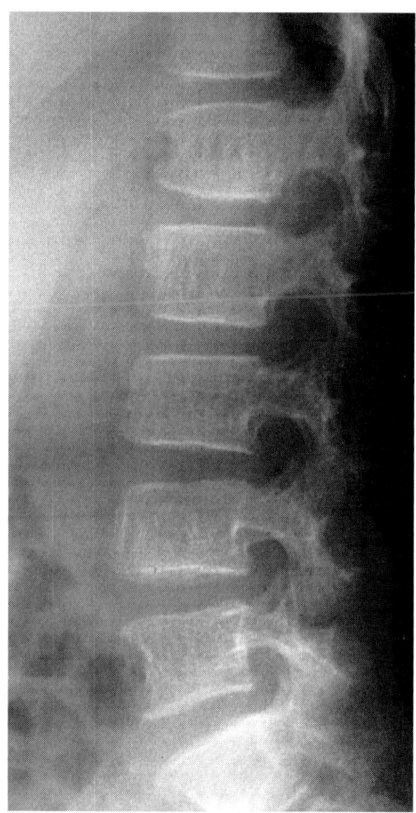

FIGURE 4–105. β-thalassemia.[128] In this 11-year-old boy, marked osteopenia and lace-like trabeculae are observed throughout the lumbar spine.

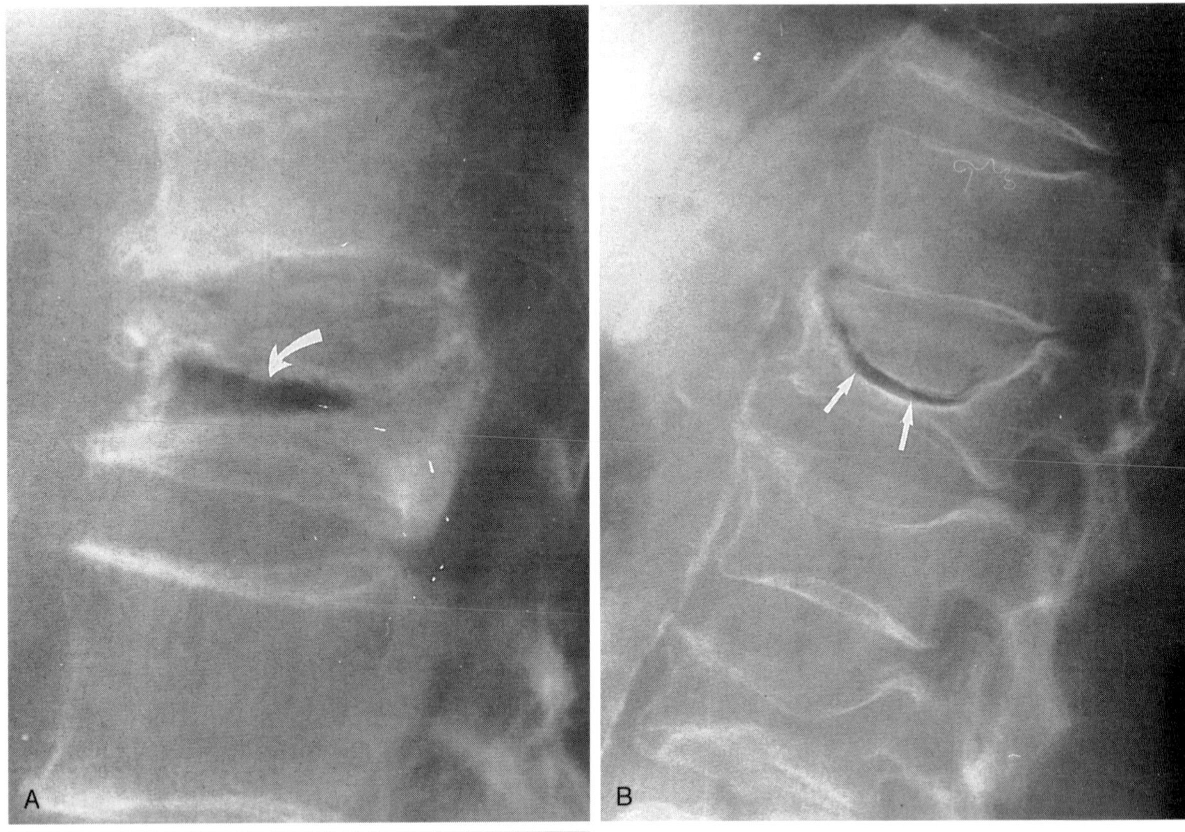

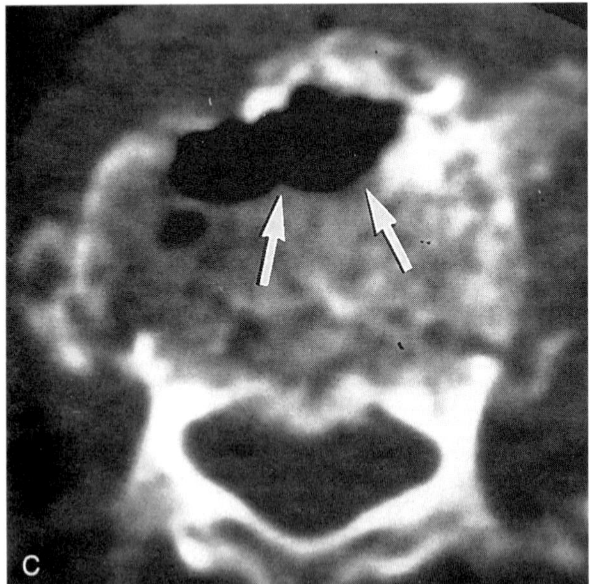

FIGURE 4–106. Corticosteroid-induced osteonecrosis and vertebral collapse.[129] A This 79-year-old woman on long-term corticosteroid medication had acute low back pain. A lateral radiograph reveals diffuse osteopenia. Upper lumbar vertebral collapse is associated with a radiolucent collection of gas within the fractured body (curved arrow). Gas within the vertebral body is termed the intravertebral vacuum cleft and is a sign of vertebral osteonecrosis, often associated with the use of corticosteroid medication. *(A, Courtesy of P. Kindynis, M.D., Geneva, Switzerland.)* B In another patient, diffuse osteopenia and multiple biconcave compression fractures are seen. A prominent intravertebral vacuum cleft is present (arrows). This finding should not be confused with intradiscal gas characteristically seen with degenerative disc disease. C In a third patient, the gas collection within the vertebral body (arrows) is well demonstrated on this transaxial CT image. *(C, Courtesy of G. Greenway, M.D., Dallas, Texas.)*

TABLE 4–20. **Lumbar Spine Surgery***

Type of Surgery	Figure(s)	Indications	Complications
Spinal fusion[130]	4–107	Pathologic disc processes Instability	Spinal cord compression Thecal sac encroachment Screw malpositioning Fracture, displacement, or malposition of screw, plate, or wire Osteomyelitis Failed interbody plug fusion Pseudarthrosis Epidural hematoma Cerebrospinal fluid leak
Laminectomy and facetectomy[131–133]	4–108, 4–109, 4–110	Decompression for spinal stenosis	Postlaminectomy instability Postlaminectomy kyphosis Epidural hematoma Osteomyelitis Neural arch stress fractures
Spinal instrumentation devices[134]	4–111	Direct current stimulators Plates, screws, and other orthopedic appliances	Instrumentation failure

*Adapted from Pathria MN, Garfin SR: Imaging after spine surgery. *In* Resnick D (ed): Diagnosis of Bone and Joint Disorders. 3rd Ed. Philadelphia, WB Saunders, 1995, p 525.

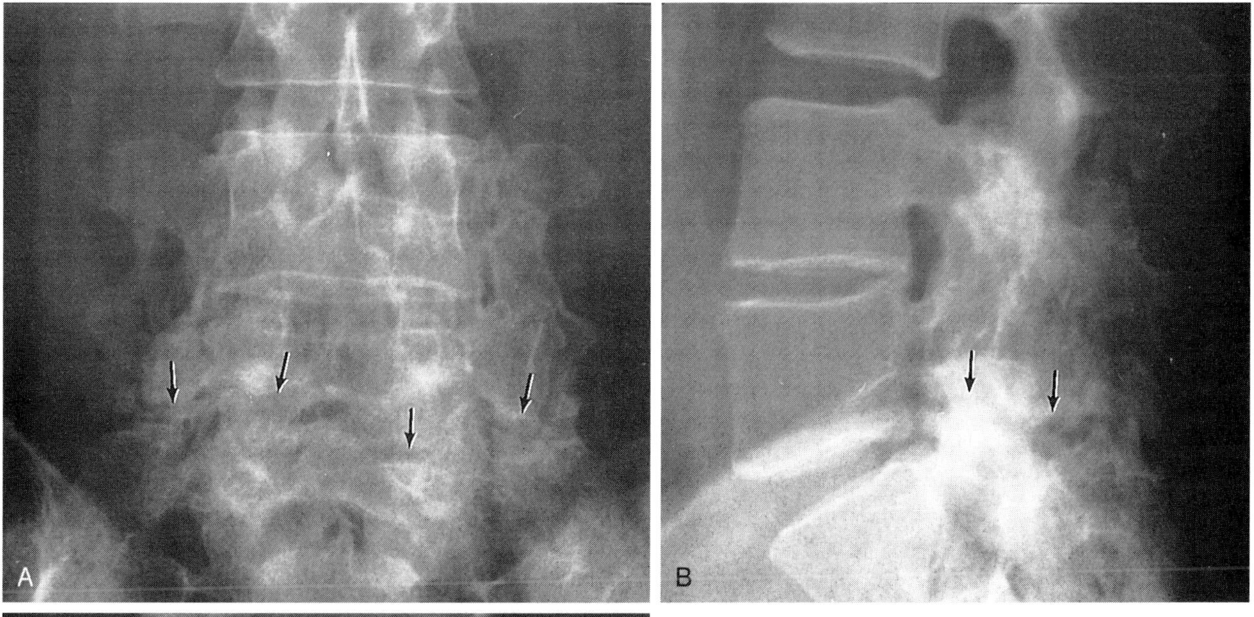

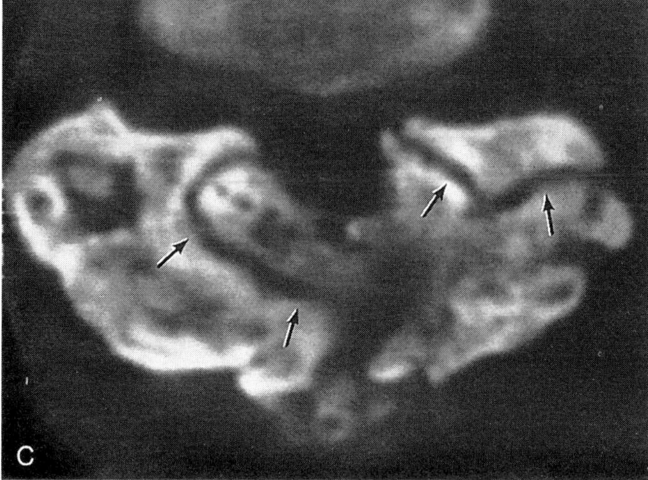

FIGURE 4–107. Spine surgery: Failed spinal fusion.[130] This 42-year-old patient had persistent pain 18 months after posterior L4-L5 and L5-S1 fusion. **A, B** Frontal (**A**) and lateral (**B**) radiographs show extensive bilateral intertransverse bone grafts at the L4-L5 and L5-S1 levels. A radiolucent defect (arrows) is seen at the L5-S1 segment and suggests both nonincorporation and nonunion of the graft. **C** Transaxial CT scan obtained at the L5-S1 level shows a radiolucent discontinuity (arrows) in the graft material, confirming the presence of nonunion and pseudarthrosis.

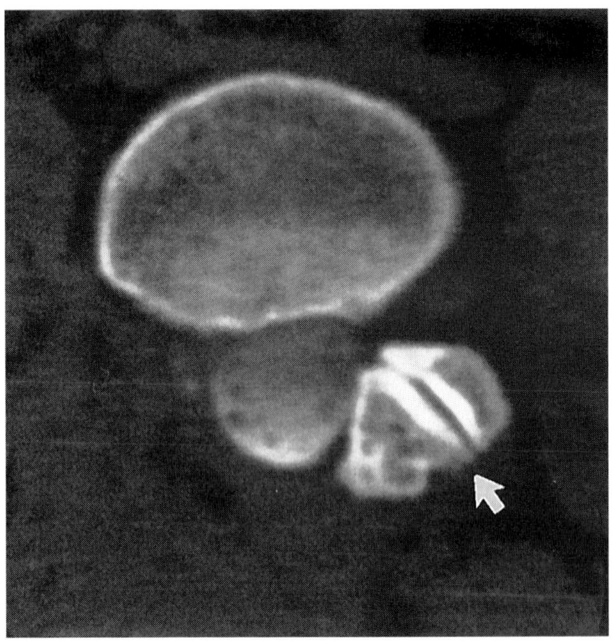

FIGURE 4–108. Spine surgery: Laminectomy and facetectomy.[131] Transaxial CT–myelogram image reveals a complete L5 laminectomy and right facetectomy in this 31-year-old woman. The left articular processes and facet joint (arrow) are intact, whereas the spinous process, right lamina, and articular processes are absent. This procedure is employed for the treatment of symptomatic lumbar stenosis. Such extensive surgeries with complete resection of the laminae and articular processes frequently result in instability unless accompanied by arthrodesis.

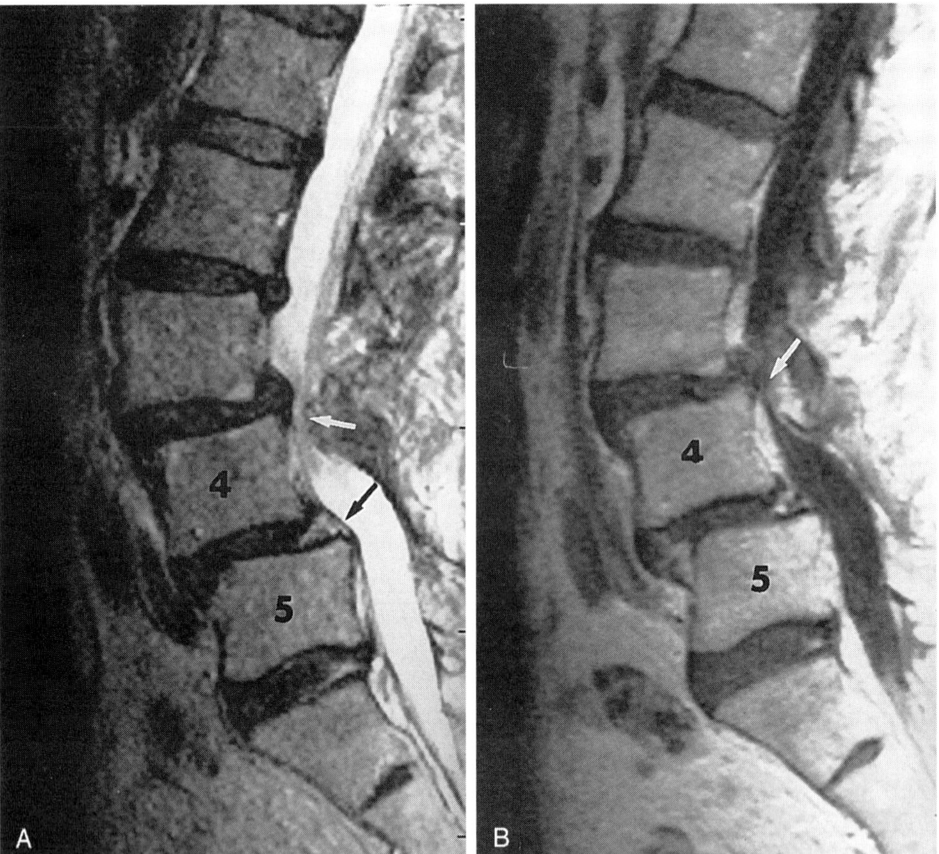

FIGURE 4–109. Postsurgical spine instability: Magnetic resonance (MR) imaging.[132] This 73-year-old woman underwent multilevel decompressive laminectomies for spinal stenosis. She had persistent postsurgical pain and disability and was sent for MR imaging. Parasagittal T2-weighted (TR/TE, 4000/100) **(A)** and postgadolinium T1-weighted (TR/TE, 650/15) **(B)** spin echo MR images reveal widespread disc degeneration with degenerative anterolisthesis of L3 and L4. The sagittal diameter of the spinal canal is severely narrowed at the L3-L4 level (white arrows). Disc protrusions are apparent at L2-L3 and L3-L4. The posterior longitudinal ligament is tethered over the posterior aspect of the L4 and L5 vertebral bodies (black arrows). Postoperative segmental instability, as demonstrated in this patient, is the most common complication encountered in patients after extensive decompressive surgery of the thoracic or lumbar region. Postoperative instability also occurs in up to 65 per cent of elderly women with preexisting degenerative spondylolisthesis. *(Courtesy of R. Lutz, D.C., Prince Rupert, British Columbia, Canada.)*

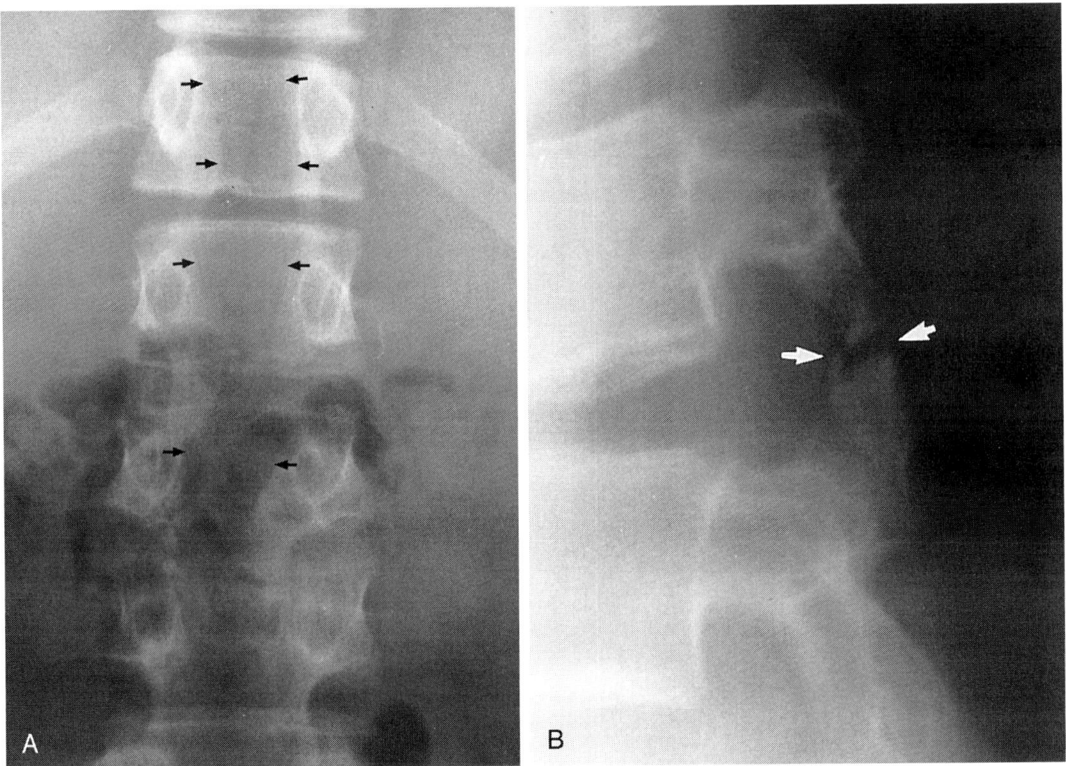

FIGURE 4–110. Stress (fatigue) fracture, postsurgical.[133] This 17-year-old male patient underwent a laminectomy extending from the T11 to L3 levels. **A** Frontal radiograph reveals the multilevel laminectomy (arrows). **B** Lateral radiograph shows a fracture through the L2 inferior articular process (arrows) and an associated flexion deformity. Fatigue fracture of the articular process is a well-recognized complication of extensive laminectomy surgery. *(Courtesy of J.A. Amberg, M.D., San Diego, California.)*

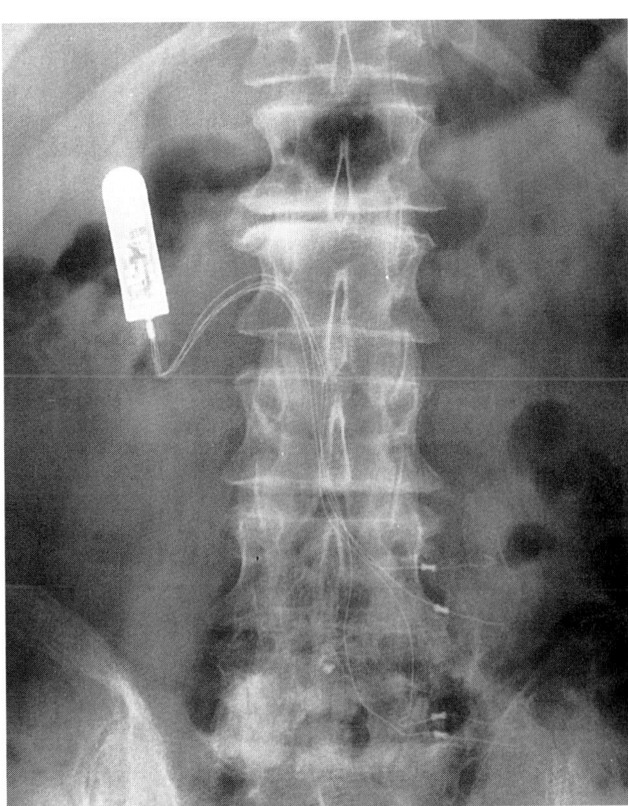

FIGURE 4–111. Direct current electrical stimulation.[134] An electrical stimulator and its electrodes have been implanted subcutaneously in the paraspinal tissues to enhance osseous incorporation of a bone graft at the L4-L5 and L5-S1 levels. *(Courtesy of F.G. Bauer, D.C., Sydney, New South Wales, Australia.)*

TABLE 4–21. Vascular Disorders

Entity	Figure(s)	Characteristics
Abdominal aortic aneurysm (AAA)[135, 136]	4–112	Patients frequently have low back pain, but 50 per cent are asymptomatic Prevalence of AAA in persons older than the age of 50 years varies from as low as 1.4 per cent in women to as high as 8.2 per cent in men Aorta is considered aneurysmal if diameter exceeds 3.8 cm; those greater than 6 cm are associated with a rupture rate of 75 per cent; surgery usually indicated in aneurysms over 5 cm Ruptured AAA accounts for 1.3 per cent of the deaths in men older than 65 years of age; risk of death as a consequence of rupture is three times that of elective surgery for repair of aneurysm Risk factors for AAA: male sex, age older than 75 years, white race, previous vascular disease, cigarette smoking, family history, and hypercholesterolemia *Diagnosis:* Physical examination: often inadequate in the diagnosis of AAA Radiography: calcification of vessel wall visible in about 75 per cent of cases; may be seen initially on abdominal or lumbar spine radiographs Diagnostic ultrasonography: method of choice for screening (98 per cent accuracy) Computed tomography (CT): also accurate in the diagnosis of AAA but more expensive and with greater radiation exposure than ultrasonography
Iliac artery aneurysm[135, 136]	4–113	Less common than AAA, but risk factors are the same Dilatation of calcified vessel wall overlying lower lumbar or sacroiliac region

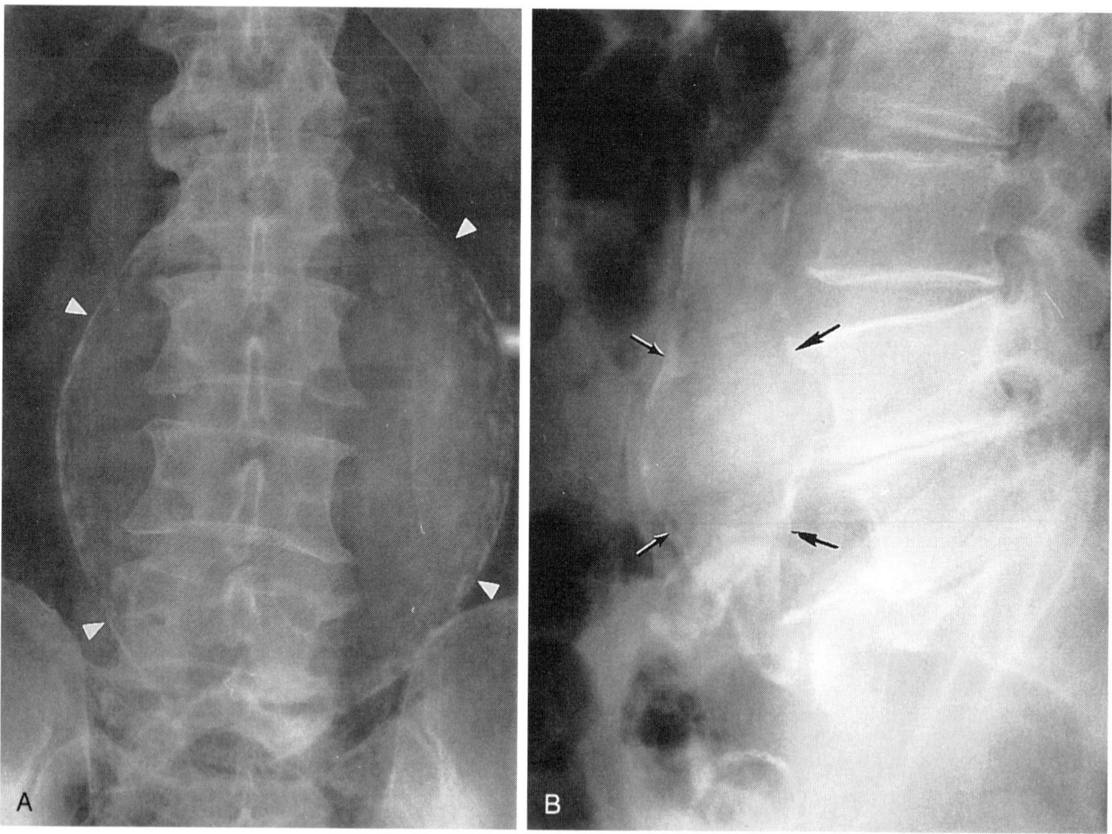

FIGURE 4–112. Abdominal aortic aneurysm.[135, 136] **A** This 74-year-old man had diffuse low back pain. Frontal radiograph shows a huge, oval, dilated abdominal aortic aneurysm (AAA). The aneurysm shows characteristic linear, plaque-like calcification (arrowheads), and measures 14.5 cm at its maximum transverse diameter. **B** In another patient, a large, atherosclerotic AAA is evident on the lateral radiograph (arrows). The curvilinear plaque-like calcification allows visualization of this life-threatening condition. *(**B**, Reprinted with permission from Taylor JAM, Hoffman LE: The geriatric patient: Diagnostic imaging of common musculoskeletal disorders. Top Clin Chiropr 3:23, © 1996, Aspen Publishers, Inc.)*

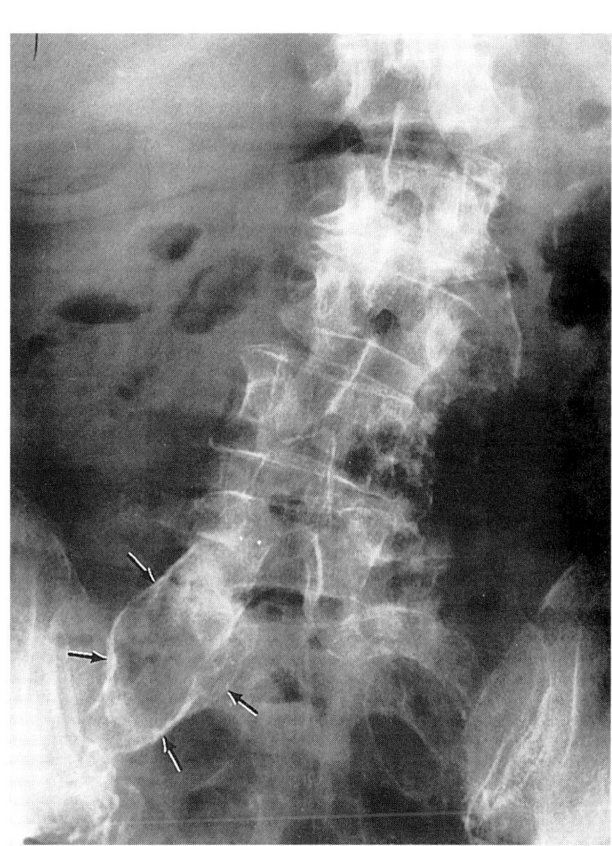

FIGURE 4–113. Iliac artery aneurysm.[135, 136] Observe the aneurysm of the atherosclerotic common iliac artery (arrows). This 81-year-old patient also has degenerative scoliosis. *(Reprinted with permission from Taylor JAM, Hoffman LE: The geriatric patient: Diagnostic imaging of common musculoskeletal disorders. Top Clin Chiropr 3:23, © 1996, Aspen Publishers, Inc.)*

REFERENCES

1. Edeiken J, Dalinka M, Karasick D: Edeiken's Roentgen Diagnosis of Diseases of Bone. 4th Ed. Baltimore, Williams & Wilkins, 1990.
2. Keats TE, Smith TH: An Atlas of Normal Developmental Roentgen Anatomy. 2nd Ed. Chicago, Year Book, 1988.
3. Greenfield GB: Radiology of Bone Diseases. 2nd Ed. Philadelphia, JB Lippincott, 1975.
4. Köhler A, Zimmer EA: Borderlands of Normal and Early Pathologic Findings in Skeletal Radiography. 4th Ed. New York, Thieme Medical Publishers, 1993.
5. Keats TE: Atlas of Normal Roentgen Variants That May Simulate Disease. 5th Ed. Chicago, Year Book Medical Publishers, 1992.
6. Magora A, Schwartz A: Relation between the low back pain syndrome and x-ray findings. 3. Spina bifida occulta. Scand J Rehabil Med 12:9, 1980.
7. Yochum TR, Rowe LJ: Essentials of Skeletal Radiology. 2nd Ed. Baltimore, Williams & Wilkins, 1996.
8. Ozonoff MB: Spinal anomalies and curvatures. *In* Resnick D (ed): Diagnosis of Bone and Joint Disorders. 3rd Ed. Philadelphia, WB Saunders, 1995, p 4245.
9. Greenspan A: Orthopedic Radiology: A Practical Approach. Philadelphia, JB Lippincott, 1988.
10. Chan KK, Sartoris DJ, Haghighi P, et al: Cupid's bow contour of the vertebral body: Evaluation of pathogenesis with bone densitometry and imaging-histopathologic correlation. Radiology 202:253, 1997.
11. Lovell WW, Winter RB: Pediatric Orthopedics, Philadelphia, JB Lippincott, 1978.
12. Cowell MJ, Cowell HR: The incidence of spina bifida occulta in idiopathic scoliosis. Clin Orthop 118:116, 1976.
13. Goobar JE, Erickson F, Pate D, et al: Symptomatic clasp-knife deformity of spinous processes. Spine 13:953, 1988.
14. Mitchell R: Congenital absence of a lumbosacral facet. Topics Diagn Radiol Adv Imaging 1:3, 1993.
15. Tini PG, Wieser C, Zinn WM: The transitional vertebra of the lumbosacral spine: Its radiological classification, incidence, prevalence, and clinical significance. Rheumatol Rehabil 16:180, 1977.
16. Kim NH, Suk KS: The role of transitional vertebrae in spondylolysis and spondylolytic spondylolisthesis. Bull Hosp Joint Dis 56:161, 1997.
17. van Tulder MW: Spinal radiographic findings and nonspecific low back pain. Spine 22:427, 1997.
18. Castillo M: MRI of diastematomyelia. MRI Decisions, Sept/Oct, 1991, p 12.
19. Langer LO, Baumann PA, Gorlin RJ: Achondroplasia. AJR 100:12, 1967.
20. Langer LO: Spondyloepiphyseal dysplasia tarda, hereditary chondrodysplasia with characteristic vertebral configuration in the adult. Radiology 82:833, 1964.
21. Watts RWE, Spellacy E, Kendall BE, et al: Computed tomography studies on patients with mucopolysaccharidosis. Neuroradiology 21:9, 1981.
22. Holzgrave W, Grobe H, von Figura K, et al: Morquio syndrome: Clinical findings of 11 patients with MPS IV-A and 2 patients with MPS IV-B. Hum Genet 57:360, 1981.
23. Kahler SG, Burns JA, Aylsworth AS: A mild autosomal recessive form of osteopetrosis. Am J Genet 17:451, 1984.
24. Kovanlikaya A, Loro ML, Gilsanz V: Pathogenesis of osteosclerosis in autosomal dominant osteopetrosis. AJR 168:929, 1997.
25. Weisz GM: Lumbar spinal canal stenosis in osteopoikilosis. Clin Orthop 166:89, 1982.
26. Benli IT, Akalin S, Boysan E, et al: Epidemiological, clinical, and radiological aspects of osteopoikilosis. J Bone Joint Surg [Br] 74:504, 1992.
27. Tallroth K, Malmivaara A, Laitinen M-L, et al: Lumbar spine in Marfan syndrome. Skeletal Radiol 24:337, 1995.
28. Mitchell GE, Lourie H, Berne AS: The various causes of scalloped vertebrae with notes on their pathogenesis. Radiology 89:67, 1967.
29. Taylor JAM, Greene-DesLauriers K, Tanaka DI: Ehlers-Danlos syndrome. J Manip Phys Therap 13:273, 1990.
30. Root L: The treatment of osteogenesis imperfecta. Orthop Clin North Am 15:775, 1984.
31. Wardinski TD, Pagon RA, Powell BR, et al: Rhizomelic chondrodysplasia punctata and survival beyond one year: A review of the literature and five case reports. Clin Genet 38:84, 1990.
32. Poussa M, Merikanto J, Ryoppy S, et al: The spine in diastrophic dysplasia. Spine 16:881, 1991.
33. Wiltse LL, Newman PH, MacNab I: Classification of spondylolysis and spondylolisthesis. Clin Orthop 117:23, 1976.
34. Myerding HW: Low backache and sciatic pain associated with spondylolisthesis and protruded intervertebral disc. J Bone Joint Surg [Am] 23:461, 1941.
35. Frederickson BE, Baker D, McHollick WJ, et al: The natural history of spondylolysis and spondylolisthesis. J Bone Joint Surg [Am] 66:699, 1984.
36. Langston JW, Gavant ML: Incomplete ring sign: A simple method for CT detection of spondylolysis. J Comput Assist Tomogr 9:728, 1985.
37. Bellah RD, Summerville DA, Treves ST, et al: Low-back pain in adolescent athletes: Detection of stress injury to the pars interarticularis with SPECT. Radiology 180:509, 1991.
38. Saifuddin A, Burnett SJD: The value of lumbar spine MRI in the assessment of the pars interarticularis. Clin Radiol 52:666, 1997.
39. Kauppila LI, Eustace S, Kiel DP, et al: Degenerative displacement of lumbar vertebrae: A 25-year follow-up study in Framingham. Spine 23:1868, 1998.
40. Khanchandani BA: Albers-Schonberg's disease with multiple-level lumbar spondylolysis: A case report. Eur J Chiropr 37:5, 1989.
41. Yochum TR, Sellers LT, Oppenheimer DA, et al: The sclerotic pedicle—how many causes are there? Skeletal Radiol 19:411, 1990.
42. Wood KB, Popp CA, Transfeldt EE, et al: Radiographic evaluation of instability in spondylolisthesis. Spine 19:1697, 1994.
43. Pitkänen M, Manninen HI, Lindgren K, et al: Limited usefulness of traction-compression films in the radiographic diagnosis of lumbar spinal instability: Comparison with flexion-extension films. Spine 22:193, 1997.
44. Friberg O: Lumbar instability: A dynamic approach by traction-compression radiography. Spine 12:119, 1987.
45. Ohmori K, Ishida Y, Tkatsu T, et al: Vertebral slip in lumbar spondylolysis and spondylolisthesis: Long-term follow-up of 22 adult patients. J Bone Joint Surg [Br] 77:771, 1995.
46. Weinstein SL, Ponseti IV: Curve progression in idiopathic scoliosis. J Bone Joint Surg [Am] 65:447, 1983.
47. Taylor JAM, Hoffman LE: The geriatric patient: Diagnostic imaging of common musculoskeletal disorders. Top Clin Chiropr 3:23, 1996.

48. Giles LGF, Taylor JR: Lumbar spine structural changes associated with leg length inequality. Spine 7:159, 1982.
49. Joseph KN, Kane HA, Milner RS, et al: Orthopedic aspects of the Marfan phenotype. Clin Orthop 277:251, 1992.
50. DeSmet AA, Robinson RG, Johnson BE, et al: Spinal compression fractures in osteoporotic women: Patterns and relationship to hyperkyphosis. Radiology 166:497, 1988.
51. Petersilge CA, Pathria MN, Emery SE, et al: Thoracolumbar burst fractures: Evaluation with MR imaging. Radiology 194:49, 1995.
52. Terk MR, Hume-Neal M, Fraipont M, et al: Injury of the posterior ligament complex in patients with acute spinal trauma: Evaluation by MR imaging. AJR 168:1481, 1997.
53. Sturm JT, Perry JF: Injuries associated with fractures of the transverse processes of lumbar vertebrae. Radiology 134:627, 1980.
54. Jackson DW: Unilateral osseous bridging of the lumbar transverse processes following trauma. J Bone Joint Surg [Am] 57:125, 1975.
55. Denis F: The three column spine and its significance in the classification of acute thoracolumbar spinal injuries. Spine 8:817, 1983.
56. Graves VB, Keene JS, Strother CM, et al: CT of bilateral lumbosacral facet dislocation. AJNR 9:809, 1988.
57. Wagner A, Albeck MJ, Madsen FF: Diagnostic imaging in fracture of lumbar vertebral ring apophyses. Acta Radiol 33:72, 1992.
58. Bonic EE, Taylor JAM, Knudsen JT: Posterior limbus fractures: Five case reports and a review of selected published cases. J Manip Phys Therap 21:281, 1998.
59. Lafforgue PF, Chagnaud CJ, Daver LMH, et al: Intervertebral disk vacuum phenomenon secondary to vertebral collapse: Prevalence and significance. Radiology 193:853, 1994.
60. Ross JS, Modic MT: Current assessment of spinal degenerative disease with magnetic resonance imaging. Clin Orthop 279:68, 1992.
61. Cohn EL, Maurer EJ, Keats TE, et al: Plain film evaluation of degenerative disk disease at the lumbosacral junction. Skeletal Radiol 26:161, 1997.
62. Modic MT, Steinberg PM, Ross JS, et al: Degenerative disc disease: Assessment of changes in vertebral body marrow with MR imaging. Radiology 166:193, 1988.
63. Firooznia H, Benjamin V, Kricheff II, et al: CT of lumbar spine disc herniation: Correlation with surgical findings. AJR 142:587, 1984.
64. Mortensen WW, Thorne RP, Donaldson WF III: Symptomatic gas-containing disc herniation: Report of four cases. Spine 16:190, 1991.
65. Thornbury JR, Fryback DG, Turski PA, et al: Disk-caused nerve compression in patients with acute low back pain: Diagnosis with MR, CT myelography, and plain CT. Radiology 186:731, 1993.
66. Stäbler A, Bellan M, Weiss M, et al: MR imaging of enhancing intraosseous disk herniation (Schmorl's nodes). AJR 168:933, 1997.
67. Yagan R: CT diagnosis of limbus vertebra. J Comput Assist Tomogr 8:149, 1984.
68. Blumenthal SL, Roach J, Herring JA: Lumbar Scheuermann's disease: A clinical series and classification. Spine 12:929, 1987.
69. Kirkaldy-Willis WH, Farfan HF: Instability of the lumbar spine. Clin Orthop 165:110, 1982.
70. Fitzgerald JAW, Newman PH: Degenerative spondylolisthesis. J Bone Joint Surg [Br] 58:184, 1976.
71. Sanderson PL, Fraser RD: The influence of pregnancy on the development of degenerative spondylolisthesis. J Bone Joint Surg [Br] 78:951, 1996.
72. Wiltse LL, Guyer RD, Spencer CW, et al: Alar transverse process impingement of the L5 spinal nerve: The far-out syndrome. Spine 9:31, 1984.
73. Dihlmann W, Delling G: Spondylosclerosis hemisphaerica. ROFO 138:592, 1983.
74. Lee CK, Rauschning W, Glenn W: Lateral lumbar spinal canal stenosis: Classification, pathologic anatomy, and surgical decompression. Spine 13:313, 1988.
75. Carrera GF, Haughton VM, Syvertsen A, et al: Computed tomography of the lumbar facet joints. Radiology 134:145, 1980.
76. Cone RO, Resnick D: Diffuse idiopathic skeletal hyperostosis (DISH). Contemp Diagn Radiol 6:1, 1983.
77. Broudeur P, Larroque CH, Passeron R, et al: The iliolumbar syndrome. Rev Rhum Mal Osteoartic 50:393, 1982.
78. Kapila A, Lines M: Neuropathic spinal arthropathy: CT and MR findings. J Comput Assist Tomogr 11:736, 1987.
79. Heywood AWB, Meyers OL: Rheumatoid arthritis of the thoracic and lumbar spine. J Bone Joint Surg [Br] 68:362, 1986.
80. Kahn MS: Pathogenesis of ankylosing spondylitis. J Rheumatol 20:1273, 1993.
81. Sparling MJ, Bartleson JD, McLeod RA, et al: Magnetic resonance imaging of arachnoid diverticula associated with cauda equina syndrome in ankylosing spondylitis. J Rheumatol 16:1335, 1989.
82. Sundaram M, Patton JT: Paravertebral ossification in psoriasis and Reiter's syndrome. Br J Radiol 48:628, 1975.
83. Park Y-H, Huang G-S, Taylor JAM, et al: Patterns of vertebral ossification and pelvic abnormalities in paralysis: A study of 200 patients. Radiology 188:561, 1993.
84. Resnick D, Pineda C: Vertebral involvement in calcium pyrophosphate dihydrate crystal deposition disease: Radiographic-pathologic correlation. Radiology 153:55, 1984.
85. Steinbach LS, Resnick D: Calcium pyrophosphate dihydrate crystal deposition disease revisited. Radiology 200:1, 1996.
86. Justesen P, Andersen PE Jr: Radiologic manifestations in alkaptonuria. Skeletal Radiol 11:204, 1984.
87. Yagan R, Khan MA: The coexistence of ochronosis and ankylosing spondylitis. J Rheumatol 18:1639, 1991.
88. Alarcón GS, Reveille JD: Gouty arthritis of the axial skeleton including the sacroiliac joints. Arch Intern Med 147:2018, 1987.
89. Dagirmanjian A, Schils J, McHenry M, et al: MR imaging of vertebral osteomyelitis revisited. AJR 167:1539, 1996.
90. Rohde V, Meyer B, Schaller C, et al: Spondylodiscitis after lumbar discectomy: Incidence and a proposal for prophylaxis. Spine 23:615, 1998.
91. Travlos J, Du Toit G: Spinal tuberculosis: Beware the posterior elements. J Bone Joint Surg [Br] 72:722, 1990.
92. Graves VB, Schrieber MH: Tuberculous psoas muscle abscess. J Can Assoc Radiol 24:268, 1973.
93. Algra PR, Bloem JL, Tissing H, et al: Detection of vertebral metastases: Comparison between MR imaging and bone scintigraphy. RadioGraphics 11:219, 1991.
94. Wong DA, Fornasier VL, MacNab I: Spinal metastases: The obvious, the occult, and the impostors. Spine 15:1, 1990.
95. Mirra JM: Lymphoma and lymphoma-like disorders. *In*

Mirra JM, Picci P, Gold RH (eds): Bone Tumors: Clinical, Radiologic, and Pathologic Considerations. Lea & Febiger, London, 1989, p 1177.
96. Algra PR, Heimans JJ, Valk J, et al: Do metastases in vertebrae begin in the body or the pedicles? Imaging study in 45 patients. AJR 158:1275, 1992.
97. Sudaresan N: Chordomas. Clin Orthop 204:135, 1986.
98. Barwick KW, Huvos AG, Smith J: Primary osteogenic sarcoma of the vertebral column: A clinicopathologic correlation of ten patients. Cancer 46:595, 1980.
99. Kyle RA: Multiple myeloma: Review of 869 cases. Mayo Clin Proc 50:29, 1975.
100. Lecouvet FE, Vande Berg BC, Maldague BE, et al: Vertebral compression fractures in multiple myeloma. Part I: Distribution and appearance at MR imaging. Radiology 204:195, 1997.
101. Franczyk J, Samuels T, Rubenstein J, et al: Skeletal lymphoma. J Can Assoc Radiol 40:75, 1989.
102. Epstein BS: Vertebral changes in childhood leukemia. Radiology 68:65, 1957.
103. Greenspan A: Bone island (enostosis): Current concept—a review. Skeletal Radiol 24:111, 1995.
104. Esposito PW, Crawford AH, Vogler C: Solitary osteochondroma occurring on the transverse process of the lumbar spine: A case report. Spine 10:398, 1985.
105. Karasick D, Schweitzer ME, Eschelman DJ: Symptomatic osteochondromas: Imaging features. AJR 168:1507, 1997.
106. De Dios AMV, Bond JR, Shives TC, et al: Aneurysmal bone cyst: A clinico-pathologic study of 238 cases. Cancer 69:2921, 1992.
107. Papagelopoulos PJ, Currier BJ, Shaughnessy WJ, et al: Aneurysmal bone cyst of the spine: Management and outcome. Spine 23:621, 1998.
108. Laredo J-D, Reizine D, Bard M, et al: Vertebral hemangiomas: Radiologic evaluation. Radiology 161:183, 1986.
109. Hadjipavlou A, Lander P: Paget disease of the spine. J Bone Joint Surg [Am] 73:1376, 1991.
110. Mirra JM, Brien EW, Tehranzadeh J: Paget's disease of bone: Review with emphasis on radiologic features, part II. Skeletal Radiol 24:173, 1995.
111. Angtuaco EJ, Binet EF, Flanigan S: Value of CT myelography in neurofibromatosis. Neurosurgery 13:668, 1983.
112. Stull MA, Kransdorf MJ, Devaney KO: Langerhans cell histiocytosis of bone. RadioGraphics 12:801, 1992.
113. Kilpatrick SE, Wenger DE, Gilchrist GS, et al: Langerhans' cell histiocytosis (histiocytosis X) of bone: A clinicopathologic analysis of 263 pediatric and adult cases. Cancer 76:2471, 1995.
114. Ryan PJ, Fogelman I: Osteoporotic vertebral fractures: Diagnosis with radiography and bone scintigraphy. Radiology 190:669, 1994.
115. Genant HK, Engelke K, Fuerst T, et al: Noninvasive assessment of bone mineral and structure: State of the art. J Bone Miner Res 11:707, 1996.
116. Resnick D: Disorders of other endocrine glands and of pregnancy. *In* Resnick D (ed): Diagnosis of Bone and Joint Disorders. 3rd Ed. Philadelphia, WB Saunders, 1995, p 2076.
117. Pacifici R, Rupich R, Griffin M, et al: Dual energy radiography versus quantitative computer tomography for the diagnosis of osteoporosis. J Clin Endocrinol Metab 70:705, 1990.
118. Mankin HJ: Rickets, osteomalacia, and renal osteodystrophy. Orthop Clin North Am 21:81, 1990.
119. Resnick D: Thyroid disorders. *In* Resnick D (ed): Diagnosis of Bone and Joint Disorders. 3rd Ed. Philadelphia, WB Saunders, 1995, p 2005.
120. Resnick D, Niwayama G: Parathyroid disorders and renal osteodystrophy. *In* Resnick D (ed): Diagnosis of Bone and Joint Disorders. 3rd Ed. Philadelphia, WB Saunders, 1995, p 2036.
121. Parikh M, Iyer K, Elias AN, et al: Spinal stenosis in acromegaly. Spine 12:627, 1987.
122. Wang Y, Yin Y, Gilula LA, et al: Endemic fluorosis of the skeleton: Radiographic features in 127 cases. AJR 162:93, 1994.
123. De Gennes C, Kuntz D, De Vernejoul MC: Bone mastocytosis: A report of nine cases with a bone histomorphometric study. Clin Orthop 279:281, 1992.
124. Schwartz AM, Homer MJ, McCauley RGK: "Step-off" vertebral body: Gaucher's disease versus sickle cell hemoglobinopathy. AJR 132:81, 1979.
125. Moseley JE: Skeletal changes in the anemias. Semin Roentgenol 9:169, 1974.
126. Marlow TJ, Brunson CY, Jackson S, et al: "Tower vertebra": A new observation in sickle cell disease. Skeletal Radiol 27:195, 1998.
127. Barton CJ, Cockshott WP: Bone changes in hemoglobin SC disease. AJR 88:523, 1962.
128. Resnick D: Hemoglobinopathies and other anemias. *In* Resnick D (ed): Diagnosis of Bone and Joint Disorders. 3rd Ed. Philadelphia, WB Saunders, 1995, p 2128.
129. Malghem J, Maldague B, Labaisse M-A, et al: Intravertebral vacuum cleft: Changes in content after supine positioning. Radiology 187:483, 1993.
130. Steinmann JC, Herkowitz HN: Pseudoarthrosis of the spine. Clin Orthop 284:80, 1992.
131. Garfin SR, Glover M, Booth RE, et al: Laminectomy: A review of the Pennsylvania hospital experience. J Spinal Disord 1:116, 1988.
132. Katz JN, Lipson SJ, Larson MG, et al: The outcome of decompressive laminectomy for degenerative lumbar stenosis. J Bone Joint Surg [Am] 73:809, 1991.
133. Rothman SLG, Glenn WV, Kerber CW: Postoperative fractures of the lumbar articular facets: Occult cause of radiculopathy. AJR 145:779, 1985.
134. Kahanovitz N, Arnoczky SP: The efficacy of direct current electrical stimulation to enhance canine spinal fusions. Clin Orthop 251:295, 1990.
135. Pleumeekers HJCM, Hoes AW, van der Does E, et al: Epidemiology of abdominal aortic aneurysms. Eur J Vasc Surg 8:119, 1994.
136. Yochum TR, Guebert GM, Kettner NW: Abdominal aortic aneurysm—the total picture. Appl Diagn Imag 1:1, 1989.
137. Kleinman PK, Marks SC: Vertebral body fractures in child abuse: Radiologic-histopathologic correlates. Invest Radiol 27:715, 1992.
138. Crock HV: Internal disc disruption. *In* Frymoyer JW (ed): The Adult Spine: Principles and Practice. New York, Raven Press, 1991, p 2015.

CHAPTER 5

Sacrococcygeal Spine and Sacroiliac Joints

- Normal Developmental Anatomy
- Developmental Anomalies, Variants, and Skeletal Dysplasias
- Physical Injury
- Articular Disorders
- Bone Tumors

Normal Developmental Anatomy

The accurate assessment of pediatric radiographs of the sacrum, coccyx, and sacroiliac joints requires a thorough knowledge of normal developmental anatomy. Table 5–1 outlines the age of appearance and fusion of the primary and secondary ossification centers. Figures 5–1 and 5–2 demonstrate the radiographic appearance of many important ossification centers and other developmental landmarks at selected ages from birth to skeletal maturity.

Developmental Anomalies, Variants, and Skeletal Dysplasias

Interpretation of radiographs of the sacrum, coccyx, and sacroiliac joint region frequently is complicated by the presence of anomalies or normal variations and occasionally by skeletal dysplasias. Many of these entities have already been presented in Chapter 4. Table 5–2 and Figures 5–3 to 5–7 illustrate additional examples of these commonly encountered processes.

When considering vertebral anomalies, it is helpful to remember some general rules:

1. Most anomalies occur at transitional areas, such as the lumbosacral and sacrococcygeal regions.
2. When one anomaly is identified, always search for more: anomalies may be multiple.
3. Anomalies may occur in isolation or be associated with more diffuse abnormalities as part of a syndrome.
4. Osseous anomalies may be associated with underlying or distant neurologic or visceral anomalies.

Physical Injury

Physical injury, including fractures and joint trauma, may involve the sacrum, coccyx, or sacroiliac joints alone, in combination with each other, or in combination with other spinal, pelvic, and abdominal visceral injuries. Some combined injuries are discussed in more detail in Chapter 6 in association with pelvic trauma. Table 5–3 lists the important injuries in this region and discusses their characteristics. Many examples are illustrated in Figures 5–8 to 5–10.

Articular Disorders

The sacroiliac joints are a frequent target site of involvement for degenerative, inflammatory, metabolic, and infectious spondyloarthropathies. Table 5–4 outlines these diseases and their characteristics, and Table 5–5 describes their anatomic distribution. Figures 5–11 to 5–22 provide examples of characteristic radiographic manifestations.

Bone Tumors

Many different malignant and benign tumors and tumor-like lesions affect the sacrum, and, to a lesser extent, the coccyx. Table 5–6 lists only those neoplasms illustrated in Figures 5–23 to 5–30. A more complete list of vertebral column neoplasms—including sacrococcygeal lesions—is found in Chapter 2 (Table 2–13).

TABLE 5–1. Sacrum and Coccyx: Approximate Age of Appearance and Fusion of Ossification Centers[1–4] (Figs. 5–1, 5–2)

Ossification Center	Primary or Secondary	No. of Centers	Age of Appearance (Years)*†	Age of Fusion* (Years)†	Comments
Sacrum					
Bodies	P	5	Birth	18–30	Fuse together in order from S5-S1
Neural arches	P	10	Birth	5	Fuse in order: S2, S1, S4, S3
Costal processes	P	4	Birth	5–18	S1-S4
Anterior costal apophyses	S	8	1–25	18–25	S1-S4
Posterior costal apophyses	S	4	1–22	18–25	S1-S2
Transverse process apophyses	S	8 or 10	1–19	5–18	Lateral sacral crest
Spinous process apophyses	S	3	5–22	5–22	S1-S3
End-plate ring apophyses	S	10	1–21	13–17	S1-S5
Mamillary process apophyses	S	2	1–4	1–18	S1
Coccyx					
Bodies	P	4	1–18	No fusion	Variable number
Neural arch or cornua	P	2	1–6	No fusion	Present at first coccygeal segment only
Transverse process apophyses	S	2		No fusion	Present at first coccygeal segment only

*Ages of appearance and fusion of ossification centers in girls typically precede those of boys. Ethnic differences also exist.
†Adapted from Broome DR, Hayman LA, Herrick RC, et al: Postnatal maturation of the sacrum and coccyx: MR imaging, helical CT, and conventional radiography. AJR 170:1061, 1998. In this study, ossification centers typically were evident on computed tomographic (CT) and magnetic resonance (MR) imaging long before they appeared radiographically.
P, Primary; S, secondary.

FIGURE 5–1. Skeletal maturation and normal development: Frontal sacrococcygeal radiographs.[1–5] A 4-year-old boy. The primary ossification centers are unfused and appear as vertical radiolucent shadows (arrows). B 8-year-old boy. The sacroiliac joints are wide, and the L5 neural arch has not yet fused (arrow). Portions of the sacrum are obscured by bowel gas. C Observe the apparent widening of the sacroiliac joints in this 9-year-old boy. D In an 11-year-old child, the S1 neural arch remains unfused. E 13-year-old boy. The sacroiliac joints have a more adult configuration in this child compared with the more juvenile appearance of the sacroiliac joints in the patient in F. Observe the bilateral ossification centers of the sacral alae (arrows). F Another 13-year-old boy. The ossification center of the S1 neural arch, which typically fuses by the age of 5 years, remains unfused in this child (arrows), a condition termed spina bifida occulta. This developmental anomaly is common at that level and usually is of no clinical significance. G 14-year-old girl. Posteroanterior radiograph obtained with caudad tube tilt. The sacroiliac joints are wide, and bilateral ossification centers are present at the sacral alae. The widening of the sacroiliac joints, seen in many of these children, is associated with blurred and poorly defined articular margins. These findings relate to the presence of thick articular cartilage and incomplete subchondral ossification. Occasionally, they are accompanied by normal subchondral sclerosis, not to be confused with the findings of sacroiliitis. H Adult configuration. In this 30-year-old man, observe the well-defined subchondral bone, uniform joint space, and the absence of adjacent sclerosis. The angulated frontal projection of the sacroiliac joints is ideal for clearly visualizing the sacroiliac joints. This projection is obtained as a posteroanterior view with 20 to 30 degrees of caudal tube angulation or as an anteroposterior view with 20 to 30 degrees of cephalad tube angulation.

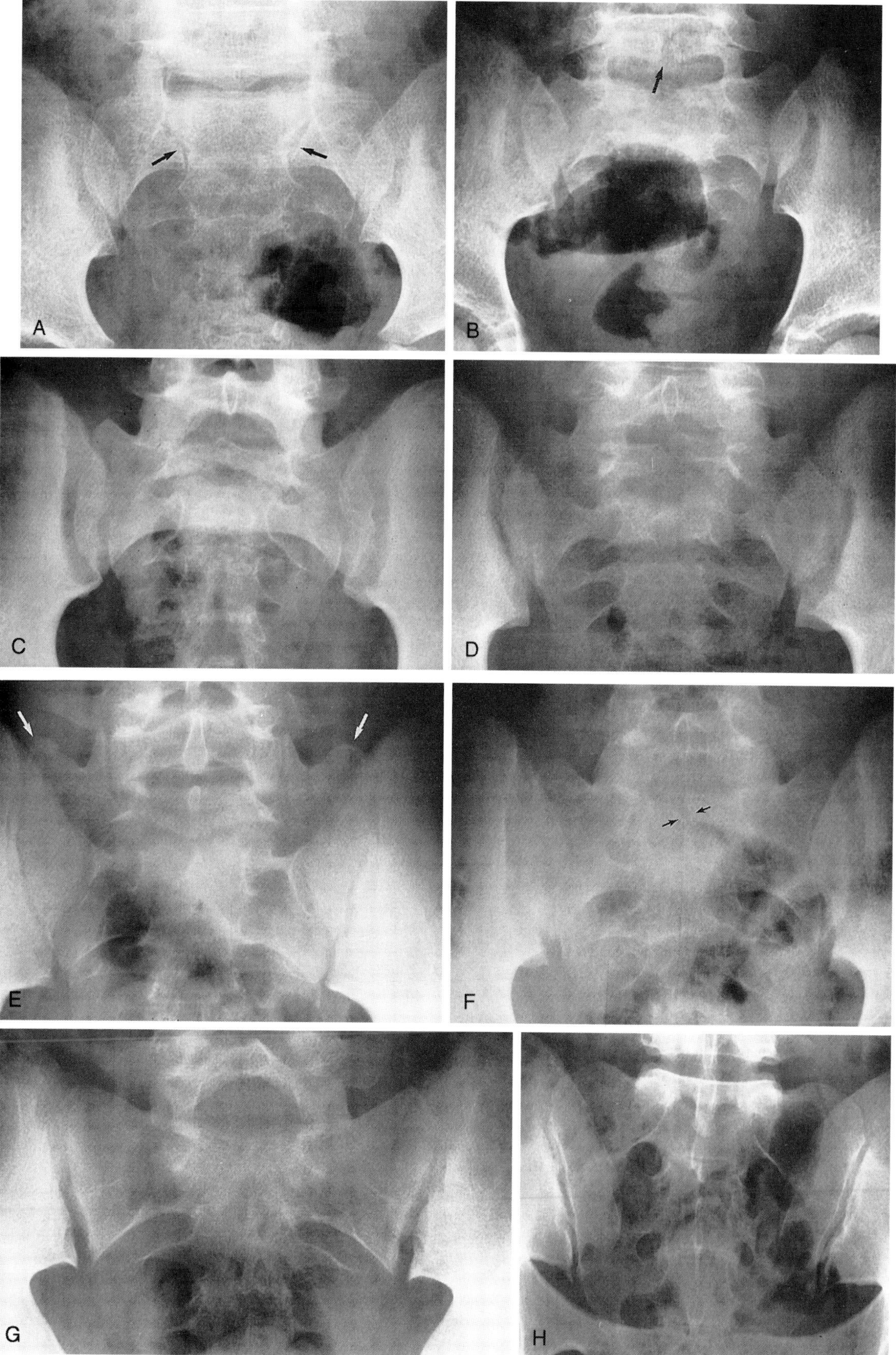

FIGURE 5–1 *See legend on opposite page*

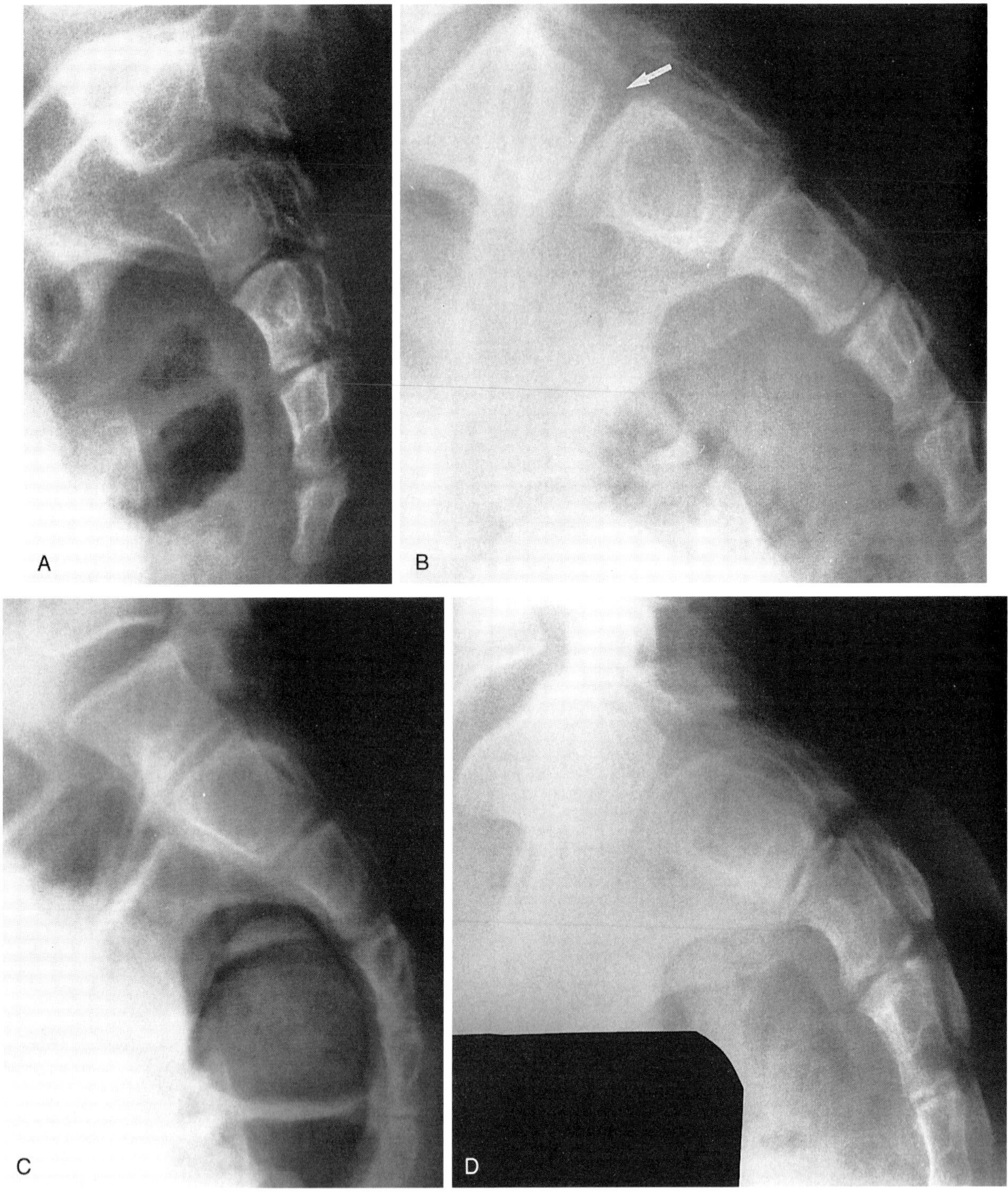

FIGURE 5–2. Skeletal maturation and normal development: Lateral sacrococcygeal radiographs.[1–4] **A** 7-year-old boy. Each individual sacral segment is well visualized. **B** 10-year-old boy. The radiolucent growth center at S1-S2 often is wedge-shaped (arrow) and may create the false appearance of spondylolisthesis at S1-S2. **C** 13-year-old boy. The individual sacral segments remain unfused. **D** 14-year-old boy. The body segments appear better defined and are beginning to fuse. These body segments usually fuse completely between the ages of 18 and 30 years, beginning at S5 and ending at S1.

TABLE 5–2. Developmental Anomalies, Anatomic Variants, and Skeletal Dysplasias Affecting the Sacrum and Coccyx*

Entity	Figure(s), Table(s)	Characteristics
Pseudonarrowing of sacroiliac joint[6]	5–3	Positional rotation of the patient in which the radiographic beam is not tangent to the joint, simulating the appearance of joint space narrowing Repositioning the patient usually results in a more adequate radiograph and corrects this potential source of misinterpretation
Sacral wing fossa[7]	5–4	Well-circumscribed circular radiolucent zone within the sacral wing, or ala, simulating an osteolytic lesion Normal variant of no clinical significance
Accessory sacroiliac articulations[8]	5–5; see 5–13D	Accessory articulation between the sacrum and the ilium; usually between the posterior superior iliac spine or iliac tuberosity of the ilium and the posterolateral aspect of the sacrum Present in as much as 30 per cent of the population In some cases, it may represent only a contact point rather than a true articulation True articulation may undergo degenerative changes
Spina bifida occulta[9, 10]	5–6	Extremely common developmental anomaly consisting of a midline defect within the neural arch in which the paired sacral arches fail to fuse in the midline Radiolucent cleft occurring most frequently at L5 and S1 segments Sacral hiatus present in 1 to 7 per cent of persons; failure of ossification of all sacral arches; no clinical significance Strong cartilage and fibrous tissues fill the cleft; anomaly generally is of no clinical consequence Isolated anomaly or occurring in conjunction with other entities, such as cleidocranial dysplasia or clasp-knife syndrome Spina bifida infrequently associated with meningomyelocele: protrusion of the meninges or spinal cord, or both; meningomyelocele may result in severe neurologic abnormalities
Clasp-knife syndrome[12]	4–9	Spina bifida occulta of S1 and elongation of the L5 spinous process During trunk extension, the L5 spinous process may impinge on the spinal canal, irritating pain-sensitive structures
Sacral agenesis[11]	5–7	Complete or partial sacral agenesis present in 0.1 to 0.2 per cent of all infants of diabetic mothers Also seen as a component of the VATER syndrome complex (vertebral, anorectal, tracheal, esophageal, renal anomalies), and may be associated with other gastrointestinal and genitourinary anomalies, or meningomyelocele Frequently accompanied by developmental acetabular dysplasia with congenital hip dislocation Flexion and extension radiographs can be performed to evaluate spinal stability
Paraglenoid sulcus[3, 5]	See Figs. 5–12, 5–13	Focal zone of bone resorption occurring in response to increased stress at the site of attachment of the inferior sacroiliac ligament, seen almost exclusively in women Bilateral grooves in inferior ilium just lateral to the sacroiliac joints Deep grooves occur only in parous women Increased prevalence is found in persons with hyperlordosis and, questionably, with osteitis condensans ilii No clinical significance
Sacrococcygeal synostosis[6]		First coccygeal segment often is fused to the lowest sacral segment, and the lower coccygeal vertebrae may be fused together; no clinical significance
Facet tropism[5, 7, 10]	4–12 Table 4–3	Asymmetric orientation of left and right lumbosacral facet joints
Transitional lumbosacral segment[12]	4–15 Table 4–3	

*See also Tables 1–1 and 1–2.

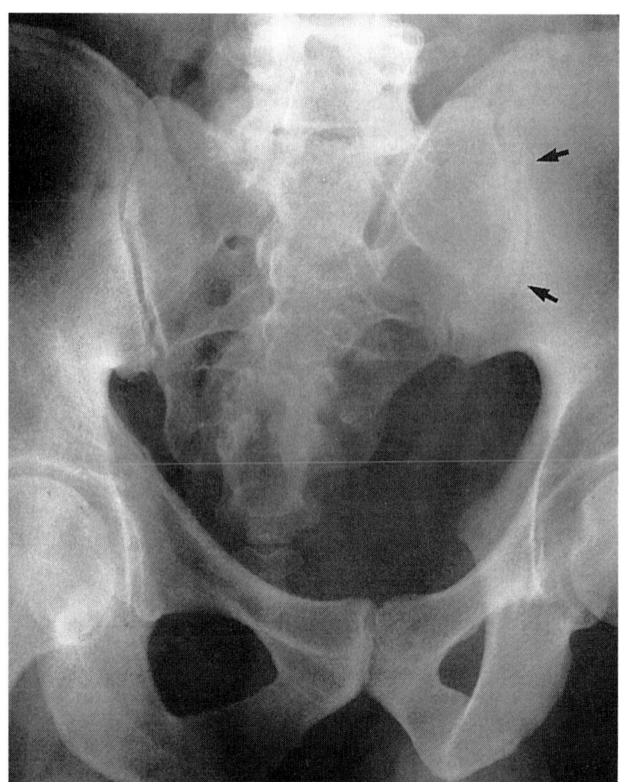

FIGURE 5–3. Pseudonarrowing of the sacroiliac joints from patient obliquity on imaging.[6] This incorrectly positioned frontal radiograph was taken with the patient rotated relative to the film. Such obliquity results in a false appearance of unilateral sacroiliac joint narrowing, ankylosis, or obliteration (arrows).

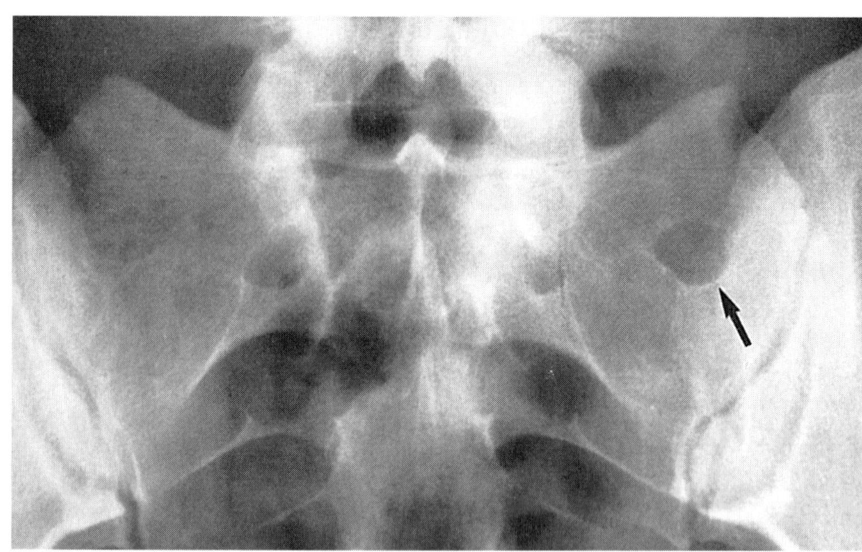

FIGURE 5–4. Sacral wing fossa.[7] Observe the well-circumscribed radiolucent shadow in the sacral wing simulating an osteolytic lesion (arrow). Such fossae are normal variants that are of no clinical significance. *(Courtesy of D. McCallum, D.C., Vancouver, British Columbia, Canada.)*

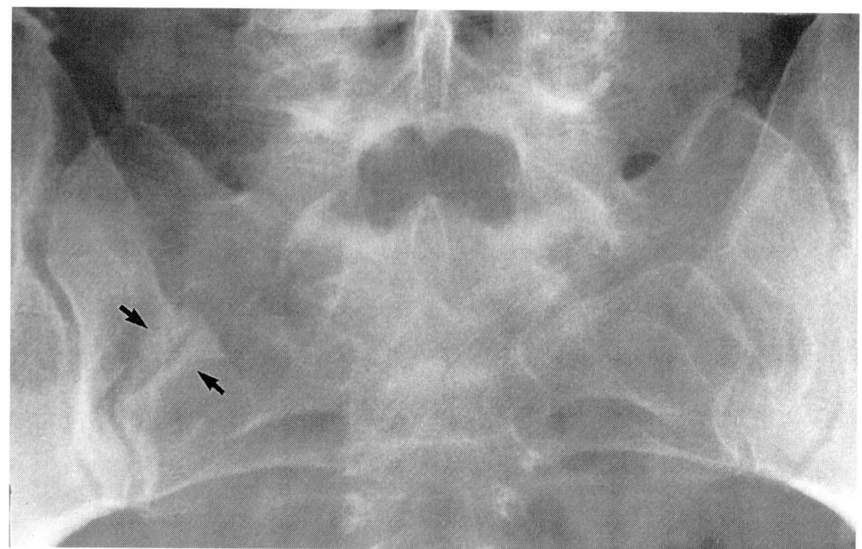

FIGURE 5–5. Accessory sacroiliac articulation.[8] An anomalous articulation between the ilium and sacrum is seen adjacent to the posterior superior iliac spine (arrows).

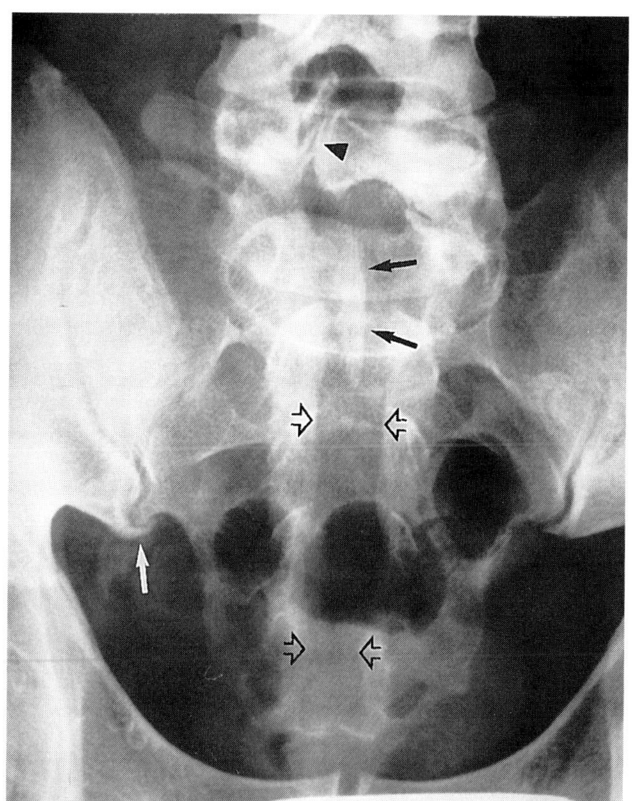

FIGURE 5–6. Spina bifida occulta.[9, 10] A long midline defect is present throughout every sacral segment (open arrows). This defect, which represents failure of ossification of all the sacral arches and has been termed a sacral hiatus, is a harmless variation found in 1 to 7 per cent of the normal population. A vertical zone of incomplete ossification is evident within the midline cleft at the S1 level (black arrows). The neural arches of L5 also are anomalous, touching in the midline, but with no evidence of fusion (arrowhead). An osteophyte spans the lower sacroiliac joint (white arrow).

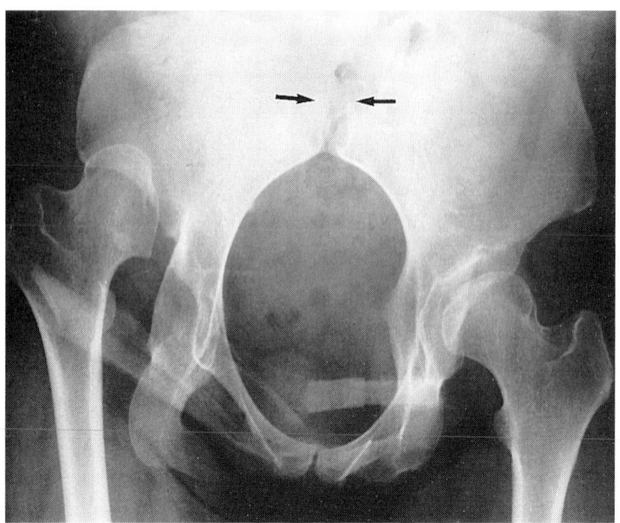

FIGURE 5–7. Sacral agenesis.[11] Frontal radiograph from a 26-year-old woman reveals complete absence of the sacrum with both ilia articulating in the midline (arrows). Acetabular dysplasia with congenital hip dislocation, present in this patient, frequently accompanies sacral agenesis.

TABLE 5–3. Injuries of the Sacrococcygeal Spine and Sacroiliac Joint*

Entity	Figure(s)	Characteristics
Fracture of the sacrum[13, 14]	5–8, 5–9	Isolated transverse fractures of the sacrum are rare but usually stable; easily overlooked on routine radiographs Vertical fractures more likely to be associated with other osseous and ligamentous injuries Associated unstable (type III) pelvic fractures and sacroiliac injury are common (see Chapter 6) Complications: 30 to 40 per cent of unstable type III injuries result in injury of the urethra or other pelvic viscera; neurologic injury of sacral nerve roots also may occur
Insufficiency fracture of the sacrum[15–17]	5–10	Sclerotic appearance with osteolysis simulating malignancy; often misdiagnosed or overlooked on routine radiographs; classic H-shaped pattern on scintigraphy; computed tomographic (CT) and magnetic resonance (MR) imaging also useful Complications: delayed union, refracture, and additional fractures
Fracture of the coccyx or sacrococcygeal dislocation[14]		Women > men Mechanism: fall on buttocks in seated position Best seen on lateral radiograph Stable injury usually with minimal complications; occasional chronic coccygodynia
Diastasis of the sacroiliac joint[14]		Isolated fractures near or diastasis of the sacroiliac joint are rare occurrences that usually result from direct trauma Isolated injury stable; diastasis combined with pelvic ring fracture is unstable (see Chapter 6)
Abused child syndrome[18]	2–30	Sacrococcygeal trauma rare in child abuse Injuries may include fracture or dislocation

*See also Tables 1–3 and 1–4.

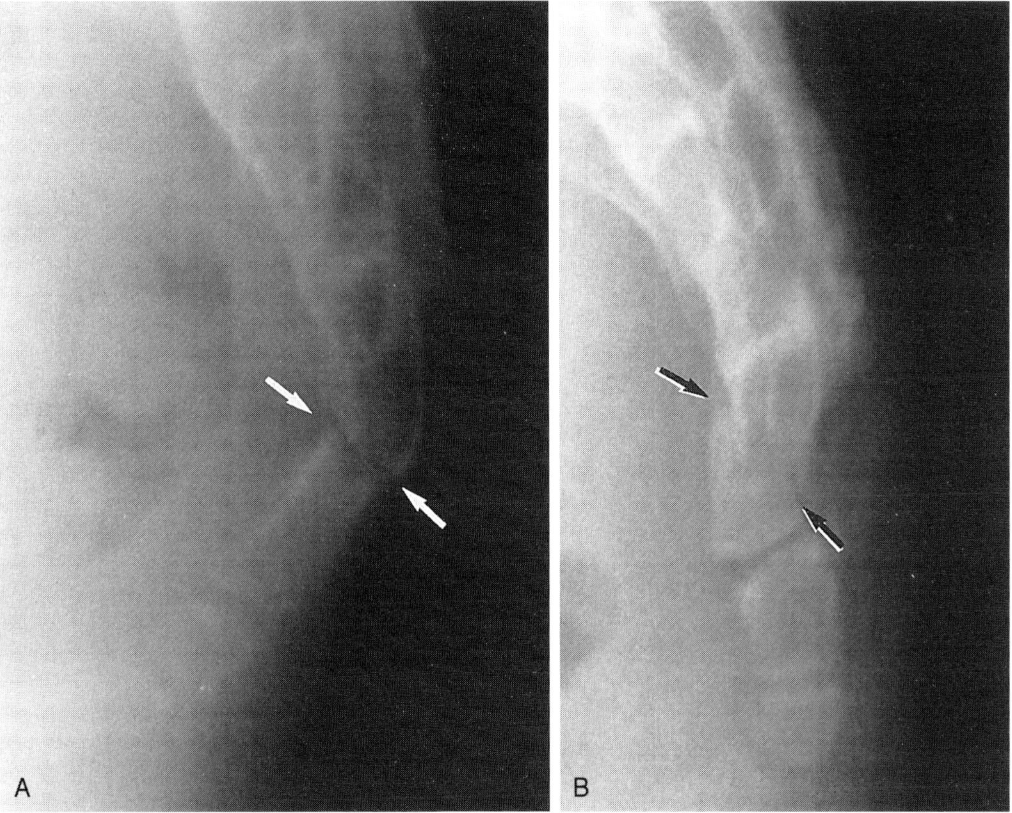

FIGURE 5–8. Sacral fractures.[13, 14] A Observe the transverse, horizontal fracture of the sacrum with anterior displacement just above the sacrococcygeal articulation (arrows). B Distal sacral fracture. This 28-year-old woman fell on her buttocks. Observe the oblique, minimally displaced fracture of the distal sacrum (arrows) on this lateral sacrococcygeal radiograph. Isolated transverse fractures of the sacrum are rare and easily overlooked on routine radiographs. Identification of such a fracture, as with other types of sacral fracture, should prompt a careful search for associated fractures of the spine and pelvis. Computed tomographic (CT) imaging and scintigraphy may be helpful in evaluating sacral fractures.

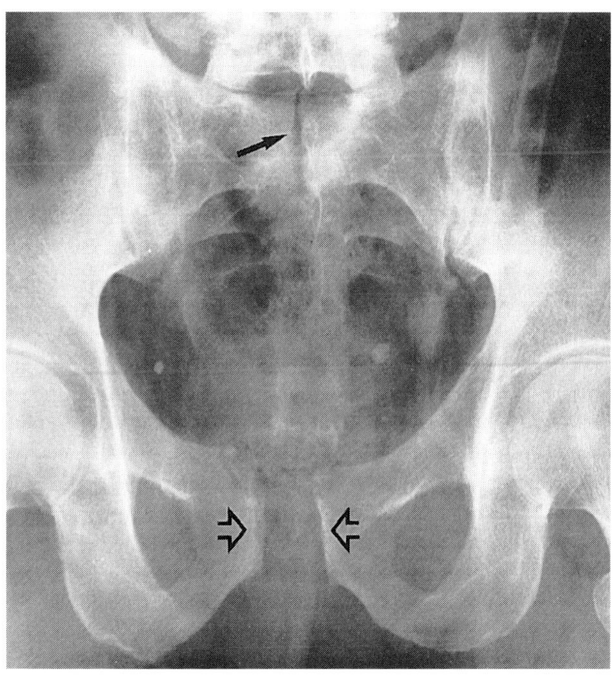

FIGURE 5–9. Sacral fracture with associated pubic diastasis.[13, 14] Frontal radiograph reveals a vertical fracture through the sacrum (arrow) and an associated diastasis of the pubic symphysis (open arrows). Injuries with double breaks (fractures or diastases) of the pelvic ring (type III injuries) are highly unstable. Type III pelvic injuries frequently are associated with injuries to the urethra or other visceral organs.

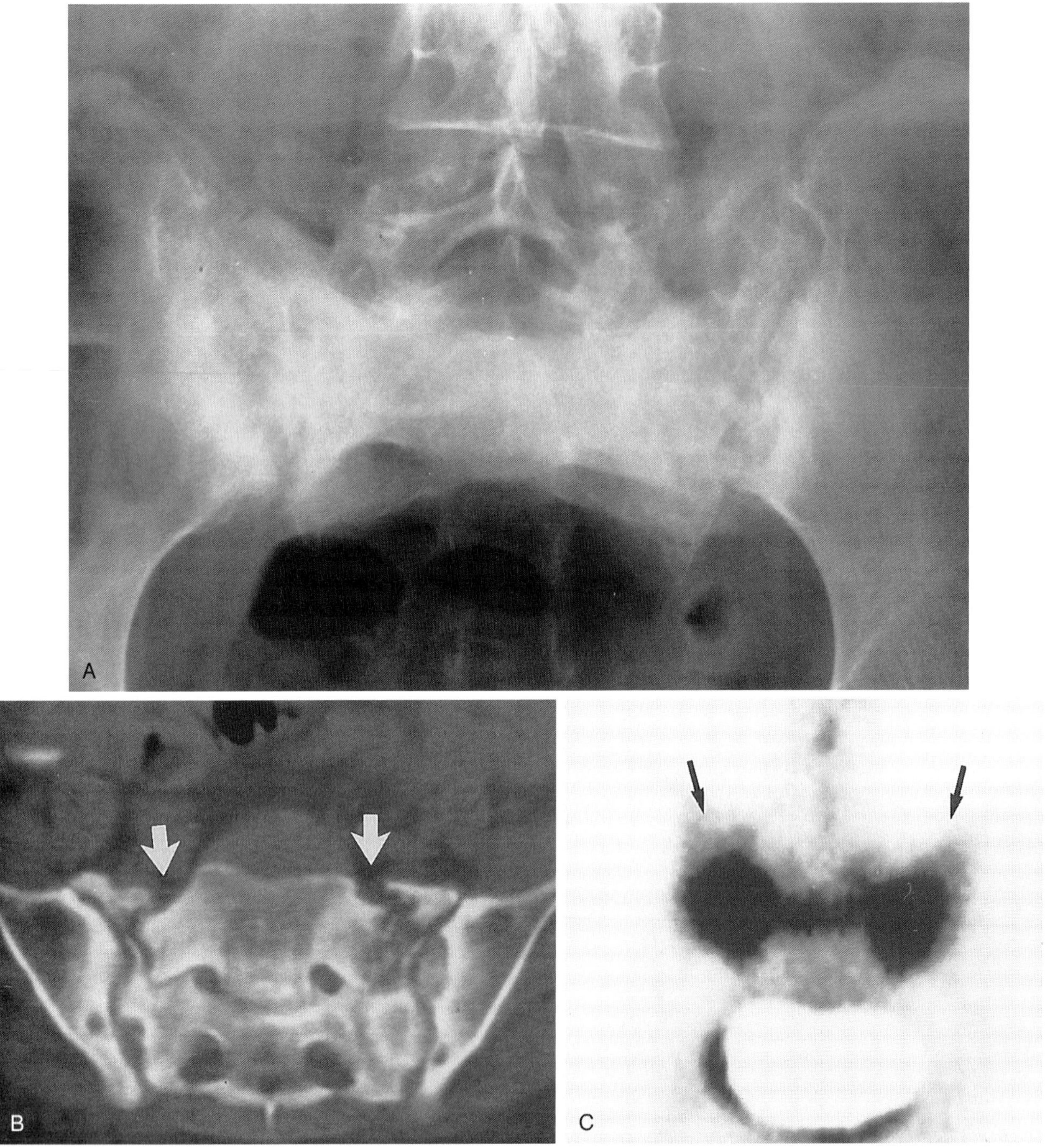

FIGURE 5–10. Insufficiency fracture: 65-year-old woman with osteoporosis.[15–17] A Frontal radiograph reveals diffuse osteosclerosis and fragmentation of the sacrum and adjacent subchondral bone of the ilium. B Transverse computed tomographic (CT) image shows bilateral fractures (arrows) and adjacent sclerosis involving the sacrum and both iliac bones. C Scintigraphy clearly demonstrates the classic H-shaped pattern of increased radionuclide activity (arrows). Sacral insufficiency fractures occur in about 20 per cent of patients undergoing pelvic radiation therapy. *(Courtesy of G. Greenway, M.D., Dallas, Texas.)*

TABLE 5–4. Sacroiliac Joint: Articular Disorders*

Entity	Figure(s)	Characteristics
Degenerative and related disorders		
Degenerative joint disease[19, 20]	5–11	Accompanies aging and is accelerated by previous injury and lumbosacral transitional segments
		Men > women
		Narrowed articular space
		Osteophytes (may simulate osteoblastic pelvic lesions)
		Subchondral bone sclerosis
		Vacuum phenomenon
Ligament calcification and ossification[19]	5–12	Calcification or ossification of the sacroiliac, sacrotuberous, or sacrospinous ligaments occurs in degenerative disease, diffuse idiopathic skeletal hyperostosis (DISH), fluorosis, or as an idiopathic phenomenon
Osteitis condensans ilii[5, 21]	5–13	Well-defined triangular sclerosis of the iliac side of the sacroiliac joints
		Most frequently bilateral and relatively symmetric process; occasionally unilateral
		Affects primarily women and frequently is associated with paraglenoid sulci
		Cause not clear; predominant theory suggests that the condition is secondary to mechanical stress across the joint coupled with increased vascularity during pregnancy
		Postulated theories include associations with urinary tract infections and ankylosing spondylitis, but these do not have widespread support
		Radiographic appearance may simulate that of ankylosing spondylitis and other seronegative spondyloarthropathies
DISH[22]	5–14	Enthesopathy of ligaments and para-articular bone excrescences predominate at the anterior, anterosuperior, or anteroinferior articular margins and tend to bridge the joint rather than cause true intra-articular ankylosis or sacroiliitis
		Bridging ossification may span the inferior sacroiliac joint or the upper ligamentous portion of the joint
Inflammatory disorders		
Rheumatoid arthritis[23]	5–15	Sacroiliac joint involvement rare and findings are mild compared with those in ankylosing spondylitis
		Unilateral or bilateral
		Sclerosis and erosions
		Osteoporosis
		Absence of osteophytes and other osseous outgrowths
Ankylosing spondylitis[24, 25]	5–16	Sacroiliitis is the hallmark of ankylosing spondylitis
		Occurs early in the disease
		Usually bilateral and symmetric in distribution
		Initial joint space widening from erosions
		Eventually results in osseous ankylosis
Enteropathic arthropathy[26]	5–17	Changes identical to those of ankylosing spondylitis
		Sacroiliitis and spondylitis account for about 20 to 30 per cent of articular involvement in ulcerative colitis, whereas peripheral involvement constitutes as much as 60 per cent
Psoriatic spondyloarthropathy[27]	5–18	Sacroiliac joint changes are found on radiographs of approximately 10 to 25 per cent of patients with moderate or severe psoriatic skin disease
		Unilateral or bilateral asymmetric pattern of sacroiliitis is typical
Reiter's syndrome[28]	5–19	Associated with sacroiliac joint changes in about 50 per cent of cases
		Unilateral or bilateral asymmetric pattern of sacroiliitis is typical
		Associated with urethritis and conjunctivitis
Metabolic disorders		
Hyperparathyroidism[29, 30]	5–20	Bilateral, symmetric subchondral bone resorption predominates on the iliac side and results in widening of the sacroiliac joints
		Minimal adjacent subchondral sclerosis
Renal osteodystrophy[30, 31]	5–21	Sacroiliac changes identical to those in hyperparathyroidism
Infection		
Pyogenic septic arthritis[32]	5–22	Septic arthritis results in unilateral sacroiliac joint widening and destruction
		Paravertebral soft tissue mass or abscess variable; osseous ankylosis rare
		Tuberculous infection of the sacroiliac joint occurs only infrequently

*See also Tables 1–6 to 1–9 and Table 1–17.

TABLE 5–5. Distribution of Sacroiliac Joint Articular Disorders

			Sacroiliac Joint Involvement			
Entity	**Figure(s)**	*Pathology*	*Intra-articular Ankylosis*	*Bilateral Symmetric**	*Bilateral Asymmetric**	*Unilateral**
Degenerative and related disorders						
Degenerative disease	5–11	Joint degeneration	Absent	+	+ +	+
Osteitis condensans ilii	5–13	Iliac sclerosis	Absent	+ +	+	+
Diffuse idiopathic skeletal hyperostosis (DISH)	5–14	Enthesopathy	Absent	+ +		
Inflammatory disorders						
Rheumatoid arthritis	5–15	Erosion, minor sclerosis	Absent		+	+
Ankylosing spondylitis	5–16	Erosion, sacroiliitis, iliac sclerosis	Common	+ +		
Enteropathic arthropathy	5–17	Erosion, sacroiliitis, iliac sclerosis	Common	+ +		
Psoriatic spondyloarthropathy	5–18	Erosion, sacroiliitis, iliac sclerosis	Uncommon	+	+ +	+
Reiter's syndrome	5–19	Erosion, sacroiliitis, iliac sclerosis	Uncommon	+	+ +	+
Metabolic disorders						
Hyperparathyroidism	5–20	Subchondral resorption, minimal sclerosis	Absent	+ +		
Renal osteodystrophy	5–21	Subchondral resorption, minimal sclerosis	Absent	+ +		
Infection						
Pyogenic septic arthritis	5–22	Septic arthritis with joint destruction	Uncommon			+ +

* +, Occasional pattern of distribution; + +, predominant pattern of distribution.

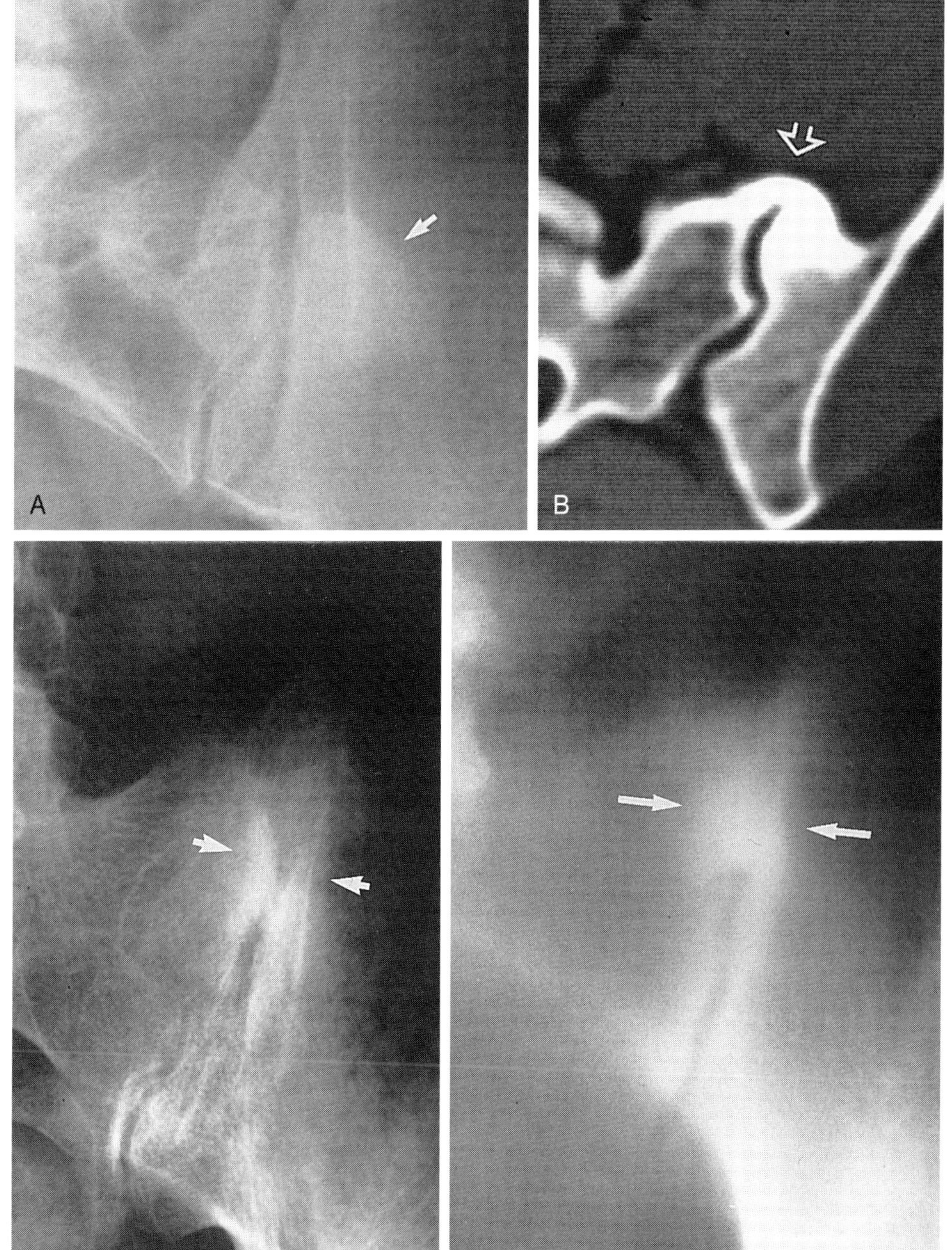

FIGURE 5–11. Degenerative joint disease.[19, 20] A, B This 39-year-old man had injured his sacroiliac joint. In A, a radiograph obtained 15 years later reveals an area of increased density overlying the left sacroiliac joint (arrow). In B, a transaxial computed tomographic (CT) scan more clearly defines the nature of this osteophyte bridging the anterior portion of the sacroiliac joint (open arrow). C, D Another patient, a 41-year-old man. In C, the routine radiograph shows sclerosis overlying the right sacroiliac joint (arrows). In D, conventional tomography reveals an osteophyte spanning the joint (arrows). Sacroiliac joint osteophytes may simulate osteoblastic lesions of bone. *(C, D, Courtesy of P. Wilson, M.D., Eugene, Oregon.)*

Illustration continued on following page

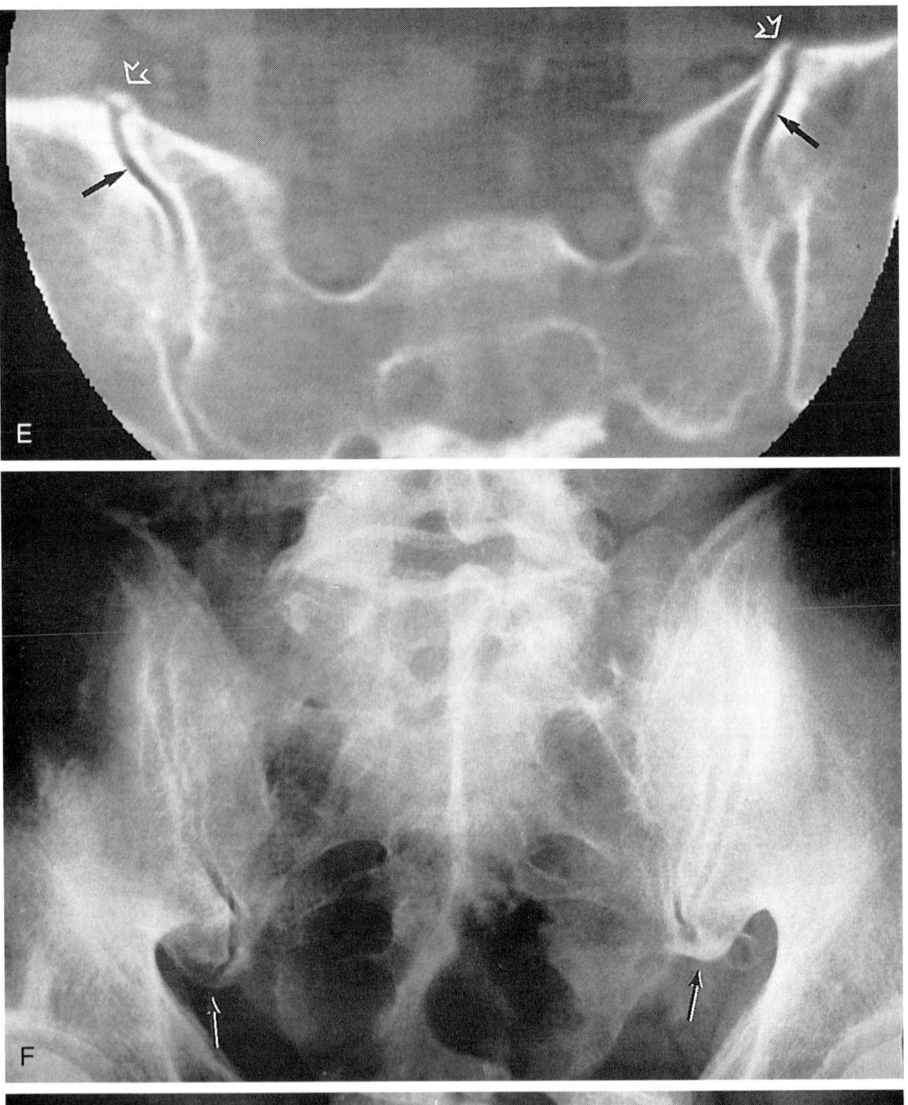

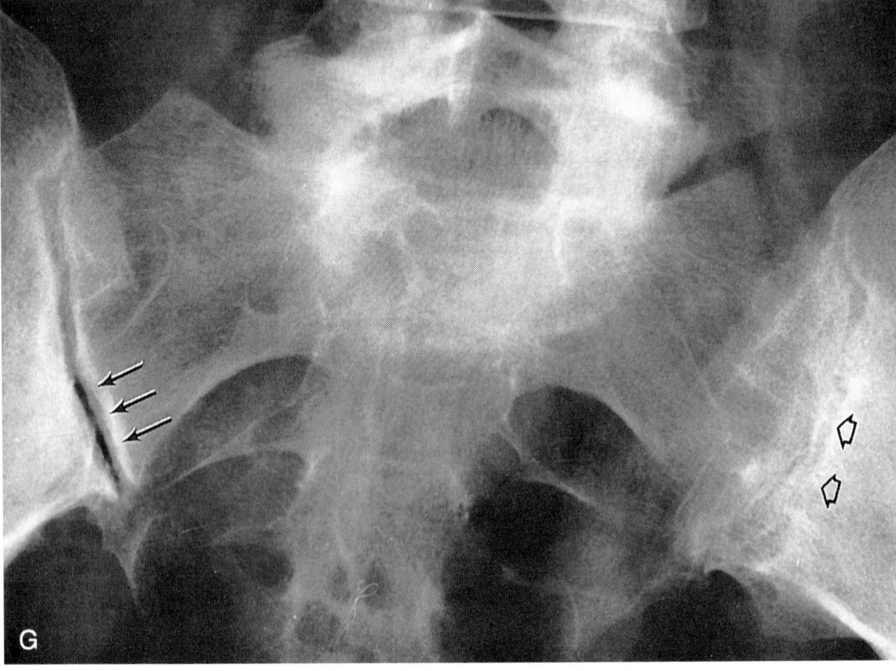

FIGURE 5–11 *Continued.* E In a third patient, a transaxial CT scan reveals bilateral subchondral sclerosis, small anterior osteophytes (open arrows), and intra-articular gas (arrows). F This 73-year-old man had back pain and stiffness. Radiograph shows bridging osteophytes spanning the inferior aspect of both sacroiliac joints (arrows). Subtle sclerosis also is seen adjacent to the middle regions of the sacroiliac joints. G In another patient, a vacuum phenomenon is evident on one side (arrows), whereas sclerosis and joint space narrowing predominate on the other side (open arrows). *(*F, G, *Reprinted wtih permission from Taylor JAM, Hoffman LE: The geriatric patient: Diagnostic imaging of common musculoskeletal disorders. Top Clin Chiropr 3:23, © 1996, Aspen Publishers, Inc.)*

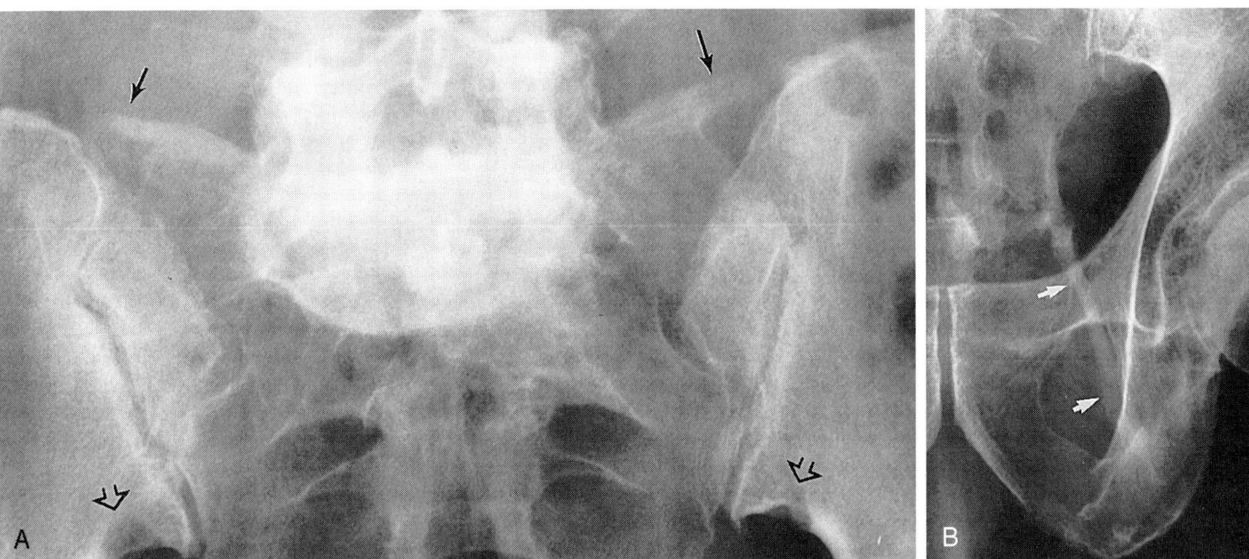

FIGURE 5–12. Ligament calcification and ossification.[19] A Observe the enthesopathic proliferation involving the superior sacroiliac ligaments (arrows). Minimal degenerative disease of the sacroiliac joints, characterized by bilateral subchondral bone sclerosis and a vacuum phenomenon within the right sacroiliac joint, also is evident. Bilateral notches within the inferior ilium adjacent to the sacroiliac joints are termed paraglenoid sulci (open arrows). These grooves represent a normal variant found almost exclusively in women. B Sacrotuberous ligament ossification is seen in this 79-year-old patient (arrows). Ligament ossification may be idiopathic or associated with degenerative disease, fluorosis, or diffuse idiopathic skeletal hyperostosis (DISH).

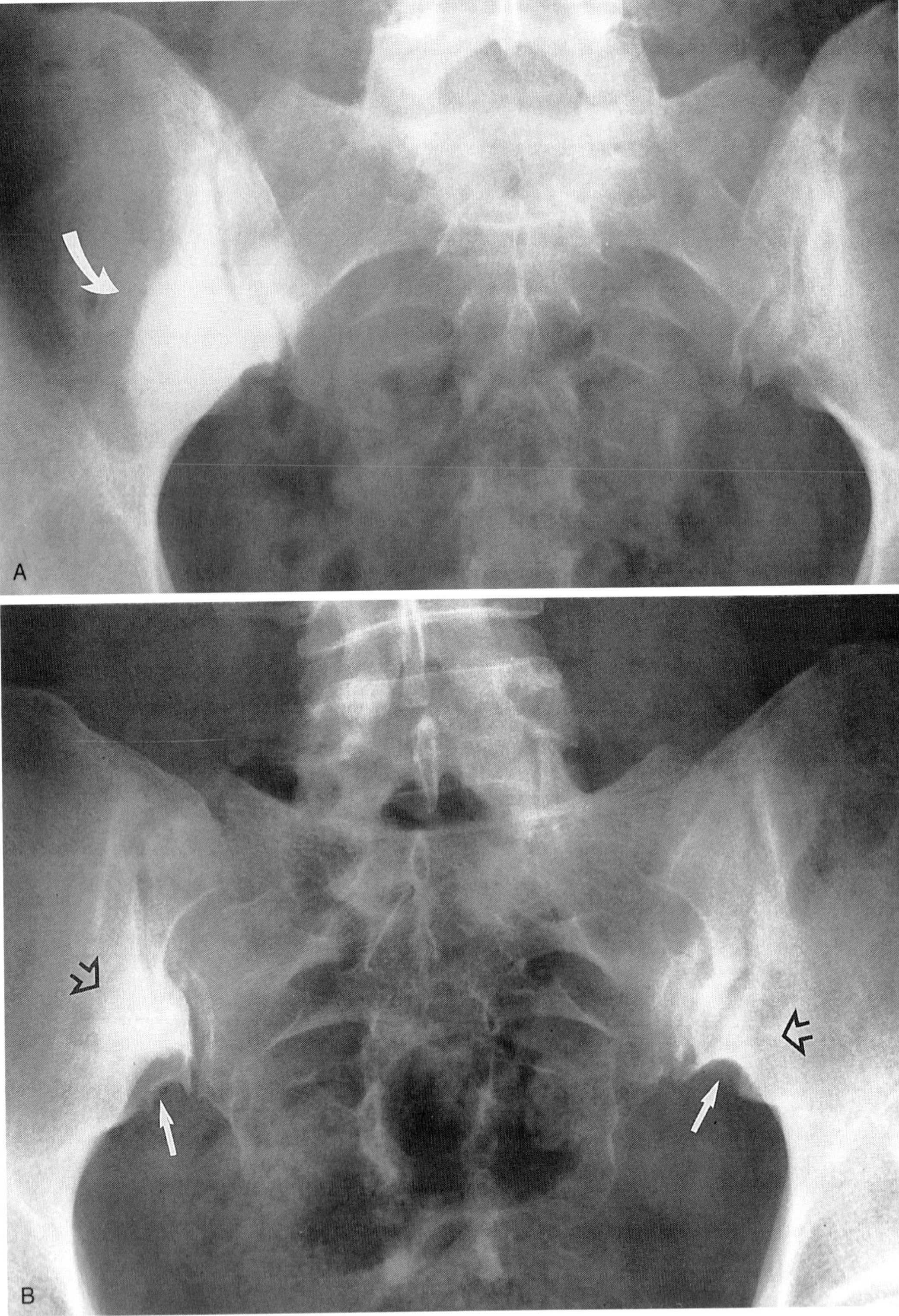

FIGURE 5–13. Osteitis condensans ilii.[21] A Unilateral triangular hyperostosis is seen (curved arrow) in the ilium of this postpartum woman. B In another patient, observe the triangular areas of ossification adjacent to the inferior portions of the sacroiliac joints (open arrows). Also noted are bilateral paraglenoid fossae (arrows).

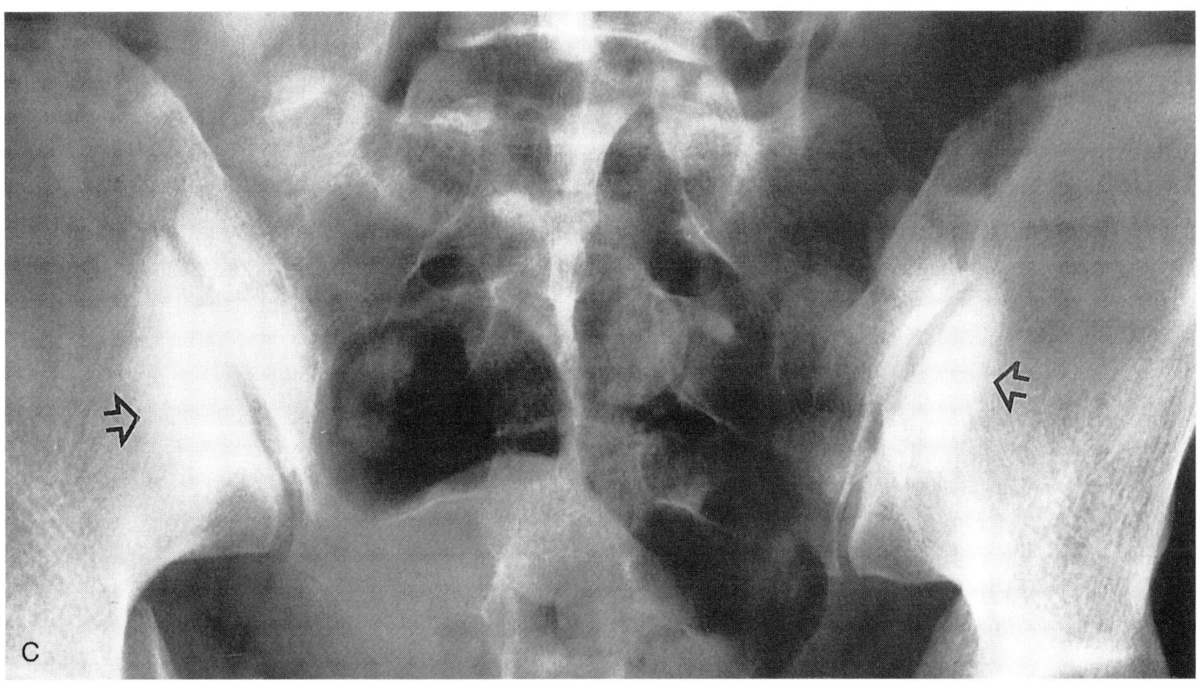

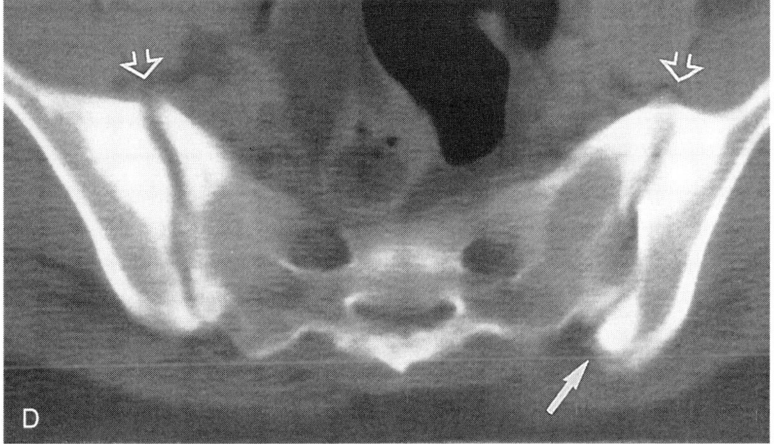

FIGURE 5–13 *Continued.* **C, D** This 23-year-old woman was involved in a motor vehicle accident and fractured her right ischium and pubis. In **C**, a radiograph reveals, as an incidental finding, bilateral, well-defined osteosclerosis (open arrows) predominating on the iliac side of the articulations. The joint spaces are well maintained and the joint margins are sharply defined. In **D**, a transaxial computed tomographic (CT) scan clearly delineates the sclerosis involving both the iliac and sacral aspects of the joint (open arrows). A small focal zone of sclerosis also is noted adjacent to an accessory sacroiliac articulation (arrow).

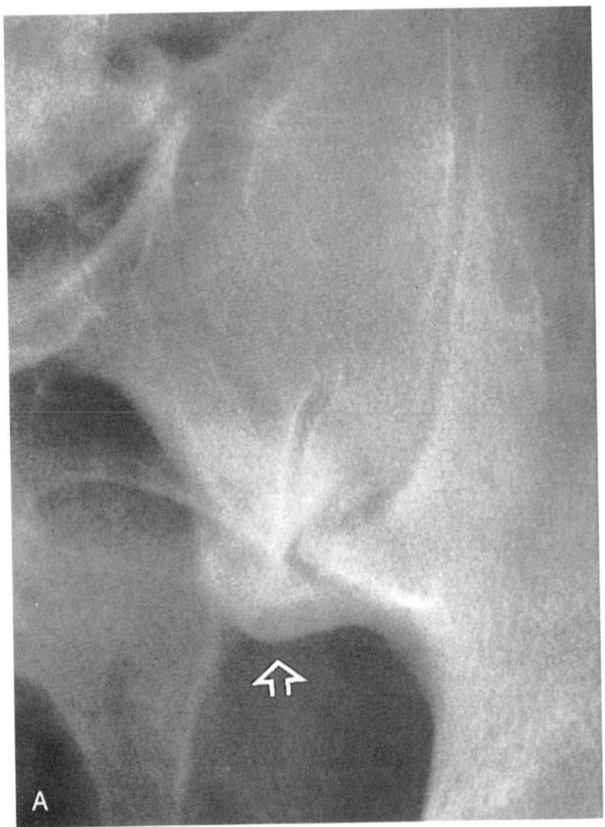

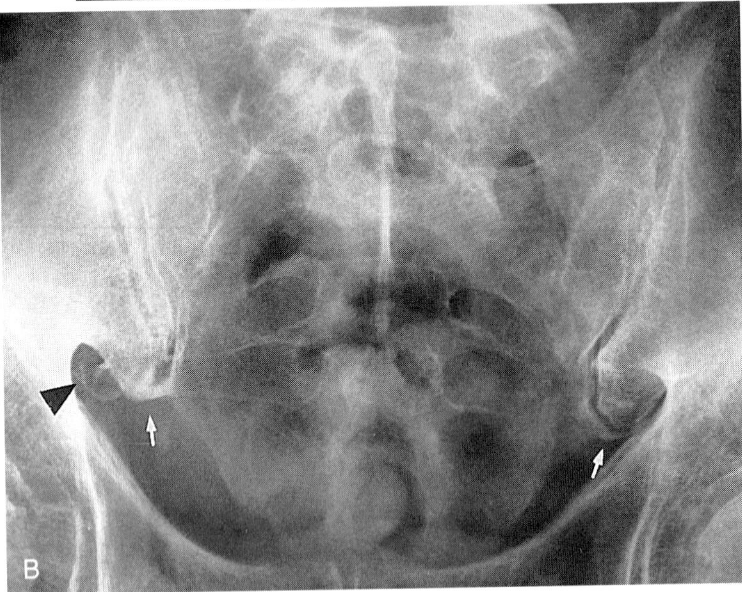

FIGURE 5–14. Diffuse idiopathic skeletal hyperostosis (DISH).[22] **A** Bridging ossification is seen at the inferior aspect of the sacroiliac joint (open arrow) in this patient with long-standing DISH. The sacroiliac joint is otherwise normal. **B** In another patient, bilateral osseous bridging (arrows) and vascular calcification (arrowhead) are evident.

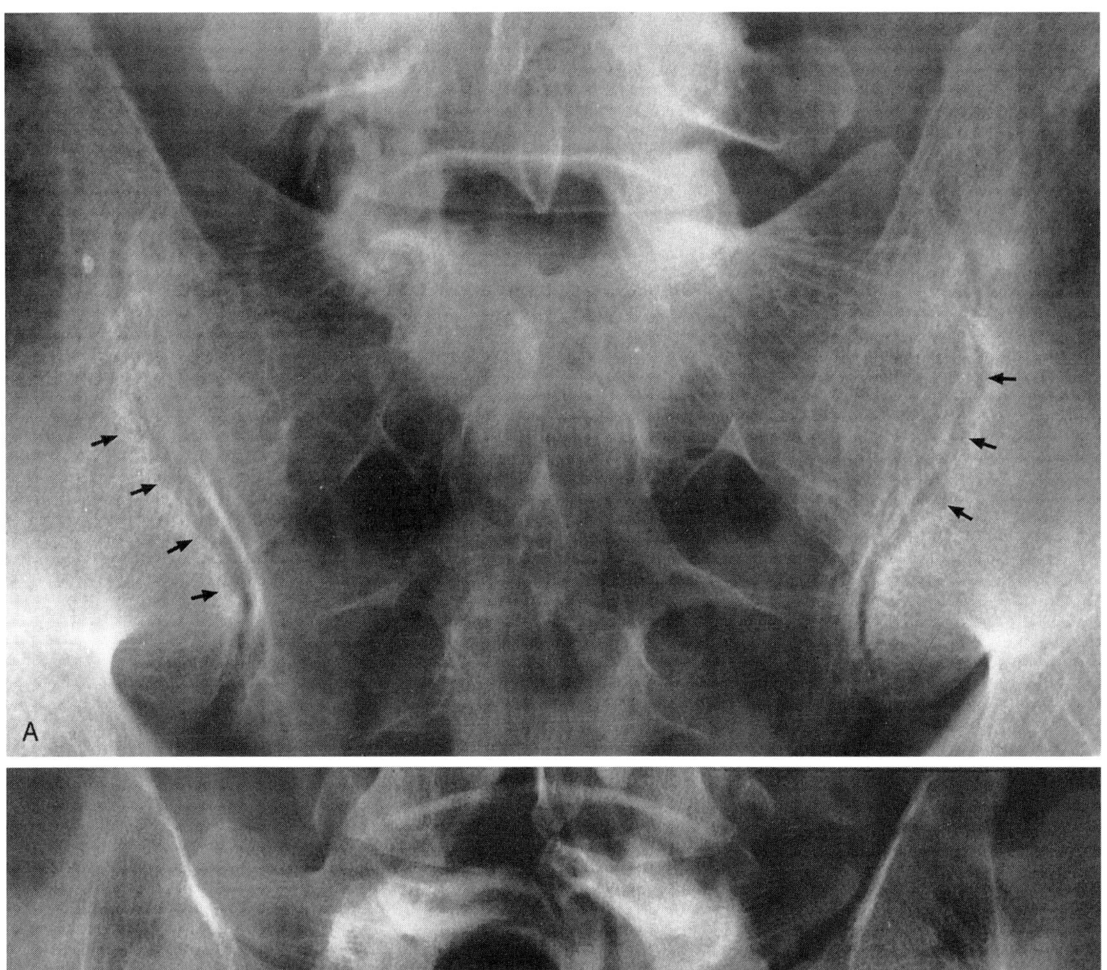

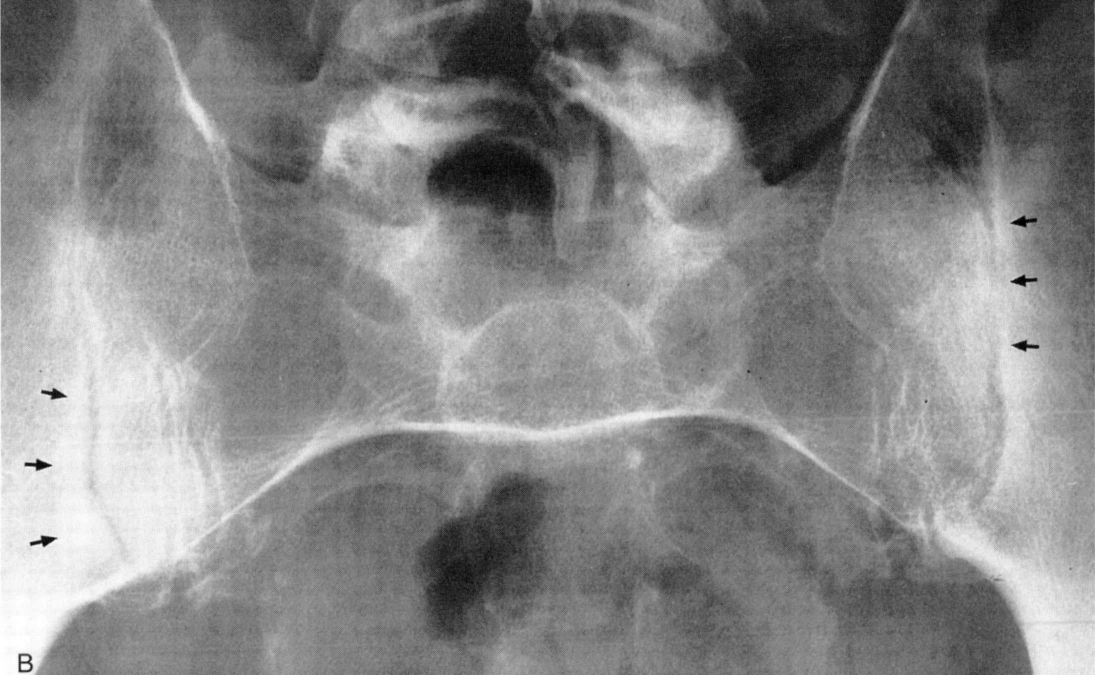

FIGURE 5–15. Rheumatoid arthritis.[23] A Subtle subchondral bone erosion mainly on the iliac side of the joints (arrows) and minimal sclerosis are seen in this patient. B In another patient with rheumatoid arthritis, mild erosive changes and minimal sclerosis involving the lower right and middle left portions of the articulations are evident (arrows).

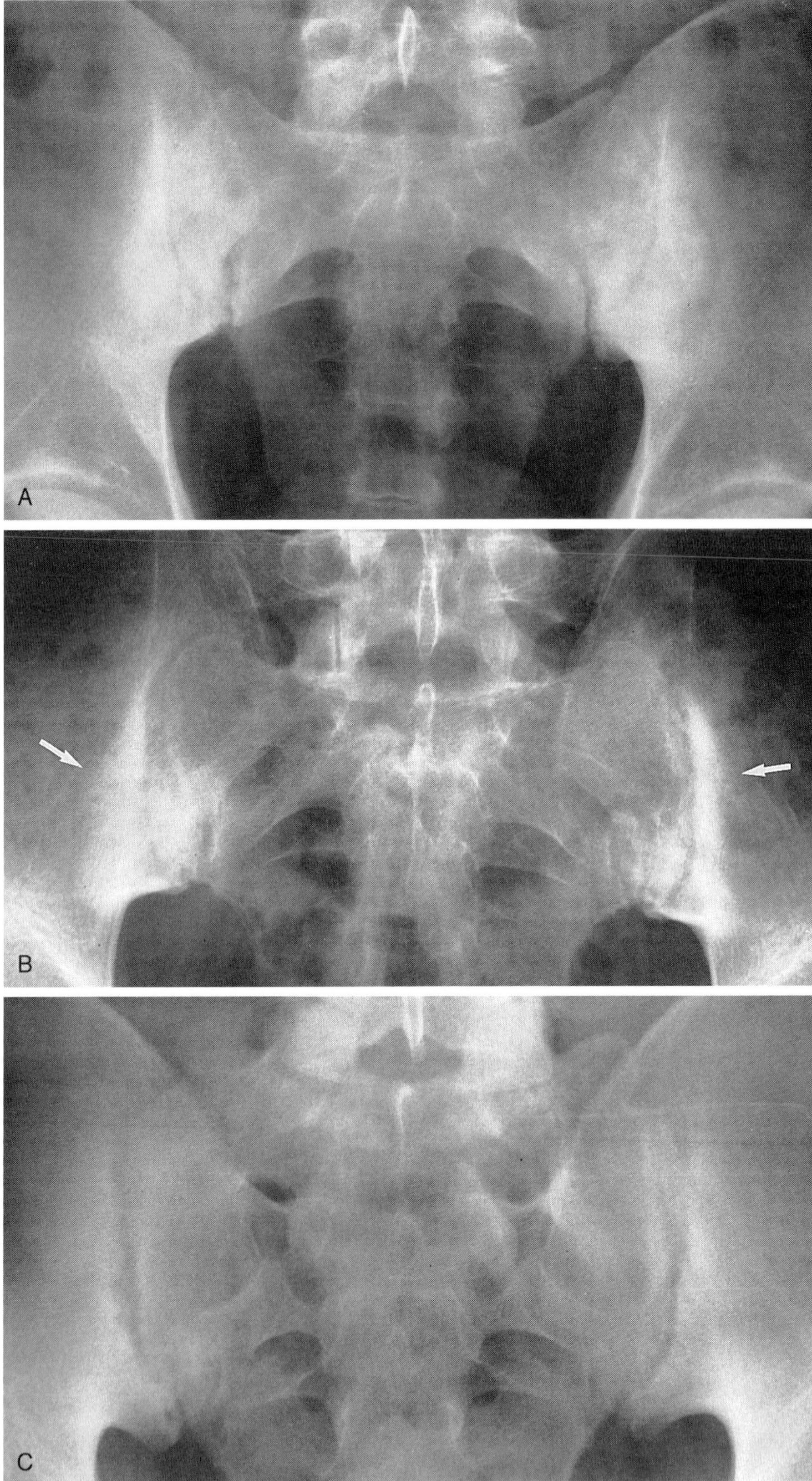

FIGURE 5–16. Ankylosing spondylitis.[24, 25] A Bilateral sacroiliitis. Blurring of the sacroiliac joint margins is associated with subchondral sclerosis, predominating on the iliac side of the sacroiliac joints in this 40-year-old man with long-standing ankylosing spondylitis. B In another patient, marked sclerosis (arrows) and blurring of the subchondral bone are noted. C In a third patient, sacroiliitis with sclerosis and subchondral bone erosion are apparent.

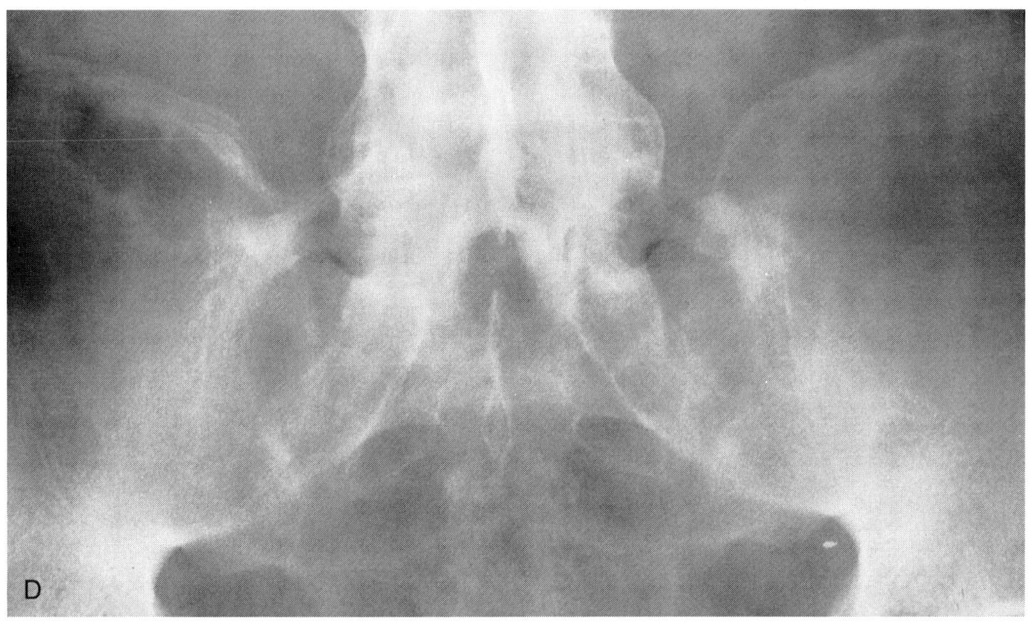

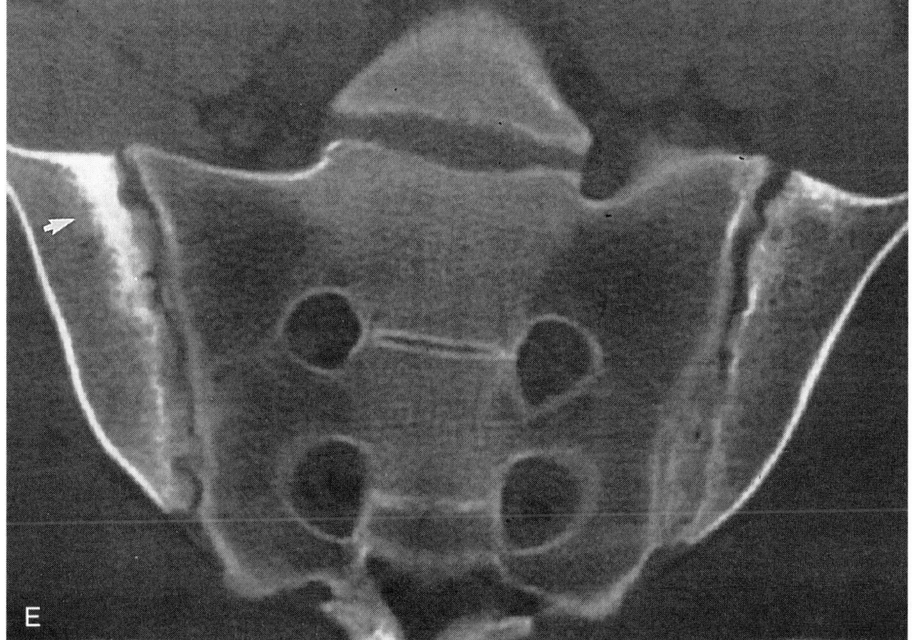

FIGURE 5–16 *Continued.* D Ankylosis. In a 65-year-old man with advanced ankylosing spondylitis, the sacroiliac joint margins are completely obliterated by osseous ankylosis. Observe the enthesopathy of the L5 transverse processes and the characteristic syndesmophytes in the lumbosacral spine. E Computed tomographic (CT) abnormalities. CT scan shows bilateral erosion of subchondral bone with asymmetric sclerosis of the iliac side of the joints, especially on the right (arrow). *(*E*, Courtesy of T. Learch, M.D., Los Angeles, California.)*

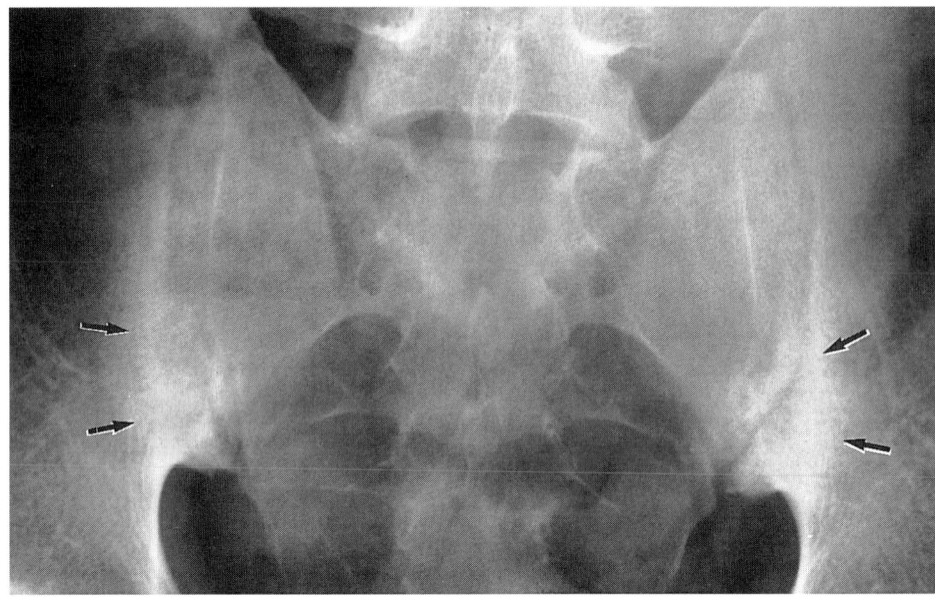

FIGURE 5–17. Ulcerative colitis: Enteropathic arthropathy.[26] Bilateral, symmetric sacroiliitis is characterized by joint space narrowing, subarticular erosions, and subchondral bone sclerosis involving the lower synovial portion of the articulations (arrows).

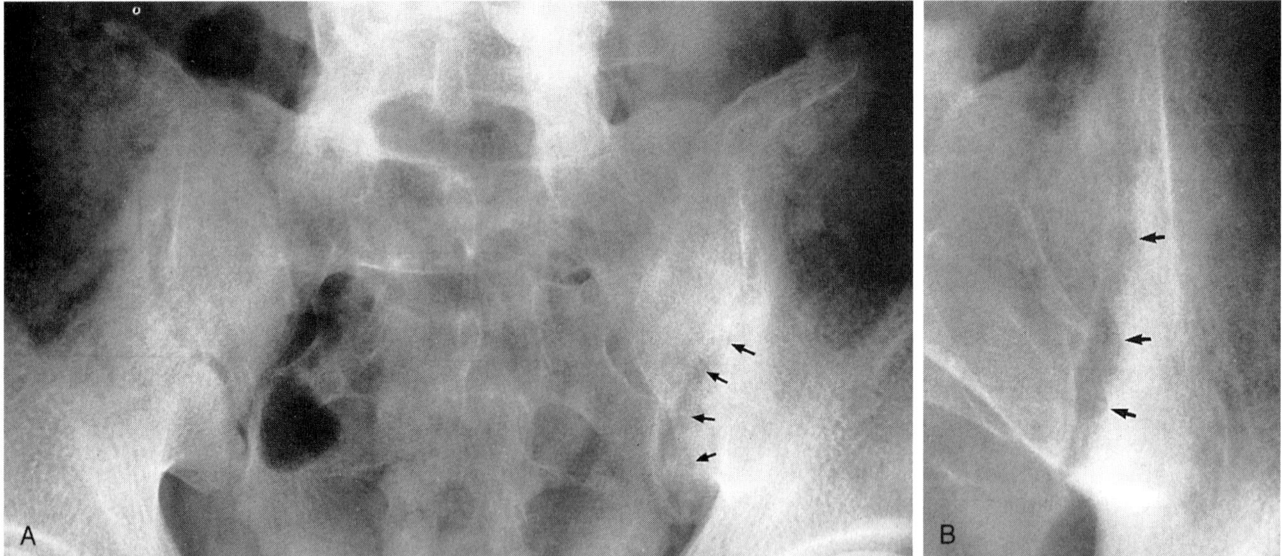

FIGURE 5–18. Psoriatic spondyloarthropathy.[27] **A** Asymmetric sacroiliac joint changes including loss of definition of the lower portion of the left sacroiliac joint (arrows) as well as subchondral sclerosis are characteristic of sacroiliitis. The margins of the right sacroiliac joint are slightly indistinct. **B** In another patient, subchondral scalloped erosions (arrows) are accompanied by sclerosis of the iliac side of the joint. The subarticular joint surface is indistinct.

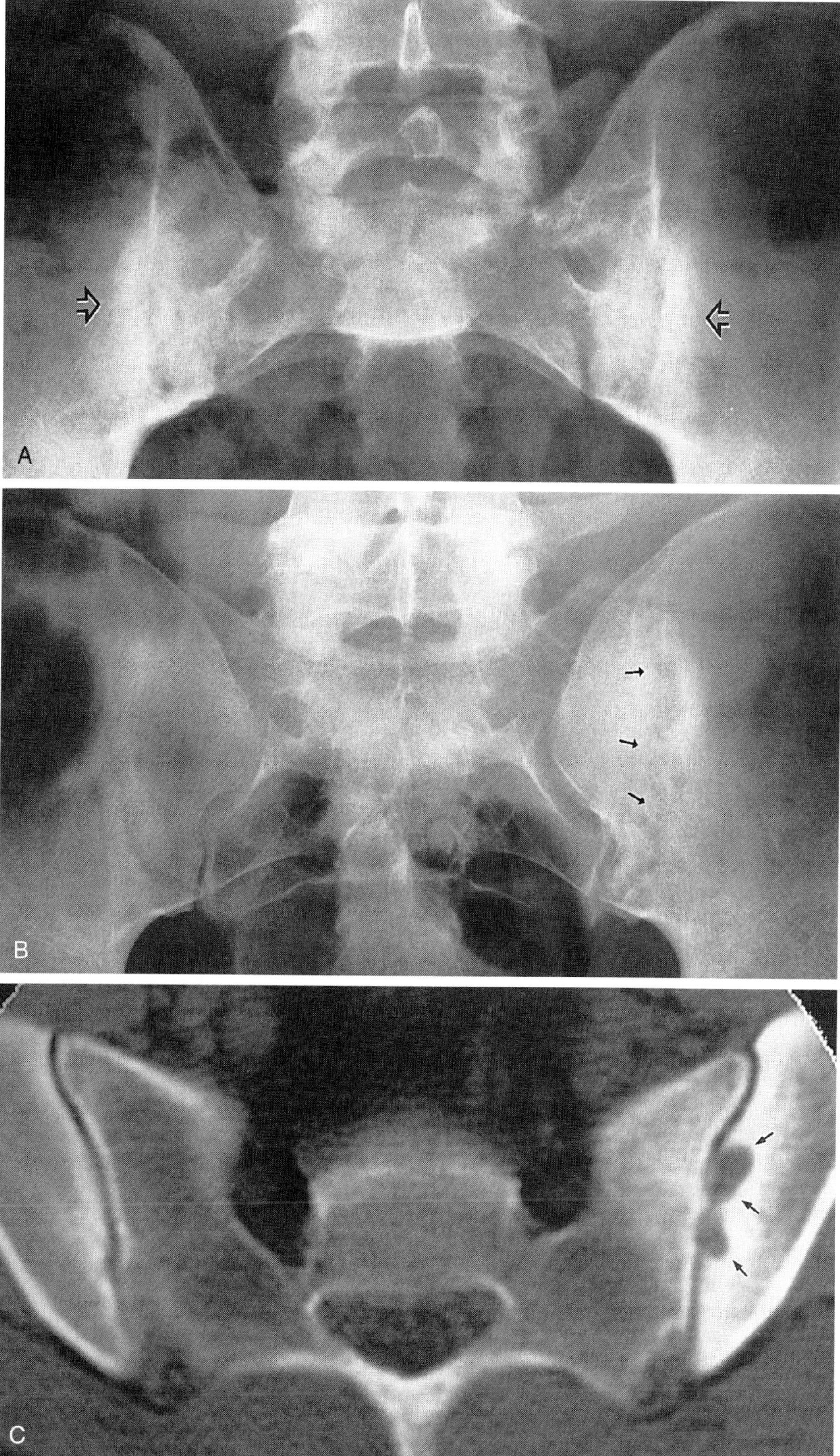

FIGURE 5–19. Reiter's syndrome.[28] **A** Bilateral symmetric sacroiliitis is evident in this 35-year-old man with urethritis, conjunctivitis, and back pain. The radiographic findings include sclerosis predominating on the iliac side of the joints (open arrows) and indistinct subchondral joint margins. A lumbosacral transitional segment with enlargement of the left L5 transverse process, which has an anomalous articulation with the sacrum, also is present. **B** In another patient, the findings, predominating on the left side, include asymmetric sclerosis and indistinct joint margins (arrows). **C** In a third patient, a transaxial computed tomographic (CT) image reveals unilateral sacroiliitis with subchondral erosions (arrows) and prominent sclerosis, especially on the iliac side of the articulation.

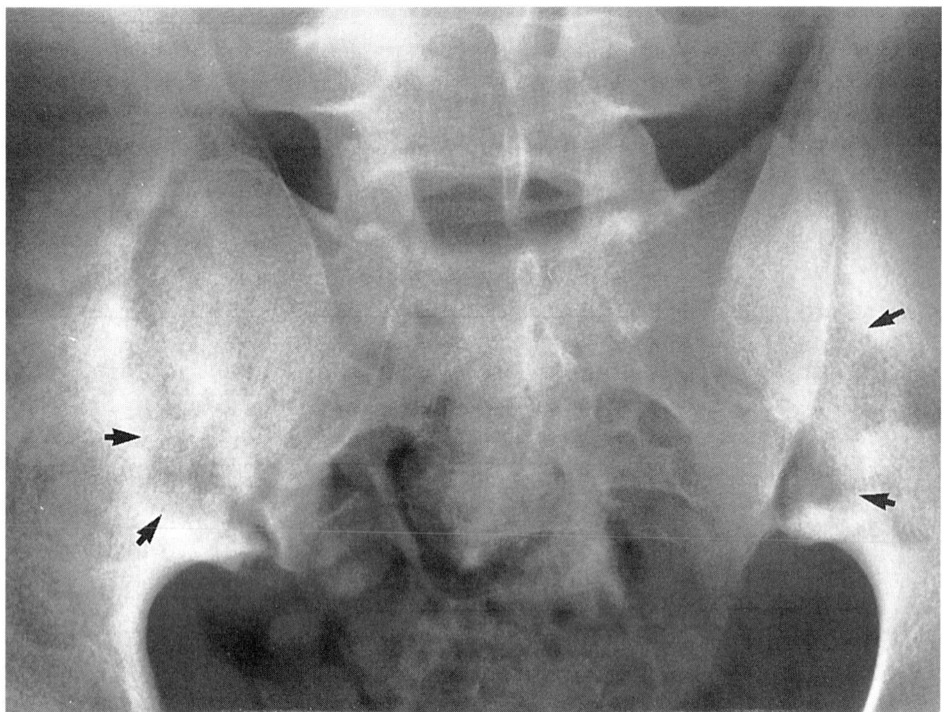

FIGURE 5–20. Hyperparathyroidism: Subchondral resorption.[29, 30] Extensive resorption of the subarticular bone is seen adjacent to the sacroiliac joints (arrows) in this 28-year-old man with renal failure and secondary hyperparathyroidism.

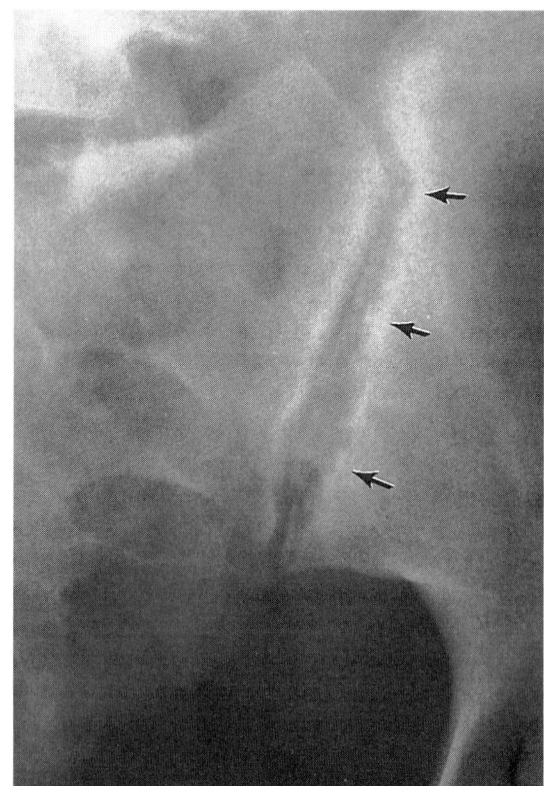

FIGURE 5–21. Renal osteodystrophy: Subchondral resorption.[30, 31] Observe the widening and indistinct margins of the subchondral bone adjacent to the sacroiliac joint (arrows) in this patient with chronic renal disease, renal osteodystrophy, and secondary hyperparathyroidism. Marked resorption of bone is present, but the amount of subchondral bone sclerosis is minimal. *(Courtesy of J.T. Knudsen, D.C., Chicago, Illinois, and C. Yomtob, D.C., Los Angeles, California.)*

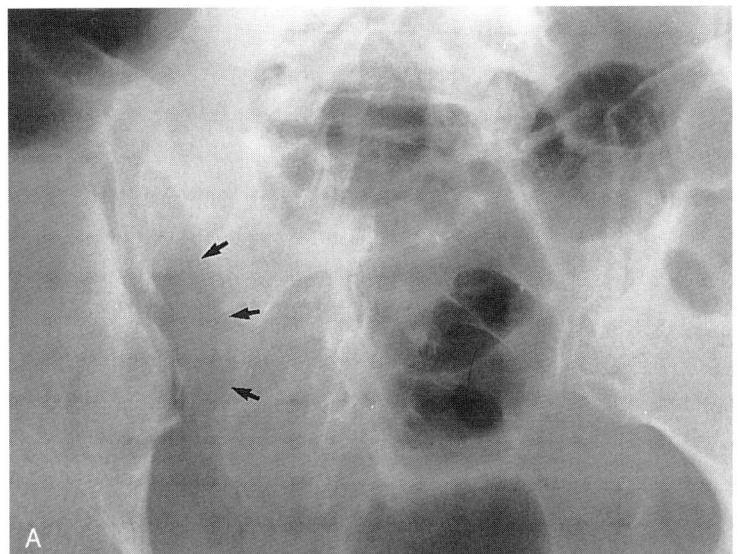

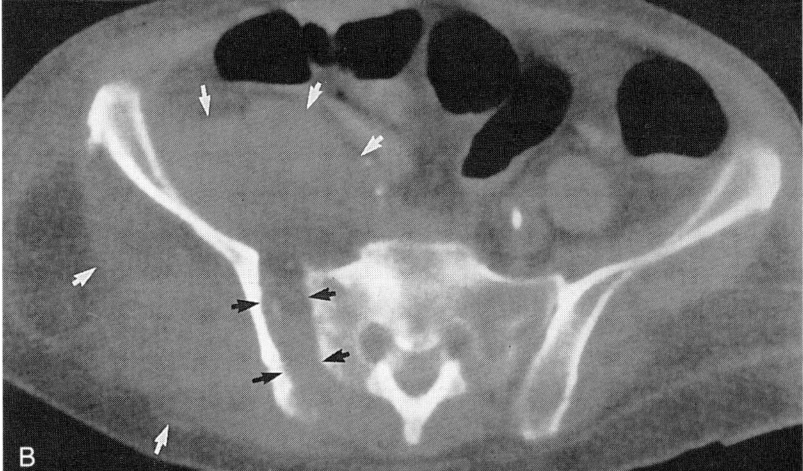

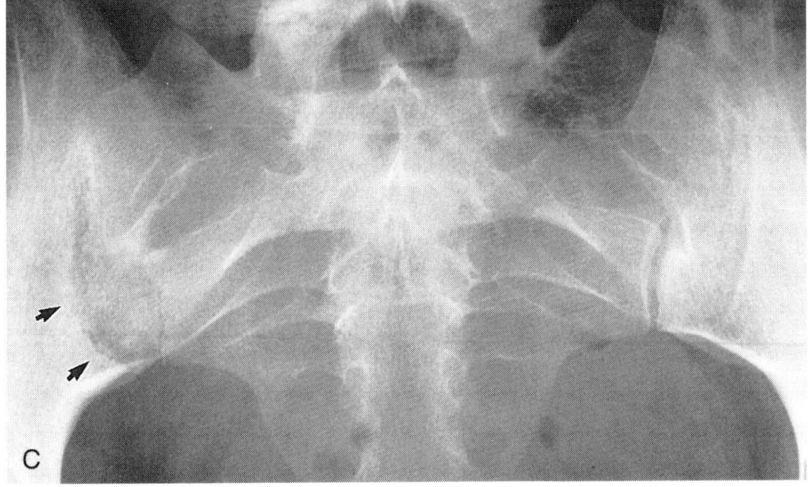

FIGURE 5–22. Pyogenic septic arthritis.[32] A, B Abscess formation. This 58-year-old woman had low back pain. In A, the routine radiograph demonstrates unilateral destruction of the subchondral bone of the sacrum adjacent to the lower sacroiliac joint (arrows). The subchondral bone of the ilium is not well visualized on this radiograph, but it also appears eroded. In B, the transaxial computed tomographic (CT) image shows joint space widening and extensive erosion of the adjacent subchondral surfaces of bone (black arrows). A huge soft tissue abscess extending from the articulation into the pelvic basin and gluteal region is seen (white arrows). C In another patient, a 28-year-old heroin addict, a routine radiograph demonstrates unilateral sacroiliitis with joint widening and obliteration of the sharp margin of the subchondral surface of the articulation (arrows). *Pseudomonas aeruginosa* was cultured from a bone biopsy specimen. Intravenous drug abusers are especially predisposed to sacroiliac joint infections. The sacroiliitis of pyogenic infection usually is monoarticular and may result in eventual osseous ankylosis.

TABLE 5–6. Sacrococcygeal Spine Neoplasms*

Entity	Figure(s)	Entity	Figure(s)
Malignant neoplasms		**Benign neoplasms**	
Skeletal metastasis		*Primary benign neoplasms*	
Osteolytic metastasis[33, 34]	5–23	Enostosis[37]	5–27
Osteoblastic metastasis[33, 34]	5–24	Giant cell tumor[38]	5–28
Primary malignant neoplasms of bone		*Tumor-like lesions*	
Chordoma[35]	5–25	Paget's disease[39, 40]	5–29
Myeloproliferative disorders		Neurofibromatosis Type I (von Recklinghausen's disease)[41]	5–30
Plasmacytoma[36]	5–26		

*This table lists only the neoplasms illustrated in this chapter; for a more complete discussion of neoplasms see Tables 1–10 to 1–12 and 2–13.

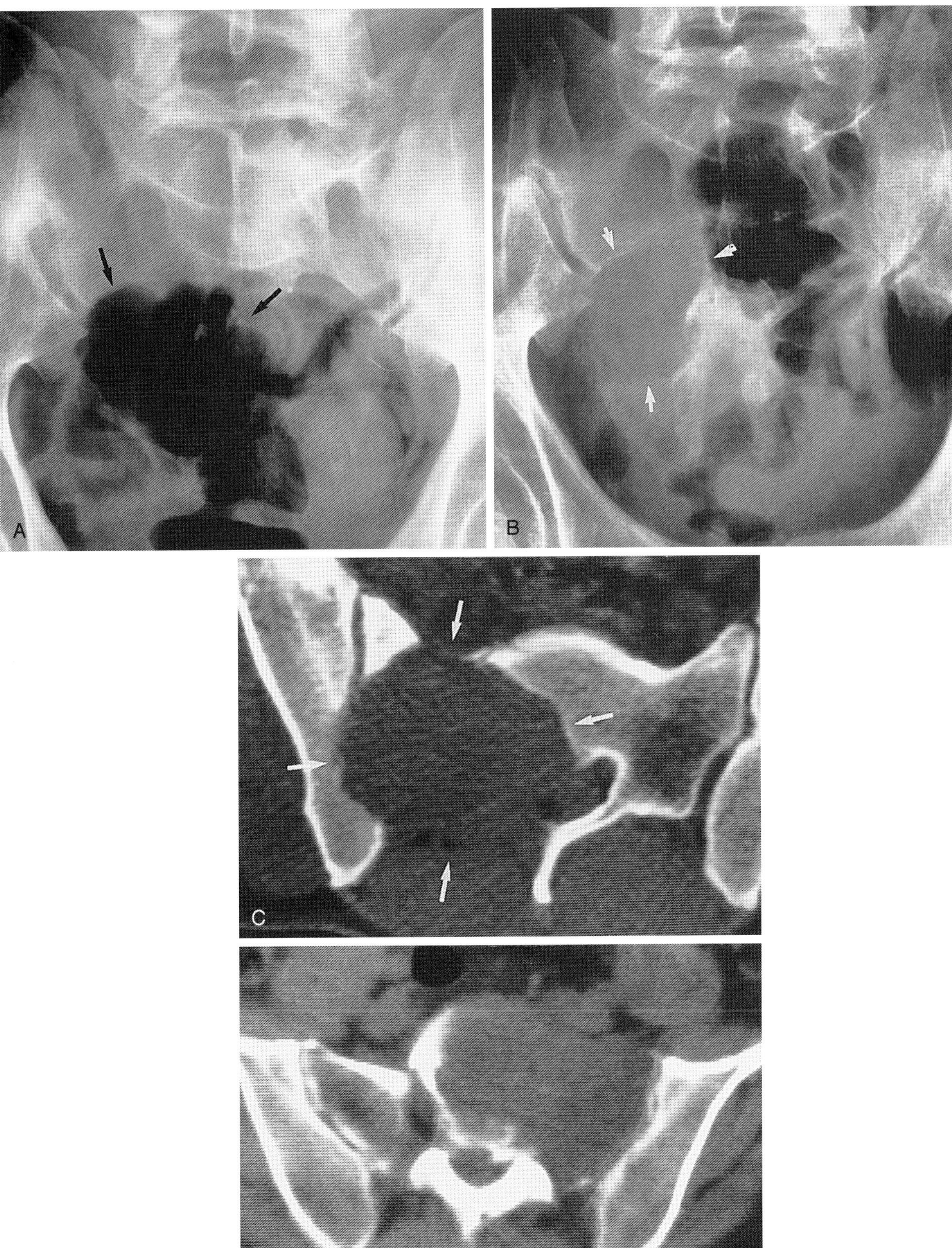

FIGURE 5–23. Skeletal metastasis: Osteolytic pattern.[33, 34] This 42-year-old man had a 6-month history of severe right leg pain. A On the initial radiograph, the lower sacrum is obscured by overlying bowel gas (arrows). B Radiograph obtained the next day reveals a large osteolytic lesion in this region (arrows). C Striking osteolysis of the sacrum and ilium is evident on the transaxial computed tomographic (CT) display (arrows). The histologic diagnosis proved to be skeletal metastasis secondary to renal cell carcinoma. *(A–C, Courtesy of G. Greenway, M.D., Dallas, Texas.)* D *In another patient, a transaxial CT scan through the sacrum delineates the extent of osteolytic destruction in this patient with skeletal metastasis. The lesion does not cross the sacroiliac joint, remaining confined to the sacrum.*

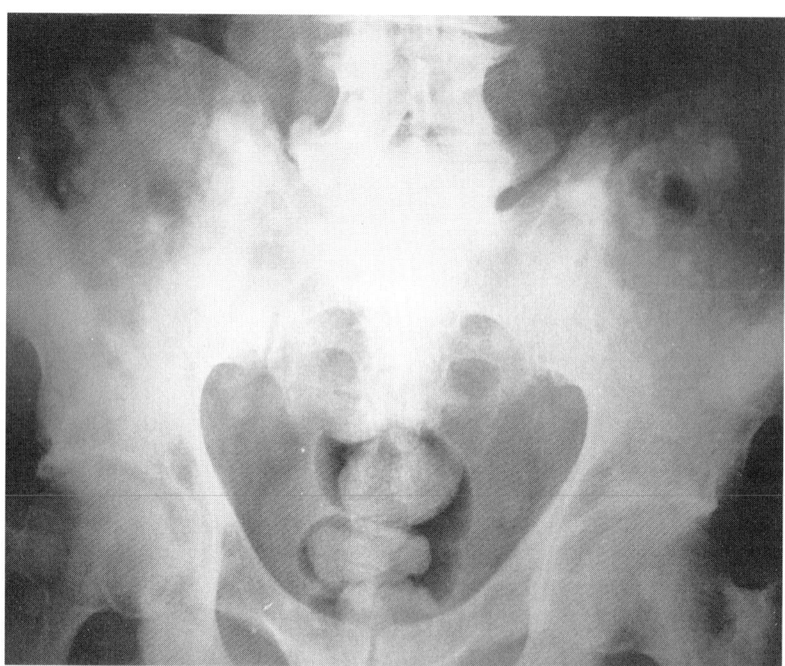

FIGURE 5–24. Skeletal metastasis: Osteosclerotic pattern.[33, 34] In this 82-year-old patient with advanced prostate carcinoma, diffuse osteoblastic skeletal metastasis is evident throughout the pelvis, sacrum, and lumbar spine. Prostate carcinoma is manifested as purely osteosclerotic metastases in approximately 80 per cent of cases.

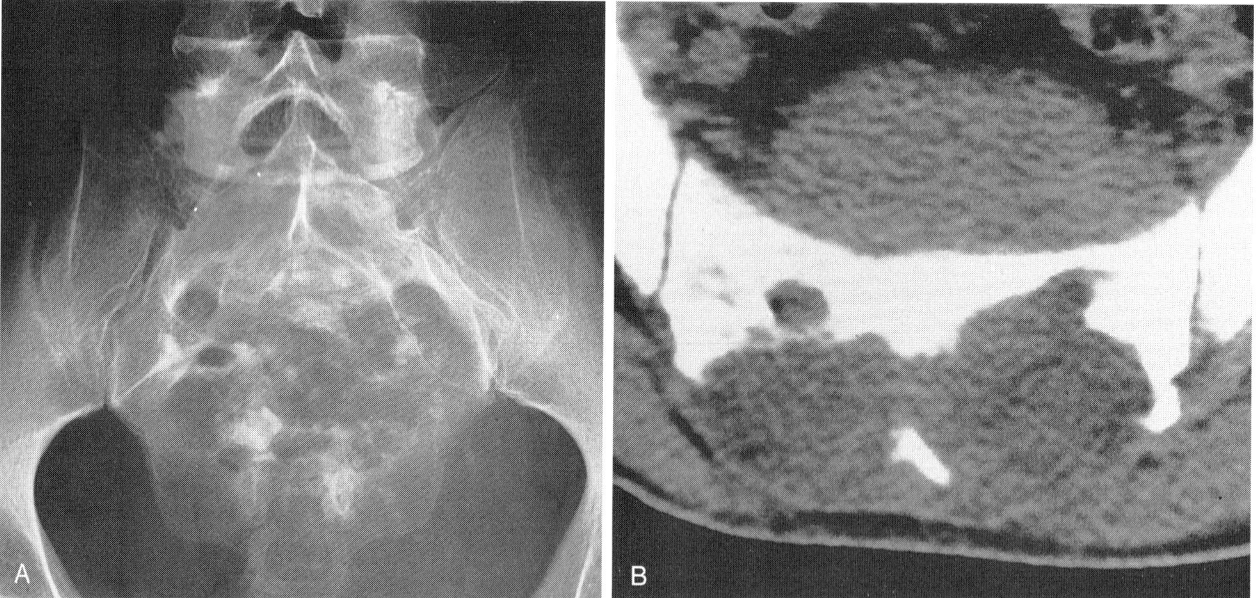

FIGURE 5–25. Chordoma.[35] A This large sacral chordoma is predominantly osteolytic with prominent punctate calcification within its matrix, a feature seen in 50 to 70 per cent of sacrococcygeal chordomas. B In another patient, radiographs from this 29-year-old man (not shown) revealed osteolytic destruction of the sacrum. The transaxial computed tomographic (CT) image shows a large destructive lesion of the sacrum with soft tissue extension. Approximately 50 per cent of all chordomas are sacrococcygeal in location. In addition to chordoma, the differential diagnosis of sacral tumors includes giant cell tumor, plasmacytoma, chondrosarcoma, neurogenic tumor, meningocele, and skeletal metastasis. *(B, Courtesy of K. Kortman, M.D., San Diego, California.)*

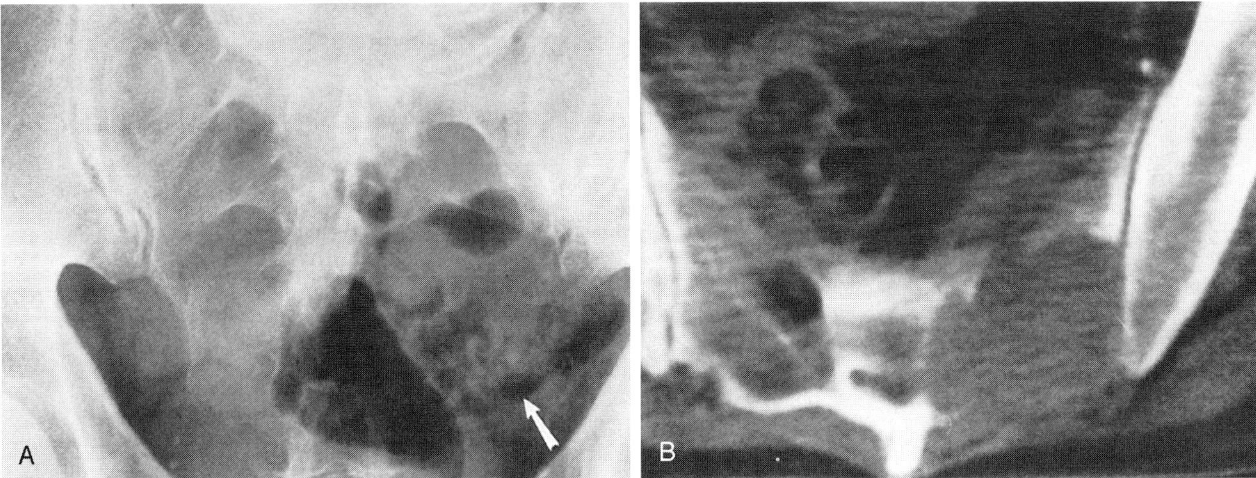

FIGURE 5–26. Plasmacytoma.[36] A 74-year-old man developed progressive pain in the lower back and left buttock over a 6-week period. The pain radiated to the left thigh and calf and was intensified when the leg was raised. The subtle osteolytic lesion in the sacrum (arrow), demonstrable on the plain radiograph (A), is readily evident on a transaxial computed tomographic (CT) image (B). A closed biopsy of the lesion confirmed the presence of a plasmacytoma. *(From Resnick D: Diagnosis of Bone and Joint Disorders. 3rd Ed. Philadelphia, WB Saunders, 1995, p 2165.)*

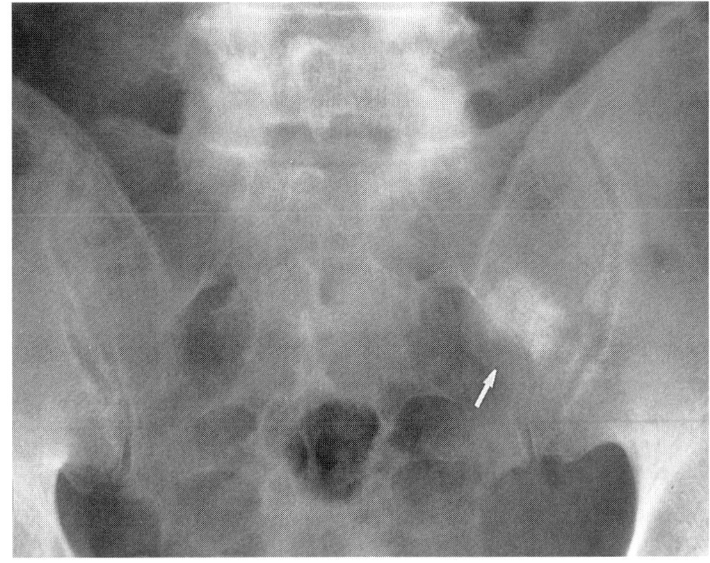

FIGURE 5–27. Enostosis (bone island).[37] Observe the solitary, circular, osteosclerotic lesion in the sacrum (arrow). The sacrum is one of the most common sites for bone islands. It is usually a solitary, discrete focus of osteosclerosis within the spongiosa of bone. It may be round, ovoid, or oblong. It often has a brush border composed of radiating osseous spicules that intermingle with the surrounding trabeculae of the spongiosa. Additionally, enostoses may increase or decrease in size and may even be positive on bone scans, especially in large or growing lesions. Enostoses in the sacrum must be differentiated from other osteosclerotic processes, such as osteoblastic metastasis, osteoma, osteoid osteoma, enchondroma, bone infarct, fibrous dysplasia, and osteopoikilosis.

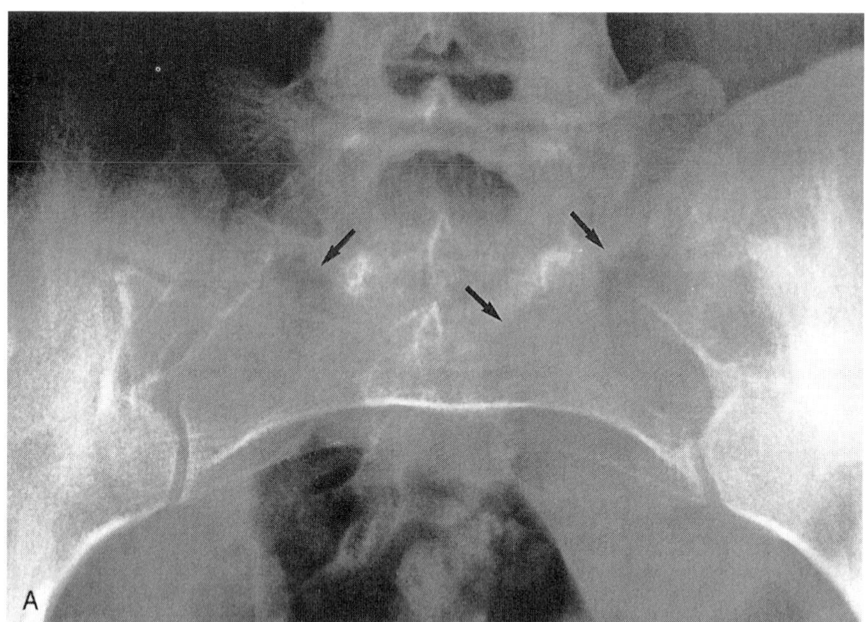

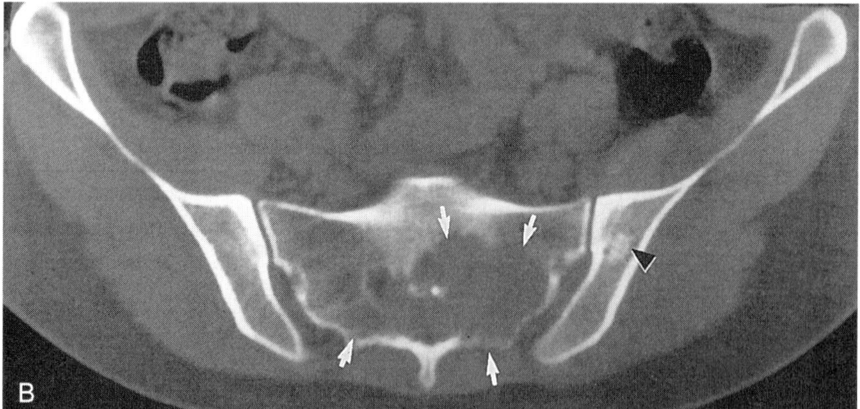

FIGURE 5–28. Giant cell tumor.[38] This 27-year-old woman had sacral pain. The anteroposterior radiograph (A) shows poorly defined radiolucency involving both sides of the sacrum (arrows). A transaxial computed tomographic (CT) image (B) more clearly delineates the extent of involvement of the large, eccentric, purely radiolucent lesion (white arrows). Fewer than 10 per cent of all giant cell tumors affect the spine, but the sacrum is the most common spinal site of involvement. About 5 to 10 per cent of giant cell tumors are malignant. Of incidental note is an enostosis (bone island) within the ilium (arrowhead).

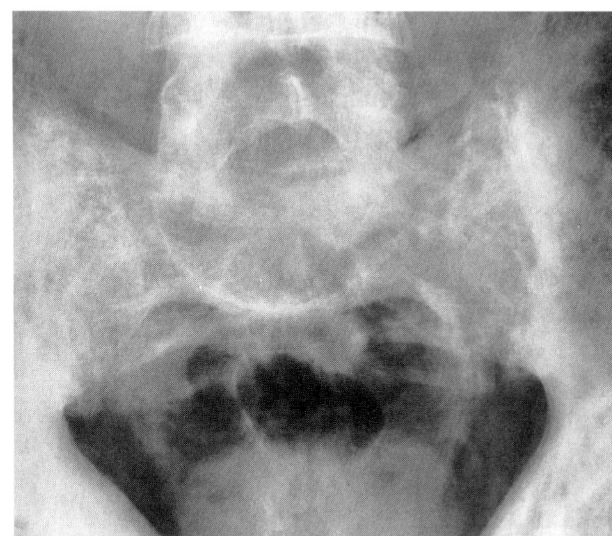

FIGURE 5–29. Paget's disease.[39, 40] Routine radiograph from this patient reveals diffuse sclerosis of the sacrum with accentuation of trabeculae and poorly defined bone expansion. The sacrum is a frequent site of involvement in Paget's disease.

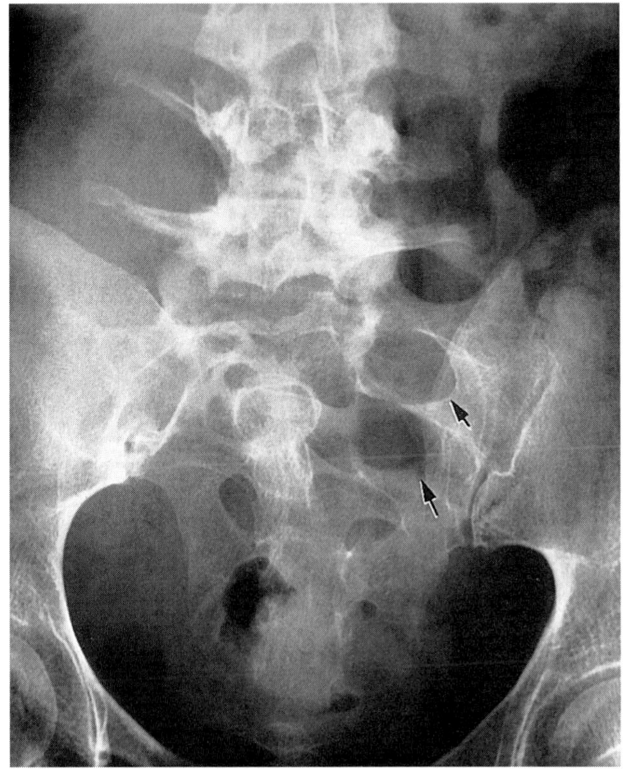

FIGURE 5–30. Neurofibromatosis Type I (von Recklinghausen's disease).[41] Observe the enlarged sacral foramina in this patient with neurofibromatosis (arrows). The transverse processes of the lower lumbar vertebrae are dysplastic and attenuated. *(Courtesy of G. Koors, D.C, Eugene, Oregon, and G. Smith, D.C., Vancouver, Washington.)*

REFERENCES

1. Edeiken J, Dalinka M, Karasick D: Edeiken's Roentgen Diagnosis of Diseases of Bone. 4th Ed. Baltimore, Williams & Wilkins, 1990.
2. Keats TE, Smith TH: An Atlas of Normal Developmental Roentgen Anatomy. 2nd Ed. Chicago, Year Book Medical Publishers, 1988.
3. Dihlmann W: Diagnostic Radiology of the Sacroiliac Joints. Chicago, Year Book Medical Publishers, 1980.
4. Broome DR, Hayman LA, Herrick RC, et al: Postnatal maturation of the sacrum and coccyx: MR imaging, helical CT, and conventional radiography. AJR 170:1061, 1998.
5. Schemmer D, White PG, Friedman L: Radiology of the paraglenoid sulcus. Skeletal Radiol 24:205, 1995.
6. Köhler A, Zimmer EA: Borderlands of Normal and Early Pathologic Findings in Skeletal Radiography. 4th Ed. New York, Thieme Medical Publishers, 1993.
7. Keats TE: Atlas of Normal Roentgen Variants That May Simulate Disease. 6th Ed. Chicago, Year Book Medical Publishers, 1996.
8. Hadley LA: Accessory sacroiliac articulations with arthritic changes. Radiology 55:403, 1950.
9. Magora A, Schwartz A: Relation between the low back pain syndrome and x-ray findings. 3. Spina bifida occulta. Scand J Rehabil Med 12:9, 1980.
10. Yochum TR, Rowe LJ: Essentials of Skeletal Radiology. 2nd Ed. Baltimore, Williams & Wilkins, 1996.
11. Renshaw TS: Sacral agenesis: A classification and review of twenty-three cases. J Bone Joint Surg [Am] 60:373, 1978.
12. Tini PG, Wieser C, Zinn WM: The transitional vertebra of the lumbosacral spine: Its radiological classification, incidence, prevalence, and clinical significance. Rheumatol Rehabil 16:180, 1977.
13. Montana MA, Richardson ML, Kilcoyne RF, et al: CT of sacral injury. Radiology 161:499, 1986.
14. Kane WJ: Fractures of the pelvis. *In* CA Rockwood Jr, DP Green (Eds): Fractures in Adults. 2nd Ed. Philadelphia, JB Lippincott, 1984, p 1093.
15. Newhouse KE, El-Khoury GY, Buckwalter JA: Occult sacral fractures in osteopenic patients. J Bone Joint Surg [Am] 74:227, 1992.
16. Dasgupta B, Shah N, Brown H, et al: Sacral insufficiency fractures: An unsuspected cause of low back pain. Br J Rheumatol 37:789, 1998.
17. Mammone JF, Schweitzer ME: MRI of occult sacral insufficiency fractures following radiotherapy. Skeletal Radiol 24:101, 1995.
18. Sty JR, Starshak RJ: The role of bone scintigraphy in the evaluation of the suspected abused child. Radiology 146:369,1983.
19. Taylor JAM, Hoffman LE: The geriatric patient: Diagnostic imaging of common musculoskeletal disorders. Top Clin Chiropr 3:23, 1996.
20. Resnick D, Niwayama G, Goergen TG: Comparison of radiographic abnormalities of the sacroiliac joint in degenerative disease and ankylosing spondylitis. AJR 128:189, 1977.
21. Olivieri I, Gemignani G, Camerini E, et al: Differential diagnosis between osteitis condensans ilii and sacroiliitis. J Rheumatol 17:1504, 1990.
22. Durback MA, Edelstein G, Schumacher HR Jr: Abnormalities of the sacroiliac joints in diffuse idiopathic skeletal hyperostosis: Demonstration by computed tomography. J Rheumatol 15:1506, 1988.
23. DeCarvalho A, Graudal H: Sacroiliac joint involvement in classical or definite rheumatoid arthritis. Acta Radiol Diagn 21:417, 1980.
24. Forrester DM: Imaging of the sacroiliac joints. Radiol Clin North Am 28:1055, 1990.
25. Murphey MD, Wetzel LH, Bramble JM, et al: Sacroiliitis: MR imaging findings. Radiology 180:239, 1991.
26. Jayson MIV, Bouchier IAD: Ulcerative colitis with ankylosing spondylitis. Ann Rheum Dis 27:219, 1968.
27. Russell AS, Suarez-Almazor ME: Sacroiliitis in psoriasis: Relationship to peripheral arthritis and HLA B27. J Rheumatol 17:804, 1990.
28. Russell AS, Davis P, Percy JS, et al: The sacroiliitis of acute Reiter's syndrome. J Rheumatol 4:293, 1977.
29. Hooge WA, Li D: CT of the sacroiliac joints in secondary hyperparathyroidism. J Can Assoc Radiol 31:42, 1981.
30. Murphy MD, Sartoris DJ, Quale JL, et al: Musculoskeletal manifestations of chronic renal insufficiency. RadioGraphics 13:357, 1993.
31. Sundaram M: Renal osteodystrophy. Skeletal Radiol 18:415, 1989.
32. Vyskocil JJ, McIlroy MA, Brennan TA, et al: Pyogenic infection of the sacroiliac joint: Case reports and review of the literature. Medicine 70:188, 1991.
33. Wong DA, Fornasier VL, MacNab I: Spinal metastases: The obvious, the occult, and the impostors. Spine 15:1, 1990.
34. Rafii M, Firooznia H, Golimbu C, et al: CT of skeletal metastasis. Semin Ultrasound CT MR 7:371, 1986.
35. Sudaresan N: Chordomas. Clin Orthop 204:135, 1986.
36. Kyle RA: Multiple myeloma: Review of 869 cases. Mayo Clin Proc 50:29, 1975.
37. Greenspan A: Bone island (enostosis): Current concept—a review. Skeletal Radiol 24:111, 1995.
38. Dahlin DC: Giant cell tumor of bone: Highlights of 407 cases. AJR 144:955, 1985.
39. Matfin G, McPherson F: Paget's disease of bone: Recent advances. J Orthop Rheumatol 6:127, 1993.
40. Mirra JM, Brien EW, Tehranzadeh J: Paget's disease of bone: Review with emphasis on radiologic features, part II. Skeletal Radiol 24:173, 1995.
41. Angtuaco EJ, Binet EF, Flanigan S: Value of CT myelography in neurofibromatosis. Neurosurgery 13:668, 1983.

CHAPTER 6

Pelvis and Symphysis Pubis

- Normal Developmental Anatomy
- Developmental Anomalies, Anatomic Variants, and Sources of Diagnostic Error
- Skeletal Dysplasias and Other Congenital Diseases
- Physical Injury
- Articular Disorders
- Neoplasms
- Metabolic, Hematologic, and Infectious Disorders

Normal Developmental Anatomy

Accurate interpretation of pediatric pelvic radiographs requires a thorough understanding of normal developmental anatomy. Table 6–1 outlines the age of appearance and fusion of the primary and secondary ossification centers. Figures 6–1 through Figures 6–5 demonstrate the radiographic appearance of many important ossification centers and other developmental landmarks at selected ages from birth to skeletal maturity.

Developmental Anomalies, Anatomic Variants, and Sources of Diagnostic Error

The pelvis is an important site of anomalies, normal variants, and other sources of diagnostic error that may simulate disease and result in misdiagnosis. Table 6–2 and Figures 6–6 to 6–11 have been selected as examples of some of the more common of these processes.

Skeletal Dysplasias and Other Congenital Diseases

Table 6–3 outlines a number of the skeletal dysplasias and congenital disorders that affect the pelvis and symphysis pubis. Figures 6–12 to 6–18 illustrate the radiographic manifestations of some of these disorders.

Physical Injury

Fractures, dislocations, and soft tissue injuries involving the pelvis and symphysis pubis often are associated with serious clinical manifestations. Table 6–4 lists the more important injuries of the pelvis and their characteristics. Figures 6–19 to 6–26 represent examples of frequently encountered pelvic injuries.

Articular Disorders

The symphysis pubis, a fibrous joint, is a site of involvement for a variety of degenerative, inflammatory, crystal-induced, and infectious articular disorders. Table 6–5 outlines these diseases and their characteristics, and Figures 6–27 to 6–37 illustrate the typical radiographic manifestations.

Neoplasms

The bones of the pelvis are a frequent site of involvement for several malignant and benign tumors and tumor-like lesions. Table 6–6 lists and characterizes the neoplasms that typically involve the pelvis. Many of these tumors are illustrated in Figures 6–38 to 6–54.

Metabolic, Hematologic, and Infectious Disorders

Many metabolic, hematologic, and infectious disorders exhibit radiographic changes in the bones of the pelvis. Table 6–7 outlines these disorders, and Figures 6–55 to 6–64 illustrate some of the more common examples.

TABLE 6–1. Pelvis: Approximate Age of Appearance and Fusion of Ossification Centers[1–5] (Figs. 6–1 to 6–5)

Ossification Center	Primary or Secondary	No. of Centers	Age of Appearance* (Years)	Age of Fusion* (Years)	Comments
Ilium	P	2	Birth	14	Fuses with ischium
				14	Fuses with pubis
Ischium	P	2	Birth	4–8	Fuses with pubis
				14	Fuses with ilium
Pubis	P	2	Birth	4–8	Fuses with ischium
				14	Fuses with ilium
Iliac crest apophysis	S	2	14–16	18–25	
Iliac spine	S	2	16	18–25	
Pubic symphysis	S	2	16	18–25	
Ischial tuberosity apophysis	S	2	16	18–25	

*Ages of appearance and fusion of ossification centers in girls typically precede those of boys. Ethnic differences also exist.
P, Primary; S, secondary.

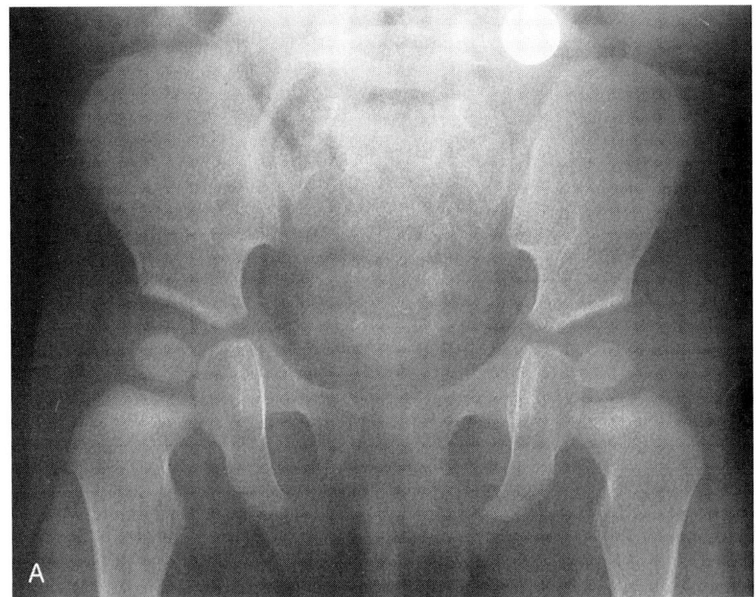

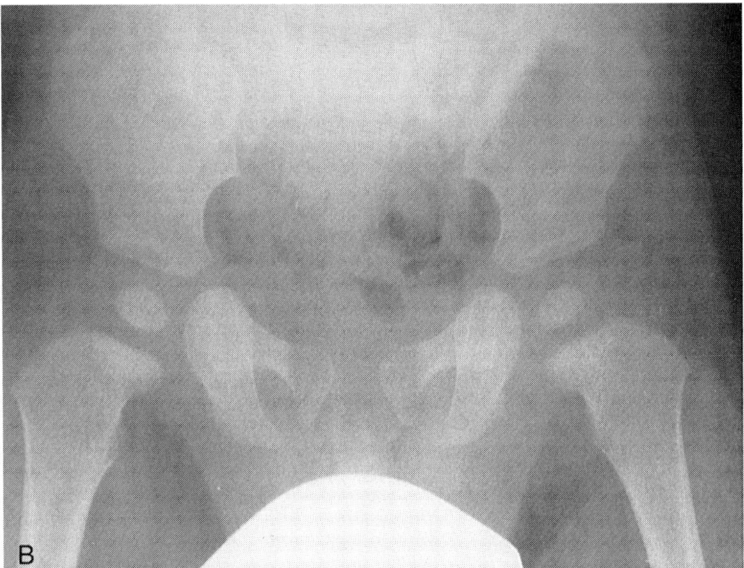

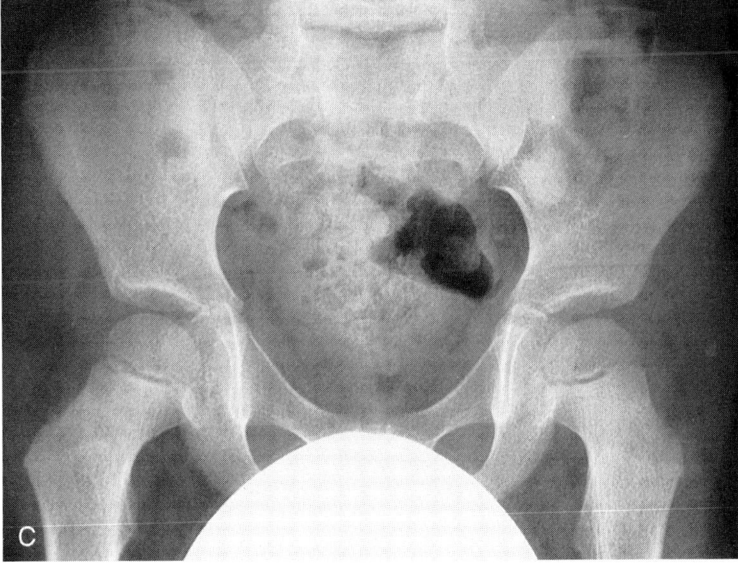

FIGURE 6–1. Skeletal maturation and normal development: Frontal pelvic radiographs.[1–4] A 6-month-old girl. The triradiate cartilage and ischiopubic synchondroses are not fused. The capital femoral epiphyses, which usually begin to ossify between the ages of 1 and 8 months, are present. At this stage, the capital femoral epiphyses are circular and small, and the iliac bones are proportionately small. B 8-month-old boy. Skeletal development approximates that of the 6-month-old girl (A). C 4-year-old boy. The iliac bones are proportionately larger, and the triradiate cartilage is diminishing in size prior to fusion. The femoral capital epiphyses are larger, and the physeal growth center is thinner, is more linear, and conforms to the shape of the femoral necks.

Illustration continued on following page

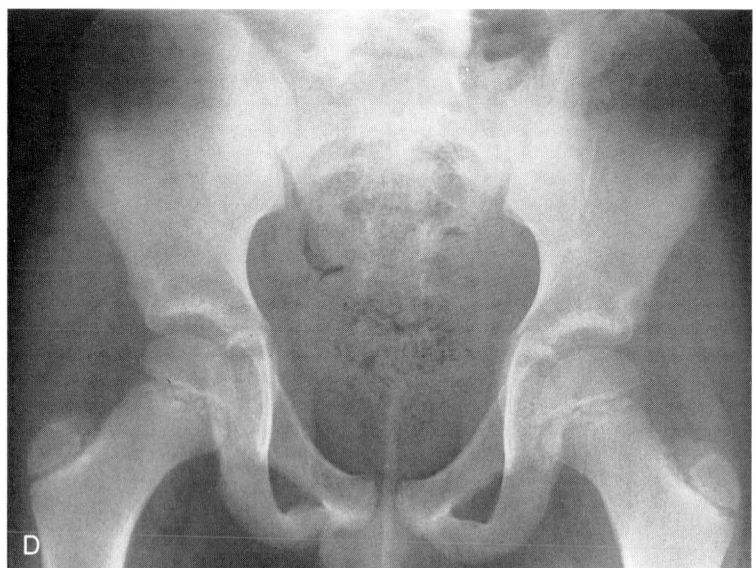

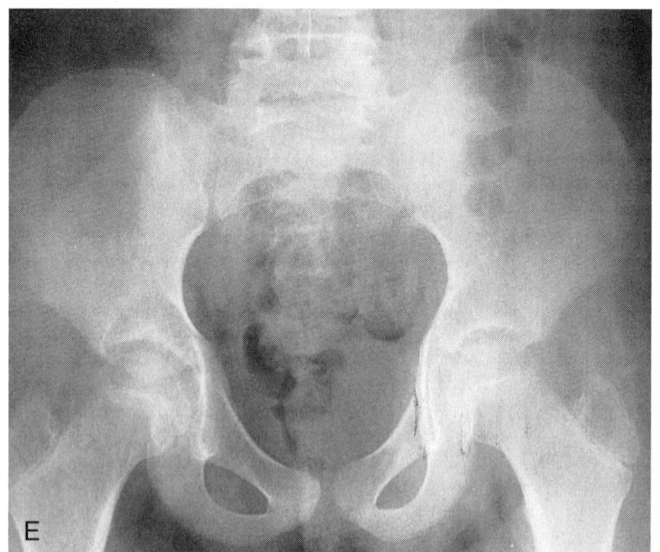

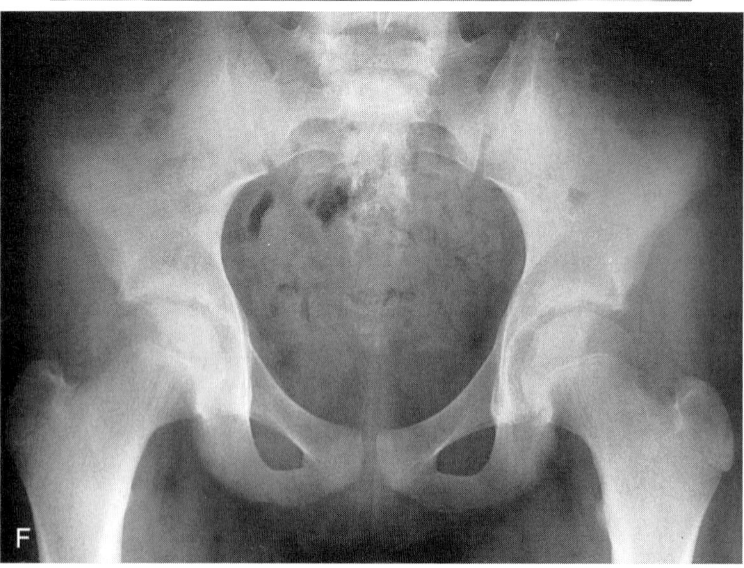

FIGURE 6–1 *Continued.* D 7-year-old boy. The triradiate cartilages remain unfused, but the ischiopubic synchondroses are fusing in an asymmetric pattern. The ossified apophyses of the greater trochanters are developing. Observe the presence of normal physiologic acetabular protrusion. This phenomenon persists until about 13 years of age in girls and 16 years of age in boys, when the pelvis adopts the adult configuration. E 9-year-old girl. The apophyses of the lesser trochanters are beginning to ossify. The femoral capital epiphyses and greater trochanter apophyses are taking on adult proportions but remain unfused. Physiologic protrusio acetabuli persists. F 13-year-old girl. The pelvis is adopting adult proportions. The greater and lesser trochanters and the femoral capital epiphyses are fusing to the femur. The triradiate cartilages and ischiopubic synchondroses are fused. The apophyses of the ischium and iliac crests have not yet appeared.

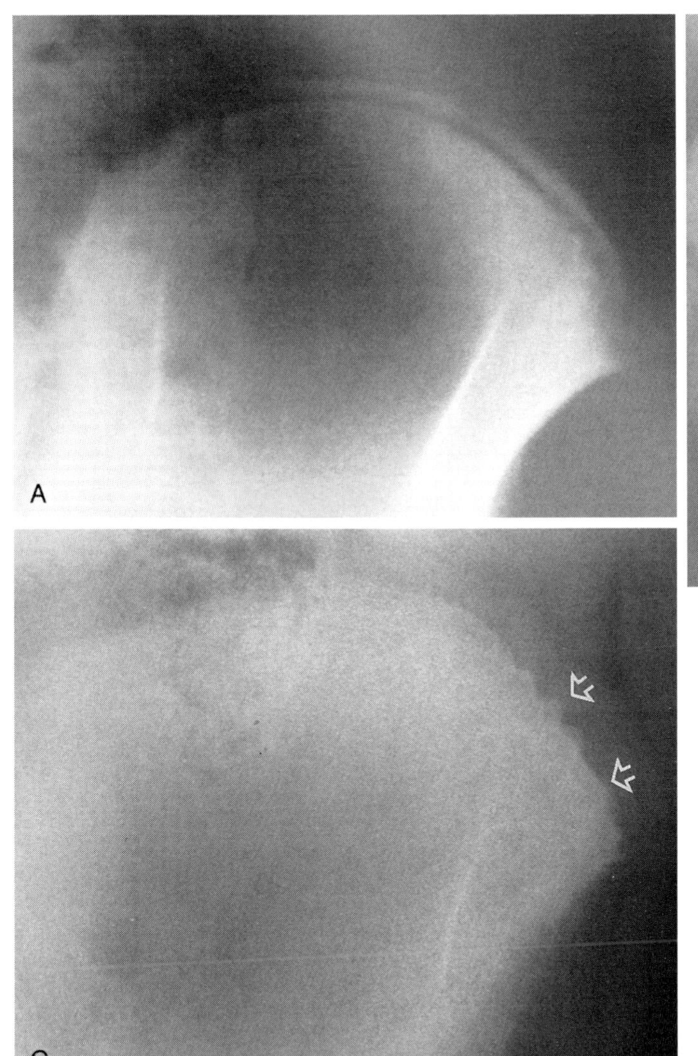

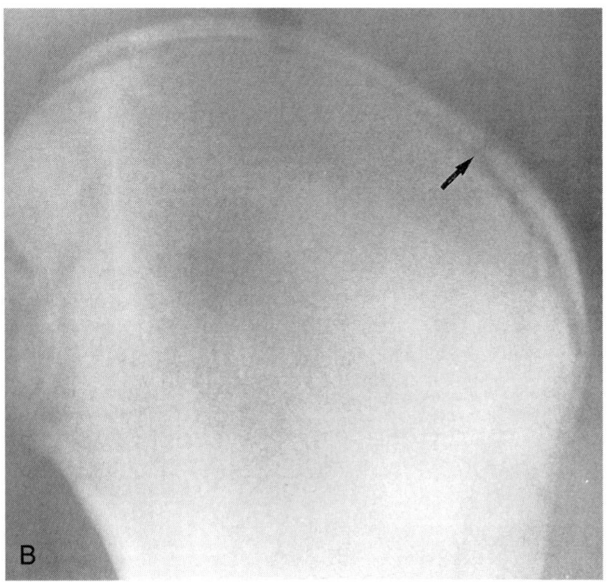

FIGURE 6–2. Skeletal maturation and normal development of the iliac crest apophysis.[1–5] **A** 13-year-old girl. Approximately 60 per cent of the iliac apophysis is ossified. **B** 14-year-old girl. The apophysis is almost completely ossified, but it has not yet fused to the ilium. Note the superolateral radiolucent disruption of the apophysis (arrow). This fragmentation is a variation of normal and is of no clinical significance. **C** 15-year-old boy. The superolateral margin of the iliac crest appears serrated (open arrows), a finding that is typical just before and during ossification of the iliac apophysis. That the iliac crest apophysis has not begun to ossify in this 15-year-old boy illustrates that between boys and girls there is variability in the onset of puberty and skeletal maturity, with boys typically showing a lag.

Illustration continued on following page

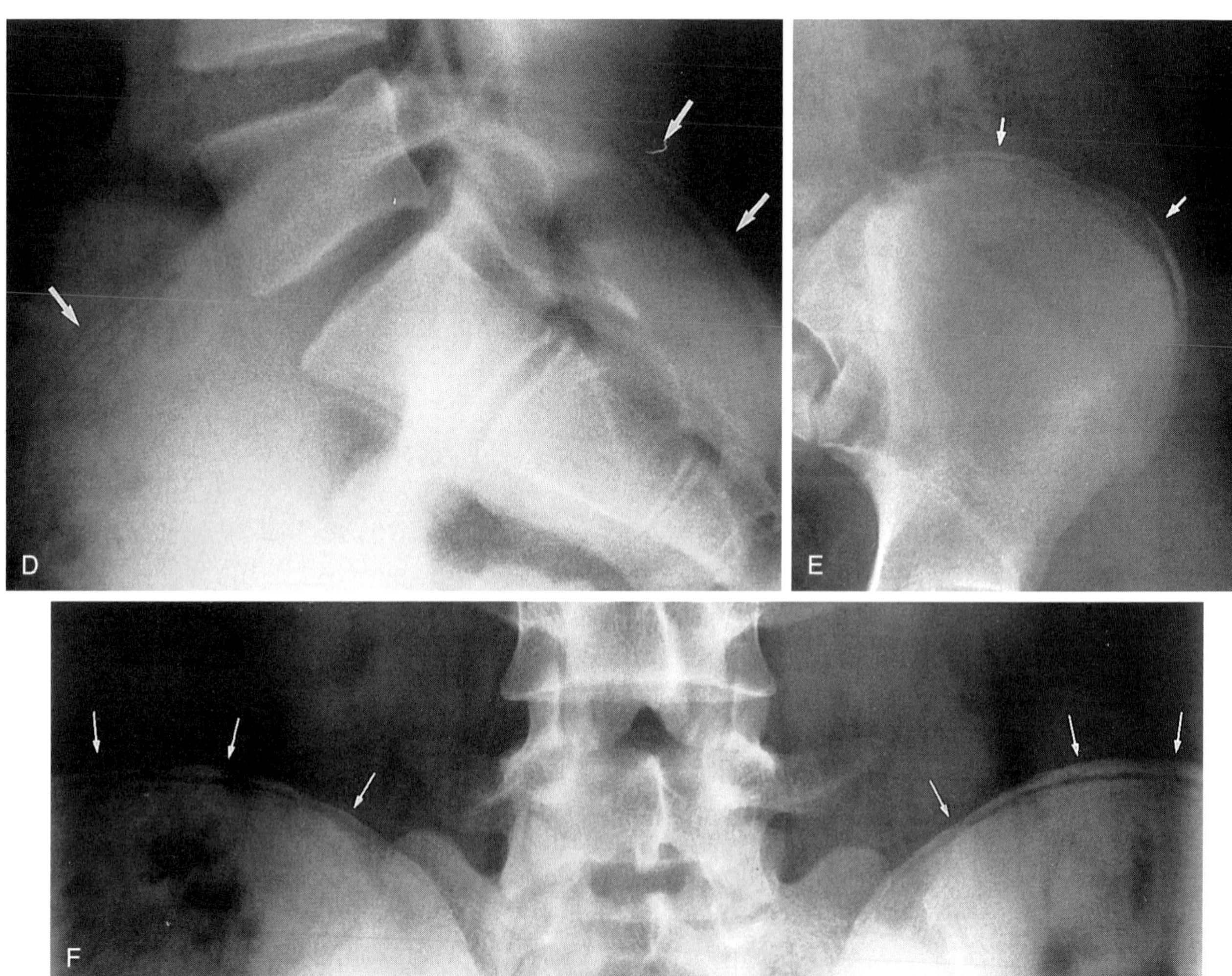

FIGURE 6–2 *Continued.* D 13-year-old boy. A lateral radiograph reveals advanced ossification of the iliac crest apophysis (arrows). E In another 14-year-old girl, observe the thin curvilinear ossifying growth center (arrows) adjacent to the iliac crest. Although the growth center is almost completely ossified, it has not fused with the ilium, indicating incomplete skeletal maturation. F Normal iliac apophysis just prior to fusion in a 19-year-old man. Note the curvilinear ossified rim along the iliac crest (arrows). The iliac crest apophysis begins to ossify at or about the onset of puberty, beginning laterally at the anterosuperior iliac spine and progressing medially toward the posterosuperior iliac spine. When the apophysis is fully ossified and fused to the ilium—usually between the ages of 20 and 25 years—it indicates that the patient is skeletally mature. This indicator, sometimes referred to as the Risser sign, is useful in the management of scoliosis.

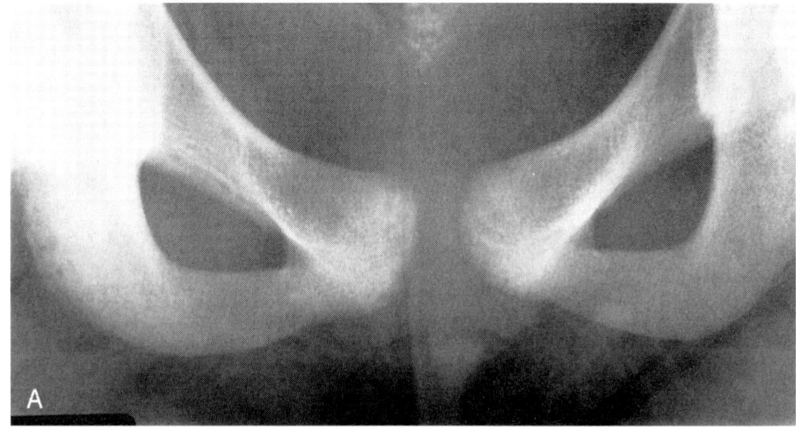

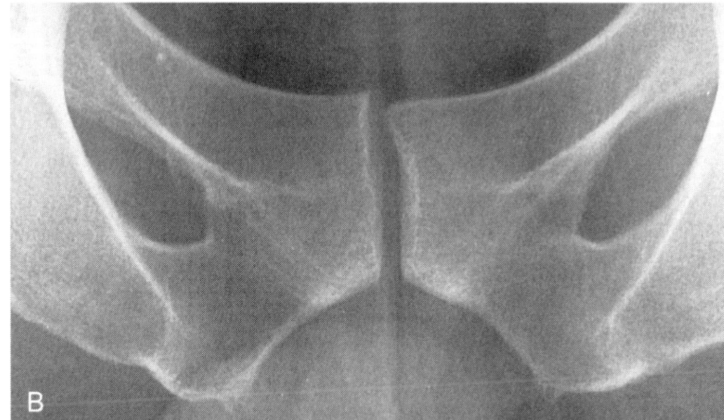

FIGURE 6–3. Skeletal maturation and normal development: Symphysis pubis.[1–4] A 13-year-old girl. Observe the rounded appearance of the articular surfaces of the symphysis pubis. Paired secondary ossification centers typically appear about the age of 16 years and fuse to the pubic bones by the age of 20 to 25 years. B 35-year-old man. In the adult, a flat, parallel configuration of the apposing joint surfaces is evident. Slight offset of the superior aspect is common and usually is of no clinical significance.

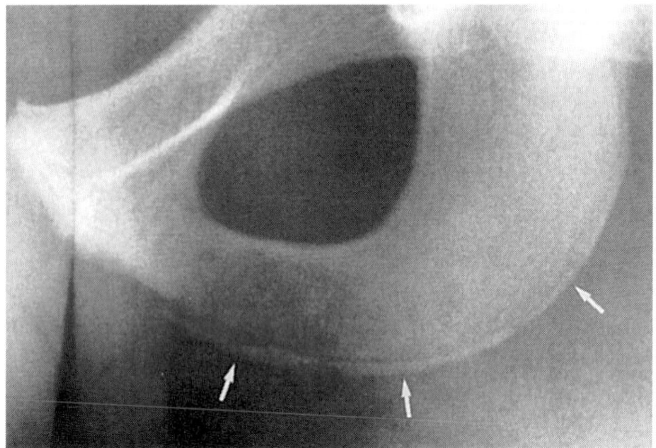

FIGURE 6–4. Skeletal maturation and normal development: Ischial apophysis.[1–4] In this 15-year-old boy, observe the linear zone of ossification adjacent to the inferior aspect of the ischium (arrows). This secondary ossification center first appears in adolescence about the age of 15 years and fuses to the ischial bone between the ages of 20 and 25 years.

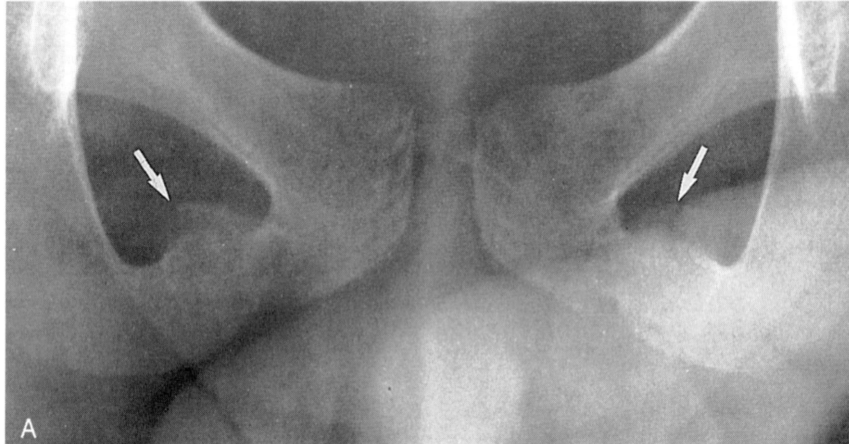

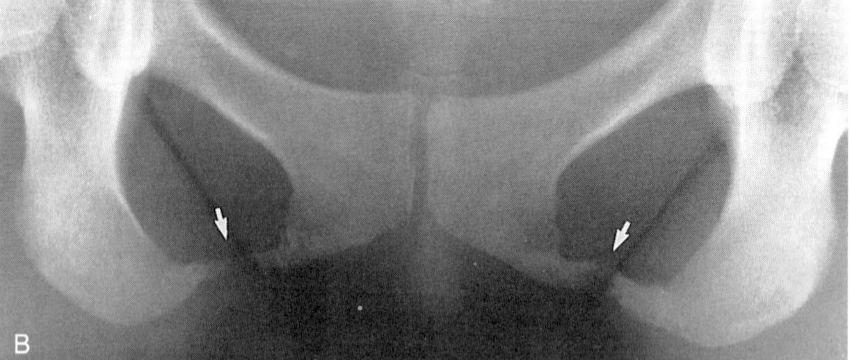

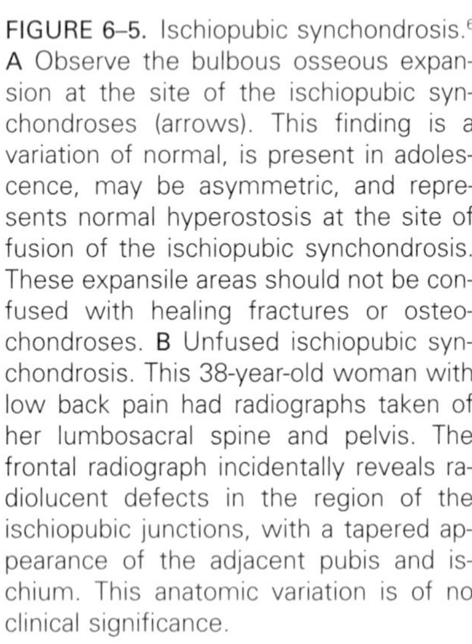

FIGURE 6–5. Ischiopubic synchondrosis.[6] A Observe the bulbous osseous expansion at the site of the ischiopubic synchondroses (arrows). This finding is a variation of normal, is present in adolescence, may be asymmetric, and represents normal hyperostosis at the site of fusion of the ischiopubic synchondrosis. These expansile areas should not be confused with healing fractures or osteochondroses. B Unfused ischiopubic synchondrosis. This 38-year-old woman with low back pain had radiographs taken of her lumbosacral spine and pelvis. The frontal radiograph incidentally reveals radiolucent defects in the region of the ischiopubic junctions, with a tapered appearance of the adjacent pubis and ischium. This anatomic variation is of no clinical significance.

TABLE 6–2. Developmental Anomalies, Anatomic Variants, and Sources of Diagnostic Error Affecting the Pelvis*

Entity	Figure(s)	Characteristics
Unfused ischiopubic synchondrosis[6]	6–5B	Failure of fusion of the synchondrosis joining the ischium and pubis No clinical significance Frequently confused with fracture These synchondroses normally fuse between the ages of 4 and 8 years and may appear bulbous and expansile, simulating callus surrounding a healing fracture May not close synchronously and may even reappear after initial closure
Pelvic digit[7]	6–6	Anomalous, elongated, rib-like or digit-like structure within pelvis Also called pelvic rib or ectopic lumbar rib May have one or more articulations and a pseudarthrotic attachment to the ilium No clinical significance
Os acetabuli marginalis superior[4]	6–7	Large or small triangular ossicle with well-corticated margins adjacent to the superior acetabular rim Present in about 5 per cent of normal persons No clinical significance but may simulate acetabular rim fracture
Grooves in ilium for nutrient artery[4, 6]	6–8	V-shaped or Y-shaped groove in iliac wing for nutrient artery Normal anatomy of no clinical significance
Calcification of the pectineal ligament[4]	6–9	Characteristic curvilinear rim of calcification parallels the superior margins of the pubic bones Normally, an aponeurotic extension of the lacunar ligament extends laterally to the iliopectineal line Calcification of this ligament is a normal variant frequently found in elderly patients Differential diagnosis: periosteal proliferation, Paget's disease Cephalad angulation of the x-ray beam also may produce a double contour of the upper margin of the pubic bone simulating this appearance
Pelvic phleboliths[8]	6–10	Pelvic vein calcification appears as multiple circular radiodense areas overlying the lower pelvic basin and the pubic rami No clinical significance
Penile implant[8]	6–11	Penile implants used for impotency overlie the lower pubic region within the penis

*See also Table 1–1.

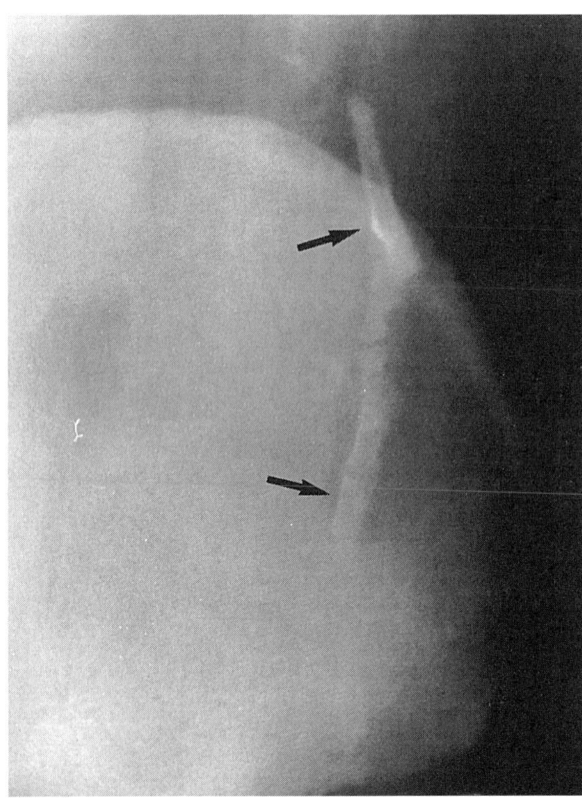

FIGURE 6–6. Pelvic digit.[7] This anomaly, also called a pelvic rib or ectopic lumbar rib, is seen as an elongated, two-part, rib-like, or digit-like, structure with a pseudarthrotic attachment overlying the ilium (arrows).

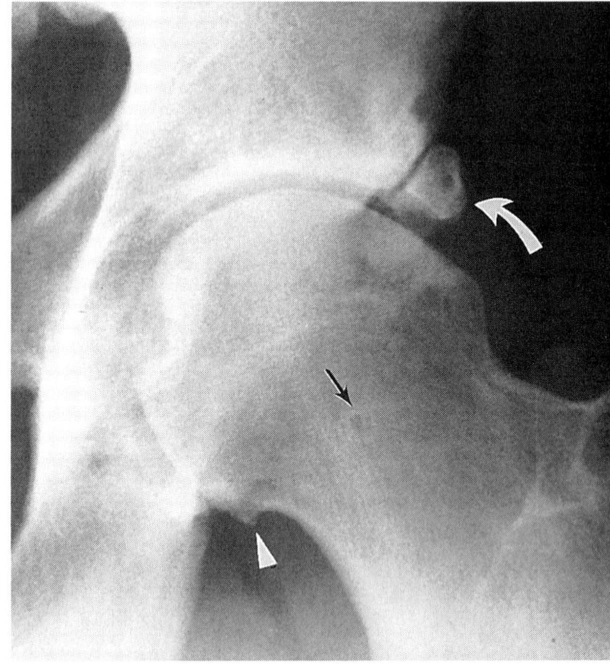

FIGURE 6–7. Os acetabuli.[4] 27-year-old man had bilateral prominent os acetabuli. These triangular ossicles with well-corticated margins adjacent to the superior acetabular rim (curved arrow) are present in about 5 per cent of the population. Note also the presence of a small herniation pit (arrow) and an osteophyte surrounding the femoral head-neck junction (arrowhead). *(From Taylor JAM, Harger BL, Resnick D: Diagnostic imaging of common hip disorders: A pictorial review. Top Clin Chiropr 1:8, 1994.)*

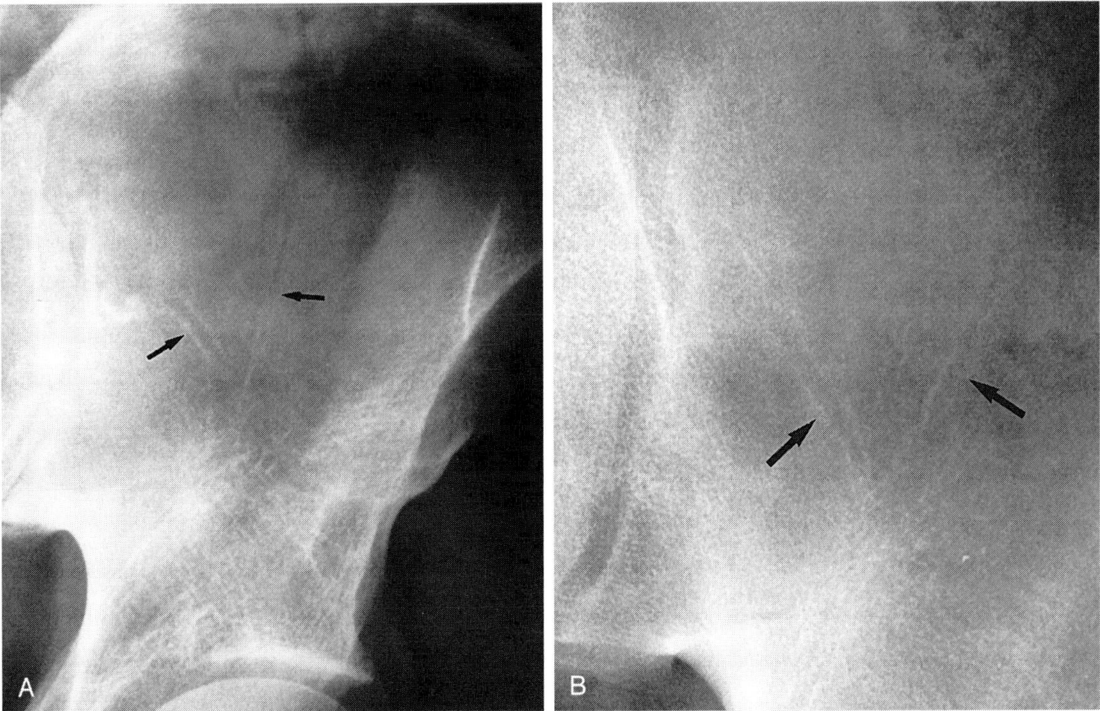

FIGURE 6–8. Grooves for the nutrient arteries of the ilium.[4, 6] A The typical Y- or V-shaped groove for the nutrient arteries in the iliac wing (arrows) is evident. B A similar groove (arrows) is seen in the ilium of another patient. This commonly encountered normal vascular channel may be prominent and should not be mistaken for a stellate fracture.

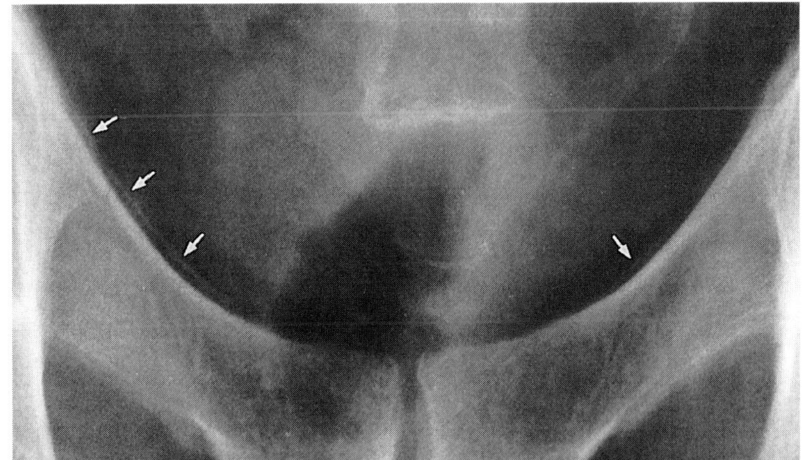

FIGURE 6–9. Calcification of the pectineal ligament.[4] In this 75-year-old man, characteristic bilateral curvilinear rims of calcification (arrows) parallel the superior margins of the pubic bones and extend laterally to the iliopectineal lines.

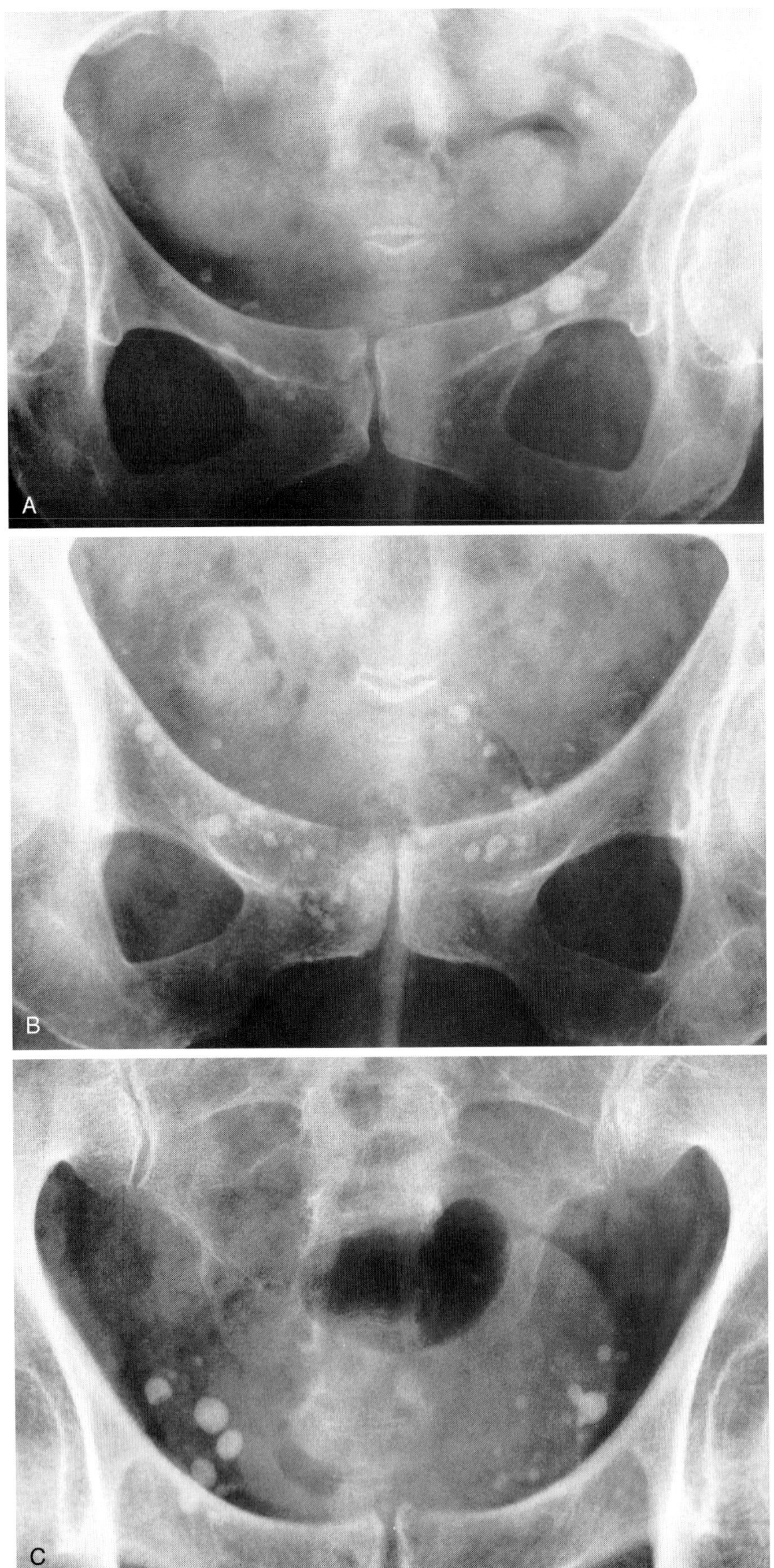

FIGURE 6–10. Pelvic phleboliths.[8] Observe the circular radiodense shadows overlying the lower pelvic basin and pubic ramus in three separate patients. These opacities, which represent calcification in pelvic veins, may contain a central radiolucent region. They are of no clinical significance.

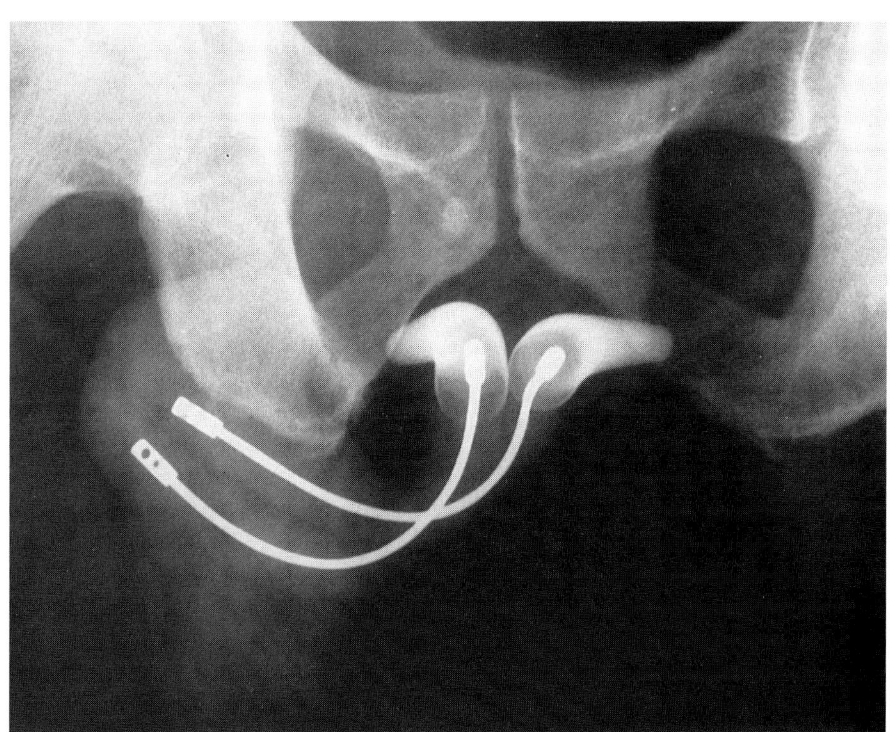

FIGURE 6–11. Penile implant[8] (metallic) in a patient being treated for impotence.

TABLE 6–3. Skeletal Dysplasias and Other Congenital Diseases Affecting the Pelvis*

Entity	Figure(s)	Characteristics
Achondroplasia[9]	6–12	"Champagne glass" pelvis: flattened pelvic opening Square appearance of iliac bones Small sacrosciatic notches Flattened acetabular angles Short femoral necks and coxa vara deformities
Down syndrome (trisomy 21)[10]	6–13	Flaring of iliac wings Flattening of acetabular roofs Decreased iliac angle Developmental hip dysplasia (40 per cent of affected persons)
Osteopetrosis[11]	6–14A	May appear as diffuse osteosclerosis or bone-within-bone appearance of ilium Bones are brittle and fracture easily
Osteopoikilosis[12]	6–14B	Multiple 2- to 3-mm circular foci of osteosclerosis Symmetric periarticular lesions predominate about the hip joints and at the periphery of the pelvic bones
Mucopolysaccharidoses (MPS)[13]	6–15	*MPS I-H (Hurler's syndrome)* Pseudoenlargement of acetabular region Wide femoral necks Coxa valga *MPS IV (Morquio's syndrome)* Flaring of the iliac wings Underdevelopment of acetabular roofs Coxa valga Dysplasia of femoral capital epiphyses
Osteogenesis imperfecta[14]	6–16	Severe osteopenia Thin cortices Multiple fractures Narrow pelvis with protrusio acetabuli Bone remodeling Altered trabecular architecture
Cleidocranial dysplasia[15]	6–17	Incomplete ossification of the pubic bones May simulate pubic diastasis or destructive osseous lesions
Hereditary osteo-onychodysostosis (HOOD syndrome)[16]	6–18	Bilateral iliac horns that arise from the posterior surface of the iliac wings and project into the buttocks Unilateral iliac horn also can be an isolated finding unassociated with other skeletal abnormalities

*See also Table 1–2.

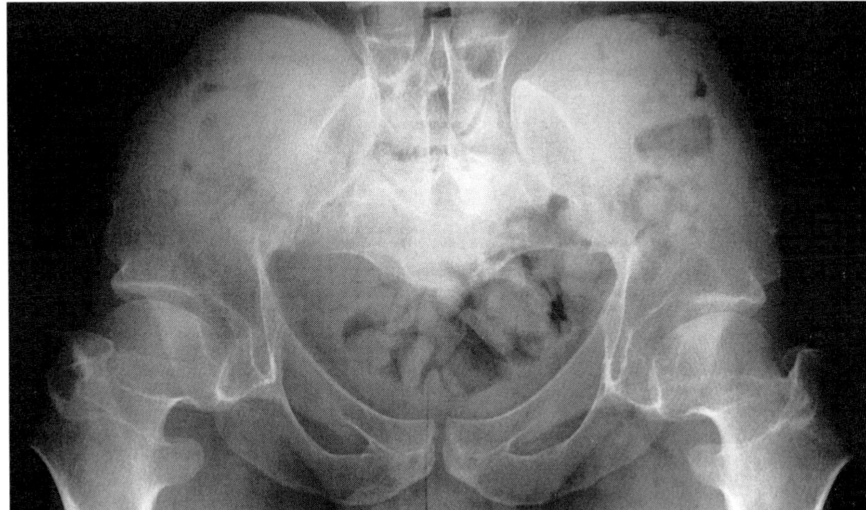

FIGURE 6–12. Achondroplasia.[9] In this adult patient, the pelvic opening is flattened, creating the "champagne glass" appearance. The iliac bones are squared and have small sacrosciatic notches and flat acetabular angles. The femoral necks are short, and coxa varus deformities are present bilaterally.

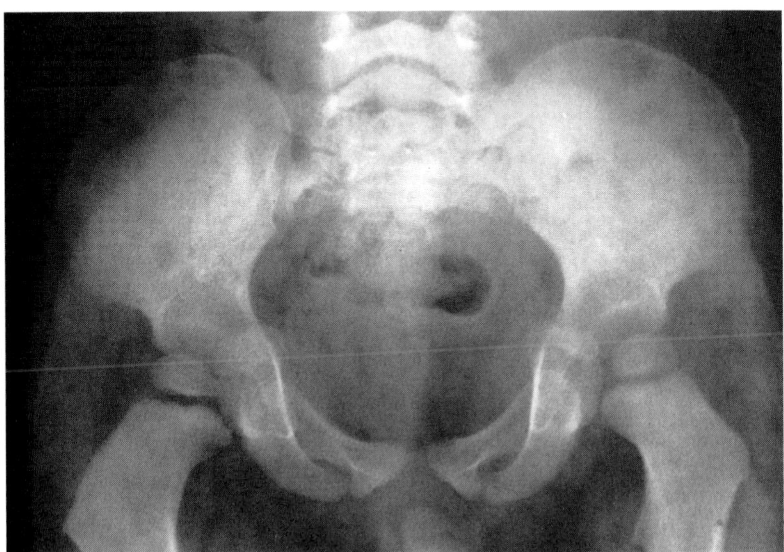

FIGURE 6–13. Down syndrome (trisomy 21).[10] Observe flaring of the iliac wings, flattening of the acetabular roofs, and decreased iliac angles in this child with Down syndrome. Developmental hip dysplasia, although absent in this patient, is present in about 40 per cent of affected persons with Down syndrome. The iliac flaring may persist into adulthood.

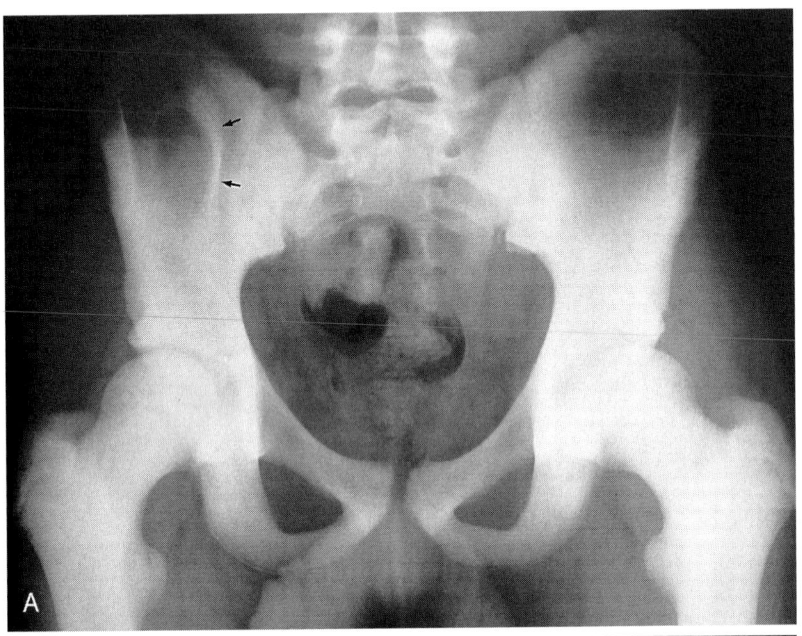

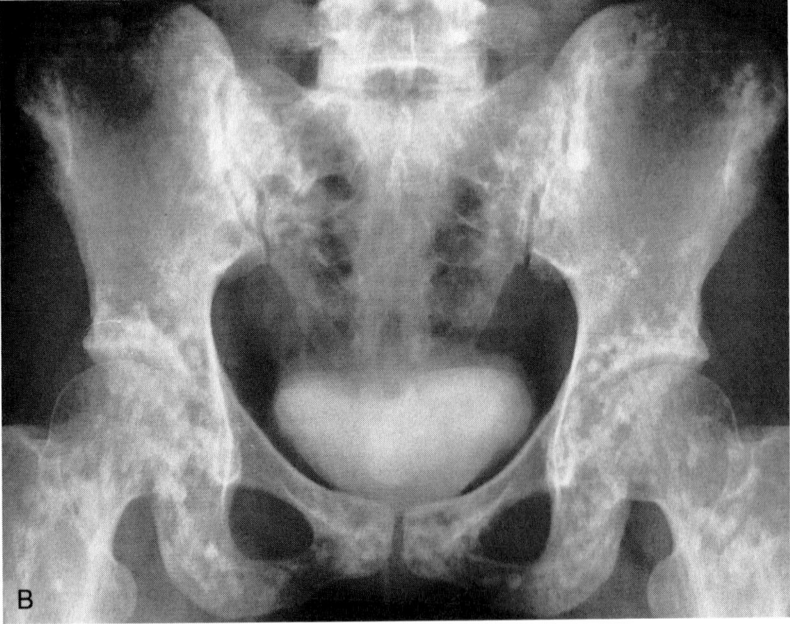

FIGURE 6–14. Sclerosing dysplasias.[11, 12] A Osteopetrosis. A routine radiograph of the pelvis in this 15-year-old boy exhibits diffuse osteosclerosis of the pelvic bones. The curvilinear opacity within the right ilium (arrows) is referred to as the "bone-within-bone" appearance. B Osteopoikilosis. Circular and ovoid osteosclerotic foci are localized in a periarticular pattern about the hip joints and at the periphery of the pelvic bones. The symmetric, periarticular distribution is characteristic of this fairly common sclerosing dysplasia. Although the epiphysis may be affected, most lesions predominate in the metaphysis. Osteopoikilosis was an incidental, asymptomatic finding in this patient who was undergoing a cystogram (note contrast in the bladder).

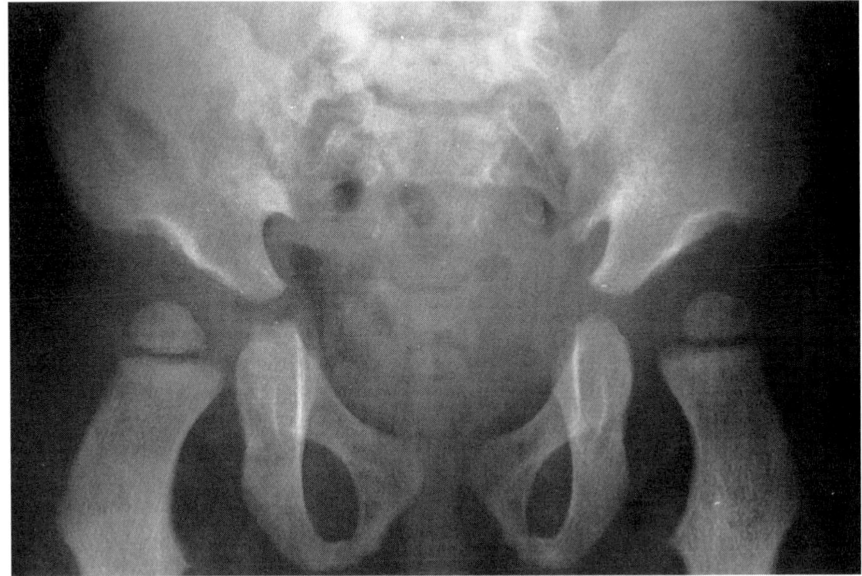

FIGURE 6–15. Hurler's syndrome (MPS 1-H).[13] Characteristic hypoplasia of the superior acetabular region, wide femoral necks, and coxa valga deformities are seen in the pelvis of this 3-year-old girl with Hurler's syndrome.

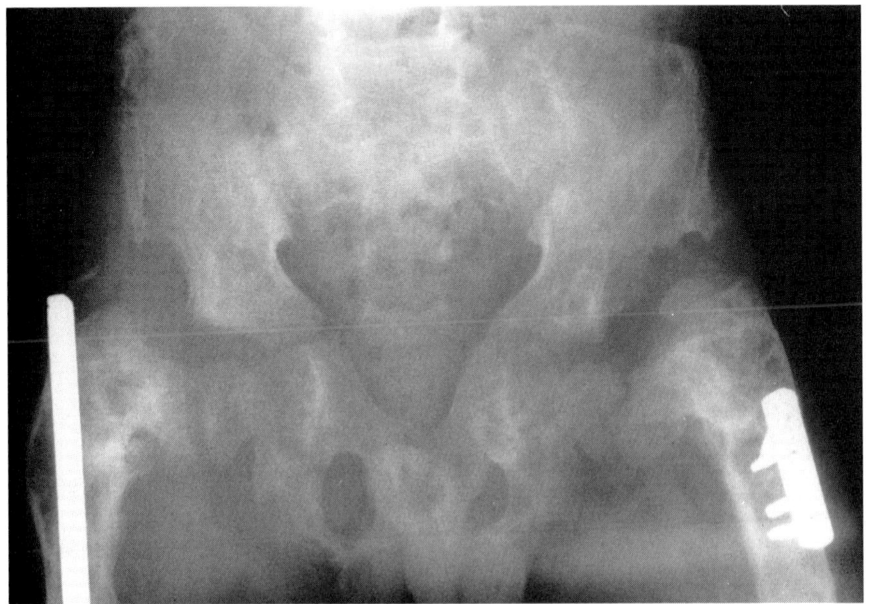

FIGURE 6–16. Osteogenesis imperfecta.[14] Routine radiograph from this 7-year-old patient reveals remodeling of bone, altered trabecular architecture, and bilateral protrusio acetabuli and coxa vara deformities. The pelvis demonstrates a triradiate shape. Femoral fixation devices are also seen.

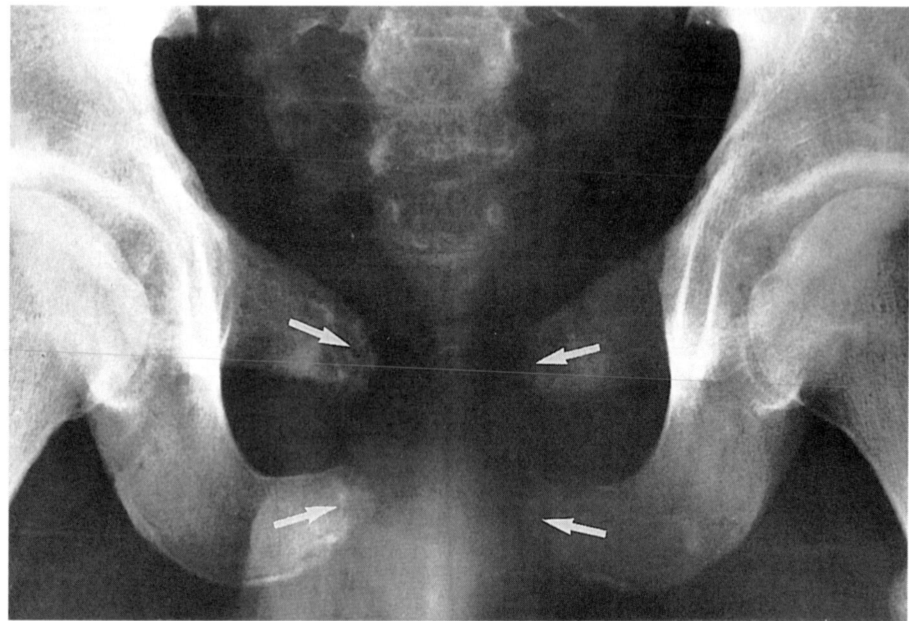

FIGURE 6–17. Cleidocranial dysplasia.[15] Incomplete ossification of the pubic bones (arrows) in this disorder may simulate destructive lesions. *(Courtesy of A.G. Bergman, M.D., Stanford, California.)*

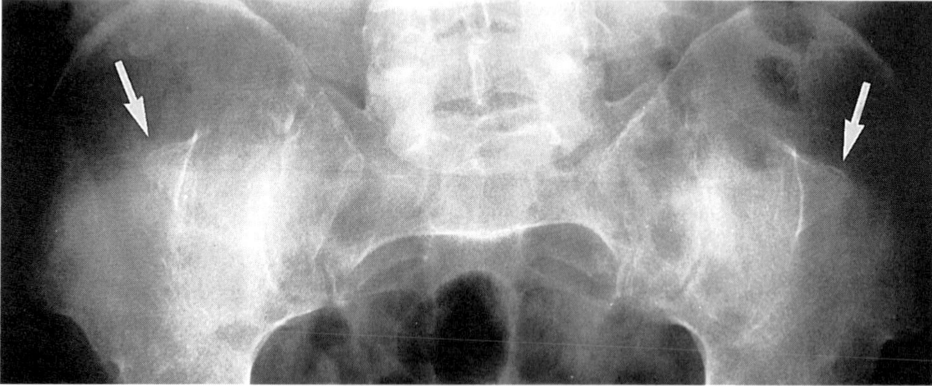

FIGURE 6–18. Hereditary osteo-onychodysostosis (HOOD) syndrome.[16] Observe the characteristic bilateral outgrowths arising from the posterior iliac wings (arrows). The presence of these iliac horns, which occasionally are capped by an epiphysis, is virtually pathognomonic of the HOOD syndrome. This patient also had associated hypoplasia and splitting of the nails of the fingers and toes, absence of the patellae, and dislocation of the radial heads.

TABLE 6–4. Injuries of the Bony Pelvis*†

Entity	Figure(s)	Characteristics
Type I: Injuries without disruption of the pelvic ring		30 per cent of all pelvic fractures
Avulsion fracture[17]		Prevalent in adolescent athletes involved in gymnastics, running, jumping, and hurdling Stable avulsion fracture of bone at muscular and tendinous insertion sites such as the following:
	6–19A	1. Anterior inferior iliac spine: rectus femoris muscle
	6–19B	2. Anterior superior iliac spine: sartorius or tensor fasciae femoris muscle
	6–19C	3. Ischial tuberosity: hamstring muscles
	6–19D	4. Iliac crest: abdominal muscles
		5. Symphysis pubis: adductor muscles Complication: bizarre skeletal overgrowth or deformity simulating neoplasm
Fracture of the pubis or ischium[18]	See Fig. 6–25	Unilateral stable fractures of a single ramus are common in the following situations: 1. Elderly patients: after a fall or hip surgery 2. Young athletes: as a stress fracture Subsequent osteolysis may simulate a neoplasm
Fracture of the iliac wing[18]	6–20	Duverney fracture is a fracture of the iliac wing that occurs as a result of direct injury Stable and infrequently displaced
Fracture of the sacrum[19–22]	5–8, 5–9	See Chapter 5 for discussion and illustrations Isolated transverse fracture of the sacrum is stable and occurs only infrequently
Fracture or dislocation of the coccyx[18]		See Chapter 5 for discussion
Type II: Injuries with single break in the pelvic ring		25 per cent of all pelvic fractures
Fractures of two ipsilateral rami[18]		Unilateral stable fractures of superior and inferior ischiopubic rami Associated fractures or ligamentous disruptions common
Single fracture near, or diastasis of, the symphysis pubis[18, 23]	6–21	Isolated stable fracture of the pubic ramus or pubic diastasis occurs infrequently The greater the degree of diastasis, the more likely is the occurrence of a second break in the pelvic ring and visceral injury Pubic diastasis exceeding 25 mm suggests a high likelihood of sacrospinous and anterior sacroiliac ligament disruption *Postpartum diastasis* Known complication of pregnancy related to increased elasticity of the pubic ligaments Usually limited to 7 mm or less In most cases it is self-limited, gradually reducing over a period of months
Single fracture near, or diastasis of, the sacroiliac joint[24]		Rare occurrence that usually results from direct trauma Stable injury

Table continued on following page

TABLE 6–4. Injuries of the Bony Pelvis*† *Continued*

Entity	Figure(s)	Characteristics
Type III: Injuries with double breaks in the pelvic ring		
Double vertical fractures of the ischiopubic ring or dislocations of the pubis[18, 25]	6–22	Straddle fracture: 20 per cent of all pelvic fractures Bilateral vertical fractures of both pubic rami or a unilateral fracture of both pubic rami combined with symphyseal diastasis Unstable *Complications* Urethral or visceral damage in 30 to 40 per cent of cases Hemorrhage and peripheral nerve injury common Associated spine and other remote fractures 10 per cent mortality rate with all pelvic fractures
Double vertical fractures or dislocations of the pelvis[25]	6–23	Malgaigne fracture: 15 per cent of all pelvic fractures *Types* 1. Vertical fracture of both pubic rami combined with either a sacroiliac joint dislocation or a fracture of the ilium or sacrum 2. Symphyseal dislocation combined with either a sacroiliac joint dislocation or a fracture of the ilium or sacrum Sacroiliac joint dislocation is twice as common as para-articular fracture Unstable fractures Hemorrhage, urinary tract injury, peripheral nerve injury common Associated spine and other remote fractures
Type IV: Injuries of the acetabulum[26–28]	6–24	*Four important bony landmarks* 1. Anterior acetabular rim 2. Posterior acetabular rim 3. Iliopubic (anterior) column 4. Ilioischial (posterior) column Fractures result from impact of the femoral head against the acetabulum May involve one or two columns Classified as wall fractures, column fractures, and transverse fractures Fracture types may overlap, fitting into more than one classification *Complications* Intra-articular osseous fragments Associated fractures of the bony pelvis Triradiate cartilage damage in children Degenerative joint disease Protrusio acetabuli Ischemic necrosis (usually associated with posterior hip dislocation) Heterotopic ossification Pelvic visceral, nerve, and vascular injury common
Stress injuries of the pelvis		
Stress (fatigue) fractures[29, 30]	6–25	Pregnant women, joggers, long distance runners, and patients with hip osteoarthrosis and hip arthroplasty are predisposed to parasymphyseal and pelvic ring fatigue fractures *Complications* Osteolysis simulating malignancy Delayed union Refracture
Insufficiency fractures[20–22, 30]	6–26	Sites include parasymphyseal, sacral, and supra-acetabular regions Osteolysis simulating malignancy *Complications* Delayed union Refracture Additional pelvic fractures

*See also Tables 1–3 to 1–5.
†Adapted from Kane WJ: Fractures of the pelvis. *In* Rockwood CA Jr, Green DP (eds): Fractures in Adults. 2nd Ed. Philadelphia, JB Lippincott, 1984, p 1112.

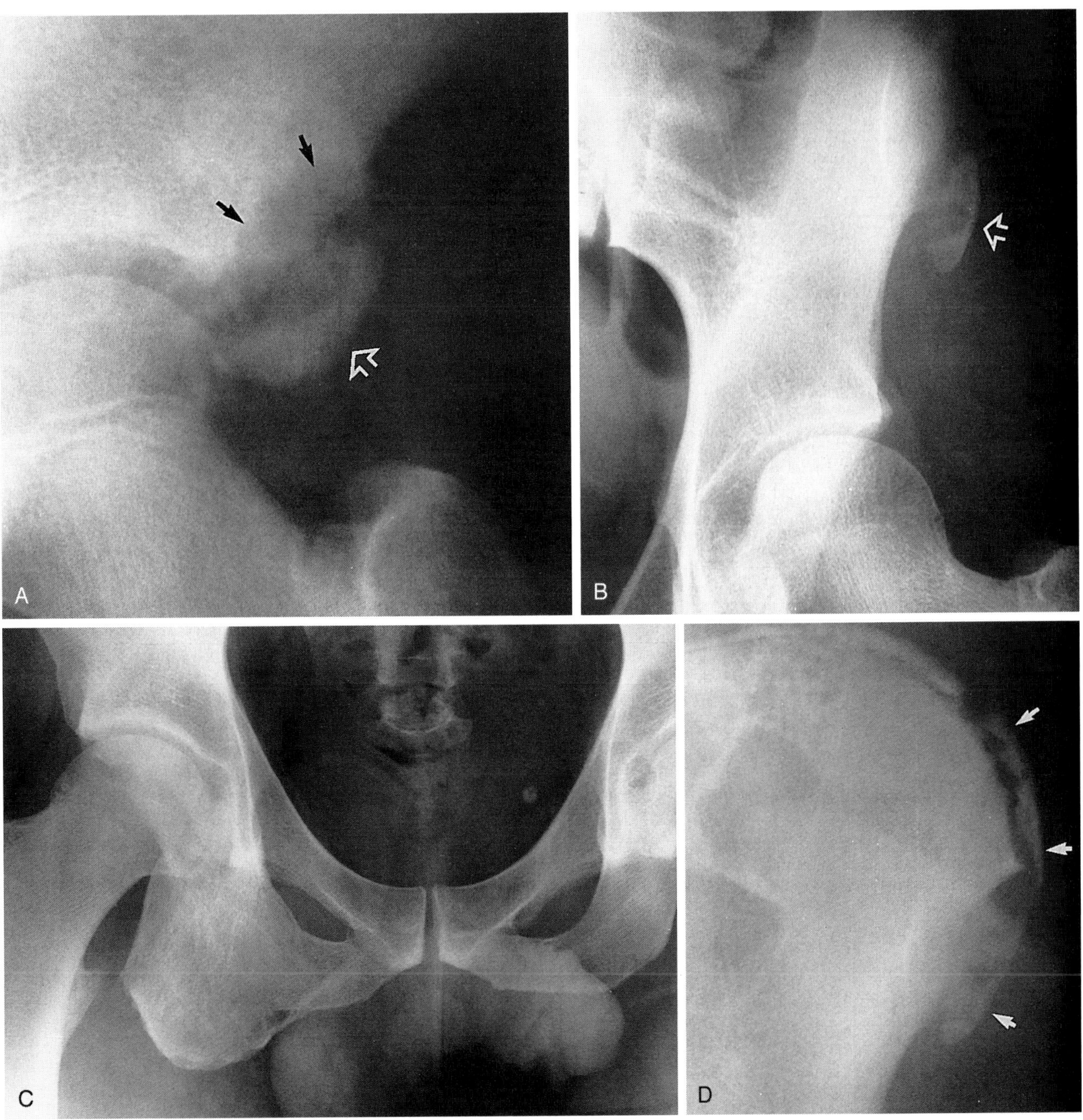

FIGURE 6–19. Pelvic avulsion injuries.[17] **A** Anteroinferior iliac spine. The avulsed fragment (open arrow) is related to muscular pull at the attachment of the rectus femoris muscle. Note the radiolucent defect adjacent to the acetabular rim (arrows). **B** Anterosuperior iliac spine. Routine radiograph shows avulsion of the anterosuperior iliac spine, the attachment site of the sartorius muscle (open arrow). *(***B***, Courtesy of W. Ewing, M.D., Pueblo, Colorado.)* **C** Ischial tuberosity. This 30-year-old man had an old avulsion fracture of the ischial tuberosity at the site of attachment of the hamstring tendons. The fracture has healed with dramatic osseous enlargement, a finding often termed "rider's bone." **D** Iliac apophysis. This 14-year-old girl felt something pop in the anterior thigh during a fight. Observe the separation of the iliac apophysis, the site of attachment of the abdominal muscles (arrows).

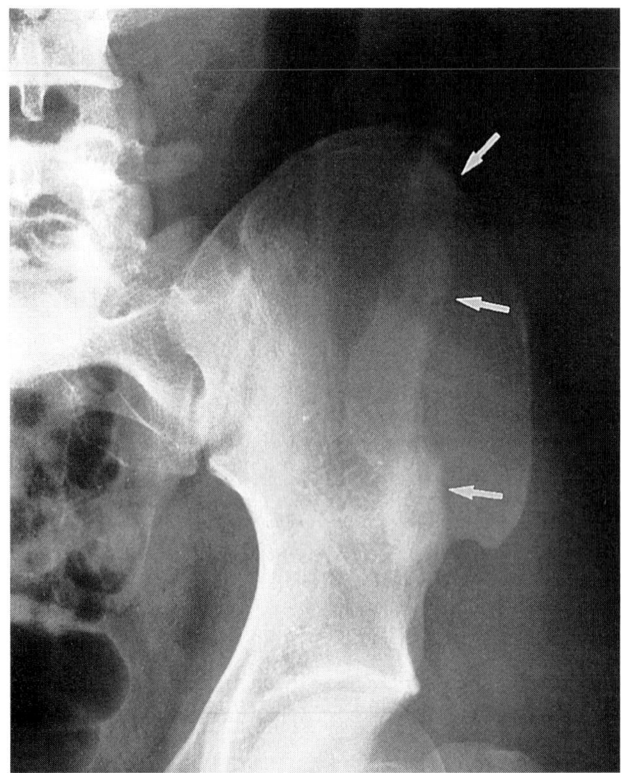

FIGURE 6–20. Type I injury: Duverney's fracture.[18] Observe the solitary fracture of the iliac wing after a direct injury in this teenager. These fractures represent about 30 per cent of all pelvic fractures. They do not disrupt the pelvic ring, and, therefore, are considered stable.

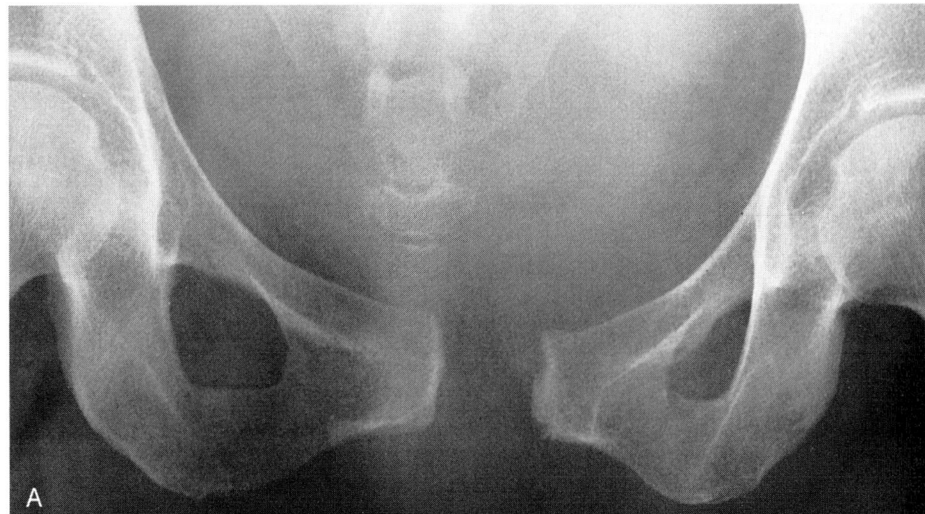

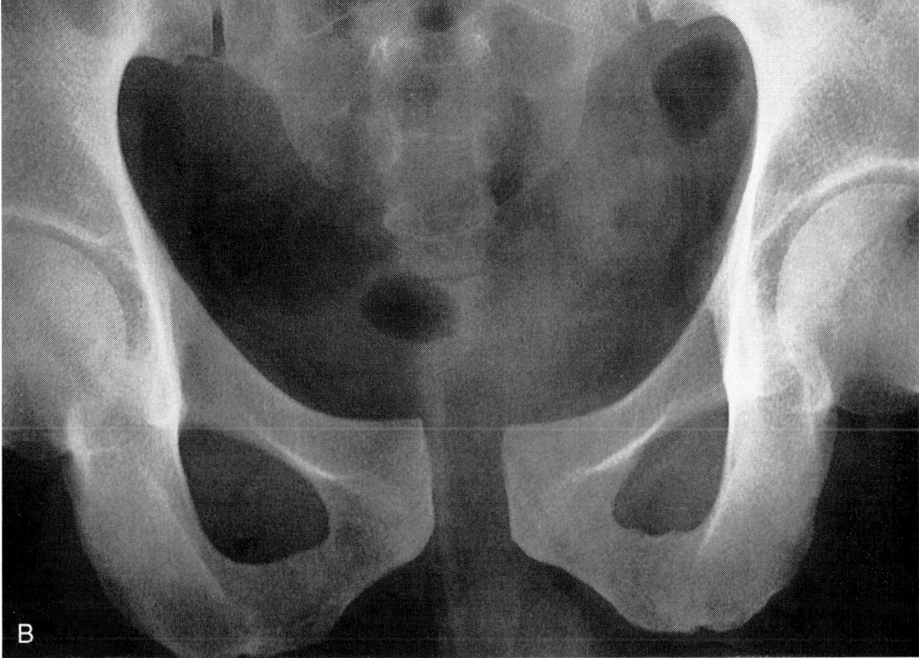

FIGURE 6–21. Diastasis of the pubic symphysis.[18, 23] A Postpartum diastasis. This 38-year-old woman had persistent pain and tenderness in the pubic region after an uncomplicated vaginal delivery. Widening of the symphysis pubis measuring 20 mm is evident. This is a self-limited condition related to increased elasticity of the pubic ligaments during pregnancy. B Type II injury. This man was involved in a motorcycle accident. The articulation measures 15 mm, and no associated sacral fractures or sacroiliac diastases were found. *Illustration continued on following page*

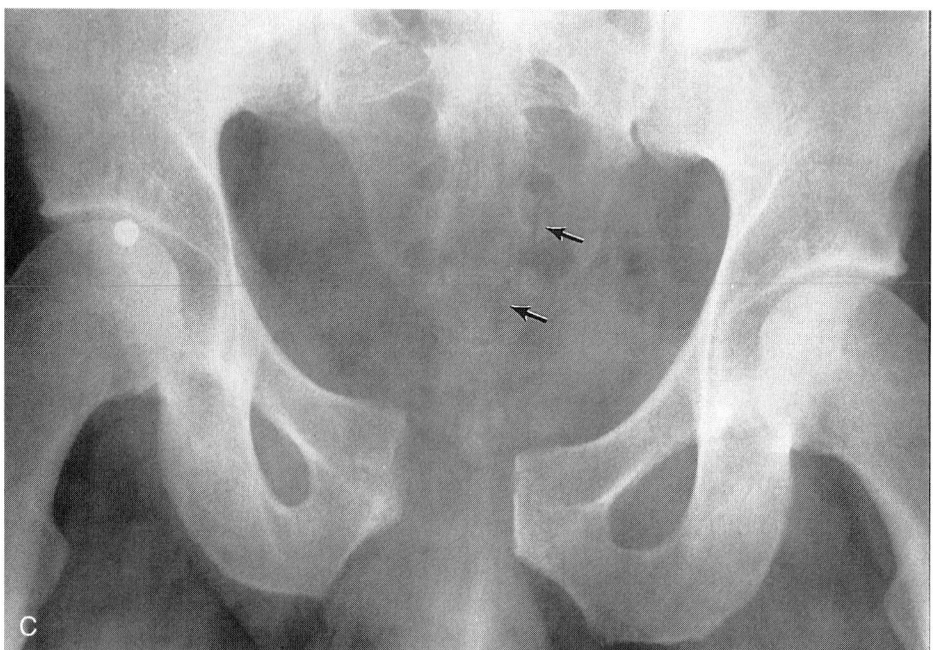

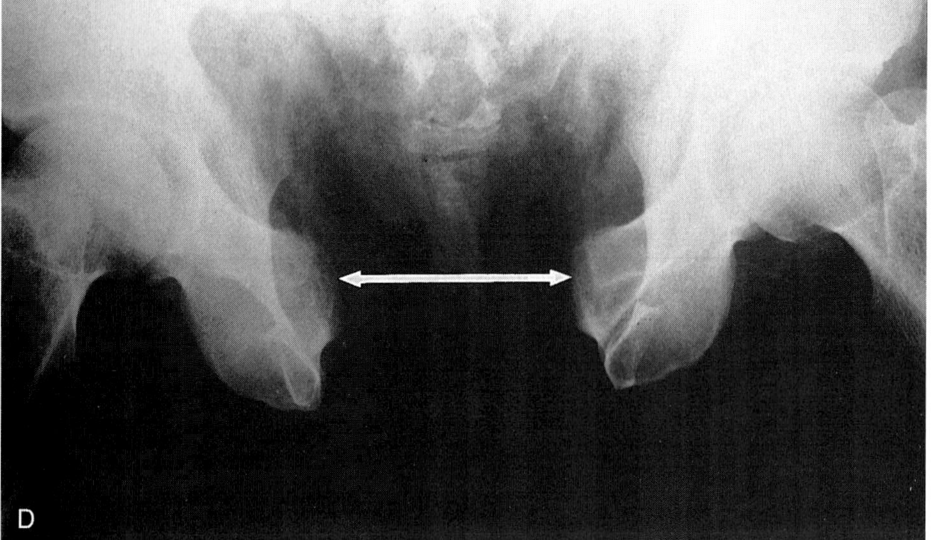

FIGURE 6–21 *Continued.* C Type III injury. A 35-mm pubic diastasis is associated with a vertical fracture of the sacrum (arrows). Diastasis of the left sacroiliac joint also was present. *(A–C, Courtesy of B.A. Howard, M.D., Charlotte, North Carolina.)* D Type III injury. Dramatic separation of the symphysis pubis is evident (double-headed arrow) in this patient, who has sustained a type III unstable pelvic injury in a motorcycle accident. A sacral fracture also was evident (not shown). This injury resulted in associated rectal laceration and denervation of the lower extremity. *(D Courtesy of F.G. Bauer, D.C., Sydney, New South Wales, Australia.)*

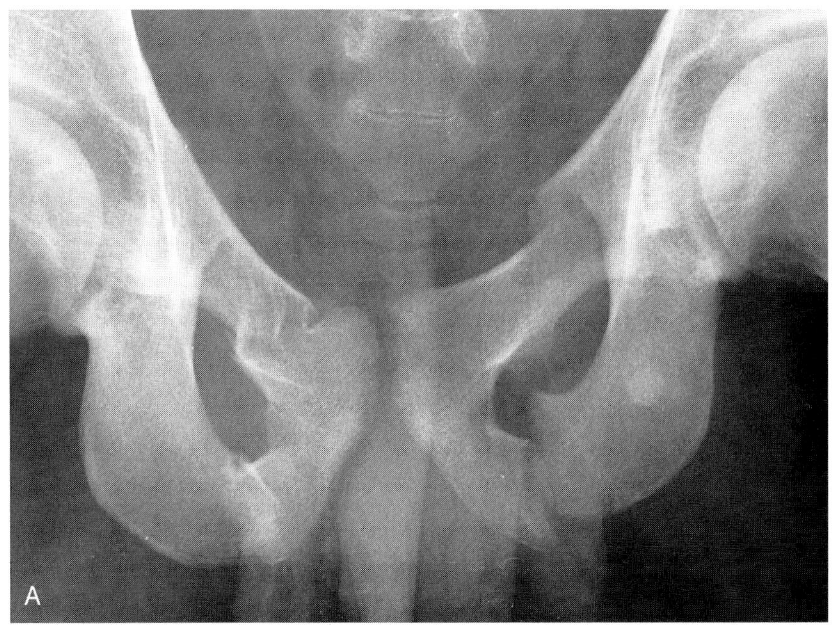

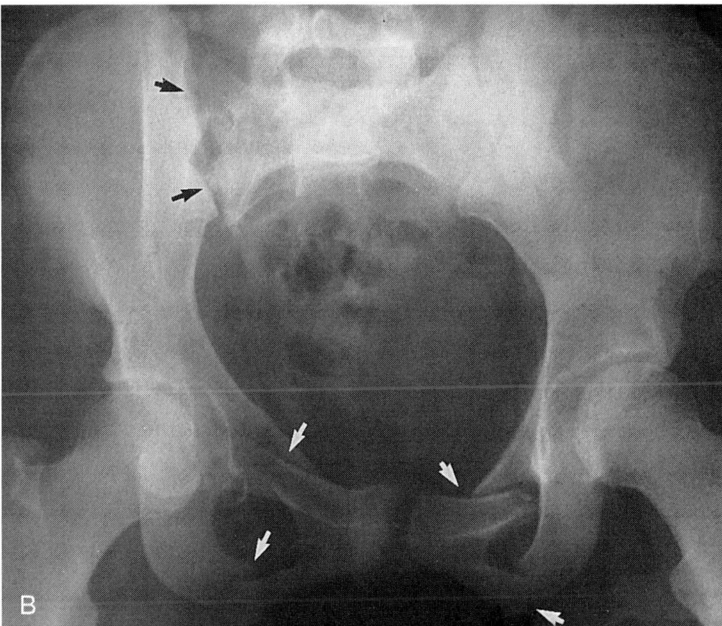

FIGURE 6–22. Type III pelvic injuries.[18] A Straddle fracture. Observe the bilateral vertical fractures of the pubic rami in this 18-year old boy. B In another patient, a 17-year-old girl, bilateral fractures of the ischiopubic rami (white arrows) are combined with diastasis of the right sacroiliac joint (black arrows).

Illustration continued on following page

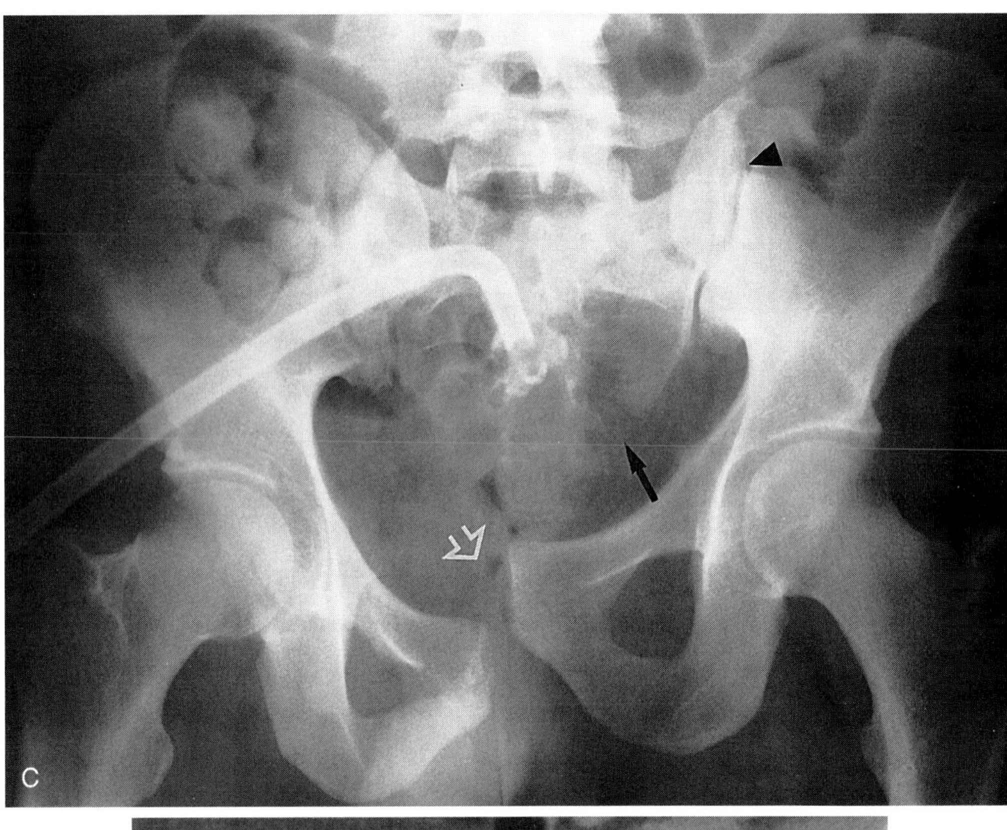

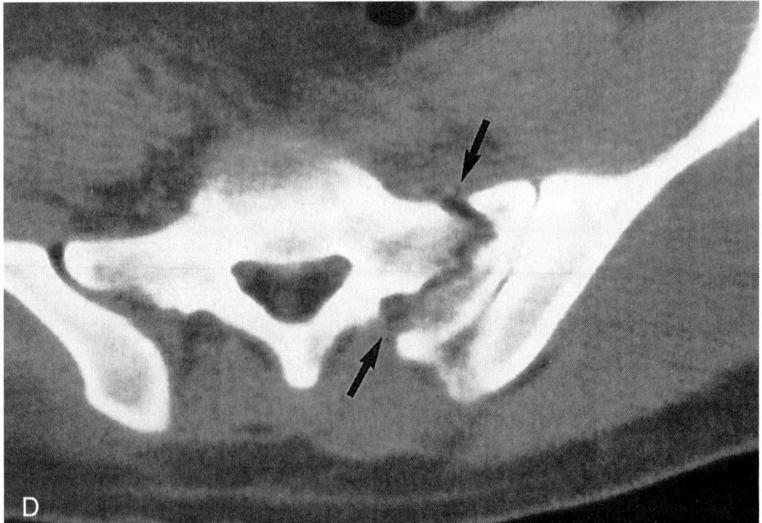

FIGURE 6–22 *Continued.* C, D Complex pelvic injury in another patient. In C, an anteroposterior radiograph of the pelvis reveals a fracture of the sacrum (black arrow), sacroiliac joint diastasis (arrowhead), and pubic diastasis (open arrow). A suprapubic catheter is in place. In D, a transaxial CT scan from the same patient as in C demonstrates the extent of the sacral fracture (arrows). Intra-articular gas within the right sacroiliac joint suggests the presence of diastasis.

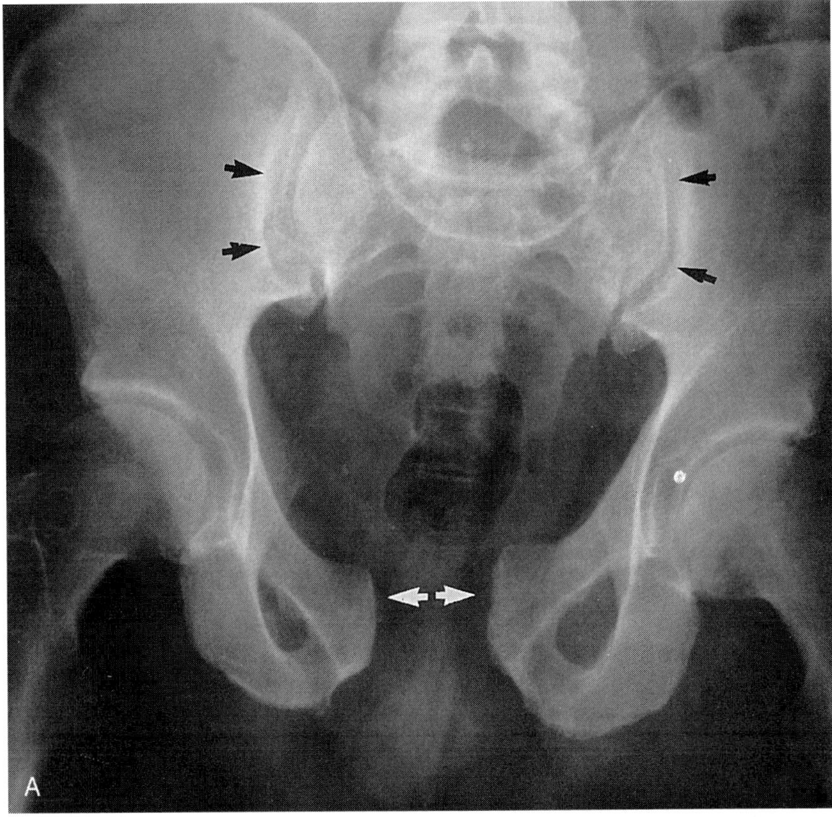

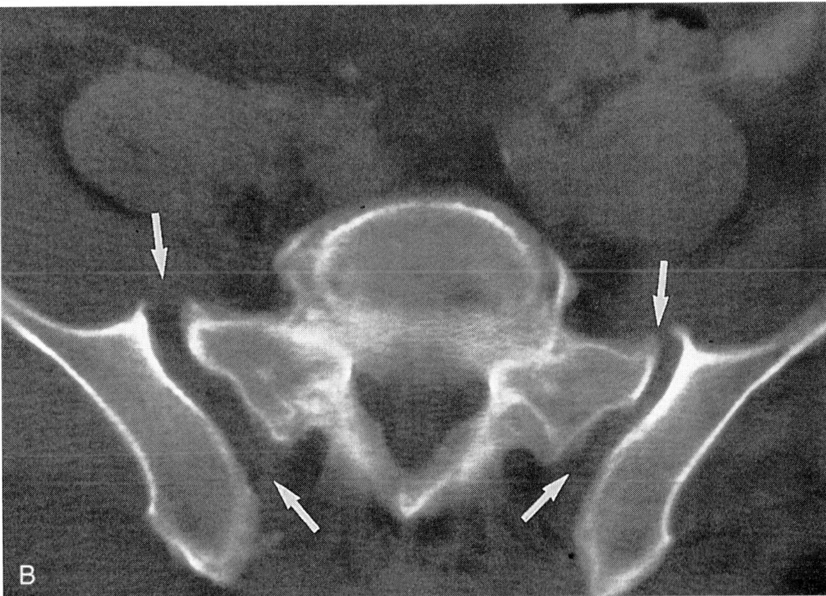

FIGURE 6–23. Complex pelvic injury: Sprung pelvis.[25] Routine radiograph (A) shows wide diastasis of the symphysis pubis (white arrows) and less obvious sacroiliac joint widening (black arrows). Transaxial computed tomographic (CT) scan (B) demonstrates the bilateral sacroiliac joint diastasis (arrows) more clearly. The sprung pelvis occurs as a result of massive crushing injuries and, as with other pelvic injuries, may be complicated by hemorrhage, urinary tract injury, peripheral nerve injury, and remote injuries.

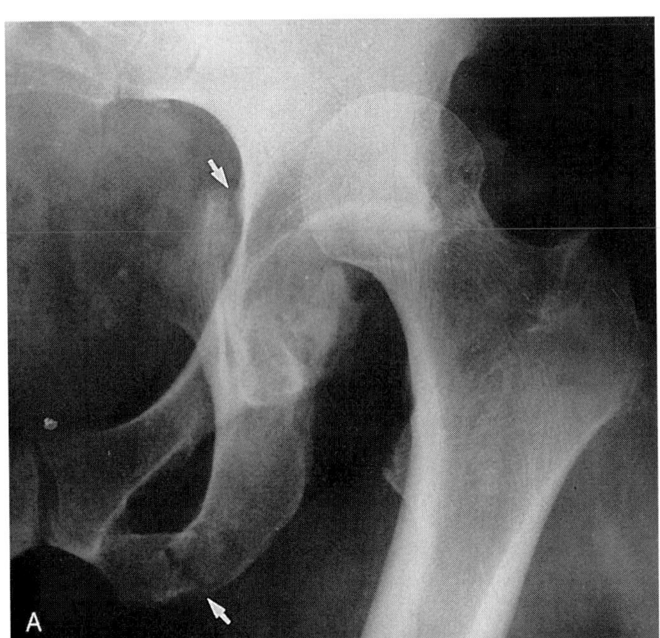

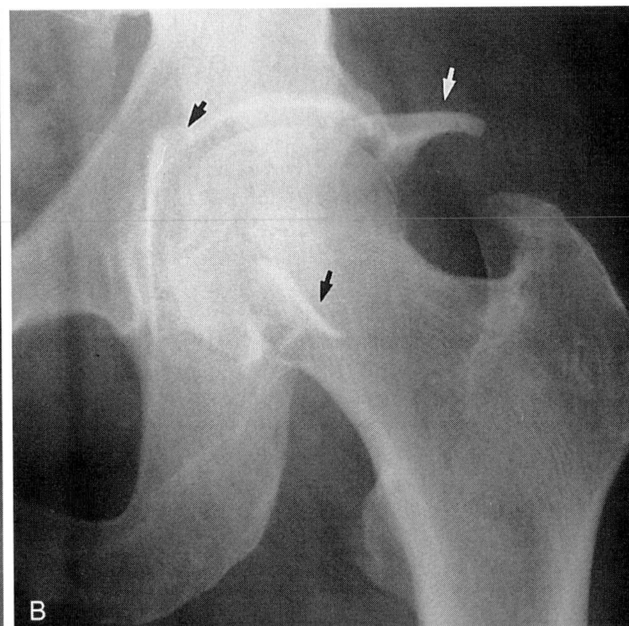

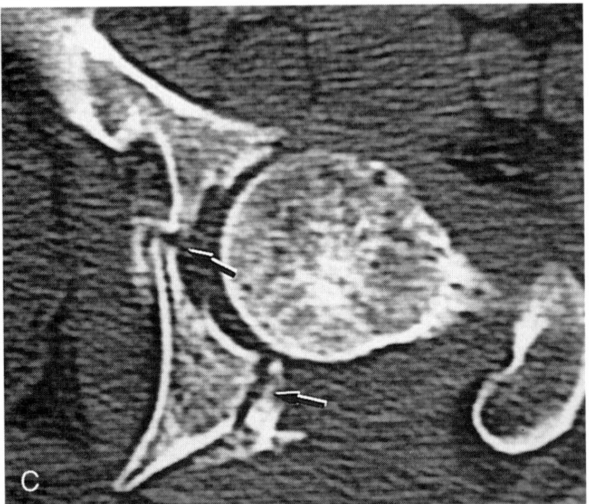

FIGURE 6–24. Acetabular fracture.[26–28] A–C This 29-year-old man sustained a posterior hip dislocation in a motor vehicle accident. In A, a prereduction radiograph shows the posterior hip dislocation and associated fracture of the acetabulum and ischium (arrows). In B, a postreduction radiograph shows the associated fracture fragments (arrows). C Postreduction, transaxial computed tomographic (CT) scan shows the extensive comminution of the acetabulum (arrows).

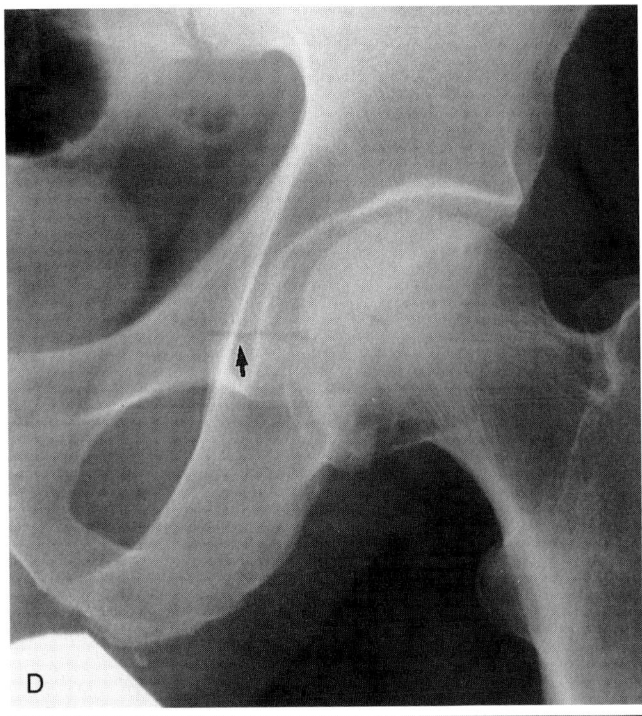

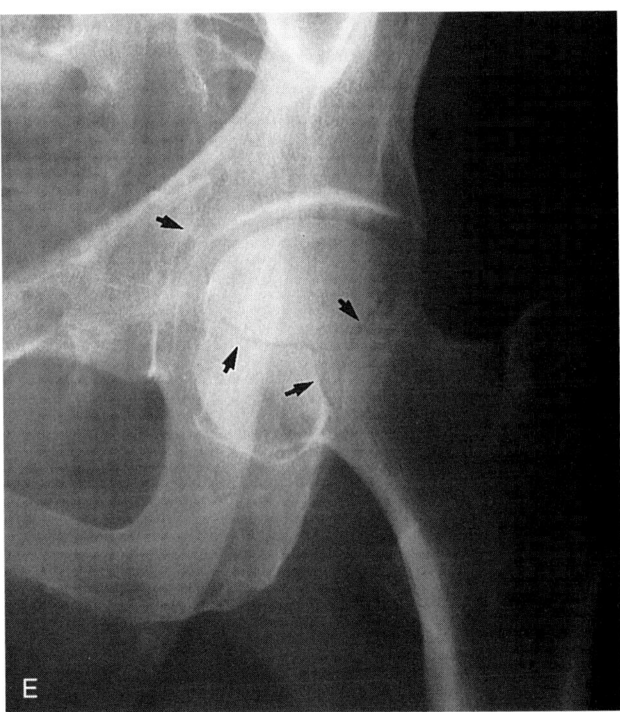

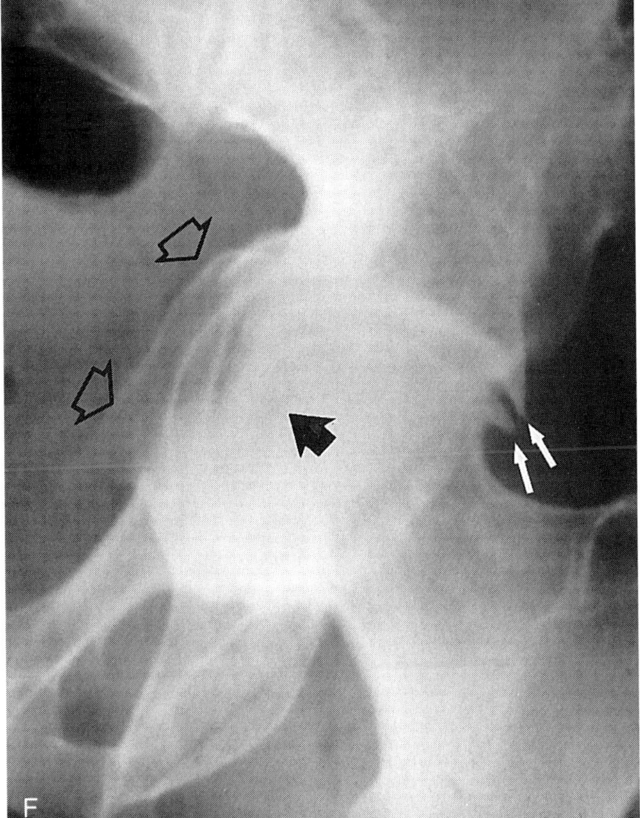

FIGURE 6–24 *Continued.* **D, E** Value of oblique projections. In another patient, routine frontal radiograph **(D)** reveals only one fracture line (arrow). In **E**, a 45-degree oblique (Judet's) projection, demonstrates more clearly the comminuted fractures of the central acetabular region and posterior acetabular rim fractures superimposed on the femoral head (arrows). **F** Postinjury complications. In a third patient, several years after sustaining an acetabular fracture, osteophytes (white arrows) and axial joint space narrowing (black arrow) characteristic of degenerative joint disease can be observed, as can persistent acetabular protrusion (open arrows). Computed tomographic (CT) imaging is indicated in most cases of pelvic trauma as it provides a cross-sectional display of the bony pelvis, identification of intra-articular fracture fragments, and evidence of hemorrhage and other soft tissue or visceral injury. Magnetic resonance (MR) imaging is useful in detecting subclinical injury of the sciatic nerve and occult injuries of the femoral head not readily visible on CT scans. MR imaging, however, is not as accurate as CT in identifying intra-articular fragments. (**F** *From Taylor JAM, Harger BL, Resnick D: Diagnostic imaging of common hip disorders: A pictorial review. Top Clin Chiropr 1:8, 1994. Reprinted with permission.)*

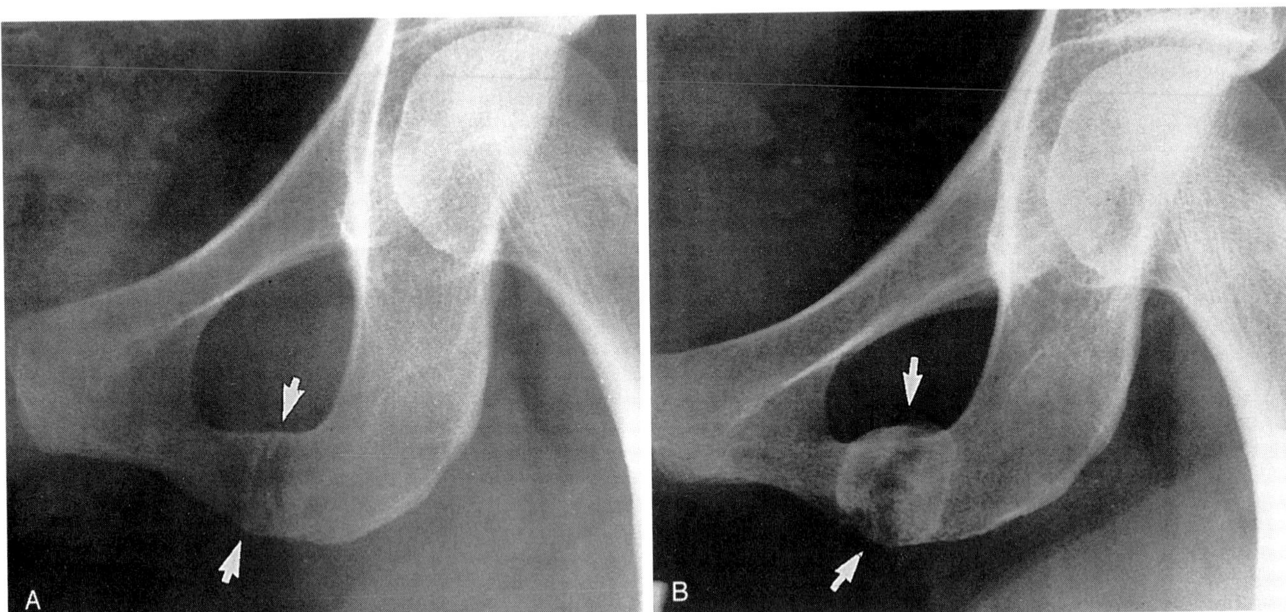

FIGURE 6–25. Stress (fatigue) fracture.[29, 30] A, B A 35-year-old female runner had a 4-week history of left hip pain. In A, an initial radiograph reveals a transverse radiolucent shadow through the inferior ischiopubic ramus (arrows). In B, a serial radiograph obtained 7 months later demonstrates bulbous callus formation at the fracture site, indicating adequate healing.

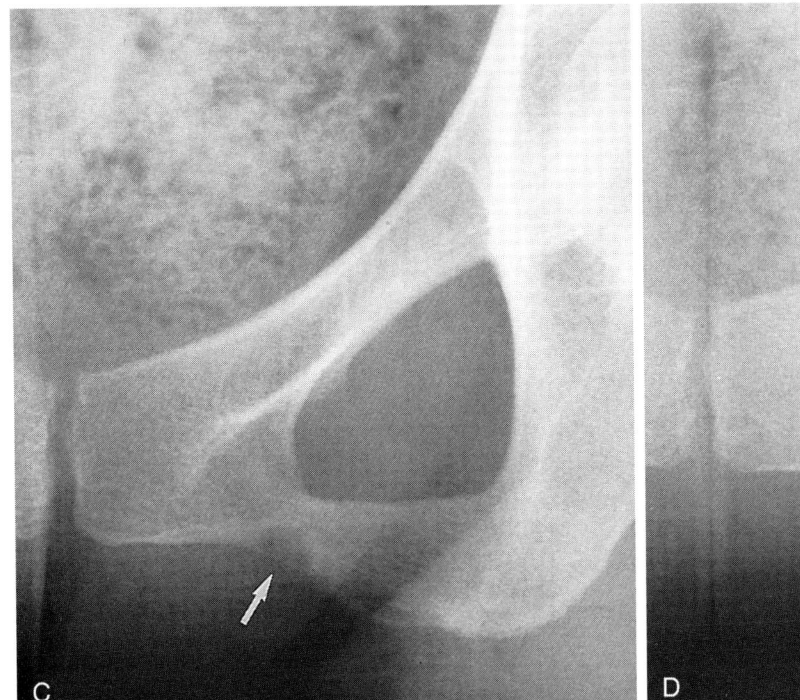

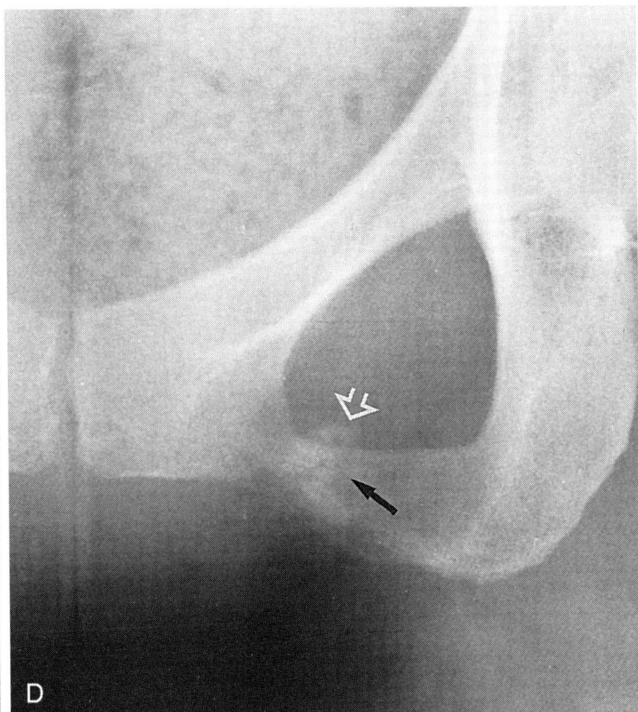

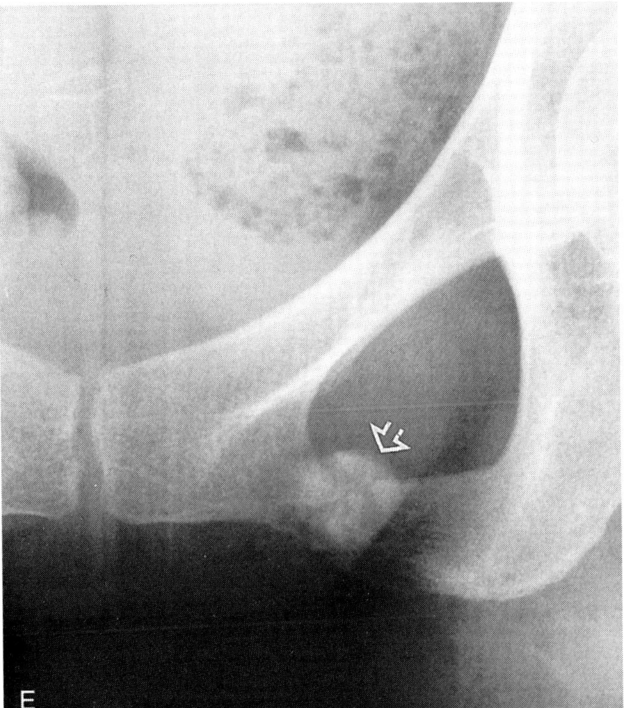

FIGURE 6–25 *Continued.* C–E This 25-year-old woman began an aggressive exercise regimen, including distance running. In **C**, the initial radiograph taken at the time of onset of pain shows a small, circular, osteolytic cortical lesion in the pubic ramus (arrow). In **D**, a serial radiograph taken 1 month later reveals evidence of a fracture line (arrow) and early callus formation (open arrow). In **E**, a third radiograph taken 3 months after the initial film (**C**) reveals abundant callus (open arrow). Fatigue fractures of the pubic ramus affect normal bone primarily in pregnant women, joggers, long-distance runners, and marathoners. (C–E, *Courtesy of S. Standish, D.C., and C. Russell, D.C., Calgary, Alberta, Canada.)*

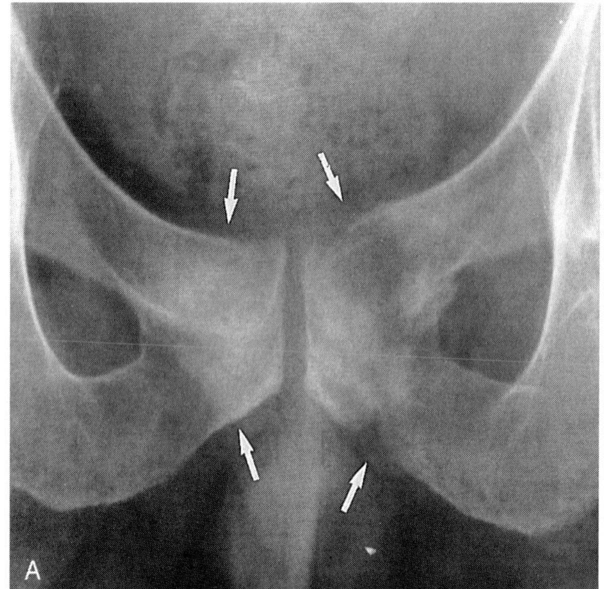

FIGURE 6–26. Insufficiency fracture.[20–22, 30] A Parasymphyseal location. Frontal radiograph of this 61-year-old man shows bilateral insufficiency fractures of bone adjacent to the pubic symphysis (arrows). The findings include osteolysis, osteosclerosis, and bone fragmentation, resembling an aggressive destructive process. B, C Supra-acetabular location. In a 76-year-old man with carcinoma of the prostate, zones of increased density are seen on the frontal radiograph (B) (arrows). Conventional tomography (C) performed 2 weeks after the radiograph was obtained shows areas of increased radiolucency and sclerosis (arrows), typical of an insufficiency fracture. Parasymphyseal and supra-acetabular insufficiency fractures occur after radiation therapy or hip arthroplasty and in patients with osteoporosis, osteoarthrosis, or rheumatoid arthritis of the hip.

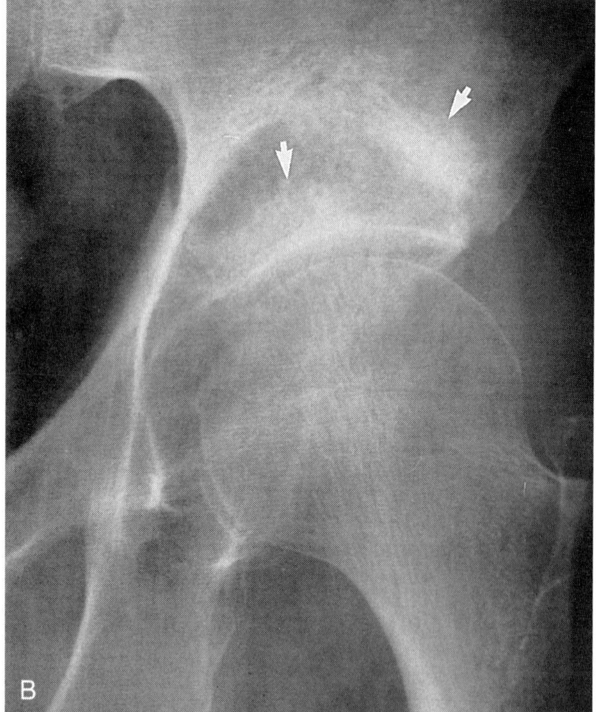

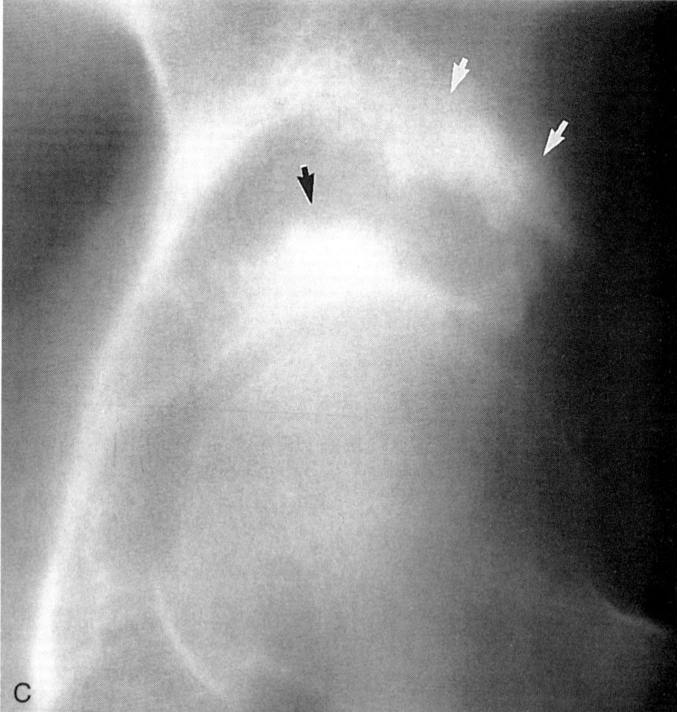

TABLE 6–5. Symphysis Pubis and Pelvis: Articular Disorders*

Entity	Figure(s)	Characteristics
Degenerative and related disorders		
Degenerative disease[31]	6–27	*Pelvis:* Degenerative enthesopathy of the pelvis is common in aging persons *Symphysis pubis:* Accompanies aging and is accelerated by childbirth and trauma Osteophytes, subchondral sclerosis, vacuum phenomenon May resemble infection and inflammatory spondyloarthropathies
Diffuse idiopathic skeletal hyperostosis (DISH)[31–33]	6–28	*Pelvis:* Extensive enthesopathy and ligament ossification
	6–29	*Symphysis pubis:* Osseous bridging of the symphysis pubis
Osteitis pubis[34, 35]	6–30	Painful, self-limited condition Women: after childbirth or pelvic surgery Men: after prostate or bladder surgery Athletes: as a result of chronic stress across the articulation or as a result of acute avulsion of muscle attachments adjacent to the joint Other injuries and low-grade infections also may precipitate these changes *Radiographic findings:* Bilateral symmetric subchondral bone sclerosis, irregularity, resorption, osteolysis Restoration of the osseous surface and disappearance of sclerosis may be associated with bony ankylosis of the joint
Inflammatory disorders		
Rheumatoid arthritis[36]		Rare involvement of symphysis pubis usually is clinically silent Subchondral erosion, mild sclerosis, joint space narrowing
Ankylosing spondylitis[37]	6–31	Symphysis pubis involved in 16 to 23 per cent of patients Erosions, sclerosis, blurring of subchondral surfaces, joint space narrowing, and eventual ankylosis of symphysis pubis
Psoriatic spondyloarthropathy and Reiter's syndrome[37]	6–32	Symphysis pubis findings similar to those of ankylosing spondylitis, but less frequently involved
Dermatomyositis and polymyositis[38]	6–33	Diffuse sheet-like calcification in soft tissues surrounding pelvis
Crystal deposition and metabolic disorders		
Calcium pyrophosphate dihydrate (CPPD) crystal deposition disease[39, 40]	6–34	Articular space narrowing, sclerosis, chondrocalcinosis within joint and, in some cases, considerable bone fragmentation
Hemochromatosis[41]	6–35	Findings identical to those of CPPD crystal deposition disease
Alkaptonuria[42]	6–36	Accelerated degenerative disease, chondrocalcinosis, joint space narrowing, sclerosis, fragmentation, and osseous bridging
Renal osteodystrophy[43, 44]	6–37	Subchondral resorption results in indistinct subchondral bone margins and widening of the symphysis pubis and sacroiliac joint
Infection		
Infective osteitis pubis[35, 45]		Occasionally, osteitis pubis is associated with a low-grade infection Predisposing factors: intravenous drug abuse and pelvic surgery More aggressive course than "sterile" osteitis pubis Antibiotics usually provide relief of symptoms

*See also Tables 1–6 to 1–9 and Table 1–17.

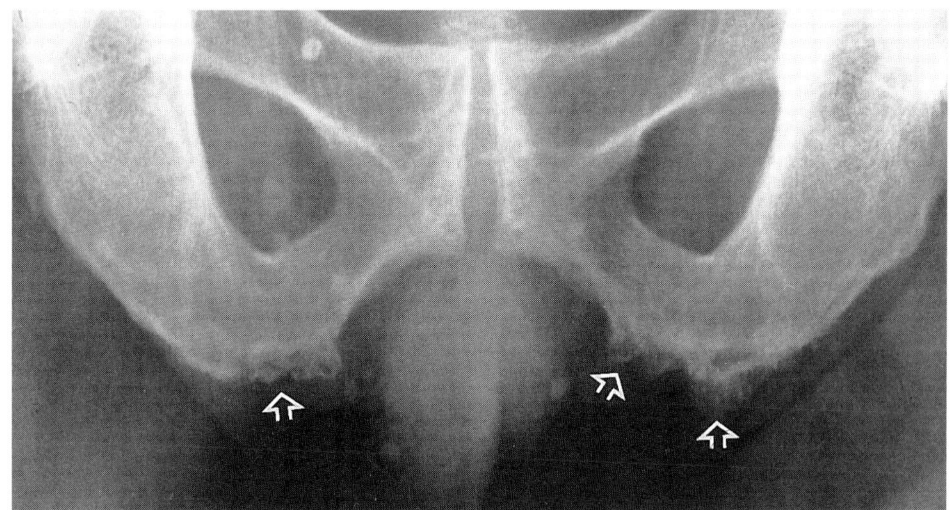

FIGURE 6–27. Degenerative enthesopathy.[31] Observe the irregular whisker-like projections of bone arising from the ischiopubic region (open arrows). Enthesophytes are bony projections at the site of attachment of ligaments and tendons, in this case where the hamstring muscles are attached to the pelvis. Such enthesophytes are seen as a result of degeneration or in patients with diffuse idiopathic skeletal hyperostosis or seronegative spondyloarthropathies. The small circular opaque shadows represent incidental pelvic phleboliths.

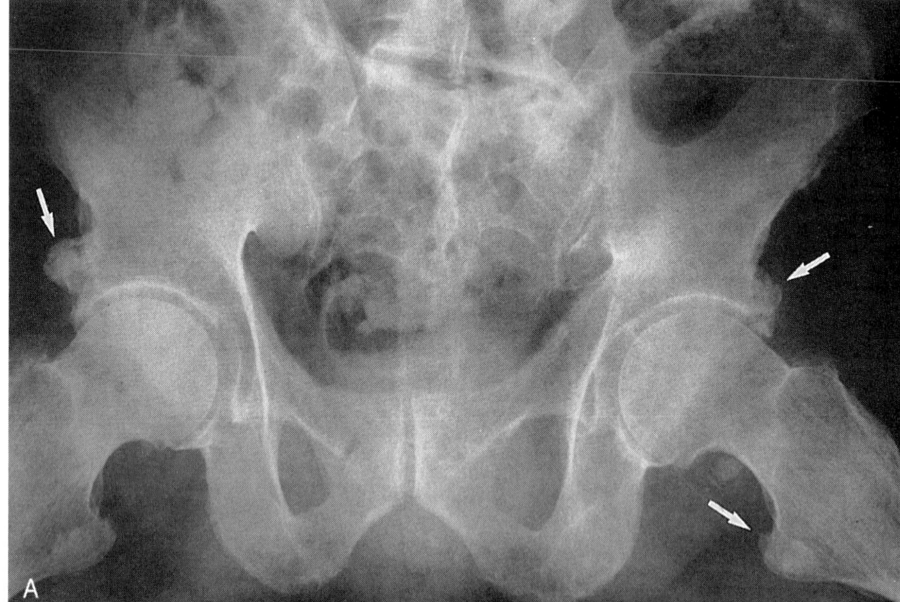

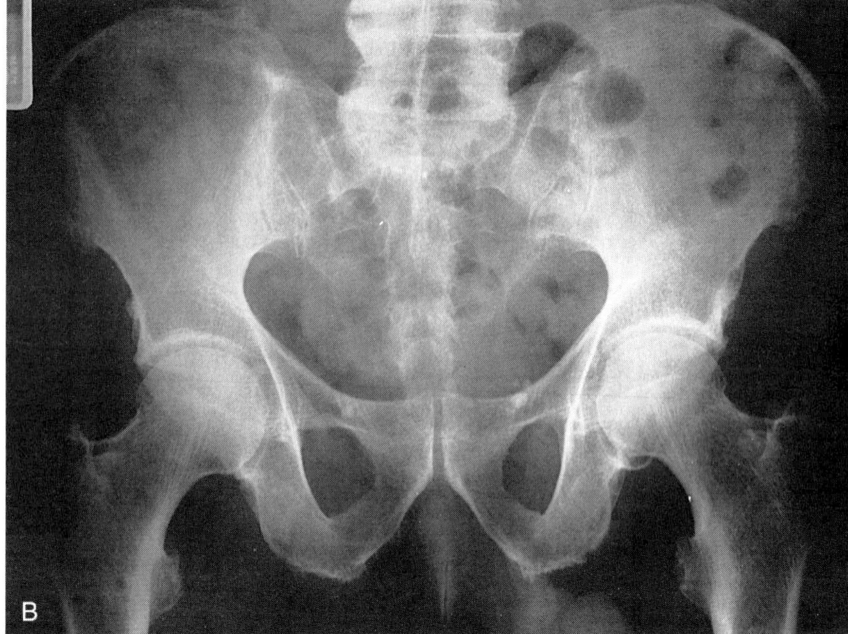

FIGURE 6–28. Diffuse idiopathic skeletal hyperostosis (DISH).[31, 32] **A** Pelvic enthesopathy. Prominent osseous excrescences are present at several characteristic sites in the pelvis (arrows). **B** In another patient, enthesopathy is seen at multiple sites of tendinous attachment.

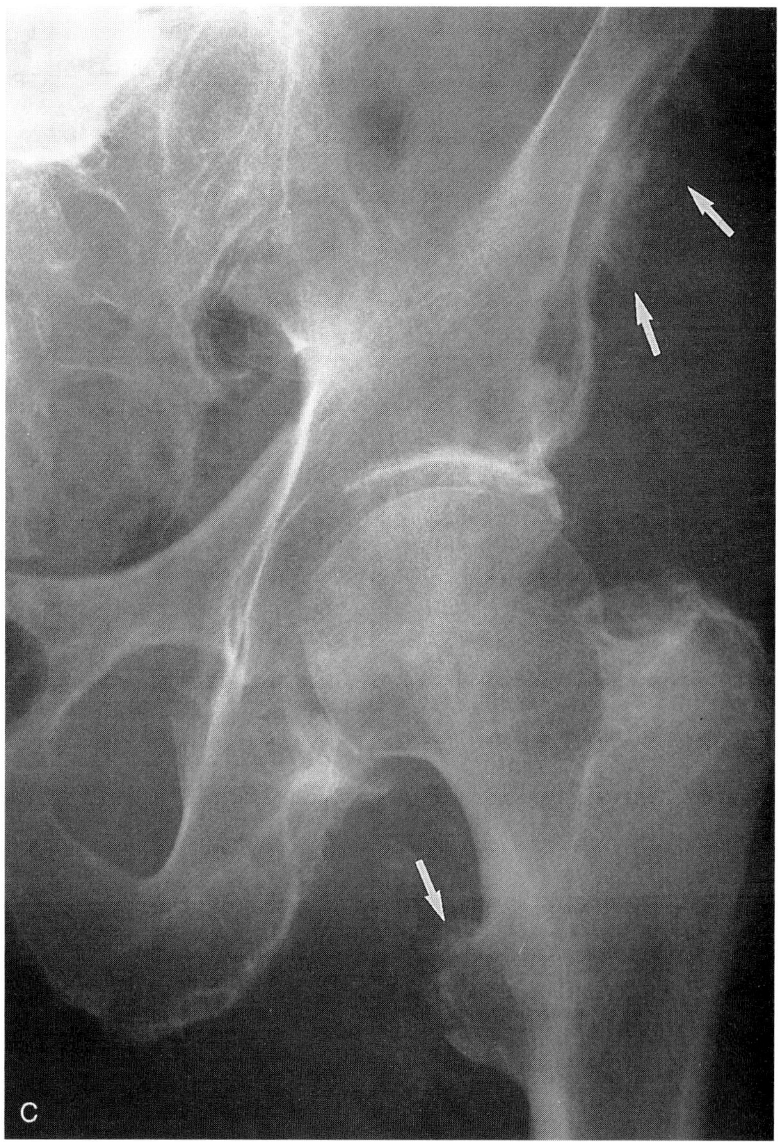

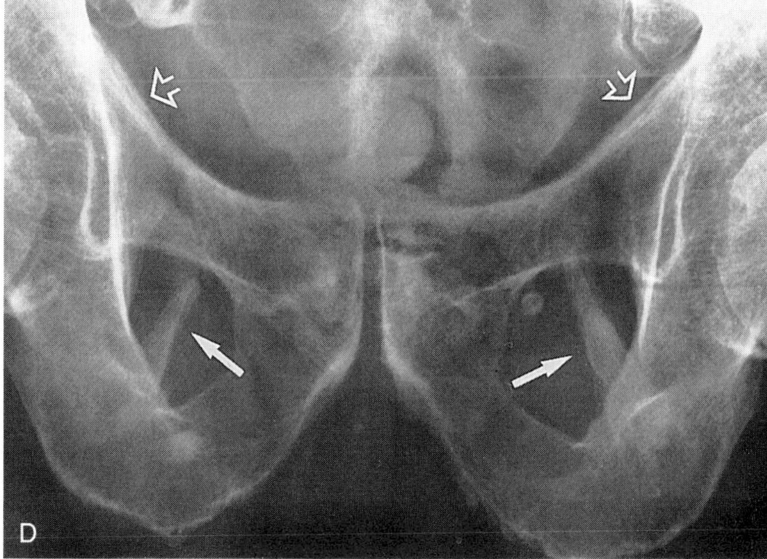

FIGURE 6–28 *Continued.* C In a third patient, ossification and para-articular osseous excrescences (whiskering) project from several sites along the margin of the innominate bones and lesser trochanter (arrows). D Ligament ossification. In this 73-year-old man with DISH, observe the extensive ossification of the sacrotuberous ligaments (arrows). Note also pectineal ligament calcification (open arrows).

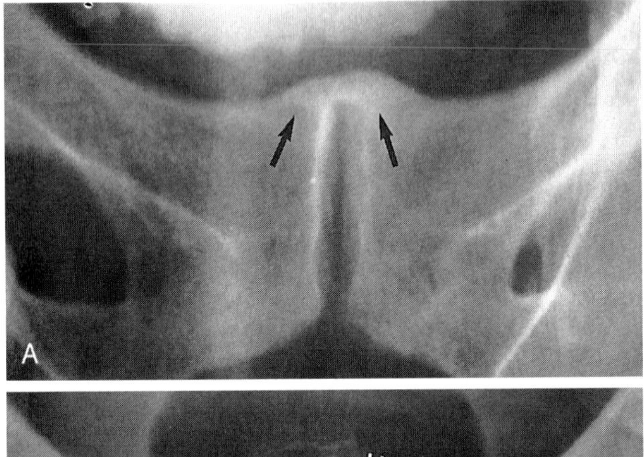

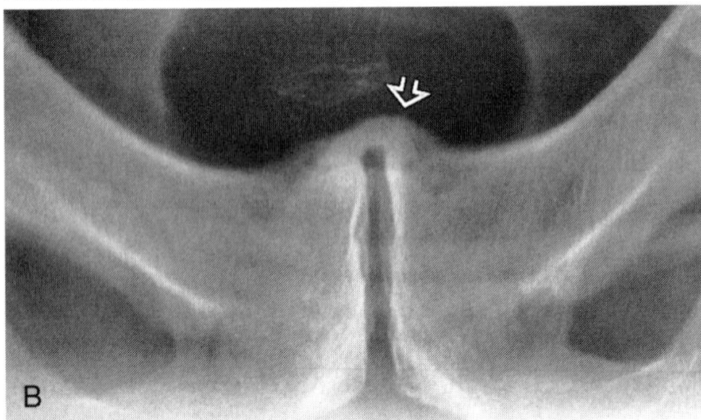

FIGURE 6–29. Diffuse idiopathic skeletal hyperostosis (DISH): Symphysis pubis abnormalities.[33] A On this postvoid intravenous urogram, observe the osseous bridging spanning the superior aspect of the symphysis pubis (arrows). B In a 78-year-old man, similar osseous bridging of the symphysis pubis is evident (open arrow).

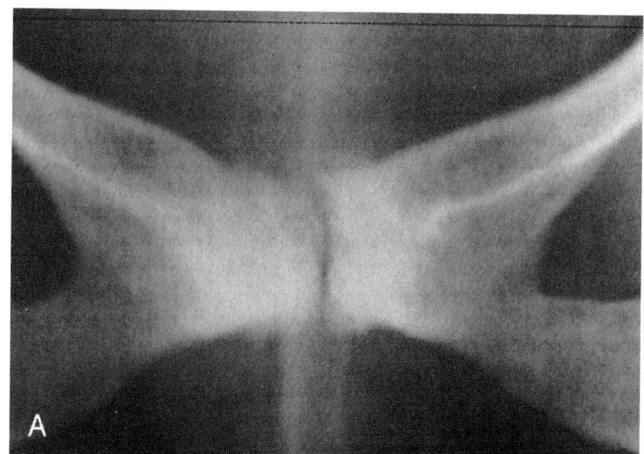

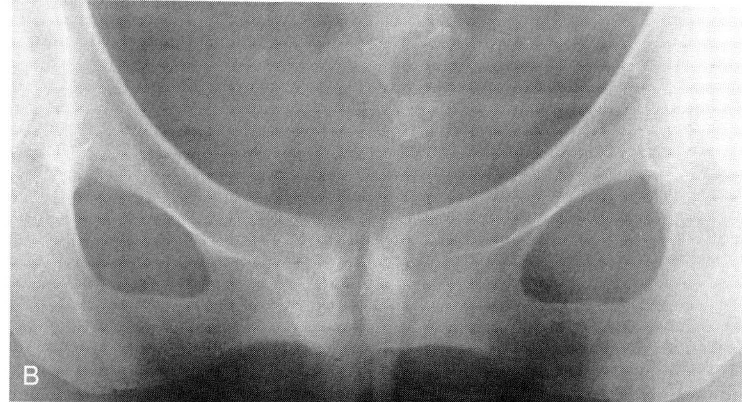

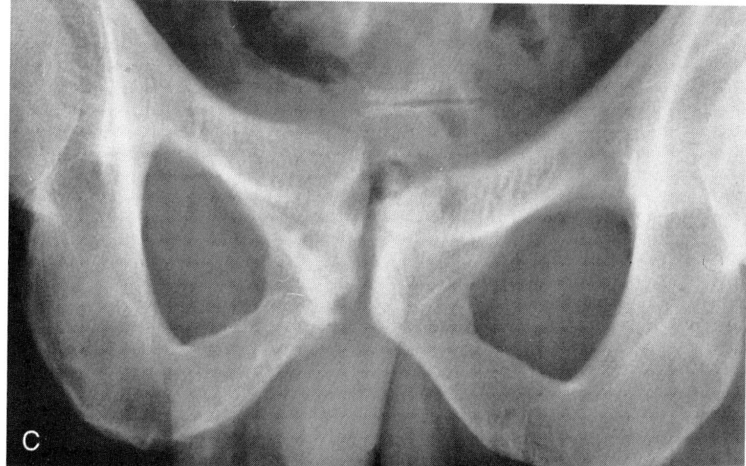

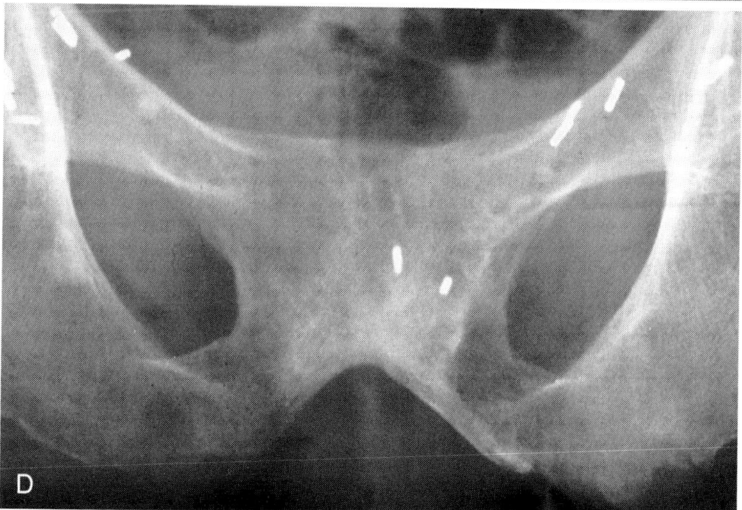

FIGURE 6–30. Osteitis pubis.[34, 35] **A** This 30-year-old woman had localized pubic pain for several months after childbirth. The radiograph reveals bilateral subchondral bone sclerosis and narrowing of the joint space. **B** A 27-year-old woman initially developed pubic pain during the third trimester of pregnancy. The radiographic findings include diffuse sclerosis of the apposing surfaces of the pubic symphysis and irregularity of the articular surfaces. Her symptoms eventually resolved and the sclerosis disappeared. (**B**, *Courtesy of V. Vint, M.D., La Jolla, California.*) **C** 32-year-old man. Posttraumatic sclerotic changes and irregularity of the joint surfaces are seen adjacent to the pubic symphysis on the frontal radiograph. Offset of the adjacent pubic bones is a frequent finding, which is attributed to pelvic obliquity or instability and is not necessarily related to osteitis pubis. **D** Ankylosis. This patient underwent a transurethral prostatectomy and developed osteitis pubis. This radiograph, obtained 2 years later, reveals complete osseous ankylosis.

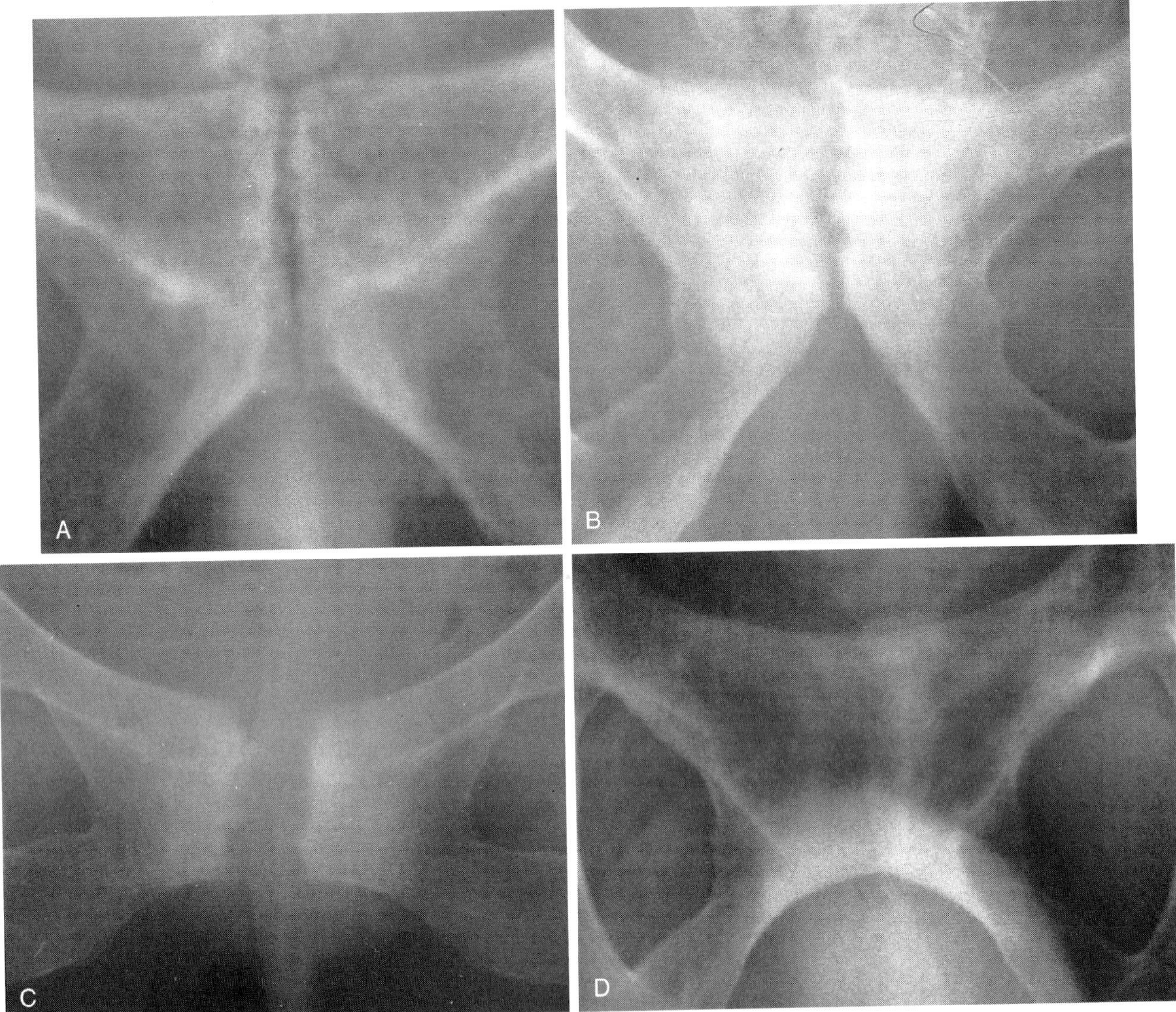

FIGURE 6–31. Ankylosing spondylitis: Spectrum of abnormalities.[37] A Observe the narrowing of the symphysis pubis and indistinct margin of the parasymphyseal subchondral bone surface. B In another patient, the joint space is narrowed and the joint surfaces are indistinct and irregular. Additionally, the subchondral bone is sclerotic. C In a 61-year-old woman with severe ankylosing spondylitis, the symphysis pubis is markedly widened, and the articular margins are indistinct and mildly sclerotic, an appearance resembling that of septic arthritis or hyperparathyroidism. D Complete ankylosis of the symphysis pubis is present in this 38-year-old man with advanced ankylosing spondylitis.

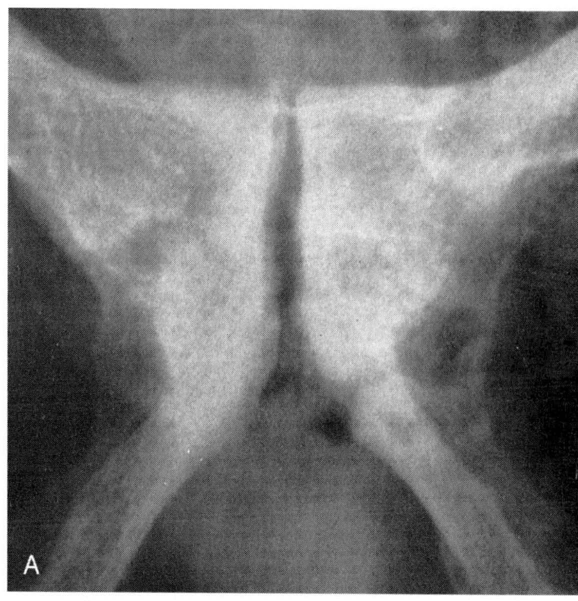

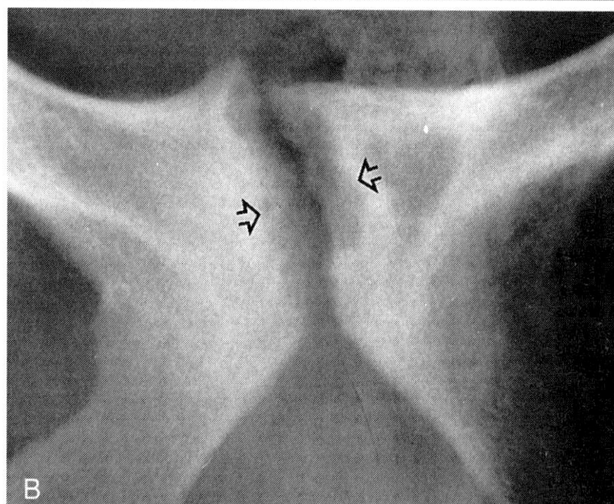

FIGURE 6–32. Psoriatic arthropathy: Pubic symphysis.[37] A The parasymphyseal subchondral bone appears sclerotic, and the articular surfaces are indistinct. B In another patient, subchondral erosions (open arrows) and parasymphyseal sclerosis are seen.

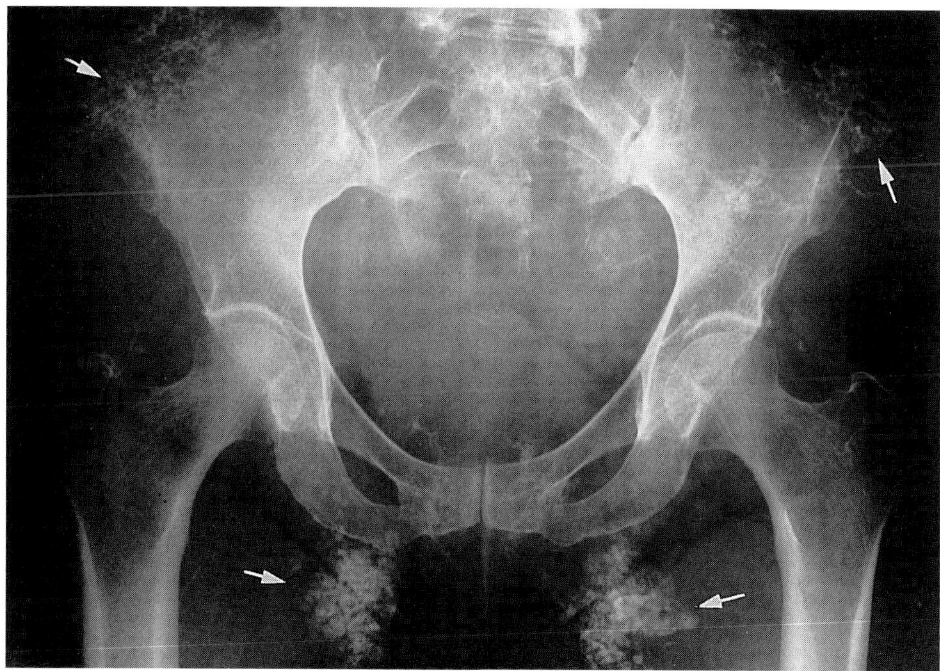

FIGURE 6–33. Dermatomyositis.[38] Multiple areas of sheet-like calcification are seen within the soft tissues of the pelvis (arrows) in this 57-year-old woman with dermatomyositis.

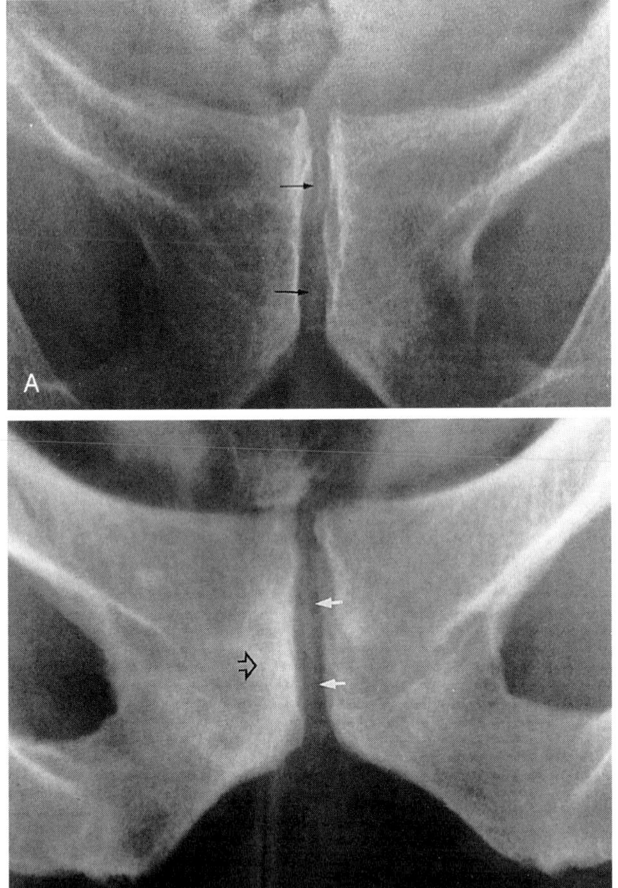

FIGURE 6–34. Calcium pyrophosphate dihydrate (CPPD) crystal deposition disease.[39, 40] A Observe the linear band of chondrocalcinosis within the symphysis pubis (arrows). B In another patient, chondrocalcinosis (arrows) and subchondral sclerosis (open arrow) are evident.

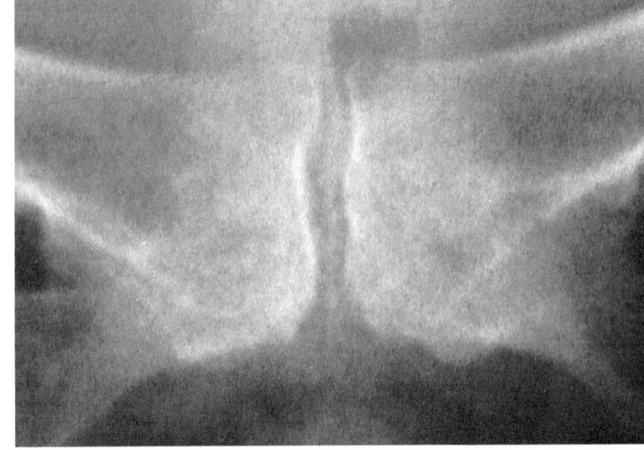

FIGURE 6–35. Hemochromatosis.[41] Observe the linear calcification within the symphysis pubis. The radiographic findings of hemochromatosis resemble those of calcium pyrophospate dihydrate (CPPD) crystal deposition disease. *(Courtesy of G. Greenway, M.D., Dallas, Texas.)*

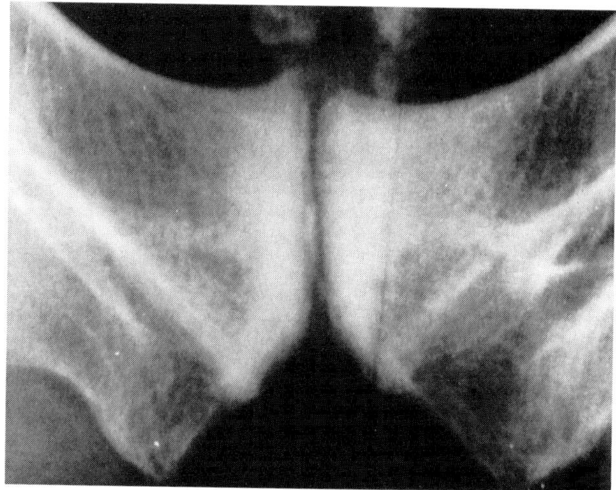

FIGURE 6–36. Alkaptonuria: Symphysis pubis.[42] Radiograph reveals severe joint space narrowing, osteophytosis, and extensive subchondral sclerosis characteristic of alkaptonuria. *(Courtesy of J. Goobar, M.D., Ostersund, Sweden.)*

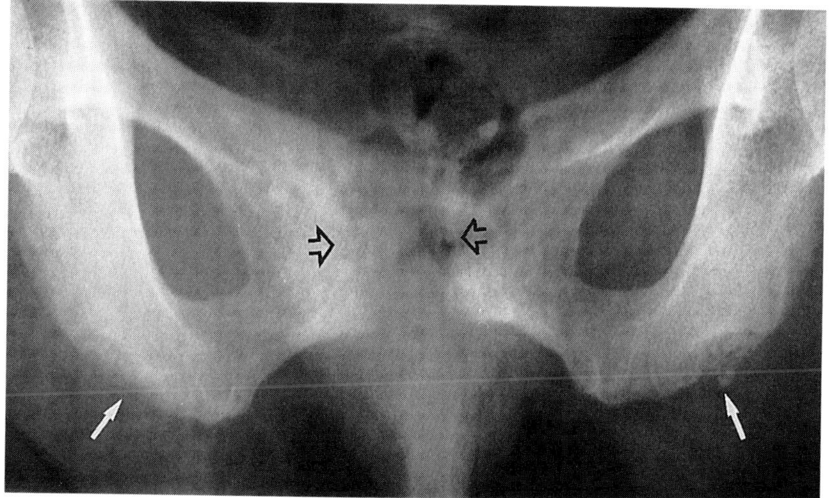

FIGURE 6–37. Renal osteodystrophy: Subchondral resorption.[43, 44] Observe the widening and indistinct margins of the subchondral bone adjacent to the symphysis pubis (open arrows) in this patient with chronic renal disease, renal osteodystrophy, and secondary hyperparathyroidism. Also evident is subtendinous resorption of the ischial tuberosities (arrows). *(Courtesy of J.T. Knudsen, D.C., Chicago, Illinois, and C. Yomtob, D.C., Los Angeles, California.)*

TABLE 6–6. Tumors and Tumor-like Lesions Affecting the Pelvis

Entity	Figure(s)	Characteristics
Malignant neoplasms		
Skeletal Metastasis[46, 47]	6–38	15 per cent of skeletal metastatic lesions affect pelvic bones
Primary Malignant Neoplasms of Bone		
Osteosarcoma[48]		7 per cent of osteosarcomas affect pelvic bones
Osteoblastoma (aggressive)[49]		13 per cent of aggressive osteoblastomas affect pelvic bones Expansile osteolytic lesion that may be partially ossified or contain calcium
Chondrosarcoma (conventional)[50, 51]	6–39	24 per cent of chondrosarcomas affect pelvic bones Peripheral chondrosarcomas arise from preexisting osteochondromas or, infrequently, as juxtacortical lesions arising from the periosteal membrane Central chondrosarcomas may contain a bulky cartilaginous cap Tend to be osteolytic lesions frequently containing calcifications Soft tissue masses common in pelvic lesions
Giant cell tumor (aggressive)[52]		Only 4 per cent of aggressive giant cell tumors involve the pelvis Eccentrically located osteolytic lesion
Fibrosarcoma[53]	6–40	10 per cent of fibrosarcomas affect the pelvic bones Purely osteolytic destruction with no associated sclerotic reaction or periostitis
Ewing's sarcoma[54]	6–41	18 per cent of Ewing's sarcomas affect the pelvic bones Aggressive permeative or moth-eaten pattern of bone destruction
Myeloproliferative Disorders		
Plasma cell (multiple) myeloma[55]	6–42	75 per cent of all patients with plasma cell myeloma have the multiple form 27 per cent of patients with myeloma have pelvic bone involvement
Solitary plasmacytoma[55]	6–43	25 per cent of all patients with plasma cell myeloma have the solitary form; 70 per cent of these eventually develop into multiple myeloma 13 per cent of solitary plasmacytomas affect the bones of the pelvis
Hodgkin's disease[56]		11 per cent of lesions in Hodgkin's disease occur in the pelvic bones
Primary lymphoma (non-Hodgkin's)[57, 58]		18 per cent of bone lesions in non-Hodgkin's lymphoma occur in the pelvic bones
Leukemia[59]	6–44	Occasional pelvic involvement
Benign neoplasms		
Primary Benign Neoplasms of Bone		
Enostosis[60]	6–45	25 per cent of enostomas occur in the pelvic bones, especially about the acetabulum
Osteoid osteoma[61]	6–46	Only 2 per cent of osteoid osteomas occur in the pelvic bones
Osteoblastoma (conventional)[62]		Rare involvement of pelvic bones (2 per cent)
Enchondroma (solitary)[51, 63]	6–47	Only 3 per cent of solitary enchondromas affect the pelvic bones
Enchondromatosis (Ollier's disease)[63]		Lesions of Ollier's disease resemble multiple enchondromas and frequently occur in the pelvis
Maffucci's syndrome[63]		More than 20 per cent of lesions in Maffucci's syndrome occur in the pelvis Multiple enchondromas and soft tissue hemangiomas
Osteochondroma (solitary)[51, 64]	6–48	Only 5 per cent of solitary osteochondromas arise from the bones of the pelvis
Hereditary multiple exostosis[51, 65]		The multiple osteochondroma-like lesions occasionally involve pelvic bones, but femoral necks are more frequently affected
Giant cell tumor (benign)[66]		Fewer than 5 per cent of benign giant cell tumors are located in the pelvic bones
Simple bone cyst[67]	6–49	2 per cent of simple bone cysts occur in the pelvis; multiloculated and eccentric
Aneurysmal bone cyst[68]	6–50	Almost 10 per cent of aneurysmal bone cysts involve the pelvic bones Eccentric, thin-walled, expansile, multiloculated osteolytic lesion

TABLE 6–6. Tumors and Tumor-like Lesions Affecting the Pelvis *Continued*

Entity	Figure(s)	Characteristics
Tumor-like lesions		
Paget's disease[69–71]	6–51, 6–52	Predilection for pelvic bones Usually polyostotic and may have unilateral involvement of one hemipelvis May result in protrusio acetabuli and osteoarthrosis of the hip
Neurofibromatosis 1 (von Recklinghausen's disease)[72]		Occasional pelvic bone involvement Dysplastic appearance with deformity and remodeling of bone and circumscribed osteolytic lesions
Monostotic fibrous dysplasia[73]	6–53A, B	Monostotic pelvic involvement rare: 7 per cent of all monostotic lesions affect the pelvis
Polyostotic fibrous dysplasia[73]	6–53C	Pelvic bone involvement is seen in 78 per cent of cases of polyostotic fibrous dysplasia Unilateral or bilateral, asymmetric involvement of the innominate bones usually associated with concomitant disease in the proximal portion of the femur Lesions contain thick rim of sclerosis surrounding a radiolucent lesion; ground-glass appearance of matrix Acetabular protrusion may occur
Langerhans' cell, histiocytosis[74, 75]	6–54	20 per cent of lesions affect the pelvic bones, most frequently eosinophilic granuloma

*See also Tables 1–10 to 1–12.

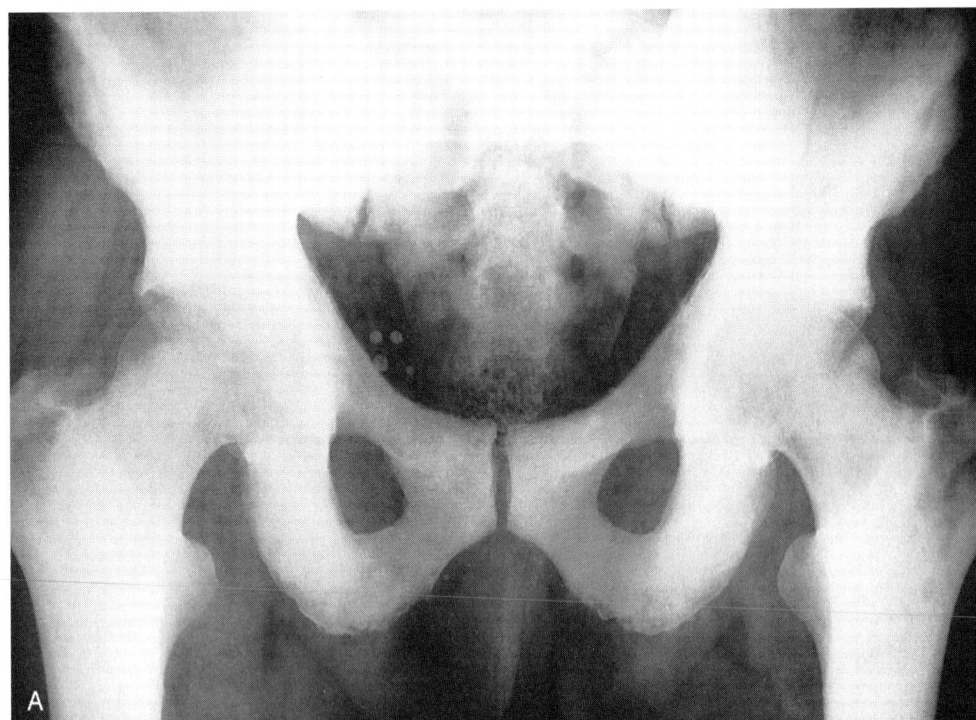

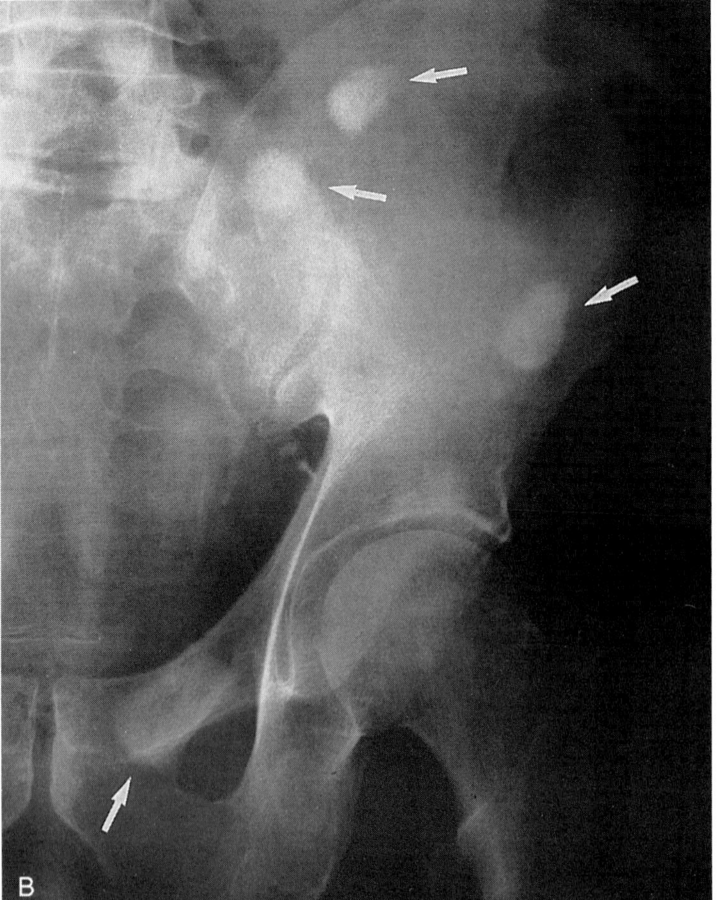

FIGURE 6–38. Skeletal metastasis: Spectrum of abnormalities.[46, 47] A Diffuse osteosclerotic pattern. Frontal pelvic radiograph of this man with prostate carcinoma shows uniform, diffuse osteosclerosis of the pelvis, sacrum, and proximal portions of the femora. B Patchy osteosclerotic pattern. In another patient with prostate carcinoma, observe the distinct, asymmetric, circular, and oval osteoblastic lesions (arrows) throughout the bones of the pelvis.

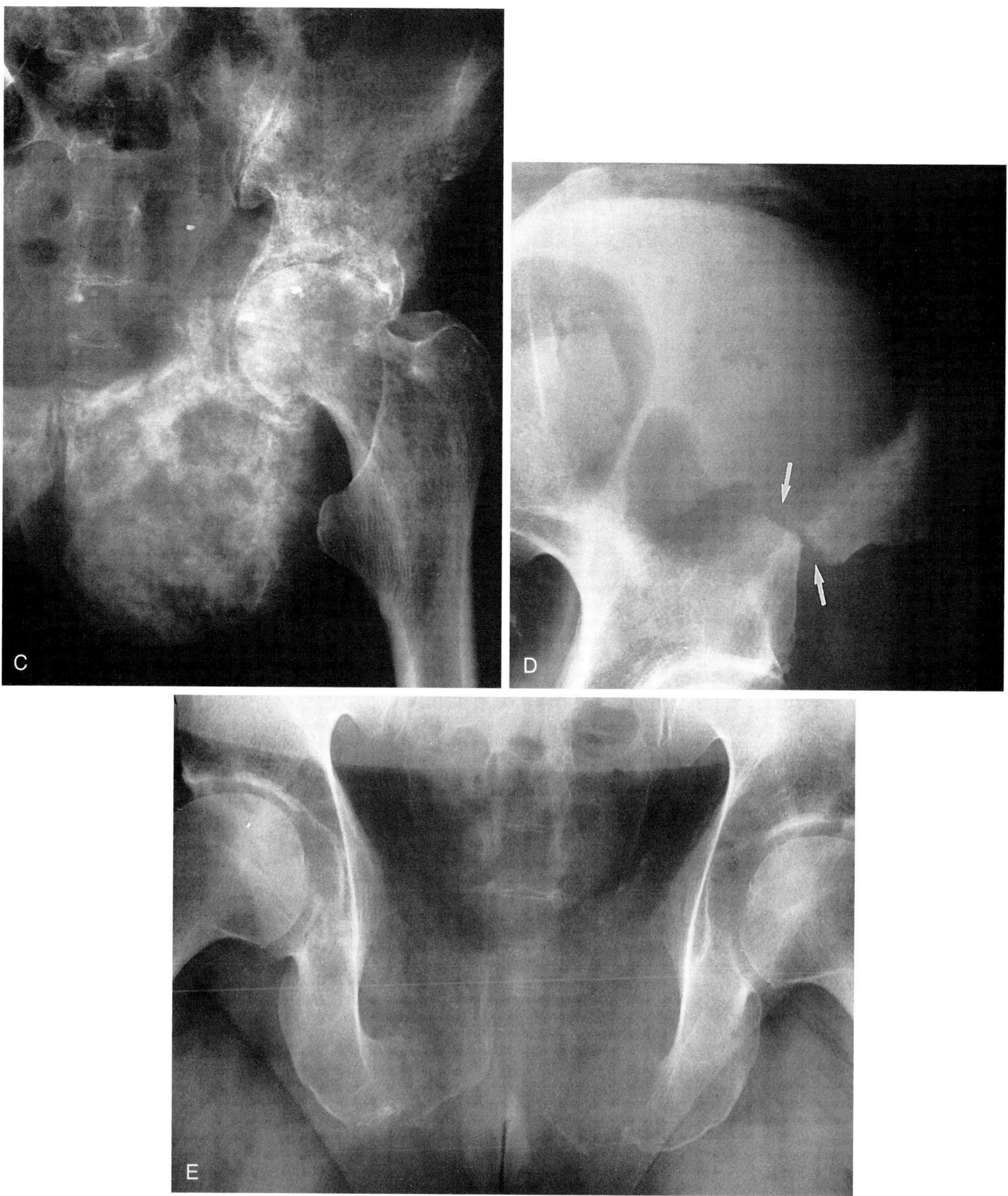

FIGURE 6–38 *Continued.* C Expansile pattern. A radiograph of the pelvis of this patient with primary bronchogenic carcinoma shows a bizarre, expansile, mixed pattern of osteolysis and osteosclerosis. The cortical margins are poorly defined, and acetabular protrusion is evident. Skeletal metastases secondary to primary carcinoma of the kidney, thyroid, and lung often exhibit a blow-out pattern of severe osteolytic destruction. D Pathologic fracture. A huge osteolytic metastatic lesion of the ilium is associated with a transverse pathologic fracture (arrows) secondary to osseous weakening. Breast metastasis is the leading cause of pathologic fracture in skeletal metastasis. E Osteolytic pattern. Widespread destruction of both pubic rami is evident in this patient with skeletal metastasis from bronchogenic carcinoma.

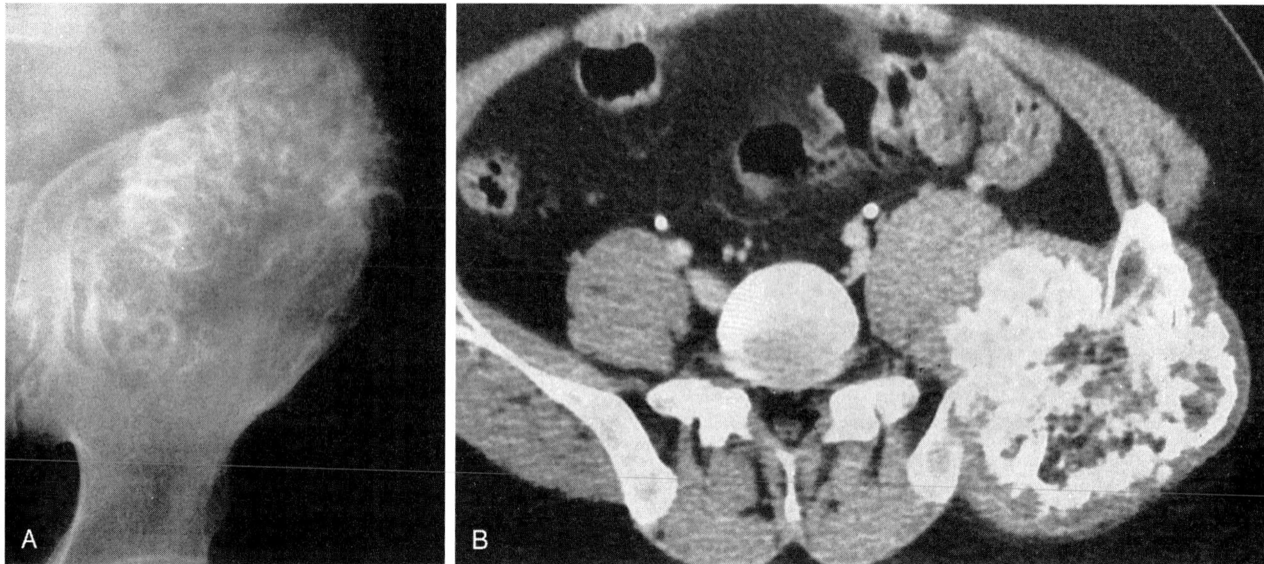

FIGURE 6–39. Chondrosarcoma.[50, 51] This 25-year-old man complained of a painful lump in the gluteal region. **A** The routine radiograph shows a bizarre, irregular, calcified excrescence resembling a cauliflower arising from the ilium. **B** Transaxial computed tomographic (CT) image depicts the lesion clearly. Observe the tumor expanding into the pelvis, displacing pelvic structures, and expanding into the buttock, displacing the gluteal musculature. These findings are visible on the CT scan but are not well seen on the radiograph. *(Courtesy of T. Mattson, M.D., Riyadh, Saudi Arabia.)*

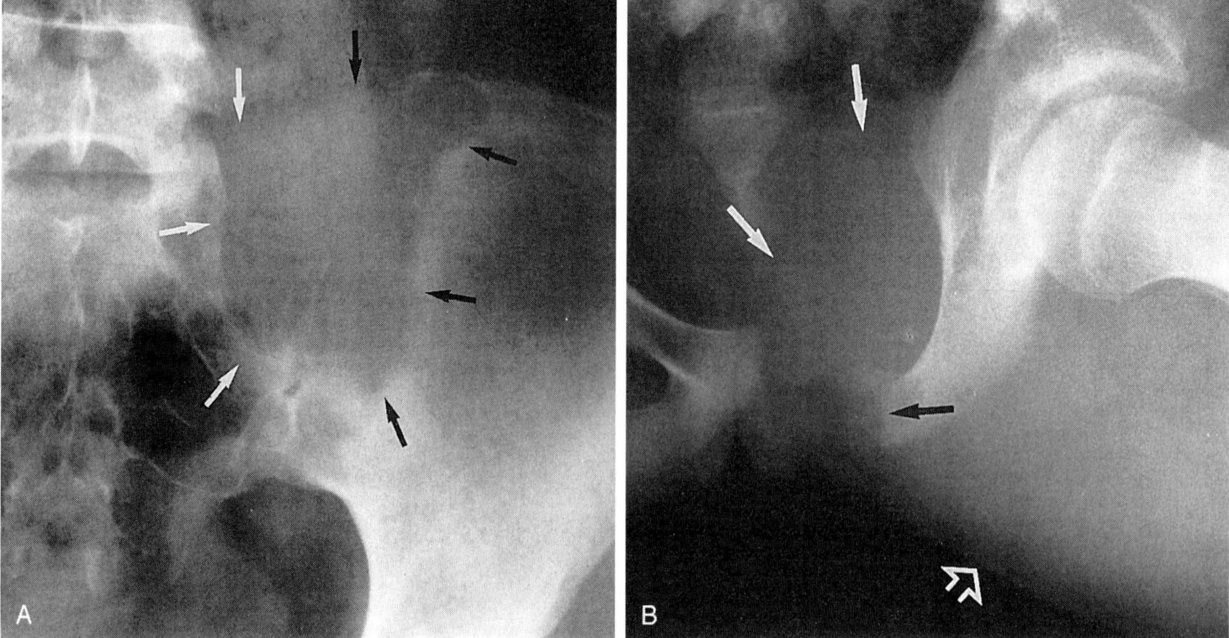

FIGURE 6–40. Fibrosarcoma.[53] **A** A purely osteolytic lesion involving both the ilium (black arrows) and the sacrum (white arrows) is seen. No reactive sclerosis is identified. **B** In a 13-year-old boy, complete osteolytic destruction of the pubic bone (arrows) is seen. No evidence of calcification or ossification is present within the lesion. Marked soft tissue swelling or a soft tissue mass is seen (open arrow). The histologic diagnosis based on biopsy results was fibrosarcoma.

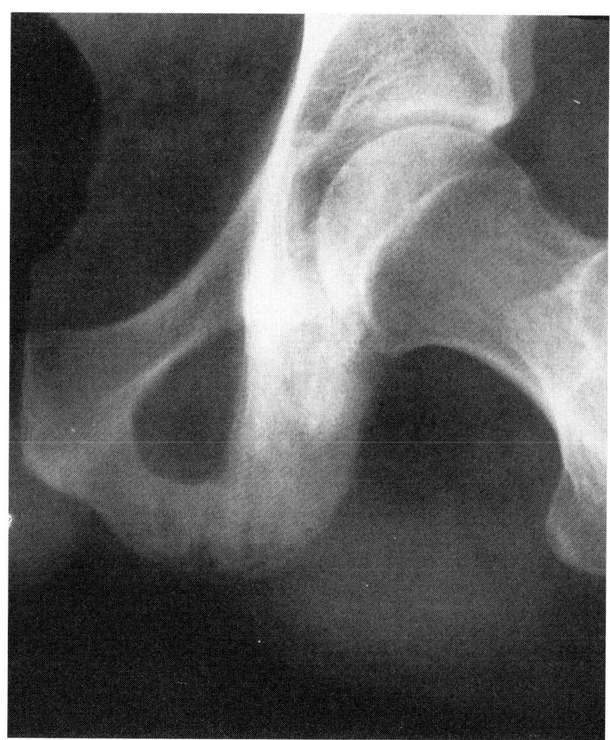

FIGURE 6–41. Ewing's sarcoma.[54] A permeative pattern of bone destruction combined with sclerosis is evident in this aggressive lesion of the ischium in a 17-year-old male patient. A laminated periosteal response is evident along the medial aspect of the ischium.

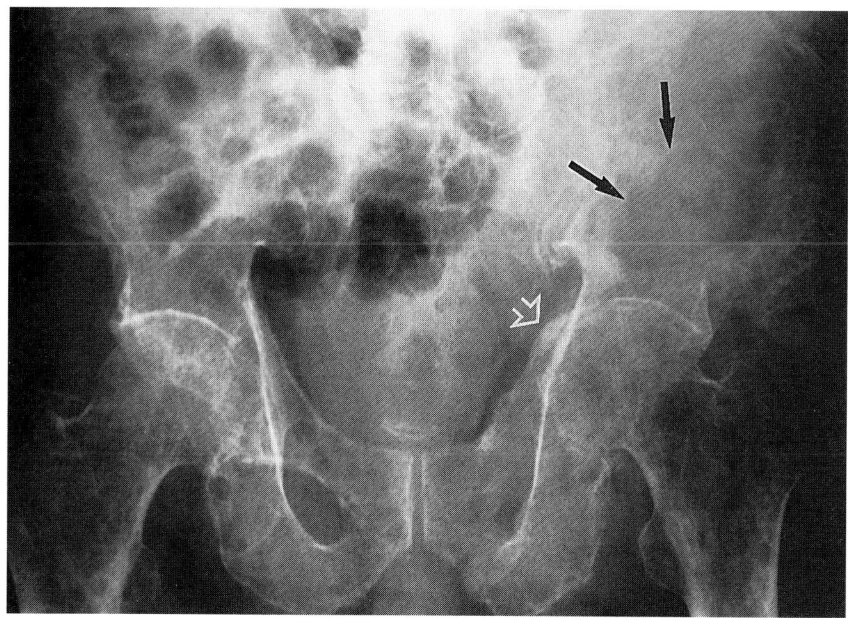

FIGURE 6–42. Plasma cell (multiple) myeloma.[55] Diffuse osteopenia and numerous osteolytic lesions permeate the bones of the pelvis and proximal femora. Pathologic collapse of the left acetabulum has resulted in acetabular protrusion (open arrow), and a large zone of osteolytic destruction is seen in the left ilium (arrows).

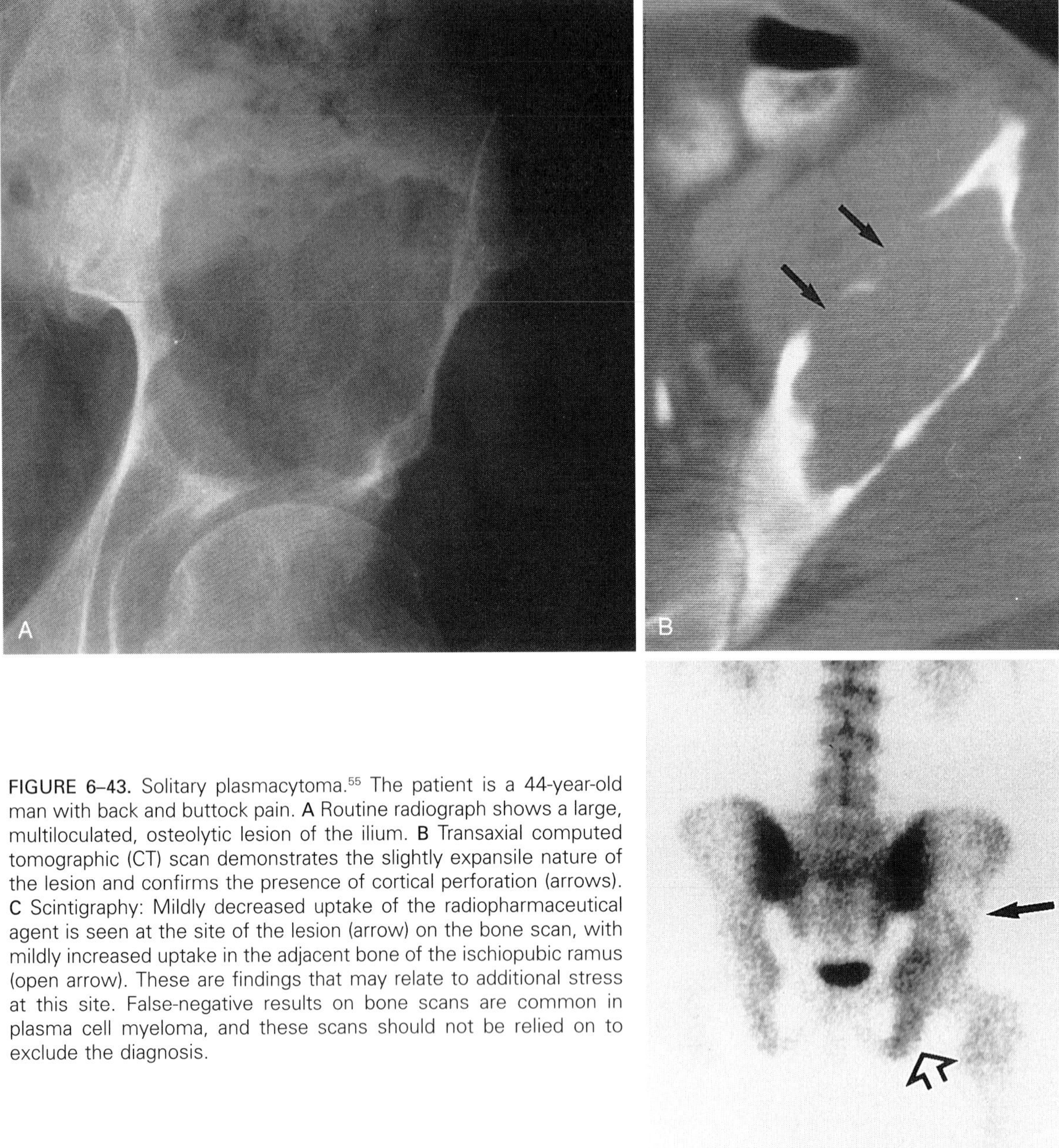

FIGURE 6–43. Solitary plasmacytoma.[55] The patient is a 44-year-old man with back and buttock pain. A Routine radiograph shows a large, multiloculated, osteolytic lesion of the ilium. B Transaxial computed tomographic (CT) scan demonstrates the slightly expansile nature of the lesion and confirms the presence of cortical perforation (arrows). C Scintigraphy: Mildly decreased uptake of the radiopharmaceutical agent is seen at the site of the lesion (arrow) on the bone scan, with mildly increased uptake in the adjacent bone of the ischiopubic ramus (open arrow). These are findings that may relate to additional stress at this site. False-negative results on bone scans are common in plasma cell myeloma, and these scans should not be relied on to exclude the diagnosis.

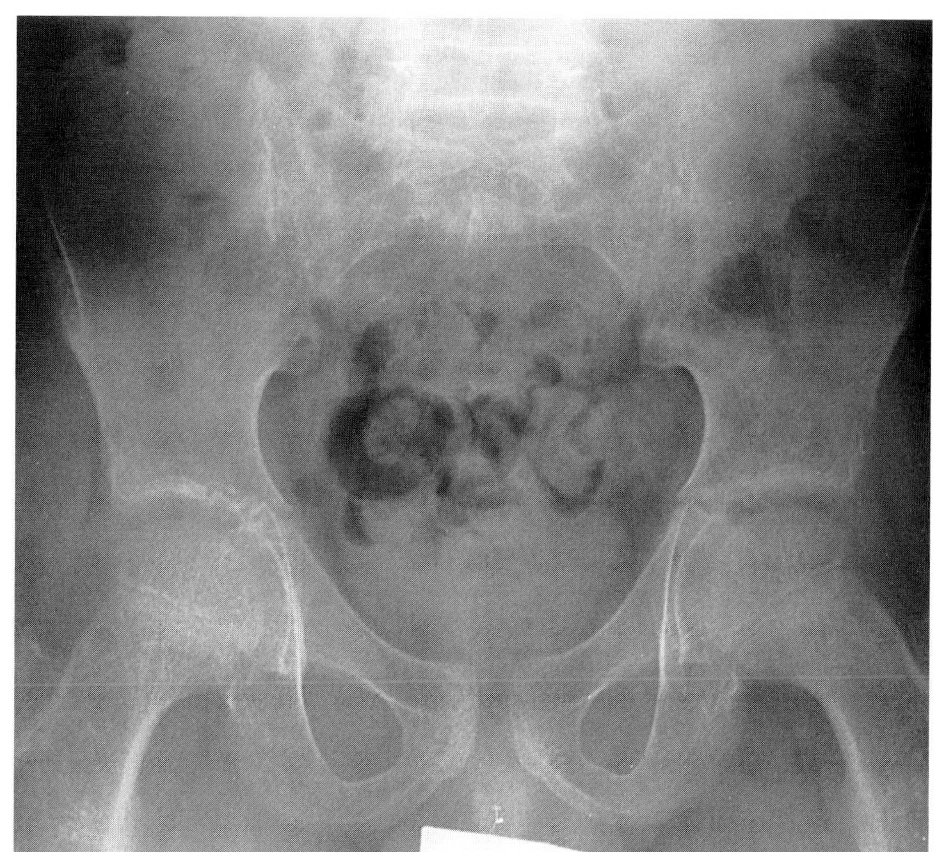

FIGURE 6–44. Acute childhood leukemia.[59] This 11-year-old boy has generalized osteopenia throughout the bones of the pelvis and proximal ends of the femora. Growth recovery lines are seen about the symphysis pubis.

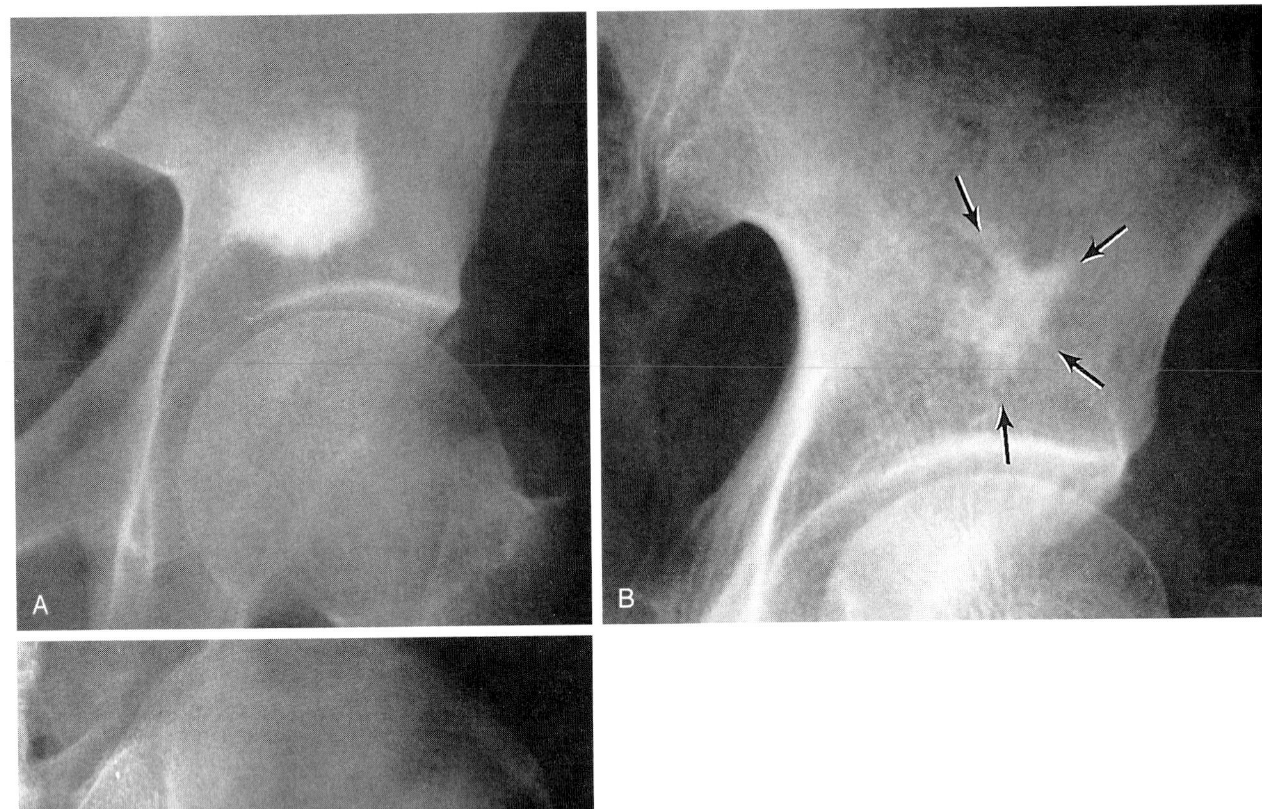

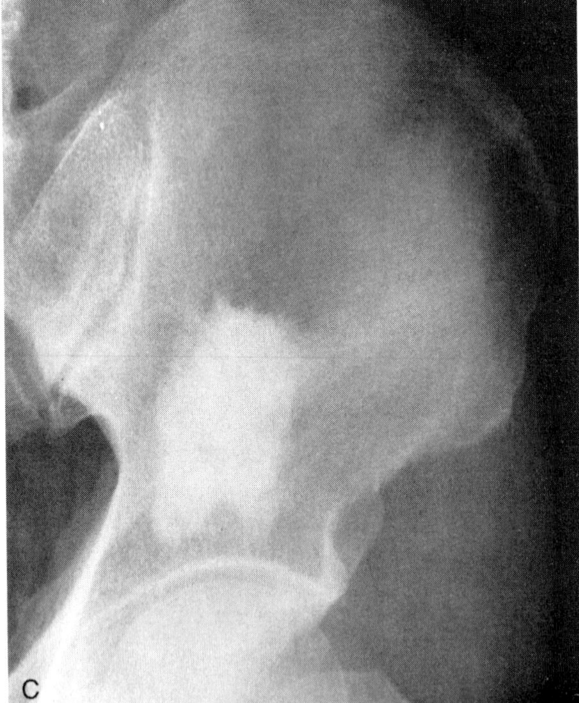

FIGURE 6–45. Enostosis (bone island).[60] **A** A large, solitary, circular, osteosclerotic lesion is located in the supra-acetabular region, a common site of bone islands. **B** This enostosis has prominent radiating spicules along its margin (arrows). **C** Giant bone island. In another patient, observe the huge osteosclerotic lesion with a spiculated margin in the supra-acetabular region. (**B**, *From Taylor JAM, Harger BL, Resnick D: Diagnostic imaging of common hip disorders: A pictorial review. Top Clin Chiropr 1:8,1994.)*

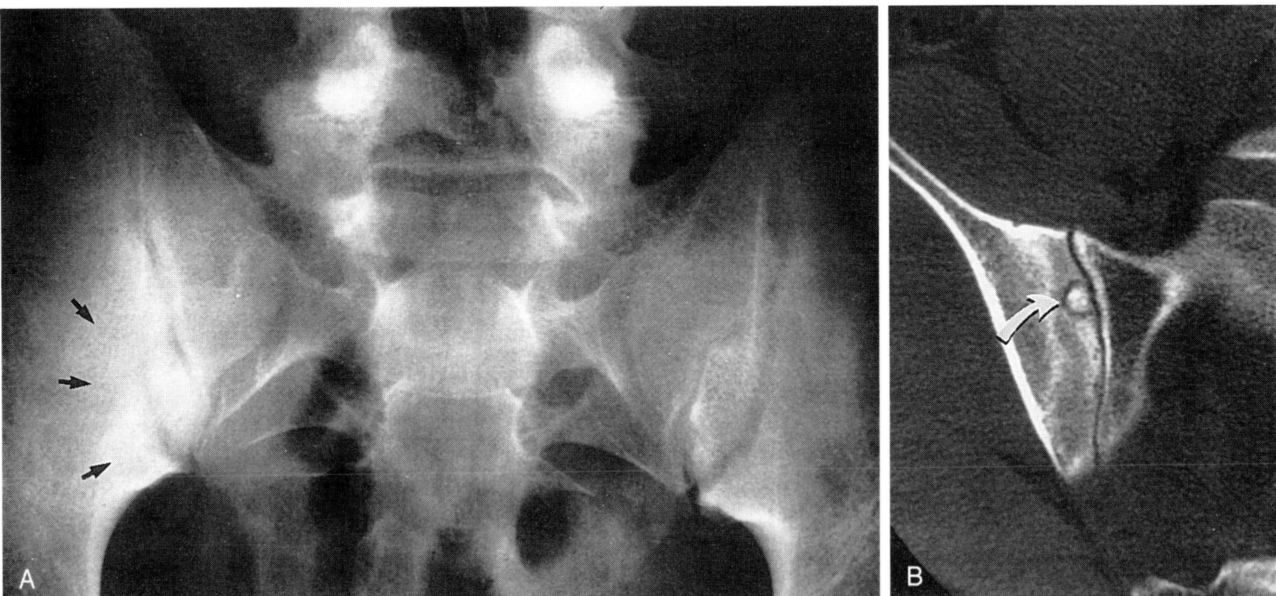

FIGURE 6–46. Osteoid osteoma.[61] **A** Frontal radiograph reveals nonspecific sclerosis of the right ilium adjacent to the sacroiliac joint (arrows). The nidus of the tumor is not visible on the plain radiograph. **B** Transaxial computed tomographic (CT) scan shows, in exquisite detail, the partially calcified nidus (curved arrow) surrounded by reactive sclerosis, a classic appearance of osteoid osteoma. *(Courtesy of A. D'Abreu, M.D., Porto Alegre, Brazil.)*

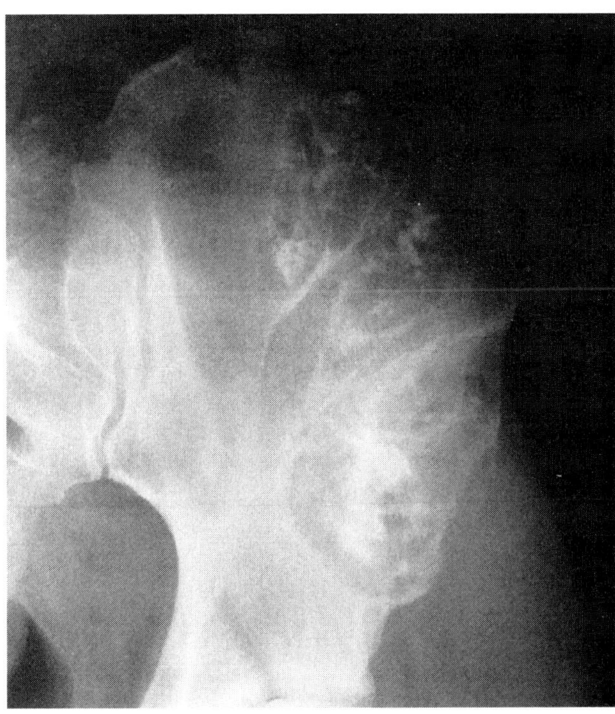

FIGURE 6–47. Enchondroma.[51, 63] In a 39-year-old woman, a large multilocular radiolucent lesion is seen. Stippled calcification within the matrix is a reliable sign of a cartilage neoplasm. *(Courtesy of R. Stonebrink, D.C., Phoenix, Arizona, and H. West, D.C., Pocatello, Idaho.)*

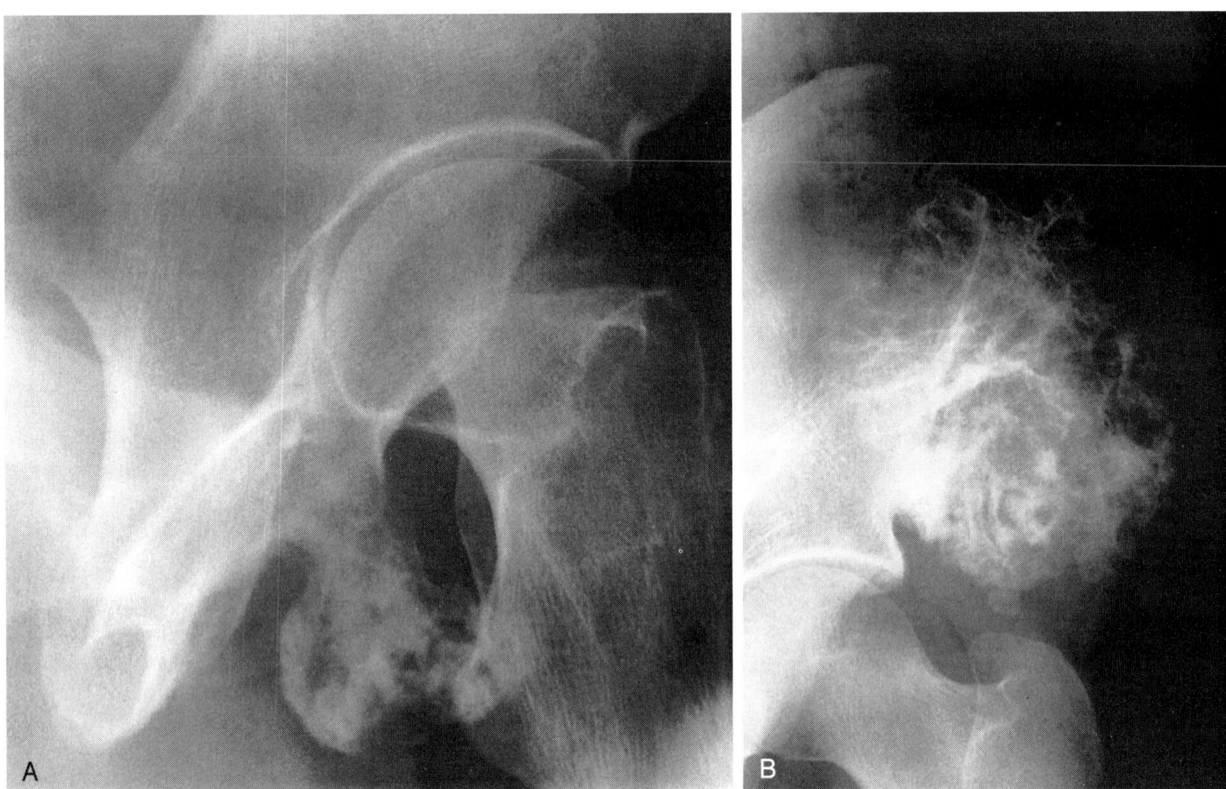

FIGURE 6–48. Solitary osteochondroma.[51, 64] A Ischium: A large pedunculated osseous outgrowth is seen arising from the ischium and projecting toward the lesser trochanter of the femur. The mass is bulbous, and the cortical margin is well defined. Small areas of radiolucency are seen within the substance of the lesion, most likely representing zones of unossified cartilage. B Ilium: Possible malignant transformation to chondrosarcoma. A cauliflower-like osseous lesion arising from the ilium appears irregular and has multiple areas of radiolucency throughout its matrix. This lesion became painful and was growing rapidly. The biopsy result was equivocal, indicating possible transformation to chondrosarcoma.

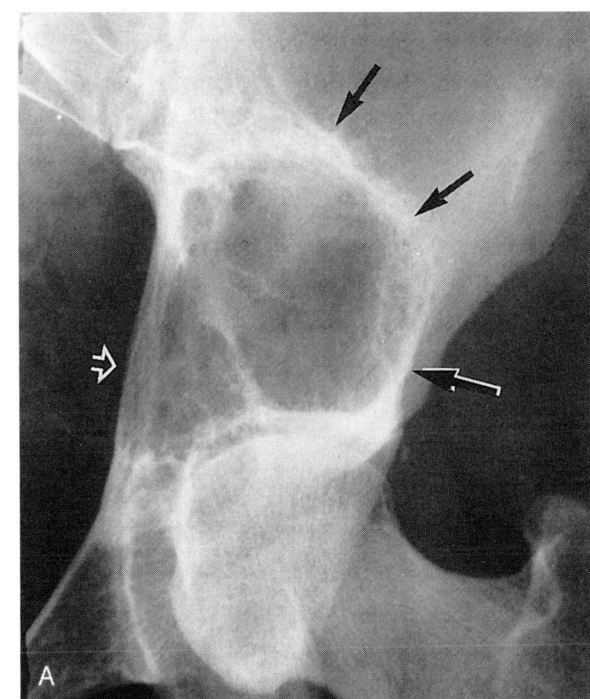

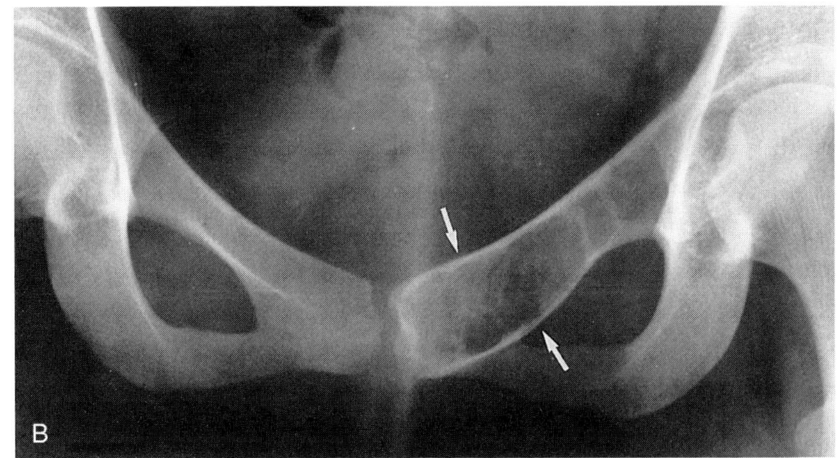

FIGURE 6–49. Simple bone cyst.[67] A This 21-year-old woman has a biopsy-proved simple bone cyst in the acetabulum, which was found incidentally on pelvic radiographs performed for trauma. Frontal radiograph reveals a geographic, radiolucent, multiloculated lesion with cortical thinning medially (open arrow) and a thin sclerotic margin surrounding its periphery (arrows). This simple bone cyst resembles fibrous dysplasia and giant cell tumor. B Simple bone cyst. Radiographs obtained from a 20-year-old woman after a fall demonstrate a radiolucent lesion within the pubic ramus. It is a centrally located, geographic, expansile, multiloculated lesion. Cortical thinning and a thin sclerotic margin (arrows) are evident. The patient had no pain over this area before the fall.

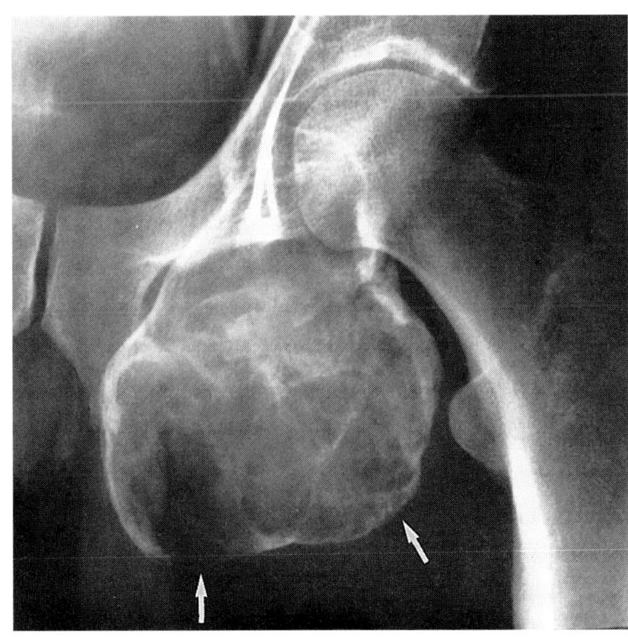

FIGURE 6–50. Aneurysmal bone cyst.[68] An expansile, multiseptated osteolytic lesion arises from the ischiopubic ramus of this 40-year-old man (arrows). The sclerotic margins are well defined. (The apparent cortical lucent shadow in the lower margin of the tumor is an artifact of photographic reproduction.) The histologic diagnosis was an aneurysmal bone cyst. *(Courtesy of R. Stiles, M.D., Atlanta, Georgia.)*

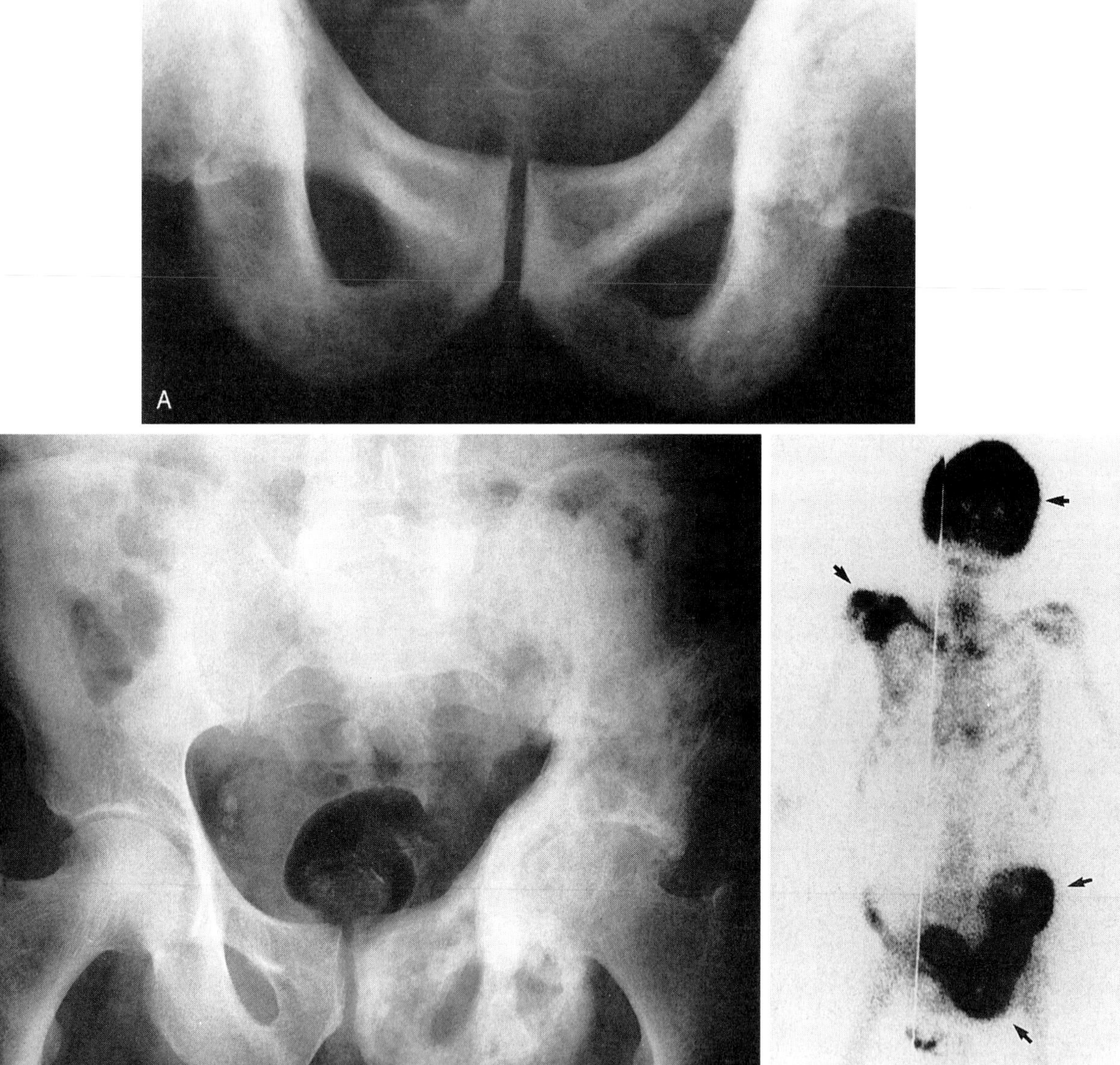

FIGURE 6–51. Paget's disease.[69, 70] A Osteosclerotic pattern. In this patient with long-standing Paget's disease, generalized osteosclerosis and trabecular thickening are evident. **B, C** Hemipelvis involvement in another patient. In **B,** diffuse osteosclerosis, trabecular and cortical bone thickening, bone enlargement, and acetabular protrusion involve only the left hemipelvis. In **C,** intense scintigraphic activity is evident in the left hemipelvis, skull, and right scapula (arrows).

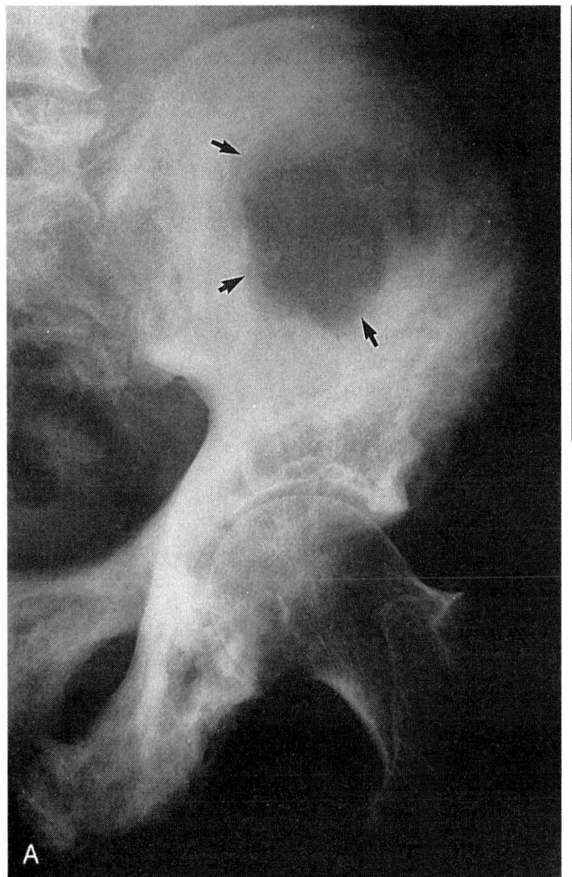

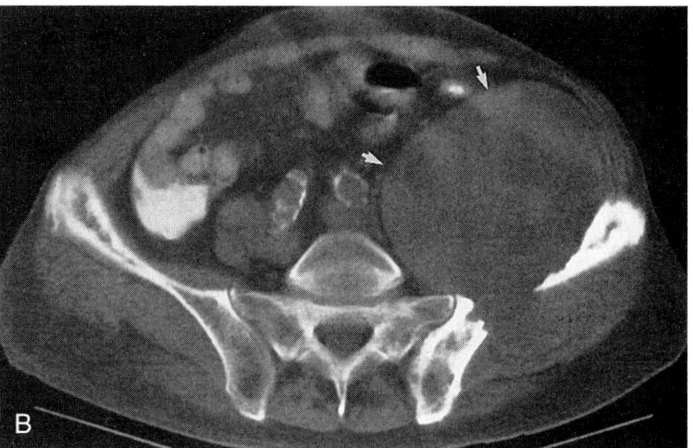

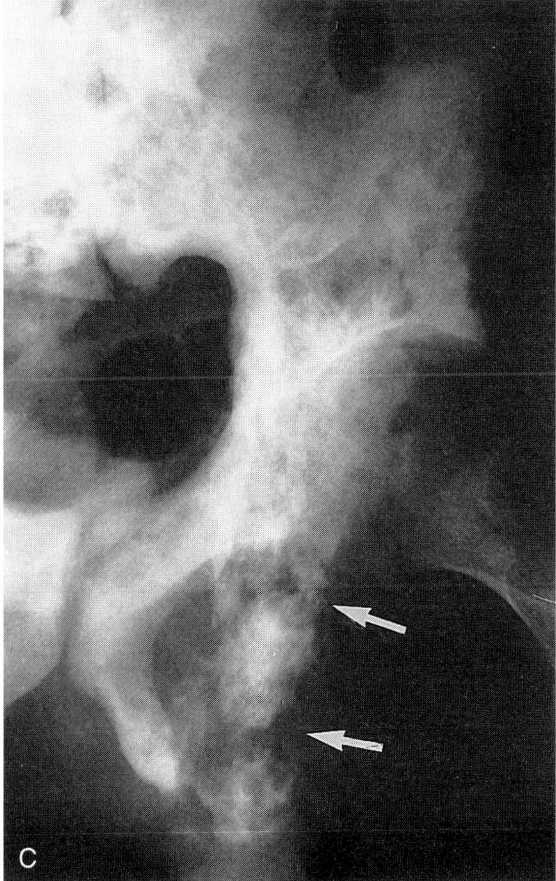

FIGURE 6–52. Paget's disease: Sarcomatous transformation.[69, 71] A Routine radiograph reveals an osteosclerotic pattern of trabecular thickening and osseous enlargement with a large osteolytic lesion in the ilium (arrows). B Transaxial computed tomographic (CT) image of the lesion displays vividly the extent of osseous destruction and a huge soft tissue mass (arrows). The lesion was biopsied, and the diagnosis was osteosarcoma within Paget's disease. *(A, B, Courtesy of P. Kaplan, M.D., Charlottesville, Virginia.)* C In another patient, extensive sarcomatous destruction of the ischium is seen at a site of previous Paget's disease (arrows).

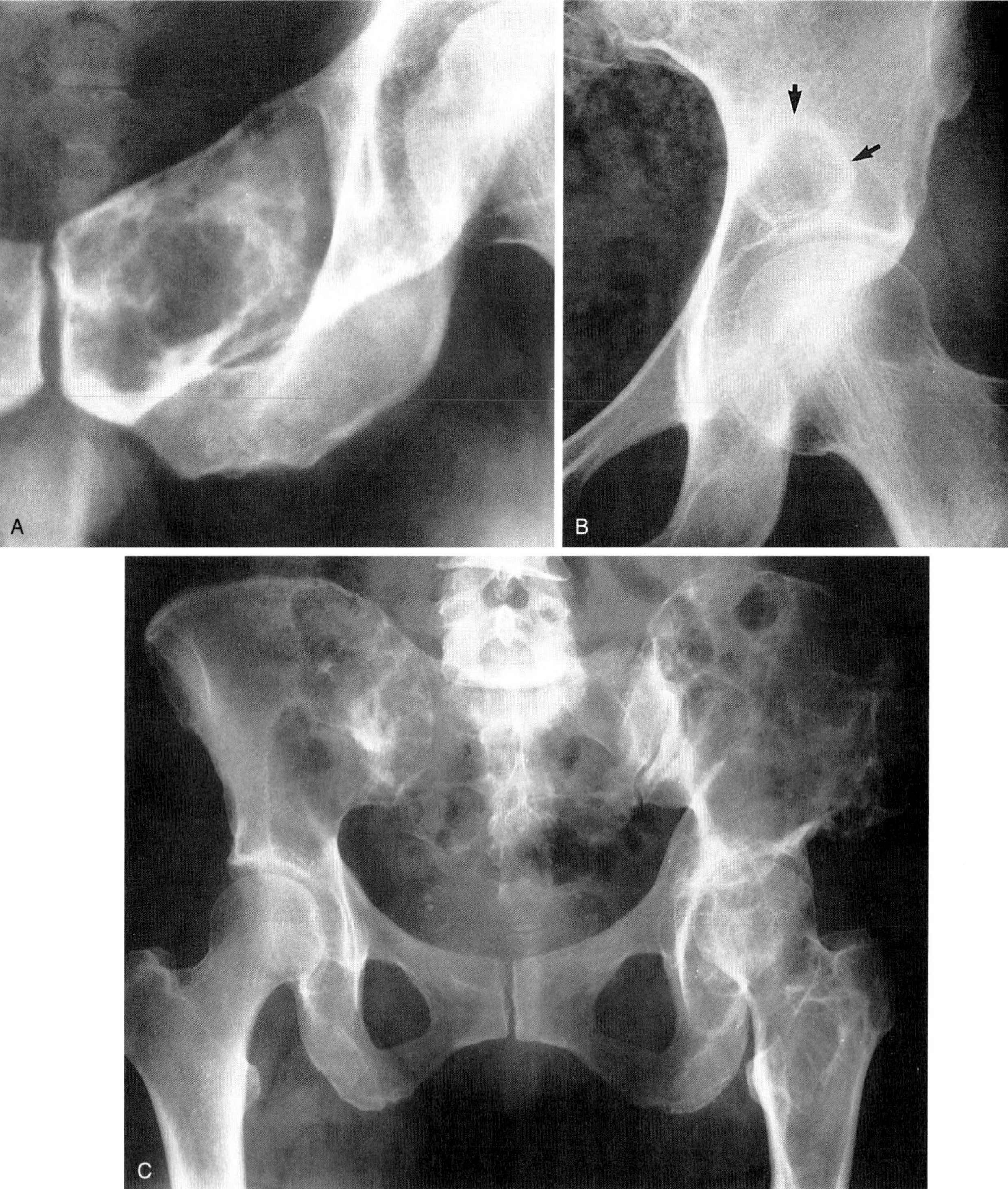

FIGURE 6–53. Fibrous dysplasia.[73] A Monostotic form. In this 54-year-old man, an expansile, multiloculated lesion in the pubic ramus demonstrates the characteristic ground-glass appearance of fibrous dysplasia. B This 49-year-old woman with monostotic fibrous dysplasia has a well-defined supra-acetabular lesion with a sclerotic margin (arrows). *(B, Courtesy of G. Greenway, M.D., Dallas, Texas.)* C Polyostotic form: Pelvis and femur. Observe the multiloculated, osteolytic, slightly expansile lesions throughout the pelvis and left femur of this 55-year-old woman. The lesions are surrounded by continuous curvilinear sclerotic margins, and the tumor matrix appears smoky or hazy, a finding termed the ground-glass appearance.

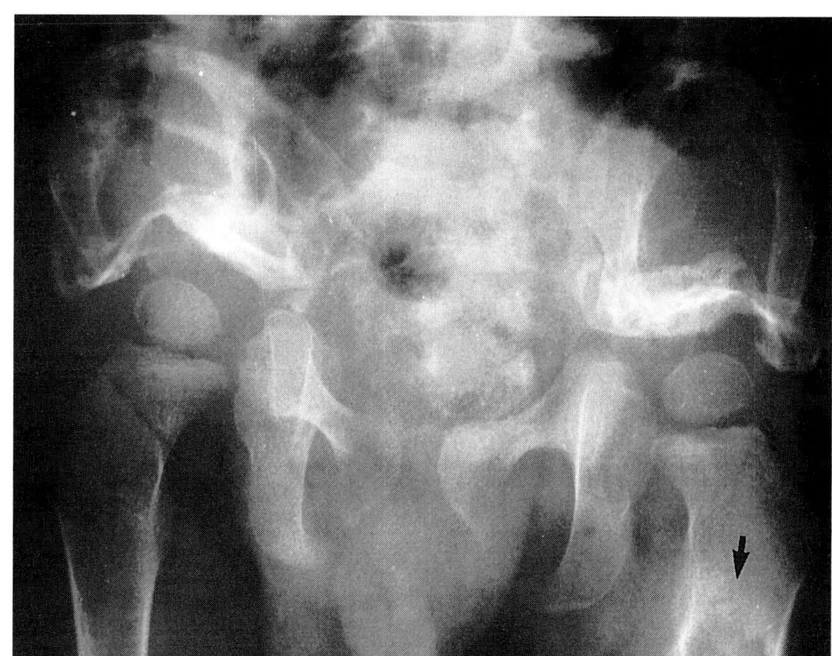

FIGURE 6–54. Langerhans' cell histiocytosis: Eosinophilic granuloma.[74, 75] Observe the large osteolytic lesions involving both innominate bones and proximal portion of the femur (arrow). Prominent acetabular remodeling and collapse also are evident.

TABLE 6–7. Metabolic, Hematologic, and Infectious Disorders Affecting the Pelvis*

Entity	Figure(s)	Characteristics
Generalized osteoporosis[76]		Uniform decrease in radiodensity, thinning of cortices, accentuation of weight-bearing trabeculae May result in parasymphyseal and supra-acetabular insufficiency fractures
Osteomalacia[77]	6–55	Diminished radiodensity and prominent coarsened trabeculae Transverse "pseudofractures" common in osteomalacia
Hyperparathyroidism and renal osteodystrophy[78]	6–56	Brown tumor (osteoclastoma): solitary or multiple expansile osteolytic lesions containing fibrous tissue and giant cells; may disappear after treatment for hyperparathyroidism Subchondral resorption about symphysis pubis and sacroiliac joints
Hypoparathyroidism[79]	6–57	Prominent enthesopathy and bone proliferation arising from pelvic bones: resembles changes of diffuse idiopathic skeletal hyperostosis (DISH) Osteosclerosis (as many as 23 per cent of patients) Painless subcutaneous calcification
Mastocytosis[80]	6–58	Resembles lymphoma and leukemia; combinations of diffuse or focal osteosclerosis or, less likely, osteopenia or osteolysis
Sickle cell anemia[81, 82]	6–59	Diffuse osteopenia or osteosclerosis and osteonecrosis
β-thalassemia[82]	6–60	Diffuse osteopenia with lace-like trabecular pattern Marrow hyperplasia, growth disturbances, fractures, crystal deposition, extramedullary hematopoiesis
Hemophilia[83, 84]	6–61	Hemophilic pseudotumor: geographic osteolytic lesions with internal trabeculation and multiloculated appearance
Osteomyelitis[85]	6–62	Poorly defined permeative bone destruction Periostitis; usually single layer or solid
Poliomyelitis[86]	6–63	Bone atrophy results in asymmetric hypoplasia and osteopenia of the hemipelvis and femur May result in scoliosis and mechanical disorders of the spine and lower extremity
Radiation changes[87, 88]	6–64	*Adults* Insufficiency fractures, osteomyelitis, bone infarcts, and radiation-induced neoplasms: osteosarcoma, malignant fibrous histiocytoma, chondrosarcoma *Children* Asymmetric hypoplasia of the pelvis and spine with scoliosis, and radiation-induced neoplasms: osteochondroma (common), enchondroma (rare), and osteoblastoma

*See also Tables 1–13, 1–14, and 1–17.

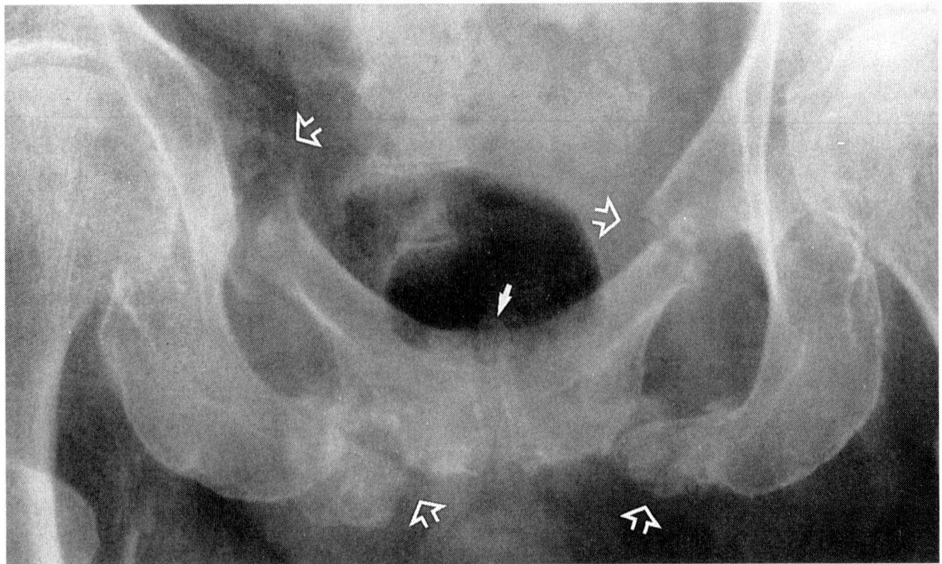

FIGURE 6–55. Osteomalacia.[77] Bilateral insufficiency fractures of the superior and inferior pubic rami (open arrows) are seen in this 85-year-old woman. The fractures occurred several months earlier, and healing appears to be delayed, with evidence of osteolysis and incomplete callus formation. Chondrocalcinosis of the symphysis pubis (arrow), related to calcium pyrophosphate dihydrate (CPPD) crystal deposition, also is evident.

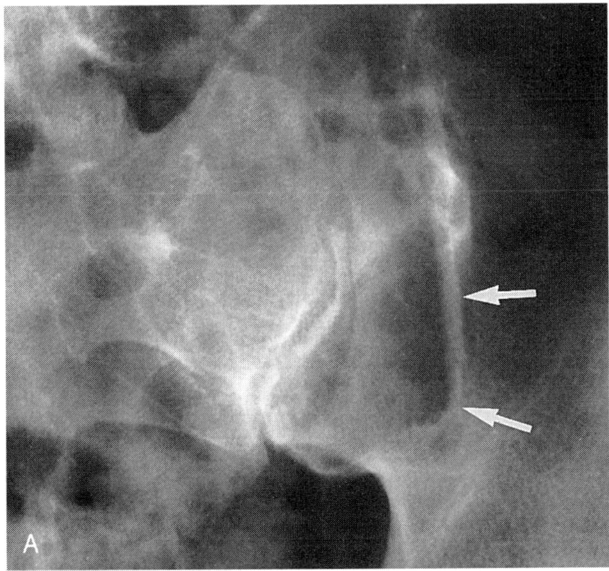

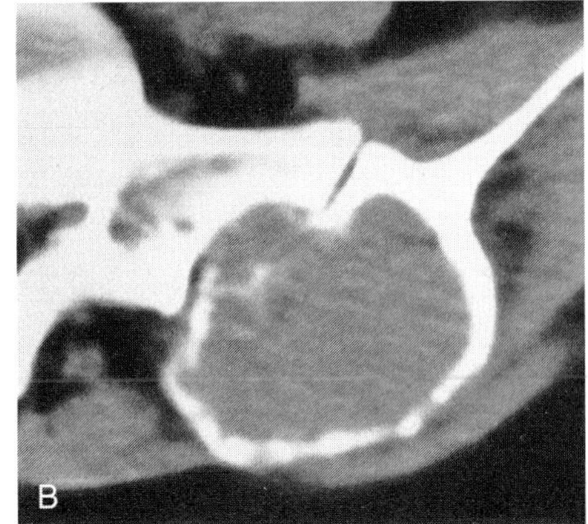

FIGURE 6–56. Renal osteodystrophy: Hyperparathyroidism with brown tumors.[78] **A** Routine radiograph shows an expansile osteolytic lesion with a thick sclerotic margin (arrows) in the subchondral region of the ilium adjacent to the sacroiliac joint. **B** Computed tomographic (CT) scan taken with a transaxial soft tissue window clearly displays the expansile nature of this lesion with a well-corticated margin. *(Courtesy of A. Newberg, M.D., Boston, Massachusetts.)*

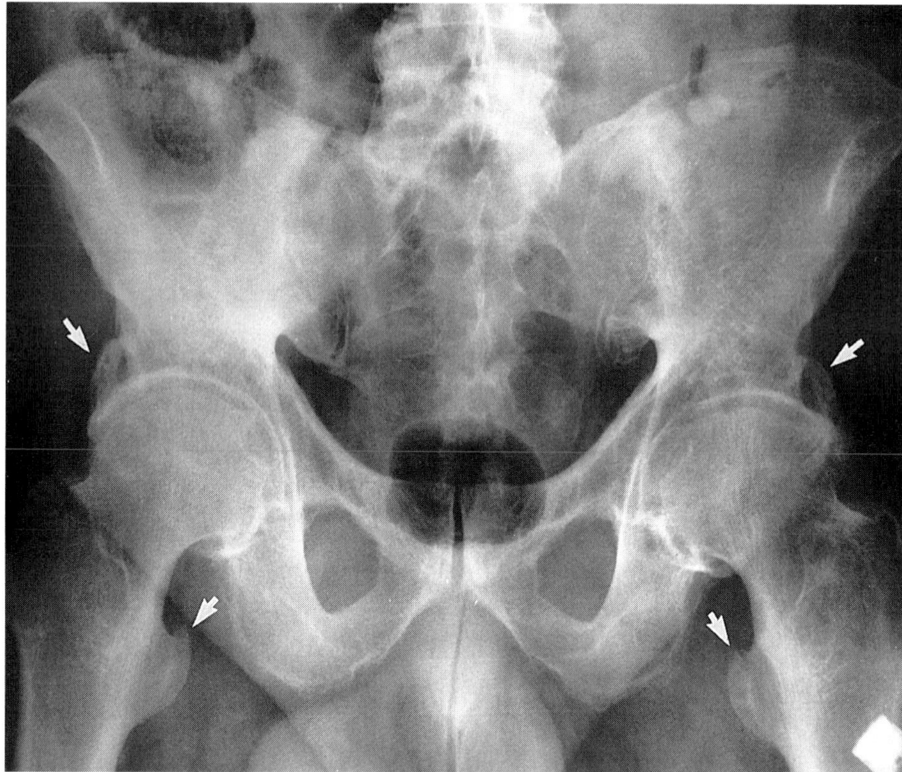

FIGURE 6–57. Hypoparathyroidism: Enthesopathy.[79] Observe the bone proliferation adjacent to the acetabulum and other surfaces of the pelvic bones (arrows) in this 49-year-old man. These changes resemble those of diffuse idiopathic skeletal hyperostosis (DISH). *(Courtesy of V. Wing, M.D., Walnut Creek, California.)*

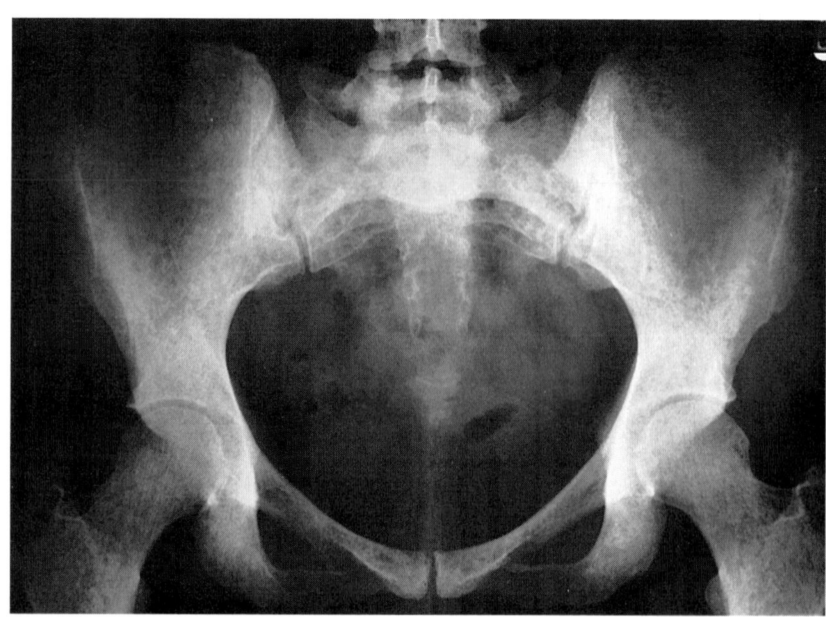

FIGURE 6–58. Mastocytosis.[80] Observe the widespread, patchy osteosclerosis throughout the pelvic bones of this 38-year-old woman. *(Courtesy of B. Holtan, M.D., Rock Springs, Wyoming.)*

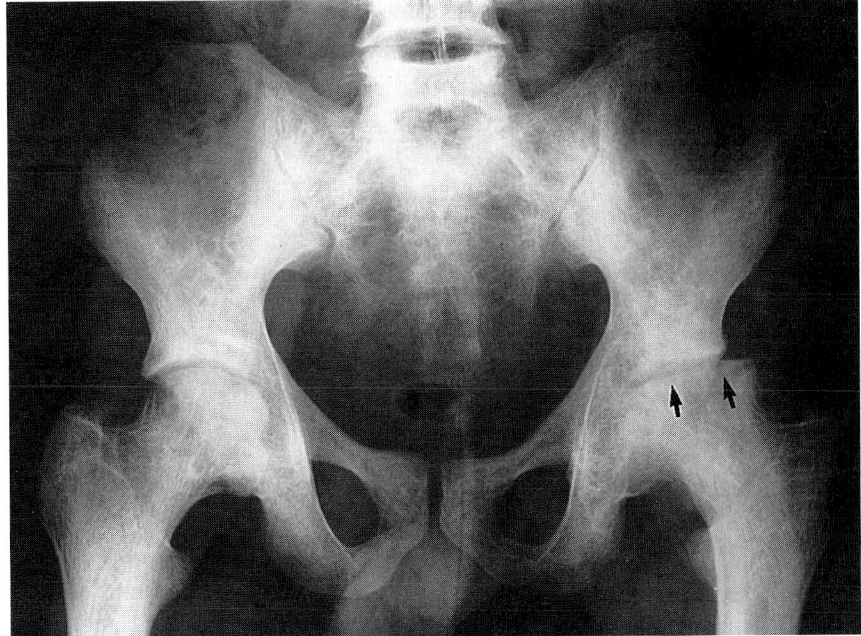

FIGURE 6–59. Sickle cell–hemoglobin C disease.[81] In this 24-year-old man, the bones are sclerotic, the trabeculae are coarsened, and the femoral heads are osteonecrotic. The left femoral head is significantly collapsed (arrows). Note deformity of the lower lumbar vertebral bodies.

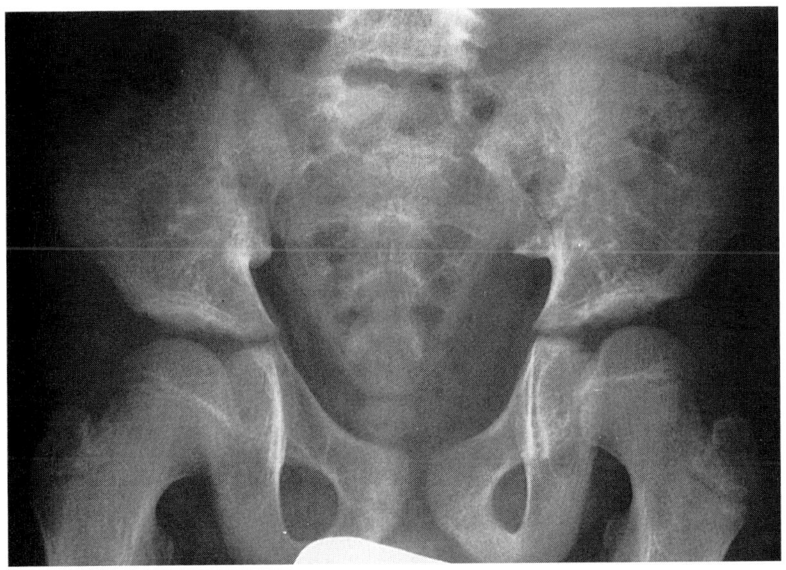

FIGURE 6–60. β-thalassemia.[82] Observe the lacy trabecular pattern, osteoporosis, and extreme thinning of cortical bone in the pelvis of this 11-year-old girl with thalassemia.

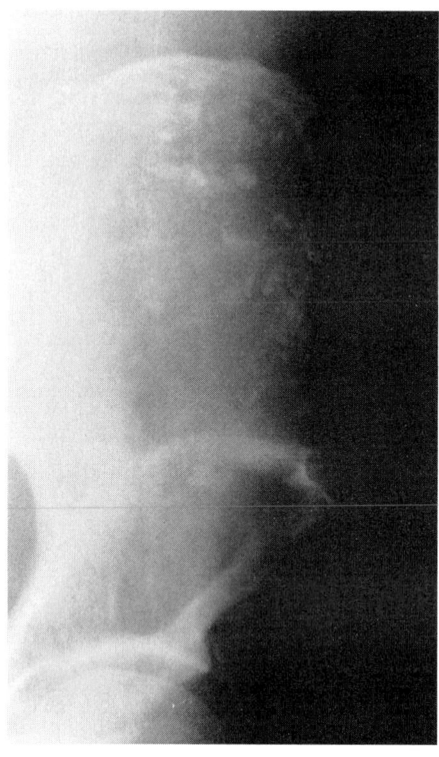

FIGURE 6–61. Hemophilia: Pseudotumor.[83, 84] A large, slightly expansile, osteolytic lesion located in the ilium is seen in this 37-year-old man with long-standing hemophilia. Osseous debris is present within the matrix of the lesion. The hemophilic pseudotumor results from intraosseous or subperiosteal hemorrhage.

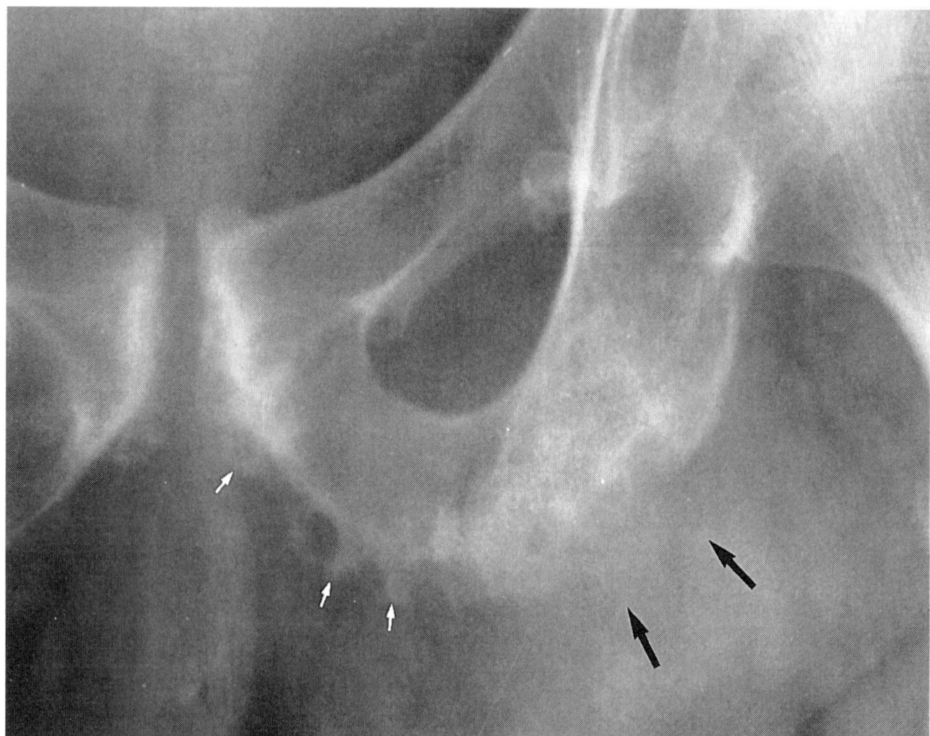

FIGURE 6–62. Osteomyelitis: Actinomycosis.[85] This 72-year-old man has a sinus draining to his buttock. Diffuse soft tissue swelling and a large erosion of the ischial tuberosity are seen. Osseous outgrowths arising from the pubic bone (small arrows) probably represent degenerative enthesopathy. Actinomycosis is a noncontagious suppurative infection that is caused by anaerobic organisms normally found in the mouth.

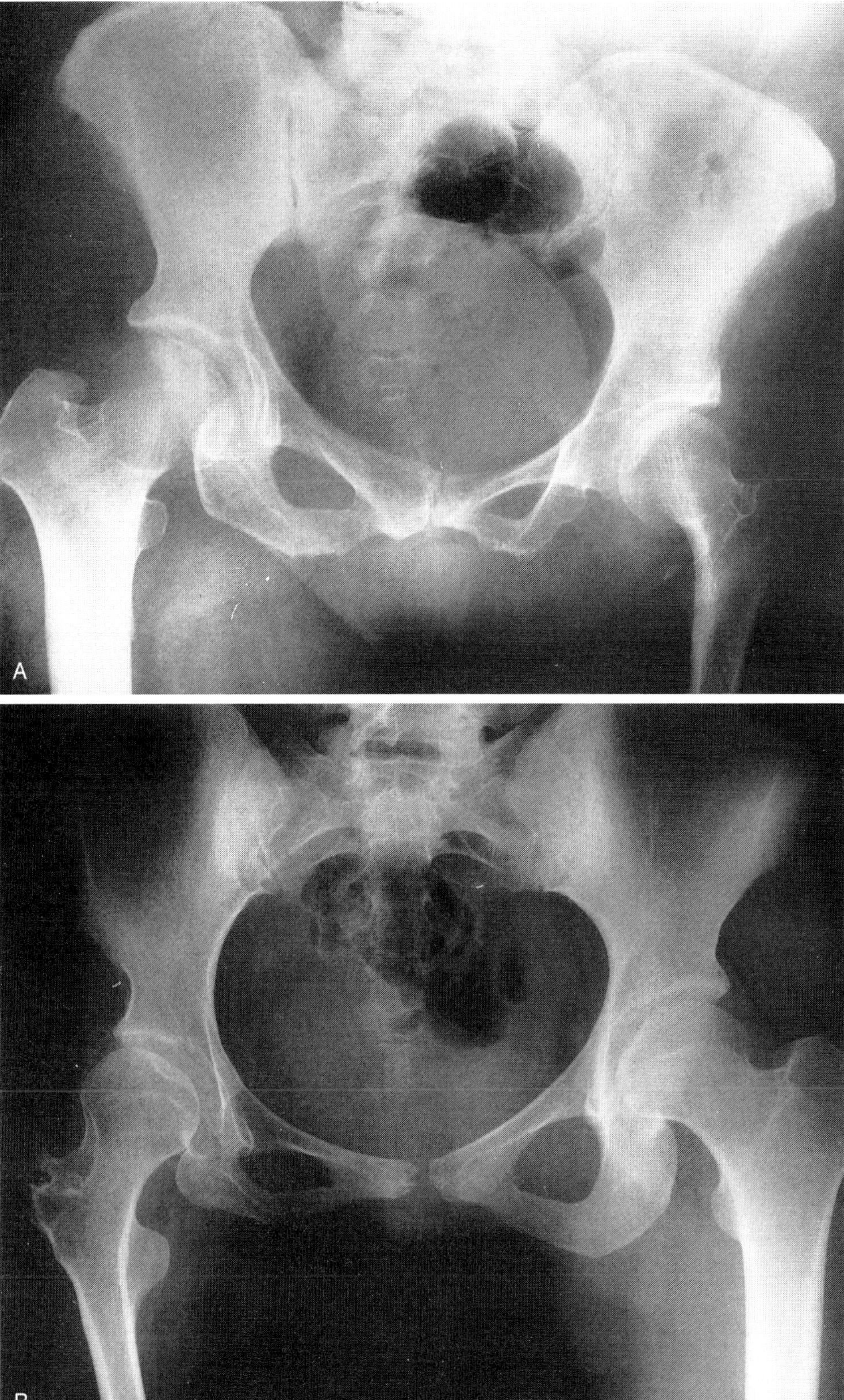

FIGURE 6–63. Poliomyelitis: Bone atrophy.[86] A Observe the coxa valga deformity as well as hypoplasia and osteopenia of the left hemipelvis, sacrum, and proximal portion of the femur in this 53-year-old woman with poliomyelitis. B In another patient, right-sided atrophy of the hemipelvis and proximal portion of the femur are associated with unilateral osteopenia.

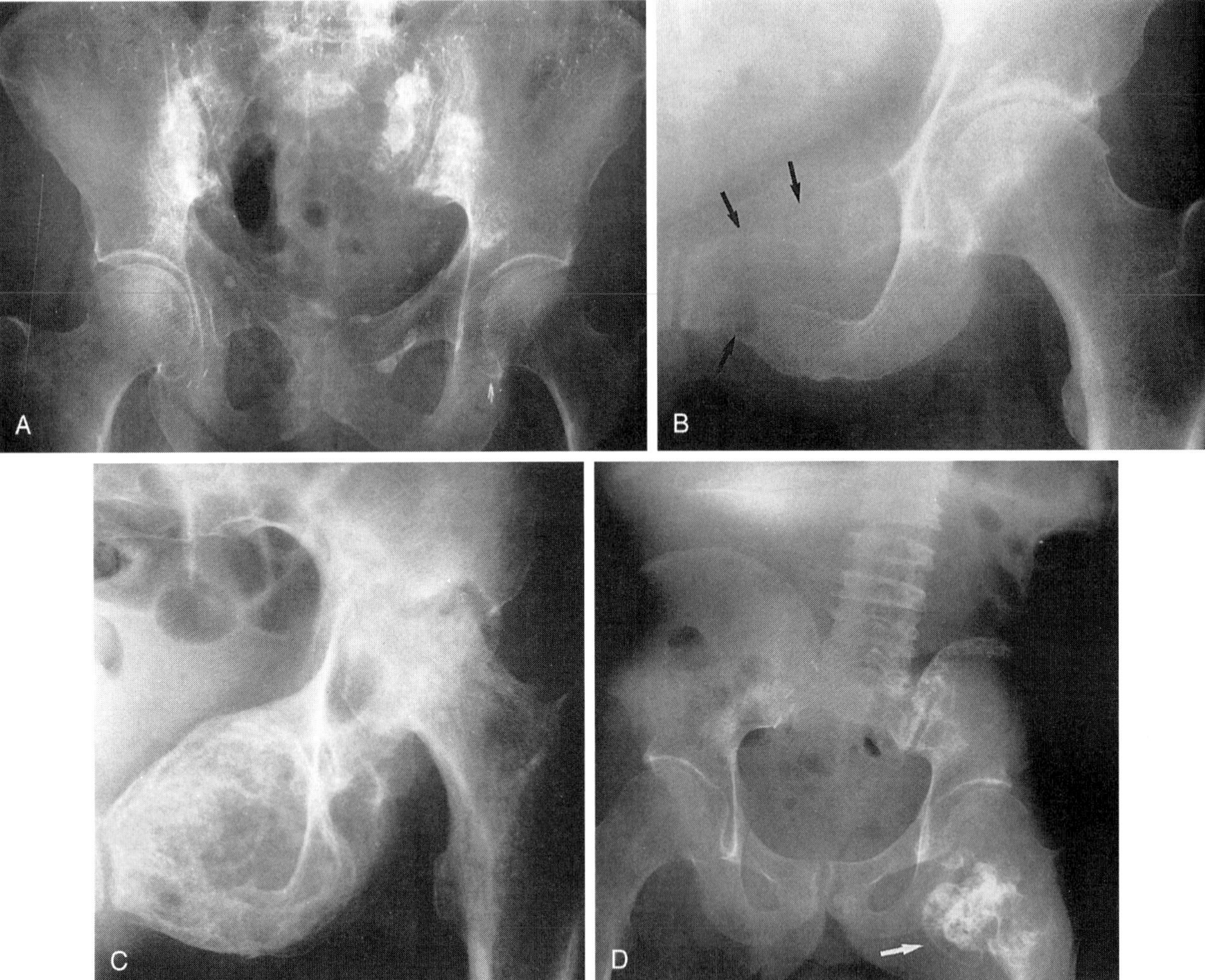

FIGURE 6–64. Radiation changes.[87, 88] A Insufficiency fractures. This 80-year-old woman underwent radiation therapy for carcinoma of the uterine cervix. Observe the multiple osteosclerotic insufficiency fractures involving the sacrum, ilia, and parasymphyseal region. Differentiation among radiation changes, skeletal metastasis, and chondrosarcoma may be difficult in such cases. B, C 55-year-old woman with endometrial carcinoma. In B, a frontal pelvic radiograph shows osteolytic metastasis involving the left pubic ramus (arrows). In C, another radiograph taken 30 months after a course of radiation therapy shows osteonecrosis of the femoral head and acetabulum. Mature ossification of the ischiopubic ramus is indicative of healing. (B, C, *Courtesy of H. Kroon, M.D., Leiden, Netherlands.*) D Effects on the immature skeleton. This young patient underwent radiation therapy for Wilms' tumor. Observe the radiation-induced osteochondroma arising from the femur (arrow), playtspondyly, and unilateral hypoplasia of the left innominate bone.

REFERENCES

1. Edeiken J, Dalinka M, Karasick D: Edeiken's Roentgen Diagnosis of Diseases of Bone. 4th Ed. Baltimore, Williams & Wilkins, 1990.
2. Keats TE, Smith TH: An Atlas of Normal Developmental Roentgen Anatomy. 2nd Ed. Chicago, Year Book, 1988.
3. Greenfield GB: Radiology of Bone Diseases. 2nd Ed. Philadelphia, JB Lippincott, 1975.
4. Köhler A, Zimmer EA: Borderlands of Normal and Early Pathologic Findings in Skeletal Radiography. 4th Ed. New York, Thieme Medical Publishers, 1993.
5. Risser JC: The iliac apophysis: An invaluable sign in the management of scoliosis. Clin Orthop 175:111, 1958.
6. Keats TE: Atlas of Normal Roentgen Variants That May Simulate Disease, 6th Ed. Chicago, Year Book Medical Publishers, 1996.
7. Greenspan A, Norman A: The "pelvic digit"—an unusual developmental anomaly. Skeletal Radiol 9:118, 1982.
8. Yochum TR, Rowe LJ: Essentials of Skeletal Radiology. 2nd Ed. Baltimore, Williams & Wilkins, 1996.
9. Langer LO, Baumann PA, Gorlin RJ: Achondroplasia. AJR 100:12, 1967.
10. Diamond LS, Lynne D, Sigman B: Orthopedic disorders in patients with Down's syndrome. Orthop Clin North Am 12:57, 1981.
11. Kovanlikaya A, Loro ML, Gilsanz V: Pathogenesis of osteosclerosis in autosomal dominant osteopetrosis. AJR 168:929, 1997.
12. Benli IT, Akalin S, Boysan E, et al: Epidemiological, clinical, and radiological aspects of osteopoikilosis. J Bone Joint Surg [Br] 74:504, 1992.
13. Watts RWE, Spellacy E, Kendall BE, et al: Computed tomography studies on patients with mucopolysaccharidosis. Neuroradiology 21:9, 1981.
14. Root L: The treatment of osteogenesis imperfecta. Orthop Clin North Am 15:775, 1984.
15. Jarvis JL, Keats TE: Cleidocranial dysostosis: A review of 40 cases. AJR 121:5, 1974.
16. Guidera KJ, Satterwhite Y, Ogden JA, et al: Nail-patella syndrome: A review of 44 orthopaedic patients. J Pediatr Orthop 11:737, 1991.
17. Sundar M, Carty H: Avulsion fractures of the pelvis in children: A report of 32 fractures and their outcome. Skeletal Radiol 23:85, 1994.
18. Kane WJ: Fractures of the pelvis. *In* CA Rockwood Jr, DP Green (eds): Fractures in Adults. 2nd Ed. Philadelphia, JB Lippincott, 1984.
19. Montana MA, Richardson ML, Kilcoyne RF, et al: CT of sacral injury. Radiology 161:499, 1986.
20. Mumber MP, Greven KM, Miner Haygood T: Pelvic insufficiency fractures associated with radiation atrophy: Clinical recognition and diagnostic evaluation. Skeletal Radiol 26:94, 1997.
21. Hosono M, et al: MR appearance of parasymphyseal insufficiency fractures of the os pubis. Skeletal Radiol 26:525, 1997.
22. Mammone JF, Schweitzer ME: MRI of occult sacral insufficiency fractures following radiotherapy. Skeletal Radiol 24:101, 1995.
23. Berg PM: Acute pelvic disruption, the bucking horse injury. Orthop Trans 3:271, 1979.
24. Failinger MS, McGanity PLJ: Unstable fractures of the pelvic ring. J Bone Joint Surg [Am] 74:781, 1992.
25. Dalal SA, Burgess AR, Siegel JH, et al: Pelvic fracture in multiple trauma: Classification by mechanism is key to pattern of organ injury, resuscitative requirements, and outcome. J Trauma 29:981, 1989.
26. Gill K, Bucholz RW: The role of computerized tomographic scanning in the evaluation of major pelvic fractures. J Bone Joint Surg [Am] 66:34, 1984.
27. Potok PS, Hopper KD, Umlauf MJ: Fractures of the acetabulum: Imaging, classification, and understanding. RadioGraphics 15:7, 1995.
28. Brandser E, Marsh JL: Acetabular fractures: Easier classification with a systematic approach. AJR 171:1217, 1998.
29. Pavlov H, Nelson TL, Warren RF, et al: Stress fractures of the pubic ramus: A report of twelve cases. J Bone Joint Surg [Am] 64:1020, 1982.
30. Otte MT, Helms CA, Fritz RC: MR imaging of supra-acetabular insufficiency fractures. Skeletal Radiol 26:279, 1997.
31. Haller J, Resnick D, Miller CW, et al: Diffuse idiopathic skeletal hyperostosis: Diagnostic significance of radiographic abnormalities of the pelvis. Radiology 172:835, 1989.
32. Prescher A, Bohndorf K: Anatomical and radiological observations concerning ossification of the sacrotuberous ligament: Is there a relation to spinal diffuse idiopathic skeletal hyperostosis (DISH)? Skeletal Radiol 22:581, 1993.
33. Resnick D, Shaul SR, Robins JM: Diffuse idiopathic skeletal hyperostosis (DISH): Forestier's disease with extraspinal manifestations. Radiology 115:513, 1975.
34. Coventry MB, Mitchell WC: Osteitis pubis: Observations based on a study of 45 patients. JAMA 178:898, 1961.
35. Fricker PA, Taunton JE, Ammann W: Osteitis pubis in athletes: Infection, inflammation or injury? Sports Med 12:266, 1991.
36. Kormano M: Symphysial changes in rheumatoid arthritis. Scand J Rheumatol 4:17, 1975.
37. Scott DL, Eastmond CJ, Wright V: A comparative radiological study of the pubic symphysis in rheumatic disorders. Ann Rheum Dis 38:529, 1979.
38. Resnick D: Dermatomyositis and polymyositis. *In* Diagnosis of Bone and Joint Disorders. 3rd Ed. Philadelphia, WB Saunders, 1995, p 1218.
39. Resnick D, Niwayama G, Georgen TG, et al: Clinical, radiographic, and pathologic abnormalities in calcium pyrophosphate dihydrate deposition disease (CPPD): Pseudogout. Radiology 122:1, 1977.
40. Steinbach LS, Resnick D: Calcium pyrophosphate dihydrate crystal deposition disease revisited. Radiology 200:1, 1996.
41. Faraawi R, Harth M, Kertesz A, et al: Arthritis in hemochromatosis. J Rheumatol 20:448, 1993.
42. Justesen P, Andersen PE Jr: Radiologic manifestations in alkaptonuria. Skeletal Radiol 11:204, 1984.
43. Sundaram M: Renal osteodystrophy. Skeletal Radiol 18:415, 1989.
44. Murphy MD, Sartoris DJ, Quale JL, et al: Musculoskeletal manifestations of chronic renal insufficiency. RadioGraphics 13:357, 1993.
45. Bouza E, Winston DJ, Hewitt WL: Infectious osteitis pubis. Urology 12:663, 1978.
46. Habermann ET, Lopez RA: Metastatic disease of bone and treatment of pathologic fractures. Orthop Clin North Am 20:469, 1989.
47. Wong DA, Fornasier VL, MacNab I: Spinal metastases: The obvious, the occult, and the impostors. Spine 15:1, 1990.
48. Dahlin DC, Unni KK: Osteosarcoma of bone and its important recognizable varieties. Am J Surg Pathol 1:61, 1977.
49. Mitchell M, Ackerman LV: Metastatic and pseudomalig-

nant osteoblastoma: A report of two unusual cases. Skeletal Radiol 15:213, 1986.
50. Henderson ED, Dahlin DC: Chondrosarcoma of bone—a study of two hundred and eighty-eight cases. J Bone Joint Surg [Am] 45:1450, 1963.
51. Brien EW, Mirra JM, Kerr R: Benign and malignant cartilage tumors of bone and joint: Their anatomic and theoretical basis with an emphasis on radiology, pathology and clinical biology. 1. The intramedullary cartilage tumors. Skeletal Radiol 26:325, 1997.
52. Eckardt JJ, Grogan TJ: Giant cell tumor of bone. Clin Orthop 204:45, 1986.
53. Huvos AG, Higinbotham NL: Primary fibrosarcoma of bone: A clinicopathologic study of 130 patients. Cancer 35:837, 1975.
54. Dahlin DC, Coventry MB, Scanlon PW: Ewing's sarcoma: A critical analysis of 165 cases. J Bone Joint Surg [Am] 43:185, 1961.
55. Kyle RA: Multiple myeloma: Review of 869 cases. Mayo Clin Proc 50:29, 1975.
56. Franczyk J, Samuels T, Rubenstein J, et al: Skeletal lymphoma. J Can Assoc Radiol 40:75, 1989.
57. Hermann G, Klein MJ, Fikry Abedlewahab I, et al: MRI appearance of primary non-Hodgkin's lymphoma of bone. Skeletal Radiol 26:629, 1997.
58. Clayton F, Butler JJ, Ayala AG, et al: Non-Hodgkin's lymphoma in bone: Pathologic, and radiologic features with clinical correlates. Cancer 60:2494, 1987.
59. Benz G, Brandeis WE, Willich E: Radiological aspects of leukemia in childhood: An analysis of 89 children. Pediatr Radiol 4:201, 1976.
60. Greenspan A: Bone island (enostosis): Current concept—a review. Skeletal Radiol 24:111, 1995.
61. Cohen MD, Harrington TM, Ginsbury WW: Osteoid osteoma: 95 cases and a review of the literature. Semin Arthritis Rheum 12:265, 1983.
62. Kroon HM, Schurmans J: Osteoblastoma: Clinical and radiologic findings in 98 new cases. Radiology 175:783, 1990.
63. Schiller AL: Diagnosis of borderline cartilage lesions of bone. Semin Diagn Pathol 2:42, 1985.
64. Karasick D, Schweitzer ME, Eschelman DJ: Symptomatic osteochondromas: Imaging features. AJR 168:1507, 1997.
65. Shapiro F, Simon S, Glimcher MJ: Hereditary multiple exostoses: Anthropometric, roentgenographic, and clinical aspects. J Bone Joint Surg [Am] 61:815, 1979.
66. Sanjay BKS, Frassica FJ, Frassica DA, et al: Treatment of giant-cell tumor of the pelvis. J Bone Joint Surg [Am] 75:1466, 1993.
67. Chigira M, Maehara S, Arita S, et al: The aetiology and treatment of simple bone cysts. J Bone Joint Surg [Br] 65:633, 1983.
68. De Dios AMV, Bond JR, Shives TC, et al: Aneurysmal bone cyst: A clinico-pathologic study of 238 cases. Cancer 69:2921, 1992.
69. Matfin G. McPherson F: Paget's disease of bone: Recent advances. J Orthop Rheumatol 6:127, 1993.
70. Mirra JM, Brien EW, Tehranzadeh J: Paget's disease of bone: Review with emphasis on radiologic features, part II. Skeletal Radiol 24:173, 1995.
71. Moore TE, King AR, Kathol MH, et al: Sarcoma in Paget disease of bone: Clinical, radiologic, and pathologic features in 22 cases. AJR 156:1199, 1991.
72. Crawford AH Jr, Bogamery N: Osseous manifestations of neurofibromatosis in childhood. J Pediatr Orthop 6:72, 1986.
73. Gibson MJ, Middlemiss JH: Fibrous dysplasia of bone. Br J Radiol 44:1, 1971.
74. Kilpatrick SE, Wenger DE, Gilchrist GS, et al: Langerhans' cell histiocytosis (histiocytosis X) of bone: A clinicopathologic analysis of 263 pediatric and adult cases. Cancer 76:2471, 1995.
75. Stull MA, Kransdorf MJ, Devaney KO: Langerhans cell histiocytosis of bone. RadioGraphics 12:801, 1992.
76. Taylor JAM, Resnick D, Sartoris J. Osteoporosis: radiologic-pathologic correlation. *In* Sartoris J (Ed): Osteoporosis: Current and Future Concepts. New York, Marcel Dekker, 1996.
77. Mankin HJ: Rickets, osteomalacia, and renal osteodystrophy. Orthop Clin North Am 21:81, 1990.
78. Chew FS, Huang-Hellinger F: Brown tumor. AJR 160:752, 1993.
79. Bronsky D, Kushner DS, Dubin A, et al: Idiopathic hypoparathyroidism and pseudohypoparathyroidism: Case reports and review of the literature. Medicine 37:317, 1958.
80. De Gennes C, Kuntz D, De Vernejoul MC: Bone mastocytosis: A report of nine cases with a bone histomorphometric study. Clin Orthop 279:281, 1992.
81. Barton CJ, Cockshott WP: Bone changes in hemoglobin SC disease. AJR 88:523, 1962.
82. Resnick D: Hemoglobinopathies and other anemias. *In* Resnick D: Diagnosis of Bone and Joint Disorders. 3rd Ed. Philadelphia, WB Saunders, 1995, p 2128.
83. Jaovisidha S, Nam Ryu K, Hodler J, et al: Hemophilic pseudotumor: Spectrum of MR findings. Skeletal Radiol 26:468, 1997.
84. Wilson DA, Prince JR: MR imaging of hemophilic pseudotumors. AJR 150:349, 1988.
85. Marcus NA, Grace TG, Hodgin UG: Osteomyelitis of the sacrum and sepsis of the hip complicating pelvic actinomycosis. Orthopedics 4:645, 1981.
86. Hancock DA, Reed GW, Atkinson PJ: Bone and soft tissue changes in paraplegic patients. Paraplegia 17:267, 1979–1980.
87. Butler MS, Robertson WW Jr, Rate W, et al: Skeletal sequelae of radiation therapy for malignant childhood tumors. Clin Orthop 251:235, 1990.
88. Blomlie V, Rofstad EK, Talle K, et al: Incidence of radiation-induced insufficiency fractures of the female pelvis: Evaluation with MR imaging. AJR 167:1205, 1996.

CHAPTER 7

Hip

- Normal Developmental Anatomy
- Developmental Anomalies, Anatomic Variants, and Sources of Diagnostic Error
- Hip Deformities
- Developmental Dysplasia of the Hip
- Physical Injury
- Articular Disorders
- Metabolic Disorders
- Osteonecrosis of the Femoral Head

Normal Developmental Anatomy

Accurate interpretation of radiographs of the pediatric hip requires a thorough understanding of normal developmental anatomy. Table 7–1 outlines the age of appearance and fusion of the primary and secondary ossification centers. Figures 7–1 and 7–2 demonstrate the radiographic appearance of many important ossification centers and other developmental landmarks at selected ages from birth to skeletal maturity.

Developmental Anomalies, Anatomic Variants, and Sources of Diagnostic Error

The hip joint and proximal portion of the femur are sites of anomalies, anatomic variations, and other sources of diagnostic error that may simulate disease and potentially result in misdiagnosis. Table 7–2 and Figures 7–3 to 7–5 represent selected examples of some of the more common processes.

Hip Deformities

The proximal portion of the femur and the acetabulum are frequent sites for deformities such as coxa vara, coxa valga, and acetabular protrusion. Table 7–3 lists the major causes of such deformities. Figures 7–6 to 7–8 illustrate some selected examples of these deformities. Other examples are displayed throughout the chapter as they are manifested in several other diseases.

Developmental Dysplasia of the Hip

Developmental dysplasia of the hip and associated instability, subluxation, and dislocation are important pediatric disorders that are described in Table 7–4. Some of the more useful radiographic measurements and their normal values are listed in Table 7–5. Figures 7–9 to 7–13 illustrate the imaging manifestations and radiographic measurements of developmental dysplasia.

Physical Injury

Physical injury to the hip region may result in a wide variety of fractures of the proximal portion of the femur and acetabulum as well as dislocations of the hip joint itself. Table 7–6 outlines three types of hip dislocation, two of which are illustrated in Figure 7–14. Table 7–7 lists the most common types of fracture in this area. (Figures 7–15 to 7–17.) Table 7–8 describes the specific classifications of fractures of the proximal portion of the femur, and Table 7–9 lists their associated complications.

Several examples of these fractures are illustrated in Figures 7–18 to 7–20. Acetabular fractures were discussed and illustrated in Chapter 6 (Fig. 6–24).

Articular Disorders

The hip joint is a frequent target site of involvement for many degenerative, inflammatory, crystal-induced, and infectious disorders of articulations. Table 7–10 outlines these diseases and their characteristics, and Table 7–11 identifies the patterns of joint space narrowing typical of these disorders. Figures 7–21 to 7–42 illustrate the typical radiographic manifestations of the most common articular disorders affecting the hip.

Metabolic Disorders

Several metabolic disorders affect the hip joint and the surrounding osseous and soft tissue structures. Table 7–12 lists some of the more common disorders and discusses their characteristics. Table 7–13 describes the Singh index, a radiographic method of analysis used in assessing osteoporosis of the proximal portion of the femur. Figures 7–43 to 7–53 illustrate the typical imaging findings of many metabolic diseases.

Osteonecrosis of the Femoral Head

The femoral head is the most common site of involvement for osteonecrosis, an ischemic condition of bone. Additionally, Legg-Calvé-Perthes disease, osteonecrosis of the immature femoral head ossification center, is a relatively common condition that results in important clinical consequences. Table 7–14 lists the most important characteristics of osteonecrosis of the femoral head. Tables 7–15 and 7–16 outline the staging of Legg-Calvé-Perthes disease and adult osteonecrosis, respectively. Several examples of these disorders are shown in Figures 7–54 to 7–57.

TABLE 7–1. Hip: Approximate Age of Appearance and Fusion of Ossification Centers[1–4] (Figs. 7–1 and 7–2)

Ossification Center	Primary or Secondary	No. of Centers Per Hip	Age of Appearance*	Age of Fusion* (Years)	Comments
Femoral capital epiphysis	P	1	1–8 months	16–20	Fuses with femoral neck
Greater trochanter	S	1	18–54 months	16–19	Fuses with femur
Lesser trochanter	S	1	9–13 years	16–18	Fuses with femur
Acetabulum	S	1	16 years	25	May persist as os acetabuli marginalis superior in adults

*Ages of appearance and fusion of ossification centers in girls typically precede those of boys. Ethnic differences also exist.
P, Primary; S, secondary.

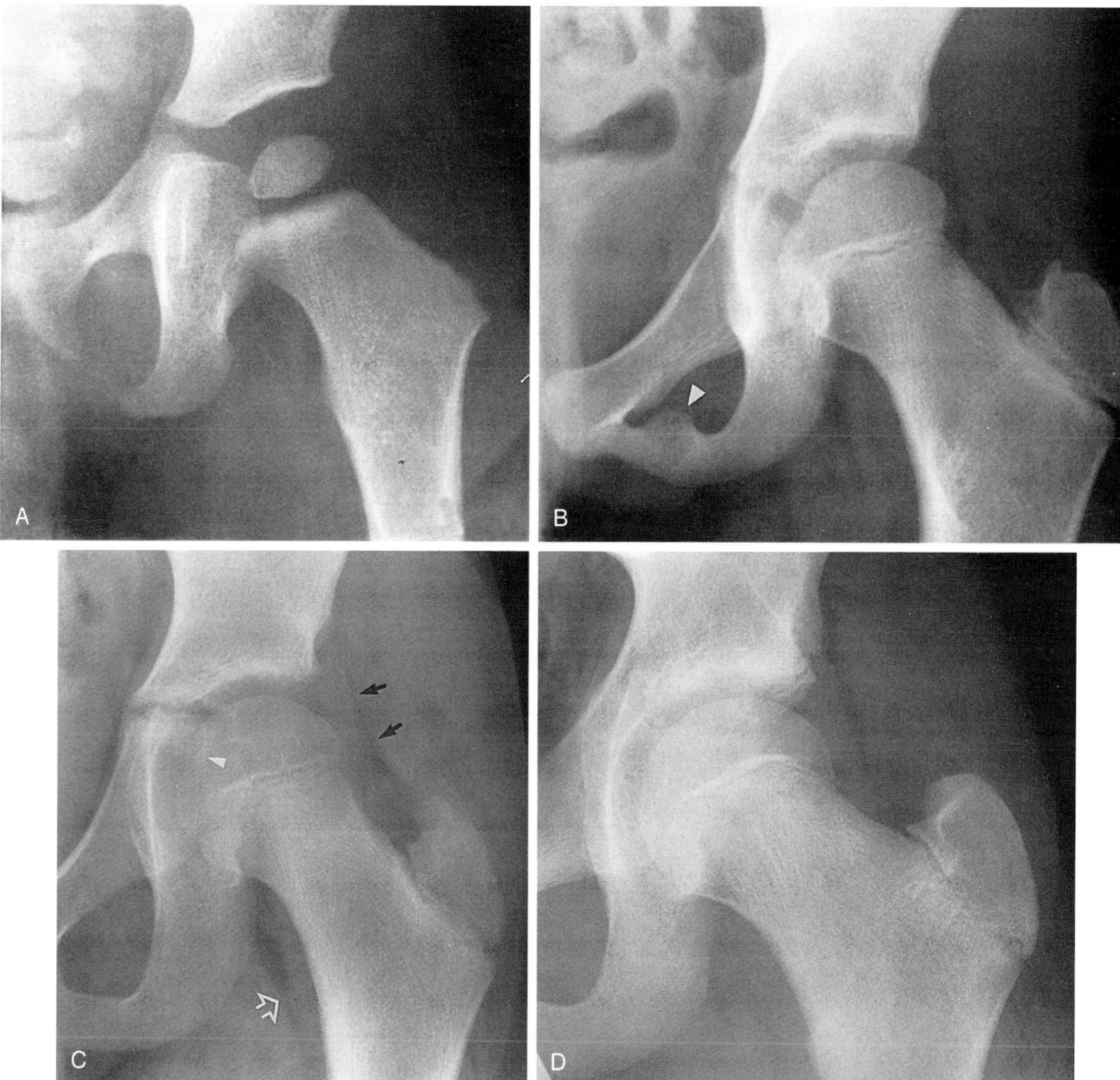

FIGURE 7–1. Skeletal maturation and normal development of the hip.[1–4] Anteroposterior radiographs. **A** In a 2-year-old boy, the femoral capital epiphysis is round and small. The triradiate cartilage and ischiopubic synchondroses are not yet fused. The femoral capital epiphysis generally begins to appear between the first and eighth months of life, allowing radiographic assessment of developmental dysplasia of the hip. **B** In a 7-year-old girl, the greater trochanter ossification center is ossified and well developed. The ischiopubic synchondrosis has fused and is seen as a normal bulbous, callus-like protrusion (arrowhead). The femoral capital epiphysis is approaching adult proportions, and the physeal growth center is thinner, is more linear, and conforms to the shape of the femoral neck. **C** In an 11-year-old boy, anatomic proportions approximate those of the adult, but the apophyses of the lesser trochanter and ischium have not yet appeared. Minimal physiologic acetabular protrusion is evident, and the fossa of the fovea capitus is apparent (arrowhead). The gluteal (arrows) and iliopsoas (open arrow) fat planes are clearly visualized. **D** In a 15-year-old boy, secondary ossification centers for the lesser trochanter and acetabulum are visible. Acetabular protrusion is not as evident as in the previous example (**C**). The femoral capital epiphysis and greater trochanter apophysis are about to fuse to the femur.

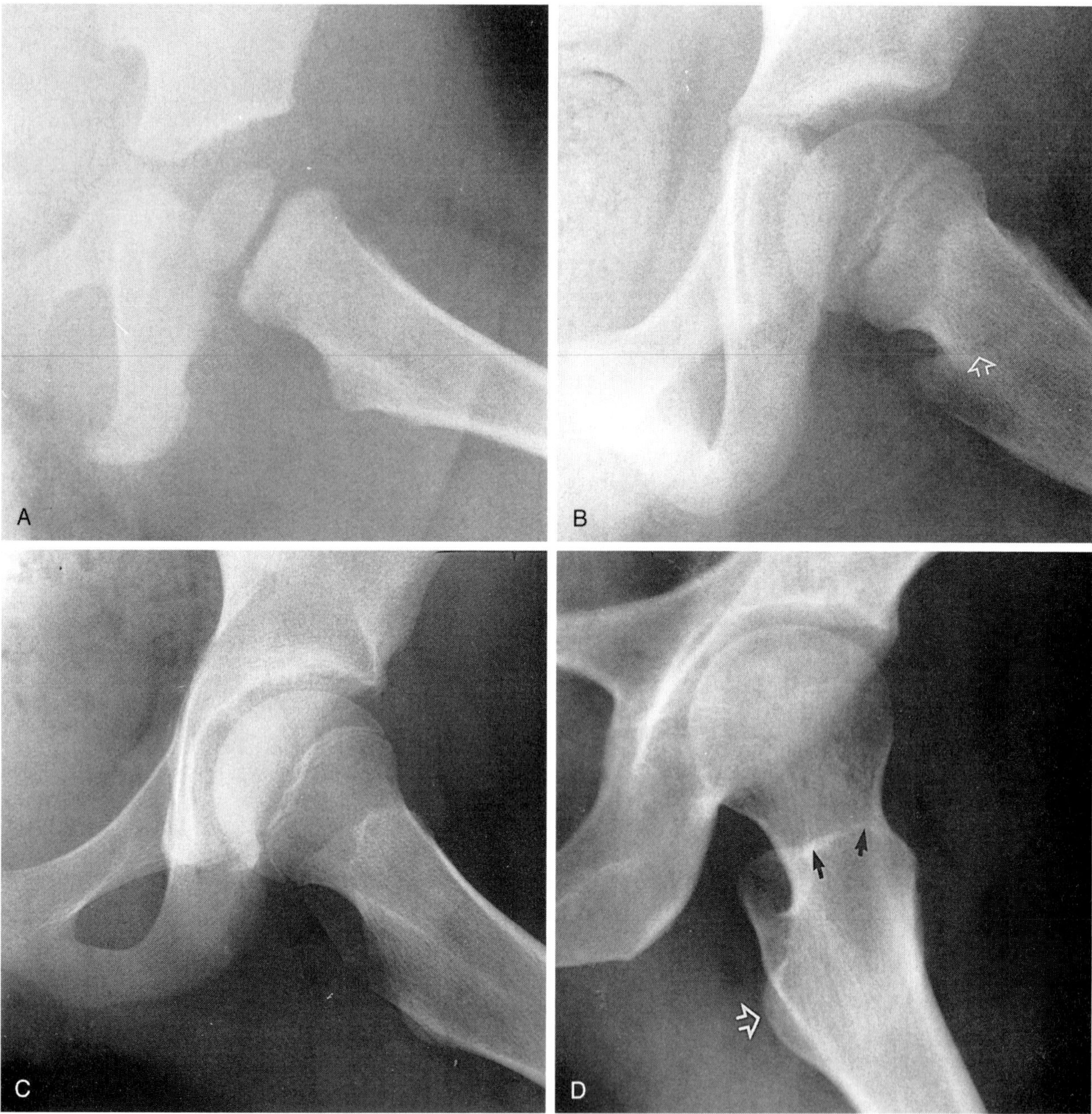

FIGURE 7–2. Skeletal maturation and normal development of the hip. Frog-leg (lateral) radiographs.[1–4] A 2-year-old boy. B 7-year-old boy. The radiolucent line represents the unfused lesser trochanter (open arrow). C 13-year-old girl. Observe the lesser trochanter apophysis. The femoral capital epiphysis appears sclerotic owing to its position overlying the acetabular margin, and this finding should not be mistaken for osteonecrosis or other osteosclerotic processes. D Adult. The apophyses of the greater (arrows) and lesser (open arrow) trochanters are fully fused.

TABLE 7–2. Developmental Anomalies, Anatomic Variants, and Sources of Diagnostic Error Affecting the Hip*

Entity	Figure(s)	Characteristics
Synovial herniation pits[5, 6]	6–7, 7–3	Also termed Pitt's pits Small, round, radiolucent area surrounded by a well-defined sclerotic margin, located in the anterior surface of the femoral neck Unilateral or bilateral ingrowth of fibrous and cartilaginous elements through a cortical perforation Occasionally painful but usually asymptomatic May enlarge and are usually negative on bone scan
Os acetabuli marginalis superior[4, 7]	6–7	Large or small triangular ossicle with well-corticated margins adjacent to the superior acetabular rim Present in about 5 per cent of normal persons No clinical significance but may simulate acetabular rim fracture
Fovea capitis[4, 7]	7–4	Normal notch in the medial aspect of the articular surface of the femoral head that accommodates the ligamentum teres femoris and its associated blood vessels Should not be mistaken for an erosion of the articular surface
Positional variations of the femoral neck[4, 7, 8]	7–5	Frontal radiographs of the hip or pelvis should be obtained with internal rotation of the femur, a position that results in an elongated appearance of the femoral neck Radiographs taken with external rotation result in a shortened appearance of the femoral neck with superimposition of the greater trochanter and femoral neck

*See also Table 1–1.

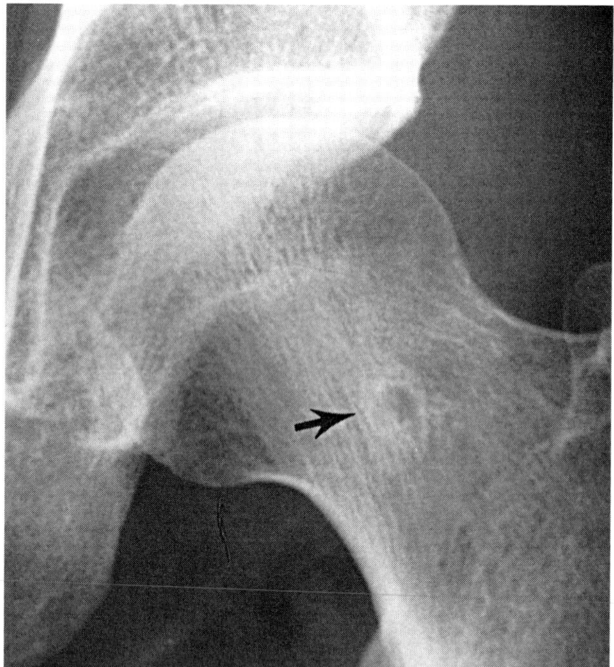

FIGURE 7–3. Synovial herniation pit.[5, 6] This variation of normal appears as a solitary, circular, well-circumscribed radiolucent lesion in the femoral neck (arrow). It represents a benign ingrowth of fibrous and cartilaginous elements through a perforation of the cortex in the anterior surface of the femoral neck. Such lesions may enlarge and occasionally are painful.

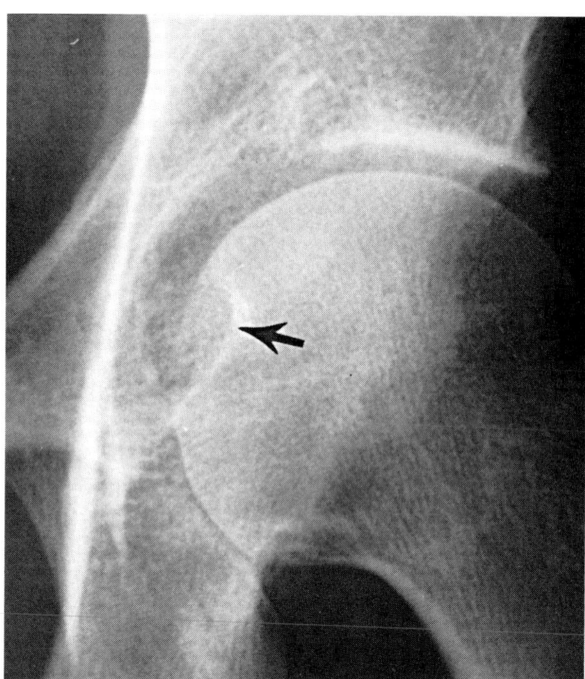

FIGURE 7–4. Fovea capitis.[4, 7] The normal notch in the medial articular surface of the femoral head (arrow) represents the site of attachment of the ligamentum teres femoris and should not be misdiagnosed as an erosion.

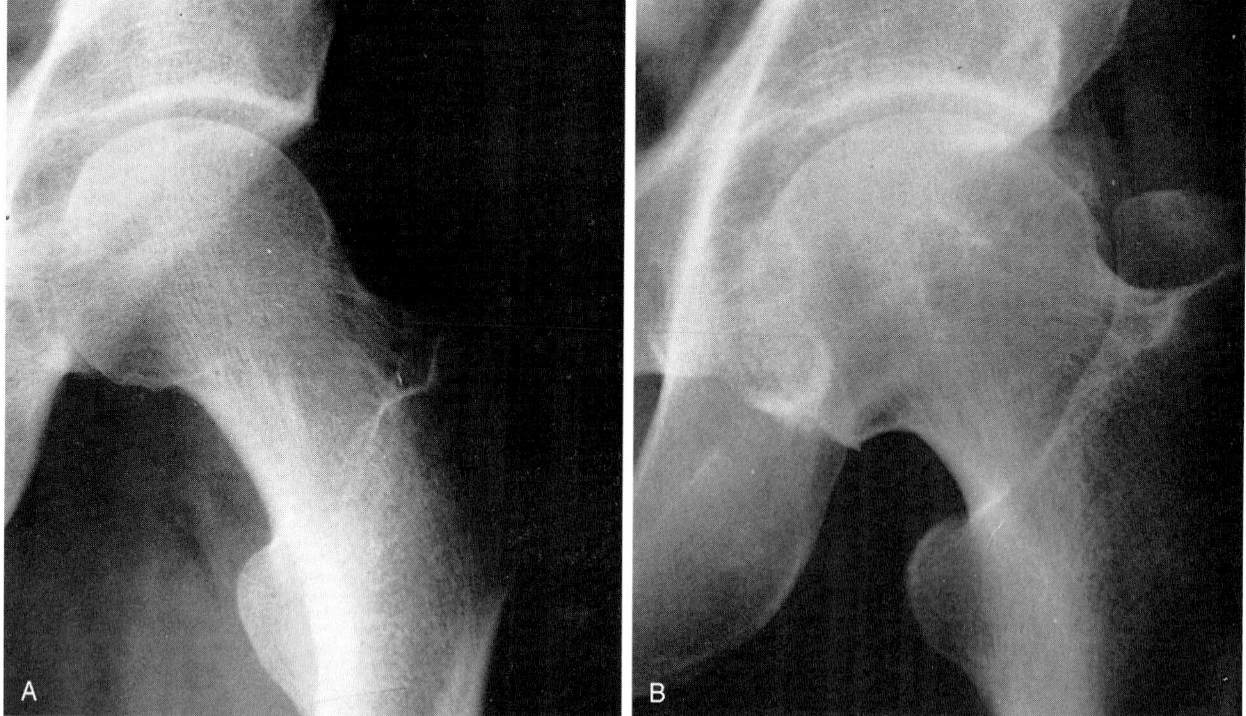

FIGURE 7–5. Positional variations of the femoral neck.[4, 7, 8] **A** Routine anteroposterior radiograph obtained with 15 degrees of internal rotation of the thigh. The femoral neck has an elongated appearance because it is more parallel to the film. **B** Improper positioning of the patient with external rotation of the thigh results in superimposition of the greater trochanter and the femoral neck. In this position, the femoral neck is more perpendicular to the film, creating a shortened appearance and making it difficult or impossible to evaluate. This patient has calcium pyrophosphate dihydrate (CPPD) crystal deposition disease.

TABLE 7–3. Hip Deformities[8–14]

Entity	Figure(s)	Entity	Figure(s)
Coxa vara		**Protrusio acetabuli**	
Legg-Calvé-Perthes disease	7–6 B; see Fig. 7–54	Acetabular fracture	6–24
Infantile (developmental) coxa vara	7–7	Rheumatoid arthritis	7–8 A
Paget's disease	7–8 C	Paget's disease	7–8 B
Slipped capital femoral epiphysis	See Figs. 7–15, 7–49	Primary protrusio acetabuli (Otto pelvis)	7–8 C
Femoral neck fracture	See Figs. 7–18, 7–33	Skeletal metastasis	7–8 D
Rickets	See Fig. 7–48	Ankylosing spondylitis	See Fig. 7–25
Cleidocranial dysplasia		Psoriatic arthropathy	See Fig. 7–26 A
Developmental dysplasia of the hip		Collagen vascular diseases	See Fig. 7–29
Meningomyelocele		Calcium pyrophosphate dihydrate	See Fig. 7–30 D
Multiple epiphyseal dysplasia		(CPPD) crystal deposition disease	See Fig. 7–35
Osteogenesis imperfecta		Alkaptonuria	See Fig. 7–40
Renal osteodystrophy		Idiopathic chondrolysis	See Fig. 7–47
Neuromuscular disorders		Osteomalacia and rickets	See Fig. 7–53
Rheumatoid arthritis		Sickle cell anemia	
Osteonecrosis		Osteoarthrosis	
Coxa valga		Radiation	
Idiopathic	7–6 C	Marfan syndrome	
Poliomyelitis	7–6 D		
Femoral neck fracture	See Fig. 7–18 C		
Abductor muscle weakness			
Hereditary multiple exostosis			
Cleidocranial dysplasia			
Hunter's syndrome			
Meningomyelocele			
Juvenile chronic arthritis			
Ollier's disease			
Neuromuscular disorders			
Diastrophic dysplasia			

Adapted from Swischuk LE: Differential Diagnosis in Pediatric Radiology, Baltimore, Williams & Wilkins, 1984; and Chapman S, Nakielny R: Aids to Radiological Differential Diagnosis. 3rd Ed. London, WB Saunders, 1995.

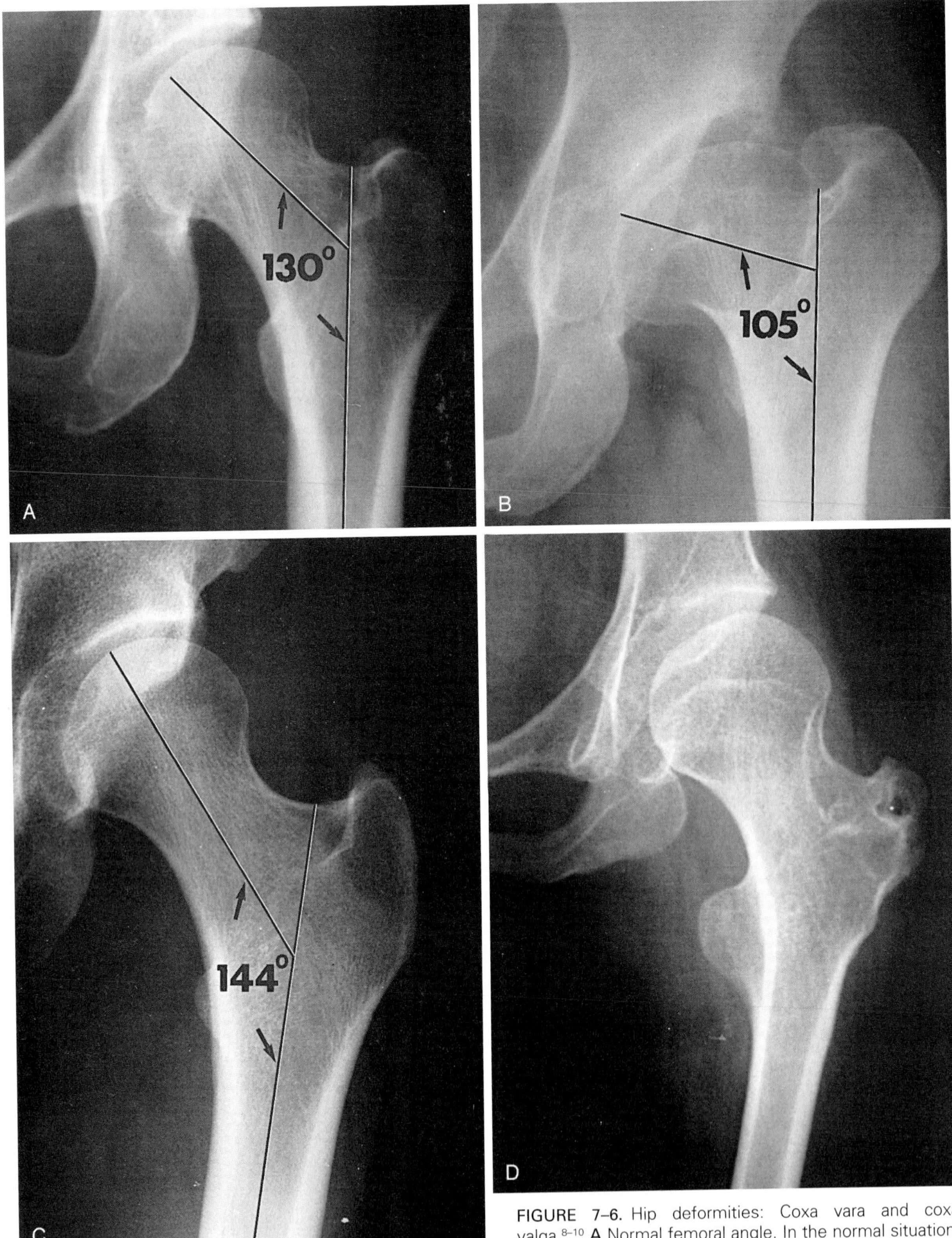

FIGURE 7–6. Hip deformities: Coxa vara and coxa valga.[8–10] A Normal femoral angle. In the normal situation, the femoral angle should measure between 120 and 130 degrees. The angle is determined by drawing two lines through the femoral shaft and the femoral neck, parallel to the midaxis of each structure. The angle is 130 degrees in this patient. B Coxa vara. In this adult patient who had had Legg-Calvé-Perthes disease as a child, a decreased femoral angle measures 105 degrees. Note also the flattening and deformity of the femoral head and shortening of the femoral neck. C Coxa valga deformity. In another adult with idiopathic coxa valga, the femoral angle measures 144 degrees. D Coxa valga deformity: poliomyelitis. Observe the valgus deformity of the proximal femur associated with hypoplasia of the femoral shaft. Many different conditions result in coxa valga and vara deformities (Table 7–3). Technical note: Accurate femoral angle measurements can be calculated only on frontal radiographs obtained with the femur internally rotated 15 degrees.

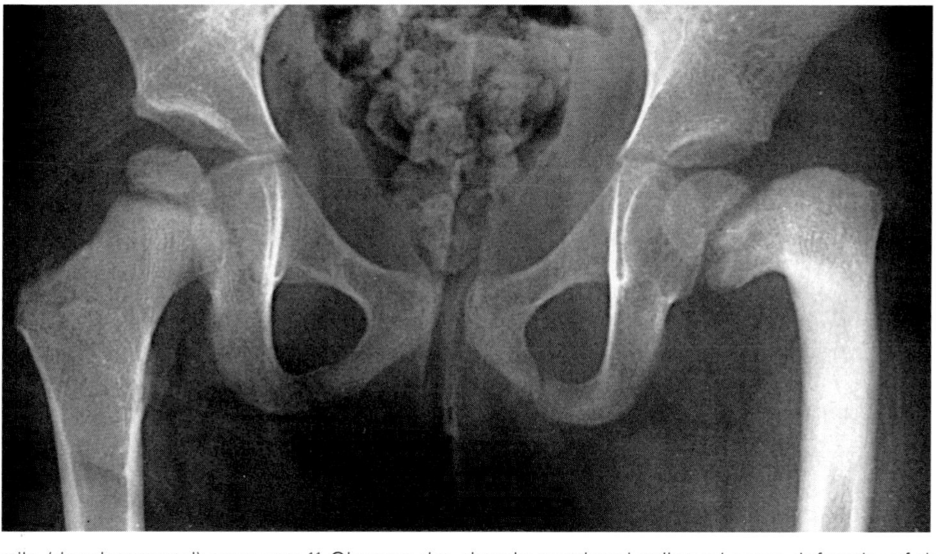

FIGURE 7–7. Infantile (developmental) coxa vara.[11] Observe the sharply angulated unilateral varus deformity of the femoral neck in relation to the femoral shaft. The infantile or developmental form of coxa vara usually becomes apparent in the first few years of life, especially as the child first begins to walk. It is unilateral in 60 to 75 per cent of cases, and the child has a lurching or "duck-waddle" gait. Radiographically, the neck-shaft angle is less than 120 degrees, the proximal femoral physis is vertically oriented, and the femoral head appears dramatically depressed relative to the greater trochanter. Differential diagnosis includes other causes of coxa vara (Table 7–3). *(Courtesy of M. N. Pathria, M.D., San Diego, California.)*

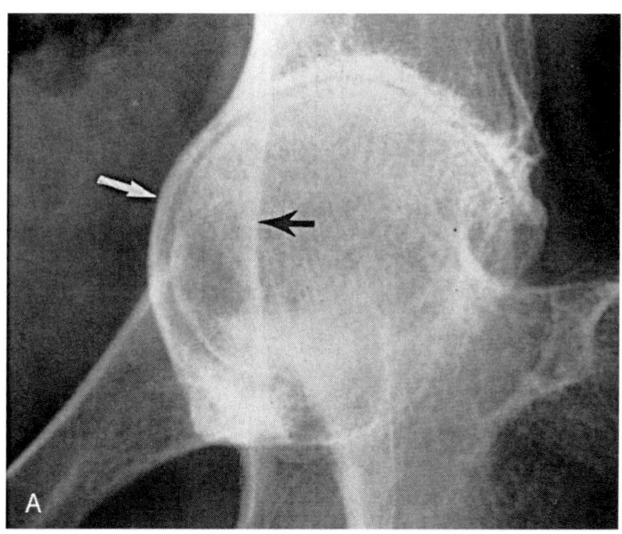

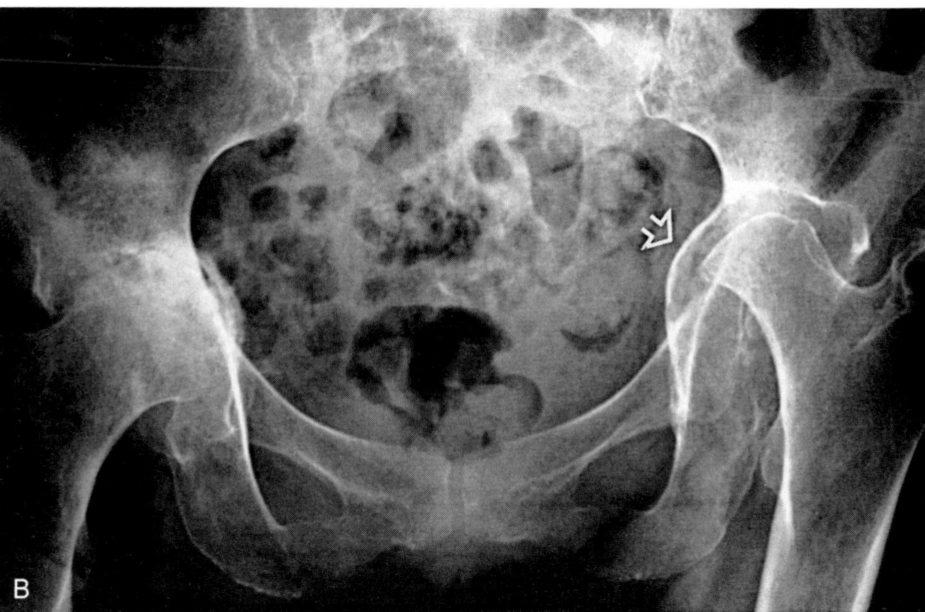

FIGURE 7–8. Protrusio acetabuli.[8–10, 12–14] **A** Measurement. A protrusio acetabuli deformity is present when the acetabular line (white arrow) projects medially to the ilioischial line (black arrow) by 3 mm or more in men and by 6 mm or more in women. **B** Rheumatoid arthritis. This 69-year-old woman with rheumatoid arthritis has asymmetric bilateral acetabular protrusion. The left femoral head is severely eroded, and the acetabulum is dramatically remodeled (open arrow). The right femoral head is not as severely damaged, but the joint space is uniformly narrowed and the acetabulum is protruding medially.

Illustration continued on following page

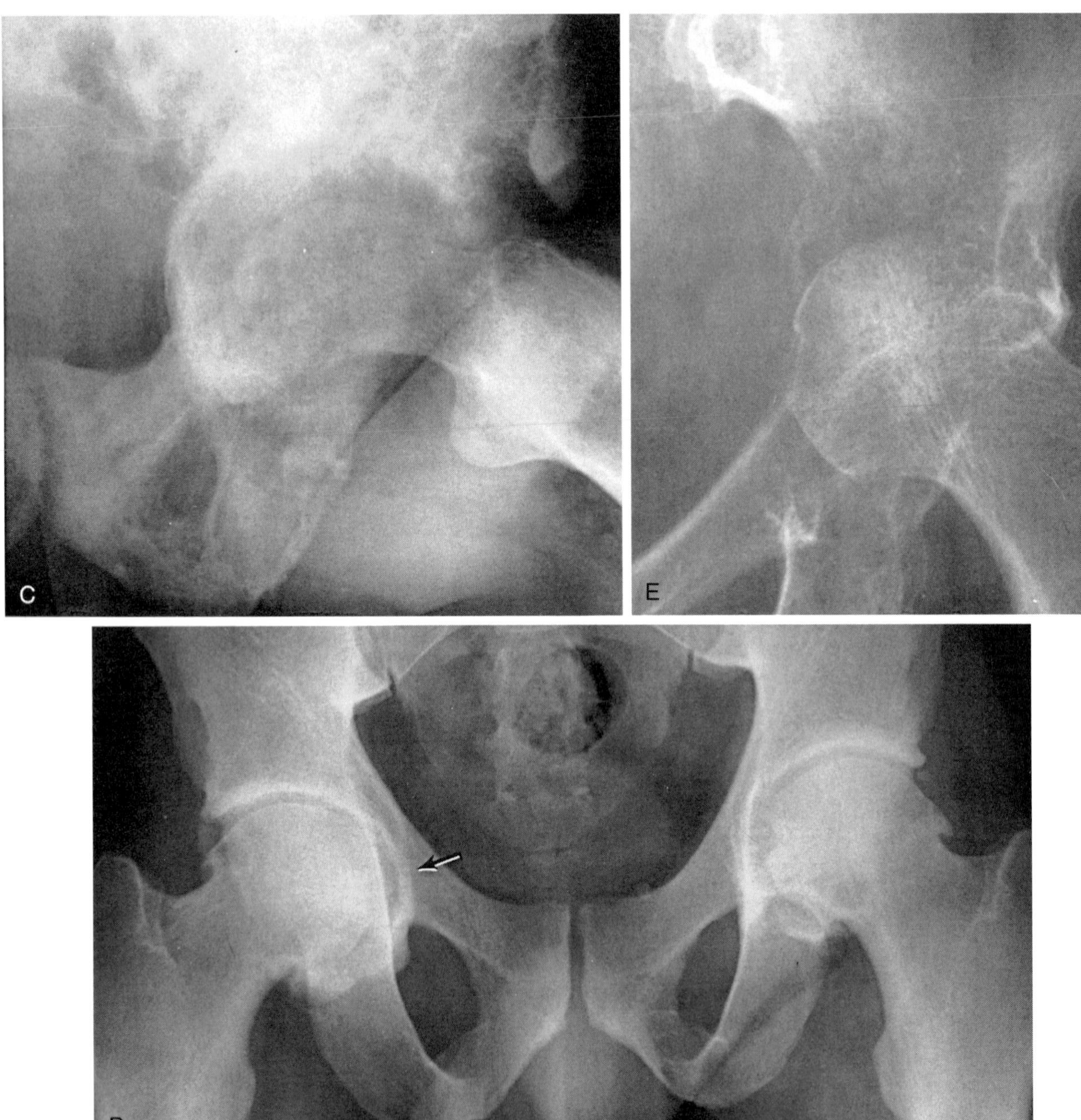

FIGURE 7–8 *Continued.* C Paget's disease. Observe the extensive acetabular protrusion in this patient with severe Paget's disease. D Primary protrusio acetabuli (Otto pelvis). A frontal pelvic radiograph of this 26-year-old man shows bilateral symmetric concentric loss of joint space with axial and medial migration of the femoral heads resulting in mild bilateral acetabular protrusion, more severe on the right (arrow). Degenerative osteophytes also are seen arising from both femoral heads and acetabula. Primary protrusio acetabuli is a familial, idiopathic condition that may lead to premature secondary degenerative joint disease of the hips. It is usually bilateral and symmetric and is much more frequent in women than in men. This condition may resemble idiopathic chondrolysis of the hip. *(D, Courtesy of R. Taketa, M.D., Long Beach, California.)* E Skeletal metastasis: Periarticular bone involvement. This 65-year-old woman developed a destructive lesion of the left hemipelvis secondary to metastasis (or direct invasion) from a clear cell carcinoma of the uterus. The loss of acetabular support has allowed inward protrusion of the femoral head. (See Table 7–3.)

TABLE 7–4. Developmental Dysplasia of the Hip[15–18]

Entity	Figure(s)	Characteristics
Terminology		
Developmental dysplasia of the hip (DDH)		Deformity of the acetabulum in which the head of the femur may be properly located or partially or completed displaced Hips that are subluxatable, dislocatable, subluxated, or dislocated Results in continuously deforming acetabular cartilage
Instability		Type I hip dysplasia pattern Subluxatable and dislocatable hips Pliable labrum may be slightly deformed
Subluxation		Type II hip dysplasia pattern Protrusion of the femoral head beyond the acetabulum with contact still maintained Fibrocartilaginous superior acetabular labrum may be everted or inverted
Dislocation		Type III hip dysplasia pattern Loss of contact between femoral head and acetabulum Frequently results in inversion and hypertrophy of the acetabular labrum, which causes an impediment to reduction
Etiology and predisposing factors		
Mechanical factors		Results from restricted space in utero with limitation of fetal motion Oligohydramnios Among newborn infants with DDH, 60 per cent are firstborns Breech presentation (30 per cent of DDH patients) Associated with torticollis (20 per cent of cases) Associated with clubfoot and metatarsus varus (2 per cent of cases) Also associated with generalized joint laxity, scoliosis, cardiac and renal anomalies, and multiple syndromes
Functional factors		Elevated estrogen levels (more common in newborn infants with DDH) block collagen maturation
Epidemiology		
Prevalence		DDH: 2–6 live newborn infants per 1000 births Complete dislocation: 1 per 1000 births Four to eight times more common in girls than boys Familial incidence in 20 per cent of patients Left hip involved in 80 per cent of patients Bilateral in 25 per cent of cases *Risk of DDH* 1. Female fetus in breech presentation: 1 in 15 2. Female fetus in nonbreech presentation: 1 in 25 3. Newborn infant with affected sibling: 6 per cent 4. Newborn infant with one affected parent: 12 per cent 5. Newborn infant with two affected parents: 36 per cent *Ethnicity* Native Americans and Lapps: 25–50 per 1000 live newborn infants Chinese and black Africans: negligible prevalence rate
Detection and evaluation		
Physical examination		Ortolani's reduction maneuver and Barlow's dislocation maneuver 1 per cent missed diagnosis based on these tests These tests are more accurate in cases of frank dislocation Long-standing dislocations with muscle spasm or formation of a pseudoacetabulum may result in false-negative tests

Table continued on following page

TABLE 7–4. Developmental Dysplasia of the Hip[15–18] *Continued*

Entity	Figure(s)	Characteristics
Routine radiography	7–9 to 7–11	Earliest radiographic signs appear at 6 weeks of age Radiographs are most useful after 2 to 8 months of age, when the cartilaginous femoral head begins to ossify Frontal views are preferred over frog-leg views because dislocations may reduce in the frog-leg position Femoral head ossification center usually is much smaller or absent in the dysplastic hip Several lines and angles are used to measure the relationship of the femur to the acetabulum (Table 7–5) *Limitations of Radiography* Cartilaginous femoral head is not visible on radiographs in the first few months of life, the most critical time in the diagnosis of DDH Frontal projections do not show anteroposterior displacement Patient positioning is demanding and often results in pelvic rotation or tilting that interferes with accurate measurements Risk of ionizing radiation
Ultrasonography	7–12	More sensitive than physical examination and far superior to radiography in the first few months of life Should be performed at 4–6 weeks in infants with any risk factor or abnormal physical findings with a stable hip; should be performed within 2 weeks in patients with abnormal physical examination results and unstable hip Measurements can be obtained for acetabular angle, acetabular coverage of the femoral head, acetabular cartilage thickness, and lateral head distance
Computed tomography (CT)		Computed tomographic (CT) scanning may be used to document the adequacy of a reduction in DDH, especially in the transverse plane, revealing anterior or posterior displacement Also useful in measuring acetabular anteversion and other preoperative and postoperative morphologic changes
Magnetic resonance (MR) imaging	7–13	Reserved for complicated cases of DDH in which initial treatment has been unsuccessful

Adapted from Gerscovich EO: A radiologist's guide to imaging in the diagnosis and treatment of developmental dysplasia of the hip. I and II. Skeletal Radiol 26:386, 447, 1997.

TABLE 7–5. Radiographic Measurements in Developmental Dysplasia of the Hip[16]

Method	Age	Normal Values (Degrees)	
		Female	*Male*
Acetabular index (AI)	Newborn infant	28.8 ± 4.8	26.4 ± 4.4
	3 months	25.0 ± 3.5	22.0 ± 4
	6 months	23.2 ± 4	20.3 ± 3.7
	1 year	21.2 ± 3.8	19.8 ± 3.6
	2 years	18.0 ± 4	19.0 ± 3.6
		A value >30–32 is abnormal at any age	
Center-edge (C-E) angle	3 months	18–20	
	2 years	30	
		Lowest limit of normal	
	5–8 years	19	
	9–12 years	25	
	13–20 years	26–30	
Medial joint space (MJS)	6 months to 11 years	5–12 mm Difference between the two hips: <1.5 mm	

Adapted from Gerscovich EO: A radiologist's guide to imaging in the diagnosis and treatment of developmental dysplasia of the hip. I. General considerations, physical examination as applied to real-time sonography and radiography. Skeletal Radiol 26:386, 1997.

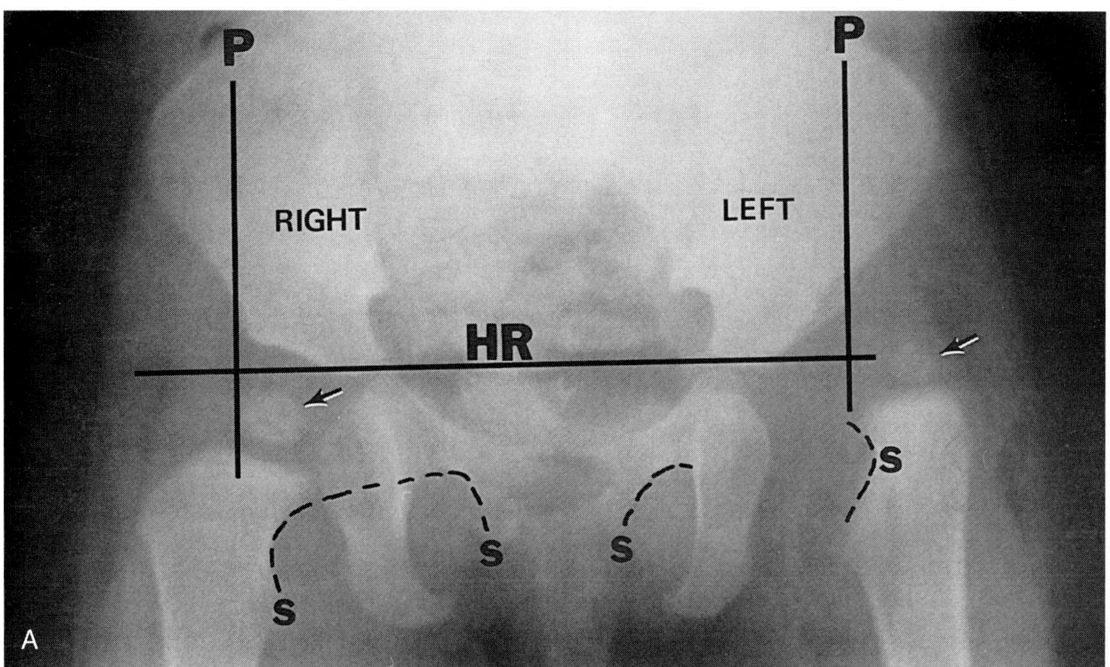

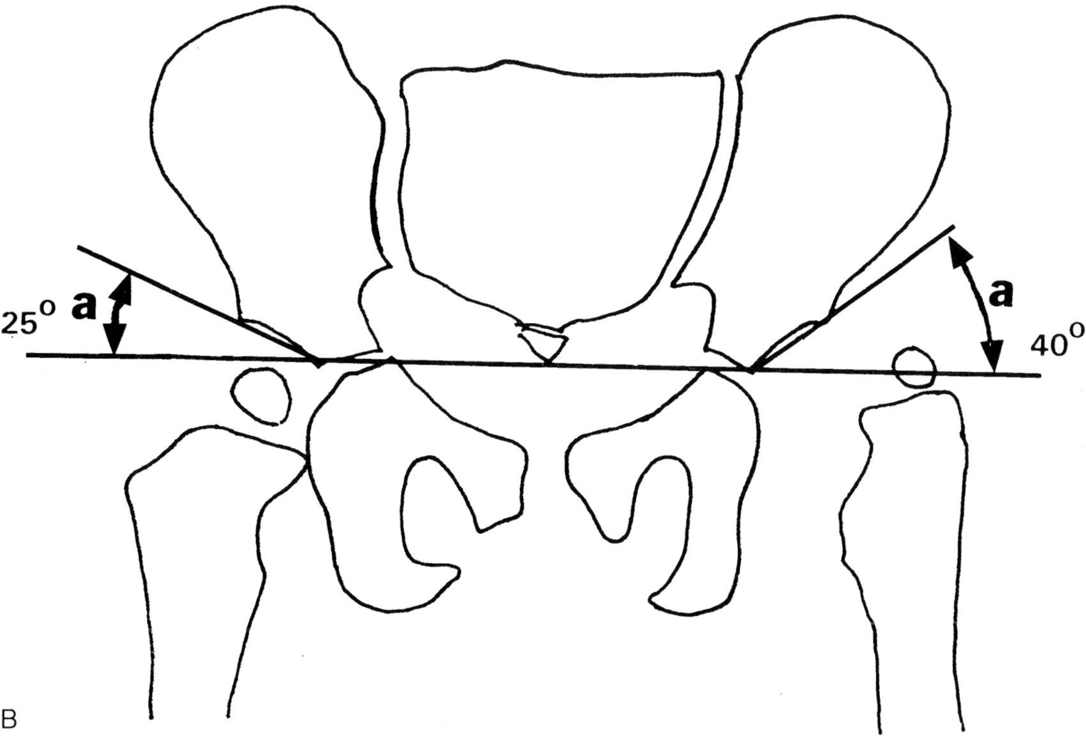

FIGURE 7–9. Developmental dysplasia of the hip (DDH): Radiographic measurements.[15, 16] (See Table 7–5 for normal values.) A Hilgenreiners' line, Perkins' line, and Shenton's line. Pelvic radiograph from an 8-month-old girl with left acetabular dysplasia and hip dislocation. Hilgenreiner's line (HR) is a transverse line intersecting the top of both triradiate cartilages. Perkins' line (P) is a vertical line perpendicular to Hilgenreiner's line that intersects the lateral acetabular margin. Normally, the femoral head ossification centers (arrows) and the upper medial corner of the femoral metaphyses should project in the lower medial quadrant of the intersection of Hilgenreiner's line and Perkins' line. The left femoral head is dislocated superiorly and laterally, and the right femoral head is located in the normal position. Shenton's line (S) is a smooth, continuous arc extending from the medial aspect of the femoral neck to the lower margin of the superior pubic ramus. In this patient, Shenton's line on the right is normal and continuous; on the left, the line is disrupted owing to superolateral dislocation of the hip. B Acetabular index. A schematic diagram illustrates the angle (a) formed between Hilgenreiner's line and the acetabular roof line. In this example, the left acetabular index measures 40 degrees in the dysplastic hip and 25 degrees in the normal right hip. In normal newborn infants, this measurement is less than 30 to 32 degrees and becomes progressively smaller in older infants.

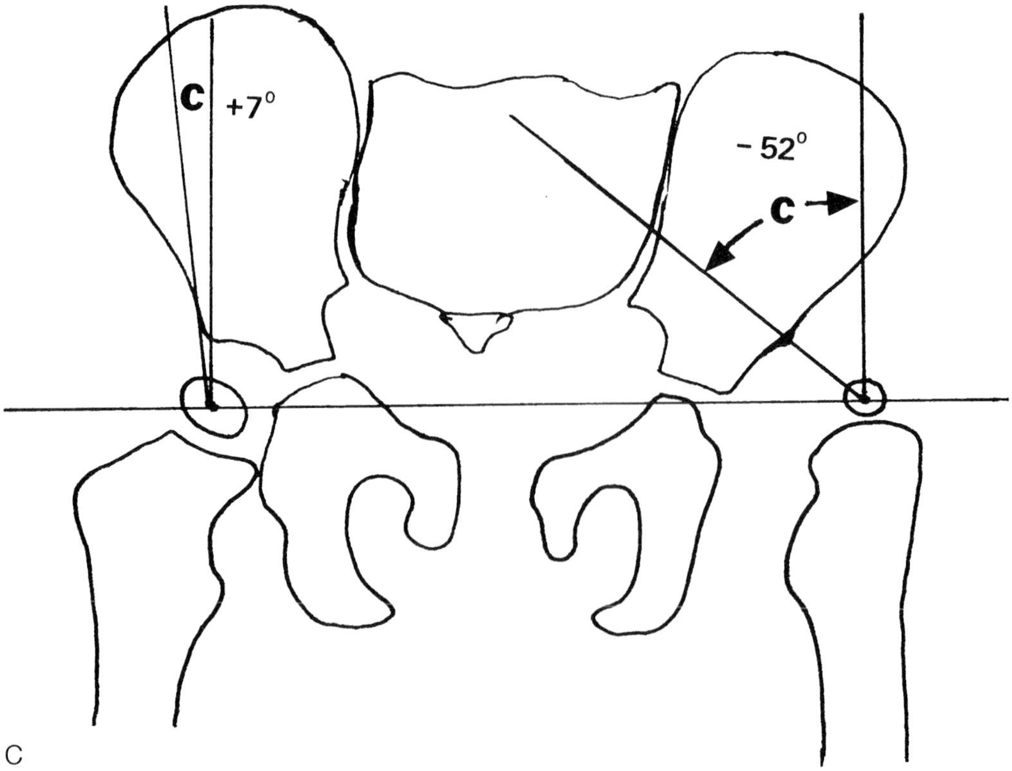

C

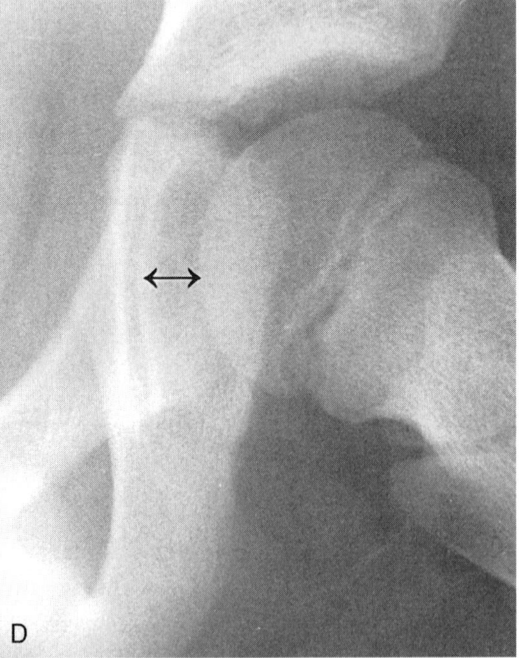

FIGURE 7–9 *Continued.* **C** Center-edge (C-E) angle. A line intersecting the centers of both femoral epiphyses is constructed. A vertical line perpendicular to the initial line is then drawn from the center of the epiphysis. A third line is drawn superiorly from the center of the epiphysis to the lateral acetabular margin. The C-E angle represents the angle between the last two lines and is measured bilaterally. In this example, the angle is +7 degrees in the normal right hip and −52 degrees in the dislocated left hip. **D** Medial joint space (MJS) width. The MJS width is the distance between the lateral aspect of the acetabular wall and the medial aspect of the ossification center of the femoral head at its widest portion (double-headed arrow). If the femoral head is not ossified, the line is drawn to the medial aspect of the metaphysis. In children aged 6 months to 11 years, this measurement should range from 5 to 12 mm, and the difference between the two hips should not exceed 1.5 mm.

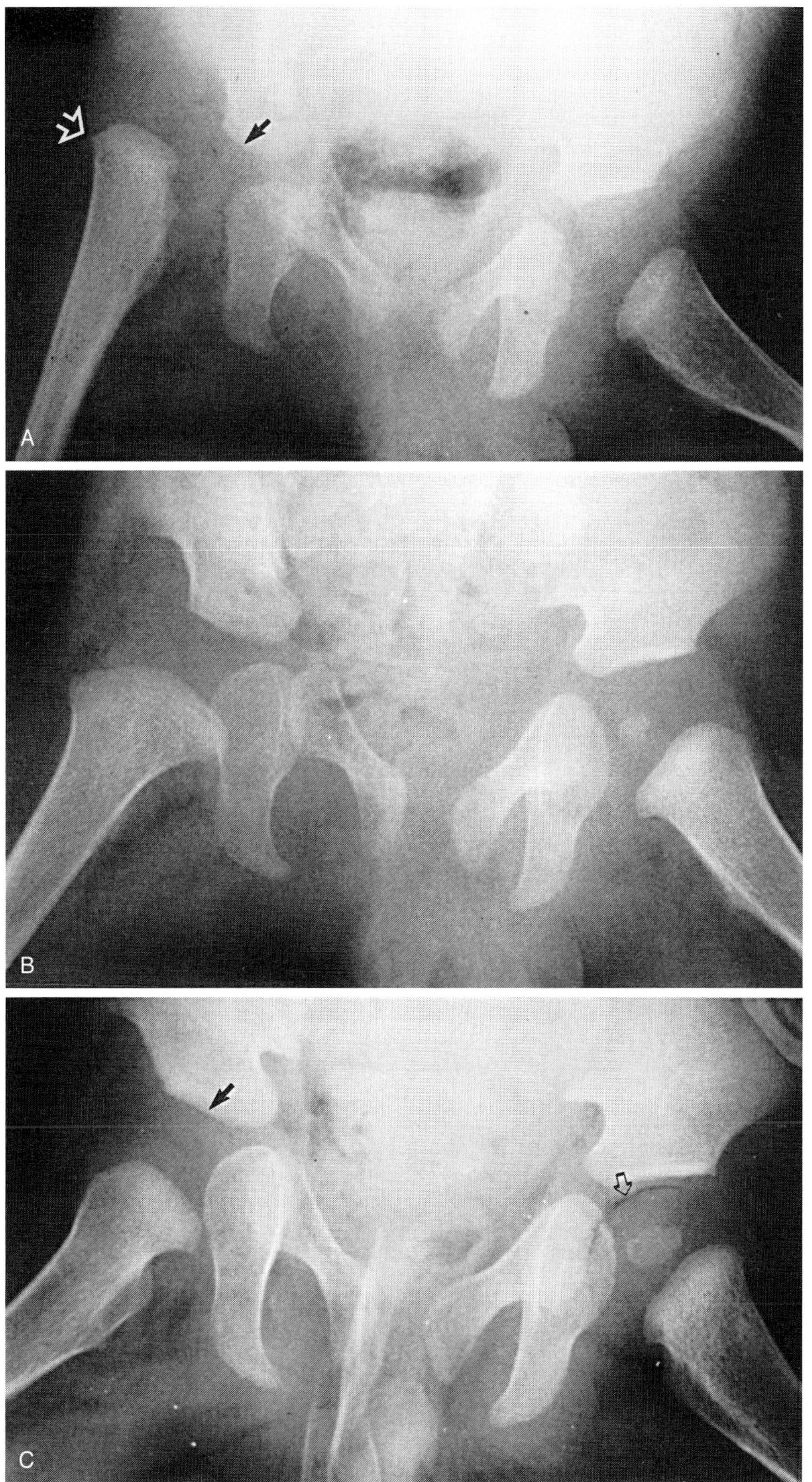

FIGURE 7–10. *See legend on following page*

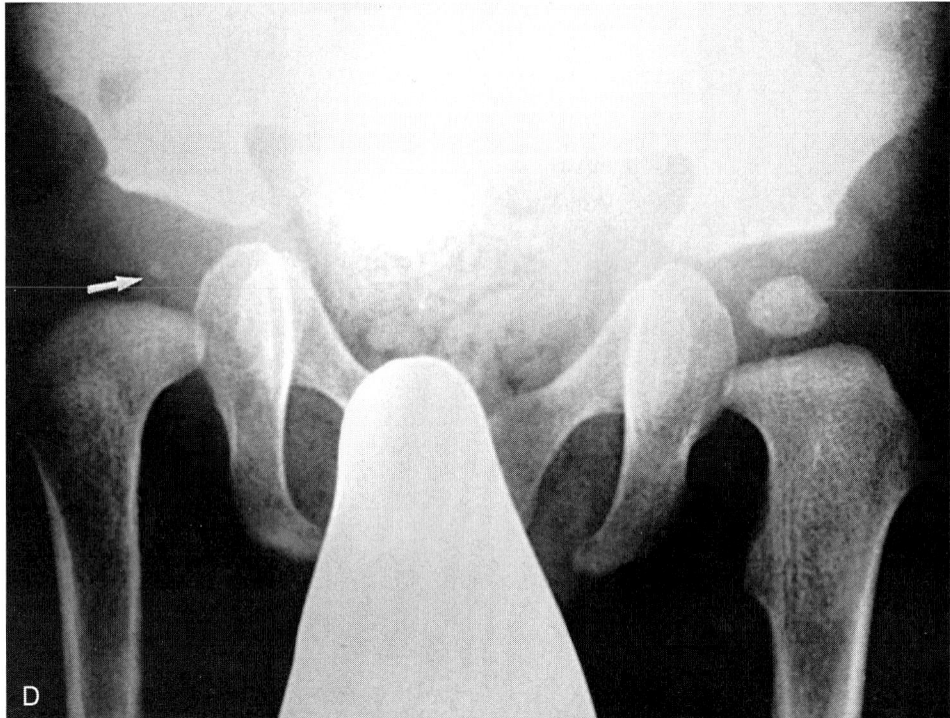

FIGURE 7–10. Developmental dysplasia of the hip (DDH).[15, 16] Serial radiographs of a boy with a clicking right hip and positive Barlow's and Ortolani's tests. **A** 5 months of age. The right acetabulum is shallow and poorly developed (arrow). The right femur is dislocated superiorly and laterally (open arrow). The femoral head epiphyses have not yet begun to ossify. **B** 9 months of age, after treatment in a harness. The left femoral head has begun to ossify normally, but the right remains unossified. The right femur is positioned more adequately than in the earlier radiograph **(A)**. **C** 11 months of age, with continued treatment in a harness. The right femoral head remains unossified, and the right acetabulum remains underdeveloped (arrow). The femur was not displaced at the time the radiograph was obtained. Intra-articular gas outlines the cartilaginous epiphysis of the left hip (open arrow) in this frog-leg view, a finding that often is present during traction of the thigh. The right epiphysis remains unossified. **D** 18 months of age. The right femoral head has begun to ossify (arrow) and is well positioned in relation to the acetabulum. *(Courtesy of B. Howard, M.D., Charlotte, North Carolina.)*

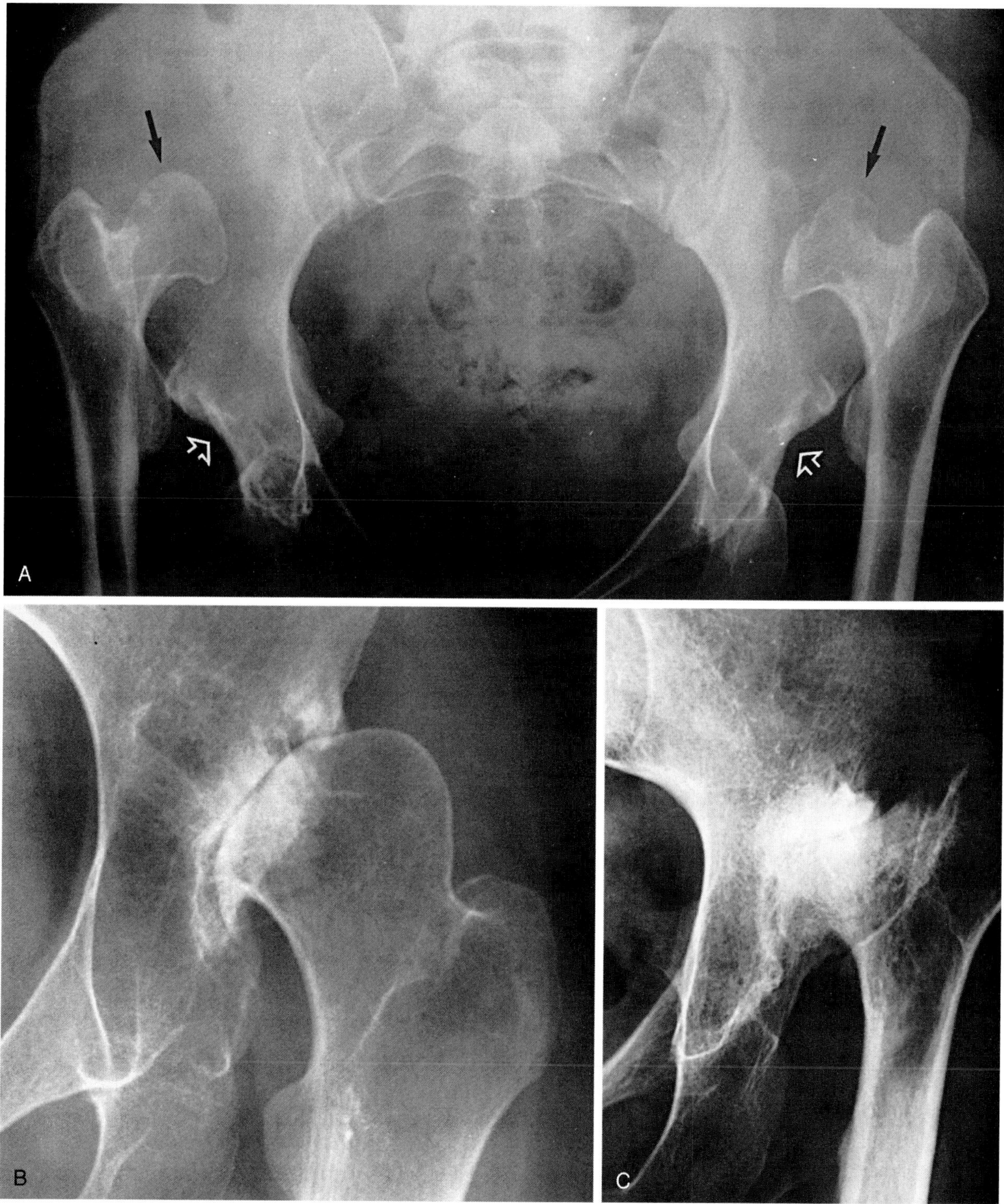

FIGURE 7–11. Developmental dysplasia of the hip (DDH) in the adult.[15] A Bilateral hip dislocations are evident on this frontal radiograph of an adult patient who had had untreated type III DDH as a child. Symmetric acetabular hypoplasia (open arrows) and abnormal articulation of the femoral heads with the posterior iliac fossae are seen (arrows). B Osteoarthrosis, secondary to DDH. Observe the subchondral sclerosis, cyst formation, joint space narrowing, and osteophytes in this 32-year-old woman with long-standing type III DDH. A pseudoacetabulum has developed in a position superior to the normal location of the acetabulum, and the femoral head is only partially covered by the acetabulum. C In a third patient, a 35-year-old man, severe degenerative changes, including sclerosis and joint space obliteration, remodeling of the femoral head, and formation of a pseudoacetabulum on the superolateral aspect of the ilium, are evident. Early detection of hip dysplasia is essential for appropriate management. *(C, From Taylor JAM, Harger BL, Resnick D: Diagnostic imaging of common hip disorders: A pictorial review. Top Clin Chiropr 1:8, 1994. Reprinted with permission.)*

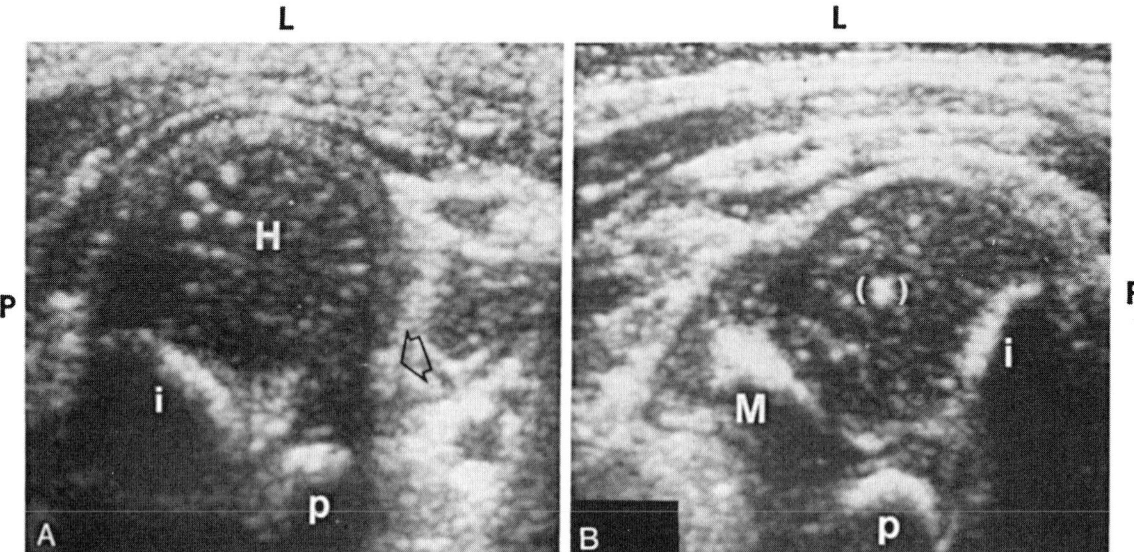

FIGURE 7–12. Developmental dysplasia of the hip (DDH): Ultrasonography.[16, 17] A Transaxial image of right subluxatable hip after stress. The femoral head (H) has subluxated posteriorly and laterally with respect to the acetabulum. B Contralateral normal left hip for comparison. More advanced maturation of the femoral head ossific nucleus (parentheses) is evident. I, Ischium; p, pubis; arrow, echogenicity within acetabular fossa; L, lateral; P, posterior; M, femoral metaphysis. *(From Resnick D, Kang SK: Internal Derangements of Joints. Philadelphia, WB Saunders, 1997, p 538.)*

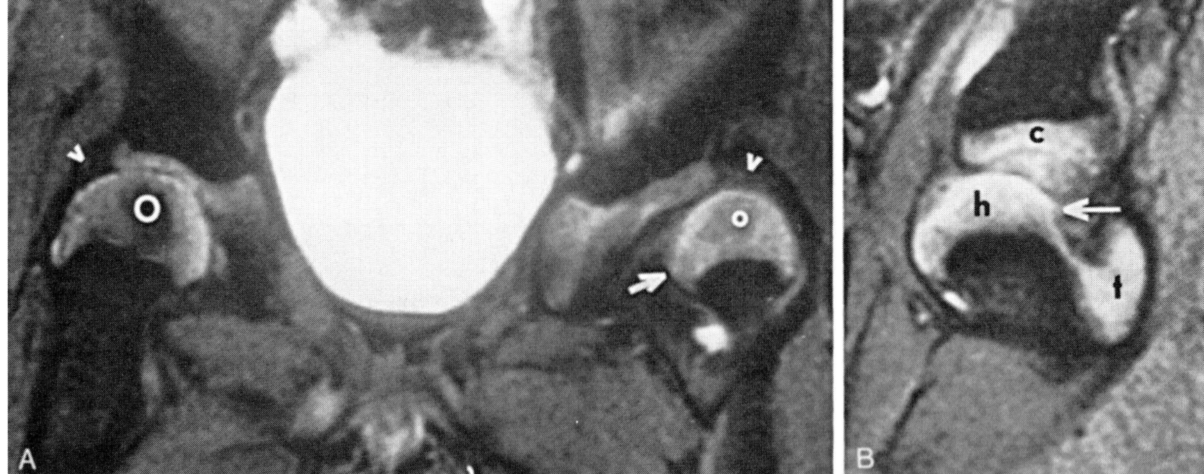

FIGURE 7–13. Developmental dysplasia of the hip: Magnetic resonance (MR) imaging.[18] A Coronal gradient echo (TR/TE, 100/25) MR image reveals lateral subluxation of the left femoral head (arrow) and presence of a secondary ossification center that is delayed in development (O > o). Both acetabular labra are in the normal everted position (arrowheads). B Sagittal MR image (TR/TE, 100/25) demonstrates mild anterior subluxation of the femoral head (arrow). Note the continuity between the cartilaginous femoral head (h) and the greater trochanter (t). c, Triradiate cartilage. *(From Resnick D, Kang SK: Internal Derangements of Joints. Philadelphia, WB Saunders, 1997, p 539.)*

TABLE 7–6. Traumatic Dislocations of the Hip*

Entity	Figure(s)	Characteristics	Complications and Related Injuries
Posterior hip dislocation[19, 77]	7–14	80–85 per cent of all hip dislocations Usually result from dashboard injury in which the flexed knee strikes the dashboard during a head-on automobile collision Motorcycle accidents also are a common cause of this injury Dislocated femoral head is seen on frontal radiograph at or above the level of the acetabulum, displaced superolaterally with the femur adducted and internally rotated	Associated trauma and fractures to the knee, femur, and acetabulum Shear fractures of femoral head (7–10 per cent of cases) Compression fractures of femoral head (13–60 per cent of cases) Osteonecrosis (25 per cent of cases) Acetabular labral tears Sciatic nerve injury Periarticular soft tissue calcification and ossification Secondary degenerative joint disease Entrapment of acetabular labrum or osseous fragment Occasional recurrence
Anterior hip dislocation[19]	7–14	10 to 11 per cent of all hip dislocations Results from forced abduction and external rotation of the thigh Two types of anterior dislocation: *Inferior (obturator) dislocation:* 90 per cent of anterior dislocations Anterior and inferomedial femoral head displacement is seen on the frontal radiograph with the femur abducted and externally rotated *Superior dislocation* 10 percent of anterior dislocations Femoral head dislocates superiorly May be confused for a posterior dislocation	Associated impaction fractures of the femoral head or other fractures of the acetabular rim, greater trochanter, or femoral neck Osteonecrosis (4 per cent of cases) Vascular injury (1 per cent of cases) Occasional recurrence
Central acetabular fracture-dislocation[20, 21]		Rare injury Results from forces applied to the lateral side of the greater trochanter and pelvis, with forces transmitted through the femoral head	Central acetabular fracture Hemorrhage into pelvis Secondary degenerative joint disease Associated visceral injury and other musculoskeletal injuries

*See also Tables 1–3 to 1–5.

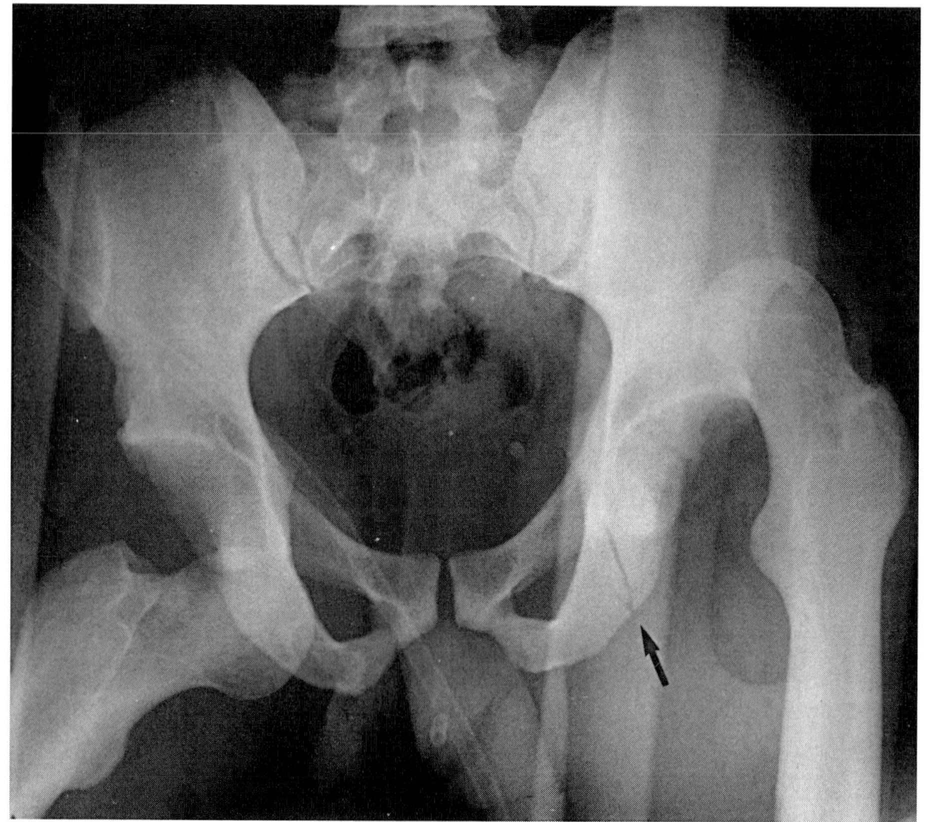

FIGURE 7–14. Bilateral hip dislocation with associated pelvic fractures.[19] This patient was involved in a motorcycle accident. Note the presence of both anterior and posterior hip dislocations with associated fractures of the acetabular margin and ischium (arrow). *(Courtesy of T. Martin, M.D., and J. Spaeth, M.D., Albuquerque, New Mexico.)*

TABLE 7–7. Fractures and Physeal Injuries About the Hip*

Entity	Figure(s), Table(s)	Characteristics
Acetabular fractures[20, 21]	6–24 Table 6–4	See Chapter 6
Slipped capital femoral epiphysis[22]	7–15; See Fig. 7–37	Salter-Harris type I growth plate injury More common in boys, African Americans, and obese children Boys: aged 10–17 years, twice as frequent on the left side Girls: aged 8–15 years, both sides affected equally 20–35 per cent of patients have bilateral involvement History of injury in fewer than 50 per cent of cases Predisposing factors: adolescent growth spurt, hormonal influences, obesity, and increased levels of physical activity Infrequently found in younger children with severe trauma, malnutrition, developmental acetabular dysplasia, Legg-Calvé-Perthes disease, tuberculosis *Radiographic findings* Decreased height of involved epiphysis in relation to contralateral side on frontal radiograph Blurring and widening of the physis Lateral cortical line of the femoral neck (Klein's line) does not intersect a portion of the epiphysis—most evident on the frog-leg projection Typical epiphyseal slippage is posteromedioinferior Varus deformity *Complications* Shortening and broadening of the femoral neck Osteonecrosis (6–15 per cent of cases) Chondrolysis (as many as 40 per cent of cases) Degenerative joint disease Persistent varus deformity
Stress (fatigue) fracture of the femoral neck[23, 24]	7–16	Activity-related onset of pain Young athletes: common activities include long-distance running, ballet dancing, gymnastics, and marching May become complete fractures with displacement *Transverse type* More frequent in older patients Radiolucent area in the superior aspect of the femoral neck *Compression type* More common in younger patients Stable in most cases Appears as haze of callus surrounding the inferior aspect of the neck
Insufficiency fracture of the femoral neck[25]	7–17	Most common in elderly patients, especially women Predisposing factors: osteoporosis, rheumatoid arthritis, corticosteroid medication, malignancy, radiation therapy History of minor trauma often is elicited Fractures tend to course horizontally across the femoral neck at angles almost perpendicular to the trabeculae
Acute fractures of the proximal portion of the femur	7–18 Tables 7–8, 7–9	

*See also Tables 1–3 and 1–4.

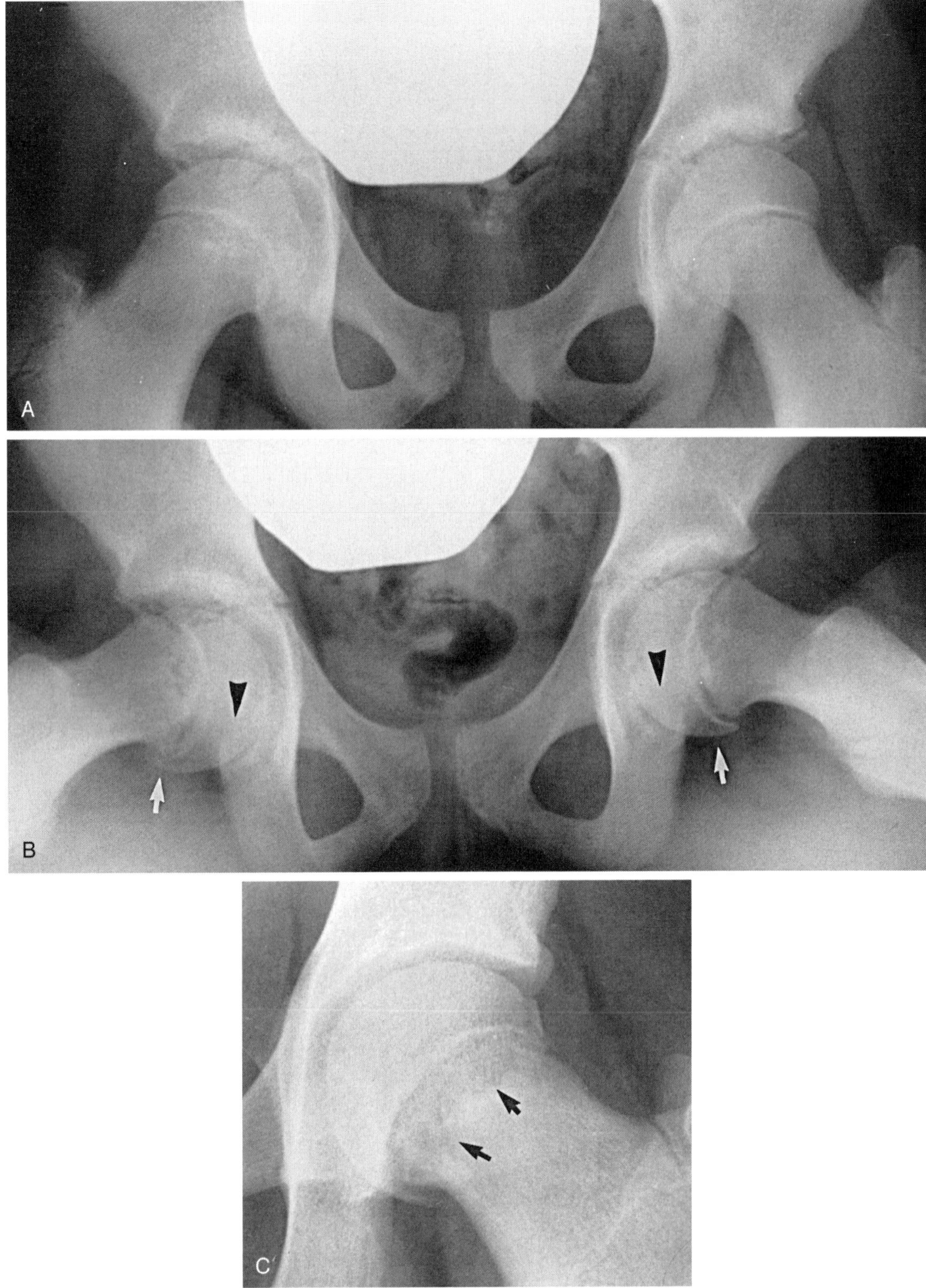

FIGURE 7–15. Slipped capital femoral epiphysis.[22] **A, B** Bilateral involvement. Frontal (**A**) and frog-leg (**B**) projections of this 11-year-old girl show posteromedial displacement of both proximal femoral epiphyses (white arrows). The arrowheads indicate the direction of displacement. The growth plates appear widened, and the osseous margins are blurred and indistinct. **C** In another patient, a frontal radiograph shows subphyseal radiolucency (arrows), widening of the physis, and minimal slippage of the femoral capital epiphysis. *(**C**, Courtesy of B. Howard, M.D., Charlotte, North Carolina.)*

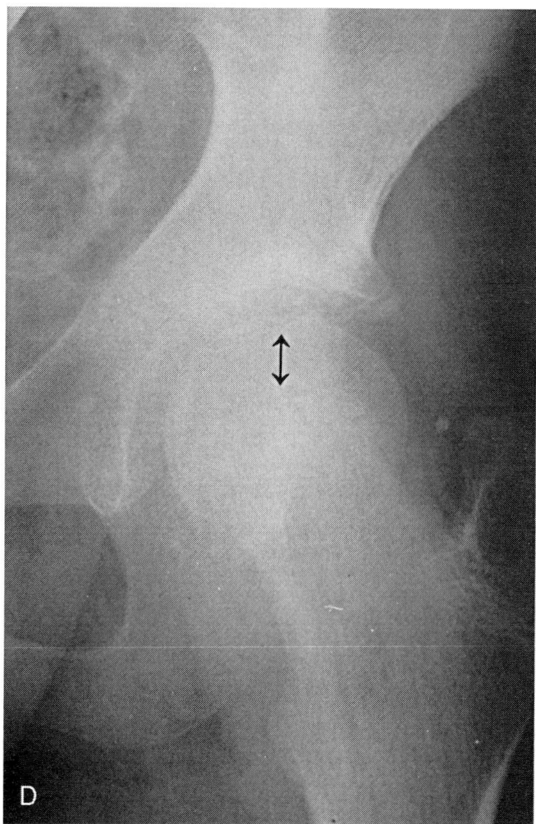

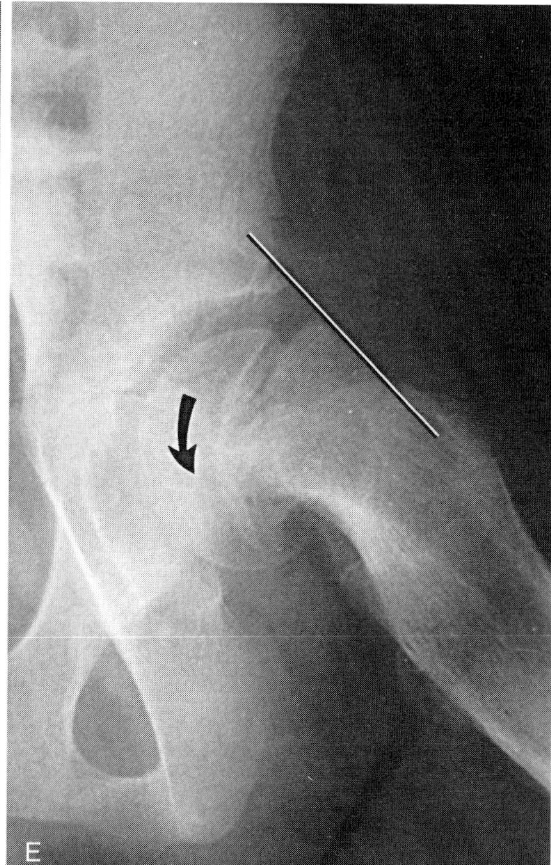

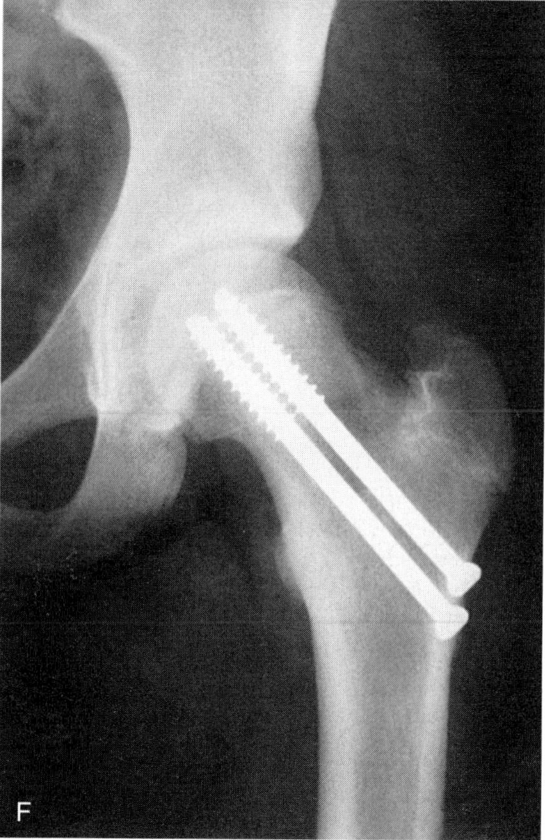

FIGURE 7–15 *Continued.* D, E This 9-year-old girl had knee pain and a limp. In D, a frontal radiograph reveals a decrease in the vertical height of the capital femoral epiphysis (double-headed arrow) but no visible misalignment because the displacement occurred predominantly in a posterior direction. In E, a lateral frog-leg projection rotates the femur, revealing medial and posterior migration of the epiphysis in the direction of the curved arrow. A line constructed along the outer margin of the femoral neck (Klein's line) should intersect the epiphysis. In this case, the line does not intersect the epiphysis. F In a fourth patient, orthopedic lag screws have been inserted in an attempt to facilitate fusion of the epiphysis to the metaphysis and to avoid further slippage. *(D–F, From Taylor JAM, Harger BL, Resnick D: Diagnostic imaging of common hip disorders: A pictorial review. Top Clin Chiropr 1:8, 1994.)*

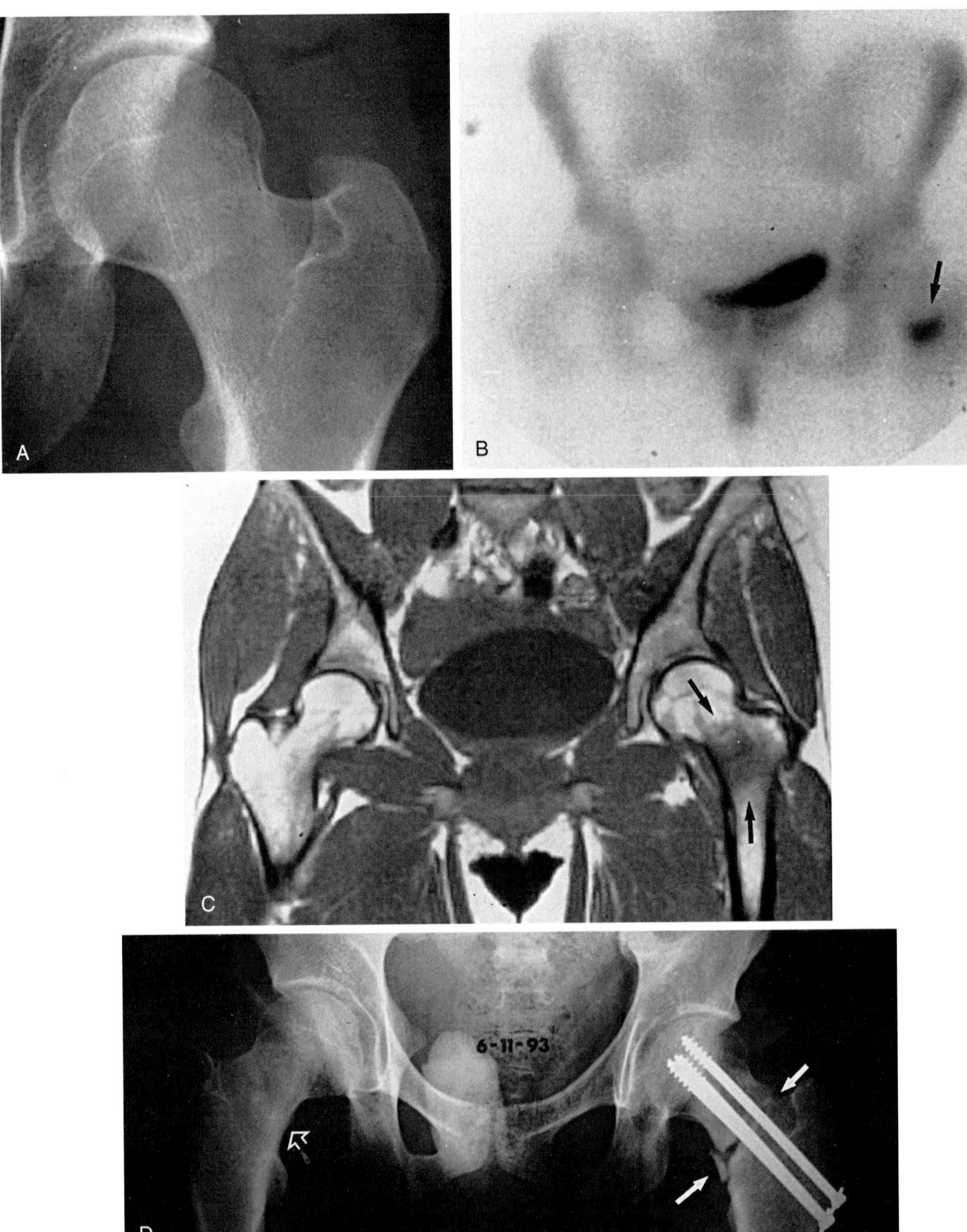

FIGURE 7–16. Stress (fatigue) fracture: Femoral neck.[23, 24] A–C This runner developed hip pain. In A, a frontal radiograph shows a radiodense line across the medial aspect of the femoral neck. In B, a bone scan obtained at the same time as the radiograph shows a zone of increased uptake of radionuclide corresponding to the fracture site (arrow). C A coronal T1-weighted (TR/TE, 500/15) spin echo magnetic resonance (MR) image demonstrates low signal intensity at the fracture site due to compression of bone and surrounding marrow edema (arrows). D Another patient. This military recruit developed bilateral stress fractures from repeated marching. The problem went undiagnosed, resulting in a complete fracture through the left femoral neck (arrows). The fracture was repaired with lag screws. A zone of sclerosis (open arrow) in the contralateral femoral neck represents the other stress fracture. (D, *From Taylor JAM, Harger BL, Resnick D: Diagnostic imaging of common hip disorders: A pictorial review. Top Clin Chiropr 1:8, 1994.* D, *Courtesy of G. S. Huang, M.D., Taipei, Taiwan.)*

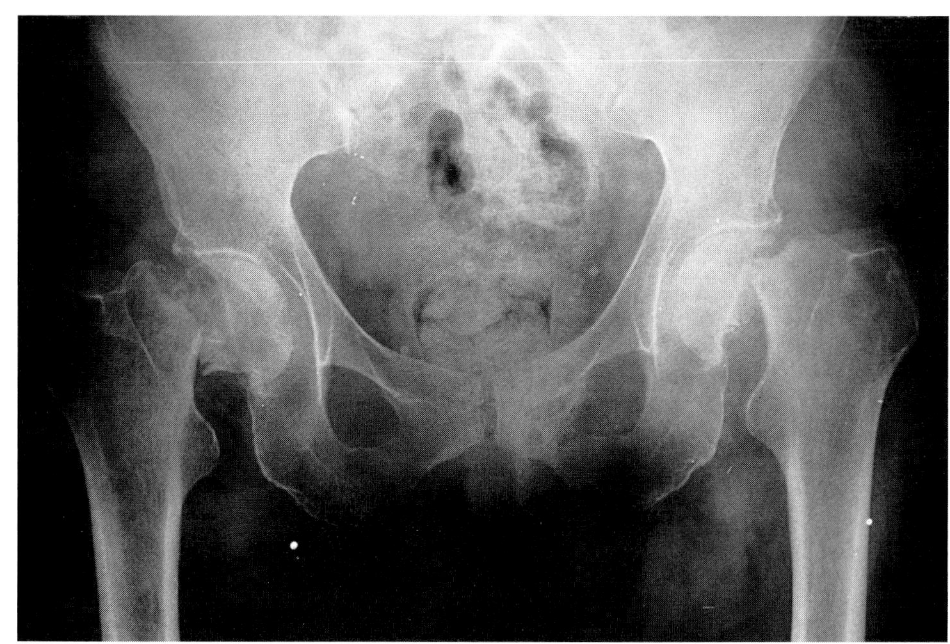

FIGURE 7–17. Stress (insufficiency) fractures.[25] In this 62-year-old woman with long-standing rheumatoid arthritis, bilateral insufficiency fractures have resulted in displacement and varus deformities. *(Courtesy of V. Vint, M.D., La Jolla, California.)*

TABLE 7–8. Classification of Fractures of the Proximal Portion of the Femur

Entity	Characteristics
A. Classified according to fracture type[79]	
Major trauma	Major direct forces along the shaft of the femur with or without a rotational component
Insufficiency fracture	Most common in elderly patients, especially women, with osteoporosis
Pathologic fracture	Uncommon Patients with skeletal metastasis, Paget's disease, and other pathologic disorders of bone
Fatigue fracture	Uncommon Young athletes
B. Classified according to anatomic location[79]	
Intracapsular fractures	Twice as common as extracapsular fractures
Subcapital	Immediately beneath the articular surface of the femoral head at the head-neck junction (Fig. 7–18)
Transcervical	Across the middle of the femoral neck
Basicervical	Across the base of the femoral neck
Extracapsular fractures	
Intertrochanteric	Across a line between the greater and lesser trochanters
Subtrochanteric	Below the intertrochanteric line
C. Classified according to degree of displacement, instability, or extent of fracture	
Intracapsular fractures[80]	*Garden system* Classified according to displacement
Type I	Incomplete or impacted fracture
Type II	Complete fracture without osseous displacement
Type III	Complete fracture with partial displacement of fracture fragments commonly associated with shortening and external rotation of the distal fragments
Type IV	Complete fracture with total displacement of the fragments
Intertrochanteric fractures[81]	*Evans's system* Classified according to the presence or absence of stability and ease of fracture reduction
Type I	Stable fractures (50 per cent) Absence of comminution of medial cortices of the proximal and distal fragments and absence of displacement of the lesser trochanter
Type II	Unstable fractures (50 per cent) 1. Fractures with reversed obliquity and marked tendency toward medial displacement of the femoral shaft due to adductor muscle pull or to comminution of the greater trochanter and adjacent posterolateral surface of the shaft 2. Fractures in which there is absence of contact between the proximal and distal fragments due to comminution or medial and posterior displacement of fracture fragments
Subtrochanteric fractures[82]	*Seinsheimer's system* Classified according to the extent of the fracture and the configuration of fracture lines
Type I	Nondisplaced fracture
Type II	Two-part fracture
Type III	Three-part fracture
Type IV	Comminuted fracture with four or more fragments
Type V	Combined subtrochanteric and intertrochanteric fractures

*See also Tables 1–3 and 1–4.

TABLE 7–9. Complications of Fractures of the Proximal Portion of the Femur*

Entity	Figure(s)	Complications	Characteristic
Intracapsular fractures[80]	7–19	Delayed union	Under normal circumstances, these fractures show evidence of healing in the first 6 months, and fractures that remain ununited beyond that time are considered delayed union
		Nonunion	Fractures that do not unite after 12 months are considered nonunion fractures 5–25 per cent of cases *Predisposing factors for delayed union and nonunion* Advancing age Osteoporosis Posterior comminution of fracture Inadequate reduction Poor internal fixation technique
		Osteonecrosis	10–30 per cent of cases *Predisposing factors for osteonecrosis* Moderate or severe displacement of fracture fragments Persistent motion with inadequate stabilization Increased intracapsular pressure from hemarthrosis Vascular injury to femoral head during trauma or attempts at reduction
		Thromboembolism	
		Postoperative infection	
Intertrochanteric fractures[81]	7–20	Varus deformity	Nonsurgical and occurring after failed internal fixation
		Secondary subcapital fracture	Occurring after internal fixation of intertrochanteric fracture
		Vessel injury	Laceration of adjacent vessels
		Nonunion	Uncommon
		Osteonecrosis	Uncommon Fewer than 1 per cent of cases
Subtrochanteric fractures[82]		Delayed union	
		Nonunion	
		Implant failure	

*See also Tables 1–3 to 1–5.

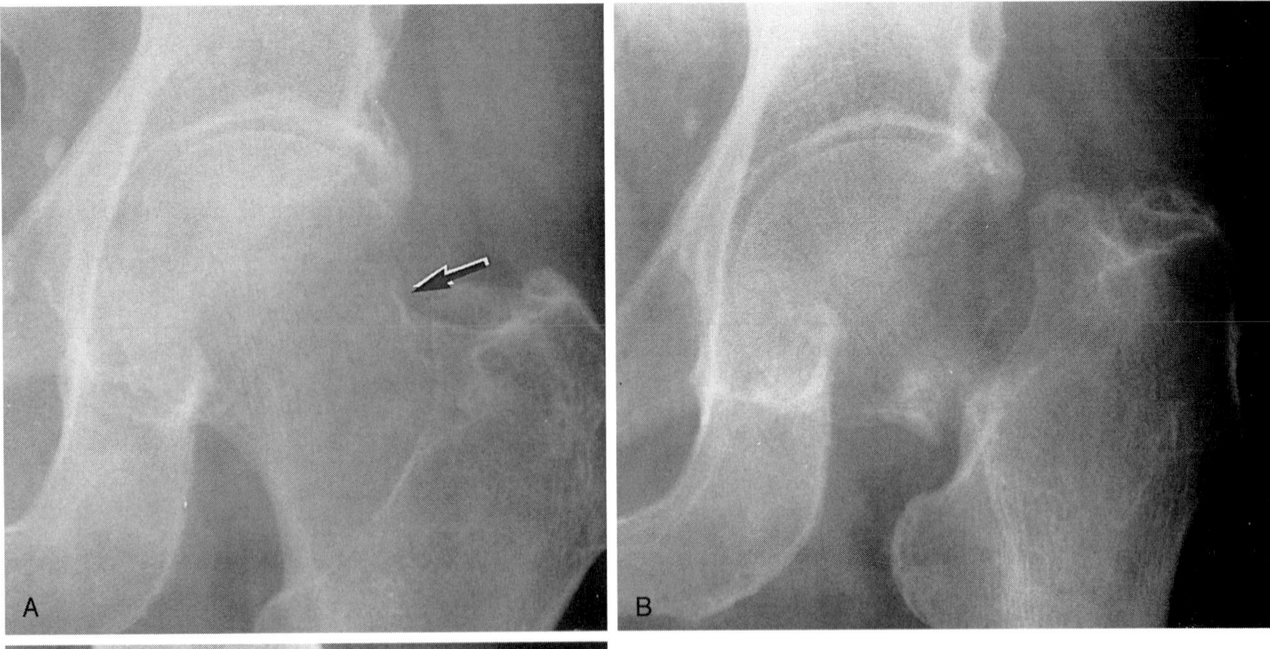

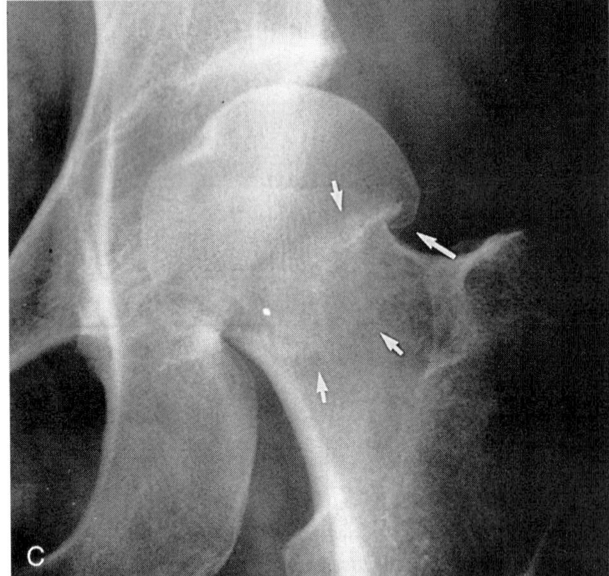

FIGURE 7–18. Intracapsular fractures of the femoral neck: Radiologic diagnosis.[26, 27, 80] **A, B** This 74-year-old osteoporotic woman sustained a minor fall. In **A,** a radiograph obtained on the day of injury reveals a subtle offset of the subcapital cortex at the head-neck junction that initially was overlooked. In **B,** a radiograph obtained 3 weeks later shows a complete intracapsular fracture, extensive resorption and rotation at the fracture site, and marked varus deformity. **C** In another patient, a 51-year-old woman, observe the impaction and valgus deformity at the site of this subcapital fracture (arrows). Slight offset in the cortex and cortical bone impaction often are difficult to see on routine radiographs.

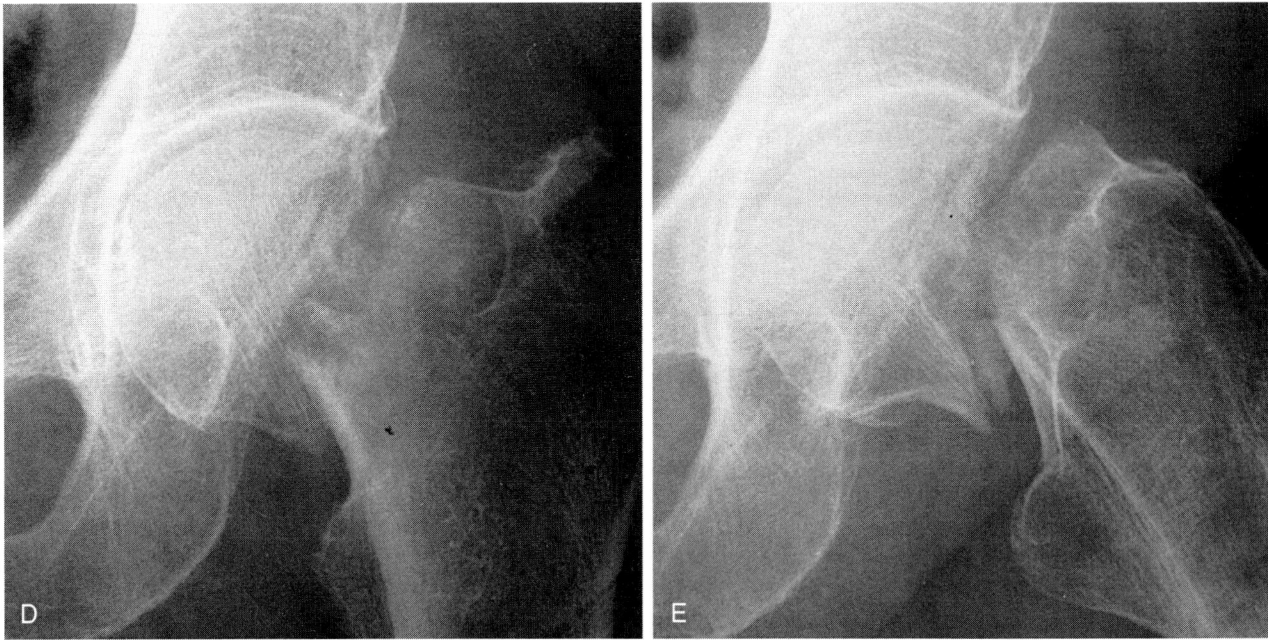

FIGURE 7–18 *Continued.* D, E 87-year-old woman. Frontal (D) and frog-leg (E) projections reveal a displaced intracapsular fracture. Magnetic resonance (MR) imaging and scintigraphy often are helpful in the early diagnosis of occult hip fractures. The radiographic appearance of subcapital fractures of the femoral neck unrelated to neoplasm often is similar to that of pathologic fractures. This appearance is caused primarily by rotation of the fracture fragments, and the finding is accentuated by displacement.

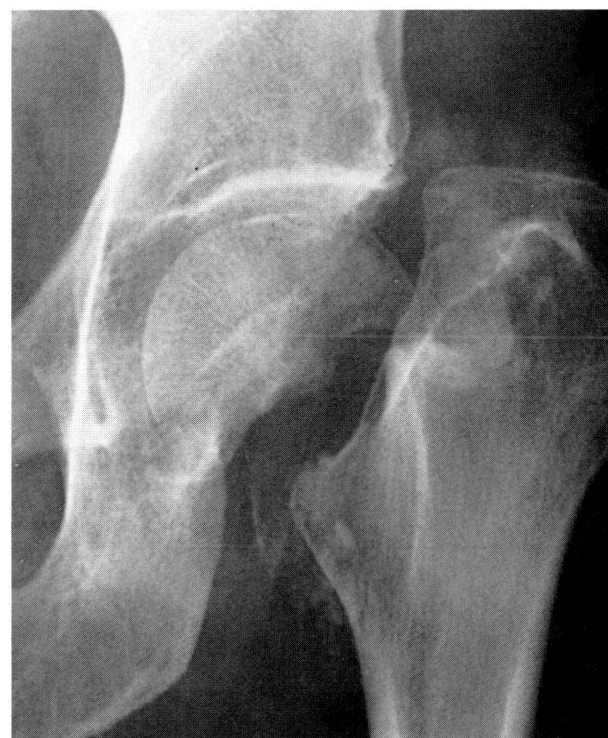

FIGURE 7–19. Intracapsular femoral neck fracture with nonunion and osteolysis.[28] Observe osteolysis of the femoral neck in this 71-year-old man with an ununited subcapital fracture. Osseous debris is seen within and around the fracture cleft, and rotation is evident at the fracture site.

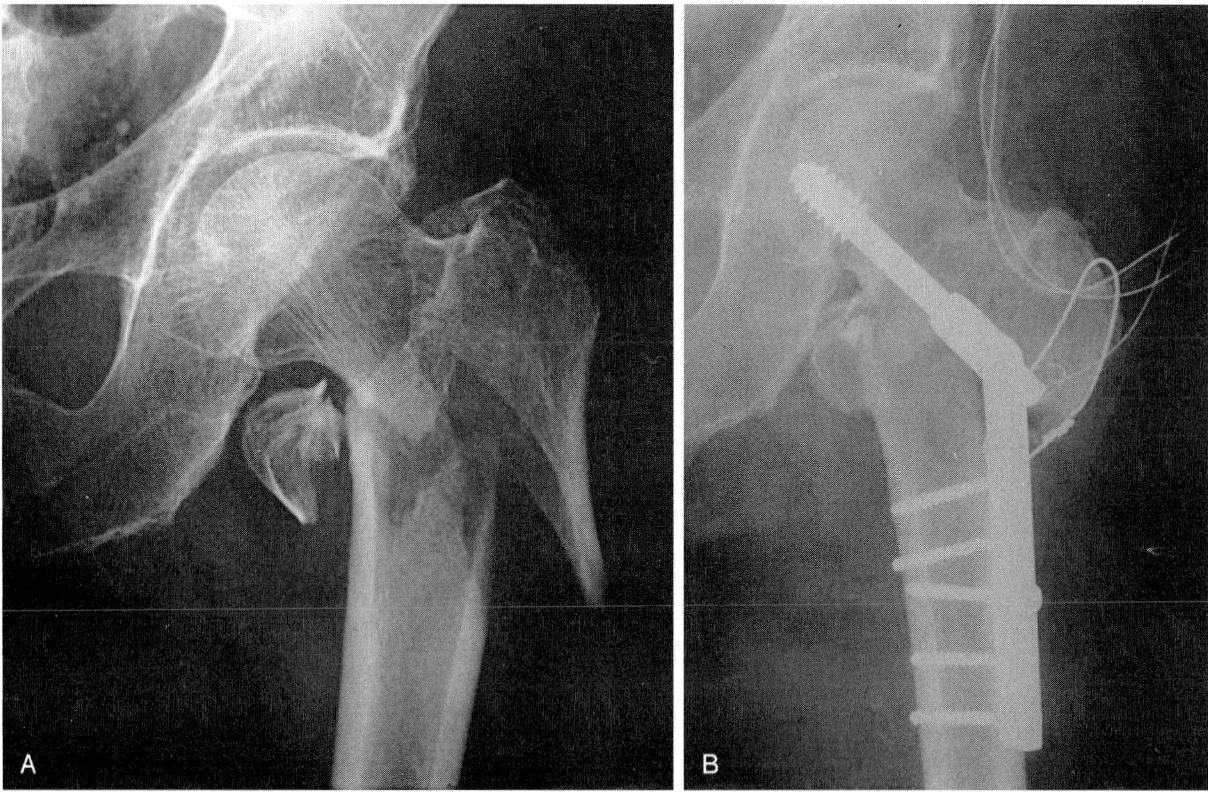

FIGURE 7–20. Intertrochanteric fracture. Surgical repair.[29] A An unstable type II comminuted intertrochanteric fracture is seen in this 69-year-old man. Marked displacement of both trochanters is evident. B A dynamic (sliding) compression screw has been used to provide fixation while allowing impaction to occur at the fracture during healing and weight-bearing. Intertrochanteric fractures predominate in elderly patients and usually result from falls.

TABLE 7–10. Articular Disorders Affecting the Hip*

Entity	Figure(s)	Characteristics
Degenerative and related disorders		
Osteoarthrosis[30–32]	7–21	*Radiographic findings* Osteophytes Subchondral sclerosis Subchondral cysts Subluxation Buttressing Intra-articular bodies: infrequently secondary synovial osteochondromatosis See Table 1–6 for causes of secondary osteoarthrosis of the hip
Diffuse idiopathic skeletal hyperostosis (DISH)[33]	7–22	Enthesopathy and ligament ossification about the acetabulum, ischiopubic region, and lesser trochanters DISH typically does not result in joint space narrowing of the hip
Inflammatory disorders		
Rheumatoid arthritis[34, 35]	7–23, 7–24	Hip involvement common in rheumatoid arthritis *Radiographic findings* Bilateral symmetric, concentric joint space narrowing with axial migration of femoral head Subchondral erosion Absent or mild sclerosis Periarticular osteoporosis Synovial cysts
Juvenile chronic arthritis[34]		Diffuse joint space loss with concentric narrowing, periarticular osteoporosis, and erosions of the femoral head and acetabulum

TABLE 7–10. Articular Disorders Affecting the Hip* *Continued*

Entity	Figure(s)	Characteristics
Ankylosing spondylitis[36]	7–25	Bilateral symmetric, concentric joint space narrowing with axial migration of the femoral heads Osteophytosis about the superolateral aspect of the femoral head may lead to a collar surrounding the head-neck junction Acetabular and femoral cysts, periarticular osteoporosis, mild acetabular protrusion; may eventually result in partial or complete intra-articular osseous ankylosis
Psoriatic arthropathy and Reiter's syndrome[37]	7–26	Hip involvement similar to but less frequent than in ankylosing spondylitis
Dermatomyositis and polymyositis[38]	7–27	Widespread sheetlike calcification in soft tissues surrounding pelvis and hip region
Progressive systemic sclerosis (scleroderma)[39]	7–28	Globular accumulations of periarticular soft tissue calcinosis
Systemic lupus erythematosus (SLE)[40]	7–29, See Fig. 7–57	Osteonecrosis of the femoral head occurs in SLE patients treated with corticosteroid therapy; also occurs in SLE patients not treated with steroid medication, possibly because of vasculitis
Mixed connective tissue disease[40]	7–29	Mixed connective tissue diseases and overlap syndromes Diseases include combinations of rheumatoid arthritis, dermatomyositis, scleroderma, systemic lupus erythematosus, or scleroderma Radiographic features variable; may result in diffuse joint space narrowing, erosions, soft tissue calcinosis, and acetabular protrusion
Crystal deposition and metabolic disorders		
Calcium pyrophosphate dihydrate (CPPD)[41, 42]	7–30	Articular space narrowing, sclerosis, cyst formation, osteophytes, as well as intra-articular and periarticular chondrocalcinosis Acetabular protrusion and considerable femoral head destruction and fragmentation resembling neuropathic osteoarthropathy may occur in severe cases
Calcific bursitis and tendinitis[43]	7–31	Calcium hydroxyapatite crystal deposition in tendons and bursae about the hip Single or multiple cloud-like linear, triangular, or circular soft tissue calcifications at the gluteal insertions in the greater trochanter and surrounding bursae; also adjacent to acetabular margin, lesser trochanter, and proximal portion of femur Occasionally, large tumor-like accumulations of calcification will also be seen about the hip in patients with chronic renal disease or collagen vascular disorders
Rapidly destructive hip disease[44]	7–32	Cause is unclear; believed to be related to a generalized process such as osteonecrosis or intra-articular deposition of calcium hydroxyapatite crystals Severe, rapid atrophic destruction of femoral head resembling septic arthritis
Gouty arthropathy[45]	7–33	Rare hip involvement Periarticular erosions predominate; soft tissue tophi may be identified
Hemochromatosis[46]	7–34	Rare disorder exhibiting findings identical to those of CPPD crystal deposition disease with prominent chondrocalcinosis
Alkaptonuria[47]	7–35	Rare hip joint involvement Accelerated degenerative disease, chondrocalcinosis, diffuse joint space narrowing, sclerosis, fragmentation, osteophytosis, mild acetabular protrusion, and eventual femoral head remodeling
Infection		
Pyogenic septic arthritis[48, 49]	7–36, 7–37	*Radiographic findings in adult septic arthritis of the hip* Rapid concentric loss of joint space Periarticular osteoporosis Loss of definition and destruction of subchondral bone Capsular distention Erosions *Radiographic findings in neonatal and childhood septic arthritis of the hip* Soft tissue swelling or capsular distention Pathologic subluxation or dislocation: lateral displacement of ossification center Slipped capital femoral epiphysis Metaphyseal osteomyelitis Concentric loss of joint space

Table continued on following page

TABLE 7–10. Articular Disorders Affecting the Hip* *Continued*

Entity	Figure(s)	Characteristics
Tuberculous arthritis[50]	7–38	Phemister's triad: juxta-articular osteoporosis, peripherally located erosions, gradual joint space narrowing Various degrees of soft tissue swelling Subchondral erosions Periarticular abscess
Miscellaneous disorders		
Neurologic injury: heterotopic ossification[51, 52]	7–39	Periarticular soft tissue ossification in paraplegic and quadriplegic patients Begins as poorly defined opaque areas; typically progresses to large accumulations possessing trabeculae and often results in complete osseous ankylosis
Idiopathic chondrolysis of the hip[53]	7–40	Idiopathic monoarticular disorder seen mainly in adolescents, especially African Americans; also seen in children with slipped capital femoral epiphysis *Clinical findings* Pain, restriction of motion, stiffness, absence of trauma history, aspiration fails to reveal presence of effusion or organisms *Radiographic findings* Osteoporosis, diffuse joint space narrowing, erosion of subchondral bone
Pigmented villonodular synovitis[54, 55]	7–41	Cystic erosions on both sides of the joint Hemorrhagic joint effusion Eventual osteoporosis Well preserved joint space until late in the disease Extra-articular process termed giant cell tumor of the tendon sheath may be related to pigmented villonodular synovitis
Idiopathic synovial osteochondromatosis[56–58]	7–42	Multiple intra-articular or periarticular collections of calcification or ossification of variable size and density Erosion of adjacent bone Secondary osteoarthrosis Noncalcified bodies are best demonstrated with arthrography or (MR) imaging Secondary synovial osteochondromatosis may occur as a result of degenerative joint disease

*See also Tables 1–6 to 1–9 and Table 1–17.

TABLE 7–11. Hip Joint Disorders: Typical Patterns of Joint Space Narrowing

	Joint Compartment			Symmetry		
Entity	*Superior*	*Medial*	*Axial*	*Unilateral*	*Bilateral Asymmetric*	*Bilateral Symmetric*
Osteoarthrosis	+	Rare		+	+	
Calcium pyrophosphate dihydrate (CPPD) crystal deposition disease	Rare		+		+	+
Rheumatoid arthritis	Rare		+			+
Juvenile chronic arthritis	Rare		+			+
Osteonecrosis (late in disease process)	+		+	+	+	
Ankylosing spondylitis	Rare		+			+
Psoriatic arthropathy and Reiter's syndrome			+		+	
Neuropathic osteoarthropathy	Rare	+	+	+	+	
Septic arthritis			+	+		
Idiopathic chondrolysis of the hip			+	+		
Alkaptonuria			+		+	+
Hemophilia			+		+	+
Osteomalacia		+	+			+
Paget's disease with secondary joint degeneration	+	+	+	+	+	

+, Predominant pattern(s); Rare, less common patterns.

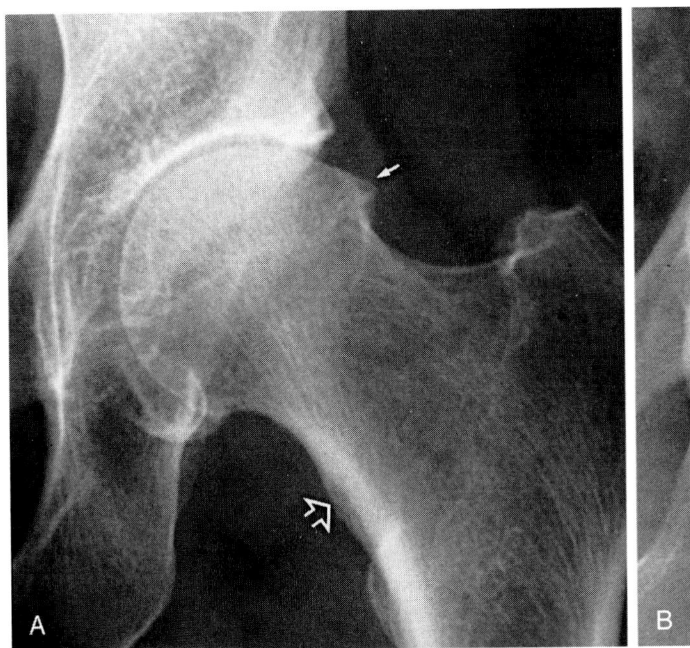

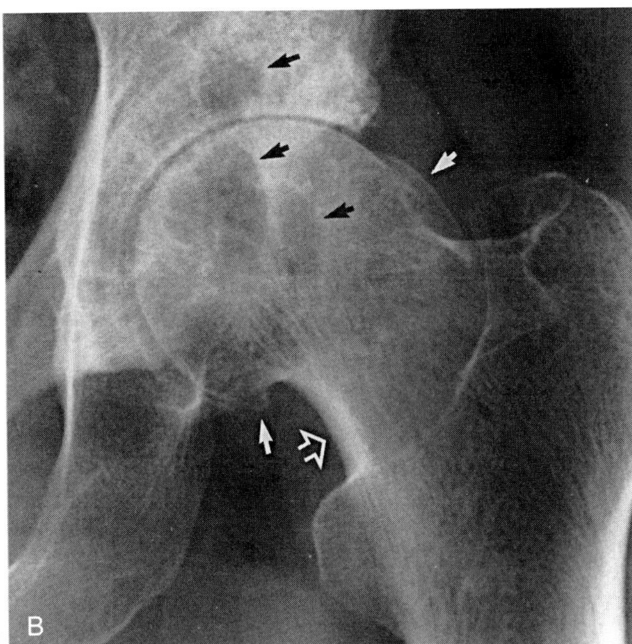

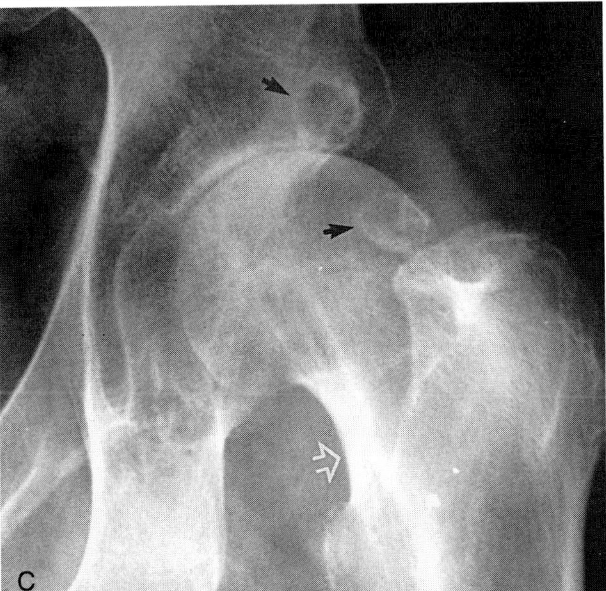

FIGURE 7–21. Osteoarthrosis: Spectrum of abnormalities.[30–32] A–D Radiographic changes of hip joint osteoarthrosis include joint space narrowing (predominantly in the superior compartment), osteophytes (white arrows), subchondral cysts (black arrows), subchondral sclerosis, and buttressing of the medial femoral neck (open arrows). In **A**, mild changes are evident. In **B**, moderate changes include more severe joint space narrowing and circumferential osteophytes at the head-neck junction (white arrows), buttressing of the femoral neck, and subchondral cysts. All of these changes are more prominent in this patient with advanced disease. In **C**, moderate changes in another patient consist of subchondral cysts, which are a prominent feature on this radiograph.

Illustration continued on following page

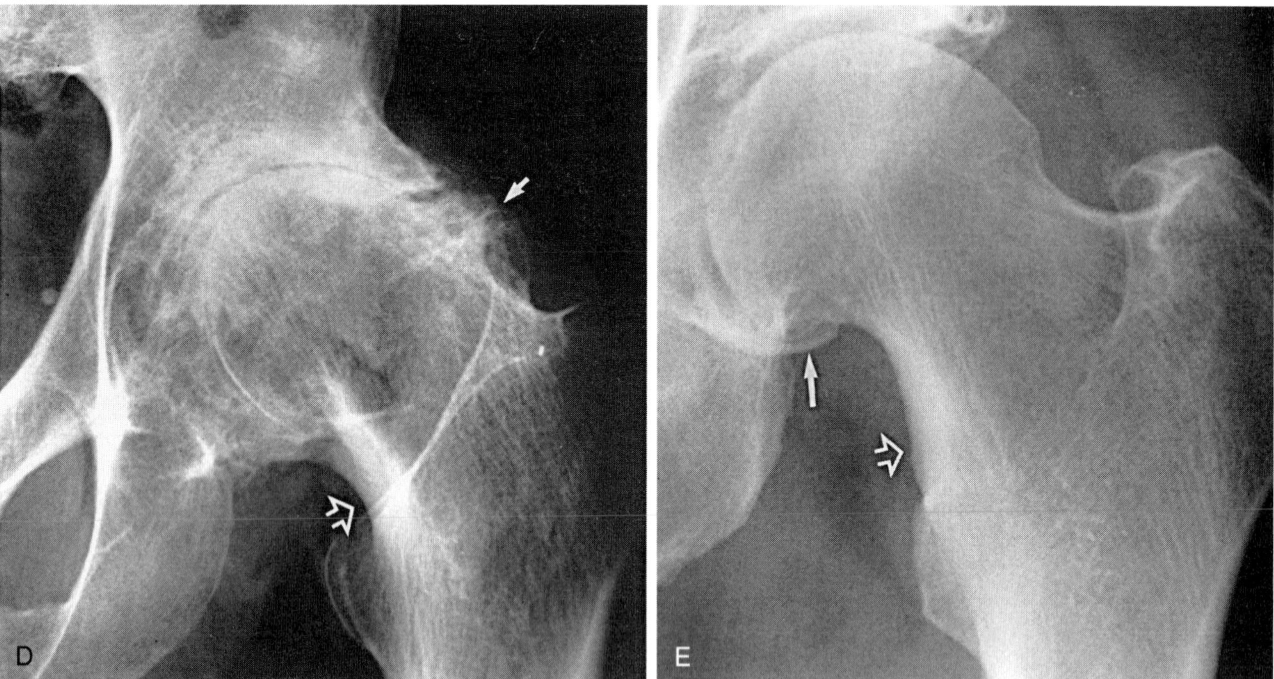

FIGURE 7–21 *Continued.* D Severe changes. Severe sclerosis, osteophyte formation, joint space obliteration, and medial buttressing are evident. E Buttressing. Observe the prominent sclerosis and hypertrophy of the medial cortex of the femoral neck (open arrow), a finding that most frequently accompanies degenerative joint disease. Buttressing also may be apparent in osteonecrosis, developmental acetabular dysplasia, rheumatoid arthritis, and ankylosing spondylitis. It likewise may be seen adjacent to an osteoid osteoma. An osteophytic rim is evident surrounding the acetabulum (arrow).

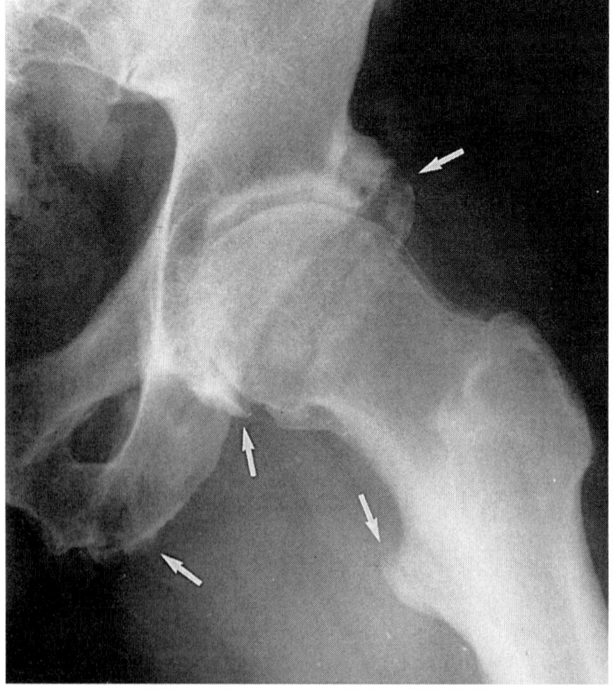

FIGURE 7–22. Diffuse idiopathic skeletal hyperostosis (DISH).[33] Observe the hypertrophic periarticular enthesopathy (arrows) affecting the acetabular, ischiopubic, and lesser trochanteric regions in this patient with long-standing DISH. Evidence of degenerative joint disease also is present.

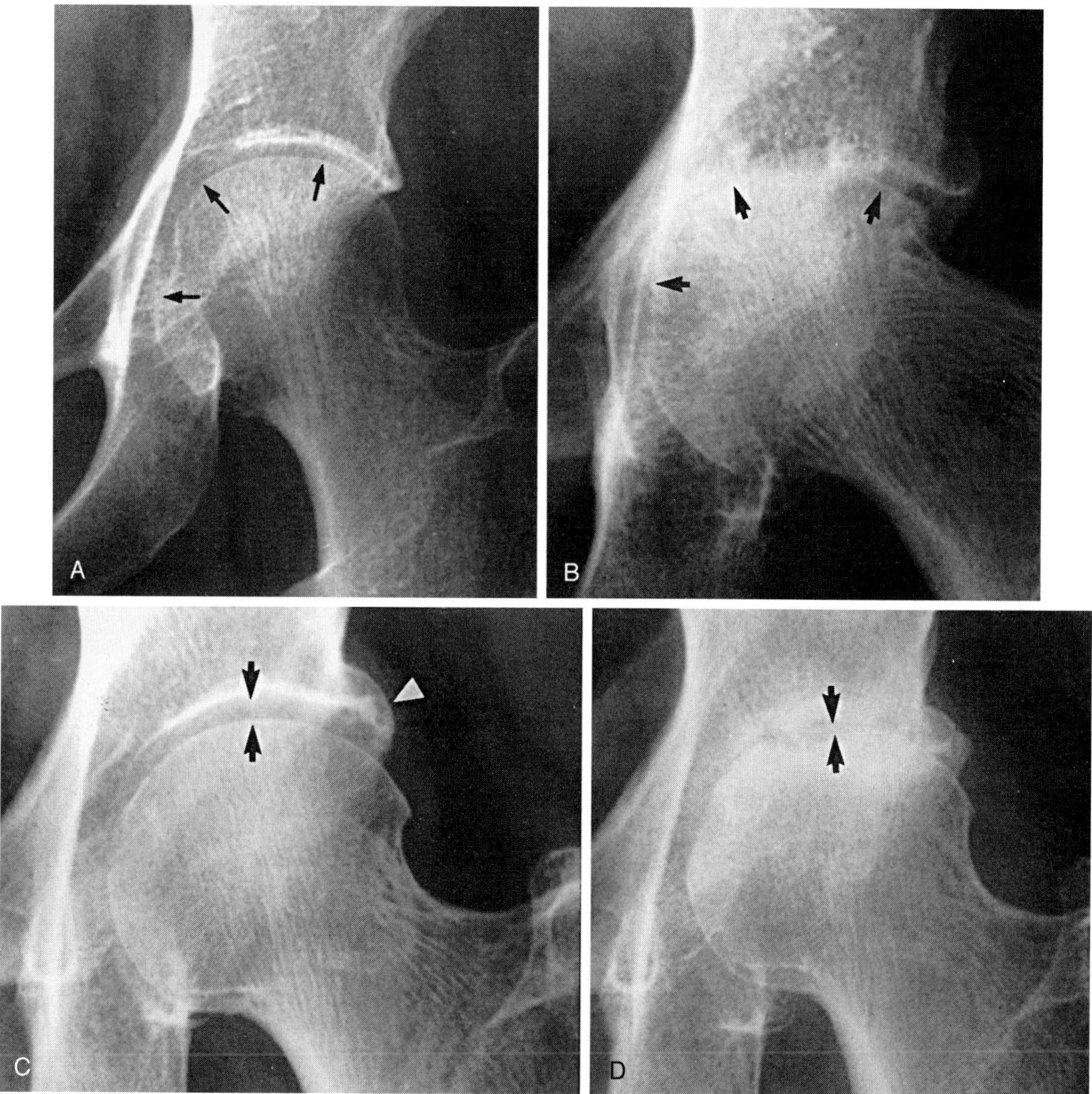

FIGURE 7–23. Rheumatoid arthritis: Hip abnormalities.[34] A Early changes. Uniform (concentric) joint space narrowing has resulted in axial migration of the femoral head in relation to the acetabulum (arrows). These changes were bilateral and symmetric. This is the most characteristic pattern of joint space narrowing in the hip in patients with rheumatoid arthritis. B Advanced changes. This man with rheumatoid arthritis had bilateral symmetric involvement (opposite hip not shown) with severe axial migration and joint space obliteration (arrows). Periarticular osteopenia and absence of productive changes, such as osteophytes and sclerosis, are characteristic signs of this inflammatory synovial process. C, D Progressive changes: Serial radiographs. In C, an initial radiograph shows early uniform joint space narrowing (arrows). An acetabular osteophyte (arrowhead) relates to superimposed degenerative joint disease. In D, a radiograph taken 5 years later demonstrates progressive joint space narrowing (arrows), subchondral erosions, and sclerosis.

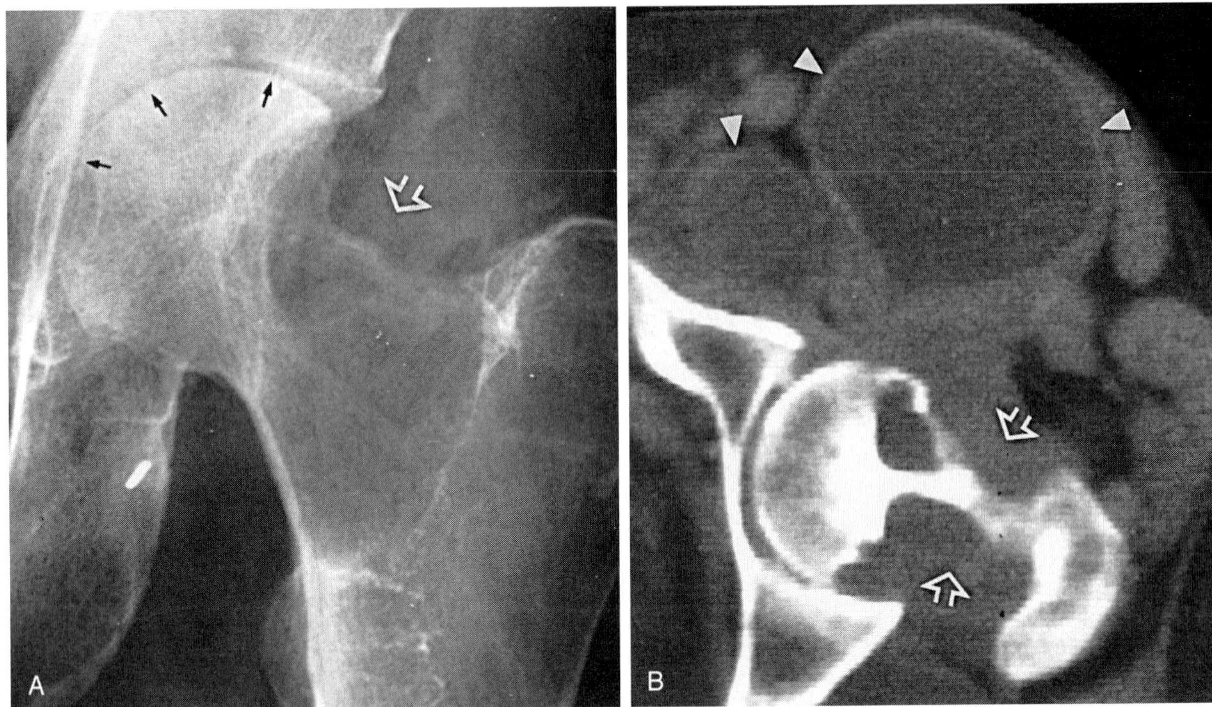

FIGURE 7–24. Rheumatoid arthritis: Synovial cyst.[35] A 54-year-old man with long-standing rheumatoid arthritis and a mass in the groin. **A** Anteroposterior radiograph shows extensive scalloped osteolytic destruction of the femoral neck (open arrow). Uniform loss of joint space with axial migration of the femoral head also is present (arrows). **B** Transaxial computed tomographic (CT) scan at the level of the femoral neck reveals a synovial cyst that is seen as two circular fluid-filled outpouchings (arrowheads) anterior to the femur. Osseous destruction of the femoral neck (open arrows) and diffuse joint space narrowing also are evident. *(Courtesy of J. Scavulli, M.D., San Diego, California.)*

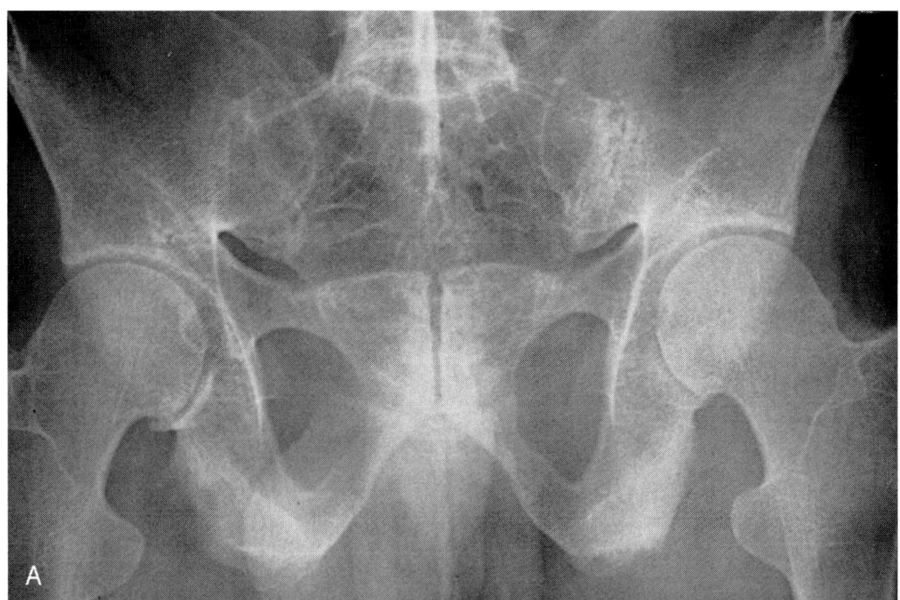

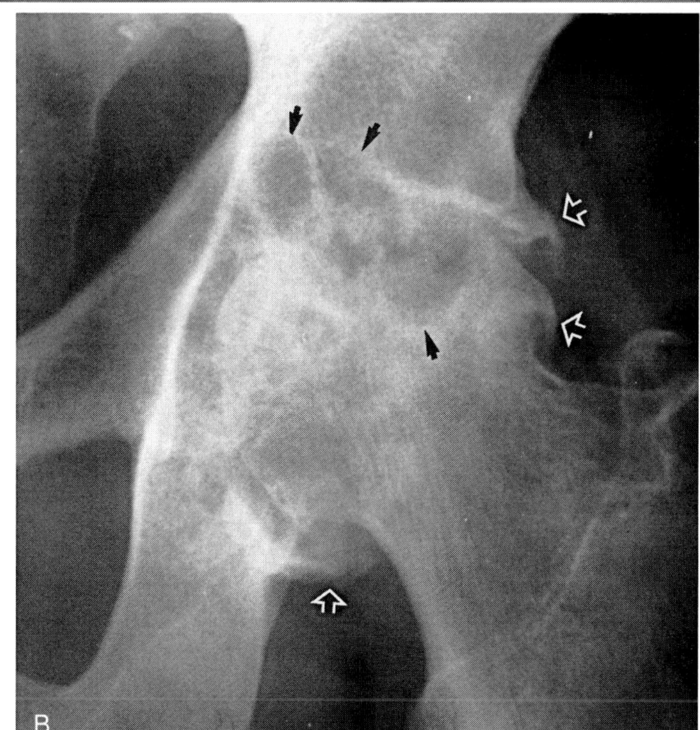

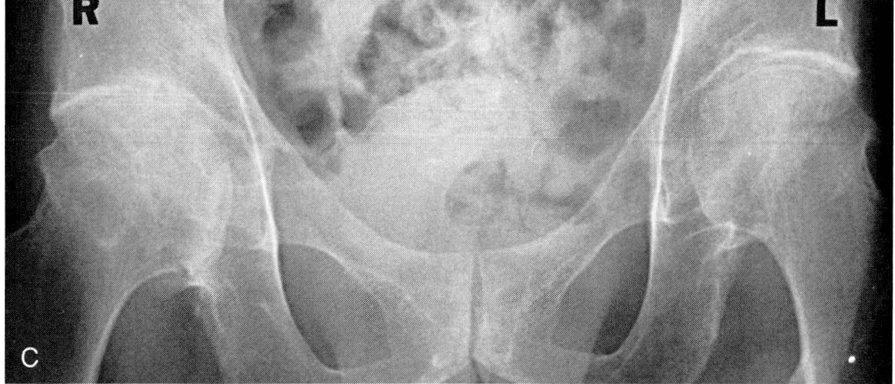

FIGURE 7–25. Ankylosing spondylitis.[36] **A** A pelvic radiograph from this 36-year-old man with long-standing ankylosing spondylitis reveals bilateral concentric narrowing of the hip joint spaces. Observe also the presence of enthesopathy adjacent to both ischial tuberosities. The sacroiliac joints are ankylosed. *(***A***, Courtesy of M.N. Pathria, M.D., San Diego, California.)* **B** In another patient with concentric loss of joint space and prominent osteophytes (open arrows), large subchondral cysts are present in the femoral head and acetabulum (arrows). **C** Bilateral, relatively symmetric involvement of both hips in a 47-year-old man with a 20-year history of ankylosing spondylitis. Observe the concentric decrease of joint space, osteophyte formation, and subchondral cyst formation that predominate on the right side. Hip involvement in ankylosing spondylitis is common and exhibits a bilateral symmetric pattern in more than 75 per cent of cases.

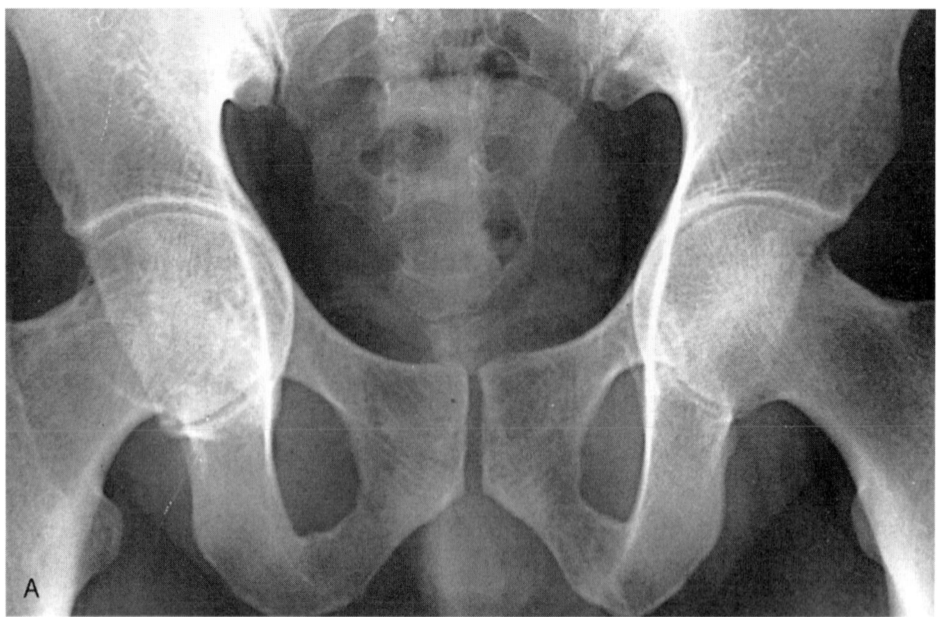

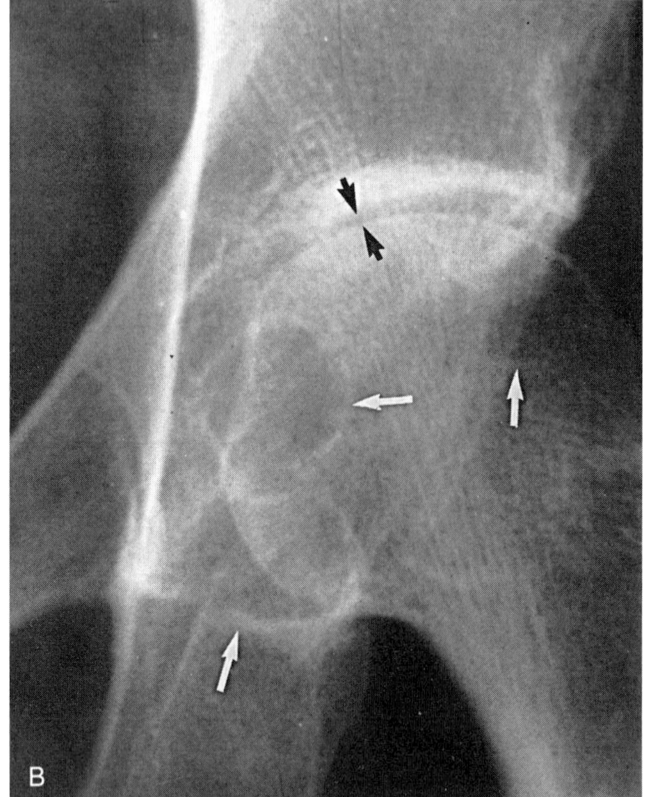

FIGURE 7–26. Psoriatic arthropathy.[37] A This patient with psoriatic skin lesions and polyarticular inflammatory disease of long duration demonstrates axial migration of the femoral heads and early acetabular protrusion. B Diffuse axial loss of joint space (black arrows) and large subchondral cysts (white arrows) are present in this patient with chronic psoriasis of the skin and joints.

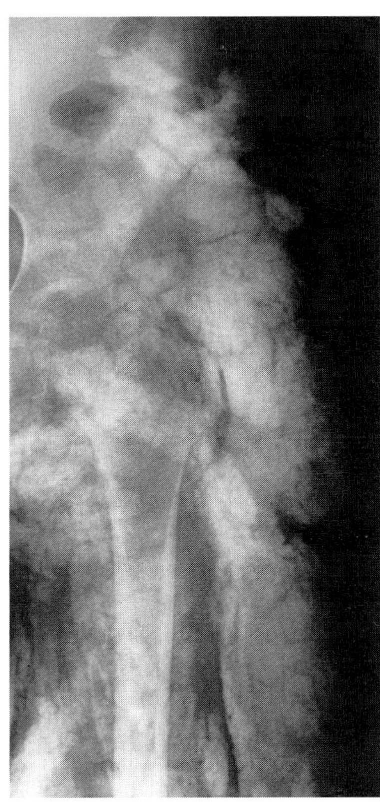

FIGURE 7–27. Dermatomyositis-polymyositis.[38] Bizarre globular calcification is present within the muscles and subcutaneous tissues of the upper thigh and hip region in this 9-year-old boy with dermatomyositis-polymyositis. *(Courtesy of T. Broderick, M.D., Orange, California.)*

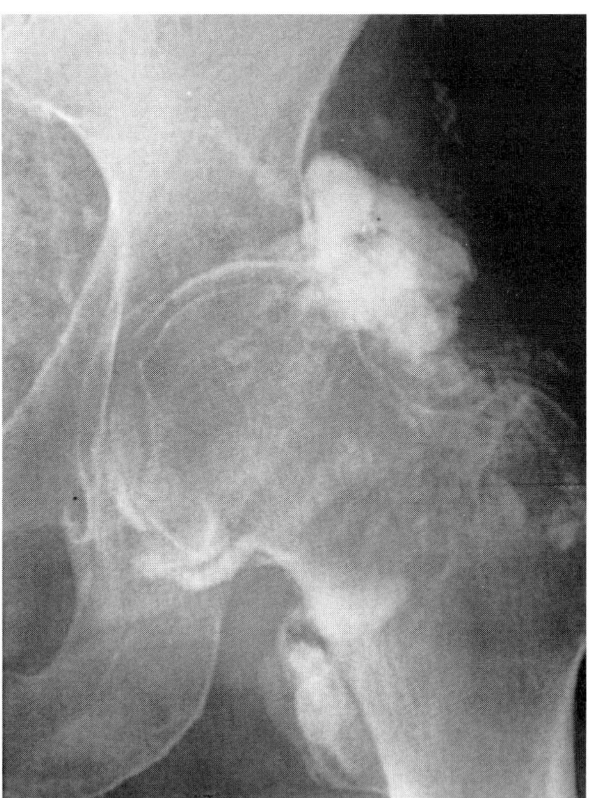

FIGURE 7–28. Progressive systemic sclerosis (scleroderma).[39] Extensive globular accumulations of periarticular soft tissue calcification are seen adjacent to the hip joint. Concentric joint space narrowing is evident. *(Courtesy of A. Nemcek, M.D., Chicago, Illinois, and L. Rogers, Winston-Salem, North Carolina.)*

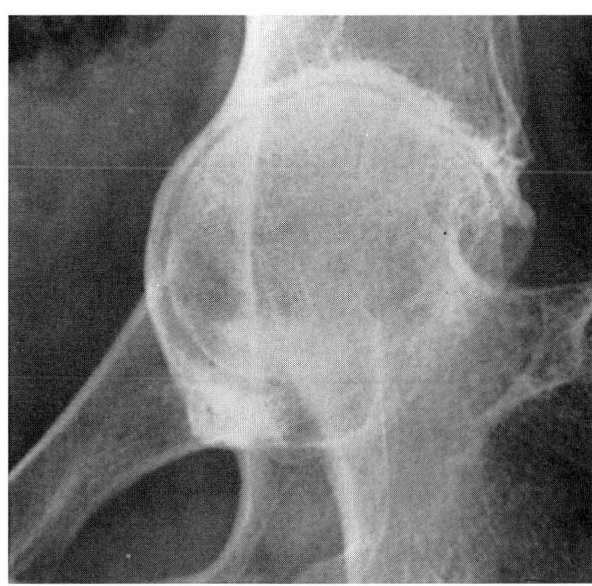

FIGURE 7–29. Collagen vascular disease: Overlap syndrome.[40] A patient with juvenile chronic arthritis subsequently developed classic systemic lupus erythematosus as an adult. Observe the symmetric joint space narrowing typical of inflammatory arthritis. Protrusio acetabuli also is seen. *(Courtesy of V. Vint, M.D., San Diego, California.)*

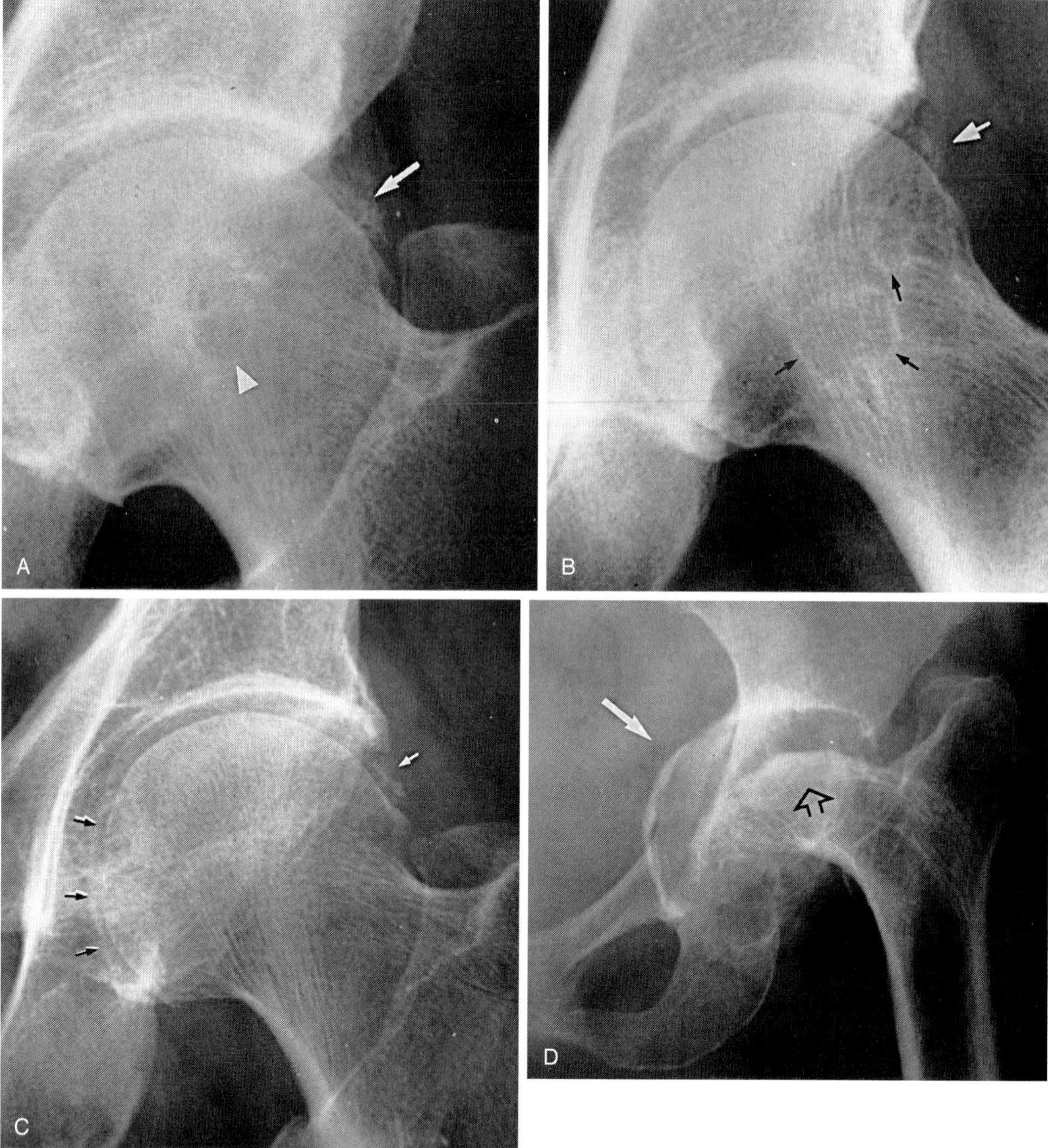

FIGURE 7–30. Calcium pyrophosphate dihydrate (CPPD) crystal deposition disease.[41, 42] A Chondrocalcinosis of the hyaline cartilage of the hip (arrow), as in this patient, is found in about 45 per cent of patients with CPPD crystal deposition disease. Observe also the subchondral cyst in the femoral head (arrowhead) and the joint space narrowing. B In another patient, subtle chondrocalcinosis (white arrow) and subchondral cysts (black arrows) are apparent. *(B, Courtesy of G. Greenway, M.D., Dallas, Texas.)* C In a 76-year-old man, chondrocalcinosis is evident (arrows). Medial and axial joint space narrowing is noted. D This 80-year-old woman has severe acetabular protrusion (arrow) and dramatic femoral head destruction (open arrow) secondary to pyrophosphate arthropathy.

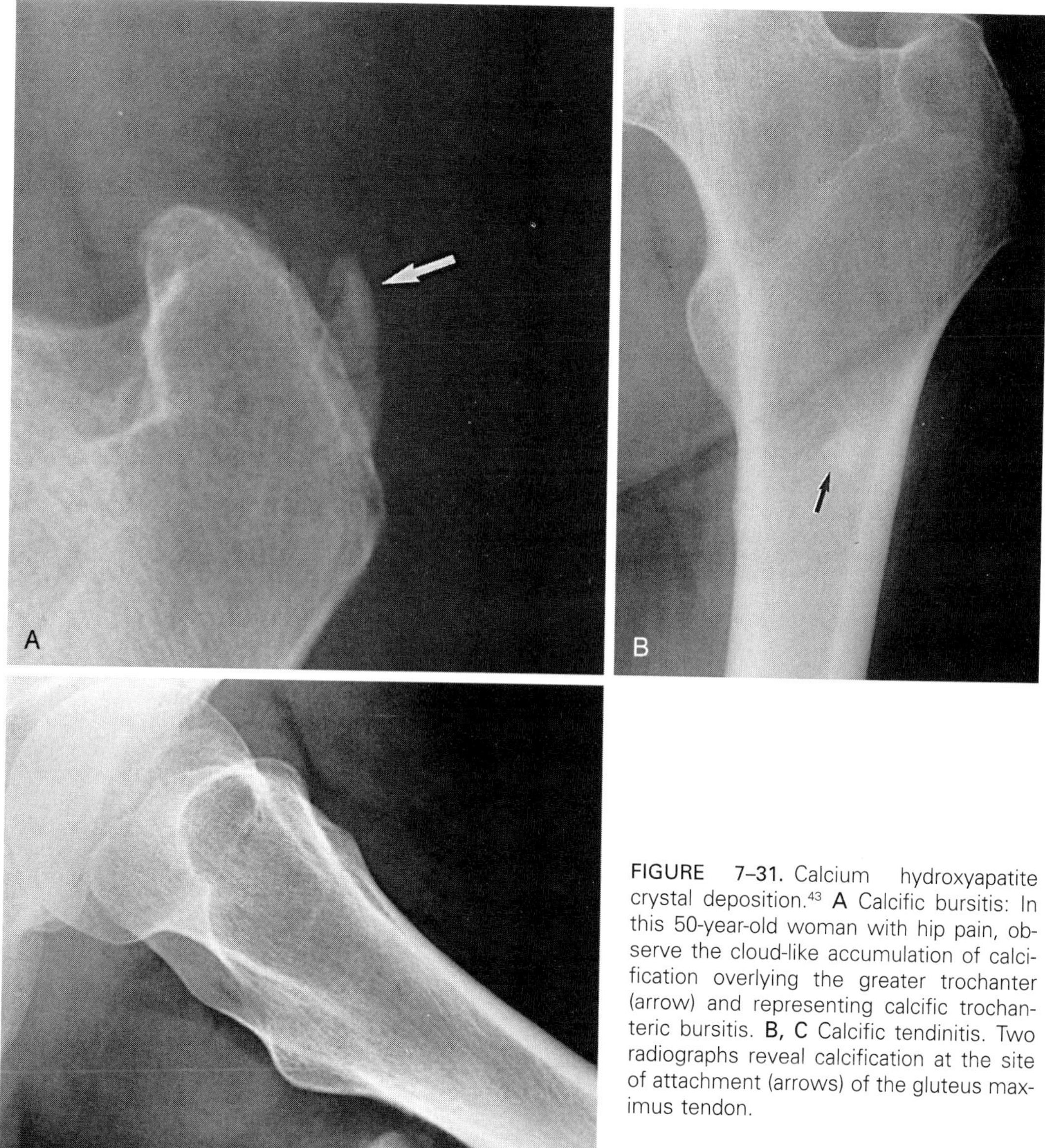

FIGURE 7–31. Calcium hydroxyapatite crystal deposition.[43] A Calcific bursitis: In this 50-year-old woman with hip pain, observe the cloud-like accumulation of calcification overlying the greater trochanter (arrow) and representing calcific trochanteric bursitis. B, C Calcific tendinitis. Two radiographs reveal calcification at the site of attachment (arrows) of the gluteus maximus tendon.

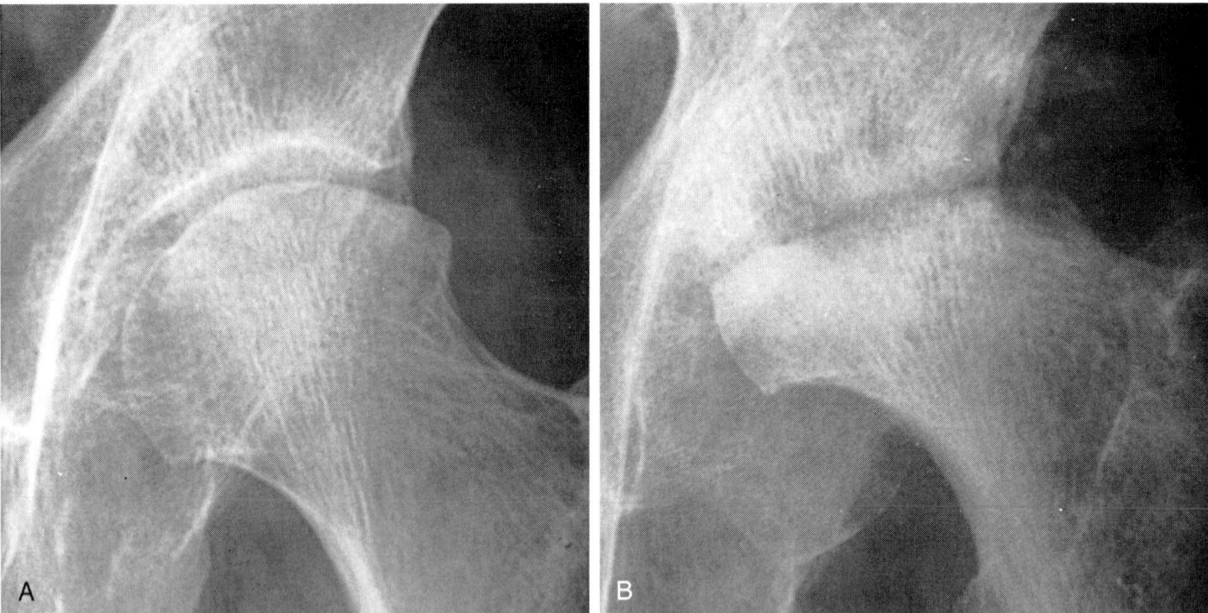

FIGURE 7–32. Rapidly destructive hip disease.[44, 78] This 74-year-old man had rapid onset of hip pain and limp. **A** Initial radiograph shows minimal joint space narrowing and irregularity of the femoral articular surface. **B** Radiograph obtained 5 months later shows dramatic dissolution and atrophic destruction of the femoral head and loss of definition of the acetabulum. Joint aspiration failed to reveal infectious organisms. The cause of these abnormalities is unclear, but they are believed to be related to a generalized process such as intra-articular deposition of calcium hydroxyapatite crystals.

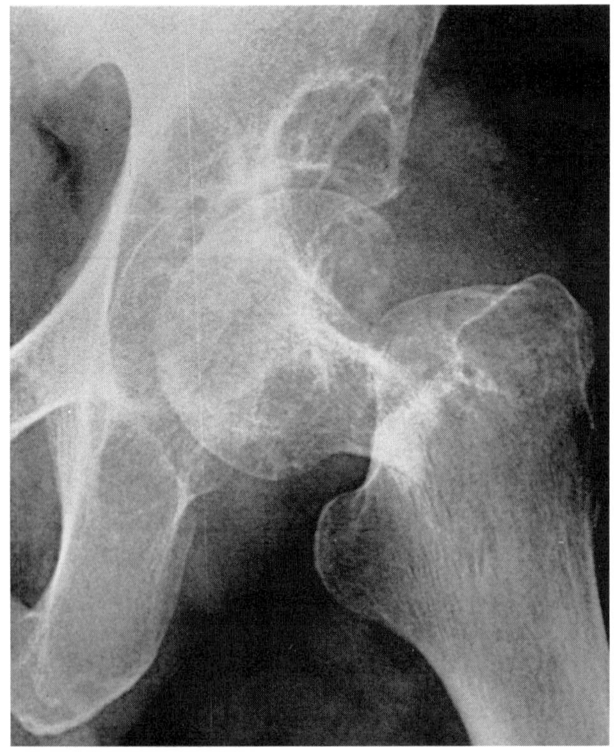

FIGURE 7–33. Gouty arthritis and coexistent chronic renal insufficiency.[45] A 53-year-old man with chronic tophaceous gout, gouty nephritis, and chronic renal insufficiency had acute onset of severe hip pain. A pathologic fracture of the femoral neck with varus angulation is evident on the frontal radiograph. Extensive periarticular erosion of the femoral neck with an overhanging margin is present. Multiple subchondral cyst-like erosions also are seen in the acetabulum. The erosive changes likely result from tophaceous deposits or deposition of amyloid secondary to chronic renal disease. *(Courtesy of C. Chen, M.D., Taipei, Taiwan, Republic of China.)*

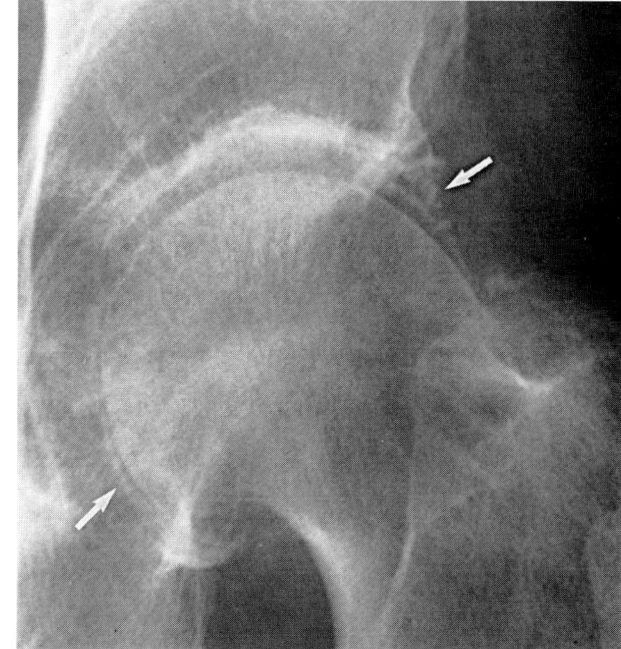

FIGURE 7–34. Hemochromatosis: Chondrocalcinosis.[46] Observe the linear calcification within the hyaline cartilage paralleling the femoral head and also within the acetabular labrum (arrows). Articular changes in hemochromatosis are indistinguishable from those of idiopathic calcium pyrophosphate dihydrate (CPPD) crystal deposition disease.

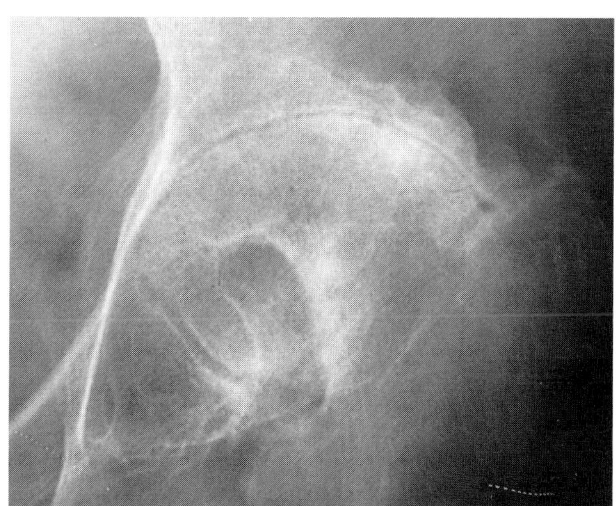

FIGURE 7–35. Alkaptonuria.[47] The radiographic changes of severe ochronotic arthropathy include diffuse joint space narrowing, osteophytosis, mild acetabular protrusion, and femoral head remodeling.

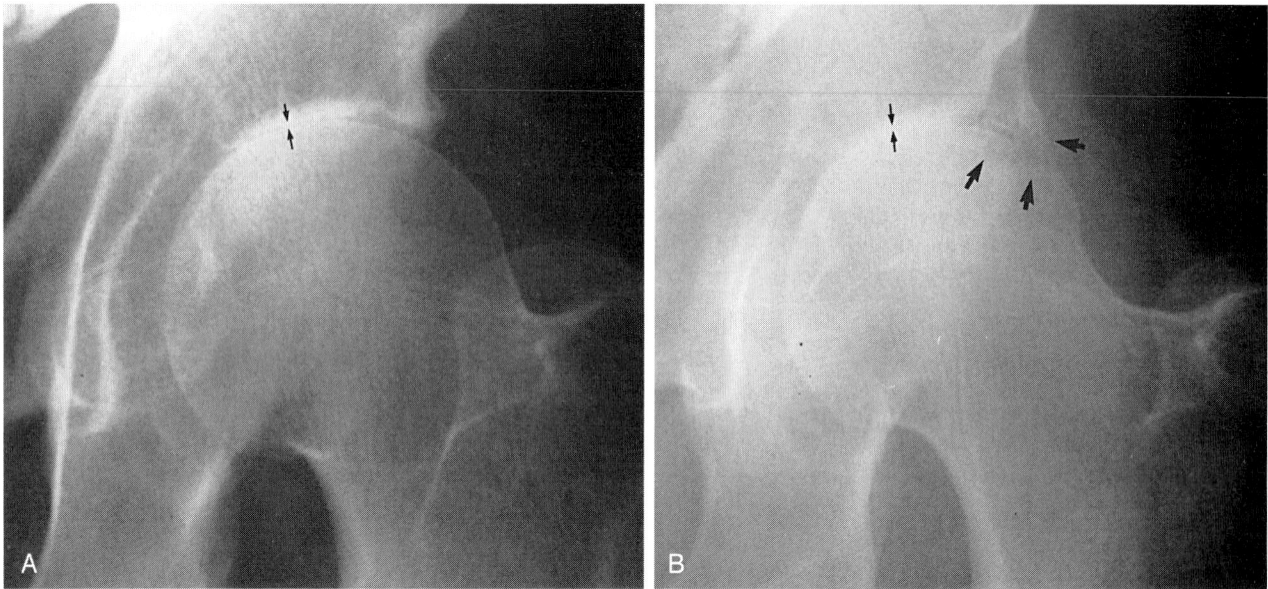

FIGURE 7–36. Septic arthritis and osteomyelitis.[48] A, B This 47-year-old man had hip pain and fever. Routine radiographs taken at initial presentation (A) and 11 days later (B) show the rapid, destructive nature of infectious arthritis. Observe the concentric loss of joint space (small arrows), periarticular osteopenia, and destruction of the femoral head and acetabulum (large arrows). The causative organism in this case was β-hemolytic streptococcus.

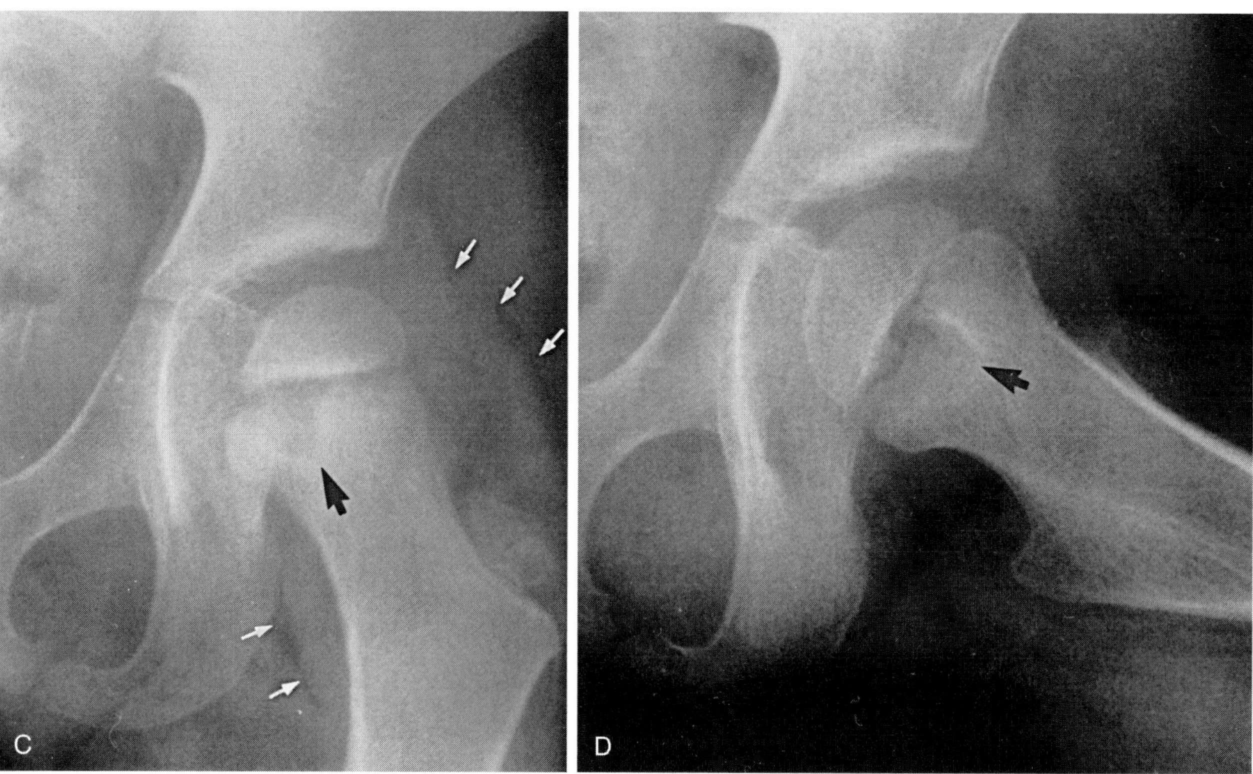

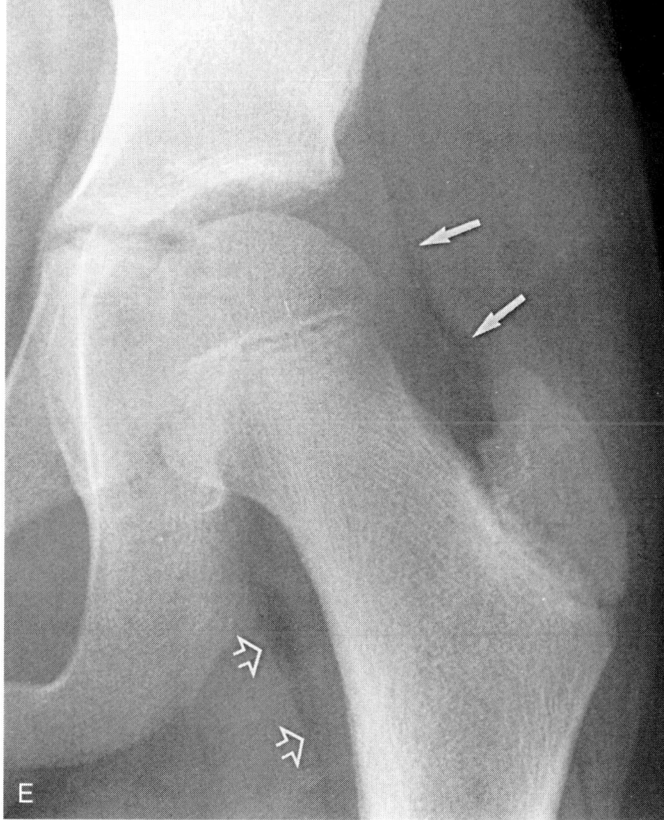

FIGURE 7–36 *Continued.* C, D Osteomyelitis with large joint effusion. Anteroposterior (C) and frog-leg (D) projections of this 3-year-old girl illustrate a well-defined osteolytic lesion within the proximal femoral metaphysis abutting on the physis (black arrows). Displacement of the capsular, iliopsoas, and gluteal fat planes of the hip joint (white arrows in C) indicates a prominent joint effusion. Metaphyseal osteomyelitis in the proximal portion of the femur may spread to the contiguous joint, resulting in septic arthritis. *(C, D, Courtesy of P. H. VanderStoep, M.D., St. Cloud, Minnesota.)* E Normal fat planes adjacent to the hip. For comparison in a normal child, the gluteal (arrows) and iliopsoas (open arrows) fat planes are seen. Note that the fat planes are curved inward, toward the joint, rather than bulged out as in C. The soft tissue findings indicative of intra-articular fluid may be more helpful in this age group than in adults.

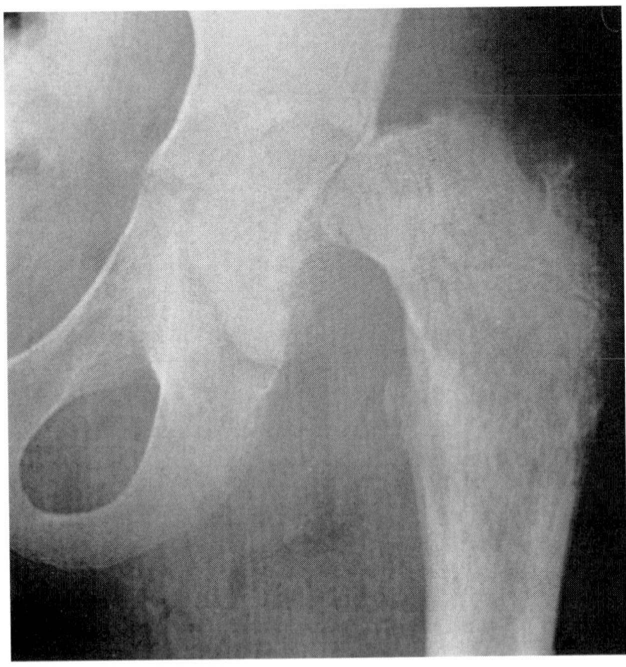

FIGURE 7–37. Septic arthritis with epiphysiolysis.[49] This young patient with pyogenic arthritis of the hip developed a slipped capital femoral epiphysis secondary to physeal destruction by infection. Note the superior displacement of the femoral neck in relation to the femoral head. *(Courtesy of B. Howard, M.D., Charlotte, North Carolina.)*

FIGURE 7–38. Tuberculous arthritis: Psoas abscess.[50] This 40-year-old woman with a history of pulmonary tuberculosis had hip pain of 2 months' duration. **A** Anteroposterior radiograph shows concentric joint space narrowing (arrowheads) and patchy areas of periarticular osteopenia (open arrows). **B** Transaxial CT image reveals narrowing of the joint posteriorly (arrowhead) and a large infected synovial cyst or abscess arising from the anterior portion of the joint (straight arrows). A small erosion also is seen within the anterior cortex of the femoral head (curved arrow). **C** A coronal (TR/TE, 2000/30) proton-density-weighted spin echo magnetic resonance (MR) image reveals the high signal intensity of an abscess or infected cyst in the vicinity of the iliopsoas tendon attachment (short white arrows) and areas of mixed signal intensity within the marrow of the proximal portion of the femur (long arrows). *Mycobacterium tuberculosis* was cultured from the abscess and joint aspirate. *(From Taylor JAM, Harger BL, Resnick D: Diagnostic imaging of common hip disorders: A pictorial review. Top Clin Chiropr 1:8, 1994. Courtesy of G. S. Huang, Taipei, Taiwan.)*

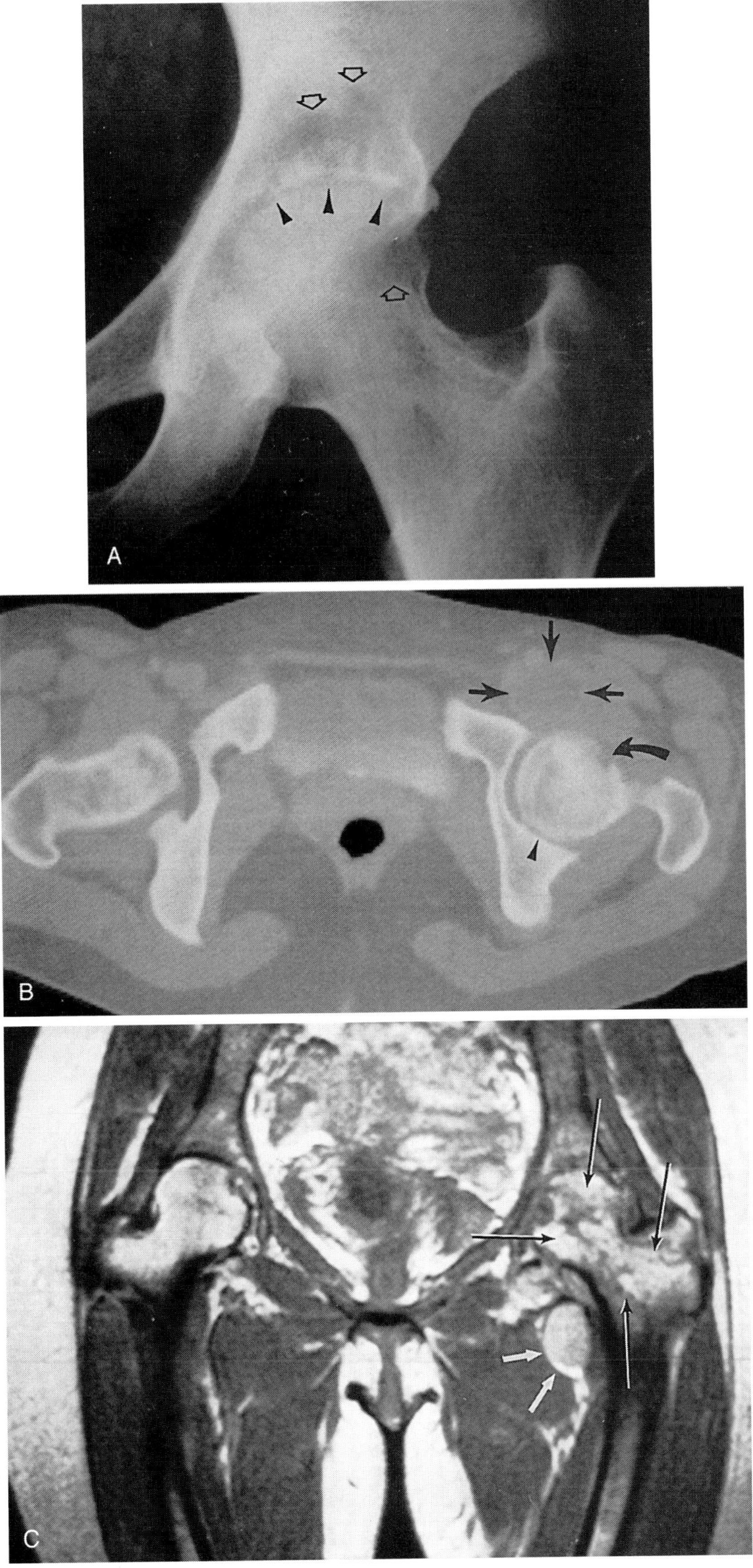

FIGURE 7–38. *See legend on opposite page*

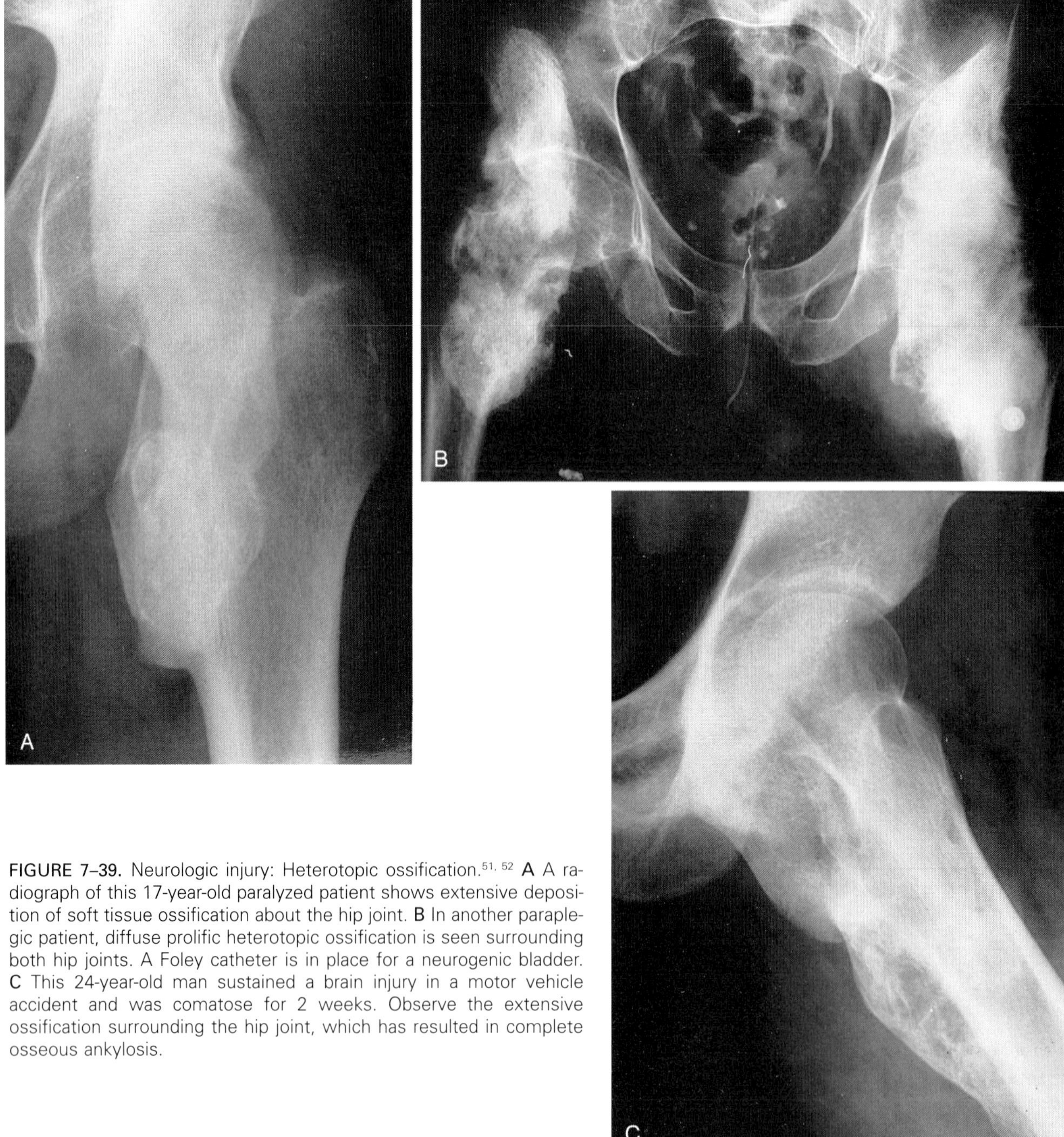

FIGURE 7–39. Neurologic injury: Heterotopic ossification.[51, 52] A A radiograph of this 17-year-old paralyzed patient shows extensive deposition of soft tissue ossification about the hip joint. B In another paraplegic patient, diffuse prolific heterotopic ossification is seen surrounding both hip joints. A Foley catheter is in place for a neurogenic bladder. C This 24-year-old man sustained a brain injury in a motor vehicle accident and was comatose for 2 weeks. Observe the extensive ossification surrounding the hip joint, which has resulted in complete osseous ankylosis.

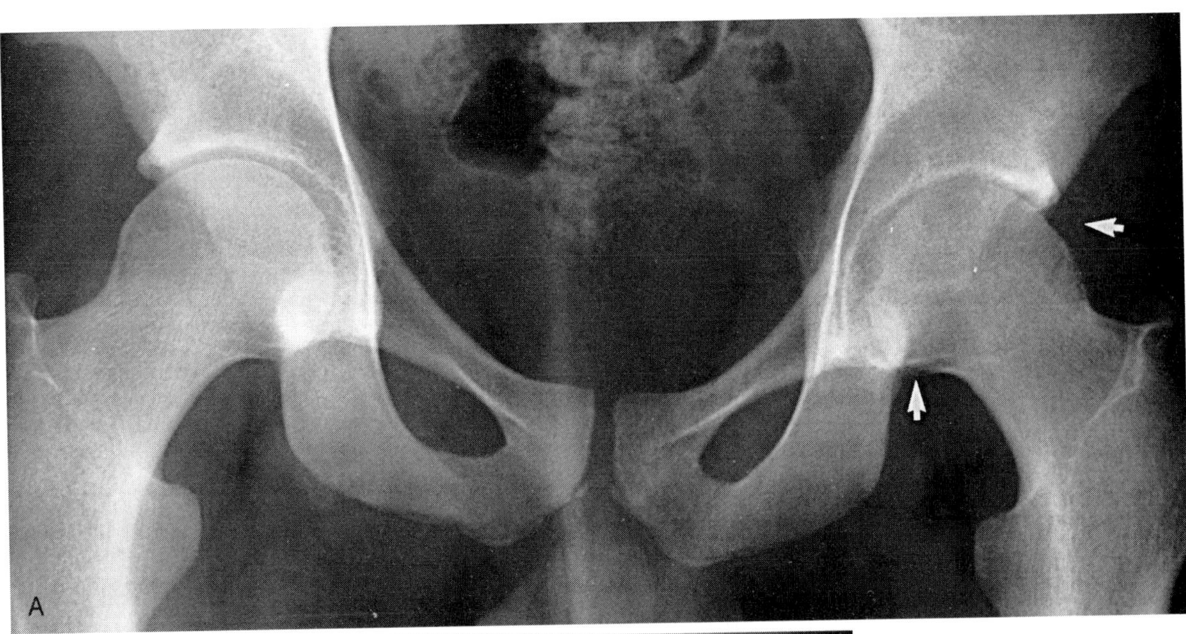

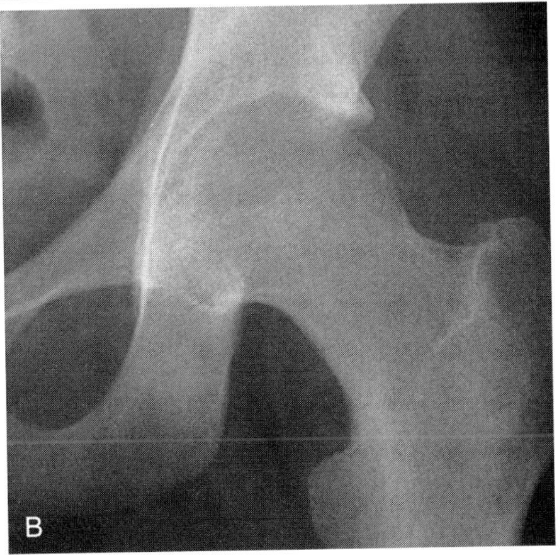

FIGURE 7–40. Idiopathic chondrolysis of the hip.[53] A Observe the unilateral osteoporosis and uniform joint space narrowing of the left hip (arrows) in this young man. The opposite hip appears normal. B Another frontal radiograph of the involved hip taken 3 weeks later shows advancing osteopenia, concentric loss of joint space, and indistinct subchondral bone surfaces. Aspiration of the joint did not reveal evidence of septic arthritis, a major diagnostic consideration.

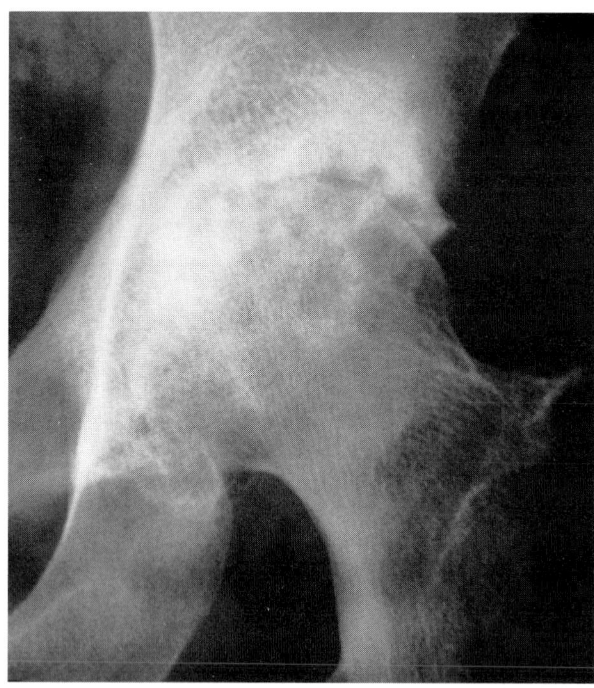

FIGURE 7–41. Pigmented villonodular synovitis.[54, 55] A 34-year-old man had groin and hip pain. Several erosions within the subchondral bone of the femoral head and acetabulum are noted. The joint space is diffusely narrowed, an inconsistent finding in this disease. Osteopenia is not prominent.

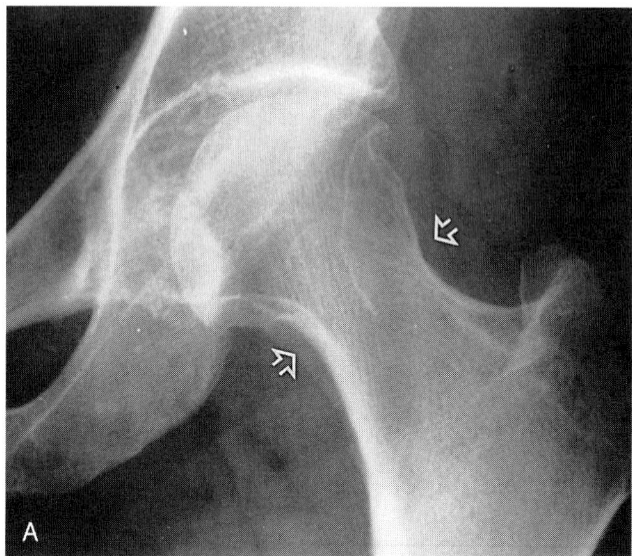

FIGURE 7–42. Idiopathic synovial osteochondromatosis.[56–58] A Observe the extensive, circumferential, scalloped erosion of the femoral neck on this anteroposterior radiograph. At surgery, multiple juxta-articular cartilaginous bodies were removed. B, C In another patient, the frontal radiograph (B) appears essentially normal. However, the arthrogram (C) demonstrates hundreds of tiny cartilaginous bodies, seen as circular filling defects displacing the contrast material. In this case, the intra-articular bodies are radiolucent owing to their cartilaginous nature. Only osteocartilaginous bodies are visible on routine radiographs. (B, C, *Courtesy of G. Greenway, M.D., Dallas, Texas.*)

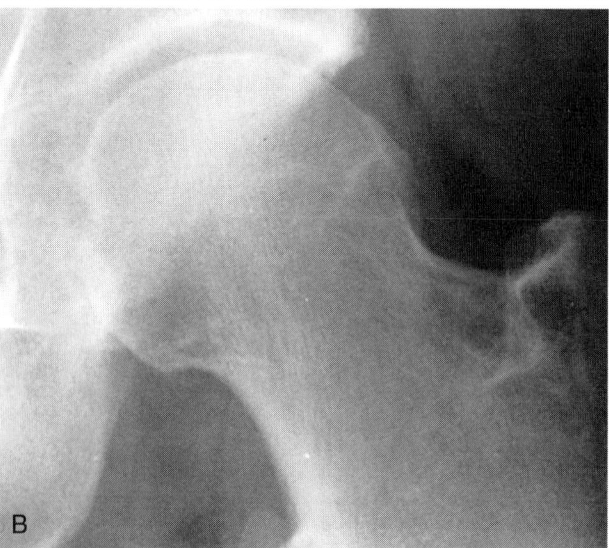

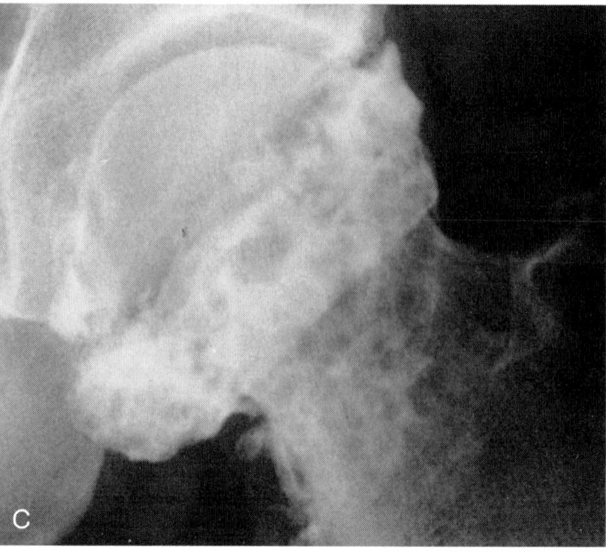

TABLE 7–12. Metabolic and Hematologic Disorders Affecting the Hip*

Entity	Figure(s), Table(s)	Characteristics
Generalized osteoporosis[59–62]	7–43 to 7–45	Singh index: predictable pattern of trabecular bone loss in the proximal portion of the femur (Table 7–13) Quantitative bone mineral analysis (densitometry) is necessary to assess the presence and extent of diminished bone mineral content accurately Dual energy X-ray absorptiometry (DXA) is the most widely used method to assess bone mineral density owing to its ease of use, high precision, and low radiation exposure to patients Major complication: fractures of the proximal portion of the femur common in 17.5 per cent of women older than age 50 years and in 6 per cent of men older than age 50 years
Transient osteoporosis of the hip[63, 64]	7–46	*Clinical findings* Young and middle-aged adults typically with no history of trauma or infection Hip pain, antalgic limp, limitation of movement Unilateral, although opposite hip may occasionally be involved later Self-limited: full recovery in 2 to 6 months *Imaging findings* Progressive, rapid, regional osteoporosis of the femoral head several weeks after onset of pain Acetabulum and femoral neck involved less extensively Positive bone scan Magnetic resonance (MR) imaging signal: decreased on T1-weighted, increased on T2-weighted images typical of bone marrow edema Joint effusion on T2-weighted images Bone density on radiographs and MR imaging signal return to normal in 1 year
Osteomalacia and rickets[65]	7–47, 7–48	*Osteomalacia* Axial and appendicular skeleton Osteopenia Decreased trabeculae; remaining trabeculae appear prominent and coarsened Looser's zones or pseudofractures (i.e., insufficiency fractures) *Rickets* Findings are most prominent in the appendicular skeleton Metaphyseal demineralization: frayed metaphysis, widened physis Bowing of bones Osteopenia
Hypothyroidism[66]	7–49	Slipped capital femoral epiphysis may be the presenting feature of the disease Delayed skeletal maturation, linear sclerosis in metaphysis, irregularity of ossification of the greater trochanter, femoral head (i.e., epiphyseal dysgenesis)
Hyperparathyroidism[67]	7–50	Subperiosteal, subchondral, subligamentous, intracortical, and endosteal bone resorption Occasional bone sclerosis (more common with renal osteodystrophy) Chondrocalcinosis (calcium pyrophosphate dihydrate [CPPD] crystal deposition) Brown tumors Severe bone remodeling with osteitis fibrosa cystica (now infrequently encountered) Acetabular protrusion in advanced cases Soft tissue calcification
Renal osteodystrophy[67, 68]	7–51	Osteosclerosis or osteopenia Similar findings to those of hyperparathyroidism, osteomalacia, and rickets Pathologic fractures Soft tissue calcification
Acromegaly[69]	7–52	Initially: cartilage hypertrophy results in hip joint space widening Later: premature degenerative disease with subchondral cysts and exuberant osteophytosis surrounding femoral head-neck junction
Sickle cell anemia[70]	7–53	Diffuse osteopenia, protrusio acetabuli, and osteonecrosis may be encountered in severe cases of sickle cell anemia and other hemoglobinopathies
Gaucher's disease[76]	See Fig. 7–57 Table 7–14	Osteonecrosis of the femoral head

*See also Tables 1–13 and 1–14.

TABLE 7–13. Osteoporosis of the Proximal Portion of the Femur: The Singh Index*[59]

Grade	Radiographic Appearance of Trabeculae in the Proximal Portion of the Femur	Grade	Radiographic Appearance of Trabeculae in the Proximal Portion of the Femur
6	*No evidence of osteoporosis* All normal trabecular groups visible Proximal portion of the femur appears to be completely occupied by cancellous bone	3	*Suggests definite osteoporosis* Break in continuity of principal tensile trabeculae opposite greater trochanter
5	*Subtle evidence of osteoporosis* Principal tensile and compressive trabeculae accentuated Ward's triangle is prominent	2	*Marked osteoporosis* Only the principal compressive trabeculae are seen No tensile trabeculae visible
4	*Equivocal evidence of osteoporosis* Principal tensile trabeculae reduced in number but continue to extend from lateral cortex to the femoral neck	1	*Severe osteoporosis* Marked reduction even in number of principal compressive trabeculae

*Adapted from Taylor JAM, Resnick D: Radiographic-pathologic correlation. *In* Sartoris DJ: Osteoporosis: Diagnosis and Management. New York, Marcel Dekker, 1996, p. 157.

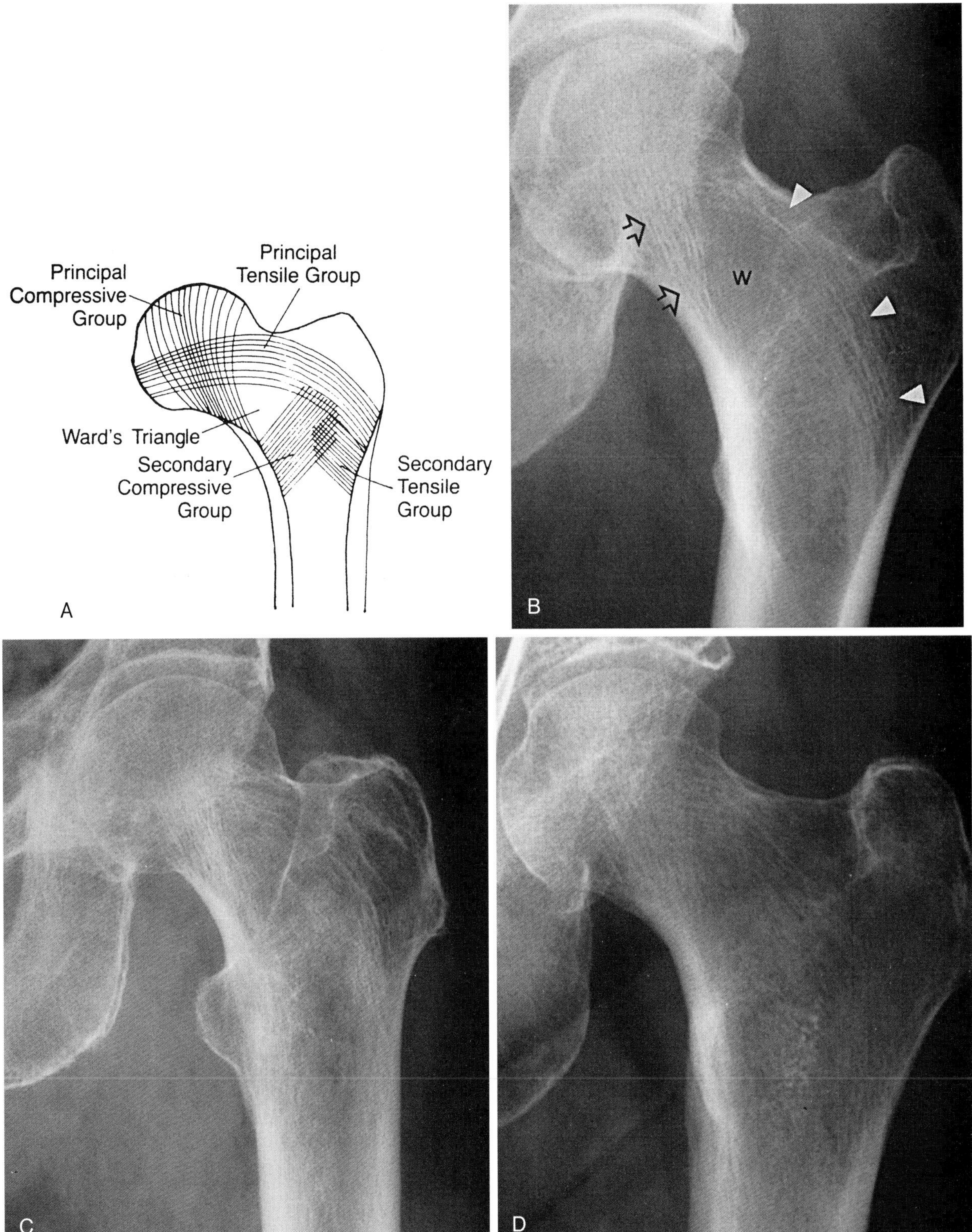

FIGURE 7–43. Osteoporosis.[59–61] **A** Normal trabecular pattern, proximal portion of femur. Four of the anatomic groups of trabeculae are indicated in this schematic drawing. Ward's triangle lies within the neutral axis, wherein compressive and tensile forces balance one another, and contains thin, widely spaced trabeculae. Analysis of these trabeculae may be used as a radiographic index (i.e., Singh index) of osteoporosis in this region (Table 7–13). *(**A**, From Resnick D: Diagnosis of Bone and Joint Disorders. Philadelphia, WB Saunders, 1995, p 1824.)* **B** Normal trabecular pattern: Radiographic appearance in a patient with minimal osteoporosis. Ward's triangle (W) is a relatively radiolucent zone located between the principal tensile (arrowheads) and principal compressive (open arrows) groups of trabeculae. **C** Osteoporosis. In this 79-year-old woman with severe corticosteroid-induced osteoporosis, note the increased radiolucency, cortical thinning, and paucity of trabeculae within the proximal portion of the femur. The osteopenia is especially prevalent within the greater and lesser trochanters as well as in Ward's triangle. **D** Mild osteoporosis secondary to hemiplegia occurring after a cerebrovascular accident. Note the increased radiolucency combined with relative loss of the primary tensile trabeculae.

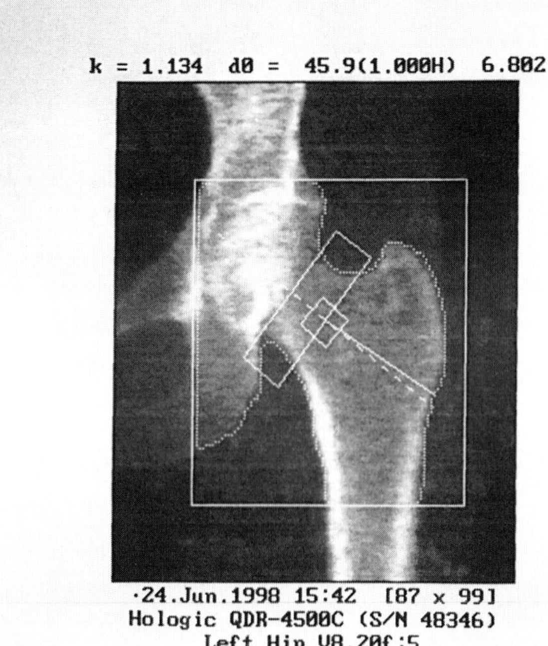

00624980C Wed 24.Jun.1998 15:40
Name:
Comment: baseline/heel bd done
I.D.: 0081 Sex: F
S.S.#: - - Ethnic: W
ZIPCode: Height: 157.00 cm
Operator: CR Weight: 67.00 kg
BirthDate: 30.Jan.47 Age: 51
Physician:
Image not for diagnostic use

TOTAL BMD CV 1.0%
C.F. 1.035 1.008 1.000

Region	Est.Area (cm^2)	Est.BMC (grams)	BMD (gms/cm^2)
Neck	4.93	3.76	0.763
Troch	10.58	6.54	0.618
Inter	16.17	14.92	0.923
TOTAL	31.68	25.22	0.796
Ward's	1.26	0.71	0.564

Midline (84,110)-(152, 58)
Neck -49 x 15 at [24, 14]
Troch 5 x 41 at [0, 0]
Ward's -11 x 11 at [5, 5]

A

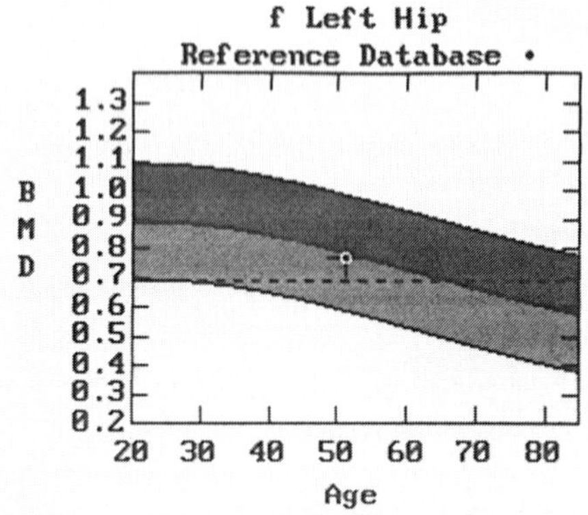

BMD(Neck[L]) = 0.763 g/cm^2

Region	BMD	T		Z	
Neck	0.763	-1.32 (22.0)	85%	-0.26	97%
Troch	0.618	-1.16 (30.0)	86%	-0.58	92%
Inter	0.923	-1.61 (29.0)	80%	-1.06	86%
TOTAL	0.796	-1.49 (28.0)	82%	-0.88	88%
Ward's	0.564	-2.11 (20.0)	71%	-0.36	94%

• Age and sex matched
T = peak bone mass

00624980C Wed 24.Jun.1998 15:40
Name:
Comment: baseline/heel bd done
I.D.: 0081 Sex: F
S.S.#: - - Ethnic: W
ZIPCode: Height: 157.00 cm
Operator: CR Weight: 67.00 kg
BirthDate: 30.Jan.47 Age: 51
Physician:

B

FIGURE 7–44. Quantitative bone mineral analysis (densitometry).[62] Dual energy X-ray absorptiometry (DXA). **A** Data are shown as depicted on a DXA display and printout for a scan of the left hip. Regions of interest (ROI) include the femoral neck, trochanter, intertrochanteric region, and Ward's triangle. For each ROI, the area (cm^2), bone mineral content (g), and bone mineral density (g/cm^2) are computed. **B** Further evaluation includes comparing the patient's bone mineral density with normal peak bone mass (T-score) and age-matched (Z-score) control populations, both of which are predetermined in a reference database. With DXA, the patient's bone mineral density is expressed in terms of standard deviations from normal, information that can be applied to management, prognosis, and estimation of fracture risk.

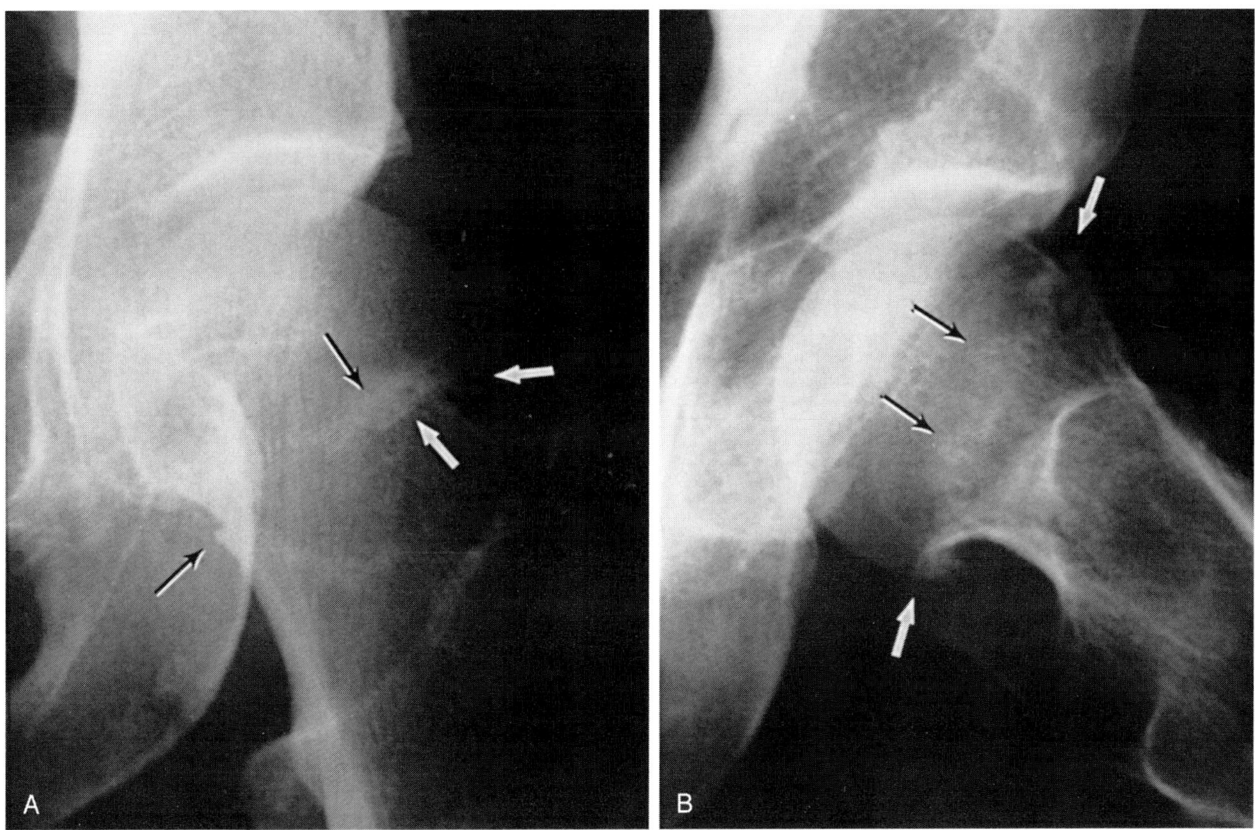

FIGURE 7–45. Osteoporosis: Complicated by subcapital fracture.[60] This 62-year-old osteoporotic woman slipped on an icy sidewalk and fractured her hip. Anteroposterior (A) and frog-leg (B) projections reveal cortical offset and slight compaction of the femoral neck at the subcapital region (arrows). Intracapsular fractures are frequent complications of osteoporosis. *(From Taylor JAM, Harger BL, Resnick D: Diagnostic imaging of common hip disorders: A pictorial review. Top Clin Chiropr 1:8, 1994. Reprinted with permission. Courtesy of T. Wei, D.C., Portland, Oregon.)*

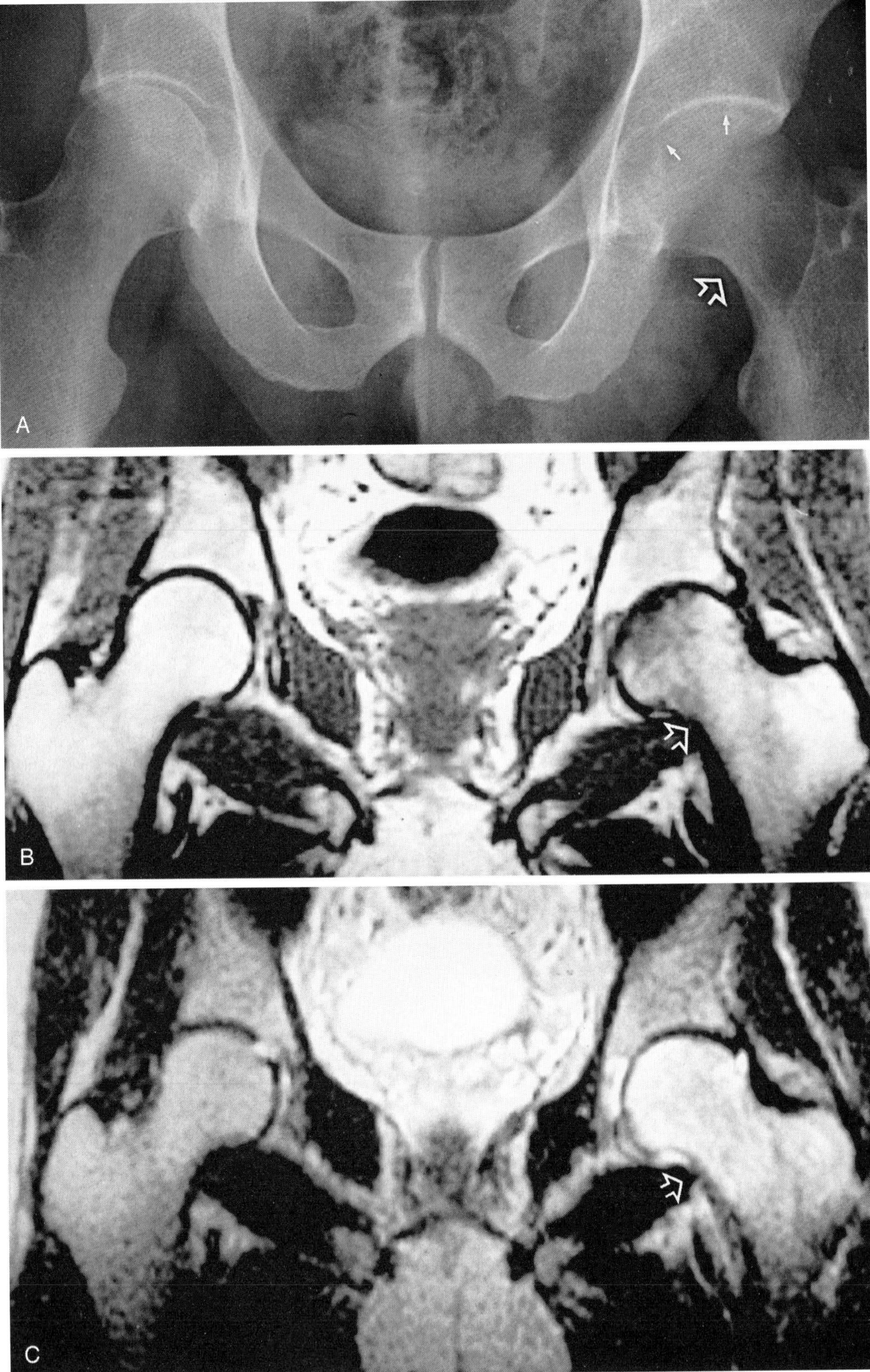

FIGURE 7–46. Transient osteoporosis of the hip.[63, 64] A–C 40-year-old man with left hip pain. In **A,** initial radiograph shows diffuse osteopenia of the proximal portion of the left femur (open arrow). In addition, the subarticular cortex is rather indistinct (arrows). In **B,** a coronal T1-weighted (TR/TE, 418/15) spin echo magnetic resonance (MR) image reveals intermediate signal intensity (open arrow) of the bone marrow in the left femoral head and neck. In **C,** a coronal T2-weighted (TR/TE, 2000/110) spin echo MR image demonstrates high signal intensity (open arrow) within the bone marrow of the left femoral head and neck. *(A–C, Courtesy of E. Bosch, M.D., Santiago, Chile.)*

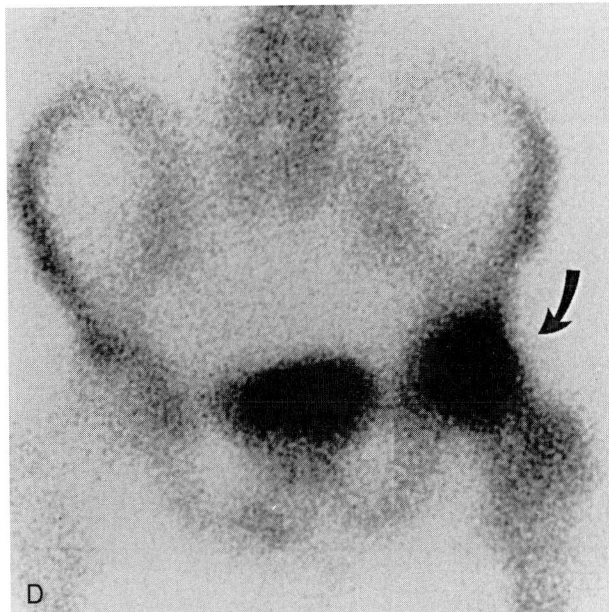

FIGURE 7–46 *Continued.* D Bone scan in another patient shows increased isotope uptake localized to the left femoral head (curved arrow), a characteristic feature of this disease. The findings illustrated in these patients are consistent with bone marrow edema characteristic of transient osteoporosis of the hip. Bone marrow edema also may be observed in cases of osteonecrosis, trauma, infection, and infiltrative neoplasms.

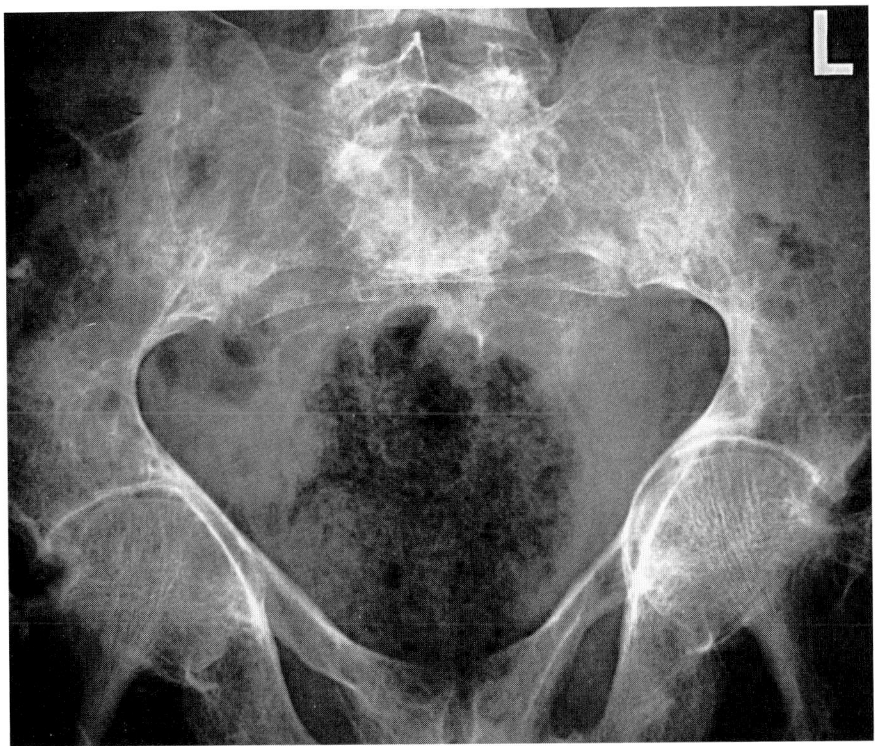

FIGURE 7–47. Osteomalacia and hyperparathyroidism.[65] In this 60-year-old woman, observe the marked osteopenia and acetabular deformity, worse on the left.

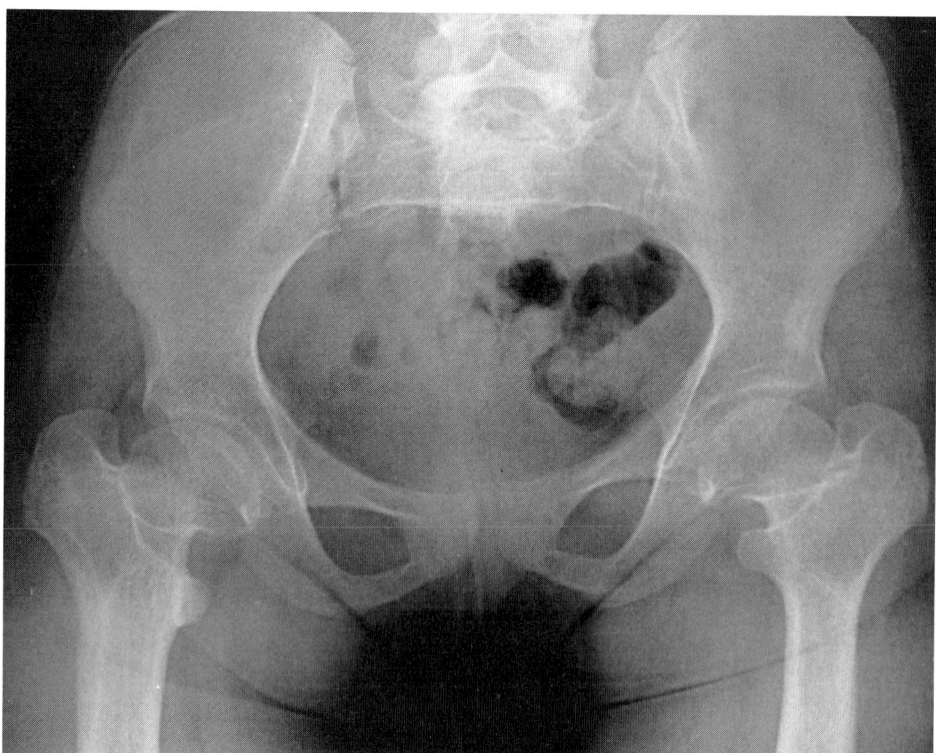

FIGURE 7–48. Rickets: Coxa vara deformities.[65] In this 15-year-old girl with long-standing vitamin D–resistant rickets, bilateral varus deformities of the hip are associated with shortening of the femoral necks.

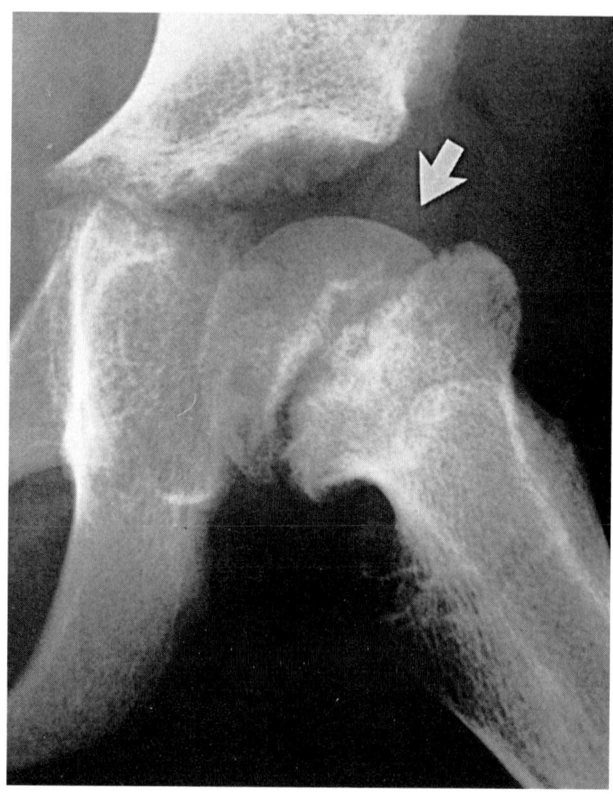

FIGURE 7–49. Hypothyroidism.[66] This 13-year-old girl had bilateral hip pain that developed over a period of 1 year. Radiographs revealed a slipped capital femoral epiphysis (arrow), which was bilateral (other hip not shown). The patient also had delayed bone age. Slipped capital femoral epiphysis, an important manifestation of hypothyroidism, can be bilateral or unilateral, and it may be the initially apparent feature of this disease. *(Courtesy of G. Greenway, M.D., Dallas, Texas.)*

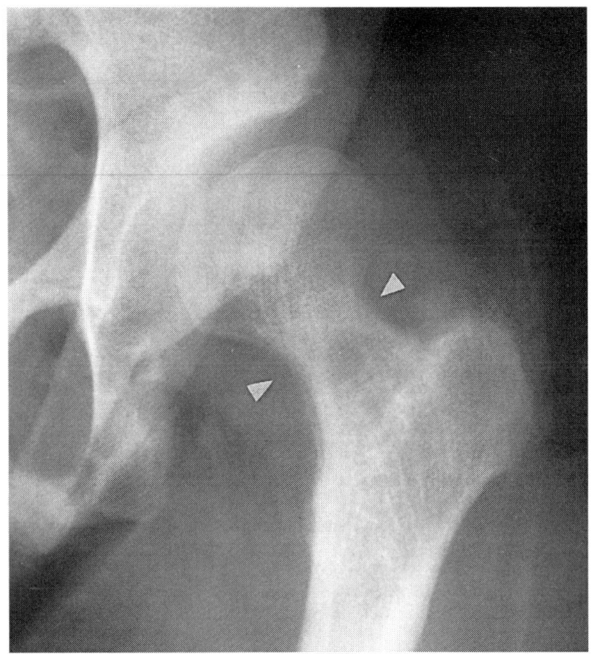

FIGURE 7–50. Hyperparathyroidism.[67, 68] A radiograph of the proximal portion of the femur in this 18-year-old woman with chronic renal failure shows subperiosteal bone resorption of the femoral neck (arrowheads). A catheter is seen overlying the pubic bone.

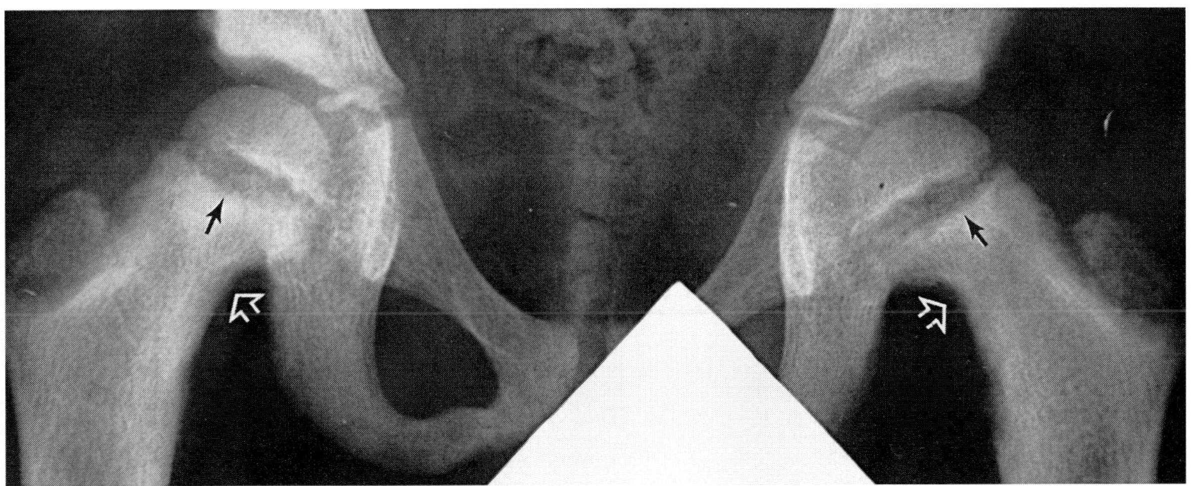

FIGURE 7–51. Renal osteodystrophy.[67, 68] Observe the generalized dense sclerosis, subchondral resorption adjacent to the femoral physes (arrows), and cortical resorption at the medial aspects of the femoral necks (open arrows) in this child with long-standing renal insufficiency. *(Courtesy of B. L. Harger, D.C., Portland, Oregon.)*

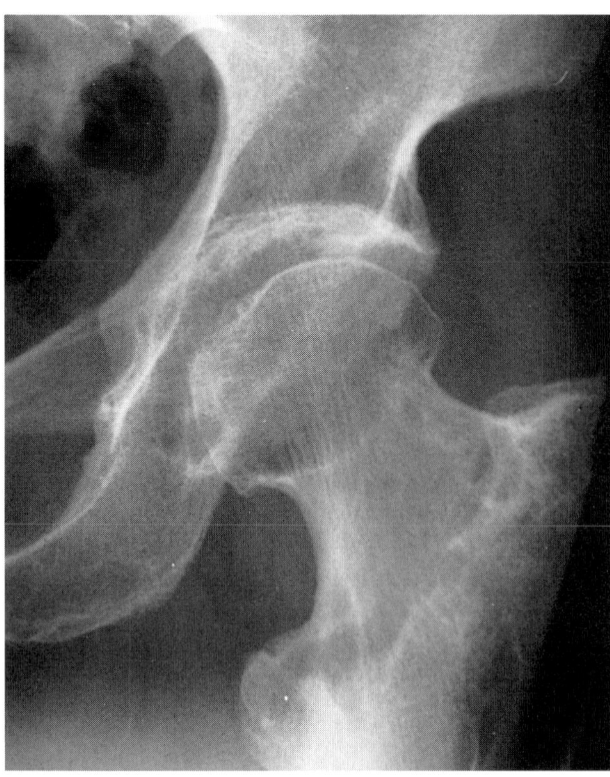

FIGURE 7–52. Acromegaly.[69] Widening of the hip joint space, prominent osteophyte formation, and irregularity of the articular surfaces are characteristic of acromegalic arthropathy. The pathogenesis of this arthropathy relates to proliferation of chondrocytes with secondary degeneration of the abnormally proliferated cartilage.

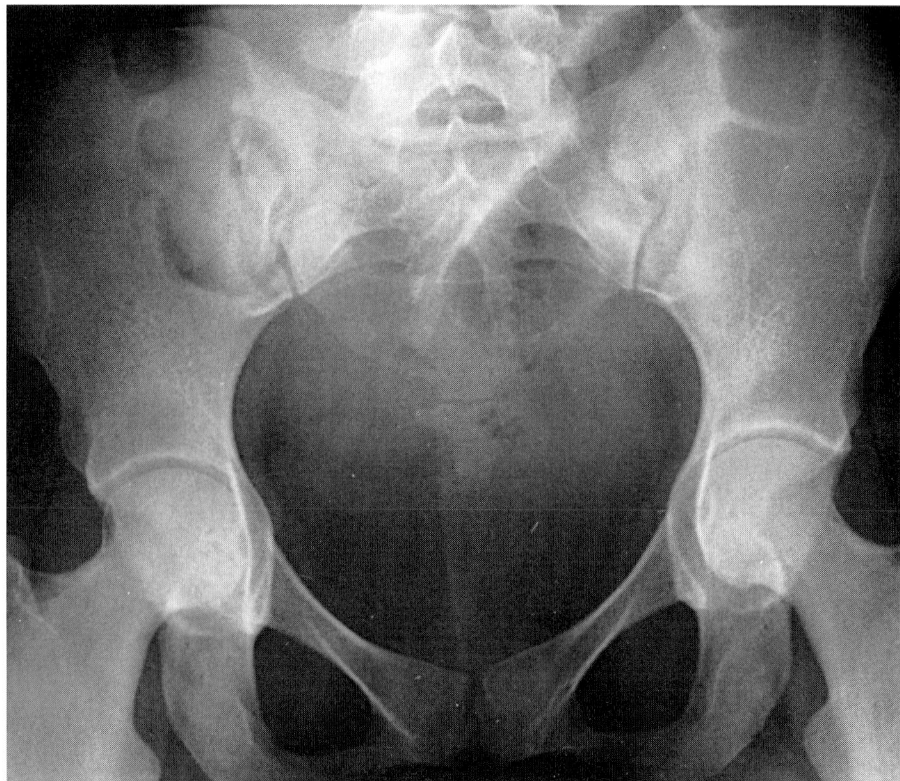

FIGURE 7–53. Sickle cell anemia: Acetabular protrusion.[70] Protrusio acetabuli is present in up to 20 per cent of patients with sickle cell anemia. The cause is unclear, but it may be related to acetabular ischemia from vascular occlusion. Epiphyseal osteonecrosis (not seen in this patient) is a frequent complication of sickle cell anemia and other hemoglobinopathies.

TABLE 7–14. Osteonecrosis of the Femoral Head*

Entity	Figure(s)	Characteristics
Legg-Calvé-Perthes disease[71]	7–54	
Definition		Osteonecrosis of the immature femoral capital epiphysis
Distribution		Bilateral in 15 per cent of patients
Typical age of onset		3–12 years of age; in most patients onset is between the ages of 5 and 9 years
Gender		Male > female
Radiographic findings		Catterall classification: grades I–IV (Table 7–15) Epiphyseal flattening, deformity, fragmentation, and osteosclerosis Crescent sign with or without subchondral collapse and sequestered bone fragments Metaphyseal sclerosis and cyst formation Eventual degenerative joint disease and mushroom appearance of femoral head Shortening of femoral neck from failure of normal growth Magnetic resonance (MR) imaging may be used to determine the extent of epiphyseal involvement and to document the presence and extent of deformity
Prognosis		Almost always remodels and heals, but may result in residual deformity in the shape of the femoral head
Differential diagnosis		Femoral head irregularity and collapse in children: Legg-Calvé-Perthes, Meyer's dysplasia, hypothyroidism, epiphyseal dysplasia, spondyloepiphyseal dysplasia, sickle cell anemia, Gaucher's disease, infection, and hemophilia
Osteonecrosis of the adult femoral head[72–76]	7–55 to 7–57	
Synonyms		Ischemic necrosis, avascular necrosis, aseptic necrosis
Distribution		Bilateral in 50 per cent of patients
Typical age of onset		20–40 years
Gender		Male = female
Imaging findings		Stages 0–V (Table 7–15) *Radiographic findings* May be negative Bone sclerosis Cysts Subchondral collapse (crescent sign) May be focal or "segmental" area of involvement Joint space narrowing in advanced cases *Scintigraphic findings* Increased radionuclide uptake in femoral head Often focal in superior portion With or without photopenic areas *CT findings* Increased density area often is wedge-shaped, corresponding to segmental region of involvement Articular collapse *MR imaging findings* Focal abnormalities of femoral head Surrounding margin of low signal in T1-weighted images with central higher signal zone consistent with fat; may exhibit high signal with acute bleeding Variable signal in T2-weighted images Diffuse abnormalities of femoral head and neck related to bone marrow edema
Prognosis		Variable, but progressive in 75 per cent of cases Often necessitates operative intervention

*See also Tables 1–15 and 1–16.

TABLE 7–15. Grades of Femoral Involvement in Legg-Calvé-Perthes Disease (Catterall Classification)

	Grade			
	I	*II*	*III*	*IV*
Anterior part of epiphysis involved	+	+	–	–
Majority of epiphysis involved	–	–	+	–
Whole epiphysis involved	–	–	–	+
Sequestrum	–	+	+	+
Anterior crescent sign	–	+	–	–
Anterior crescent sign extends posteriorly	–	–	+	–
Anterior and posterior crescent sign	–	–	–	+
Articular collapse	–	+	+	+
Localized metaphyseal abnormalities	–	+	–	–
Diffuse metaphyseal abnormalities	–	–	+	+

+, Present; –, absent.

TABLE 7–16. Staging of Osteonecrosis in the Adult Femoral Head

	Stage of Osteonecrosis					
Characteristics	*0*	*I*	*II*	*III*	*IV*	*V*
Clinical assessment						
Suspected necrosis	+	+	+	+	+	+
Clinical findings	–	+	+	+	+	+
Advanced imaging						
Bone scan	–	+	+	+	+	+
Magnetic resonance (MR) imaging	–	+	+	+	+	+
Radiographic findings						
Osteopenia	–	–	+	+	+	+
Cystic areas	–	–	+	+	+	+
Bone sclerosis	–	–	+	+	+	+
Crescent sign	–	–	–	+	+	+
Subchondral collapse	–	–	–	–	+	+
Flattening of femoral head	–	–	–	–	+	+
Joint space narrowing	–	–	–	–	–	+
Acetabular abnormalities	–	–	–	–	–	+

+, Present; –, absent.

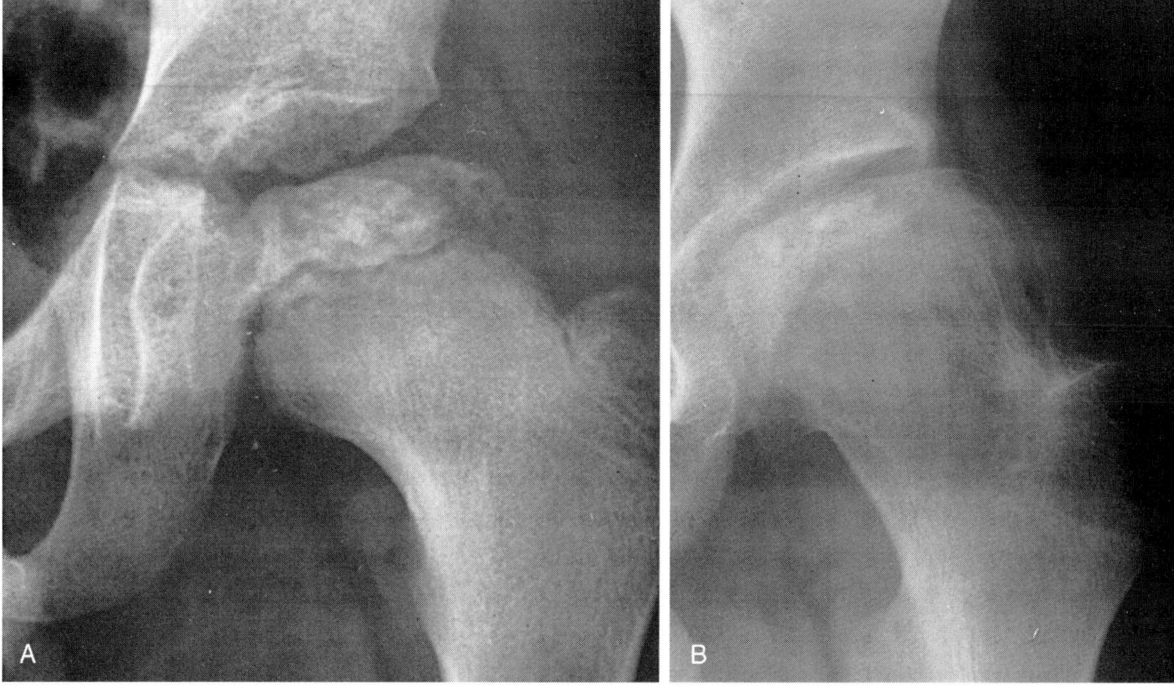

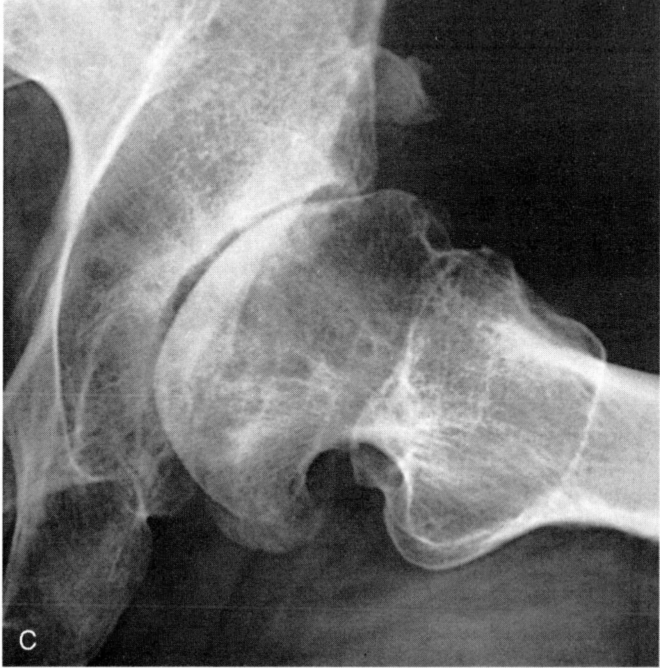

FIGURE 7–54. Legg-Calvé-Perthes disease.[71] **A** Sclerosis, flattening, fragmentation, and deformity of the proximal femoral epiphysis are noted in this 8-year-old boy. *(**A**, Courtesy of P. VanderStoep, M.D., St. Cloud, Minnesota.)* **B** In a 16-year-old boy with long-standing Legg-Calvé-Perthes disease, observe the flattening of the femoral head, osseous fragmentation of the subchondral bone, overall widening of the femoral neck, and deformity of the acetabulum. **C** In a 60-year-old man who had had Legg-Calvé-Perthes disease as a child, observe the nonuniform joint space narrowing, subchondral sclerosis, subchondral cysts, and osteophytes indicative of secondary degeneration, a frequent complication of this childhood disease. The mushroom-shaped femoral head is characteristic. (See also Fig. 7–6 **B**.)

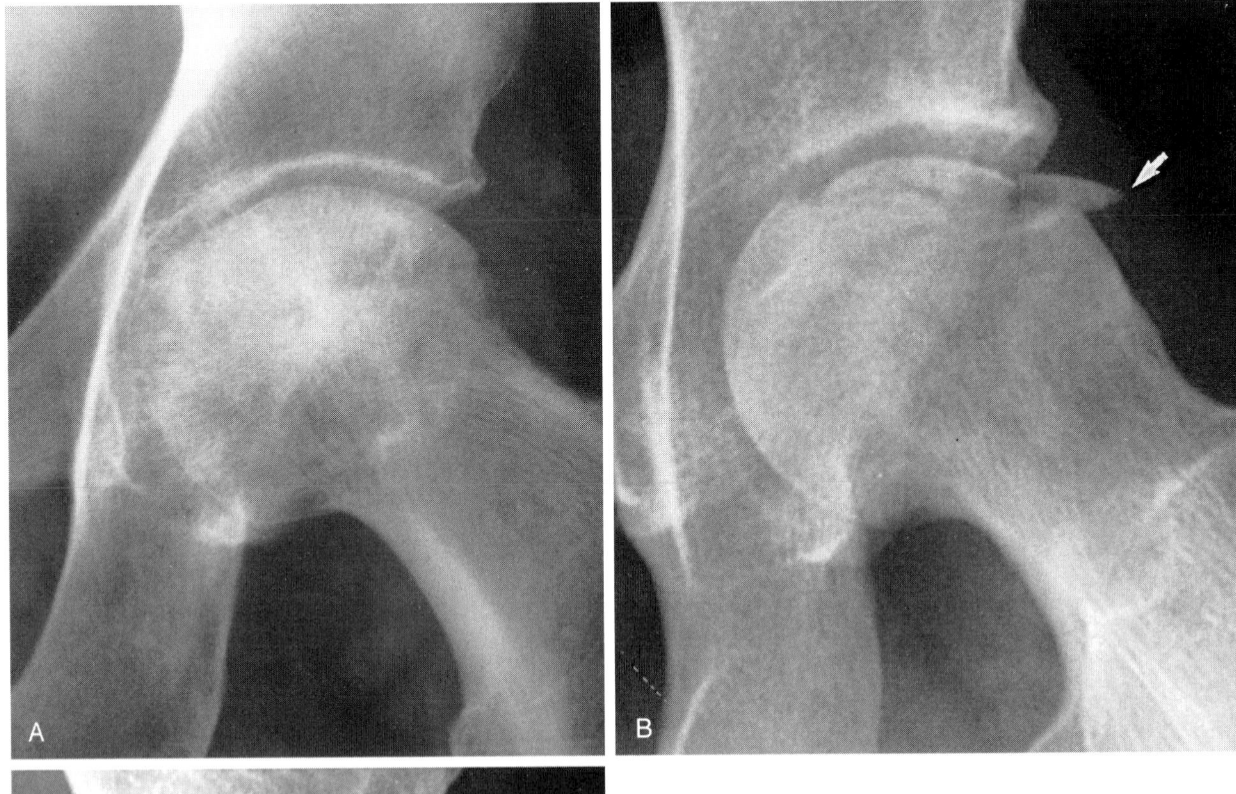

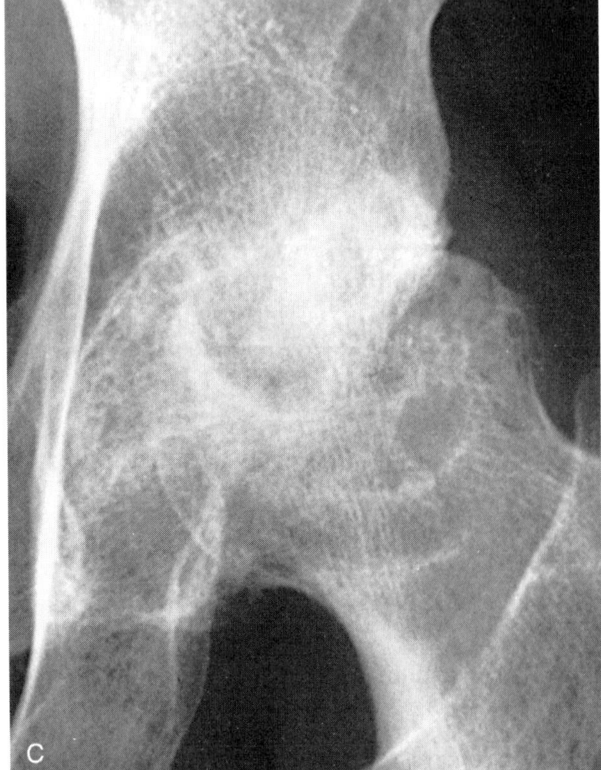

FIGURE 7–55. Osteonecrosis: Routine radiography.[72, 73] **A** Early involvement (stage II). Subchondral cyst-like lucent areas and sclerosis are seen in the femoral head of this 47-year-old man. Note the relative preservation of joint space, a feature typical of early osteonecrosis. **B** Moderate disease (stage IV). In a 27-year-old intravenous drug abuser, a radiograph reveals marked subchondral collapse, femoral head flattening, and a displaced osseous fragment (arrow). **C** Advanced disease (stage V). This 52-year-old man worked in a decompression chamber. Observe the marked collapse of the femoral head, cyst-like femoral and acetabular radiolucent areas, patchy sclerosis, and joint space narrowing. This patient eventually developed bilateral involvement.

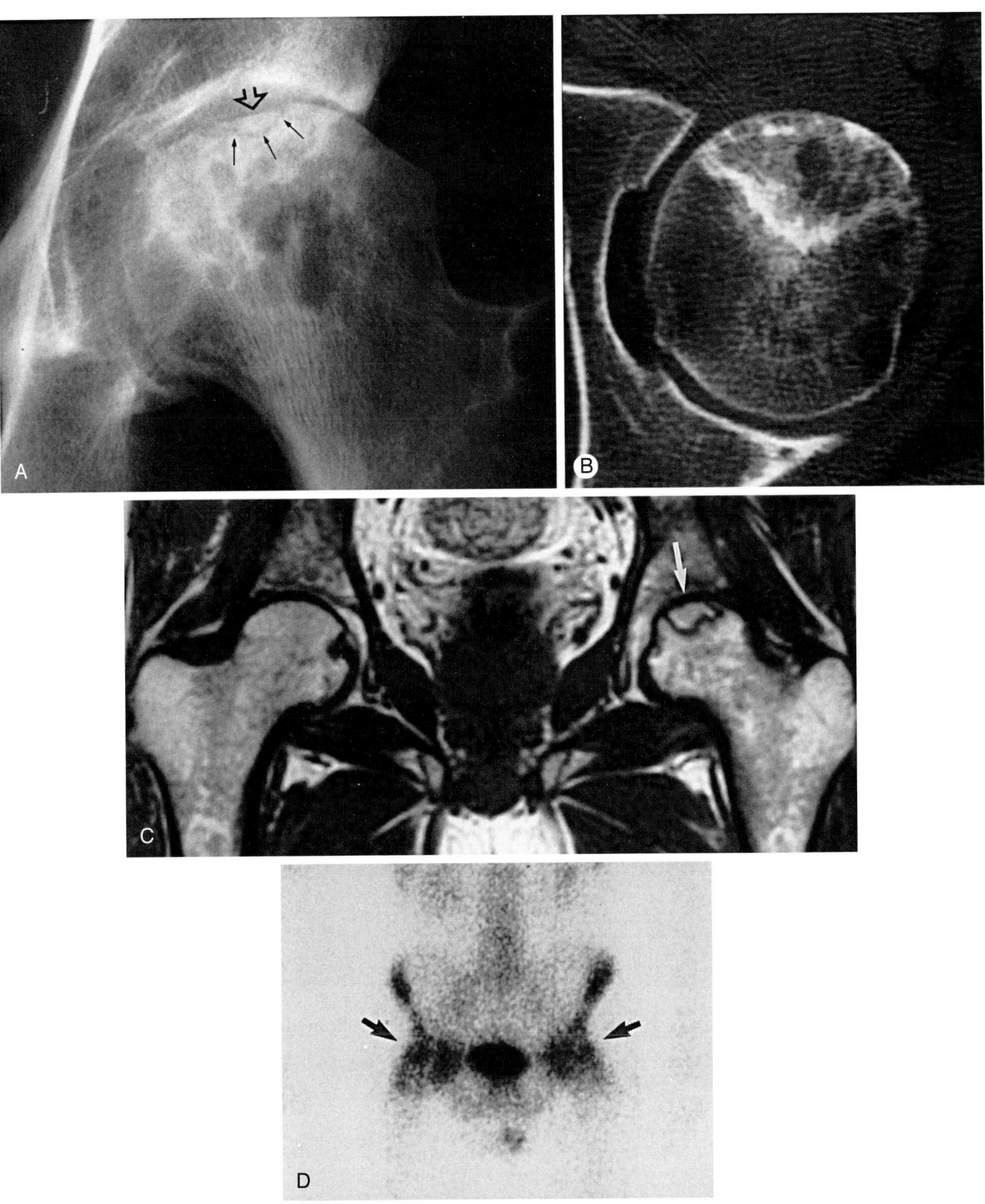

FIGURE 7–56. Osteonecrosis: Imaging abnormalities.[72, 73] A The classic radiographic findings of stage V osteonecrosis include a subchondral radiolucent line (crescent sign) (arrows), collapse and flattening of the femoral head articular surface (open arrow), large subchondral radiolucent areas surrounded by sclerosis, and the absence of osteophytes. This patient exhibits some superolateral joint space narrowing and sclerosis, indicating that this is a long-standing process. B Computed tomography (CT). In another patient, a transaxial CT scan shows a well-localized focus of osteonecrosis confined to the anterior aspect of the femoral head, a pattern termed segmental osteonecrosis. The cyst-like radiolucent areas are bordered by a well-defined zone of osteosclerosis. C MR imaging. In a third patient, a coronal T1-weighted (TR/TE, 600/20) spin echo magnetic resonance (MR) image shows a curvilinear zone of low signal intensity surrounding a zone of intermediate signal intensity within the left femoral head (arrow). MR imaging is ideal for evaluating osteonecrosis and is more sensitive to early changes than routine radiography. D Bone scan. In a fourth patient with bilateral osteonecrosis, increased uptake is seen in both femoral heads (arrows).

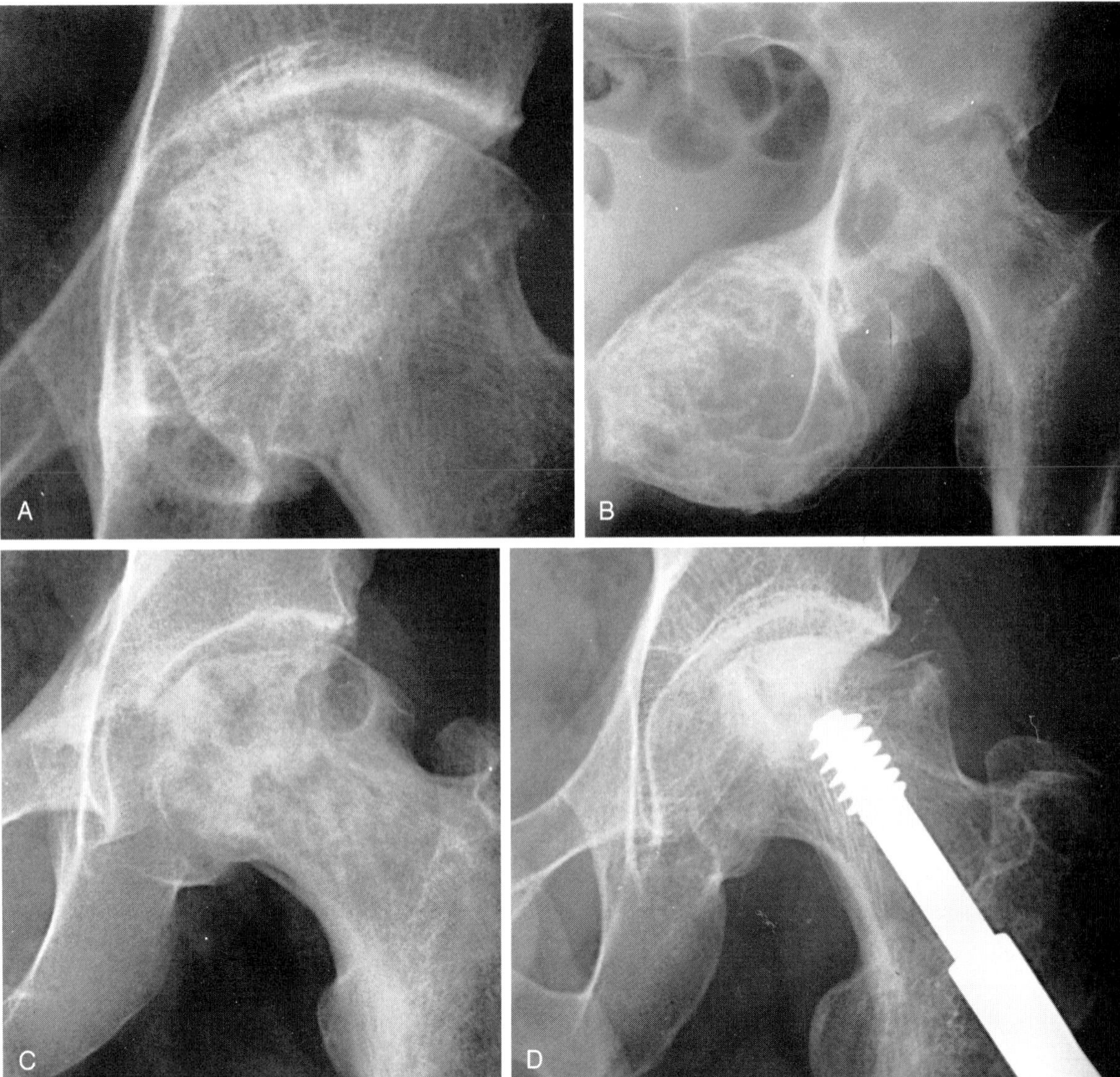

FIGURE 7–57. Osteonecrosis: Some associated disorders.[74–76] A Systemic lupus erythematosus. This 35-year-old woman had been taking corticosteroid medication for 5 years for long-standing systemic lupus erythematosus. Articular collapse of the femoral head is associated with cyst-like radiolucent areas and surrounding sclerosis typical of osteonecrosis. Secondary degenerative changes also are evident. The osteonecrosis was bilateral. The femoral head is the most common site of osteonecrosis in patients with systemic lupus erythematosus. B Radiation-induced osteonecrosis. In this 55-year-old woman with endometrial carcinoma, a radiograph obtained after a course of radiation therapy shows osteonecrosis of the femoral head, destruction of the acetabulum, joint space loss, and a large sclerotic metastatic lesion involving the ischiopubic ramus. C Gaucher's disease. Observe the multiple cystic subchondral lesions, articular collapse, and punctate sclerosis in the femoral head and neck of this patient with Gaucher's disease complicated by osteonecrosis. (C, *Courtesy of V. Vint, M.D., La Jolla, California.*) D Postsurgical osteonecrosis. In this patient with a previous intertrochanteric fracture treated with a dynamic hip screw, evidence of type IV osteonecrosis is seen. This complication is less frequent in intertrochanteric fractures than in subcapital fractures. (D, *From Taylor JAM, Harger BL, Resnick D: Diagnostic imaging of common hip disorders: A pictorial review. Top Clin Chiropr 1:8, 1994.*)

REFERENCES

1. Edeiken J, Dalinka M, Karasick D: Edeiken's Roentgen Diagnosis of Diseases of Bone. 4th Ed. Baltimore, Williams & Wilkins, 1990.
2. Keats TE, Smith TH: An Atlas of Normal Developmental Roentgen Anatomy. 2nd Ed. Chicago, Year Book, 1988.
3. Greenfield GB: Radiology of Bone Diseases. 2nd Ed. Philadelphia, JB Lippincott, 1975.
4. Köhler A, Zimmer EA: Borderlands of Normal and Early Pathologic Findings in Skeletal Radiography. 4th Ed. New York, Thieme Medical Publishers, 1993.
5. Pitt MJ, Graham AR, Shipman JH, et al: Herniation pit of the femoral neck. AJR 138:1115, 1982.
6. Daenen B, Preidler KW, Padmanabhan S, et al: Symptomatic herniation pits of the femoral neck: Anatomic and clinical study. AJR 168:149, 1997.
7. Keats TE: Atlas of Normal Roentgen Variants That May Simulate Disease. 6th Ed. Chicago, Year Book Medical Publishers, 1996.
8. Yochum TR, Rowe LJ: Essentials of Skeletal Radiology. 2nd Ed. Baltimore, Williams & Wilkins, 1996.
9. Swischuk LE: Differential Diagnosis in Pediatric Radiology. Baltimore, Williams & Wilkins, 1984.
10. Chapman S, Nakielny R: Aids to Radiological Differential Diagnosis. 3rd Ed. London, WB Saunders, 1995.
11. Weinstein JN, Kuo KN, Millar EA: Congenital coxa vara: A retrospective review. J Pediatr Orthop 4:70, 1984.
12. D'Arcy K, Ansell BM, Bywaters EGL: A family with primary protrusio acetabuli. Ann Rheum Dis 37:53, 1978.
13. Meals RA, Hungerford DS, Stevens MB: Malignant disease mimicking arthritis of the hip. JAMA 239:1070, 1978.
14. Armbruster TG, Guerra J Jr, Resnick D, et al: The adult hip: An anatomic study. Part I. The bony landmarks. Radiology 128:1, 1978.
15. Poul J, Bajerova J, Sommernitz M, et al: Early diagnosis of congenital dislocation of the hip. J Bone Joint Surg [Br] 74:695, 1992.
16. Gerscovich EO: A radiologist's guide to the imaging in the diagnosis and treatment of developmental dysplasia of the hip. I. General considerations, physical examination as applied to real-time sonography and radiography. Skeletal Radiol 26:386, 1997.
17. Gerscovich EO: A radiologist's guide to the imaging in the diagnosis and treatment of developmental dysplasia of the hip. II. Ultrasonography: Anatomy, technique, acetabular angle measurements, acetabular coverage of femoral head, acetabular cartilage thickness, three-dimensional technique, screening of newborns, study of older children. Skeletal Radiol 26:447, 1997.
18. Resnick D, Kang SK: Pelvis and hip. *In* Resnick D, Kang SK (eds.): Internal Derangements of Joints. Philadelphia, WB Saunders, 1997, p 473.
19. Erb RE, Steele JR, Nance EP Jr, et al: Traumatic anterior dislocation of the hip: Spectrum of plain film and CT findings. AJR 165:1215, 1995.
20. Potok PS, Hopper KD, Umlauf MJ: Fractures of the acetabulum: Imaging, classification, and understanding. RadioGraphics 15:7, 1995.
21. Brandser E, Marsh JL: Acetabular fractures: Easier classification with a systematic approach. AJR 171:1217, 1998.
22. Cooperman DR, Charles LM, Pathria MN, et al: Postmortem description of slipped capital femoral epiphysis. J Bone Joint Surg [Br] 74:595, 1992.
23. Tountas AA, Waddell JP: Stress fractures of the femoral neck: A report of seven cases. Clin Orthop 210:160, 1986.
24. Anderson MW, Greenspan A: Stress fractures. Radiology 199:1, 1996.
25. Reading JM, Sheehan NJ: Spontaneous fractures of the lower limb in chronic rheumatoid arthritis. J Orthop Rheumatol 4:173, 1991.
26. Haramati N, Staron RB, Barax C, et al: Magnetic resonance imaging of occult fractures of the proximal femur. Skeletal Radiol 23:19, 1994.
27. Schwappach JR, Murphey MD, Kokmeyer SF, et al: Subcapital fractures of the femoral neck: Prevalence and cause of radiographic appearance simulating pathologic fracture. AJR 162:651, 1994.
28. Roback DL: Posttraumatic osteolysis of the femoral neck. AJR 134:1243, 1980.
29. DeLee JC: Fractures and dislocations of the hip. *In* CA Rockwood Jr, DP Green (Eds): Fractures in Adults. 2nd Ed. Philadelphia, JB Lippincott Co, 1984, p 1211.
30. Altman R, Alarcón G, Appelrouth D, et al: The American College of Rheumatology criteria for the classification and reporting of osteoarthritis of the hip. Arthritis Rheum 34:505, 1991.
31. Preidler KW, Resnick D: Imaging of osteoarthritis. Radiol Clin North Am 34:259, 1996.
32. Martel W, Braunstein EM: The diagnostic value of buttressing of the femoral neck. Arthritis Rheum 21:161, 1978.
33. Haller J, Resnick D, Miller CW, et al: Diffuse idiopathic skeletal hyperostosis: Diagnostic significance of radiographic abnormalities of the pelvis. Radiology 172:835, 1989.
34. Resnick D, Niwayama G: Rheumatoid arthritis. *In* Resnick D (ed): Diagnosis of Bone and Joint Disorders. 3rd Ed. Philadelphia, WB Saunders, 1995, p 866.
35. Pellman E, Kumari S, Greenwald R: Rheumatoid iliopsoas bursitis presenting as unilateral leg edema. J Rheumatol 13:197, 1986.
36. Dwosh IL, Resnick D, Becker MA: Hip involvement in ankylosing spondylitis. Arthritis Rheum 19:683, 1976.
37. Scarpa R, Oriente P, Pucino A, et al: Psoriatic arthritis in psoriatic patients. Br J Rheumatol 23:246, 1984.
38. Pachman LN: Juvenile dermatomyositis. Pediatr Clin North Am 33:1097, 1986.
39. Czirjak L, Nagy Z, Szegedi G: Systemic sclerosis in the elderly. Clin Rheumatol 11:483, 1992.
40. Olivieri I, Gemignani G, Balagi M, et al: Concomitant systemic lupus erythematosus and ankylosing spondylitis. Ann Rheum Dis 49:323, 1990.
41. Resnick D, Niwayama G, Goergen TG, et al: Clinical, radiographic and pathologic abnormalities in calcium pyrophosphate dihydrate deposition disease (CPPD): Pseudogout. Radiology 122:1, 1977.
42. Steinbach LS, Resnick D: Calcium pyrophosphate dihydrate crystal deposition disease revisited. Radiology 200:1, 1996.
43. Archer BD, Friedman L, Stilgenbauer S, et al: Symptomatic calcific tendinitis at unusual sites. J Can Assoc Radiol 43:203, 1992.
44. Bock GW, Garcia A, Weisman MH, et al: Rapidly destructive hip disease: Clinical and imaging abnormalities. Radiology 186:461, 1993.
45. Borg EJT, Rasker JJ: Gout in the elderly, a separate entity? Ann Rheum Dis 46:72, 1987.
46. Faraawi R, Harth M, Kertesz A, et al: Arthritis in hemochromatosis. J Rheumatol 20:448, 1993.
47. Justesen P, Andersen PE Jr: Radiologic manifestations in alkaptonuria. Skeletal Radiol 11:204,1984.
48. Vincent GM, Amirault JD: Septic arthritis in the elderly. Clin Orthop 251:241, 1990.

49. Betz RR, Cooperman DR, Wopperer JM, et al: Late sequelae of septic arthritis of the hip in infancy and childhood. J Pediatr Orthop 10:365, 1990.
50. Torres GM, Cernigilaro JG, Abbitt PL, et al: Iliopsoas compartment: Normal anatomy and pathologic processes. RadioGraphics 15:1285, 1995.
51. Garland DE, Blum CE, Waters RL: Periarticular heterotopic ossification in head-injured adults: Incidence and location. J Bone Joint Surg [Am] 62:1143, 1980.
52. Garland DE: A clinical perspective on common forms of acquired heterotopic ossification. Clin Orthop 263:13, 1991.
53. van der Hoeven H, Keesen W, Kuis W: Idiopathic chondrolysis of the hip. A distinct clinical entity? Acta Orthop Scand 60:661, 1989.
54. Cotton A, Flipo R-M, Chastanet P, et al: Pigmented villonodular synovitis of the hip: Review of radiographic features in 58 patients. Skeletal Radiol 24:1, 1995.
55. Hughes TH, Sartoris DJ, Schweitzer ME, et al: Pigmented villonodular synovitis: MRI characteristics. Skeletal Radiol 24:7, 1995.
56. Thomas S: Synovial chondromatosis of the hip: Case with long-term follow up. SD J Med 30:7, 1977.
57. Prager RJ, Mall JC: Arthrographic diagnosis of synovial chondromatosis. AJR 127:344, 1976.
58. Kramer J, Recht M, Deely DM, et al: MR appearance of idiopathic synovial osteochondromatosis. J Comput Assist Tomogr 17:772, 1993.
59. Singh M, Nagrath AR, Maini PS: Changes in the trabecular pattern of the upper end of the femur as an index of osteoporosis. J Bone Joint Surg [Am] 52:457, 1970.
60. Schwappach JR, Murphey MD, Kokmeyer SF, et al: Subcapital fractures of the femoral neck: Prevalence and cause of radiographic appearance simulating pathologic fracture. AJR 162:651, 1994.
61. Kerr R, Resnick D, Sartoris DJ, et al: Computed tomography of proximal femoral trabecular patterns. J Orthop Res 4:45, 1986.
62. Grampp S, Jergas M, Lang P, et al: Quantitative assessment of osteoporosis: Current and future status. *In* Sartoris DJ (ed): Osteoporosis: Diagnosis and Treatment. New York, Marcel Dekker, 1996, p 233.
63. Potter H, Moran M, Schneider R, et al: Magnetic resonance imaging in diagnosis of transient osteoporosis of the hip. Clin Orthop 280:223, 1992.
64. Hayes CW, Conway WF, Daniel WW: MR imaging of bone marrow edema pattern: Transient osteoporosis, transient bone marrow edema syndrome, or osteonecrosis. RadioGraphics 13:1001, 1993.
65. Mankin HJ: Rickets, osteomalacia, and renal osteodystrophy. Orthop Clin North Am 21:81, 1990.
66. Heyerman W, Weiner D: Slipped epiphysis associated with hypothyroidism. J Pediatr Orthop 4:569, 1984.
67. Resnick D., Niwayama G: Parathyroid disorders and renal osteodystrophy. *In* Resnick D (ed): Diagnosis of Bone and Joint Disorders. 3rd Ed. Philadelphia, WB Saunders, 1995, p 2012.
68. Tigges S, Nance EP, Carpenter WA, et al: Renal osteodystrophy: Imaging findings that mimic those of other diseases. AJR 165:143, 1995.
69. Johanson NA, Vigorita VH, Goldman AB, et al: Acromegalic arthropathy of the hip. Clin Orthop 173:130, 1983.
70. Hernigou P, Galacteros F, Bachir D, et al: Deformities of the hip in adults who have sickle-cell disease and had avascular necrosis in childhood: A natural history of fifty-two patients. J Bone Joint Surg [Am] 73:81, 1991.
71. Wenger DR, Ward WT, Herring JA: Legg-Calvé-Perthes disease. J Bone Joint Surg [Am] 73:778, 1991.
72. Takatori Y, Kokubo T, Ninomiya S, et al: Avascular necrosis of the femoral head: Natural history and magnetic resonance imaging. J Bone Joint Surg [Br] 75:217, 1993.
73. Van de Berg BE, Malghem JJ, Labaisse M-A, et al: MR imaging of avascular necrosis and transient marrow edema of the femoral head. RadioGraphics 13:501, 1993.
74. Dalinka MK, Edeiken J, Finkelstein JB: Complications of radiation therapy: Adult bone. Semin Roentgenol 9:29, 1974.
75. Weiner ES, Abeles M: Aseptic necrosis and glucocorticosteroids in systemic lupus erythematosus: A reevaluation. J Rheumatol 16:604, 1989.
76. Amstutz HC: The hip in Gaucher's disease. Clin Orthop 90:83, 1973.
77. Laorr A, Greenspan A, Anderson MW, et al: Traumatic hip dislocation: Early MRI findings. Skeletal Radiol 24:239, 1995.
78. Ryu KN, Kim EJ, Yoo MC, et al: Ischemic necrosis of the entire femoral head and rapidly destructive hip disease: Potential causative relationship. Skeletal Radiol 26:143, 1997.
79. Askin SR, Bryan RS: Femoral neck fractures in young adults. Clin Orthop 114:259, 1976.
80. Garden RS: Reduction and fixation of subcapital fractures of the femur. Orthop Clin North Am 5:683, 1974.
81. Evans EM: The treatment of trochanteric fractures of the femur. J Bone Joint Surg [Br] 31:190, 1949.
82. Seinsheimer F: Subtrochanteric fractures of the femur. J Bone Joint Surg [Am] 60:300, 1978.

CHAPTER 8

Femur

- Developmental Anomalies, Anatomic Variants, Skeletal Dysplasias, and Other Congenital Diseases
- Physical Injury
- Neoplasms
- Metabolic, Hematologic, and Infectious Disorders

Developmental Anomalies, Anatomic Variants, Skeletal Dysplasias, and Other Congenital Diseases

A wide variety of developmental anomalies, anatomic variants, skeletal dysplasias, and other congenital conditions affect the femur and its surrounding structures. Table 8–1 and Figures 8–1 to 8–5 represent selected examples of some of the more common of such processes.

Physical Injury

The femoral diaphysis may be a site of acute fracture, fatigue fracture, and insufficiency fracture. Additionally, the muscles of the thigh are a frequent site of posttraumatic heterotopic ossification. These conditions are described in Table 8–2 and are illustrated in Figures 8–6 and 8–7. Injuries to the proximal and distal portions of the femur are discussed in Chapters 7 and 9, respectively.

Neoplasms

The femur is the bone most frequently affected by malignant and benign neoplasms and tumor-like processes. Tables 8–3 to 8–5 list some of the characteristics of these disorders. Their radiographic manifestations are illustrated in Figures 8–8 to 8–33.

Metabolic, Hematologic, and Infectious Disorders

Several metabolic, hematologic, and infectious disorders involve the femur. Table 8–6 lists some of the more common disorders and describes their characteristics. The radiographic features of these disorders are illustrated in Figures 8–34 to 8–44. Additional manifestations of the disorders within the proximal and distal portions of the femur are discussed in Chapters 7 and 9, respectively.

TABLE 8–1. Developmental Anomalies, Anatomic Variants, Skeletal Dysplasias, and Other Congenital Diseases*

Entity	Figure(s)	Characteristics
Limb length inequality[1–3]	8–1	Synonyms: anisomelia, leg length discrepancy, short leg syndrome *Etiology* Congenital disorders, paralysis, infection, trauma, neoplasm, joint replacement surgery Accurate assessment aids in treatment planning Three imaging techniques are used for measuring the length of the femur and tibia: 1. Orthoradiograph: single exposure of entire length of both lower extremities on a long film; may be obtained supine or standing 2. Scanogram: three separate exposures are obtained of the hips, knees, and ankles; the patient is immobilized in a supine position, and the x-ray tube and cassettte are moved to expose all three anatomic regions on one film 3. Computed tomographic (CT) scanogram: an anteroposterior scout scanogram of both lower extremities is obtained; cursors are placed at the superior tip of the capital femoral epiphysis and the most distal portion of the lateral femoral condyle and measurements are obtained; tibial length is determined in a similar manner; lateral views of the femur also may be obtained and measured to account for limb flexion CT scanograms are accurate and result in less radiation exposure than radiographic techniques; this is particularly useful in patients with joint contractures
Proximal femoral focal deficiency (PFFD)[4]	8–2	Spectrum of conditions characterized by partial absence and shortening of the proximal portion of the femur Disorder is congenital but not inherited Usually PFFD is an isolated anomaly, unilateral in 90% of affected patients *Radiographic findings* Femoral head may be present or absent; may be just a small ossicle Acetabulum: variable degree of dysplasia Femoral shaft: short, often deformed Sometimes no connection exists between femur and acetabulum
Osteopetrosis[5]		Diffuse osteosclerosis results in brittle bones and predisposition to pathologic fracture of femur
Osteopoikilosis[6]	8–3	Mutiple 2- to 3-mm circular foci of osteosclerosis Symmetric periarticular lesions resembling bone islands predominate about hip and knee articulations
Osteopathia striata[7]	8–4	Regular, linear, vertically oriented bands of osteosclerosis extending from the metaphysis for variable distances into the diaphysis Longest lesions frequently are found in the femur Metaphyseal flaring of the femur also may be seen with osteopathia striata
Melorheostosis[8, 9]	8–5	Usual pattern: hemimelic involvement of a single femur Peripherally located cortical hyperostosis resembling "flowing candle wax" on the surface of bones Para-articular soft tissue calcification and ossification may occur and may even lead to joint ankylosis May be positive on bone scans
Mixed sclerosing bone dystrophy[10]	8–3	Combinations of various sclerosing dysplasias

*See also Tables 1–1 and 1–2.

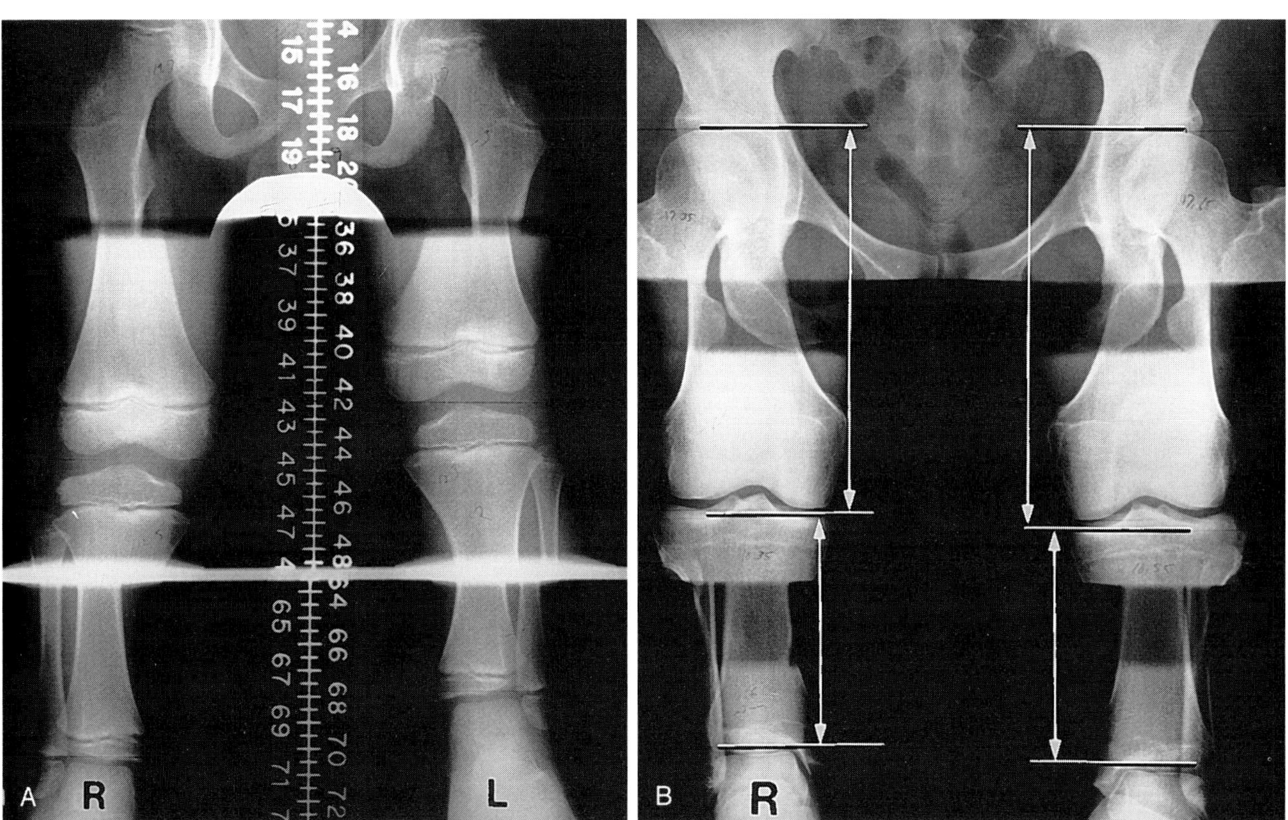

FIGURE 8–1. Limb length inequality: measurement techniques.[1-3] **A, B** Radiographic scanogram. In **A,** a scanogram from a 12-year-old child with a noticeable limp and short leg reveals a 3-cm deficiency of the left femur and a 0.2-cm deficiency of the left tibia. In **B,** an adult patient, the landmarks for the measurements of the tibia and fibula are illustrated. In this example, the right femur had a 0.3-cm deficiency and the right tibia had a 0.2-cm deficiency. In this procedure, the patient remains stationary in a supine position on the radiographic table, and three separate exposures of the hips, knees, and ankles are taken on one film. The accurate measurement of the length of the femur and tibia assists in management planning.

Illustration continued on following page

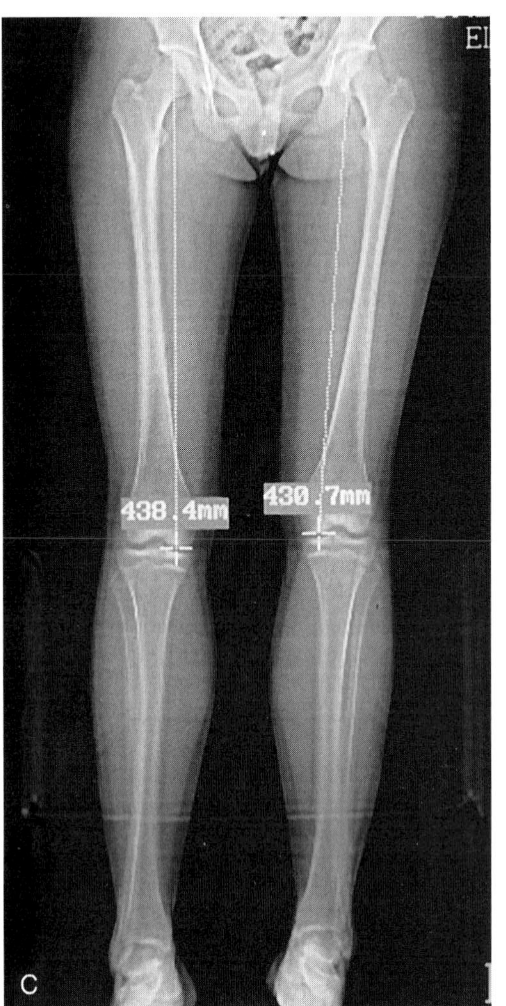

FIGURE 8–1 *Continued.* C–E computed tomographic (CT) scanogram. In **C,** a frontal CT image of the entire lower extremities is obtained with the patient in the supine position, and precise anatomic measurements of each extremity are made. In this patient, the left femur is 7.7 mm shorter than the right. Similar measurements of the tibiae are also obtained, and an overall leg length is determined. In **D,** another patient, the left femur (474 mm) is 10 mm shorter than the right (484 mm). In **E,** a computerized display of the same patient as in **D** shows the precise length of tibia, femur, and total lower extremity bilaterally.

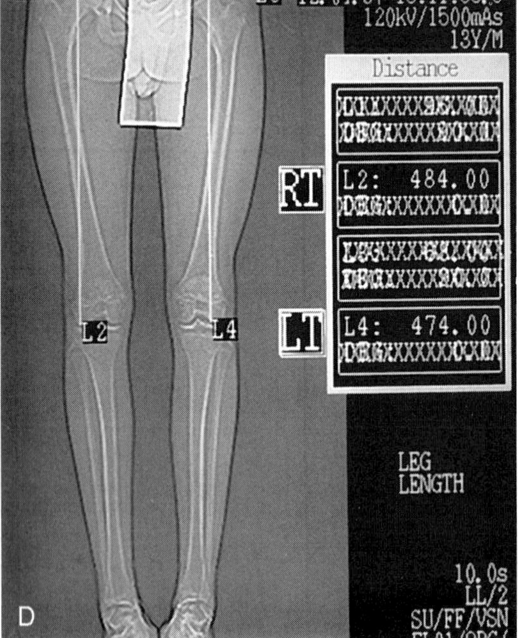

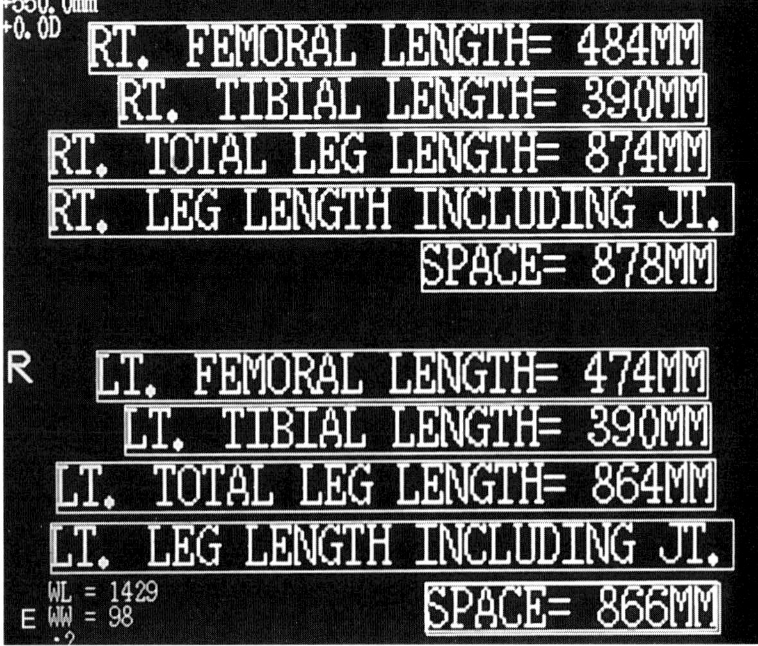

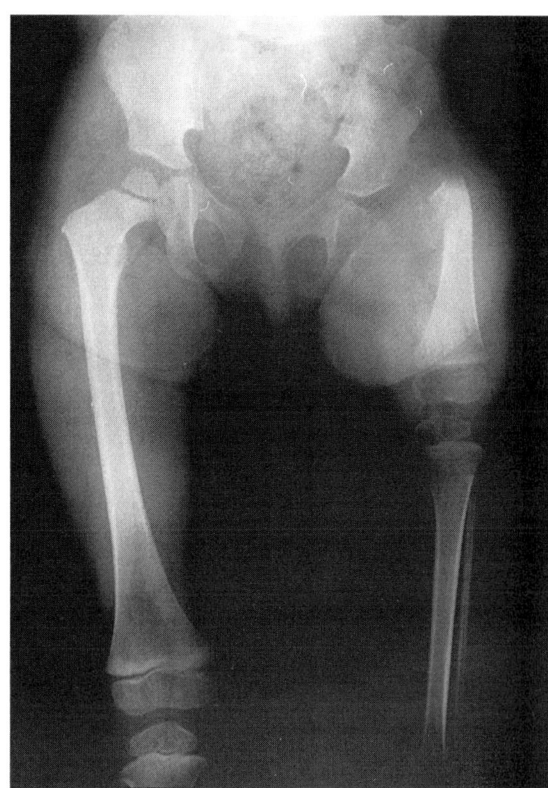

FIGURE 8–2. Proximal femoral focal deficiency (PFFD).[4] In this 4-year-old girl, the proximal portion of the left femur is shortened and tapered. No evidence of ossification of the proximal femoral epiphysis is present, and unilateral hip dislocation is evident. *(Courtesy of J. Spaeth, M.D., Albuquerque, New Mexico.)*

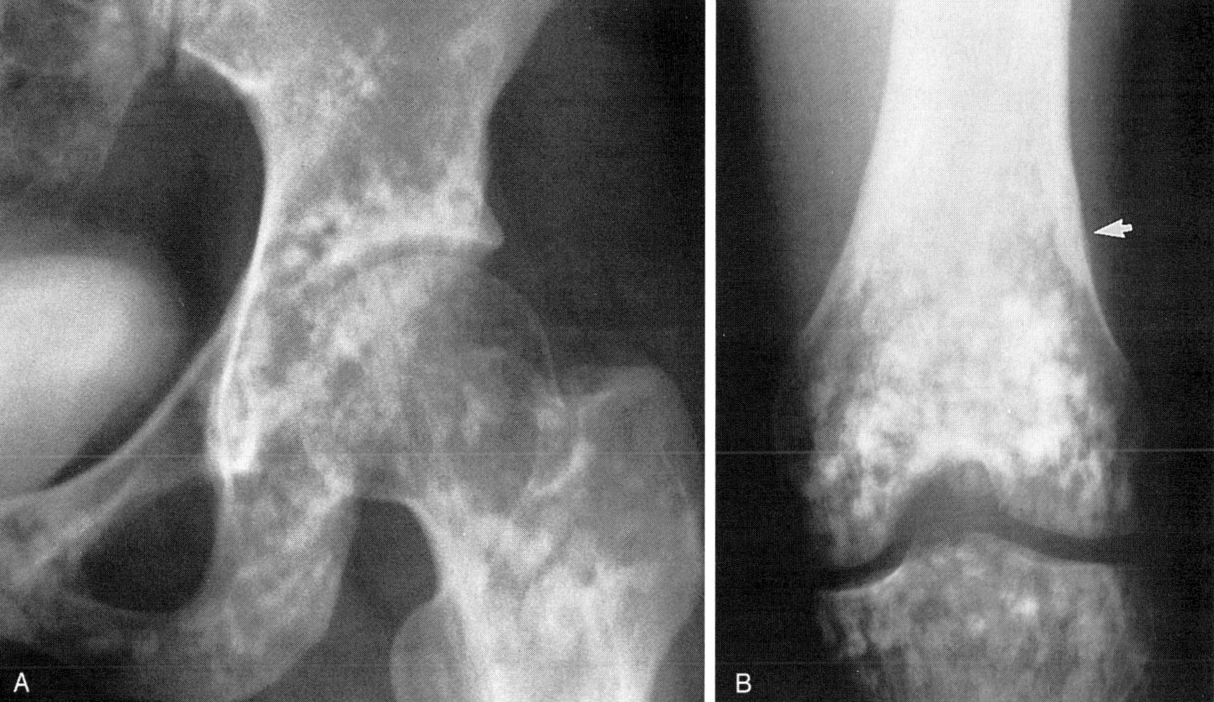

FIGURE 8–3. Osteopoikilosis.[6] A Note the circular and ovoid osteosclerotic foci localized in a periarticular distribution within the femur and pelvic bones. The symmetric, periarticular distribution is characteristic of this fairly common sclerosing dysplasia. Although the epiphysis may be affected, most lesions predominate in the metaphysis. Osteopoikilosis was an incidental asymptomatic finding in this patient, who was undergoing cystography (note contrast agent in the bladder). B Mixed sclerosing bone dystrophy.[10] Evidence of both punctate zones of sclerosis (typical of osteopoikilosis), and linear hyperostosis (characteristic of melorheostosis) (arrows) is seen in the distal end of the femur and proximal portion of the tibia in this patient. Mixed sclerosing bone dystrophy is a condition characterized by radiologic features of more than one of the sclerosing dysplasias, including osteopoikilosis, osteopathia striata, and melorheostosis. *(***B***, Courtesy of C. Resnik, M.D., Baltimore, Maryland.)*

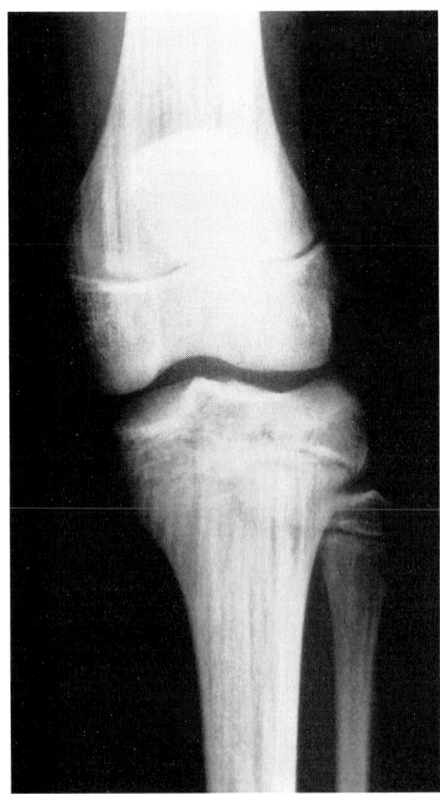

FIGURE 8–4. Osteopathia striata.[7] Linear regular bands of increased radiodensity are seen extending vertically from the metaphyses into the diaphyses of the femur, tibia, and fibula. The skeletal manifestations of this rare sclerosing dysplasia are usually bilateral.

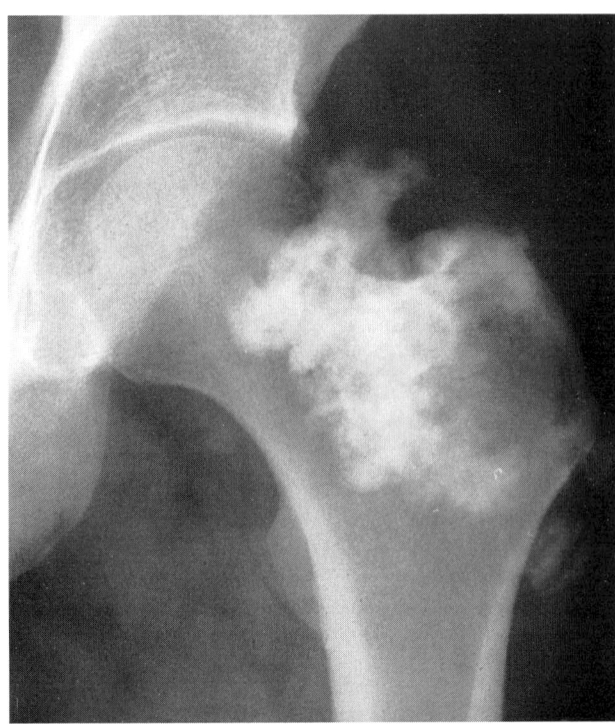

FIGURE 8–5. Melorheostosis.[8, 9] A cloud-like accumulation of ossification is seen adjacent to the proximal portion of the femur. The characteristic radiographic abnormalities of melorheostosis include asymmetric hyperostosis simulating flowing candle wax, which typically affects only one side of an extremity. *(Courtesy of A. Newberg, M.D., Boston, Massachusetts.)*

TABLE 8–2. Fractures of the Femoral Diaphysis and Soft Tissue Injury*

Entity	Figure(s)	Characteristics	Complications and Related Injuries
Acute fractures[11]			
Any level		Major trauma with associated injuries of tibia, patella, acetabulum, hip, or knee Open or closed Spiral, oblique, or transverse fracture with possible butterfly fragment and comminution	Refracture Peroneal nerve injury resulting from skeletal traction Thrombophlebitis Nonunion (1 per cent of cases), malunion, or delayed union Infection Fat embolization (approximately 10 per cent of cases)
Proximal		Less common than midshaft fractures Commonly extend into subtrochanteric region	Malalignment
Middle		Most common site Transverse fracture at this location is most typical	Nonunion
Distal and supracondylar		Less common than midshaft fractures	Malalignment Arterial injury
Stress fractures[12, 13]	8–6	Fatigue fracture: Ballet and long distance running Insufficiency fracture: Paget's disease Commonly proximal portion of femur	May result in complete fracture with or without displacement May result in complete pathologic fracture with or without displacement
Posttraumatic heterotopic ossification[14]	8–7	Ossifying hematoma in muscle after direct trauma such as "charley horse" injury Faint calcific intermuscular or intramuscular shadow may appear within 2 to 6 weeks of injury Well-defined region of ossification aligned parallel to the long axis of the femur may be evident within 6 to 8 weeks Most frequent location: quadriceps muscle Associated periostitis may relate to subperiosteal hemorrhage	Limitation of motion May result in abnormal hip or knee biomechanics and lead to premature joint degeneration May resemble aggressive neoplasms, such as osteosarcoma or Ewing's sarcoma

*See also Tables 1–3 to 1–5.

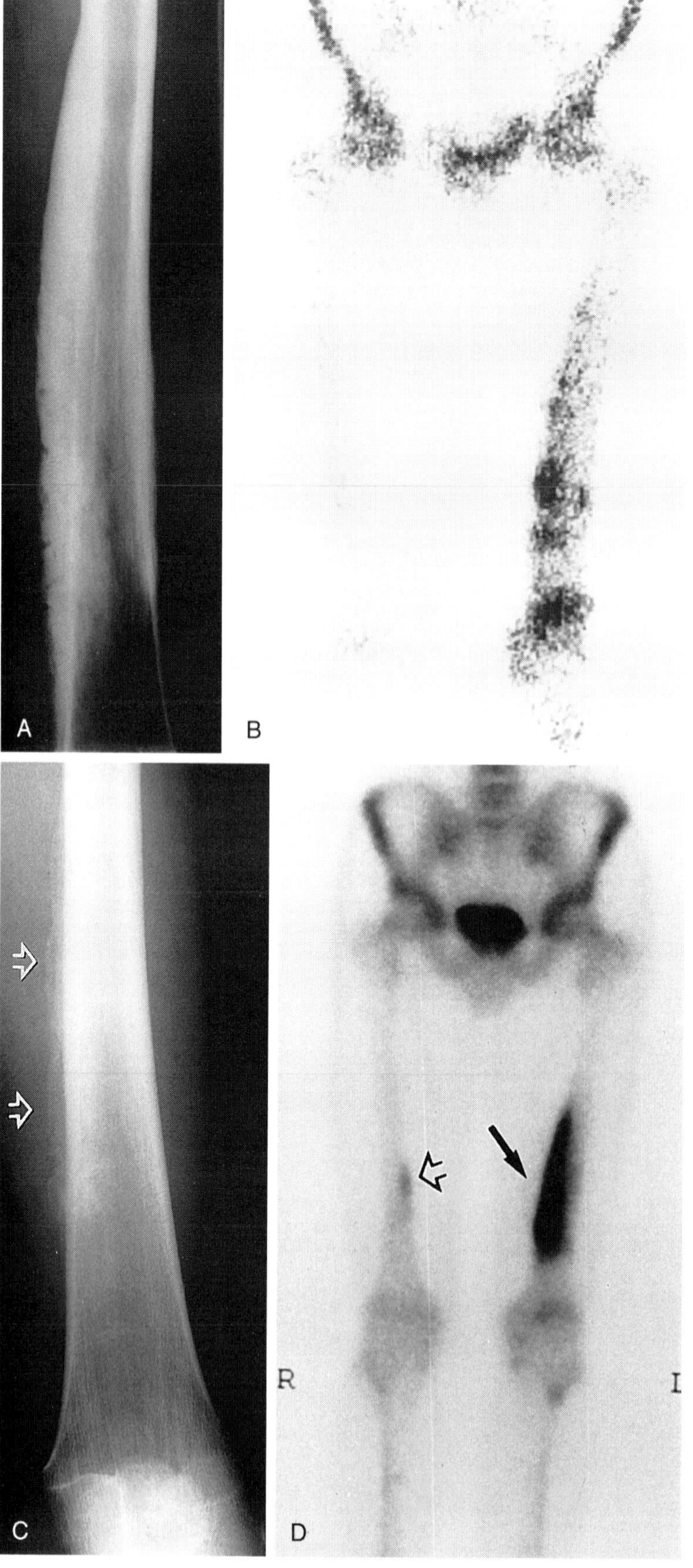

FIGURE 8–6. Stress (fatigue) fracture.[12, 13] A, B 53-year-old woman. In A, a routine radiograph shows marked periosteal and endosteal new bone formation with thickening and hyperostosis of the shaft of the femur. Multiple irregular, transverse, radiolucent striations are evident. In B, a bone scan shows increased uptake throughout the medial shaft of the femur corresponding to the zones of hyperostosis and radiolucent striations. *(A, B, Courtesy of A. Newberg, M.D., Boston, Massachusetts.)* C, D This 19-year-old marine recruit had bilateral thigh pain, worse on the left. In C, a frontal radiograph shows thick periostitis along the medial aspect of the femoral diaphysis (open arrows). In D, scintigraphic examination reveals prominent radionuclide activity at the medial aspect of the left femur (arrow). Mild increased focal uptake in the right femoral shaft (open arrow) represents an early stress reaction. Scintigraphy and magnetic resonance (MR) imaging often are helpful in the early diagnosis of stress reactions and fractures in bone.

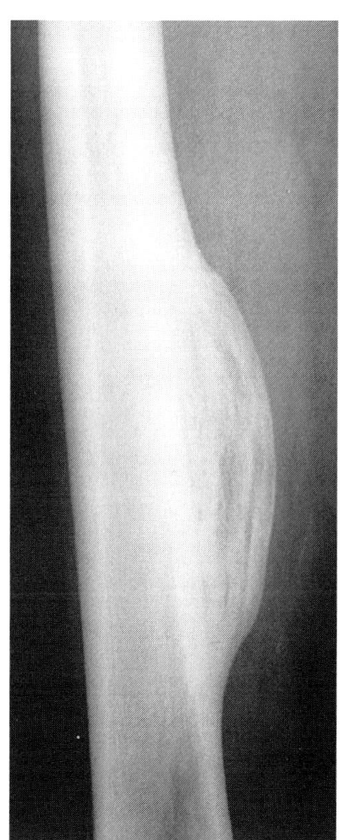

FIGURE 8–7. Heterotopic ossification: posttraumatic myositis ossificans.[14] This 56-year-old man had sustained an injury 2 months earlier. A radiograph shows a zone of well-organized ossification arising from the surface of the femur. *(Courtesy of G. Scher, M.D., San Diego, California.)*

TABLE 8–3. Malignant Tumors Affecting the Femur*

Entity	Figure(s)	Characteristics
Skeletal metastasis[15–17]	8–8 to 8–10	Fewer than 10 per cent of skeletal metastatic lesions affect the femur 75 per cent permeative or moth-eaten osteolysis 25 per cent diffuse or patchy osteosclerosis or mixed pattern of lysis and sclerosis Usually multiple sites of involvement Pathologic fracture Predilection for the lesser trochanter
		Cortical metastasis Prevalent in the long bones of patients with metastasis, especially from bronchogenic carcinoma Small radiolucent, eccentric, saucer-shaped, scalloped erosions are referred to as "cookie-bite" lesions
Primary malignant tumors of bone		
Osteosarcoma (conventional)[18]	8–11	50–75 per cent of osteosarcomas occur in the femur and tibia about the knee Osteolytic, osteosclerotic, or mixed patterns of medullary and cortical destruction Prominent periosteal reaction common Preferential involvement of the metaphysis
Osteosarcoma (parosteal)[19]	8–12	64 per cent of parosteal osteosarcomas occur in the femur Most common site: posterior surface of distal end of the femur Osteosclerotic surface lesion of bone Large radiodense, oval, sessile mass with smooth or irregular margins Peripheral portion of lesion may have plane separating it from the femur Ossification begins centrally and progresses outwardly as opposed to heterotopic bone formation (myositis ossification)
Osteoblastoma (aggressive)[20]		11 per cent of aggressive osteoblastomas occur in the femur Expansile osteolytic lesion that may be partially ossified or contain calcium Metaphyseal location Aggressive osteoblastomas have histologic and radiographic characteristics suggestive of malignancy and can be difficult to differentiate from osteosarcoma
Chondrosarcoma (conventional)[21, 22]	8–13	24 per cent of chondosarcomas occur in the femur Tend to be osteolytic lesions, sometimes containing a bulky cartilaginous cap and frequently contain calcifications May have a soft tissue mass
Giant cell tumor (aggressive)[23]	8–14	More than 40 per cent of aggressive giant cell tumors occur in the femur Involve the knee and less commonly the hip Eccentrically located, subarticular osteolytic lesion extending into the metaphysis Cortical destruction and soft tissue mass are variable findings Radiographic appearance is an inaccurate guide to determining malignancy of lesion; biopsy necessary

TABLE 8–3. Malignant Tumors Affecting the Femur* *Continued*

Entity	Figure(s)	Characteristics
Fibrosarcoma[24]		39 per cent of fibrosarcomas involve the femur Purely osteolytic destruction with no associated sclerotic reaction or periostitis Most common in distal portion of the femur
Malignant fibrous histiocytoma[24]		44 per cent of malignant fibrous histiocytomas involve the femur Pathologic fracture in 30 to 50 per cent of cases Metaphyseal location with frequent spread to epiphysis and diaphysis Moth-eaten or permeative osteolysis, frequently resembling fibrosarcoma
Ewing's sarcoma[25]	8–15	22 per cent of Ewing's sarcomas occur in the femur Permeative or moth-eaten osteolysis, aggressive cortical erosion or violation, laminated or spiculated periostitis and soft tissue masses Most lesions central and diametaphyseal in location
Myeloproliferative disorders		
Multiple myeloma[26]	8–16	16 per cent of multiple myeloma lesions occur in the femur Early: normal radiographs or diffuse osteopenia Later: widespread well-circumscribed osteolytic lesions with discrete margins, which appear uniform in size 97 per cent osteolytic; 3 per cent osteosclerotic False-negative bone scans common
Solitary plasmacytoma[26]	8–17	18 per cent of solitary plasmacytomas occur in the femur Solitary, geographic, expansile, osteolytic lesion that frequently results in pathologic fracture 70 per cent of cases eventually develop into multiple myeloma
Hodgkin's disease[27]		10 per cent of osseous involvement occurs in the femur 75 per cent of lesions are osteolytic; permeative or moth-eaten osteolysis 25 per cent of lesions are osteosclerotic More than 60 per cent of patients have multiple sites of involvement
Primary lymphoma (non-Hodgkin's)[28, 29]	8–18	Approximately 24 per cent of lesions in primary lymphoma occur in the femur Multiple moth-eaten or permeative osteolytic lesions Diffuse or localized sclerotic lesions are rare Common cause of pathologic fracture
Leukemia[30]	8–19	Diffuse osteopenia, radiolucent or radiodense transverse metaphyseal bands, osteolytic lesions, periostitis, and, infrequently, osteosclerosis Radiodense metaphyses more frequently in patients undergoing chemotherapy for leukemia; may resemble lead poisoning

*See also Table 1–10.

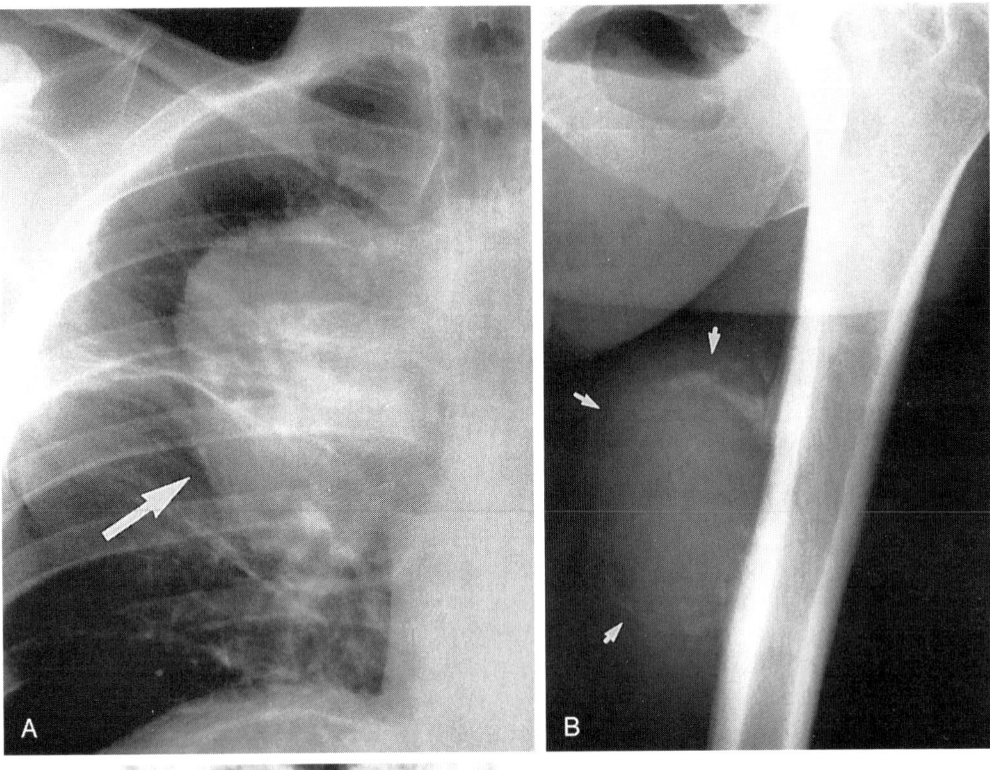

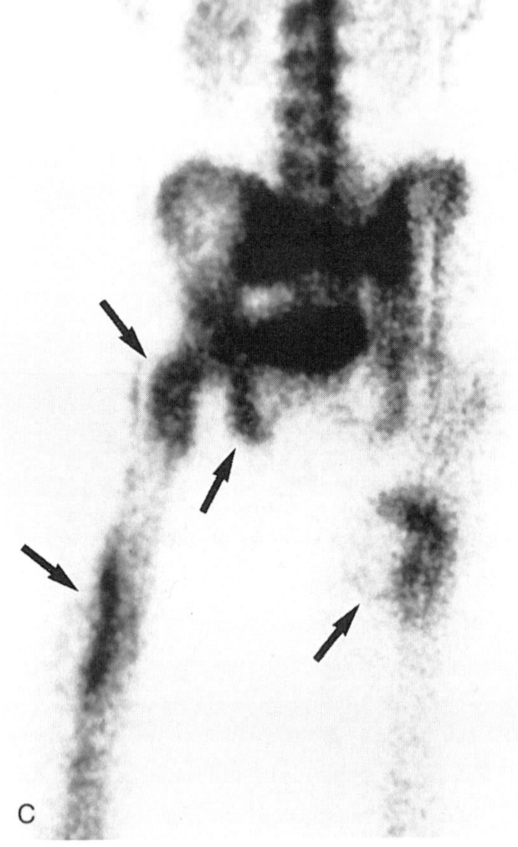

FIGURE 8–8. Skeletal metastasis: Osteolytic pattern.[15] This 40-year-old man with bronchogenic carcinoma had widespread metastasis throughout his skeleton. A Posteroanterior chest radiograph demonstrates a large pulmonary mass representing the primary tumor (arrow). B Frontal radiograph of the femur shows an osteolytic cortical lesion with a thin-shelled, calcified soft tissue mass (arrows). C Bone scan shows several sites of increased uptake of radionuclide (arrows) and specifically outlines the osseous shell surrounding the soft tissue mass.

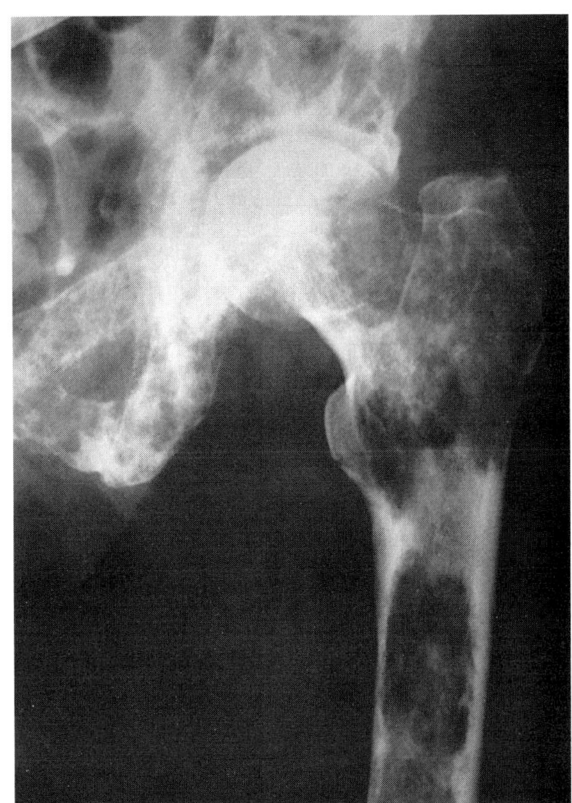

FIGURE 8–9. Skeletal metastasis: mixed pattern.[16] This 56-year-old woman had a history of breast carcinoma and diffuse bone pain. A combined pattern of osteolytic destruction and osteosclerosis is evident throughout the proximal portion of the femur and pelvis. *(From Taylor AM, Harger BL, Resnick D: Diagnostic imaging of common hip disorders: A pictorial review. Top Clin Chiropr 1:8, 1994. Courtesy of F. G. Bauer, Sydney, Australia.)*

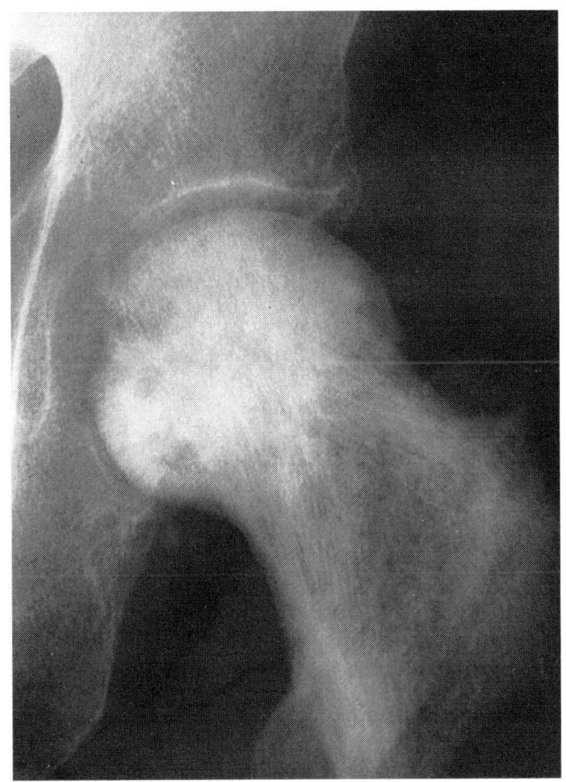

FIGURE 8–10. Skeletal metastasis: Osteoblastic pattern.[17] This patient with prostate carcinoma developed metastasis to bone. Radiographs show a diffuse pattern of osteosclerosis that extends to the subarticular region of the femoral head. Sclerosis and prominence of the primary weight-bearing trabeculae and subarticular involvement resemble the changes of Paget's disease.

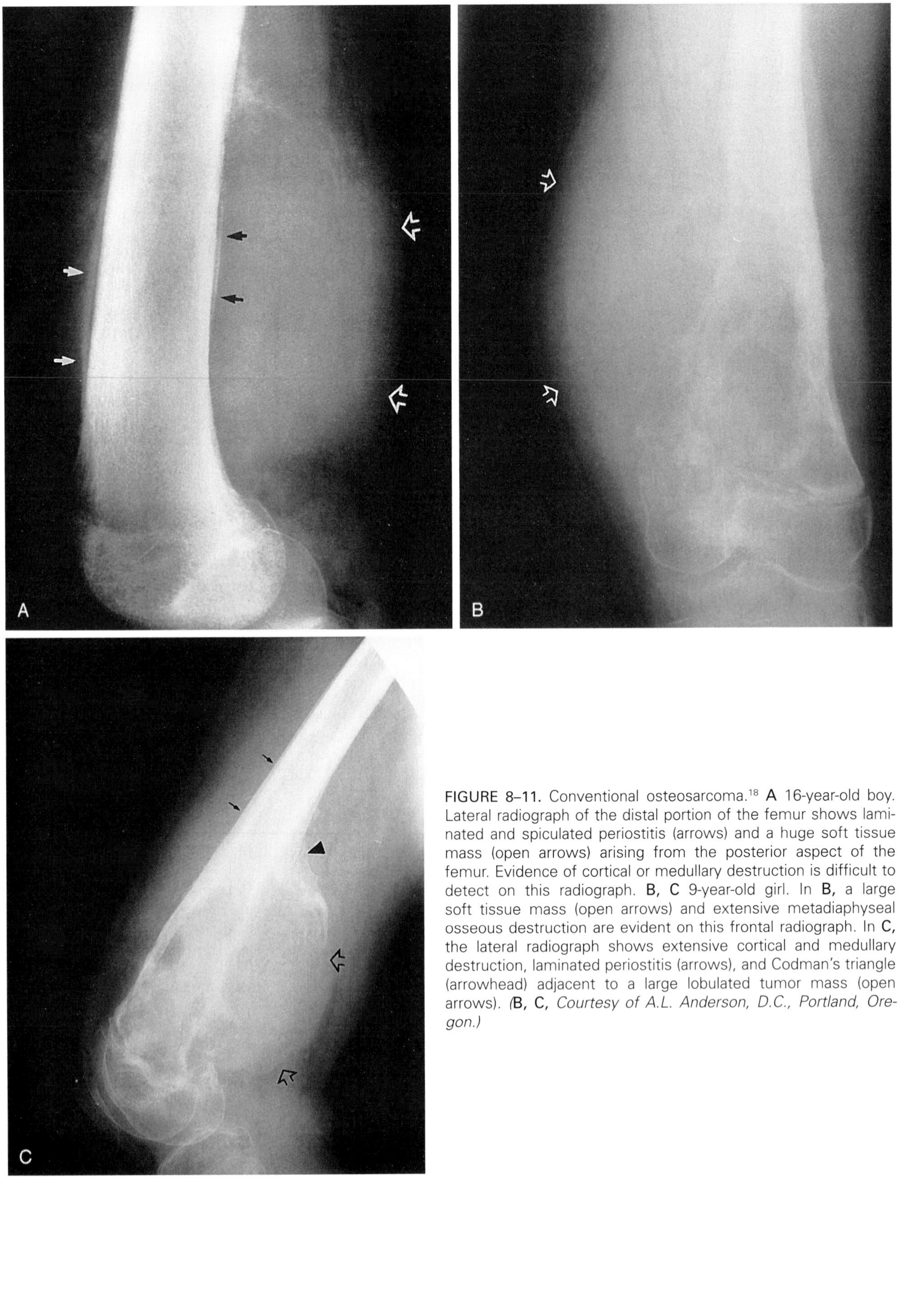

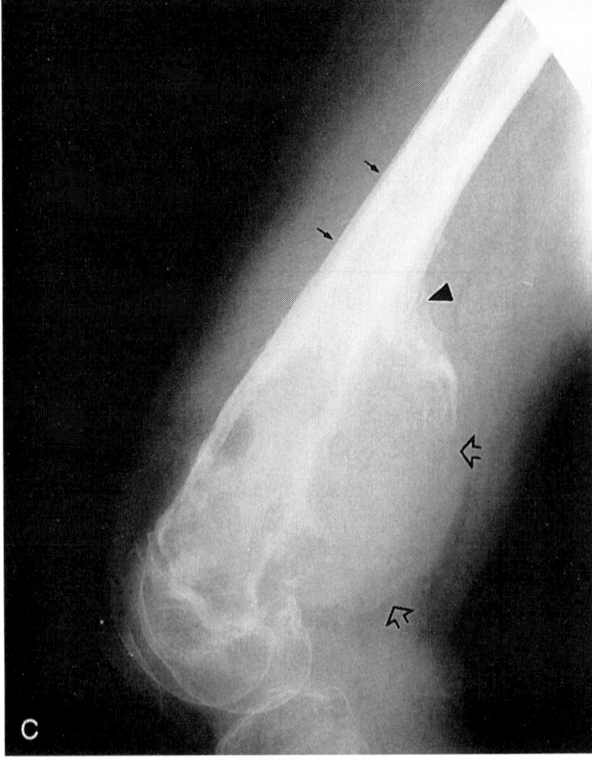

FIGURE 8–11. Conventional osteosarcoma.[18] **A** 16-year-old boy. Lateral radiograph of the distal portion of the femur shows laminated and spiculated periostitis (arrows) and a huge soft tissue mass (open arrows) arising from the posterior aspect of the femur. Evidence of cortical or medullary destruction is difficult to detect on this radiograph. **B, C** 9-year-old girl. In **B**, a large soft tissue mass (open arrows) and extensive metadiaphyseal osseous destruction are evident on this frontal radiograph. In **C**, the lateral radiograph shows extensive cortical and medullary destruction, laminated periostitis (arrows), and Codman's triangle (arrowhead) adjacent to a large lobulated tumor mass (open arrows). *(**B, C,** Courtesy of A.L. Anderson, D.C., Portland, Oregon.)*

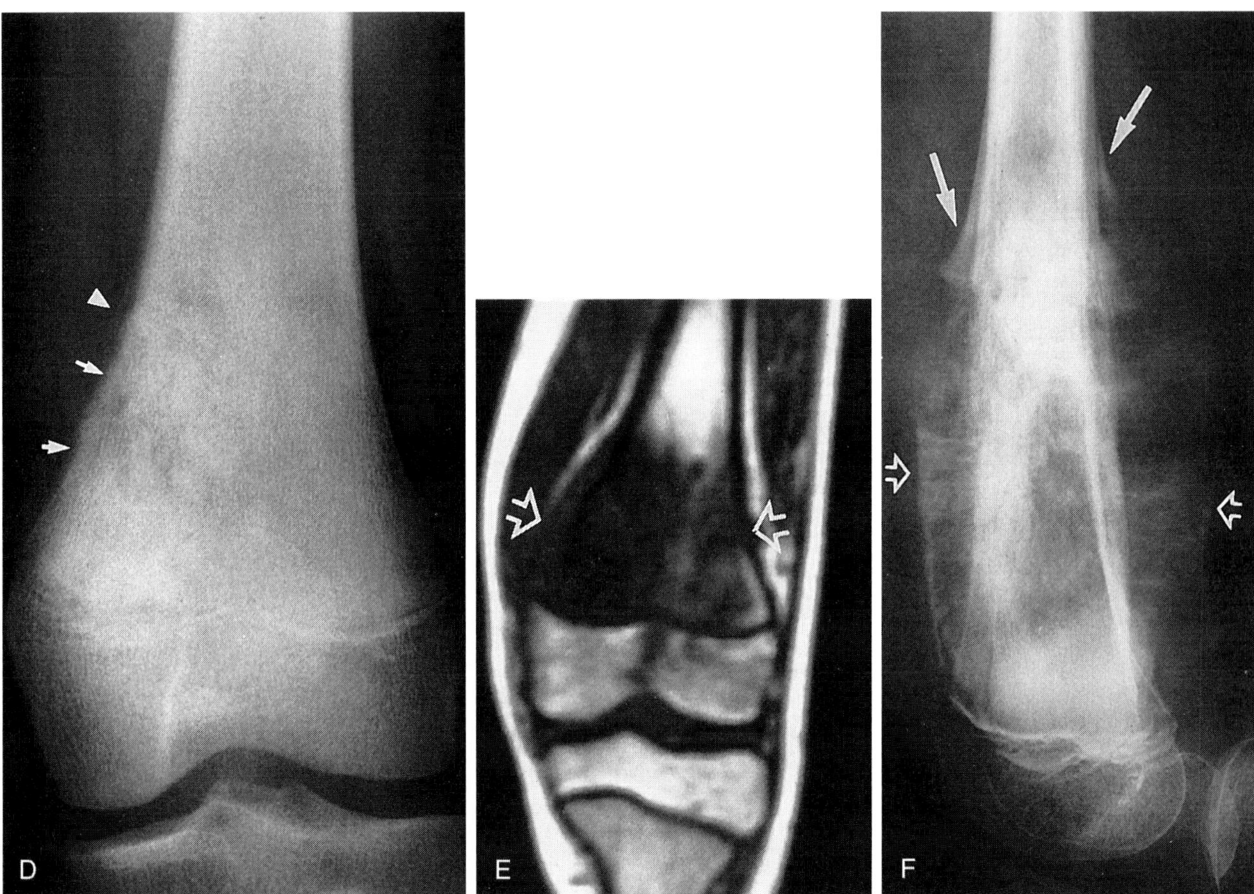

FIGURE 8–11 *Continued.* **D, E** 12-old girl with leg pain. In **D,** an anteroposterior radiograph shows an osteosclerotic metaphyseal lesion. The cortical margin of the medial aspect of the metaphysis is indistinct (arrows). A barely perceptible periosteal reaction is also seen (arrowhead). In **E,** a coronal T1-weighted (TR/TE, 600/20) spin echo magnetic resonance (MR) image shows an area of low signal intensity corresponding to the metaphyseal region of osteosclerosis (open arrows). *(***D, E,** *Courtesy of R. Kerr, M.D., Los Angeles, California.)* **F** Periosteal reaction patterns. Radiograph of another patient with osteosarcoma demonstrates typical patterns of aggressive periosteal reaction. Codman's triangle is seen as a triangular buttress appearing to arise from the surface of bone at the tumor margins (arrows). The spiculated periosteal reaction is evident as a series of parallel horizontal spicules emanating from the underlying bone (hair-on-end pattern) at the site of the tumor (open arrows).

Illustration continued on following page

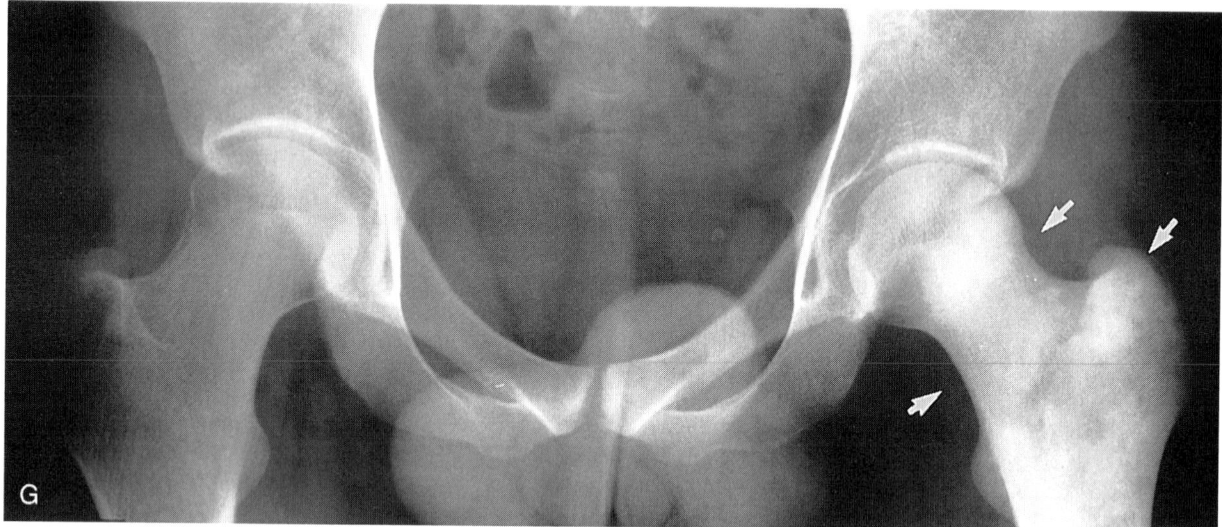

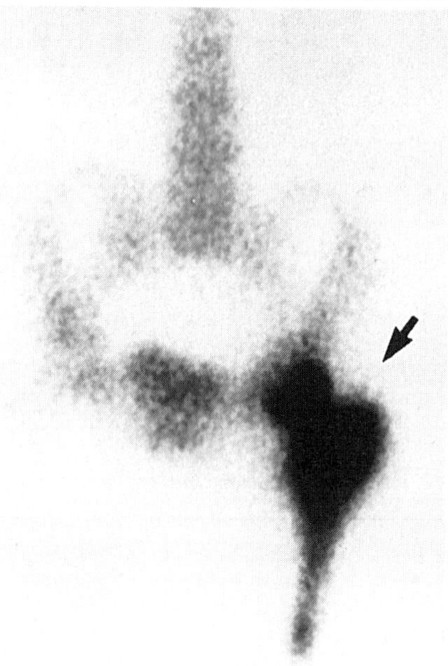

FIGURE 8–11 *Continued.* G, H Conventional osteosarcoma in a 19-year-old man: Osteoblastic pattern. In G, a frontal pelvic radiograph reveals patchy osteosclerosis in the proximal portion of the left femur (arrows). In H, a bone scan obtained the same day shows intense increased uptake of the bone-seeking radiopharmaceutical agent at the site of the lesion (arrow). (G, H, *Courtesy of T. Broderick, M.D., Orange, California.*)

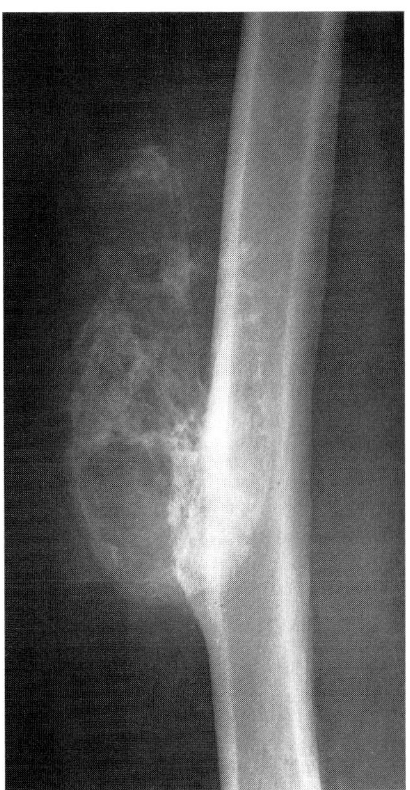

FIGURE 8–12. Parosteal osteosarcoma.[19] A large osteosclerotic parosteal osteosarcoma is seen arising from the surface of the femoral diaphysis. The pedunculated attachment to the surface of the femur is helpful in differentiating this malignant neoplasm from more benign processes, such as posttraumatic myositis ossificans.

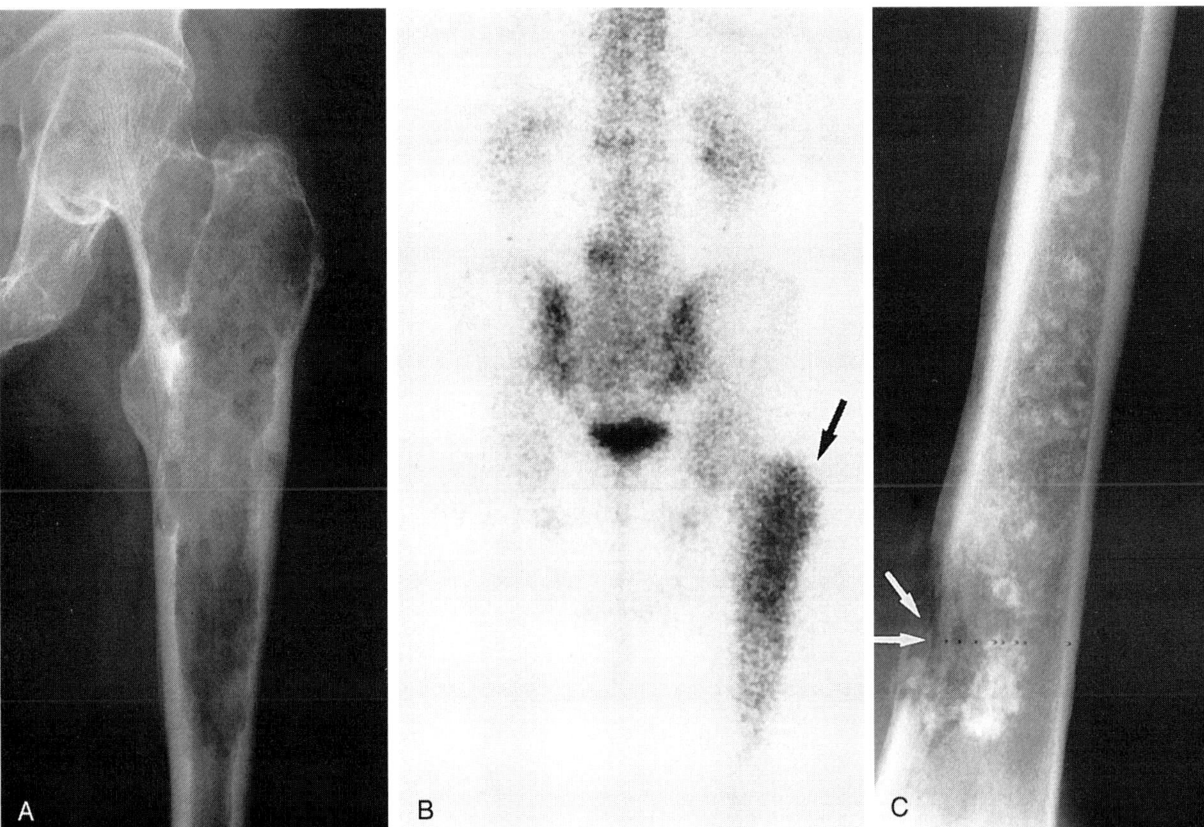

FIGURE 8–13. Conventional chondrosarcoma, 63-year-old male patient.[21, 22] A Routine frontal radiograph demonstrates a moth-eaten destructive appearance of the proximal portion of the femur extending from the femoral neck into the mid-diaphysis. Extensive endosteal scalloping is noted. B Radionuclide bone scan reveals intense homogeneous increased uptake at the site of the lesion (arrow). C Routine radiograph of the femur in another patient shows a long metadiaphyseal lesion with extensive stippled calcification, endosteal scalloping, and cortical perforation (arrows). *(Courtesy of J. Schils, M.D., Cleveland, Ohio.)*

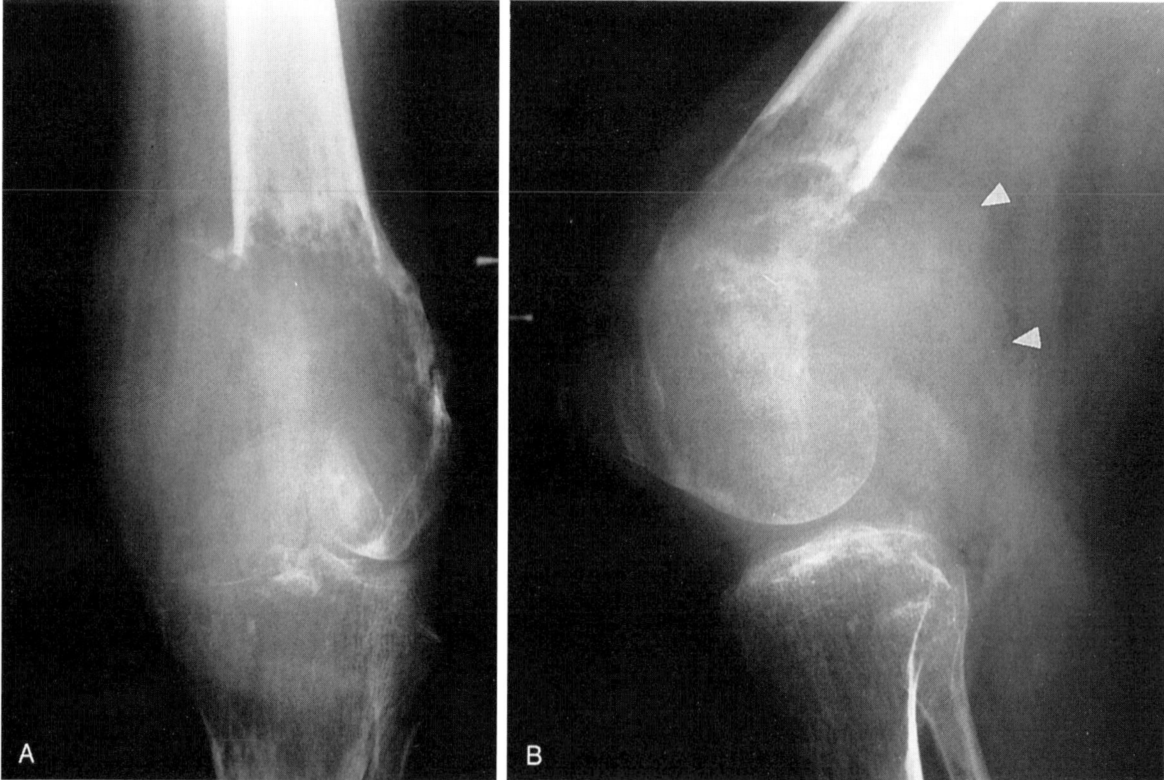

FIGURE 8–14. Aggressive giant cell tumor.[23] This 33-year-old man had a history of several months' duration of an increasingly painful, expanding mass near his knee. A Frontal radiograph. B Lateral radiograph. A highly destructive osteolytic lesion obliterates the cortical and medullary bones of the entire metaphysis and subchondral region of the distal portion of the femur. The matrix of the lesion is purely osteolytic, and a pathologic fracture with angulation is seen on the lateral view. A large soft tissue mass is evident (arrowheads). Marked osteopenia secondary to disuse is seen in the proximal portions of the tibia and fibula. The tumor was biopsied, analyzed, and reported to be a malignant (aggressive) giant cell tumor.

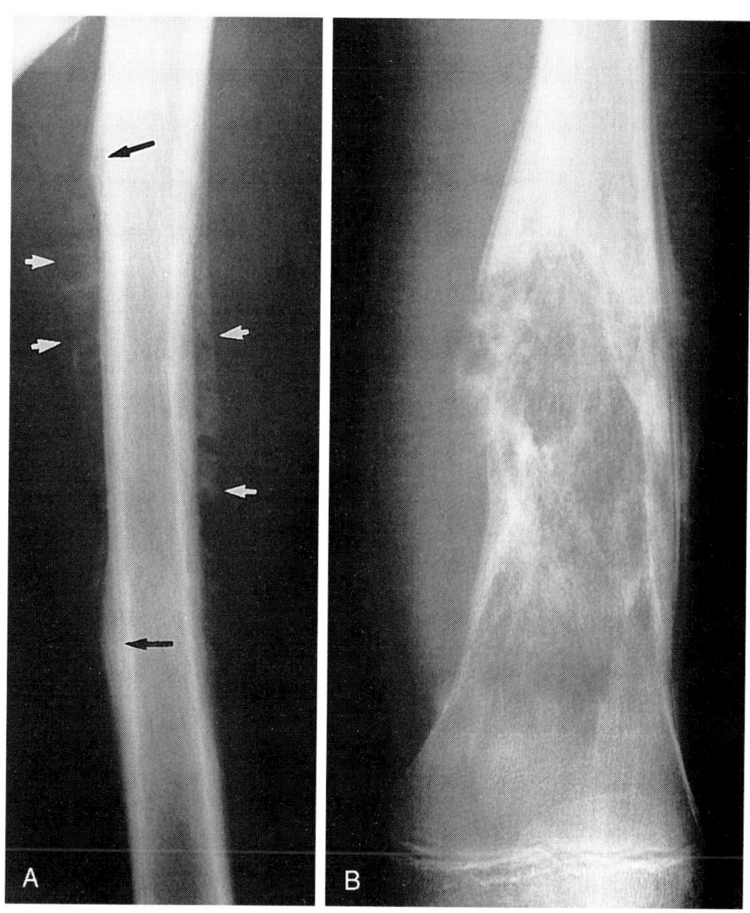

FIGURE 8–15. Ewing's sarcoma.[25] **A** Routine radiograph of this 12-year-old boy with biopsy-proved Ewing's sarcoma demonstrates spiculated periostitis (white arrows) and Codman's triangles (black arrows) involving the femoral diaphysis. **B** In this 9-year-old boy, permeative osteolytic destruction of the metadiaphysis of the distal end of the femur is associated with aggressive, laminated periostitis and cortical destruction. Biopsy revealed Ewing's sarcoma. (*B, Courtesy of T. Broderick, M.D., Orange, California.*)

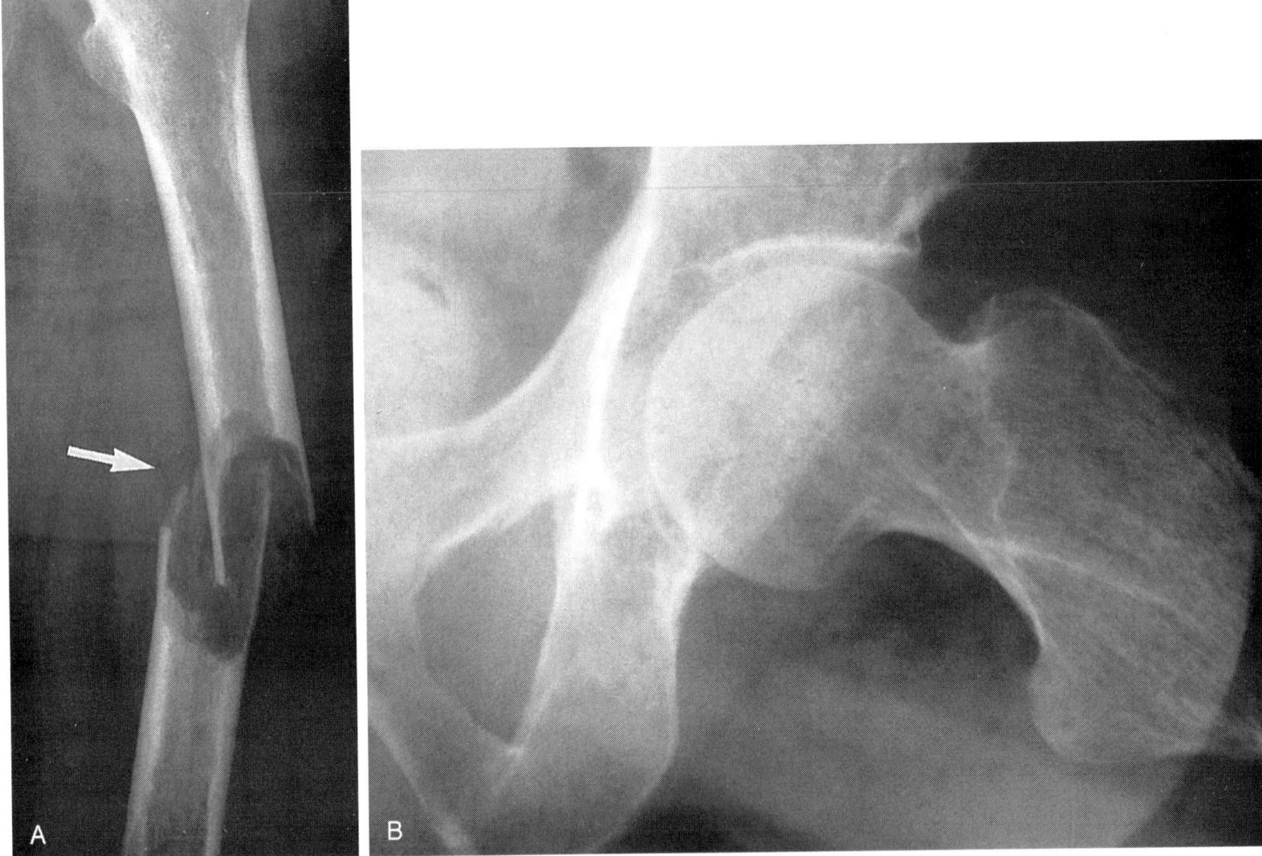

FIGURE 8–16. Plasma cell (multiple) myeloma.[26] A Pathologic fracture has occurred through a large radiolucent lesion in the mid-diaphysis of the femur (arrow) in this patient with a histologic diagnosis of multiple myeloma. (A, *Courtesy of V. Wing, M.D., Danville, California.*) B In another patient with multiple myeloma, a permeative pattern of diffuse osteopenia is the only radiographic manifestation. (B, *From Taylor JAM, Harger BL, Resnick D: Diagnostic imaging of common hip disorders: A pictorial review. Top Clin Chiropr 1:8, 1994.*)

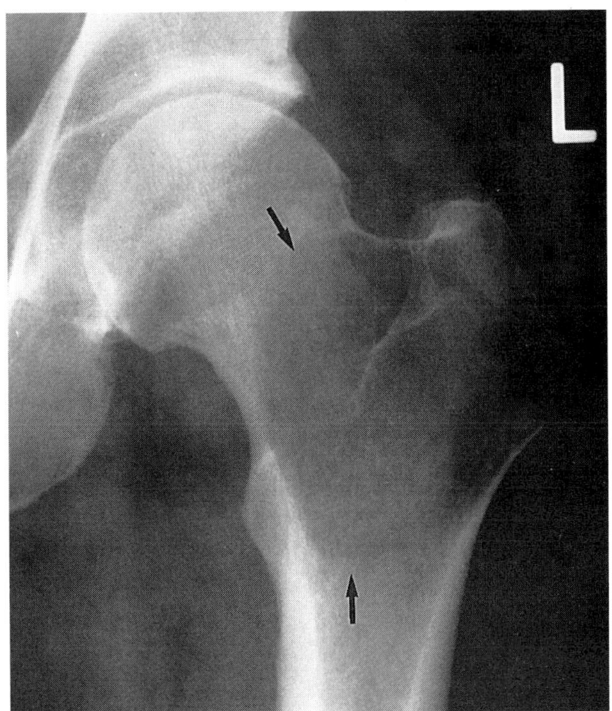

FIGURE 8–17. Solitary plasmacytoma.[26] This 37-year-old man had a 4-month history of hip pain and a limp. A large, solitary osteolytic lesion (arrows) is evident in the intertrochanteric region of the proximal portion of the femur. *(Courtesy of G. Greenway, M.D., Dallas, Texas.)*

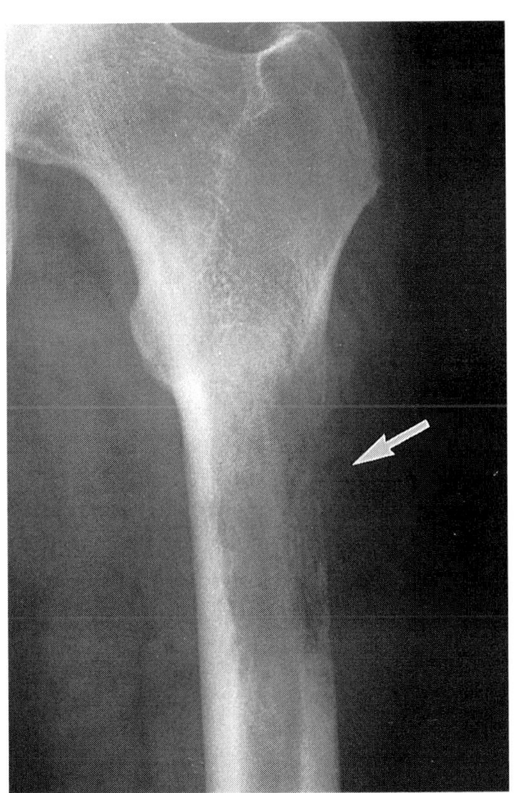

FIGURE 8–18. Non-Hodgkin's lymphoma: histiocytic type.[28, 29] Observe the eccentric moth-eaten osteolysis and cortical penetration (arrow) of the femoral diaphysis in this 47-year-old man.

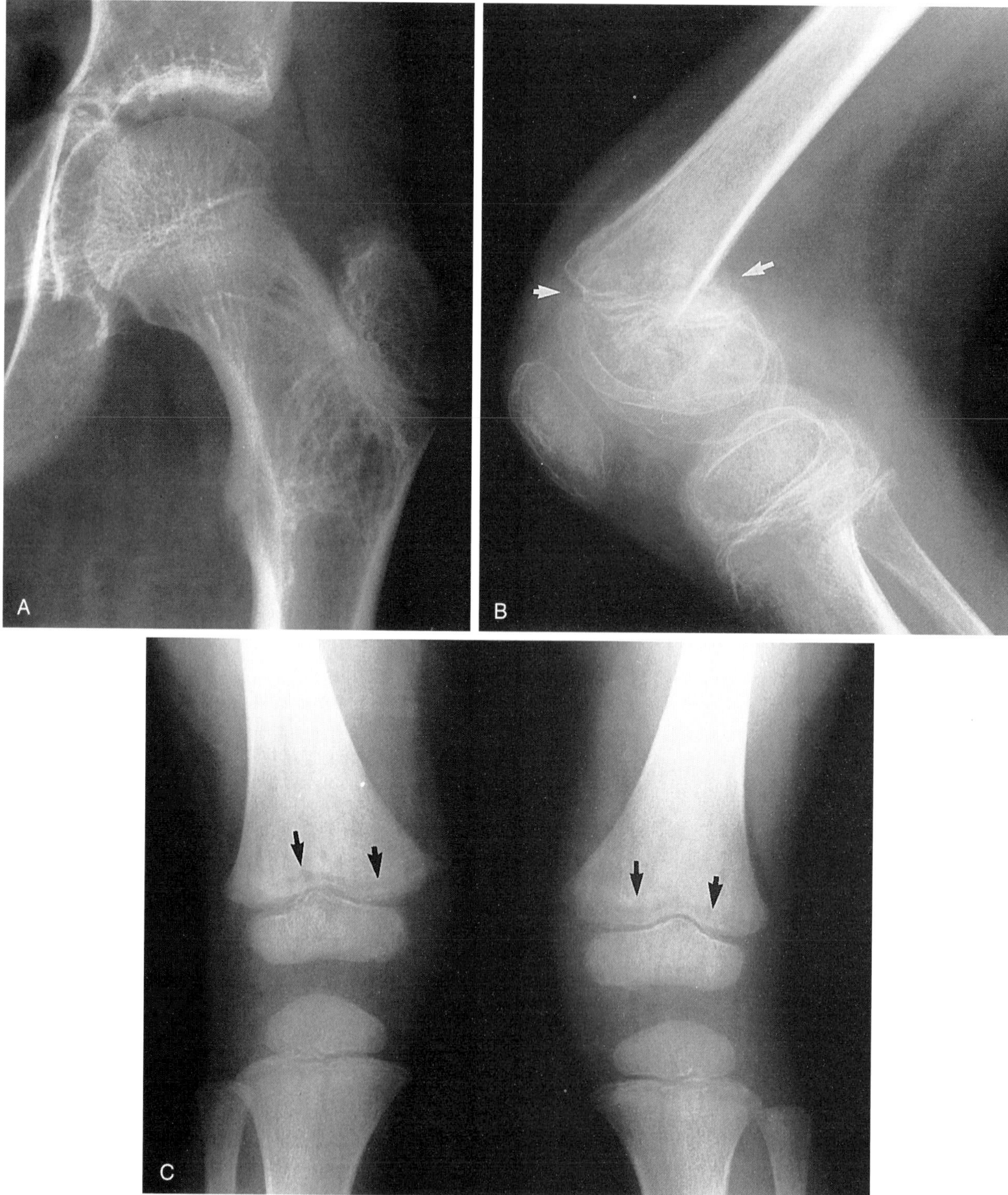

FIGURE 8–19. Leukemia.[30] A–C Acute lymphocytic leukemia. In a 14-year-old boy (A, B), a radiograph (A) of the proximal portion of the femur demonstrates diffuse osteopenia and apparent trabecular accentuation. Observe the increased radiolucency and prominence of the primary weight-bearing trabeculae. In B, diffuse osteopenia and a displaced pathologic fracture through the distal femoral physis (arrows) are evident. Excessive radiolucency is seen in the epiphyses and metaphyses. C In another patient, observe the bilateral radiolucent metaphyseal bands involving the distal portions of the femora (arrows).

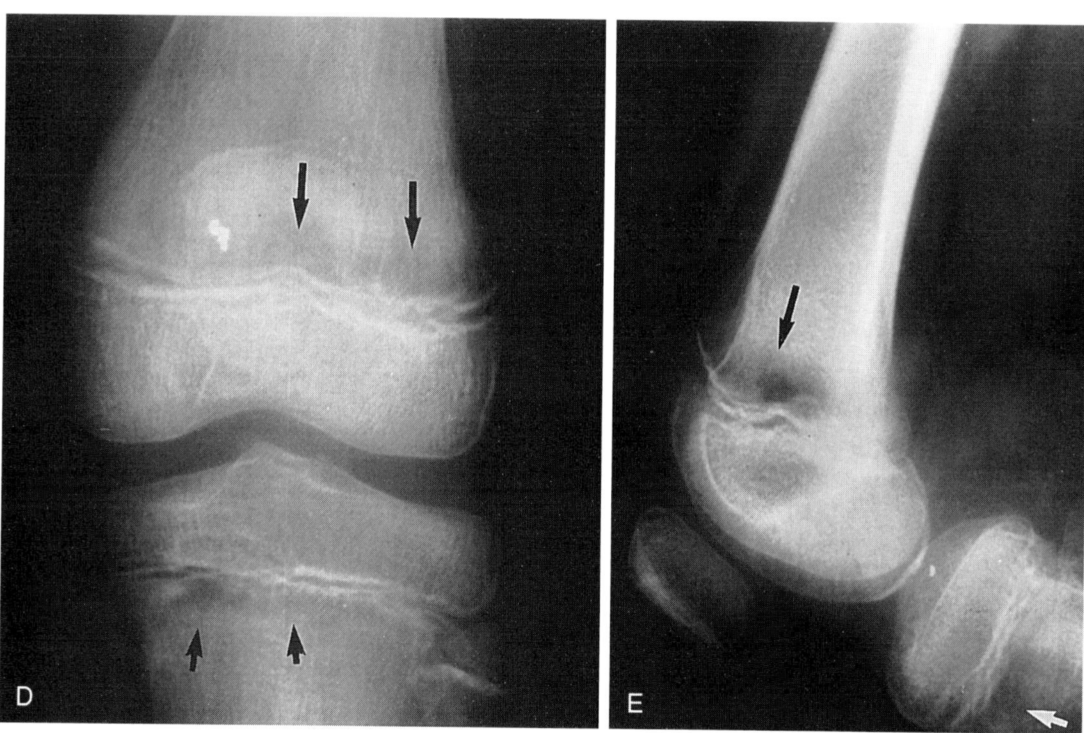

FIGURE 8–19 *Continued.* D, E Acute childhood leukemia. Anteroposterior and lateral radiographs of the knee in this 8-year-old girl with acute leukemia reveal transverse radiolucent bands in the metaphyses of the femur and tibia (arrows).

TABLE 8–4. Benign Tumors Affecting the Femur*

Entity	Figure(s)	Characteristics
Enostosis[31]	8–20	25 per cent of enostoses (bone islands) occur in the femur Solitary, painless, infrequently multiple, discrete focus of osteosclerosis within the spongiosa of bone Round, ovoid, or oblong with brush border composed of radiating osseous spicules that interdigitate with the surrounding trabeculae of the spongiosa
Osteoid osteoma[32–34]	8–21	32 per cent of osteoid osteomas occur in the femur Solitary cortical or subperiosteal lesion with reactive sclerosis surrounding central radioluent nidus Nidus is less than 1 cm in diameter and usually not visible on routine radiographs Intracapsular lesions provoke less reactive sclerosis and are more likely to cause joint pain
Osteoblastoma (conventional)[35]		Fewer than 15 per cent of conventional osteoblastomas involve the femur Osteolytic, osteosclerotic, or both Solitary expansile lesion that may be subperiosteal Partially calcified matrix in many cases Cortical thinning Often resembles large osteoid osteoma
Enchondroma (solitary)[36]	8–22	Approximately 10 per cent of solitary enchondromas involve the femur Central or eccentric medullary osteolytic lesion Lobulated endosteal scalloping Approximately 50 per cent of lesions have stippled calcification within the matrix
Enchondromatosis (Ollier's disease)[36]		Multiple enchondromas; frequently involve the femur
Maffucci's syndrome[36]		Over 50 per cent of cases involve the femur Multiple enchondromas and soft tissue hemangiomas Unilateral distribution in 50 per cent of cases
Chondroblastoma[37, 38]	8–23	Approximately one third of chondroblastomas affect the femur Solitary circular osteolytic lesion affecting femoral capital epiphyses, trochanteric apophyses, and distal femoral epiphyses May exhibit calcification in matrix Occasionally periosteal reaction and edema may be seen on magnetic resonance (MR) imaging
Chondromyxoid fibroma[39]		17 per cent of chondromyxoid fibromas occur in the femur Solitary eccentric, elongated metaphyseal lesion 2–10 cm in length Cortical expansion, coarse trabeculation, endosteal sclerosis Calcification is rare (5–27 per cent of cases) May appear aggressive with large "bite" lesion penetrating cortex
Osteochondroma (solitary)[40, 41]	8–24	More than 30 per cent of solitary osteochondromas arise from the femur Pedunculated or sessile cartilage-covered osseous excrescence arising from the surface of the metaphysis of the distal or proximal portion of the femur Cortex and medulla are continuous with the host bone Typically, grow away from the adjacent joint
Hereditary multiple exostosis[42–44]	8–25	Multiple osteochondromas, sometimes numbering in the hundreds Femoral neck frequently involved; also occur about the knee Results in valgus deformity of hip and widening of the femoral neck
Nonossifying fibroma and fibrous cortical defect[45]	8–26	Almost 40 per cent of nonossifying fibromas and fibrous cortical defects involve the femur Solitary eccentric, multiloculated osteolytic lesion arising from the metaphyseal cortex Resemble a well-circumscribed blister-like shell of bone arising from the cortex Cortical thinning often is present
Giant cell tumor (benign)[46]	8–27	Approximately one third of benign giant cell tumors occur in the femur; most commonly in the distal portion of the femur; also found at the proximal region near the hip Solitary eccentric osteolytic neoplasm with a predilection for the subarticular region Often multiloculated and expansile Radiographs are inaccurate in distinguishing benign from aggressive giant cell tumors

TABLE 8–4. Benign Tumors Affecting the Femur* *Continued*

Entity	Figure(s)	Characteristics
Intraosseous lipoma[47]	8–28	15 per cent of intraosseous lipomas occur in the femur Intertrochanteric region and femoral neck are common sites of involvement Solitary osteolytic lesion surrounded by a thin, well-defined sclerotic border Occasional central calcified or ossified nidus Osseous expansion occurs infrequently Cortical destruction and periostitis absent
Simple bone cyst[48]	8–29	Approximately 25 per cent of all simple bone cysts occur in the femur Mildly expansile, solitary osteolytic lesion within medullary cavity of proximal portion of femur May be multiloculated
Aneurysmal bone cyst[49]	8–30	Approximately 15 per cent of aneurysmal bone cysts occur in the femur Eccentric, thin-walled, expansile osteolytic lesion of the metaphysis Thin trabeculation with multiloculated appearance Buttressing at edge of lesion Typically more expansile than osteoblastoma Fluid levels may be seen with computed tomographic (CT) scan or magnetic resonance (MR) imaging

*See also Table 1–11.

TABLE 8–5. Tumor-Like Lesions Affecting the Femur*

Entity	Figure(s)	Characteristics
Paget's disease[50, 51]	8–31	Femur is one of the most commonly involved bones Usually polyostotic and may be unilateral Coarsened trabeculae and bone enlargement Stages of involvement: osteolytic (50 per cent), osteosclerotic (25 per cent), mixed (25 per cent), and malignant transformation (less than 2 per cent) Pathologic fracture, coxa vara (shepherd's crook) deformities, insufficiency fractures in convex surface of bowed bones, acetabular protrusion
Neurofibromatosis 1 (von Recklinghausen's disease)[52]		Femur involved only occasionally Dysplastic appearance of femur with overconstriction, deformity, remodeling of bone, and circumscribed osteolytic lesions
Monostotic fibrous dysplasia[53]	8–32	15 per cent of monostotic lesions affect the femur Predilection for the intertrochanteric region Thick rim of sclerosis surrounding radiolucent lesion Ground-glass appearance of fibrous matrix Acetabular protrusion may occur
Polyostotic fibrous dysplasia[53]		92 per cent of patients have femoral lesions Unilateral or bilateral, asymmetric femoral involvement Usually associated with concomitant disease in the innominate bone Lesions appear the same as those in monostotic form but frequently are larger, more expansile, and more multiloculated than monostotic lesions
Langerhans' cell histiocytosis[54, 55]	8–33	Femur is involved in 15 per cent of cases Osteolytic lesions may be multiloculated and expansile

*See also Table 1–12.

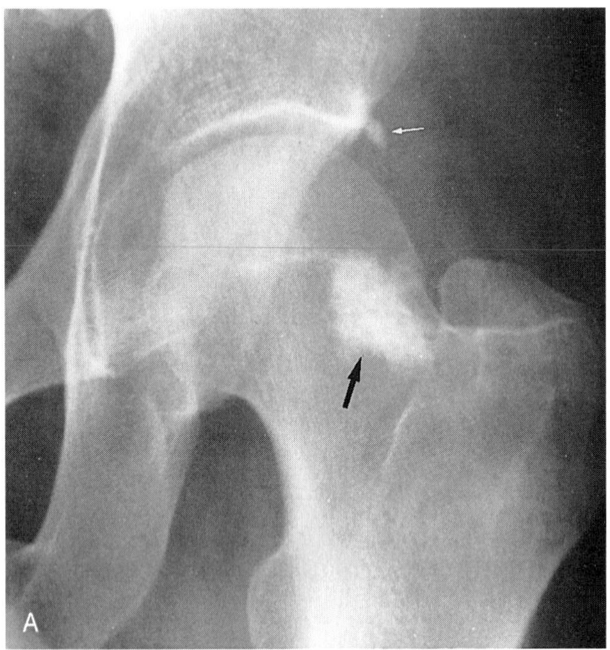

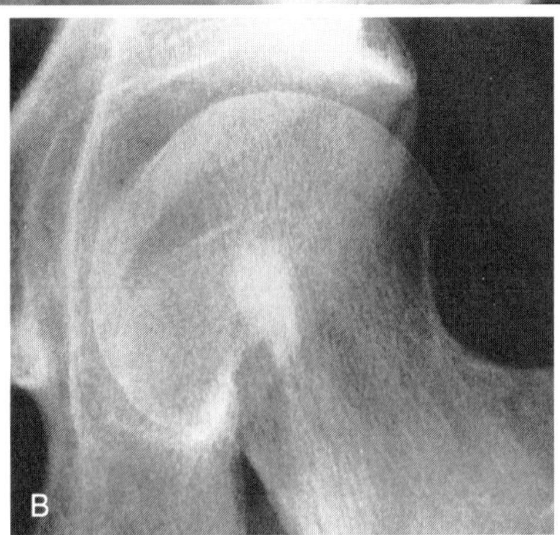

FIGURE 8–20. Enostosis (bone island). A Observe the solitary, circular osteosclerotic lesion that is aligned with the long axis of trabecular architecture in the femoral neck (black arrow). Note the irregular margins of the lesion. Incidentally, a small os acetabuli (white arrow) is present. B In another patient, note that the enostosis is oriented along the long axis of the principal compressive trabeculae.

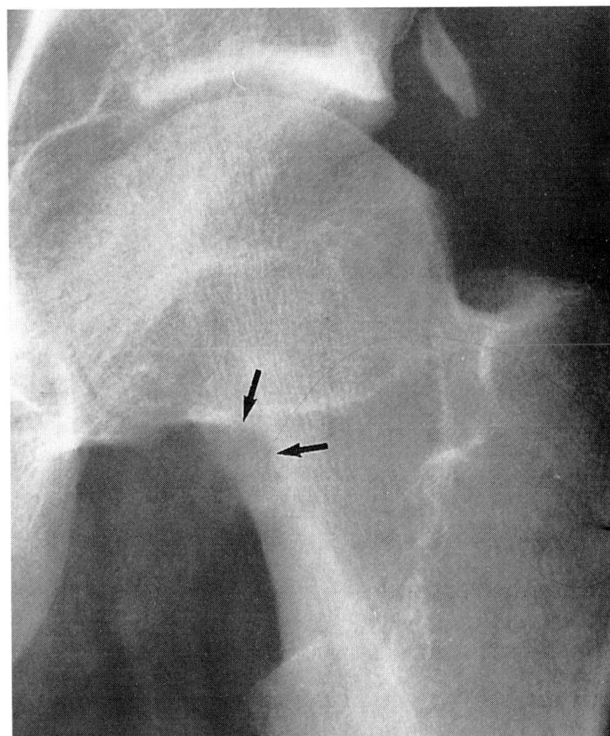

FIGURE 8–21. Osteoid osteoma.[32–34] A painful intracapsular osteoid osteoma in this 22-year-old man is seen as a circular radiolucent area within the cortex of the medial femoral neck (arrows). In addition, this patient has findings consistent with degenerative disease of the hip joint. The femur is the bone that is affected most commonly by osteoid osteoma (32 per cent occur in the femur), although epiphyseal or intracapsular lesions such as in this patient are rare. Intracapsular osteoid osteomas do not characteristically provoke severe reactive sclerosis.

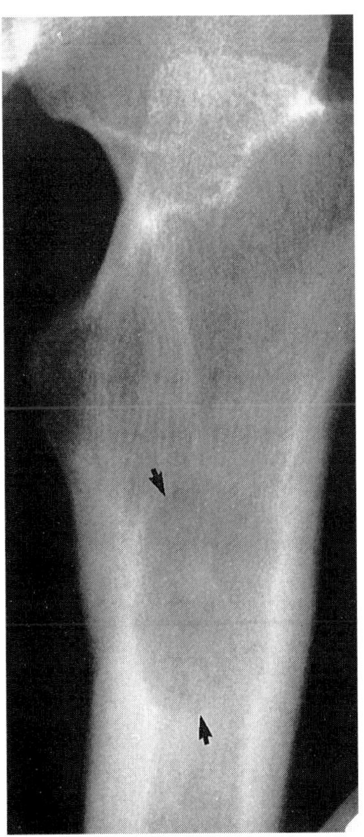

FIGURE 8–22. Enchondroma.[22, 36] This painless, oval, geographic osteolytic lesion has resulted in minimal endosteal scalloping of the proximal femoral diaphysis (arrows). *(Courtesy of R. Kerr, M.D., Los Angeles, California.)*

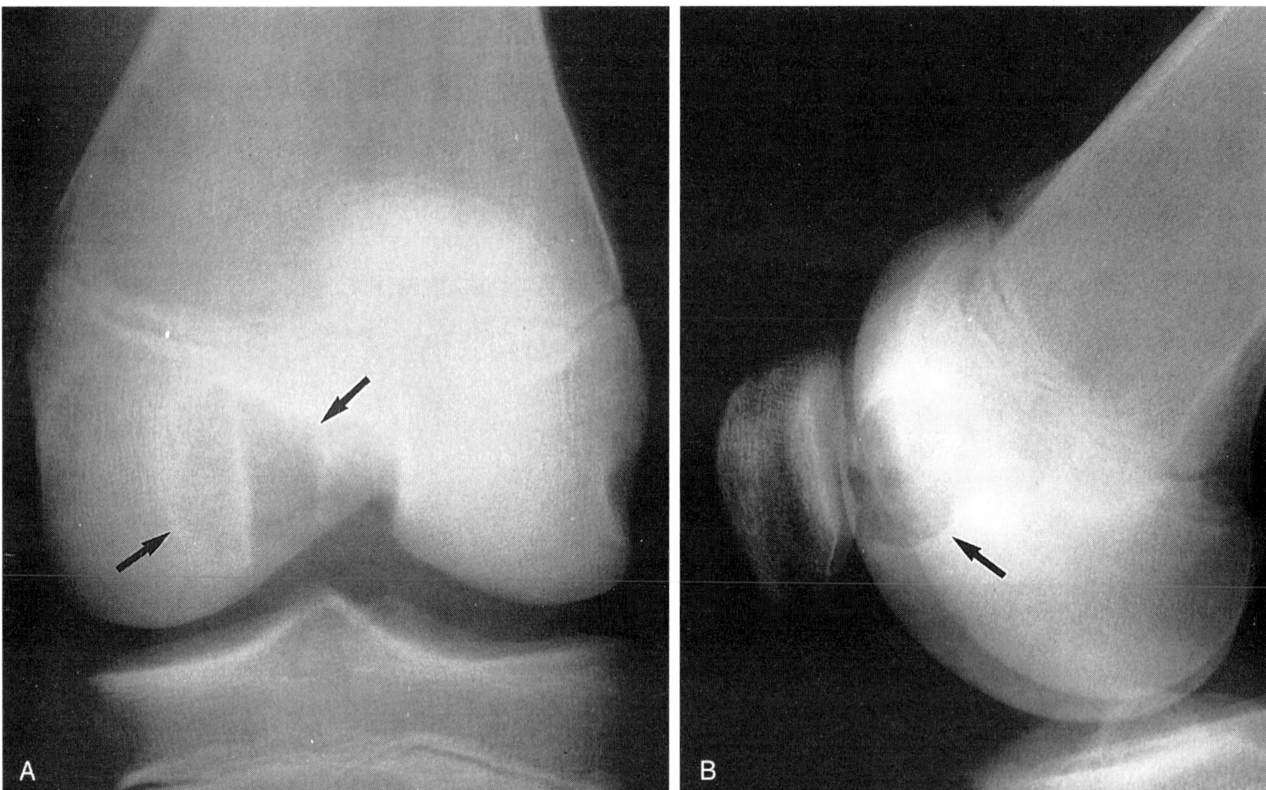

FIGURE 8–23. Chondroblastoma.[37, 38] This 16-year-old boy had knee pain for 4 months. Anteroposterior (A) and lateral (B) radiographs show a well-defined, geographic osteolytic lesion involving the distal femoral epiphysis (arrows). *(Courtesy of G. Greenway, M.D., Dallas, Texas.)*

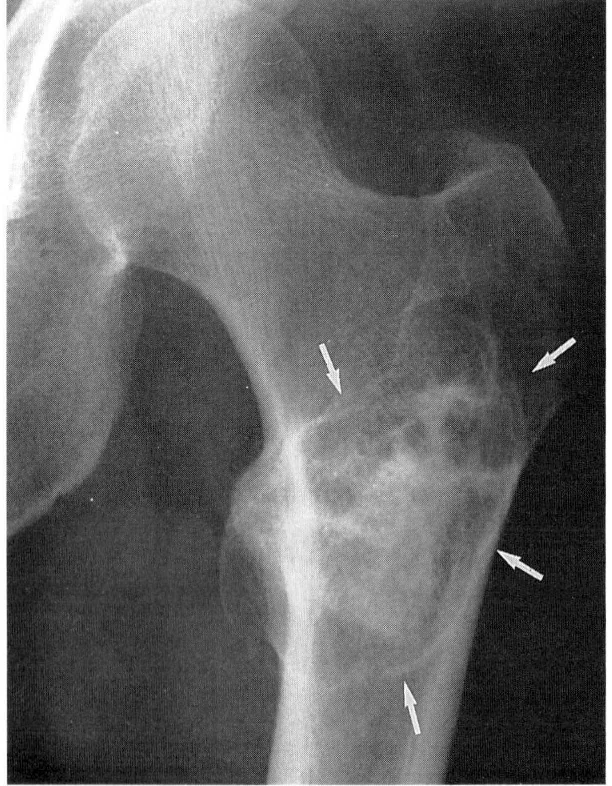

FIGURE 8–24. Solitary osteochondroma.[40, 41] A large osteochondroma arising from the intertrochanteric region of the femur is seen en face (arrows), with zones of increased and decreased radiodensity. In this location, fibrous dysplasia and intraosseous lipoma should be considered in the differential diagnosis.

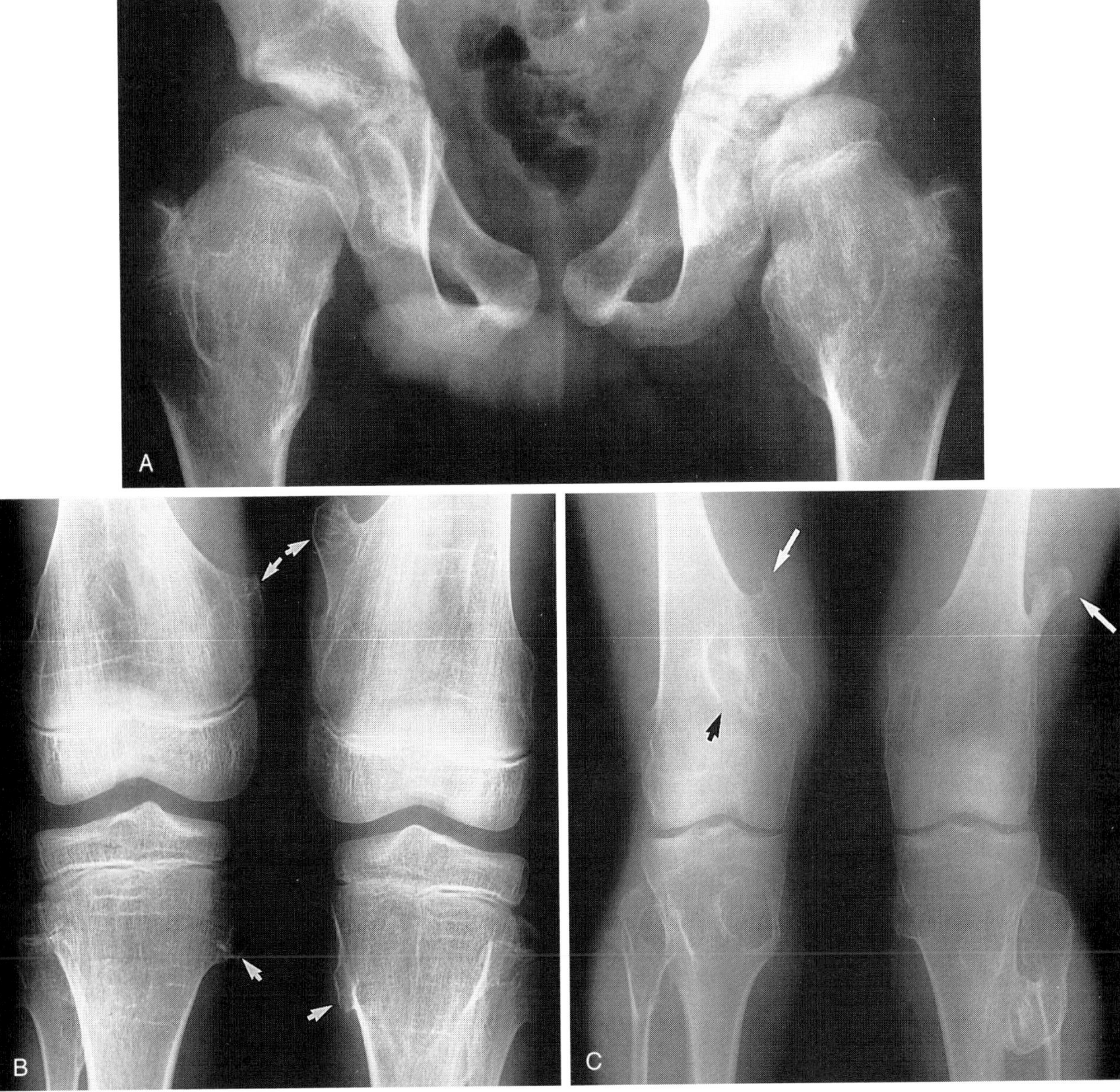

FIGURE 8–25. Hereditary multiple exostoses.[42–44] A Marked deformity and expansion of the femoral necks are apparent in this 14-year-old boy with hereditary multiple exostosis. B Observe the pedunculated exostoses (arrows) involving the distal end of the femur and proximal portion of the tibia in this 11-year-old boy. C In a third patient, large bilateral pedunculated and sessile osseous outgrowths are seen arising from the metaphyses of the femur (arrows), tibia, and fibula.

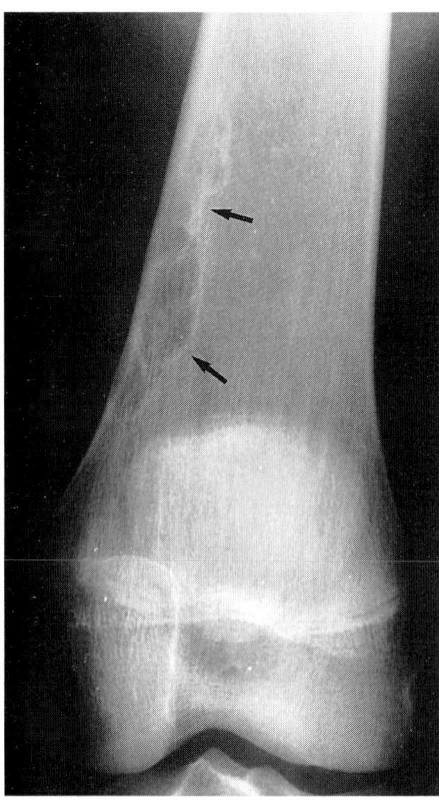

FIGURE 8–26. Nonossifying fibroma.[45] Routine radiograph shows an eccentric, multiloculated geographic lesion (arrows) in the metadiaphysis of the distal portion of the femur. The cortical margin appears lobulated, and evidence of cortical thinning is present.

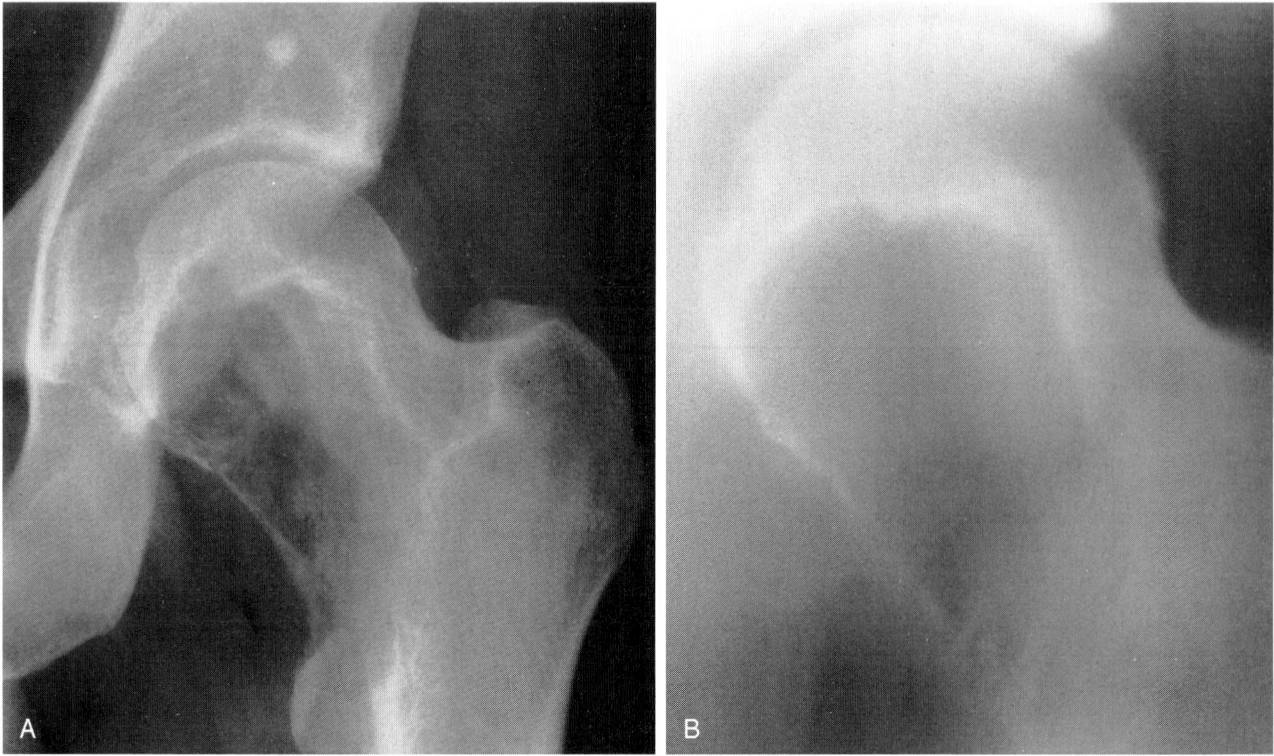

FIGURE 8–27. Giant cell tumor.[46] Frontal radiograph (A) and conventional tomogram (B) of the proximal end of the femur reveal an eccentric, osteolytic geographic lesion extending into the subchondral region of the femoral head, resulting in cortical thinning and minimal expansion. *(Courtesy of G. Greenway, M.D., Dallas, Texas.)*

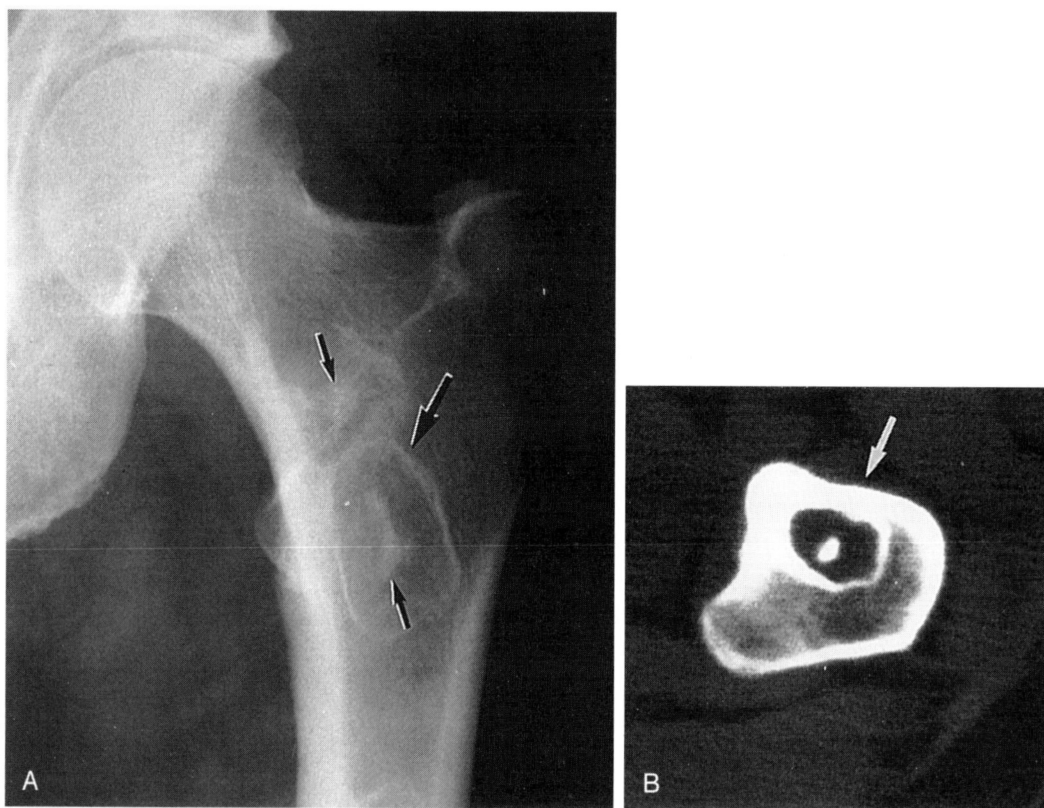

FIGURE 8–28. Intraosseous lipoma.[47] A Routine frontal radiograph of this 57-year-old man reveals a geographic lesion with a faint rim of sclerosis (large arrow) and two foci of sclerosis (small arrows) in the femoral neck. B Transaxial computed tomographic (CT) image confirms the fatty nature of the lesion by measurements of attenuation values derived from CT data. Lipomas of bone often possess a small, central, radiodense focus (arrow).

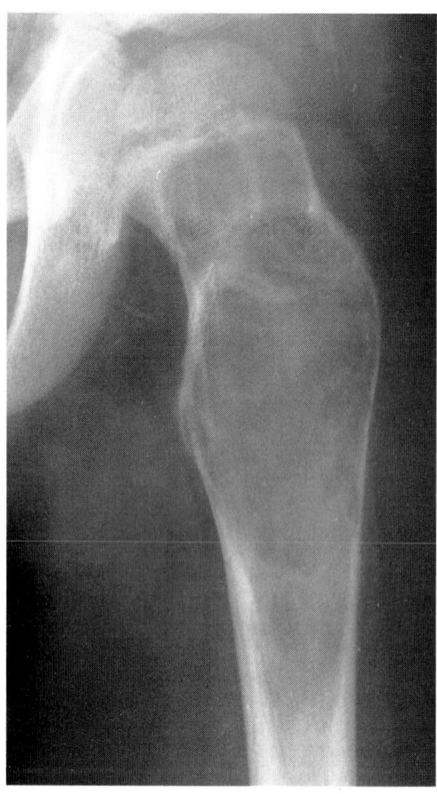

FIGURE 8–29. Simple bone cyst.[48] Routine radiograph of the proximal portion of the femur in this child reveals a centrally located, geographic, multiloculated metadiaphyseal lesion. Cortical thinning, a thin sclerotic margin, and mild osseous expansion are evident.

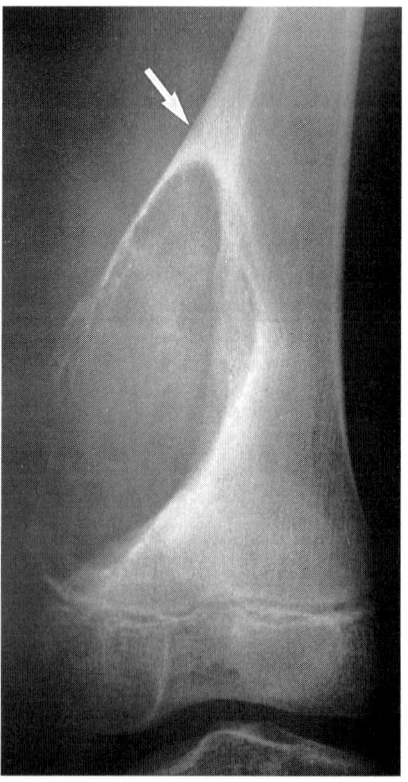

FIGURE 8–30. Aneurysmal bone cyst.[49] This aneurysmal bone cyst was found in the distal portion of the femur in a 10-year-old boy. Observe the eccentric, expansile appearance of the lesion. Evidence of buttressing is seen at the margin of the lesion (arrow), a feature characteristic of aneurysmal bone cysts. The matrix often contains fine trabeculation. *(Courtesy of A. Newberg, M.D., Boston, Massachusetts.)*

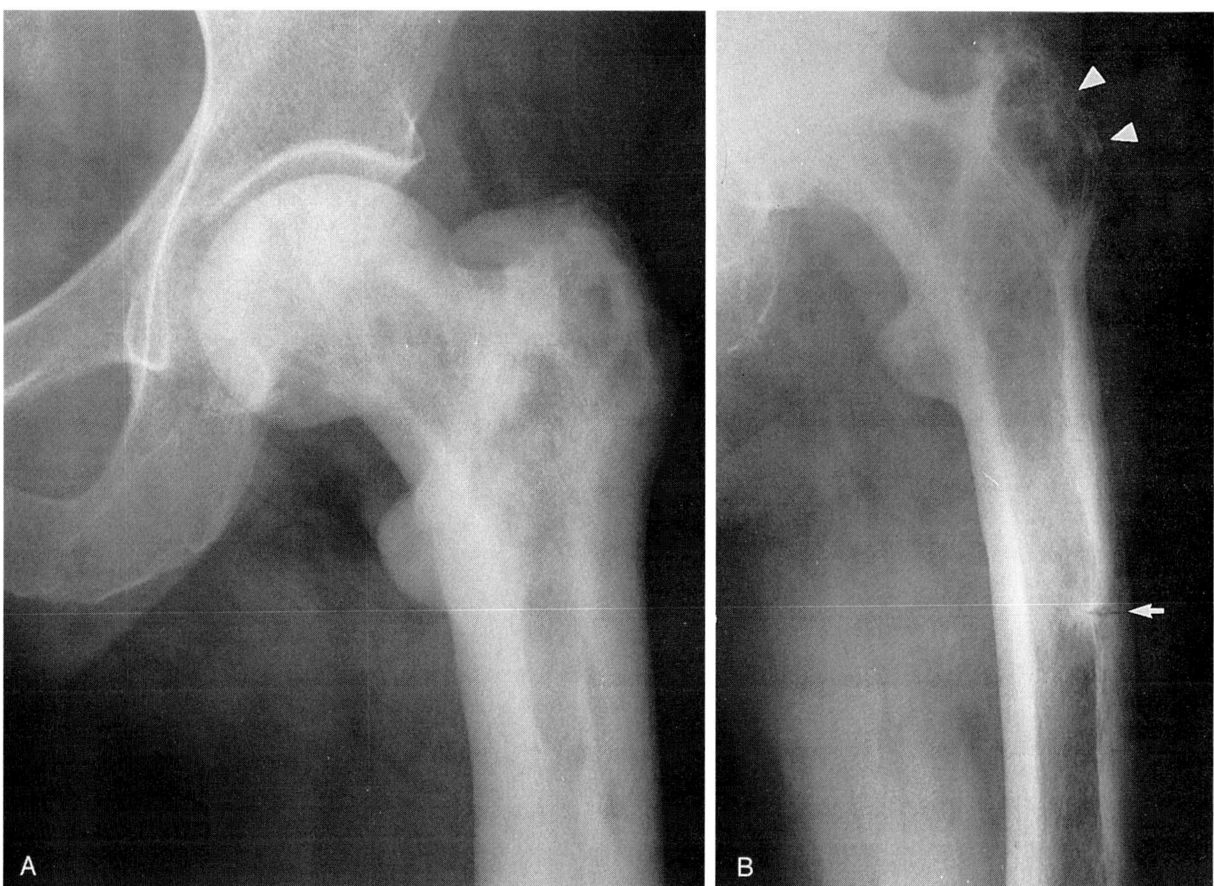

FIGURE 8–31. Paget's disease.[50, 51] A The osteosclerotic pattern of Paget's disease is seen involving the proximal portion of the femur. Observe the characteristic subarticular distribution and the coarsened, thickened, and sclerotic appearance of the cortex and trabeculae. B In another patient, diaphyseal involvement predominates. An area of osteolysis is seen involving the greater trochanteric region (arrowheads). An insufficiency fracture (arrow) and minimal bowing of the femur accompany the characteristic findings of thickened cortex and coarsened trabeculae. In Paget's disease, such incomplete fractures usually appear on the convex side of the bone and may progress to extend across the entire bone to become complete fractures.

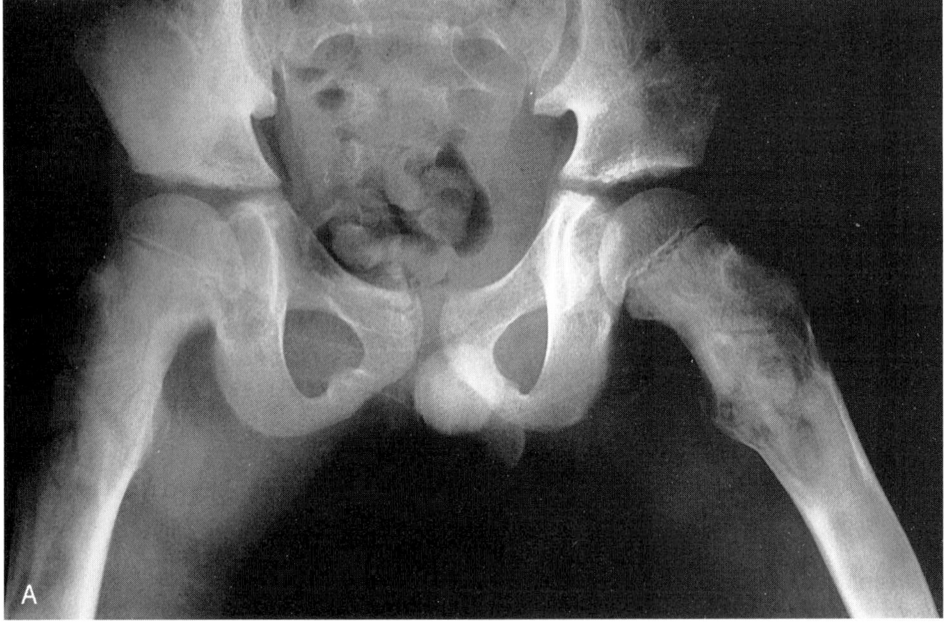

FIGURE 8–32. Fibrous dysplasia.[53] A Polyostotic involvement. Radiograph of this 10-year-old boy reveals bilateral femoral involvement in polyostotic fibrous dysplasia. The lesions are predominantly osteolytic, and the matrix appears hazy, a feature referred to as the ground-glass appearance. No osseous expansion is evident in this patient. The right ilium also is involved.

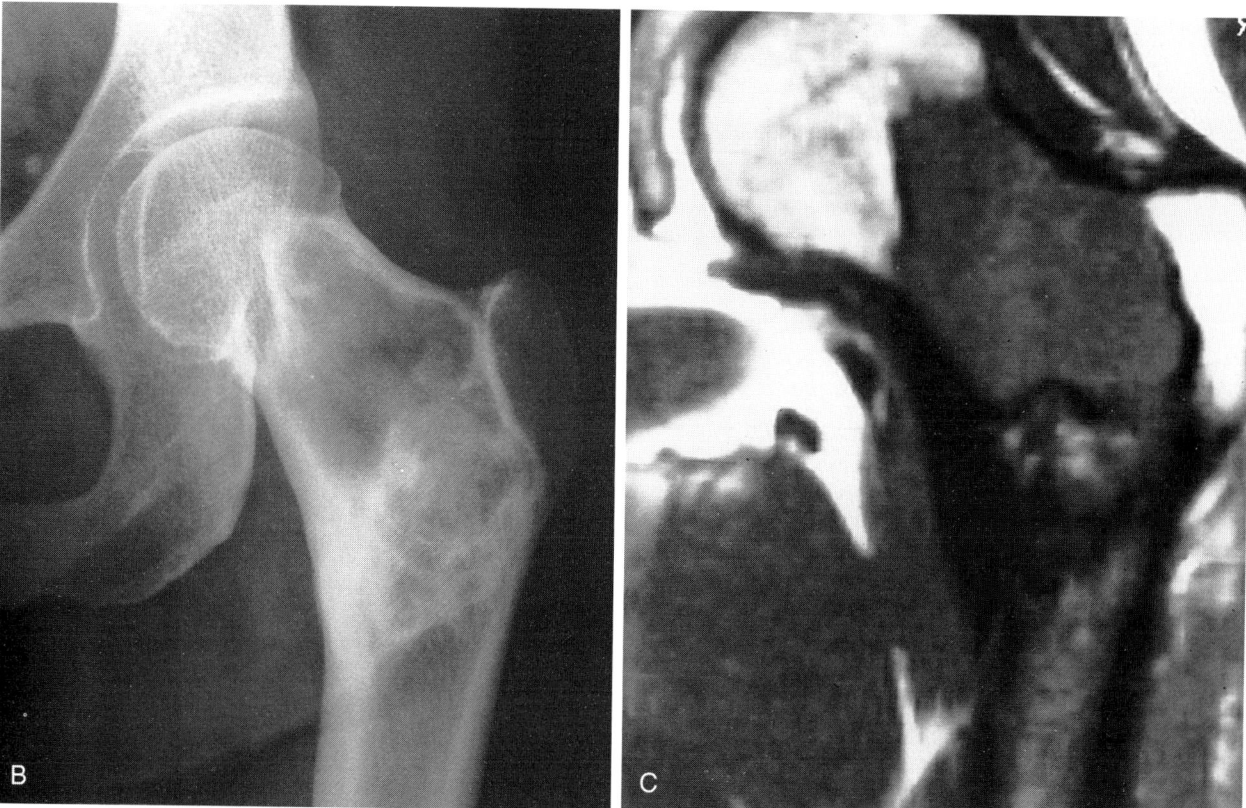

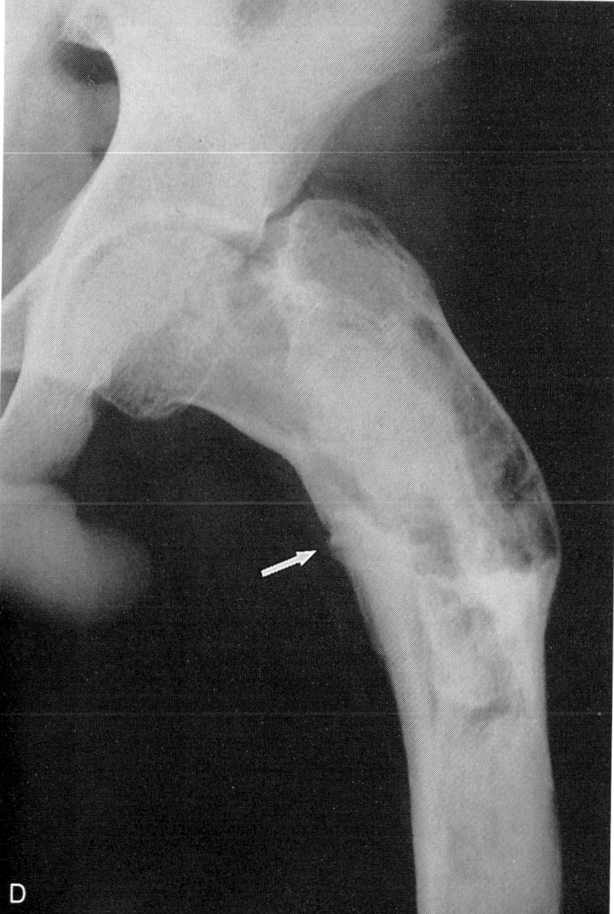

FIGURE 8–32 *Continued.* B, C Monostotic involvement in a 50-year-old woman. In B, a routine radiograph demonstrates an osteolytic lesion occupying a large portion of the femoral neck and intertrochanteric region. The predominantly osteolytic lesion has a sclerotic margin and a ground-glass matrix. In C, a coronal T1-weighted (TR/TE, 500/15) spin echo magnetic resonance (MR) image reveals low signal intensity within the lesion. *(B, C, Courtesy of J. Kramer, M.D., Vienna, Austria.)* D Pathologic fracture in a 48-year-old man with monostotic fibrous dysplasia. A transverse pathologic fracture (arrow) in the medial femoral cortex is seen. Prominent coxa valga deformity and bowing of the femur are evident. *(D, From Taylor JAM, Harger BL, Resnick D: Diagnostic imaging of common hip disorders: A pictorial review. Top Clin Chiropr 1:8, 1994.)*

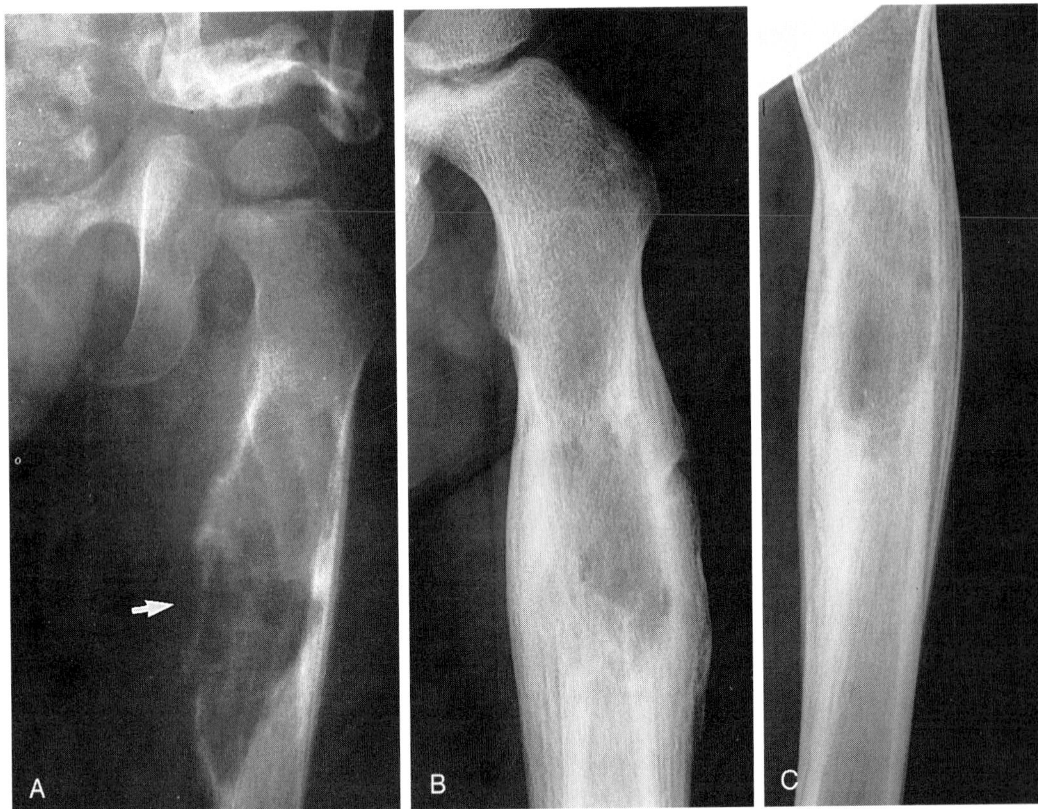

FIGURE 8–33. Langerhans' cell histiocytosis: Eosinophilic granuloma.[54, 55] **A** Observe the large multilocular osteolytic lesion (arrow) involving the femoral diaphysis with acetabular remodeling and collapse. Extensive involvement of the innominate bones was also present. **B, C** Frontal **(B)** and lateral **(C)** radiographs of the proximal portion of the femur show a geographic lesion with prominent, laminated, organized periostitis. Eosinophilic granuloma of bone is the most frequent and mildest form of Langerhans' cell histiocytosis, a disease characterized by histiocytic infiltration of tissues. *(**B, C,** Courtesy of U. Mayer, M.D., Klagenfurt, Austria.)*

TABLE 8–6. Metabolic, Hematologic, and Infectious Disorders*

Entity	Figure(s)	Characteristics
Generalized osteoporosis[56]	7–43 to 7–45	Uniform decrease in radiodensity, thinning of cortices, accentuation of weight-bearing trabeculae May result in insufficiency fractures of the femoral neck See Chapter 7
Osteogenesis imperfecta[68]	8–34	Osteoporosis and bone fragility Thin, gracile appearance of entire skeleton Severe deformities and fractures commonly affect the femur
Osteomalacia and rickets[69]	8–35	*Osteomalacia* Diffuse osteopenia Decreased trabeculae; remaining trabeculae appear prominent and coarsened Looser's zones (pseudofractures) *Rickets* Findings are most prominent in the appendicular skeleton Metaphyseal demineralization resulting in frayed metaphyses Bowing deformities Osteopenia Looser's zones
Hyperparathyroidism and renal osteodystrophy[57]	8–36	Brown tumor (osteoclastoma): solitary or multiple expansile osteolytic lesions containing fibrous tissue and giant cells; may disappear after treatment for hyperparathyroidism Osteosclerosis more common in renal osteodystrophy
Gaucher's disease[58]	8–37	Marrow infiltration results in osteopenia, osteolytic lesions, cortical diminution, and medullary widening Osseous weakening results in pathologic fractures Modeling deformities: Erlenmeyer flask deformity (widening of the distal diametaphysis of the femur) Osteonecrosis of the femoral head
Myelofibrosis[59, 60]	8–38	Chief radiographic finding: osteosclerosis Occasional periosteal bone apposition or periostitis, osteolysis, or osteopenia
Secondary hypertrophic osteoarthropathy[61]	8–39	Syndrome characterized by digital clubbing, arthritis, and bilateral symmetric periostitis of femur and other tubular bones Complication of many diseases including bronchogenic carcinoma, mesothelioma, and other intrathoracic and intra-abdominal diseases
Hypovitaminosis C (scurvy)[62]	8–40	Radiographic evidence of skeletal changes in scurvy is seen only in advanced long-standing disease *Infantile scurvy* Periostitis secondary to subperiosteal hemorrhage Transverse radiodense zone of provisional calcification (white line of Frankel) Transverse radiolucent metaphyseal line (scurvy line, Trümmerfeldzone) Beak-like metaphyseal excrescences (corner or angle sign or Pelken's spurs) Radiodense shell surrounding epiphyses (Wimberger's sign of scurvy) Healing scurvy may result in increased radiodensity of the metaphyses and epiphyses
Meningomyelocele[63]	8–41	Prominent bilateral periosteal new bone formation Epiphyseal fragmentation and physeal widening
Growth recovery lines[64]	8–42	Transverse radiodense lines representing a sign of new or increased growth in children, presumably after a period of inhibited bone growth from a previous episode of trauma, infection, malnutrition, or other chronic disease states Also seen in normal children without episodes of trauma or disease
Osteomyelitis[65]	8–43	Acute pyogenic osteomyelitis frequently involves the metaphysis in children Poorly defined permeative bone destruction Chronic osteomyelitis most frequently involves the femur: poorly defined areas of sclerosis and osteolysis, thin linear periostitis, and sequestration
Chronic recurrent multifocal osteomyelitis (CRMO)[66]		Occurs mainly in children and adolescents Initial lytic destruction of metaphysis adjacent to growth plate with no periosteal bone formation or sequestration
Collagen vascular disease: soft tissue calcification[67]	8–44	Dermatomyositis, polymyositis, scleroderma, and other collagen vascular diseases may result in soft tissue calcinosis in the thigh Differential diagnosis: hyperparathyroidism, neurologic injury, melorheostosis, posttraumatic heterotopic ossification, soft tissue neoplasms

*See also Tables 1–13, 1–14, and 1–17.

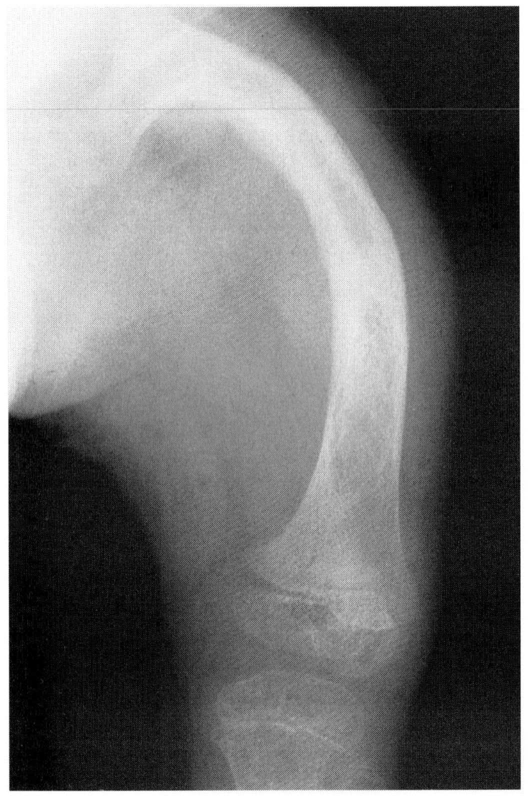

FIGURE 8–34. Osteogenesis imperfecta.[68] Dramatic bowing and coxa vara deformity involving the femur are seen in this young patient. Generalized osteopenia was observed throughout the skeleton, but this appearance is masked by increased density from cortical thickening as a result of bowing deformities and previous trauma.

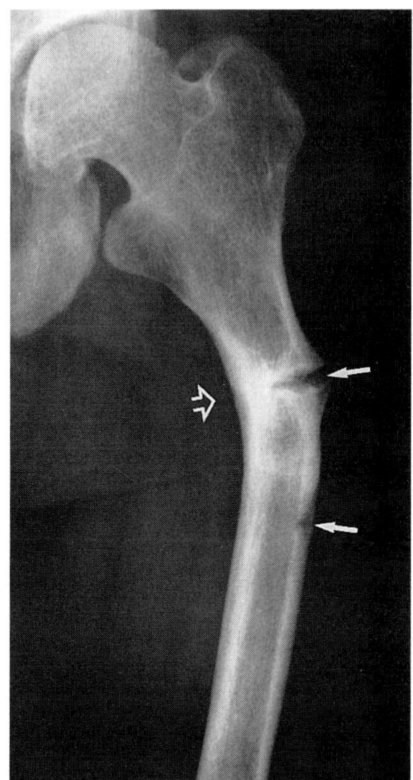

FIGURE 8–35. Hypophosphatemic rickets.[69] In this patient with long-standing hypophosphatemia, diffuse osteopenia, two incomplete transverse fractures (arrows), and bowing deformity (open arrow) involving the femoral diaphysis are present. *(Courtesy of C. Pineda, M.D., Mexico City, Mexico.)*

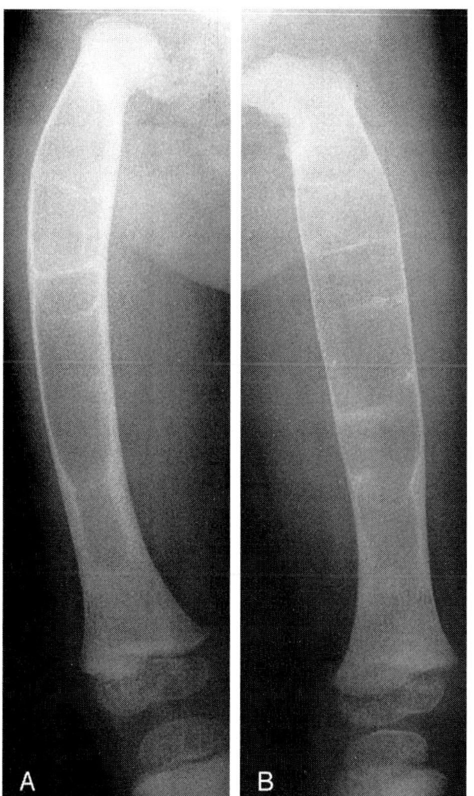

FIGURE 8–36. A, B Hyperparathyroidism: Brown tumors.[57] Bilateral radiographs of this 5-year-old girl with secondary hyperparathyroidism reveal multiple septated, osteolytic brown tumors in the femoral shafts. Marked femoral bowing also is present. *(Courtesy of T. Broderick, M.D., Orange, California.)*

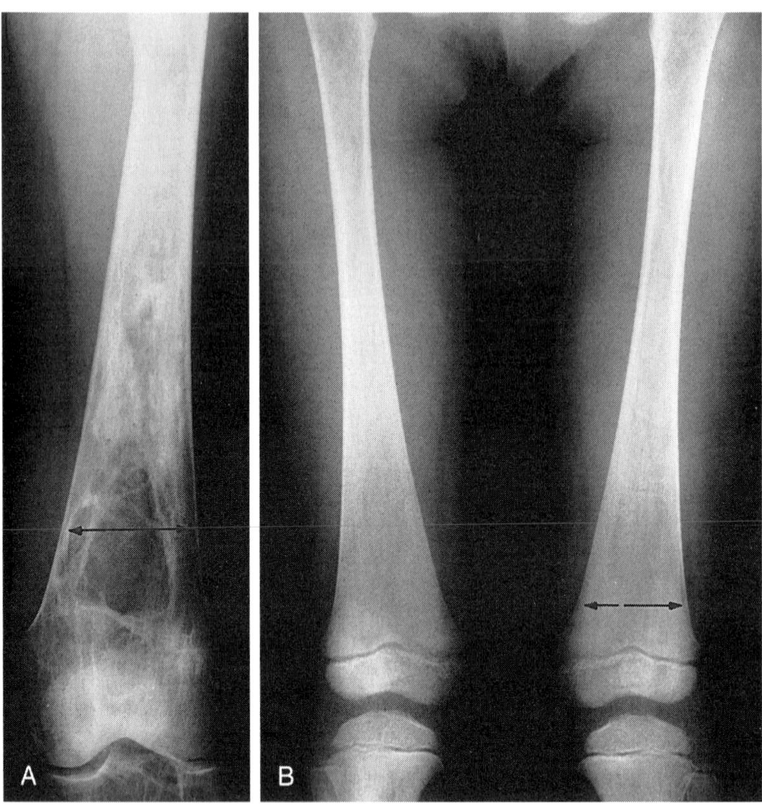

FIGURE 8–37. Gaucher's disease.[58] A Radiograph of this 26-year-old man with Gaucher's disease demonstrates large septated osteolytic lesions due to extensive marrow replacement. Observe also the presence of undertubulation (Erlenmeyer flask deformity) (double-headed arrow) and osteosclerotic intraosseous infarcts throughout the diaphysis. B In a child, bilateral femoral undertubulation is seen as widening of the metaphyses (double-headed arrow). Severe cortical thinning also is evident. Gaucher's disease additionally may be characterized by osteopenia, osteonecrosis, cortical erosion, and coarsened trabecular pattern.

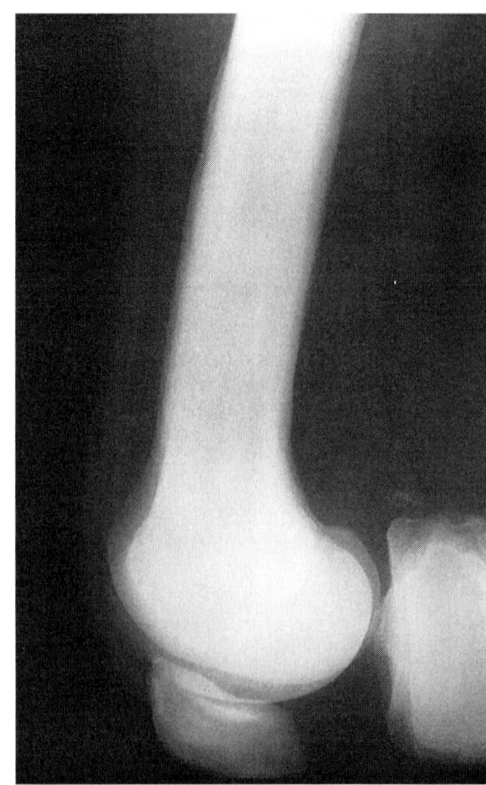

FIGURE 8–38. Myelofibrosis.[59, 60] Diffuse osteosclerosis involving the entire femur is characteristic of myelofibrosis. *(Courtesy of G. Greenway, M.D., Dallas, Texas.)*

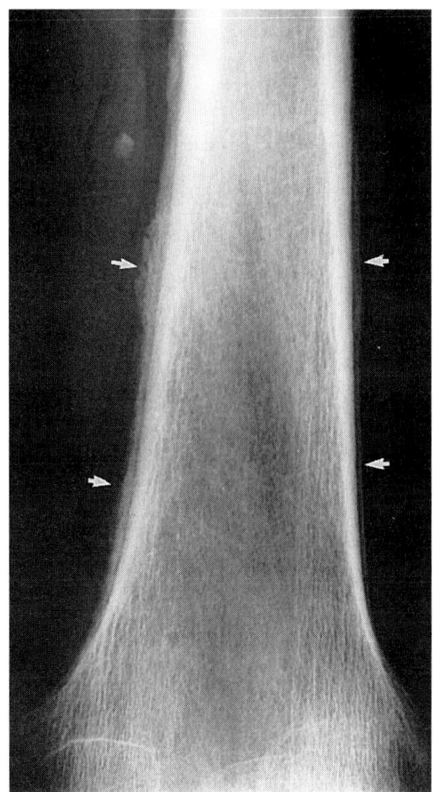

FIGURE 8–39. Secondary hypertrophic osteoarthropathy.[61] Bilateral symmetric periostitis involving the distal portion of the femur (arrows) was present in this patient with bronchogenic carcinoma. Observe the thick solid layer of new bone formation characteristic of hypertrophic osteoarthropathy. *(Courtesy of U. Mayer, M.D., Klagenfurt, Austria.)*

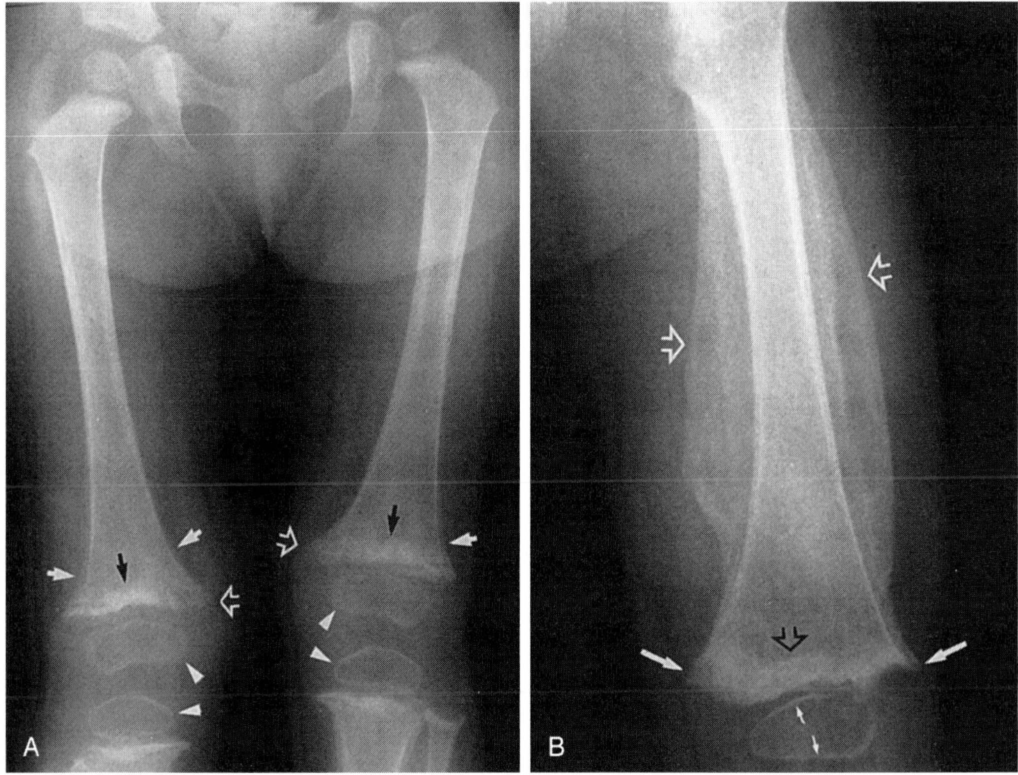

FIGURE 8–40. Hypovitaminosis C (scurvy).[62] **A** In this infant, bilateral femoral radiographs demonstrate subtle periostitis caused by subperiosteal hemorrhage (white arrows). In addition, thick, sclerotic metaphyseal lines (black arrows), beak-like excrescences (Pelken's spurs) (open arrows), and radiodense shells around the epiphyses (Wimberger's ring) (arrowheads) are seen. These findings are all consistent with long-standing scurvy. **B** This patient exhibits classic radiographic findings of chronic ascorbic acid deficiency, including thick periostitis from subperiosteal hemorrhage (white open arrows), a sclerotic metaphyseal line (black open arrow), Pelken's spurs (large arrows), radiolucent epiphysis surrounded by a sclerotic shell (Wimberger's ring) (small arrows), and generalized osteopenia.

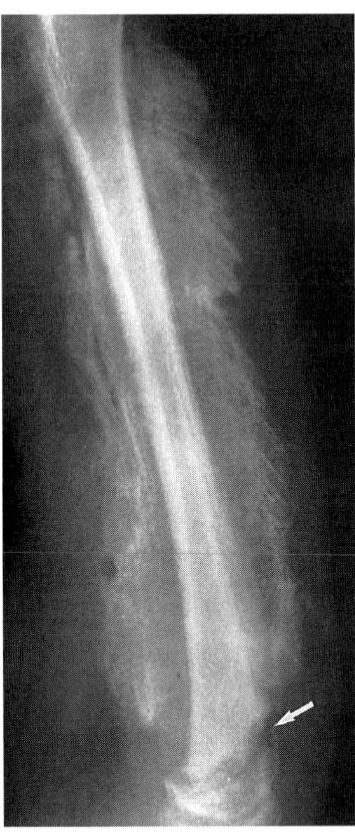

FIGURE 8–41. Meningomyelocele.[63] In this 6-year-old boy born with a meningomyelocele, exuberant periosteal new bone formation was present bilaterally. Widened, fragmented distal femoral growth plates also are evident (arrow). *(Courtesy of J.E.L. Desautels, M.D., Calgary, Alberta, Canada.)*

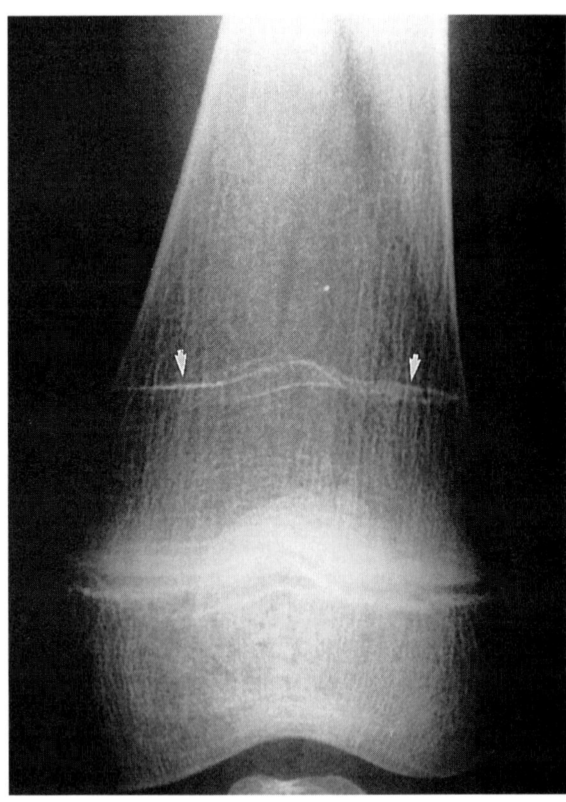

FIGURE 8–42. Growth recovery lines.[64] In this chronically ill 6-year-old child with juvenile rheumatoid arthritis, prominent transverse sclerotic bands are seen in the distal femoral metaphysis (arrows).

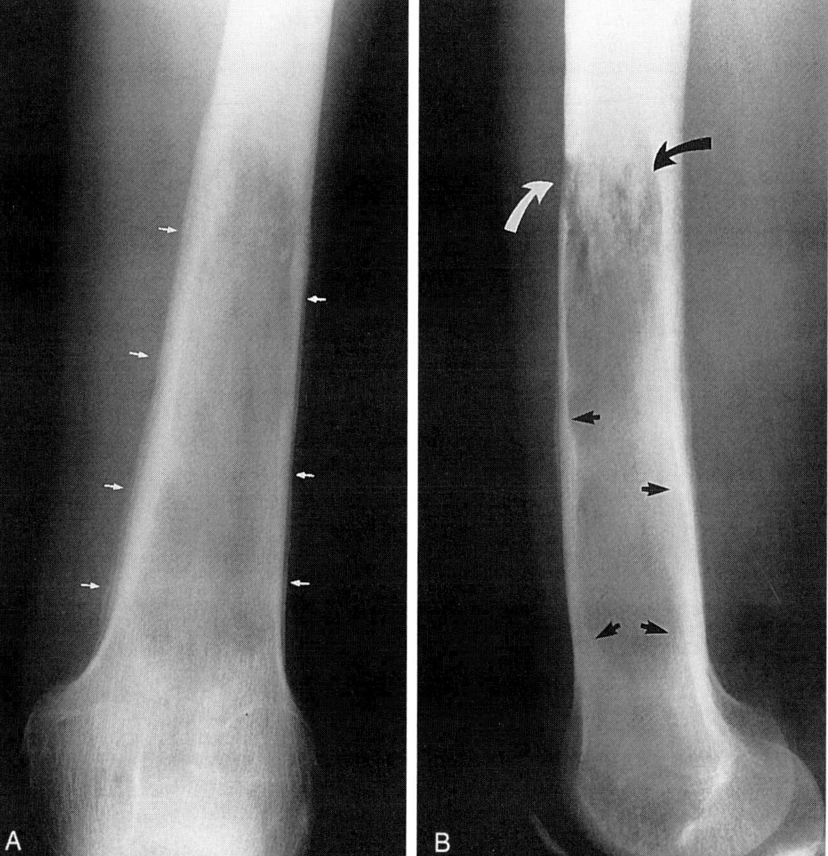

FIGURE 8–43. Pyogenic osteomyelitis: *Staphylococcus aureus.*[65] This 23-year-old man had pain of 4 months' duration. Frontal (A) and lateral (B) radiographs demonstrate a large, elongated radiolucent lesion with endosteal scalloping of the medullary cavity of the femoral diaphysis (black arrows). A thin layer of periosteal reaction is seen on the frontal view (white arrows). A more aggressive zone of permeative destruction is present at the superior aspect of the lesion (curved arrows). A well-defined radiolucent channel was evident at the bottom of the lesion, typical of infection, but it is not well seen in these photographs. *(Courtesy of G. Greenway, M.D., Dallas, Texas.)*

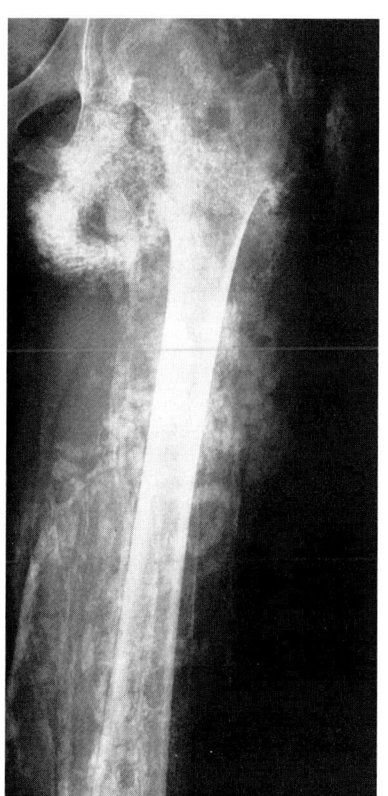

FIGURE 8–44. Collagen vascular disease: Dermatomyositis and polymyositis.[67] Observe the globular, sheet-like, and amorphous calcification within the muscles and subcutaneous tissues adjacent to the femur in this 16-year-old girl with dermatomyositis-polymyositis. Dermatomyositis and polymyositis are diseases of striated muscle characterized by diffuse, nonsuppurative inflammation and degeneration. Dermatomyositis affects skin and muscle and polymyositis affects only muscle. The cause is unknown, and it affects patients of all ages. About one third of patients also have Raynaud's phenomenon, and up to 50 per cent have arthralgia. *(Courtesy of C. Van Lom, M.D., San Diego, California.)*

REFERENCES

1. Horsfield D, Jones SN: Assessment of inequality in length of the lower limb. Radiography 52:233, 1986.
2. Huurman WW, Jacobsen FS, Anderson JC, et al: Limb-length discrepancy measured with computerized axial tomographic equipment. J Bone Joint Surg [Am] 69:699, 1987.
3. Mannello DM: Leg length inequality. J Manip Physiol Ther 15:576, 1992.
4. Levinson ED, Ozonoff MB, Royers PM: Proximal femoral focal deficiency (PFFD). Radiology 125:197, 1977.
5. Kovanlikaya A, Loro ML, Gilsanz V: Pathogenesis of osteosclerosis in autosomal dominant osteopetrosis. AJR 168:929, 1997.
6. Benli IT, Akalin S, Boysan E, et al: Epidemiological, clinical, and radiological aspects of osteopoikilosis. J Bone Joint Surg [Br] 74:504, 1992.
7. Bass HN, Weiner JR, Goldman A, et al: Osteopathia striata syndrome: Clinical, genetic, and radiologic considerations. Clin Pediatr 19:369, 1980.
8. Campbell CJ, Papademetriou T, Bonfiglio M: Melorheostosis: A report of the clinical, roentgenographic, and pathological findings in fourteen cases. J Bone Joint Surg [Am] 50:1281, 1968.
9. Yu JS, Resnick D, Vaughan LM, et al: Melorheostosis with an ossified soft tissue mass. Skeletal Radiol 24:367, 1995.
10. Whyte MP, Murphy WA, Fallon MD, et al: Mixed-sclerosing-bone-dystrophy: Report of a case and review of the literature. Skeletal Radiol 6:95, 1981.
11. Rogers LF: Radiology of Skeletal Trauma. 2nd Ed. New York, Churchill Livingstone, 1992.
12. Johansson C, Ekenman I, Tönkvist H, et al: Stress fractures of the femoral neck in athletes: The consequence of a delay in diagnosis. Am J Sports Med 18:524, 1990.
13. Anderson MW, Greenspan A: Stress fractures. Radiology 199:1, 1996.
14. Nuovo MA, Norman A, Chumas A, et al: Myositis ossificans with atypical clinical, radiographic, or pathologic findings: A review of 23 cases. Skeletal Radiol 21:87, 1992.
15. Greenspan A, Norman A: Osteolytic cortical destruction: An unusual pattern of skeletal metastasis. Skeletal Radiol 17:402, 1988.
16. Taylor JAM, Harger BL, Resnick D: Diagnostic imaging of common hip disorders: A pictorial review. Top Clin Chiropr 1:8,1994.
17. Resnik C, Garver P, Resnick D: Bony expansion in skeletal metastasis from carcinoma of the prostate as seen by bone scintigraphy. South Med J 77:1331, 1984.
18. Dahlin DC, Unni KK: Osteosarcoma of bone and its important recognizable varieties. Am J Surg Pathol 1:61, 1977.
19. Ritschl P, Wurnig C, Lechner G, et al: Parosteal osteosarcoma. 2-23-year follow-up of 33 patients. Acta Orthop Scand 62:195, 1991.
20. Mitchell M, Ackerman LV: Metastatic and pseudomalignant osteoblastoma: A report of two unusual cases. Skeletal Radiol 15:213, 1986.
21. Henderson ED, Dahlin DC: Chondrosarcoma of bone—a study of two hundred and eighty-eight cases. J Bone Joint Surg [Am] 45:1450, 1963.
22. Brien EW, Mirra JM, Kerr R: Benign and malignant cartilage tumors of bone and joint: Their anatomic and theoretical basis with an emphasis on radiology, pathology and clinical biology. 1. The intramedullary cartilage tumors. Skeletal Radiol 26:325, 1997.
23. Dahlin DC: Giant cell tumor of bone: Highlights of 407 cases. AJR 144:955, 1985.
24. Taconis WK, Mulder JD: Fibrosarcoma and malignant fibrous histiocytoma of long bones: Radiographic features and grading. Skeletal Radiol 11:237, 1984.
25. Dahlin DC, Coventry MB, Scanlon PW: Ewing's sarcoma: A critical analysis of 165 cases. J Bone Joint Surg [Am] 43:185, 1961.
26. Kyle RA: Multiple myeloma: Review of 869 cases. Mayo Clin Proc 50:29, 1975.
27. Franczyk J, Samuels T, Rubenstein J, et al: Skeletal lymphoma. J Can Assoc Radiol 40:75, 1989.
28. Hermann G, Klein MJ, Fikry Abedlewahab I, et al: MRI appearance of primary non-Hodgkin's lymphoma of bone. Skeletal Radiol 26:629, 1997.
29. Clayton F, Butler JJ, Ayala AG, et al: Non-Hodgkin's lymphoma in bone: Pathologic and radiologic features with clinical correlates. Cancer 60:2494, 1987.
30. Benz G, Brandeis WE, Willich E: Radiological aspects of leukemia in childhood: An analysis of 89 children. Pediatr Radiol 4:201, 1976.
31. Greenspan A: Bone island (enostosis): Current concept–a review. Skeletal Radiol 24:111, 1995.
32. Kattapuram SV, Kushner DC, Phillips WC, et al: Osteoid osteoma: An unusual cause of articular pain. Radiology 147:383, 1983.
33. Shankman S, Desai P, Beltran J: Subperiosteal osteoid osteoma: Radiographic and pathologic manifestations. Skeletal Radiol 26:457, 1997.
34. Kayser F, Resnick D, Haghighi P, et al: Evidence of the subperiosteal origin of osteoid osteomas in tubular bones: Analysis by CT and MR imaging. AJR 170:609, 1998.
35. Lichtenstein L, Sawyer WF: Benign osteoblastoma: Further observations and report of twenty additional cases. J Bone Joint Surg [Am] 46:755, 1964.
36. Schiller AL: Diagnosis of borderline cartilage lesions of bone. Semin Diagn Pathol 2:42, 1985.
37. Bloem JL, Mulder JD: Chondroblastoma: A clinical and radiological study of 104 cases. Skeletal Radiol 14:1, 1985.
38. Weatherall PT, Maale GE, Mendelsohn DB, et al: Chondroblastoma: Classic and confusing appearance at MR imaging. Radiology 190:467, 1994.
39. Wilson AJ, Kyriakos M, Ackerman LV: Chondromyxoid fibroma: Radiographic appearance in 38 cases and in a review of the literature. Radiology 179:513, 1991.
40. Milgram JW: The origins of osteochondromas and enchondromas: A histopathologic study. Clin Orthop 174:264, 1983.
41. Karasick D, Schweitzer ME, Eschelman DJ: Symptomatic osteochondromas: Imaging features. AJR 168:1507, 1997.
42. Shapiro F, Simon S, Glimcher MJ: Hereditary multiple exostoses: Anthropometric, roentgenologic and clinical aspects. J Bone Joint Surg [Am] 61:815, 1979.
43. Solomon L: Chondrosarcoma in hereditary multiple exostosis. S Afr Med J 48:671, 1974.
44. Schmale GA, Conrad EV, Raskind WH: The natural history of hereditary multiple exostosis. J Bone Joint Surg [Am] 76:986, 1994.
45. Ritschl P, Karnel F, Hajek P: Fibrous metaphyseal defects—determination of their origin and natural history using a radiomorphological study. Skeletal Radiol 17:8, 1988.
46. McInerney DP, Middlemiss JH: Giant-cell tumour of bone. Skeletal Radiol 2:195, 1978.
47. Milgram JW: Intraosseous lipoma: A clinicopathologic study of 66 cases. Clin Orthop 231:277, 1988.
48. Chigira M, Maehara S, Arita S, et al: The aetiology and

treatment of simple bone cysts. J Bone Joint Surg [Br] 65:633, 1983.
49. De Dios AMV, Bond JR, Shives TC, et al: Aneurysmal bone cyst: A clinico-pathologic study of 238 cases. Cancer 69:2921, 1992.
50. Matfin G, McPherson F: Paget's disease of bone: Recent advances. J Orthop Rheumatol 6:127, 1993.
51. Mirra JM, Brien EW, Tehranzadeh J: Paget's disease of bone: Review with emphasis on radiologic features. Part II. Skeletal Radiol 24:173, 1995.
52. Crawford AH Jr, Bogamery N: Osseous manifestations of neurofibromatosis in childhood. J Pediatr Orthop 6:72, 1986.
53. Gibson MJ, Middlemiss JH: Fibrous dysplasia of bone. Br J Radiol 44:1, 1971.
54. Stull MA, Kransdorf MJ, Devaney KO: Langerhans cell histiocytosis of bone. RadioGraphics 12:801, 1992.
55. Kilpatrick SE, Wenger DE, Gilchrist GS, et al: Langerhans' cell histiocytosis (histiocytosis X) of bone: A clinicopathologic analysis of 263 pediatric and adult cases. Cancer 76:2471, 1995.
56. Kerr R, Resnick D, Sartoris DJ, et al: Computed tomography of proximal femoral trabecular patterns. J Orthop Res 4:45, 1986.
57. Chew FS, Huang-Hellinger F: Brown tumor. AJR 160:752, 1993.
58. Greenfield GB: Bone changes in chronic adult Gaucher's disease. AJR 110:800, 1970.
59. Bouroncle BA, Doan CA: Myelofibrosis: clinical, hematologic and pathologic study of 110 patients. Am J Med Sci 243:697, 1962.
60. Yu JS, Greenway G, Resnick D: Myelofibrosis associated with prominent periosteal bone apposition: Report of two cases. Clin Imaging 18:89, 1994.
61. Pineda C: Diagnostic imaging in hypertrophic osteoarthropathy. Clin Exp Rheumatol 10:27, 1992.
62. Nerubay J, Pilderwasser D: Spontaneous bilateral distal femoral physiolysis due to scurvy. Acta Orthop Scand 55:18, 1984.
63. Westcott MA, Dynes MC, Remer EM, et al: Congenital and acquired orthopedic abnormalities in patients with myelomeningocele. RadioGraphics 12:1155, 1992.
64. Ogden JA: Growth slowdown and arrest lines. J Pediatr Orthop 4:409, 1984.
65. Gold RH, Hawkins RA, Katz RD: Bacterial osteomyelitis: Findings on plain radiography, CT, MR, and scintigraphy. AJR 157:365, 1991.
66. Jurik AG, Egund N: MRI in chronic recurrent multifocal osteomyelitis. Skeletal Radiol 26:230, 1997.
67. Pachman LN: Juvenile dermatomyositis. Pediatr Clin North Am 33:1097, 1986.
68. Root L: The treatment of osteogenesis imperfecta. Orthop Clin North Am 15:775, 1984.
69. Mankin HJ: Rickets, osteomalacia, and renal osteodystrophy. Orthop Clin North Am 21:81, 1990.

CHAPTER 9

Knee

Normal Developmental Anatomy

Accurate interpretation of radiographs of the pediatric knee requires a thorough understanding of normal developmental anatomy. Tables 9–1 and 9–2 outline the age of appearance and fusion of the primary and secondary ossification centers. Figures 9–1 and 9–2 demonstrate the radiographic appearance of many important ossification centers and other developmental landmarks at selected ages from birth to skeletal maturity.

Developmental Anomalies, Anatomic Variants, and Sources of Diagnostic Error

The knee and patella are sites of anomalies, anatomic variations, and other sources of diagnostic error that may simulate disease and potentially result in misdiagnosis. Table 9–2 and Figures 9–3 to 9–5 address some of the more common processes.

Skeletal Dysplasias and Other Congenital Diseases

Table 9–3 outlines a number of skeletal dysplasias and congenital disorders that affect the knee and patella. Figures 9–6 and 9–7 illustrate the radiographic manifestations of some of these disorders.

Alignment Abnormalities

Several alignment abnormalities affect the knee and patella. Tables 9–4 and 9–5 outline a number of potential causes of genu valgum, genu varum, genu recurvatum, patella alta, patella baja, and lateral patellar displacement. These malalignments are illustrated throughout this chapter as they are manifested in many disorders.

Physical Injury

Physical injury to the knee results in a wide variety of fractures and dislocations. Table 9–6 describes fractures of the distal portion of the femur, proximal end of the tibia, and the patella. Dislocations of the knee joint itself, the patella, and the proximal tibiofibular articulation are described in Table 9–7. These conditions are illustrated in Figures 9–8 to 9–22. Fractures of the diaphyses of the femur, the tibia, and the fibula are described and illustrated in Chapters 8 and 10, respectively.

Internal Derangements and Soft Tissue Disorders

The soft tissues within and around the knee are complex and may be involved in a variety of inherited and acquired disorders. This chapter describes internal derangements and soft tissue disorders of the synovial structures (Table 9–8), the menisci (Tables 9–9 and 9–10), the ligaments and tendons (Table 9–11), and the patellofemoral articulation (Table 9–12). Figures 9–23 to 9–45 illustrate many features of these conditions, with an emphasis on radiographic and magnetic resonance(MR) imaging findings.

Articular Disorders

The knee is a frequent target site of involvement for many degenerative, inflammatory, crystal-induced, and infectious articular disorders. Table 9–13 outlines these diseases and their chief characteristics. Table 9–14 provides a compartmental analysis emphasizing the pattern of joint space narrowing typical of these disorders. Figures 9–46 to 9–60 illustrate the typical radiographic manifestations of the most common articular disorders affecting the knee.

Neoplasms

The patella and the knee joint itself are infrequent sites of involvement for malignant and benign tumors and tumor-like lesions. Table 9–15 lists and characterizes the neoplasms that typically involve the patella. Figure 9–61 illustrates an example of skeletal metastasis invading the articulation and its surrounding bones. Many of the more common patellar tumors are illustrated in Figures 9–62 to 9–65.

Metabolic, Hematologic, and Vascular Disorders

Several metabolic, hematologic, and vascular disorders affect the knee and the surrounding osseous and soft tissue structures. Table 9–16 lists some of the more common disorders and describes their characteristics. Figures 9–66 to 9–73 illustrate the typical imaging findings of several of these disorders.

TABLE 9–1. Knee: Approximate Age of Appearance and Fusion of Ossification Centers[1–4] (Figs. 9–1 and 9–2)

Ossification Center	Primary or Secondary	No. of Centers Per Knee	Age of Appearance* (Years)	Age of Fusion* (Years)
Patella	P	1	Girls: 1.5–3.5 Boys: 3–5	
Distal femoral epiphysis	S	1	Birth	19–22
Proximal tibial epiphysis	S	1	Birth	18–23
Proximal fibular epiphysis	S	1	2–5	21–24
Tibial tubercle apophysis	S	1	10–13	18–24

*Ages of appearance and fusion of ossification centers in girls typically precede those of boys. Ethnic differences also exist.
P, Primary; S, secondary.

TABLE 9–2. Developmental Anomalies, Anatomic Variants, and Sources of Diagnostic Error Affecting the Knee*

Entity	Figure(s)	Characteristics
Accessory ossification centers[5, 6]		Accessory ossification centers in the inferior pole of the patella may simulate fractures or Sinding-Larsen-Johansson disease Usually asymptomatic
Bipartite patella[5–8]	9–3	Developmental anomaly in which the ossification center of the patella may be fragmented or fail to unite Bilateral in 80 per cent of cases and may occasionally be accompanied by mild pain Located at superolateral aspect of patella Bone edges are smoothly corticated and not displaced from the parent bone Fragment usually is connected to the patella by fibrous tissue Two separate pieces of bone—bipartite patella; three pieces of bone—tripartite patella; more than 3 pieces—multipartite patella Typical location, absence of severe pain, and characteristic appearance allow differentiation from acute fractures, which usually are horizontal (transverse) or stellate and possess jagged, irregular edges
Dorsal defect of the patella[9]	9–4	Variant in ossification Circular radiolucent defect in superolateral pole of patella May simulate a neoplasm May be related to bipartite patella Usually a self-limited, incidental finding in children
Juxtacortical desmoid[10, 11]	9–5	Also termed periosteal desmoid, avulsive cortical irregularity, cortical irregularity syndrome, cortical desmoid, and distal metaphyseal femoral defect Normal variant believed to be a benign reaction to stress or trauma occurring at the musculotendinous insertion site of the adductor magnus muscle or, less commonly, of the medial head of the gastrocnemius muscle Occurs only in children, adolescents, or young adults Male > female Histologic and imaging findings simulate malignancy Usually asymptomatic *Radiographic findings* Irregular periosteal new bone formation Cortical irregularity and saucering Soft tissue swelling also is often seen in this condition *MR imaging findings* Low signal intensity on T1-weighted images High signal intensity on T2-weighted images Surrounding rim of low signal intensity on all sequences
Hypoplastic or aplastic patellae[5]	9–6	Rare condition usually seen in association with hereditary osteo-onychodysostosis (nail-patella syndrome) and other congenital syndromes
Patellar duplication[12]		Coronal cleft between two separate patellae has been referred to as double patella, a rare anomaly that may be associated with multiple epiphyseal dysplasia Transverse cleft may separate the patella into two separate pieces; usually associated with trauma or cerebral palsy
Lateral dystopia of the patella[5]		Lateral malposition of patella, hypoplasia of lateral femoral condyle, prominent medial femoral condyle, small patella with flattened ridge between medial and lateral facets Frequently associated with congenital patellar dislocation with habitual patellar dislocation—"slipping patella"

*See also Table 1–1.

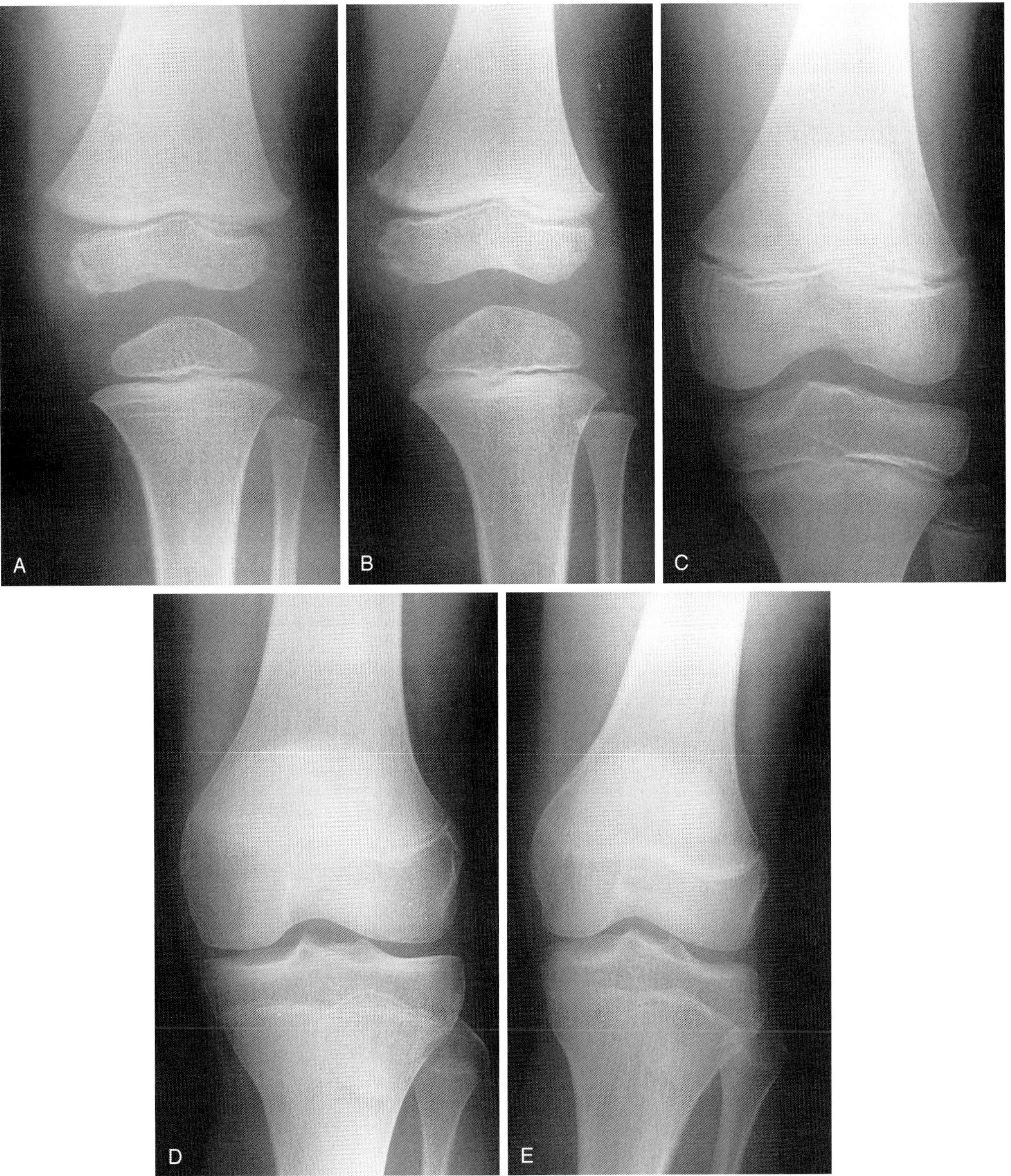

FIGURE 9–1. Skeletal maturation and normal development: Anteroposterior knee radiographs.[1–4] A 2-year-old girl. The secondary ossification center of the proximal end of the fibula is barely visible, typically appearing between the ages of 18 months and 5 years. The proximal tibial epiphysis is ossified, but it is much smaller than the metaphysis. A normal, irregular, serrated appearance of the medial aspect of the distal femoral epiphysis is evident. The zones of provisional calcification are radiodense. Beaking of the distal femoral metaphysis is prominent laterally. B 4-year-old boy. The tibial and femoral epiphyses are approaching the size of the metaphyses. The medial aspect of the femoral epiphysis remains irregular, and the proximal fibular epiphysis is barely visible. The zones of provisional calcification remain sclerotic. Beaking of the distal lateral femoral metaphysis persists. C 10-year-old boy. The widths of the tibial and femoral epiphyses have exceeded the widths of the adjacent metaphyses. The fibular epiphysis and patella are well developed and resemble the adult configuration. D 13-year-old girl. The distal femoral epiphysis and proximal tibial epiphysis are fusing to their adjacent metaphyses. The patella has adopted adult proportions. E 15-year-old girl. The femoral, tibial, and fibular epiphyses have fused to their respective metaphyses, but the physeal lines are still clearly visible.

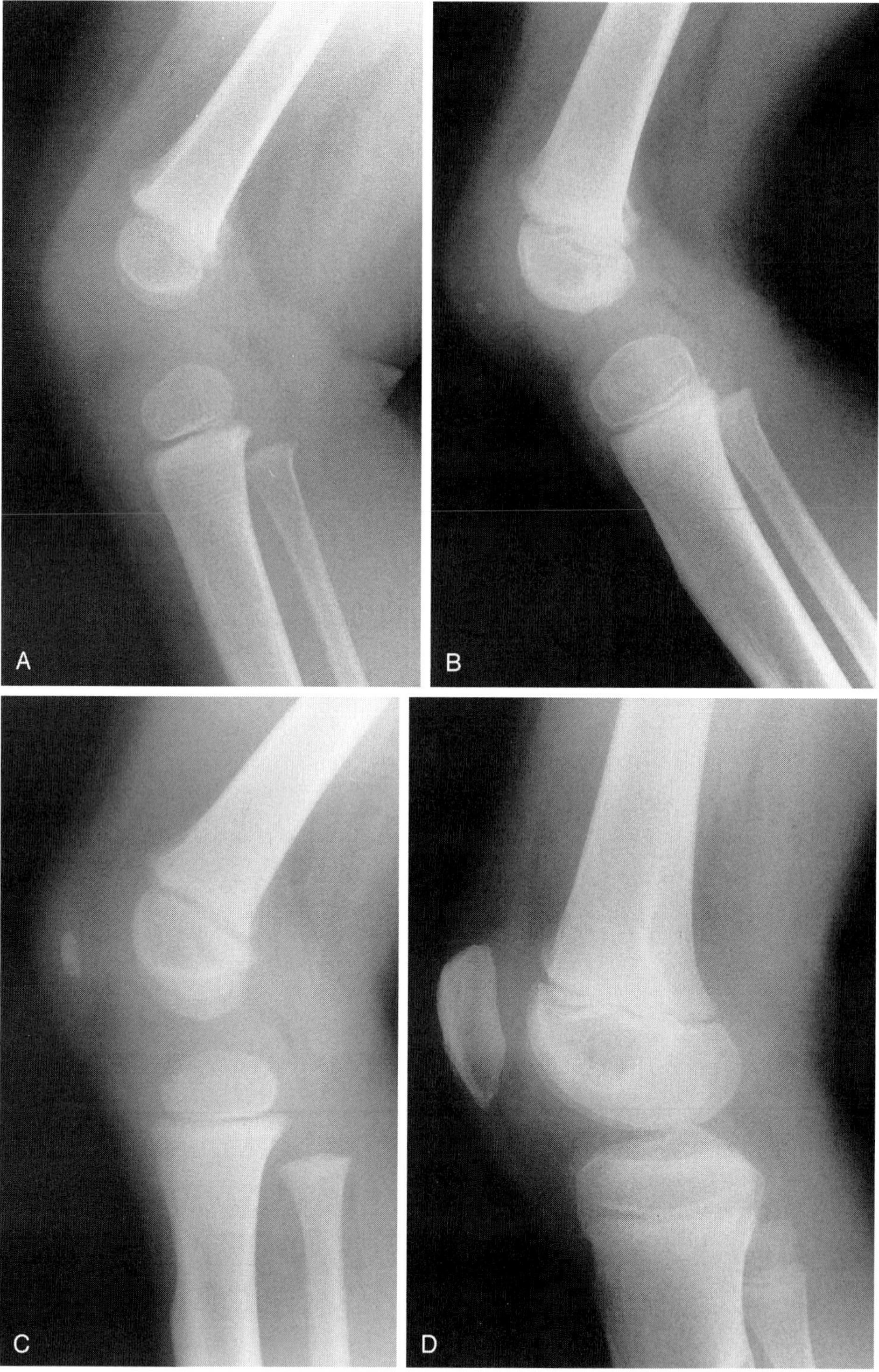

FIGURE 9–2. Skeletal maturation and normal development: Lateral knee radiographs.[1–4] A 18-month-old boy. The patellar and fibular head ossification centers have not ossified. The femoral and tibial epiphyses are ossified and round, and the zones of provisional calcification are radiodense. B 4-year-old boy. The primary center of ossification for the patella has begun to ossify. The femoral epiphysis is irregular. C 5-year-old boy. The patellar ossification center is more prominent, and a normal pronounced indentation is evident at the anterior portion of the tibia at the eventual site of the tibial tubercle. The fibular epiphyseal center is barely visible. D 9-year-old boy. The patella and the epiphyses are more fully ossified and have grown in size.

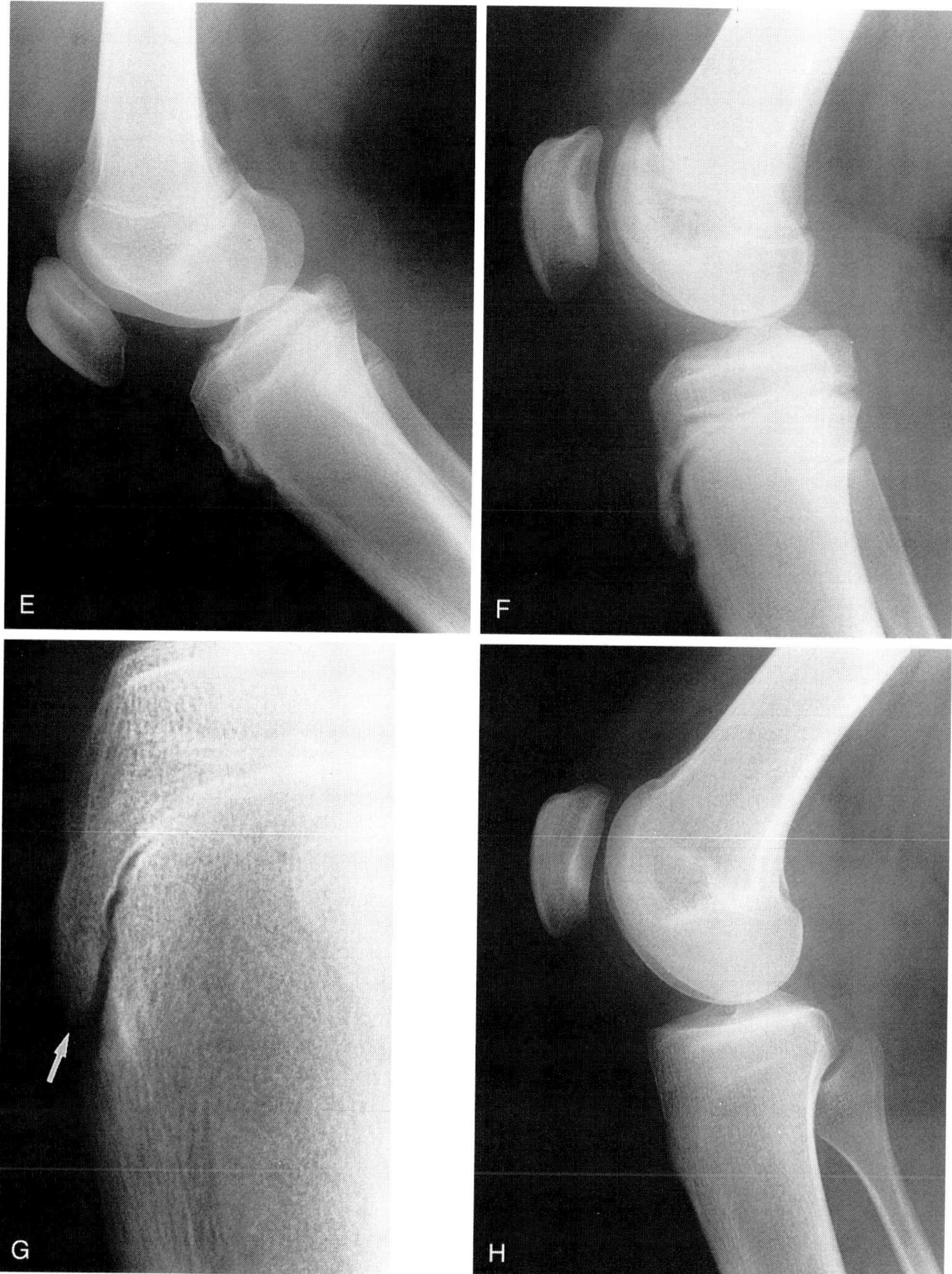

FIGURE 9–2 *Continued.* **E** 12-year-old girl. The zones of provisional calcification are not as radiodense. The patella is approaching adult proportions, and the epiphyses of the femur, tibia, and fibula are conforming to the shape of their respective metaphyses and are beginning to fuse. The tibial tubercle, arising from the anterior aspect of the proximal tibial epiphysis, is undergoing ossification and projects inferiorly along the shaft of the tibia. **F** 14-year-old boy. The tibial tubercle, now quite prominent, remains separated from the tibial shaft by a radiolucent cartilaginous cleft. Fusion of the epiphyses of the femur, the tibia, and the fibula lags behind that in the 12-year-old girl (**E**), a typical occurrence around this age. **G** 14-year-old girl. Radiograph shows the normal appearance of the apophysis of the tibial tubercle before fusion (arrow). **H** 15-year-old girl. The tibial tubercle apophysis has been incorporated into the tibial shaft. All epiphyses have fused, and the physeal lines remain barely visible.

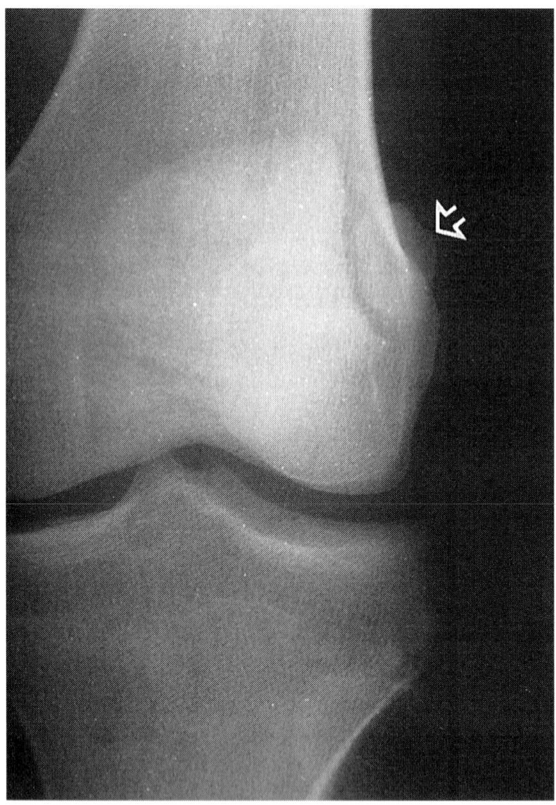

FIGURE 9–3. Bipartite patella.[5–8] Observe the characteristic radiolucency separating a circular ossified region at the superolateral aspect of the patella (open arrow).

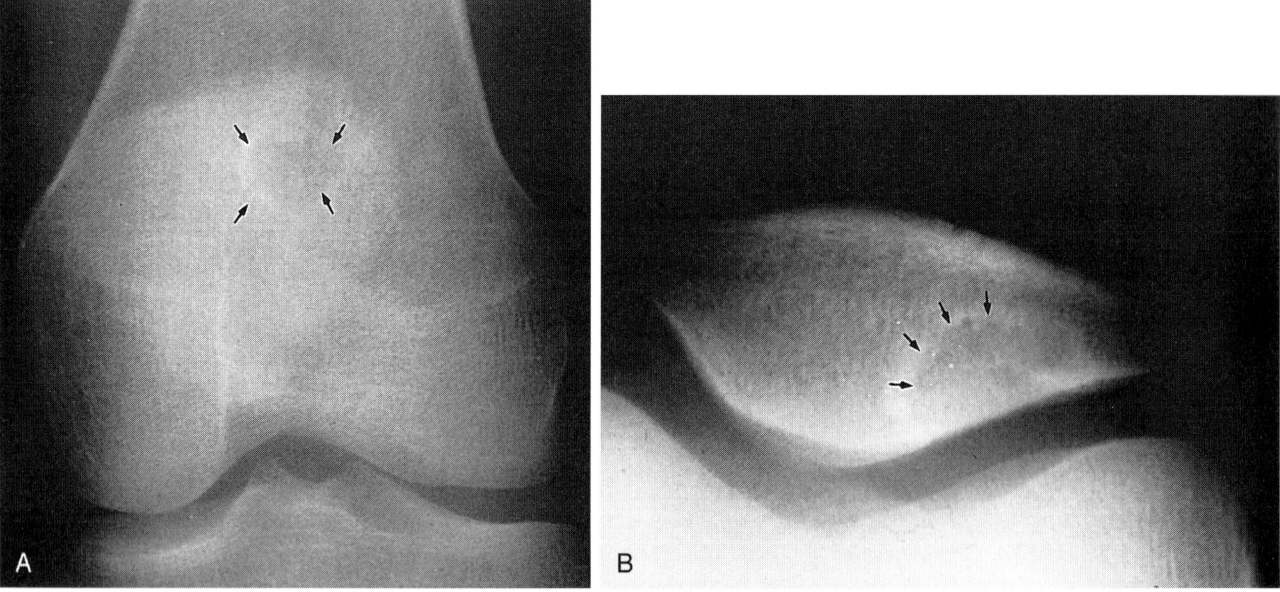

FIGURE 9–4. Dorsal defect of the patella.[9] A well-circumscribed radiolucent defect (arrows) is seen on frontal (A) and tangential (B) radiographs in the superior pole on the dorsal surface of the patella. This variant in ossification usually is a self-limited, incidental finding in children.

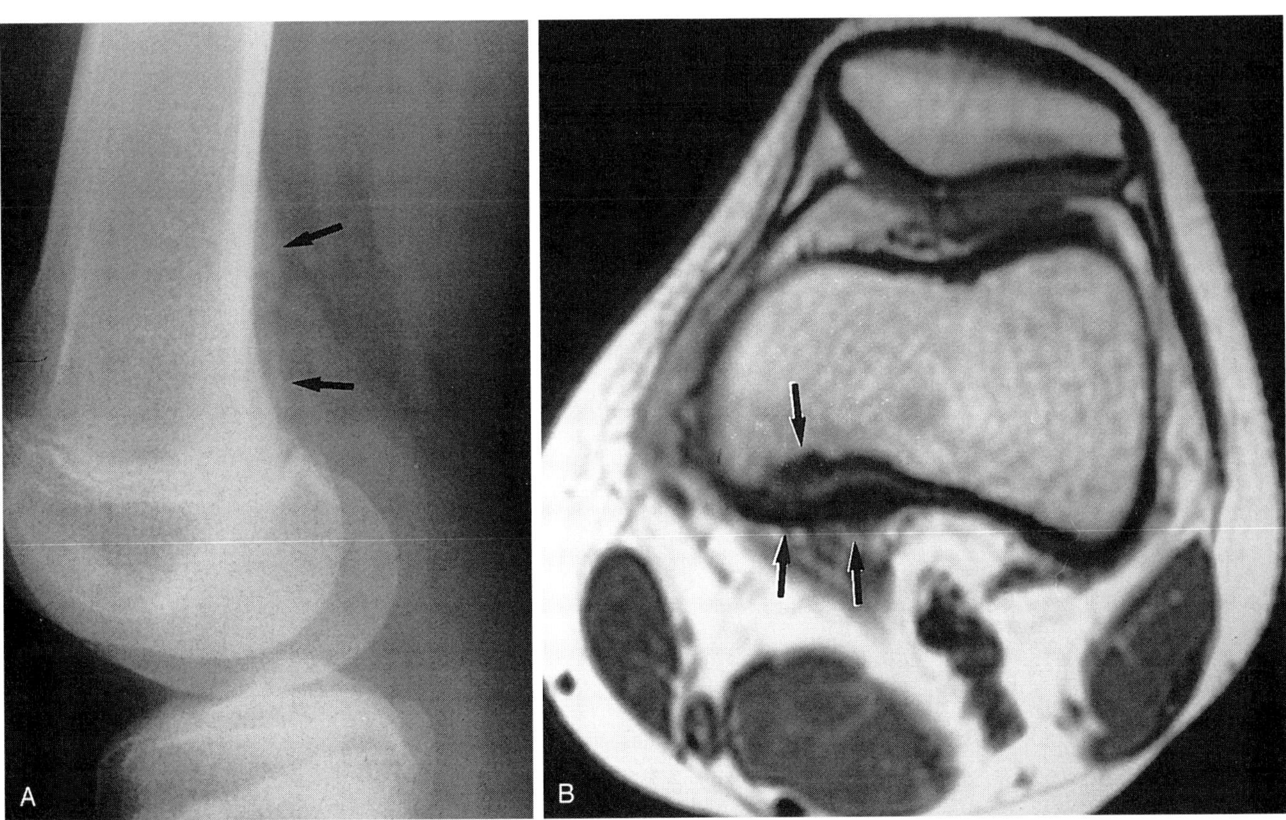

FIGURE 9–5. Juxtacortical desmoid (avulsive cortical irregularity).[10, 11] This 12-year-old swimmer had knee pain. A lateral radiograph (**A**) and a transaxial T1-weighted (TR/TE, 400/20) spin echo magnetic resonance (MR) image (**B**) show irregular periosteal new bone formation and cortical irregularity along a segment of the posteromedial cortex (arrows). The MR image localizes the lesion precisely. This classic location and appearance allow differentiation from a malignant process such as osteosarcoma. *(Courtesy of D. Witte, M.D., Memphis, Tennessee.)*

TABLE 9–3. Skeletal Dysplasias and Other Congenital Diseases Affecting the Knee*

Entity	Figure(s)	Characteristics
Hereditary osteo-onychodysostosis[13]	9–6	Absent or hypoplastic patellae
Dysplasia epiphysealis hemimelica[14, 15]	9–7	Asymmetric cartilaginous overgrowth in one or more epiphyses
		Radiographically resembles large eccentric osteochondroma arising from tibial or femoral epiphyses
		Bulky irregular ossification extending into soft tissues
Ehlers-Danlos syndrome[16]		Genu recurvatum
		Joint laxity
		Soft tissue hemangiomas appear as phleboliths on radiographs
Chondrodysplasia punctata[17]		Rare condition
		Stippled calcification in the immature cartilaginous skeleton: epiphyses of the femur and tibia and within the patella

*See also Table 1–2.

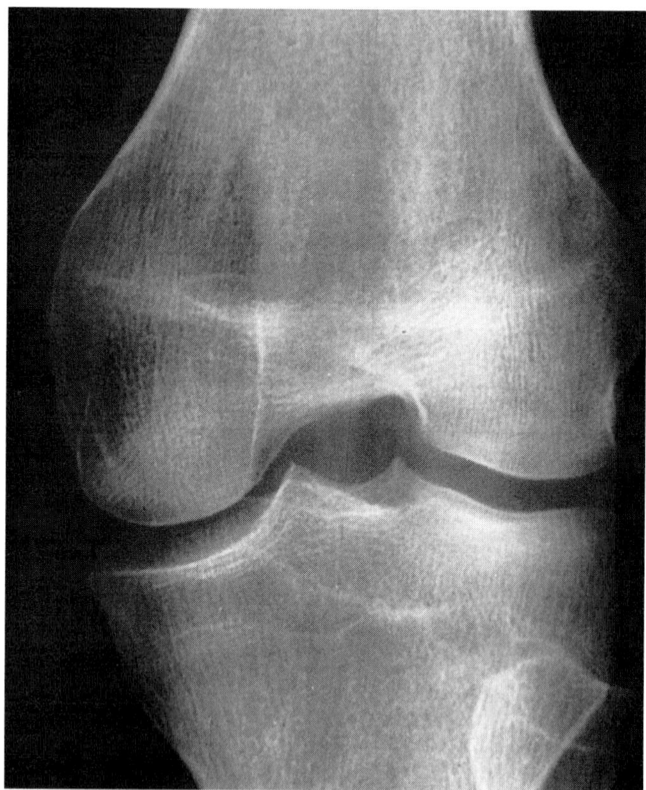

FIGURE 9–6. Hereditary osteo-onychodysostosis (HOOD syndrome).[13] Observe the characteristic absence of the patella.

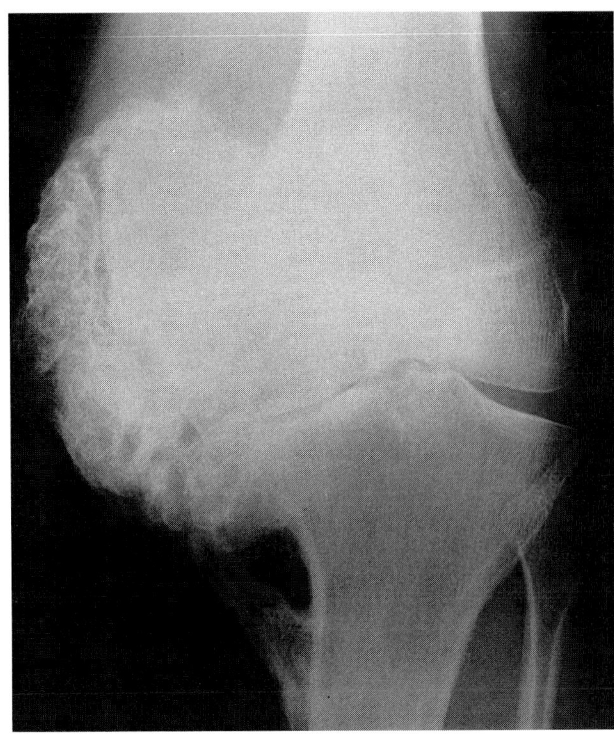

FIGURE 9–7. Dysplasia epiphysealis hemimelica (Trevor's disease).[14, 15] A huge cloud-like accumulation of ossification is seen arising from the medial aspect of the tibia and femur, spanning the medial aspect of the knee. A small osseous bridge also connects the mass to the proximal tibial shaft. These changes have resulted in a mild varus deformity. *(Courtesy of J. Schils, M.D., Cleveland, Ohio.)*

TABLE 9–4. **Alignment Abnormalities: Knee**

Entity	Figure(s)
Genu valgum (knock-knees)	
Osteo-onychodysostosis	See Fig. 9–6
Tibial plateau fracture	See Fig. 9–11
Medial collateral ligament tear	See Fig. 9–36
Rheumatoid arthritis	See Fig. 9–48
Flatfeet (pronation)	
Neuromuscular disease	
Achondroplasia	
Osteoarthrosis	
Multiple epiphyseal dysplasia	
Neurofibromatosis	
Osteogenesis imperfecta	
Homocystinuria	
Proximal tibial metaphyseal fracture	
Genu varum (bowlegs)	
Dysplasia epiphysealis hemimelica	See Fig. 9–7
Osteoarthrosis	See Fig. 9–46
Rheumatoid arthritis	See Fig. 9–48
Neuropathic osteoarthropathy	See Fig. 9–60
Rickets	See Fig. 9–66
Idiopathic	
Physiologic prenatal bowing	
Tibia vara (Blount disease)	See Fig. 10–2
Achondroplasia	
Premature partial growth arrest	
Multiple epiphyseal dysplasia	
Genu recurvatum (hyperextended knees)	
Osgood-Schlatter disease	See Fig. 9–18
Knee dislocation	See Fig. 9–21
Neuropathic osteoarthropathy	See Fig. 9–60
Ehlers-Danlos syndrome	
Premature partial growth arrest	
Posterior cruciate ligament tear	
Neuromuscular disease	

TABLE 9–5. **Alignment Abnormalities: Patella**

Entity	Figure(s)
Patella baja (inferiorly displaced patella)	
Neuromuscular disease	See Fig. 9–10
Osgood-Schlatter disease	See Fig. 9–18
Quadriceps tendon tear	See Fig. 9–42
Achondroplasia	
Surgery involving transfer of tibial tubercle	
Patella alta (superiorly displaced patella)	
Joint effusion	See Figs. 9–19, 9–23
Patellar tendon tear	See Figs. 9–41, 9–52
Chondromalacia patella	See Fig. 9–45
Patellar subluxation & dislocation	
Osgood-Schlatter disease	
Neuromuscular disease	
Homocystinuria	
Patellar sleeve fracture	
Sinding-Larsen-Johansson disease	
Lateral patellar displacement	
Patellar dislocation	See Fig. 9–22
Patellofemoral instability	See Fig. 9–44
Developmental lateral dystopia	

TABLE 9–6. Fractures About the Knee*

Entity	Figure(s)	Characteristics	Complications and Related Injuries
Fractures of the distal portion of the femur			
All types[18, 19]		Most injuries result from axial loading combined with varus, valgus, or rotational stress	Ligament disruption Patellar fracture Other associated fractures
Supracondylar[18, 19]		Extra-articular, transverse, or slightly oblique orientation May be displaced, comminuted, impacted, open, or closed	Displaced fragments Popliteal artery injury
Intercondylar[18, 19]		Intra-articular extension Supracondylar fracture combined with vertical component Y or T configuration	Incongruity of femorotibial or patellofemoral articular surfaces Degenerative joint disease Patellofemoral tracking disorders
Condylar[20]	9–8	Sagittal or coronal fracture lines isolated to the region of a single condyle	
Patellar fractures			
All types[21, 22]		Direct injury from fall or direct blow or indirect injury related to contraction of the quadriceps mechanism Unilateral injuries predominate	Osteochondral fracture Displaced fragments Ischemic necrosis involving proximal fragment 1–3 months after injury
Transverse[21, 22]	9–9A	50–80 per cent of cases Indirect force most common mechanism	
Longitudinal[21]	9–9B	25 per cent of cases Direct injury such as striking knee on dashboard of car	
Stellate or comminuted[21]		20–35 per cent of cases	
Stress (fatigue) fracture[22]		Rare occurrence of spontaneous displaced or nondisplaced fracture Usually transverse fracture of middle or distal third of patella Occur most frequently in young athletes	
Patellar sleeve fracture[23]		Rare cartilaginous avulsion from the lower pole of the patella in children Results from hyperextension injuries *Radiographic findings* Radiographs may be normal Avulsed fragment from inferior pole of patella Joint effusion with patella alta *MR imaging findings* Marrow edema in patella Peripatellar soft tissue edema Osteochondral fracture through cartilage-bone interface Joint effusion or lipohemarthrosis Thickening of patellar tendon	Severity of avulsion often underestimated on routine radiography
Spastic paralysis[24]	9–10	Fragmentation or separation of the inferior pole of the patella Seen in patients with cerebral palsy and other causes of spastic paralysis Related to a traction phenomenon with contusion or tendinitis in the proximal attachment of the patellar tendon with subsequent calcification or ossification May also represent an avulsion injury	

TABLE 9–6. Fractures About the Knee* *Continued*

Entity	Figure(s)	Characteristics	Complications and Related Injuries
Fractures of the proximal portion of the tibia			
Tibial plateau fractures			
All types[25–27]	9–11	Vertical compression, valgus, varus, and rotational forces May be intra- or extra-articular	Cruciate and collateral ligament injuries and avulsion fractures Meniscal injuries Depression of plateau Lipohemarthrosis Peroneal nerve or artery injury Degenerative joint disease
Isolated lateral plateau[25–27]	9–11	75–80 per cent of all plateau fractures Valgus stress predominates *Type I* Wedge-shaped pure cleavage or fracture that splits the lateral plateau *Type II* Combined cleavage and compression fracture *Type III* Pure compression fracture	Valgus deformity Fibular head and neck fractures
Isolated medial plateau[25–27]		5–10 per cent of all plateau fractures Varus forces predominate *Type IV* May be split, wedge-shaped, or depressed and comminuted; may involve associated fractures of tibial eminences	
Combined medial and lateral plateau[25–27]		10–15 per cent of all plateau fractures *Type V* Bicondylar fracture	Fibular head and neck fractures
Fractures of the tibial eminences[28]	9–12	Result from violent twisting, abduction-adduction injury, or direct contact with the femoral condyle Avulsion from cruciate ligament Intra-articular fracture fragment may be undisplaced, hinged, detached, or detached and inverted	Associated cruciate ligament injury Intra-articular fracture fragment
Segond injury[29]	9–13	Segond fracture: avulsion fracture of the proximal portion of the tibia at the attachment of the lateral joint capsule Occurs as a result of internal rotation of the tibia with the knee in flexion Acute avulsion appears as thin, vertically oriented sliver of bone just distal to the joint line on the lateral tibia Fracture fragment eventually merges with the lateral tibial margin, producing an outgrowth that simulates an osteophyte	Anterior cruciate ligament disruption (75–100 per cent of cases) Meniscal tears (more than 60 per cent of cases)
Fractures of the proximal portion of the fibula[19]		Fractures of fibular head or neck result from direct or indirect forces: Direct blows Varus forces associated with avulsion of proximal pole or styloid process Valgus force associated with lateral plateau fracture Twisting forces at ankle may cause high fibular fracture (Maisonneuve fracture)	Contusion or traction of the biceps tendon Peroneal nerve injury Anterior tibial artery rupture Associated collateral ligament injury and lateral tibial plateau fracture Avulsion of fibular head with possible intra-articular entrapment Associated ankle injuries

Table continued on following page

TABLE 9–6. Fractures About the Knee* *Continued*

Entity	Figure(s)	Characteristics	Complications and Related Injuries
Child abuse[30, 31]	9–14	Most frequent in children 1–4 years of age Metaphyseal corner fractures of femur and tibia Physeal injuries Fractures in various stages of healing Acute fractures of the tibia and femur Subperiosteal hemorrhage with periosteal reaction	Associated injuries elsewhere
Growth plate injuries			
Distal femoral physis[32]	9–15	1.2 per cent of growth plate injuries Most common age: 10 to 15 years Trauma from birth, athletic, or automobile injuries Child catches legs between spokes of a wagon or bicycle wheel Clipping injury in adolescent football Type II and III injuries common	Shortening and angulation of the femur Prognosis guarded
Proximal tibial physis[32]	9–16	Proximal tibial physis injuries are rare Type III lesions predominate	Approximately 20 per cent of patients develop partial or complete growth arrest Popliteal artery injury
Tibial tubercle apophysis[33, 34]	9–17	Rare injury Violent avulsion at quadriceps attachment Fracture may extend vertically into proximal tibial epiphysis	Disruption of quadriceps mechanism
Posttraumatic osteochondroses			
Osgood-Schlatter disease[5, 35]	9–18	Acute or chronic repetitive trauma resulting in various degrees of avulsion of the apophysis of the tibial tubercle at the distal attachment of the patellar tendon *Clinical findings* Local pain, tenderness, swelling, and palpable mass over tibial tubercle Symptoms aggravated with activity and alleviated with rest Most frequently appears initially between the ages of 10 and 17 years Male > female (3:1 to 10:1 ratio) Related to participation in sports that involve kicking, jumping, and squatting Usually self-limited with symptoms resolving when the tibial apophysis fuses between 18 and 24 years of age Bilateral in as many as 60 per cent of cases *Soft tissue radiographic findings* Swelling and irregularity of the soft tissues anterior to tibial tubercle Thickening of the patellar tendon Loss of sharpness or obliteration of the inferior angle of the infrapatellar fat pad Widening of soft tissues bordering the anterior articular surface of the tibia *Osseous radiographic findings* Inconsistent and unreliable Irregularity, fragmentation, and displacement of the tibial tubercle ossification center Ossicles may persist into adulthood	Normal ossification of the tibial tubercle apophysis may resemble Osgood-Schlatter disease with amorphous calcification, fragmentation, rarefaction, and sclerosis
Sinding-Larsen-Johansson disease[5]		Painful fragmentation or avulsion of the inferior pole of the patella Self-limited condition that may result in permanent irregularity of patellar margin Pathogenesis disputed: may represent traction apophysitis or posttraumatic osteonecrosis	

TABLE 9–6. Fractures About the Knee* *Continued*

Entity	Figure(s)	Characteristics	Complications and Related Injuries
Osteochondral fracture[36, 37]	9–19	Momentary, persistent, or recurrent dislocations and subluxations of the patella may result in injury to the patella or lateral femoral condyle or both Acute injury to the articular surface can result in cartilaginous or osteocartilaginous fracture fragments within the joint	Associated with painful joint effusion or hemarthrosis, joint locking, clicking, and limitation of motion
Osteochondritis dissecans[38–41]	9–20	Fragmentation and possible separation of a portion of the articular surface Adolescent onset most frequent, but occurs from childhood to middle age Symptoms and signs usually begin between 15 and 20 years of age Men > women Significant history of trauma in only 50 per cent of cases Femoral condyles are the most typical location: medial condyle 85 per cent of cases and lateral condyle 15 per cent of cases Magnetic resonance (MR) arthrography and computed tomographic (CT) arthrography are the most useful imaging techniques Patellar involvement is rare	Painful or painless joint effusion Joint locking, clicking, and limitation of motion

*See Tables 1–3 and 1–4.

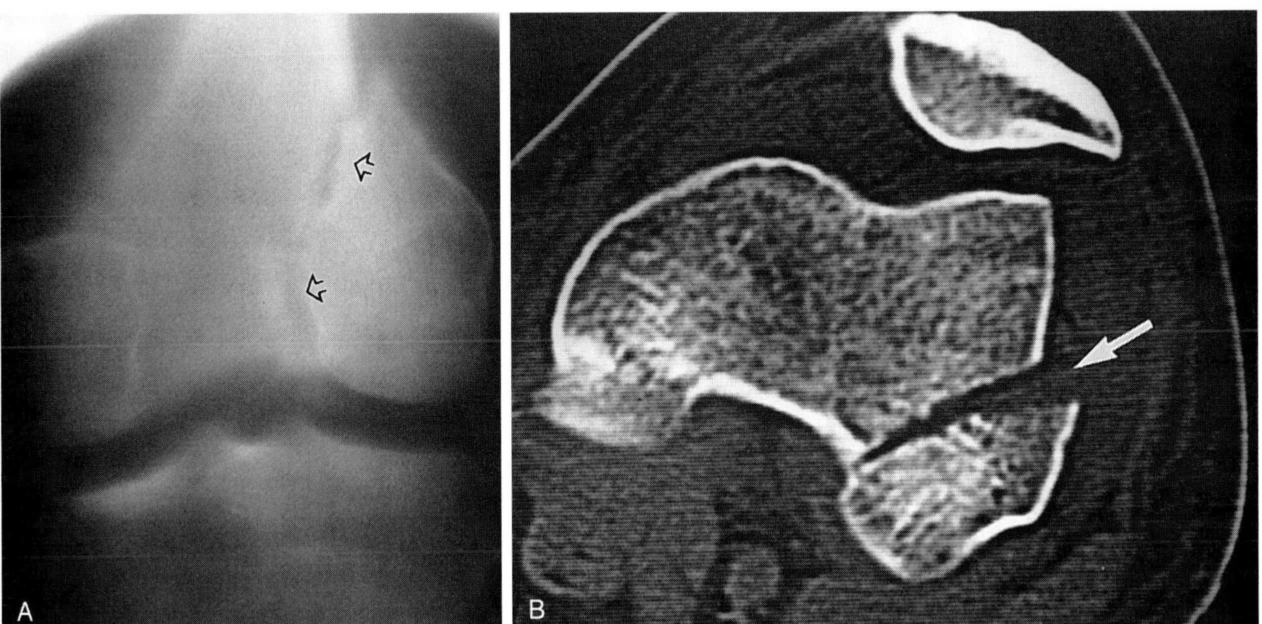

FIGURE 9–8. Fracture of the lateral femoral condyle.[20] **A** Coronal conventional tomogram shows a sagittally oriented vertical intra-articular fracture involving the lateral femoral condyle (open arrows). **B** Transaxial computed tomographic (CT) scan shows minimal displacement of the fracture fragment (arrow). Condylar fractures, in which sagittal fracture lines are isolated to a single condyle, may be difficult to detect on routine radiographs and often, as in this case, require conventional tomography or CT.

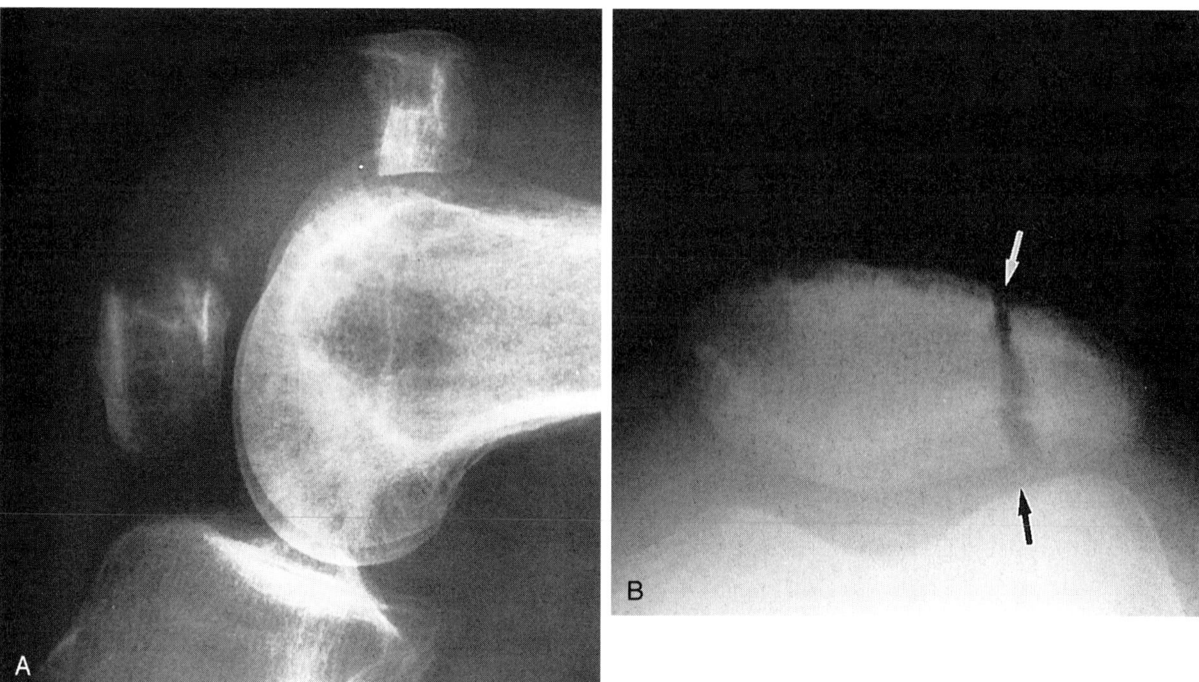

FIGURE 9–9. Patellar fracture.[21, 22] A Transverse fracture of the patella with wide displacement of the fracture fragments. B Tangential radiography from another patient shows a jagged, minimally displaced longitudinal fracture of the patella (arrows).

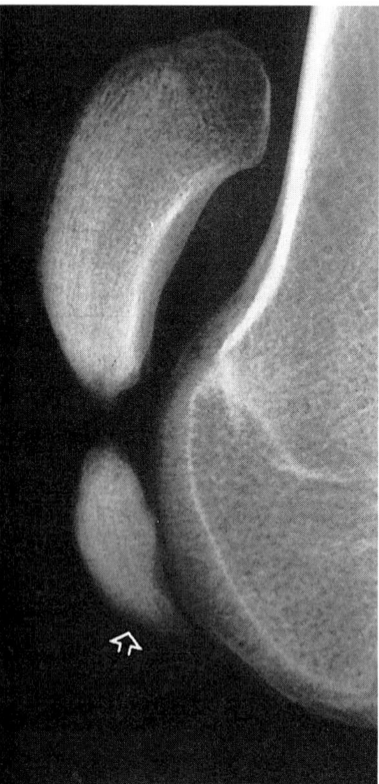

FIGURE 9–10. Spastic paralysis: patella.[24] Observe the fragmentation of the inferior pole of the patella (open arrow) in this 17-year-old patient with cerebral palsy. The lesion, frequently associated with spastic paralysis, probably is related to a traction phenomenon.

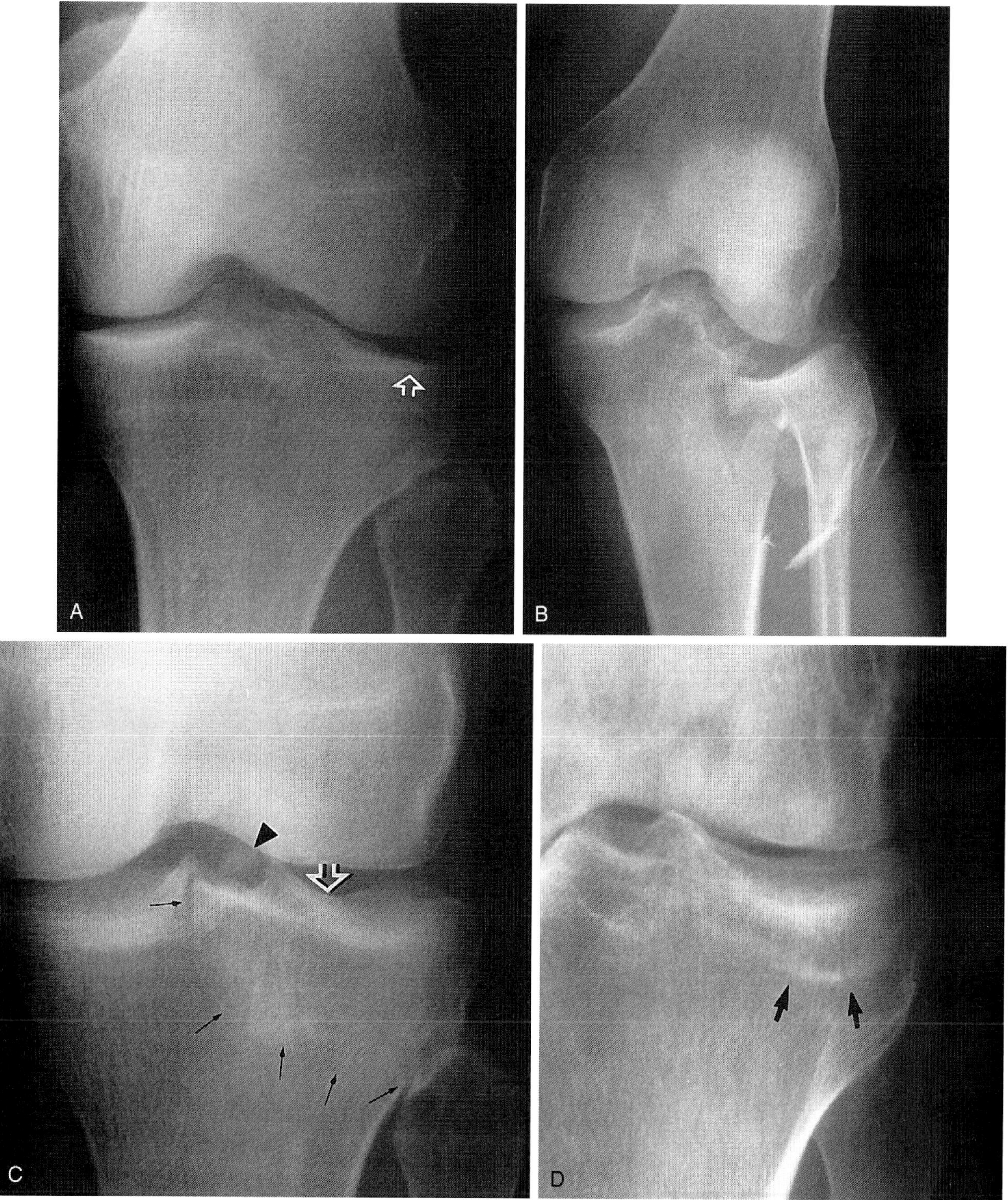

FIGURE 9–11. Tibial plateau fracture.[25–27] A Acute fracture: Type III. A 47-year-old man was involved in a motor vehicle collision. Frontal radiograph reveals minimal depression of the lateral tibial plateau (open arrow). B Acute comminuted fracture: Type II. In another patient, observe the severely comminuted lateral plateau and lateral displacement of the proximal tibiofibular articulation. C In another patient with a type III fracture, the radiograph shows depression of the lateral tibial articular surface (open arrow) and compaction of the fracture fragments (arrows). An intra-articular fragment also is seen (arrowhead). D Stress (fatigue) fracture. This 50-year-old woman developed pain after embarking on a rigorous program of running after years of inactivity. Observe the transverse zone of sclerosis (arrows) characteristic of a fatigue fracture of the lateral tibial plateau (arrows).

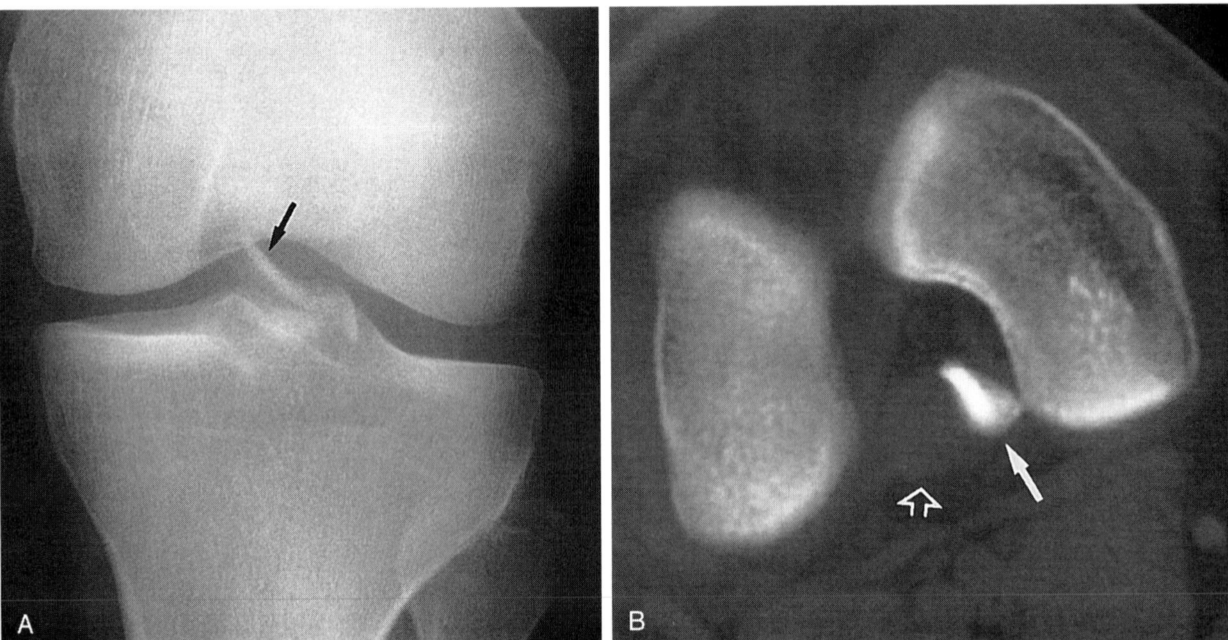

FIGURE 9–12. Avulsion fracture of the tibial eminence: posterior cruciate ligament tear.[28] A Frontal radiograph of this 18-year-old boy reveals a displaced bone fragment (arrow) within the knee joint related to an avulsion of the tibial eminence. B Axial computed tomographic (CT) scan shows the osseous fragment (arrow) attached to the circular posterior cruciate ligament (open arrow).

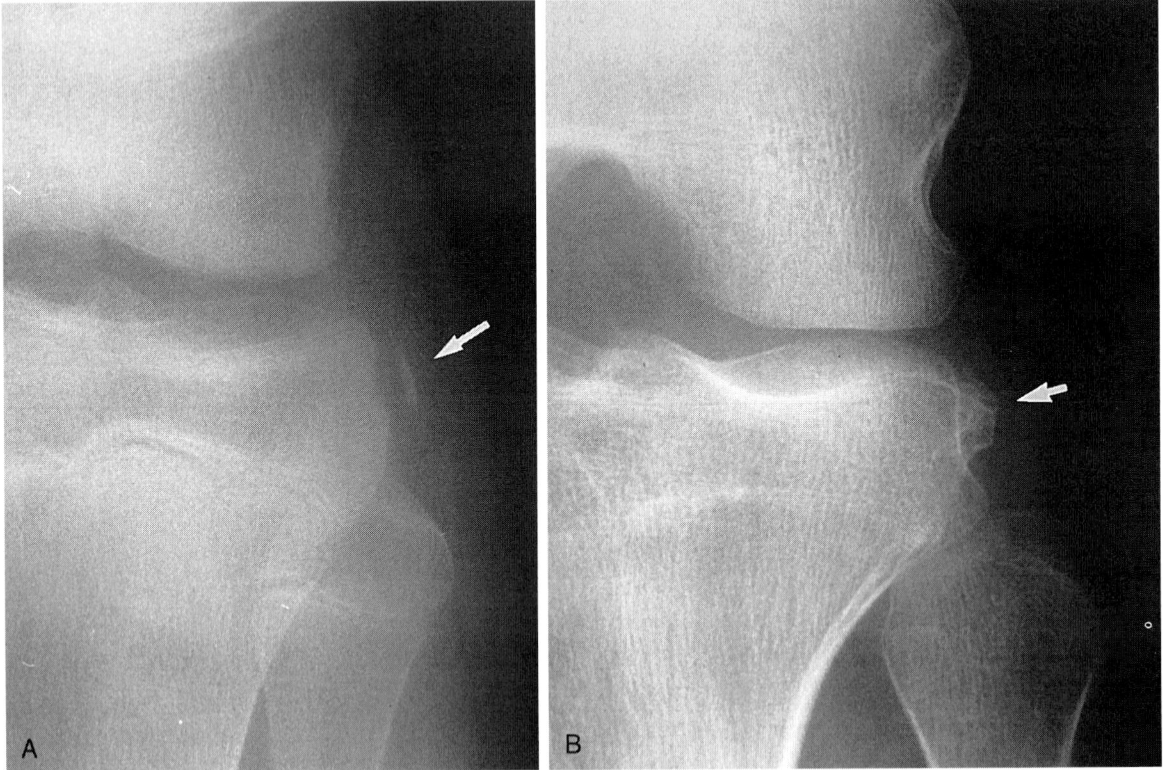

FIGURE 9–13. Segond injury: lateral capsular avulsion.[29] A Acute situation. A thin, vertically oriented linear avulsion fracture is seen at the superolateral aspect of the lateral tibial condyle. B Chronic situation. Anteroposterior intercondylar view in a 33-year-old man shows a well-defined bony excrescence arising from the lateral tibial rim proximal to the head of the fibula (arrow). This appearance of an irregular outgrowth of bone is typical of a healed Segond injury, indicating a previous avulsion and disruption of the lateral joint capsule.

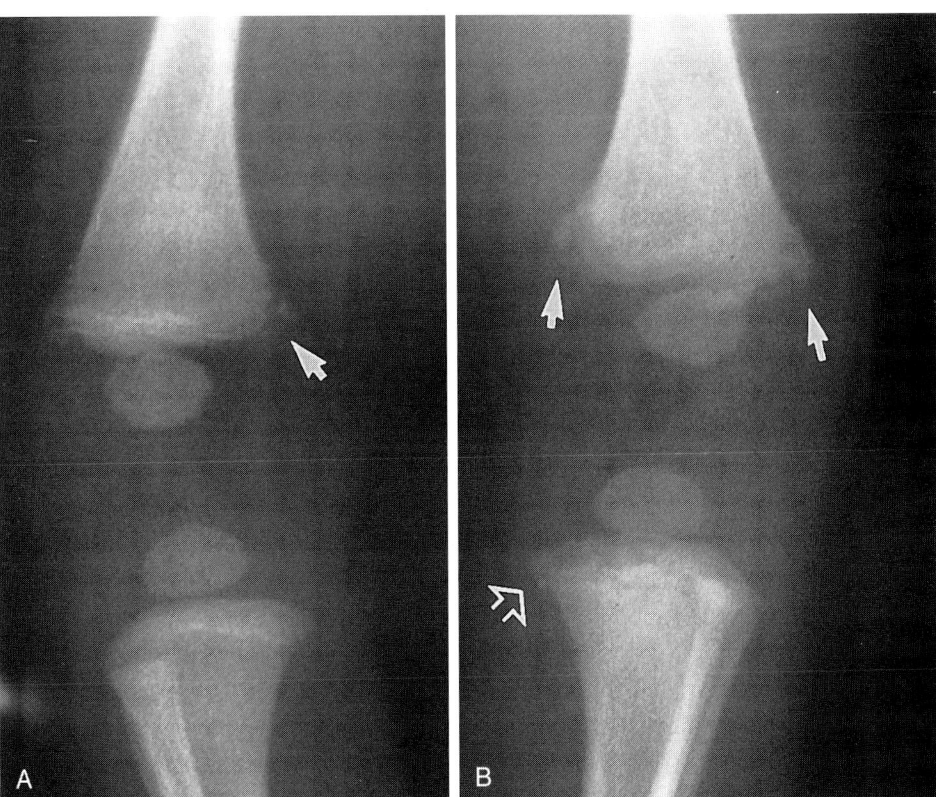

FIGURE 9–14. A, B Child abuse.[30, 31] Observe the irregularities and corner fractures of the proximal tibial metaphyseal margin (open arrow) and both distal femoral metaphyseal margins (arrows). Metaphyseal lesions of child abuse classically involve the knee. These fractures tend to be less conspicuous when they are acute, and become more visible with healing. *(Courtesy of D. Edwards, M.D., San Diego, California.)*

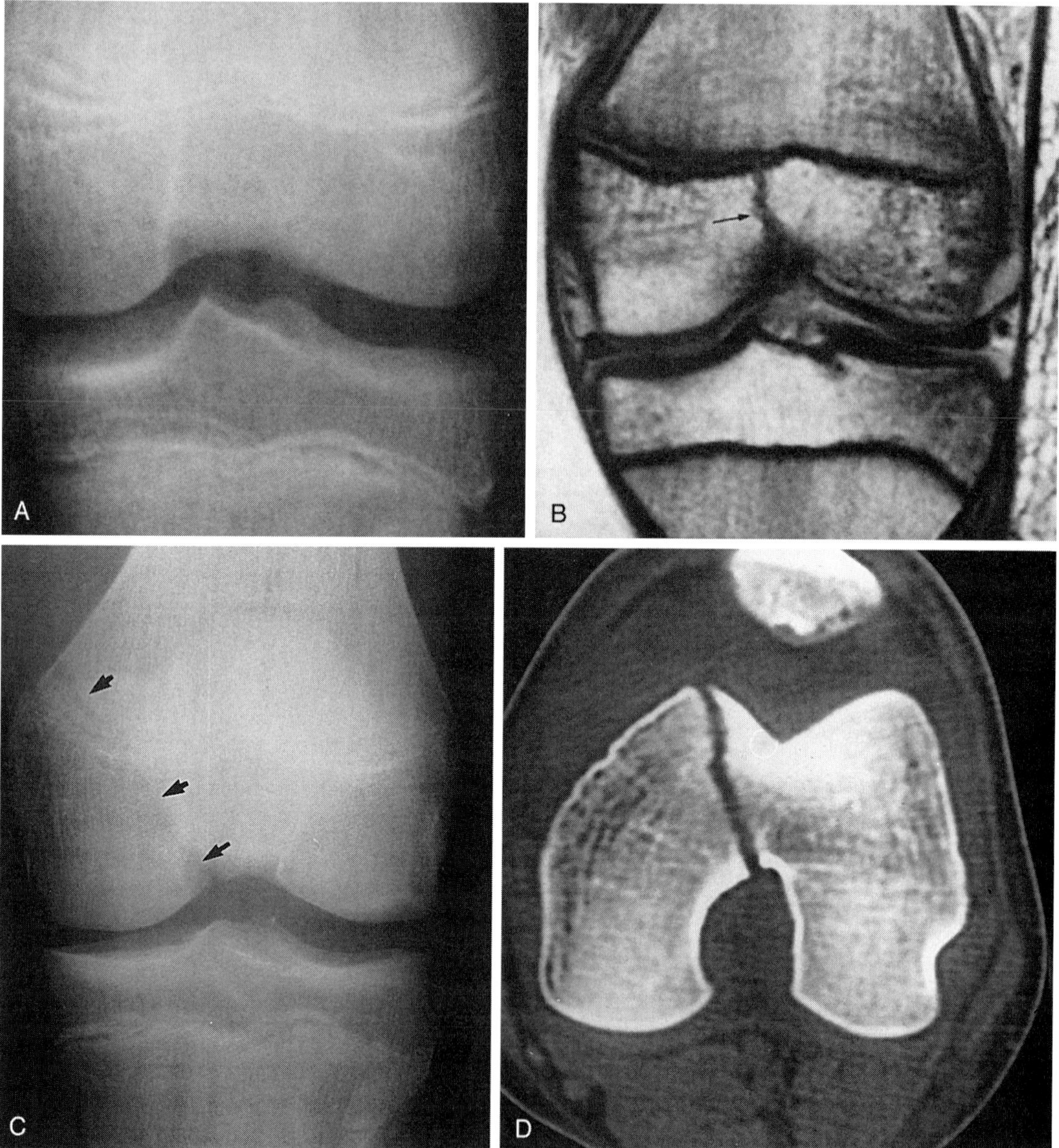

FIGURE 9–15. Growth plate injuries: Magnetic resonance (MR) imaging—distal portion of the femur.[32] **A, B** In a 13-year-old boy, a frontal radiograph (**A**) reveals no significant abnormality. A coronal T1-weighted (TR/TE, 800/20) spin echo MR image (**B**) shows a vertical fracture line (arrow) in the distal femoral epiphysis, indicative of a Salter-Harris type III physeal injury. Bone contusions appear as regions of diminished signal intensity in the metaphysis and epiphysis of the distal portion of the femur and in the epiphysis of the proximal end of the tibia. (**A, B,** *From Resnick D [ed]: Diagnosis of Bone and Joint Disorders. 3rd Ed. Philadelphia, WB Saunders, 1995, p 2646.*) **C, D** Salter-Harris type III injury. In **C,** a routine radiograph of a 15-year-old boy shows an intercondylar fracture through the medial condylar growth plate as well as the metaphysis and epiphysis of the distal portion of the femur (arrows). In **D,** a transaxial computed tomographic (CT) scan shows the extent of the complete nondisplaced fracture. (**C, D,** *Courtesy of G. Greenway, M.D., Dallas, Texas.*)

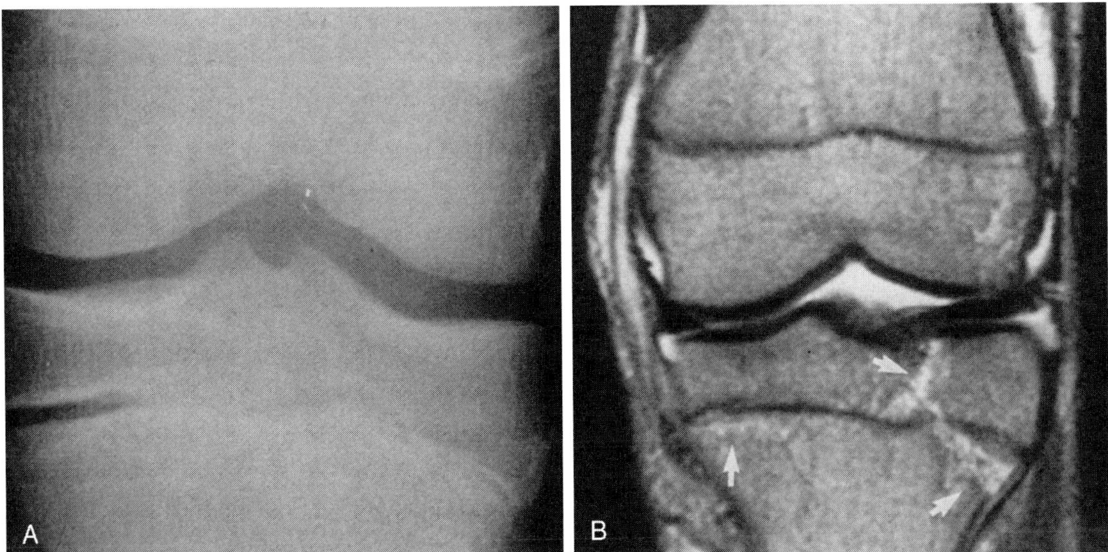

FIGURE 9–16. Growth plate injuries: Magnetic resonance (MR) imaging—proximal portion of the tibia.[32] This young boy suffered an injury to the knee while playing soccer. A Routine radiograph shows widening of the medial portion of the proximal tibial physis, suggesting a Salter-Harris type I injury. B Coronal T2-weighted (TR/TE, 2000/80) spin echo MR image reveals high signal intensity (arrows) in the tibial epiphysis and metaphysis, consistent with a Salter-Harris type IV injury. High signal intensity also is seen in a bone contusion of the lateral portion of the distal femoral epiphysis and in and about the medial collateral ligament, indicating ligament disruption and soft tissue edema. A joint effusion is present. *(From Resnick D [ed]: Diagnosis of Bone and Joint Disorders. 3rd Ed. Philadelphia, WB Saunders, 1995, p 2646.)*

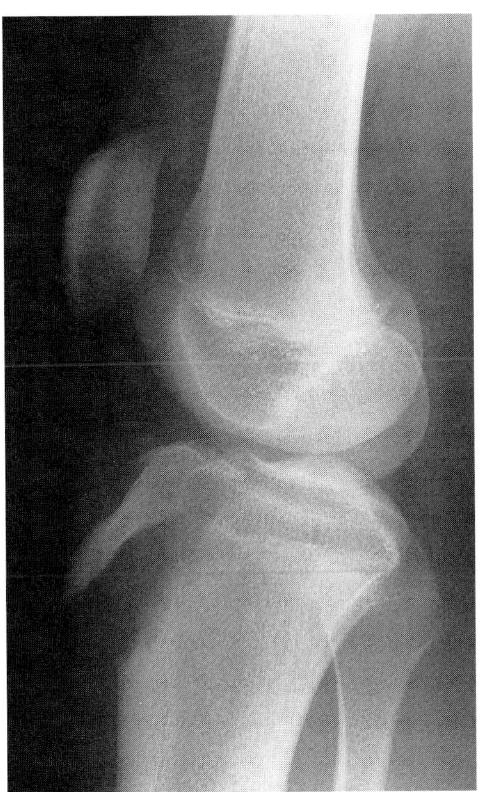

FIGURE 9–17. Avulsion fracture: Tibial tubercle apophysis.[33, 34] A lateral radiography of the knee in this 14-year-old boy shows an extensive avulsion of a large segment of the tibial tubercle at the attachment of the patellar tendon. The fracture extends through the proximal tibial epiphysis into the articulation.

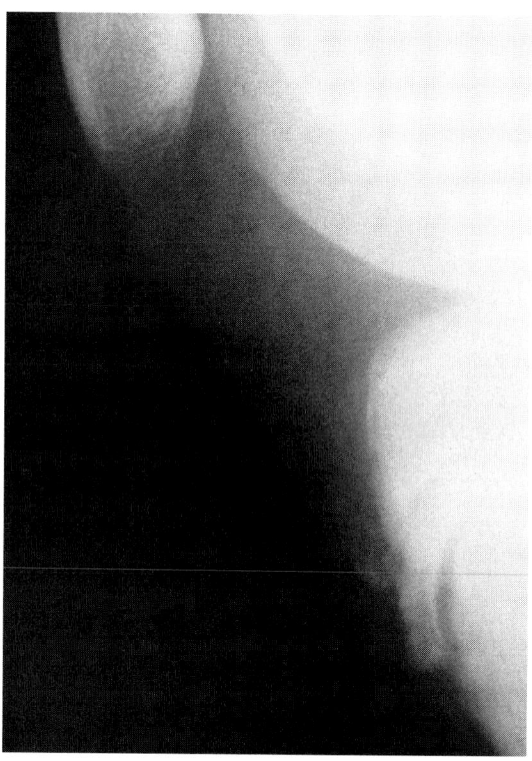

FIGURE 9–18. Osgood-Schlatter disease.[35] A lateral radiograph of an 11-year-old girl shows thickening of the patellar tendon (seen as soft tissue swelling) and loss of definition and fragmentation of the tibial tubercle. *(Courtesy of S.K. Brahme, M.D., San Diego, California.)*

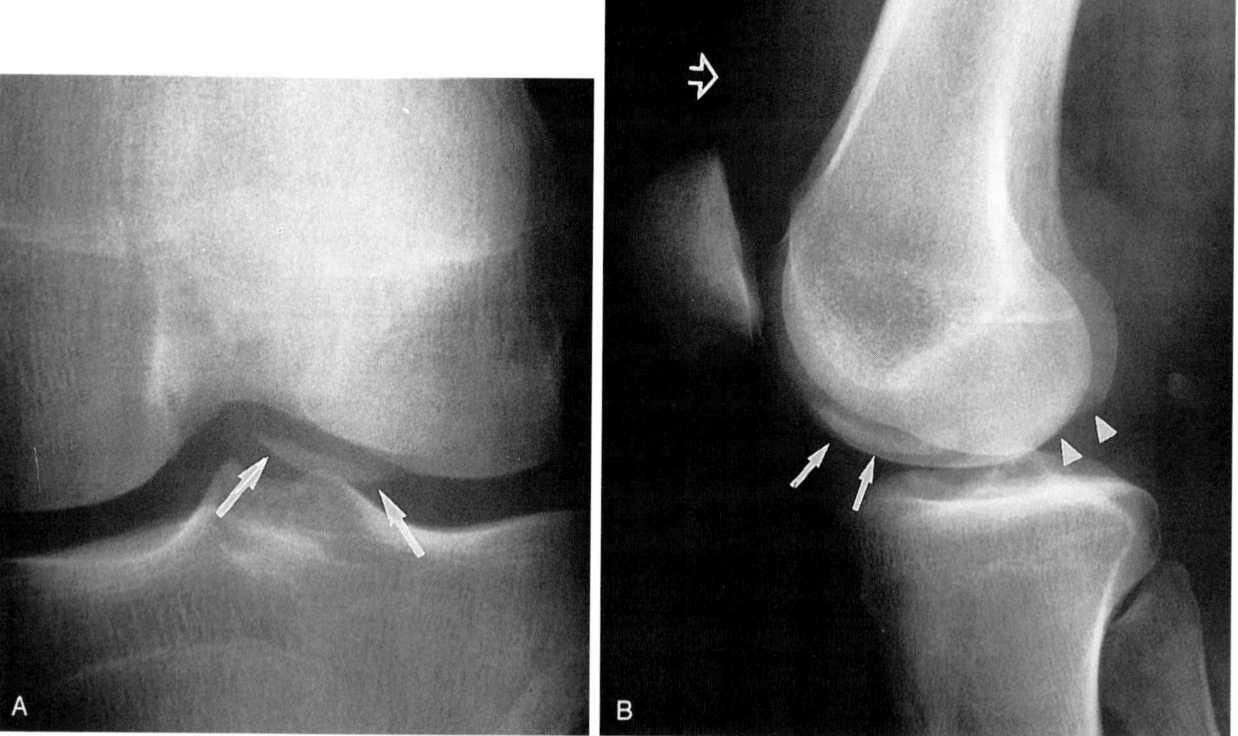

FIGURE 9–19. Osteochondral fracture.[36, 37] Frontal (A) and lateral (B) radiographs of this 23-year-old man show a crescent-shaped osseous fragment (arrows) and a corresponding radiolucent defect in the posterior aspect of the lateral femoral condyle (arrowheads). A large joint effusion (open arrow) displaces the superior portion of the patella.

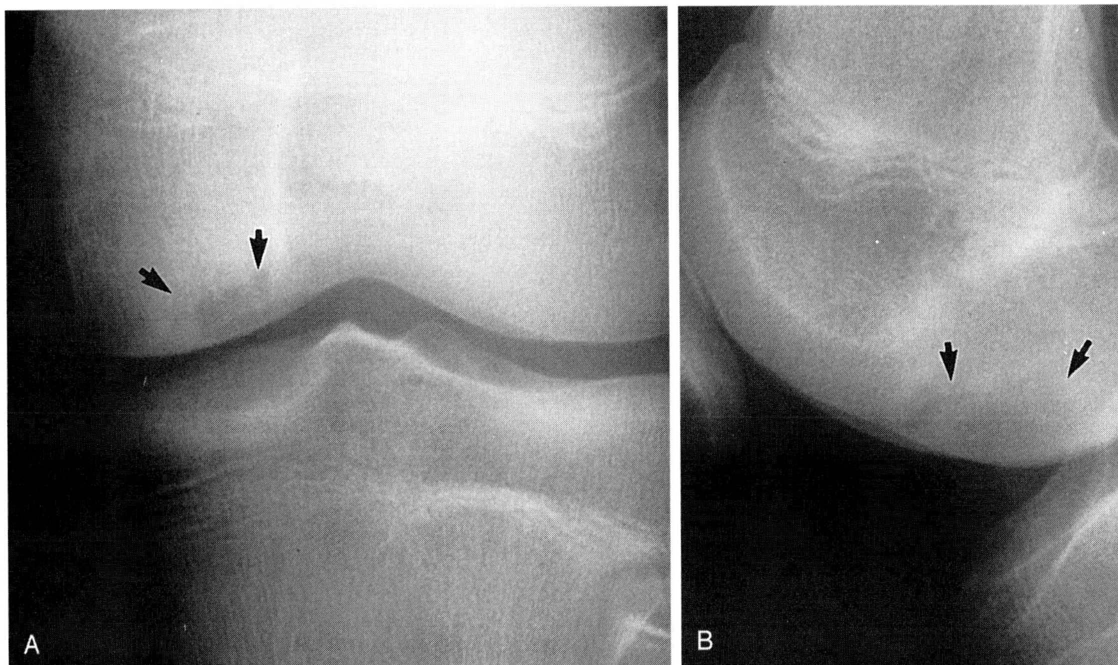

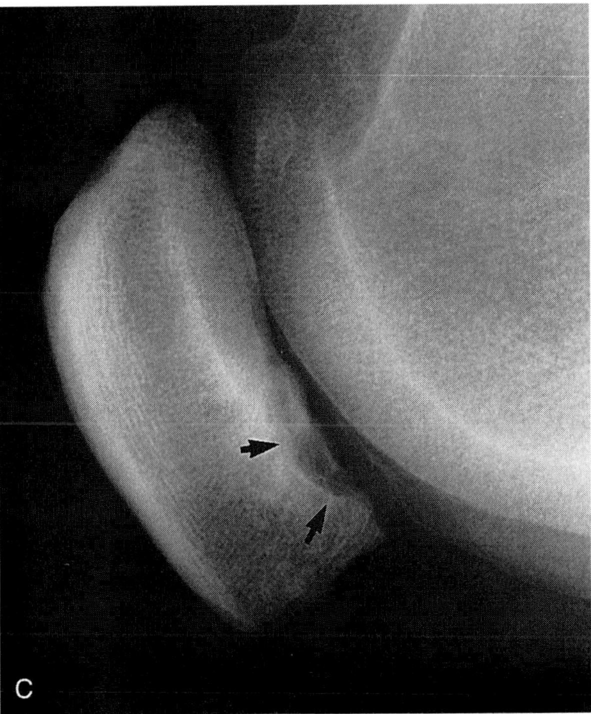

FIGURE 9–20. Osteochondritis dissecans.[38–41] A, B Distal portion of the femur. Frontal (A) and lateral (B) radiographs of this 15-year-old patient show a classic subchondral radiolucent defect in the lateral aspect of the medial femoral condyle (arrows). Eighty-five per cent of cases of osteochondritis dissecans affect the medial femoral condyle, most commonly at the lateral aspect. C Patella. Lateral radiograph shows a radiolucent defect in the articular surface of the patella (arrows). Degenerative changes also are noted in the superior aspect of the patellofemoral joint. The patella is a rare site for osteochondritis dissecans. The medial patellar facet is involved most frequently.

TABLE 9–7. Dislocations About the Knee*

Entity	Figure(s)	Characteristics	Complications and Related Injuries
Femorotibial dislocation			
All types[42, 43]		Rare but serious injury High-energy trauma from automobile collisions, industrial injuries, or falls from a considerable height Occasionally occurs with sports injuries Closed injuries more common than open injuries	Associated fractures Visceral and head injuries Popliteal artery laceration or thrombosis (25–50 per cent of cases) Popliteal vein and peroneal nerve injury Capsular, meniscal, and ligamentous injury Disruption of four major knee ligaments or both cruciate ligaments implies that a dislocation has occurred
Anterior	9–21	30–50 per cent of all knee dislocations Hyperextension injury Tearing of posterior capsule, posterior cruciate ligament, and anterior cruciate ligament	
Posterior		Next in frequency to anterior dislocations Crushing blows to the anterior surface of the proximal end of the tibia	Injury of extensor mechanism of knee
Lateral, medial, and rotary		Uncommon Valgus, varus, or torsional injury	Collateral ligament damage
Patellar dislocation[44]	9–22	Direct blow or exaggerated contraction of quadriceps mechanism Lateral displacement predominates Patellar subluxation or dislocation often is a transient, recurrent problem Spontaneous reduction usually occurs *Predisposing factors* Patella alta Deficient height of lateral femoral condyle Shallowness of the patellofemoral groove Genu valgum or genu recurvatum Lateral insertion of patellar tendon Muscular weakness (vastus medialis muscle) Excessive tibial torsion	Osteochondral fracture of medial patellar facet and lateral femoral condyle Patellar tracking disorders Retinacular injury of femoral or patellar site of attachment (76 per cent of cases) Contusions of femoral condyle and patella
Proximal tibiofibular joint dislocation[19]		Rare injury Seen in parachuting and horseback riding injuries Adduction of the knee in the flexed position Anterior dislocation twice as common as posterior dislocation Subtle radiographic findings of anterior dislocation include anterior and lateral fibular displacement	Common peroneal nerve injury

*See also Table 1–5.

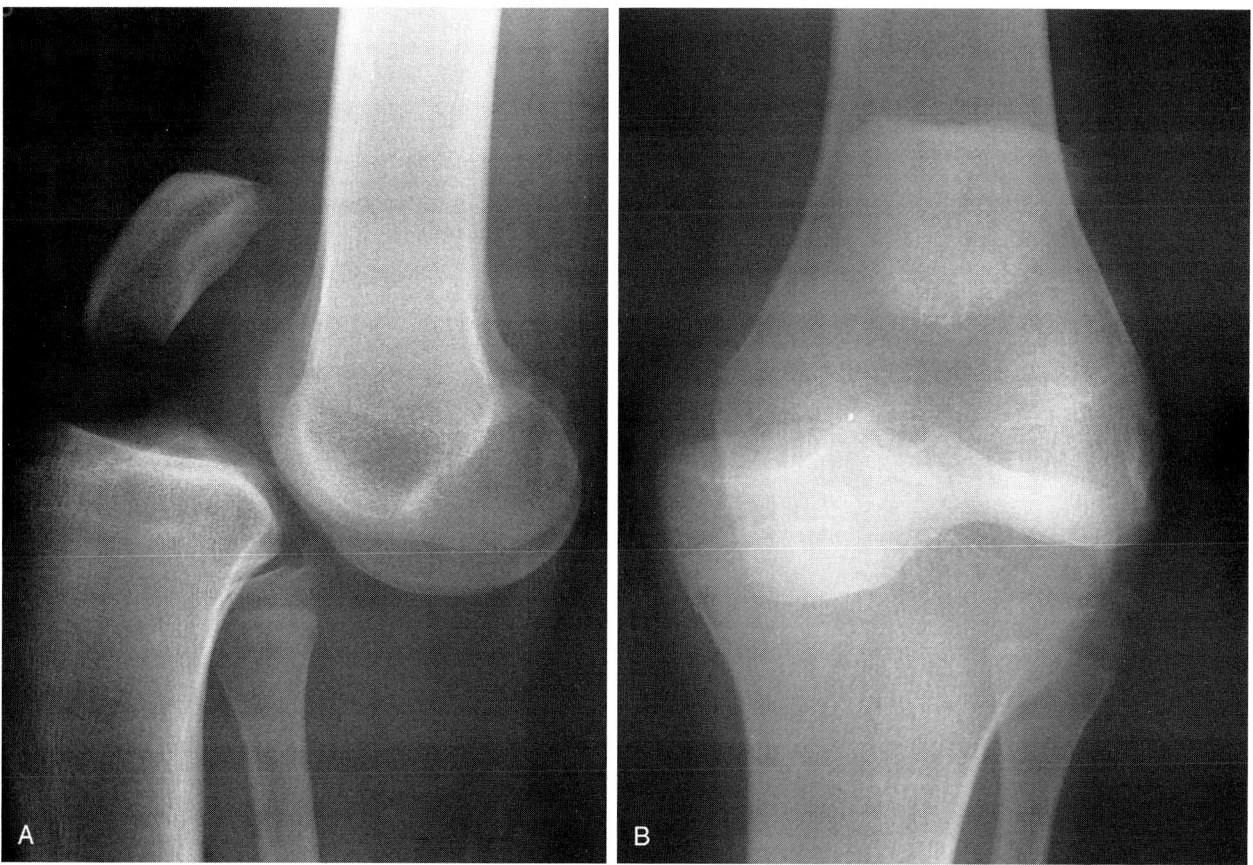

FIGURE 9–21. Acute femorotibial dislocation.[42, 43] A Lateral radiograph of the knee in this 18-year-old man shows anterior dislocation of the tibia and fibula. B Anteroposterior radiograph shows marked overlap of the tibia and femur as well as medial dislocation of the tibia with respect to the femur. Nearly all cases of such dislocation result in complete disruption of the cruciate ligaments, and many also result in injury to the menisci, collateral ligaments, peroneal tendon, and popliteal artery.

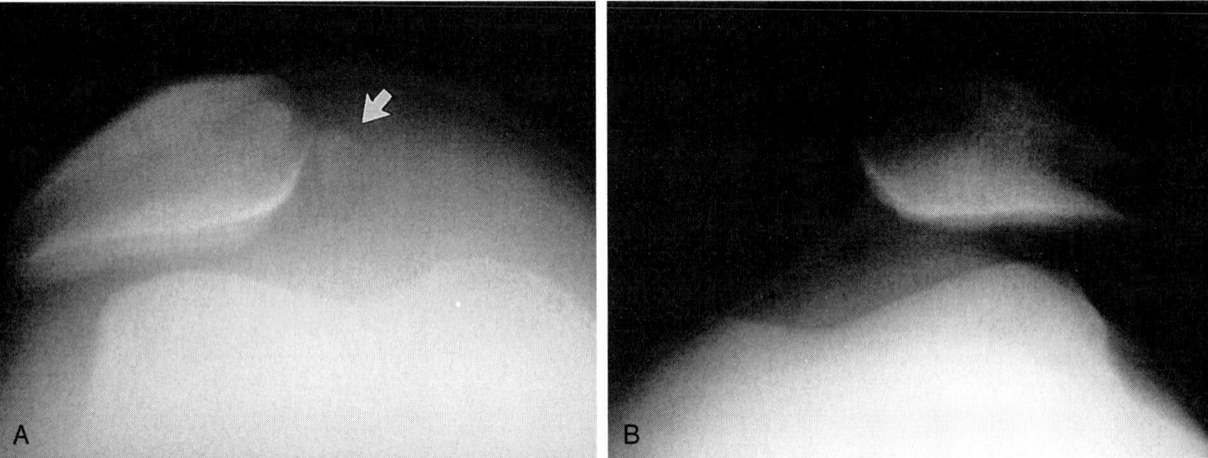

FIGURE 9–22. A, B Bilateral patellar dislocation.[44] Axial radiographs of the knee in this 25-year-old woman reveal bilateral lateral patellar dislocations. Observe the fracture of the right medial patellar facet resulting from avulsion at the site of attachment of the medial retinaculum (arrow). Note also the straight line appearance of the lateral patellar facet and the gentle slope of the lateral femoral condyle, both of which predispose to patellofemoral instability with subluxation and dislocation. Lateral patellar dislocation often is a transient phenomenon, with spontaneous reduction.

TABLE 9–8. Internal Derangements—Synovial Disorders*

Entity	Figure(s), Table(s)	Characteristics	Complications and Related Disorders
Joint effusion[45, 46]	9–23; see Figs. 9–16, 9–19, 9–29A, 9–38B, 9–46C, 9–49D, 9–55D, 9–59, 9–61, 9–64, 9–69B	Accumulation of excessive synovial fluid within joint Enlargement of the suprapatellar recess seen on lateral radiographs, computed tomograph (CT), magnetic resonance (MR) and ultrasonogram *MR imaging findings* Low signal intensity on T1-weighted and high signal intensity on T2-weighted spin echo MR images Absence of effusion with severe trauma may indicate capsular rupture of such a degree that fluid extravasates into the soft tissues surrounding the knee	Bland effusion associated with acute injury or internal joint derangement Differential diagnosis: pyarthrosis, hemathrosis, or effusion associated with proliferative synovitis
Hemarthrosis[47]	See Figs. 9–58E, F, 9–61, 9–69B	Accumulation of blood within joint Hemarthroses usually result in joint effusion within the first few hours after injury As many as 75 per cent of acute traumatic hemarthroses are associated with anterior cruciate ligament injuries With MR imaging, single fluid level may be seen in acute stage and hemosiderin deposition of low signal intensity in the chronic stage	
Lipohemarthrosis[48–50]	9–24	Accumulation of blood and lipid material within synovial fluid Fat-blood interface seen on cross-table, horizontal beam lateral radiographs as well as transaxial and sagittal MR images Double fluid-fluid levels on MR images are more specific for lipohemarthrosis than a single fluid-fluid level	Usually related to acute intra-articular fracture May accompany fractures of the tibial plateau, fibula, patella, or distal portion of femur as well as injury to cartilage, ligaments, fat pads, or synovium
Synovial cysts[51, 52]	9–25	Most common in popliteal region Also termed Baker's cysts Communiction between the synovial cavities and bursae Enlarged palpable mass with or without pain Ruptures can simulate thrombophlebitis MR, CT, ultrasonography, or arthrography will demonstrate synovial cysts	Any inflammatory, degenerative, traumatic or neoplastic condition that produces knee effusion may lead to synovial cysts: rheumatoid arthritis, degenerative joint disease, gout, villonodular synovitis, synovial osteochondromatosis, and other articular diseases
Periarticular ganglion cysts[53]		Loculated or septated cysts containing jelly-like viscous fluid Adjacent to fibular head or proximal tibiofibular joint May also occur at the tibial insertion of the pes anserinus tendons, where it has been referred to as pes anserinus bursitis	May lead to common peroneal nerve compression May rarely result in anterior compartment syndrome
Intra-articular ganglion cysts[54]	9–26	Infrequent Arise adjacent to the infrapatellar fat bodies and the cruciate ligaments	May result in knee pain similar to that of meniscal tears
Synovial plicae[55]		Remnants of embryonic synovial tissue that divided the joint into three separate compartments during early development May be a normal finding in adults Occasionally these membranes become pathologically thickened, leading to symptoms referred to as the plica syndrome Three most common plicae: infrapatellar, suprapatellar, and medial patellar	Symptoms may mimic those of arthritis, meniscal injury, and other internal derangements of the knee Occasional flexion contractures of the knee

Table continued on following page

TABLE 9–8. Internal Derangements—Synovial Disorders* *Continued*

Entity	Figure(s), Table(s)	Characteristics	Complications and Related Disorders
Bursitis[56]	9–27	Any bursa about the knee may become inflamed Prepatellar bursitis (housemaid's knee), deep or superficial infrapatellar bursitis, pes anserinus bursitis, and suprapatellar bursitis Ultrasonography and MR imaging are best techniques for evaluating bursitis High signal intensity on T2-weighted images	Prepatellar bursitis may develop from chronic stress with prolonged kneeling Other causes of burisitis include infection, synovial inflammatory disease, and gouty arthropathy
Pigmented villonodular synovitis[57, 58]	9–28 Table 1–9	Knee is most frequent site of involvement *Radiographic findings* Cystic erosions on both sides of the joint Hemorrhagic joint effusion Eventual osteoporosis Well-preserved joint space until late in the disease	
Idiopathic synovial osteochondromatosis[59]	9–29, 9–30 Table 1–9	*Radiographic findings* Multiple intra- or periarticular collections of calcification of variable size and density Erosion of adjacent bone Noncalcified bodies are best demonstrated with arthrography or MR imaging	Primary idiopathic synovial osteochondromatosis leads to secondary osteoarthrosis and, infrequently, to malignant transformation (fewer than 5 per cent of cases) Secondary synovial osteochondromatosis may occur as a result of osteoarthrosis

*See also Tables 1–5 and 1–9.

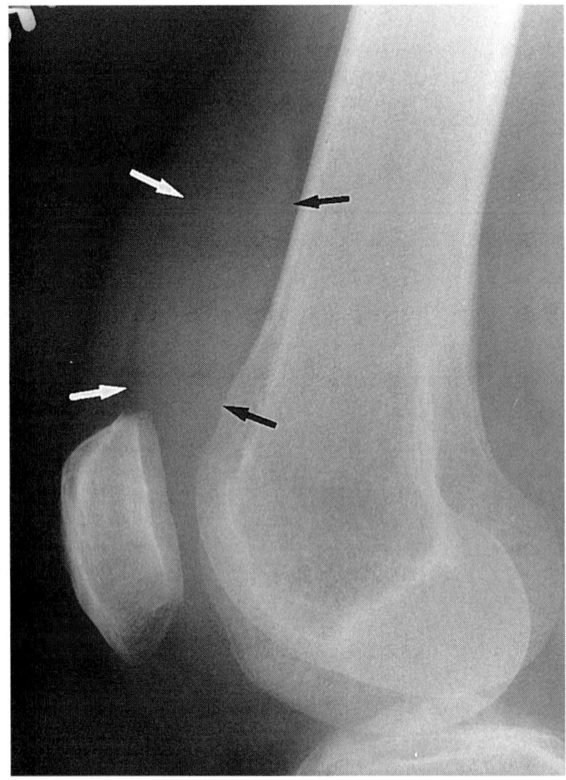

FIGURE 9–23. Joint effusion.[45, 46] Observe the distention of the suprapatellar pouch (arrows) in this patient with an injury to the knee. Bloody effusions (hemarthroses) generally appear within the first few hours after injury, and nonbloody effusions usually appear 12 to 24 hours after injury.

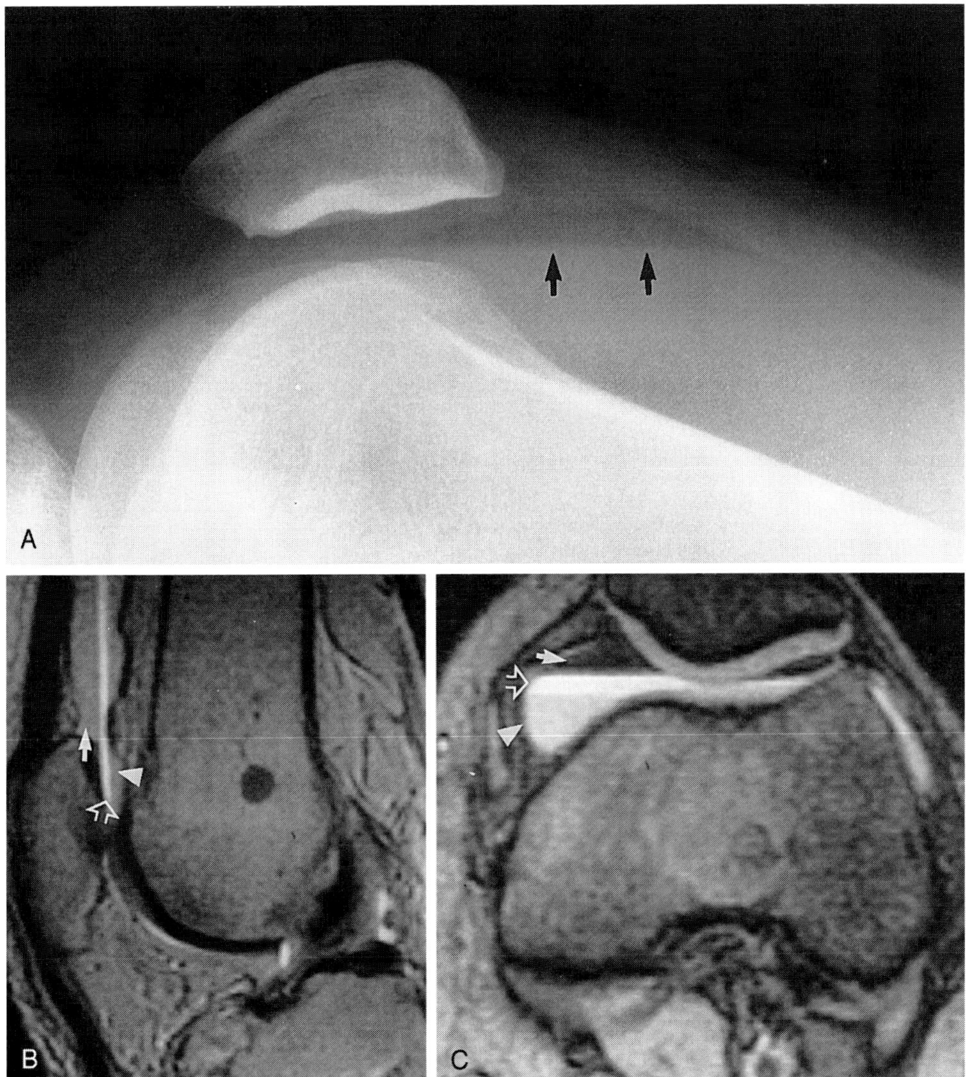

FIGURE 9–24. Lipohemarthrosis.[48–50] A Routine radiography. This cross-table, horizontal-beam lateral radiograph shows a straight radiodense fluid line at a fat-blood interface (arrows). This finding strongly suggests an intra-articular fracture, the fat and blood being released from bone marrow after cortical fracture. B, C magnetic resonance (MR) imaging. In B, a different patient, a sagittal T2-weighted (TR/TE, 2000/70) spin echo MR image shows three distinct layers. The uppermost layer (solid arrow) represents fat, the middle layer (open arrow) contains serum, and the lowest layer (arrowhead) contains erythrocytes. A band representing chemical shift artifact at the interface of serum and fat is difficult to identify. In C, a transaxial multiplanar gradient recalled (MPGR) (TR/E, 500/11; flip angle, 15 degrees) MR image reveals these same layers (solid and open arrows, arrowhead) and a band representing chemical shift artifact. *(B, C, From Resnick D, Kang HS: Internal Derangements of Joints. Philadelphia, WB Saunders, 1997, p 581.)*

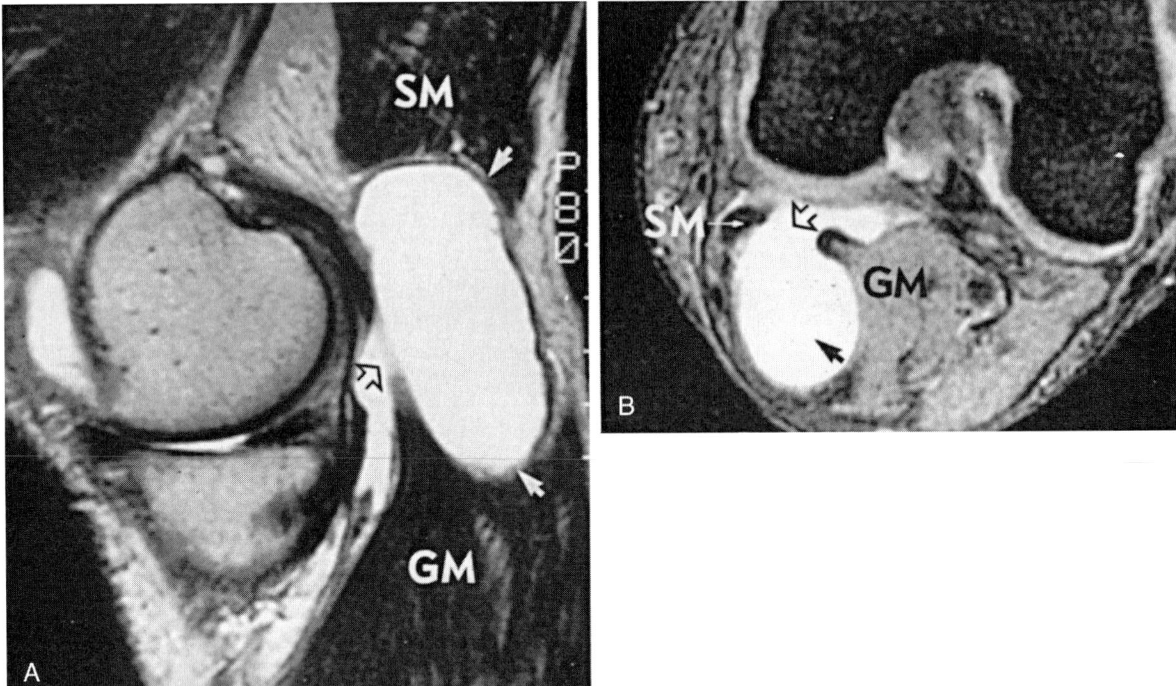

FIGURE 9–25. Synovial cysts: magnetic resonance (MR) imaging.[51, 52] A Sagittal T2-weighted (TR/TE, 4000/76) fast spin echo MR image shows a channel (open arrow) leading from the joint into a large synovial cyst (solid arrows) located between the semimembranosus muscle (SM) and the medial head of the gastrocnemius muscle (GM). B Transaxial MPGR (TR/E, 500/11; flip angle, 15 degrees) MR image shows the communicating channel (open arrow) and the synovial cyst (solid arrow) located between the semimembranosus muscle (SM) and the medial head of the gastrocnemius muscle (GM). *(From Resnick D, Kang HS: Internal Derangements of Joints. Philadelphia, WB Saunders, 1997, p 588.)*

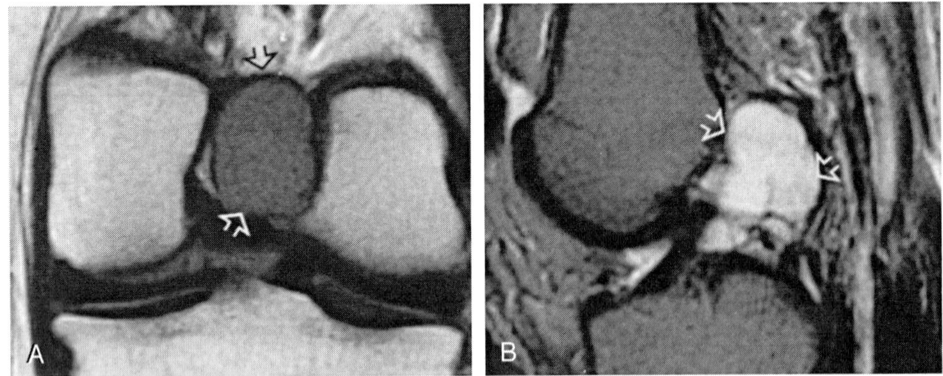

FIGURE 9–26. Intra-articular ganglion cysts: magnetic resonance (MR) imaging—posterior cruciate ligament.[54] Coronal T1-weighted (TR/TE, 800/25) spin echo MR image (**A**) and sagittal T2-weighted (TR/TE, 2000/80) spin echo MR image (**B**) show the large ganglion cyst (open arrows) adjacent to the posterior cruciate ligament. *(From Resnick D, Kang HS: Internal Derangements of Joints. Philadelphia, WB Saunders, 1997 p 588.)*

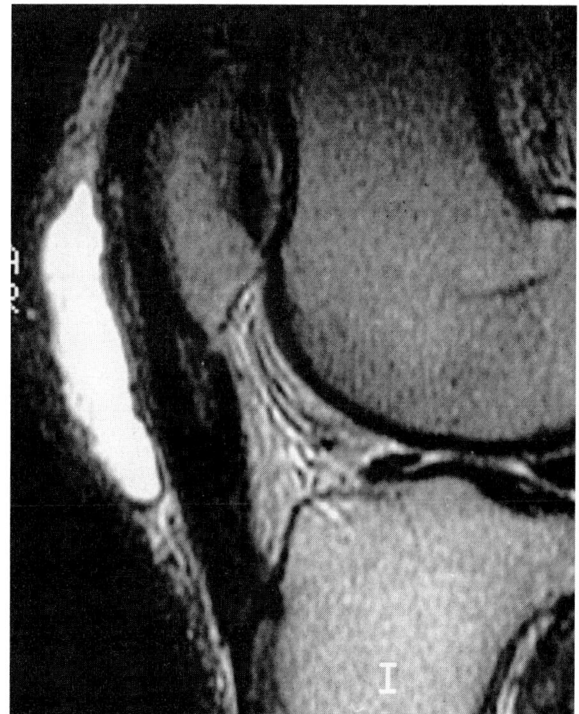

FIGURE 9–27. Prepatellar bursitis (housemaid's knee): Magnetic resonance (MR) imaging.[56] Sagittal T2-weighted (TR/TE, 2200/80) spin echo MR image shows the fluid-filled bursa and a thickened, partially torn patellar tendon. *(From Resnick D, Kang HS: Internal Derangements of Joints. Philadelphia, WB Saunders, 1997, p 590.)*

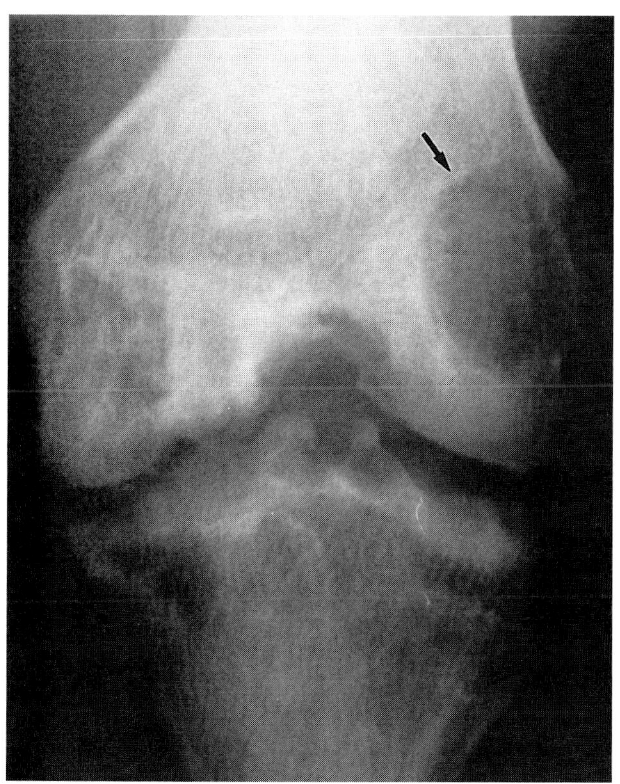

FIGURE 9–28. Pigmented villonodular synovitis.[57, 58] Multiple erosions are seen within the subchondral bone of the femur and the tibia, creating an irregular appearance of the articular surfaces. A large cyst is present in the lateral femoral condyle (arrow). The knee is the most common articulation to be affected in pigmented villonodular synovitis. *(Courtesy of H. Griffiths, M.D., Minneapolis, Minnesota.)*

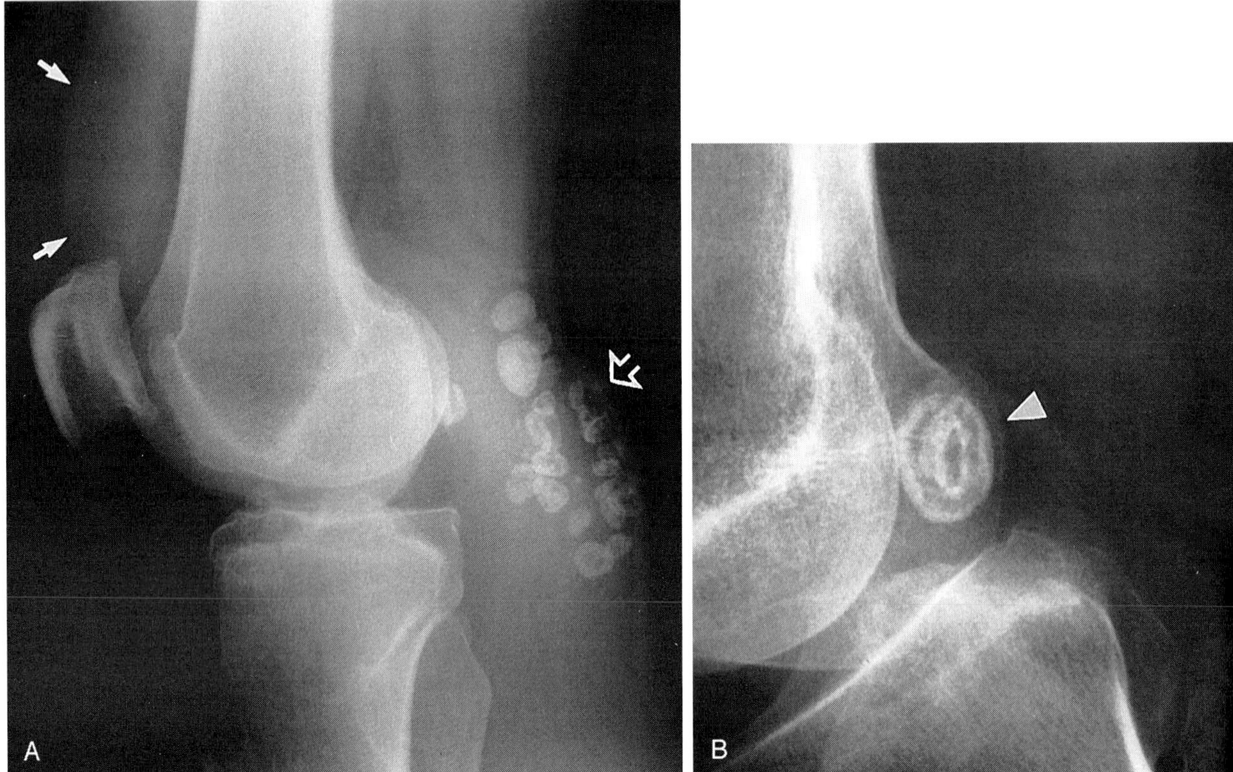

FIGURE 9–29. Secondary synovial osteochondromatosis: Intra-articular osteochondral bodies.[59] A Multiple round and ovoid osseous bodies (open arrow) are evident posterior to the knee within a synovial (Baker's) cyst. The bodies have a somewhat stippled or laminated appearance. Degenerative changes and a large joint effusion (arrows) are also present. B In another patient, a solitary oval, laminated intra-articular body is seen (arrowhead). These osteochondral bodies are usually degenerative or posttraumatic. A primary idiopathic form of synovial osteochondromatosis also occurs in which cartilage is formed by the synovium.

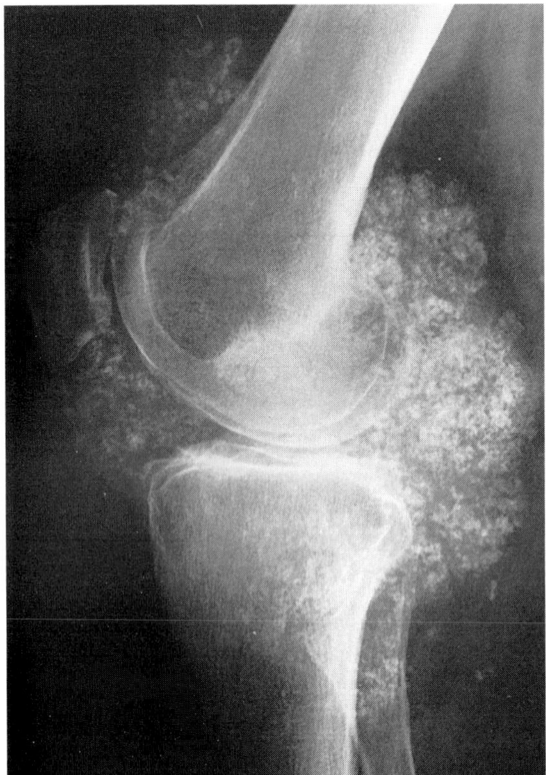

FIGURE 9–30. Recurrent idiopathic synovial osteochondromatosis.[59] Observe the multiple juxta-articular radiodense, osteocartilaginous bodies within the joint cavity, especially in the infrapatellar, suprapatellar, and popliteal regions. This patient already has had two operations to remove osteocartilaginous bodies. Idiopathic synovial osteochondromatosis represents metaplastic or neoplastic proliferation of cartilaginous bodies by the synovial membrane. Noncalcified lesions are best evaluated by arthrography. *(Courtesy of A.G. Bergman, M.D., Stanford, California.)*

TABLE 9–9. Internal Derangements—Meniscal Disorders

Entity	Figure(s), Table(s)	Characteristics	Complications and Related Disorders
Meniscal degeneration[60]		Encountered in elderly patients Mucinous or eosinophilic degeneration *Radiographic findings (rare)* Intrameniscal gas Meniscal chondrocalcinosis: calcium hydroxyapatite or calcium pyrophosphate dihydrate crystal deposition *MR imaging findings* Increased signal intensity on magnetic resonance (MR) images Areas of grade 1 and 2 intrameniscal signal intensity that do not communicate with the articular surface of the meniscus Often difficult to differentiate from meniscal tear	Age-related changes aggravated or precipitated by the following: Physical injury Osteoarthrosis Intrameniscal crystal deposition Association with meniscal tears is unclear
Discoid meniscus[61]		Broad, disc-like meniscus lacking the normal semilunar appearance Lateral >> medial Found in up to 2.7 per cent of population Most patients presenting with torn meniscus are between 15 and 35 years of age *Classified according to shape* Slab—flat, circular Biconcave—biconcave disc thinner in its central portion Wedge—large but normally tapered Anterior—enlarged anterior horn Forme fruste—slightly enlarged Grossly torn—too deformed for accurate classification *MR imaging* Visualization of bowtie appearance on at least three contiguous 5 mm sagittal sections, or an abnormally thickened bowtie appearance Discoid appearance rather than wedge-shaped appearance on coronal images	High prevalence of associated meniscal tear
Meniscal cysts[62]	9–31	Multiloculated collections of mucinous material that occur at the periphery of the meniscus Found in 1 per cent of meniscectomies Three to seven times more frequent adjacent to the lateral meniscus May be discovered as a focal mass or swelling at the joint line Also referred to as ganglion cysts Usually high signal intensity on T2-weighted images	Frequently associated with myxoid degeneration and horizontal cleavage tears of the adjacent meniscus Irritation of the common peroneal nerve may occur
Meniscal ossicles[63, 64]	9–32	Abnormal foci of ossification within the menisci Most common site: posterior horn of medial meniscus Cause unclear: represent either vestigial structures or acquired after trauma May be asymptomatic or associated with local pain	Meniscus usually is normal, but associated findings include tears of discoid meniscus
Meniscal tears[65–68]	9–33 to 9–35 See Table 9–10		

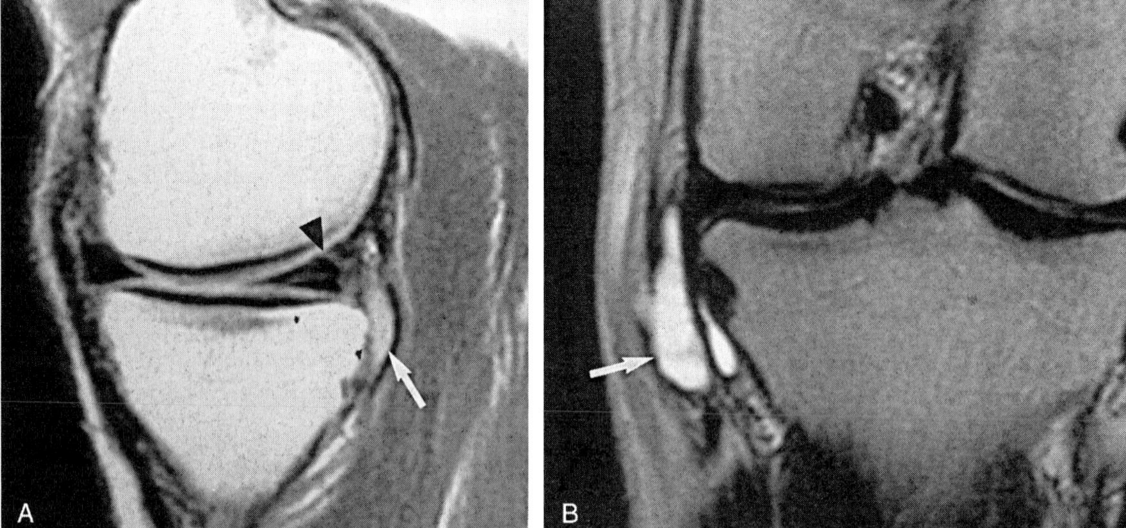

FIGURE 9–31. Meniscal cysts: magnetic resonance (MR) imaging—medial meniscus.[62] A large meniscal cyst (arrows) associated with a tear (arrowhead) of the posterior horn of the medial meniscus is well demonstrated on sagittal proton density–weighted (TR/TE, 2000/32) spin echo (**A**) and coronal fast spin echo (TR/TE, 3300/100) (**B**) MR images. Observe the intimate relationship between the cyst and the superficial portion of the medial collateral ligament in **B**. *(From Resnick D, Kang HS: Internal Derangements of Joints. Philadelphia, WB Saunders, 1997, p 626.)*

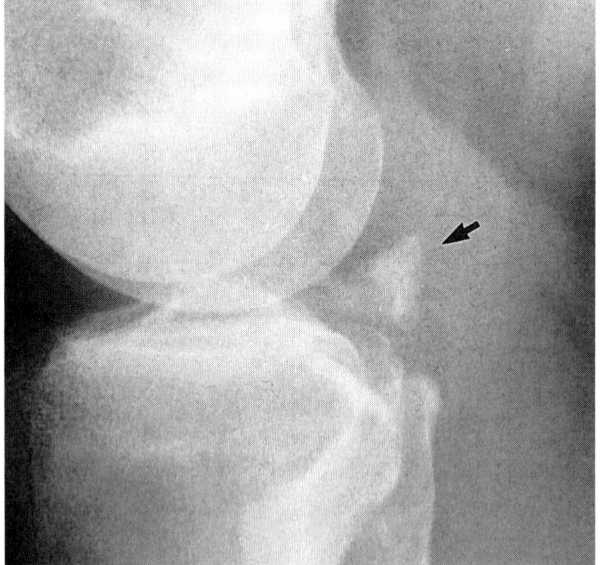

FIGURE 9–32. Meniscal ossicle.[63, 64] On a lateral radiograph, observe the triangular ossification in the posterior horn of the meniscus (arrow) in this 51-year-old man.

TABLE 9–10. Internal Derangements—Meniscal Tears[65–68]

Entity	Figure(s)	Characteristics
Pathogenesis		Traumatic: acute injuries in young persons Degenerative: more in older patients in association with osteoarthrosis
Clinical findings		Symptoms: pain and tenderness overlying affected meniscus, effusion, joint locking Signs: positive McMurray's test with snapping or popping
Classification	9–33	Longitudinal and radial Longitudinal tears are vertical or horizontal
General		Medial tears more common than lateral tears
Longitudinal tears		90 to 95 per cent of all meniscal tears *Vertical longitudinal tears* Three times more common in medial than lateral meniscus Peripheral or central Posterior horn, midportion, anterior horn, or combinations Bucket handle tear—inner portion displaced into the central portion of the joint *Horizontal longitudinal tears* Cleavage lesions common in degenerated menisci in older patients May be oblique and extend to superior or inferior surface Medial, lateral, or both Often associated with meniscal cyst
Radial tears		5–10 per cent of all meniscal tears Vertical tear of the inner margin of the meniscus Most frequently involves middle third of lateral meniscus Parrot beak or flap tears extend anterolaterally or posterolaterally Extensive radial tears may divide the meniscus into anterior and posterior portions
MR imaging features	9–34, 9–35	Sagittal T1-weighted and proton density–weighted spin echo magnetic resonance (MR) images most useful for detecting high signal intensity characteristic of tears Coronal, transaxial, and T2-weighted images not as valuable in detecting tears Sensitivity, specificity, and accuracy of MR imaging for meniscal tears: 85–90 per cent Tears of the posterior horn of the lateral meniscus and small tears of the inner edge of each meniscus are often overlooked on MR imaging studies
MR imaging grading system	9–34, 9–35	Classified according to changes in signal intensity and changes of morphology: grades 0 through 3
Grade 0		Normal: uniform low signal intensity
Grade 1		Indicative of degenerative changes One or several punctate regions of intermediate signal intensity not contiguous with an articular surface of the meniscus (capsular margin not considered an articular surface)
Grade 2		Indicative of more advanced degenerative changes Linear regions of intermediate signal intensity without extension to the articular surface of the meniscus
Grade 3		Indicative of fibrocartilaginous tear Regions of intermediate signal intensity with extension to the articular surface of the meniscus When grade 3 signal is seen on only one image, it should be designated "possible tear" as opposed to "definite tear"

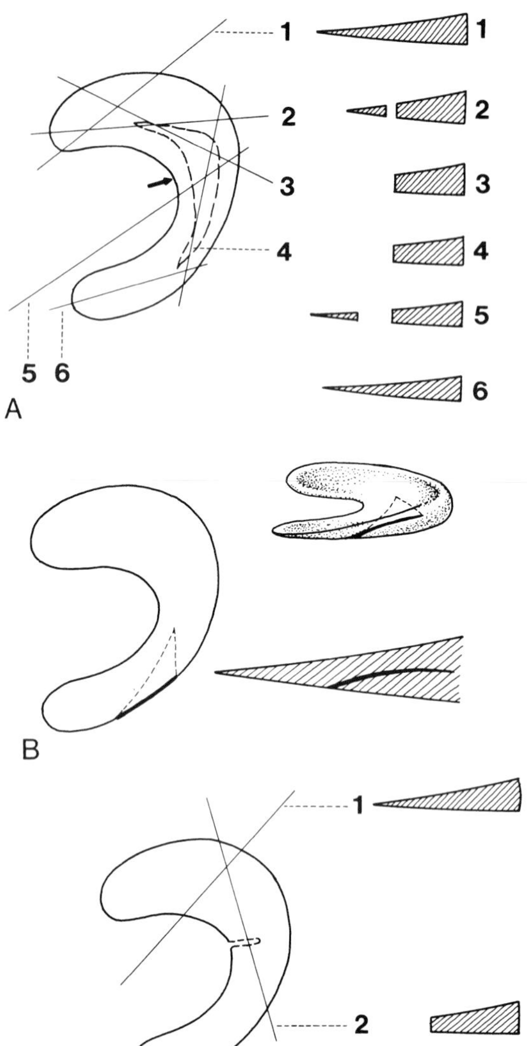

FIGURE 9–33. Meniscal tears: classification.[65, 66] A Longitudinal vertical tears (with displacement). The medial meniscus is viewed from above with the posterior horn located superiorly. The longitudinal vertical tear can be seen, and the inner fragment is displaced centrally (arrow). The appearance in radial sections obtained with magnetic resonance (MR) imaging depends on the specific site of the tear. A view of the posterior aspect of the meniscus (position 1) is normal. Slightly more anteriorly (position 2), a vertical tear is apparent with minimal displacement of the fragment. At positions 3 and 4, an amputated meniscal morphology can be seen. At position 5, significant displacement of the inner fragment is observed. The anterior horn of the meniscus (position 6) appears normal. B Longitudinal horizontal tears. The medial meniscus is viewed from above (left), in front (top right), and in longitudinal section (bottom right). The extent and appearance of the tear can be appreciated. Such cleavage lesions tend to occur more in older patients with meniscal degeneration. C Radial tear. The medial meniscus is viewed from above, with its posterior horn located superiorly. A radial tear is evident on the inner contour of the meniscus. Some radial sections provided by MR imaging will appear normal (position 1), whereas others passing through the tear (position 2) will reveal a blunted or truncated inner meniscal contour. *(From Resnick D, Kang HS: Internal Derangements of Joints. Philadelphia, WB Saunders, 1997, p 610.)*

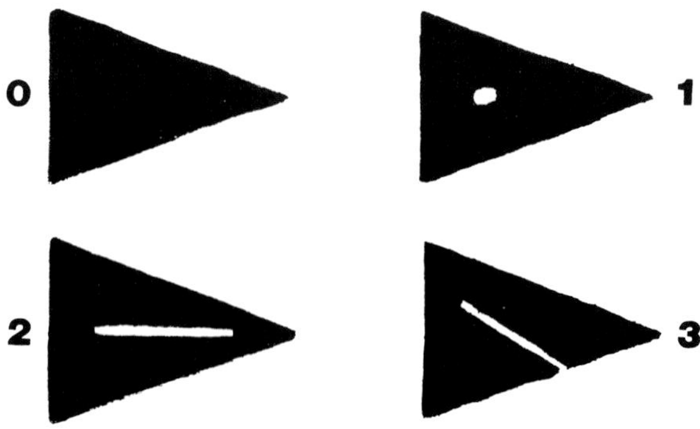

FIGURE 9–34. Grades of intrameniscal signal intensity: magnetic resonance (MR) imaging.[65] Grade 0: The normal meniscus appears as uniform low signal intensity. Grade 1: The meniscus may contain one or several circular foci of intermediate signal intensity. Grade 2: The meniscus may contain a linear region of intermediate signal intensity that does not extend to an articular surface of the meniscus. Grade 3: The meniscus may contain linear or irregular regions of intermediate signal intensity that extend to one or both articular surfaces. *(From Resnick D, Kang HS: Internal Derangements of Joints. Philadelphia, WB Saunders, 1997, p 617.)*

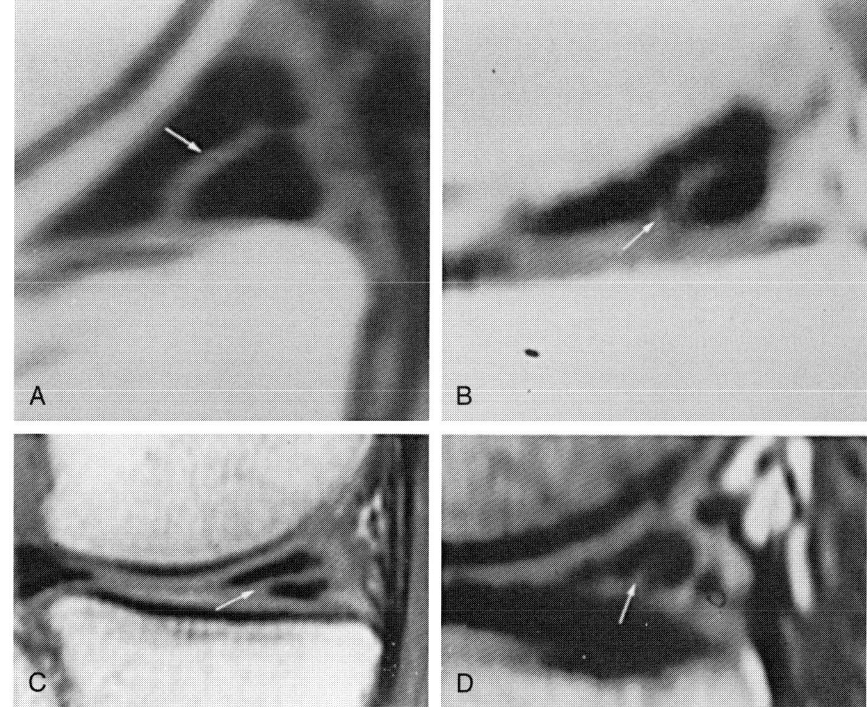

FIGURE 9–35. Meniscal tears: Abnormalities of intrameniscal signal intensity and meniscal morphology.[65–68] Sagittal proton density–weighted (TR/TE, 2000/20) spin echo magnetic resonance (MR) images. **A** Posterior horn of the medial meniscus. A grade 3 pattern of intrameniscal signal intensity (arrow) that communicates with the inferior articular surface of the meniscus is evident. **B** Posterior horn of the medial meniscus. A grade 3 pattern of intrameniscal signal intensity (arrow) and irregularity of the inferior meniscal surface are seen. **C** Posterior horn of the medial meniscus. A grade 3 pattern of increased signal intensity (arrow) and altered meniscal morphology are evident. **D** Posterior horn of the lateral meniscus. A grade 3 pattern of intrameniscal signal intensity (arrow) and an irregular inferior and inner meniscal surface are seen. *(From Resnick D, Kang HS: Internal Derangements of Joints. Philadelphia, WB Saunders, 1997, p 620.)*

TABLE 9–11. Internal Derangements—Ligament and Tendon Disorders*

Entity	Figure(s), Table(s)	Characteristics	Complications and Related Disorders
Ligament abnormalities			
Medial collateral ligament (MCL) tears[69–71]	9–36, 9–37	Valgus injuries *Radiographic findings* Joint effusion Rare avulsion fracture Medial joint space widening on valgus stress Pellegrini-Stieda syndrome: ossification of proximal attachment of MCL in chronic tears	Lateral tibial plateau fracture Associated tears of the menisci, cruciate ligaments, or lateral collateral ligament
		Magnetic resonance (MR) imaging findings Acute sprain: subcutaneous edema, hemorrhage, joint effusion, and slight contour irregularity of MCL fibers Acute partial tear: same as sprain with discontinuity and increased signal intensity (T2-weighted images) of some MCL fibers Acute complete tear: same findings as partial tear, but also frank discontinuity of all fibers of the MCL Chronic: intraligamentous ossification (Pellegrini-Stieda syndrome)	Bone infractions of femoral condyles or tibial plateaus
Lateral collateral ligament tears[71]	9–38	Varus injuries *Radiographic findings* Focal soft tissue swelling and possible avulsion of fibular head and styloid process *MR imaging findings* Interruption or waviness of the lateral collateral ligament or tendon of the biceps femoris tendon; or regions of high signal intensity within or adjacent to these structures on T2-weighted images	Fibular head avulsion fracture Rupture of biceps femoris tendon Iliotibial tract rupture Lateral displacement of the lateral meniscus Popliteus muscle and tendon injuries Cruciate ligament injuries
Lateral capsular ligament avulsion fracture[29]	9–13 Table 9–6	Segond injury: avulsion fracture of tibial rim	
Anterior cruciate ligament tears[72–75]	9–39	One of the most frequent sequelae of knee trauma *Radiographic findings* Avulsion fracture of anterior tibial eminence Segond fracture Posterior fracture of lateral tibial plateau Osteochondral fracture of lateral femoral condyle *MR imaging findings* Sensitivity, specificity, and accuracy from 90–100 per cent for tears of the anterior cruciate ligament Acute injuries: High signal intensity on T2-weighted spin echo images with inhomogeneous appearance on sagittal images Empty notch sign on coronal images from retraction of torn ligament Disruption or wavy contour of fibers Chronic injuries: alterations in angulation of ligament with scar tissue formation Many indirect signs also evident	O'Donoghue's triad: Simultaneous tears of the medial meniscus and anterior cruciate and medial collateral ligaments Chronic instability of the anterior cruciate ligament predisposes to additional injuries such as meniscal tears *Indirect signs* Segond fractures Bone bruises Deep notch in lateral femoral condyle Buckling of posterior cruciate ligament (PCL) Posterior PCL line Coronal PCL line Coronal fibular collateral ligament (FCL) sign Buckling of patellar tendon Anterior translation of tibia (drawer sign) Shearing of infrapatellar fat body

TABLE 9–11. Internal Derangements—Ligament and Tendon Disorders* *Continued*

Entity	Figure(s), Table(s)	Characteristics	Complications and Related Disorders
Posterior cruciate ligament (PCL) tears[76]	9–40	Less common than anterior cruciate ligament tears Force applied to the anterior aspect of the proximal portion of the tibia with the knee flexed Extreme flexion, extension, rotation, or valgus forces also may result in this injury Usually occurs during a fall or from striking the knee against the dashboard during a motor vehicle collision *Radiographic findings* Joint effusion Rare avulsion fracture of tibial site of insertion Radiography usually not helpful in diagnosis *MR imaging findings* Tears usually occur in the midsubstance, but occasionally at distal or proximal end Acute or subacute: high signal intensity on T2-weighted images Discontinuity of fibers	Isolated injury (30 per cent of cases) Combined with other injuries (70 per cent of cases) Complete tear (45 per cent of cases) Partial tear (47 per cent of cases) Bone avulsions (8 per cent of cases) Associated ligament injuries (38 per cent of cases) Associated meniscal injuries (47 per cent of cases) Bone contusions or fractures (36 per cent of cases)
Tendon abnormalities			
Patellar tendinitis[77, 78]		Jumper's knee Overuse syndrome related to sudden and repetitive extension of the knee Most common in athletes: running, kicking, jumping *Radiographic findings* Usually normal, but may show thickening of the patellar tendon and obscuration of portions of the infrapatellar fat body *MR imaging findings* Sagittal images are most useful Thickening and indistinct posterior margin of the tendon Increased signal intensity at inferior or superior end of tendon indicative of superimposed tear	May result in patellofemoral pain, patellar tracking disorders, or complete patellar tendon rupture
Tears of the quadriceps mechanism[79, 80]		*General* Indirect forces applied to the extensor mechanism may result in ruptures of the patellar or quadriceps tendons (or fractures of the patella)	
Patellar tendon tear[79, 94]	9–41	Failure occurs at the junction with the patella or, less commonly, the tibial tubercle *Radiographic findings* Complete tears result in patella alta Incomplete tears are associated with normal patellar position Prominent soft tissue swelling *MR imaging findings* Thickening and complete or incomplete disruption of the tendon In recent tears, high signal intensity of the tendon and its surrounding structures is evident on T2-weighted spin echo, certain gradient echo, and short-τ inversion-recovery (STIR) images	May occur spontaneously or after vigorous exercise in patients with chronic patellar tendinitis Rheumatoid arthritis, chronic renal disease, corticosteroid use, and systemic lupus erythematosus all may predispose to rupture

Table continued on following page

TABLE 9–11. **Internal Derangements—Ligament and Tendon Disorders*** *Continued*

Entity	Figure(s), Table(s)	Characteristics	Complications and Related Disorders
Quadriceps tendon tear[79, 80]	9–42	Partial or complete tears result from injury invoving a direct blow to the tendon or forceful flexion of the knee *Radiographic findings* Patella baja position in complete tears Soft tissue swelling, distortion of soft tissue planes above the patella, avulsed patellar fragment, and buckled or undulating appearance of patellar tendon *MR imaging findings* Partial or complete discontinuity of the tendon Undulating or buckled appearance of patellar tendon In acute tears, hemorrhage and edema result in high signal intensity on T2-weighted spin echo and some gradient echo images	Rheumatoid arthritis, chronic renal disease, corticosteroid use, and systemic lupus erythematosus all may predispose to rupture

*See also Table 1–5.

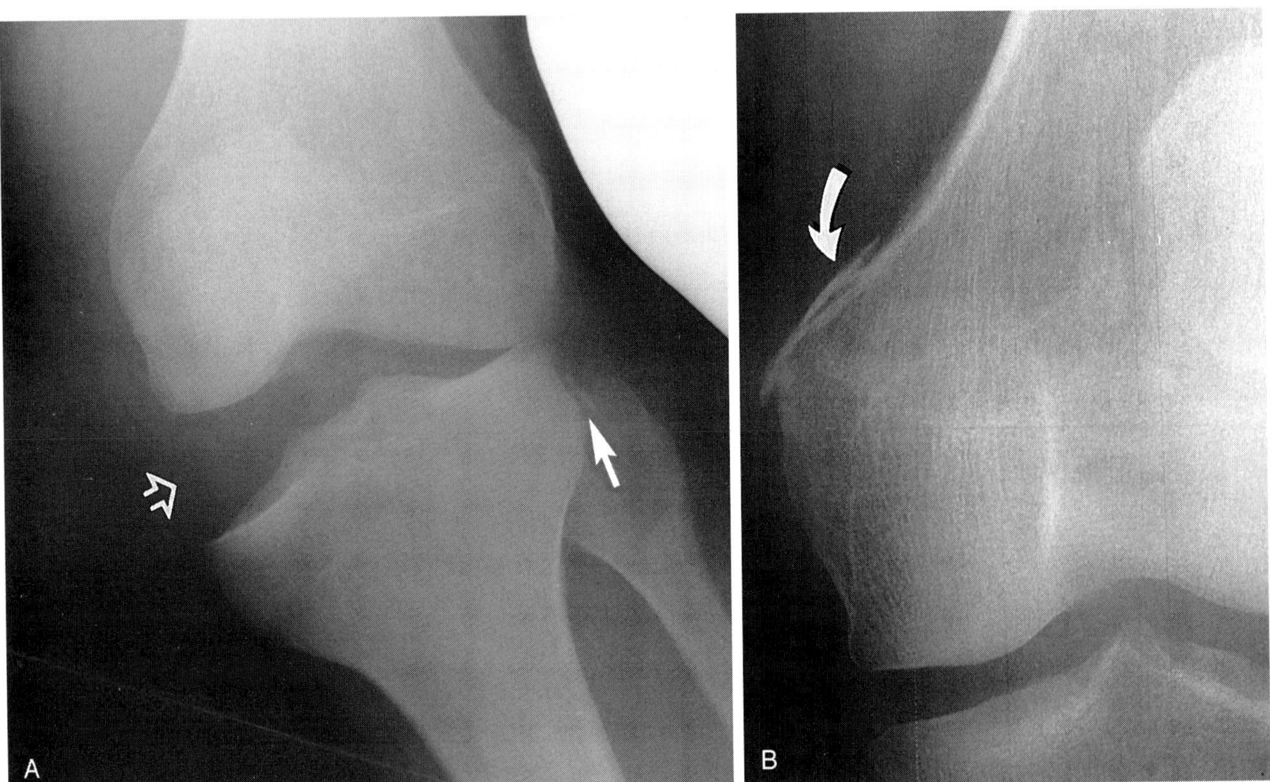

FIGURE 9–36. Medial collateral ligament injury. Acute and chronic radiographic appearance.[69, 70] **A** Acute injury. Valgus stress radiograph shows severe widening of the medial joint compartment (open arrow) in this 24-year-old man with complete (grade III) rupture of the medial collateral ligament. A bone fragment related to avulsion of the lateral capsular ligament is shown (arrow). Isolated injuries of the medial collateral ligament are rare and usually are accompanied by associated internal derangements, which should be evaluated by magnetic resonance (MR) imaging. **B** Chronic injury: Pellegrini-Stieda syndrome. Observe the thin layer of ossification or calcification (curved arrow) characteristic of a long-standing injury at the proximal attachment of the medial collateral ligament.

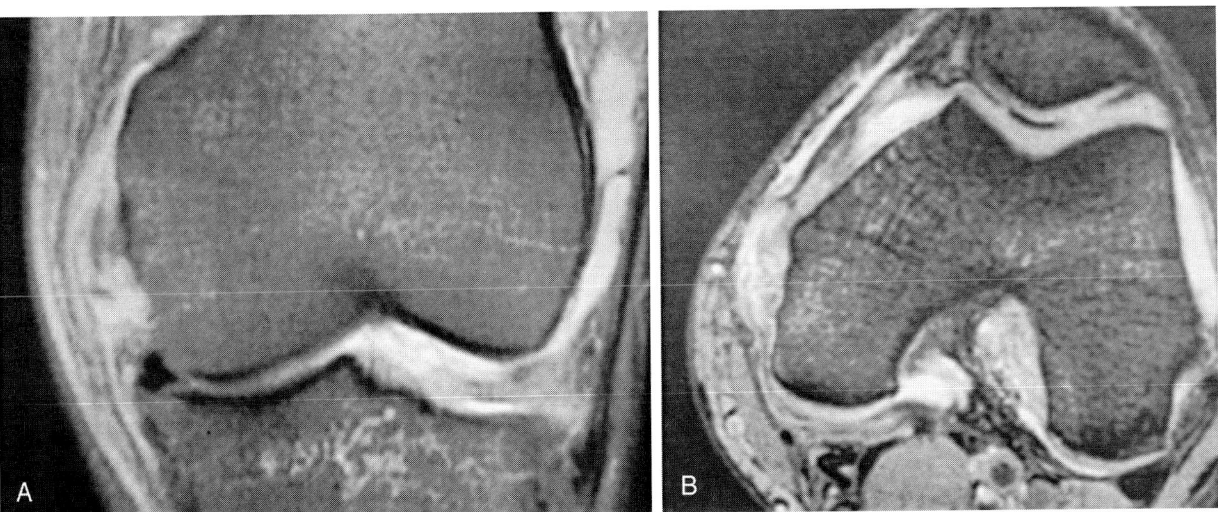

FIGURE 9–37. Complete tear of the medial collateral ligament: Magnetic resonance (MR) imaging.[69–71] **A** Coronal fast spin echo (TR/TE, 4000/18) MR image. **B** Transaxial MPGR (TR/TE, 400/16; flip angle, 30 degrees) MR image. A poorly demarcated, elongated area of high signal intensity adjacent to the medial femoral condyle is consistent with an acute tear of the medial collateral ligament. The anterior portion of the medial patellar retinaculum appears intact. *(From Resnick D, Kang HS: Internal Derangements of Joints. Philadelphia, WB Saunders, 1997, p 644.)*

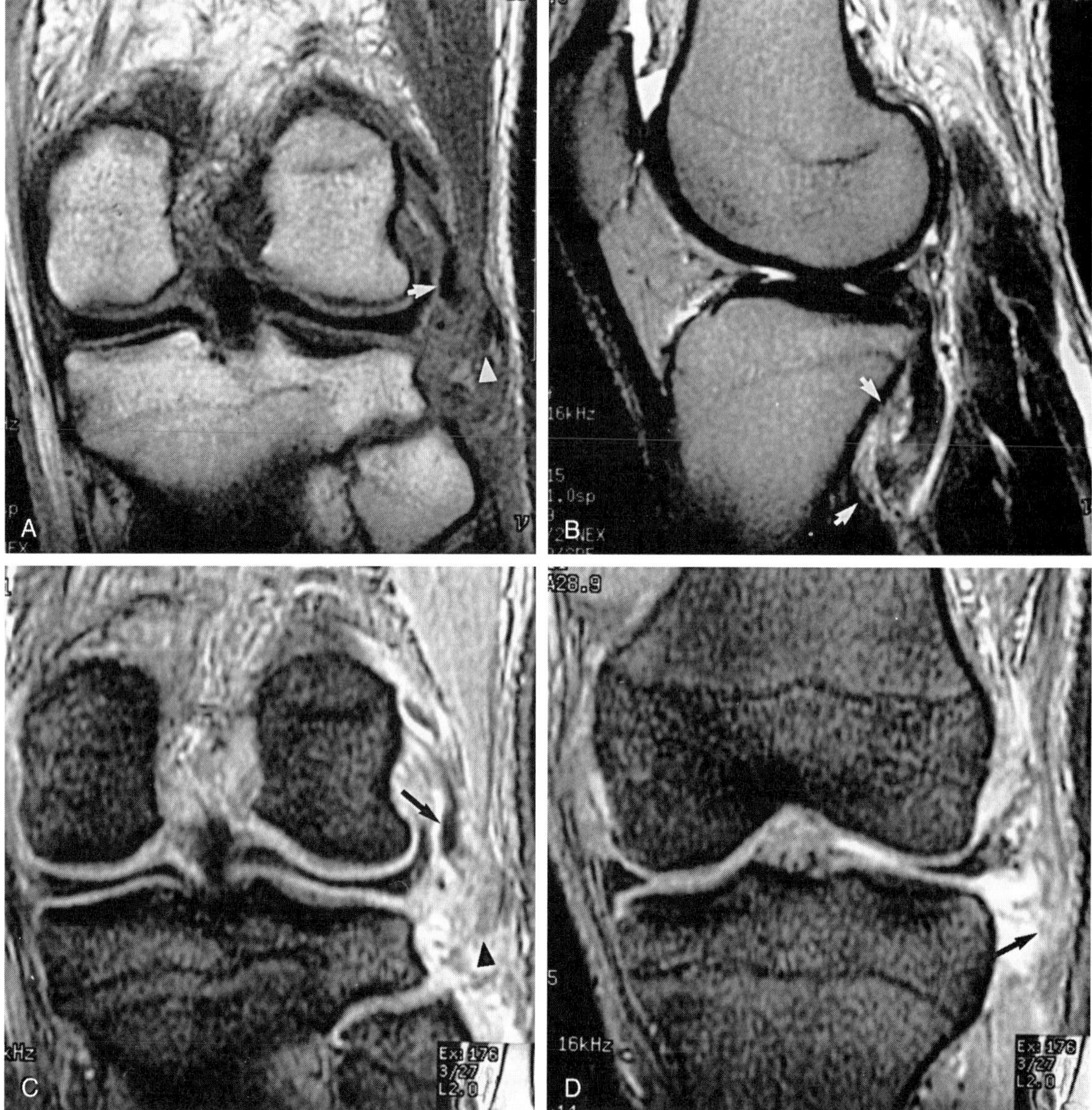

FIGURE 9–38. Injuries of the lateral collateral ligament, biceps femoris muscle and tendon, iliotibial tract, and popliteus muscle: magnetic resonance (MR) imaging.[71] This 21-year-old man developed severe knee instability after a recent injury. Although not shown on these images, the anterior cruciate ligament also was disrupted. A The coronal T1-weighted (TR/TE, 749/18) spin echo MR image shows avulsion of the biceps femoris tendon (arrowhead) and waviness of the lateral collateral ligament (arrow). B On a sagittal fast spin echo (TR/TE, 4466/90) MR image, note abnormal signal intensity and morphology of the popliteus muscle (arrows), joint effusion, and soft tissue edema. C Coronal MPGR (TR/TE, 500/15; flip angle, 25 degrees) MR image of the posterior aspect of the joint again shows avulsion of the biceps femoris tendon (arrowhead) and an abnormal lateral collateral ligament (arrow). Note the high signal intensity of the adjacent soft tissues. D More anteriorly, a coronal MPGR (TR/TE, 500/15; flip angle 25 degrees) MR image shows disruption of the iliotibial tract (arrow), lateral displacement of the lateral meniscus, and lateral and, to a lesser extent, medial soft tissue edema. The anterior cruciate ligament appears abnormal, although this was more evident in other images. *(From Resnick D, Kang HS: Internal Derangements of Joints. Philadelphia, WB Saunders, 1997, p 653.)*

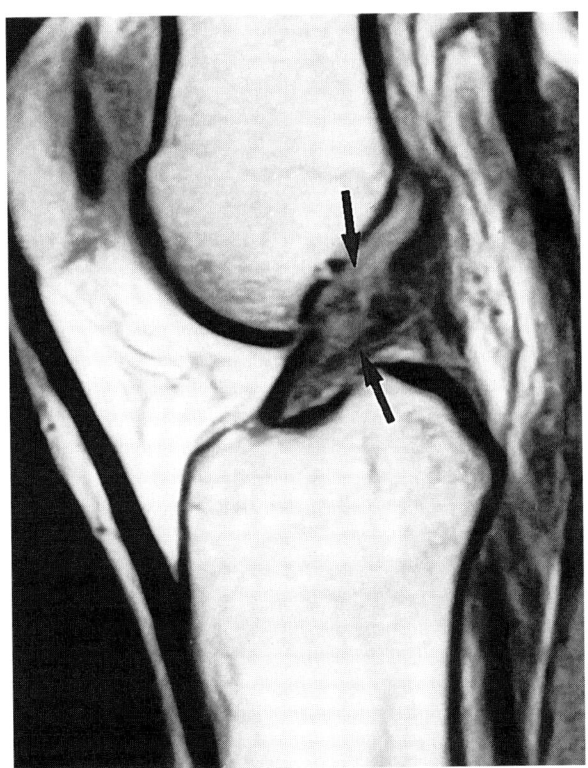

FIGURE 9–39. Acute anterior cruciate ligament tear.[72–75] This 31-year-old woman injured her knee while running. A sagittal proton density–weighted (TR/TE, 1100/25) spin echo magnetic resonance (MR) image reveals discontinuity and inhomogeneous intermediate signal intensity within the midportion of the anterior cruciate ligament (arrows). The patellar tendon is intact and shows no evidence of buckling. *(Courtesy of L. Beinekis, D.C., Portland, Oregon.)*

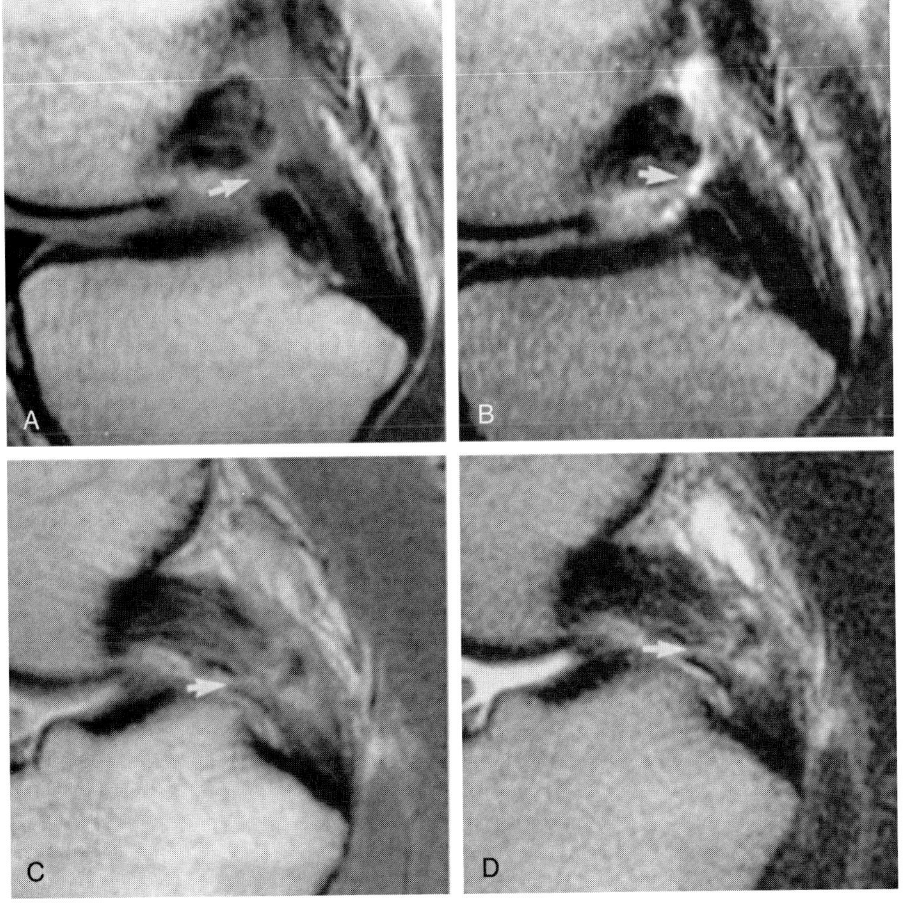

FIGURE 9–40. Acute complete posterior cruciate ligament tears: magnetic resonance (MR) imaging.[76] **A, B** Sagittal proton density–weighted (TR/TE, 2000/30) (**A**) and T2-weighted (TR/TE, 2000/80) (**B**) spin echo MR images reveal complete disruption (arrows) of the posterior cruciate ligament, with an increase in signal intensity in **B**. **C, D** Sagittal proton density–weighted (TR/TE, 2200/20) (**C**) and T2-weighted (TR/TE, 2200/80) (**D**) spin echo MR images in a second patient again show complete disruption (arrows) of the posterior cruciate ligament, with an increase in signal intensity in **D**. *(From Resnick D, Kang HS: Internal Derangements of Joints. Philadelphia, WB Saunders, 1997, p 701.)*

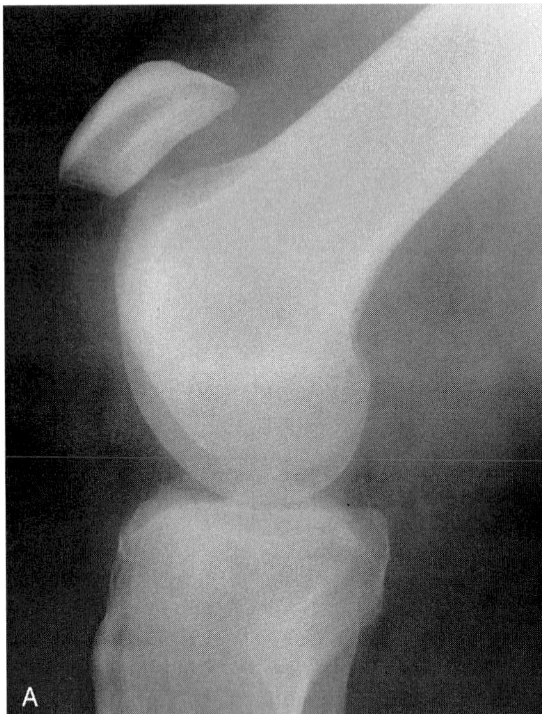

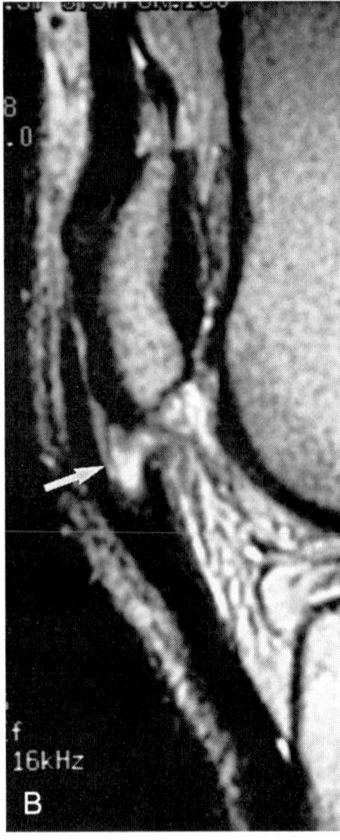

FIGURE 9–41. Patellar tendon tears.[78, 79] A Radiographic features. Observe the superior displacement of the patella (patella alta) in this patient with a complete tear of the patellar tendon. *(**A**, From Siweck CW, Rao JP: Ruptures of the extensor mechanism of the knee joint. J Bone Joint Surg [Am] 63:932, 1981.)* **B** Magnetic resonance (MR) imaging features. In another patient, a sagittal T2-weighted (TR/TE, 4466/90) spin echo MR image clearly displays the site of tendon disruption (arrow). Observe the high signal intensity within the ruptured tendon. *(**B**, From Resnick D, Kang HS: Internal Derangements of Joints. Philadelphia, WB Saunders, 1997, p 665.)*

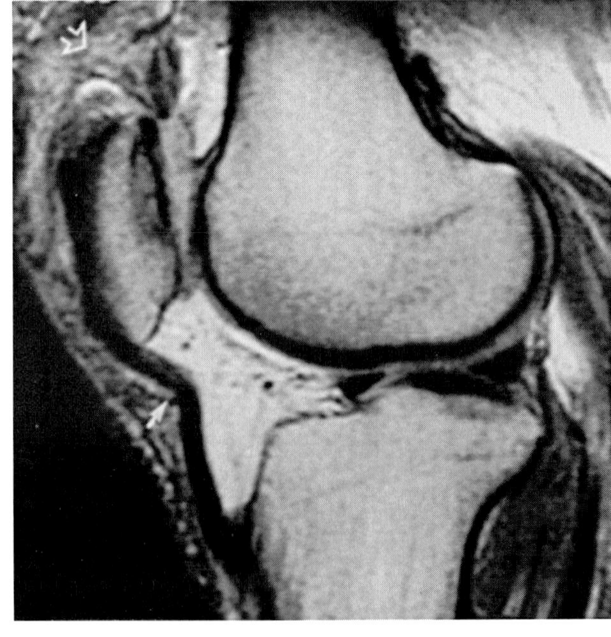

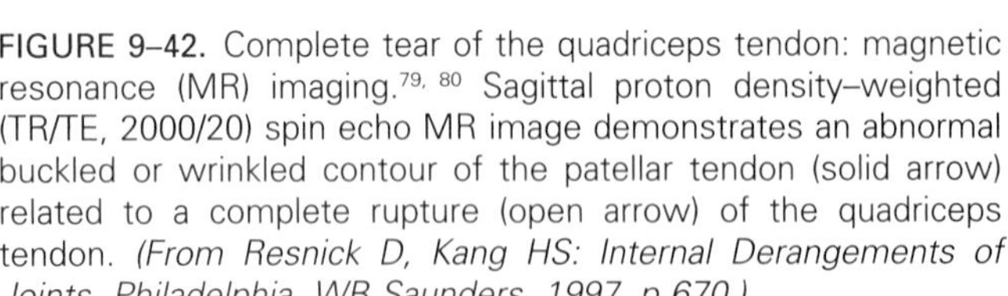

FIGURE 9–42. Complete tear of the quadriceps tendon: magnetic resonance (MR) imaging.[79, 80] Sagittal proton density–weighted (TR/TE, 2000/20) spin echo MR image demonstrates an abnormal buckled or wrinkled contour of the patellar tendon (solid arrow) related to a complete rupture (open arrow) of the quadriceps tendon. *(From Resnick D, Kang HS: Internal Derangements of Joints. Philadelphia, WB Saunders, 1997, p 670.)*

TABLE 9–12. Internal Derangements—Patellofemoral Disorders

Entity	Figure(s), Table(s)	Characteristics	Complications and Related Disorders
Patella alta[81]	9–43 Table 9–5	Superior patellar position best seen on lateral radiographs Insall-Salvati ratio—measurement method Height of the patella and height of patellar tendon are determined on lateral radiograph; ratio of these heights should be approximately 1:1; in patella alta, the patellar tendon is longer than the height of the patella	Associated with patellar tendon rupture, recurrent lateral patellar subluxation or dislocation, Sinding-Larsen-Johansson disease, and joint effusions
Patella baja[81]	9–43 Table 9–5	Inferior patellar position best seen on lateral radiographs Insall-Salvati ratio is abnormal: the patellar height is longer than the patellar tendon	Associated with neuromuscular disorders and achondroplasia; also may be present after surgery involving transfer of the tibial tubercle
Patellofemoral instability[82, 83]	9–44	Patellofemoral tracking disorder in which the patella moves abnormally with respect to the femur during flexion and extension Radiography, computed tomographic (CT), magnetic resonance (MR), and kinematic MR imaging are all used to assess the patellofemoral relationship Patellofemoral tracking is affected by the configuration of the trochlea, the patellar shape, and the relationship of the patella to the femur Excessive lateral pressure syndrome: abnormal lateral tilt of the patella with respect to the femur; this leads to patellofemoral pain	May result in or be associated with the following: Transient, recurrent, lateral subluxation or dislocation of the patella Excessive lateral pressure syndrome Chondromalacia patellae Osteochondral fractures Avulsion fractures Medial retinacular injury
Chondromalacia patellae[84, 85]	9–45	Synonym: patellofemoral pain syndrome Cartilage loss involving one or more portions of the patella; this leads to patellofemoral pain, crepitus, and synovitis Imaging techniques generally are inadequate to assess cartilage loss CT arthrography can be useful in cases with advanced cartilage loss	Cause is unclear: may be related to single or recurrent episodes of acute trauma, as in excessive lateral pressure syndrome, patellofemoral instability, and anatomic variations in bone morphology

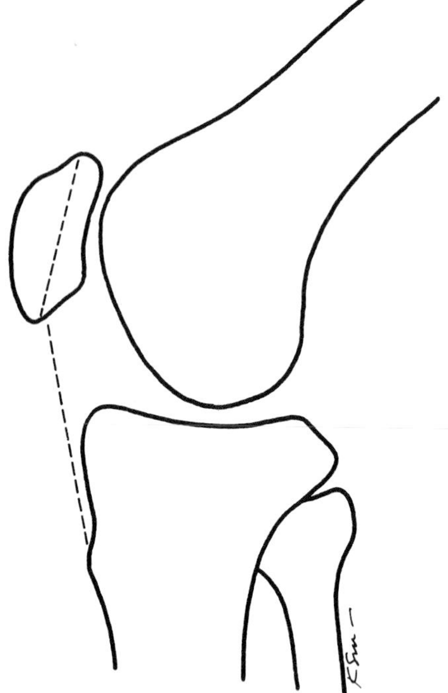

FIGURE 9–43. Patellar position: Insall-Salvati method.[81] The ratio of patellar tendon length to the greatest diagonal length of the patella should be approximately 1:1. This method may be used to diagnose patella alta and patella baja. In patella alta, the patellar tendon length exceeds that of the patellar length; in patella baja, the length of the patella exceeds that of the tendon. *(From Resnick D, Kang HS: Internal Derangements of Joints. Philadelphia, WB Saunders, 1997, p 670.)*

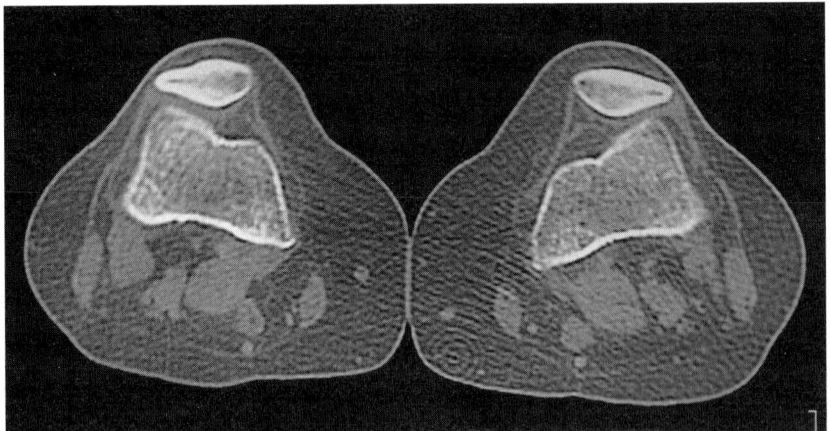

FIGURE 9–44. Patellofemoral instability: computed tomographic (CT) scanning.[82–84] Transaxial CT scan, obtained with the knees flexed 20 degrees, shows lateral subluxation of both patellae. *(From Resnick D, Kang HS: Internal Derangements of Joints. Philadelphia, WB Saunders, 1997, p 671.)*

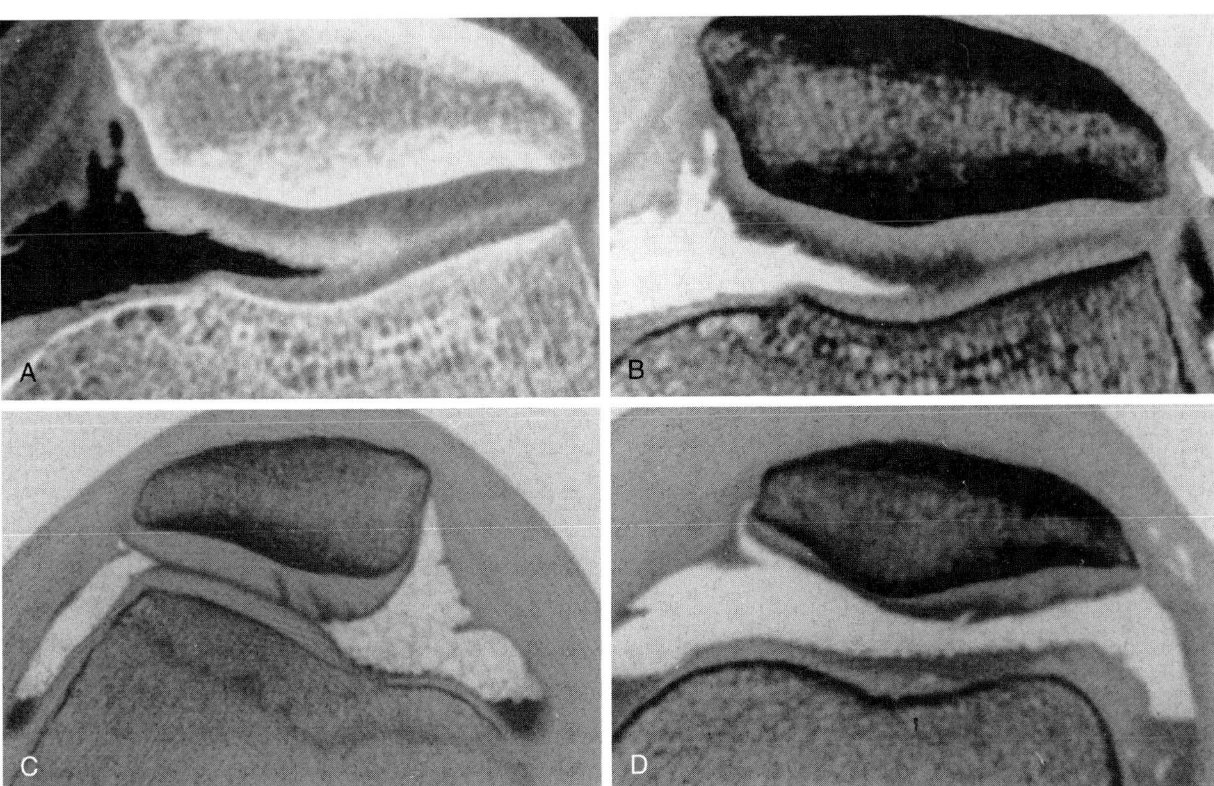

FIGURE 9–45. Chondromalacia patellae: computed tomographic (CT) arthrography.[85] A, B Transaxial CT arthrographic images (using double-contrast technique) filmed without (A) and with (B) subtraction technique show imbibition of radiopaque contrast material and cartilage fibrillation and ulceration. C, D Two additional subtracted CT arthrographic images of other patients reveal cartilage fissuring and contrast material imbibition. *(From Resnick D, Kang HS: Internal Derangements of Joints. Philadelphia, WB Saunders, 1997, p 675. Courtesy of A. D'Abreau, M.D., Porto Alegre, Brazil.)*

TABLE 9–13. Articular Disorders Affecting the Knee*

Entity	Figure(s)	Characteristics
Degenerative and related disorders		
Osteoarthrosis[86, 87]	9–46	Findings predominate in the medial femorotibial compartment in men; distribution more variable in women Osteophytes Subchondral sclerosis Subchondral cysts Subluxation Intra-articular bodies: infrequently, secondary synovial osteochondromatosis
Diffuse idiopathic skeletal hyperostosis (DISH)[88]	9–47	Occasional enthesopathy and ligament ossification about the knee
Inflammatory disorders		
Rheumatoid arthritis[89]	9–48	Knee involvement common in rheumatoid arthritis Bilateral symmetric, concentric joint space narrowing of medial and lateral joint spaces and of patellofemoral joint Subchondral erosion Absent or mild sclerosis Periarticular osteoporosis
Juvenile chronic arthritis[90–91]	9–49	Knee involvement common Soft tissue swelling and joint effusion Epiphyseal overgrowth (ballooning) Squaring of inferior pole of patella Widening of the intercondylar notch Diffuse, bilateral symmetric joint space loss Periarticular osteoporosis Erosions of the femoral condyles and tibial surfaces Closely resembles findings in hemophilic arthropathy
Ankylosing spondylitis[92]	9–50	Bilateral symmetric, joint space narrowing of all three compartments Erosions Joint effusion Enthesopathy of quadriceps and patellar tendons at the anterior aspect of the patellae Rarely, may eventually result in partial or complete intra-articular osseous ankylosis
Reiter's syndrome and psoriatic arthropathy[93]	9–51	Knee involvement similar to but less frequent than ankylosing spondylitis
Systemic lupus erythematosus (SLE)[94]	9–52	Osteonecrosis of the femoral condyles in SLE patients treated with or without corticosteroid therapy Patellar and quadriceps tendon ruptures
Dermatomyositis and polymyositis[95]	9–53	Widespread sheet-like calcification in skin and muscle about the knee
Mixed connective tissue disease[96, 97]	9–54	Radiographic features variable; may result in diffuse joint space narrowing, erosions, and soft tissue calcinosis
Crystal deposition and metabolic disorders		
Calcium pyrophosphate dihydrate (CPPD) crystal deposition disease[98–100]	9–55	Knee is most commonly involved articulation Differs from osteoarthrosis in its prominent involvement of the patellofemoral and lateral tibiofemoral joint compartments and its high rate of chondrocalcinosis *Radiographic findings* Prominent joint effusion during acute episode Articular space narrowing, sclerosis, cyst formation, and osteophytes Intra- and periarticular chondrocalcinosis of hyaline cartilage and fibrocartilage, calcification of capsule and synovium Advanced, severe disease: considerable osseous destruction and fragmentation resembling neuropathic osteoarthropathy
Gouty arthropathy[101]	9–56	Rare knee involvement Periarticular erosions Soft tissue tophi and joint effusions Intraosseous tophi result in osteolytic cyst-like lesions in patella
Hemochromatosis[102]	9–57	Arthropathy identical to that of CPPD crystal deposition disease Prominent chondrocalcinosis

TABLE 9–13. Articular Disorders Affecting the Knee* *Continued*

Entity	Figure(s)	Characteristics
Acromegalic arthropathy[89]		Hyperostosis and ossification of the patellar attachments of the quadriceps and patellar tendons Cartilage hypertrophy may initially result in joint space widening Degenerative joint disease later results in cartilage thinning, sclerosis, and osteophytes
Hemophilic arthropathy[102, 103]	9–58	Knee is the joint affected most commonly in hemophilia Typical pattern: bilateral symmetric joint involvement Findings closely resemble the changes in juvenile chronic (rheumatoid) arthritis *Radiographic findings* Dense joint effusions Periarticular osteoporosis: radiolucent epiphyses Articular surface irregularity and flattening Subchondral cysts Overgrowth of epiphyses (ballooning) Widening of the intercondylar notch Squaring of inferior pole of patella Fixed flexion deformity
Infection		
Pyogenic septic arthritis[104]		Rapid loss of joint space usually begins in femorotibial compartments; may eventually involve patellofemoral joint Periarticular osteoporosis Loss of definition and destruction of subchondral bone Capsular distention Erosion May disseminate from site of metaphyseal osteomyelitis
Tuberculous arthritis[105]	9–59	Various degrees of soft tissue swelling Gradual joint space narrowing Periarticular osteoporosis Peripherally located erosions Subchondral erosions Periarticular abscess Patellar involvement: osteolytic lesions with sequestrum
Miscellaneous disorder		
Neuropathic osteoarthropathy[89]	9–60	Most frequent causes of knee involvement: tabes dorsalis and diabetes mellitus; less common causes are amyloidosis and congenital indifference to pain *Radiographic findings* Large joint effusions Joint space narrowing and obliteration Joint subluxation, disorganization, and destruction Bone fragmentation, destruction, and sclerosis

*See also Tables 1–6 to 1–9 and Table 1–17.

TABLE 9–14. Articular Disorders of the Knee: Compartmental Analysis

Entity	Figure(s)	Femorotibial Compartments	Patellofemoral Compartment
Osteoarthrosis	9–46	Medial > lateral	Commonly involved in conjunction with medial or lateral femorotibial disease
Rheumatoid arthritis	9–48	Medial = lateral	Commonly involved in conjunction with medial or lateral femorotibial disease
Calcium pyrophosphate dihydrate (CPPD) crystal deposition disease	9–55	Medial < lateral	Commonly involved alone or in conjunction with medial or lateral femorotibial disease
Infectious arthritis	9–59	Medial = lateral	May involve any compartment, but more frequent in femorotibial joints
Hyperparathyroidism	See Fig. 9–69	Medial = lateral	Subchondral resorption, crystal-induced arthropathies, or unknown mechanism

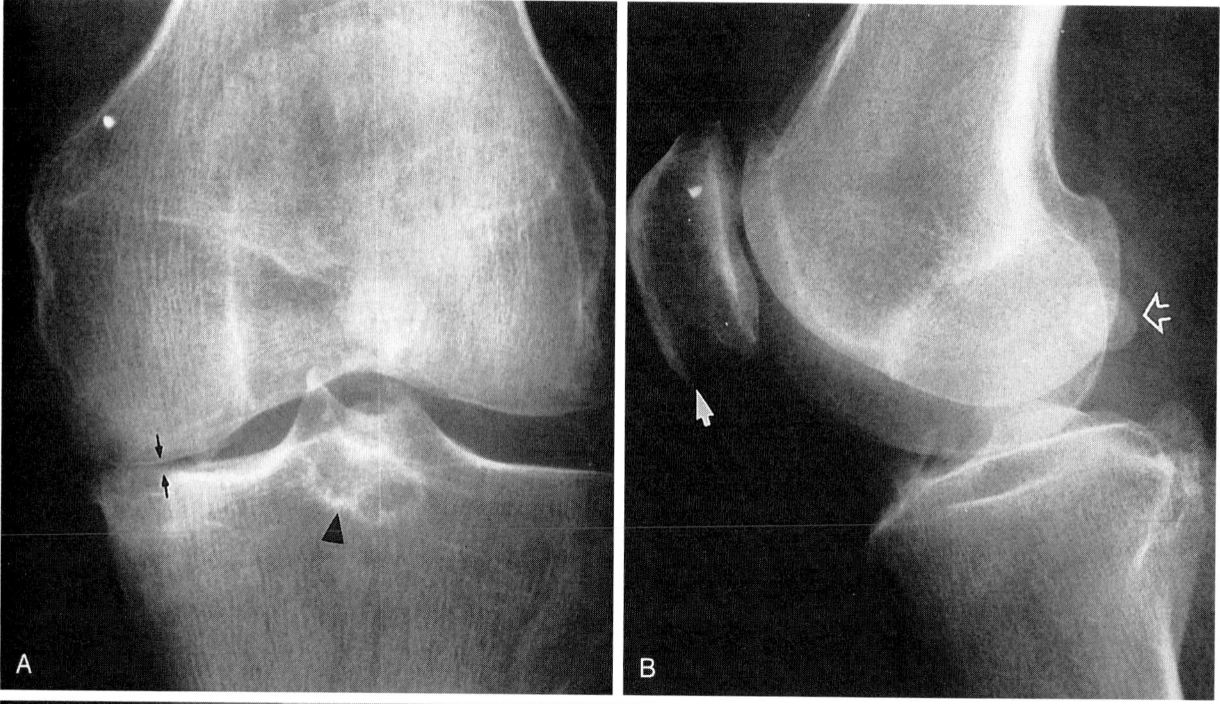

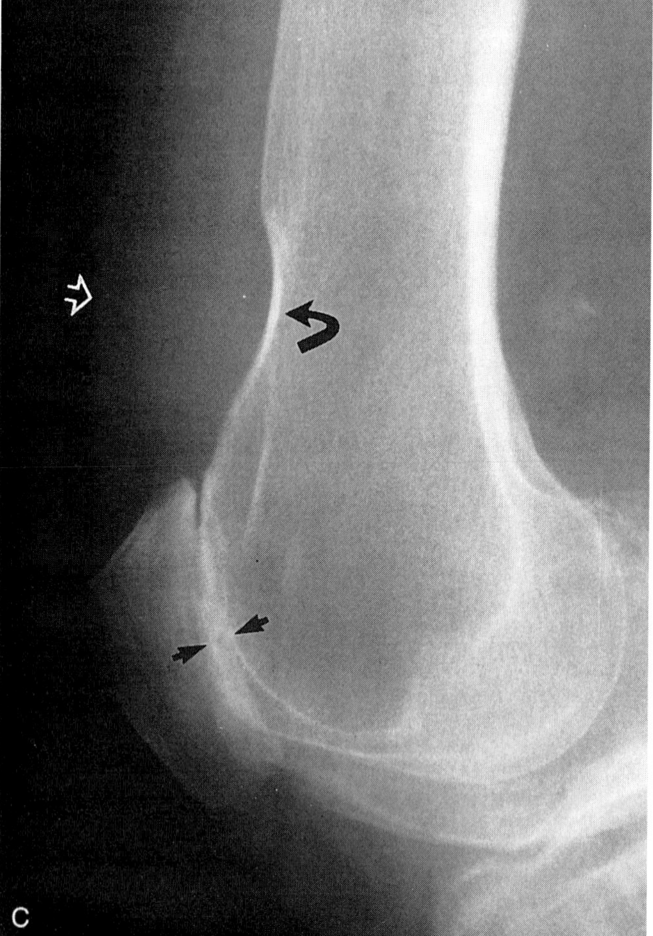

FIGURE 9–46. Osteoarthrosis (degenerative joint disease).[86, 87] A, B Frontal (A) and lateral (B) radiographs show medial femorotibial joint space narrowing (black arrows), patellar enthesophyte (white arrow), subchondral cyst formation (arrowhead), and a large laminated intra-articular osseous body (open arrow). C In another patient, patellofemoral joint abnormalities predominate. Extensive narrowing of the patellofemoral compartment (arrows) and a joint effusion (open arrow) are present. Anterior scalloping of the distal portion of the femur (curved arrow) is a result of mechanical irritation from repeated contact with the patella. Similar scalloped defects may be observed in hyperparathyroidism and calcium pyrophosphate dihydrate (CPPD) crystal deposition disease.

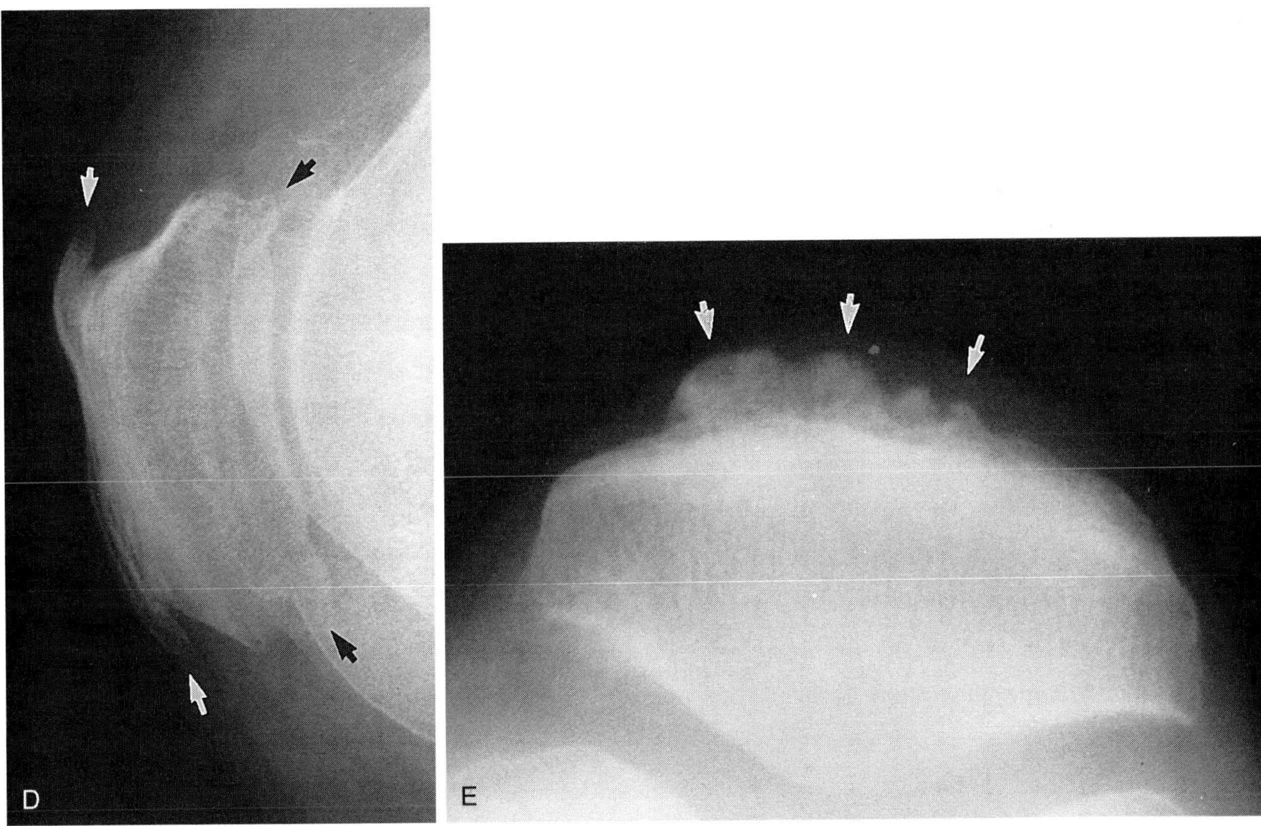

FIGURE 9–46 *Continued.* **D, E** Patellar enthesopathy. In **D**, bony excrescences (enthesophytes) arising from the anterior aspect of the patella (white arrows) at the site of attachment of the quadriceps mechanism are evident on this lateral radiograph. Note also the patellofemoral joint space narrowing and osteophytes (black arrows) arising from the posterior margins of the patella. **E** On this tangential radiograph, observe the typical tooth-like osseous excrescences at the quadriceps attachment to the anterior surface of the patella (arrows), a finding sometimes referred to as the patellar tooth sign. Enthesophytes are probably related to abnormal stress at the ligamentous or tendinous connection of the quadriceps mechanism to the bone and are not a manifestation of osteoarthrosis. Such enthesopathy is common in elderly patients and in patients with diffuse idiopathic skeletal hyperostosis.

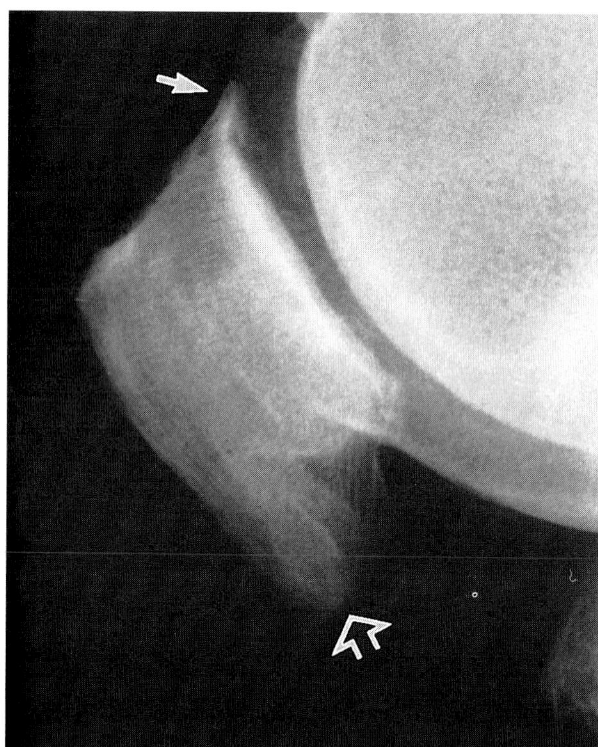

FIGURE 9–47. Diffuse idiopathic skeletal hyperostosis (DISH).[88] Radiograph of this 69-year-old man with long-standing DISH reveals prominent, thick patellar enthesopathy (open arrow), a feature characteristic in the peripheral skeleton. A small osteophyte (arrow), probably related to degenerative disease, also is present. Knee involvement is seen in about 29 per cent of DISH patients.

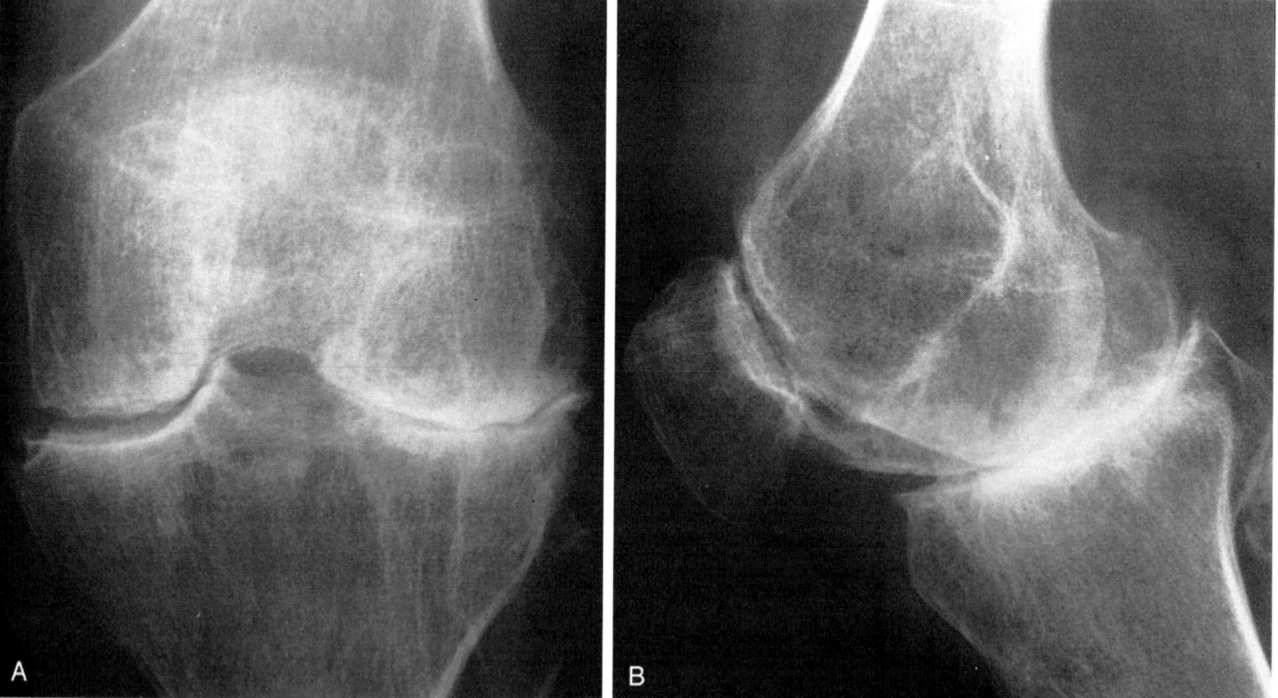

FIGURE 9–48. Rheumatoid arthritis.[89] A 59-year-old woman with early-onset, adult-type rheumatoid arthritis. Frontal (A) and lateral (B) radiographs show signs of both inflammatory disease and degenerative disease. The uniform loss of the patellofemoral and the medial and lateral joint spaces, along with relative absence of osteophytes, is characteristic of rheumatoid arthritis. The other knee (not shown) was equally affected. The subchondral sclerosis and lateral tibial osteophyte are characteristic of superimposed degenerative joint disease.

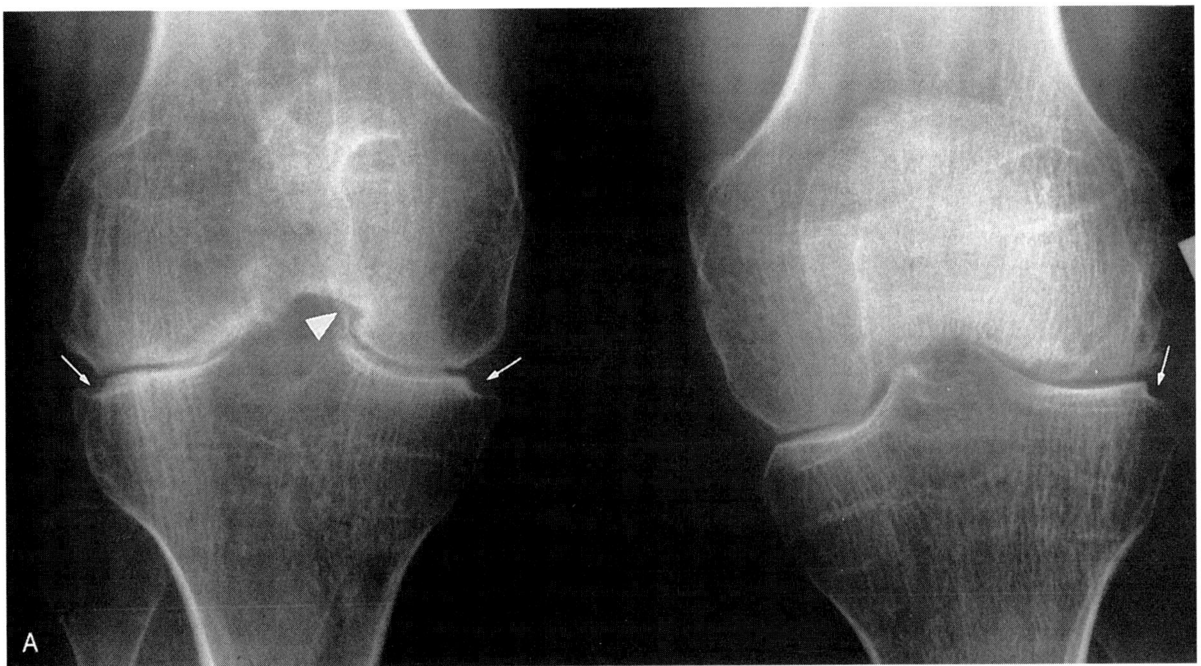

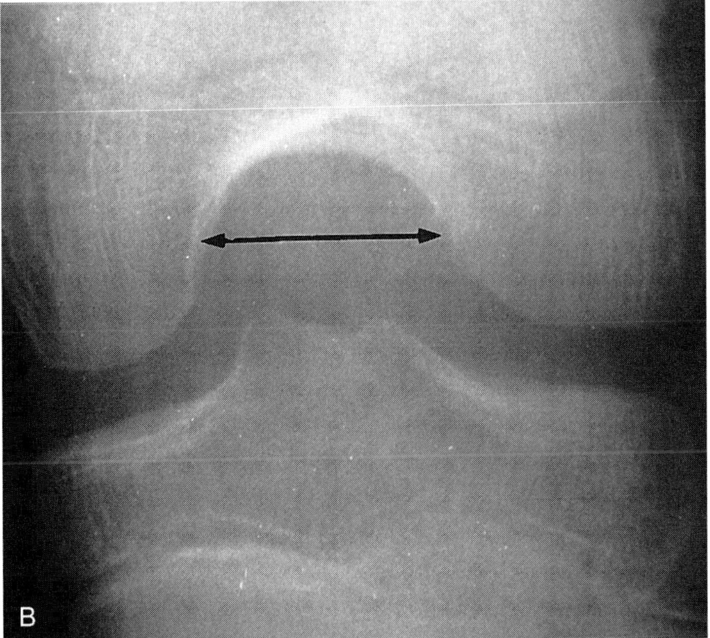

FIGURE 9–49. Juvenile chronic arthritis: Knee abnormalities.[90, 91] A Osteoporosis, marginal erosions (arrows), bilateral symmetric joint space narrowing, widening of the intercondylar notch (arrowhead), and overgrowth of the medial femoral condyles are evident in this 22-year-old woman with long-standing juvenile rheumatoid arthritis. B Widening of the intercondylar notch (double-headed arrow) is a common finding in juvenile chronic arthritis, illustrated on this routine frontal radiograph of another patient.

Illustration continued on following page

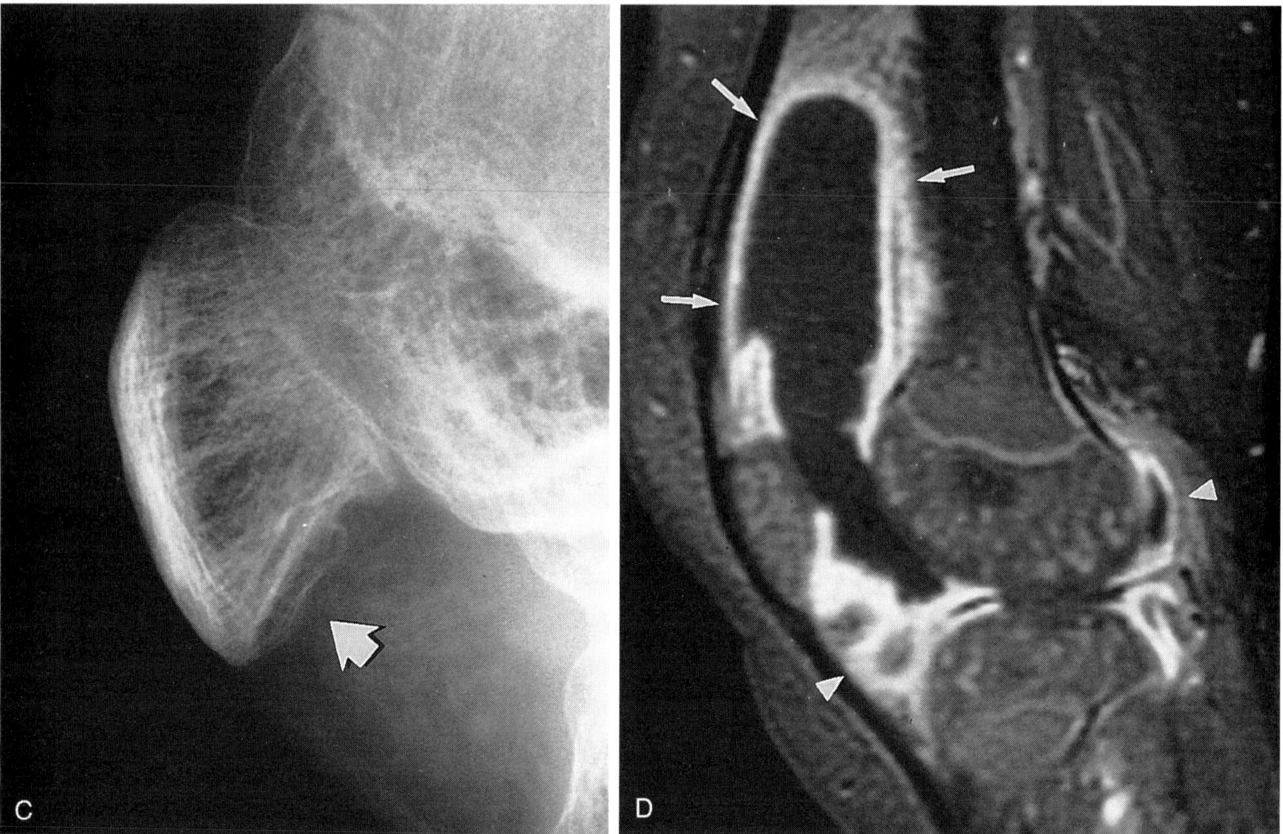

FIGURE 9–49 *Continued.* C Flattening of the inferior portion of the patella results in a characteristic squared patellar configuration (arrow). D A sagittal T1-weighted (TR/TE, 550/11) spin echo magnetic resonance (MR) image after administration of gadolinium contrast agent shows a large, low signal intensity suprapatellar joint effusion surrounded by an enhancing zone of high signal intensity characteristic of inflamed, hypertrophic synovial membrane (arrows). Similar synovial changes are observed in the posterior and infrapatellar synovial compartments (arrowheads). *(D, Courtesy of B. Coley, M.D., Columbus, Ohio.)* The radiographic findings of juvenile chronic arthritis closely resemble those of hemophilia.

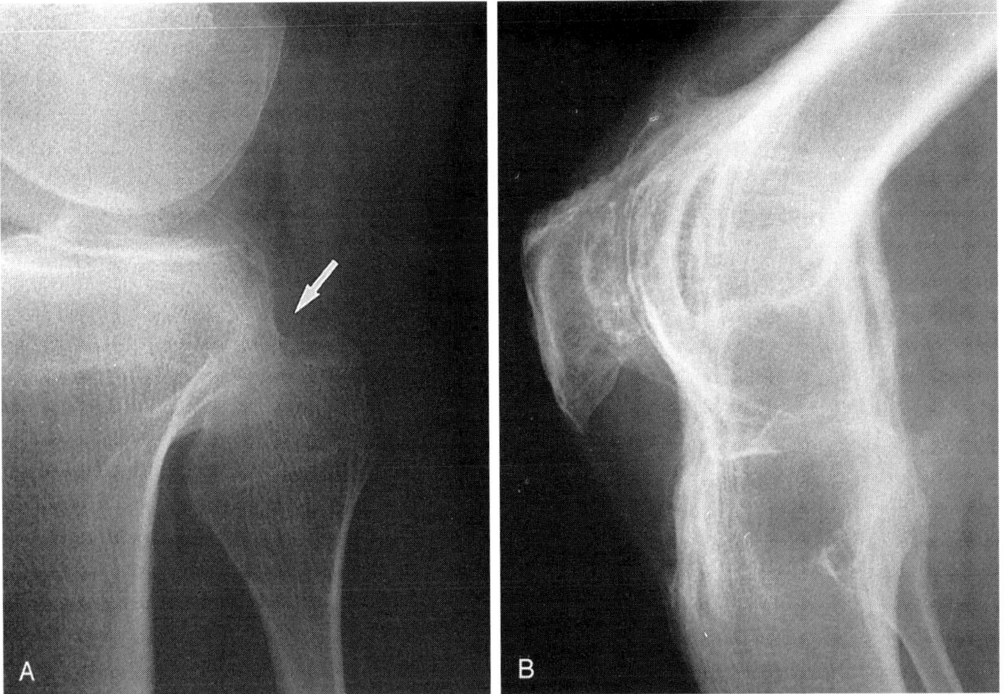

FIGURE 9–50. Ankylosing spondylitis.[92] A This 20-year-old man had a 4-year history of juvenile onset ankylosing spondylitis. Observe partial osseous ankylosis of the proximal tibiofibular joint (arrow). B In another patient, a 67-year-old man with a 40-year history of adult-onset ankylosing spondylitis, observe the osseous ankylosis of the femorotibial joint, diffuse muscle atrophy, and patellofemoral joint space narrowing. Radiographic abnormalities in the knees are found in about 30 per cent of persons with severe ankylosing spondylitis.

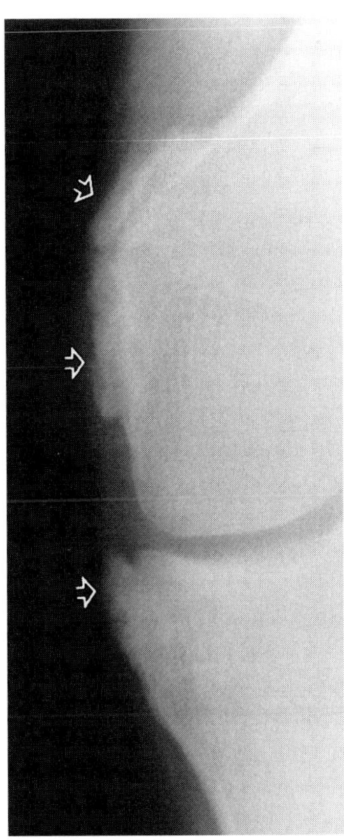

FIGURE 9–51. Reiter's syndrome.[93] In this 24-year-old man with Reiter's syndrome and HLA B27 antigen, observe the prominent, irregular periarticular osseous proliferation arising from the medial tibia and femur (open arrows). Such fluffy enthesopathy is characteristic of the seronegative spondyloarthropathies. *(Courtesy of R. Shapiro, M.D., Sacramento, California.)*

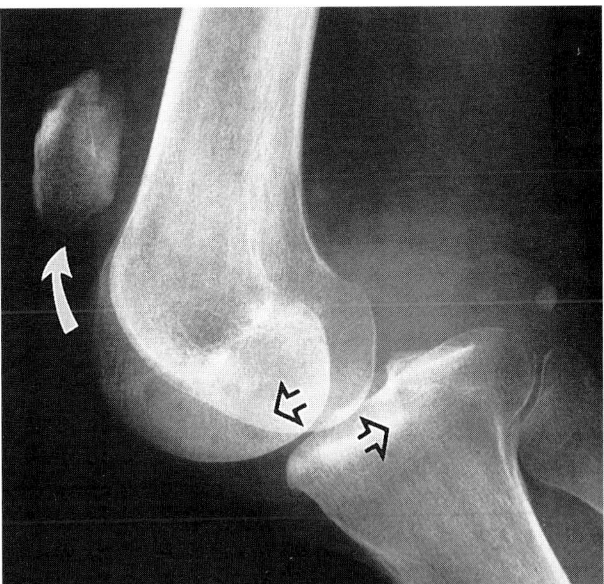

FIGURE 9–52. Systemic lupus erythematosus.[94] Lateral radiograph of the knee reveals superior patellar displacement (patella alta) as a result of spontaneous rupture of the patellar tendon (curved arrow). Posterior subluxation of the tibia in relation to the femur also is present (open arrows). Spontaneous tendon rupture in systemic lupus erythematosus almost invariably is associated with corticosteroid administration. *(Courtesy of A.G. Bergman, M.D., Stanford, California.)*

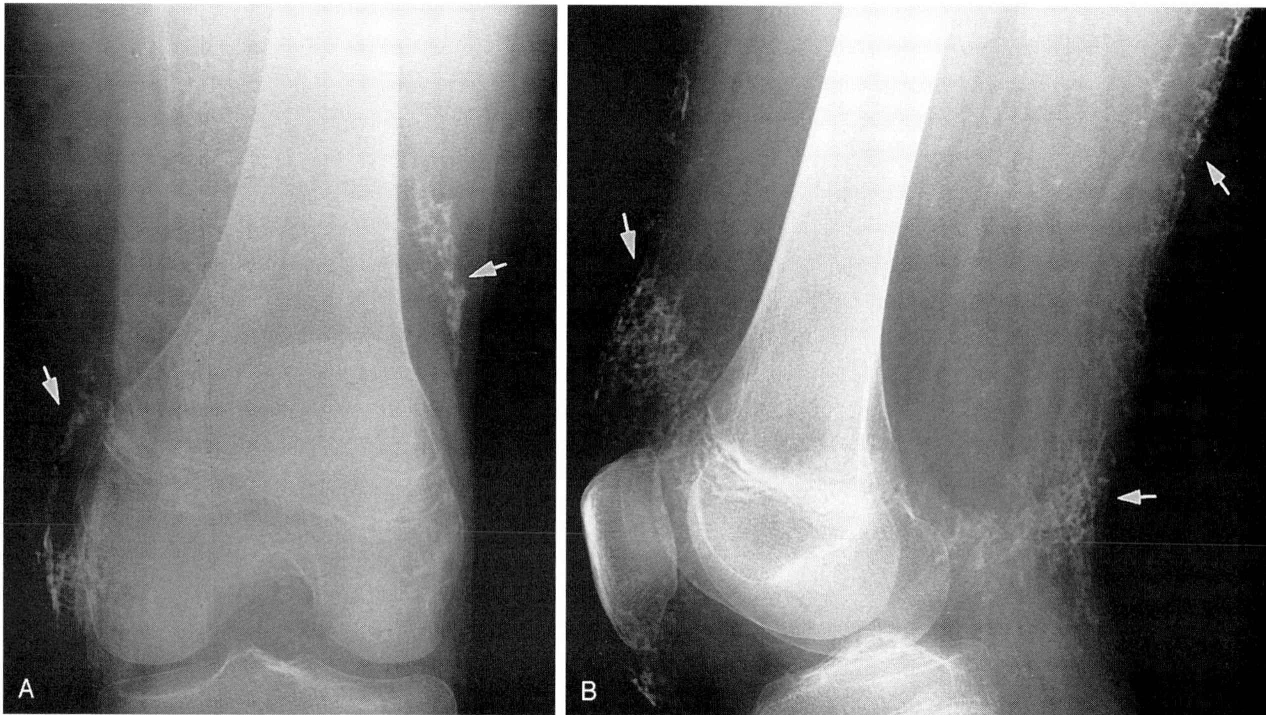

FIGURE 9–53. Dermatomyositis and polymyositis.[95] Frontal (A) and lateral (B) radiographs of this 13-year-old girl reveal a characteristic sheet-like calcinosis within the subcutaneous tissues about the knee and thigh (arrows).

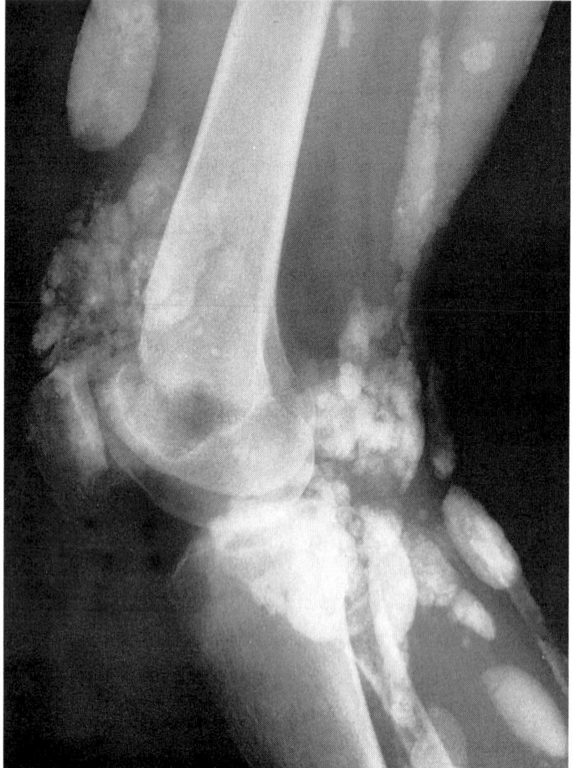

FIGURE 9–54. Mixed connective tissue disease.[96, 97] This patient with bizarre globular accumulations of periarticular calcification exhibits clinical and radiographic findings of combined dermatomyositis, scleroderma, and systemic lupus erythematosus.

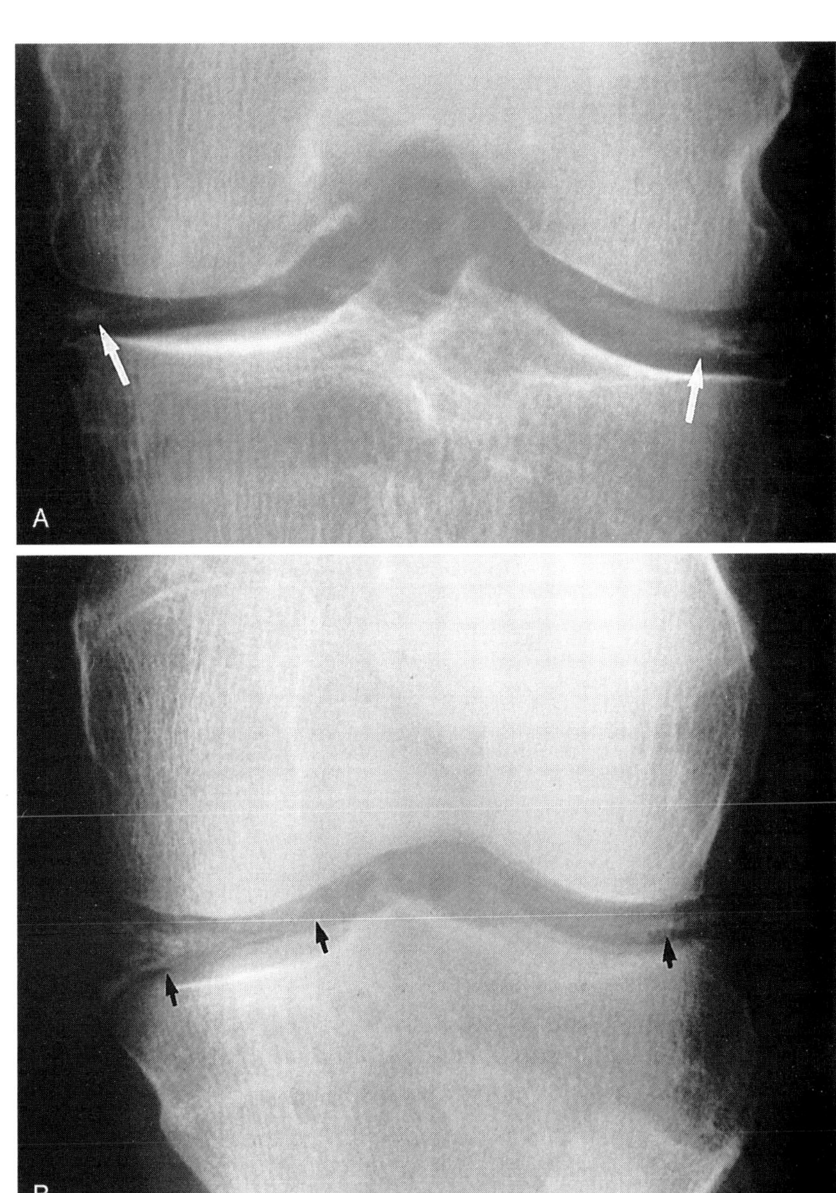

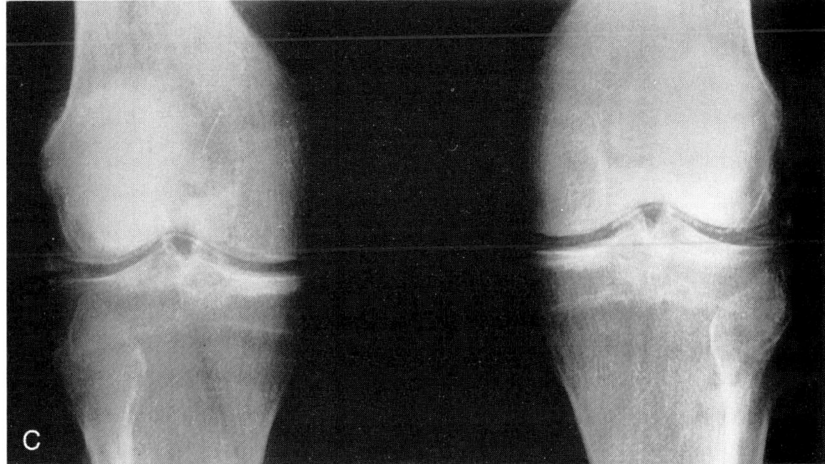

FIGURE 9–55. Calcium pyrophosphate dihydrate (CPPD) crystal deposition disease.[98–100] A In this 75-year-old man, observe chondrocalcinosis within the hyaline cartilage lining the tibial and femoral articular surfaces and the meniscal fibrocartilage (arrows). B In another patient, linear calcification is seen in the meniscal fibrocartilage and hyaline cartilage of the tibiofemoral articulation (arrows). C Bilateral narrowing of the medial and lateral compartments and extensive chondrocalcinosis is characteristic of CPPD crystal deposition disease.

Illustration continued on following page

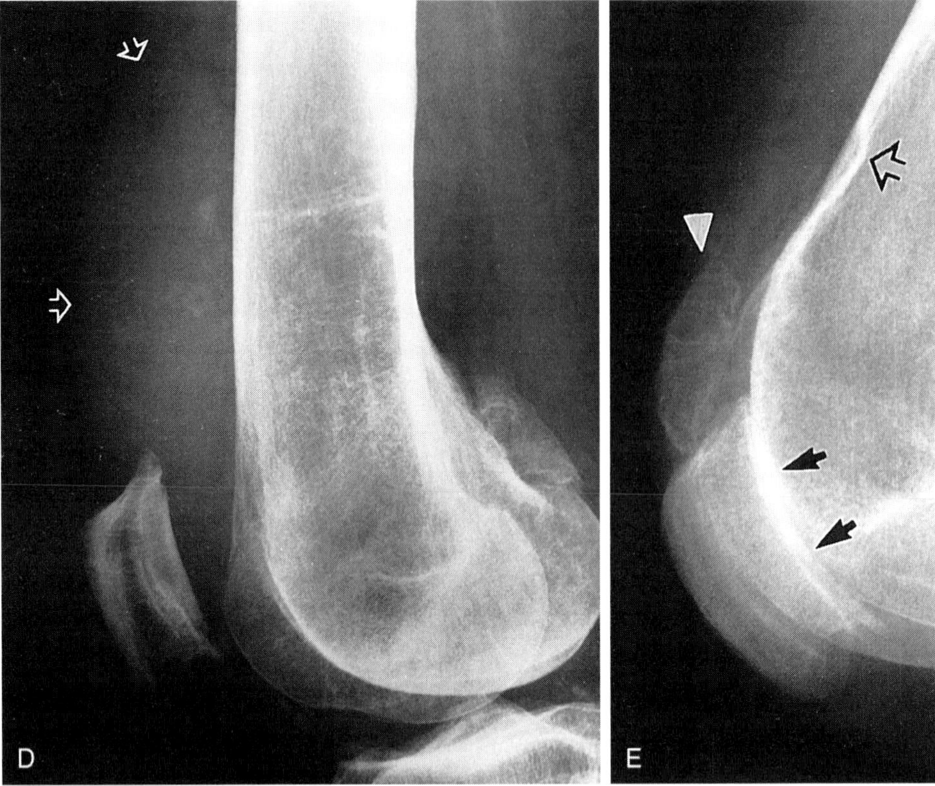

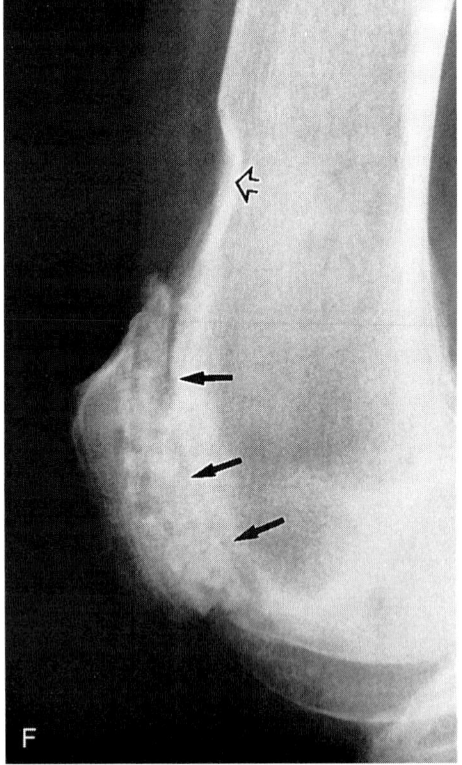

FIGURE 9–55 *Continued.* D Radiograph taken during an acute episode of pseudogout reveals anterior displacement of the patella caused by a huge suprapatellar effusion (open arrows). Synovial calcification is also evident. E Patellofemoral joint involvement predominates in this patient. Findings include extensive compartmental narrowing (arrows) and a suprapatellar femoral erosion (open arrow). An intra-articular body within the suprapatellar pouch (arrowhead) is also apparent. F In another patient, destructive patellofemoral arthropathy with joint space narrowing (arrows) and femoral erosion (open arrow) are seen.

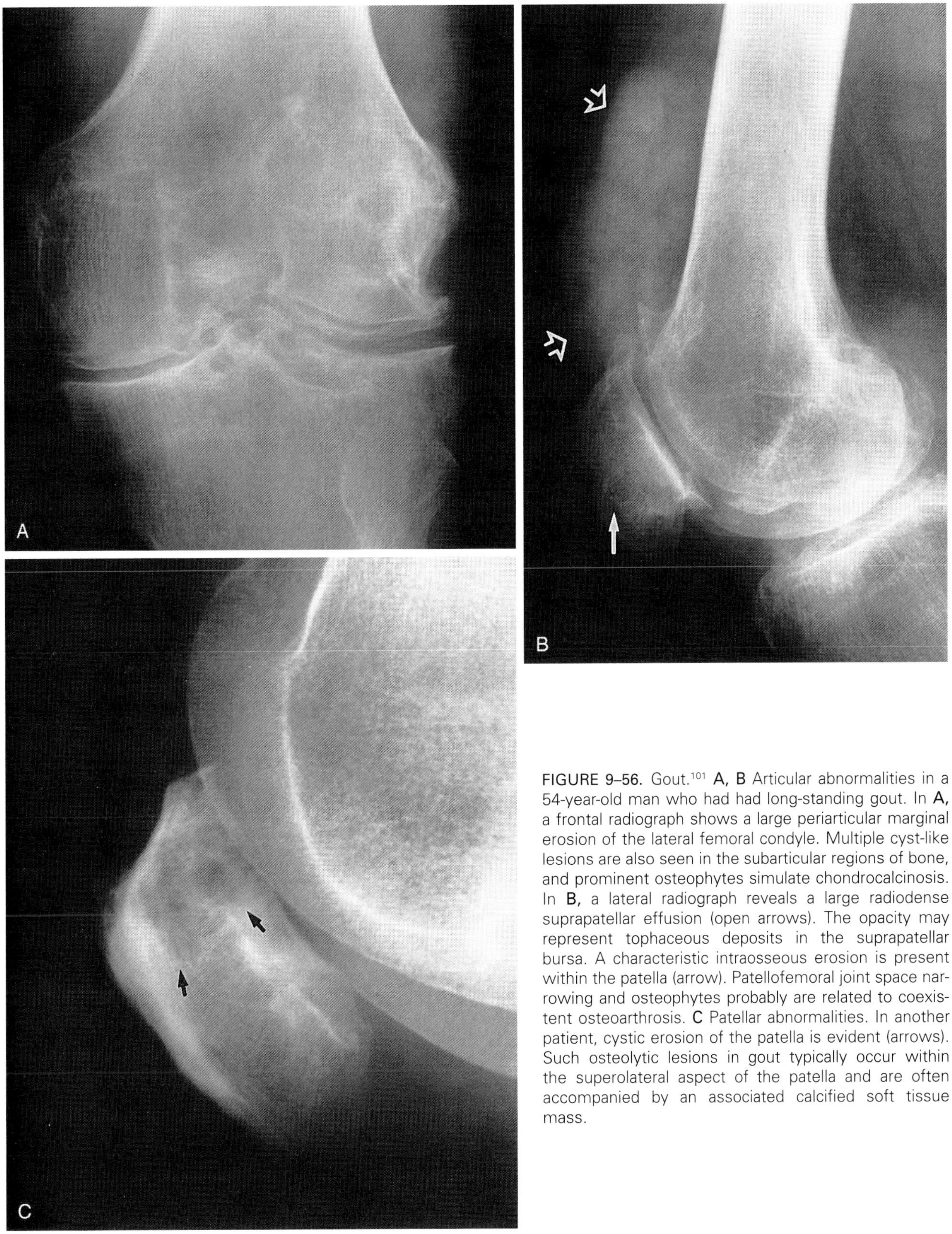

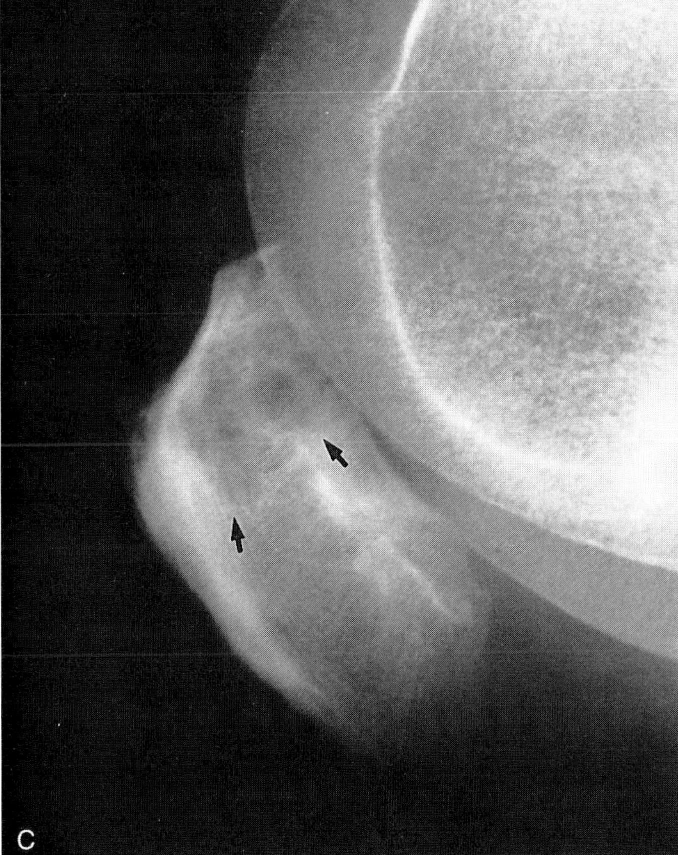

FIGURE 9–56. Gout.[101] A, B Articular abnormalities in a 54-year-old man who had had long-standing gout. In A, a frontal radiograph shows a large periarticular marginal erosion of the lateral femoral condyle. Multiple cyst-like lesions are also seen in the subarticular regions of bone, and prominent osteophytes simulate chondrocalcinosis. In B, a lateral radiograph reveals a large radiodense suprapatellar effusion (open arrows). The opacity may represent tophaceous deposits in the suprapatellar bursa. A characteristic intraosseous erosion is present within the patella (arrow). Patellofemoral joint space narrowing and osteophytes probably are related to coexistent osteoarthrosis. C Patellar abnormalities. In another patient, cystic erosion of the patella is evident (arrows). Such osteolytic lesions in gout typically occur within the superolateral aspect of the patella and are often accompanied by an associated calcified soft tissue mass.

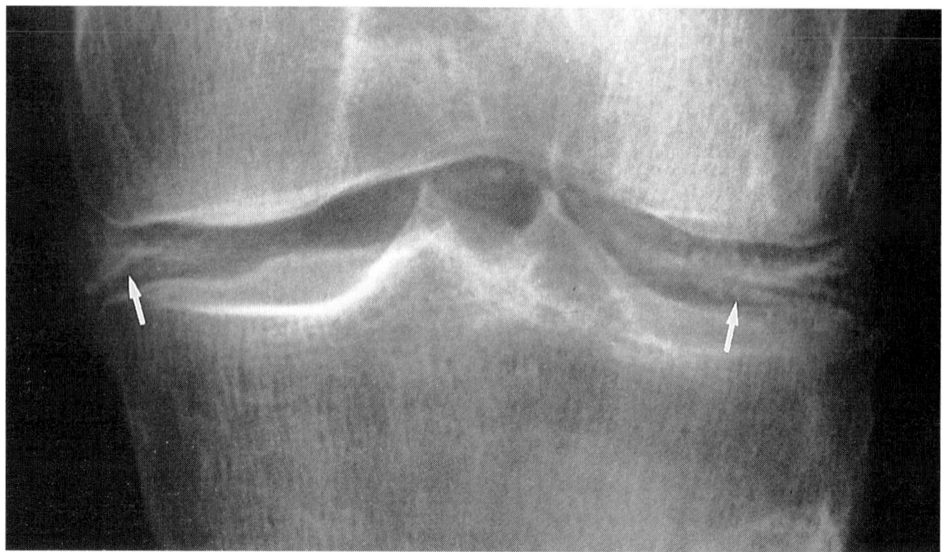

FIGURE 9–57. Hemochromatosis: Chondrocalcinosis.[102] Observe the linear calcification within the fibrocartilage of the medial and lateral menisci (arrows).

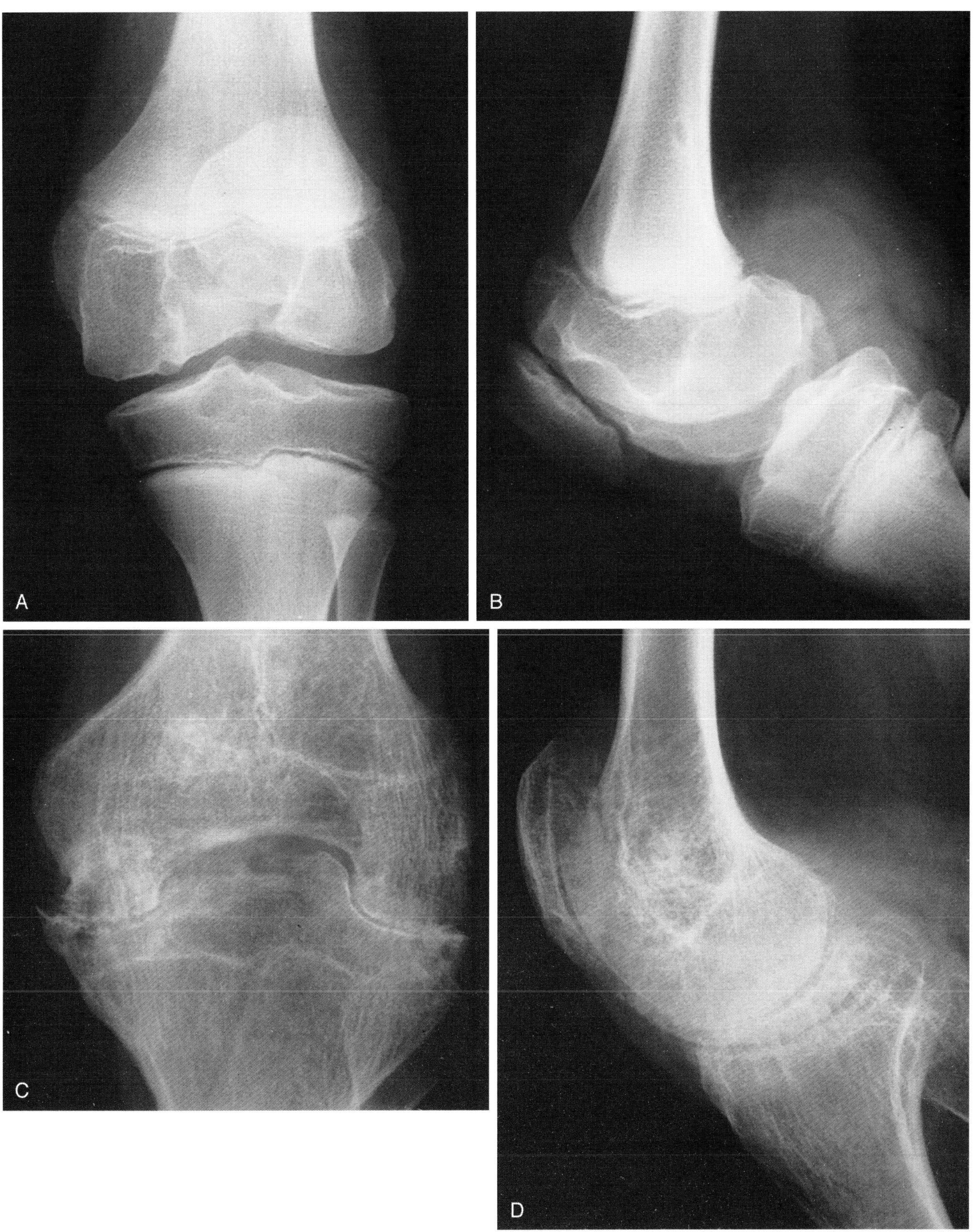

FIGURE 9–58. Hemophilic arthropathy: Radiographic abnormalities.[103] A, B Frontal (A) and lateral (B) radiographs of this boy with hemophilia reveal well-defined subchondral erosions resulting in an undulating appearance of the joint surfaces. Epiphyseal hyperplasia, squaring of the distal end of the femur, patellofemoral joint space narrowing, and a radiodense joint effusion are also evident. C, D In another patient, a 40-year-old man, frontal (C), and lateral (D) radiographs reveal the characteristic widening of the intercondylar notch, osteopenia, enlargement and ballooning of the epiphyses, dramatic joint space narrowing, and flattening of the articular surfaces of bone. The patella is eroded and the patellofemoral joint is obliterated.

Illustration continued on following page

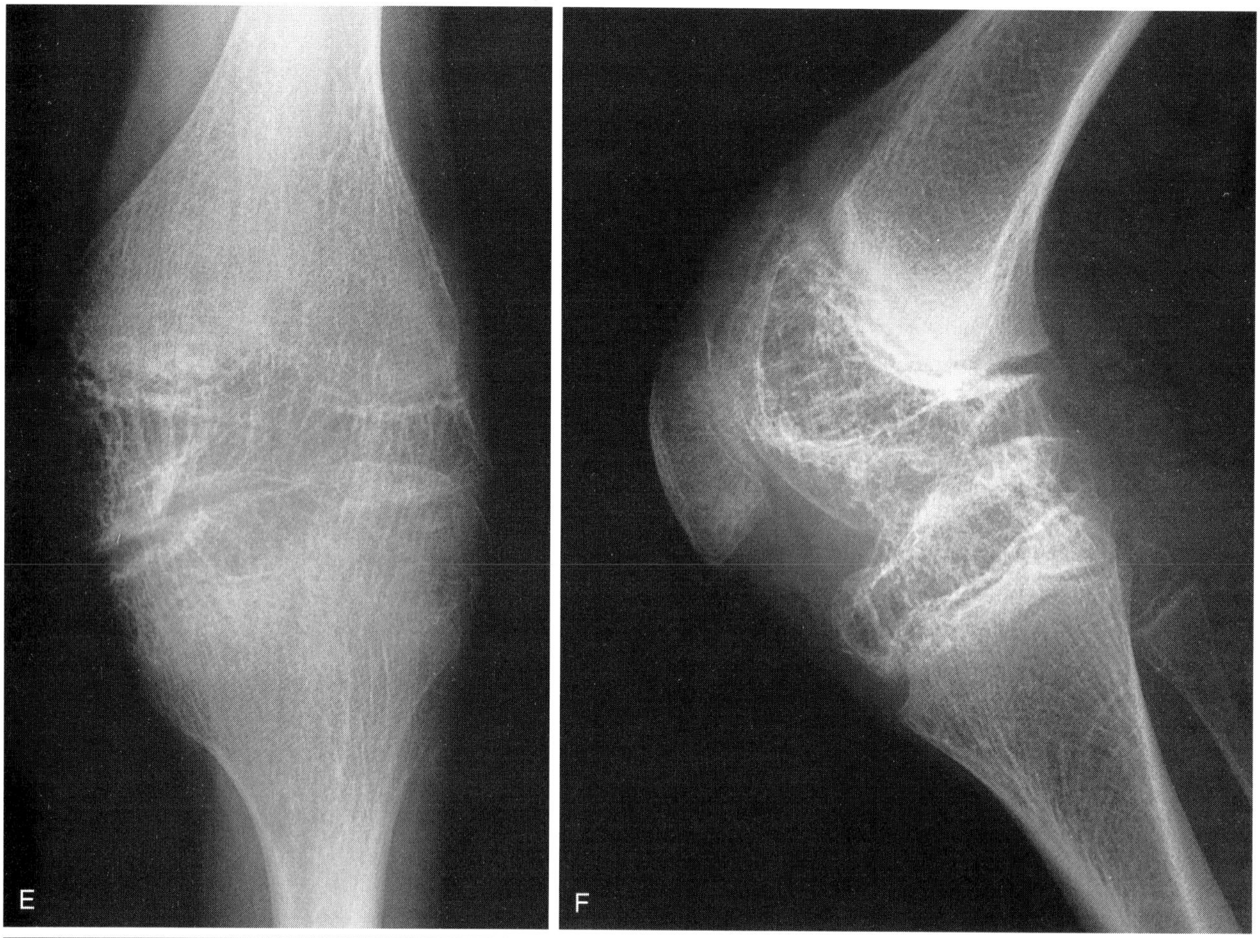

E

F

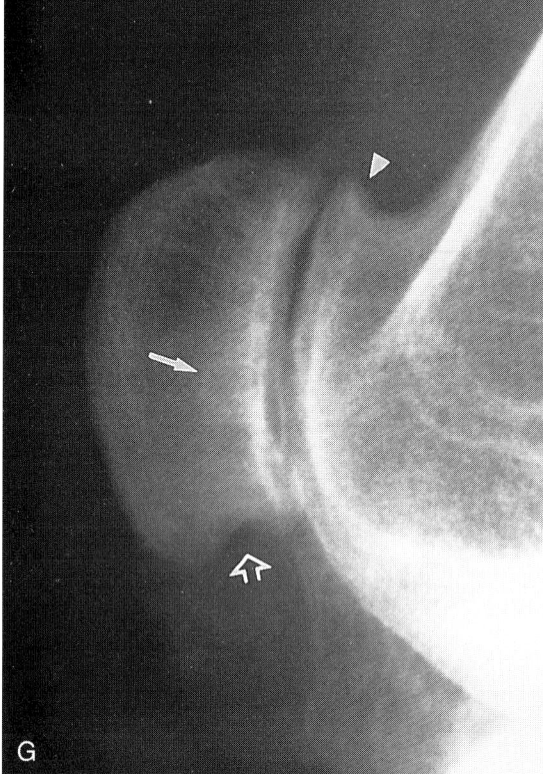

FIGURE 9–58 *Continued.* E, F This 17-year-old boy has had long-standing hemophilia and has sustained several episodes of hemarthrosis involving several joints. Frontal (E) and lateral (F) radiographs reveal severe articular destruction, advanced diffuse osteopenia, enlargement of the medial femoral condyle, squaring of the inferior aspect of the patella, and severe muscle atrophy. G In a fourth patient, patellofemoral changes include joint space narrowing, osteophytes (arrowhead), cyst formation (arrow), and prominent squaring of the inferior margin of the patella (open arrow).

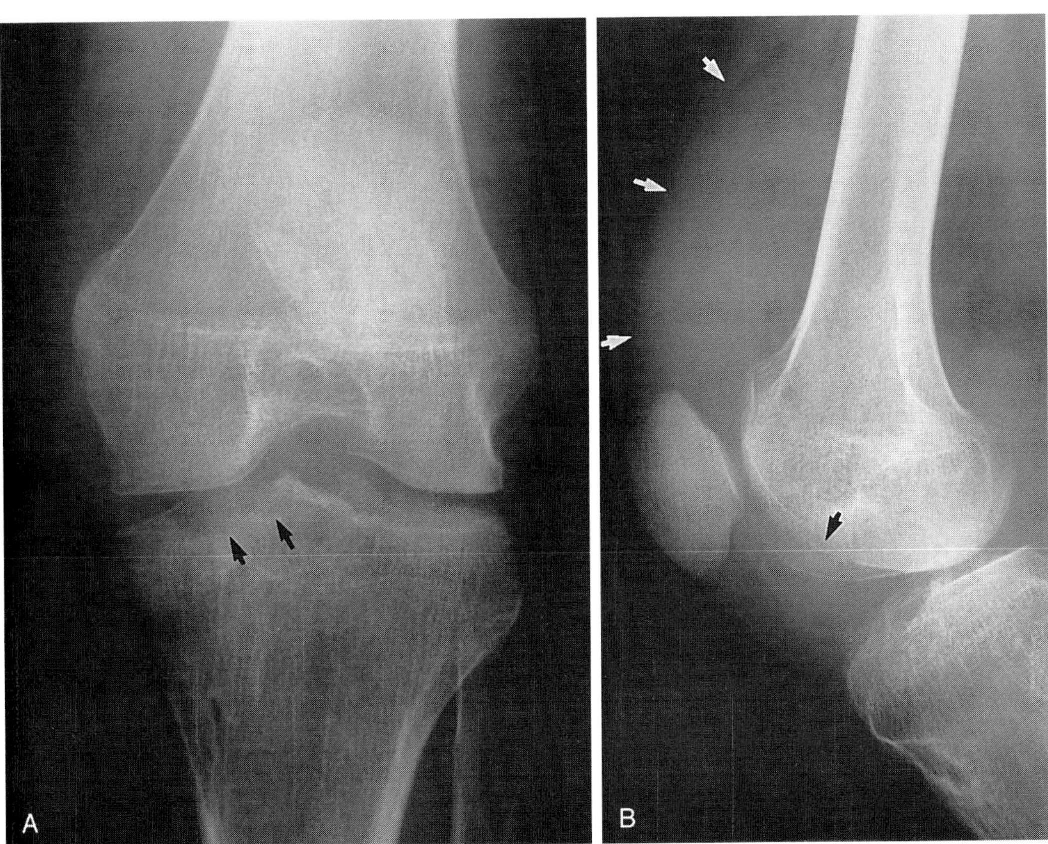

FIGURE 9–59. Tuberculous arthritis.[105] Routine frontal (A) and lateral (B) radiographs of the knee in this 19-year-old patient reveal the characteristic findings of joint infection. Marginal and central erosions (black arrows), minimal periarticular osteoporosis, and a huge joint effusion distending the suprapatellar bursa and displacing the patella (white arrows) are evident. *Mycobacterium tuberculosis* was cultured from the joint aspirate.

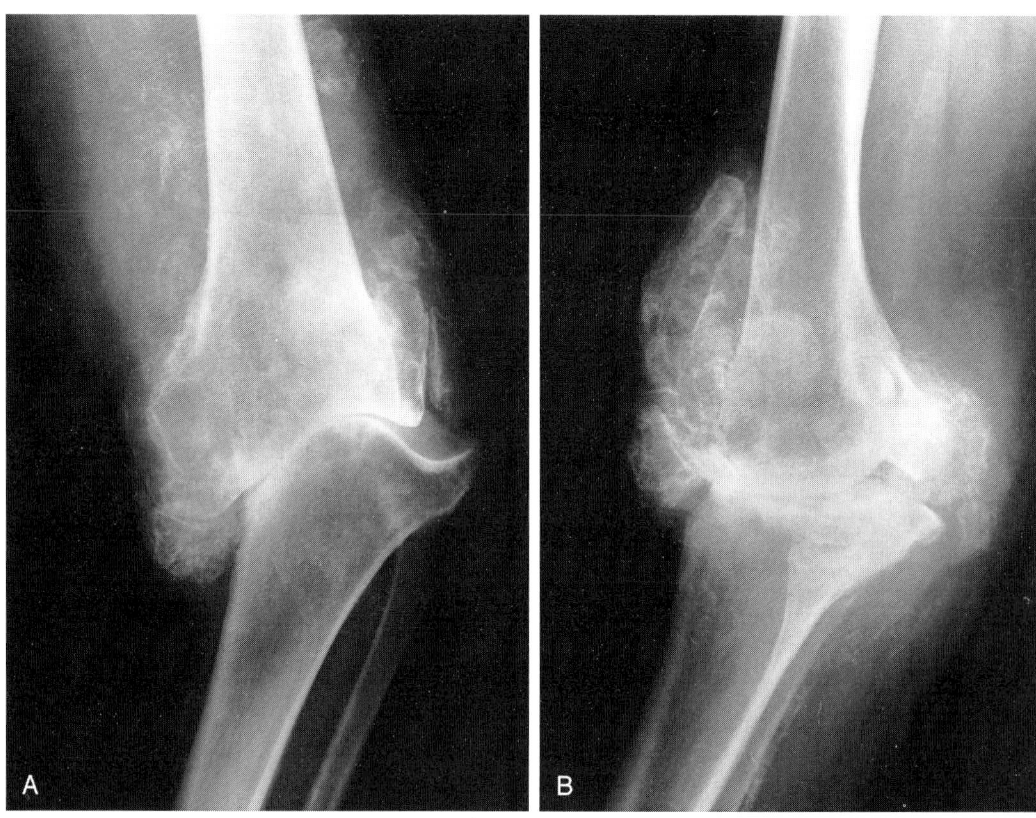

FIGURE 9–60. Neuropathic osteoarthropathy: Neurosyphilis.[89] This 67-year-old man with long-standing syphilis had no pain in his knees but complained of deformities, unsteadiness while walking, and limitation of motion. A Frontal radiograph of the left knee reveals a striking pattern of exuberant new bone formation, fragmentation, varus angulation, subluxation, destruction, and remodeling of the joint surfaces. B Lateral radiograph of the opposite knee shows marked genu recurvatum and changes similar to those on the left side. Note also the extensive vascular calcification. (A, *Courtesy of P. VanderStoep, M.D., St. Cloud, Minnesota.*)

TABLE 9–15. Neoplasms and Other Lesions Affecting the Knee and Patella*

Entity	Figure(s)	Characteristics
Malignant		
Skeletal Metastasis[106]	9–61	Most common in the axial skeleton; rare occurrence about the knee 75 per cent of cases exhibit permeative or moth-eaten osteolysis Articular involvement: may involve both sides of the articulation with widespread destruction
Myeloproliferative disorders		
Plasma cell myeloma[107]	9–62	Bones about the knee are an uncommon site for multiple myeloma Early diffuse osteopenia or later widespread well-circumscribed osteolytic lesions with discrete margins, which appear uniform in size
Benign		
Chondroblastoma[108, 109]	9–63	Predilection for the epiphyses and apophyses—the patella is an "epiphyseal equivalent" structure Circular osteolytic lesion less than 5 or 6 mm in diameter May exhibit calcification in matrix Occasionally periosteal reaction in adjacent metaphysis with corresponding marrow edema seen on magnetic resonance (MR) images
Giant cell tumor[89]	7–27	Eccentric osteolytic neoplasm with a predilection for the subarticular region Often multiloculated expansile lesion Radiographs are inaccurate in distinguishing benign from aggressive giant cell tumors
Aneurysmal bone cyst[110]	9–64	Eccentric, thin-walled, expansile osteolytic lesion Thin trabeculation with multiloculated appearance
Tumor-like lesions		
Paget's disease[111, 112]	9–65	Usually polyostotic and may have unilateral involvement Coarsened trabeculae and bone enlargement Patterns of involvement: osteolytic (50 per cent), osteosclerotic (25 per cent), and mixed (25 per cent)
Other patellar lesions		
Hemangioma		Osteolytic, prominent trabeculae
Lipoma		Osteolytic
Enchondroma		Osteolytic, matrix calcification
Plasmacytoma		Osteolytic, expansile
Aggressive giant cell tumor		Osteolytic, cortical destruction
Primary lymphoma		Osteolytic or osteosclerotic
Osteosarcoma		Osteolytic or osteosclerotic
Chondrosarcoma		Osteolytic, soft tissue mass, matrix calcification
Degenerative cyst		Osteolytic, associated degenerative changes
Brodie's abscess		Osteolytic, sclerotic margin
Intraosseous ganglion		Osteolytic

*See also Tables 1–10 to 1–12.

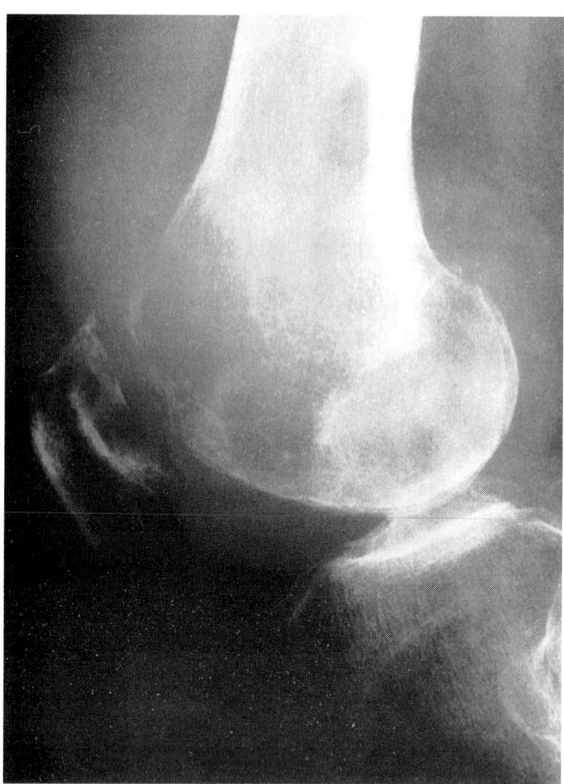

FIGURE 9–61. Skeletal metastasis. Articular involvement.[106] In this patient with skeletal metastasis from an unknown primary source, a large osteolytic pattern of destruction involving the distal end of the femur is evident. A large suprapatellar joint effusion or mass is also present. Biopsy indicated anaplastic carcinoma involving bone and extending into the articular cavity with hemarthrosis. *(Courtesy of V. Vint, M.D., La Jolla, California.)*

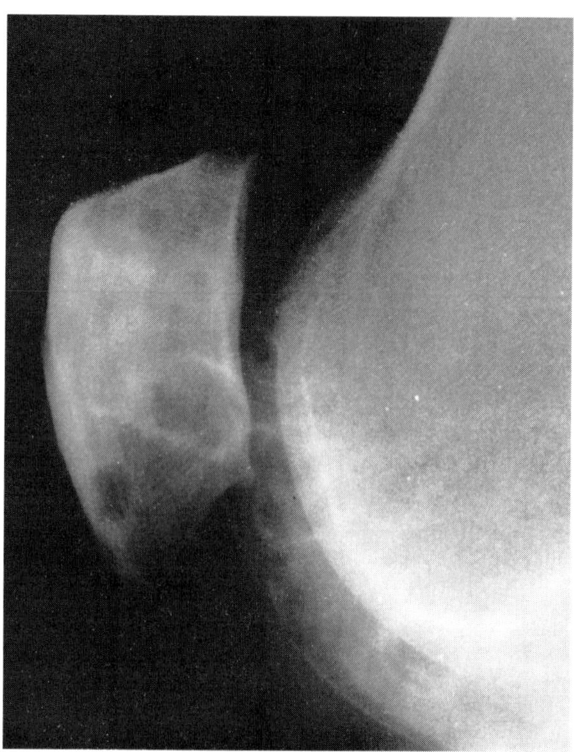

FIGURE 9–62. Plasma cell myeloma.[107] Multiple geographic lesions are evident in the patella and the femoral condyles in this patient with multiple myeloma. Classically, myeloma is first manifested as widespread osteolytic lesions with discrete margins, which appear uniform in size. Alternatively, diffuse osteopenia may be the only radiographic finding.

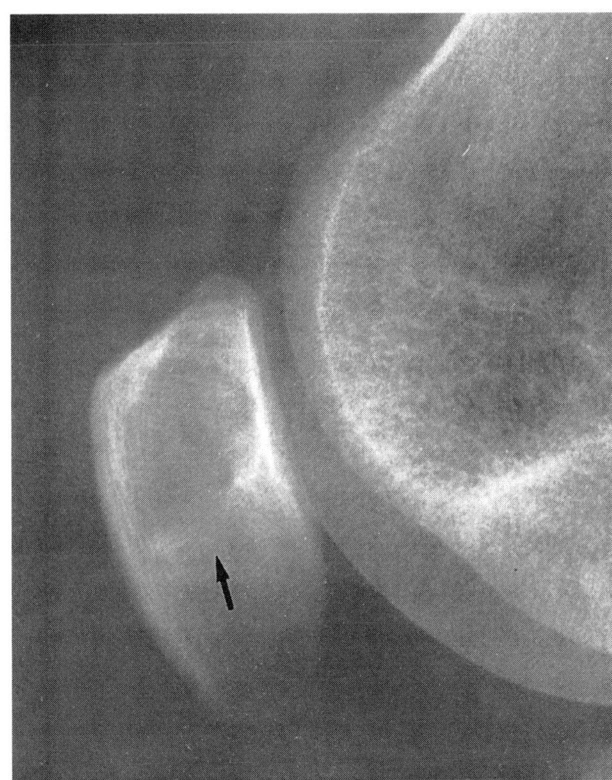

FIGURE 9–63. Chondroblastoma.[108, 109] This 19-year-old man with a 6-month history of patellar pain had a solitary radiolucent lesion within the patella (arrow). The lesion is well defined, possesses a sclerotic margin, and is associated with extensive soft tissue swelling overlying the patella.

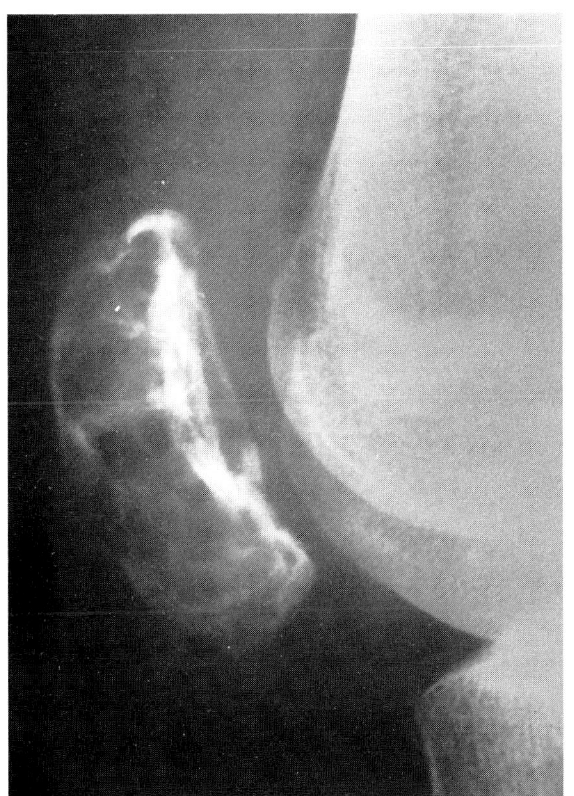

FIGURE 9–64. Aneurysmal bone cyst.[110] An expansile osteolytic lesion is seen involving the patella. The radiographic appearance of a multiseptated osteolytic lesion in the patella is nonspecific, and biopsy was required to confirm the diagnosis of aneurysmal bone cyst in this patient. A joint effusion is also present, displacing the superior pole of the patella anteriorly. *(Courtesy of R. Stiles, M.D., Atlanta, Georgia.)*

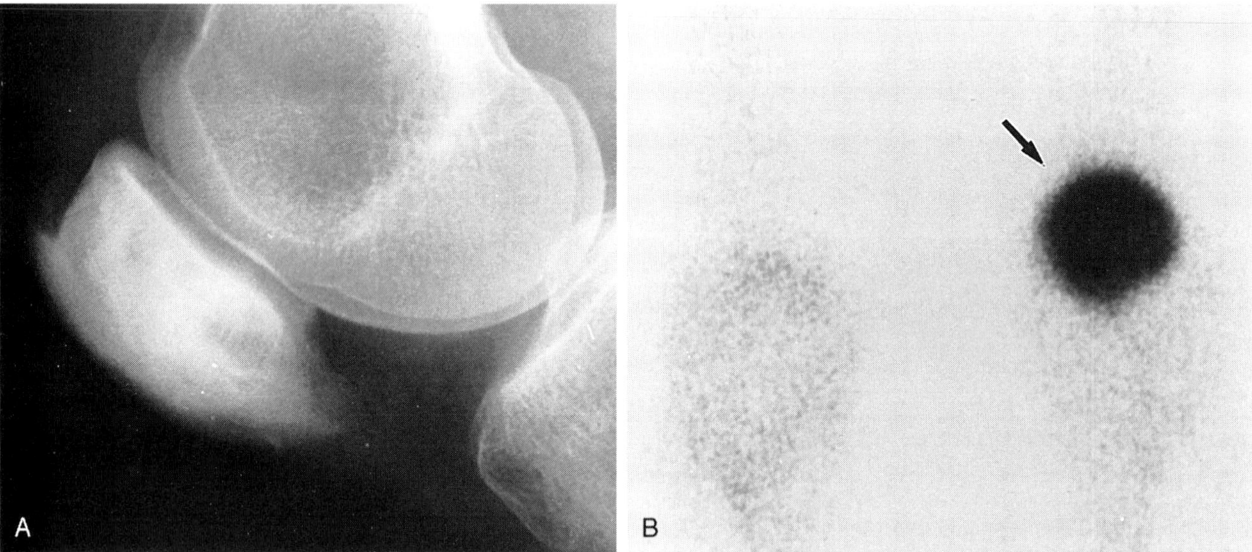

FIGURE 9–65. Paget's disease.[111, 112] A Lateral radiograph reveals coarsely trabeculated osteoblastic involvement of the patella. B Bone scan reveals intensely increased uptake of bone-seeking radiopharmaceutical agent (arrow).

TABLE 9–16. Metabolic, Hematologic, and Vascular Disorders*

Entity	Figure(s)	Characteristics
Generalized osteoporosis[89]		Increased radiolucency Trabecular accentuation
Rickets[113]	9–66	Metaphyseal demineralization: frayed metaphysis Bowing of bones Osteopenia
Primary hypertrophic osteoarthropathy[114]	9–67	Pachydermoperiostosis: primary form (3–5 per cent of all cases) of hypertrophic osteoarthropathy Rare autosomal dominant disease characterized by enlargement of the hands and feet, digital clubbing, convexity of the nails, cutaneous abnormalities, and joint pains *Radiologic findings* Bilateral symmetric periostitis of the long tubular bones
Hypovitaminosis C (scurvy)[115]		Radiographic evidence of skeletal changes in scurvy is seen only in advanced long-standing disease Periostitis secondary to subperiosteal hemorrhage Sclerotic metaphyseal lines Beak-like metaphyseal excrescences Radiodense shell surrounding epiphyses Healing scurvy may result in increased radiodensity of the metaphyses and epiphyses
Hyperparathyroidism[116–119]	9–68	Subperiosteal bone resorption of medial tibial metaphysis Occasional bone sclerosis (more common with renal osteodystrophy) Chondrocalcinosis ([calcium pyrophosphate dihydrate] CPPD crystal deposition) Brown tumors Severe bone remodeling with osteitis fibrosa cystica (now infrequently encountered) Soft tissue calcification
Renal osteodystrophy[116–119]	9–69, 9–70	Similar findings to those in hyperparathyroidism, osteomalacia, and rickets Pathologic fractures
Osteonecrosis[120, 121]	9–70 to 9–72	*Secondary epiphyseal osteonecrosis and medullary osteonecrosis* See Table 1–15 for predisposing causes and associations *Spontaneous osteonecrosis* Idiopathic osteonecrosis may occur spontaneously in the absence of any risk factors; most common in women older than 60 years of age; sudden onset of localized tenderness, stiffness, effusion and restriction of motion; usually unilateral; most frequently affects the weight-bearing surface of the medial femoral condyle; initial radiographs frequently normal *Radiographic findings* Bone sclerosis, subchondral cysts, subchondral collapse *Magnetic resonance (MR) imaging findings* Subchondral collapse and associated meniscal and articular cartilage abnormalities
Popliteal artery aneurysm[52, 122]	9–73	May appear as a pulsatile mass in the popliteal fossa Often posttraumatic Complications include leaking, embolism, and thrombus

*See also Tables 1–13 to 1–15.

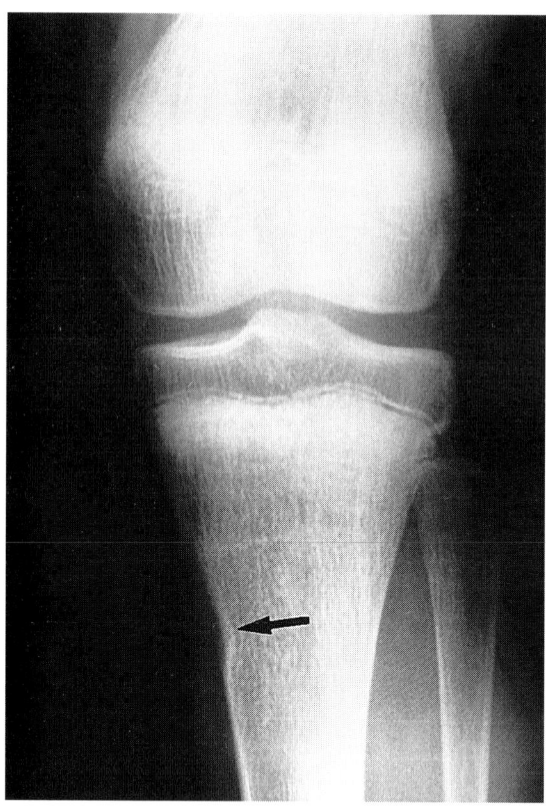

FIGURE 9–66. Rickets.[113] Renal rickets. A knee radiograph of this 19-year-old woman with rickets and chronic renal disease shows metaphyseal sclerosis and erosion of the medial tibial metaphysis (arrow), characteristic of renal rickets.

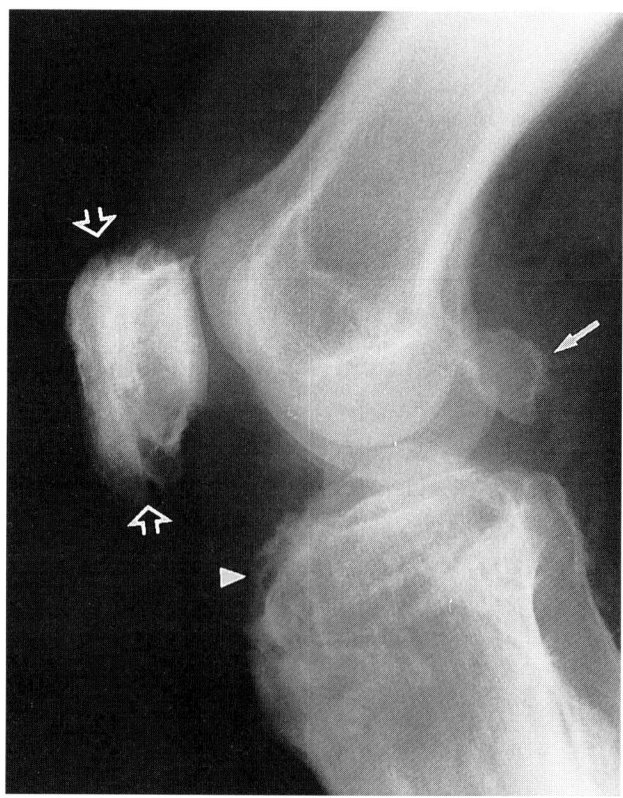

FIGURE 9–67. Primary hypertrophic osteoarthropathy: Pachydermoperiostosis.[114] Observe the widespread prominent enthesophytes arising from the patella (open arrows), fabella (arrow), and anterior surface of the tibia (arrowhead). The findings in this patient were bilateral and symmetric and affected several bones throughout the skeleton. *(Courtesy of C. Chen, M.D., Kaohsiung, Taiwan.)*

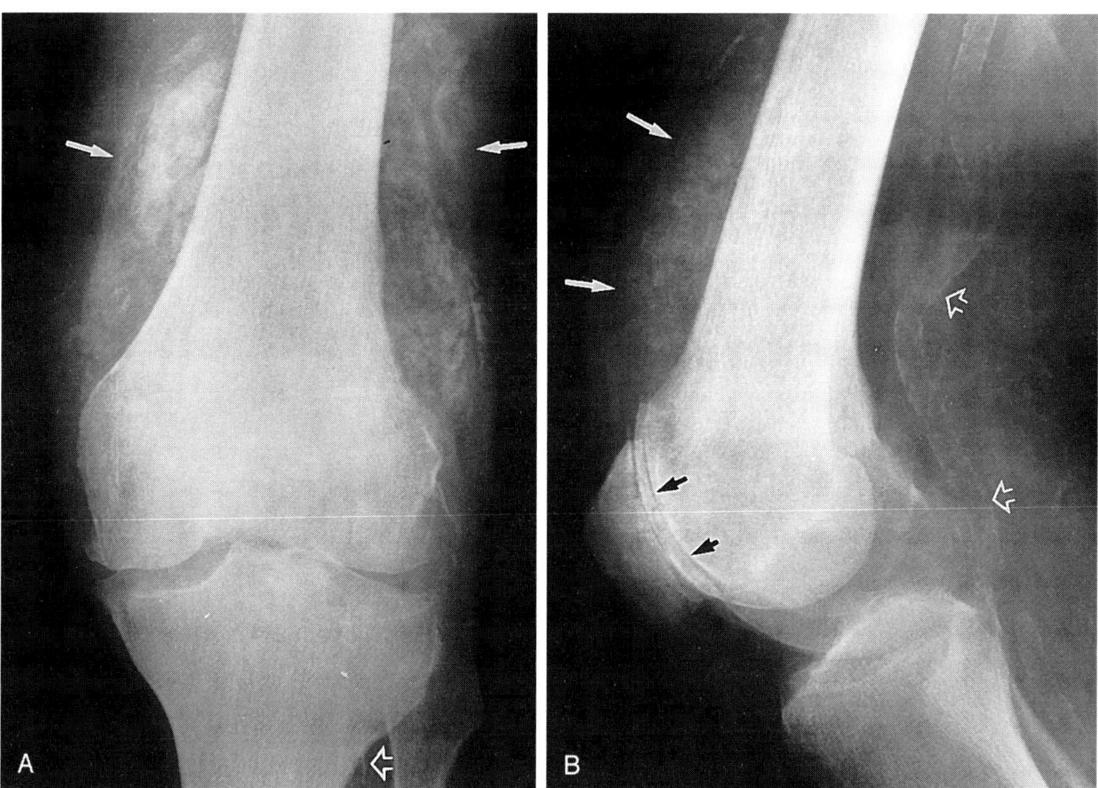

FIGURE 9–68. Hyperparathyroidism.[116, 117] Frontal (A) and lateral (B) radiographs show extensive intra-articular soft tissue calcification involving the synovium, suprapatellar bursa (white arrows), and vasculature (open arrows) about the knee. Observe also the dramatic erosion and deformity of the posterior surface of the patella (black arrows).

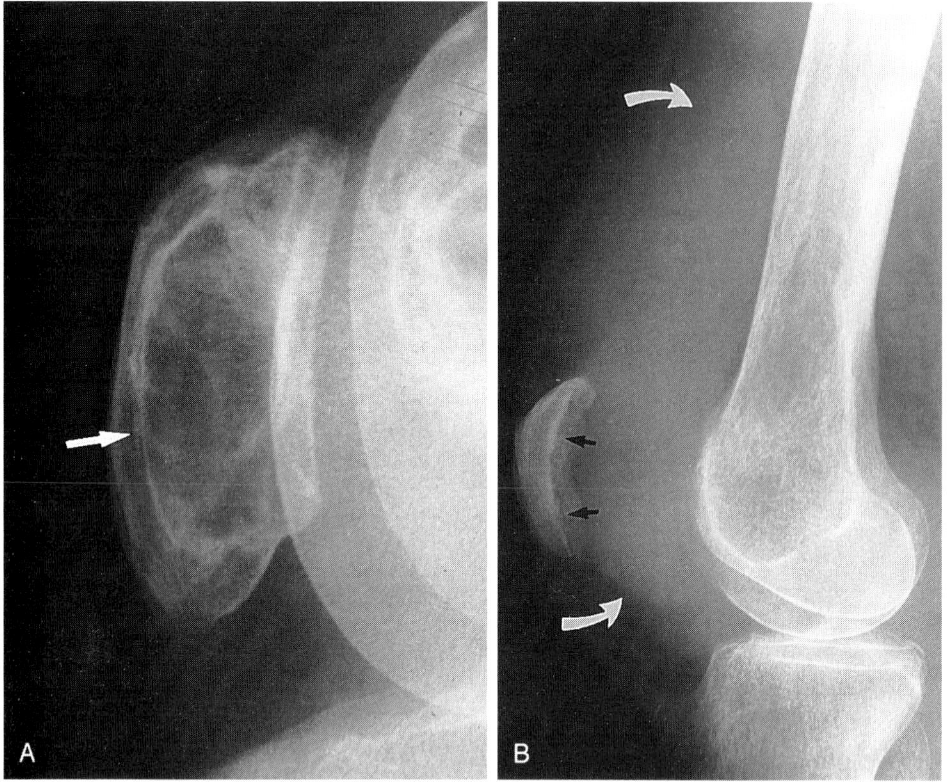

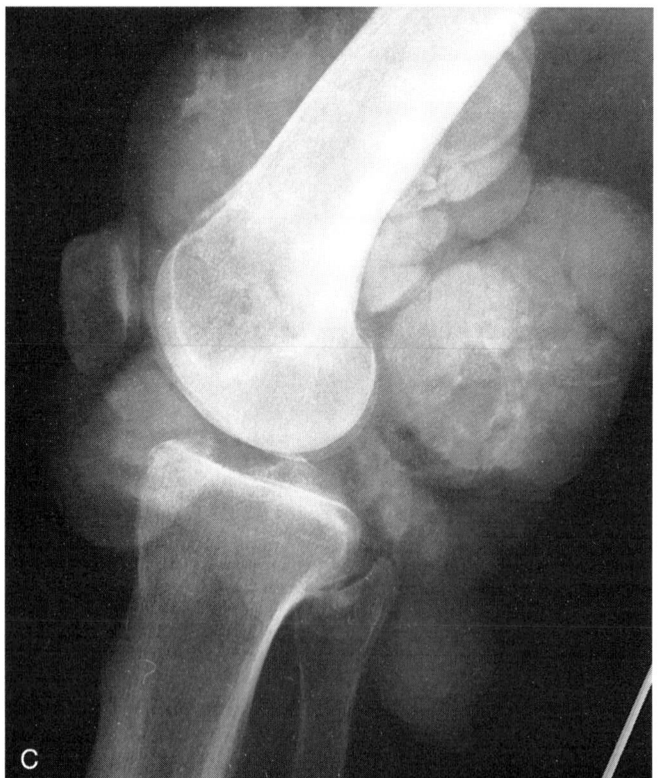

FIGURE 9–69. Renal osteodystrophy: Radiographic abnormalities.[116–120] **A** Brown tumor. Routine radiograph reveals an osteolytic lesion affecting the patella (arrow) in this patient with chronic renal failure and secondary hyperparathyroidism. Brown tumors or osteoclastomas represent localized accumulations of fibrous tissue and giant cells, which can replace bone and may produce expansion. They may be single or multiple and may disappear after treatment of the underlying cause of hyperparathyroidism. **B** Patellofemoral erosion and hemarthrosis. In a 68-year-old woman, observe the presence of a large suprapatellar effusion (curved arrows) and subchondral erosion and deformity of the undersurface of the patella (small arrows). **C** In a third patient with secondary hyperparathyroidism, observe the presence of intra-articular and intrabursal tumoral calcification. *(**C**, Courtesy of J. Goobar, M.D., Ostersund, Sweden.)*

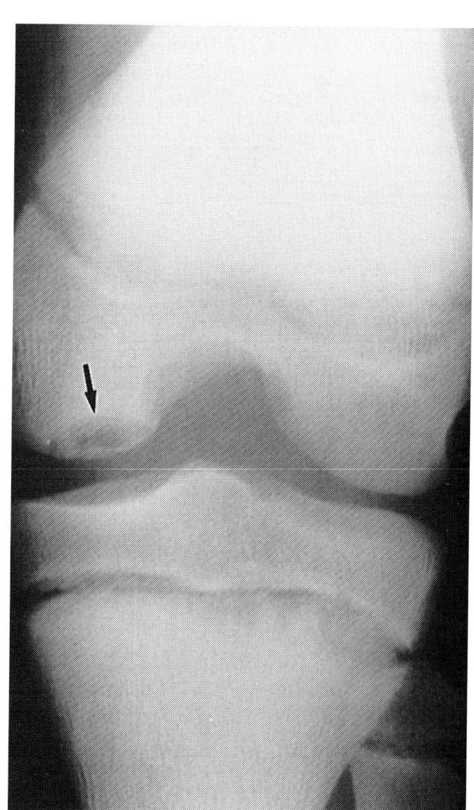

FIGURE 9–70. Osteonecrosis: Chronic renal disease.[120, 121] In a 15-year-old boy with renal osteodystrophy, observe the generalized osteosclerosis, physeal widening and itrregularity, and evidence of osteonecrosis of the medial femoral condyle (arrow). Osteonecrosis has been reported in patients with chronic renal failure treated with and without dialysis or transplantation.

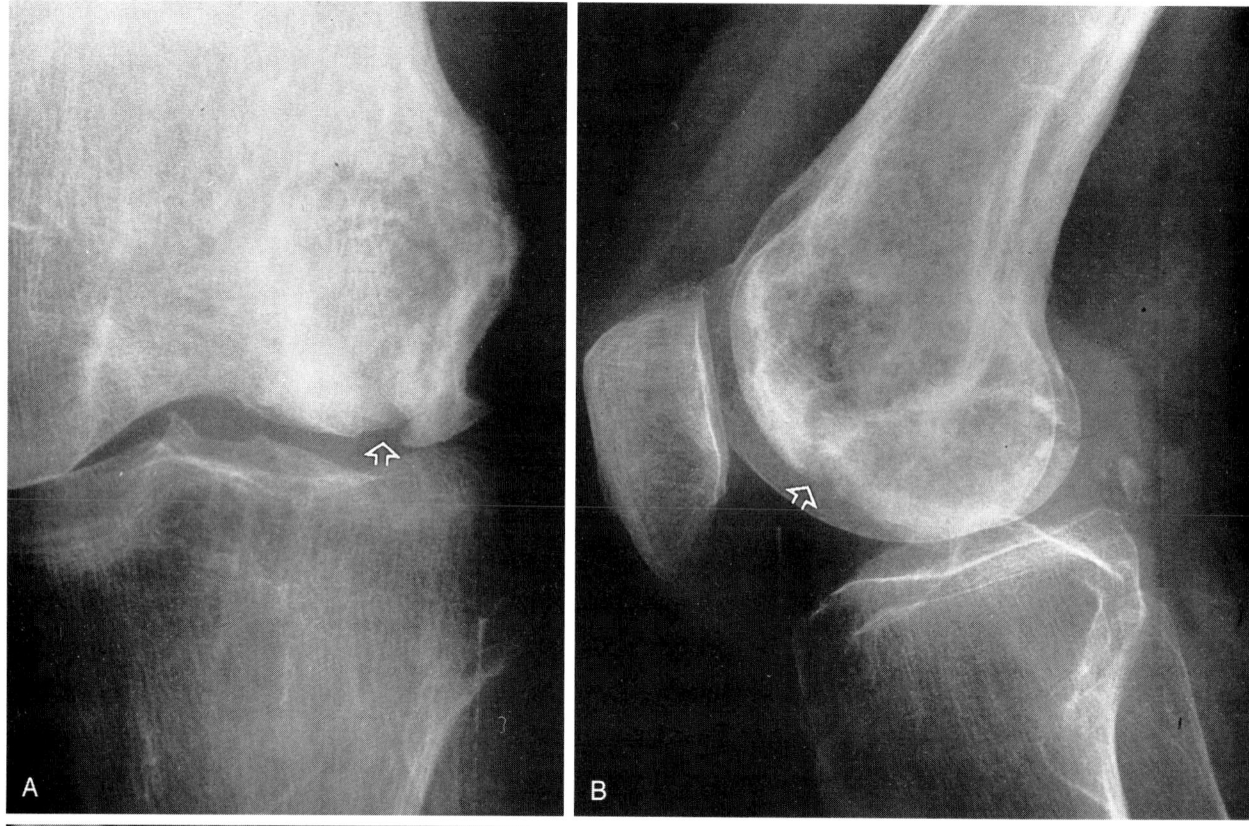

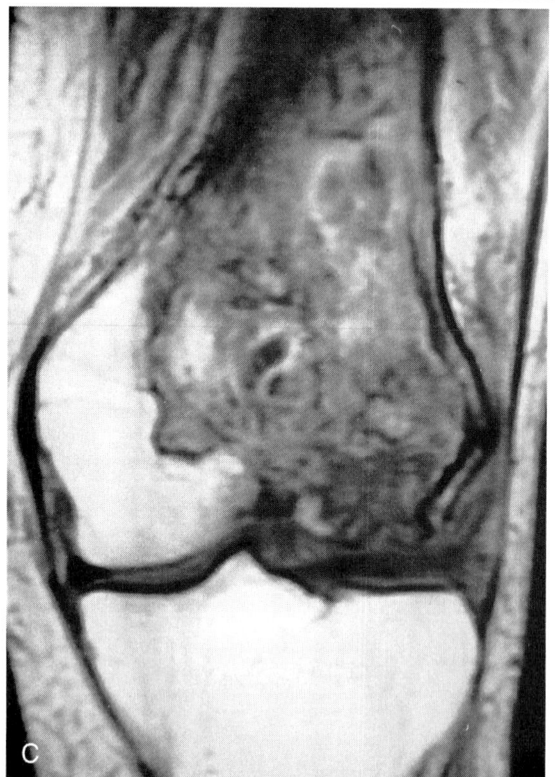

FIGURE 9–71. Spontaneous osteonecrosis about the knee.[120, 121] This 73-year-old woman had no risk factors for osteonecrosis, and no underlying cause for these changes was found. A Routine frontal radiograph shows increased density of the lateral femoral condyle. The articular surface has collapsed (open arrow), and areas of osteolysis also are seen. B Lateral radiograph shows collapse of the articular surface of the lateral condyle (open arrow) combined with areas of osteolysis and osteosclerosis. C Coronal T1-weighted (TR/TE, 600/22) spin echo magnetic resonance (MR) image shows extensive mixed intermediate to low signal intensity characteristic of widespread osteonecrosis in the lateral femoral condyle and femoral metaphysis. MR imaging is ideally suited for evaluating osteonecrosis. *(Courtesy of D. Artenian, M.D., Fresno, California.)*

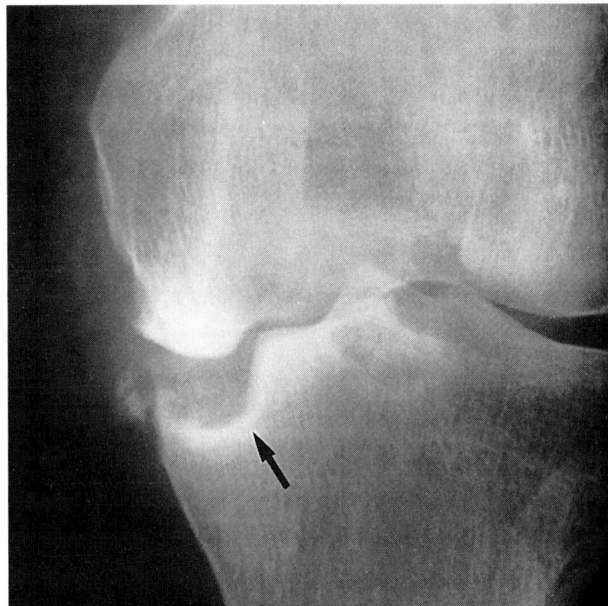

FIGURE 9–72. Corticosteroid-induced osteonecrosis.[121] Observe, in this patient on long-term corticosteroid therapy, joint space narrowing and collapse of the articular surface of the tibial plateau (bite sign) (arrow). Typical radiographic features of osteonecrosis include subchondral curvilinear radiolucent shadows (crescent sign), osteopenia, osteosclerosis, bony collapse and fragmentation, and a relatively normal articular space early in the disease process. Osteonecrosis may occur with exogenous corticosteroid administration or excessive endogenous corticosteroid secretion.

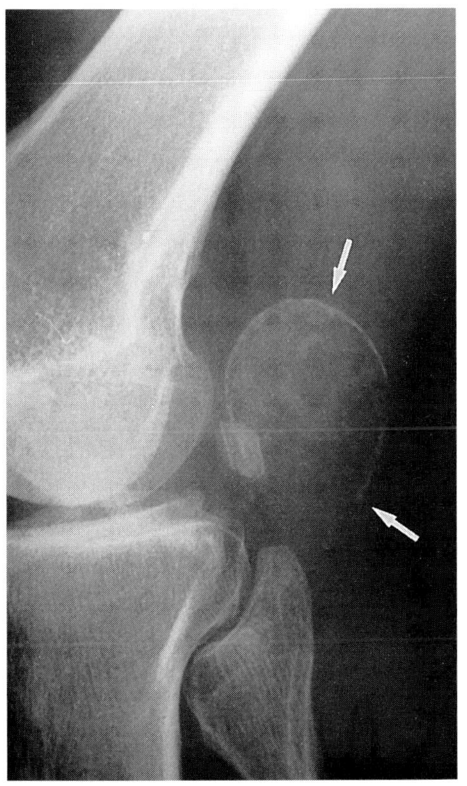

FIGURE 9–73. Posttraumatic popliteal artery aneurysm.[52, 122] This 61-year-old man had a pulsatile mass in the popliteal fossa several months after fracturing the shaft of his femur. A large ovoid mass with a calcified rim is evident behind the knee (arrows). The differential diagnosis includes synovial cyst, calcified soft tissue neoplasm, or popliteal vein aneurysm. *(Courtesy of A. Orloff, M.D., San Diego, California.)*

REFERENCES

1. Edeiken J, Dalinka M, Karasick D: Edeiken's Roentgen Diagnosis of Diseases of Bone. 4th Ed. Baltimore, Williams & Wilkins, 1990.
2. Ogden JA: Radiology of postnatal skeletal development. X. Patella and tibial tuberosity. Skeletal Radiol 11:246, 1984.
3. Keats TE, Smith TH: An Atlas of Normal Developmental Roentgen Anatomy. 2nd Ed. Chicago, Year Book Medical Publishers, 1988.
4. Greenfield GB: Radiology of Bone Diseases. 2nd Ed. Philadelphia, JB Lippincott, 1975.
5. Köhler A, Zimmer EA: Borderlands of Normal and Early Pathologic Findings in Skeletal Radiography. 4th Ed. New York, Thieme Medical Publishers, 1993.
6. Keats TE: Atlas of Normal Roentgen Variants That May Simulate Disease, 6th Ed. Chicago, Year Book Medical Publishers, 1996.
7. Yochum TR, Rowe LJ: Essentials of Skeletal Radiology. 2nd Ed. Baltimore, Williams & Wilkins, 1996.
8. Ogden JA, McCarthy SM, Jokl P: The painful bipartite patella. J Pediatr Orthop 2:263, 1982.
9. van Holsbeeck M, Vandamme B, Marchal G, et al: Dorsal defect of the patella: Concept of its origin and relationship with bipartite and multipartite patella. Skeletal Radiol 16:304, 1987.
10. Resnick D, Greenway G: Distal femoral cortical defects, irregularities, and excavations: A critical review of the literature with the addition of histologic and paleopathologic data. Radiology 143:345, 1982.
11. Yamazaki T, Maruoka S, Takahashi S, et al: MR findings of avulsive cortical irregularity of the distal femur. Skeletal Radiol 24:43, 1995.
12. Yochum TR, Sprowl CG, Barry MS: Double patella syndrome with a form of multiple epiphyseal dysplasia. J Manip Physiol Ther 18:407, 1995.
13. Guidera KJ, Satterwhite Y, Ogden JA, et al: Nail patella syndrome: A review of 44 orthopaedic patients. J Pediatr Orthop 11:737, 1991.
14. Keret D, Spatz DK, Caro PA, et al: Dysplasia epiphysealis hemimelica: Diagnosis and treatment. J Pediatr Orthop 12:365, 1992.
15. Lang IM, Azouz EM: MRI appearances of dysplasia epiphysealis hemimelica of the knee. Skeletal Radiol 26:226, 1997.
16. Taylor JAM, Greene-DesLauriers K, Tanaka DI: Ehlers-Danlos syndrome. J Manip Physiol Therap 13:273, 1990.
17. Wardinski TD, Pagon RA, Powell BR, et al: Rhizomelic chondrodysplasia punctata and survival beyond one year: A review of the literature and five case reports. Clin Genet 38:84, 1990.
18. Helfet DL: Fractures of the distal femur. *In* Browner BD, Jupiter JB, Levine AM, et al (eds): Skeletal Trauma: Fractures, Dislocations, Ligamentous Injuries. Philadelphia, WB Saunders, 1992, p 1643.
19. Hohl M, Larson RL, Jones DC: Fractures and dislocations of the knee. *In* Rockwood CA Jr, Green DP (eds): Fractures in Adults. 2nd Ed. Philadelphia, JB Lippincott, 1984, p 1429.
20. Lewis SL, Pozo JL, Muirhead-Allwood WFG: Coronal fractures of the lateral femoral condyle. J Bone Joint Surg [Br] 71:118, 1989.
21. Lotke PA, Ecker ML: Transverse fractures of the patella. Clin Orthop 158:180, 1981.
22. Mason RW, Moore TE, Walker CW, et al: Patellar fatigue fractures. Skeletal Radiol 25:329, 1996.
23. Bates DG, Hresko MT, Jaramillo D: Patellar sleeve fracture: Demonstration with MR imaging. Radiology 193:825, 1994.
24. Lloyd-Roberts GC, Jackson AM, Albert JS: Avulsion of the distal pole of the patella in cerebral palsy: A cause of deteriorating gait. J Bone Joint Surg [Br] 67:252, 1985.
25. Anglen JO, Healy WL: Tibial plateau fractures. Orthopedics 11:1527, 1988.
26. Tscherne H, Lobenhoffer P: Tibial plateau fractures: Management and expected results. Clin Orthop 292:87, 1993.
27. Barrow BA, Fajman WA, Parker LM, et al: Tibial plateau fractures: Evaluation with MR imaging. RadioGraphics 14:553, 1994.
28. Sonin AH, Fitzgerald SW, Hoff FL, et al: MR imaging of the posterior cruciate ligament: Normal, abnormal, and associated injury patterns. RadioGraphics 15:551, 1995.
29. Bock GW, Bosch E, Mishra DK, et al: The healed Segond fracture: A characteristic residual bone excrescence. Skeletal Radiol 23:555, 1994.
30. Kleinman PK, Marks SC Jr: A regional approach to the classic metaphyseal lesion in abused infants: The distal femur. AJR 170:43, 1998.
31. Kleinman PK, Marks SC Jr: A regional approach to the metaphyseal lesion in abused infants: Proximal tibia. AJR 166:421, 1996.
32. Harcke HT, Snyder M, Caro PA, et al: Growth plate of the normal knee: Evaluation with MR imaging. Radiology 183:119, 1992.
33. Frankl U, Waisilewski SA, Healy WL: Avulsion fracture of the tibial tubercle with avulsion of the patellar ligament: Report of two cases. J Bone Joint Surg [Am] 72:1411, 1990.
34. Ogden JA, Tross RB, Murphy MJ: Fractures of the tibial tuberosity in adolescents. J Bone Joint Surg [Am] 62:205,1980.
35. Kujala UM, Kvist M, Heinonen O: Osgood-Schlatter's disease in adolescent athletes: Retrospective study of incidence and duration. Am J Sports Med 13:236, 1985.
36. Milgram JW: Injury to articular cartilage joint surfaces: Displaced fractures of underlying bone. Clin Orthop 206:236, 1986.
37. Hodler J, Resnick D: Current status of imaging of articular cartilage. Skeletal Radiol 25:703, 1996.
38. Milgram JW: Radiological and pathological manifestations of osteochondritis dissecans of the distal femur: A study of 50 cases. Radiology 126:305, 1978.
39. Brossman J, Preidler K-W, Baenen B, et al: Imaging of osseous and cartilaginous intraarticular bodies in the knee: Comparison of MR imaging and MR arthrography with CT and CT arthrography in cadavers. Radiology 200:509, 1996.
40. DeSmet AA, Ilahi OA, Graf BK: Untreated osteochondritis dissecans of the femoral condyles: Prediction of patient outcome using radiographic and MR findings. Skeletal Radiol 26:463, 1997.
41. Pfeiffer WH, Gross ML, Seeger LL: Osteochondritis dissecans of the patella: MRI evaluation and a case report. Clin Orthop 271:207, 1991.
42. Kaufman SL, Martin LG: Arterial injuries associated with complete dislocation of the knee. Radiology 184:153, 1992.
43. Yu JS, Goodwin D, Salonen D, et al: Complete dislocation of the knee: Spectrum of associated soft-tissue injuries depicted by MR imaging. AJR 164:135, 1995.
44. Kirsch MD, Fitzgerald SW, Friedman H, et al: Transient

lateral patellar dislocation: Diagnosis with MR imaging. AJR 161:109, 1993.
45. Kaneko K, De Mony EH, Robinson AE: Distribution of joint effusion in patients with knee joint disorders: MRI assessment. Clin Imaging 17:176, 1993.
46. Butt WP, Lederman H, Chuang S: Radiology of the suprapatellar region. Clin Radiol 34:511, 1983.
47. Maffulli N, Binfield PM, King JB, et al: Acute hemarthrosis of the knee in athletes: A prospective study of 106 cases. J Bone Joint Surg [Br] 75:945, 1993.
48. Kier R, McCarthy SM: Lipohemarthrosis of the knee: MR imaging. J Comput Assist Tomogr 14:395, 1990.
49. Lugo-Olivieri CH, Scott WW Jr, Zerhouni EA: Fluid-fluid levels in injured knees: Do they always represent lipohemarthrosis? Radiology 198:499, 1996.
50. Ryu KN, Jaovisidha S, De Maeseneer M, et al: Evolving stages of lipohemarthrosis of the knee: Sequential magnetic resonance imaging findings in cadavers with clinical correlation. Invest Radiol 32:7, 1997.
51. Janzen DL, Peterfy CG, Forbes JR, et al: Cystic lesions around the knee joint: MR imaging findings. AJR 163:155, 1994.
52. Butler MG, Fuchigami KD, Chako A: MRI of posterior knee masses. Skeletal Radiol 25:309, 1996.
53. Ward WG, Eckardt JJ: Ganglion cyst of the proximal tibiofibular joint causing anterior compartment syndrome: A case report and anatomical study. J Bone Joint Surg [Am] 76:1561, 1994.
54. Nokes SR, Koonce TW, Montanez J: Ganglion cysts of the cruciate ligaments of the knee: Recognition on MR images and CT-guided aspiration. AJR 162:1503, 1994.
55. Johnson DP, Eastwood DM, Witherow PJ: Symptomatic synovial plicae of the knee. J Bone Joint Surg [Am] 75:1485, 1993.
56. Myllymäki T, Tikkakoski T, Typpö T, et al: Carpet-layer's knee: An ultrasonographic study. Acta Radiol Diagn 34:496, 1993.
57. Flandry F, McCann SB, Hughston JC, et al: Roentgenographic findings in pigmented villonodular synovitis of the knee. Clin Orthop 247:208, 1989.
58. Hughes TH, Sartoris DJ, Schweitzer ME, et al: Pigmented villonodular synovitis: MRI characteristics. Skeletal Radiol 24:7, 1995.
59. Kramer J, Recht M, Deely DM, et al: MR appearance of idiopathic synovial osteochondromatosis. J Comput Assist Tomogr 17:772, 1993.
60. Hodler J, Haghighi P, Pathria MN, et al: Meniscal changes in the elderly: Correlation of MR imaging and histologic findings. Radiology 184:221, 1992.
61. Stark JE, Siegel MJ, Weinberger E, et al: Discoid menisci in children: MR features. J Comp Assist Tomogr 19:608, 1995.
62. Tyson LL, Daughters TC Jr, Ryu RKN, et al: MRI appearance of meniscal cysts. Skeletal Radiol 24:421, 1995.
63. Yu JS, Resnick D: Meniscal ossicle: MR imaging appearance in three patients. Skeletal Radiol 23:637, 1994.
64. Schnarkowski P, Tirman PFJ, Fuchigama KD, et al: Meniscal ossicle: Radiographic and MR imaging findings. Radiology 196:47, 1995.
65. Stoller DW, Martin C, Crues JV III, et al: Meniscal tears: Pathologic correlation with MR imaging. Radiology 163:731, 1987.
66. Mesgarzadeh M, Moyer R, Leder DS, et al: MR imaging of the knee: Expanded classification and pitfalls in the interpretation of meniscal tears. RadioGraphics 13:489, 1993.
67. Firooznia H, Golimbu C, Rafii M: MR imaging of the menisci: Fundamentals of anatomy and pathology. MRI Clin North Am 2:325, 1994.
68. Wright DH, De Smet AA, Norris M: Bucket-handle tears of the medial and lateral menisci of the knee: Value of MR imaging in detecting displaced fragments. AJR 165:621, 1995.
69. Schweitzer ME, Tran D, Deely DM, et al: Medial collateral ligament injuries: Evaluation of multiple signs, prevalence and location of associated bone bruises, and assessment with MR imaging. Radiology 194:825, 1995.
70. Garvin GJ, Munk PL, Vellet AD: Tears of the medial collateral ligament: Magnetic resonance imaging findings and associated injuries. J Can Assoc Radiol 44:199, 1993.
71. Ruiz ME, Erickson SJ: Medial and lateral supporting structures of the knee: Normal MR imaging anatomy and pathologic findings. MRI Clin North Am 2:381, 1994.
72. Speer KP, Warren RF, Wickiewicz TL, et al: Observations on the injury mechanism of anterior cruciate ligament tears in skiers. Am J Sports Med 23:77, 1995.
73. Liu SH, Osti L, Henry M, et al: The diagnosis of acute complete tears of the anterior cruciate ligament: Comparison of MRI, arthrometry, and clinical examination. J Bone Joint Surg [Br] 77:586, 1995.
74. Yu JS, Bosch E, Pathria MN, et al: Deep lateral femoral sulcus: Study of 124 patients with anterior cruciate ligament tear. Emerg Radiol 2:129, 1995.
75. Brandser EA, Riley MA, Berbaum KS, et al: MR imaging of anterior cruciate ligament injury: Independent value of primary and secondary signs. AJR 167:121, 1996.
76. Sonin AH, Fitzgerald SW, Friedman H, et al: Posterior cruciate ligament injury: MR imaging diagnosis and patterns of injury. Radiology 190:455, 1994.
77. Johnson DP, Wekely CJ, Watt I: Magnetic resonance imaging of patellar tendinitis. J Bone Joint Surg [Br] 78:452, 1996.
78. Yu JS, Popp JE, Kaeding CC, et al: Correlation of MR imaging and pathologic findings in athletes undergoing surgery for patellar tendinitis. AJR 165:115, 1995.
79. Siwek CW, Rao JP: Ruptures of the extensor mechanism of the knee joint. J Bone Joint Surg [Am] 74:435, 1992.
80. Kuivila TE, Brems JJ: Diagnosis of acute rupture of the quadriceps tendon by magnetic resonance imaging: A case report. Clin Orthop 262:236, 1991.
81. Berg EE, Mason SL, Lucas MJ: Patellar height ratios: A comparison of four measurement methods. Am J Sports Med 24:218, 1996.
82. Shellock FG, Mink JH, Deutsch AL, et al: Patellofemoral joint: Identification of abnormalities with active-movement, "unloaded" versus "loaded" kinematic MR imaging techniques. Radiology 188:575, 1993.
83. Brossman J, Muhle C, Büll CC, et al: Evaluation of patellar tracking in patients with suspected patellar malalignment: Cine MR imaging vs. arthroscopy. AJR 162:361, 1994.
84. Ficat RP, Hungerford DS: Disorders of the Patello-Femoral Joint. Baltimore, Williams & Wilkins, 1977.
85. Conway WF, Hayes CW, Loughran T, et al: Cross-sectional imaging of the patellofemoral joint and surrounding structures. RadioGraphics 11:195, 1991.
86. Barrett JP Jr, Rashkoff E, Sirna EC, et al: Correlation of roentgenographic patterns and clinical manifestations of symptomatic idiopathic osteoarthritis of the knee. Clin Orthop 253:179, 1990.
87. Preidler KW, Resnick D: Imaging of osteoarthritis. Radiol Clin North Am 34:259, 1996.
88. Resnick D, Shaul SR, Robins JM: Diffuse idiopathic

skeletal hyperostosis (DISH): Forestier's disease with extraspinal manifestations. Radiology 115:513, 1975.
89. Resnick D: Diagnosis of Bone and Joint Disorders. 3rd Ed. Philadelphia, WB Saunders, 1995.
90. Fiszman P, Ansell BM, Renton P: Radiological assessment of knees in juvenile chronic arthritis (juvenile rheumatoid arthritis). Scand J Rheumatol 10:145, 1981.
91. Azouz EM, Duffy CM: Juvenile spondyloarthropathies: Clinical manifestations and medical imaging. Skeletal Radiol 24:399, 1995.
92. Schurman JR II, Wilde AH: Total knee replacement after spontaneous osseous ankylosis: A report of three cases. J Bone Joint Surg [Am] 72:455, 1990.
93. Martel W, Braunstein EM, Borlaza G, et al: Radiologic features of Reiter's syndrome. Radiology 132:1, 1979.
94. Pritchard CH, Berney S: Patellar tendon rupture in systemic lupus erythematosus. J Rheumatol 16:786, 1989.
95. Pachman LN: Juvenile dermatomyositis. Pediatr Clin North Am 33:1097, 1986.
96. Shiokawa S, Yasuda M, Kikuchi M, et al: Mixed connective tissue disease associated with lupus lymphadenitis. J Rheumatol 20:147, 1993.
97. Basanti M, Hardin JG: Undifferentiated, overlapping, and mixed connective tissue diseases. Am J Med Sci 305:114, 1993.
98. Resnick D, Niwayama G, Georgen TG, et al: Clinical, radiographic and pathologic abnormalities in calcium pyrophosphate dihydrate deposition disease (CPPD): Pseudogout. Radiology 122:1, 1977.
99. Mitrovic DR, Stankovic A, Iriarte-Borda O, et al: The prevalence of chondrocalcinosis in the human knee joint: An autopsy survey. J Rheumatol 15:633, 1988.
100. Steinbach LS, Resnick D: Calcium pyrophosphate dihydrate crystal deposition disease revisited. Radiology 200:1, 1996.
101. Recht MP, Seragini F, Kramer J, et al: Isolated or dominant lesions of the patella in gout: A report of seven patients. Skeletal Radiol 23:113, 1994.
102. Faraawi R, Harth M, Kertesz A, et al: Arthritis in hemochromatosis. J Rheumatol 20:448, 1993.
103. Handelsman JE: The knee joint in hemophilia. Orthop Clin North Am 10:139, 1979.
104. Vincent GM, Amirault JD: Septic arthritis in the elderly. Clin Orthop 251:241, 1990.
105. Haygood TM, Williamson SL: Radiographic findings of extremity tuberculosis in childhood: Back to the future? RadioGraphics 14:561, 1994.
106. Rougraff BT, Kneisl JS, Simon MA: Skeletal metastases of unknown origin: A prospective study of a diagnostic strategy. J Bone Joint Surg [Am] 75:1276, 1993.
107. Kyle RA: Multiple myeloma: Review of 869 cases. Mayo Clin Proc 50:29, 1975.
108. Bloem JL, Mulder JD: Chondroblastoma: A clinical and radiological study of 104 cases. Skeletal Radiol 14:1, 1985.
109. Weatherall PT, Maale GE, Mendelsohn DB, et al: Chondroblastoma: Classic and confusing appearance at MR imaging. Radiology 190:467, 1994.
110. De Dios AMV, Bond JR, Shives TC, et al: Aneurysmal bone cyst: A clinico-pathologic study of 238 cases. Cancer 69:2921, 1992.
111. Stuhl MA, Moser RP Jr, Vinh TN, et al: Paget's disease of the patella. Skeletal Radiol 19:407, 1990.
112. Mirra JM, Brien EW, Tehranzadeh J: Paget's disease of bone: Review with emphasis on radiologic features. Part II. Skeletal Radiol 24:173, 1995.
113. Mankin HJ: Rickets, osteomalacia, and renal osteodystrophy. Orthop Clin North Am 21:81, 1990.
114. Pineda C: Diagnostic imaging in hypertrophic osteoarthropathy. Clin Exp Rheumatol 10:27, 1992.
115. Sprague PL: Epiphyseo-metaphyseal cupping following infantile scurvy. Pediatr Radiol 4:122, 1976.
116. Kricun ME, Resnick D: Patellofemoral abnormalities in renal osteodystrophy. Radiology 143:667, 1982.
117. Tigges S, Nance EP, Carpenter WA, et al: Renal osteodystrophy: Imaging findings that mimic those of other diseases. AJR 165:143, 1995.
118. Chew FS, Huang-Hellinger F: Brown tumor. AJR 160:752, 1993.
119. Wolfson BH, Capitanio MA: The wide spectrum of renal osteodystrophy in children. CRC Crit Rev Diagn Imaging 27:297, 1987.
120. Bjorkengren AG, AlRowaih A, Lindstrand A, et al: Spontaneous osteonecrosis of the knee: Value of MR imaging in determining prognosis. AJR 154:331, 1990.
121. Phillips KA, Nance EP Jr, Rodriguez RM, et al: Avascular necrosis of bone: A manifestation of Cushing's disease. South Med J 79:825, 1986.
122. Lee KR, Cox GG, Neff JR, et al: Cystic masses of the knee: Arthrographic and CT evaluation. AJR 148:329, 1987.

CHAPTER 10

Tibia and Fibula

- Anatomic Variants, Skeletal Dysplasias, and Other Congenital Diseases
- Physical Injury
- Neoplasms
- Metabolic and Hematologic Disorders
- Infectious Disorders

Anatomic Variants, Skeletal Dysplasias, and Other Congenital Diseases

A number of anatomic variants, skeletal dysplasias, and other congenital conditions affect the tibia and its surrounding structures. Table 10–1 and Figures 10–1 to 10–6 represent selected examples of some of the more common processes.

Physical Injury

The tibial and fibular diaphyses and metaphyses are sites of acute fracture, fatigue fracture, and insufficiency fracture. Additionally, the muscles of the leg are a frequent site for posttraumatic heterotopic ossification. These conditions and others are described in Table 10–2 and are illustrated in Figures 10–7 to 10–12. Injuries of the proximal and distal portions of the tibia and the fibula are discussed in Chapters 9 and 11, respectively.

Neoplasms

The tibia and the fibula frequently are affected by malignant and benign tumors and tumor-like processes. Tables 10–3 to 10–5 list some of the characteristics of these disorders. Their radiographic manifestations are illustrated in Figures 10–13 to 10–36.

Metabolic and Hematologic Disorders

Several metabolic and hematologic disorders involve the tibia and fibula and their related soft tissues. Table 10–6 lists some of the more common disorders and describes their characteristics. Their radiographic features are illustrated in Figures 10–37 to 10–50. Further manifestations of these disorders within the proximal and distal portions of the tibia and the fibula are described in Chapters 9 and 11, respectively.

Infectious Disorders

The tibia is one of the most common sites of osteomyelitis. Table 10–7 lists some of the more typical forms of osteomyelitis that affect the tibia and fibula and describes their characteristics. The radiographic features of these disorders are illustrated in Figures 10–51 to 10–57. Further manifestations of infection within the proximal and distal portions of the tibia and the fibula are described in Chapters 9 and 11, respectively.

TABLE 10–1. Anatomic Variants, Skeletal Dysplasias, and Other Congenital Diseases Affecting the Tibia and the Fibula*

Entity	Figure(s)	Characteristics
Limb length inequality[1–3]	10–1	Synonyms: anisomelia, leg length discrepancy, short leg syndrome Etiology: developmental, paralysis, infection, trauma, neoplasm, joint replacement surgery Accurate assessment aids in treatment planning Three imaging techniques may be used for measuring the length of the femur and tibia: 1. Orthoradiograph: single exposure of entire length of both lower extremities on a long film; may be obtained supine or standing 2. Radiographic scanogram: three separate exposures are obtained of the hips, knees, and ankles; the patient is immobilized in a supine position, and the x-ray tube and cassettte are moved to expose all three anatomic regions on one film 3. Computed tomographic (CT) scanogram: an anteroposterior scout scanogram of both lower extremities is obtained; cursors are placed at the superior tip of the capital femoral epiphysis and the most distal portion of the lateral femoral condyle and measurements are obtained; tibial length is determined in a similar manner by measuring from the tibial plateau to the tibial plafond; lateral views of the femur and tibia also may be obtained and measured to account for limb flexion; CT scanograms are accurate and result in less radiation exposure than radiographic techniques, and they are particularly useful in patients with joint contractures
Infantile tibia vara (Blount's disease)[4]	10–2	Painless local disturbance of growth usually is first recognized between the ages of 1 and 3 years Less commonly, an adolescent type is encountered in which the deformity appears between the ages of 8 and 15 years Affects the medial aspect of the proximal portion of the tibia, resulting in tibial bowing within the first few years of life More common in black persons Believed to be more prevalent in children who begin to walk at an early age
Focal fibrocartilaginous dysplasia[95]		Synonym: focal fibrocartilaginous dysplasia associated with tibia vara Rare dysplasia involving fibrous and cartilaginous tissue at the pes anserinus insertion into the tibia Results in a unilateral deformity of the proximal end of the tibia with a prominent cortical defect within the medial proximal tibial metaphysis and varus deformity of the diametaphyseal portion of the tibia Deformity appears as early as 2 months of age and resembles the deformity of Blount's disease
Osteopetrosis[5]		Diffuse osteosclerosis results in brittle bones and predisposition to pathologic fracture
Osteopoikilosis[6]		Mutiple 2- to 3-mm circular foci of osteosclerosis Symmetric periarticular lesions resembling bone islands predominate about the knee
Osteopathia striata[7]		Regular, linear, vertically oriented bands of osteosclerosis extending from the metaphysis for variable distances into the diaphysis Long lesions frequently are found in the tibia Metaphyseal flaring of the tibia also may be seen with osteopathia striata
Melorheostosis[8, 9]	10–3	Hemimelic distribution of peripherally located cortical hyperostosis resembling flowing candle wax on the surface of the tibia or fibula Para-articular soft tissue calcification and ossification may occur and may even lead to joint ankylosis
Mixed sclerosing bone dystrophy[10]	10–4	Rare condition in which patients have radiologic findings characteristic of more than one and occasionally all of the sclerosing dysplasias
Osteogenesis imperfecta[11]	10–5	Severe osteoporosis Pencil-thin cortices Multiple fractures Bowing of long bones Rare cystic form—ballooning of bone, metaphyseal flaring, and honeycombed appearance of thick trabeculae
Progressive diaphyseal dysplasia[12]	10–6	Camurati-Engelmann disease Bilateral fusiform thickening of the diaphyses of the tibia and fibula Cortical thickening and hyperostosis result in increased diaphyseal radiodensity

*See also Tables 1–1 and 1–2.

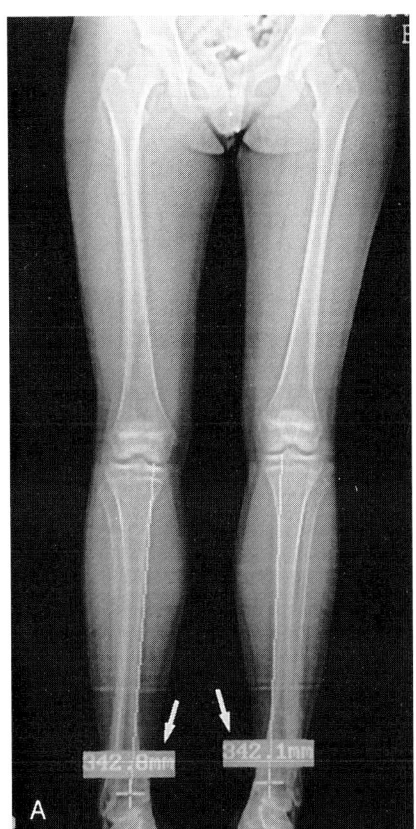

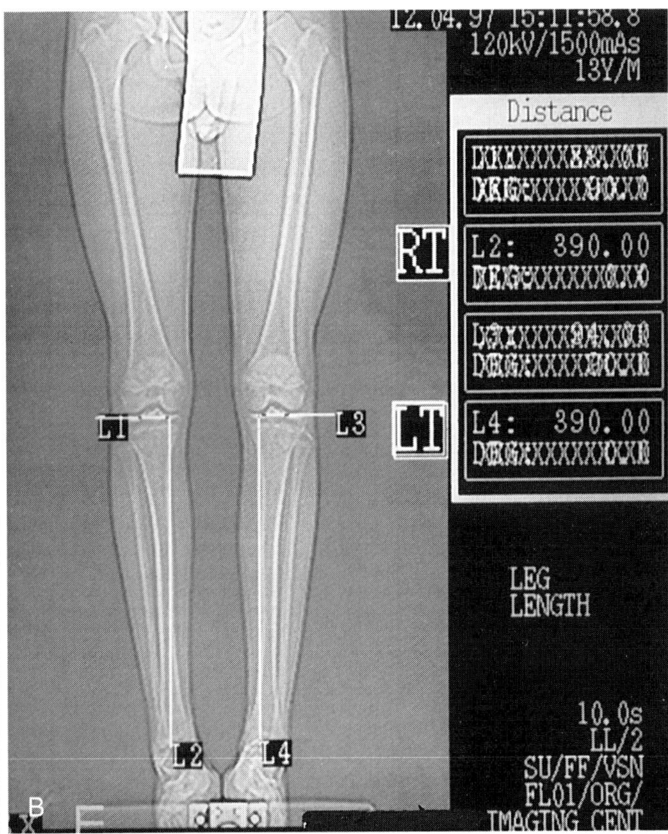

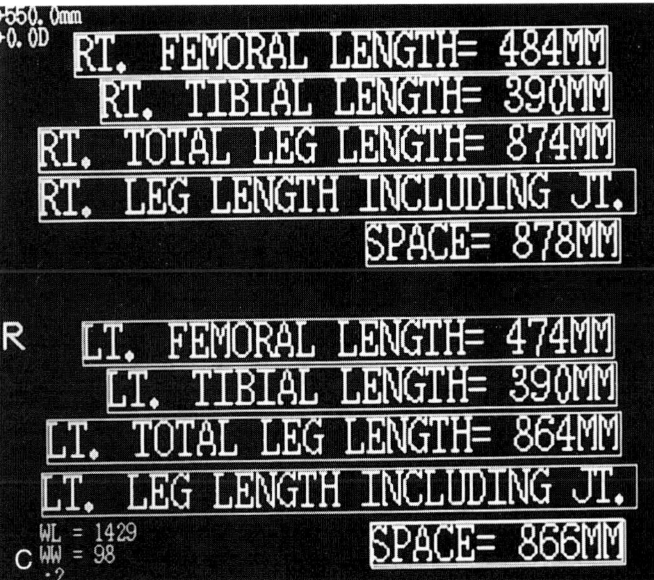

FIGURE 10–1. Limb length inequality: measurement with computed tomographic (CT) scanogram.[1–3] In this procedure, both lower extremities are imaged in the supine position, and precise anatomic measurements of the tibiae and fibulae are made. **A** In this patient, the left tibia measures 342.1 mm and the right tibia measures 342.8 mm (arrows). The left tibia, therefore, is only 0.7 mm shorter than the right tibia. Similar measurements of the femur and entire lower extremity also are obtained. **B** In another patient, the tibiae are equal in length (390 mm). **C** A computerized display in the same patient (**B**) displays the precise length measurements of tibia, femur, and total leg bilaterally.

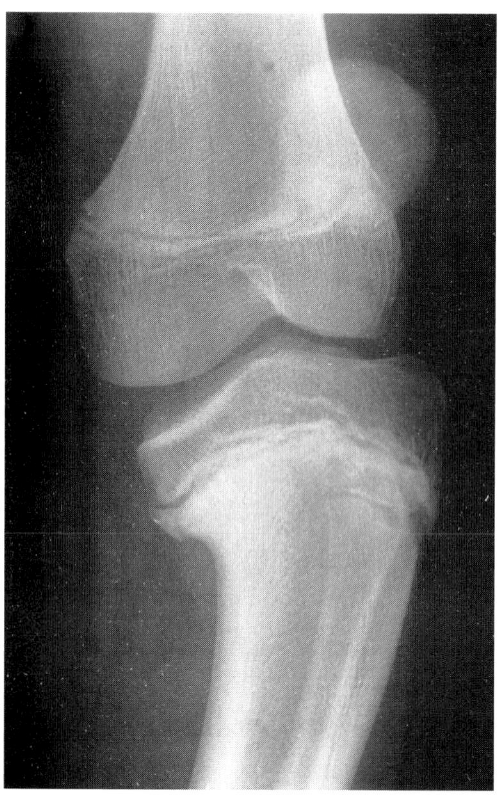

FIGURE 10–2. Blount's disease: Infantile tibia vara.[4] In this 11-year-old girl, observe the varus deformity of the tibia with epiphyseal deformity and prominence and sclerosis of the proximal medial tibial metaphyses. Prominent tibial torsion is also present.

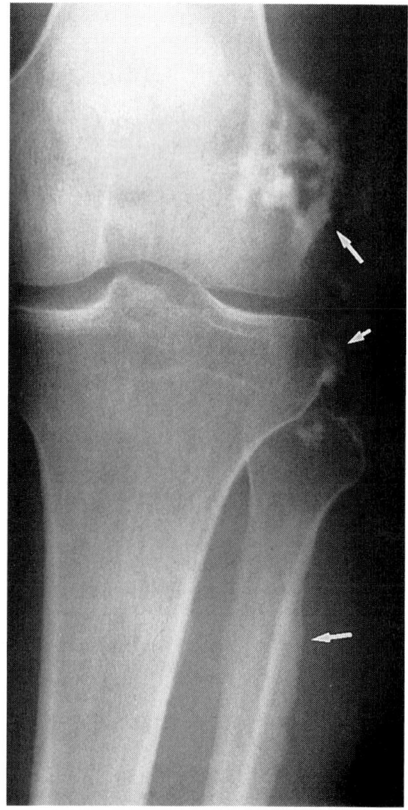

FIGURE 10–3. Melorheostosis.[8, 9] Observe the characteristic radiographic abnormalities of asymmetric hyperostosis simulating flowing candle wax affecting the proximal portion of the fibula. Cloud-like accumulations of hyperostosis and soft tissue ossification also are seen adjacent to the distal portion of the femur and the proximal portion of the tibia (arrows). *(Courtesy of A. Newberg, M.D., Boston, Massachusetts.)*

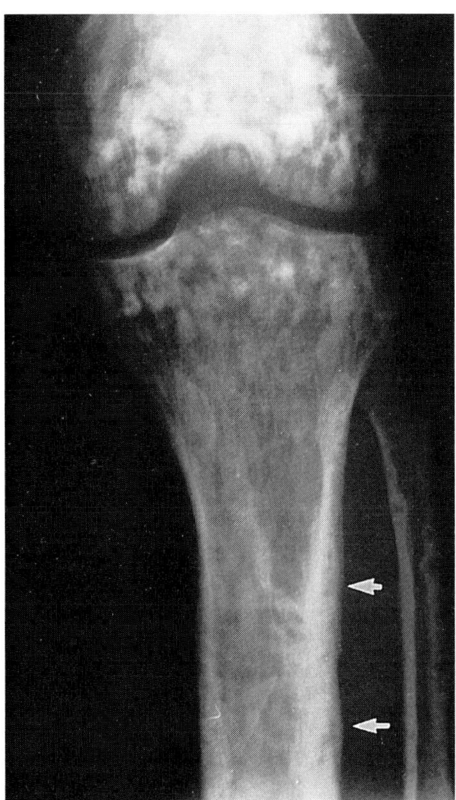

FIGURE 10–4. Mixed sclerosing bone dystrophy.[10] Evidence of both linear hyperostosis characteristic of melorheostosis (arrows) and punctate zones of sclerosis typical of osteopoikilosis are seen in the proximal part of the tibia and the distal end of the femur in this patient. *(Courtesy of C. Resnik, M.D., Baltimore, Maryland.)*

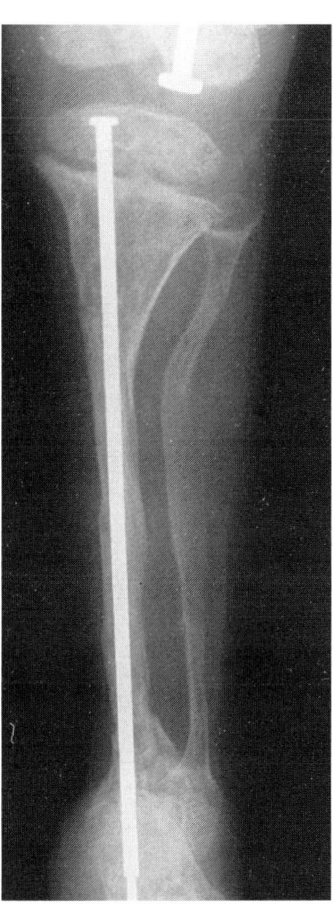

FIGURE 10–5. Osteogenesis imperfecta.[11] Characteristic radiographic findings in the tibia and the fibula include severe bowing of the osteoporotic, thin, and gracile bones. Multiple fractures in various stages of healing and intramedullary rods are seen.

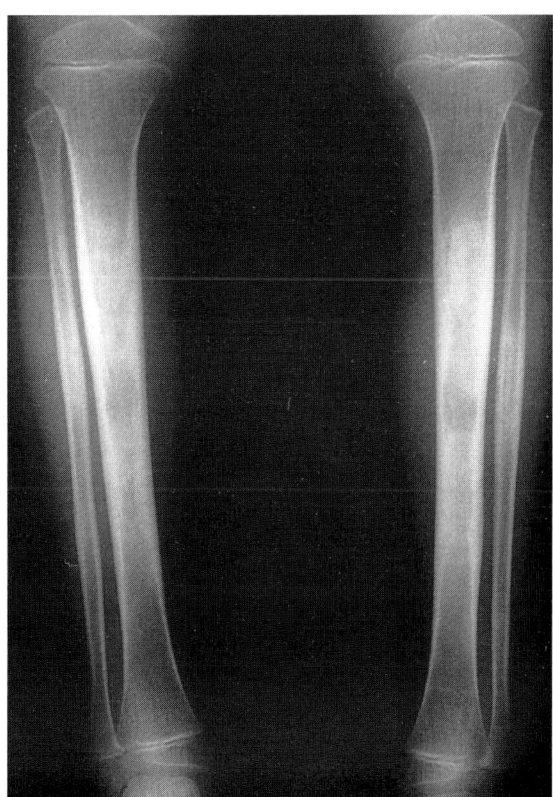

FIGURE 10–6. Progressive diaphyseal dysplasia (Camurati-Engelmann disease).[12] Observe the exuberant fusiform, hyperostotic bone formation and cortical thickening within the diaphyses of the tibiae and fibulae.

TABLE 10–2. Fractures of the Tibial and Fibular Diaphyses and Soft Tissue Injury*

Entity	Figure(s)	Characteristics	Complications and Related Injuries
Tibia			
Acute tibial fractures[13, 14]	10–7	Direct trauma: transverse or comminuted fracture Indirect trauma: oblique, spiral, or segmental fractures Middle and distal thirds > proximal third Prognosis related to amount of displacement, degree of comminution, open or closed fracture, and infection Proximal metaphyseal fracture may be associated with genu valgum deformity in children Uncomplicated tibial shaft fractures should heal within 16 to 18 weeks in adults and more quickly in children	Associated fractures of the fibula, especially in direct and severe trauma Delayed union (5–15 per cent of cases) Nonunion (most common in distal third of tibia) Infection with or without nonunion Vascular injury (to anterior tibial artery or, less commonly, posterior tibial artery) Compartment syndrome (anterior > posterior or lateral compartment) Nerve injury (uncommon, peroneal and posterior tibial nerves) Refracture (especially in athletes) Leg shortening Reflex sympathetic dystrophy Fat embolism
Acute childhood fractures[15]	10–8	Toddler fracture: nondisplaced spiral fracture in children 1 to 3 years of age May be occult on initial radiographs and may require bone scintigraphy or serial radiographs to reveal the fracture	
Stress injuries			
Fatigue fractures[16–20]	10–9	Stress fractures of the proximal portion of the tibia usually are fatigue fractures and occur in children as a result of running activities Transverse and, less commonly, longitudinal fractures may be identified Fractures often are occult on radiographs	May result in complete fracture with or without displacement
Insufficiency fractures[21, 22]	10–10	Predisposing disorders: osteoporosis, rheumatoid arthritis, osteomalacia, rickets, and other bone diseases	
Shin splints[96]		Synonyms: shin soreness, shin splint syndrome, medial tibial stress syndrome, soleus syndrome Usually related to athletic activity, especially running Pathophysiology is controversial—postulates include: 1. Fatigue damage in bone (atypical fatigue fracture) 2. Traction periostitis at origin of tibialis posterior muscle or insertion of crural fascia (soleus bridge) 3. Compartment syndrome Radiographs usually are normal Magnetic resonance (MR) imaging more useful in acute cases; may result in false negative results in patients with chronic symptoms Three-phase radionuclide bone scan may reveal abnormal linear longitudinal uptake	The relationship of shin splints and fatigue fractures is controversial, but both may represent fatigue damage to bone
Fibula			
Acute fibular fractures[23]	10–11	Isolated fractures related to direct injury are rare Maisonneuve fracture: fracture of the proximal portion of the fibula associated with severe ankle injuries; because of dramatic ankle symptoms, the proximal fibular fracture may initially be overlooked	Often associated with fractures of the tibia and injuries of the ankle
Posttraumatic heterotopic ossification[24]	10–12	Faint calcific intermuscular or intramuscular shadow may appear within 2 to 6 weeks of injury Well-defined region of ossification aligned parallel to the long axis of the tibia or fibula may be evident within 6 to 8 weeks Usually involves gastrocnemius and tibialis anterior muscles Associated periostitis may relate to subperiosteal hemorrhage	Limitation of motion Compartment syndromes May result in abnormal knee biomechanics and lead to premature degeneration May resemble aggressive neoplasms such as osteosarcoma or Ewing's sarcoma

*See also Tables 1–3 and 1–5.

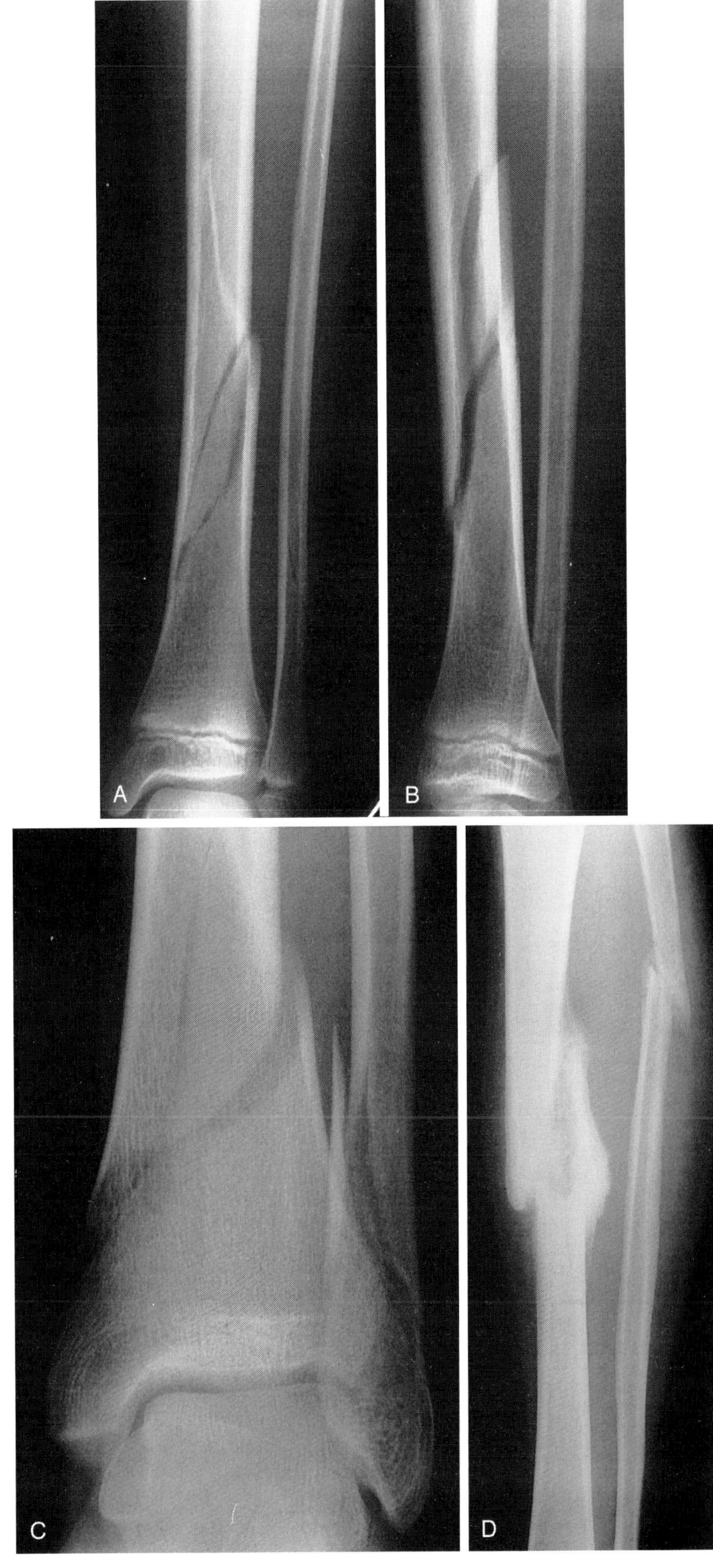

FIGURE 10–7. Tibial diaphysis fractures.[13, 14] A, B Frontal (A) and lateral (B) radiographs of this 10-year-old boy reveal a minimally displaced spiral fracture of the distal tibial diaphysis. C In another patient, a 33-year-old man, spiral fractures of both the tibia and fibula are seen. D In yet another patient with healing fractures of the mid-diaphyses of the tibia and fibula, evidence of callus formation, persistent malalignment, and limb shortening are seen. Spiral tibial (and fibular) fractures are generated by twisting forces applied during falls or sporting activities, such as skiing.

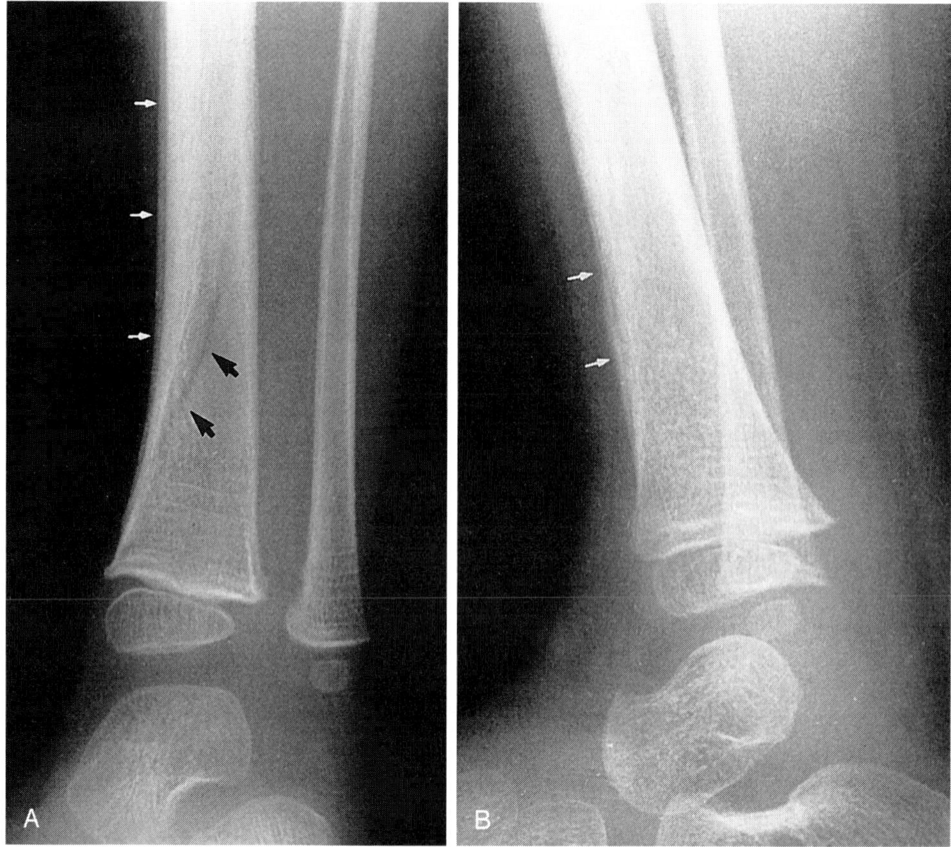

FIGURE 10–8. Toddler's fracture.[15] Two-year-old child with 10-day history of a painful limp. **A** Nondisplaced oblique fracture of the distal end of the tibia is seen on this frontal radiograph (black arrows). An extensive zone of periostitis (white arrows) indicates that healing is taking place. **B** Lateral radiograph reveals periostitis (arrows), but the fracture line is not visible. *(Courtesy of B.L. Harger, D.C., Portland, Oregon.)*

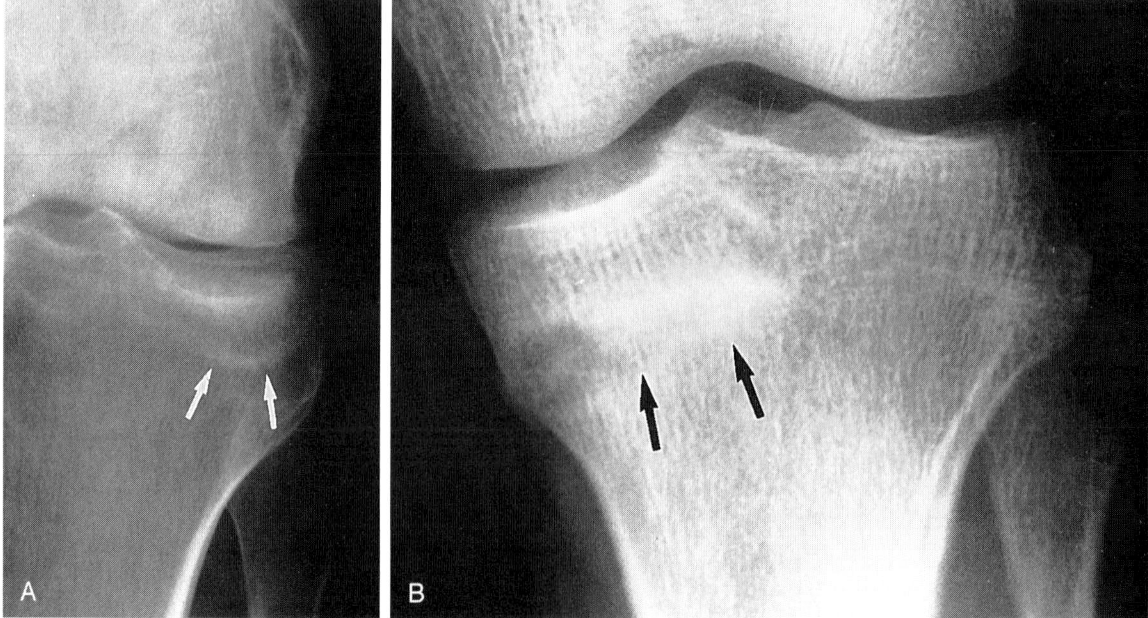

FIGURE 10–9. Stress (fatigue) fractures.[16–20] **A** This 27-year-old woman developed tibial pain after long distance running. Observe the transverse zone of sclerosis within the tibial plateau (arrows) characteristic of a stress fracture. **B** In this 58-year-old woman, a band of increased density (arrows) is apparent in the proximal tibial metaphysis.

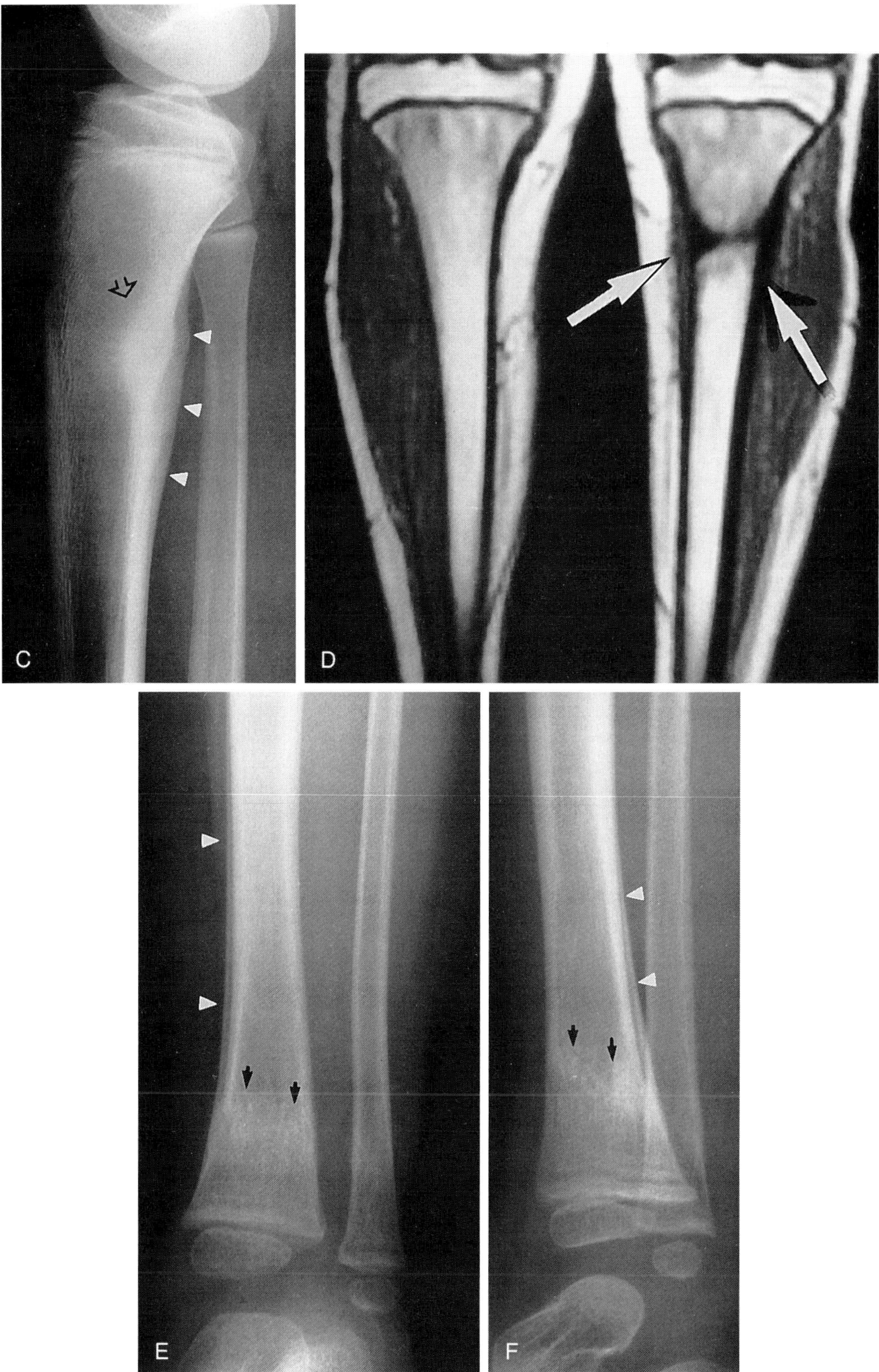

FIGURE 10–9 *Continued.* C, D 12-year-old boy. In C, a transverse zone of sclerosis (open arrow) with a collar of periostitis (arrowheads) is evident on a routine radiograph. In D, a transverse band of low signal intensity on a coronal T1-weighted (TR/TE, 617/20) spin echo magnetic resonance (MR) image also is accompanied by diffuse periosteal new bone formation (arrows). *(C, D, Courtesy of K. Van Lom, M.D., San Diego, California.)* E, F Radiographs of the distal portion of the tibia in this infant reveal a transverse zone of sclerosis (arrows) and extensive periostitis (arrowheads) typical of a fatigue fracture.

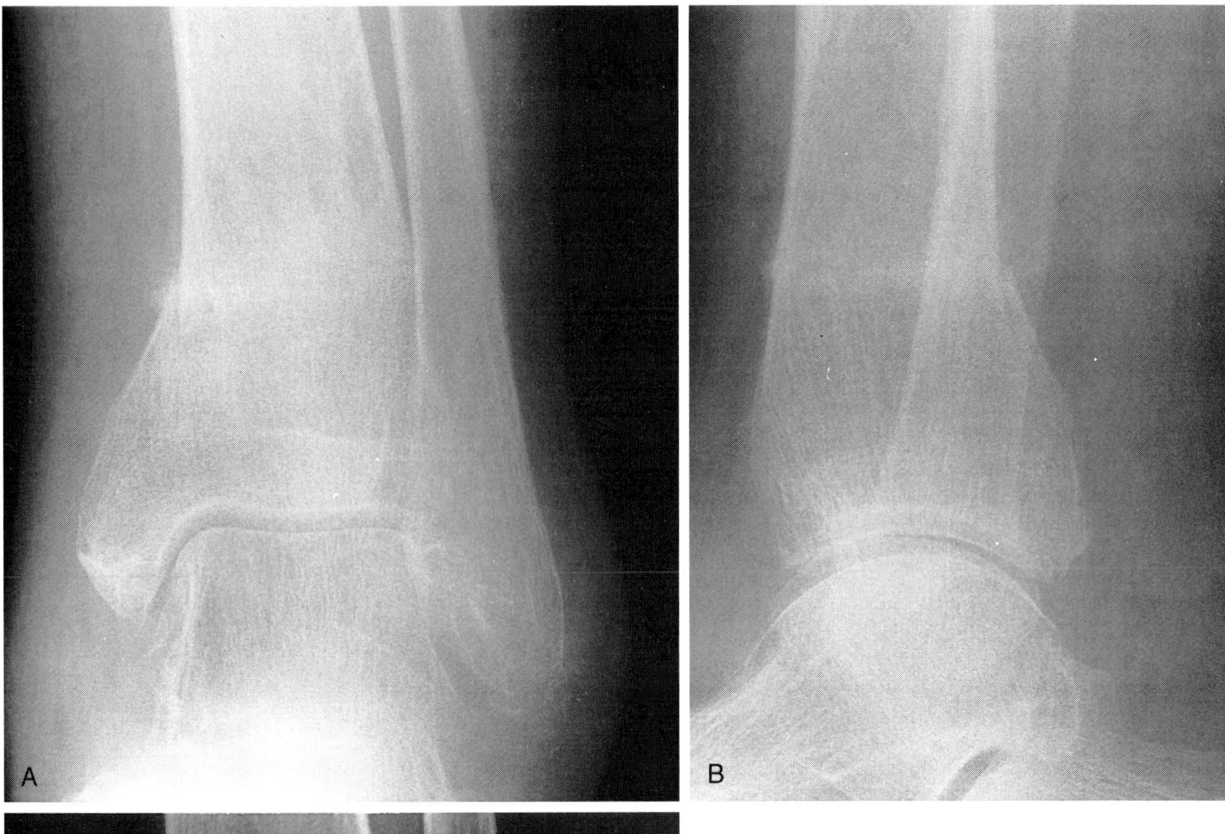

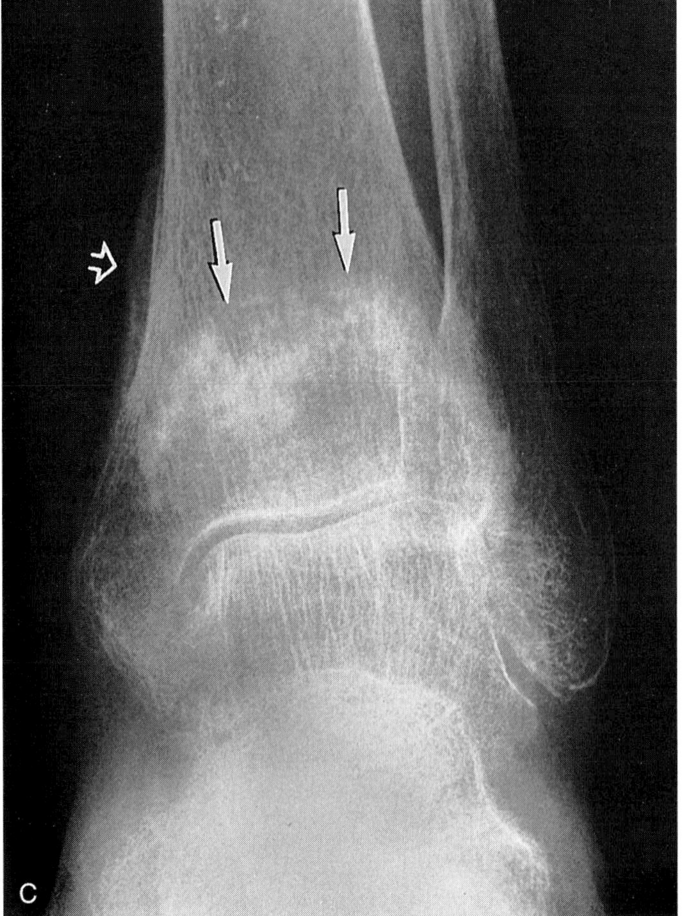

FIGURE 10–10. Insufficiency fractures.[21, 22] A, B Frontal (A) and lateral (B) radiographs of this 62-year-old woman with long-standing rheumatoid arthritis and corticosteroid-induced osteoporosis reveal a transverse insufficiency fracture involving the distal portion of the tibia. Marked soft tissue swelling and minimal offset are noted. C Frontal radiograph of this 58-year-old woman shows an insufficiency fracture through the distal portion of the tibia, a consequence of long-standing rheumatoid arthritis and osteoporosis. Observe the poorly defined zone of mottled sclerosis (arrows) and associated periostitis (open arrow).

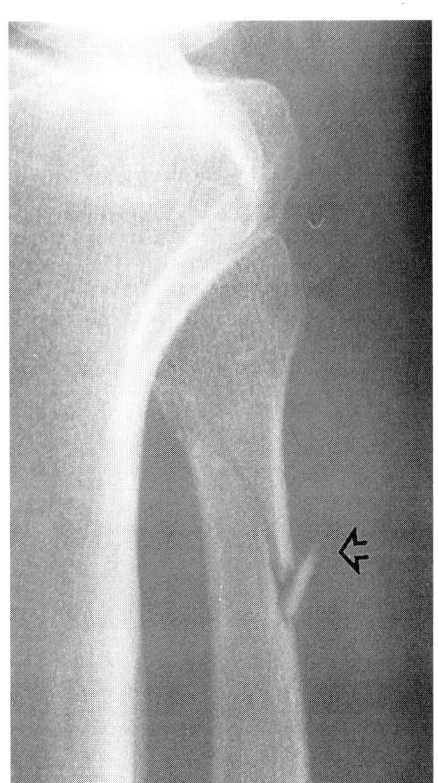

FIGURE 10–11. Proximal fibular fracture: Maisonneuve fracture.[23] This patient sustained a pronation–external rotation stage IV ankle injury rupturing the anterior talofibular ligament and fracturing the proximal portion of the fibula (arrow). This fracture is referred to as a Maisonneuve fracture and usually is associated with severe ankle injuries. Because of the dramatic symptoms about the ankle, the proximal fibular fracture may initially be overlooked.

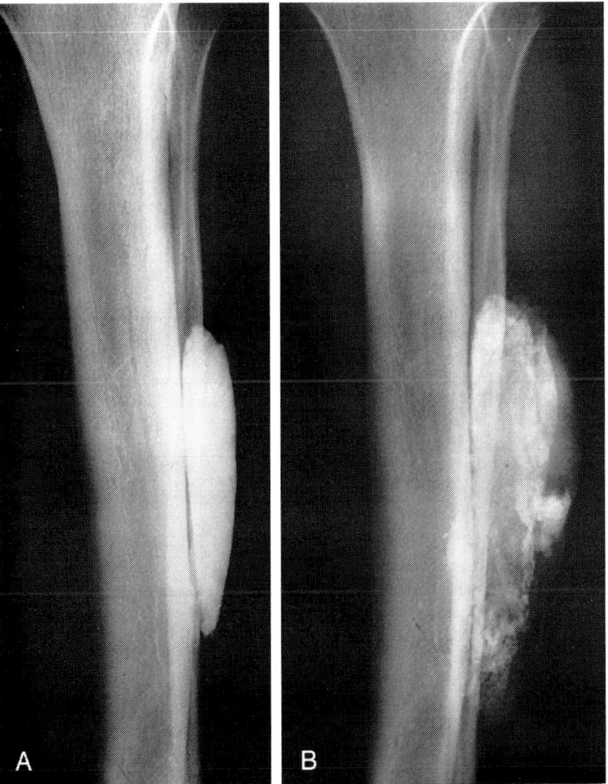

FIGURE 10–12. Posttraumatic heterotopic ossification: Myositis ossificans.[24] Serial radiographs of a 46-year-old man with painful swelling of the leg and a history of repeated injuries. A Initial radiograph reveals a homogeneous, densely sclerotic osseous mass with regular margins in the soft tissues adjacent to the lateral surface of the diaphyseal portion of the tibia, separated from the normal underlying bone by a radiolucent cleft. B Radiograph taken 15 years later demonstrates that the lesion has grown and has become more irregular. Although the underlying bone is grossly normal, a suggestion of mild cortical bulging and endosteal thickening is evident. This case is unusual, because, generally, areas of myositis ossificans merge with the adjacent bone and decrease in size over a varying period of time. The differential diagnosis of myositis ossificans must include aggressive neoplasms such as parosteal, periosteal, and soft tissue osteosarcoma, as well as Ewing's sarcoma.

TABLE 10–3. Malignant Tumors Affecting the Tibia and the Fibula*

Entity	Figure(s)	Characteristics
Skeletal metastasis[25–27]		
Lung, prostate, breast, kidney, thyroid gland	10–13, 10–14	Fewer than 5 per cent of metastatic lesions affect the tibia or fibula Occasional site of cortical metastasis, especially in patients with bronchogenic carcinoma; small radiolucent, eccentric, saucer-shaped, scalloped cortical erosions are referred to as "cookie-bite" lesions
Primary malignant tumors of bone		
Osteosarcoma (conventional)[28]	10–15	Twenty-one per cent of osteosarcomas affect the tibia; 3 per cent affect the fibula Preference for metaphyses Osteolytic, osteosclerotic, or mixed patterns of medullary and cortical destruction Laminated, spiculated, or Codman's triangle periosteal reactions common
Osteosarcoma (parosteal)[29]	10–16	Approximately 10 per cent of parosteal osteosarcomas affect the tibia; 3 per cent affect the fibula Osteosclerotic surface lesion of bone Large radiodense, oval, sessile mass arising from the surface of bone; smooth or irregular margins Peripheral portion of lesion may have cleavage plane separating it from the tibia or fibula Ossification begins centrally and progresses outward, opposite that of benign heterotopic bone formation (myositis ossification)
Osteoblastoma (aggressive)[30]	10–17	Approximately 13 per cent of aggressive osteoblastomas involve the tibia; 6 per cent involve the fibula Expansile osteolytic metaphyseal lesion that may be partially ossified or contain calcium Difficult to differentiate from osteosarcoma or benign osteoblastoma
Chondrosarcoma (conventional)[31]		Fewer than 10 per cent of chondrosarcomas affect the tibia and fibula Lesions tend to be osteolytic; sometimes have a bulky cartilaginous cap and frequently contain calcification May have soft tissue mass
Giant cell tumor (aggressive)[32]		Approximately 17 per cent of aggressive giant cell tumors involve the tibia; 2 per cent involve the fibula Eccentrically located, subarticular osteolytic lesion extending into the metaphysis Cortical destruction and soft tissue mass are variable findings
Fibrosarcoma[33, 34]	10–18	About 16 per cent of fibrosarcomas involve the tibia; 3 per cent involve the fibula Purely osteolytic destruction, soft tissue mass, and no associated sclerotic reaction or periostitis
Malignant fibrous histiocytoma[34]		Approximately 20 per cent affect the tibia; less than 2 per cent affect the fibula Moth-eaten or permeative osteolysis of the metaphysis with frequent spread to epiphysis and diaphysis Pathologic fracture common
Adamantinoma (angioblastoma)[35]	10–19	Tibia is the site of involvement in over 80 per cent of adamantinomas; the fibula is a rare primary site, but it may be involved with adjacent tibial lesions Central or eccentric, multilocular, slightly expansile, sharply or poorly delineated osteolytic lesion with reactive bone sclerosis Periostitis rare May be related to ossifying fibroma (osteofibrous dysplasia) in children and adolescents
Ewing's sarcoma[36]	10–20	Approximately 10 per cent of Ewing's sarcomas involve the tibia and another 10 per cent involve the fibula Permeative or moth-eaten osteolysis, aggressive cortical erosion or violation, laminated or spiculated periostitis and soft tissue masses Most lesions are central and diametaphyseal
Myeloproliferative disorders		
Plasma cell (multiple) myeloma[37]		Fewer than 5 per cent of myeloma lesions occur in the tibia and fibula Early: normal radiographs or diffuse osteopenia Later: widespread, well-circumscribed osteolytic lesions with discrete margins, which usually appear uniform in size
Hodgkin's disease[38]		Infrequent involvement of tibia and fibula 75 per cent of lesions are osteolytic; 25 per cent are osteosclerotic Permeative or moth-eaten osteolysis affecting multiple bones
Primary lymphoma (non-Hodgkin's)[39, 40]	10–21	Of all skeletal lesions in primary lymphoma, about 9 per cent occur in the tibia, and about 2 per cent occur in the fibula Multiple moth-eaten or permeative osteolytic lesions and pathologic fracture Diffuse or localized sclerotic lesions are rare
Leukemia[41]	10–22	Diffuse osteopenia, radiolucent or radiodense transverse metaphyseal bands, osteolytic lesions, periostitis, and, infrequently, osteosclerosis Radiodense metaphyses more frequently in patients undergoing chemotherapy for leukemia; may resemble lead poisoning

*See also Table 1–10.

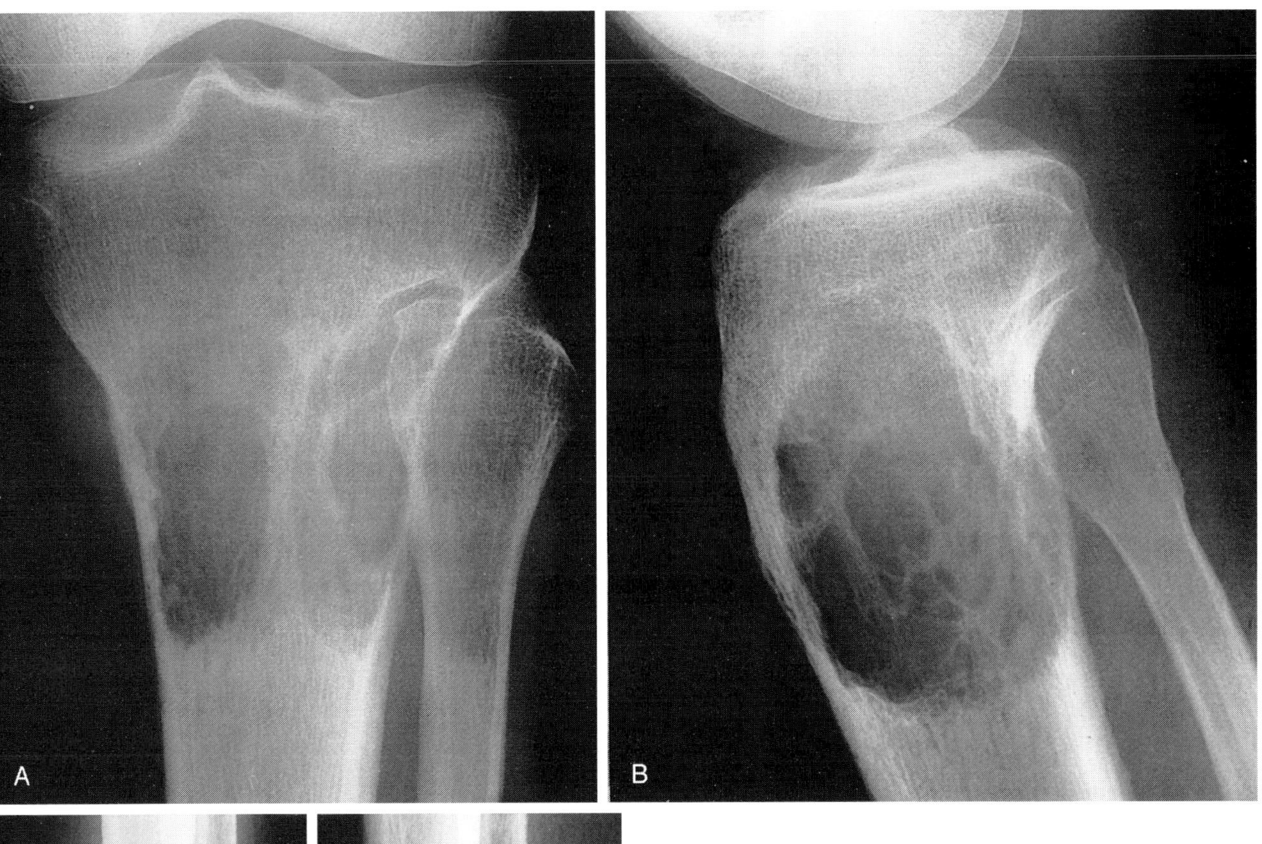

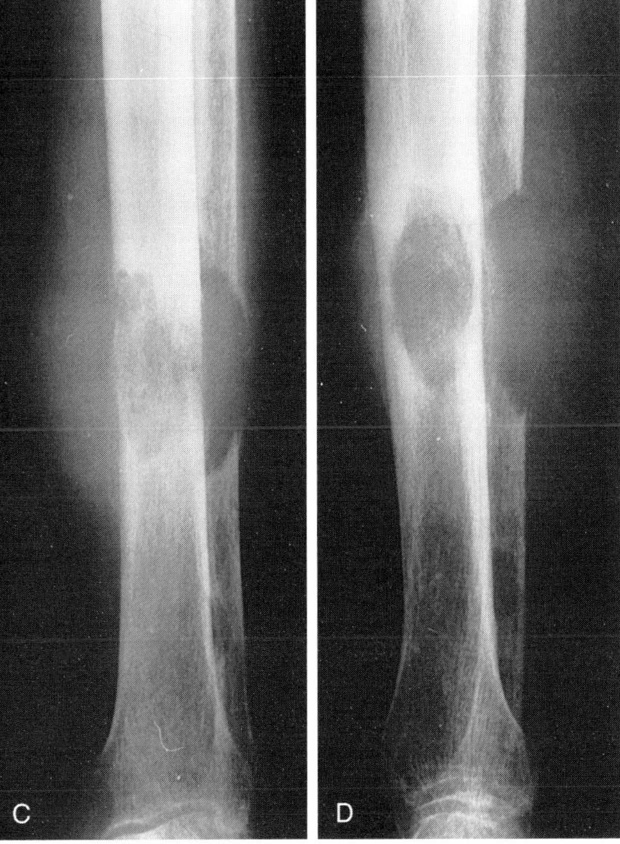

FIGURE 10–13. Skeletal metastasis.[25, 26] A, B Frontal (A) and lateral (B) radiographs of this man with renal cell carcinoma show a large, multiloculated, osteolytic lesion within the proximal tibial metadiaphysis. *(A, B, Courtesy of G. Greenway, M.D., Dallas, Texas.)* C, D Cortical pattern of osteolytic destruction. This patient with primary ovarian carcinoma developed metastasis to bone. Frontal (C) and lateral (D) radiographs demonstrate scalloped erosions of the distal tibial and fibular cortices (cookie-bite lesions). *(C, D, Courtesy of A. D'Abreu, M.D., Porto Alegre, Brazil.)* Although cortical involvement with cookie-bite lesions typically is seen in bronchogenic metastasis, these lesions also may be found with other primary tumors. Ovarian cancer rarely metastasizes to bone.

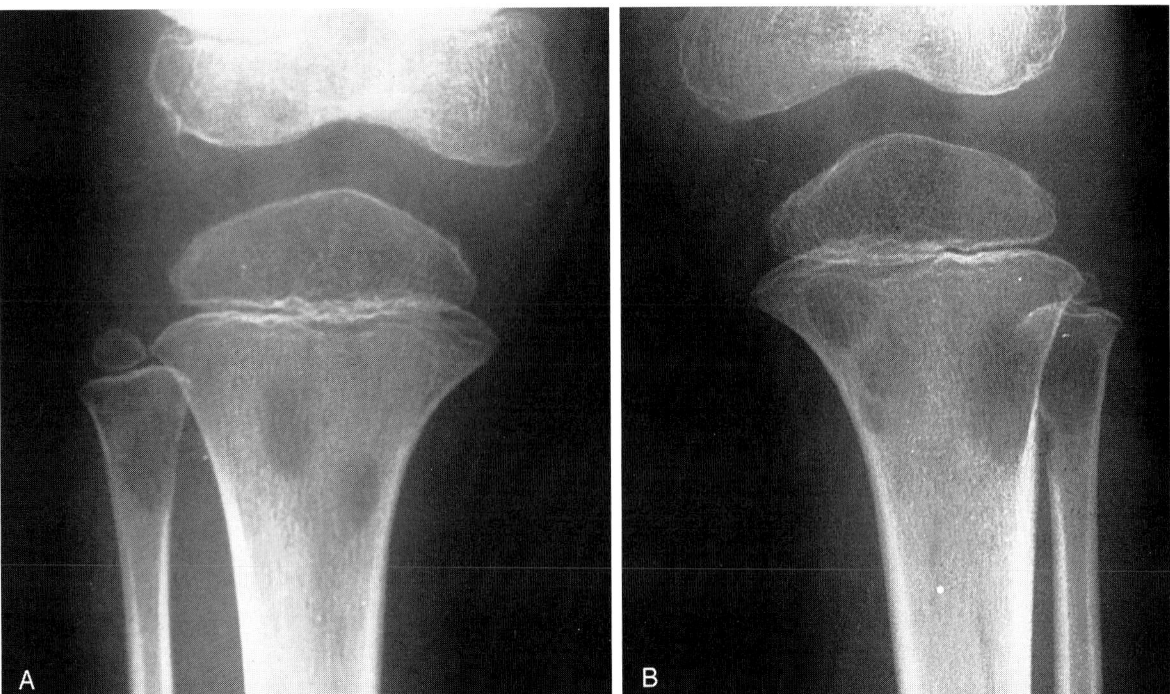

FIGURE 10–14. A, B Skeletal metastasis: Wilms' tumor.[27] This child developed bilateral leg pain. Bilateral frontal radiographs show multiple osteolytic metaphyseal lesions of the proximal portions of the tibiae and fibulae. Wilms' tumor, or nephroblastoma, is the most common abdominal tumor of infancy and childhood. It metastasizes to bone in fewer than 5 per cent of cases, and in those cases it usually is osteolytic.

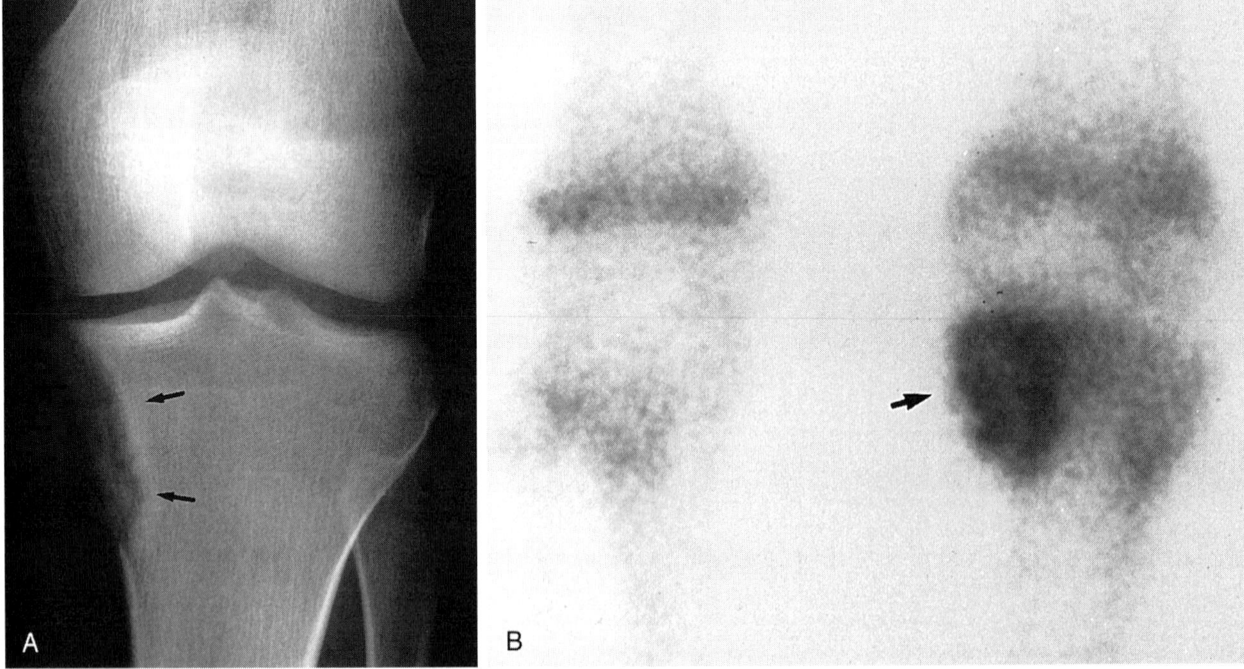

FIGURE 10–15. Conventional osteosarcoma: Osteolytic pattern.[28] This 16-year-old girl complained of long-standing knee pain. A Routine radiograph demonstrates aggressive osteolytic destruction of the proximal tibial metaphysis (arrows). B Bone scan reveals homogeneous, intense, increased uptake of the bone-seeking radionuclide at the site of the lesion (arrow) compared with the minimal uptake at the contralateral tibia. The latter is characteristic of normal growth centers.

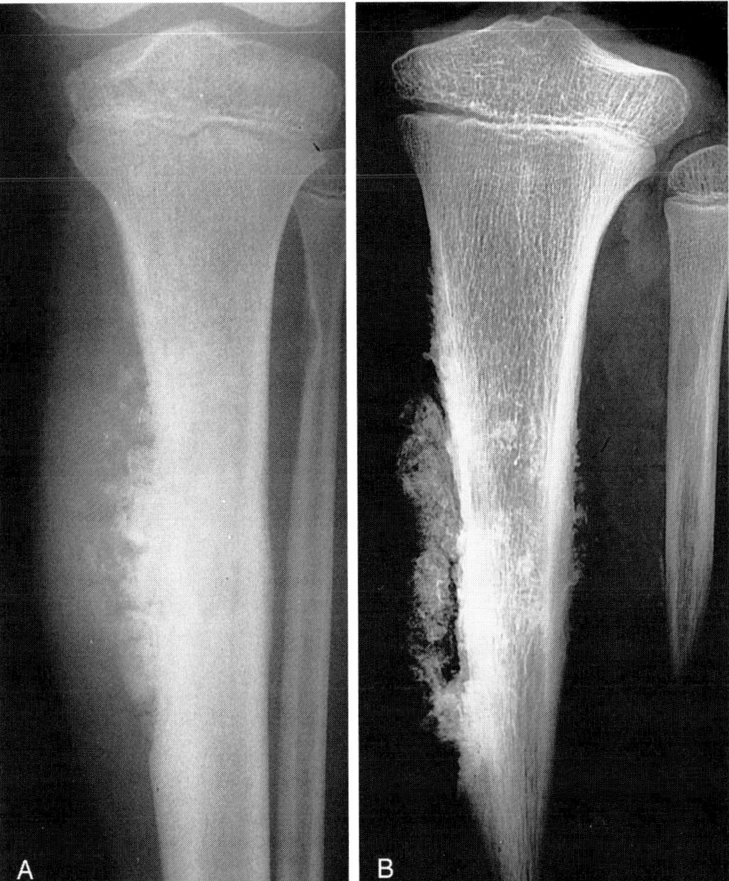

FIGURE 10–16. Parosteal osteosarcoma.[29] This 10-year-old boy underwent amputation for treatment of his sarcoma. **A,** Routine frontal radiograph of the knee shows an aggressive pattern of cortical thickening and radiating cloud-like osseous proliferation on the surface of the medial tibial cortex. A large soft tissue mass overlies the lesion. **B,** Section radiograph of the amputated segment shows similar findings in better detail.

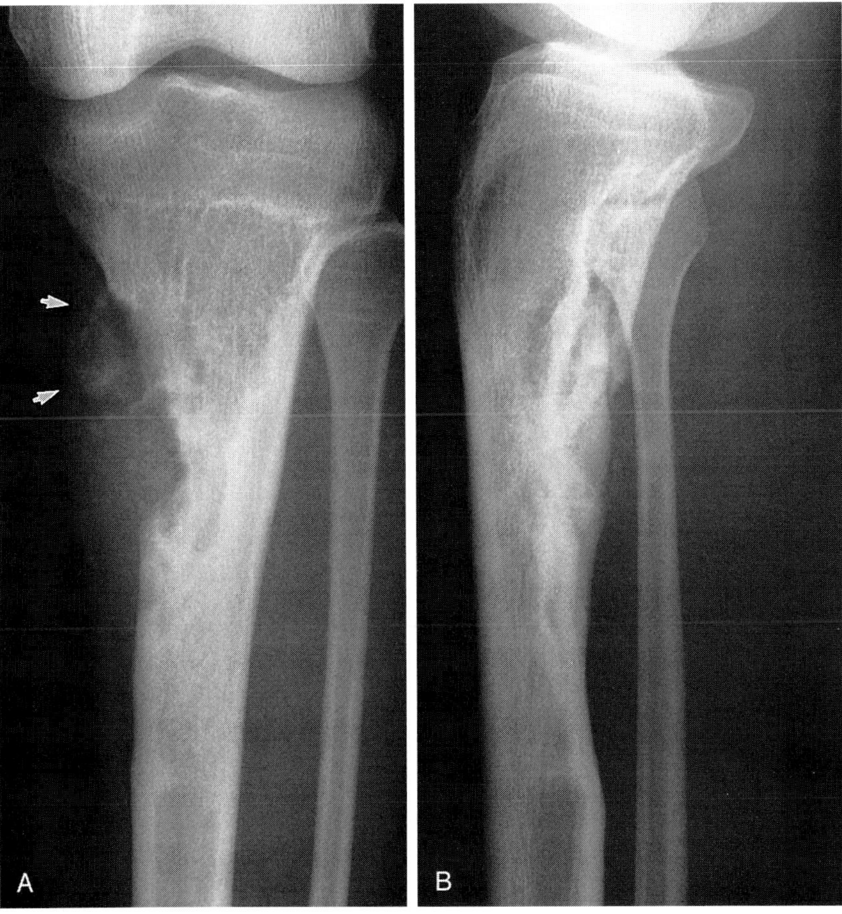

FIGURE 10–17. Aggressive (malignant) osteoblastoma.[30] This 25-year-old woman underwent multiple operations from the age of 16 years for recurrence of her biopsy-confirmed osteoblastoma. Frontal (**A**) and lateral (**B**) radiographs show an aggressive pattern of bone destruction of the medial cortex of the proximal tibial metaphysis. Note the soft tissue extension of the tumor with extraosseous ossification (arrows).

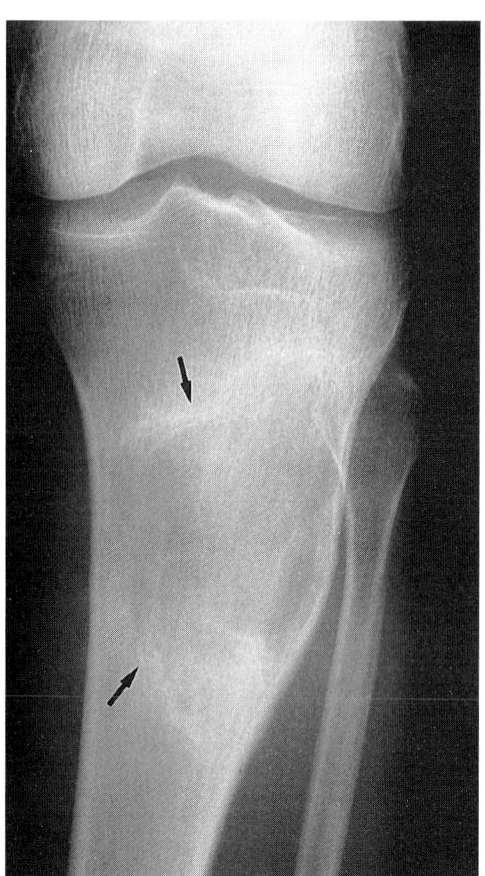

FIGURE 10–18. Fibrosarcoma.[33, 34] An osteolytic lesion within the proximal tibial metaphysis has a deceptively benign appearance, exhibiting a sharp sclerotic zone of transition (arrows) between normal and abnormal bone. Minimal osseous expansion and cortical thinning are evident, but no obvious cortical destruction can be detected. Biopsy revealed a fibrosarcoma of bone. This case illustrates that aggressive malignant tumors can exhibit a relatively benign radiographic appearance.

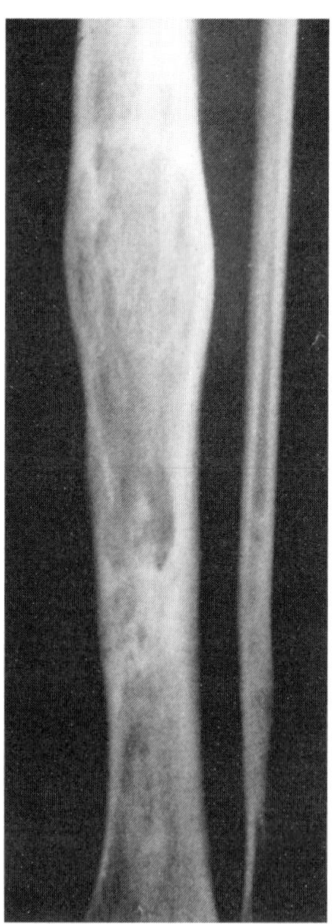

FIGURE 10–19. Adamantinoma (angioblastoma).[35] Lesions accompanied by both sclerosis and osteolysis are evident in the tibia and the fibula. The tibial lesion is slightly expansile, and the margins are poorly defined. *(From Resnick D: Diagnosis of Bone and Joint Disorders. 3rd Ed. Philadelphia, WB Saunders, 1995, p 388.)*

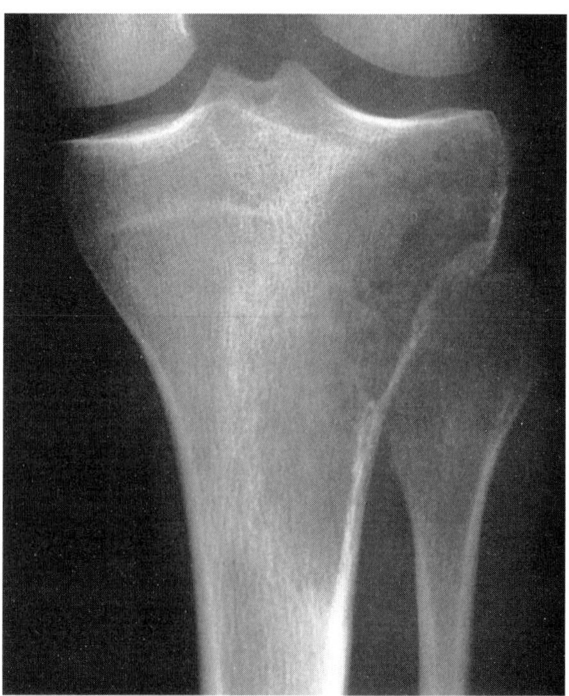

FIGURE 10–20. Ewing's sarcoma.[36] Radiograph of the knee in this 18-year-old woman shows a permeative pattern of purely osteolytic destruction affecting the proximal tibial metaphysis. The lesion extends into the subchondral region and also erodes the cortex of the lateral tibia.

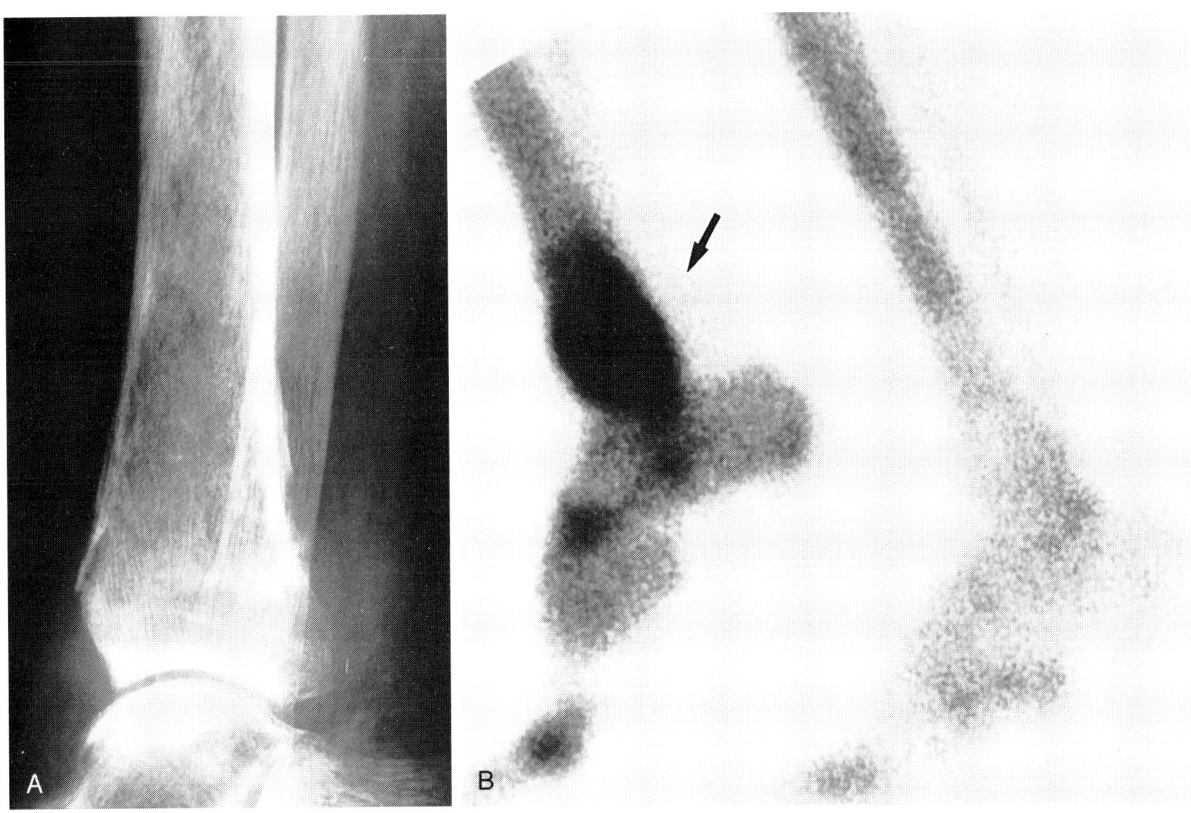

FIGURE 10–21. Non-Hodgkin's lymphoma: Histiocytic type.[39, 40] A Radiograph of this 72-year-old woman reveals diffuse, permeative osteolysis and cortical destruction of the distal end of the tibia. B Bone scan comparing both extremities reveals intense radionuclide accumulation at the involved site (arrow). *(Courtesy of G. Greenway, M.D., Dallas, Texas.)*

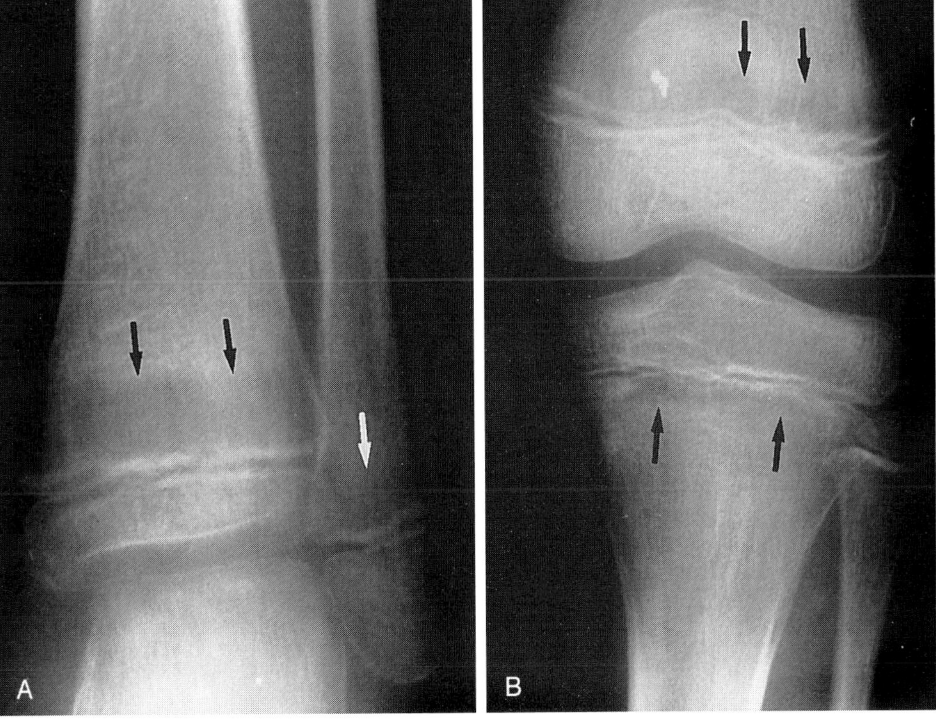

FIGURE 10–22. Acute childhood leukemia.[41] This 8-year-old girl was diagnosed as having acute leukemia. A Radiograph of the distal ends of the tibia and fibula reveals transverse radiolucent bands through the metaphyses (arrows). B Similar radiolucent bands (arrows) are seen in the distal femoral and the proximal tibial metaphyses.

TABLE 10–4. Primary Benign Tumors Affecting the Tibia and the Fibula*

Entity	Figure(s)	Characteristics
Enostosis[42]		Bone island Fewer than 10 per cent of enostoses occur in the tibia and fibula Solitary or multiple circular or oblong discrete foci of osteosclerosis within the spongiosa of bone
Osteoid osteoma[43–45]	10–23	Twenty-four per cent of osteoid osteomas occur in the tibia; 4 per cent occur in the fibula Cortical or subperiosteal lesion; reactive sclerosis surrounding central radiolucent nidus Nidus usually less than 1 cm in diameter and often not visible on routine radiographs
Osteoblastoma (conventional)[46]		Approximately 15 per cent of conventional osteoblastomas occur in the tibia and fibula Osteolytic, osteosclerotic, or both Expansile lesion with cortical thinning Partially calcified matrix in many cases Often resembles large osteoid osteoma May be subperiosteal
Ossifying fibroma[47]	10–24	Also termed osteofibrous dysplasia Rare fibro-osseous lesion of tubular bones occurs almost exclusively in the tibia (and, infrequently, the ipsilateral fibula) Long diaphyseal lesion with intracortical osteolysis clearly marginated by a band of osteosclerosis Hazy or ground-glass appearance reminiscent of fibrous dysplasia Occasionally purely osteosclerotic Osseous expansion Bowing, deformity, and pathologic fracture
Enchondroma (solitary)[48]		Tibia and fibula are infrequent sites of solitary enchondromas Solitary, central, or eccentric medullary osteolytic lesion with lobulated endosteal scalloping Stippled calcification (50 per cent of lesions)
Enchondromatosis (Ollier's)[48]	10–25	Multiple enchondromas Commonly affect the fibula and tibia
Maffucci's syndrome[48]		Multiple enchondromas and soft tissue hemangiomas More than half of patients with Maffucci's syndrome have tibial and fibular involvement Unilateral distribution in 50 per cent of cases
Chondroblastoma[49, 50]		Approximately 18 per cent of chondroblastomas involve the tibia Circular osteolytic lesion affecting the proximal tibial epiphysis, or apophysis of the tibial tubercle May exhibit calcification in matrix
Chondromyxoid fibroma[51]	10–26	Approximately 40 per cent of chondromyxoid fibromas involve the tibia; 8 per cent involve the fibula Eccentric, elongated metaphyseal lesion 2–10 cm in length Cortical expansion, coarse trabeculation, endosteal sclerosis Calcification is rare (5–27 per cent of cases) May appear aggressive with large "bite" lesion penetrating cortex
Osteochondroma (solitary)[52, 53]	10–27	Eighteen per cent of solitary osteochondromas involve the tibia; 4 per cent involve the fibula Pedunculated or sessile cartilage-covered osseous excrescence arising from the surface of the metaphysis of the proximal or distal portion of the tibia or fibula
Hereditary multiple exostosis[54]	10–28	Commonly involves tibia and fibula Multiple sessile and pedunculated osteochondromas
Nonossifying fibroma and fibrous cortical defect[55, 56]	10–29	Forty-three per cent occur in the tibia; 8 per cent occur in the fibula Eccentric, multiloculated osteolytic lesion arising from the metaphyseal cortex Resembles a well-circumscribed blister-like shell of bone arising from the metaphyseal cortex; often bilateral and symmetric May migrate away from the physis with longitudinal metaphyseal growth
Giant cell tumor (benign)[57]	10–30	More than 25 percent of benign giant cell tumors occur in the tibia; 4 per cent occur in the fibula Eccentric osteolytic neoplasm with a predilection for the subarticular region of the proximal portion of the tibia Often multiloculated expansile lesion

TABLE 10–4. Primary Benign Tumors Affecting the Tibia and the Fibula* *Continued*

Entity	Figure(s)	Characteristics
Intraosseous lipoma[58]	10–31	Osteolytic lesion surrounded by a thin, well-defined sclerotic border Central calcified or ossified nidus is common Osseous expansion occasionally Cortical destruction and periostitis absent
Hemangioma (solitary)[59]		Rare in the tibia and fibula Radiolucent, slightly expansile intraosseous lesion Radiating, lattice-like or web-like trabecular pattern Occasional cortical thinning Rarely periostitis, soft tissue mass, or osteosclerosis Intracortical and periosteal forms of hemangioma are extremely rare, but predominate in the tibia and fibula
Simple bone cyst[60]	10–32	Also termed solitary, or unicameral, bone cyst Six per cent of simple bone cysts affect the tibia; 5 per cent affect the fibula Mildly expansile solitary osteolytic lesion within medullary cavity of tibial or fibular metaphyses Multiloculated; may migrate away from the physis with normal longitudinal metaphyseal growth Fallen-fragment sign in patients with pathologic fracture
Aneurysmal bone cyst[61]	10–33	Fifteen per cent of aneurysmal bone cysts involve the tibia; 7 per cent involve the fibula Eccentric, thin-walled, expansile osteolytic lesion of the metaphysis; thin trabeculation with multiloculated appearance Buttressing at edge of lesion

*See also Table 1–11.

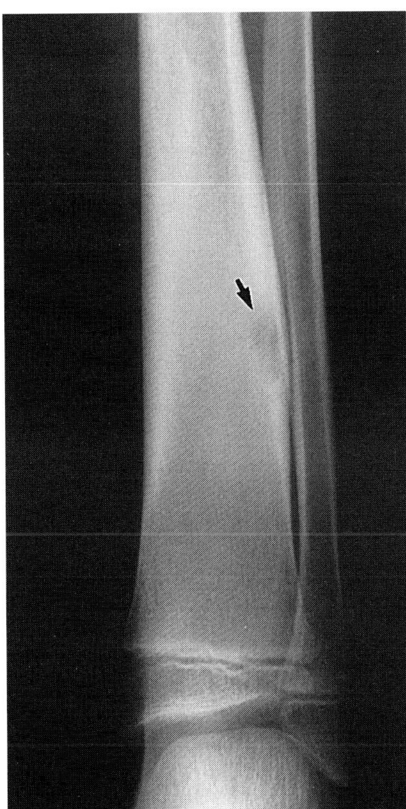

FIGURE 10–23. Osteoid osteoma.[43–45] This 7-year-old boy had a 1-year history of lower leg and ankle pain. The pain was present with activity, worse at night, and relieved by salicylates. Observe the diffuse reactive sclerosis and minimal bone expansion surrounding an eccentric, oval, radiolucent nidus (arrow) within the distal tibial diaphysis. *(Courtesy of G. Greenway, M.D., Dallas, Texas.)*

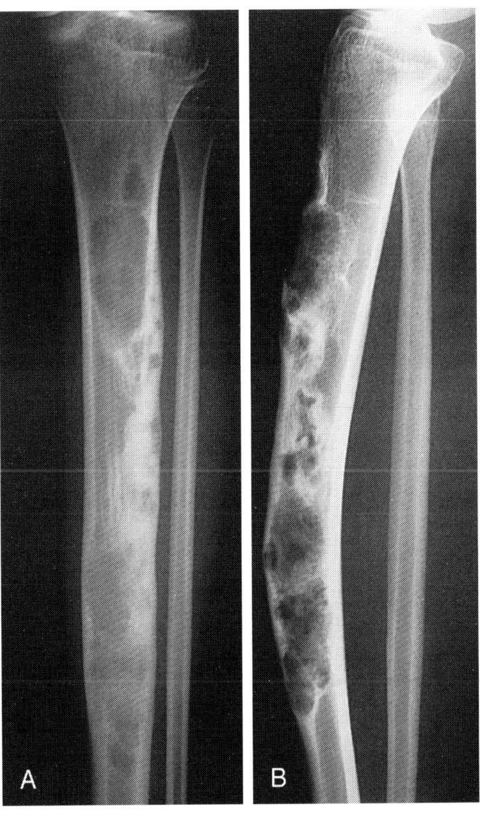

FIGURE 10–24. Ossifying fibroma.[47] Anteroposterior **(A)** and lateral **(B)** radiographs show a sharply marginated, multilocular, radiolucent lesion with associated bone sclerosis, bowing, and osseous expansion involving the tibial diaphysis. The lesions closely resemble those of polyostotic fibrous dysplasia.

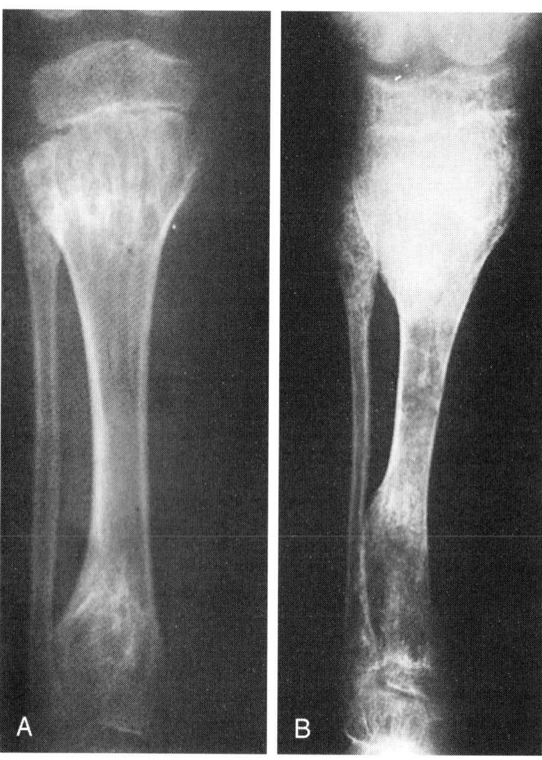

FIGURE 10–25. Enchondromatosis (Ollier's disease).[48] Progressive changes are evident within the tibia and the fibula in a child from the ages of 2 years (A) to 12 years (B). Findings include metaphyseal expansion, stippled calcification, and osseous deformity. Alternatively, lesions may appear multiloculated with endosteal scalloping. *(From Resnick D: Diagnosis of Bone and Joint Disorders. 3rd Ed. Philadelphia, WB Saunders, 1995, p 4214.)*

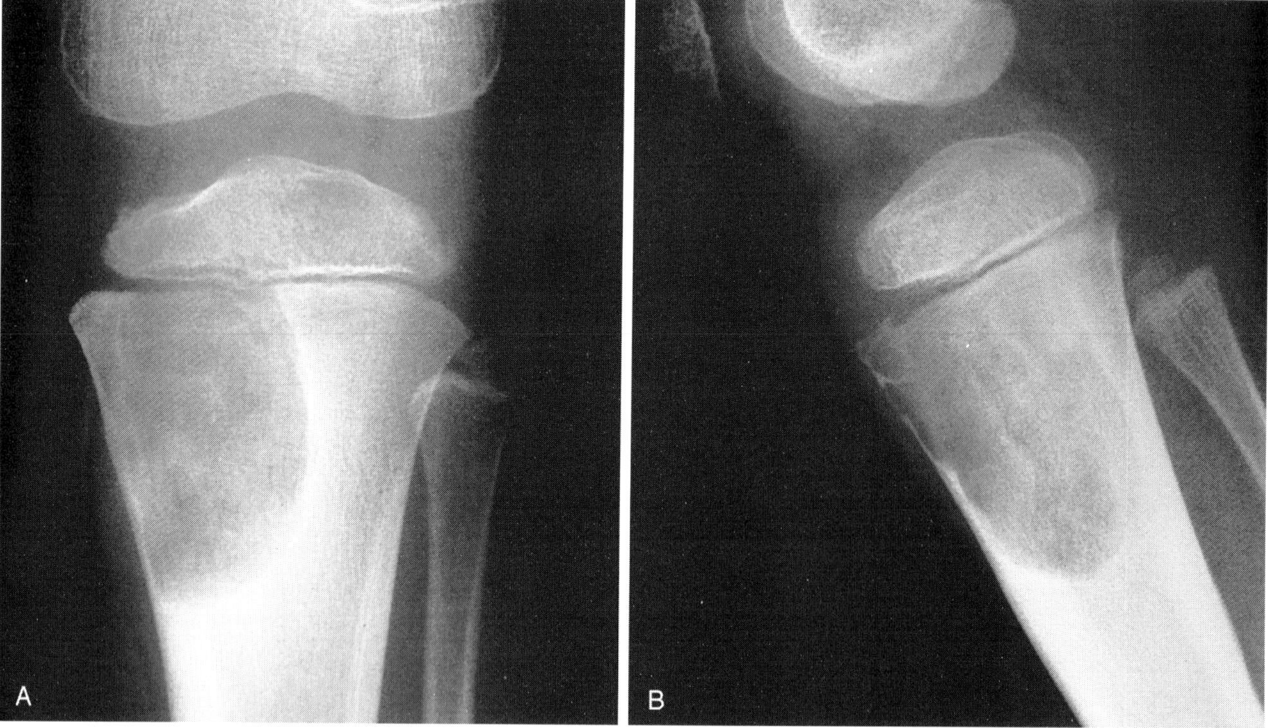

FIGURE 10–26. A, B Chondromyxoid fibroma.[51] Radiographs of the knee in a 6-year-old boy show an eccentric, osteolytic lesion in the proximal tibial metaphysis. A well-defined, sclerotic margin is present. *(Courtesy of D. Goodwin, M.D., Lebanon, New Hampshire.)*

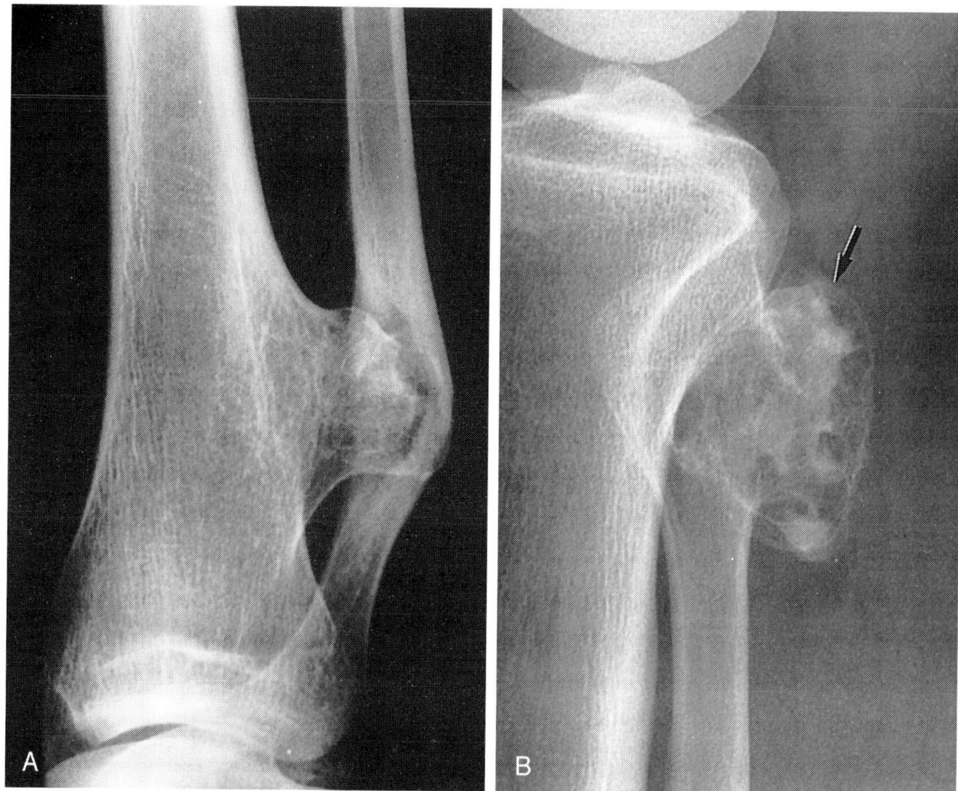

FIGURE 10–27. Solitary osteochondroma.[52, 53] A Tibia. A large pedunculated osteochondroma has resulted in dramatic fibular deformity and remodeling. Almost 20 per cent of osteochondromas occur in the tibia. *(A, Courtesy of J. Slivka, M.D., San Diego, California.)* B Fibula. Lateral radiograph of this 31-year-old man shows a large, expansile cauliflower-shaped osteocartilaginous lesion arising from the proximal metaphysis of the fibula (arrow). Fewer than 5 per cent of osteochondromas arise from the fibula. *(B, Courtesy of R. Thomas, M.D., Santa Ana, California.)*

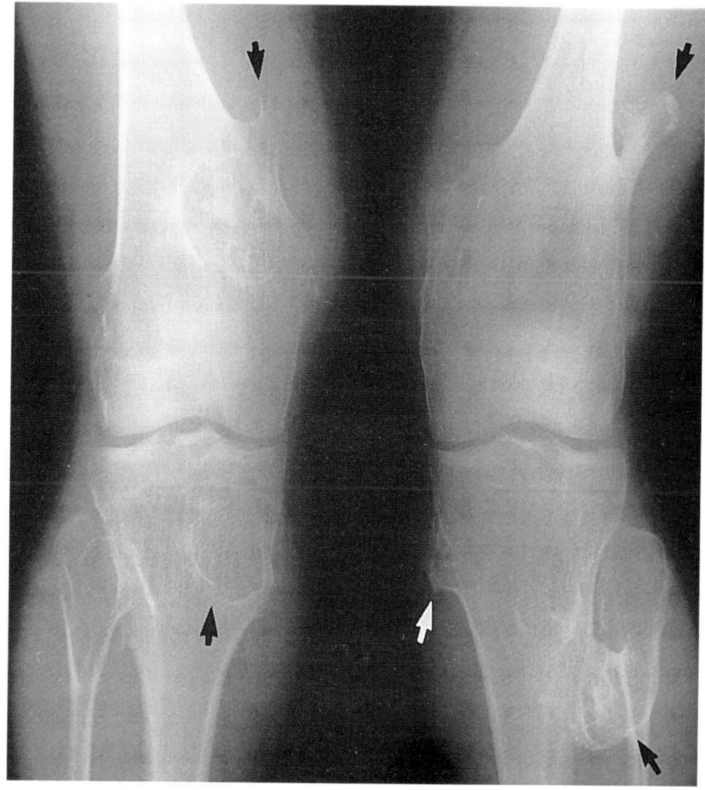

FIGURE 10–28. Hereditary multiple exostosis.[54] Large bilateral sessile and pedunculated osseous outgrowths are seen arising from the metaphyses of the femurs, the tibias, and the fibulas (arrows).

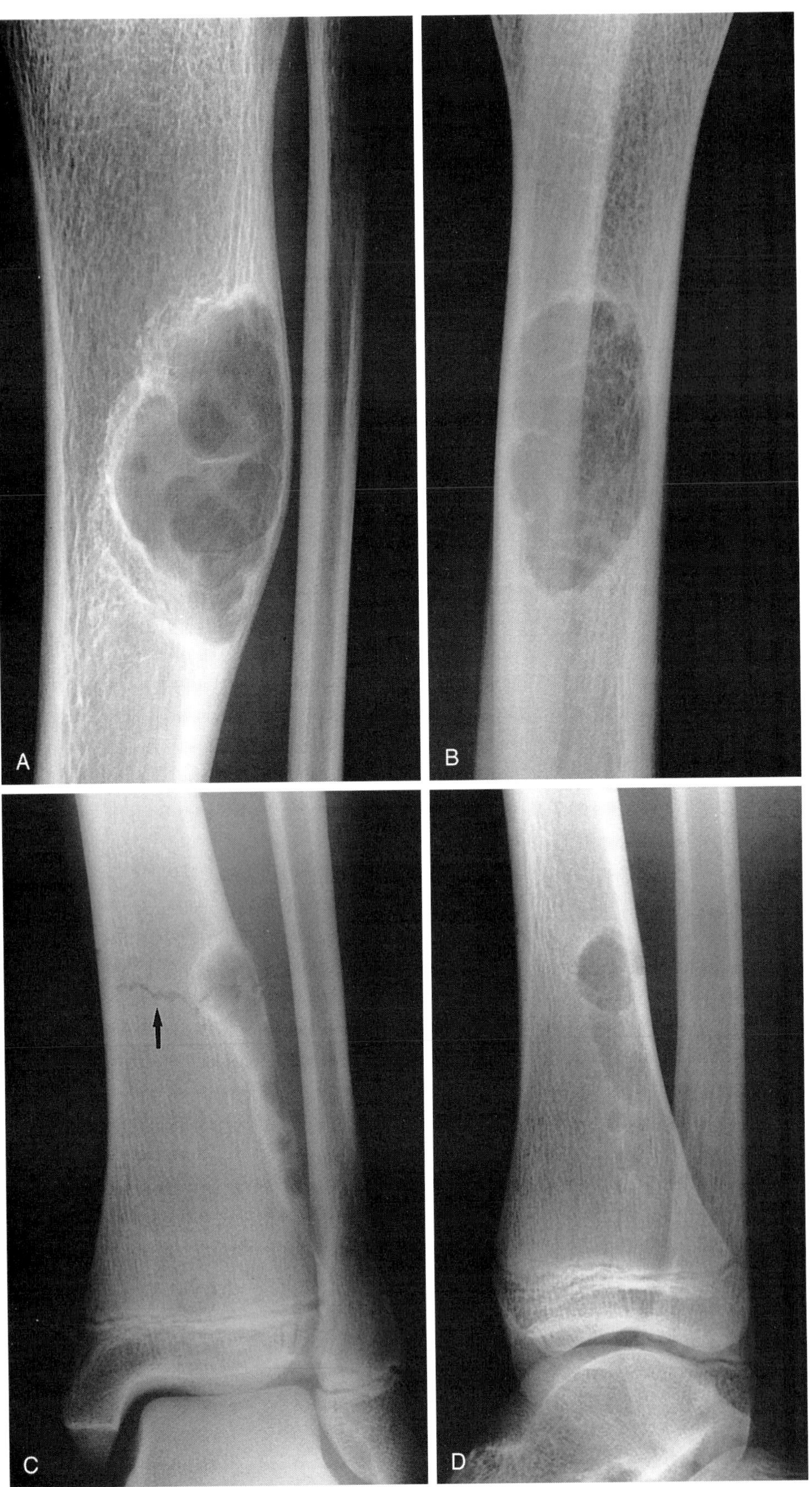

FIGURE 10–29. Nonossifying fibroma.[55, 56] A, B Anteroposterior (A) and lateral (B) magnification radiographs of the tibia show a large, eccentric, slightly expansile, multiloculated, geographic, osteolytic lesion. Observe the cortical thinning and endosteal scalloping. (*A, B, Courtesy of U. Mayer, M.D., Klagenfurt, Austria.*) Routine frontal (C) and oblique (D) radiographs of another patient, a 15-year-old boy, show a typical metaphyseal nonossifying fibroma. A transverse pathologic fracture (arrow) is visible predominantly on the anteroposterior view (C). Observe the somewhat "blistered" appearance of the cortex, a common finding in this condition.

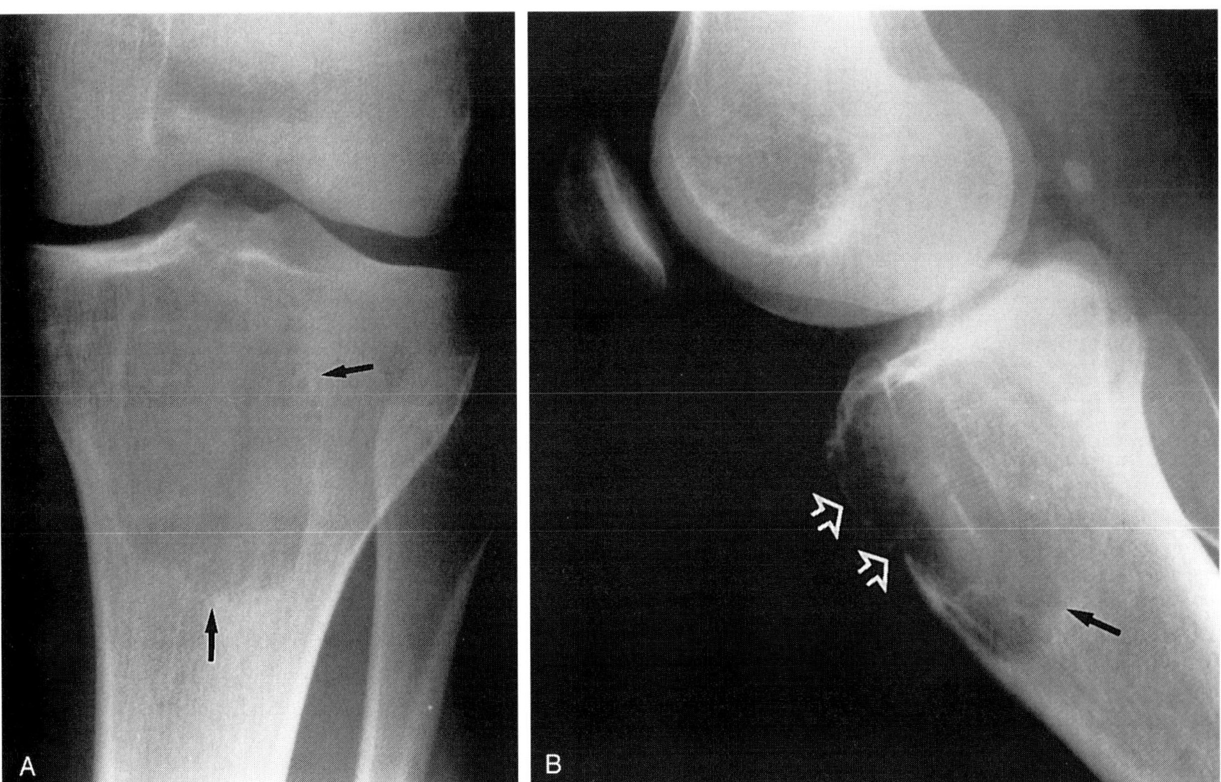

FIGURE 10–30. Giant cell tumor.[57] Frontal (A) and lateral (B) radiographs of the knee in a 19-year-old woman with a 2-year history of knee pain. An eccentric, osteolytic, geographic lesion extending into the subchondral region of the proximal portion of the tibia (arrows) is revealed. The tumor produces thinning and destruction of the anterior tibial cortex (open arrows). Slight bone expansion is present, and the lesion possesses a delicate trabecular pattern. The radiographic appearance of the giant cell tumor is an inaccurate guide to the histologic composition and clinical behavior of the lesion: Benign lesions may appear aggressive and aggressive lesions may appear benign. *(Courtesy of G. Greenway, M.D., Dallas, Texas.)*

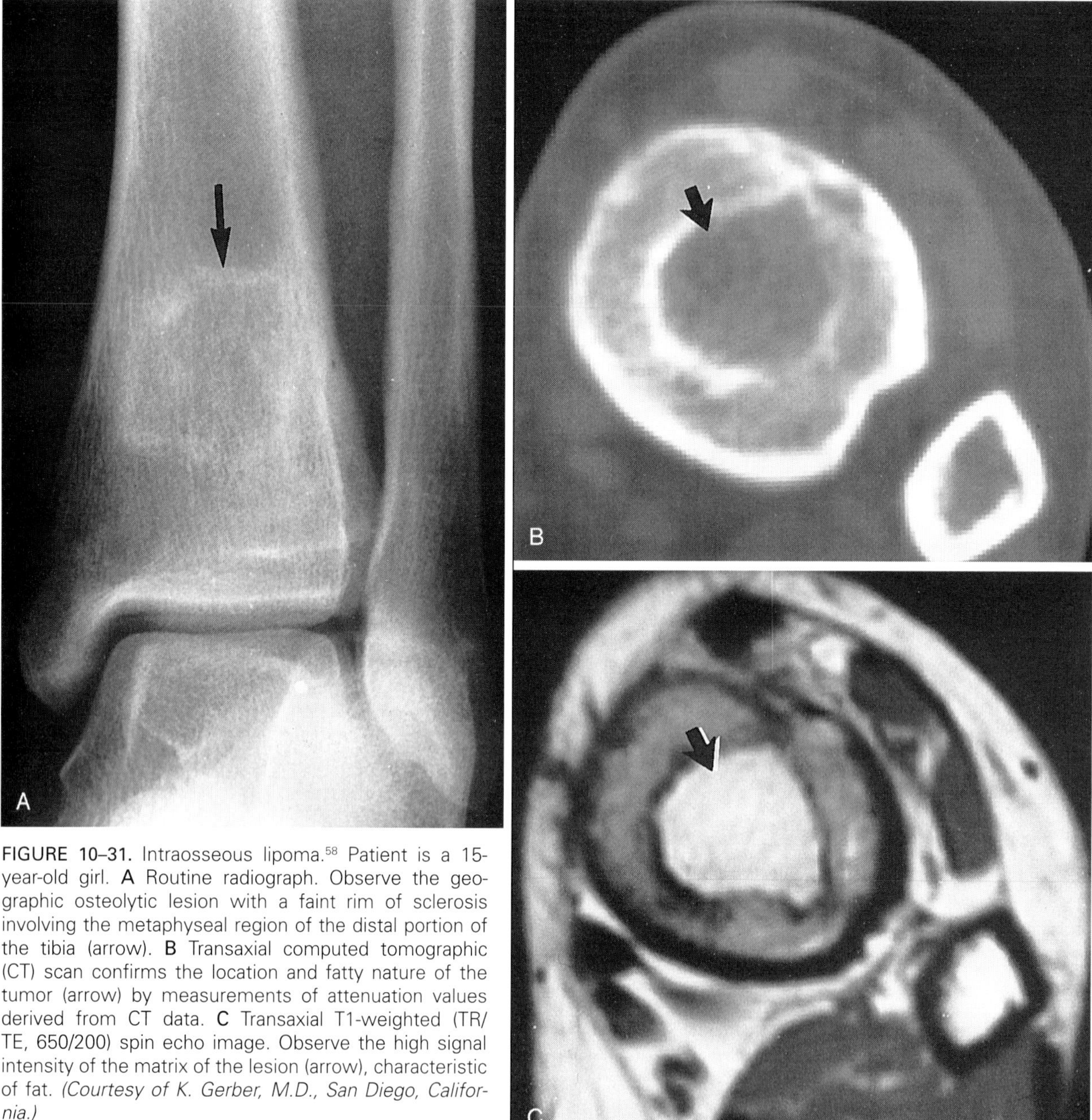

FIGURE 10–31. Intraosseous lipoma.[58] Patient is a 15-year-old girl. A Routine radiograph. Observe the geographic osteolytic lesion with a faint rim of sclerosis involving the metaphyseal region of the distal portion of the tibia (arrow). B Transaxial computed tomographic (CT) scan confirms the location and fatty nature of the tumor (arrow) by measurements of attenuation values derived from CT data. C Transaxial T1-weighted (TR/TE, 650/200) spin echo image. Observe the high signal intensity of the matrix of the lesion (arrow), characteristic of fat. *(Courtesy of K. Gerber, M.D., San Diego, California.)*

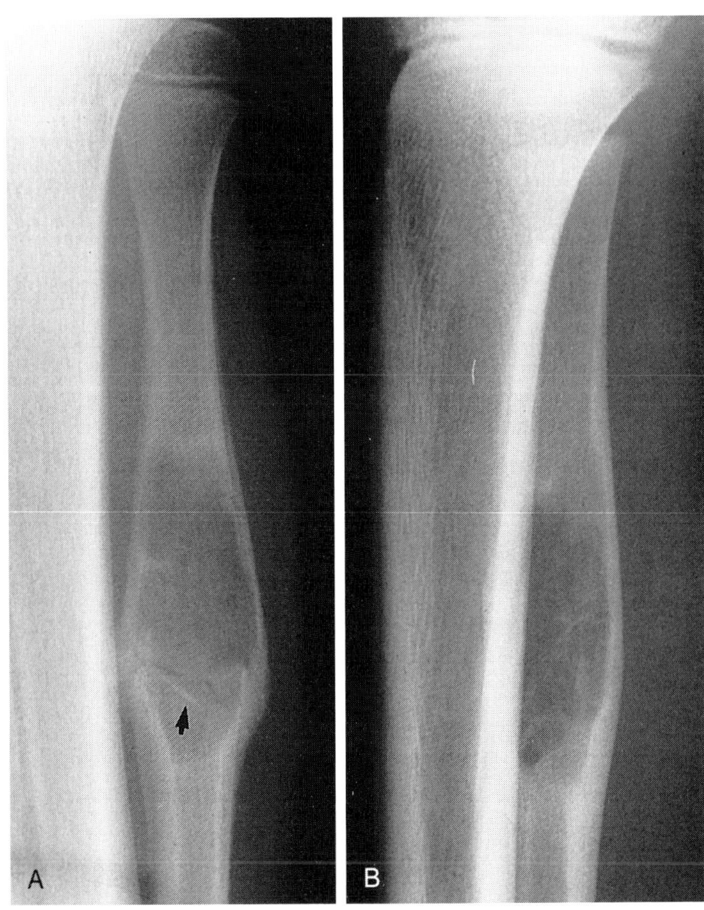

FIGURE 10–32. Simple bone cyst.[60] A 12-year-old girl noticed sudden leg pain after a minor fall. Frontal (A) and lateral (B) films of the fibula show a pathologic fracture through a cyst-like, slightly expansile diaphyseal lesion. Endosteal scalloping is present, and periostitis, probably from fracture healing, is seen adjacent to the lesion. A "fallen fragment" is seen as a tiny piece of comminuted bone that is resting in a dependent position within the fluid-filled matrix (arrow). *(Courtesy of V. Vint, M.D., La Jolla, California.)*

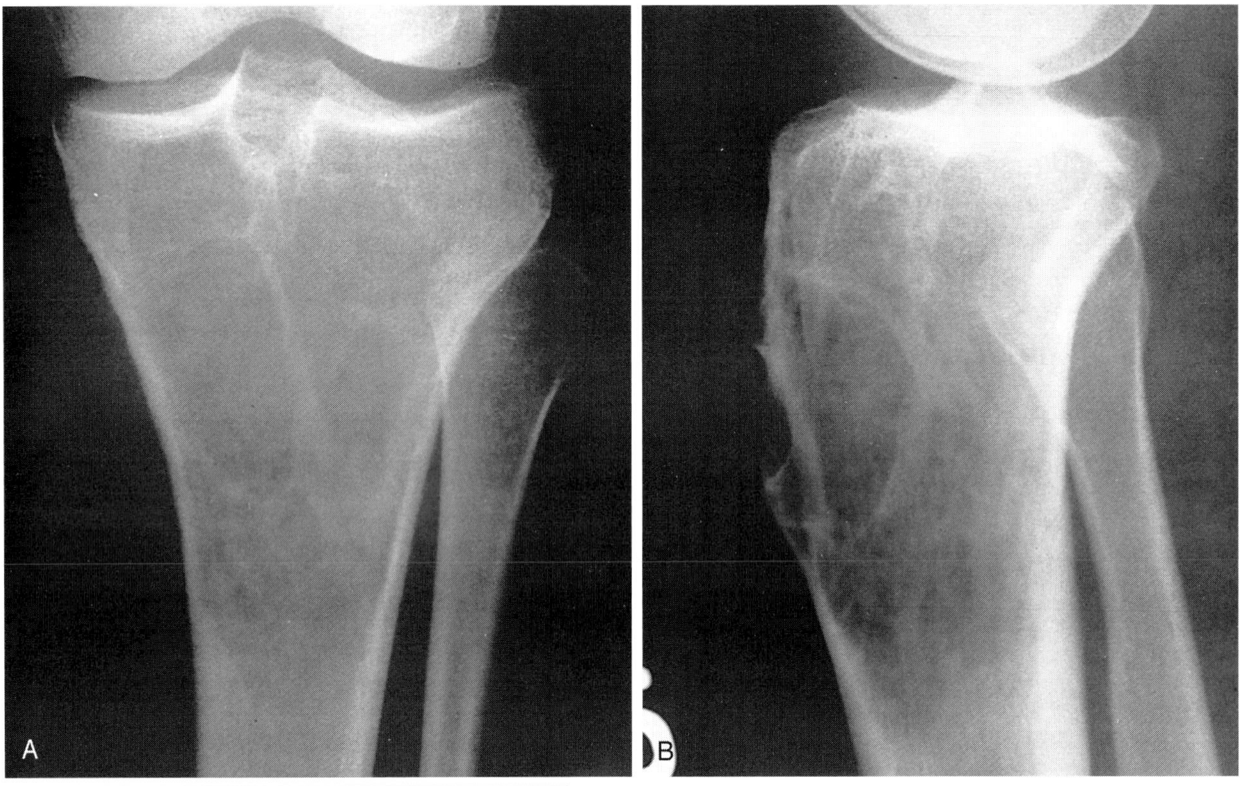

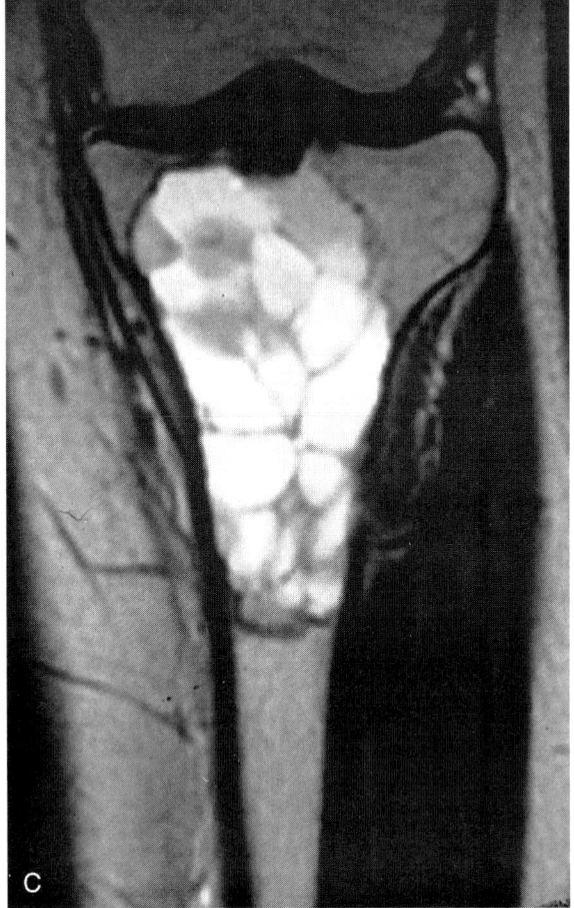

FIGURE 10–33. Aneurysmal bone cyst.[61] Routine frontal (A) and lateral (B) radiographs of the knee show an expansile, eccentrically located osteolytic metaphyseal lesion involving the proximal portion of the tibia. A coronal T2-weighted (TR/TE, 3000/104 Ef) fast spin echo magnetic resonance (MR) image (C) reveals the multichambered, fluid-filled matrix. Transaxial MR images (not shown) demonstrated fluid-fluid levels within this aneurysmal bone cyst. *(Courtesy of A. Newberg, M.D., Boston, Massachusetts.)*

TABLE 10–5. Tumor-Like Lesions of Bone Affecting the Tibia and the Fibula*

Entity	Figure(s)	Characteristics
Paget's disease[62–64]	10–34	The tibia is the fourth most common site of involvement (after the pelvis, femur, and skull) The fibula is one of the least likely bones to be involved Usually polyostotic and may have unilateral involvement Coarsened trabeculae and bone enlargement Pathologic fracture Pseudofractures of convex surface of bowed bones Saber-shin deformity (anterior tibial bowing) Blade of grass appearance (flame-shaped advancing edge of osteolysis) common in tibia
Neurofibromatosis 1 (von Recklinghausen's disease)[65, 66]	10–35	Tibia and fibula involvement common Dysplastic bones with overconstriction, deformity, and remodeling Circumscribed cyst-like intraosseous lesions The tibia and fibula are common sites for pseudarthroses: deformed bones fracture and heal incompletely
Monostotic fibrous dysplasia[67]	10–36	Fewer than 10 per cent of monostotic lesions involve the tibia; 2 per cent involve the fibula Thick rim of sclerosis surrounding radiolucent lesion; hazy ground-glass appearance of matrix Tibial or fibular bowing may occur
Polyostotic fibrous dysplasia[67]		More than 80 per cent of patients have tibial involvement; more than 60 per cent have fibula involvement Polyostotic lesions tend to be more expansile and multiloculated than monostotic lesions Bowing also is more prominent in polyostotic form
Langerhans' cell histiocytosis[68]		Tibial and fibular involvement is extremely uncommon Osteolytic lesions may be multiloculated and expansile

*See also Table 1–12.

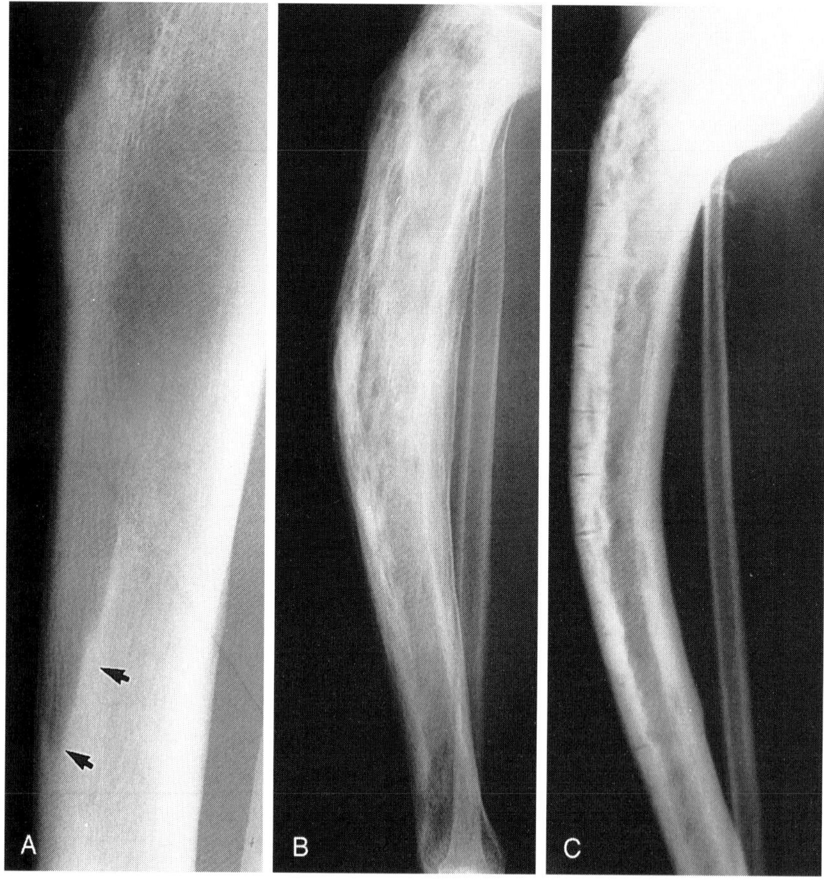

FIGURE 10–34. Paget's disease.[62–64] A Osteolytic pattern. Osteolytic destruction is seen as a wedge-shaped, radiolucent edge (blade-of-grass or flame-shaped appearance) within the tibial diaphysis (arrows). B Combined pattern. In another patient with long-standing Paget's disease, the combined pattern of osteolytic and osteosclerotic disease predominates. Anterior bowing of the tibia also is evident, a complication termed saber-shin deformity. C Osteosclerotic pattern. In a third patient, diffuse osteosclerosis, cortical thickening, pseudofractures, and anterior bowing are the predominant findings. The fibula, which is unaffected, is one of the bones involved least commonly in Paget's disease.

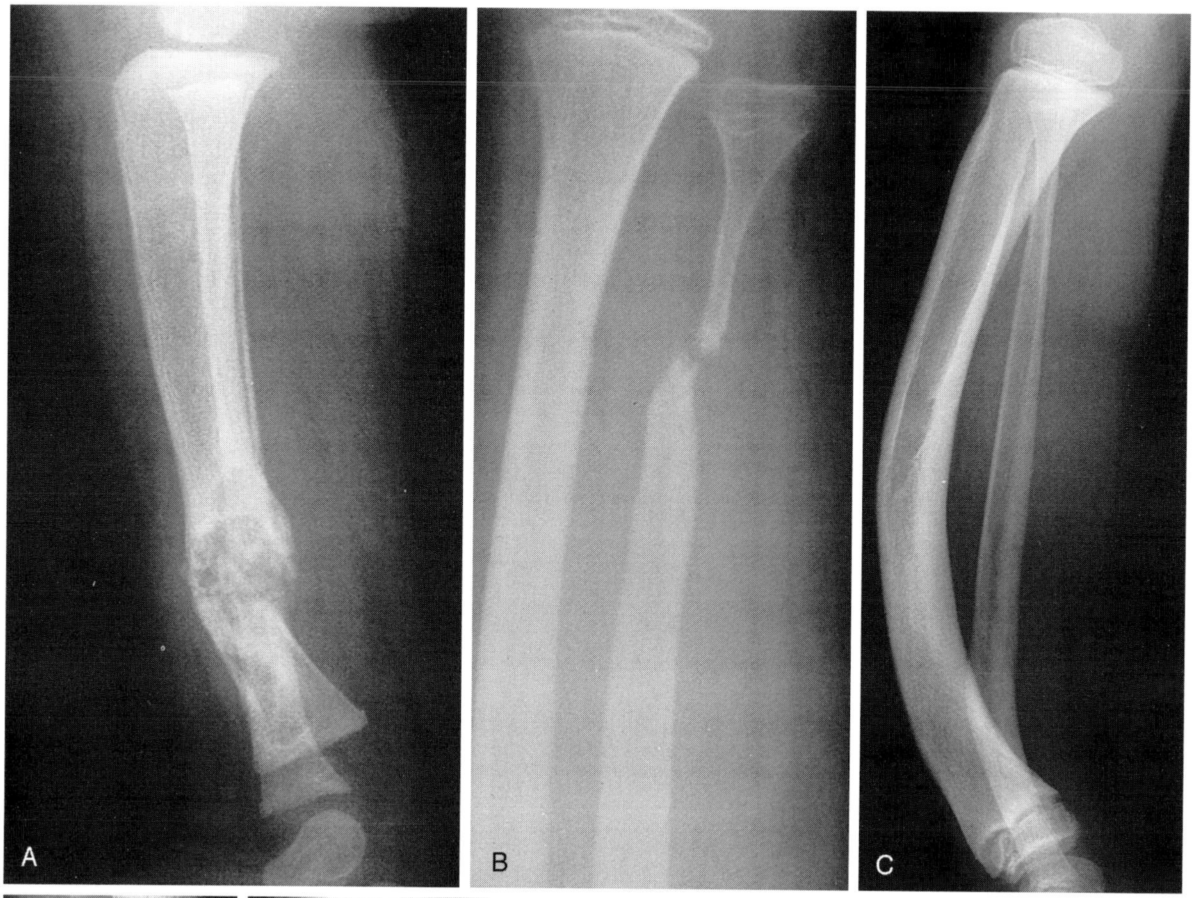

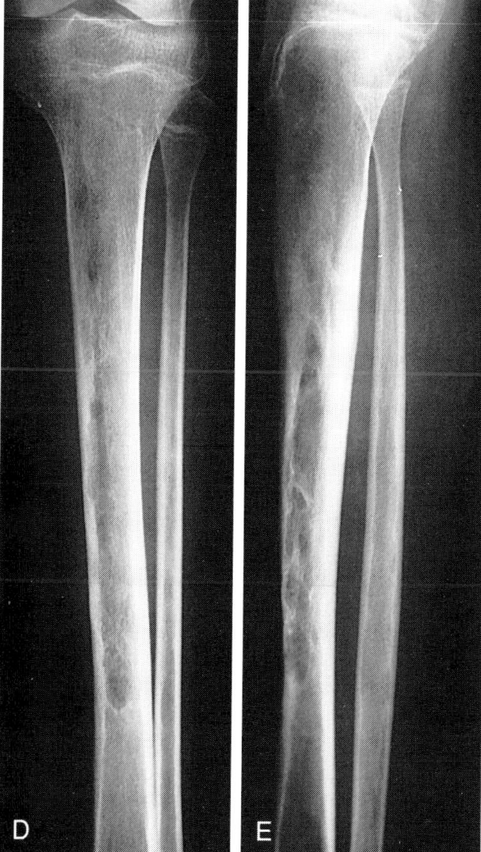

FIGURE 10–35. Neurofibromatosis.[65, 66] **A** Observe the pseudarthrosis in the diaphysis of the tibia in this patient with neurofibromatosis. *(A, Courtesy of M.N. Pathria, M.D., San Diego, California.)* **B** In another patient, a pseudarthrosis in the diaphysis of the fibula is seen. **C** Prominent bowing of the tibia is evident in a third child with neurofibromatosis. Tibial bowing, which usually becomes apparent in the first year of life, is a frequent finding in neurofibromatosis. **D, E** In an older child, frontal (**D**) and lateral (**E**) radiographs of the tibia reveal serpentine osteolytic bone destruction with endosteal scalloping and a multiloculated appearance resembling fibrous dysplasia or osteofibrous dysplasia.

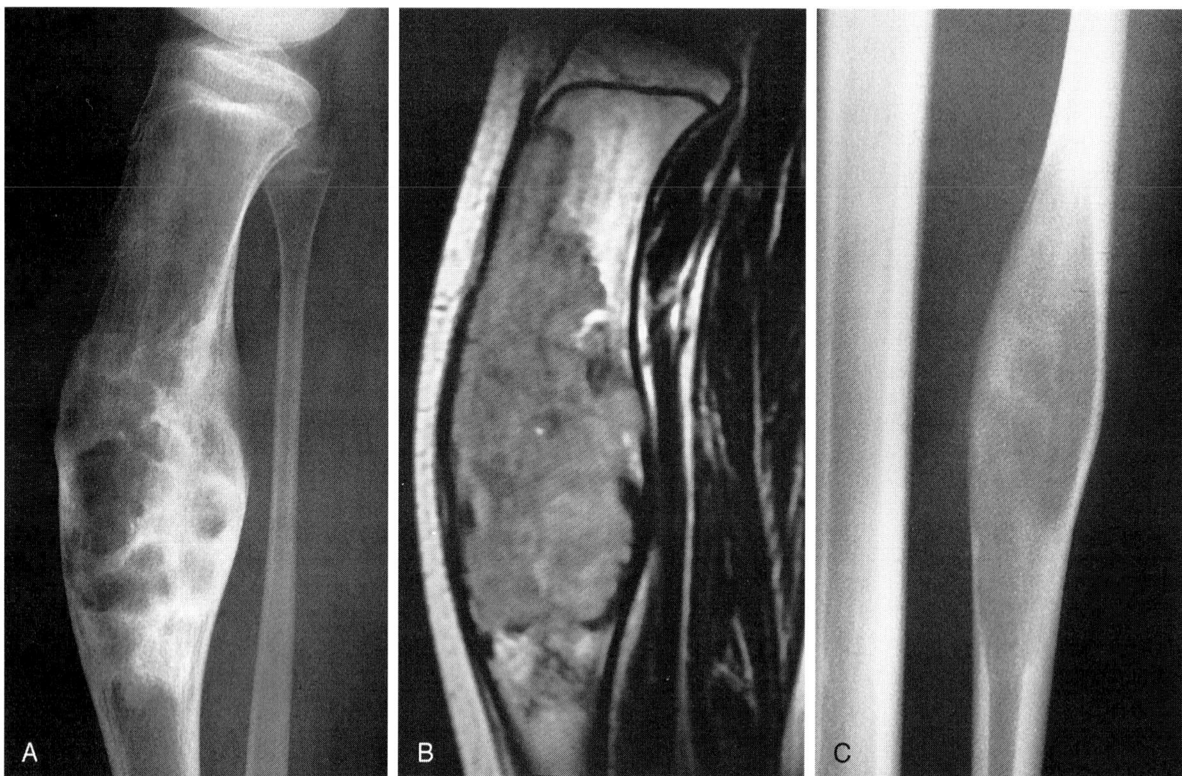

FIGURE 10–36. Monostotic fibrous dysplasia.[67] **A, B** Tibial involvement in a 14-year-old boy. In **A,** a lateral radiograph of the tibia demonstrates an expansile, multilocular diaphyseal lesion. It is characterized by endosteal scalloping, undulating zones of sclerosis, and a hazy osteolytic matrix. Tibial bowing also is apparent. In **B,** a fast spin echo (TR/TE, 4,000/75) magnetic resonance (MR) image shows an inhomogeneous hypointense signal within the matrix. *(**A, B,** Courtesy of B.Y. Yang, M.D., Kaohsiune Hsien, Taiwan.)* **C** Fibula. A characteristic ground-glass appearance with cortical endosteal scalloping is seen in this lesion in the fibular diaphysis. The fibula is infrequently affected by fibrous dysplasia. *(**C,** Courtesy of G. Greenway, M.D., Dallas, Texas.)*

TABLE 10–6. Metabolic, Hematologic, and Vascular Disorders Affecting the Tibia and the Fibula*

Entity	Figure(s)	Characteristics
Generalized osteoporosis[69]		Uniform decrease in radiodensity, thinning of cortices, accentuation of weight-bearing trabeculae Occasionally may result in insufficiency fractures of the tibia and fibula
Regional osteoporosis[69, 70]	10–37	May occur as a result of disuse and immobilization after a fracture or other injury or in reflex sympathetic dystrophy Findings may be more widespread in paralyzed patients Band-like, patchy, spotty, or periarticular osteopenia Subperiosteal (rare) and intracortical bone resoprtion Subchondral and juxta-articular cyst-like lesions Occasional scalloping of tibia
Osteogenesis imperfecta[11]	10–5	See Table 10–1
Osteomalacia and rickets[71]	10–38, 10–39	*Osteomalacia* Osteopenia; decreased trabeculae; remaining trabeculae appear prominent and coarsened Looser's zones (pseudofractures) *Rickets* Metaphyseal demineralization: frayed metaphysis Bowing deformities Osteopenia Looser's zones
Hyperparathyroidism and renal osteodystrophy[72–74]	10–40, 10–41	Brown tumor (osteoclastoma): solitary or multiple expansile osteolytic lesions containing fibrous tissue and giant cells; may disappear after treatment for hyperparathyroidism Occasionally severe tibial and fibular bowing occurs Osteosclerosis more common in renal osteodystrophy
Hypoparathyroidism[75, 76]	10–42	Osteosclerosis Subcutaneous calcification Premature physeal fusion Periarticulr bone proliferation—enthesopathy
Hypovitaminosis C (scurvy)[77, 78]	10–43	Radiographic evidence of skeletal changes in scurvy is seen only in advanced, long-standing disease Periostitis secondary to subperiosteal hemorrhage Sclerotic metaphyseal lines Beak-like metaphyseal excrescences Radiodense shell surrounding epiphyses Healing scurvy may result in increased radiodensity of the metaphyses and epiphyses
Gaucher's disease[79]	10–44	Osteopenia, septated osteolytic lesions, cortical diminution, and diametaphyseal widening (Erlenmeyer flask deformity) Osseous weakening may result in pathologic fractures Coarsened trabecular pattern
Venous insufficiency[80]	10–45	Thick, undulating periosteal reaction along the tibia and fibula seen in as many as 60 per cent of patients with chronic disabling venous stasis Associated calcification and ossification in soft tissue
Primary hypertrophic osteoarthropathy[81]	10–46	Also termed pachydermoperiostosis: primary form of hypertrophic osteoarthropathy Only 3–5 per cent of all cases of hypertrophic osteoarthropathy Bilateral symmetric tibial and fibular periostitis
Secondary hypertrophic osteoarthropathy[81, 82]	10–47	Syndrome characterized by digital clubbing, arthritis, and periostitis Complication of many diseases, including bronchogenic carcinoma, mesothelioma, and other intrathoracic and intra-abdominal diseases Bilateral symmetric periostitis of tibiae and fibulae
Growth recovery lines[83]	10–48	Transverse radiodense lines in the tubular bones of children representing a sign of new or increased growth; presumably after a period of inhibited bone growth from a previous episode of trauma, infection, malnutrition, or other chronic disease states
Collagen vascular disease: soft tissue calcification[84]	10–49	Dermatomyositis, polymyositis, scleroderma, and other collagen vascular diseases may result in soft tissue calcinosis in the leg or calf Differential diagnosis: hyperparathyroidism, neurologic injury, melorheostosis, posttraumatic heterotopic ossification, soft tissue neoplasms
Medullary osteonecrosis[85]	10–50	Also termed intramedullary bone infarct or metadiaphyseal osteonecrosis Patchy intramedullary sclerosis with areas of radiolucency Irregular calcific deposits Closely resembles appearance of enchondroma

*See also Tables 1–13 to 1–15.

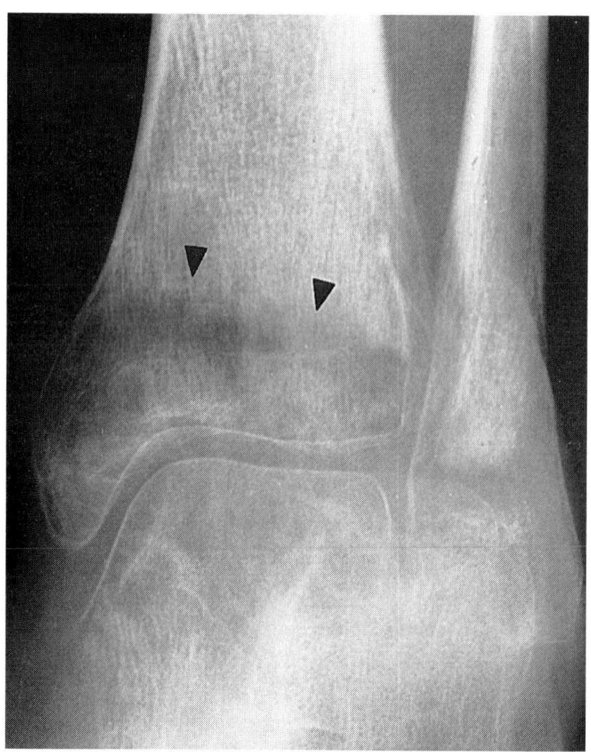

FIGURE 10–37. Regional osteoporosis: Reflex sympathetic dystrophy.[69, 70] After a minor foot injury, this patient developed progressive pain and disability. Observe the band-like and patchy metaphyseal osteopenia (arrowheads) and the subarticular loss of bone density within the talus and distal end of the tibia. Spotty, patchy, and band-like bone resorption is typical of rapid-onset osteoporosis, such as that seen in disuse, burns, frostbite, paralysis, or, as in this case, reflex sympathetic dystrophy. Such an appearance may simulate that of an aggressive neoplasm.

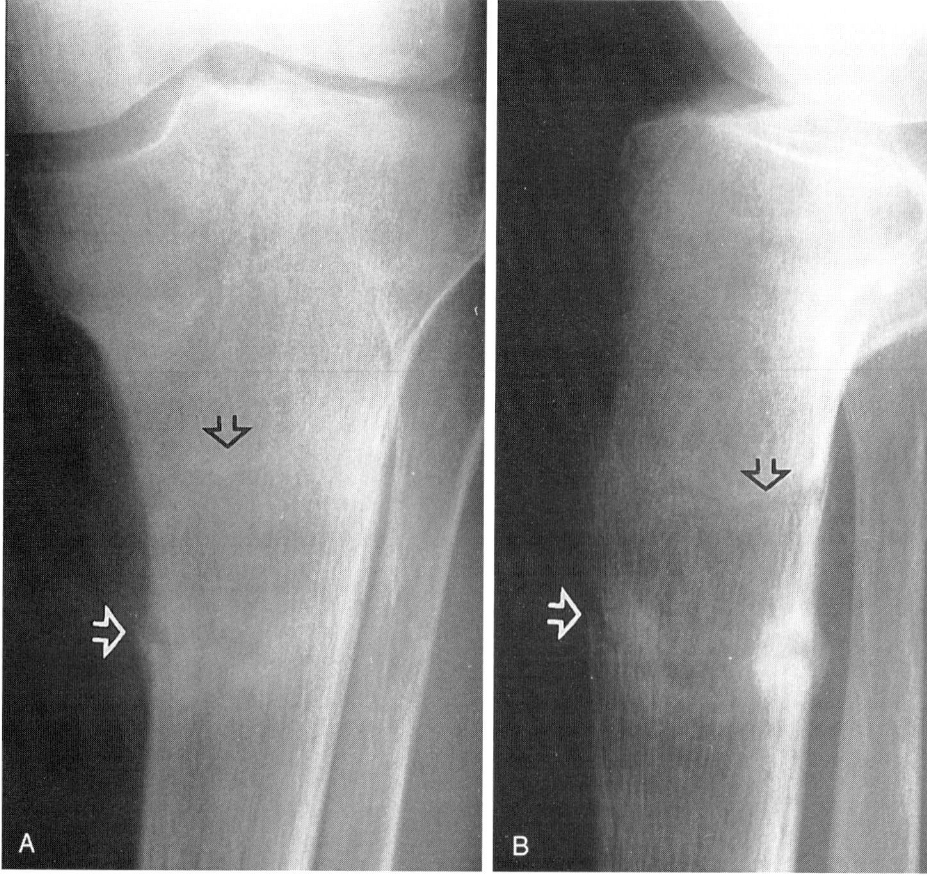

FIGURE 10–38. Osteomalacia.[71] Frontal (A) and lateral (B) radiographs of a 53-year-old man who had long-standing vitamin D–resistant osteomalacia. Diffuse osteopenia and two transverse insufficiency fractures are evident in the metadiaphysis of the tibia (open arrows). A thin veil of callus is apparent at the margin of the lower fracture.

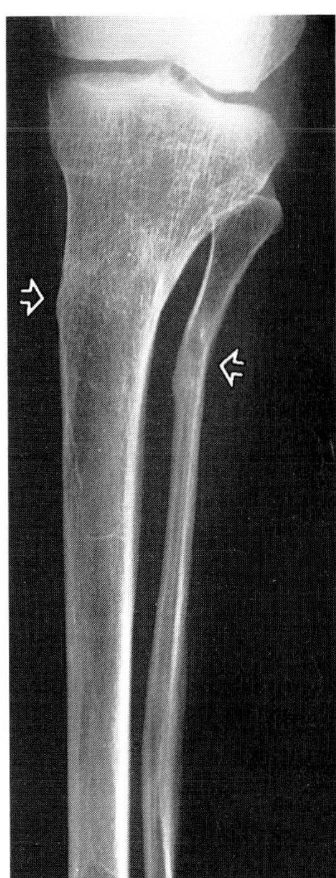

FIGURE 10–39. Rickets[71] (hypophosphatemic). In this patient with long-standing hypophosphatemia, diffuse osteopenia and bowing deformities of the tibia and fibula are present (open arrows). *(Courtesy of C. Pineda, M.D., Mexico City, Mexico.)*

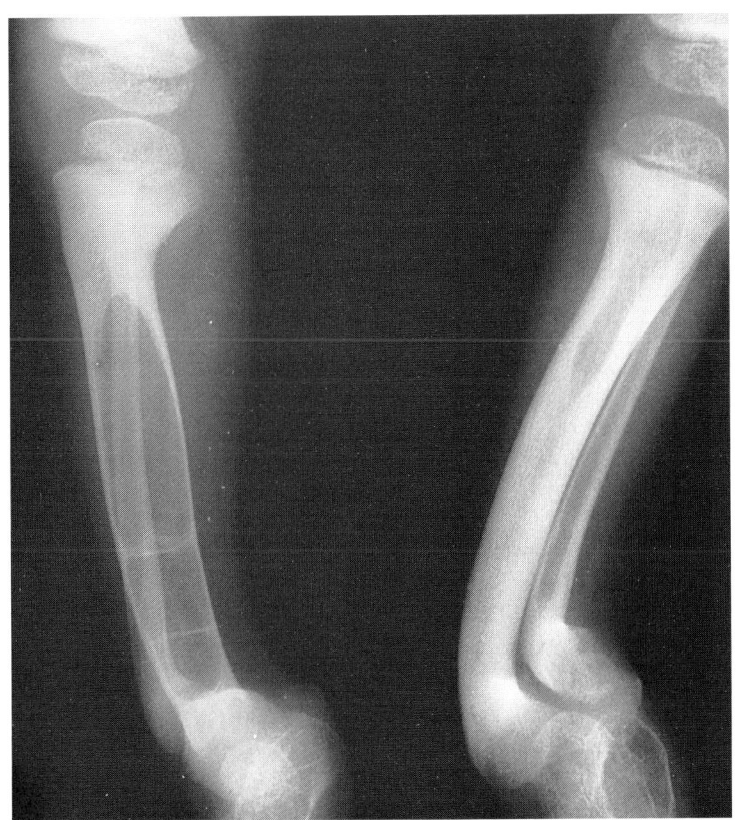

FIGURE 10–40. Secondary hyperparathyroidism: Brown tumors.[72] Observe the multiple, septated brown tumors in both tibiae of this 5-year-old girl with secondary hyperparathyroidism. Dramatic tibial bowing from bone softening also is present. Such severe skeletal involvement with brown tumors and deformities has been referred to as osteitis fibrosa cystica. *(Courtesy of T. Broderick, M.D., Orange, California.)*

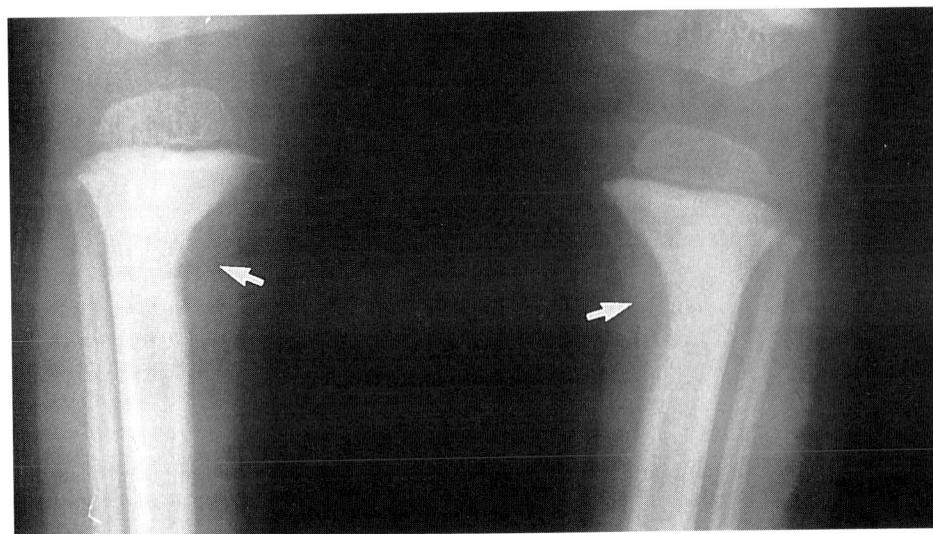

FIGURE 10–41. Renal osteodystrophy.[73, 74] In a 4-year-old boy with secondary hyperparathyroidism, observe the generalized osteosclerosis and the characteristic subperiosteal resorption of the medial aspect of the proximal tibial metaphyses (arrows).

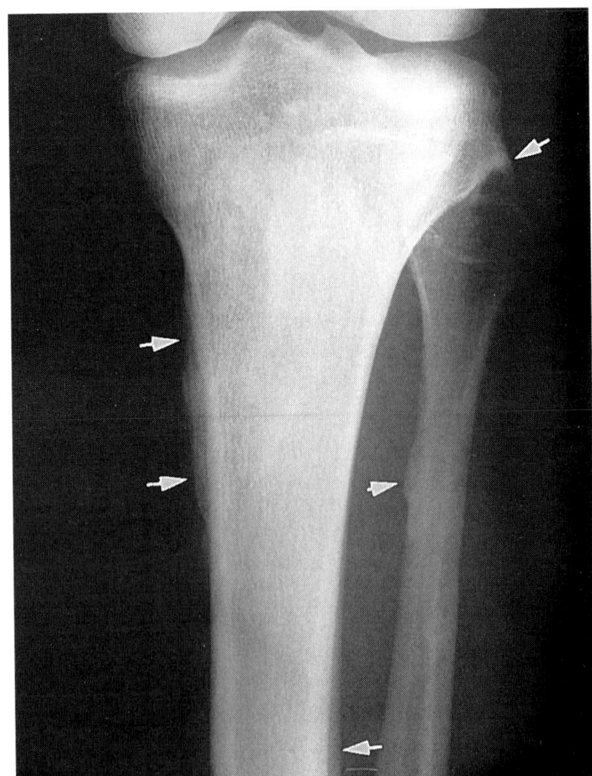

FIGURE 10–42. Hypoparathyroidism.[75, 76] Osseous proliferation is seen as prominent excrescences in the proximal portion of the tibia (arrows) in this man with hypoparathyroidism.

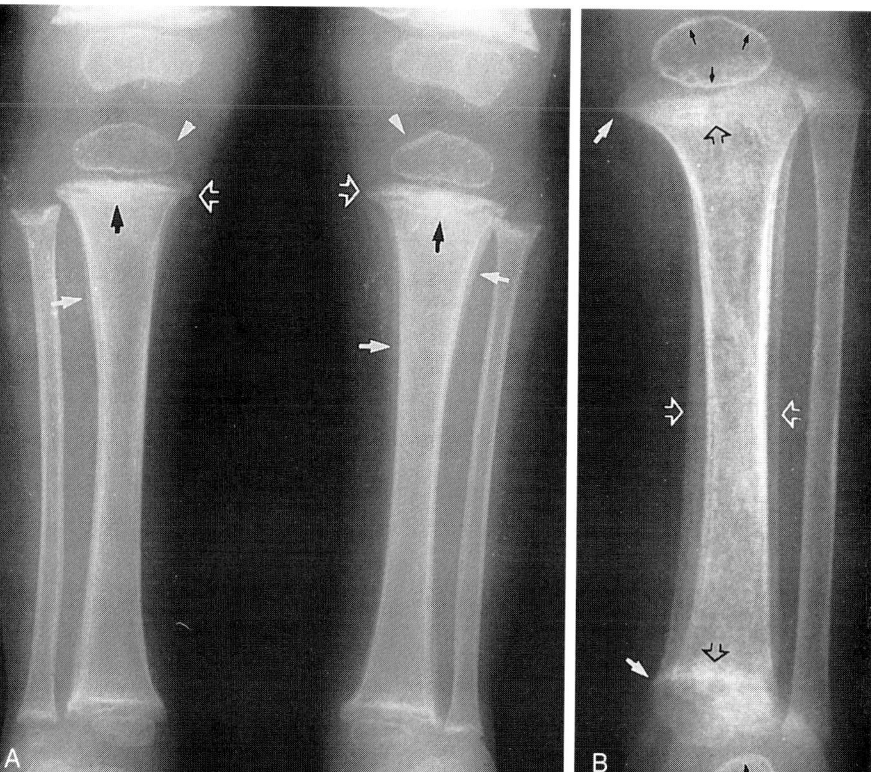

FIGURE 10–43. Hypovitaminosis C (scurvy).[77, 78] A In this infant, bilateral radiographs of the tibias and fibulas demonstrate periostitis caused by subperiosteal hemorrhage (white arrows), thick sclerotic metaphyseal lines (black arrows), beak-like excrescences (open arrows), and radiodense shells around the epiphyses (Wimberger's ring) (arrowheads). These findings all are consistent with scurvy. B In another child with chronic ascorbic acid deficiency, observe the thick periostitis from subperiosteal hemorrhage (white open arrows), sclerotic metaphyseal line (black open arrows), beak-like metaphyseal excrescences (Pelken's spurs) (white arrows), radiolucent epiphysis surrounded by a sclerotic shell (Wimberger's ring) (black arrows), and generalized osteopenia.

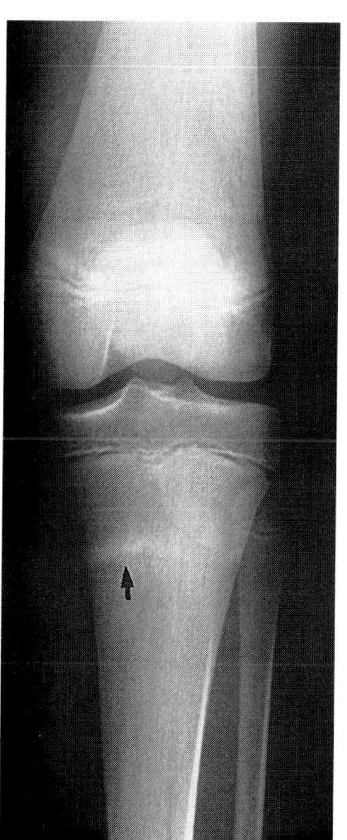

FIGURE 10–44. Gaucher's disease.[79] Undertubulation (Erlenmeyer flask deformity) and cortical thinning are associated with an insufficiency fracture (arrow) of the tibia of this 13-year-old girl with Gaucher's disease. *(Courtesy of G. Greenway, M.D., Dallas, Texas.)*

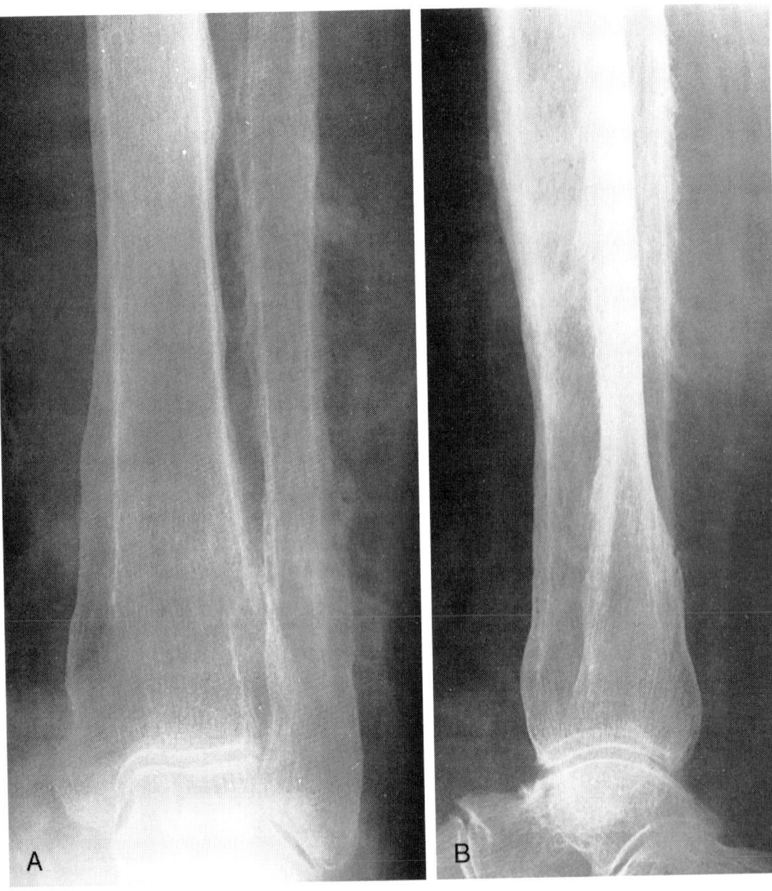

FIGURE 10–45. Venous insufficiency: Periosteal reaction.[80] Frontal (A) and lateral (B) radiographs show a thick, undulating, single-layer periosteal reaction along the shafts of the tibia and the fibula in this patient with chronic venous stasis. Such changes predominate in the lower extremity and occur in 10 to 60 per cent of patients with chronic disabling venous stasis.

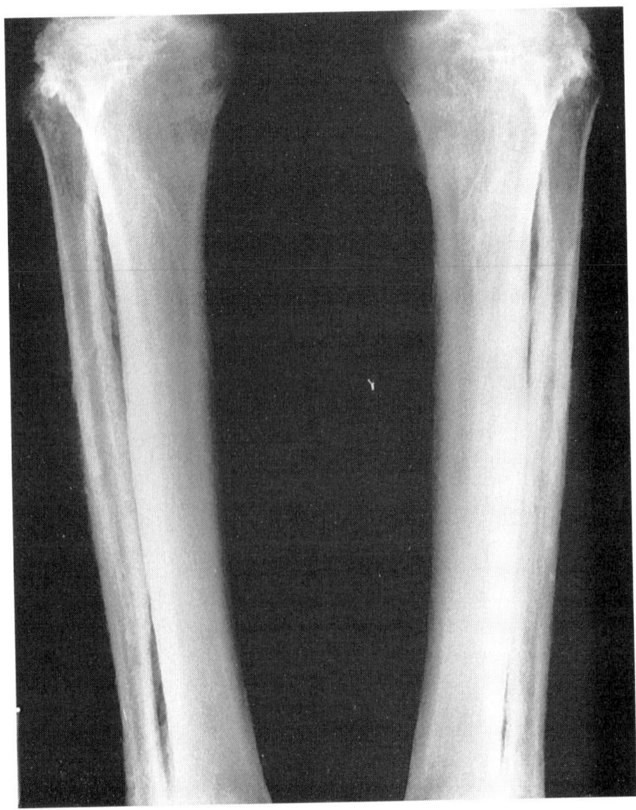

FIGURE 10–46. Primary hypertrophic osteoarthropathy: Pachydermoperiostosis.[81] Observe the widespread prominent periostitis affecting the tibiae and fibulae. The findings in this patient were bilateral and symmetric and affected several tubular bones throughout the skeleton. *(Courtesy of C. Chen, M.D., Kaohsiung, Taiwan.)*

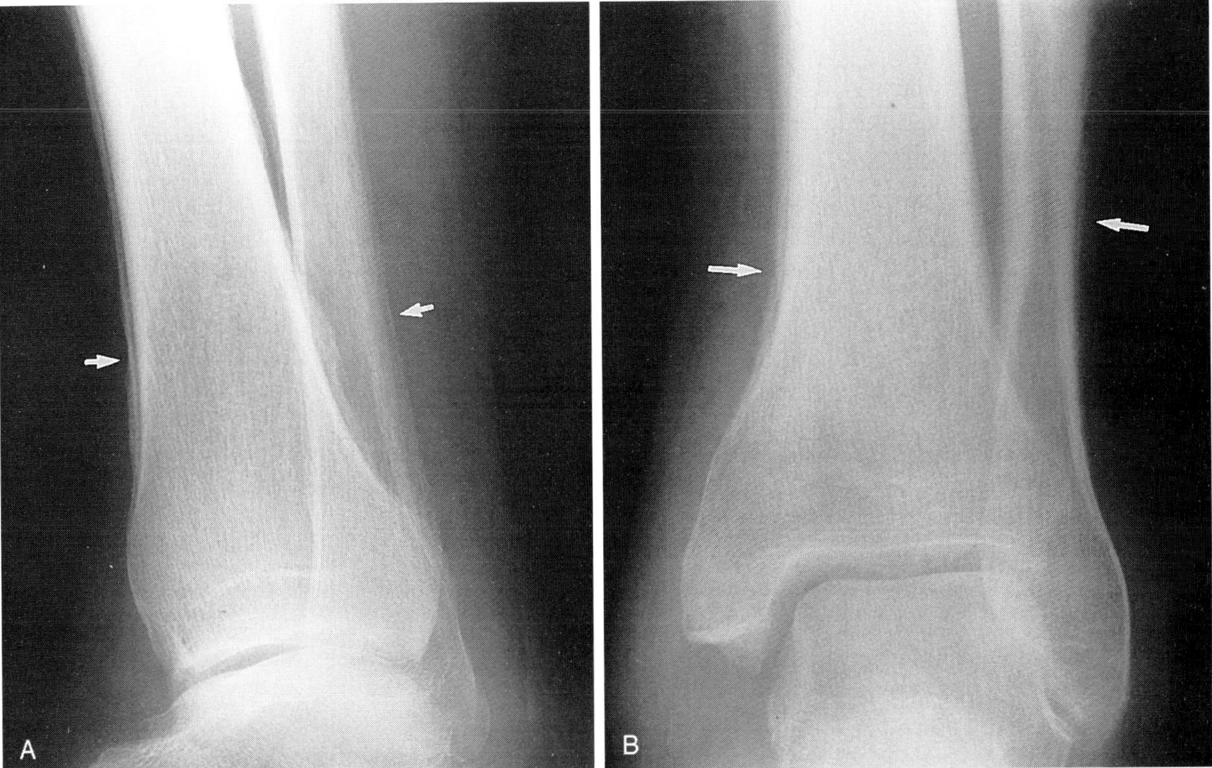

FIGURE 10–47. Secondary hypertrophic osteoarthropathy.[81, 82] A Periostitis of the tibia and the fibula is seen in this patient with bronchogenic carcinoma. B Radiograph of the distal portions of the tibia and fibula (arrows) in this 60-year-old man with bronchogenic carcinoma reveals periostitis of the distal diaphysis and metaphysis of the tibia and fibula. Soft tissue swelling also is prominent. Both patients had bilateral symmetric periostitis.

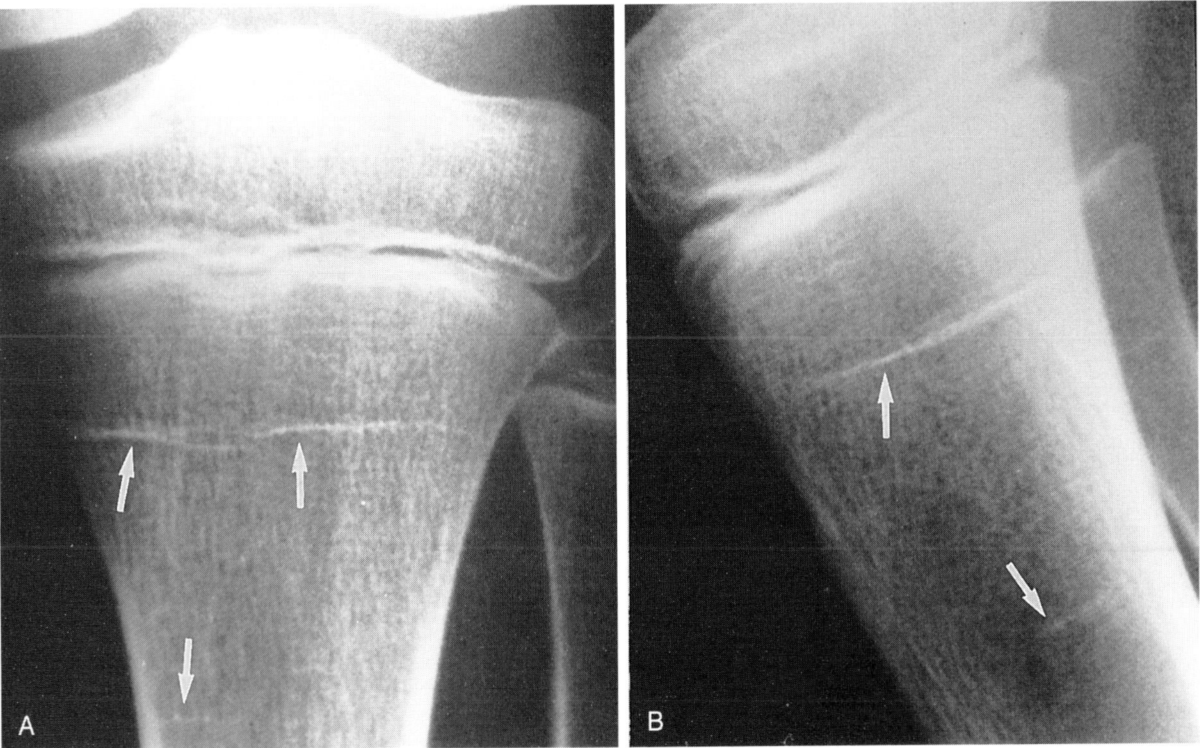

FIGURE 10–48. A, B Growth resumption lines.[83] In this chronically ill 6-year-old child with juvenile rheumatoid arthritis, prominent transverse sclerotic bands are seen in the proximal tibial metaphysis and diaphysis (arrows). These transverse radiodense lines represent a sign of new or increased growth, presumably after a period of inhibited bone growth.

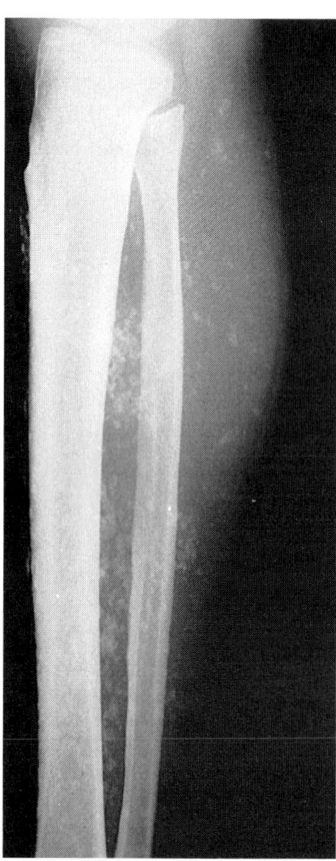

FIGURE 10–49. Collagen vascular disease: Systemic lupus erythematosus.[84] Diffuse soft tissue calcification is seen in this patient with long-standing systemic lupus erythematosus.

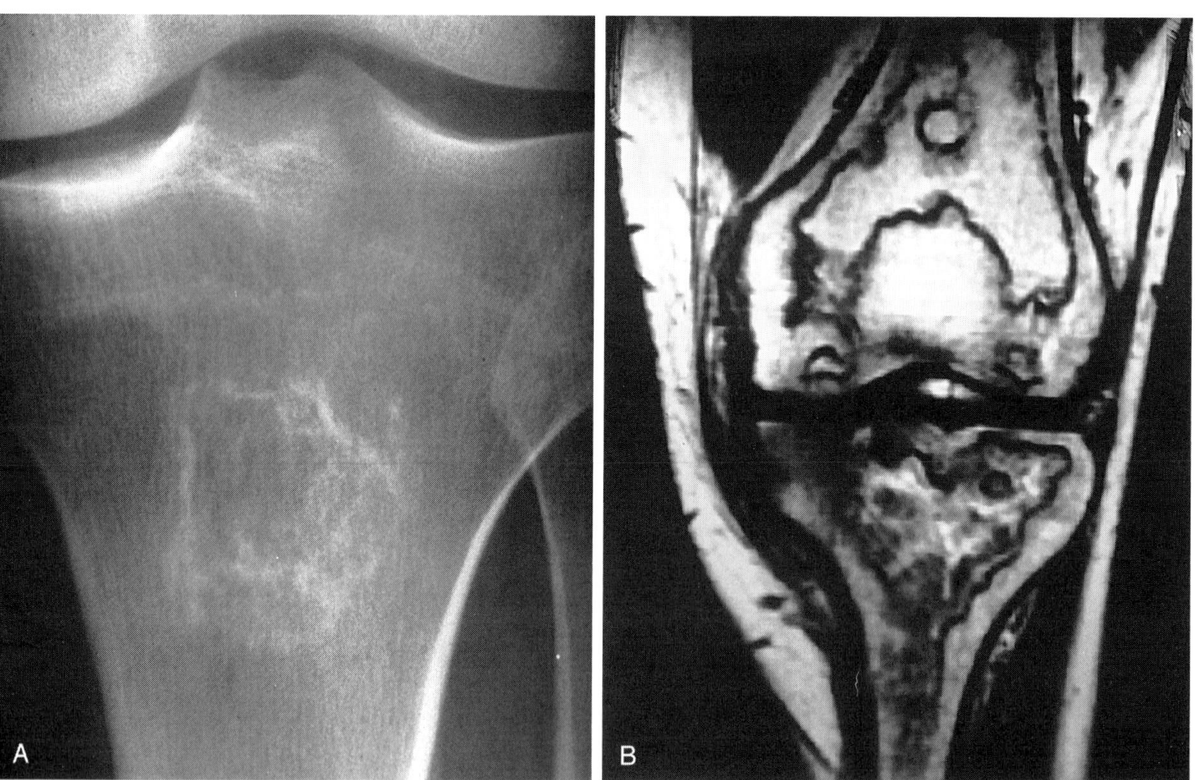

FIGURE 10–50. Medullary osteonecrosis: Bone infarct.[85] A This 46-year-old alcoholic man had bilateral osteonecrosis of the femoral heads. Radiograph of the knee reveals a circular zone of osteosclerosis in the proximal tibial metaphysis, characteristic of a medullary bone infarct. Differentiating these lesions radiographically from chondrogenic neoplasms such as enchondroma and chondrosarcoma is often difficult. B In another patient, a coronal T1-weighted (TR/TE, 600/20) spin echo magnetic resonance (MR) image reveals extensive replacement of normal marrow with mixed signal intensity surrounded by a well-defined undulating rim of low signal intensity in the subchondral region, metaphysis, and diaphysis of the proximal end of the tibia and the distal portion of the femur. This appearance is typical of medullary infarct. *(B, Courtesy of L. Pertcheck, M.D., Denver, Colorado.)*

TABLE 10–7. Infectious Disorders Affecting the Tibia and the Fibula*

Entity	Figure(s)	Characteristics
Acute pyogenic osteomyelitis[86]	10–51	Tibia is a frequent site of infection Metaphysis in children Also seen in intravenous drug abusers, diabetic persons, and immunocompromised patients Poorly defined permeative bone destruction
Chronic osteomyelitis[87]	10–52	Tibia is a frequent site Osteosclerosis and cortical thickening Thick, single layer periosteal bone proliferation Areas of osteolysis and poorly defined areas of sclerosis Sequestrum and involucrum Cloaca formation
Brodie's abscess[88]	10–53	Most frequently found in children The tibia is the most common site of Brodie's abscess Circular, geographic zone of osteolysis Sharply circumscribed sclerotic margin Metaphyseal location Radiolucent channel (i.e., tract sign) may communicate with growth plate, joint, or surface of bone
Chronic recurrent multifocal osteomyelitis (CRMO)[89, 90]	10–54	Unknown cause Occurs mainly in children and adolescents Radiographic findings suggesting acute or subacute osteomyelitis Initial osteolytic destruction of metaphysis adjacent to growth plate with no periosteal bone formation or sequestration May be associated with pustular skin lesions
Tuberculous osteomyelitis[91]	10–55	Osteolytic lesions may be accompanied by surrounding sclerosis, periostitis, and sequestrum Intracortical lesions are rare Cystic tuberculosis: disseminated lesions throughout the skeleton (rare) Often begins in epiphysis and spreads to adjacent joint Metaphyseal lesions in children may violate the growth plate (helping to differentiate tuberculous osteomyelitis from pyogenic osteomyelitis)
Congenital syphilis[92, 93]	10–56	Symmetric, transverse, radiolucent, metaphyseal bands or linear, longitudinal, alternating lucent and sclerotic bands ("celery stalk" appearance) Other osseous abnormalities include osteochrondritis, diaphyseal osteomyelitis, and gumma formation
Leprous osteomyelitis[94]	10–57	Multiple osteolytic lesions surrounded by sclerosis

*See also Table 1–17.

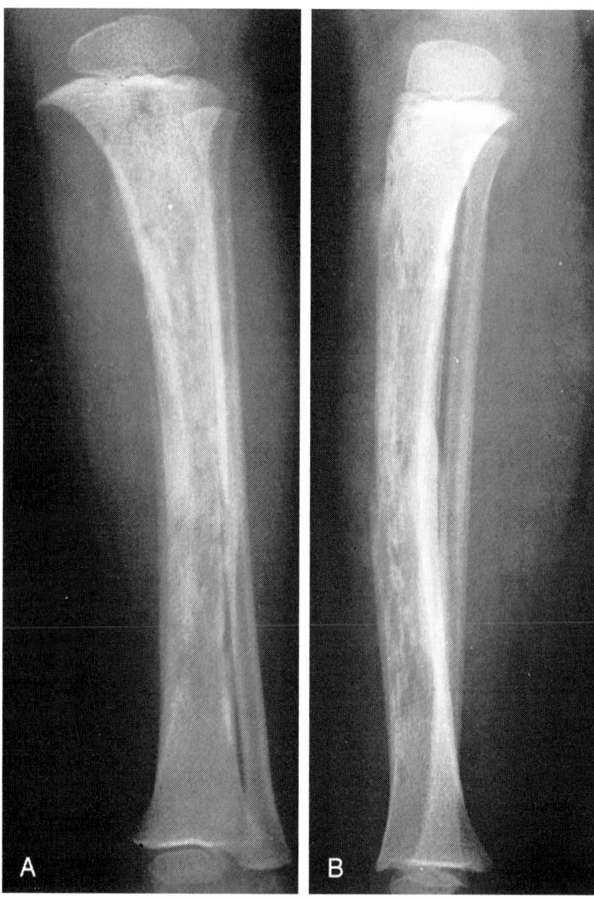

FIGURE 10–51. Acute staphylococcus osteomyelitis.[86] This young patient had a 2-week history of pain, warmth, and tenderness over the tibia. Frontal (A) and lateral (B) radiographs show poorly defined osteolysis throughout the diaphyses and proximal tibial metaphysis. Exuberant periosteal new bone formation appears as generalized increased radiodensity.

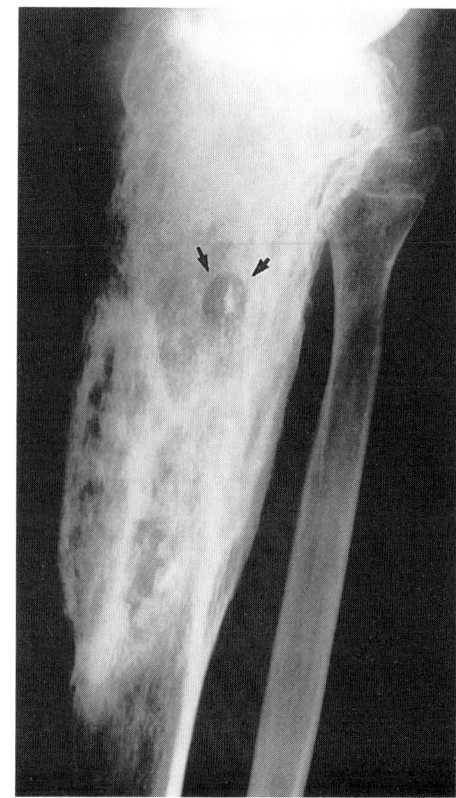

FIGURE 10–52. Chronic osteomyelitis: *Staphylococcus aureus.*[87] This patient with chronic osteomyelitis developed pain in the tibia. Widespread sclerosis, bone expansion from periosteal bone proliferation, and areas of osteolysis in the proximal portion of the tibia are characteristic of chronic osteomyelitis. A circular radiolucent cavity containing a sharply marginated, radiodense focus (arrows) represents a sequestrum, one sign of activity in osteomyelitis. *(Courtesy of C. Pineda, M.D., Mexico City, Mexico.)*

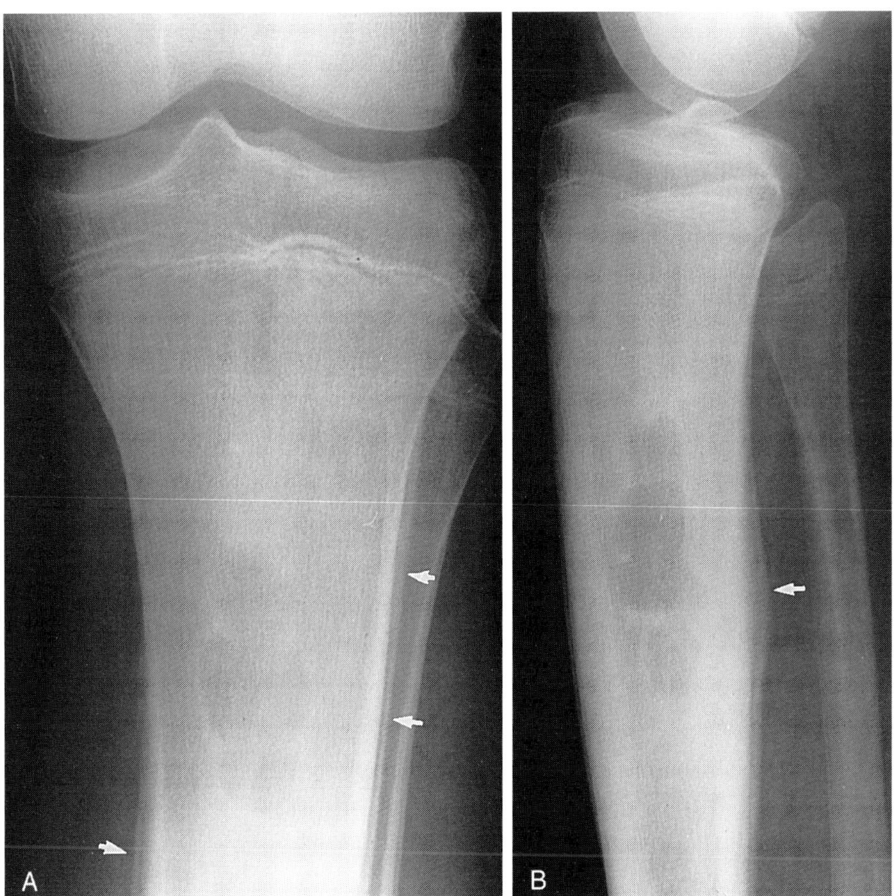

FIGURE 10–53. Brodie's abscess: Subacute osteomyelitis.[88] A, B This 13-year-old girl complained of knee pain. Frontal (A) and lateral (B) radiographs of the tibia reveal a multiloculated, elongated, well-circumscribed osteolytic lesion with surrounding sclerosis involving the proximal diaphysis of the tibia. A single-layer periosteal reaction envelops the tibia (arrows).

Illustration continued on following page

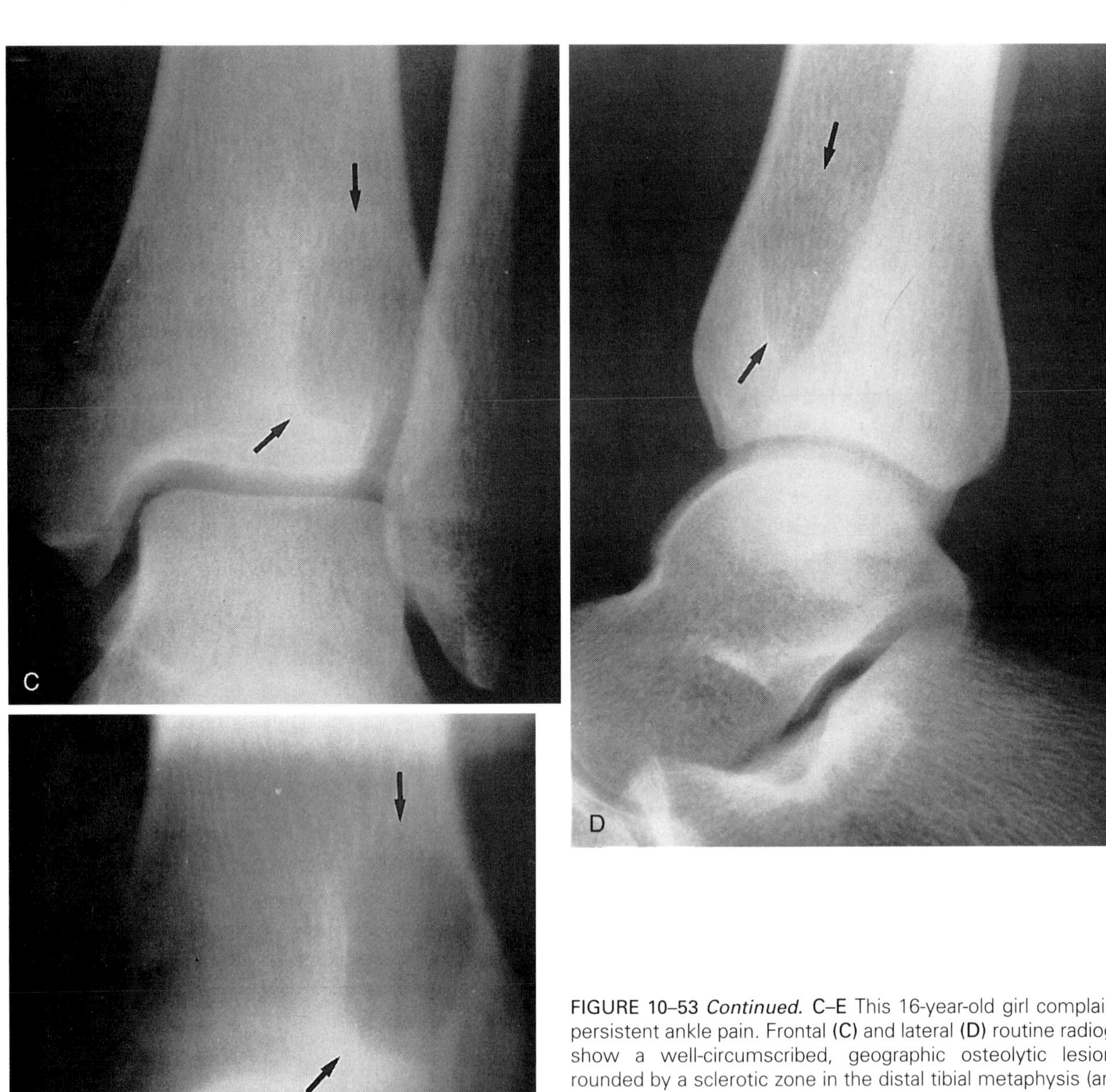

FIGURE 10–53 *Continued.* C–E This 16-year-old girl complained of persistent ankle pain. Frontal (C) and lateral (D) routine radiographs show a well-circumscribed, geographic osteolytic lesion surrounded by a sclerotic zone in the distal tibial metaphysis (arrows). The lesion is delineated more clearly with conventional tomography (E). The causative organism in both patients was *Staphylococcus aureus.*

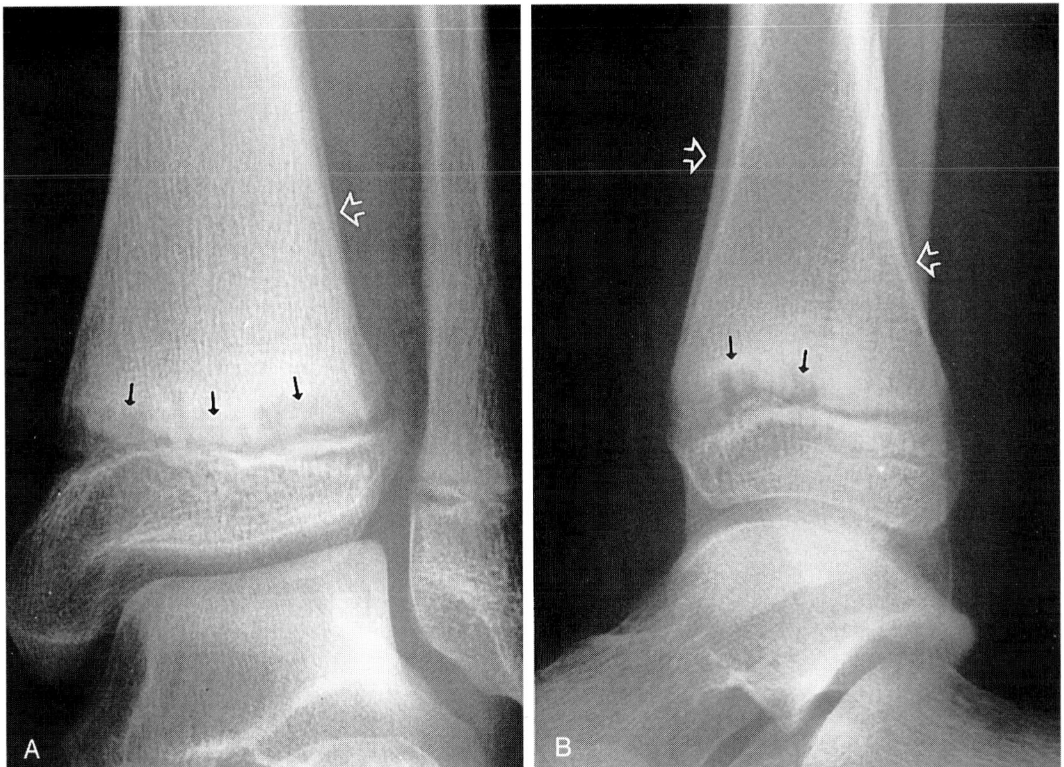

FIGURE 10–54. Chronic recurrent multifocal osteomyelitis.[89, 90] This 12-year-old boy had unilateral ankle swelling and pain for 4 months. Eight months earlier, he had had unilateral wrist pain and swelling. The erythrocyte sedimentation rate was slightly elevated, but all other serologic tests had normal results. Radiographs revealed similar changes at both sites. The findings on oblique (**A**) and lateral (**B**) radiographs include periostitis (open arrows), widening of the distal tibial physis, metaphyseal sclerosis, and subchondral osteolysis of the metaphysis adjacent to the growth plate (arrows). This unusual entity is controversial, and it is not certain whether it is truly infectious in nature. It typically causes significant symptoms but regresses without residual change. The metaphyses of long bones are the most frequent sites of involvement. *(Courtesy of S. Cassell, M.D., Eugene, Oregon.)*

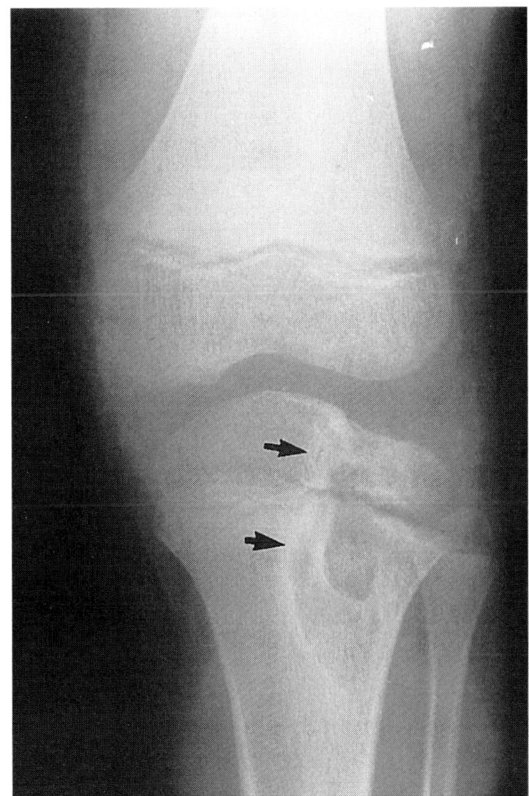

FIGURE 10–55 Tuberculous osteomyelitis: Transphyseal spread.[91] This 6-year-old girl has an atypical presentation of tuberculous osteomyelitis. A large, well-circumscribed osteolytic lesion (arrows) beginning in the metaphysis has spread across the physis to involve the epiphysis.

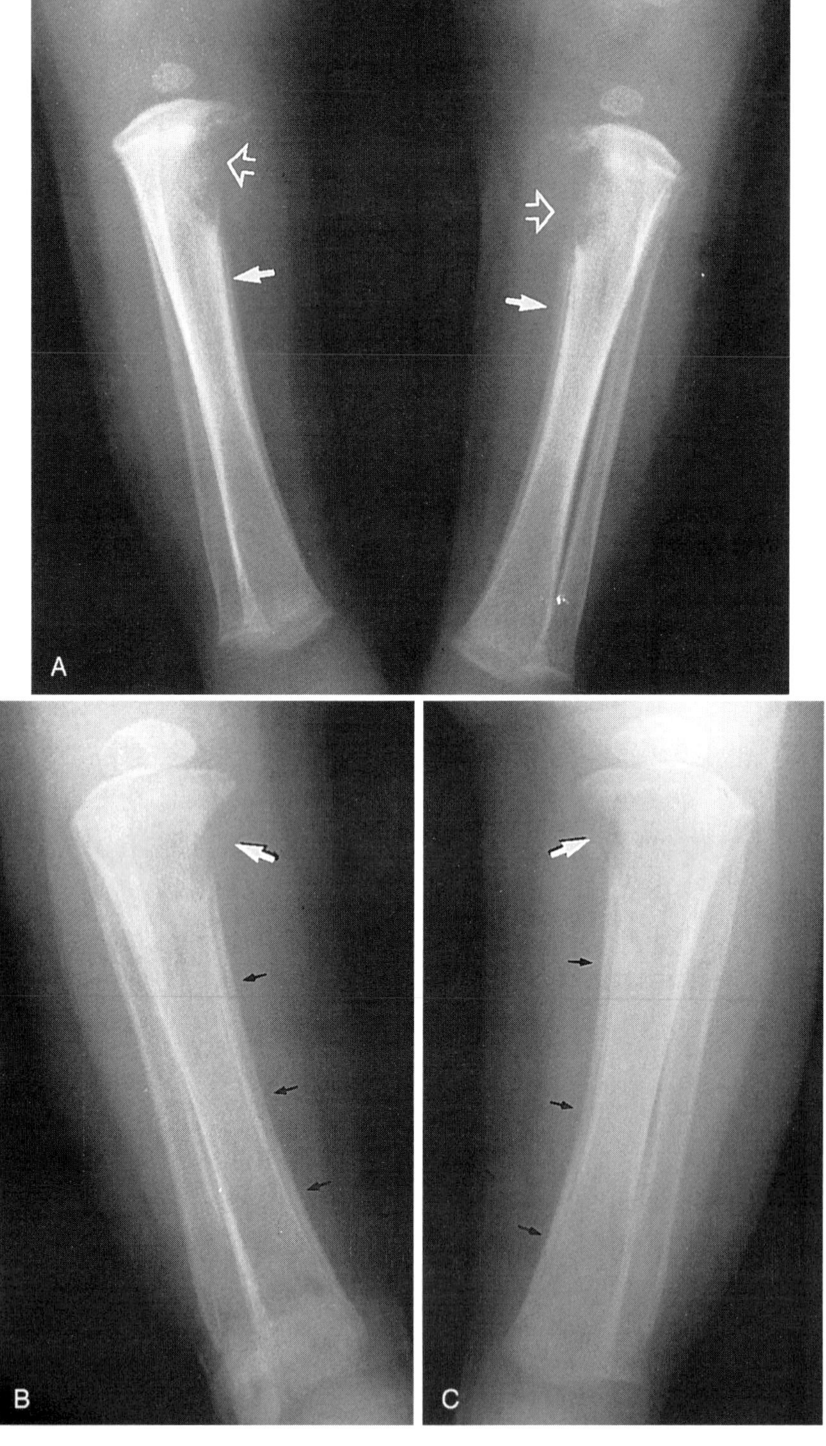

FIGURE 10–56. Congenital syphilis.[92, 93] **A** A radiograph of this 2-month-old baby demonstrates bilateral periostitis (arrows) and defects in the proximal medial tibial metaphyses (Wimberger's sign) (open arrows). **B, C** In another patient, radiographs of the lower extremities reveal extensive bilateral periostitis (small arrows) and osseous erosions of the medial tibial metaphysis (Wimberger's sign) (large arrows).

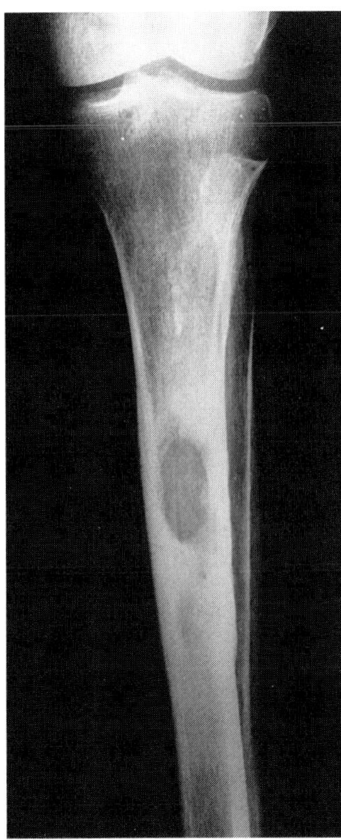

FIGURE 10–57. Leprous osteomyelitis.[94] In this patient with known leprosy, multiple osteolytic lesions surrounded by dense sclerosis were found to be related to hematogenous spread of infection, a rare manifestation of leprosy. The lesions were evident bilaterally. *(Courtesy of J. Schils, M.D., Cleveland, Ohio.)*

REFERENCES

1. Horsfield D, Jones SN: Assessment of inequality in length of the lower limb. Radiography 52:233, 1986.
2. Huurman WW, Jacobsen FS, Anderson JC, et al: Limb-length discrepancy measured with computerized axial tomographic equipment. J Bone Joint Surg [Am] 69:699, 1987.
3. Mannello DM: Leg length inequality. J Manipulative Physiol Ther 15:576, 1992.
4. Greene WB: Infantile tibia vara. J Bone Joint Surg [Am] 75:130, 1993.
5. Kovanlikaya A, Loro ML, Gilsanz V: Pathogenesis of osteosclerosis in autosomal dominant osteopetrosis. AJR 168:929, 1997.
6. Benli IT, Akalin S, Boysan E, et al: Epidemiological, clinical, and radiological aspects of osteopoikilosis. J Bone Joint Surg [Br] 74:504, 1992.
7. Bass HN, Weiner JR, Goldman A, et al: Osteopathia striata syndrome: Clinical, genetic, and radiologic considerations. Clin Pediatr 19:369, 1980.
8. Campbell CJ, Papademetriou T, Bonfiglio M: Melorheostosis: A report of the clinical, roentgenographic, and pathological findings in fourteen cases. J Bone Joint Surg [Am] 50:1281, 1968.
9. Yu JS, Resnick D, Vaughan LM, et al: Melorheostosis with an ossified soft tissue mass. Skeletal Radiol 24:367, 1995.
10. Whyte MP, Murphy WA, Fallon MD, et al: Mixed-sclerosing-bone-dystrophy: Report of a case and review of the literature. Skeletal Radiol 6:95, 1981.
11. Hanscom DA, Winter RB, Lutter L, et al: Osteogenesis imperfecta: Radiographic classification, natural history and treatment of spinal deformity. J Bone Joint Surg [Am] 74:598, 1992.
12. Kumar B, Murphy WA, Whyte MP: Progressive diaphyseal dysplasia (Englemann disease): Scintigraphic-radiographic-clinical correlations. Radiology 140:87, 1981.
13. Gershuni DH, Skyhar MJ, Thompson B, et al: A comparison of conventional radiography and computed tomography in the evaluation of spiral fractures of the tibia. J Bone Joint Surg [Am] 67:1388, 1985.
14. Sarmiento A, Gersten LM, Sobol PA, et al: Tibial shaft fractures treated with functional brace: Experience with 780 fractures. J Bone Joint Surg [Br] 71:602, 1989.
15. Conway JJ, Poznanski AP: Acute compression injuries of bone, or the toddler's fracture revisited. Pediatr Radiol 17:85, 1987.
16. Daffner RH, Martinez S, Gehweiler JA Jr, et al: Stress fractures of the proximal tibia in runners. Radiology 142:63, 1982.
17. Anderson MW, Greenspan A: Stress fractures. Radiology 199:1, 1996.
18. Mulligan ME, Shanley DJ: Supramalleolar fatigue fractures of the tibia. Skeletal Radiol 25:325, 1996.
19. Davies AM, Evans N, Grimer RJ: Fatigue fractures of the proximal tibia simulating malignancy. Br J Radiol 61:903, 1988.
20. Umans HR, Kaye JJ: Longitudinal stress fractures of the tibia: Diagnosis by magnetic resonance imaging. Skeletal Radiol 25:319, 1996.
21. Reading JM, Sheehan NJ: Spontaneous fractures of the lower limb in chronic rheumatoid arthritis. J Orthop Rheumatol 4:173, 1991.
22. Schneider R, Kaye JJ: Insufficiency fractures and stress fractures of the long bones occurring in patients with rheumatoid arthritis. Radiology 116:595, 1975.
23. Lock TR, Schaffer JJ, Manoli A II: Maisonneuve fracture: Case report of a missed diagnosis. Ann Emerg Med 16:805, 1987.
24. Nuovo MA, Norman A, Chumas A, et al: Myositis ossificans with atypical clinical, radiographic, or pathologic findings: A review of 23 cases. Skeletal Radiol 21:87, 1992.
25. Neugut AI, Casper ES, Godwin A, et al: Osteoblastic metastases in renal cell carcinoma. Br J Radiol 54:1002, 1981.
26. Greenspan A, Norman A: Osteolytic cortical destruction: An unusual pattern of skeletal metastasis. Skeletal Radiol 17:402, 1988.
27. Eklof O, Mortensson W, Sandstedt B, et al: Bone metastases in Wilm's tumor: Occurrence and radiological appearance. Ann Radiol 27:97, 1984.
28. Dahlin DC, Unni KK: Osteosarcoma of bone and its important recognizable varieties. Am J Surg Pathol 1:61, 1977.
29. Ritschl P, Wurnig C, Lechner G, et al: Parosteal osteosarcoma: 2–23-year follow-up of 33 patients. Acta Orthop Scand 62:195, 1991.
30. Mitchell M, Ackerman LV: Metastatic and pseudomalignant osteoblastoma: A report of two unusual cases. Skeletal Radiol 15:213, 1986.
31. Henderson ED, Dahlin DC: Chondrosarcoma of bone—a study of two hundred and eighty-eight cases. J Bone Joint Surg [Am] 45:1450, 1963.
32. Dahlin DC: Giant cell tumor of bone: Highlights of 407 cases. AJR 144:955, 1985.
33. Huvos AG, Higinbotham NL: Primary fibrosarcoma of

bone: A clinicopathologic study of 130 patients. Cancer 35:837, 1975.
34. Taconis WK, Mulder JD: Fibrosarcoma and malignant fibrous histiocytoma of long bones: Radiographic features and grading. Skeletal Radiol 11:237, 1984.
35. Keeney GL, Unni KK, Beabout JW, et al: Adamantinoma of long bones: A clinicopathologic study of 85 cases. Cancer 64:730, 1989.
36. Dahlin DC, Coventry MB, Scanlon PW: Ewing's sarcoma: A critical analysis of 165 cases. J Bone Joint Surg [Am] 43:185, 1961.
37. Kyle RA: Multiple myeloma: Review of 869 cases. Mayo Clin Proc 50:29, 1975.
38. Franczyk J, Samuels T, Rubenstein J, et al: Skeletal lymphoma. J Can Assoc Radiol 40:75, 1989.
39. Hermann G, Klein MJ, Abdelwahab IF, et al: MRI appearance of primary non-Hodgkin's lymphoma of bone. Skeletal Radiol 26:629, 1997.
40. Clayton F, Butler JJ, Ayala AG, et al: Non-Hodgkin's lymphoma in bone: Pathologic and radiologic features with clinical correlates. Cancer 60:2494, 1987.
41. Benz G, Brandeis WE, Willich E: Radiological aspects of leukemia in childhood: An analysis of 89 children. Pediatr Radiol 4:201, 1976.
42. Greenspan A: Bone island (enostosis): Current concept—a review. Skeletal Radiol 24:111, 1995.
43. Cohen MD, Harrington TM, Ginsbury WW: Osteoid osteoma: 95 cases and a review of the literature. Semin Arthritis Rheum 12:265, 1983.
44. Shankman S, Desai P, Beltran J: Subperiosteal osteoid osteoma: Radiographic and pathologic manifestations. Skeletal Radiol 26:457, 1997.
45. Kayser F, Resnick D, Haghighi P, et al: Evidence of the subperiosteal origin of osteoid osteomas in tubular bones: Analysis by CT and MR imaging. AJR 170:609, 1998.
46. Lichtenstein L, Sawyer WF: Benign osteoblastoma: Further observations and report of twenty additional cases. J Bone Joint Surg [Am] 46:755, 1964.
47. Wang J-W, Shih C-H, Chen W-J: Osteofibrous dysplasia (ossifying fibroma of long bones): A report of four cases and review of the literature. Clin Orthop 278:235, 1992.
48. Schiller AL: Diagnosis of borderline cartilage lesions of bone. Semin Diagn Pathol 2:42, 1985.
49. Bloem JL, Mulder JD: Chondroblastoma: A clinical and radiological study of 104 cases. Skeletal Radiol 14:1, 1985.
50. Weatherall PT, Maale GE, Mendelsohn DB, et al: Chondroblastoma: Classic and confusing appearance at MR imaging. Radiology 190:467, 1994.
51. Wilson AJ, Kyriakos M, Ackerman LV: Chondromyxoid fibroma: Radiographic appearance in 38 cases and in a review of the literature. Radiology 179:513, 1991.
52. Milgram JW: The origins of osteochondromas and enchondromas: A histopathologic study. Clin Orthop 174:264, 1983.
53. Karasick D, Schweitzer ME, Eschelman DJ: Symptomatic osteochondromas: Imaging features. AJR 168:1507, 1997.
54. Schmale GA, Conrad EV, Raskind WH: The natural history of hereditary multiple exostosis. J Bone Joint Surg [Am] 76:986, 1994.
55. Ritschl P, Karnel F, Hajek P: Fibrous metaphyseal defects—determination of their origin and natural history using a radiomorphological study. Skeletal Radiol 17:8, 1988.
56. Ehara S, Tamakawa Y, Nishida J, et al: Cortical defect of the distal fibula: Variant of ossification. Radiology 197:447, 1995.
57. Tehranzadeh J, Murphy BJ, Mnaymneh W: Giant cell tumor of the proximal tibia: MR and CT appearance. J Comput Assist Tomogr 13:282, 1989.
58. Milgram JW: Intraosseous lipoma: A clinicopathologic study of 66 cases. Clin Orthop 231:277, 1988.
59. Kenan S, Abdelwahab IF, Klein MJ, et al: Hemangiomas of the long tubular bones. Clin Orthop 280:256, 1992.
60. Chigira M, Maehara S, Arita S, et al: The aetiology and treatment of simple bone cysts. J Bone Joint Surg [Br] 65:633, 1983.
61. De Dios AMV, Bond JR, Shives TC, et al: Aneurysmal bone cyst: A clinico-pathologic study of 238 cases. Cancer 69:2921, 1992.
62. Bone HG, Kleerekoper M: Paget's disease of bone. J Clin Endocrinol Metab 7:1179, 1992.
63. Mirra JM, Brien EW, Tehranzadeh J: Paget's disease of bone: Review with emphasis on radiologic features, part II. Skeletal Radiol 24:173, 1995.
64. Yochum TR, Rowe LJ: Essentials of Skeletal Radiology. 2nd Ed. Baltimore, Williams & Wilkins, 1996.
65. Crawford AH Jr, Bogamery N: Osseous manifestations of neurofibromatosis in childhood. J Pediatr Orthop 6:72, 1986.
66. Morrissy RT: Congenital pseudoarthrosis of the tibia. Clin Orthop 166:14, 1982.
67. Gibson MJ, Middlemiss JH: Fibrous dysplasia of bone. Br J Radiol 44:1, 1971.
68. Kilpatrick SE, Wenger DE, Gilchrist GS, et al: Langerhans' cell histiocytosis (histiocytosis X) of bone: A clinicopathologic analysis of 263 pediatric and adult cases. Cancer 76:2471, 1995.
69. Taylor JAM, Resnick D, Sartoris DJ: Radiographic-pathologic correlation. *In* Sartoris DJ (ed): Osteoporosis: Diagnosis and Treatment. New York, Marcel Dekker, 1996, p 147.
70. Schwarzman RJ, McLellan TL: Reflex sympathetic dystrophy: A review. Arch Neurol 44:555, 1987.
71. Mankin HJ: Rickets, osteomalacia, and renal osteodystrophy. Orthop Clin North Am 21:81, 1990.
72. Chew FS, Huang-Hellinger F: Brown tumor. AJR 160:752, 1993.
73. Resnick D, Niwayama G: Parathyroid disorders and renal osteodystrophy. *In* Resnick D (ed): Diagnosis of Bone and Joint Disorders. 3rd Ed. Philadelphia, WB Saunders, 1995, p 2014.
74. Tigges S, Nance EP, Carpenter WA, et al: Renal osteodystrophy: Imaging findings that mimic those of other diseases. AJR 165:143, 1995.
75. Bronsky D, Kushner DS, Dubin A, et al: Idiopathic hypoparathyroidism and pseudohypoparathyroidism: Case reports and review of the literature. Medicine 37:317, 1958.
76. Lambert RGW, Becker EJ: Diffuse skeletal hyperostosis in idiopathic hypoparathyroidism. Clin Radiol 40:212, 1989.
77. Nerubay J, Pilderwasser D: Spontaneous bilateral distal femoral physiology due to scurvy. Acta Orthop Scand 55:18, 1984.
78. Sprague PL: Epiphyseo-metaphyseal cupping following infantile scurvy. Pediatr Radiol 4:122, 1976.
79. Bell RS, Mankin HJ, Doppelt SH: Osteomyelitis in Gaucher's disease. J Bone Joint Surg [Am] 68:1380, 1986.
80. Resnick D, Niwayama G: Enostosis, hyperostosis, and periostitis. *In* Resnick D (ed): Diagnosis of Bone and Joint Disorders. 3rd Ed. Philadelphia, WB Saunders, 1995, p 4434.
81. Pineda C: Diagnostic imaging in hypertrophic osteoarthropathy. Clin Exp Rheumatol 10:27, 1992.

82. Schumacher HR Jr: Hypertrophic osteoarthropathy: Rheumatologic manifestations. Clin Exp Rheumatol 10:35, 1992.
83. Ogden JA: Growth slowdown and arrest lines. J Pediatr Orthop 4:409, 1984.
84. Weinberger A, Kaplan JG, Myers AR: Extensive soft tissue calcification (calcinosis universalis) in systemic lupus erythematosus. Ann Rheum Dis 38:384, 1979.
85. Davidson JK: Dysbaric disorders: Aseptic bone necrosis in tunnel workers and divers. Clin Rheumatol 3:1, 1989.
86. Gold RH, Hawkins RA, Katz RD: Bacterial osteomyelitis: Findings on plain radiography, CT, MR, and scintigraphy. AJR 157:365, 1991.
87. Tumeh SS, Aliabadi P, Weissman BN, et al: Disease activity in osteomyelitis: Role of radiography. Radiology 165:781, 1987.
88. Stephens MM, MacAuley P: Brodie's abscess: A long-term review. Clin Orthop 234:211, 1988.
89. Rosenberg ZS, Shankman S, Klein M, et al: Chronic recurrent multifocal osteomyelitis. AJR 151:142, 1988.
90. Jurik AG, Egund N: MRI in chronic recurrent multifocal osteomyelitis. Skeletal Radiol 26:230, 1997.
91. Haygood T, Williamson SL: Radiographic findings of extremity tuberculosis in childhood: Back to the future? Radiographics 14:561, 1994.
92. Sachdev M, Bery K, Chawla S: Osseous manifestations in congenital syphilis: A study of 55 cases. Clin Radiol 33:319, 1982.
93. Dunn RA, Zenker PN: Why radiographs are useful in evaluation of neonates suspected of having congenital syphilis. Radiology 182:639, 1992.
94. Karat S, Karat ABA, Foster R: Radiological changes in the bones of the limbs in leprosy. Lepr Rev 39:147, 1968.
95. Cockshott WP, Martin R, Friedman L, et al: Focal fibrocartilaginous dysplasia and tibia vara: A case report. Skeletal Radiol 23:333, 1994.
96. Anderson MW, Ugalde V, Batt M, et al: Shin splints: MR appearance in a preliminary study. Radiology 204:177, 1997.

CHAPTER 11

Ankle and Foot

- Normal Developmental Anatomy
- Deformities of the Ankle and Foot
- Developmental Anomalies, Anatomic Variants, and Sources of Diagnostic Error
- Skeletal Dysplasias and Other Congenital Diseases
- Physical Injury
- Articular Disorders
- Infectious Disorders
- Tumors and Tumor-like Lesions
- Metabolic, Hematologic, and Vascular Disorders
- Osteonecrosis and Osteochondroses

Normal Developmental Anatomy

A thorough understanding of normal developmental anatomy is essential for accurate interpretation of radiographs of the pediatric ankle and foot. Table 11–1 outlines the age of appearance and fusion of the primary and secondary ossification centers. Figures 11–1 to 11–3 demonstrate the radiographic appearance of many important ossification centers and other developmental landmarks at selected ages from birth to skeletal maturity.

Deformities of the Ankle and Foot

Several congenital and pathologic processes result in alignment deformities about the ankle and foot. Table 11–2 describes a number of these deformities, many of which are illustrated in Figures 11–4 to 11–10; others are illustrated throughout the chapter as they are manifested in many disorders.

Developmental Anomalies, Anatomic Variants, and Sources of Diagnostic Error

The ankle and foot are frequent sites of anomalies, anatomic variants, and other sources of diagnostic error that may simulate disease and potentially result in misdiagnosis. Table 11–3 and Figures 11–11 to 11–20 represent selected examples of some of the more common processes.

Skeletal Dysplasias and Other Congenital Diseases

Table 11–4 outlines a number of the skeletal dysplasias and congenital disorders that affect the ankle and foot. Figures 11–21 to 11–24 illustrate the radiographic manifestations of some of these disorders.

Physical Injury

Physical injury to the ankle and foot results in a wide variety of fractures and dislocations. Fractures and dislocations of the ankle (Tables 11–5 and 11–6), the tarsal bones (Table 11–7), and the metarsals and phalanges (Table 11–8) are listed and discussed in this section. Soft tissue injuries are described in Table 11–9. Many of these traumatic conditions are illustrated in Figures 11–25 to 11–53. Fractures of the diaphyses of the tibia and fibula are described and illustrated in Chapter 10.

Articular Disorders

The articulations of the ankle and foot are frequent target sites for degenerative, inflammatory, crystal-induced, and infectious disorders. Table 11–10 outlines these diseases and their radiographic characteristics. Table 11–11 represents a compartmental analysis emphasizing the target sites of joint involvement typical of some of the more common disorders. Table 11–12 outlines the differential diagnosis of articular disorders that result in calcaneal changes. Figures 11–54 to 11–71 illustrate the typical radiographic manifestations of the most common articular disorders affecting the ankle and foot.

Infectious Disorders

The soft tissues, bones, and joints of the ankle and foot are frequent sites of involvement for infectious disorders. Table 11–13 describes the major types of infection. These disorders are illustrated in Figures 11–72 to 11–74.

Tumors and Tumor-like Lesions

Table 11–14 lists and characterizes the neoplasms that typically involve the bones of the foot, many of which are illustrated in Figures 11–75 to 11–88.

Metabolic, Hematologic, and Vascular Disorders

Several metabolic, hematologic, and vascular disorders affect the bones of the foot and the surrounding soft tissue structures. Table 11–15 lists some of the more common disorders and describes their characteristics. Figures 11–89 to 11–95 illustrate the typical imaging findings of several of these disorders.

Osteonecrosis and Osteochondroses

Osteonecrosis of the bones about the ankle and foot may occur spontaneously or result from trauma or other predisposing factors. Furthermore, several epiphyseal disorders termed osteochondroses may involve the bones of the foot. Table 11–16 describes these disorders, and Figures 11–96 to 11–100 illustrate typical examples of their radiographic appearance.

TABLE 11–1. Ankle and Foot: Approximate Age of Appearance and Fusion of Ossification Centers[1-4] (Figs. 11–1 to 11–3)

Ossification Center	Primary or Secondary	No. of Centers	Age of Appearance*	Age of Fusion* (Years)
Distal tibial epiphysis	S	1	2–3 years	14–18
Distal fibular epiphysis	S	1	2–3 years	14–18
Talus	P	1	Birth	
Calcaneus	P	1	Birth	
Calcaneal apophysis (girls)	S	1	7–9 years	14–18
Calcaneal apophysis (boys)	S	1	10–12 years	18–22
Cuboid bone	P	1	Birth	
Navicular bone	P	1	1.5–4 years	
Cuneiforms 1 and 2	P	1 each	3–4 years	
Cuneiform 3 (lateral)	P	1	5–6 months	
First phalangeal base	S	1	3–4 years	14–20
First metatarsal base	S	1	3–4 years	14–20
Second to fifth metatarsal heads	S	1 each	3–4 years	14–20

*Ages of appearance and fusion of ossification centers in girls typically precede those of boys. Ethnic differences also exist.
P, Primary; S, secondary.

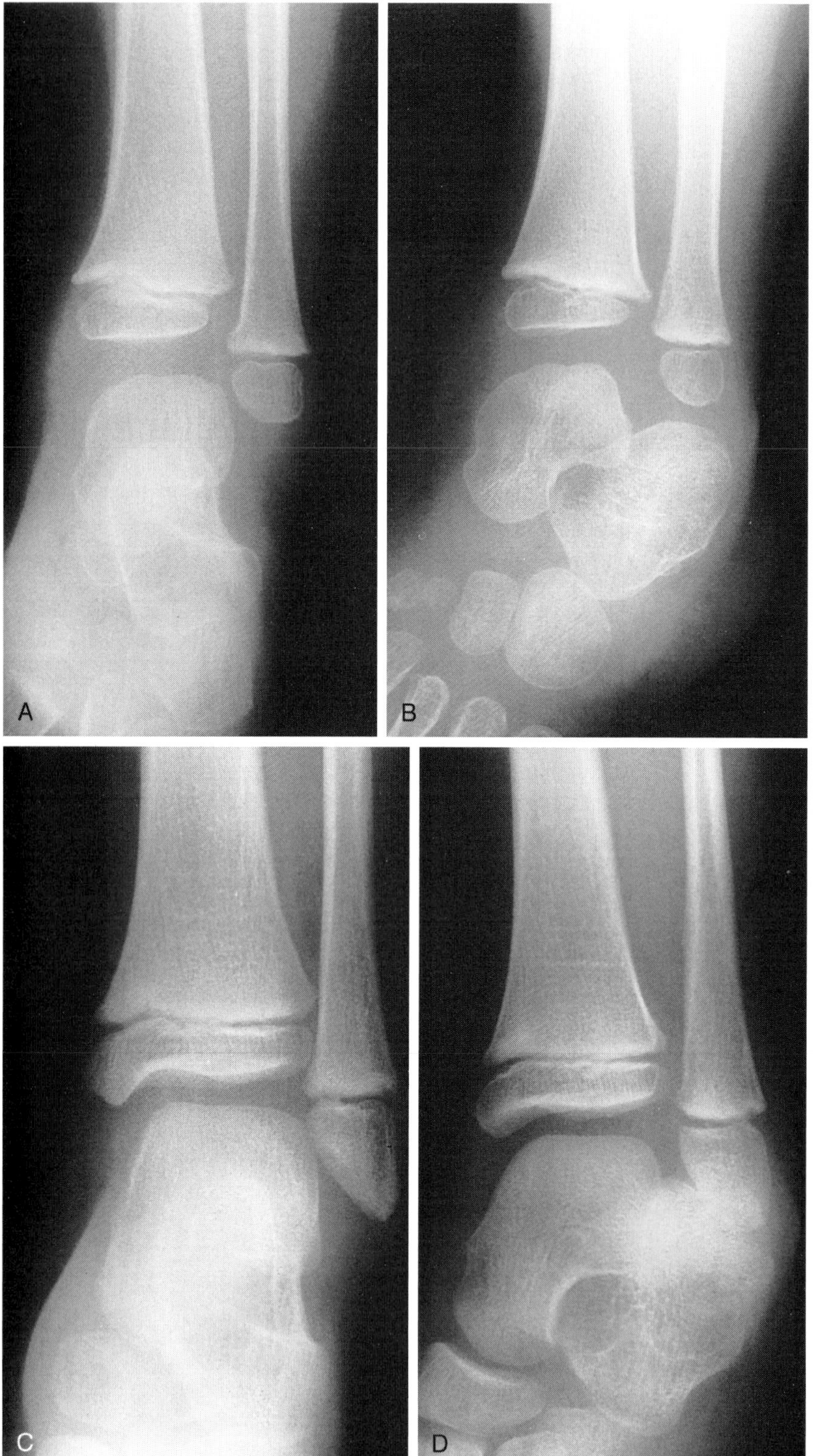

FIGURE 11–1. Skeletal maturation and normal development: Anteroposterior and oblique ankle radiographs.[1–4] A, B 3-year-old boy. The tibial and fibular epiphyses are rounded and small in relation to the adjacent metaphyses. The talus is incompletely ossified, the superior margins are rounded and undulating, and the tibiotalar joint space appears wide. The zones of provisional calcification within the tibia and fibula are sclerotic, and the metaphyses are beak-like. C, D 7-year-old girl. The superior talar surface is flatter and the tibiotalar joint space is narrower. The tibial and fibular epiphyses conform to and approximate the width of the metaphyses. The zones of provisional calcification remain radiodense. Irregular ossification of the medial aspect of the tibial and fibular epiphyses is common during normal development.

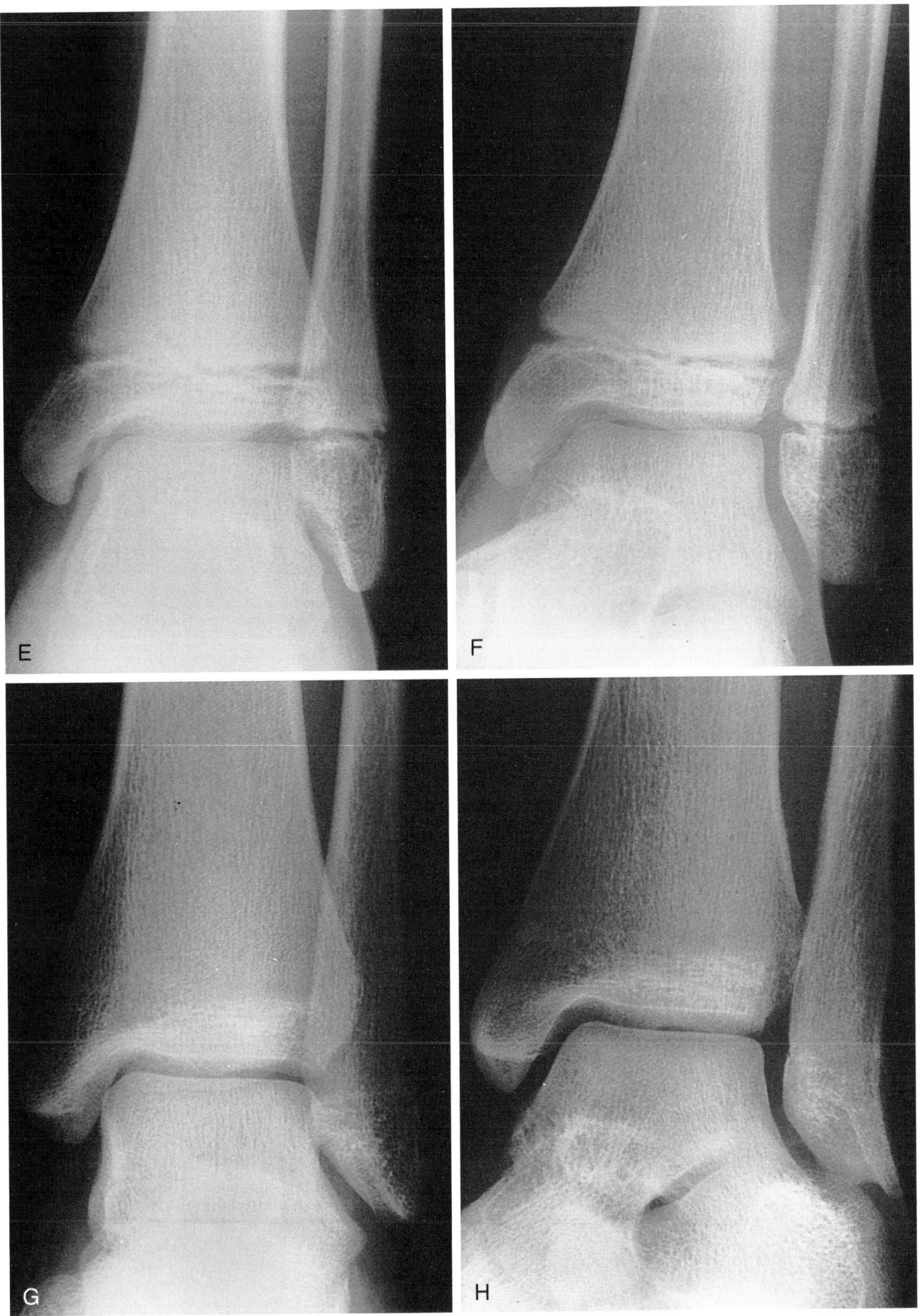

FIGURE 11–1 *Continued.* E, F 9-year-old girl. The tibial and fibular epiphyses are wider than their adjacent metaphyses. The physeal line is narrowed, and the zone of provisional calcification is less dense than previously. The talus and mortise joints exhibit an adult configuration. G, H 13-year-old girl. The epiphyses of the tibia and fibula have fused, and the physeal scars are barely visible.

Illustration continued on following page

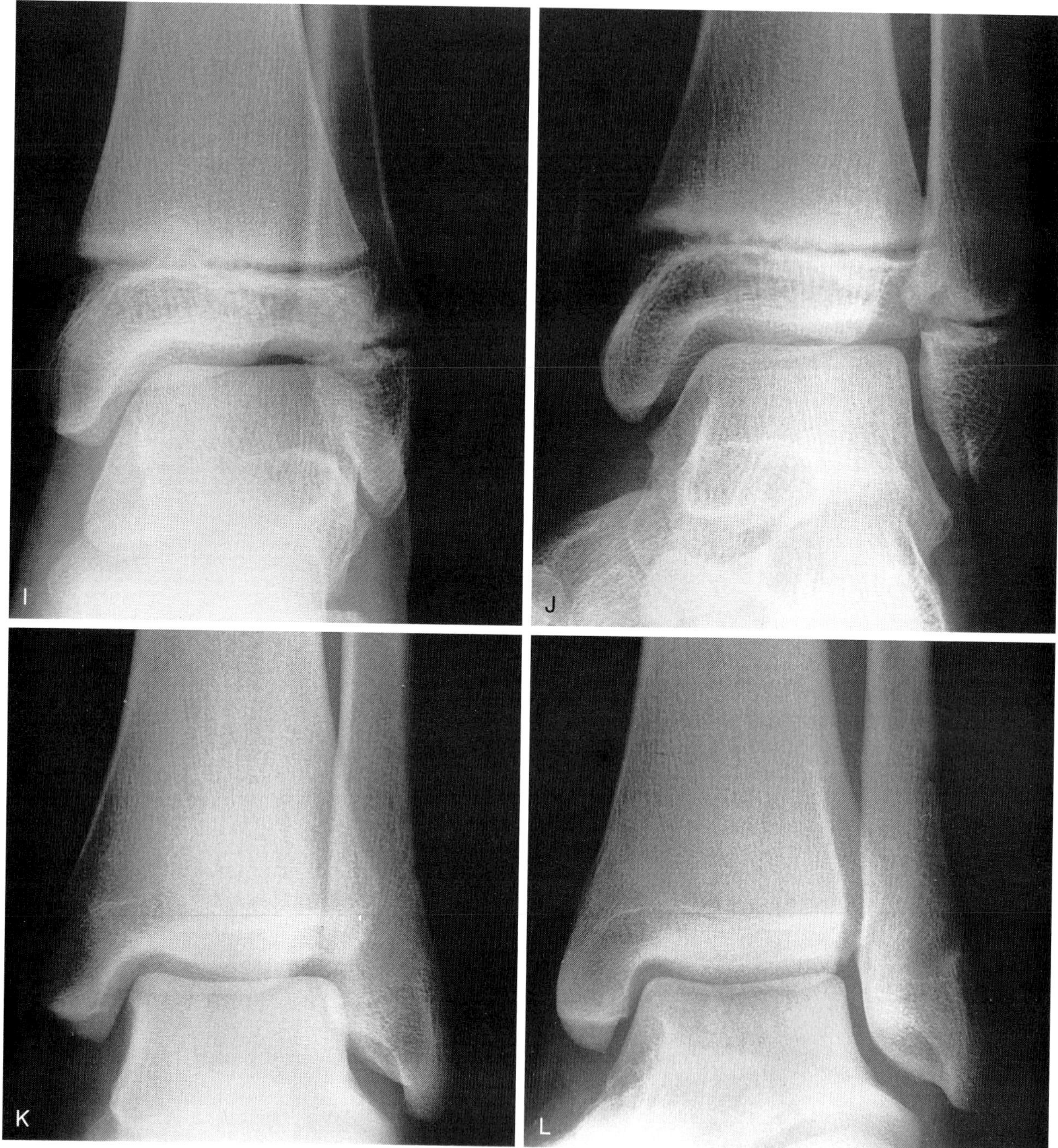

FIGURE 11–1 *Continued.* I, J 14-year-old boy. Development in the male skeleton lags behind that of the female (compare to G and H). In this case, the physes remain open, the zones of provisional calcification are radiodense, and the metaphyseal margins are irregular just before fusion. K, L 16-year-old boy. Complete epiphyseal fusion is evident. The physeal scars remain visible. Skeletal maturation in a boy of this age corresponds approximately to that of a 13-year-old girl (G, H).

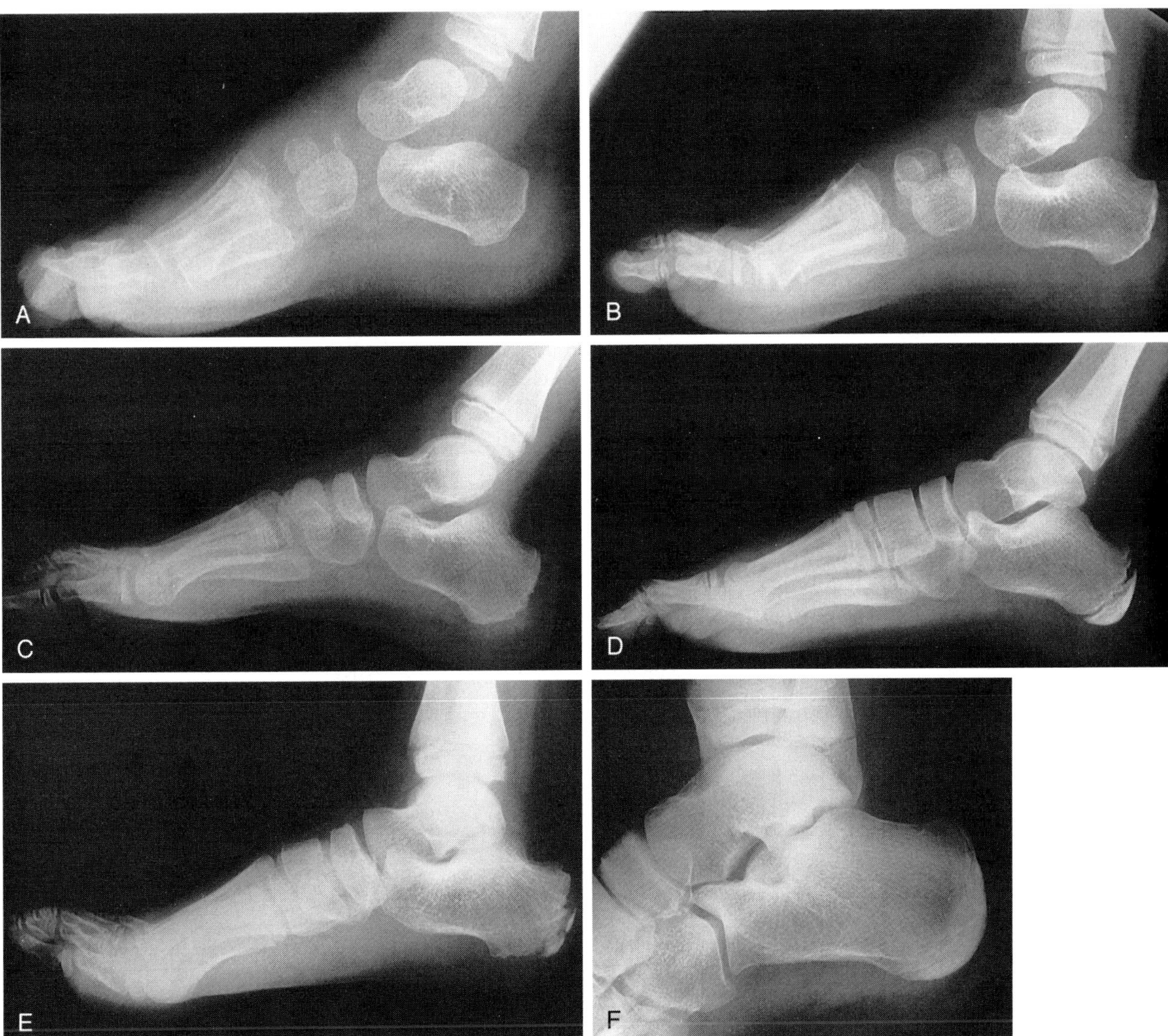

FIGURE 11–2. Skeletal maturation and normal development: Lateral radiographs of the foot and ankle.[1–4] A 2-year-old girl. The tibial and fibular epiphyses and the talus, calcaneus, cuboid, third cuneiform, and navicular bones are ossified. B 4-year-old boy. The first and second cuneiform bones are now also ossified. C 6-year-old boy. The tibial and fibular epiphyses are approaching the width of their respective metaphyses, and the zones of provisional calcification are radiodense. The posterior margin of the calcaneus is serrated. D 9-year-old girl. The tarsal bones have an adult configuration. The sclerotic calcaneal apophysis is evident, and the apposing margins are serrated. The zone of provisional calcification of the distal end of the tibia remains radiodense. E 11-year-old boy. The calcaneal apophysis is sclerotic and fragmented, and the adjacent calcaneus has a normal sawtooth appearance. Skeletal development in boys lags behind that of girls, as evidenced by comparison with the 9-year-old girl in D. F 15-year-old boy. The calcaneal apophysis is partially fused with the adjacent calcaneus. The tibial and fibular epiphyses are beginning to fuse, and the zones of provisional calcification are less sclerotic than previously.

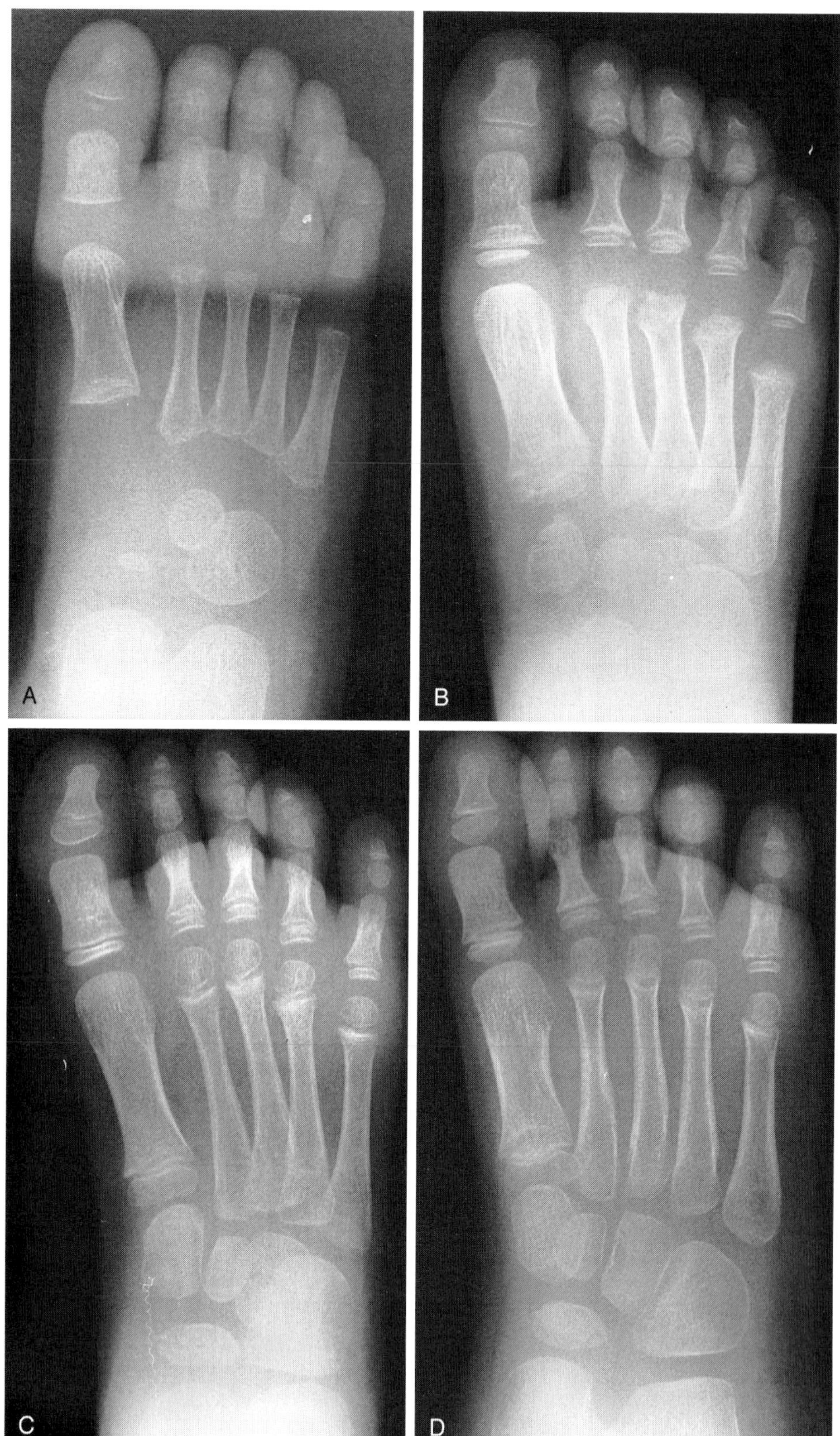

FIGURE 11–3. Skeletal maturation and normal development: Radiographs of the forefoot.[1–4] A 21-month-old boy. The cuboid, third cuneiform, and navicular bones are ossified. The epiphysis of the first distal phalanx has appeared, but no other metatarsal or phalangeal epiphyses are visible. B 31-month-old girl. The remaining two cuneiform bones are now ossified, and the metatarsal and phalangeal epiphyses are beginning to appear. C, D 4-year-old girl. Epiphyseal development is progressing, especially in the metatarsal centers.

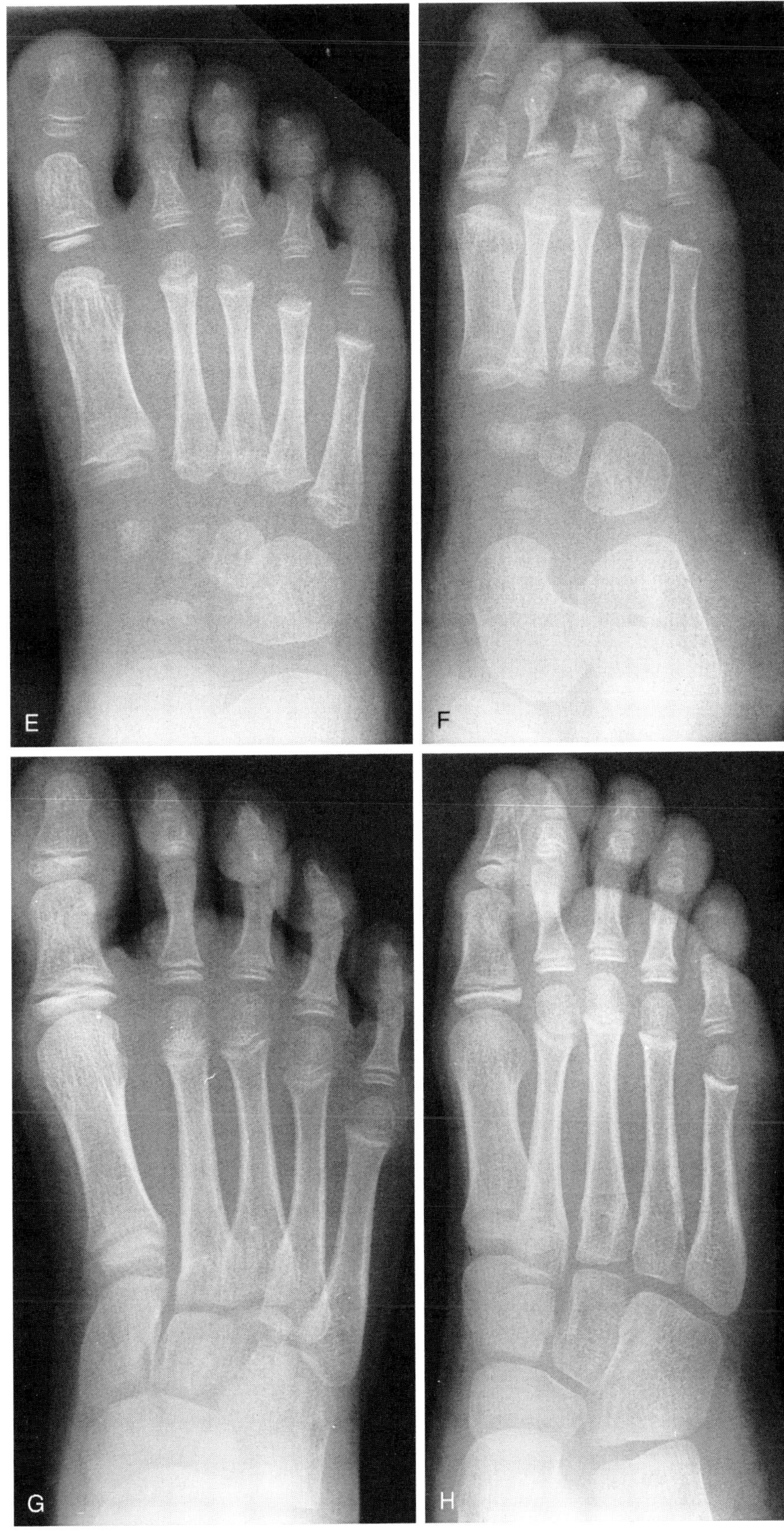

FIGURE 11–3 *Continued.* E, F 5-year-old boy. Epiphyseal development and ossification of the tarsal bones of this boy (E, F) lag behind those of the 4-year-old girl (C, D). G, H 7-year-old girl. The tarsal bones have approximated the adult configuration. The metatarsal and phalangeal epiphyseal centers have grown to adult proportions but have not yet fused.

Illustration continued on following page

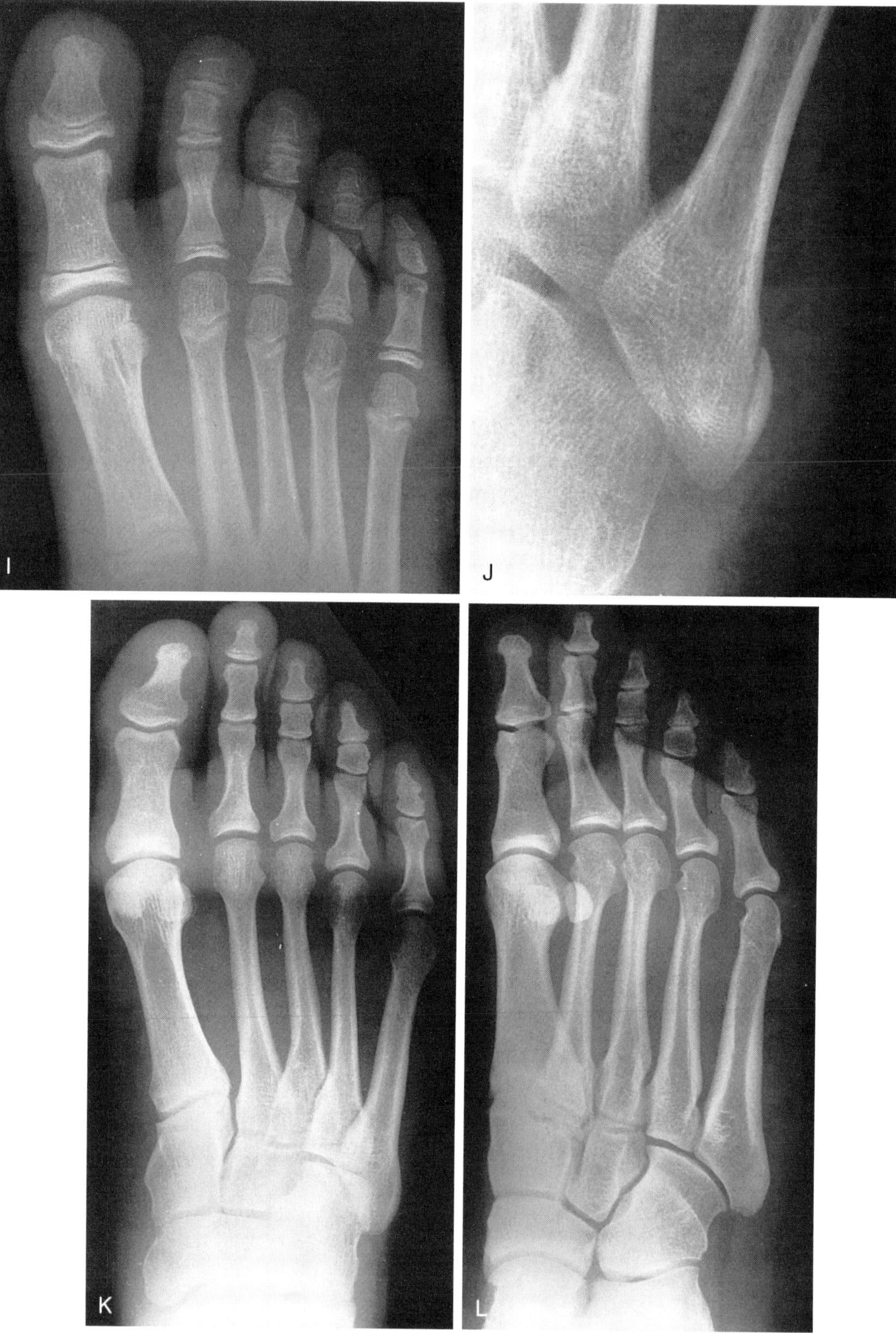

FIGURE 11–3 *Continued.* I 11-year-old boy. The radiodensity of the first and fifth proximal phalangeal epiphyseal centers is a normal finding just before fusion. The hallux sesamoid bones are ossified and clearly visible. J 13-year-old boy. Observe the longitudinal secondary ossification center of the fifth metatarsal styloid process. This should not be mistaken for a fracture. K, L 15-year-old girl. The metatarsal and phalangeal epiphyseal centers have all fused. The tarsal bones are well developed and their configuration resembles that of adults. Of incidental note is a synostosis of the fifth distal interphalangeal joint.

TABLE 11–2. Deformities of the Ankle and Foot

Entity	Figure(s)	Characteristics	Comments
Tibiotalar slant[5–6]	11–4; see Figs 11–57 B, 11–67 A	Angular joint surfaces of the tibial plafond and talar dome seen on anteroposterior views of the ankle	Improper radiographic positioning (pseudotibiotalar slant) Hemophilia Juvenile chronic arthritis Sickle cell anemia Multiple epiphyseal dysplasia Hereditary multiple exostoses
Ball-and-socket ankle joint[8]	11–5	Convex configuration of the proximal talar articular surface and associated concave configuration of the distal tibial articular surface	Talocalcaneal coalition Adaptation of joint to facilitate inversion and eversion motions that are restricted by talocalcaneal fusion
Varus deformity of foot[7]		Heel is inverted Forefoot is adducted and inverted	Usually developmental Often combined with other deformities
Valgus deformity of foot[7]		Heel is everted Forefoot is abducted and everted	Usually developmental Often combined with other deformities
Equinus deformity of foot[7]		Foot is plantar flexed Toes are lower than heel	Usually developmental Often combined with other deformities
Calcaneus deformity of foot[7]		Foot is dorsiflexed Toes are higher than heel	Usually developmental Often combined with other deformities
Talipes equinovarus[7]		Congenital clubfoot Plantar flexion of foot Hindfoot equinus Cavus deformity Parallel long axis of talus and calcaneus Metatarsus varus	Usually isolated abnormality May be associated with the following: Arthrogryposis Meningomyelocele Developmental hip dysplasia Tibial hypoplasia
Talipes calcaneovalgus[7]		Common disorder Usually bilateral Severe dorsiflexion of foot Calcaneus and valgus deformity of heel Abduction and planus deformity of forefoot	Developmental
Congenital vertical talus[7]	11–6	Rocker-bottom foot Rare rigid form of congenital flatfoot Talus oriented vertically and caudally Equinus deformity of heel Dorsiflexion and valgus deformity of forefoot Navicular bone dislocated dorsally Talus in varus position and only posterior portion articulates with tibia	Developmental Trisomy 13-15 or trisomy 18 Eighty per cent of patients have associated disorders such as the following: Scoliosis Dysraphism Syndactyly Developmental hip dysplasia Congenital heart disease
Hereditary pes planus[4, 7]	11–7	Flatfoot deformity Present in as much as 10 per cent of population Foot functions normally and is flexible Talus may be plantar flexed (vertical talus) in severe cases	Hereditary variation of normal
Acquired pes planus[4, 7]		Flatfoot deformity develops secondary to underlying disorder	Arthritis Neuropathic osteoarthropathy Posterior tibial tendon weakness or rupture Tarsal coalition Ehlers-Danlos syndrome Osteogenesis imperfecta
Pes planovalgus[4, 7]		More severe form of flatfoot typically associated with underlying disorders	Neuromuscular disorders Posterior tibial tendon rupture
Cavus deformity[9]	11–8	Elevation of the longitudinal arch Occasional equinus deformity	Developmental Acquired: neurologic disorders
Metatarsus varus (adductus)[7]	11–9	Adduction and varus position of all metatarsals at the tarsometatarsal articulations Heel in normal position Fifty per cent of cases are bilateral	Unknown cause Present at birth; usually detected during the second to third months of age Associated with stress fracture of the lateral metatarsal bones

Table continued on following page

TABLE 11–2. Deformities of the Ankle and Foot *Continued*

Entity	Figure(s)	Characteristics	Comments
Hallux valgus[10–12]	11–10	One of the most common toe deformities Lateral deviation (valgus deformity) of the first proximal phalanx in relation to the first metatarsal Often associated with lateral subluxation of the hallux sesamoid bones Women >men; bilateral asymmetric May be aggravated by advancing age, obesity, and physiologically inappropriate footwear	Developmental: often coexists with metatarsus varus Osteoarthrosis of the first MTP joint Inflammatory arthropathies Crystal deposition arthropathies Fibrodysplasia ossificans progressiva
Hallux rigidus[10]	See Fig. 11–54 D	Painful restriction of dorsiflexion at the first MTP joint	Advanced osteoarthrosis of the first MTP joint
Hallux varus[7]	See Figs. 11–20 A, 11–56 C	Rare deformity Medial deviation (varus deformity) of the first proximal phalanx in relation to the first metatarsal	Developmental; often in conjunction with polydactyly and syndactyly Infrequent finding in rheumatoid arthritis
Hammer toe[4, 7]		Dorsiflexion deformity of MTP joint with possible subluxation or dislocation of the proximal phalanx Plantar flexion of the PIP joint Dorsiflexion of DIP joint Most commonly involves second and fifth toes	Secondary to acquired or congenital foot deformities
Claw toe[4, 7]		Dorsiflexion of MTP joint Plantar flexion of PIP and DIP joints dorsiflexed Proximal phalanx is oriented vertically	Secondary to acquired or congenital foot deformities
Mallet toe[4, 7]		Plantar flexion of DIP joint	Secondary to acquired or congenital foot deformities
Curly toe[4, 7]		No deformity of MTP joint Plantar flexion of PIP and DIP joints	Secondary to acquired or congenital foot deformities

MTP, Metatarsophalangeal; PIP, proximal interphalangeal; DIP, distal interphalangeal.

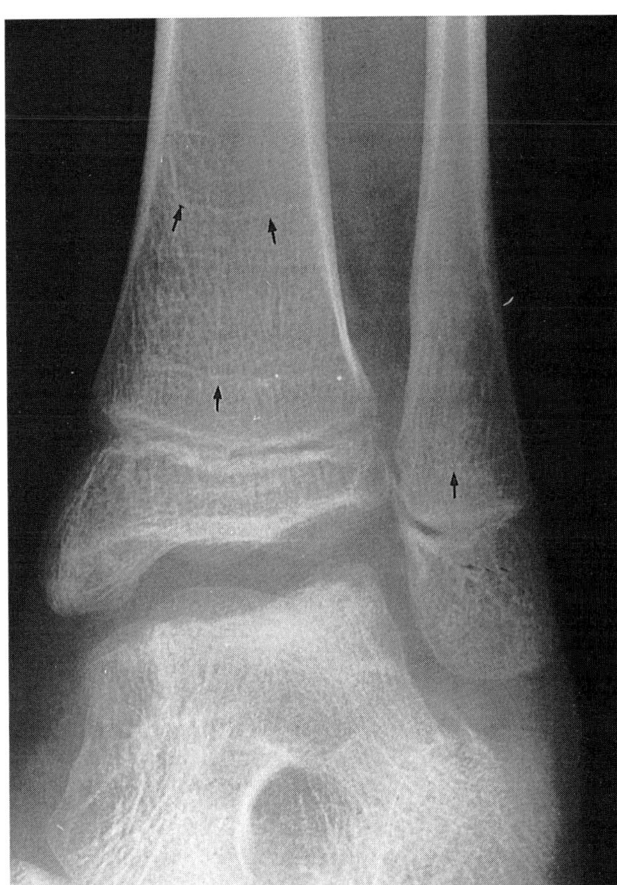

FIGURE 11–4. Tibiotalar slant: Hemophilic arthropathy.[5, 6] Oblique radiograph of the ankle in a 9-year-old boy with hemophilia reveals flattening and erosion of the superior surface of the talus with a characteristic tibiotalar slant. Prominent growth recovery lines (arrows) also are evident within the tibia and fibula. The joint space is relatively well preserved. Tibiotalar slant also occurs in juvenile chronic arthritis, Trevor's disease, fibrous dysplasia, and many other disorders. Additionally, pseudotibiotalar slant may result from improper positioning of the patient.

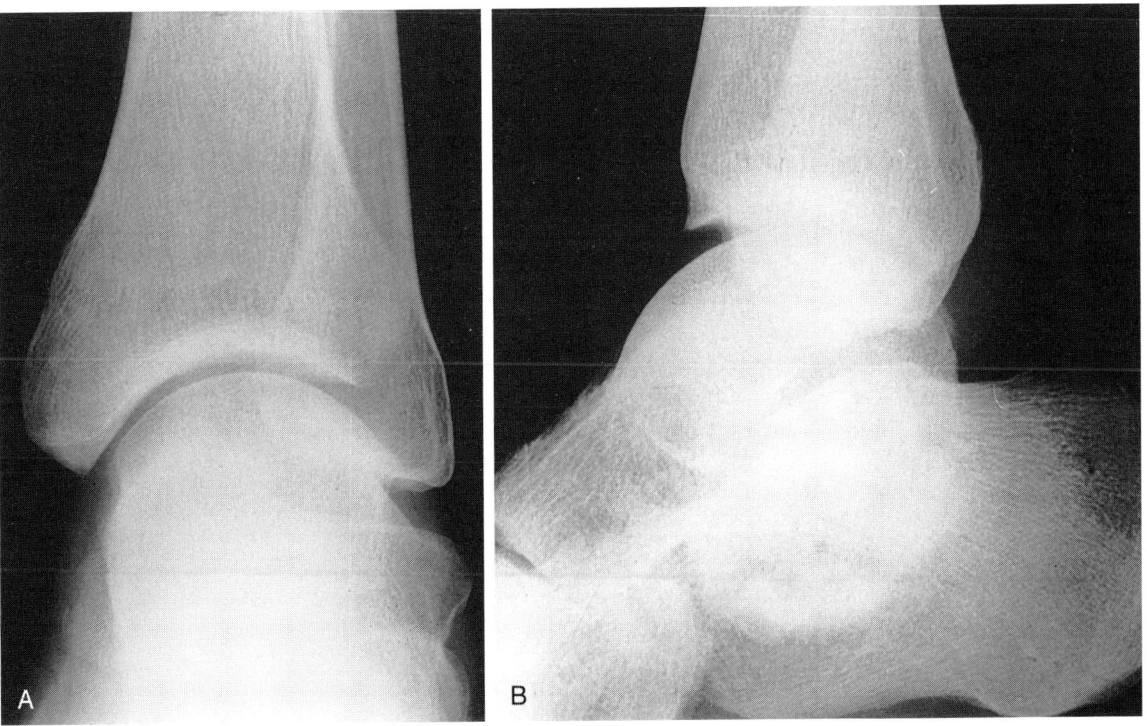

FIGURE 11–5. Ball-and-socket ankle joint: Talocalcaneal coalition.[8] Frontal (A) and lateral (B) radiographs of the ankle in this patient with congenital talocalcaneal coalition reveal a rounded convex appearance of the proximal talar articular surface and a concave appearance of the distal end of the tibia. The ball-and-socket ankle joint presumably represents an adaptation of the tibiotalar joint to provide inversion and eversion motion, which is restricted owing to the talocalcaneal fusion.

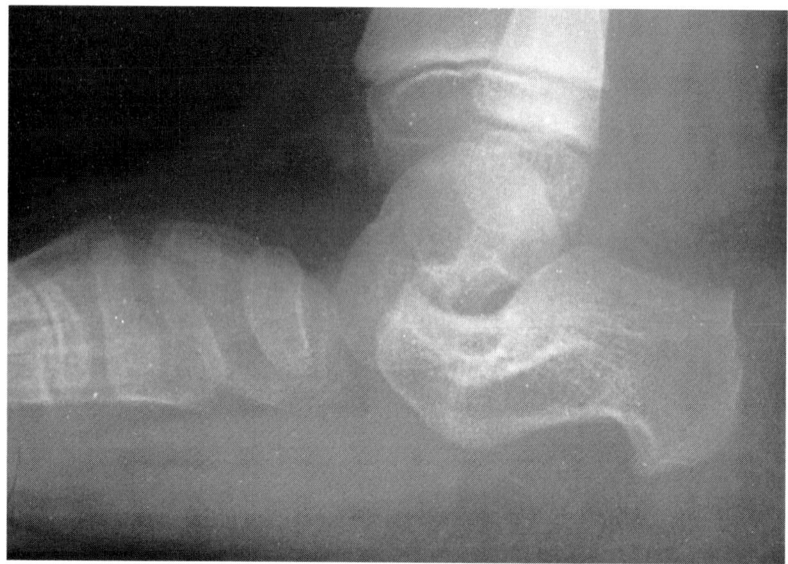

FIGURE 11–6. Congenital vertical talus (rocker-bottom foot).[7] The talus is vertically oriented on the lateral radiograph, and the longitudinal arch appears flattened. In this rare congenital deformity, the talonavicular joint is dislocated and the foot is rigid, creating a fixed deformity. More than 80 per cent of cases have associated abnormalities, such as congenital hip dislocation, scoliosis, dysraphism, ventricular septal defect, syndactyly, or one of the trisomy syndromes.

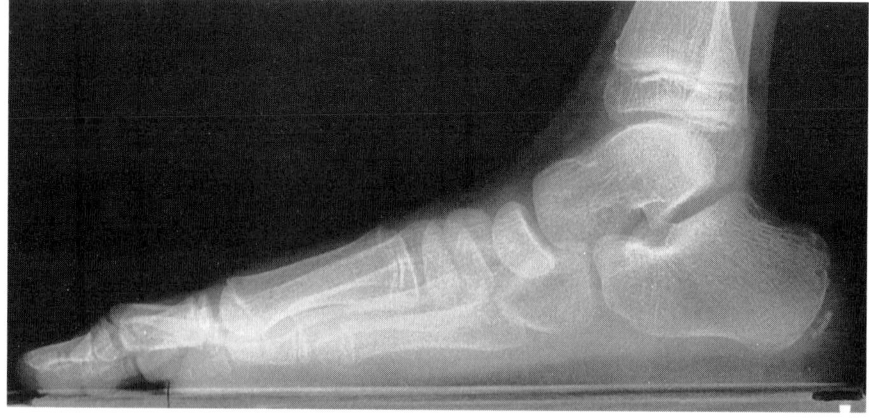

FIGURE 11–7. Pes planus (flatfoot deformity).[4, 7] Standing radiograph of the foot in this 9-year-old boy shows a characteristic reduction in the height of the longitudinal arch. This hereditary form of flatfoot, present in about 10% of the population, is considered a variation of normal in which the foot functions normally and is flexible. A more severe form of flatfoot associated with neuromuscular disorders is termed pes planovalgus. Additionally, adults may develop flatfoot secondary to severe arthritis, neuropathic joint disease, or rupture of the posterior tibial tendon.

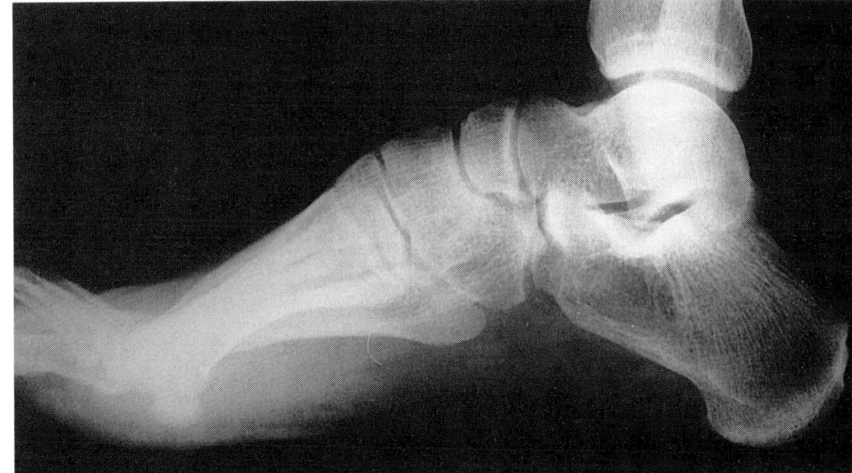

FIGURE 11–8. Cavus deformity.[9] Elevation of the longitudinal arch is seen in this radiograph of a 28-year-old man. This deformity, characterized by an unusually high longitudinal arch, may be congenital or acquired. Acquired cases usually are associated with a neurologic disorder.

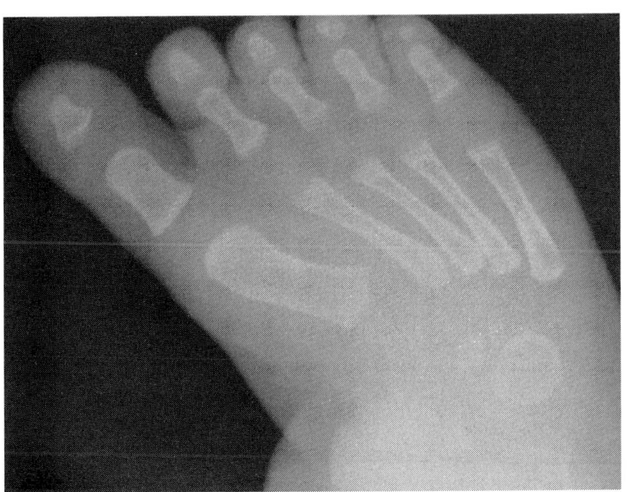

FIGURE 11–9. Metatarsus varus (adductus) deformity.[7] Observe the adduction and varus position of all the metatarsal bones at the tarsometatarsal articulations. The heel typically is in a normal position. This common deformity is of unknown cause.

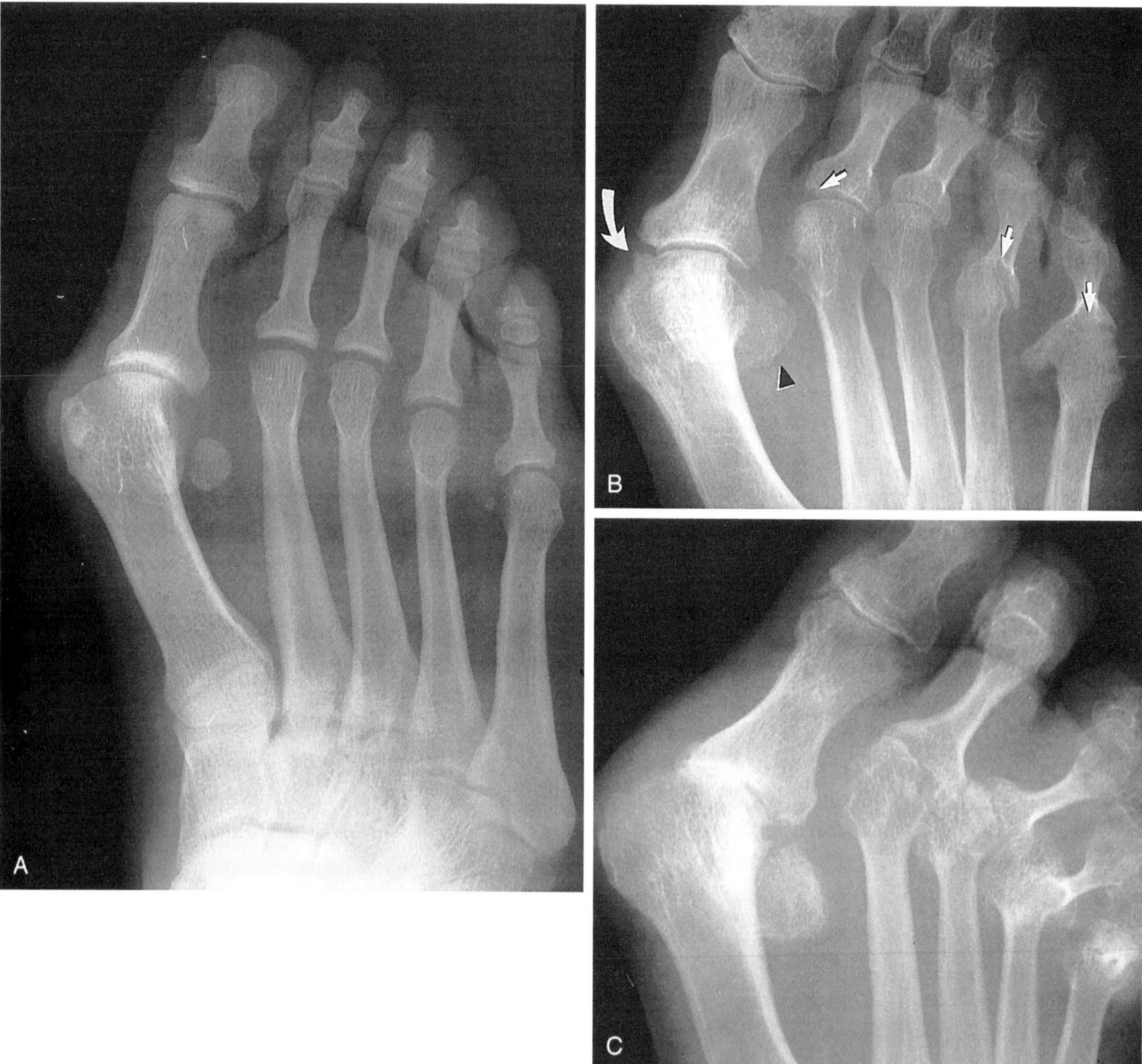

FIGURE 11–10. Hallux valgus: Differential diagnosis.[10–12] A Osteoarthrosis. Marked degenerative joint disease (osteoarthrosis) of the first metatarsophalangeal joint has resulted in severe valgus deformity with prominence of the soft tissues overlying the medial aspect of the articulation (bunion). Other findings include considerable nonuniform joint space narrowing, subchondral sclerosis, osteophyte formation, and osseous hypertrophy of the medial aspect of the metatarsal head. Note also the lateral subluxation of the sesamoid bones. B Ankylosing spondylitis. Marked hallux valgus is associated with multiple juxta-articular and intra-articular erosions (arrows), metatarsophalangeal joint space narrowing, fluffy periostitis (curved arrow), and sesamoid bone subluxation (arrowhead). C Rheumatoid arthritis. Striking valgus deformity of the great toe accompanies valgus deformities of the lateral four metatarsophalangeal joints. Observe also the widespread periarticular erosions and the lateral subluxation of the hallux sesamoid bones.

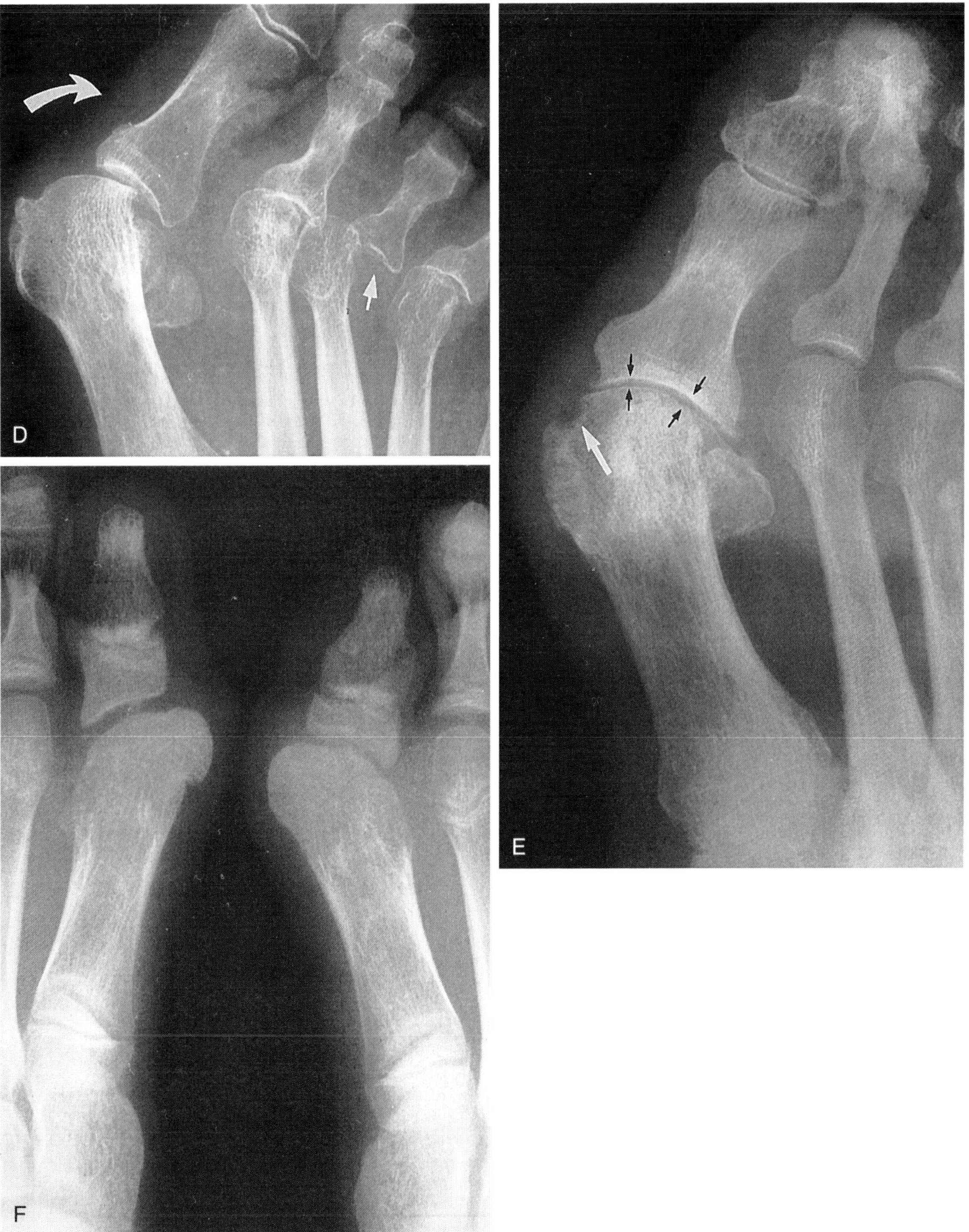

FIGURE 11–10 *Continued.* D Calcium pyrophosphate dihydrate (CPPD) crystal deposition disease. Lateral deviation of the metatarsophalangeal joint (curved arrow) is associated with a dislocation of the third metatarsophalangeal joint (arrow) in this patient. E Gout. Hallux valgus deformity, joint space narrowing (black arrows), soft tissue swelling, and erosions (white arrow) are seen in this man with long-standing gout. F Fibrodysplasia (myositis) ossificans progressiva. Frontal radiograph of both feet shows bilateral hallux valgus deformities with angulation of the distal metatarsal articular surfaces, a characteristic finding in this ossifying diathesis. Note also the abnormal shortening of the first proximal phalanges.

TABLE 11–3. Developmental Anomalies, Anatomic Variants, and Sources of Diagnostic Error Affecting the Ankle and Foot

Entity	Figure(s)	Characteristics
Tarsal coalition (developmental)		Fibrous, cartilaginous, or osseous congenital fusion of two or more tarsal bones Ossification of fibrous or cartilaginous fusions occurs during the second decade and may result in the onset of symptoms
1. Calcaneonavicular[13, 14]	11–11	May represent 50 per cent of all cases of tarsal coalition Occasionally bilateral Asymptomatic or associated with rigid flatfoot Best radiographic view: 45-degree oblique foot Fibrous and cartilaginous fusions not directly visible Secondary signs: Close approximation of the calcaneus and navicular Irregular cortical surfaces Hypoplastic head of talus Enlargement of anterior process of calcaneus ("anteater nose" sign)
2. Talocalcaneal[13–16]	11–5, 11–12	Approximately 35 to 50 per cent of all cases of tarsal coalition Twenty per cent of cases are bilateral Signs and symptoms tend to be more severe than in calcaneonavicular coalition Best radiographic view: 45-degree axial view of calcaneus; computed tomography (CT) and arthrography often diagnostic Secondary signs seen on a lateral radiograph: Talar break Widening of the lateral talar process Nonvisualization of middle subtalar joint C-sign: curvilinear radiopacity overlying the sustentaculum tali Asymmetric anterior subtalar joint Ball-and-socket ankle joint CT scanning or magnetic resonance (MR) imaging may be useful diagnostically
3. Talonavicular[13]		Rare form of coalition Best seen on dorsoplantar radiograph
4. Calcaneocuboid[13]		Infrequent form of coalition Readily visible on routine radiographs
Accessory ossicles[4]		Unfused ossicles (accessory bones) represent normal anatomic variants that usually are of no clinical significance (only the most commonly named ossicles are listed below) Rarely result in symptoms; frequently simulate fractures Typical location and smooth, well-corticated margins help to distinguish ossicles from fractures
1. Os trigonum[4, 17, 18]	11–13	Adjacent to posterior process of talus Best seen on lateral radiograph Simulates fracture of the posterior process of the talus May be associated with the os trigonum syndrome: painful condition in ballet dancers, aggravated by prolonged or repeated forced plantar flexion
2. Accessory talus[4]		Adjacent to the medial aspect of talus, just anterior to site of os trigonum Best seen on lateral radiograph
3. Calcaneus secondarium[4]	11–14	Adjacent to the anterior process of the calcaneus Round or triangular ossicle within the gap of the calcaneus, cuboid, talus, and navicular bones Best seen on oblique radiograph of midfoot
4. Os intermetatarseum[19]	11–15	Variable shaped ossicle located dorsally between the bases of the first and second metatarsals; may be elongated Best seen on oblique or dorsoplantar views May be painful

TABLE 11–3. Developmental Anomalies, Anatomic Variants, and Sources of Diagnostic Error Affecting the Ankle and Foot *Continued*

Entity	Figure(s)	Characteristics
5. Os vesalianum[20]	11–16	Situated at the insertion of the peroneus brevis tendon at the base of the fifth metatarsal Often confused with an os peroneum May be painful
6. Os peroneum[4]		Situated within the peroneus longus tendon adjacent to the cuboid bone Often multicentric Typically located more proximally than the os vesalianum May fracture or become displaced with rupture of the peroneus longus muscle or tendon
7. Os tibiale externum[21, 22]	11–17	Accessory navicular: two types Type I: circular sesamoid bone embedded within posterior tibial tendon Type II: triangular ossicle adjacent to the medial aspect of the navicular bone at the navicular tubercle May be painful
8. Os supranaviculare[4]		Small triangular ossicle adjacent to the dorsal surface of the proximal portion of the navicular bone Should not be confused for avulsion fractures that usually involve the distal aspect of the dorsal surface of the navicular bone and are common
9. Os subfibulare[4]		Circular ossicle adjacent to the inferior tip of the fibula May resemble avulsed fracture fragment
Sesamoid bones		Smooth ossicles embedded within tendons on the plantar side of the foot, usually just proximal to the adjacent joint
1. Hallux sesamoids[23]	11–18 A,B; see Fig. 11–46	Medial and lateral sesamoids are invariably present at the first MTP joint; congenital absence extremely rare; when absent, they usually have been surgically resected Situated within the flexor hallucis brevis tendons and are covered with hyaline cartilage Usually arise from a single ossification center; bipartite (4 per cent), tripartite, and multipartite sesamoids arise from multiple centers and involve the medial sesamoid more commonly May fracture or dislocate (Table 11–8)
2. Other sesamoids[4]	11–18 C	Frequent locations of single or double sesamoids: second and fifth metatarsal heads Infrequent locations: third and fourth metatarsal heads, first proximal phalanx, and second middle phalanx
Normal pseudocystic radiolucent area in calcaneus[4, 5]	11–19	Normal triangular radiolucent area frequently is seen within the calcaneus Represents an area relatively devoid of trabeculae within the normal trabecular arrangement of the spongiosa portion of bone May simulate a simple bone cyst or intraosseous lipoma Presence of a nutrient foramen within the lucent area is useful in confirming a pseudocyst as opposed to a true cyst or tumor
Talar beak[24]		Osseous prominence on superior aspect of the anterior process of the talus Normal variant simulating degenerative osteophytes Also seen in osteoarthrosis and talocalcaneal coalition
Epiphyseal variations[25]		Normal metacarpal and phalangeal epiphyses may be radiodense, irregular, asymmetric, divided by a cleft, or cone-shaped

Table continued on following page

TABLE 11–3. Developmental Anomalies, Anatomic Variants, and Sources of Diagnostic Error Affecting the Ankle and Foot *Continued*

Entity	Figure(s)	Characteristics
Syndactyly[7]		Developmental lack of differentiation between two or more digits Fusion of two digits may be partial or complete Osseous or soft tissue involvement Occurs as an isolated anomaly or in association with a generalized syndrome Syndactyly of the second and third digits is most likely an isolated anomaly Nonsegmentation of the metatarsals is termed synmetatarsalism
Macrodactyly[26]		Localized overgrowth of both soft tissues and osseus elements of a digit Congenital form is present at birth Also associated with neurofibromatosis, soft tissue hemangiomas, macrodystrophia lipomatosa, and lymphangioma
Polydactyly[7, 27, 28]	11–20	Developmental duplication of a digit Most frequently an isolated anomaly but may be related to a generalized syndrome Duplication of a great toe (preaxial polydactyly) is more likely syndrome-related than duplication of the fifth toe (postaxial polydactyly)
Symphalangism[7]	11–3 K,L	Developmental lack of differentiation of one phalanx to another within the same digit, usually related to absence of ossification centers Fusion of middle and distal phalanges of the fifth toe is a common isolated anomaly; at other sites, it may be a component of a generalized syndrome

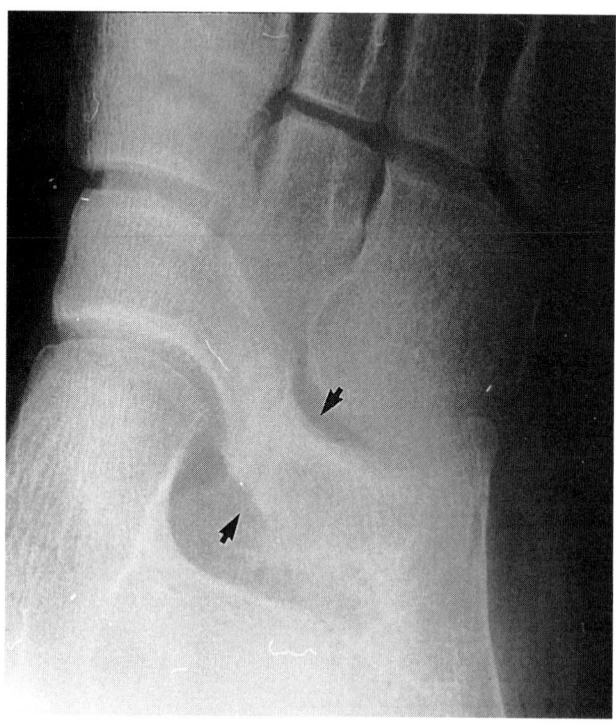

FIGURE 11–11. Tarsal coalition (fusion): Calcaneonavicular articulation.[13, 14] A 45-degree medial oblique radiograph of the foot in this 12-year-old boy demonstrates osseous coalition of the calcaneonavicular articulation (arrows), the most frequent site of tarsal coalition. The fusion is sometimes bilateral and may be either asymptomatic or associated with a rigid flatfoot deformity. The abnormality may be overlooked on frontal and lateral radiographs. The ankylosis can be osseous, fibrous, or cartilaginous.

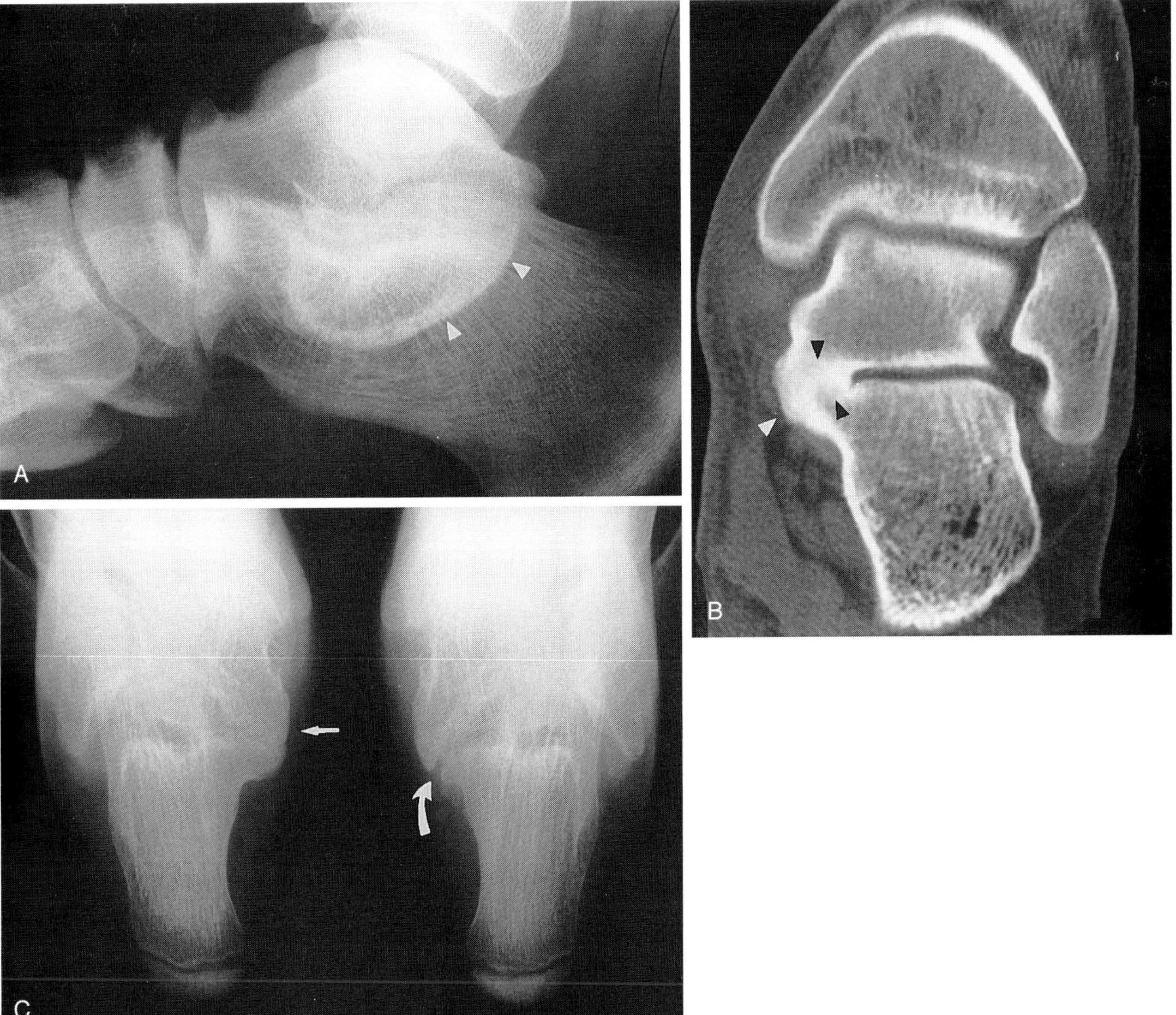

FIGURE 11–12. Tarsal coalition (fusion): Talocalcaneal articulation.[13–16] **A, B** 36-year-old man. In **A,** a routine lateral radiograph reveals a curvilinear radiodensity overlying the sustentaculum tali (C-sign) (arrowheads). In **B,** a coronal computed tomographic (CT) scan shows osseous fusion of the talocalcaneal articulation (arrowheads). **C** 8-year-old girl. A fully penetrated axial radiograph (Harris-Beath projection) may be required in addition to routine frontal and lateral projections to visualize the middle facet ankylosis. On the right (straight arrow), almost complete osseous fusion is seen. On the left (curved arrow), the radiolucent joint space is seen, indicating incomplete fusion of the medial talocalcaneal articulation.

The ankylosis typically occurs at the middle facet between the talus and the sustentaculum tali and is bilateral in 20 to 25 per cent of affected persons. In many cases, CT **(B)**, arthrography, or CT combined with arthrography is necessary to evaluate fibrous or osseous fusions adequately.

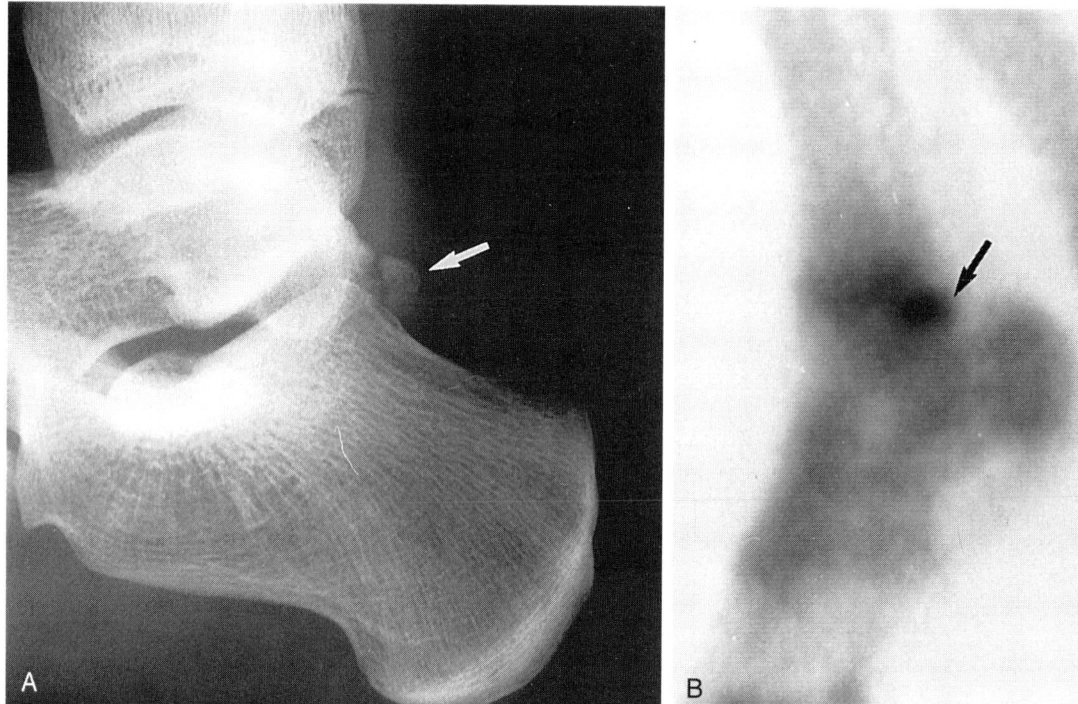

FIGURE 11–13. Os trigonum syndrome: Posterior impingement syndrome.[4, 17, 18] A Radiograph of this 14-year-old ballet dance student reveals the presence of an os trigonum (arrow). B Scintigraphy shows marked increased uptake localized in the os trigonum (arrow) as well as mild uptake at the growing physes about the ankle and foot. Surgical excision of the os trigonum relieved the pain. This condition, more common in athletes such as professional ballet dancers, is aggravated by forced plantar flexion of the ankle. *(Courtesy of G. Greenway, M.D., Dallas, Texas.)*

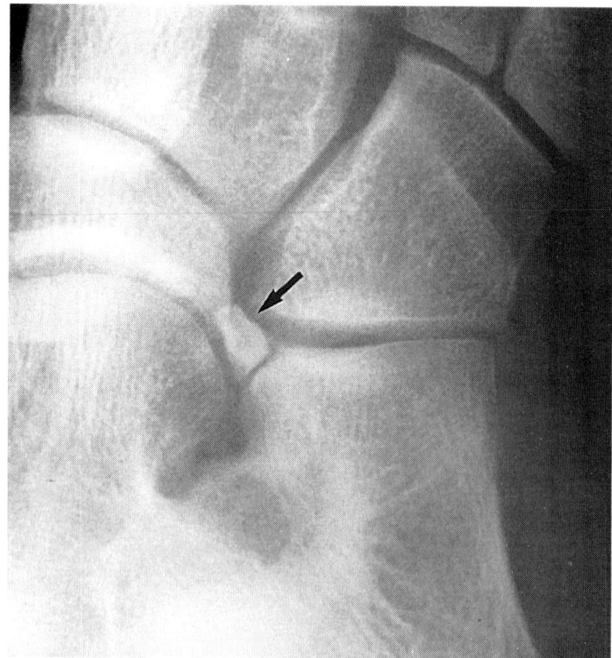

FIGURE 11–14. Calcaneus secundarium.[4] This ossicle (arrow), arising from the anterior process of the calcaneus and best seen on an oblique radiograph, should not be mistaken for an avulsion fracture.

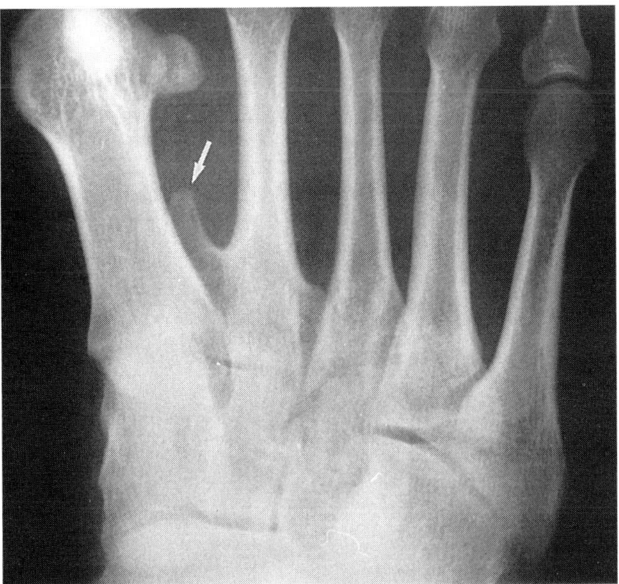

FIGURE 11–15. Os intermetatarseum.[19] A curvilinear flange of bone is seen arising from the base of the second metatarsal bone in the space between the first and second metatarsal bones (arrow). The appearance of these ossicles is highly variable, and they may be painful.

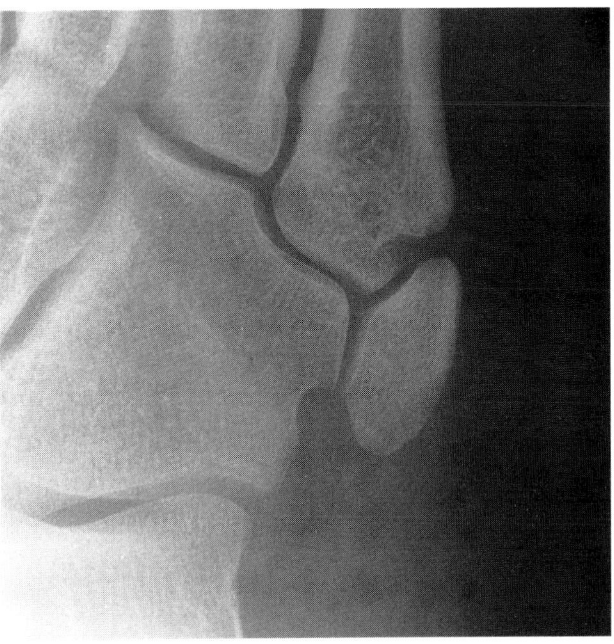

FIGURE 11–16. Os vesalianum.[20] This ossicle, situated adjacent to the base of the fifth metatarsal and cuboid bones, is widely separated from the bone and is completely corticated, with a smooth sclerotic margin. This normal variant may be painful and should not be confused with an ununited fracture.

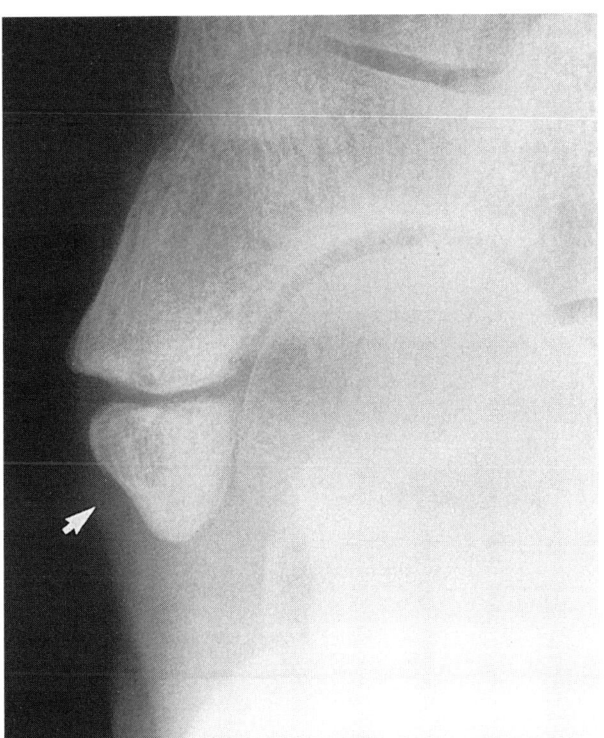

FIGURE 11–17. Os tibialis externa (accessory navicular).[21, 22] A well-corticated triangular ossicle of bone (arrow) is clearly separated from the proximal portion of the medial aspect of the navicular bone (navicular tubercle). Two types of accessory navicular have been described: type I is a circular sesamoid bone embedded within the posterior tibial tendon; type II is a separate triangular ossification center at the navicular tubercle, as seen in this patient.

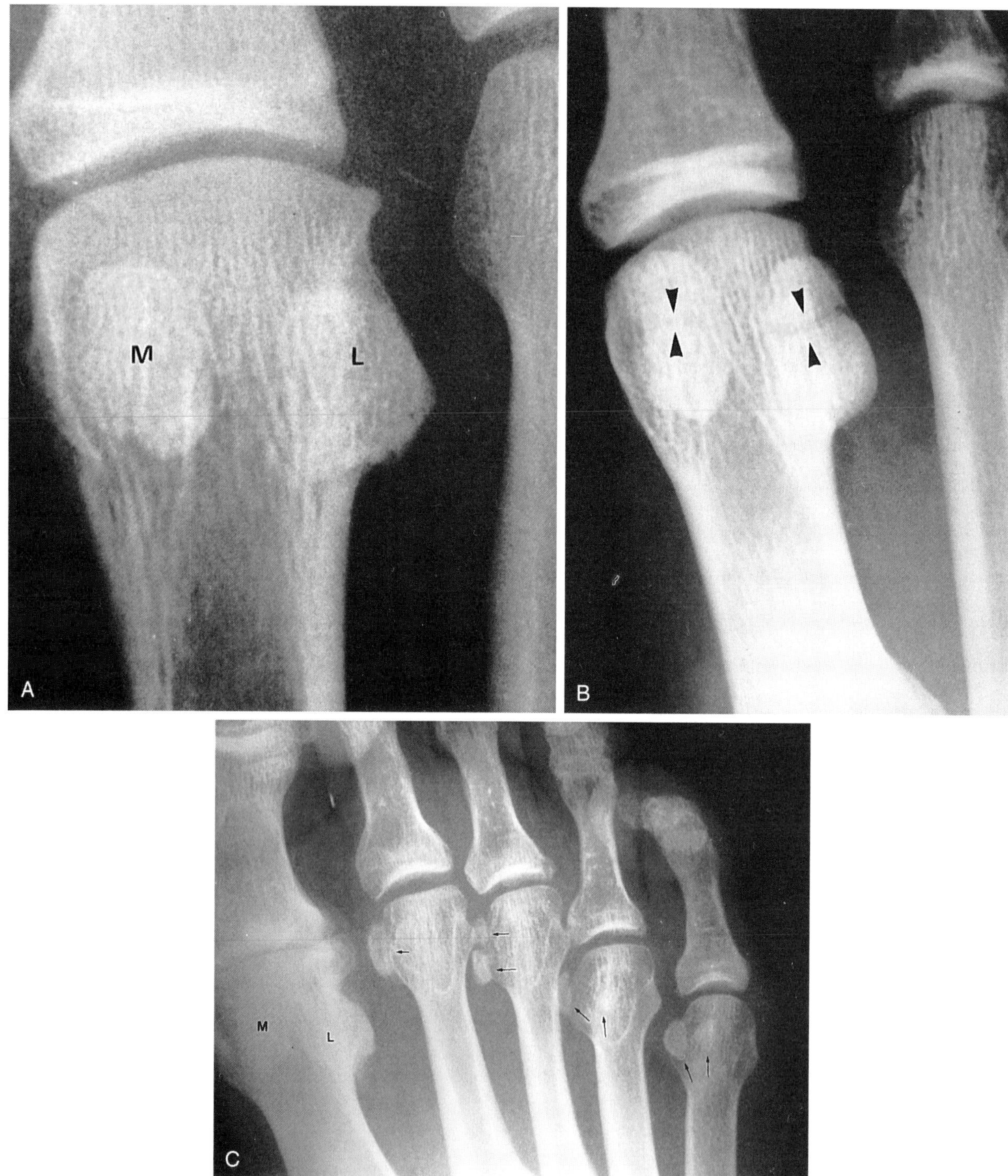

FIGURE 11–18. Sesamoid bones: Normal anatomy and anatomic variations.[23] A Normal hallux sesamoid bones. The medial (M) and lateral (L) hallux sesamoids are invariably present embedded in the flexor hallucis brevis tendons of the great toe. B Bipartite hallux sesamoid bones. Transverse radiolucent regions are evident through both medial and lateral hallux sesamoid bones (arrowheads). Observe the smooth, well-corticated margins, a feature that allows differentiation from a fracture. C Multiple sesamoid bones are seen adjacent to all metatarsal heads. Sesamoid bones adjacent to the second through fifth metatarsal heads (arrows) are variable in appearance. Marked degenerative changes are seen at the first metatarsophalangeal joint in this patient. M, Medial; L, lateral. (A, *Courtesy of G. Bustin, D.C., San Dimas, California.)*

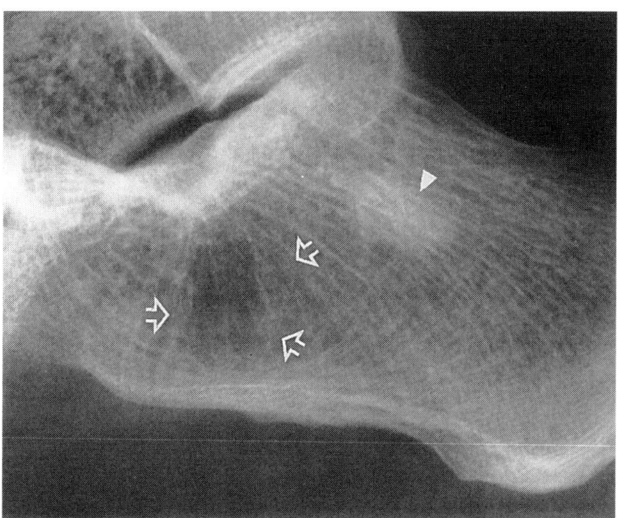

FIGURE 11–19. Normal pseudocystic radiolucency in calcaneus.[4, 5] Observe the triangular region of radiolucency (open arrows) within the normal trabecular pattern of spongiosa bone. This area, relatively devoid of trabeculae, is clearly seen in some patients and is less conspicuous in others. It may simulate a simple bone cyst, lipoma, or other tumor. Note also the presence of a radiodense enostosis (arrowhead).

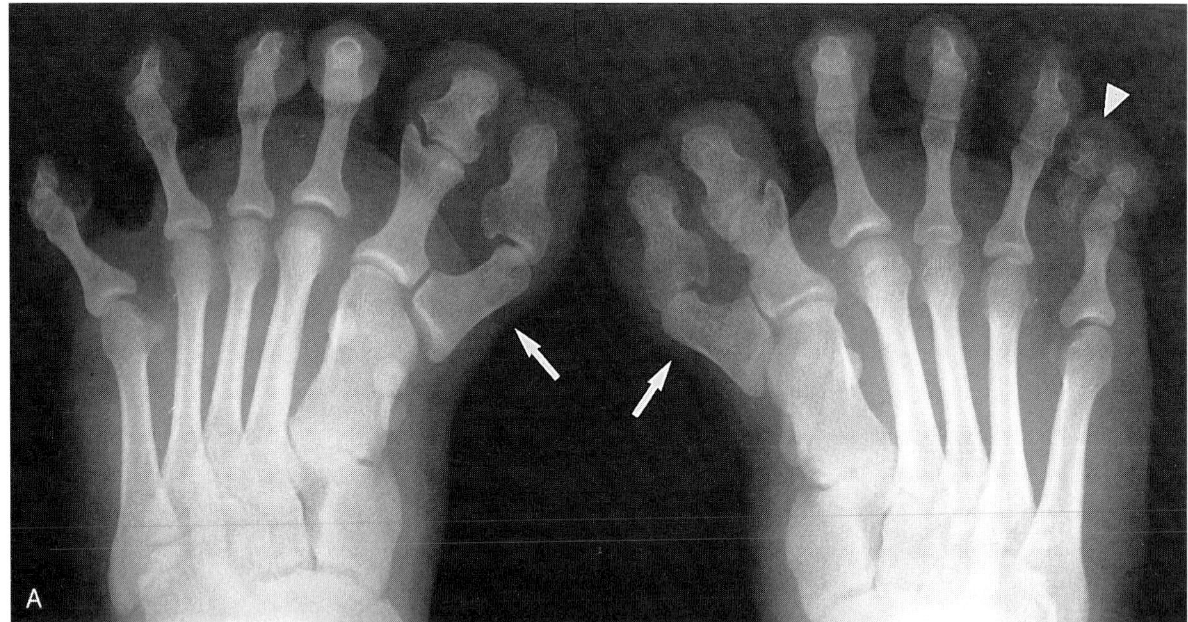

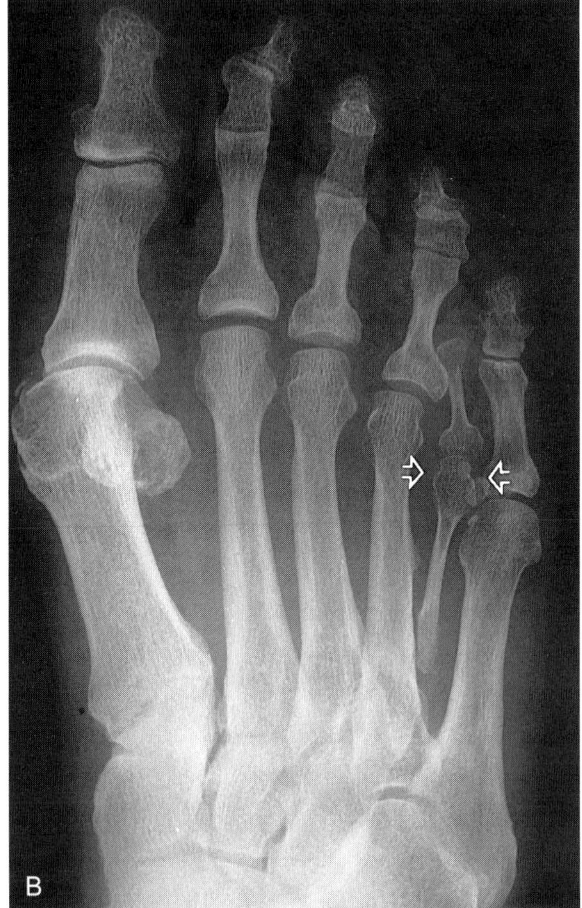

FIGURE 11–20. Polydactyly.[7, 27, 28] A Supernumerary digits are seen medial to the great toes bilaterally (arrows) and between the fourth and fifth toes unilaterally (arrowhead). Deformities of the adjacent phalanges and metatarsals also are present. B In another patient, an extra digit is interposed between the two most lateral matatarsals and phalanges (open arrows). Polydactyly in the foot usually involves the fifth digit and may be syndrome-related.

TABLE 11–4. Skeletal Dysplasias and Other Congenital Diseases Affecting the Ankle and Foot

Entity	Figure(s)	Characteristics
Fibrodysplasia (myositis) ossificans progressiva[12]	11–10 F	Multiple congenital anomalies: polydactyly, syndactyly, hypoplasia of great toe, hallux valgus, and symphalangism
Dysplasia epiphysealis hemimelica[29]	11–21	Asymmetric cartilaginous overgrowth in one or more epiphyses Radiographically resembles large eccentric osteochondroma arising from distal tibial epiphysis or tarsal bones Bulky irregular ossification extending into soft tissues
Osteogenesis imperfecta[30]	11–22	Severe osteoporosis with pencil-thin cortices Multiple fractures and bowing Rare cystic form—ballooning of bone, metaphyseal flaring, and honeycombed appearance of thick trabeculae
Osteopoikilosis[31]	11–23	Predilection for tarsal bones Multiple round or oval radiodense areas within spongiosa bone
Melorheostosis[32, 33]	11–24	Occasional involvement of feet Unilateral, hemimelic involvement is typical Cortical thickening and flowing hyperostosis resembling flowing candle wax
Marfan syndrome[34]		Arachnodactyly Hallux valgus Pes planus
Ehlers-Danlos syndrome[35]		Hallux valgus Pes planovalgus with joint laxity
Macrodystrophia lipomatosa[36]		Rare condition of unknown cause Bizarre digital overgrowth of fatty tissue within the soft tissues of the foot

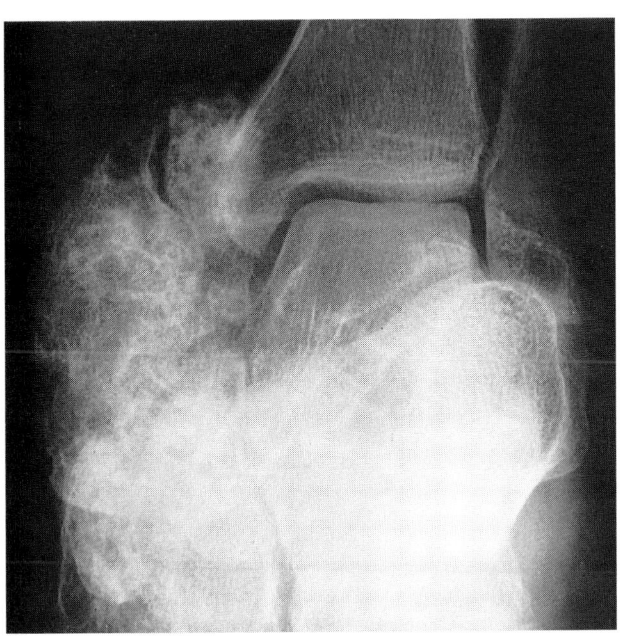

FIGURE 11–21. Dysplasia epiphysealis hemimelica (Trevor's disease).[29] A large lobulated accumulation of ossification is seen arising from the medial aspect of the distal end of the tibia and tarsal bones spanning the medial aspect of the ankle. This uncommon developmental disorder characterized by asymmetric cartilaginous overgrowth in one or more epiphyses can be localized, classic, or generalized. Joint dysfunction, pain, limitation of motion, and a mass may accompany the disease. *(Courtesy of J. Schils, M.D., Cleveland, Ohio.)*

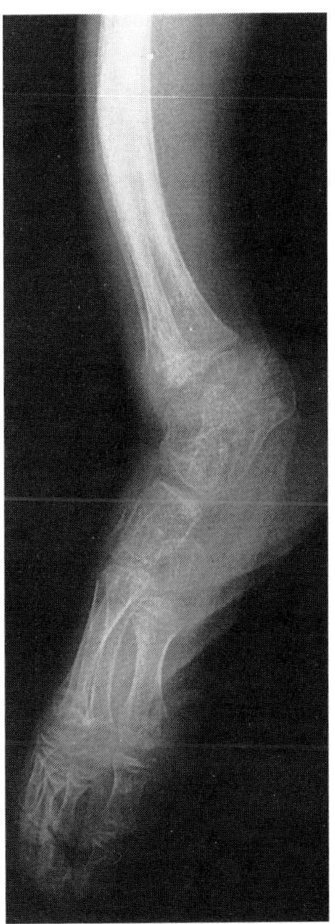

FIGURE 11–22. Osteogenesis imperfecta.[30] Severe osteopenia and thin gracile cortical bones are present in the foot and ankle in this infant with osteogenesis imperfecta. Bowing of the tibia also is evident. Pes planus deformities may be seen on weight-bearing radiographs (not shown).

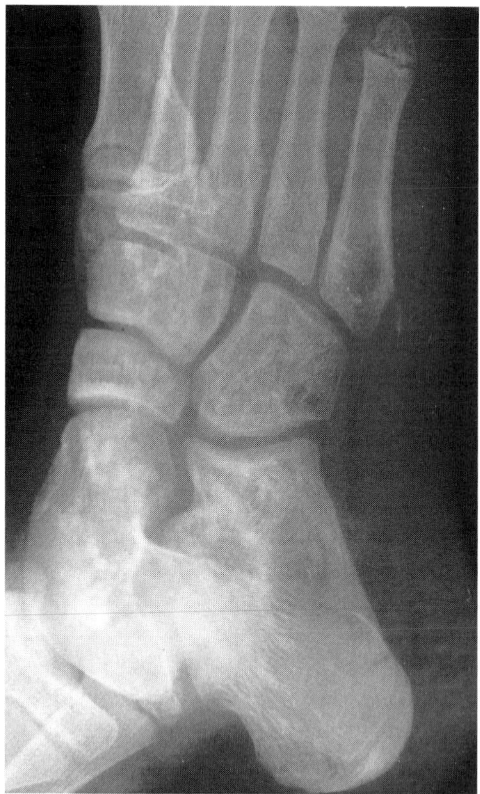

FIGURE 11–23. Osteopoikilosis.[31] Note the circular and ovoid osteosclerotic foci localized within a number of bones of the foot in a periarticular distribution.

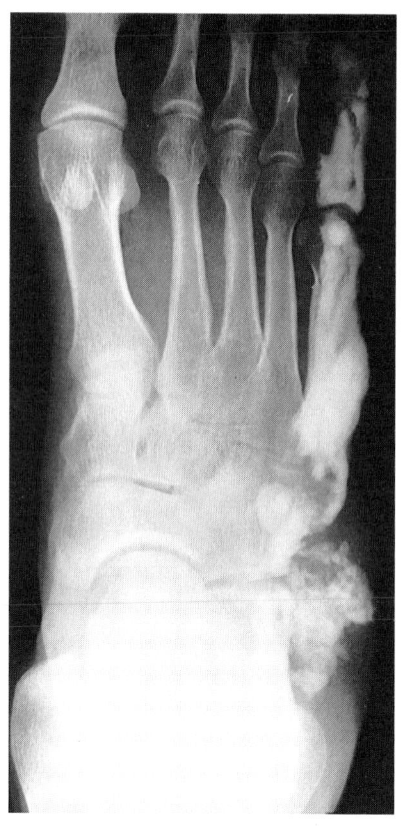

FIGURE 11–24. Melorheostosis.[32, 33] Findings include prominent soft tissue ossification and the characteristic pattern of hemimelic hyperostosis involving the lateral aspect of the fifth metatarsal, phalanges, and lateral tarsal bones. Note the absence of involvement of the medial four digits of the foot.

Melorheostosis is a sclerosing dysplasia of bone that can result in joint swelling and contracture, pain, restriction of motion, growth disturbances, muscle weakness and atrophy, and skin changes. It may be positive on bone scans.

TABLE 11–5. Acute Fractures About the Ankle: Lauge-Hansen Classification*

Fracture Type	Stage	Figure(s)	Characteristics
Supination–external rotation fractures (SER)[37, 38]			Sixty per cent of all fractures about the ankle Mechanism: external rotation of the supinated foot forces the talus against the fibula Progression of events occurs, beginning with stage I and continuing through stage IV with increasing severity of injury
	SER I		Rupture of anterior talofibular ligament or avulsion fracture of the anterior surface of the fibula or tibia (Tillaux fracture) Ligamentous injuries often not detected on radiographs
	SER II		Short oblique fracture of the distal end of the fibula within 1.5 to 2.5 cm from the tibiotalar joint
	SER III		Fracture of posterior aspect of the tibia
	SER IV	11–25	Fracture of medial malleolus or rupture of deltoid ligament Widening of the medial tibiotalar articulation with deltoid ligament rupture

TABLE 11–5. Acute Fractures About the Ankle: Lauge-Hansen Classification* *Continued*

Fracture Type	Stage	Figure(s)	Characteristics
Supination-adduction fractures (SAD)[37]			Twenty per cent of all fractures about the ankle Mechanism: medially directed adduction forces acting upon the supinated foot Two stages are identified: Stage I resulting from less force than that sustained in a stage II injury
	SAD I	11–26 A	Rupture of the lateral ligaments or a transverse (traction or avulsion) fracture of the distal portion of the fibula adjacent to the tibiotalar articulation
	SAD II	11–26 B	Fracture of medial malleolus resulting from continued pressure from the medial displacement of the talus
Pronation-external rotation fractures (PER)[37, 39–40]		11–27, 11–28	PER and PAB stages I and II are radiographically indistinguishable, and combined, represent 20 per cent of all fractures about the ankle Mechanism: external rotation forces acting upon the pronated foot As forces increase, the injuries progress to higher stages
	PER I		Deltoid ligament rupture in 60 per cent of cases Fracture of the medial malleolus in 40 per cent of cases
	PER II		Rupture of the distal tibiofibular syndesmosis (interosseous ligament) or avulsion fracture of the anterior or posterior tubercle
	PER III		Injuries of stages I and II combined with a transverse supramalleolar fracture of the fibula $>$ 2.5 cm (usually 6 to 8 cm) above the tibiotalar articulation
	PER IV		Injuries of stages I to III combined with a fracture of the posterior tibial margin
Pronation-abduction fracture (PAB)[37]			Mechanism: abduction forces acting upon the pronated foot PER and PAB stages I and II are radiographically indistinguishable As forces increase, the injuries progress to higher stages
	PAB I		Deltoid ligament rupture (60 per cent of cases) Fracture of the medial malleolus (40 per cent of cases)
	PAB II		Rupture of the distal tibiofibular syndesmosis (interosseous ligament) or an avulsion fracture of the anterior or posterior tubercle
	PAB III		Injuries of stage I and II combined with a transverse supramalleolar fiber fracture
Pronation-dorsiflexion fracture (PDF)[37]			Pilon fracture Rare: less than 0.5 per cent of all fractures about the ankle Mechanism: axial loading forces predominate Forced dorsiflexion on a pronated foot, often occurring in a fall from a height that drives the talus into the ankle mortise
	PDF I		Fracture of medial malleolus
	PDF II		Anterior tibial fracture
	PDF III		Supramalleolar fracture of the fibula
	PDF IV		Transverse fracture of the posterior aspect of the tibia, which communicates with the anterior tibial fracture

*The Lauge-Hansen classification system is based on the position of the foot (e.g., supination or pronation) relative to the body at the time of injury and the direction of talus displacement or rotation (e.g., abduction, external rotation) in relation to the ankle mortise.

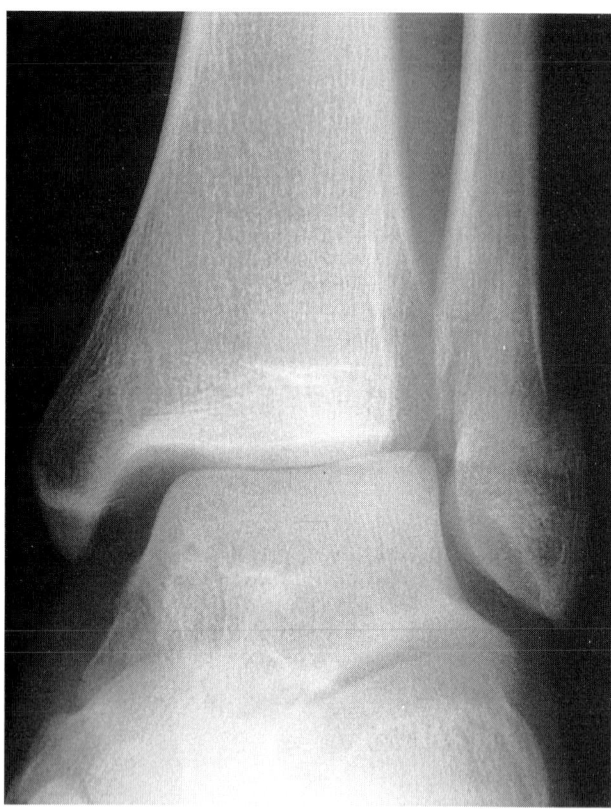

FIGURE 11–25. Ankle fracture-dislocation: Supination-external rotation fracture, stage IV.[37, 38] This radiograph shows an oblique fracture of the distal portion of the fibula and rupture of the deltoid ligament (manifested by widening of the medial clear space).

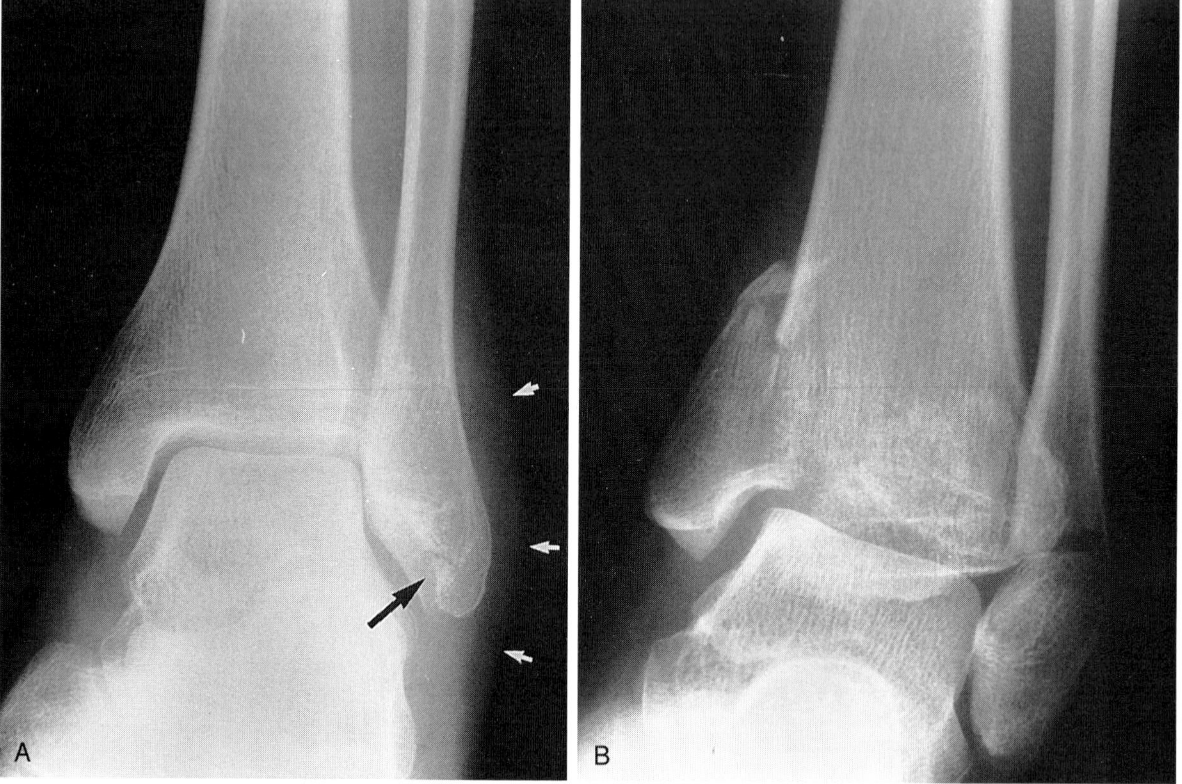

FIGURE 11–26. Ankle injury: Supination-adduction fractures.[37] A Stage I injury. Note the simple nondisplaced avulsion fracture of the fibula (black arrow) and the associated soft tissue swelling (white arrows) over the lateral side of the ankle. B Stage II injury. A bimalleolar fracture is evident on this radiograph.

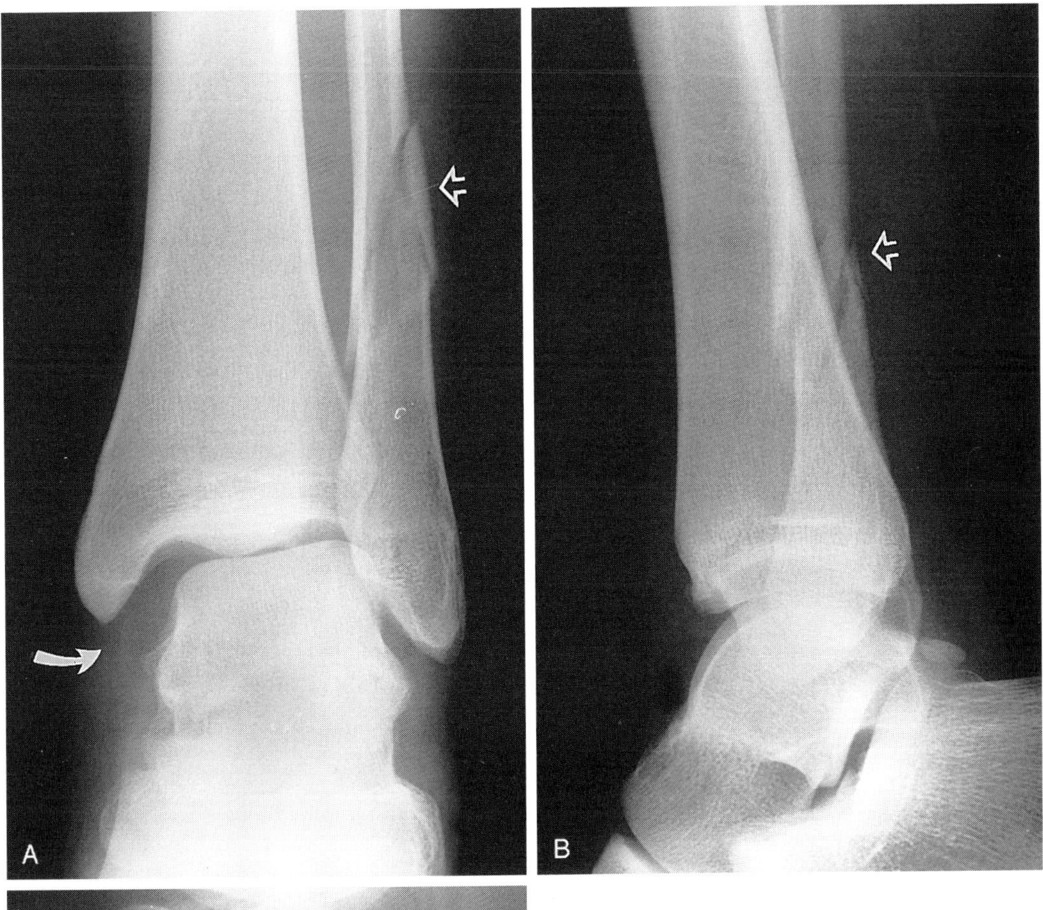

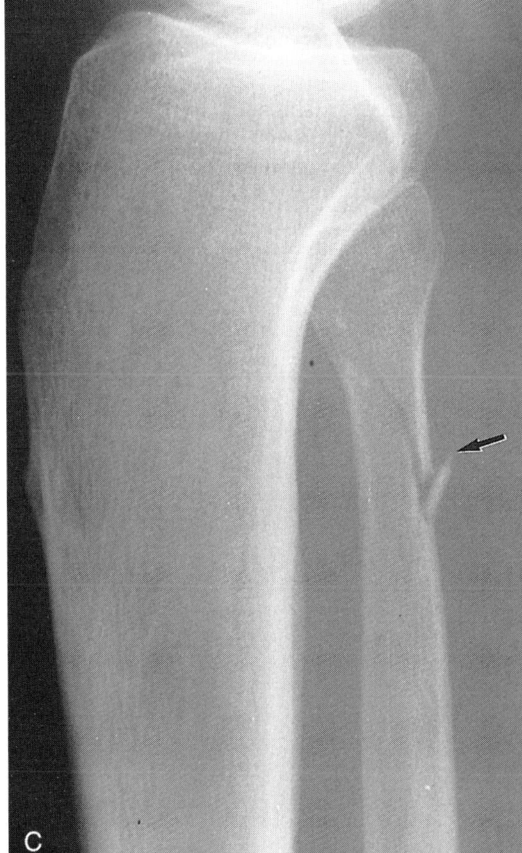

FIGURE 11–27. Ankle injury: Pronation-external rotation injury.[37, 39] A, B Stages II–III. Observe the comminuted fracture of the fibula (open arrow) and widening of the medial clear space (curved arrow), indicating rupture of the deltoid ligament. In this case, no avulsion fracture of the medial malleolus or fracture of the posterior tibial margin has occurred. C This patient sustained a pronation–external rotation injury of his ankle, rupturing the anterior talofibular ligament and fracturing the proximal portion of the fibula. This fracture is referred to as a Maisonneuve fracture (arrow) and usually is associated with disruption of the distal tibiofibular syndesmosis and interosseous membrane, a medial malleolar fracture, or a tear of the deltoid ligament. Because of the dramatic symptoms about the ankle, the proximal fibular fracture may initially be overlooked.

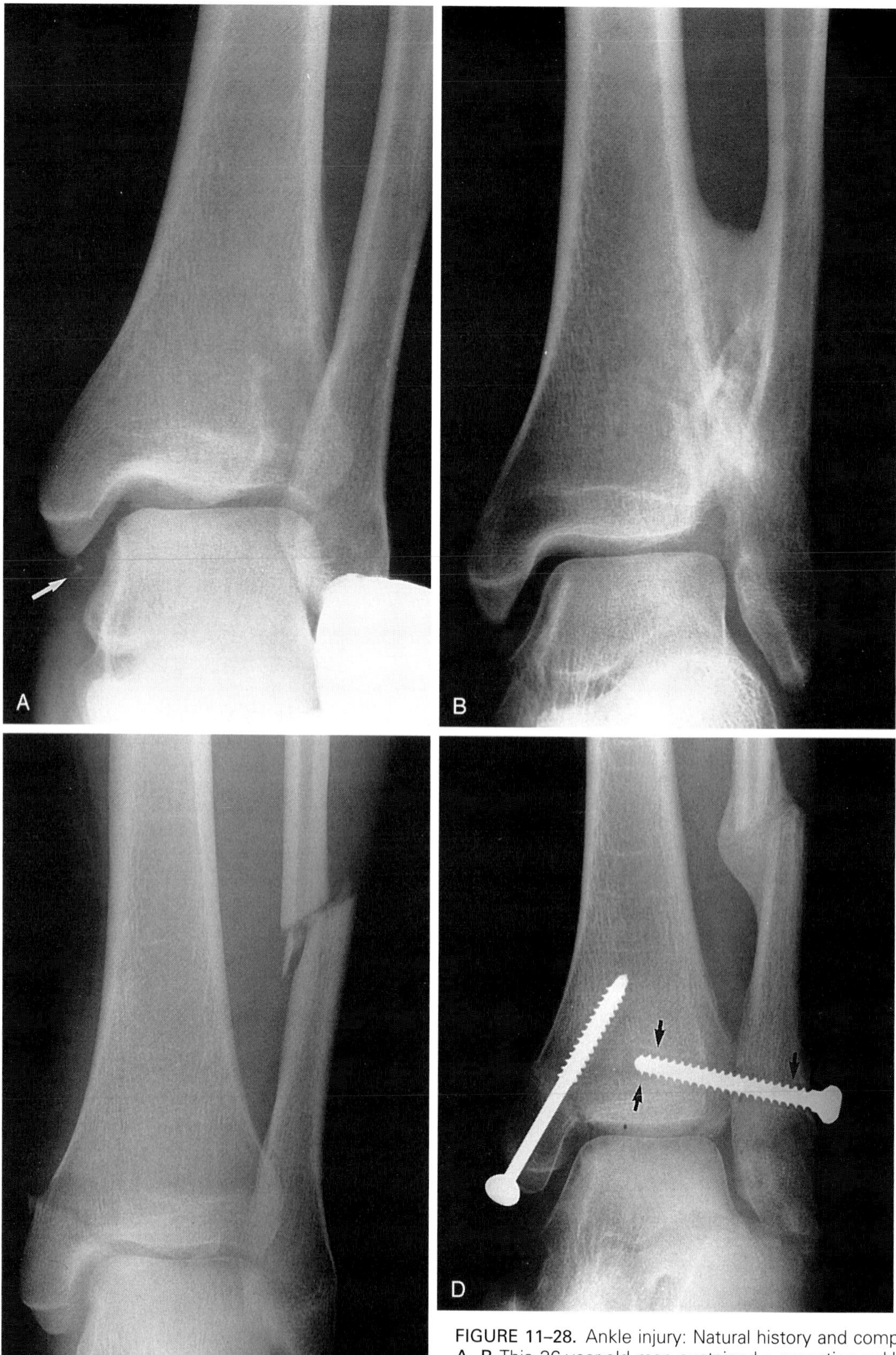

FIGURE 11–28. Ankle injury: Natural history and complications.[40] A, B This 36-year-old man sustained a pronation ankle injury. In A, an initial eversion stress radiograph obtained at the time of injury reveals widening of the medial clear space and a tiny flake of bone (arrow) representing an avulsion of the medial malleolus. In B, another radiograph obtained 2 years later demonstrates dramatic posttraumatic ossification of the interosseous membrane of the distal tibiofibular articulation. C, D Surgical repair with complications. This 33-year-old woman sustained a pronation–external rotation type IV injury In C, the initial radiograph shows a medial malleolar fracture and a displaced, comminuted oblique fracture of the fibula well above the ankle joint. In D, a radiograph taken 4 months postoperatively shows loosening of the cannulated screws used for interfragmentary compression and persistent deformity of the healed fibula. Loosening is seen as a radiolucent area surrounding the screws (arrows) and as pulling out of the screws.

TABLE 11–6. Fractures and Dislocations About the Ankle

Entity	Stage	Figure(s)	Characteristics
Acute fractures about the ankle[37–40]		11–25 to 11–28	See Table 11–5: Lauge-Hansen classification Often associated with osteochondritis dissecans or osteochondral fracture of the talus (Table 11–7)
Distal portion of the tibia[40]			Isolated fractures rare; result from ankle injuries involving impaction of talus on tibial plafond
Intra-articular osteochondral bodies[41]		11–29	Osteochondral bodies within the ankle joint may arise from osteochondral fractures or osteochondritis dissecans Best imaging methods: computed tomographic (CT) arthrography and magnetic resonance (MR) imaging Osteochondral bodies often migrate to the anterior or posterior recess, where they may become embedded in the synovial membrane Differential diagnosis: primary or secondary idiopathic synovial osteochondromatosis
Unclassified fractures			
Isolated fracture of the posterior tibial margin[40]			Posterior malleolar fracture: rare injury Mechanism: compression by the talar dome; may occur while kicking an object with the ankle in neutral or plantar flexed positions Lateral view with slight external rotation reveals the fracture
Isolated fracture of the anterior tibial margin[40]			Rare injury *Two types:* 1. Compression forces from a dorsiflexed talus Comminuted fracture of anterior margin of distal end of the tibia 2. Fall on the calcaneus with the talus being forced upward and forward Large fragment of anterior margin is fractured
Child abuse[42]		11–30	Most frequent in children 1 to 4 years of age Metaphyseal corner fractures of the distal end of the tibia Growth plate injuries Fractures in various stages of healing Acute fractures of the tibia and fibula Subperiosteal hemorrhage with periosteal reaction Associated injuries elsewhere
Growth plate injuries			
Distal portion of the tibia[43–45]		11–31	Eleven per cent of all Salter-Harris fractures of the skeleton Most common between ages 9 and 14 years Salter-Harris type II injury most frequent at this site; types III, IV, and I also occur in order of decreasing frequency Primary mechanism appears to be external rotation or plantar flexion of the foot Ten to 12 per cent of these injuries result in growth disturbances Type II injury may be complicated by anterior tibial neurovascular bundle interposition, preventing reduction and compromising blood supply Two-plane fracture (Tillaux or Kleiger fracture) involves only the epiphysis Triplane fracture includes also a metaphyseal fracture, physeal injury, articular surface involvement, and transverse, sagittal, and coronal components and represents a variant of a type IV injury
Distal portion of the fibula[40]			Nine per cent of all Salter-Harris fractures of the skeleton Salter-Harris types I and II are most frequent at this site Mechanism: supination-inversion Commonly results in a minimally displaced fracture of the distal fibular epiphysis

Table continued on following page

TABLE 11–6. Fractures and Dislocations About the Ankle *Continued*

Entity	Stage	Figure(s)	Characteristics
Stress fractures			
Fatigue fracture[40]		10–9 E,F	Distal end of the tibia: long-distance running in young athletes, prolonged walking in golfers, and in persons with osteoarthritis Subtle fissure develops at the junction of the medial malleolus and medial tibial plafond Distal portion of the fibula: heavyweight training, ballet dancing, and long-distance running; also secondary to traumatic tibiofibular synostosis
Insufficiency fracture[46]		11–32	Distal portion of the tibia or fibula Osteoporosis from rheumatoid arthritis or corticosteroid abuse in older patients
Dislocations			
Tibiotalar joint dislocation[47]		11–33	Medial dislocation of the talus is the most common type Anterior, posterior, and other displacements also occur in association with other injuries Often associated with fractures and ligamentous injuries about the ankle

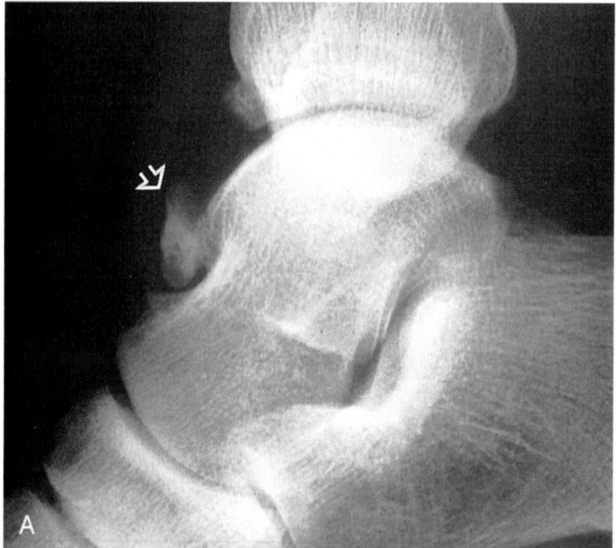

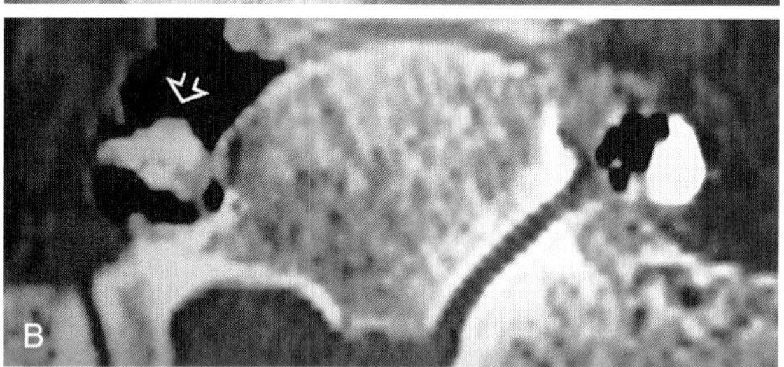

FIGURE 11–29. Intra-articular osteochondral body.[41] This 44-year-old woman had had chronic ankle pain for 4 years. **A** Routine radiograph shows an osseous fragment anterior to the articular surface of the talus (open arrow). **B** Computed tomographic (CT) arthrography. A reformatted sagittal CT scan after introduction of air and iodinated contrast material reveals an osteochondral body (open arrow) attached to the synovium of the anterior portion of the joint.

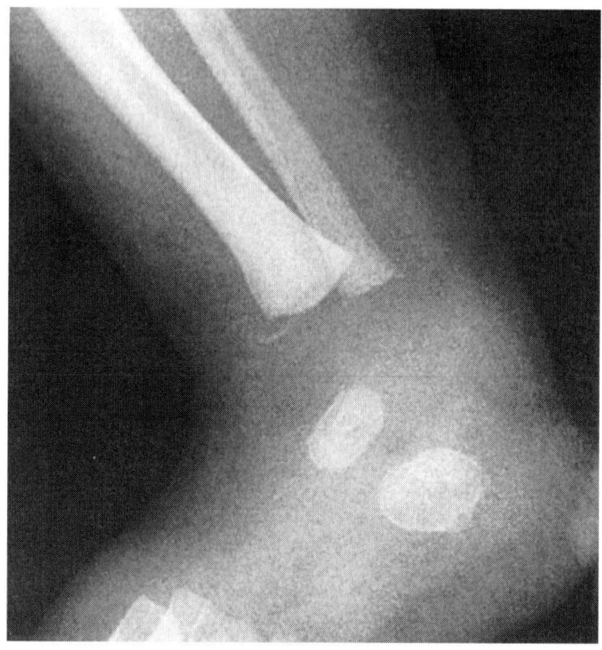

FIGURE 11–30. Child abuse: Classic metaphyseal injury.[42] The lateral view of the ankle demonstrates metaphyseal injuries of the distal ends of the tibia and fibula. Observe the normal skeleton and the absence of periosteal new bone formation. Most of these fractures are unilateral and involve the left side, but they also may be bilateral. These fractures are less conspicuous when acute and more conspicuous when they begin to heal. *(From Hilton SVW, Edwards DK. Practical Pediatric Radiology. 2nd Ed. Philadelphia, WB Saunders, 1994, p 398.)*

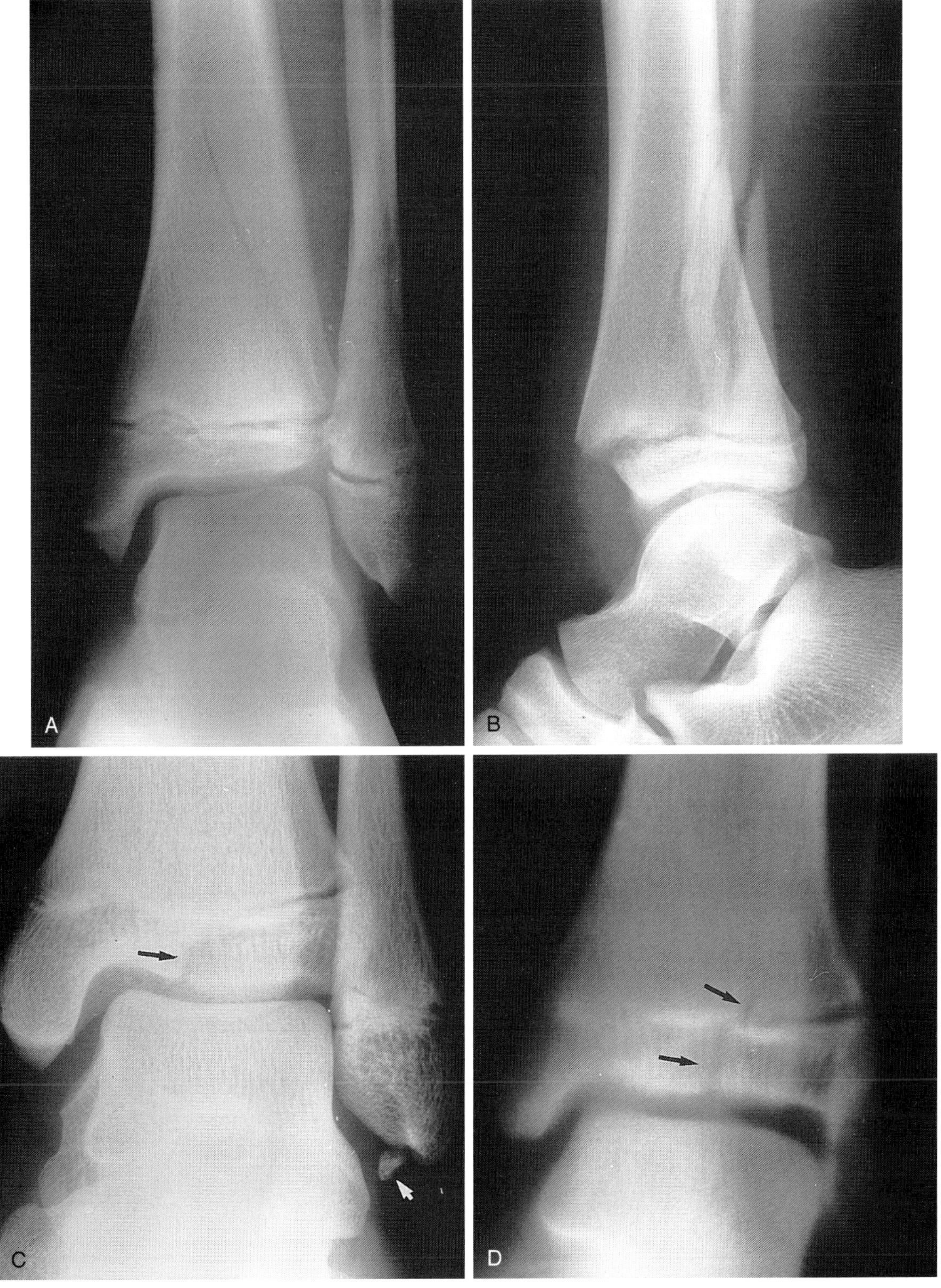

FIGURE 11–31. Growth plate injuries.[43–45] A, B Type II physeal injury. Frontal (A) and lateral (B) radiographs of the ankle in this 14-year-old boy show a fracture through the distal tibial physeal plate and extending into the metaphysis. A large metaphyseal fragment, posterior displacement of the epiphysis, and an oblique fracture of the fibula also are present. C, D Type IV physeal injury. Frontal radiograph (C) and conventional tomogram (D) of the ankle in a 13-year-old boy demonstrate fractures through the epiphysis, physis, and metaphysis (black arrows). The radiograph does not show the metaphyseal component. An avulsion of the distal end of the fibula also is apparent (white arrow).

Growth plate injuries about the ankle are common, type II injuries being the most frequent. These injuries may be accompanied by neurovascular entrapment and growth disturbances, complications that occur in 10 to 12 per cent of physeal injuries at this site.

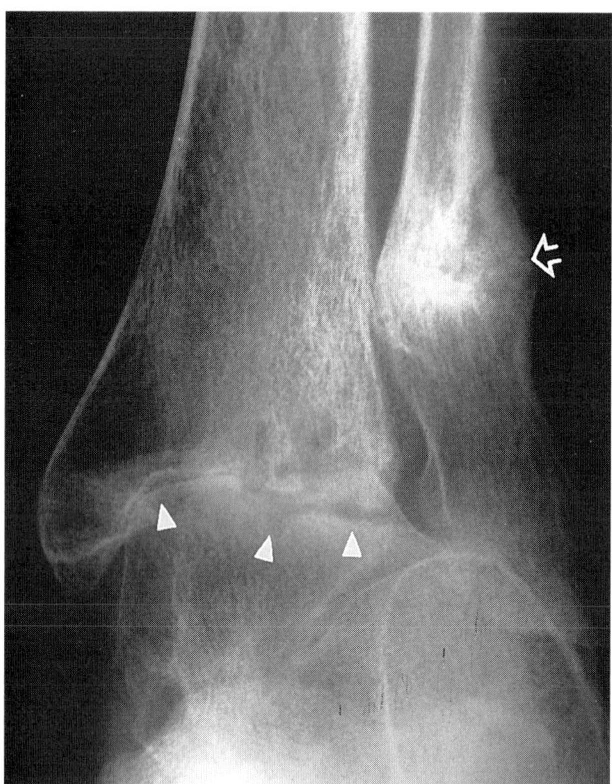

FIGURE 11–32. Stress (insufficiency) fracture.[46] This 62-year-old woman with long-standing rheumatoid arthritis and osteoporosis has sustained an insufficiency fracture through the distal portion of the fibula (open arrow). The tibiotalar joint is diffusely narrowed and extensively eroded and deformed (arrowheads) as a result of rheumatoid arthritis. This patient had sustained a similar fracture of the opposite fibula several years earlier. *(Courtesy of J. Rubinstein, M.D., Ph.D., Reno, Nevada.)*

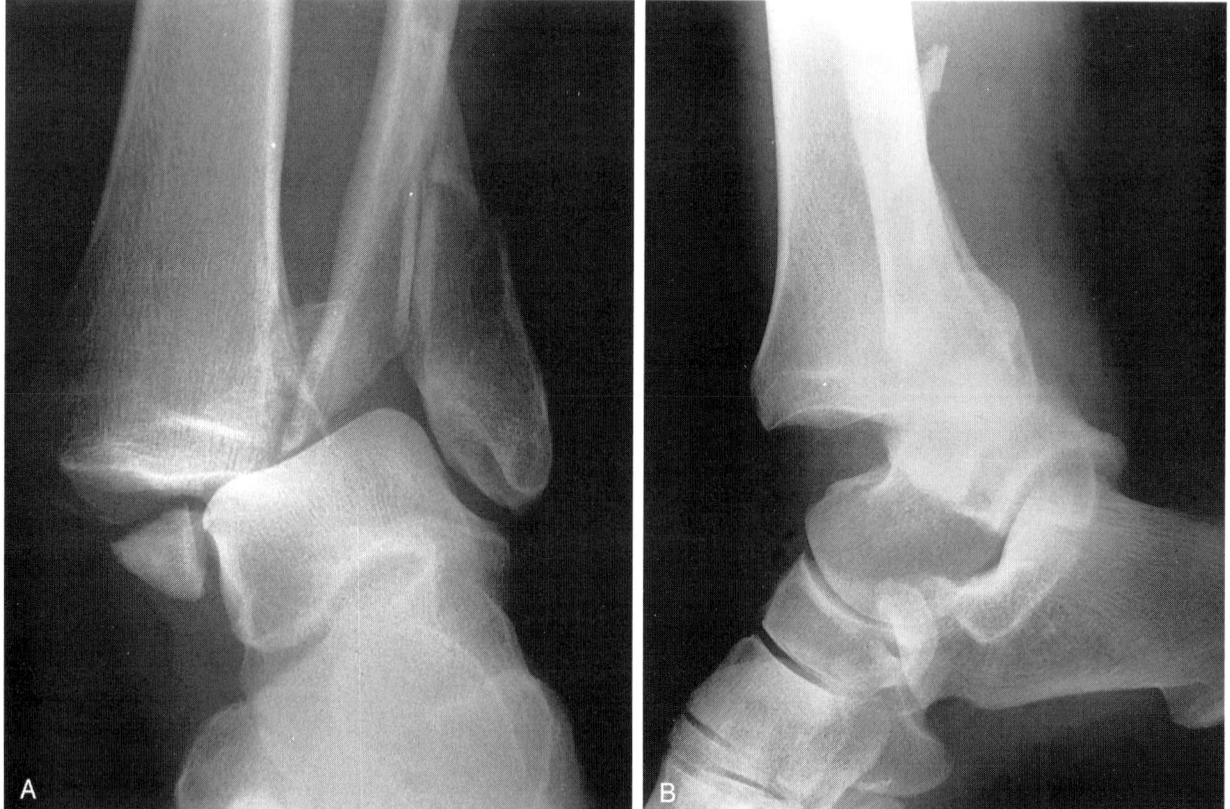

FIGURE 11–33. Fracture-dislocation: Tibiotalar joint.[47] Frontal **(A)** and lateral **(B)** radiographs reveal fracture-dislocation of the tibiotalar joint. The posteriorly dislocated fibula was trapped behind the tibia, requiring open reduction. This rare injury typically results from severe external rotation of the foot and has been called the Bosworth fracture-dislocation of the ankle.

TABLE 11–7. Fractures and Dislocations of the Tarsal Bones

Entity	Figure(s)	Characteristics	Complications and Related Injuries
Fractures of the calcaneus[48–50]	11–34	Most frequent tarsal bone to fracture *Intra-articular fracture:* 75 per cent of all calcaneus fractures Poorer prognosis than for extra-articular fracture Comminution and rotation of fragments are common and disrupt the subtalar joint Vertical falls in which the talus is driven into the cancellous bone of the calcaneus Computed tomography (CT) important in evaluation *Extra-articular fracture:* 25 per cent of all calcaneus fractures Twisting forces are most important Fractures of any part of the bone, including avulsions of the calcaneal tuberosity and the anterior process *Stress (fatigue) fracture:* common in military recruits *Stress (insufficiency) fracture:* rheumatoid arthritis, neurologic disorders, and other diseases	Displaced fragments Subtalar degenerative joint disease Malunion Peroneal tendon dislocation and entrapment Usually uncomplicated May become complete fracture May become complete fracture
Fractures of the talus[51, 52]	11–35	Second most frequent tarsal bone to fracture Sudden hyperextension of the forefoot, such as in the forceful application of automobile brakes (aviator's astragalus) *Talar neck:* eversion stress causes avulsion at site of attachment of deep fibers of the deltoid ligament to the body of the talus *Talar body:* infrequent fracture resulting from severe dorsiflexion and external rotation impacts the body on the lateral malleolus May affect the lateral process, posterior process, articular surface, or all regions *Posterior process:* severe plantar flexion of the foot causes compression of talus between tibia and calcaneus *Head of talus:* rare fracture related to longitudinal compression combined with plantar flexion of the foot	May be associated with dislocations of the tibiotalar or subtalar joints Neck: delayed union, nonunion, infection, degenerative joint disease, ischemic necrosis especially of the proximal portion of the bone (up to 90 per cent of displaced fractures) Body: ischemic necrosis, degenerative joint disease, and delayed union Posterior process: may be confused with os trigonum
Osteochondritis dissecans of the talus[53]	11–36	Osteochondritis dissecans and osteochondral fractures of the talar dome are common after ankle injury Osseous defect may be quite subtle or invisible on radiographs, and CT, arthrography, or magnetic resonance (MR) imaging may be necessary to delineate the fracture site Men > women; ages 10 to 40 years Two major anatomic sites: *Medial talar dome:* believed to be related to a combination of plantar flexion of the foot with inversion, followed by rotation of the tibia on the talus Typically involves posterior third of medial border *Lateral talar dome:* results from inversion injuries of the ankle in which the lateral margin of the talus impacts upon the fibula Fragment may remain in place or it may displace Typically involves middle third of lateral border	Pain aggravated by motion, limitation of motion, clicking, locking and swelling

Table continued on following page

TABLE 11–7. Fractures and Dislocations of the Tarsal Bones *Continued*

Entity	Figure(s)	Characteristics	Complications and Related Injuries
Dislocations of the talus[54]	11–37	Usually accompanied by fractures of bone but may be isolated injuries	
		Subtalar dislocation: disruption of the talocalcaneal and talonavicular articulations	Ischemic necrosis
		As many as 80 per cent of cases are medial subtalar dislocations	
		Forceful inversion of the foot, most typically a basketball injury	
		Total talar dislocation: infrequent and serious injury	Ischemic necrosis and infection
Fractures of the navicular bone[55–58]	11–38, 11–39	Acute fractures occur infrequently Most likely sites: dorsal surface, tuberosity, and body	Often initially overlooked Associated fractures or dislocations
	11–40	Stress (fatigue) fracture: sagittally oriented fracture observed in physically active persons, especially basketball players and runners	Can result in complete fracture
Fractures of the cuboid and cuneiform bones[40]		Acute fractures infrequent Stress fractures also infrequently encountered	Often initially overlooked Associated fractures and dislocations
Tarsal dislocations[59, 60]	11–41; see Fig. 11–68 C	Lisfranc's fracture-dislocation of the tarsometatarsal joints Direct or more commonly indirect high-energy trauma Mechanism includes plantar hyperflexion with forced supination or pronation resulting in fractures of the metatarsal bases or injury of the ligaments Indirect: violent abduction of the forefoot leads to lateral displacement of the four lateral metatarsal bones with or without a fracture of the base of the second metatarsal and cuboid bone; the first metatarsal bone may dislocate in the same (homolateral) or opposite (divergent) direction as the other metatarsals Routine radiographs useful in depicting obvious fractures MR imaging allows the detection of disruption of Lisfranc's ligament as well as tarsal and metatarsal fractures Other tarsal subluxations and dislocations are rare	Degenerative joint disease Ankylosis

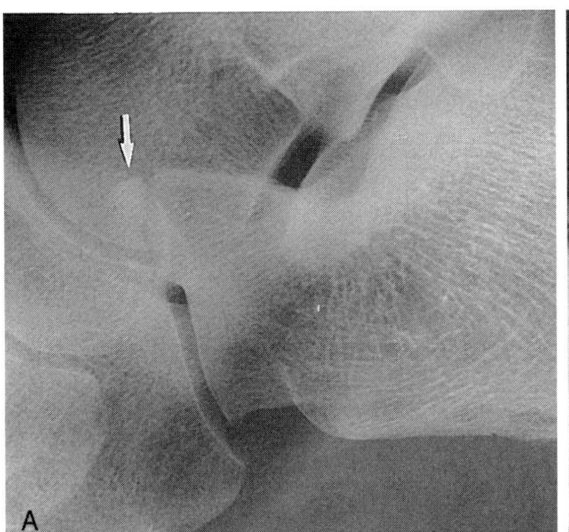

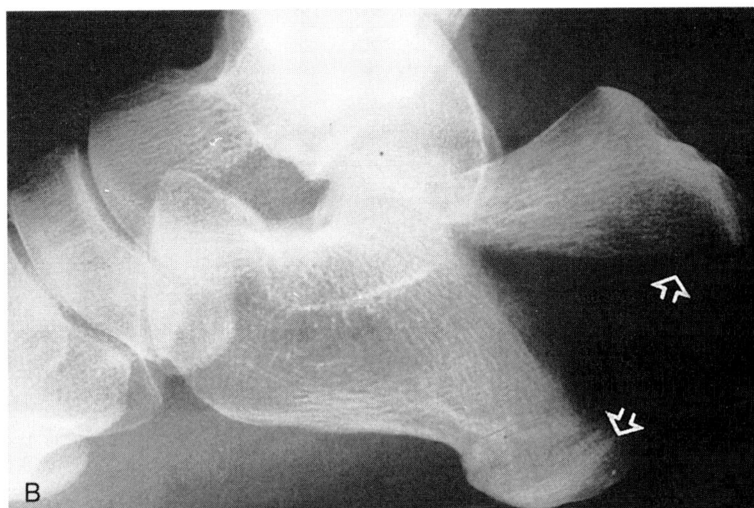

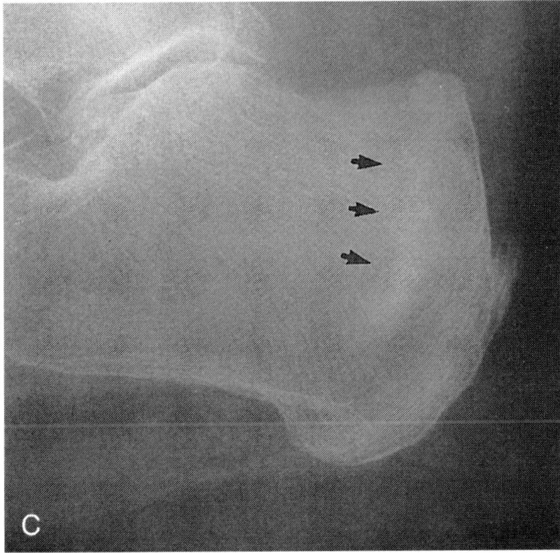

FIGURE 11–34. Fractures of the calcaneus.[48–50] **A** Anterior process avulsion. A fracture of the anterior process of the calcaneus is seen (arrow). This extra-articular fracture, which can be difficult to detect on routine radiographs, results most commonly from twisting injuries and occurs at the site of attachment of the ligamentum bifurcatum. It may resemble the calcaneus secundarium, a normal ossicle. **B** Calcaneal tuberosity avulsion. Observe the superior displacement of the fracture fragment (open arrows), which has been avulsed by the Achilles tendon. **C** Stress (fatigue) fracture. Observe the vertically oriented sclerotic zone (arrows) in the posterior aspect of the calcaneus. This radiographic appearance is characteristic of stress fractures. Calcaneal fatigue fractures have been reported after jumping, parachuting, prolonged standing, and recent immobilization. These fractures are common in military recruits.

Illustration continued on following page

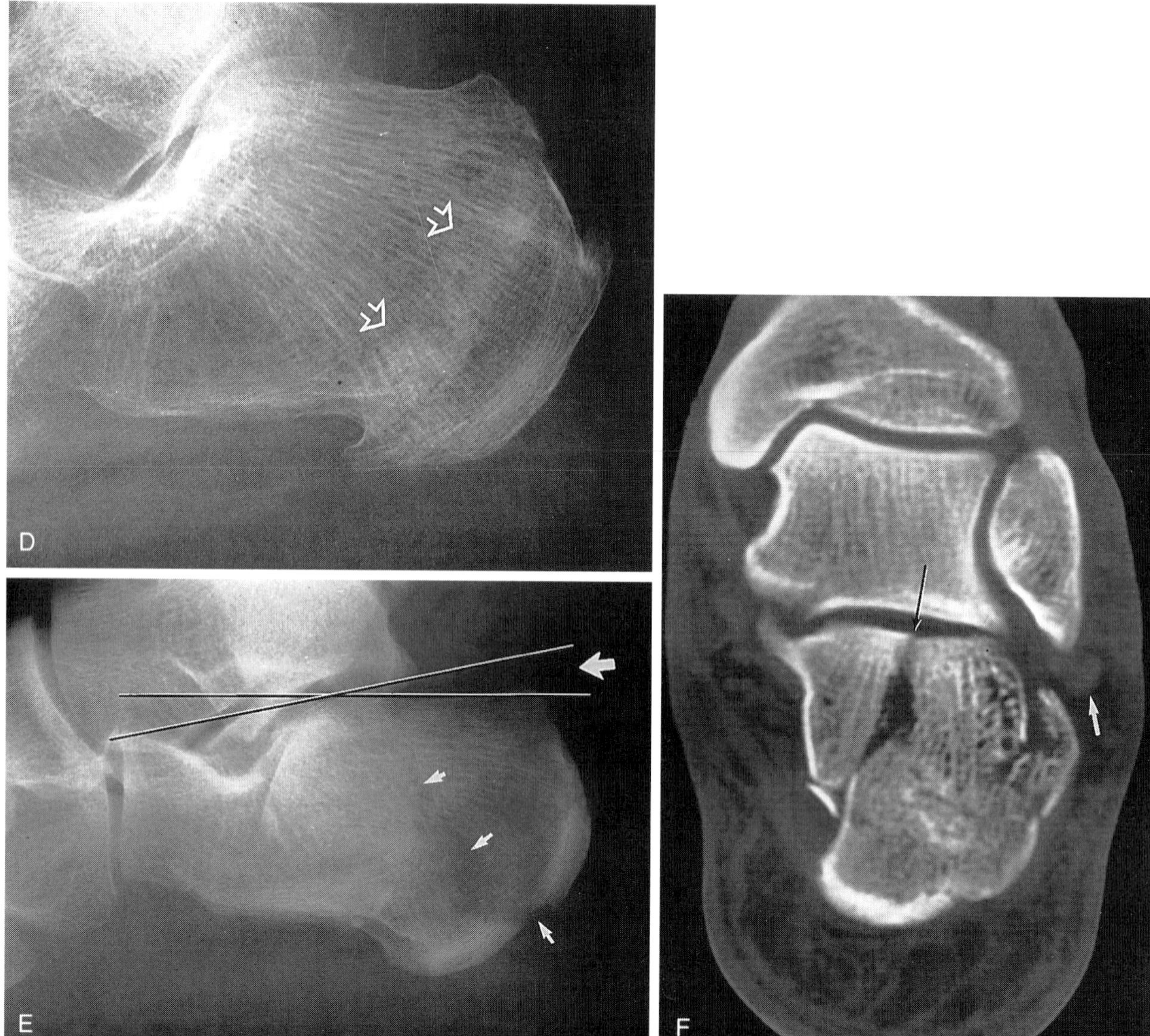

FIGURE 11–34 *Continued.* **D** Stress (insufficiency) fracture. In a 58-year-old woman with rheumatoid arthritis, a vertically oriented zone of sclerosis is seen (open arrows). This is a classic appearance of calcaneal insufficiency fracture, a frequent complication of rheumatoid arthritis. **E, F** Intra-articular fracture: Böhler's angle and computed tomographic (CT) examination. In **E,** a routine lateral radiograph shows a fracture of the calcaneus (small arrows). A useful measurement is Böhler's angle, which is formed by the intersection of two lines. The first line is constructed between the highest point of the anterior process of the calcaneus and the highest point of the posterior articular surface; the second line is constructed between the latter point and the most superior part of the calcaneal tuberosity. In a normal calcaneus, Böhler's angle measures between 25 and 40 degrees. In this patient, it measures 10 degrees (large arrow) owing to a complex intra-articular fracture. In **F,** a direct-acquisition coronal CT image shows the complexity of this comminuted, intra-articular fracture. Findings include marked lateral displacement of the lateral portion of the calcaneus, abutment of this region of the calcaneus and the distal portion of the fibula, displacement of the peroneal tendons (white arrow), and communication of the fracture line with the subtalar joint (long arrow).

The calcaneus is the most common site of tarsal fracture. Fractures are bilateral in about 10 per cent of cases and usually result from a vertical fall, such as a jump from a height. Many of these fractures may be seen on lateral radiographs as a decrease in Böhler's angle. Intra-articular fractures are more complex, are associated with a poorer prognosis, and are best evaluated with CT. *(**B, E, F,** Courtesy of M.N. Pathria, M.D., San Diego, California.)*

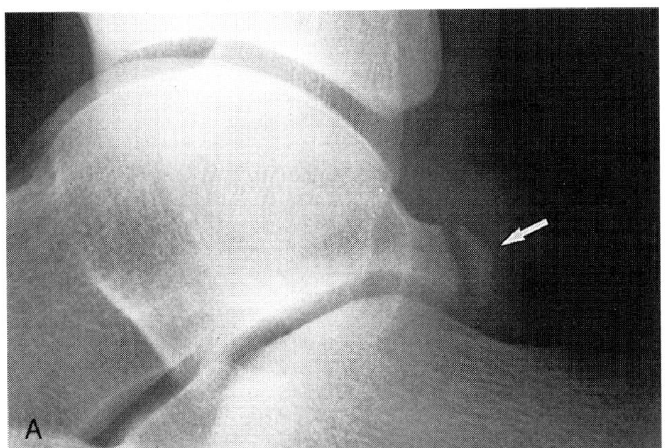

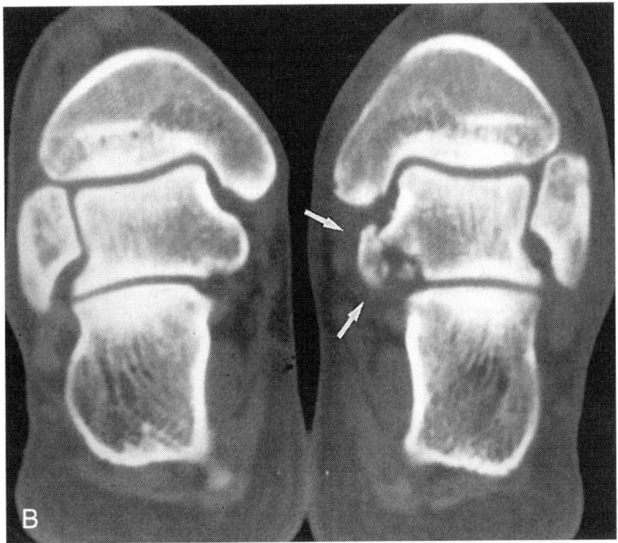

FIGURE 11–35. Fractures of the talus.[51, 52] **A** Posterior process (arrow). This fracture usually occurs during severe plantar flexion of the foot, owing to compression between the posterior surface of the tibia and the calcaneus. The posterior process may be difficult to differentiate from an os trigonum, a normal ossicle that also may be painful. **B** Talar body. Coronal computed tomographic (CT) scan accurately reveals an avulsion fracture of the medial portion of the talus (arrows). Observe the normal opposite talus. The routine radiograph (not shown) appeared normal in this 29-year-old man who injured his ankle in a jump from a 7-foot wall. Such fractures usually occur after eversion stress with osseous avulsion at the site of attachment of the deep fibers of the deltoid ligament.

A frontal radiograph obtained with external rotation of the ankle (not shown) is the best projection for demonstrating fractures of the medial process of the talus. *(**B**, Courtesy of G. Greenway, M.D., Dallas, Texas.)*

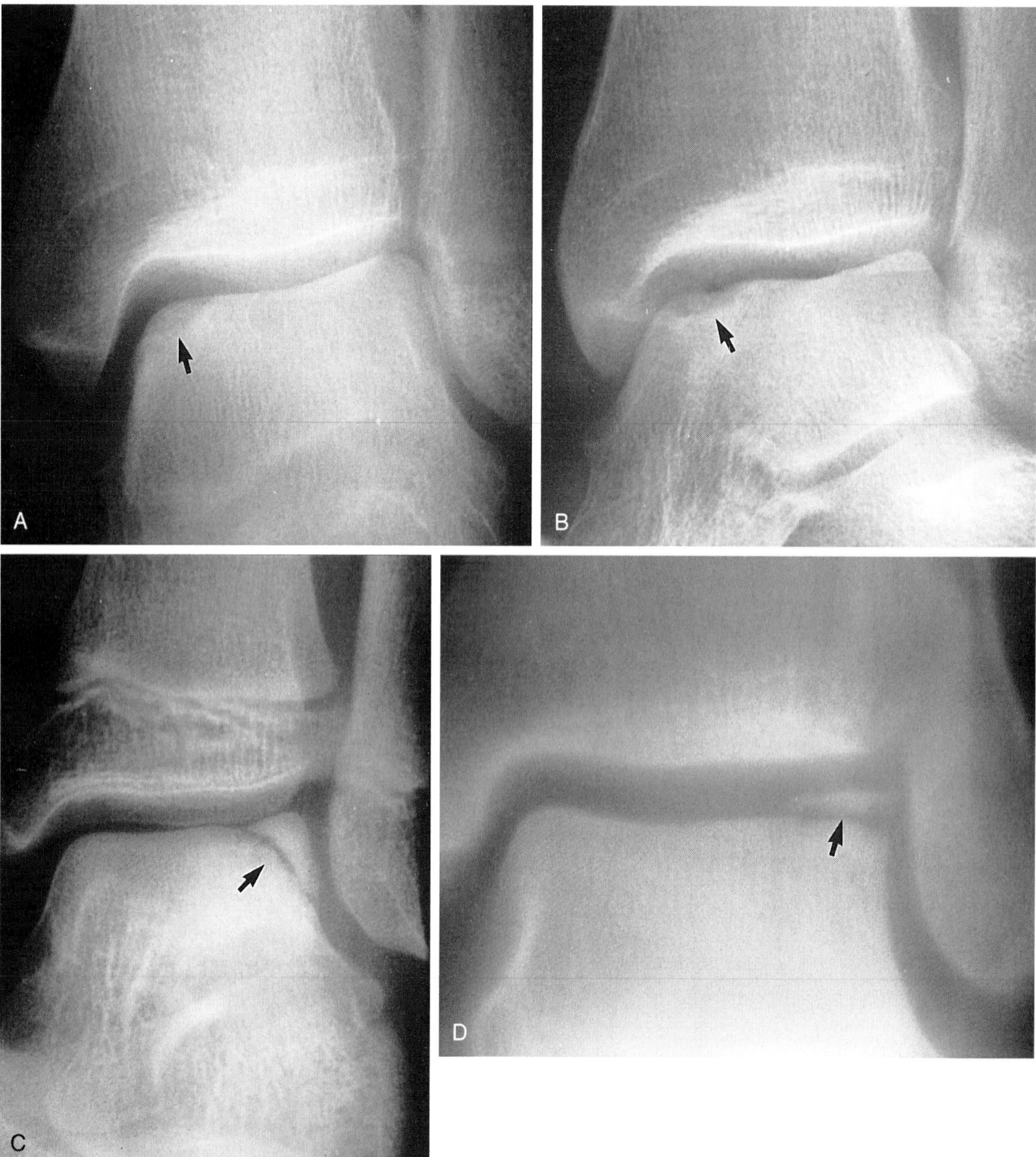

FIGURE 11–36. Osteochondritis dissecans.[53] A, B Medial talar dome. Anteroposterior (A) and medial oblique (B) radiographs show a radiolucent osteochondral defect on the medial talar dome (arrows). No associated bone fragment is seen. Such osseous and osteocartilaginous bodies are better seen with computed arthrotomography or magnetic resonance (MR) imaging. (*A, B, Courtesy of R. Kerr, M.D., Los Angeles, California.*) C, D Lateral talar dome. In C, a 10-year-old female gymnast, observe the osteosclerotic, triangular osseous fragment adjacent to the lateral articulating surface of the talar dome (arrows). The underlying bone also appears osteosclerotic. The lesions were bilateral (other side not shown). In D, another patient, a conventional tomograph clearly identifies an osseous fragment separated from a similar location on the talar dome. (*C, Courtesy of G. Greenway, M.D., Dallas, Texas.*)

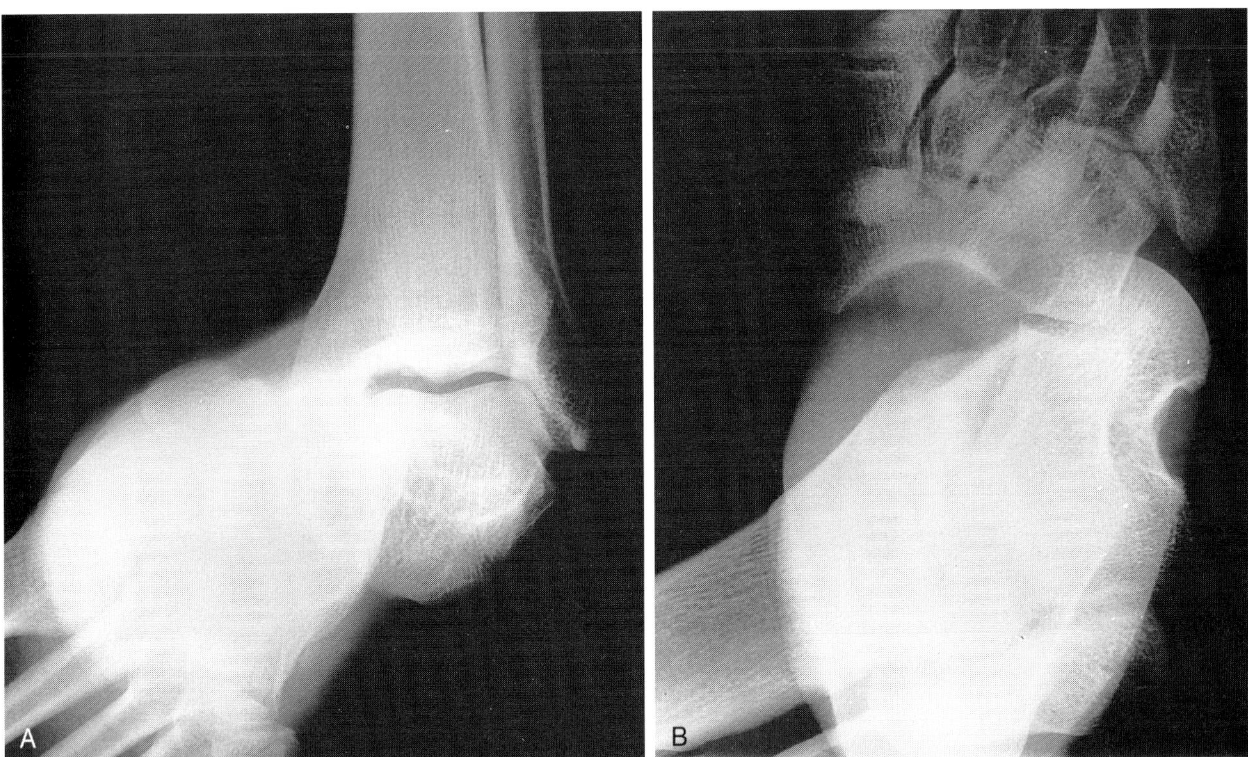

FIGURE 11–37. A, B Subtalar and talocalcaneonavicular dislocation.[54] Note the dislocation of the anterior talocalcaneonavicular and posterior subtalar joints and a relatively normal alignment of the calcaneocuboid joint. *(From Resnick D: Diagnosis of Bone and Joint Disorders. 3rd Ed. Philadelphia, WB Saunders, 1995, p 2791.)*

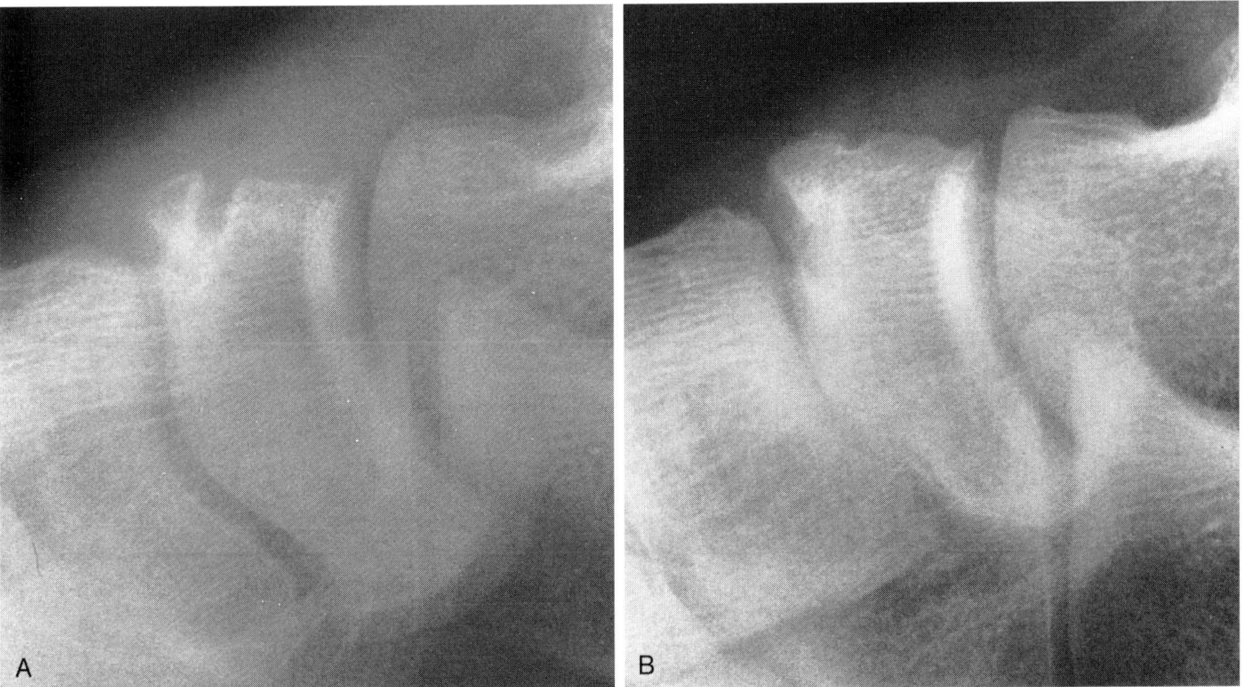

FIGURE 11–38. Healing navicular fracture.[55] This 18-year-old woman had pain on the dorsum of the foot after a soccer injury. The initial diagnosis was a painful os supranaviculare, seen on a radiograph taken several months after the injury (A). The pain persisted and another radiograph was obtained 1 year later (B), which showed fusion of the triangular fracture fragment.

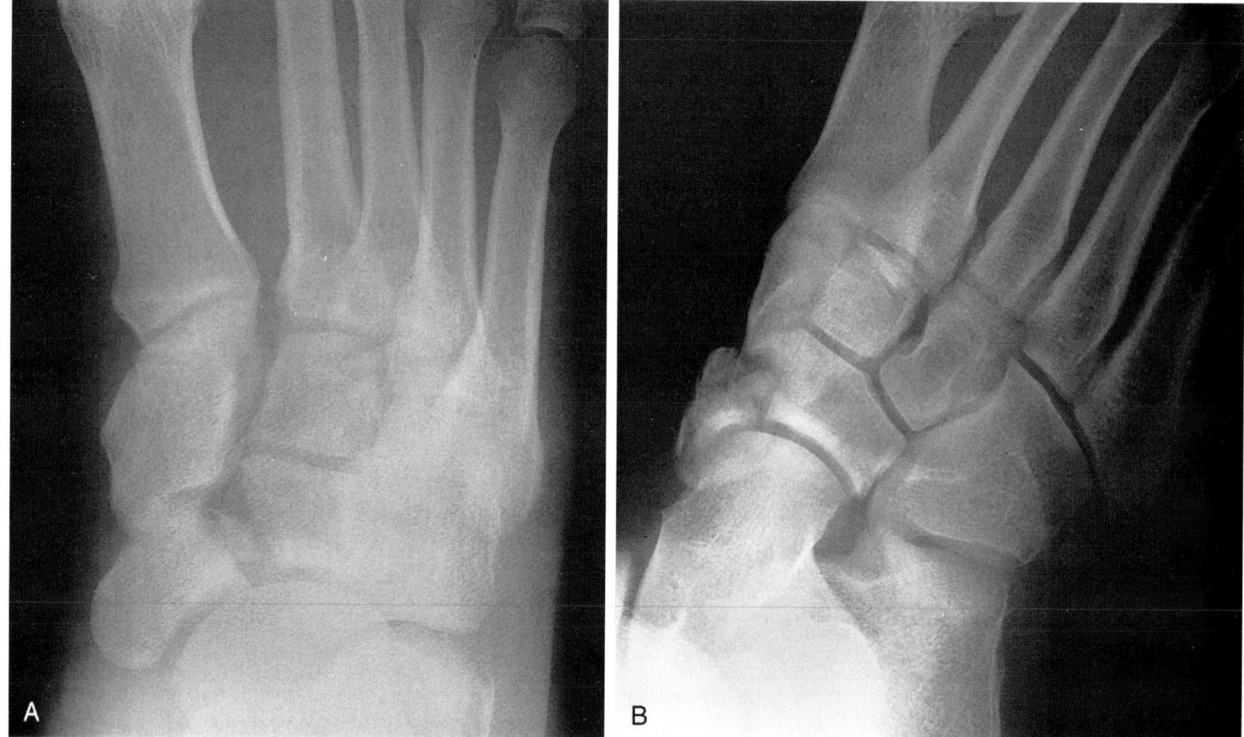

FIGURE 11–39. A, B Navicular fracture with dissociation of medial and intermediate cuneiform bones.[56] This 21-year-old man was involved in a motorcycle accident. Radiographs reveal a longitudinal fracture of the navicular bone, which is aligned with the space between the widened medial and intermediate cuneiform bones. This is an unstable injury requiring surgical reduction.

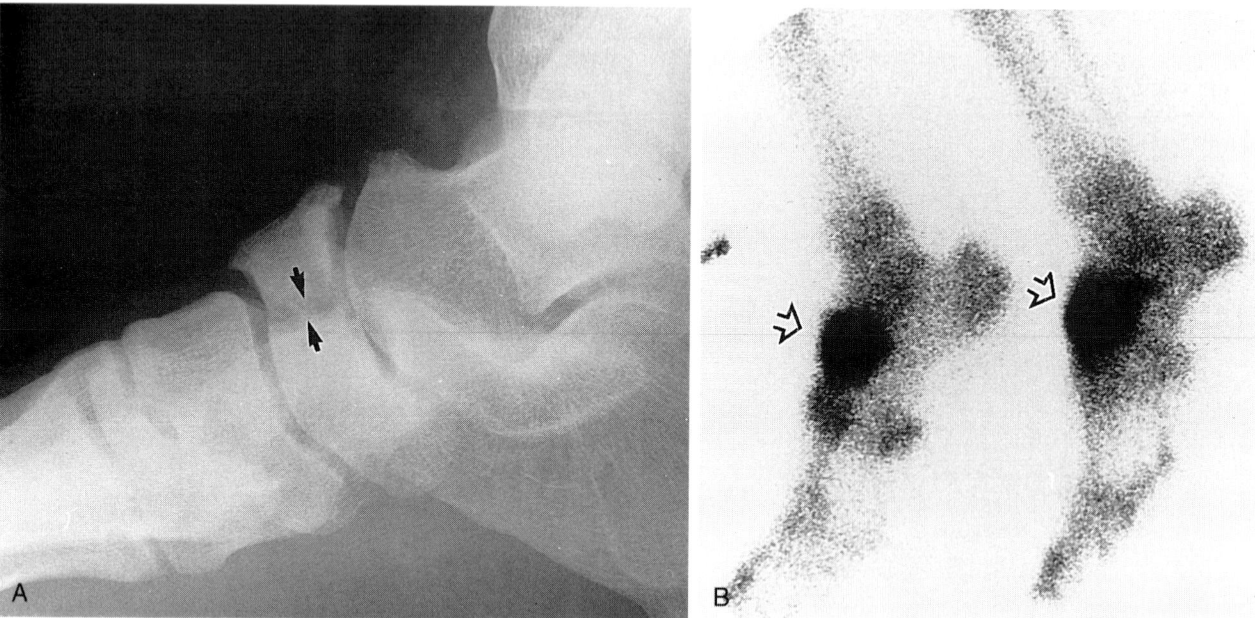

FIGURE 11–40. Stress (fatigue) fracture of tarsal navicular.[57, 58] A Lateral radiograph of this 21-year-old female physical education student shows a linear sagittal lucent area surrounded by marginal sclerosis within the navicular bone (arrows). B Bone scan demonstrates bilateral increased uptake of the bone-seeking pharmaceutical agent, revealing stress fractures of both navicular bones (arrows). The first fracture apparently was undiagnosed until the time of this examination.

Stress fractures of the navicular bone are associated with activities involving stomping on the ground, marching, and long-distance running. They are especially common in basketball players and runners. Such fractures often are not seen on conventional radiographs, and accurate diagnosis requires further evaluation by clinical examination, computed tomography (CT), scintigraphy, and magnetic resonance (MR) imaging. *(Courtesy of M. Mitchell, M.D., Halifax, Nova Scotia, Canada.)*

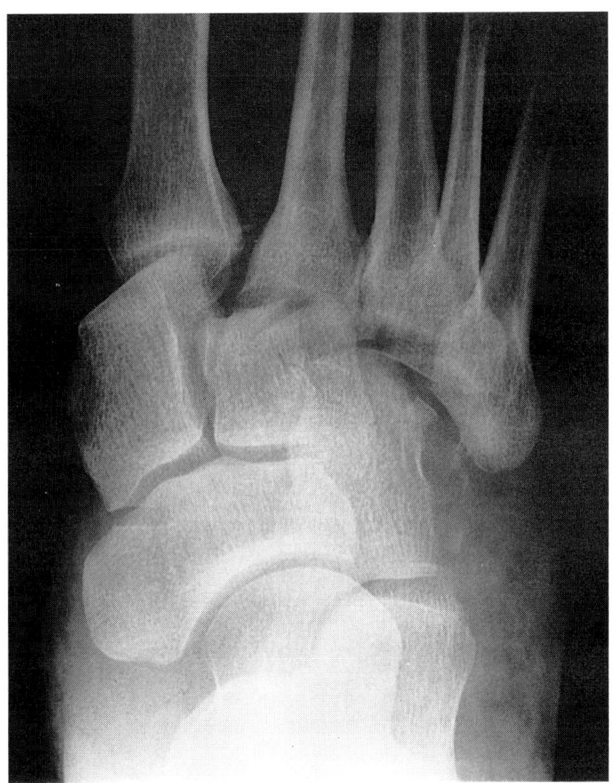

FIGURE 11–41. Lisfranc's fracture-dislocation of the tarsometatarsal joints.[59, 60] Observe the lateral dislocation of all the metatarsal bones. Fractures of the cuboid and bases of the metatarsal bones also are seen.

TABLE 11–8. Fractures and Dislocations of the Metatarsals and Phalanges

Entity	Figure(s)	Characteristics	Complications and Related Injuries
Acute metatarsal fracture[40, 61–63]	11–42	Caused by direct and indirect forces Transverse, oblique, spiral, or comminuted Shaft and neck: heavy object falling on foot Rare fractures: first metatarsal bone and the metatarsal heads Base of the fifth metatarsal: Two types	
		1. Avulsion of the tuberosity: sudden inversion results in avulsion of a portion of the styloid process by the attachment of the peroneus brevis or the lateral cord of the plantar aponeurosis Transverse orientation of fracture helps to differentiate it from a normal longitudinal growth center	Fragment may enter cuboid–metatarsal joint space
		2. Jones fracture: transverse fracture of the proximal portion of the diaphysis	Frequently associated with delayed union, nonunion, and refracture
Metatarsal stress (fatigue) fracture[64–66]	11–43	Second and third metatarsal shafts (march fracture) or metatarsal bases are common sites of fatigue fractures, but any metatarsal can be affected Often caused by marching, ballet dancing, prolonged standing, foot deformities, and surgical resection of adjacent metatarsal bones Stress fracture infrequently affects the metatarsal heads, simulating Freiberg's infraction or diabetic neuropathic osteoarthropathy	May result in complete fracture Recurrence if the stressful activity is not discontinued
Phalangeal fracture[44, 67, 68]	11–44	Frequently occurring fractures Common mechanism is the stubbed toe	Osteomyelitis in children with physeal damage from nail-bed injury
	11–45	Growth plate injuries in children	Residual deformity
Sesamoid bone fracture[23]	11–46	Hallux sesamoid bones fracture most frequently	Osteonecrosis Osteoarthrosis and hallux rigidus
Metatarsophalangeal (MTP) joint dislocation[69]		First MTP joint commonly is affected Can occur in any direction related to mechanism of injury Turf toe: hyperextension of the first MTP joint with disruption of the plantar aspect of the joint and joint capsule, which tears away from the metatarsal head; may be associated with sesamoid bone fracture	Complications of any type of hyperextension injury of the great toe Chondromalacia of the first metatarsal head Hallux rigidus Hallux valgus Dorsal osteophytes Periarticular calcification
		Sesamoid bone dislocations, with or without intra-articular entrapment, may rarely occur, especially at the first toe	May interfere with closed reduction
Interphalangeal (IP) joint dislocation[69]	11–47	The first IP joint is commonly affected	Complications similar to those of MTP joint dislocations

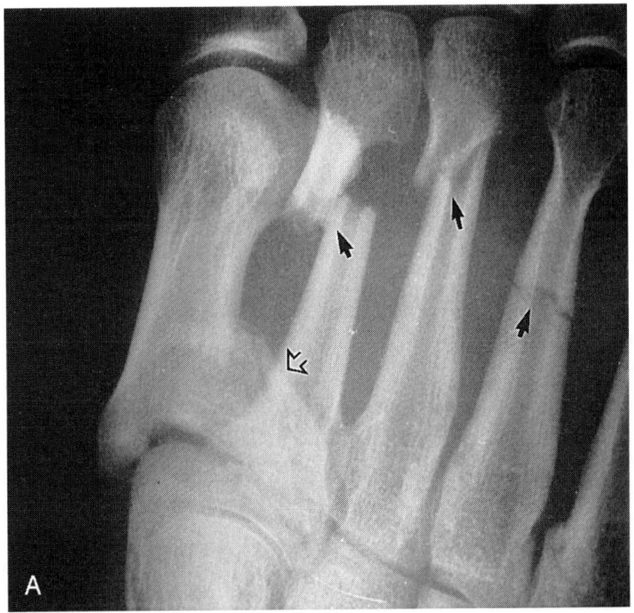

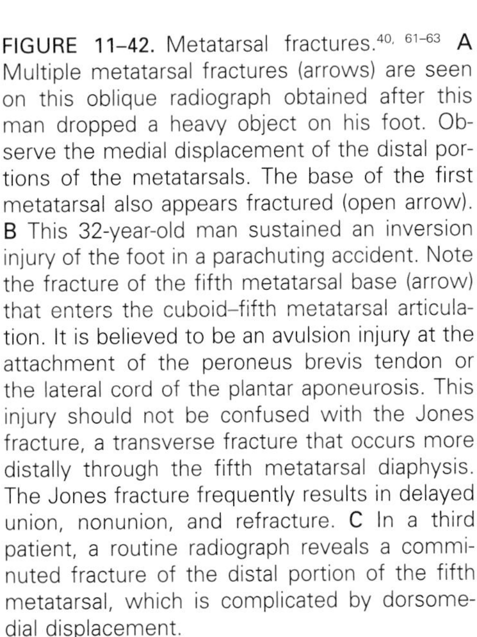

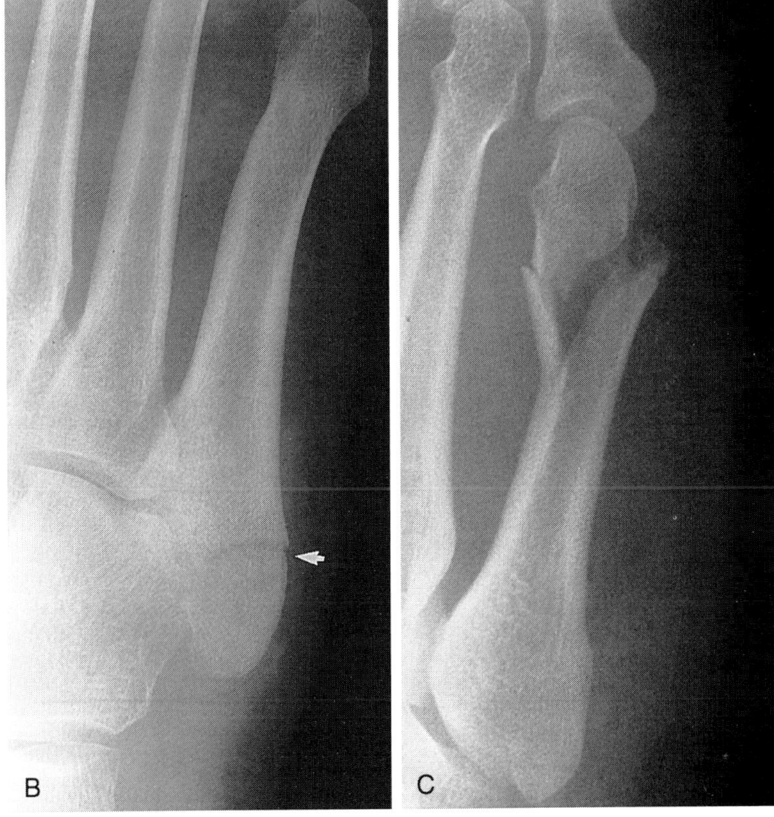

FIGURE 11–42. Metatarsal fractures.[40, 61–63] A Multiple metatarsal fractures (arrows) are seen on this oblique radiograph obtained after this man dropped a heavy object on his foot. Observe the medial displacement of the distal portions of the metatarsals. The base of the first metatarsal also appears fractured (open arrow). B This 32-year-old man sustained an inversion injury of the foot in a parachuting accident. Note the fracture of the fifth metatarsal base (arrow) that enters the cuboid–fifth metatarsal articulation. It is believed to be an avulsion injury at the attachment of the peroneus brevis tendon or the lateral cord of the plantar aponeurosis. This injury should not be confused with the Jones fracture, a transverse fracture that occurs more distally through the fifth metatarsal diaphysis. The Jones fracture frequently results in delayed union, nonunion, and refracture. C In a third patient, a routine radiograph reveals a comminuted fracture of the distal portion of the fifth metatarsal, which is complicated by dorsomedial displacement.

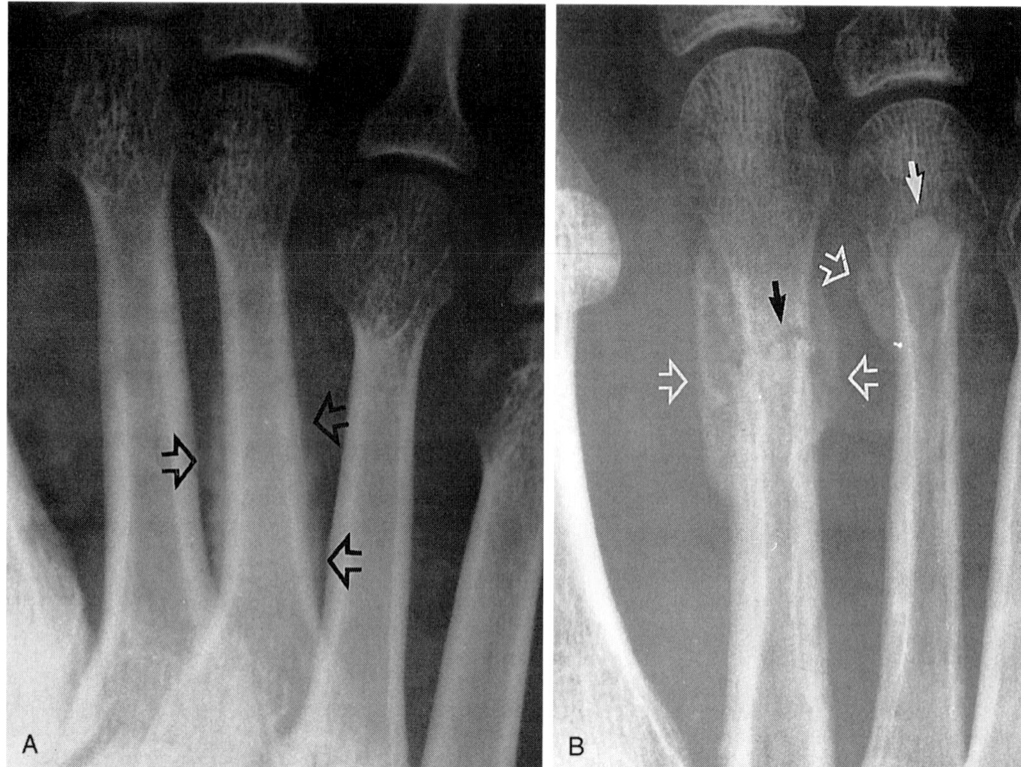

FIGURE 11–43. Metatarsal stress (fatigue) fracture: March fracture.[64–66] A Early findings. In this patient with exercise-induced foot pain, periosteal new bone formation envelops the third metatarsal diaphysis (open arrows). No fracture line is seen. B Later findings. In this 34-year-old woman who recently began a jogging program, observe the fatigue fractures of the second and third metatarsal shafts. The findings include transverse radiolucent fracture lines (arrows) with surrounding periostitis (open arrows).

Stress fractures commonly affect the metatarsal bones and accompany marching, ballet dancing, prolonged standing, foot deformities, and foot surgery. The middle and distal portions of the second and third metatarsals are most commonly affected. Such fractures, referred to as march fractures, may be imperceptible radiographically in the early stages. Bone scans, magnetic resonance (MR) images, or serial radiographs often are necessary to confirm the diagnosis. Stress fractures of the metatarsal heads are less common than those of the shaft and neck and are more frequently overlooked.

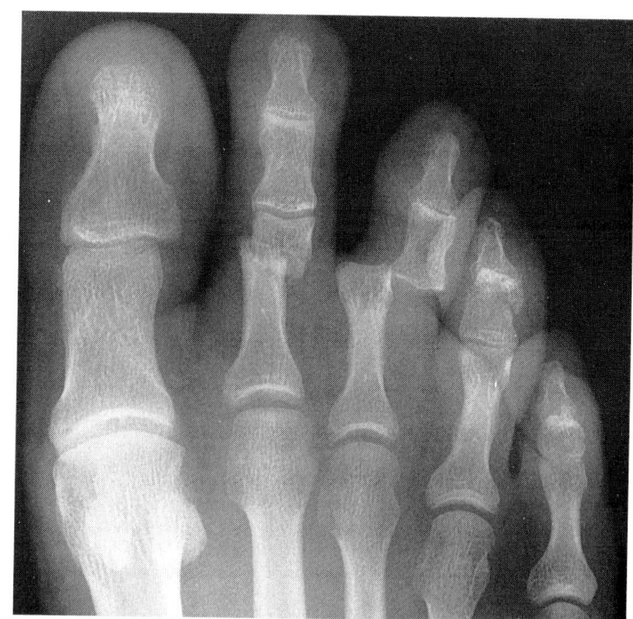

FIGURE 11–44. Fracture-dislocation.[67] Frontal radiograph reveals a fracture of the second proximal phalanx and a dislocation of the third proximal interphalangeal joint in this 37-year-old man who had dropped a heavy safe on his foot.

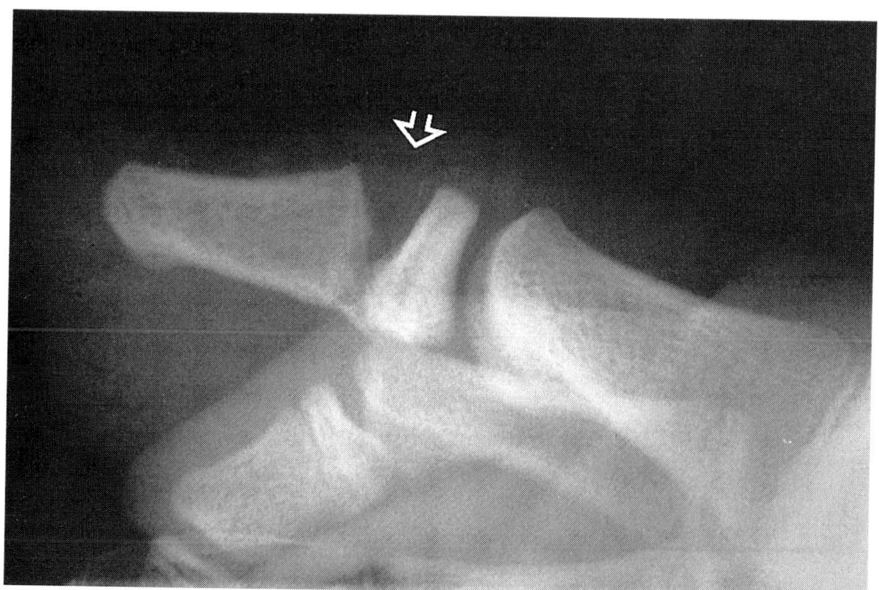

FIGURE 11–45. Salter-Harris type I injury.[44, 68] Observe the wide separation of the distal phalangeal epiphysis and metaphysis in this child after he had stubbed his toe (open arrow). Such injuries commonly violate the nail bed, creating an open injury and increasing the likelihood of osteomyelitis or septic arthritis.

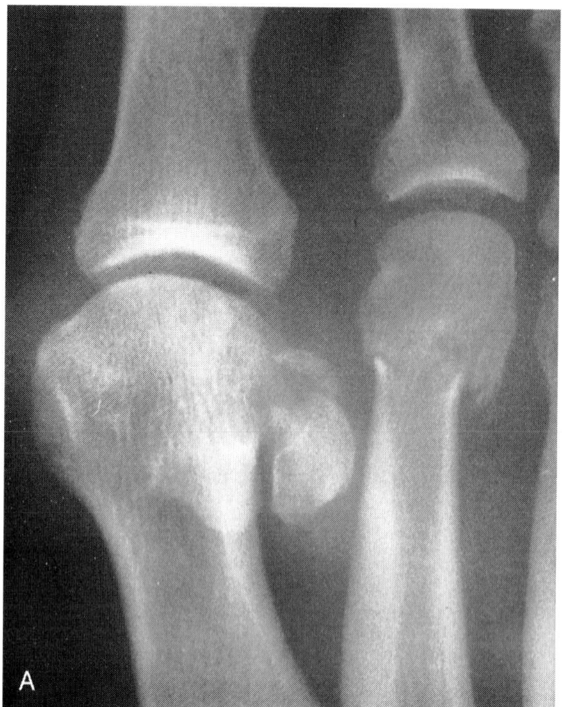

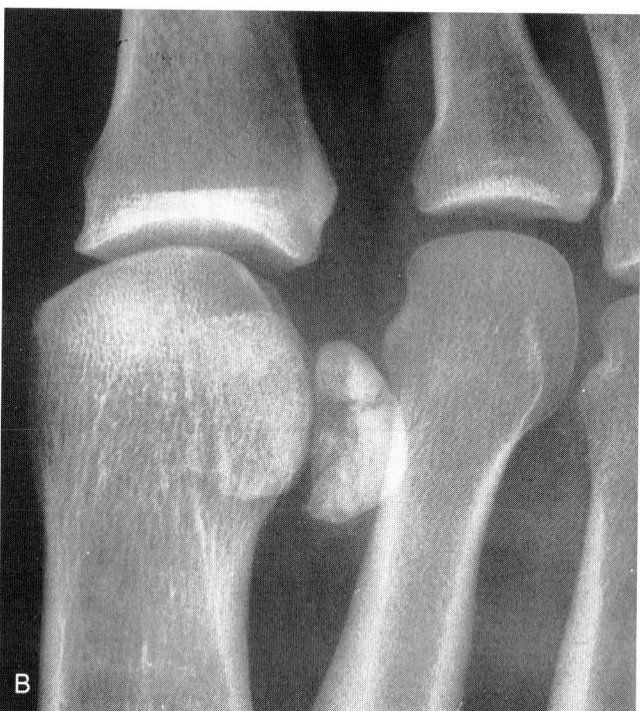

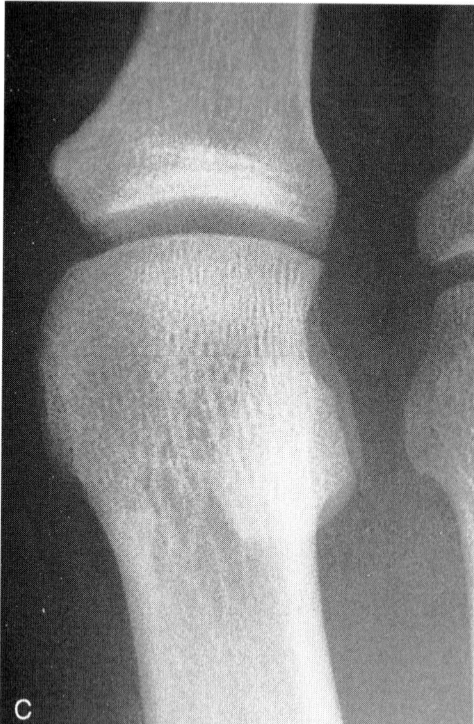

FIGURE 11–46. Hallux sesamoid bone fracture.[23] **A** This patient's foot was run over by an automobile. Observe the fracture of the hallux sesamoid bone as well as a fracture of the second metatarsal bone. **B** In another patient, the lateral hallux sesamoid bone is fractured. Fracture fragments typically have jagged edges, lack a corticated margin, and may be displaced. These features usually allow differentiation from painful bipartite sesamoid bones, which appear smooth, well-corticated, and nondisplaced. **C** Sesamoidectomy. This patient had surgical removal of the tibial hallux sesamoid after a fracture.

Congenital absence of the hallux sesamoid bones occurs rarely, and when one or both of these bones is absent, surgical removal is the most likely cause.

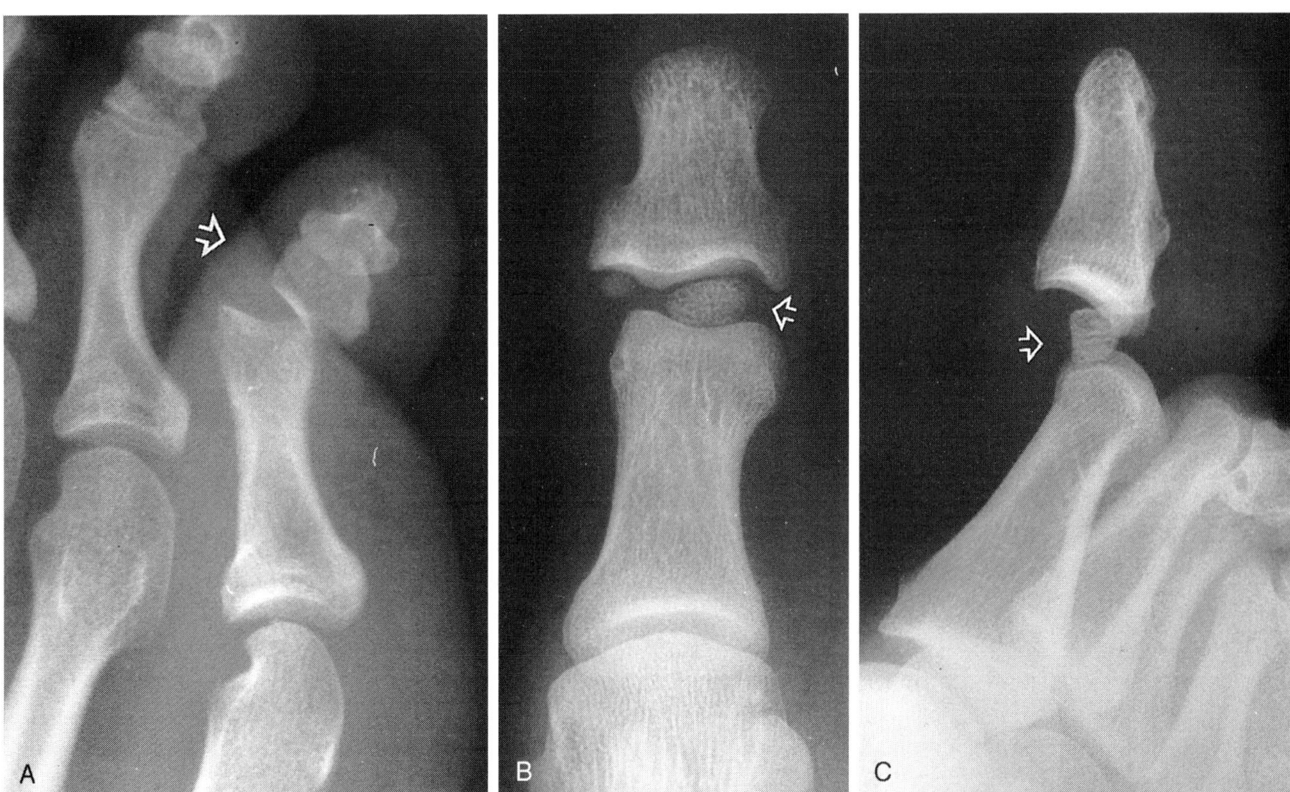

FIGURE 11–47. Dislocation: Interphalangeal joints.[69] A Observe the dislocation of the fifth proximal interphalangeal joint with lateral displacement of the middle phalanx (open arrow). B Dislocation of the interphalangeal joint of the great toe with intra-articular entrapment of the sesamoid bone (open arrow) is evident. C In another patient, radiographs taken after attempts at reduction show persistent entrapment of the sesamoid bone (open arrow), necessitating open reduction.

TABLE 11–9. Soft Tissue Injuries About the Ankle and Foot

Entity	Figure(s)	Characteristics
Joint effusion[70]	11–48	Accumulation of excessive synovial fluid within joint Usually seen as a bulging of the anterior capsule on lateral radiographs Bland effusion associated with acute injury, or internal joint derangement Proliferative effusion associated with synovial proliferation as in inflammatory arthropathy and villonodular synovitis Pyarthrosis: purulent material in joint from pyogenic septic arthritis Hemathrosis: accumulation of blood within joint: hemophilia, villonodular synovitis
Ligament injuries[71]	11–49	Severe ligament injuries may result in chronic ankle instability Classified as acute, subacute, or chronic Lateral complex: most commonly injured; inversion sprains Medial complex: deltoid ligaments; eversion sprains Tibiofibular complex: tibiofibular syndesmosis; least commonly injured Radiographs obtained with the application of inversion stress, eversion stress, and anterior stress (anterior drawer) may reveal excessive motion indicating disruption of ligaments Magnetic resonance (MR) imaging also useful
Tendon injuries[72–75]		Most common tendons to be injured:
	11–50	Achilles tendon
	11–51	Tibialis anterior tendon
	11–52	Tibialis posterior tendon
	11–53	Peroneus longus and brevis tendon
		Spectrum of injuries: Tendinitis: inflammation of a tendon (more proper term is tendinosis or tendinopathy, indicating degeneration rather than inflammation) Tenosynovitis: inflammation of a tendon sheath Tendon rupture: Type I: partial disruption with vertical splits and bulbous hypertrophy Type II: partial disruption with attenuation Type III: complete disruption and retraction of torn ends MR imaging is the most useful imaging study

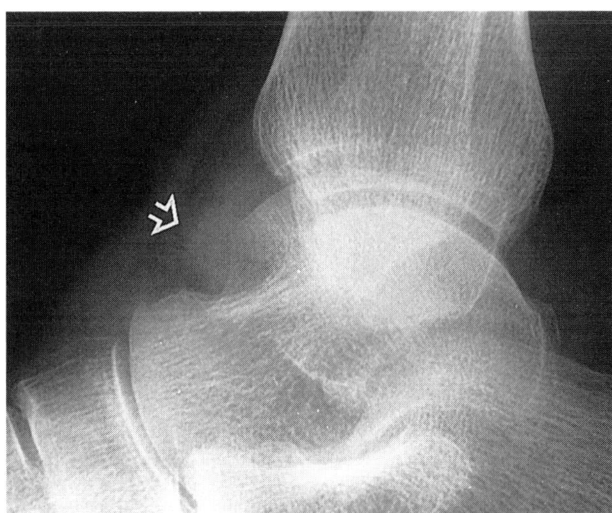

FIGURE 11–48. Joint effusion.[70] Observe the radiodense distention of the anterior capsule (arrow), indicative of a large effusion or hemarthrosis. Radiographically, it is impossible to differentiate between bloody effusions (hemarthroses), which generally appear within the first few hours of injury, and nonbloody effusions, which usually appear 12 to 24 hours after injury.

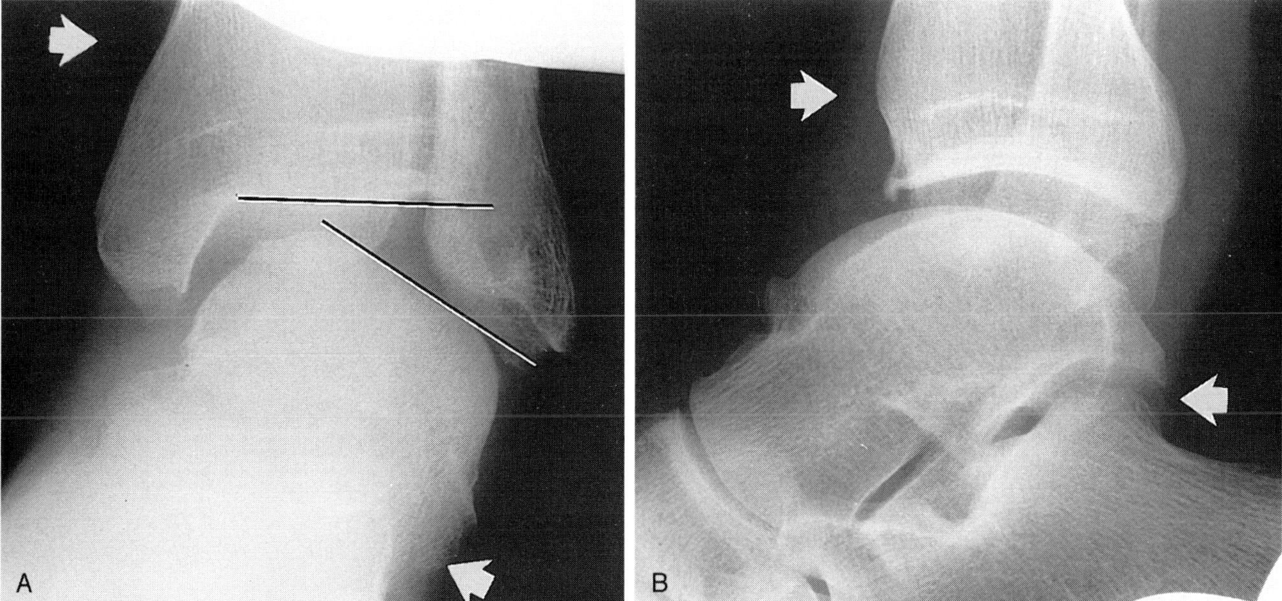

FIGURE 11–49. Ankle ligament instability: Stress radiography.[71] **A** Frontal varus (inversion) stress radiograph obtained with the foot in neutral position shows marked separation of the lateral portion of the talocrural joint, indicating some degree of lateral ligament disruption. The divergent lines along the tibial plafond and the superior talar articular surface illustrate the extent of displacement. The arrows demonstrate the direction of force applied by the examiner. **B** Lateral radiograph obtained with the application of anterior stress to the calcaneus and posterior stress to the tibia (arrows). This procedure, termed the anterior drawer test, shows anterior displacement of the talus on the tibia, indicative of lateral ligament injury.

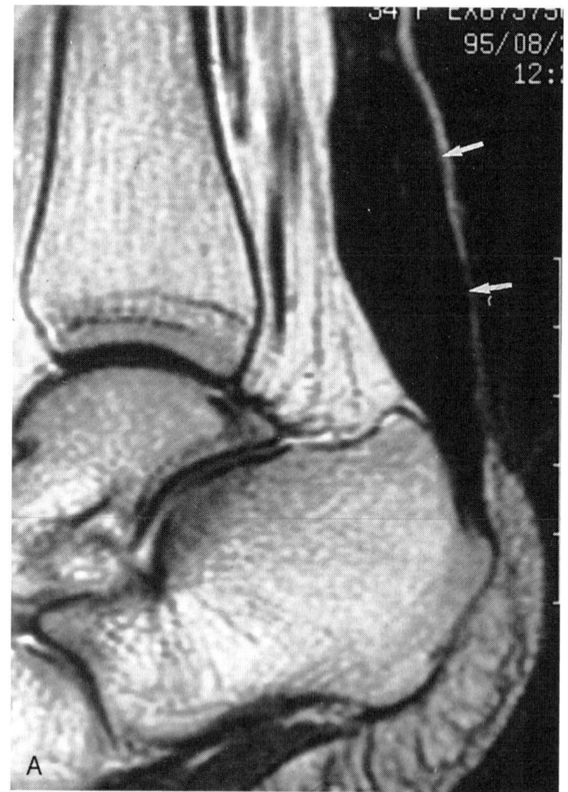

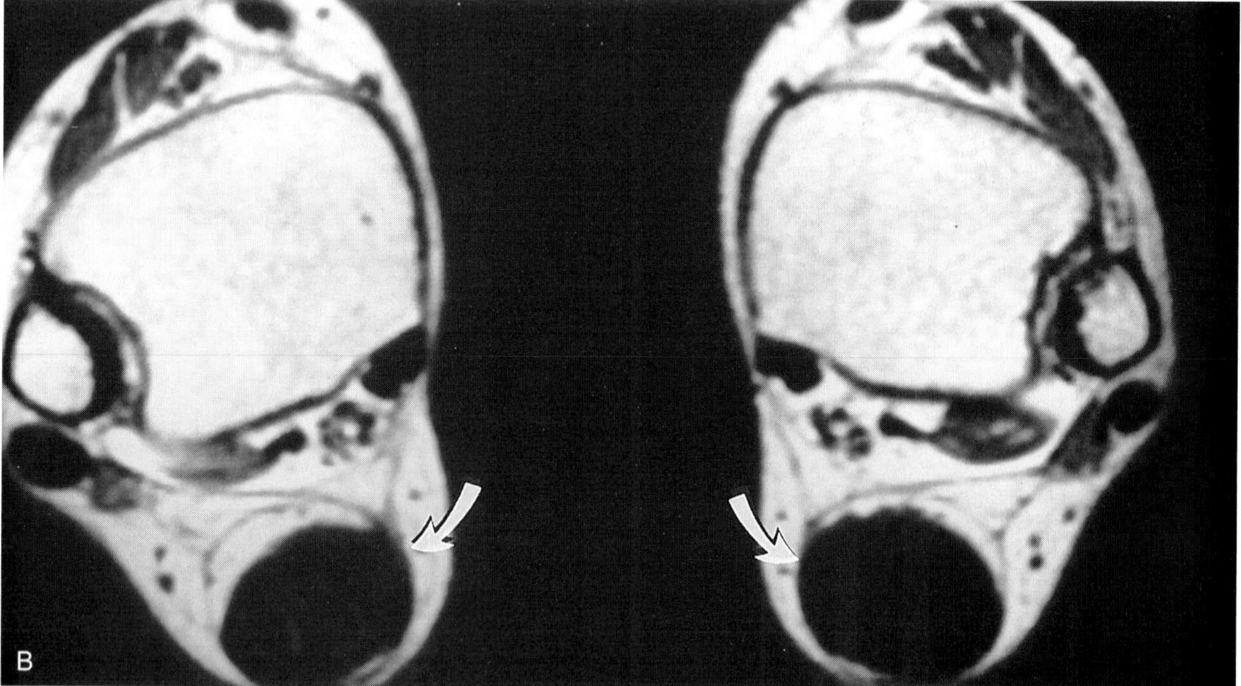

FIGURE 11–50. Achilles tendinitis: Bilateral.[72] This 34-year-old woman had bilateral pain and swelling of the Achilles tendons. A Sagittal (TR/TE, 3000/84) fast spin echo magnetic resonance (MR) image shows bulbous hypertrophy of the distal aspect of the Achilles tendon (arrows). B Bilateral transaxial T1-weighted (TR/TE, 549/16) spin echo MR image reveals the extreme hypertrophy of both Achilles tendons immediately above their attachment to the calcaneus (curved arrows). *(Courtesy of B.Y. Yang, M.D., Kaoshiung, Taiwan.)*

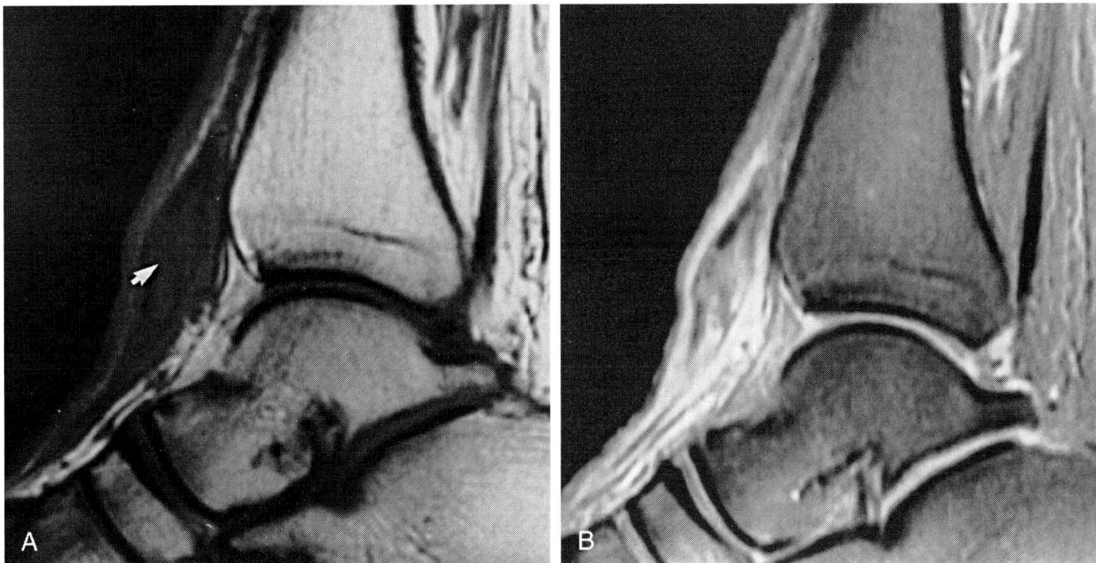

FIGURE 11–51. Injuries of the tibialis anterior tendon: magnetic resonance (MR) imaging—chronic partial tear.[73] Sagittal T1-weighted (TR/TE, 750/15) spin echo MR image **(A)** shows an enlarged tendon (arrow), which is inhomogeneous in signal intensity. After intravenous injection of a gadolinium compound, a sagittal fat-suppressed T1-weighted (TR/TE, 550/15) spin echo MR image **(B)** reveals enhancement of signal intensity within and around the abnormal tendon. *(From Resnick D, Kang HS: Internal Derangements of Joints. Philadelphia, WB Saunders, 1997, p 870.)*

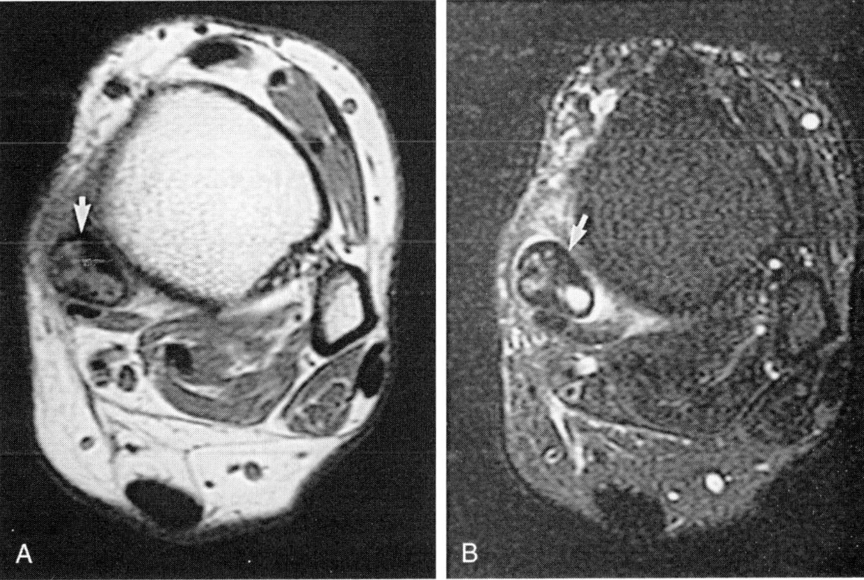

FIGURE 11–52. Injuries of the tibialis posterior tendon: Magnetic resonance (MR) imaging—chronic partial tear.[74] **A** Transaxial T1-weighted (TR/TE, 500/17) spin echo MR image shows an enlarged tibialis posterior tendon (arrow), which is inhomogeneous in signal intensity. **B** Transaxial fat-suppressed fast spin echo MR image (TR/TE, 4500/114) reveals the hypertrophied tendon (arrow) containing longitudinal splits. Fluid is present in the surrounding tendon sheath, and soft tissue edema also is evident. *(From Resnick D, Kang HS: Internal Derangements of Joints. Philadelphia, WB Saunders, 1997, p 866.)*

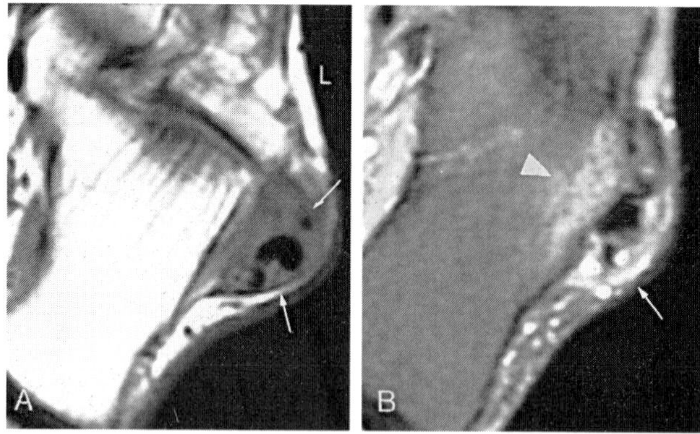

FIGURE 11–53. Injuries of the peroneal tendon and sheath: Peroneal tendinitis and tenosynovitis.[75] Transaxial T1-weighted (TR/TE, 400/17) spin echo (**A**) and transaxial T2-weighted (TR/TE, 3300/100) fast spin echo (**B**) magnetic resonance (MR) images show a fluid-filled mass (arrows) about the peroneus longus and peroneus brevis tendons. Note the reactive edema in the marrow of the calcaneus (arrowhead) in **B**. *(From Resnick D, Kang HS: Internal Derangements of Joints. Philadelphia, WB Saunders, 1997, p 874.)*

TABLE 11–10. Articular Disorders of the Ankle and Foot

Entity	Figure(s)	Characteristics
Degenerative and related disorders		
Osteoarthrosis[76–78]	11–54	Predilection for first metatarsophalangeal (MTP) joint; progresses to hallux valgus and hallux rigidus Secondary osteoarthrosis may involve any joint previously injured
Diffuse idiopathic skeletal hyperostosis (DISH)[79]	11–55	Enthesophytes: osseous excrescences arise from the surfaces of the talus, navicular, and cuboid bones, the base of fifth metatarsal, and the posterior and plantar aspects of the calcaneus
Inflammatory disorders		
Rheumatoid arthritis[80, 81]	11–56	Bilateral symmetric, concentric joint space narrowing, erosion, and subluxation
Juvenile chronic arthritis[6, 82, 83]	11–57	Soft tissue swelling Diffuse, bilateral symmetric joint space loss and erosion Periarticular osteoporosis
Ankylosing spondylitis[83, 84]	11–58	Approximately 15 per cent of patients with ankylosing spondylitis develop abnormalities of the feet Calcaneal erosions and enthesopathy Rarely may eventually result in partial or complete intra-articular osseous ankylosis
Psoriatic arthropathy[77, 85–87] and Reiter's syndrome[77, 88]	11–59, 11–60	Findings similar to those of ankylosing spondylitis Ray pattern: involvement of several joints within the same digit Diffuse soft tissue swelling: sausage digit Fluffy, poorly defined periarticular periostitis
Systemic lupus erythematosus[89]		Deforming nonerosive arthropathy Hallux valgus, MTP joint subluxation, widening of forefoot Rarely, osteonecrosis of tarsal bones
Dermatomyositis and polymyositis[90]	11–61	Diffuse soft tissue calcification
Scleroderma (progressive systemic sclerosis)[91]	11–62	Achilles tendon calcification Soft tissue, periarticular, and intra-articular calcification about the MTP joints Hallux valgus deformity

TABLE 11–10. Articular Disorders of the Ankle and Foot *Continued*

Entity	Figure(s)	Characteristics
Crystal deposition and metabolic diseases		
Calcium pyrophosphate dihydrate (CPPD) crystal deposition disease[92, 93]	11–63	Periarticular and intra-articular calcification Arthropathy is rare; affects talonavicular joint
Calcium hydroxyapatite crystal deposition disease[94]	11–64	Calcific deposits within tendons and bursae occasionally seen about ankle, foot, and heel First MTP joint involvement may resemble gout
Gouty arthropathy[95]	11–65	First MTP and IP joints most common sites but may involve any joint in ankle or foot Periarticular erosions and soft tissue tophi
Hemochromatosis[96]		Rare involvement of ankle and foot Findings resemble those of CPPD crystal deposition disease and predominate in the tibiotalar and MTP joints
Miscellaneous disorders		
Idiopathic synovial osteochondromatosis[97, 98]	11–66	Multiple intra-articular or periarticular collections of intracapsular osteochondral or chondral bodies of variable size and density within the tibiotalar joint May result in erosion of adjacent bone Idiopathic form more common than secondary form
Hemophilic arthropathy[6, 99]	11–67	Hemophilic arthropathy: tibiotalar and talocalcaneal joints Tibiotalar slant Subtalar joint osseous ankylosis may occur Occasional deformities and osteonecrosis of talus
Neuropathic osteoarthropathy[100–104]	11–68, 11–69	Ankle involvement: tabes dorsalis, amyloidosis, diabetes mellitus, and congenital indifference to pain Foot involvement: diabetes mellitus, leprosy, alcoholism, congenital insensitivity to pain, peripheral nerve injury *Radiographic findings:* Large joint effusions Joint space narrowing and obliteration Joint subluxation, disorganization, and destruction Bone fragmentation, destruction, and sclerosis
Frostbite[105]	11–70	Local tissue damage from cellular injury as a result of the freezing process itself or from the vascular insufficiency it produces Soft tissue swelling, osteoporosis, periostitis, secondary infection, arthritis secondary to cartilage injury, terminal tuft resorption, epiphyseal abnormalities, and premature physeal fusion in children
Silicone synovitis[106]	11–71	Complication of silicone arthroplasty Believed to be a reaction to shedded silicone particles embedded within the synovium with resultant synovial hypertrophy, and chronic inflammatory and giant cell infiltration of the synovial membrane Associated soft tissue swelling and preservation of cartilage spaces often is found

TABLE 11–11. Distribution, Symmetry, and Preferential Target Sites of Articular Disorders of the Ankle and Foot

	Distribution and Symmetry			Articular Compartments*									
Entity	*Bilateral Symmetric*	*Bilateral Asymmetric*	*Unilateral*	*TT*	*TCN*	*ST*	*CN*	*CC*	*TMT*	*First MTP*	*Second to Fifth MTP*	*First IP*	*Second to Fifth IP*
Osteoarthrosis		+	+						+	+			
Neuropathic osteoarthropathy		+			+	+	+	+	+		+		
Rheumatoid arthritis	+			+	+	+	+	+	+	+	+	+	
Gout	+	+		+	+	+	+	+	++	++	+	++	+

*TT, Tibiotalar; TCN, talocalcaneonavicular; ST, posterior subtalar; CN, cuneonavicular; CC, calcaneocuboid; TMT, tarsometatarsal; MTP, metatarsophalangeal; IP, interphalangeal.

TABLE 11–12. Differential Diagnosis: Calcaneal Involvement in Articular Disorders[77]

Entity	Figure(s)	Characteristics
Degenerative enthesopathy	11–54 E	Well-defined, sharply marginated osseous excrescences (heel spurs) arising from the site of attachment of the plantar aponeurosis on the calcaneus May be associated with plantar fasciitis
Diffuse idiopathic skeletal hyperostosis	11–55	Prominent, bilateral symmetric, well-defined enthesophyte proliferation at sites of attachment of the Achilles tendon and plantar aponeurosis
Rheumatoid arthritis		Well-defined posterior and plantar enthesophytes Retrocalcaneal bursitis results in unilateral or bilateral erosions of calcaneus Achilles tendinitis and soft tissue mass in preachilles fat pad Minimal or no reactive sclerosis
Ankylosing spondylitis and psoriatic arthropathy	11–58 D,E, 11–59 B	Well-defined enthesophytes at the Achilles tendon attachment Poorly defined enthesophytes at plantar aspect of bone Retrocalcaneal bursitis results in erosions at posterosuperior aspect of calcaneus Erosions may be associated with reactive sclerosis Outgrowths more irregular and fuzzy than those in rheumatoid arthritis
Reiter's syndrome	11–60 B–D	Poorly defined plantar and posterosuperior enthesophytes Retrocalcaneal bursitis results in unilateral or bilateral erosions on plantar and posterosuperior aspects of calcaneus Enthesophytes less well defined than in rheumatoid arthritis
CPPD crystal deposition disease		Bilateral or unilateral linear, calcific collections within the Achilles tendon and plantar aponeurosis
Calcium hydroxyapatite crystal deposition disease		Bilateral or unilateral linear, calcific collections within the Achilles tendon and plantar aponeurosis
Gout		Tophaceous nodules in and about the Achilles tendon may result in erosions of the posterior aspect of the calcaneus
Acromegaly	See Fig. 11–94	Prominent enthesophyte proliferation at attachments of the Achilles tendon and plantar aponeurosis Heel pad thickening (men > 23 mm; women > 21.5 mm)
Hyperparathyroidism		Bilateral, symmetric subligamentous erosions at attachment of plantar aponeurosis, or less commonly, at the posterosuperior aspect of the calcaneus

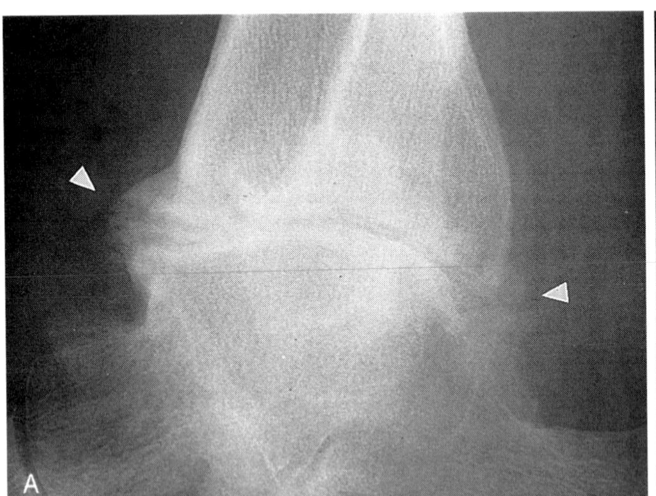

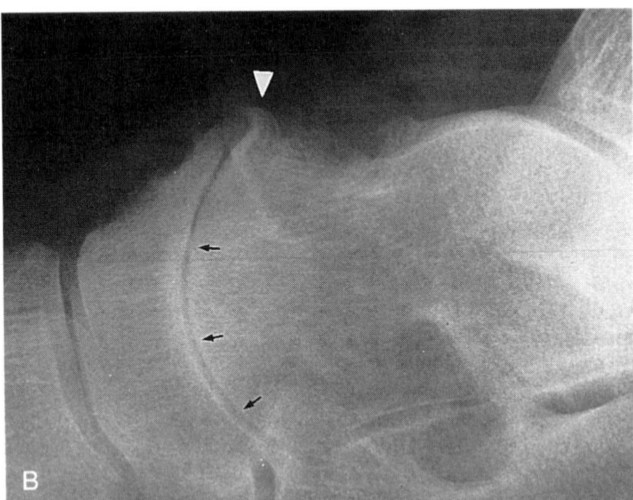

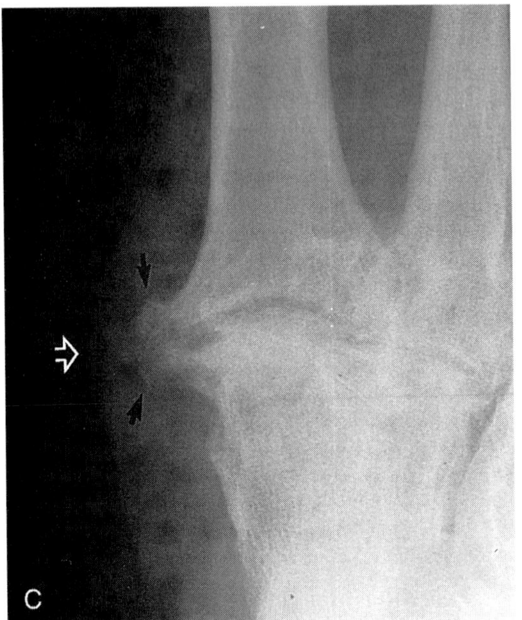

FIGURE 11–54. Osteoarthrosis.[76–78] A Tibiotalar joint. Joint space narrowing, osteophyte formation, and subchondral sclerosis (arrowheads) characterize this degenerative ankle joint. Degenerative disease of the ankle typically occurs after ligament injury, fracture, repetitive trauma, or sports injury. B Talonavicular joint. Marked joint space narrowing (arrows), dorsal osteophyte formation (arrowhead), and subchondral bone sclerosis are evident in the talonavicular articulation of this 41-year-old man. C First tarsometatarsal joint. Prominent osteophytes (arrows), subchondral sclerosis, and nonuniform joint space narrowing are signs of degenerative joint disease at this location in a 59-year-old man. Soft tissue prominence also is noted overlying the joint (open arrow).

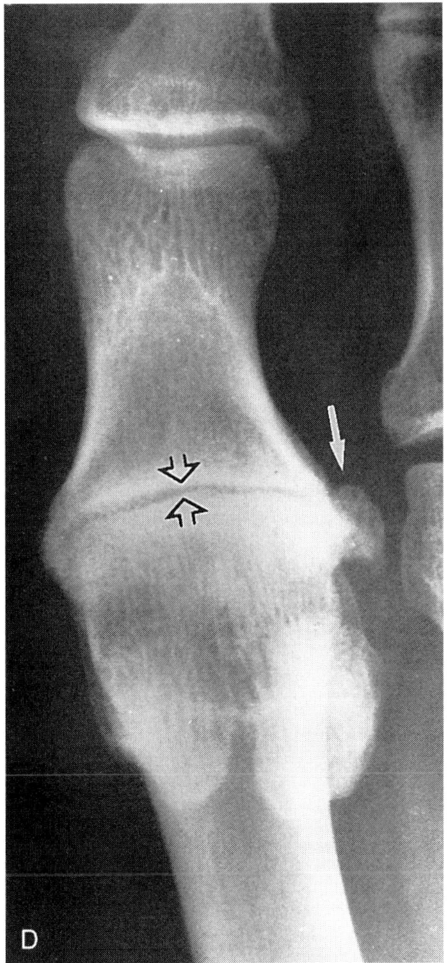

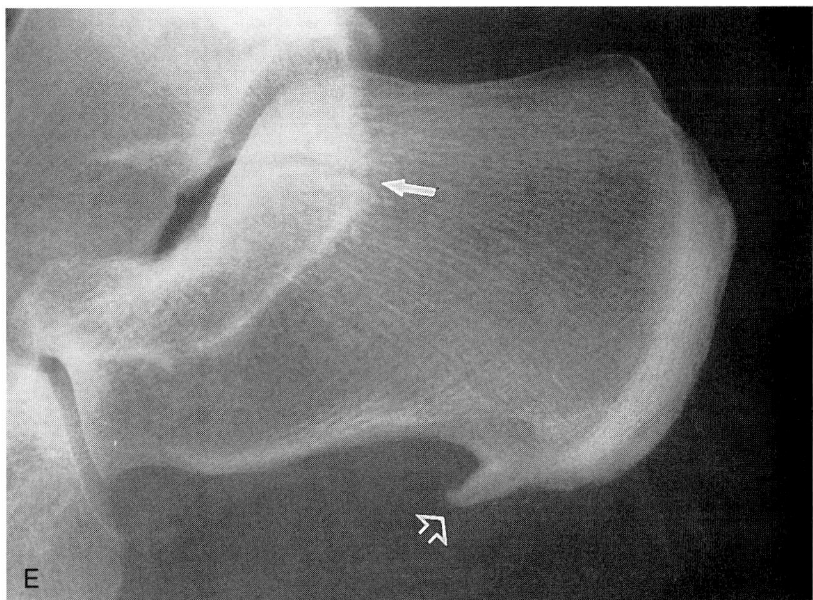

FIGURE 11–54 *Continued.* D Hallux rigidus. Degenerative joint disease of the first metatarsophalangeal joint has resulted in joint space narrowing (open arrows), subchondral sclerosis, and osteophytes (arrow). This condition often accompanies a hallux valgus deformity and bunion formation and is characterized by painful degenerative rigidity of the first metatarsophalangeal joint of the great toe. E Degenerative plantar enthesophyte. Observe the well-defined, sharply marginated osseous excrescence arising from the site of attachment of the plantar aponeurosis on the calcaneus (open arrow) in this 53-year-old woman with plantar fasciitis. Such degenerative "heel spurs" often are painful. Of incidental note is the presence of talocalcaneal coalition (white arrow).

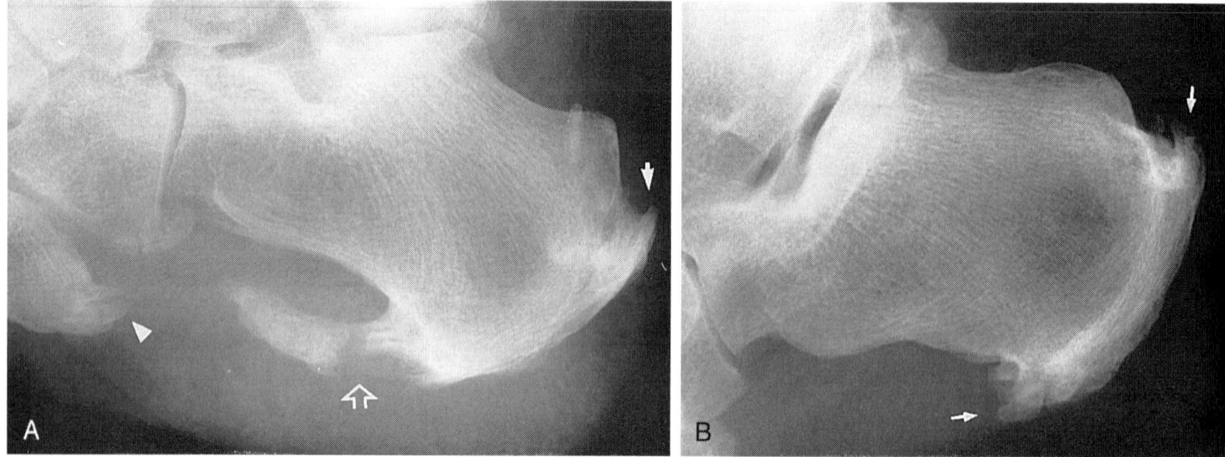

FIGURE 11–55. Diffuse idiopathic skeletal hyperostosis (DISH): Calcaneal enthesopathy.[77, 79] **A** Prominent osseous excrescences arising from the sites of attachment of the Achilles tendon (arrow), plantar aponeurosis, and peroneus brevis tendon attachment (arrowhead) represent characteristic enthesophytes seen frequently in patients with DISH. The large plantar enthesophyte is fractured (open arrow). **B** In another patient, prominent enthesophytes at the attachments of the Achilles tendon and plantar aponeurosis are noted (arrows). Enthesopathy of the calcaneus is present in about 76 per cent of patients with DISH.

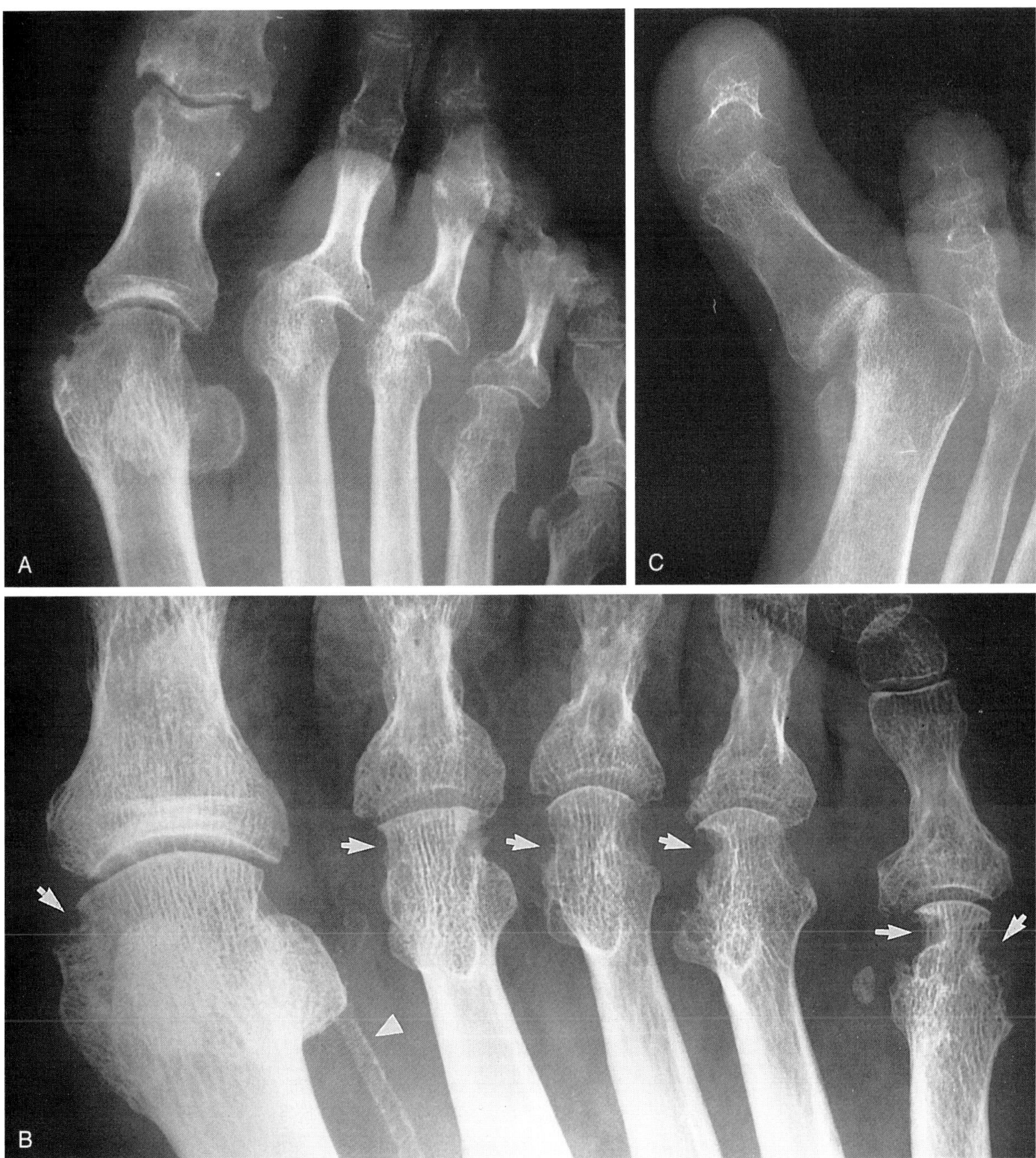

FIGURE 11–56. Rheumatoid arthritis[80, 81]: Forefoot abnormalities. A In a patient with advanced rheumatoid arthritis, the findings include marginal erosions adjacent to the metatarsophalangeal joints, joint dislocations, periarticular osteopenia, and soft tissue swelling. Involvement of the hallux interphalangeal joint also is present. B In another patient, extensive rheumatoid erosions are seen in characteristic locations (arrows). Vascular calcification also is clearly visualized (arrowhead). C Severe and unusual hallux varus deformity and subluxation are present at the first metatarsophalangeal joint. Periarticular osteopenia, sesamoid subluxation, and erosions also are present.

Clinical abnormalities of the forefoot are present in up to 90 per cent of patients with long-standing rheumatoid arthritis and are the initial manifestation of the disease in 10 to 20 per cent of patients.

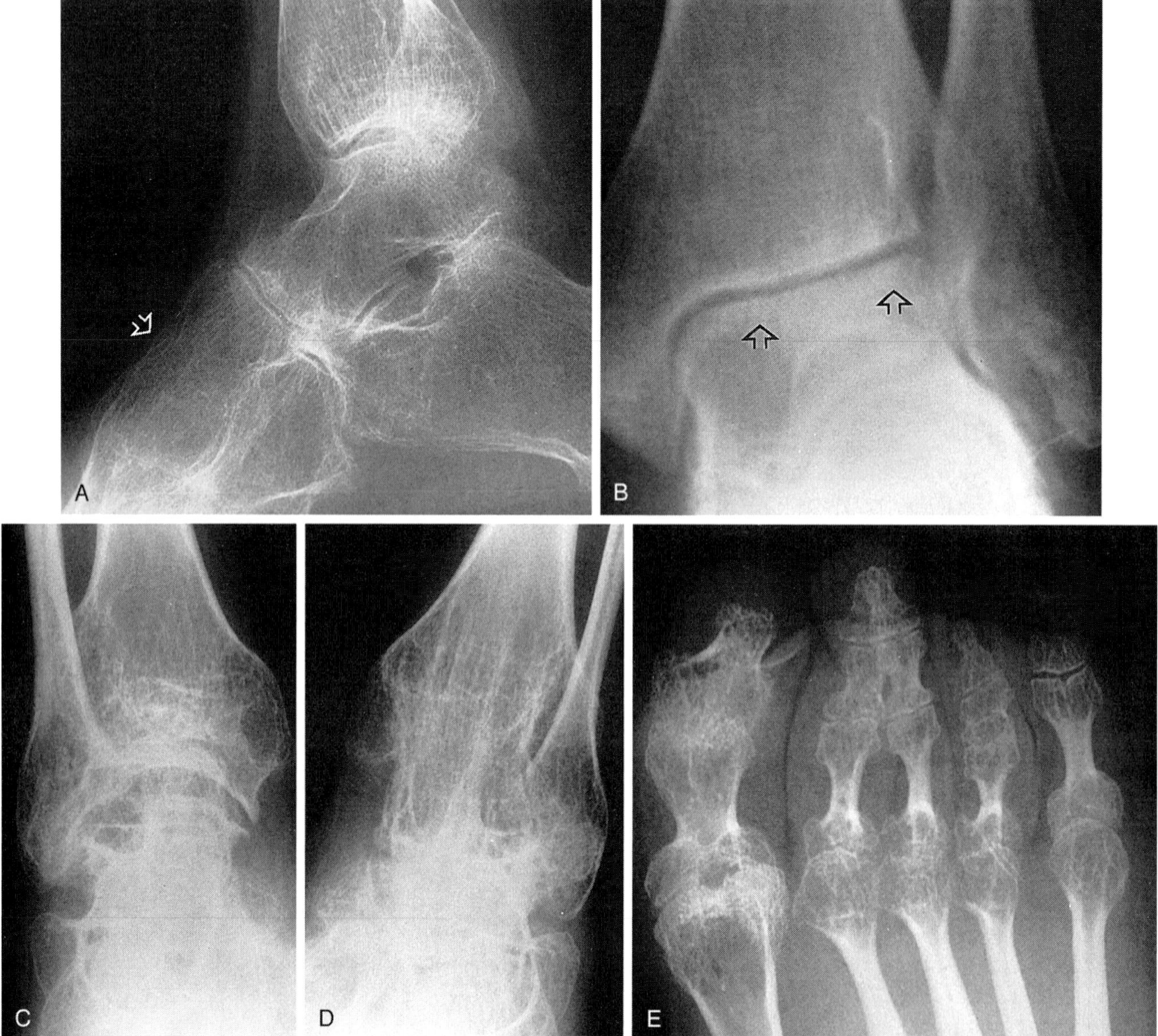

FIGURE 11–57. Juvenile chronic (rheumatoid) arthritis.[6, 82, 83] A, B Ankle abnormalities. In A, osteoporosis, uniform joint space narrowing, widespread tarsal ankylosis (open arrow), and soft tissue atrophy are present in this 22-year-old woman with long-standing juvenile rheumatoid arthritis. In B, another patient, observe the tibiotalar slant (open arrows), a sign found in juvenile chronic arthritis, hemophilia, Trevor's disease, and many other conditions. *(B, Courtesy of A. Brower, M.D., Norfolk, Virginia.)* C, D Ankle abnormalities—advanced changes. Osteoporosis, epiphyseal overgrowth, joint space erosions, and ankylosis involve both ankles in a relatively symmetric pattern in this 36-year-old woman. E Foot abnormalities—advanced changes. Osteoporosis, epiphyseal overgrowth, joint space erosions, and ankylosis appear in this 36-year-old woman. The findings were bilateral and symmetric. *(C–E, Courtesy of V. Vint, M.D., San Diego, California.)*

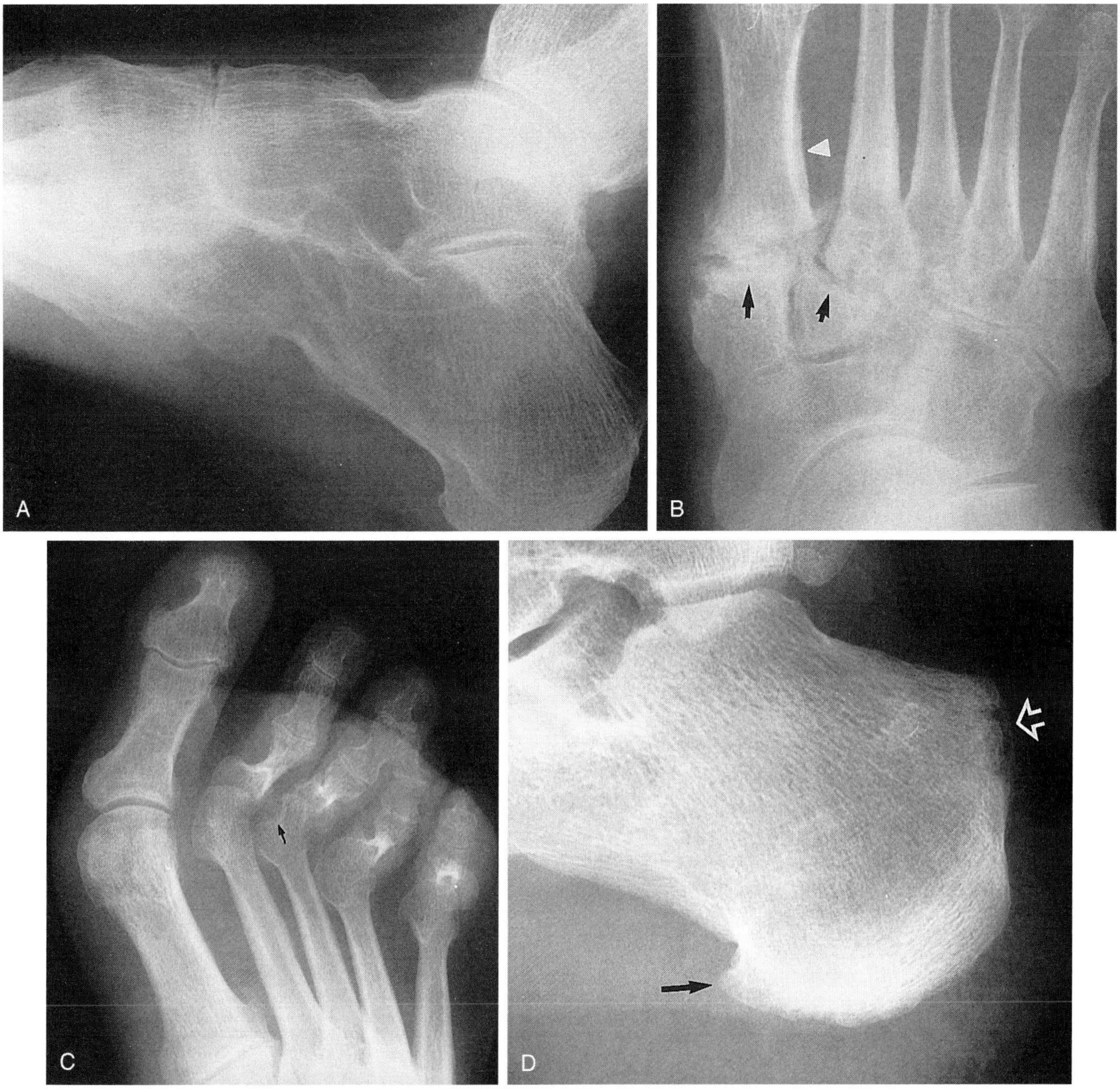

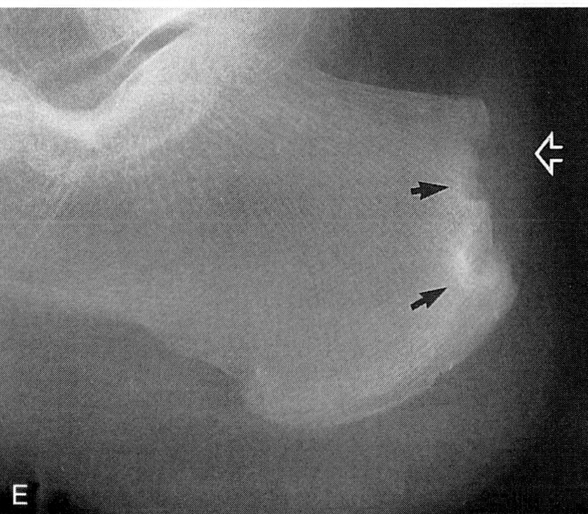

FIGURE 11–58. Ankylosing spondylitis.[83, 84] A Juvenile-onset ankylosing spondylitis. Observe the widespread and diffuse intertarsal ankylosis in this 26-year-old man. (*A, Courtesy of R. Shapiro, M.D., Sacramento, California.*) B–C Adult-onset ankylosing spondylitis. In B, observe the soft tissue swelling, tarsometatarsal joint space narrowing (arrows), periostitis (arrowhead), and marked erosions of the adjacent tarsals and metatarsals. In C, another patient with bilateral symmetric involvement, marked metatarsophalangeal joint space narrowing, erosions (arrow), and fibular deviation with subluxations are evident. In D, a 20-year-old man with a 4-year history of juvenile-onset ankylosing spondylitis, abnormalities of the calcaneus include erosion adjacent to the retrocalcaneal bursa (open arrow) and a plantar enthesophyte (arrow). In E, a 53-year-old man with adult-onset ankylosing spondylitis, large calcaneal erosions (arrows) related to retrocalcaneal bursitis are present. Soft tissue swelling in the Achilles tendon also is evident (open arrow).

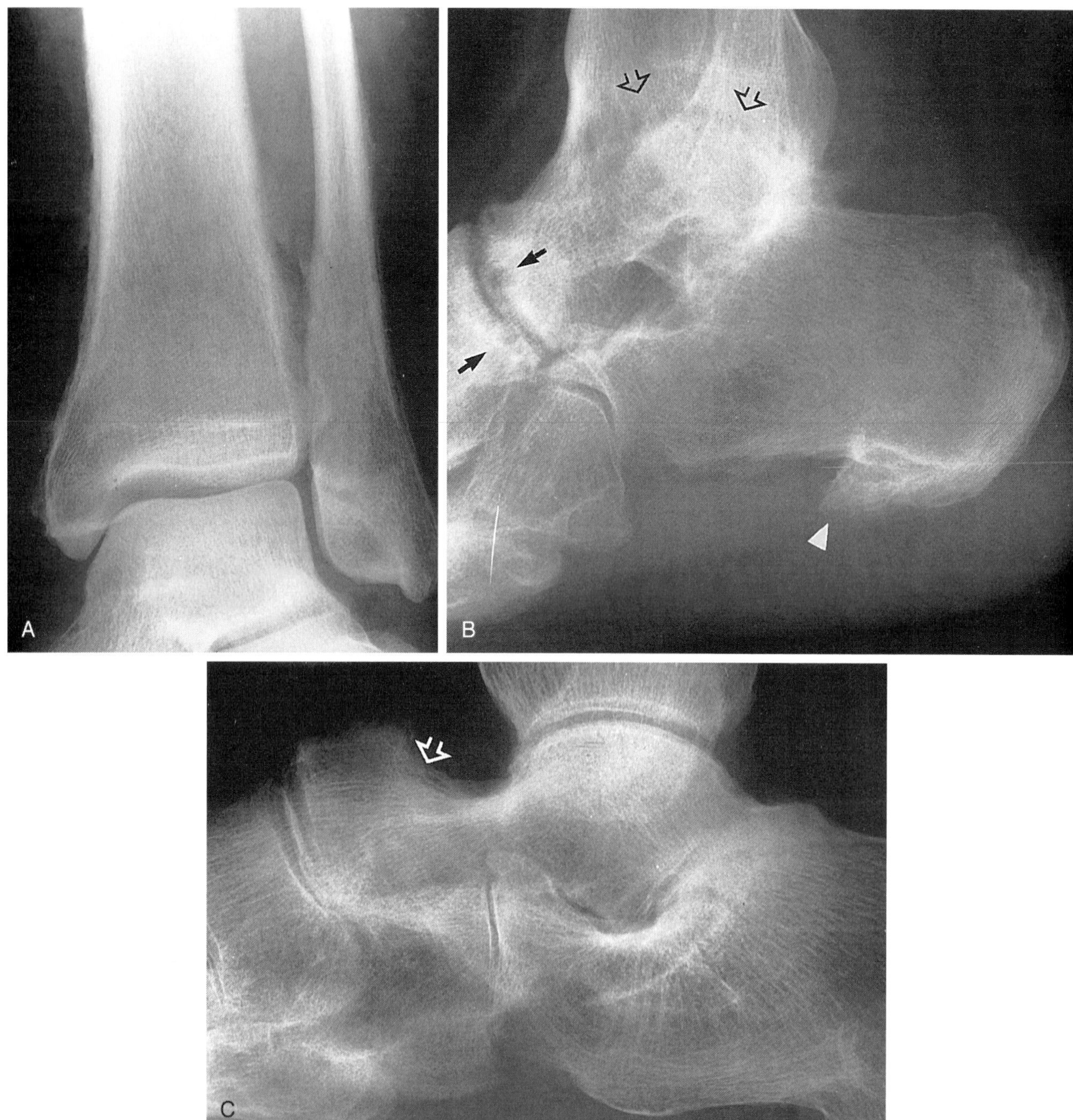

FIGURE 11–59. Psoriatic arthropathy.[77, 85–87] A Ankle involvement. Observe the exuberant fluffy periostitis arising from the distal ends of the tibia and fibula in this 47-year-old man with psoriasis. Although he has no evidence of joint space narrowing or erosions, typical psoriatic arthropathy was seen in the hand. Periarticular periostitis is frequently encountered in patients with seronegative spondyloarthropathies; however, special care should be taken to differentiate this from hypertrophic osteoarthropathy. *(A, Courtesy of T. Marklund, M.D., Linköping, Sweden.)* B Calcaneal involvement. In a 49-year-old man with psoriatic skin disease and polyarticular joint disease, a lateral ankle radiograph reveals a fluffy bony enthesophyte at the site of attachment of the plantar fascia on the calcaneus (arrowhead). Erosive changes at the talonavicular joint (arrows) and bony ankylosis of the tibiotalar joint (open arrows) are seen. C Midfoot involvement. Complete osseous ankylosis of the talonavicular joint (open arrow) is observed in this 61-year-old man with chronic psoriatic skin disease and polyarticular joint disease. Before ankylosis, a talonavicular dislocation had occurred, accounting for the inferior displacement of the talus in relation to the navicular bone. Of interest, a developmental talocalcaneal coalition also is noted.

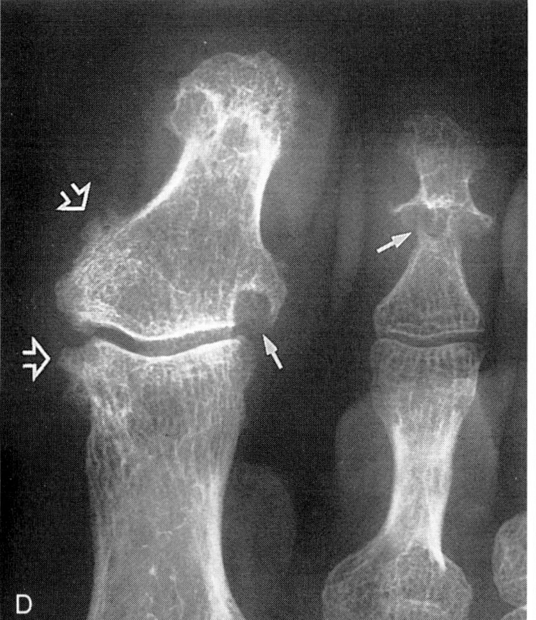

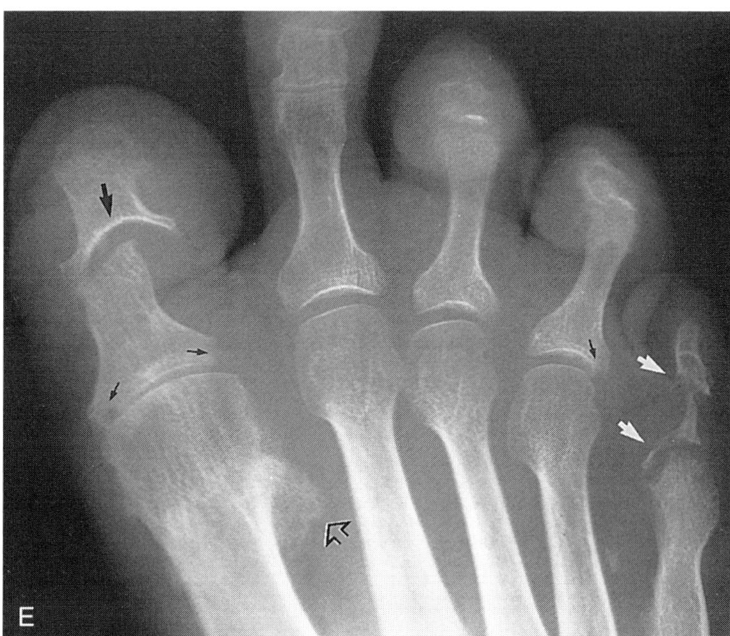

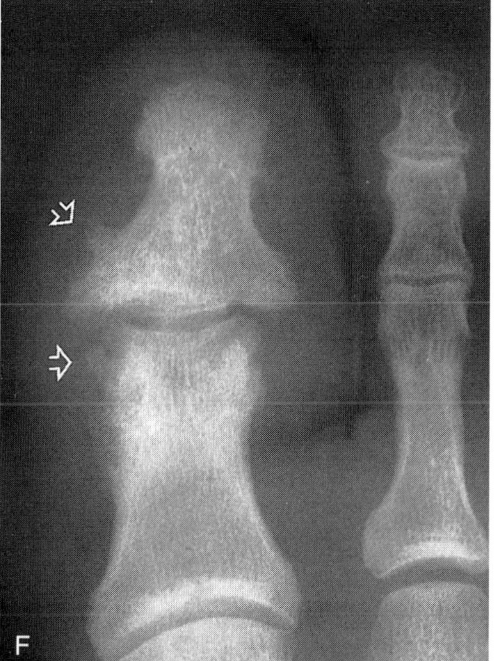

FIGURE 11–59 *Continued.* D–F Forefoot involvement. In **D**, intra-articular erosions are seen at the terminal interphalangeal joints of the first and second digits (arrows). Fluffy periostitis (open arrows), characteristic of seronegative spondyloarthropathies, also is present. In **E**, another patient, central erosions of the first and fifth terminal phalangeal articular surfaces and resorption of the distal end of the proximal phalanx and metatarsal bone are characteristic of inflammatory arthropathies, termed pencil-and-cup erosions (large black and white arrows). Note also the dramatic soft tissue swelling, marginal erosions (small black arrows), and periostitis involving the hallux sesamoid bone (open arrow). In **F**, a third patient, prominent soft tissue swelling, central erosions, "whiskering" or periostitis, and absence of osteoporosis are classic changes in psoriatic arthritis. The joints of the adjacent digit appear unaffected.

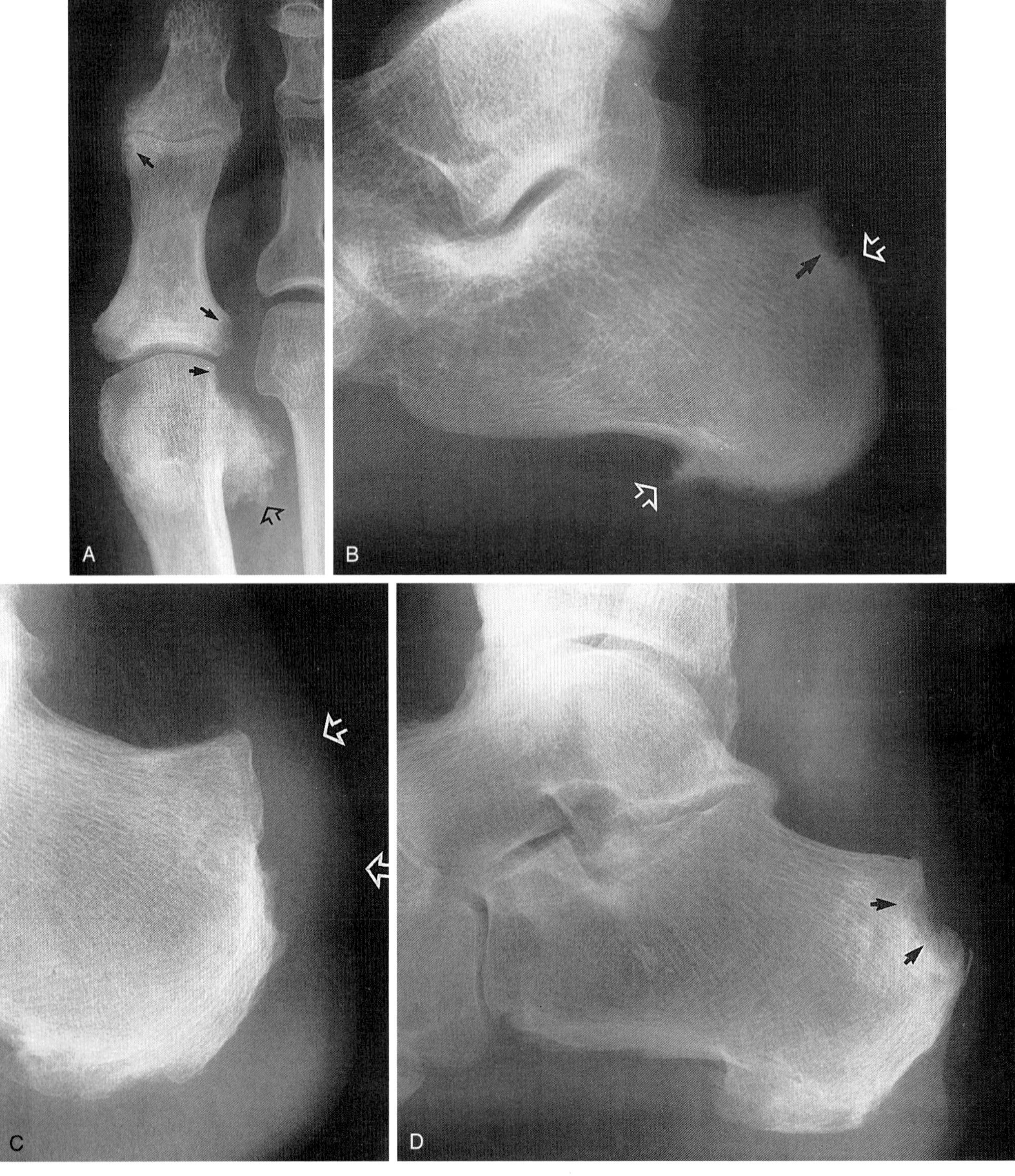

FIGURE 11–60. Reiter's syndrome.[77, 88] A Forefoot abnormalities. Prominent fluffy bone proliferation with poorly defined osseous outlines is evident at the hallux sesamoid (open arrow) and adjacent to the articulations. Diffuse soft tissue swelling and marginal erosions (arrows) also are seen. B–D Calcaneal abnormalities. In B, a fluffy pattern of enthesopathy is seen arising from the plantar and posterior aspects of the calcaneus (open arrows). A prominent erosion also is seen adjacent to the retrocalcaneal bursa (arrow). In C, another patient, osseous proliferation and soft tissue swelling of the Achilles tendon (open arrows) are evident. In D, advanced changes in a third patient include a posterior erosion (arrows) secondary to retrocalcaneal bursitis and prominent enthesopathy.

Calcaneal changes are evident in 25 to 50 per cent of patients with Reiter's syndrome.

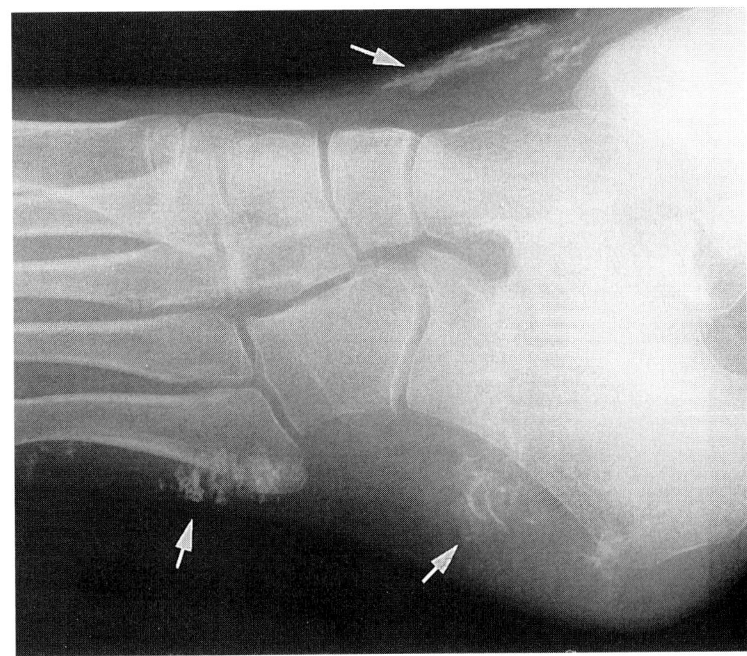

FIGURE 11–61. Dermatomyositis and polymyositis.[90] Observe the sheet-like subcutaneous calcinosis (arrows) in this 13-year-old girl with long-standing dermatomyositis.

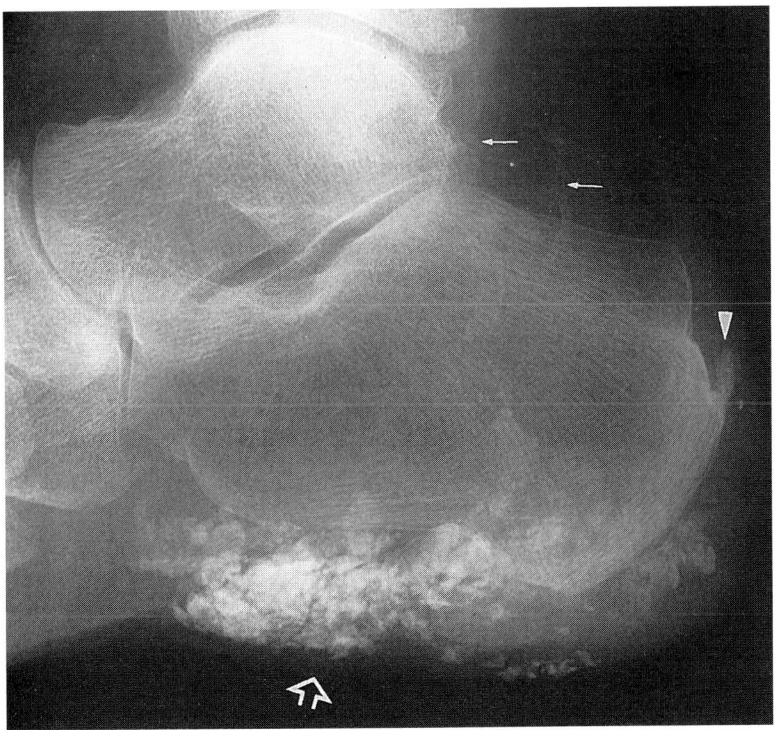

FIGURE 11–62. Scleroderma (progressive systemic sclerosis).[91] Extensive soft tissue calcification (open arrow) is seen in the heel pad of this patient with long-standing scleroderma. An Achilles tendon enthesophyte (arrowhead) and vascular calcification (arrows) also are evident.

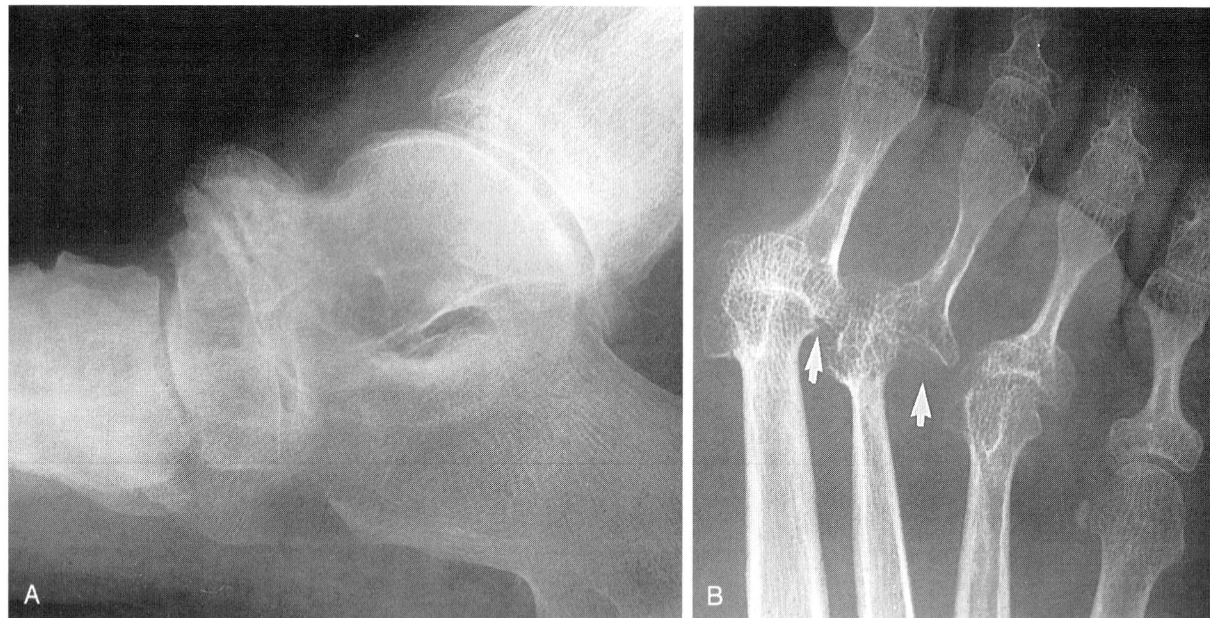

FIGURE 11–63. Calcium pyrophosphate dihydrate (CPPD) crystal deposition disease.[92, 93] A Midfoot and hindfoot involvement. Extensive hypertrophic osteophytes are seen about the talonavicular articulation in this 82-year-old man with CPPD crystal deposition disease. B Forefoot involvement. Observe the dislocations of the second, third, and fourth metatarsophalangeal joints (arrows).

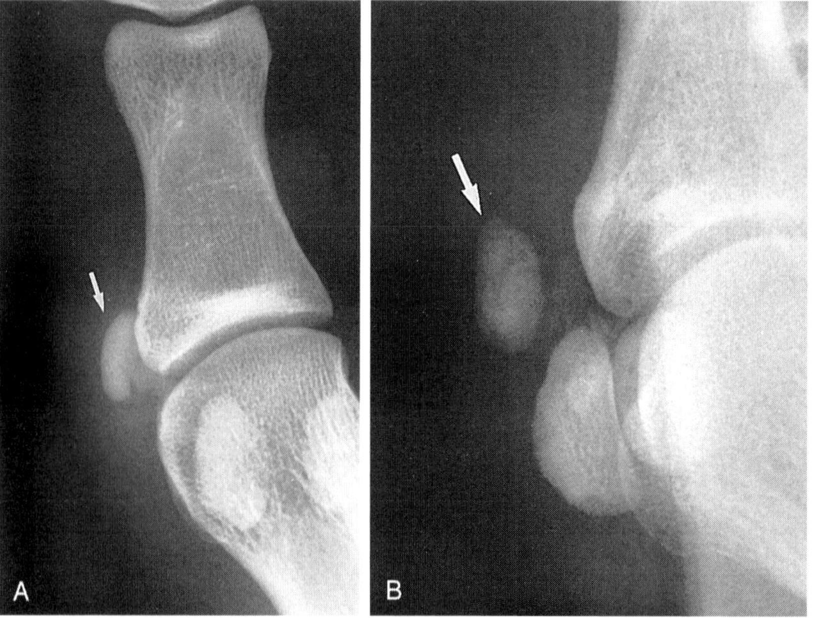

FIGURE 11–64. Calcific bursitis: Calcium hydroxyapatite crystal deposition.[94] Frontal (A) and lateral (B) radiographs show cloud-like accumulations of calcification (arrow) overlying the first metatarsophalangeal joint. Periarticular hydroxyapatite crystals may be deposited in tendons, bursae, or soft tissues.

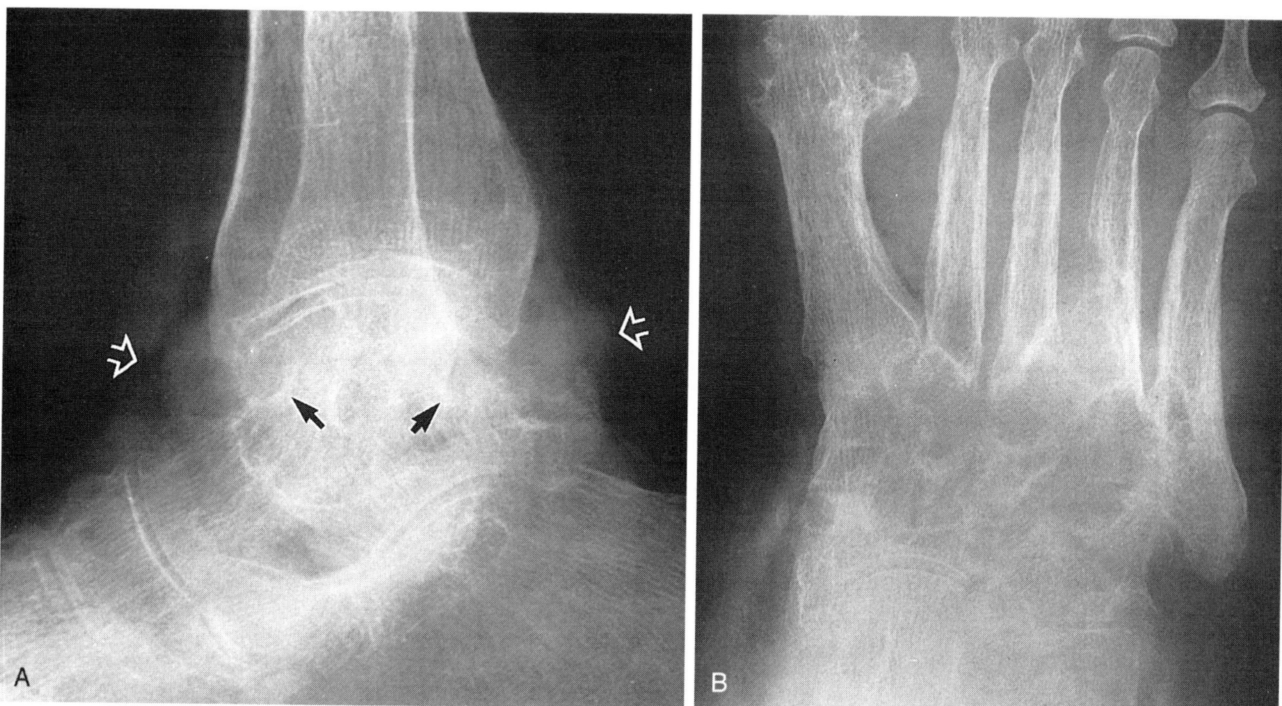

FIGURE 11–65. Gouty arthropathy.[95] A Ankle involvement. Observe the radiodense joint effusion anterior and posterior to the ankle joint (open arrows) of this 65-year-old man with polyarticular gouty arthritis. Erosions of the talus exhibit an overhanging margin (arrows). B Midfoot abnormalities. Extensive erosions are seen about the tarsometatarsal articulations in this patient with long-standing gout.

Illustration continued on following page

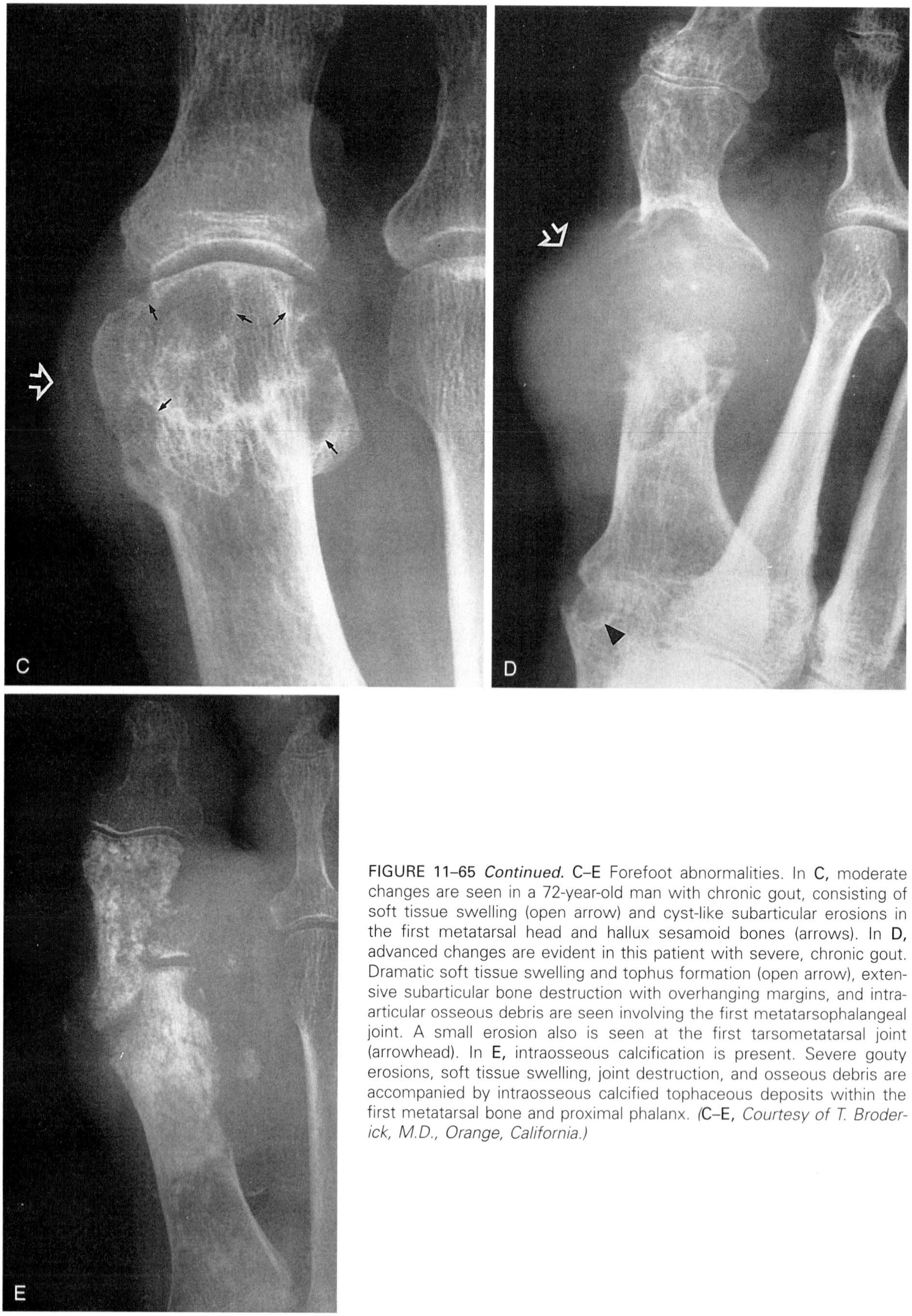

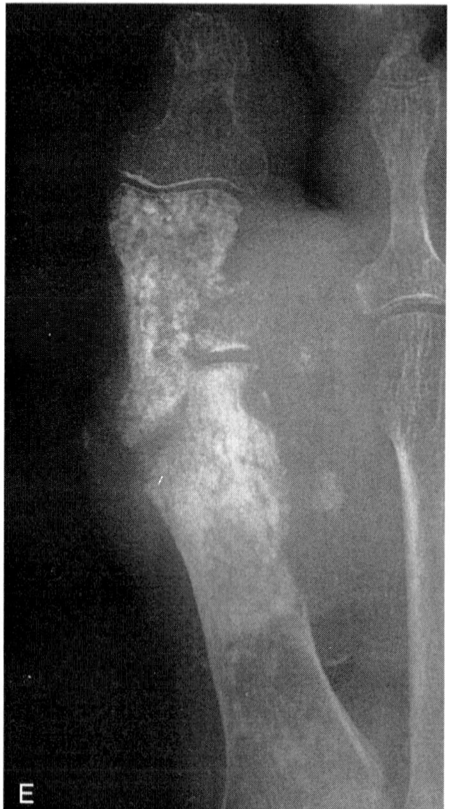

FIGURE 11–65 *Continued.* C–E Forefoot abnormalities. In **C**, moderate changes are seen in a 72-year-old man with chronic gout, consisting of soft tissue swelling (open arrow) and cyst-like subarticular erosions in the first metatarsal head and hallux sesamoid bones (arrows). In **D**, advanced changes are evident in this patient with severe, chronic gout. Dramatic soft tissue swelling and tophus formation (open arrow), extensive subarticular bone destruction with overhanging margins, and intra-articular osseous debris are seen involving the first metatarsophalangeal joint. A small erosion also is seen at the first tarsometatarsal joint (arrowhead). In **E**, intraosseous calcification is present. Severe gouty erosions, soft tissue swelling, joint destruction, and osseous debris are accompanied by intraosseous calcified tophaceous deposits within the first metatarsal bone and proximal phalanx. *(*C–E, *Courtesy of T. Broderick, M.D., Orange, California.)*

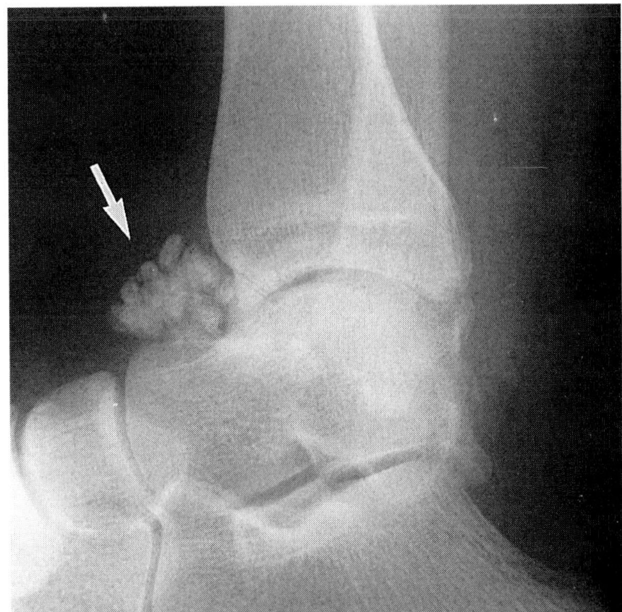

FIGURE 11–66. Idiopathic synovial osteochondromatosis. Multiple intra-articular radiodense osteocartilaginous bodies have accumulated in the anterior recess of the joint capsule of the tibiotalar joint (arrow). Idiopathic synovial osteochondromatosis represents metaplastic or neoplastic proliferation of cartilaginous bodies by the synovial membrane. Secondary synovial osteochondromatosis also may occur as a result of degenerative joint disease. Noncalcified lesions are best evaluated with arthrography.

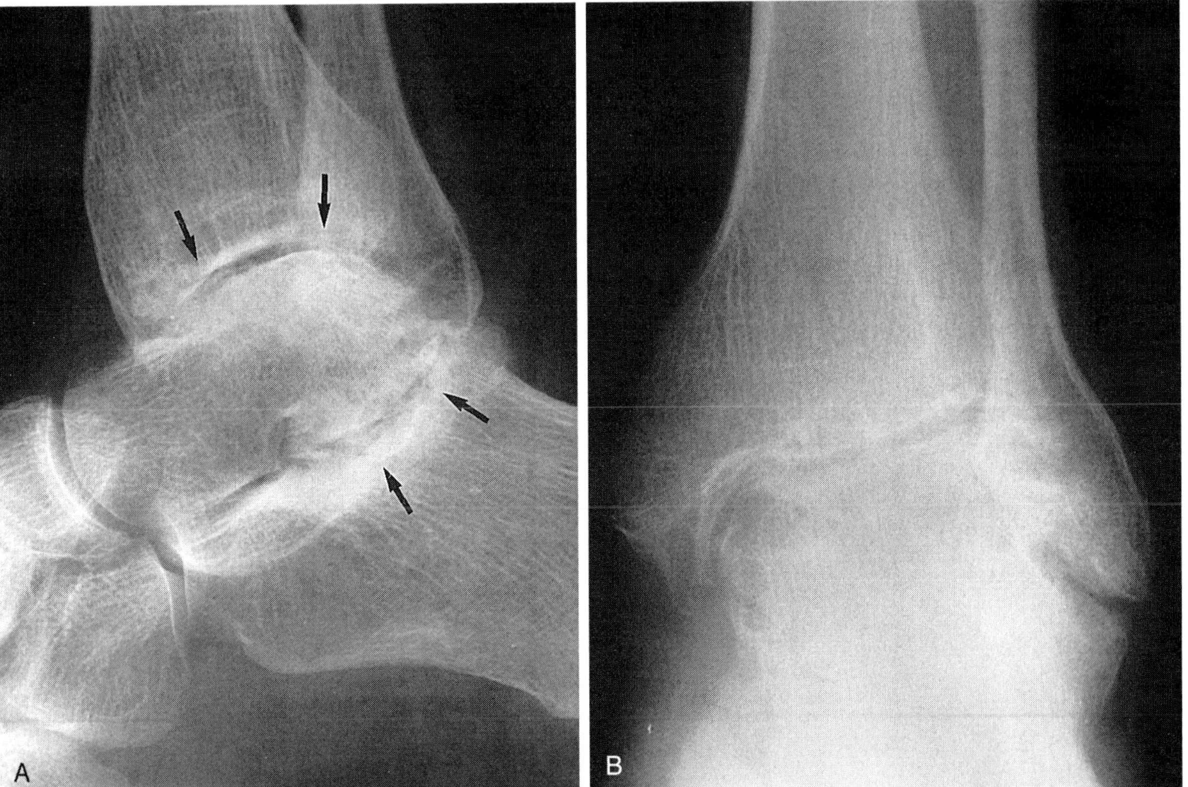

FIGURE 11–67. Hemophilic arthropathy: Ankle abnormalities.[6, 99] A In a 28-year-old man, joint space narrowing, osteopenia, and tibiotalar slant from osseous overgrowth all are characteristic findings in this bleeding disorder. Growth recovery lines also are evident within the tibia. B In a 31-year-old man, tibiotalar and subtalar joint space narrowing, sclerosis, and subchondral collapse are seen (arrows).

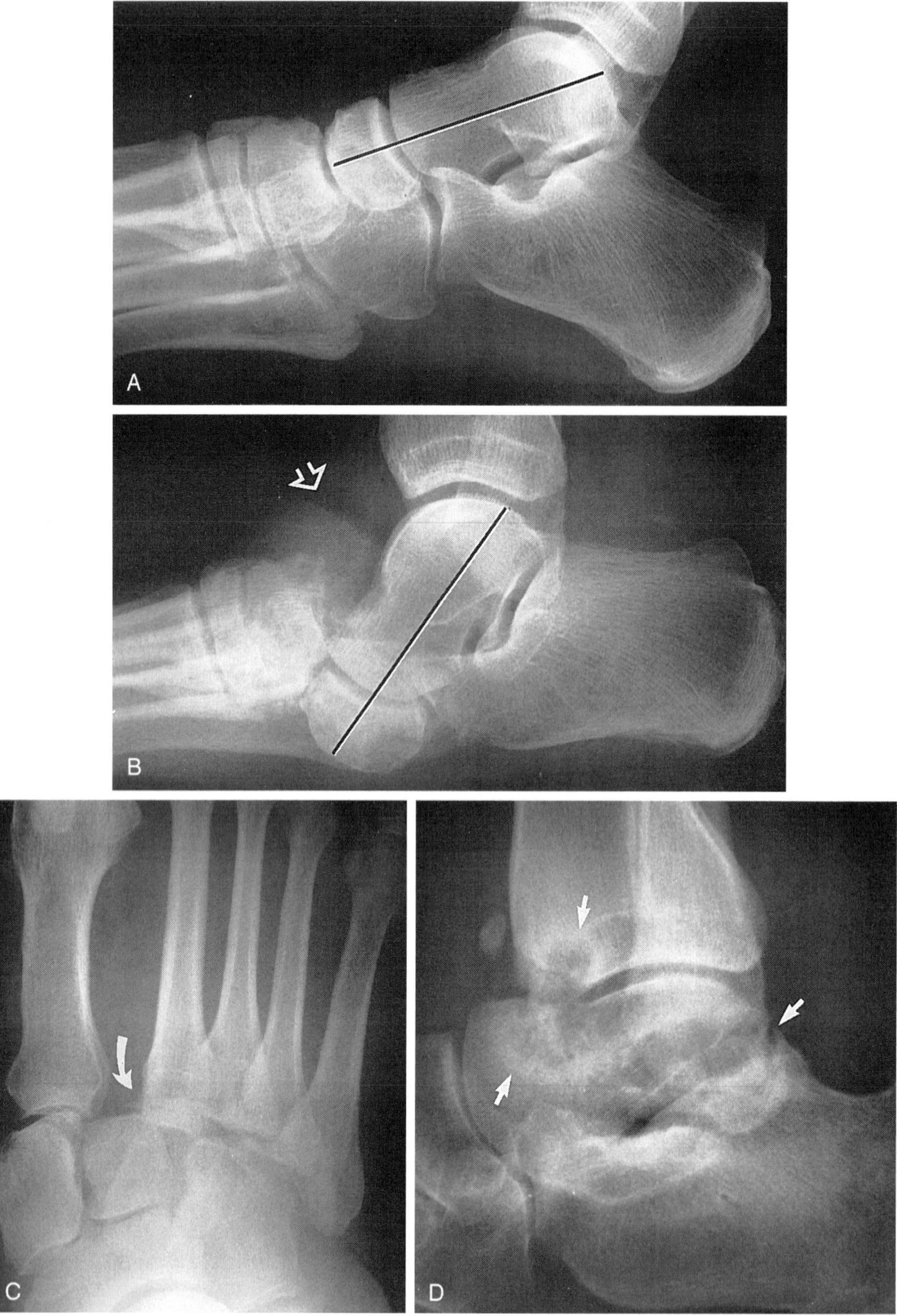

FIGURE 11–68. Neuropathic osteoarthropathy[100, 101]: Diabetes mellitus. **A, B** Serial progression in a patient with poorly controlled insulin-dependent diabetes. In **A**, an initial radiograph taken in a recumbent non–weight-bearing position is essentially normal. In **B**, a weight-bearing radiograph taken 5 years later reveals dramatic destruction of the midtarsal articulations with midfoot collapse (open arrow). The naviculocuneiform joint is disarticulated, and the patient is bearing weight directly on the navicular bone. Osseous debris also is seen associated with these changes. The lines indicate the orientation of the long axis of the talus and navicular bones before and after the midfoot collapse. Such midfoot collapse in diabetic neuropathic joint disease is associated with rupture of the tibialis posterior tendon. **C** In another patient, lateral dislocations of the tarsometatarsal joints (curved arrow) represent a neuropathic Lisfranc fracture-dislocation. Spontaneous fractures and dislocations occur frequently with diabetic neuroarthropathy, and the Lisfranc's pattern is common. **D** Juvenile-onset diabetes. An ankle radiograph of this 22-year-old patient with diabetes mellitus shows collapse of the talus with osteolytic erosive changes of the tibia and talus (arrows). Aspiration of the joint revealed blood but no evidence of infectious organisms. (**D**, *Courtesy of L. Danzig, M.D., Santa Ana, California.)*

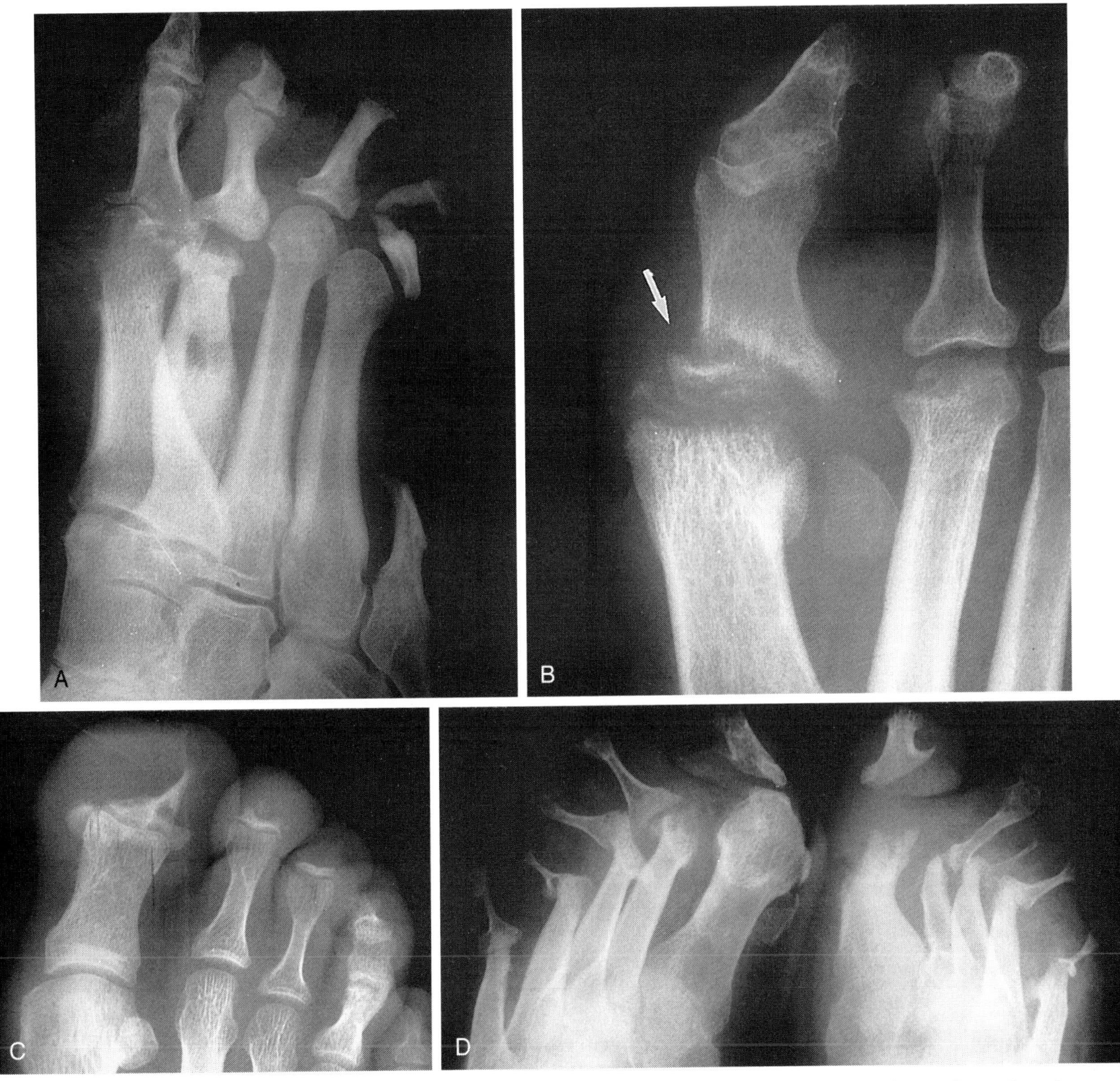

FIGURE 11–69. Neuropathic osteoarthropathy.[102–104] **A** Congenital insensitivity to pain. Atrophic resorption and tapering of several metatarsal bones and phalanges are associated with periostitis, sclerosis, and fragmentation. In this case, neuropathic osteoarthropathy is probably complicated by osteomyelitis. (**A** Courtesy of M. Pallayew, M.D., Montreal, Quebec, Canada.) **B** Alcoholism. A 35-year-old alcoholic man had increasing pain and swelling over the great toe. An oblique radiograph shows dissolution and fragmentation of the articular surfaces of the first metatarsal bone and proximal phalanx (arrow) with considerable soft tissue swelling and ulceration overlying the joint. Milder but similar changes are seen at the second metatarsophalangeal articulation. **C, D** Leprosy. In **C**, acro-osteolysis is evident. Observe the tapered, atrophic resorption of the terminal phalanges of the first three digits in this patient with leprous acro-osteolysis. The soft tissues of the terminal tufts are foreshortened and swollen. In **D**, advanced changes in another patient consist of diffuse osteolysis, bone atrophy, and tapering involving several phalanges and metatarsal bones. Marked disorganization and soft tissue deformity also are seen. Bilateral symmetric involvement is characteristic in leprosy. Other musculoskeletal abnormalities associated with leprosy include periostitis, osteitis, osteomyelitis, leprous arthritis, and secondary infection. *(**C**, Courtesy of W. Coleman, D.P.M., Carville, Louisiana; **D**, courtesy of J. Haller, M.D., Vienna, Austria.)*

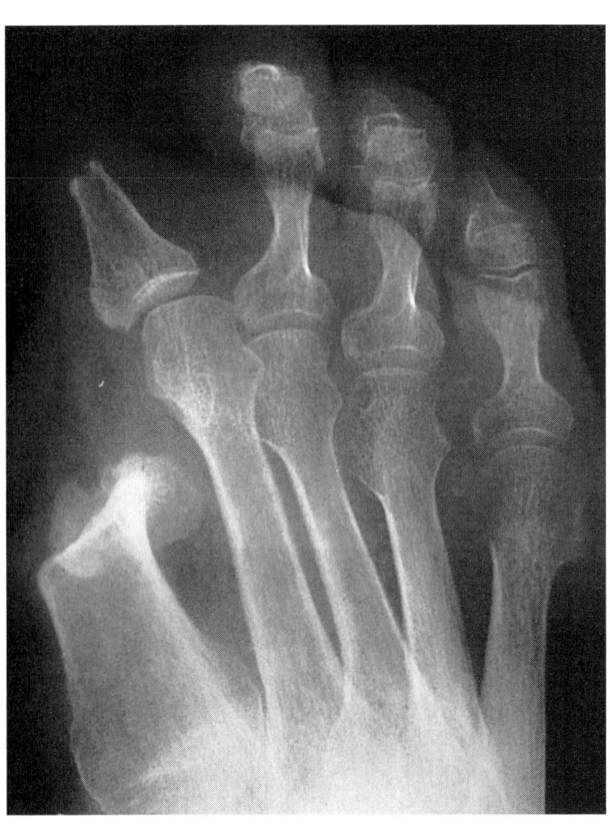

FIGURE 11–70. Frostbite.[105] This man sustained frostbite of his feet. Radiograph reveals osteoporosis, acro-osteolysis, and contractures of the toes. Amputation of the first and second toes is consistent with frostbite itself, surgical amputation, or both. *(Courtesy of R. Fellows, M.D., Fairbanks, Alaska.)*

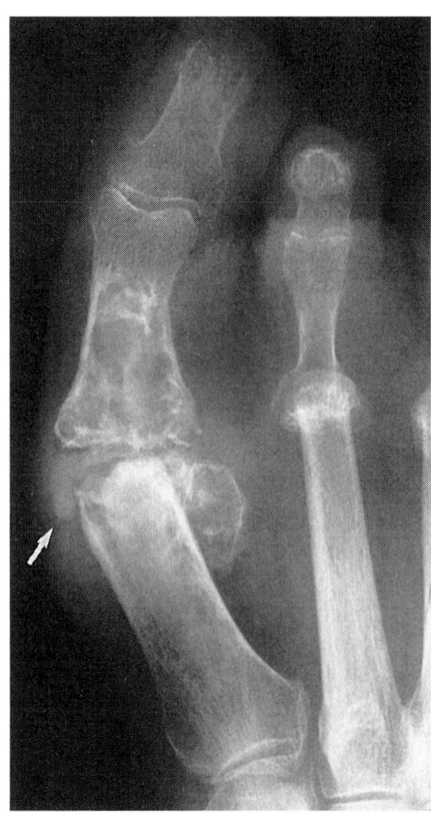

FIGURE 11–71. Silicone synovitis.[106] This patient with severe rheumatoid arthritis has a silicone prosthesis in the first metatarsophalangeal joint (white arrow). Well-defined radiolucent defects and erosions are present in the adjacent bones, characteristic of silicone synovitis, a well-known complication of silicone arthroplasty. In this case, the prosthesis also is deformed.

TABLE 11–13. Infectious Disorders of the Ankle and Foot

Entity	Figure(s)	Characteristics
Cellulitis[107]	11–72	Soft tissue infection usually as a result of stasis ulcers and vascular insufficiency Frequent complication of diabetes mellitus, foreign bodies, puncture wounds, or skin ulceration Cellulitis is a clinical diagnosis: radiographs not helpful, except in identifying gas in the soft tissues in gas-forming infections Gas-forming organisms include *Escherichia coli, Aerobacter aerogenes,* and *Bacteroides;* clostridial infection may result in extensive gas formation (gas gangrene), often necessitating amputation *Pseudomonas aeruginosa* frequently cultured from puncture wounds Spread of infection typically occurs along the plantar compartments of the foot, leading to contamination of adjacent bones and joints
Pyogenic osteomyelitis and septic arthritis[108–111]	11–72, 11–73, 11–74	Pyogenic infection of bones and joints usually spreads from contiguous sources of cellulitis Especially prevalent in patients with diabetes mellitus Difficult to differentiate from neuropathic osteoarthropathy, a coexistent condition in many diabetic patients Osteomyelitis: soft tissue swelling, osteolytic destruction Septic arthritis: most joint infections begin as a monoarticular arthritis but frequently spread to adjacent bones and joints in the foot Rapid loss of joint space and destruction of subchondral bone Periarticular osteopenia, joint subluxation, and periostitis
Tuberculous osteomyelitis and arthritis[112]		Tuberculous infection is much less common than pyogenic infection in the ankle and foot; when it does occur, it has a predilection for the ankle joint Mild symptoms and indolent course Most common organism: *Mycobacterium tuberculosis* Osteomyelitis: usually begins in epiphysis as an osteolytic lesion; may spread to metaphysis and diaphysis as moth-eaten or permeative pattern of destruction; may involve several bones of the foot Spina ventosa: tuberculous dactylitis; soft tissue swelling, bone destruction, periostitis, and bone expansion involving one or several digits; children > adults Arthritis: Juxta-articular osteoporosis, joint space narrowing, joint effusion, and periarticular erosions
Unusual and atypical infections[113]		Coccidioidomycosis: fungal disorder occurring in Mexico and southwestern United States; results in osteolytic lesions; may be disseminated; predilection for the calcaneus Congenital syphilis: *Treponema pallidum;* diametaphyseal gummas result in periostitis and aggressive bone destruction Madura foot: rare fungal disease due to *Madurella* and the actinomycetes; extensive soft tissue necrosis and widespread bone destruction

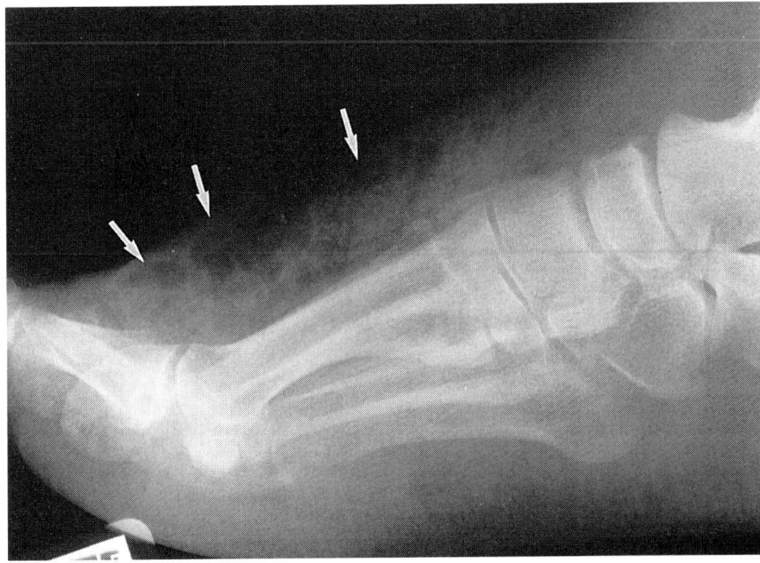

FIGURE 11–72. Cellulitis and osteomyelitis: Gas gangrene.[107] This 56-year-old insulin-dependent diabetic patient developed an ulcer on her foot that drained pus for 2 weeks. Observe the diffuse soft tissue swelling and streaky soft tissue emphysema (arrows) from a gas-forming organism. Laboratory culture yielded β-hemolytic and non–β-hemolytic streptococcus and *Bacteroides* organisms. Most gas-producing organisms are anaerobes.

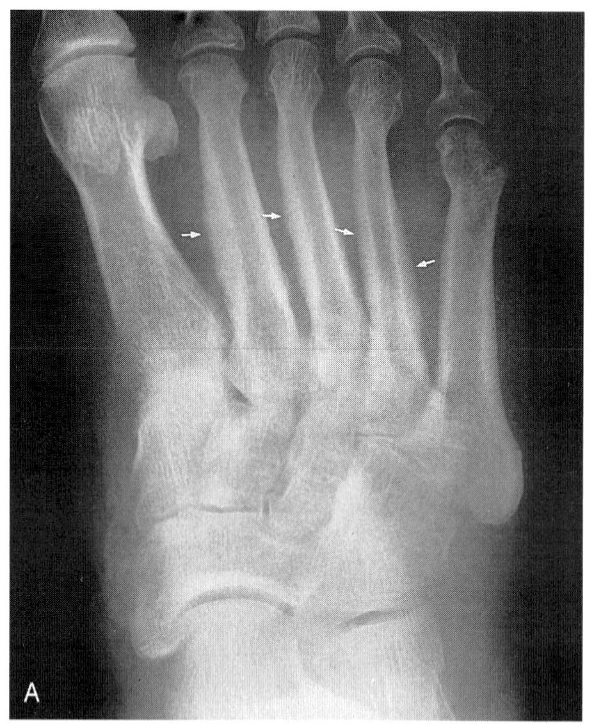

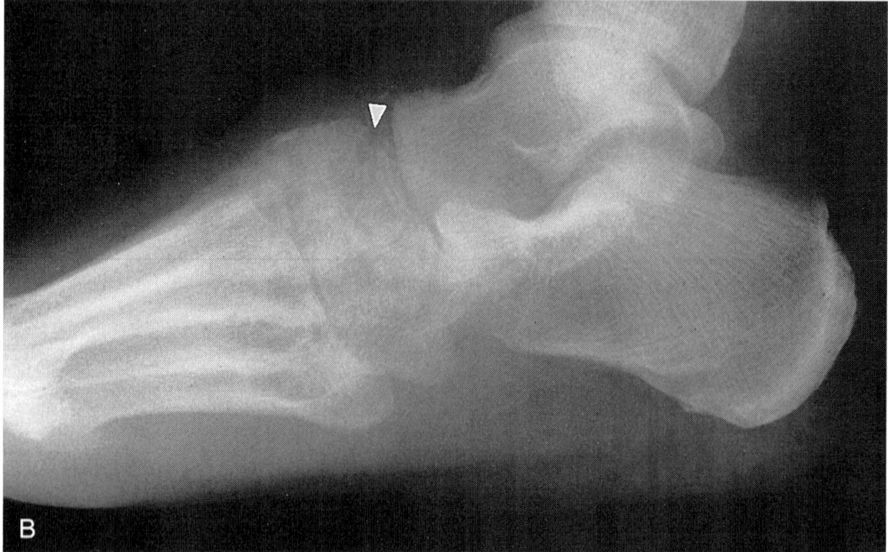

FIGURE 11–73. Pyogenic osteomyelitis and septic arthritis: Diabetes mellitus.[108–111] A, B 41-year-old insulin-dependent diabetic patient. Frontal (A) and lateral (B) radiographs of the foot demonstrate diffuse osteolysis and indistinct cortical margins of the distal row of tarsal bones and metatarsal bases. A large erosion of the superior aspect of the navicular bone (arrowhead) and periosteal new bone formation in the shafts of the metatarsals (arrows) are well visualized. Joint space narrowing of several intertarsal and tarsometatarsal articulations also is seen.

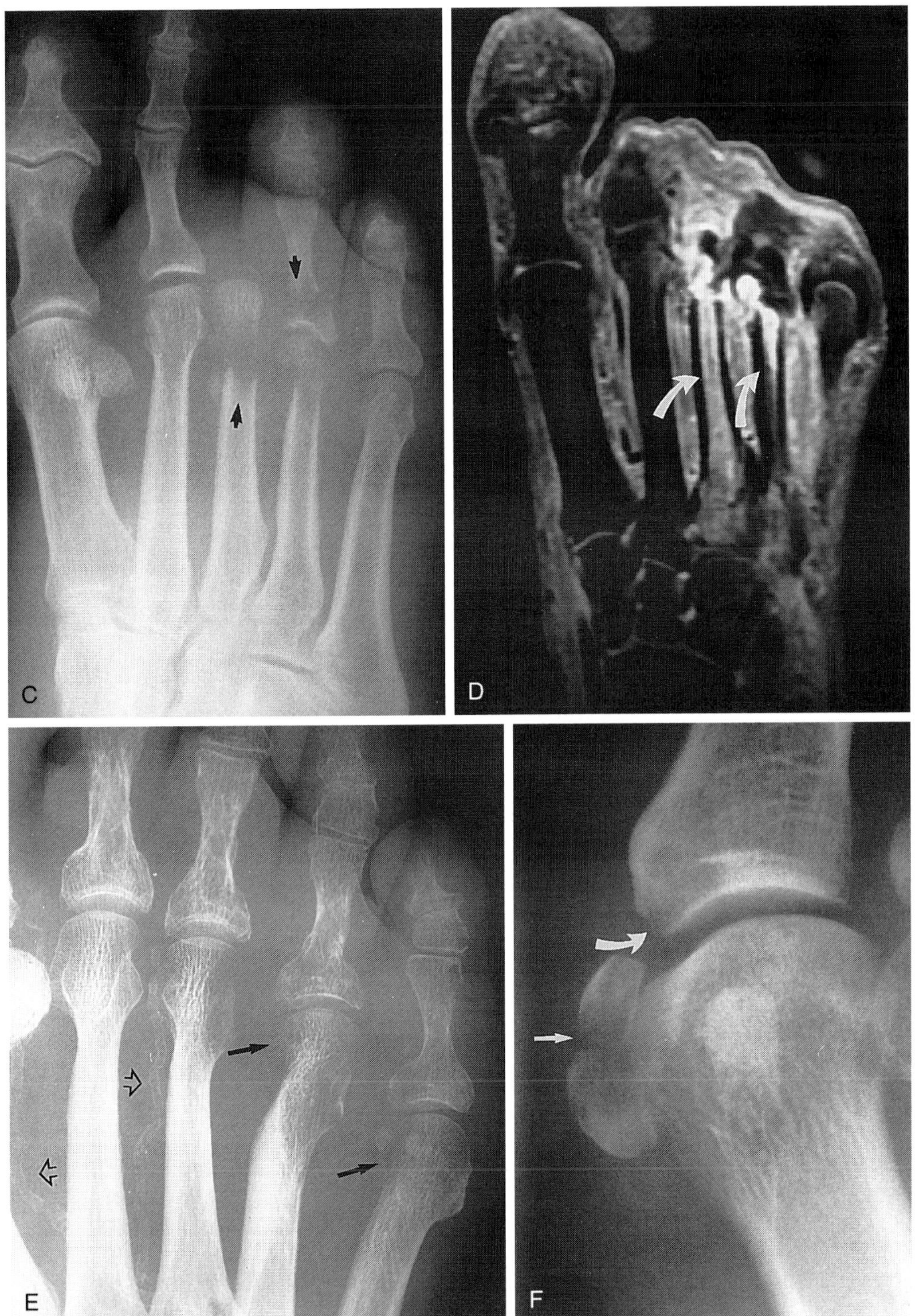

FIGURE 11–73 *Continued.* **C, D** A 63-year-old man with poorly controlled diabetes. In **C**, a routine radiograph demonstrates previous surgical amputation of the phalanges of the third toe. Permeative osteolysis involving the three lateral metatarsals and phalanges is evident. In addition, pathologic fractures or zones of osteolysis are seen in the distal third metatarsal and fourth proximal phalanx (arrows). Observe also the soft tissue swelling involving the fourth digit. In **D**, a coronal T1-weighted (TR/TE, 900/13) fat-suppressed magnetic resonance (MR) image obtained after intravenous gadolinium contrast agent administration reveals high signal intensity within the marrow of the third and fourth metatarsal shafts (curved arrows), confirming the presence of osteomyelitis. High signal intensity in the surrounding soft tissues indicates hyperemia, edema, and possible soft tissue infection. **E** In a third patient, a radiograph of the foot reveals diffuse periarticular osteopenia and erosions of the fourth and fifth metatarsal heads (arrows). Note also the diffuse vascular calcification (open arrows) typically encountered in the foot of the diabetic patient. **F** This fourth patient developed pain about the first metatarsophalangeal joint. A radiograph demonstrates diffuse osteolysis and pathologic fracture (arrow) of the medial hallux sesamoid bone. Another erosion of the proximal phalanx also is evident (curved arrow). A subsequent biopsy revealed evidence of *Staphylococcus aureus*.

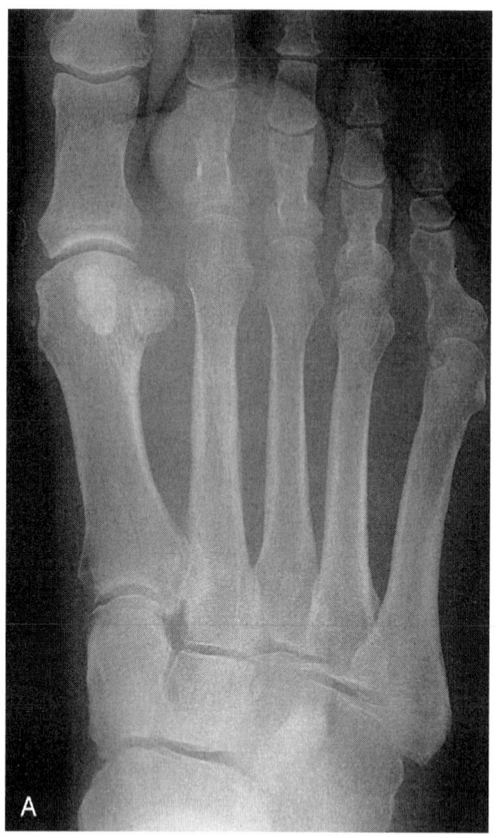

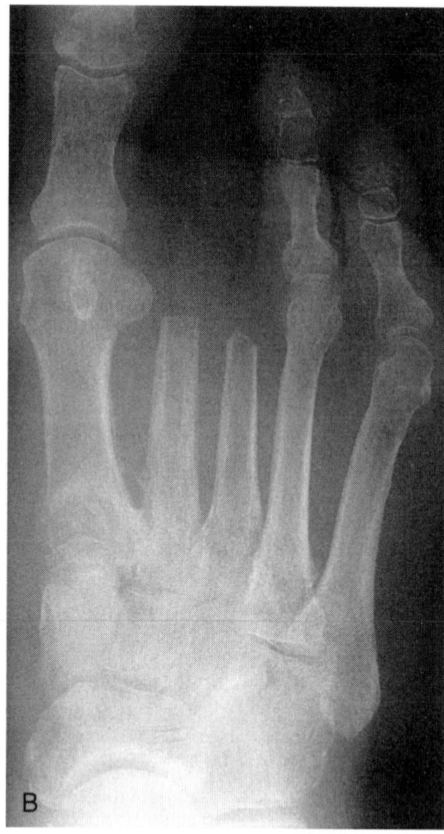

FIGURE 11–74. Osteomyelitis and septic arthritis: Tarsal involvement.[108–111] Serial radiographs (A, B) taken 4 months apart show rapidly progressive osteomyelitis of the tarsal bones and destruction of the intertarsal articulations by septic arthritis. The second and third phalanges and distal metatarsals have been surgically amputated in the interim for progressive infection.

TABLE 11–14. Tumors and Tumor-like Lesions Affecting the Bones of the Foot

Entity	Figure(s)	Characteristics
Malignant neoplasms		
Secondary malignant tumors of bone		
Skeletal metastasis[114]	11–75	Fewer than 1 per cent of metastatic lesions affect the bones of the foot Acral metastases most frequently occur in patients with carcinoma of the lung, bronchus, and kidney
Primary malignant tumors of bone		
Osteoblastoma (aggressive)[115]		Eleven per cent of aggressive osteoblastomas affect the bones of the foot Expansile osteolytic lesion that may be partially ossified or contain calcium
Fibrosarcoma[116]	11–76	Two per cent of fibrosarcomas affect the bones of the foot Purely osteolytic destruction with no associated sclerotic reaction or periostitis
Ewing's sarcoma[117]	11–77	Three per cent of Ewing's sarcomas affect the bones of the foot Aggressive permeative or motheaten pattern of bone destruction Central diaphyseal lesions of the tubular bones predominate
Synovial sarcoma[118]	11–78	Uncommon malignant neoplasms frequently found in the soft tissues in extra-articular locations More common in lower extremity Frequent recurrence and metastases, especially to the lung Poor prognosis Aggressive osteolytic destruction Approximately 20 to 30 per cent contain calcification
Myeloproliferative disorders of bone		
Plasma cell (multiple) myeloma[119]	11–79	Two per cent of multiple myeloma lesions occur in the bones of the foot Diffuse osteopenia or discrete osteolytic lesions

TABLE 11–14. Tumors and Tumor-like Lesions Affecting the Bones of the Foot *Continued*

Entity	Figure(s)	Characteristics
Benign tumors of bone		
Enostosis[120]	11–80	Five per cent of enostoses affect the bones of the foot
Osteoid osteoma[121]		Eleven per cent of osteoid osteomas occur in the bones of the foot
Subungual exostosis[122]		Solitary osteochondroma-like lesion arising from the dorsal surface of the distal phalanx Pressure on the undersurface of the nail may cause severe pain Lesion possesses smooth continuation of cortical and medullary bone Most frequently affects great toe
Enchondroma (solitary)[123]	11–81	About 7 per cent of solitary enchondromas affect the bones of the foot Lesions in the foot are more common in Ollier's disease and Maffucci's syndrome (> 60 per cent of patients with Maffucci's syndrome)
Chondroblastoma[124, 125]	11–82	Approximately 10 per cent of chondroblastomas occur in the bones of the foot Eccentric osteolytic lesion that involves epiphyses, apophyses, or epiphyseal equivalents; predilection for talus and calcaneus
Giant cell tumor (benign)[126]	11–83	Fewer than 2 per cent of benign giant cell tumors are located in the bones of the foot
Simple bone cyst[127]	11–84	Only 1 per cent of simple bone cysts occur in the bones of the foot Multiloculated and eccentric lesion usually affecting the calcaneus
Intraosseous lipoma[128]	11–85	Approximately 15 per cent of intraosseous lipomas occur in the calcaneus Geographic osteolytic lesion with sclerotic margins, often containing a central calcified or ossified nidus
Aneurysmal bone cyst[129]	11–86	Approximately 8 per cent of aneurysmal bone cysts involve the bones of the foot Eccentric, thin-walled, expansile, multiloculated osteolytic lesion Fluid levels seen with magnetic resonance (MR) imaging
Tumor-like lesions		
Paget's disease[130, 131]	11–87	Occasional involvement of the bones of the foot Usually polyostotic
Fibrous dysplasia[132]	11–88	Involvement of the bones of the foot is rare in the monostotic form but present in about 75 per cent of patients with polyostotic disease

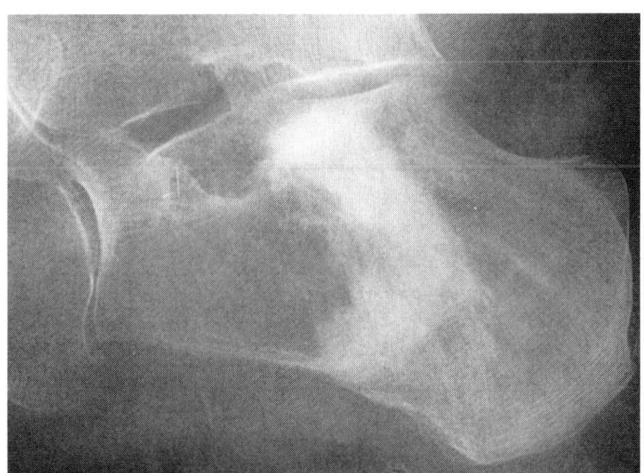

FIGURE 11–75. Skeletal metastasis.[114] Lateral radiograph of the calcaneus in this 76-year-old woman with a history of breast carcinoma reveals a mixed pattern of osteoblastic and osteolytic metastasis. Skeletal metastasis from the breast may be manifested as lytic, blastic, or mixed lesions.

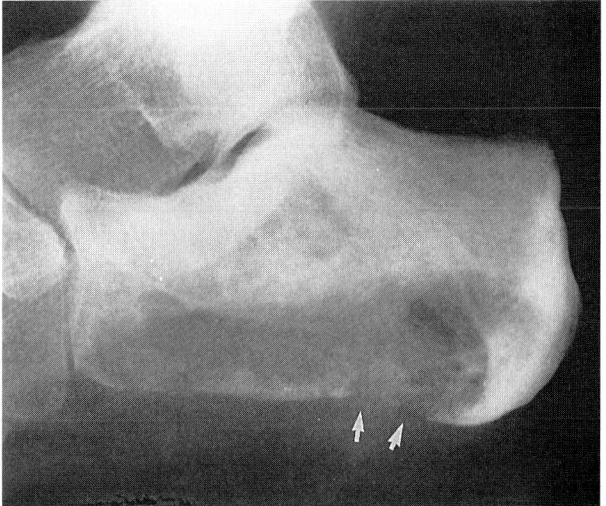

FIGURE 11–76. Fibrosarcoma.[116] A large, purely osteolytic lesion permeates the plantar aspect of the calcaneus in this 21-year-old woman. Minimal surrounding bone sclerosis is evident, but no periosteal reaction can be detected. Cortical perforation is seen (arrows).

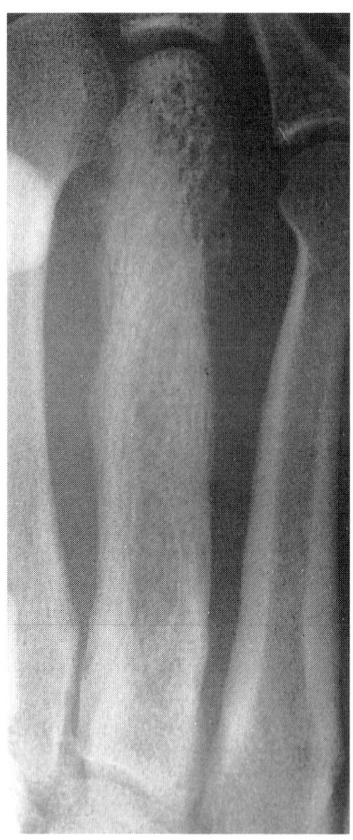

FIGURE 11–77. Ewing's sarcoma.[117] A permeative pattern of osteolytic destruction with indistinct cortical margins is evident in the third metatarsal bone of this 21-year-old man. The lesion involves the full length of the bone.

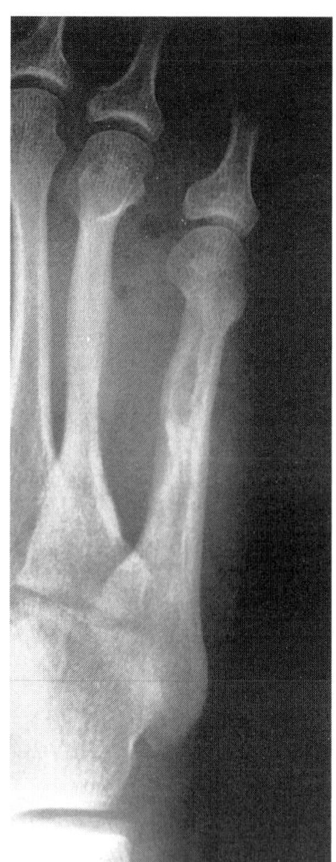

FIGURE 11–78. Synovial sarcoma.[118] This 23-year-old woman complained of a painful soft tissue mass on the lateral aspect of her foot. Permeative destruction involving the fifth metatarsal diaphysis with erosion of the adjacent fourth metatarsal bone is noted. The histologic diagnosis was synovial sarcoma.

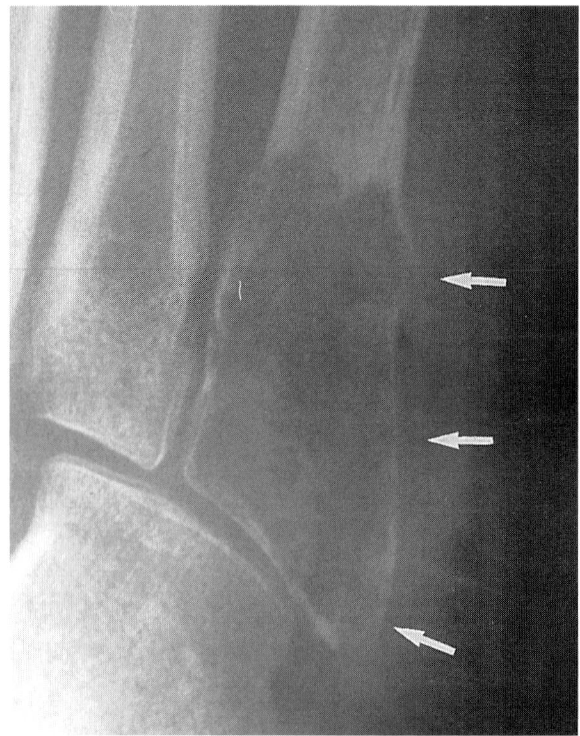

FIGURE 11–79. Plasma cell myeloma[119]; 48-year-old woman. Osteolytic destruction, cortical thinning, and disruption all are evident in the base of the fifth metatarsal bone (arrows).

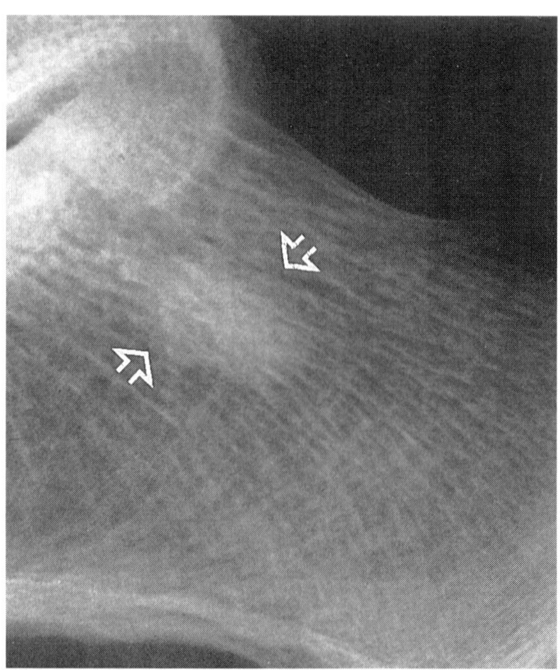

FIGURE 11–80. Enostosis (bone island).[120] An ovoid osteosclerotic focus (open arrows) is seen within the calcaneus. The long axis of the enostosis is oriented parallel to the axis of the major trabeculae.

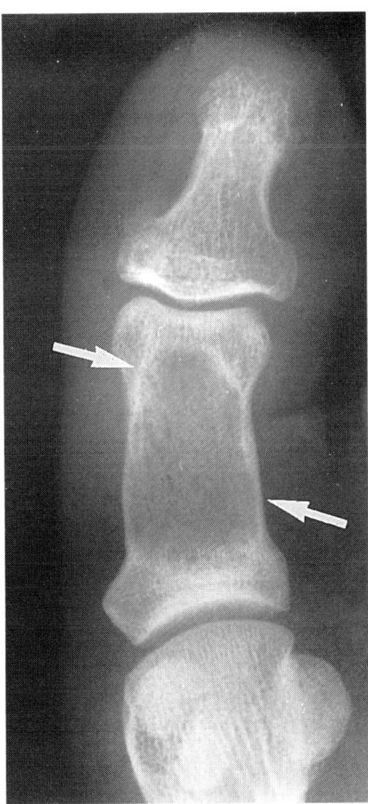

FIGURE 11–81. Enchondroma.[123] A large, purely osteolytic, geographic lesion with endosteal scalloping is seen in the metaphysis and diaphysis of the proximal phalanx of the great toe (arrows). Solitary enchondroma is a benign neoplasm composed of hyaline cartilage that develops in the medullary cavity and usually is discovered in the third or fourth decade of life. Most lesions are painless, and the presence of painful lesions should arouse the suspicion of malignant transformation, a complication that occurs only rarely in solitary lesions and in as many as 20 to 30 per cent of cases of multiple lesions (Ollier's disease and Maffucci's syndrome).

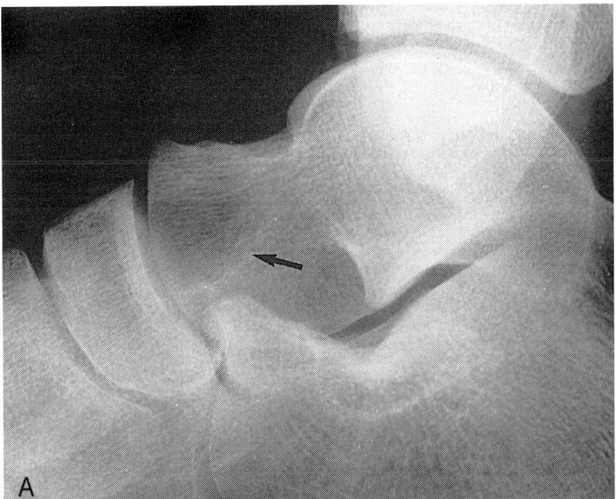

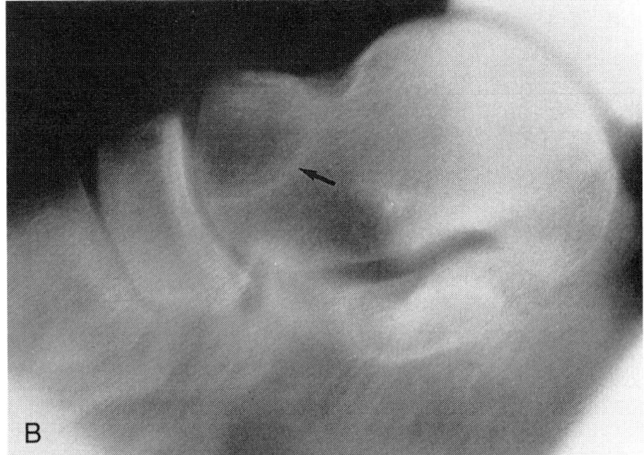

FIGURE 11–82. Chondroblastoma.[124, 125] Twenty-year-old man with ankle pain. **A** Lateral radiograph shows an osteolytic lesion in the talus. It is subchondral in location (an "epiphyseal equivalent" site) and geographic in appearance. **B** Conventional tomography confirms the findings (arrow). *(Courtesy of T. Goergen, M.D., San Diego, California.)*

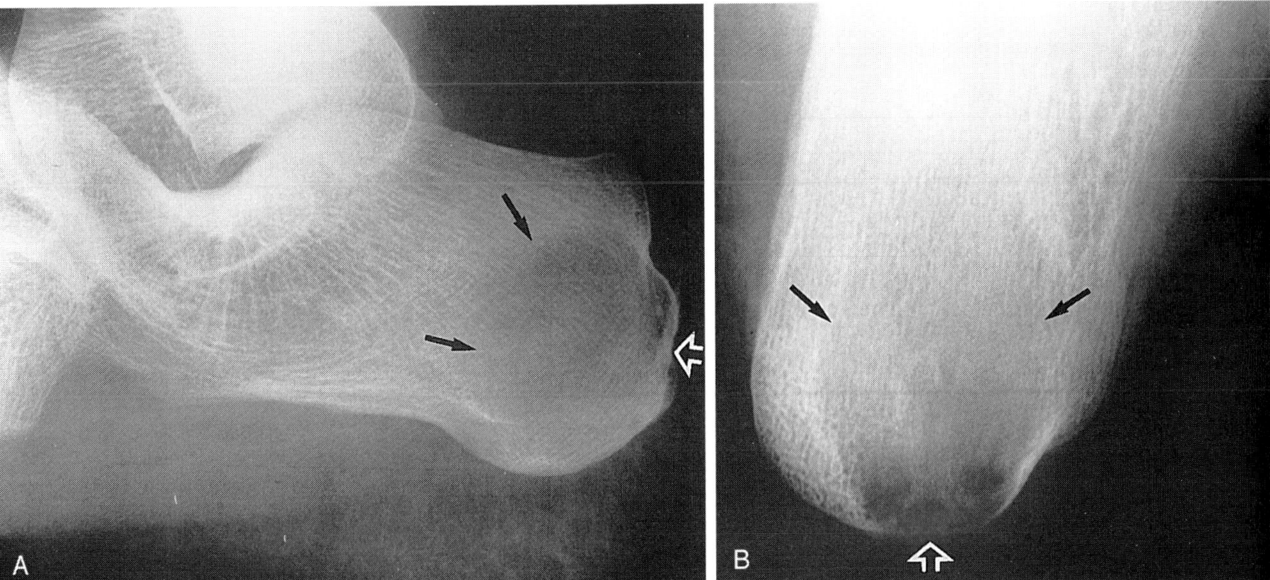

FIGURE 11–83. Giant cell tumor.[126] Lateral **(A)** and axial **(B)** radiographs of the calcaneus in this 33-year-old man show a circular, well-defined osteolytic lesion (arrows), which is eccentrically located, abutting on the posterior aspect of the calcaneus (open arrows). The calcaneus is an infrequent site for giant cell tumor. *(Courtesy of G. Greenway, M.D., Dallas, Texas.)*

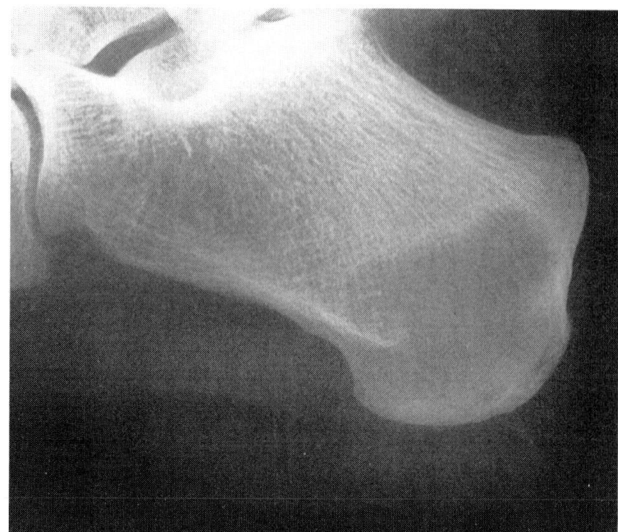

FIGURE 11–84. Simple bone cyst.[127] Lateral radiograph of the calcaneus in this 16-year-old woman with a biopsy-proved simple bone cyst reveals a geographic radiolucent lesion with a barely perceptible sclerotic margin. Approximately 3 per cent of all simple bone cysts occur in the calcaneus. Typically, they are solitary, and they are asymptomatic unless a pathologic fracture has occurred. Simple bone cysts usually are found more anteriorly in the calcaneus. *(Courtesy of R.J. Binden, M.D., Oakland, California.)*

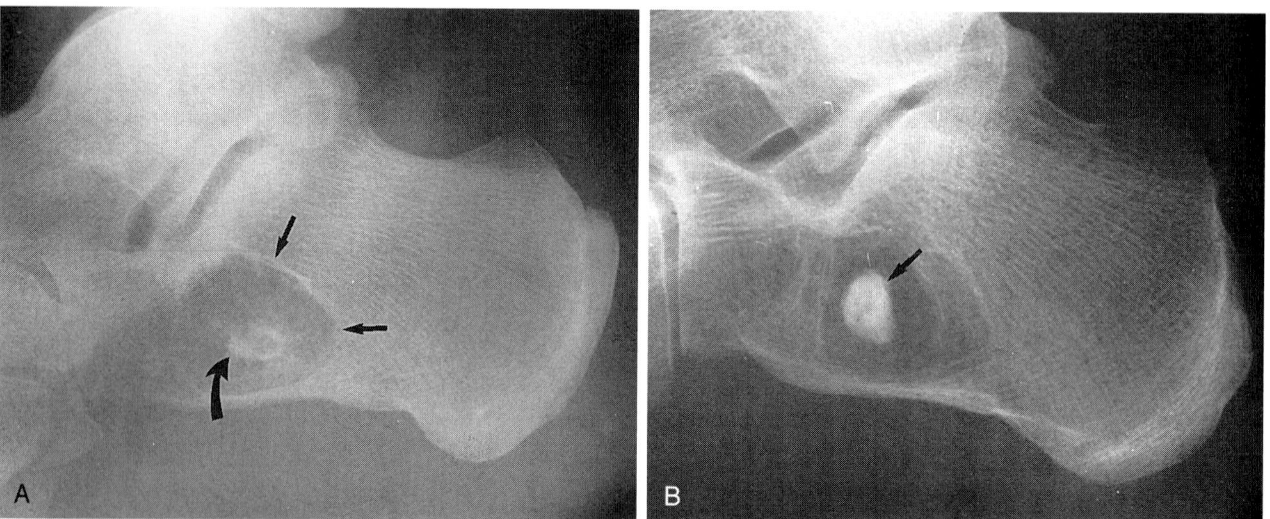

FIGURE 11–85. Intraosseous lipoma.[128] A Observe the classic appearance of a large, circular, radiolucent calcaneal lesion (arrows) containing a central fleck of calcification (curved arrow). *(A, Courtesy of P.H. VanderStoep, M.D., St. Cloud, Minnesota.)* B In another patient, a lateral radiograph of the calcaneus shows the classic appearance of an intraosseous lipoma. Observe the localization of the lesion in the triangular area between the major trabecular groups at the junction of the anterior and middle thirds of the calcaneus. The lesion is geographic and contains a central sclerotic focus (arrow). Simple bone cysts, which also are radiolucent, often occupy the same location in the calcaneus but rarely possess the central focus of calcification. *(B, Courtesy of A.H. Newberg, M.D., Boston, Massachusetts.)*

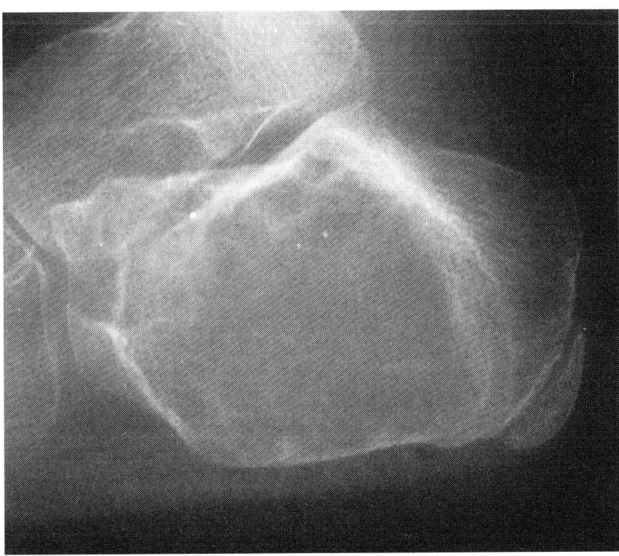

FIGURE 11–86. Aneurysmal bone cyst.[129] Lateral radiograph of the calcaneus in this 11-year-old boy shows osseous expansion of this osteolytic trabeculated lesion. The cortex is not disrupted. Computed tomographic (CT) images (not shown) demonstrated the extent of the lesion. *(Courtesy of T. Broderick, M.D., Orange, California.)*

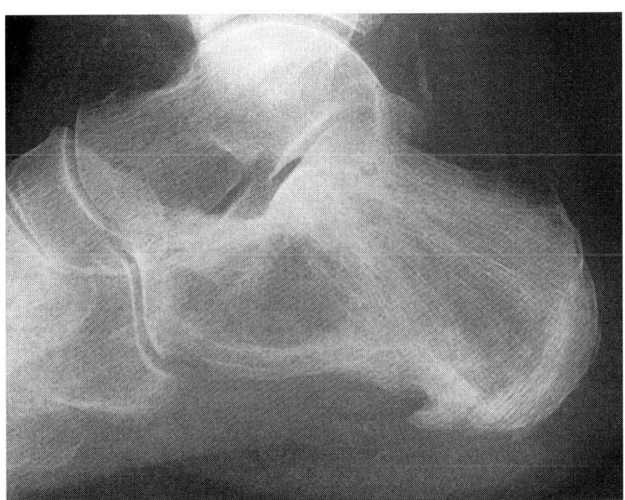

FIGURE 11–87. Paget's disease: Calcaneus.[130, 131] In this patient with the combined osteolytic and osteosclerotic pattern of Paget's disease, observe the areas of thickened, coarsely trabeculated bone with radiolucent regions of varying size. Minimal bone enlargement also is present.

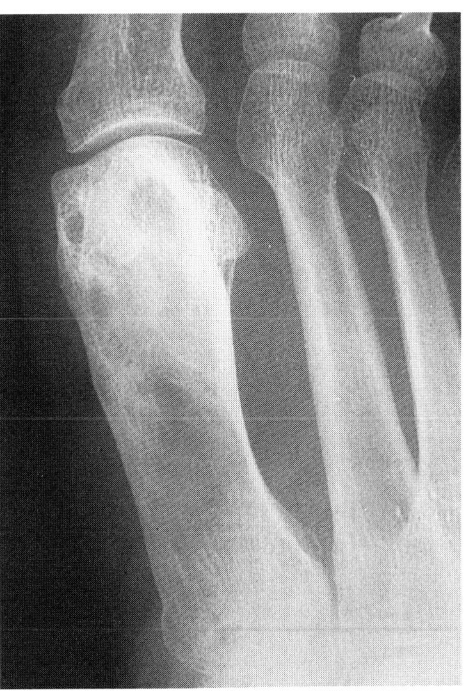

FIGURE 11–88. Fibrous dysplasia.[132] Observe the characteristic poorly defined trabeculae, hazy ground-glass appearance, and slight expansion of the first metatarsal bone in this radiograph of a 60-year-old man.

TABLE 11–15. Metabolic, Hematologic, and Vascular Disorders Affecting the Ankle and Foot

Entity	Figure(s)	Characteristics
Generalized osteoporosis[133]		Uniform decrease in radiodensity, thinning of cortices Occasionally may predispose to insufficiency fractures of the calcaneus and metatarsals
Regional osteoporosis[134]	11–89	May occur as a result of disuse and immobilization after a fracture or other injury; also seen in reflex sympathetic dystrophy, burns, frostbite, and paralysis; may occur as an idiopathic painful condition that later may migrate to other locations Findings may be more widespread in paralyzed patients Bandlike, patchy, spotty, or periarticular osteopenia Subperiosteal and intracortical bone resorption Subchondral and juxta-articular erosions
Poliomyelitis[135]	11–90	Diffuse bone and soft tissue atrophy Regional osteoporosis
Hyperparathyroidism and renal osteodystrophy[136, 137]	11–91, 11–92	Brown tumors (osteoclastomas) Subperiosteal resorption Metastatic soft tissue calcification
Vascular calcification[138]	11–93	Linear vessel wall calcification readily visible on routine radiographs Calcification within the tunica media of arterial walls occurs in patients with diabetes mellitus and hyperparathyroidism and is termed Mönckeberg's atherosclerosis Frequently affects the tibialis anterior artery, dorsalis pedis artery, and smaller arteries of the foot The clinical significance of such atherosclerosis is unclear; regarded by some physicians as insignificant
Acromegaly[139, 140]	11–94	Soft tissue overgrowth: heel pad thickening, joint space widening, and clubbing of toes Osseous overgrowth: enlargement of sesamoid bones and terminal tufts, periarticular excrescences Acromegalic arthropathy with eventual secondary osteoarthrosis
Gaucher's disease[141]	11–95	Osteopenia, septated osteolytic lesions, cortical diminution, and diametaphyseal widening (Erlenmeyer flask deformity) Osseous weakening may result in pathologic fractures Coarsened trabecular pattern May result in osteonecrosis

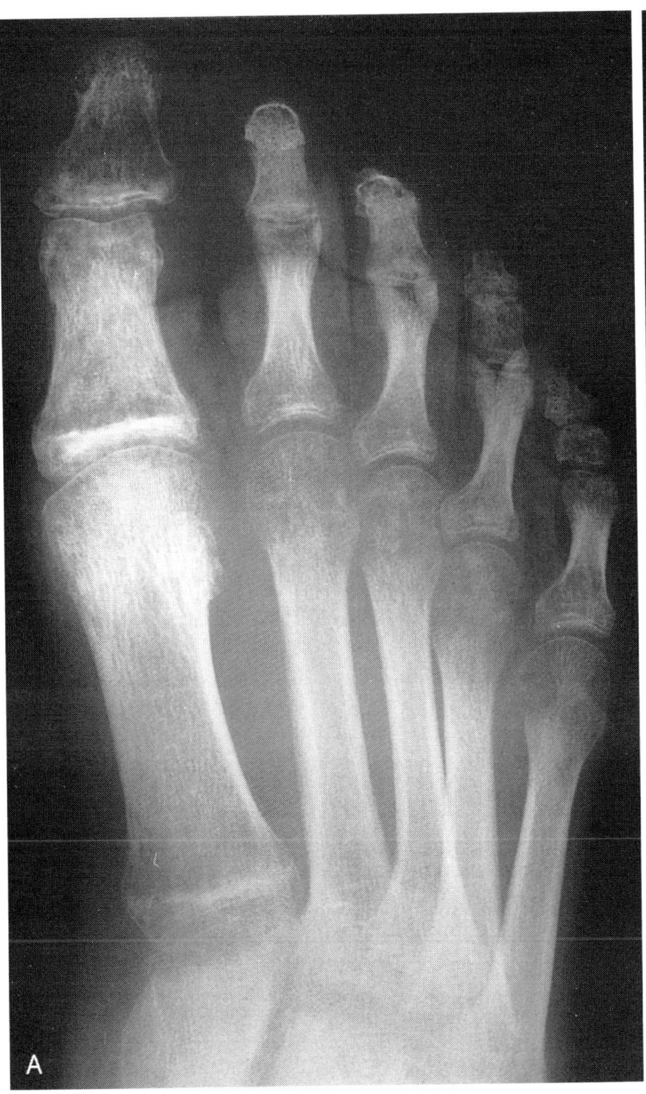

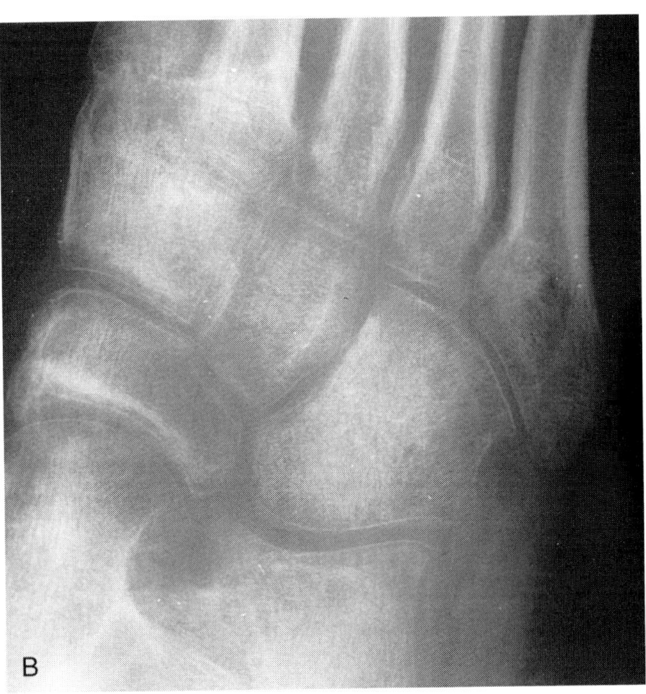

FIGURE 11–89. Regional osteoporosis.[134] A, B Disuse osteoporosis. This 22-year-old man sustained a proximal tibial fracture and was immobilized in a cast for 8 weeks. In A, subcortical, periarticular, patchy, and spotty loss of bone density is evident throughout the tarsal and metatarsal bones and the phalanges, which is characteristic of the osteoporosis of immobilization. In B, an oblique radiograph of the midfoot in the same patient shows the patchy subarticular distribution typical of regional osteoporosis. Spotty, patchy, and band-like bone resorption is typical of rapid-onset osteoporosis, such as that seen in disuse, burns, frostbite, paralysis, or reflex sympathetic dystrophy, an appearance that may simulate an aggressive neoplasm.

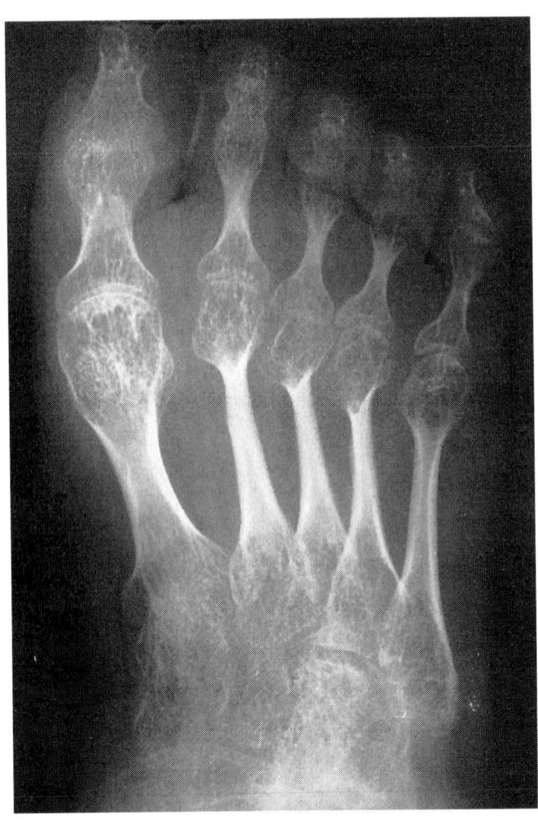

FIGURE 11–90. Poliomyelitis.[135] Observe the soft tissue atrophy, diffuse regional osteopenia, and atrophy of bone in this patient with long-standing poliomyelitis. The diaphyses of the long bones appear thin and atrophic, creating an expanded appearance of the distal ends of the bones.

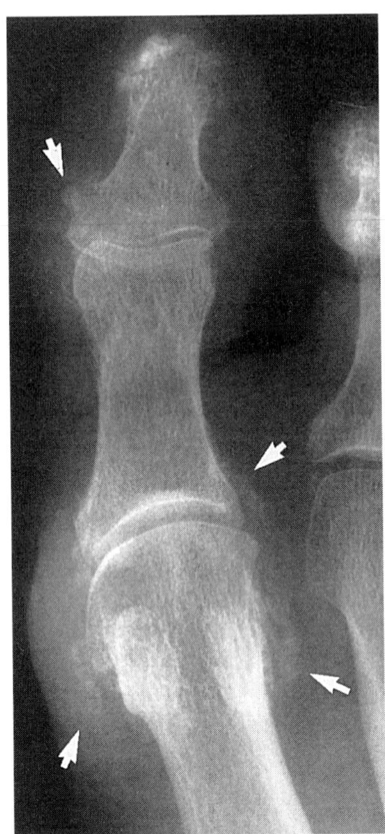

FIGURE 11–91. Hyperparathyroidism.[136, 137] Observe the extensive periarticular calcification (arrows) in this 64-year-old woman with chronic renal failure.

This form of metastatic soft tissue calcification is related to a disturbance in calcium or phosphorus metabolism and is seen in hyperparathyroidism and renal osteodystrophy. *(Courtesy of T. Broderick, M.D., Orange, California.)*

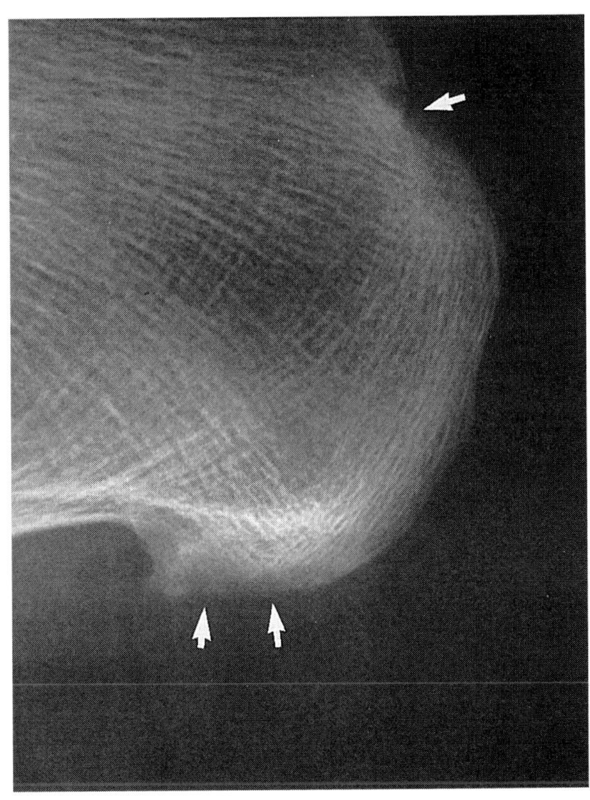

FIGURE 11–92. Renal osteodystrophy.[136, 137] Indistinct cortical margins (arrows) represent subligamentous resorption of the calcaneus, a known finding in renal osteodystrophy.

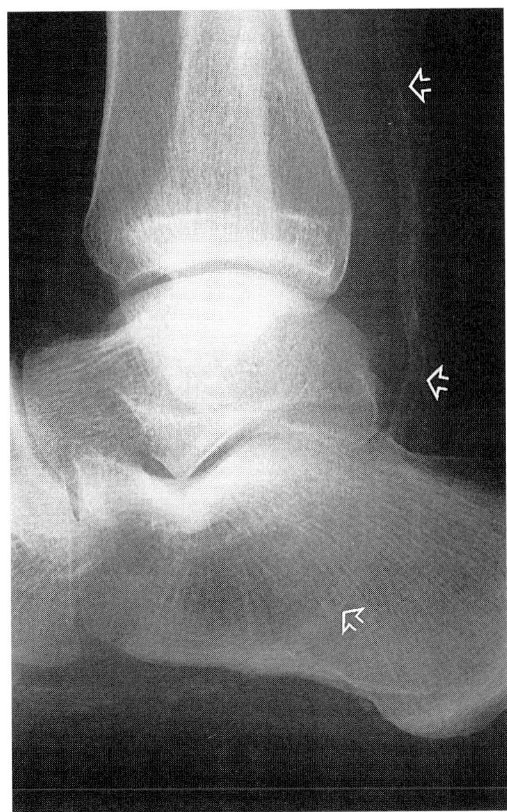

FIGURE 11–93. Vascular calcification: Diabetes mellitus.[138] Extensive arterial wall calcification (Mönckeberg's atherosclerosis) involving the posterior tibial artery (open arrows) is seen in this patient with long-standing diabetes mellitus. Calcification of the tunica media of the arteries is a well-recognized complication of diabetes mellitus.

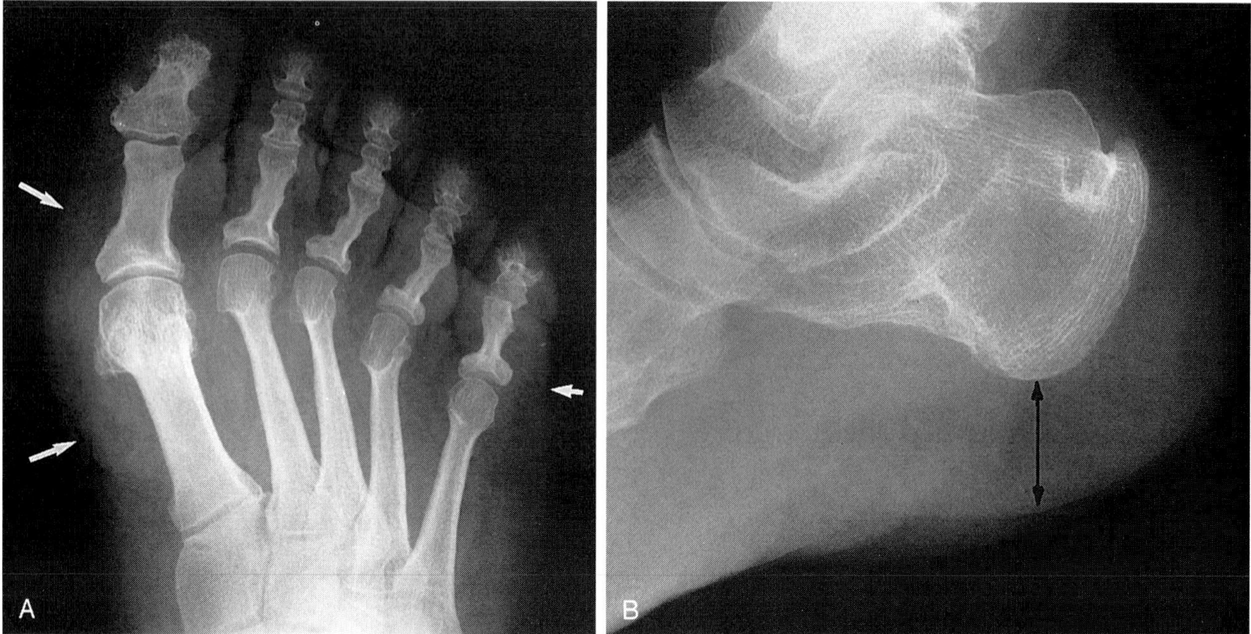

FIGURE 11–94. Acromegaly.[139, 140] A Acromegalic arthropathy. Prominent soft tissues (arrows), widened joint spaces, periarticular excrescences, and prominence of the terminal tufts are characteristic findings in this patient with acromegaly. B Thickening of the heel pad. Normally, the heel pad thickness should be no more than 23 mm in men and 21.5 mm in women. The heel pad is considerably more prominent (double-headed arrow) in this patient with long-standing acromegaly.

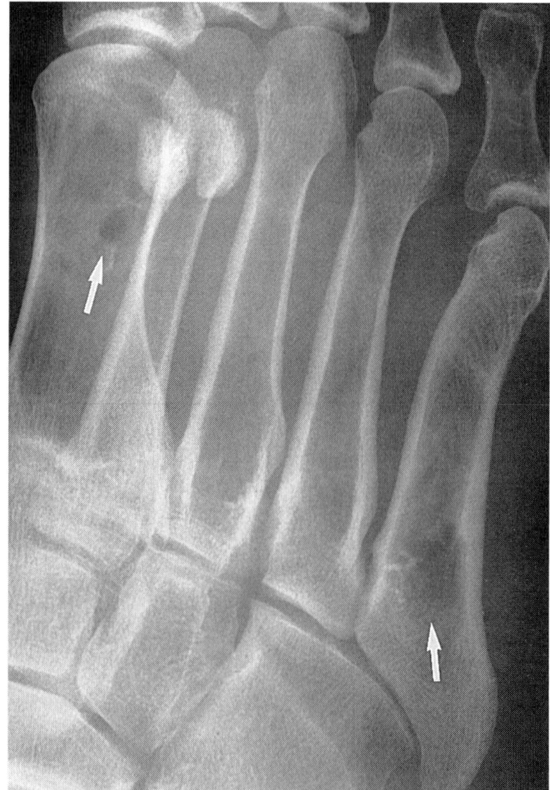

FIGURE 11–95. Gaucher's disease.[141] Observe the multiple osteolytic lesions (arrows) within the metatarsal bones in this 51-year-old woman with extensive marrow infiltration. *(Courtesy of M.N. Pathria, M.D., San Diego, California.)*

TABLE 11–16. Osteonecrosis and Osteochondroses Affecting the Ankle and Foot

Entity	Figure(s)	Characteristics
Sickle cell anemia[142]	11–96	Hand-foot syndrome or sickle cell dactylitis Typically affects children between the ages of 6 months and 2 years Osteonecrosis of the small bones of the hand and foot results from vascular occlusion Affects 20 to 50 per cent of children with sickle cell anemia Soft tissue swelling, osteolysis, and diffuse periostitis
Osteonecrosis of the talus[143, 144]	11–97	Disabling complication of corticosteroid use as well as fractures and dislocations of the talus Radiographic findings may not be present for 1 to 3 months: surrounding disuse osteopenia creates a relative increase in the density of the talar body that may be combined with collapse of the articular surface Hawkins sign: a subchondral radiolucent band seen in the dome of the talus on anteroposterior ankle radiographs 6 to 8 weeks after disuse or immobilization; radiolucent band results from active hyperemia of bone and is a reliable sign that the blood supply to the talar dome is preserved, and that ischemic necrosis likely will not occur Magnetic resonance (MR) imaging is useful in defining the extent of osteonecrosis
Köhler's disease[145]	11–98 A	Fragmentation, flattening, irregularity, and sclerosis of the tarsal navicular bone in children Boys > girls; 3 to 7 years of age Local pain, tenderness, swelling, and limitation of motion Self-limited condition; over a period of 2 to 4 years, the bone may regain its normal size, density, and trabecular structure. Possible causes: 1. Osteonecrosis secondary to mechanical forces 2. Manifestation of normal or altered ossification
Mueller-Weiss syndrome[146]	11–98 B,C	Painful spontaneous osteonecrosis of the tarsal navicular bone in adults Believed to be due to osteonecrosis related to previous injury or chronic stress
Freiberg's infraction[147]	11–99	Abnormality of the metatarsal head secondary to osteonecrosis resulting from repeated trauma Second metatarsal bone most frequent site Women > men Patients wearing high-heeled shoes are predisposed to Freiberg's infraction Articular surface fragmentation and collapse; initial joint space widening; eventual osteoarthrosis and sclerotic stress reaction of metatarsal
Normal calcaneal apophysis (Sever's "disease")[4]	11–100	Calcaneal apophysis in children normally is sclerotic, may be fragmented, and is associated with a serrated appearance of the posterior margin of the calcaneus These widely variable normal findings should not be misdiagnosed as osteochondrosis, osteonecrosis, or fracture Frequently mislabeled as Sever's disease

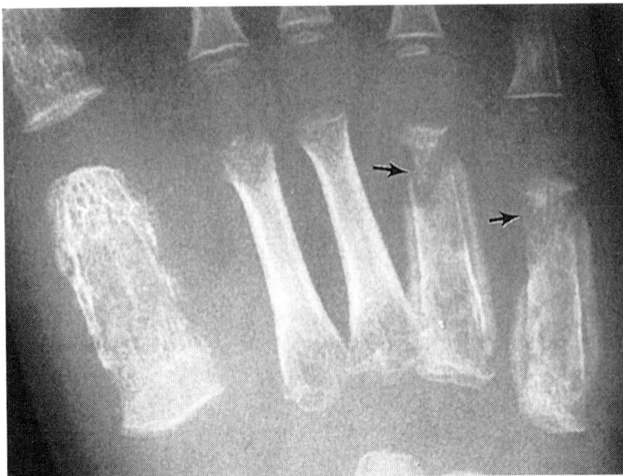

FIGURE 11–96. Sickle cell anemia: Sickle cell dactylitis.[142] Soft tissue swelling, permeative destruction, large areas of osteolysis (arrows), and diffuse periostitis involving several metatarsal bones are evident in this patient with sickle cell dactylitis. *(Courtesy of P. Kaplan, M.D., Charlottesville, Virginia.)*

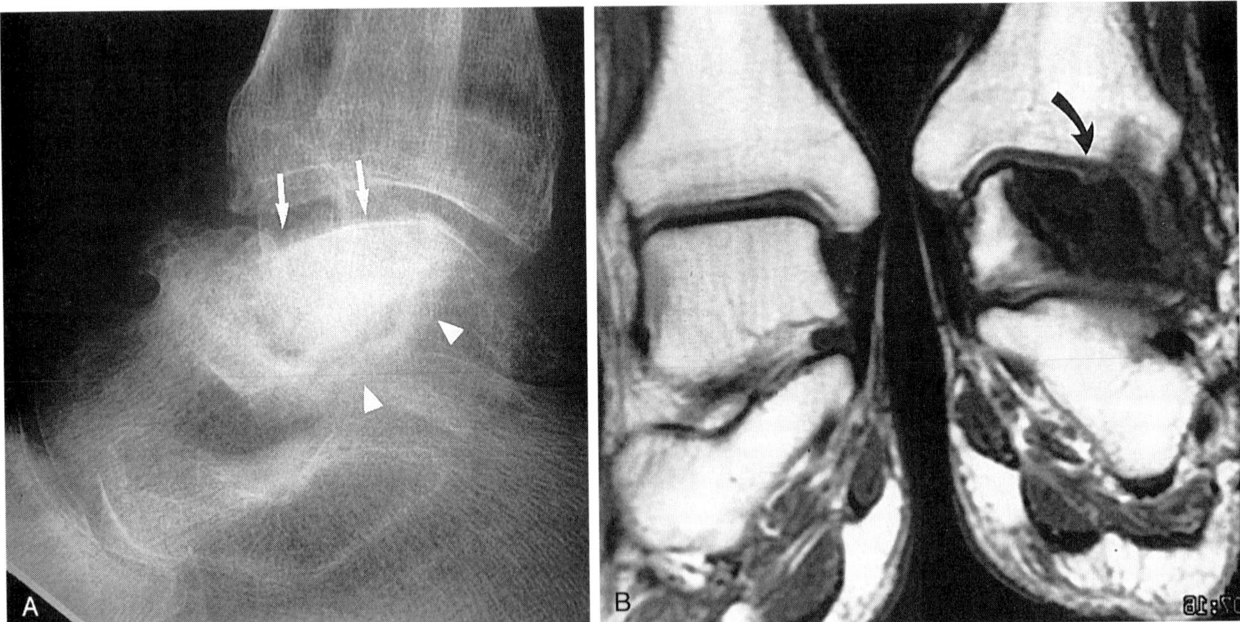

FIGURE 11–97. Osteonecrosis: Talus.[143, 144] Fifty-five-year-old man with ankle pain. **A** Lateral radiograph shows central collapse (arrows) and increased density (arrowheads) of the talus. **B** Coronal T1-weighted (TR/TE, 700/16) spin echo magnetic resonance (MR) image of both ankles shows an abnormal left talus with a well-defined zone of decreased signal intensity and associated collapse of the articular surface (curved arrow). Normal high signal intensity marrow is evident in the opposite talus.

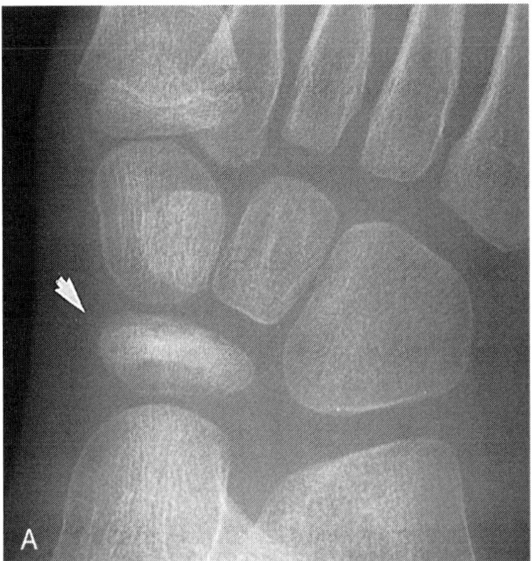

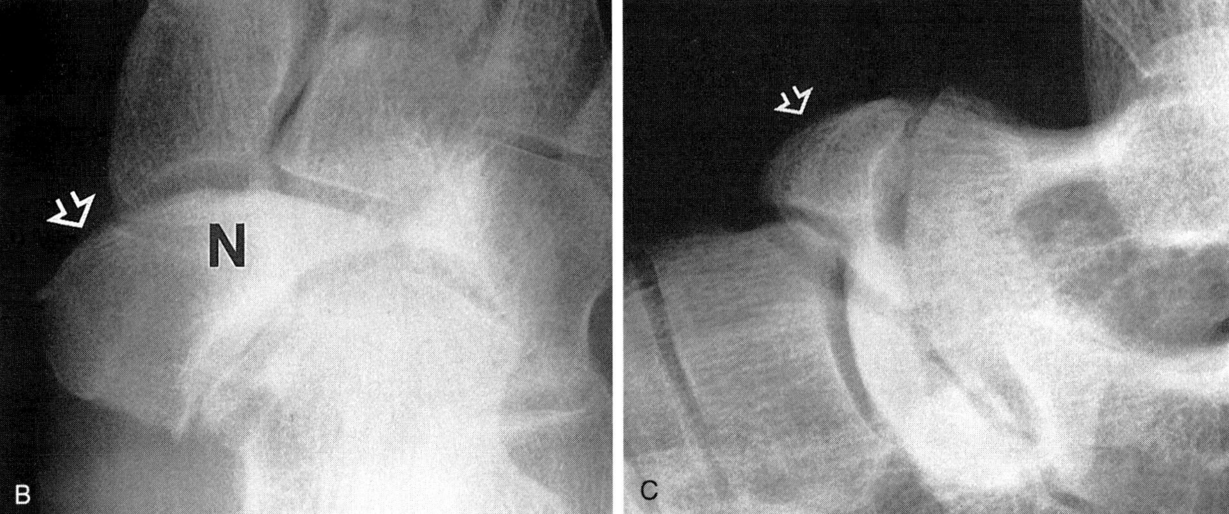

FIGURE 11–98. Osteonecrosis and osteochondrosis: Tarsal navicular bone.[145, 146] A Köhler's disease. An oblique radiograph of the foot in this 5-year-old boy with a painful limp demonstrates osteosclerosis and collapse of the tarsal navicular bone (arrow). The disease, more common in boys, usually occurs between the ages of 3 and 7 years, with an onset of local pain, tenderness, swelling, and limitation of motion. It is believed by some authorities that Köhler's disease represents osteonecrosis possibly secondary to mechanical forces. Other investigators, however, regard the condition as a manifestation of normal or altered ossification. The disease is self-limited in that over a period of 2 to 4 years, the bone may become normal in size, density, and trabecular structure. **B, C** Mueller-Weiss syndrome: Spontaneous osteonecrosis of the tarsal navicular bone. In **B**, a frontal radiograph shows a medially displaced (open arrow), comma-shaped navicular bone (N). The lateral portion of the bone is collapsed. In **C**, a lateral radiograph, the navicular bone appears triangular and is minimally displaced dorsally (open arrow). The Mueller-Weiss syndrome is a painful condition in adults, more common in women, that is believed to be due to osteonecrosis related to previous injury or chronic stress. The differential diagnosis includes osteonecrosis associated with other conditions, such as systemic lupus erythematosus and corticosteroid use, fatigue fracture, or insufficiency fracture related to rheumatoid arthritis, chronic renal disease, or diabetes mellitus. (**B, C**, *Courtesy of E. Bosch, M.D., Santiago, Chile.*)

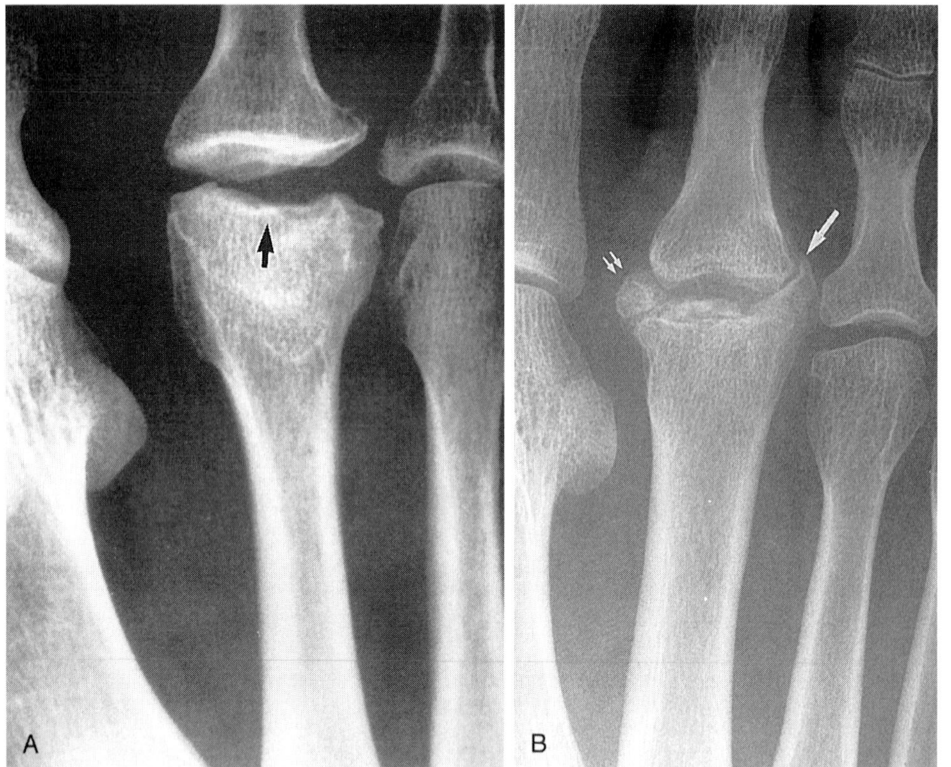

FIGURE 11–99. Freiberg's infraction.[147] A Flattening and deformity of the subchondral surface of the second metatarsal head is seen (arrow). The metatarsophalangeal joint appears widened owing to collapse of the subchondral bone. Note also the osteophytes adjacent to the articulation. *(A, Courtesy of M.N. Pathria, M.D., San Diego, California.)* B In another patient, osteophytes (arrow), subarticular collapse, and intra-articular osseous bodies (double arrows) are noted, likewise involving the second metatarsal head. Observe also the widening and cortical thickening of the second metatarsal shaft.

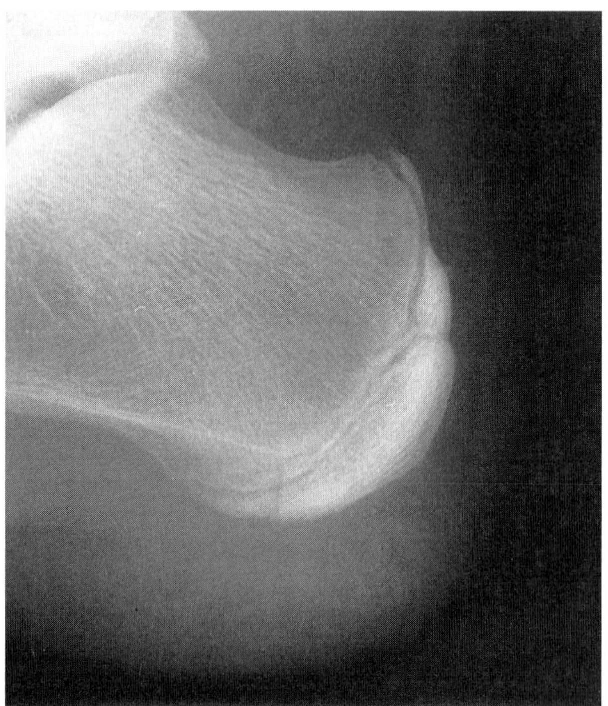

FIGURE 11–100. Normal calcaneal apophysis (Sever's "disease").[4] The calcaneal apophysis in this child is sclerotic and fragmented, and the posterior edge of the calcaneus is somewhat ragged in appearance. Sclerosis often is present as a result of weight-bearing in children who walk; the apparent fragmentation is a result of ossification occurring at multiple sites; and the posterior surface of the immature calcaneus frequently appears irregular. All of these findings are normal and should not be mistaken for osteochondrosis, osteonecrosis, or fracture. This finding has, in the past, been incorrectly designated Sever's disease.

REFERENCES

1. Edeiken J, Dalinka M, Karasick D: Edeiken's Roentgen Diagnosis of Diseases of Bone. 4th Ed. Baltimore, Williams & Wilkins, 1990.
2. Keats TE, Smith TH: An Atlas of Normal Developmental Roentgen Anatomy. 2nd Ed. Chicago, Year Book, 1988.
3. Greenfield GB: Radiology of Bone Diseases. 2nd Ed. Philadelphia, JB Lippincott, 1975.
4. Köhler A, Zimmer EA: Borderlands of Normal and Early Pathologic Findings in Skeletal Radiography. 4th Ed. New York, Thieme Medical Publishers, 1993.
5. Keats TE: Atlas of Normal Roentgen Variants That May Simulate Disease, 6th Ed. Chicago, Year Book Medical Publishers, 1996.
6. Griffiths H, Wandtke J: Tibiotalar tilt—a new slant. Skeletal Radiol 6:193, 1981.
7. Forrester DM, Kricun ME, Kerr R: Imaging of the Foot and Ankle. Rockville, MD, Aspen, 1988.
8. Takakura Y, Tamai S, Masuhara K: Genesis of the ball-and-socket ankle. J Bone Joint Surg [Br] 68:834, 1986.
9. Wesely MS, Barenfeld PA, Shea JM, et al: The congenital cavus foot: A follow-up report. Bull Hosp Joint Dis 47:217, 1982.
10. Scott G, Wilson DW, Bentley G: Roentgenographic assessment in hallux valgus. Clin Orthop 267:143, 1991.
11. Eustace S, Williamson D, Wilson M, et al: Tendon shift in hallux valgus: Observations at MR imaging. Skeletal Radiol 25:519, 1996.
12. Bridges AL, Kou-Ching H, Singh A, et al: Fibrodysplasia (myositis) ossificans progressiva. Semin Arthritis Rheum 24:155, 1994.
13. Stormont DM, Peterson HA: The relative incidence of tarsal coalition. Clin Orthop 181:28, 1983.
14. Wechsler RJ, Schweitzer ME, Deely DM, et al: Tarsal coalition: Depiction and characterization with CT and MR imaging. Radiology 193:447, 1994.
15. Kumar SJ, Guille JT, Lee MS, et al: Osseous and non-osseous coalition of the middle facet of the talocalcaneal joint. J Bone Joint Surg [Am] 74:529, 1992.
16. Lateur LM, Van Hoe LR, Van Ghillewe KV, et al: Subtalar coalition: Diagnosis with the C sign on lateral radiographs of the ankle. Radiology 193:847, 1994.
17. Wakeley CJ, Johnson DP, Watt I: The value of MR imaging in the diagnosis of the os trigonum syndrome. Skeletal Radiol 25:133, 1996.
18. Karasick D, Schweitzer ME: The os trigonum syndrome: Imaging features. AJR 166:125, 1996.
19. Reichmister JP: The painful os intermetatarseum: A brief overview and case reports. Clin Orthop 153:201, 1980.
20. Smith AD, Carter JR, Marcus RE: The os vesalianum: An unusual cause of lateral foot pain: A case report and review of the literature. Orthopedics 7:86, 1984.
21. Lawson JP, Ogden JA, Sella E, et al: The painful accessory navicular. Skeletal Radiol 12:250, 1984.
22. Miller TT, Staron RB, Feldman F, et al: The symptomatic accessory tarsal navicular bone: Assessment with MR imaging. Radiology 195:849, 1995.
23. Taylor JAM, Sartoris DJ, Huang GS, et al: Painful conditions affecting the first metatarsal sesamoid bones. RadioGraphics 13:817, 1993.
24. Resnick D: Talar ridges, osteophytes, and beaks: A radiologic commentary. Radiology 151:329, 1984.
25. Lyritis G: Developmental disorders of the proximal epiphysis of the hallux. Skeletal Radiol 10:250, 1983.
26. Turra S, Frizziero P, Cagnoni G, et al: Macrodactyly of the foot associated with plexiform neurofibroma of the medial plantar nerve. J Pediatr Orthop 6:489, 1986.
27. Nogami H: Polydactyly and polysyndactyly of the fifth toe. Clin Orthop 204:261, 1986.
28. Laurent Y, Brombart M: Variation trés rare de l'ossification des phalanges des orteils. J Belge Radiol 36:102, 1953.
29. Keret D, Spatz DK, Caro PA, et al: Dysplasia epiphysealis hemimelica: Diagnosis and treatment. J Pediatr Orthop 12:365, 1992.
30. Root L: The treatment of osteogenesis imperfecta. Orthop Clin North Am 15:775, 1984.
31. Benli IT, Akalin S, Boysan E, et al: Epidemiological, clinical, and radiological aspects of osteopoikilosis. J Bone Joint Surg [Br] 74:504, 1992.
32. Campbell CJ, Papademetriou T, Bonfiglio M: Melorheostosis: A report of the clinical, roentgenographic, and pathological findings in fourteen cases. J Bone Joint Surg [Am] 50:1281, 1968.
33. Yu JS, Resnick D, Vaughan LM, et al: Melorheostosis with an ossified soft tissue mass. Skeletal Radiol 24:367, 1995.
34. Joseph KN, Kane HA, Milner RS, et al: Orthopedic aspects of the Marfan phenotype. Clin Orthop 277:251, 1992.
35. Ainsworth SR, Aulicino PL: A survey of patients with Ehlers-Danlos syndrome. Clin Orthop 286:250, 1993.
36. Goldman AB, Kaye JJ: Macrodystrophia lipomatosa: Radiographic diagnosis. AJR 128:101, 1977.
37. Nielsen JØ, Dons-Jenson H, Sørensen HT: Lauge-Hansen classification of malleolar fractures: An assessment of the reproducibility in 118 cases. Acta Orthop Scan 61:385, 1990.
38. Verma S, Hamilton K, Hawkins HH, et al: Clinical application of the Ottawa ankle rules for the use of radiography in acute ankle injuries: An independent site assessment. AJR 169:825, 1997.
39. Lock TR, Schaffer JJ, Manoli A II: Maisonneuve fracture: Case report of a missed diagnosis. Ann Emerg Med 16:805, 1987.
40. Rogers LF: Radiology of Skeletal Trauma. 2nd Ed. New York, Churchill Livingstone, 1992.
41. Resnick D: Diagnosis of Bone and Joint Disorders. 3rd Ed. Philadelphia, WB Saunders, 1995.
42. Kleinman PK, Marks SC Jr: A regional approach to classic metaphyseal lesions in abused infants: The distal tibia. AJR 166:1207, 1996.
43. MacNealy GA, Rogers LF, Hernandez R, et al: Injuries of the distal tibial epiphysis: Systematic radiographic evaluation. AJR 138:683, 1982.
44. Rogers LF, Poznanski AK: Imaging of epiphyseal injuries. Radiology 191:297, 1994.
45. Petite P, Panuel M, Faure F, et al: Acute fracture of the distal tibial physis: Role of gradient-echo MR imaging versus plain film examination. AJR 166:1203, 1996.
46. Reading JM, Sheehan NJ: Spontaneous fractures of the lower limb in chronic rheumatoid arthritis. J Orthop Rheumatol 4:173, 1991.
47. Molinari M, Bertoldi L, De March L: Fracture-dislocation of the ankle with the fibula trapped behind the tibia: A case report. Acta Orthop Scand 61:471, 1990.
48. Wechsler RJ, Schweitzer ME, Karasick D, et al: Helical CT of calcaneal fractures: Technique and imaging features. Skeletal Radiol 27:1, 1998.
49. Renfrew DL, El-Khoury GY: Anterior process fractures of the calcaneus. Skeletal Radiol 14:121, 1985.
50. Brijs S, Brijs A: Calcaneal avulsion: A frequent traumatic foot lesion. Fortschr Rontgenstr 156:495, 1992.

51. Sneppen O, Christensen SB, Krogsoe O, et al: Fracture of the body of the talus. Acta Orthop Scand 48:317, 1977.
52. Wechsler RJ, Schweitzer ME, Karasick D, et al: Helical CT of talar fractures. Skeletal Radiol 26:137, 1997.
53. Loomer R, Fisher C, Lloyd-Smith R, et al: Osteochondral lesions of the talus. Am J Sports Med 21:13, 1993.
54. Zimmer TJ, Johnson KA: Subtalar dislocations. Clin Orthop 238:190, 1989.
55. Rogers LF, Campbell RE: Fractures and dislocations of the foot. Semin Roentgenol 12:157, 1978.
56. Dines DM, Hershon SJ, Smith N, et al: Isolated dorsomedial dislocation of the first ray at the medial cuneonavicular joint of the foot: A rare injury to the tarsus. Clin Orthop 186: 162, 1984.
57. Kiss ZS, Khan KM, Fuller PJ: Stress fractures of the tarsal navicular bone: CT findings in 55 cases. AJR 160:111, 1993.
58. Anderson MW, Greenspan A: Stress fractures. Radiology 199:1, 1996.
59. Faciszewski T, Burks RT, Manaster BJ: Subtle injuries of the Lisfranc joint. J Bone Joint Surg [Am] 72:1519, 1990.
60. Preidler KW, Brossman J, Daenen B, et al: MR imaging of the tarsometatarsal joint: Analysis of injuries in 11 patients. AJR 167:1217, 1996.
61. Richli WR, Rosenthal DI: Avulsion fracture of the fifth metatarsal: Experimental study of pathomechanics. AJR 143:889, 1984.
62. Torg JS, Balduini FC, Zelko RR, et al: Fractures of the base of the fifth metatarsal distal to the tuberosity: Classification and guidelines for non-surgical and surgical management. J Bone Joint Surg [Am] 66:209, 1984.
63. Galant JM, Spinosa FA: Digital fractures: A comprehensive review. J Am Podiatr Assoc 81:593, 1991.
64. Eisele SA, Sammarco GJ: Fatigue fractures of the foot and ankle in the athlete. J Bone Joint Surg [Am] 75:290, 1993.
65. Chowchuen P, Resnick D: Stress fractures of the metatarsal heads. Skeletal Radiol 27:22, 1998.
66. Anderson MW, Greenspan A: Stress fractures. Radiology 199:1, 1996.
67. Galant JM, Spinosa FA: Digital fractures: A comprehensive review. J Am Podiatr Assoc 81:593, 1991.
68. Pinckney LE, Currarino G, Kennedy LA: The stubbed great toe: A cause of occult compound fracture and infection. Radiology 138:375, 1981.
69. Katayama M, Murakami Y, Takahashi H: Irreducible dorsal dislocation of the toe: Report of three cases. J Bone Joint Surg [Am] 70:769, 1988.
70. Towbin R, Dunbar JS, Towbin J, et al: Teardrop sign: Plain film recognition of ankle effusion. AJR 134:985, 1980.
71. Karlsson J, Lansinger O: Lateral instability of the ankle joint. Clin Orthop 276:253, 1992.
72. Weinstabl R, Stiskal M, Neuhold A, et al: Classifying calcaneal tendon injury according to MRI findings. J Bone Joint Surg [Br] 73:683, 1991.
73. Ouzounaian TJ, Anderson R: Anterior tibial tendon rupture. Foot Ankle 16:406, 1995.
74. Karasick D, Schweitzer ME: Tear of the posterior tibial tendon causing asymptomatic flatfoot: Radiologic findings. AJR 161:1237, 1993.
75. Sammarco GJ: Peroneus longus tendon tears: Acute and chronic. Foot Ankle 16:245, 1995.
76. Innis PC, Krackow KH: Weightbearing roentgenograms in arthritis of the ankle: A case report. Foot Ankle 9:54, 1988.
77. Resnick D, Feingold ML, Curd J, et al: Calcaneal abnormalities in articular disorders: Rheumatoid arthritis, ankylosing spondylitis, psoriatic arthritis and Reiter's syndrome. Radiology 125:355, 1977.
78. Karasick D, Wapner KL: Hallux rigidus deformity: Radiologic assessment. AJR 157:1029, 1991.
79. Malhotra CM, Lally EV, Buckley WM: Ossification of the plantar fascia and peroneus longus tendons in diffuse idiopathic skeletal hyperostosis (DISH). J Rheumatol 13:215, 1986.
80. Kirkup JR: Ankle and tarsal joints in rheumatoid arthritis. Scand J Rheumatol 3:50, 1974.
81. Kirkup JR, Vidigal E, Jacoby RK: The hallux and rheumatoid arthritis. Acta Orthop Scand 48:527, 1977.
82. Garcia-Morteo O, Gusis SE, Somma LF, et al: Tarsal ankylosis in juvenile and adult onset rheumatoid arthritis. J Rheumatol 15:298, 1988.
83. Azouz EM, Duffy CM: Juvenile spondyloarthropathies: Clinical manifestations and medical imaging. Skeletal Radiol 24:399, 1995.
84. Resnick D: Patterns of peripheral joint disease in ankylosing spondylitis. Radiology 110:523, 1974.
85. Martel W, Stuck KJ, Dworin AM, et al: Erosive osteoarthritis and psoriatic arthritis: A radiologic comparison in the hand, wrist, and foot. AJR 134:125, 1980.
86. Resnick D, Niwayama G: On the nature and significance of bony proliferation in "rheumatoid variant" disorders. AJR 129:275, 1977.
87. Forrester DM, Kirkpatrick J: Periostitis and pseudoperiostitis. Radiology 118:597, 1976.
88. Martel W, Braunstein EM, Borlaza G, et al: Radiologic features of Reiter's syndrome. Radiology 132:1, 1979.
89. Mizutani W, Quismorio FP: Lupus foot: Deforming arthropathy of the feet in systemic lupus erythematosus. J Rheumatol 11:80, 1984.
90. Pachman LN: Juvenile dermatomyositis. Pediatr Clin North Am 33:1097, 1986.
91. Czirjak L, Nagy Z, Szegedi G: Systemic sclerosis in the elderly. Clin Rheumatol 11:483, 1992.
92. Resnick D, Niwayama G, Georgen TG, et al: Clinical, radiographic and pathologic abnormalities in calcium pyrophosphate dihydrate deposition disease (CPPD): Pseudogout. Radiology 122:1, 1977.
93. Steinbach LS, Resnick D: Calcium pyrophosphate dihydrate crystal deposition disease revisited. Radiology 200:1, 1996.
94. Archer BD, Friedman L, Stigenbauer S, et al: Symptomatic calcific tendinitis at unusual sites. J Can Assoc Radiol 43:203, 1992.
95. Resnick D: Gouty arthritis. *In* Diagnosis of Bone and Joint Disorders. 3rd Ed. Philadelphia, WB Saunders, 1995, p 1511.
96. Jonge-Bok JMD, Macfarlane JD: The articular diversity of early haemochromatosis. J Bone Joint Surg [Br] 69:41, 1987.
97. Holm CL: Primary synovial chondromatosis of the ankle: A case report. J Bone Joint Surg [Am] 58:878, 1976.
98. Kramer J, Recht M, Deely DM, et al: MR appearance of idiopathic synovial osteochondromatosis. J Comput Assist Tomogr 17:772, 1993.
99. Gamble JG, Bellah J, Rinsky LA, et al: Arthropathy of the ankle in hemophilia. J Bone Joint Surg [Am] 73:1008, 1991.
100. Jensen BN, Christensen KS: Diabetic osteoarthropathy: Rapid osteoarthropathic progression in the tarsal and tarso-metatarsal joints. J Orthop Rheumatol 5:179, 1992.

101. Gold RH, Tong DJF, Crim JR, et al: Imaging of the diabetic foot. Skeletal Radiol 24:563, 1995.
102. Hasegawa Y, Ninomiya M, Yamada Y, et al: Osteoarthropathy in congenital sensory neuropathy with anhidrosis. Clin Orthop 258:232, 1990.
103. Horibe S, Tada K, Nagano J: Neuroarthropathy of the foot in leprosy. J Bone Joint Surg [Br] 70:481, 1988.
104. Bjorkengren AG, Weisman M, Pathria MN, et al: Neuroarthropathy associated with chronic alcoholism. AJR 151:743, 1988.
105. Brown FE, Spiegel PK, Boyle WE Jr: Digital deformity: An effect of frostbite in children. Pediatrics 71:955, 1983.
106. Atkinson RE, Smith RJ: Silicone synovitis following silicone implant arthroplasty. Hand Clin 2:291, 1986.
107. Bornstein DL, Weinberg AN, Swartz MN, et al: Anaerobic infections—review of current experience. Medicine 43:207, 1964.
108. Morrison WB, Schweitzer ME, Wapner KL, et al: Osteomyelitis in feet of diabetics: Clinical accuracy, surgical utility, and cost-effectiveness of MR imaging. Radiology 196:557, 1995.
109. Beltran J, Campanini DS, Knight C, et al: The diabetic foot: Magnetic resonance imaging evaluation. Skeletal Radiol 19:37, 1990.
110. Mendelson EB, Fisher MR, Deschler TW, et al: Osteomyelitis in the diabetic foot: A difficult diagnostic challenge. RadioGraphics 3:248, 1983.
111. Gold RH, Hawkins RA, Katz RD: Bacterial osteomyelitis: Findings on plain radiography, CT, MR, and scintigraphy. AJR 157:365, 1991.
112. Feldman F, Auerbach R, Johnston A: Tuberculous dactylitis in the adult. AJR 112:460, 1971.
113. Resnick D, Niwayama G: Osteomyelitis, septic arthritis, and soft tissue infection: Organisms. *In* Resnick D: Diagnosis of Bone and Joint Disorders. 3rd Ed. Philadelphia, WB Saunders, 1995, p 2448.
114. Libson E, Bloom RA, Husband JE, et al: Metastatic tumours of bones of the hand and foot: A comparative review and report of 43 additional cases. Skeletal Radiol 16:387, 1987.
115. Miyayama H, Sakamoto K, Ide M, et al: Aggressive osteoblastoma of the calcaneus. Cancer 71:346, 1993.
116. Huvos AG, Higinbotham NL: Primary fibrosarcoma of bone: A clinicopathologic study of 130 patients. Cancer 35:837, 1975.
117. Dahlin DC, Coventry MB, Scanlon PW: Ewing's sarcoma: A critical analysis of 165 cases. J Bone Joint Surg [Am] 43:185, 1961.
118. Buck P, Mickelson MR, Bonfiglio M: Synovial sarcoma: A review of 33 cases. Clin Orthop 156:211, 1981.
119. Kyle RA: Multiple myeloma: Review of 869 cases. Mayo Clin Proc 50:29, 1975.
120. Greenspan A: Bone island (enostosis): Current concept—a review. Skeletal Radiol 24:111, 1995.
121. Loizaga JM, Calvo M, Barea FL, et al: Osteoblastoma and osteoid osteoma: Clinical and morphological features of 162 cases. Pathol Res Pract 189:33, 1993.
122. Muse G, Rayan G: Subungual exostosis. Orthopedics 9:997, 1986.
123. Brien EW, Mirra JM, Kerr R: Benign and malignant cartilage tumors of bone and joint: Their anatomic and theoretical basis with an emphasis on radiology, pathology and clinical biology. 1. The intramedullary cartilage tumors. Skeletal Radiol 26:325, 1997.
124. Moore TM, Roe JB, Harvey JP: Chondroblastoma of the talus: A case report. J Bone Joint Surg [Am] 59:830, 1977.
125. Weatherall PT, Maale GE, Mendelsohn DB, et al: Chondroblastoma: Classic and confusing appearance at MR imaging. Radiology 190:467, 1994.
126. Dahlin DC: Giant cell tumor of bone: Highlights of 407 cases. AJR 144:955, 1985.
127. Södegard J, Karaharju EO: Calcaneal cysts: Diagnosis and treatment. Fr J Orthop Surg 4:424, 1990.
128. Milgram JW: Intraosseous lipoma: A clinicopathologic study of 66 cases. Clin Orthop 231:277, 1988.
129. De Dios AMV, Bond JR, Shives TC, et al: Aneurysmal bone cyst: A clinico-pathologic study of 238 cases. Cancer 69:2921, 1992.
130. Matfin G. McPherson F: Paget's disease of bone: Recent advances. J Orthop Rheumatol 6:127, 1993.
131. Mirra JM, Brien EW, Tehranzadeh J: Paget's disease of bone: Review with emphasis on radiologic features. Part II. Skeletal Radiol 24:173, 1995.
132. Gibson MJ, Middlemiss JH: Fibrous dysplasia of bone. Br J Radiol 44:1, 1971.
133. Taylor JAM, Resnick D, Sartoris DJ: Radiographic-pathologic correlation. *In* Sartoris DJ: Osteoporosis: Diagnosis and Treatment. New York, Marcel Dekker, 1996, p 147.
134. Clouston WM, Lloyd HM: Immobilization-induced hypercalcemia and regional osteoporosis. Clin Orthop 216:247, 1987.
135. Resnick D: Neuromuscular disorders. *In* Resnick D: Diagnosis of Bone and Joint Disorders. 3rd Ed. Philadelphia, WB Saunders, 1995, p 3365.
136. Mankin HJ: Metabolic bone disease. J Bone Joint Surg [Am] 76:760, 1994.
137. Tigges S, Nance EP, Carpenter WA, et al: Renal osteodystrophy: Imaging findings that mimic those of other diseases. AJR 165:143, 1995.
138. Edmondson ME, Morrison N, Laws JW, et al: Medial arterial calcification and diabetic neuropathy. Br Med J 284:928.
139. Lang EK, Bessler WT: The roentgenologic features of acromegaly. AJR 86:321, 1961.
140. Gonticas SK, Ikkos DG, Stergiou LH: Evaluation of the diagnostic value of heel-pad thickness in acromegaly. Radiology 92:304, 1969.
141. Greenfield GB: Bone changes in chronic adult Gaucher's disease. AJR 110:800, 1970.
142. Stevens MCG, Padwick GR, Serjeant GR: Observations on the natural history of dactylitis in homozygous sickle cell disease. Clin Pediatr 20:311, 1981.
143. Morris HD: Aseptic necrosis of the talus following injury. Orthop Clin North Am 5:177, 1974.
144. Donnelly EF: The Hawkins sign. Radiology 210:195, 1999.
145. Williams GA, Cowell HR: Köhler's disease of the tarsal navicular. Clin Orthop 158:53, 1981.
146. Haller J, Sartoris DJ, Resnick D, et al: Spontaneous osteonecrosis of the tarsal navicular in adults: Imaging findings. AJR 151:355, 1988.
147. Hoskinson J: Freiberg's disease: A review of long-term results. Proc R Soc Med 67:106, 1974.

CHAPTER 12

Ribs, Sternum, and Sternoclavicular Joints

- Normal Developmental Anatomy
- Developmental Anomalies, Anatomic Variants, and Skeletal Dysplasias
- Physical Injury
- Articular Disorders
- Neoplasms
- Metabolic, Hematologic, and Infectious Disorders

Normal Developmental Anatomy

The accurate assessment of pediatric radiographs of the ribs, sternum, and sternoclavicular joints requires a thorough knowledge of normal developmental anatomy. Table 12–1 outlines the ages of appearance and fusion of the primary and secondary ossification centers. Figures 12–1 and 12–2 demonstrate the radiographic appearance of the development of the thoracic cage at different ages from infancy to skeletal maturity.

Developmental Anomalies, Anatomic Variants, and Skeletal Dysplasias

Developmental anomalies, normal variations, and, occasionally, skeletal dysplasias affect the ribs, sternum, and sternoclavicular joints. Table 12–2 and Figures 12–3 to 12–7 illustrate some of the more commonly encountered processes. Table 12–3 lists the major causes of rib notching.

Physical Injury

Physical injury, including fractures and joint trauma, may involve the ribs, sternum, and sternoclavicular joints alone, in combination with each other, or in combination with other spinal, pelvic, abdominal, and thoracic visceral injuries. Some combined injuries are discussed in more depth in Chapters 3 and 13 in association with the thoracic spine and shoulder, respectively. Table 12–4 lists the important injuries in this region and describes their characteristics. Many examples of these injuries are illustrated in Figures 12–9 to 12–17. Table 12–5 lists some of the causes of an extrapleural mass.

Articular Disorders

The sternoclavicular, costovertebral, manubriosternal, and sternocostal joints are frequent target sites of involvement for degenerative, inflammatory, metabolic, and infectious arthropathies. Table 12–6 outlines these diseases and their characteristics, and Figures 12–18 to 12–24 provide examples of the typical radiographic manifestations.

Neoplasms

Many different malignant, benign, and tumor-like lesions affect the ribs. The most common neoplasms are listed in Table 12–7, many of which are illustrated in Figures 12–25 to 12–38.

Metabolic, Hematologic, and Infectious Disorders

Table 12–8 describes a wide variety of metabolic, hematologic, and infectious disorders that may involve the ribs and sternum. The radiographic manifestations of many of these conditions are illustrated in Figures 12–39 to 12–43.

TABLE 12–1. Ribs and Sternum: Approximate Age of Appearance and Fusion of Ossification Centers[1–3] (Figs. 12–1 and 12–2)

Ossification Center	Primary or Secondary	No. of Centers (Per Rib)	Age of Appearance* (Year)	Age of Fusion* (Year)	Comments
Ribs					
Body	P	1	Birth	22–25	Head and tubercle fuse to body
Head	S	1	14	22–25	Fuses to body
Tubercle	S	1 or 2	14	22–25	Fuses to body Ribs 1 to 10 only
Sternum					
Manubrium	P	1	Birth	No fusion	Infrequently fuses to body in old age
Body of first segment	P	1	Birth	8–25	Fuses to second segment
Body of second segment	P	1	Birth	8–25	Fuses to third segment
Body of third segment	P	1	Birth	4–8	Fuses to fourth segment
Body of fourth segment	P	1	Birth		
Xiphoid process	S	1	3–4	No fusion	Infrequently fuses to fourth segment in old age

*Ages of appearance and fusion of ossification centers in girls typically precede those of boys. Ethnic differences also exist.
P, Primary; S, secondary.

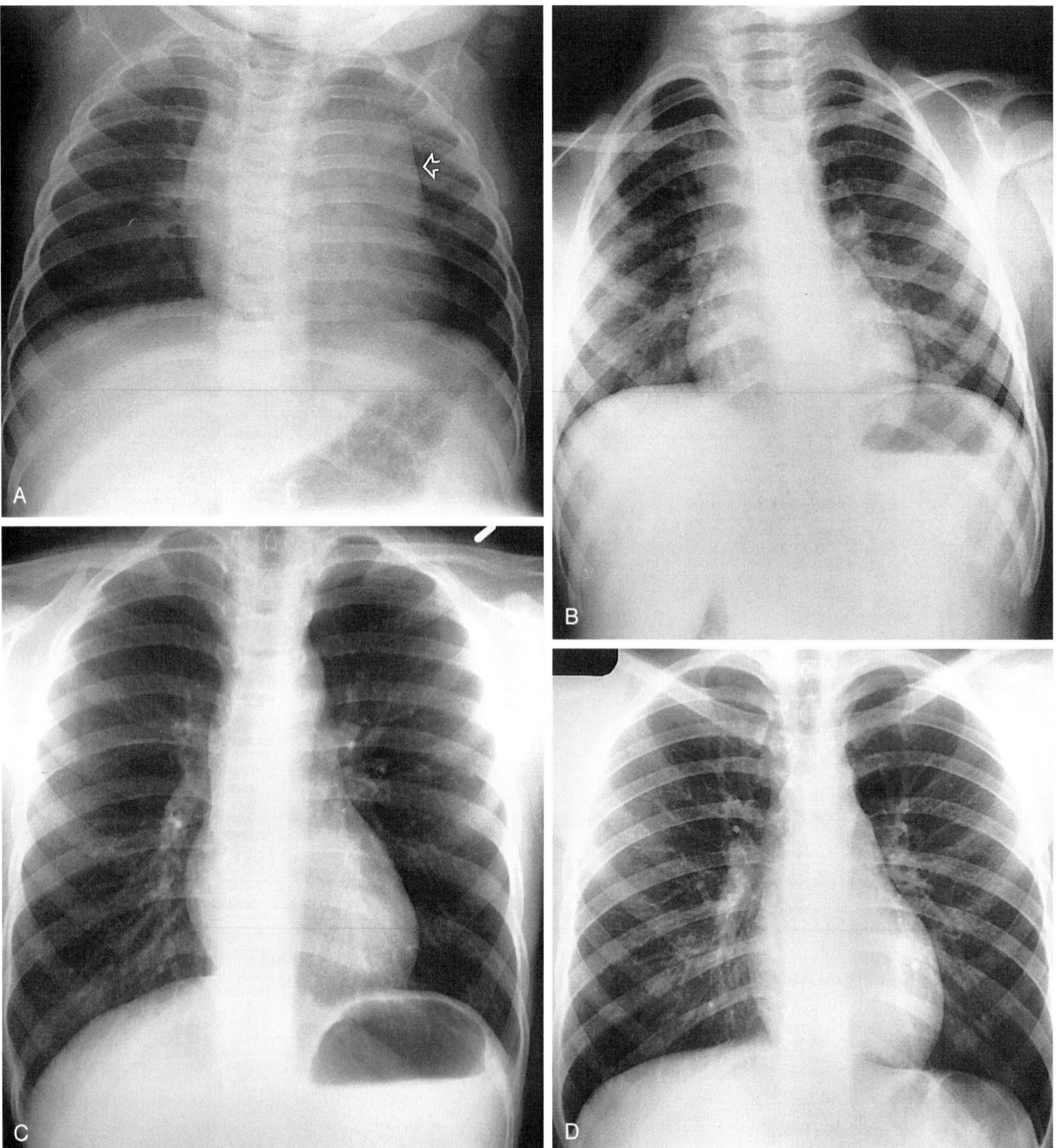

FIGURE 12–1. Skeletal maturation and normal development: Frontal radiographs of the thoracic cage.[1–3] A 7-month-old girl. The cardiac silhouette is disproportionately large in relation to the size of the thoracic cage. A prominent thymus gland (open arrow), a normal finding in infants, also is apparent in this patient. B 3-year-old girl. C 8-year-old girl. D 14-year-old boy. The heart and mediastinum are of adult proportions. Secondary ossification centers of the rib heads and tubercles usually appear between the ages of 14 to 16 years and fuse to the body of the rib by the age of 25 years (not shown). Rib tubercles typically do not develop on the eleventh and twelfth ribs.

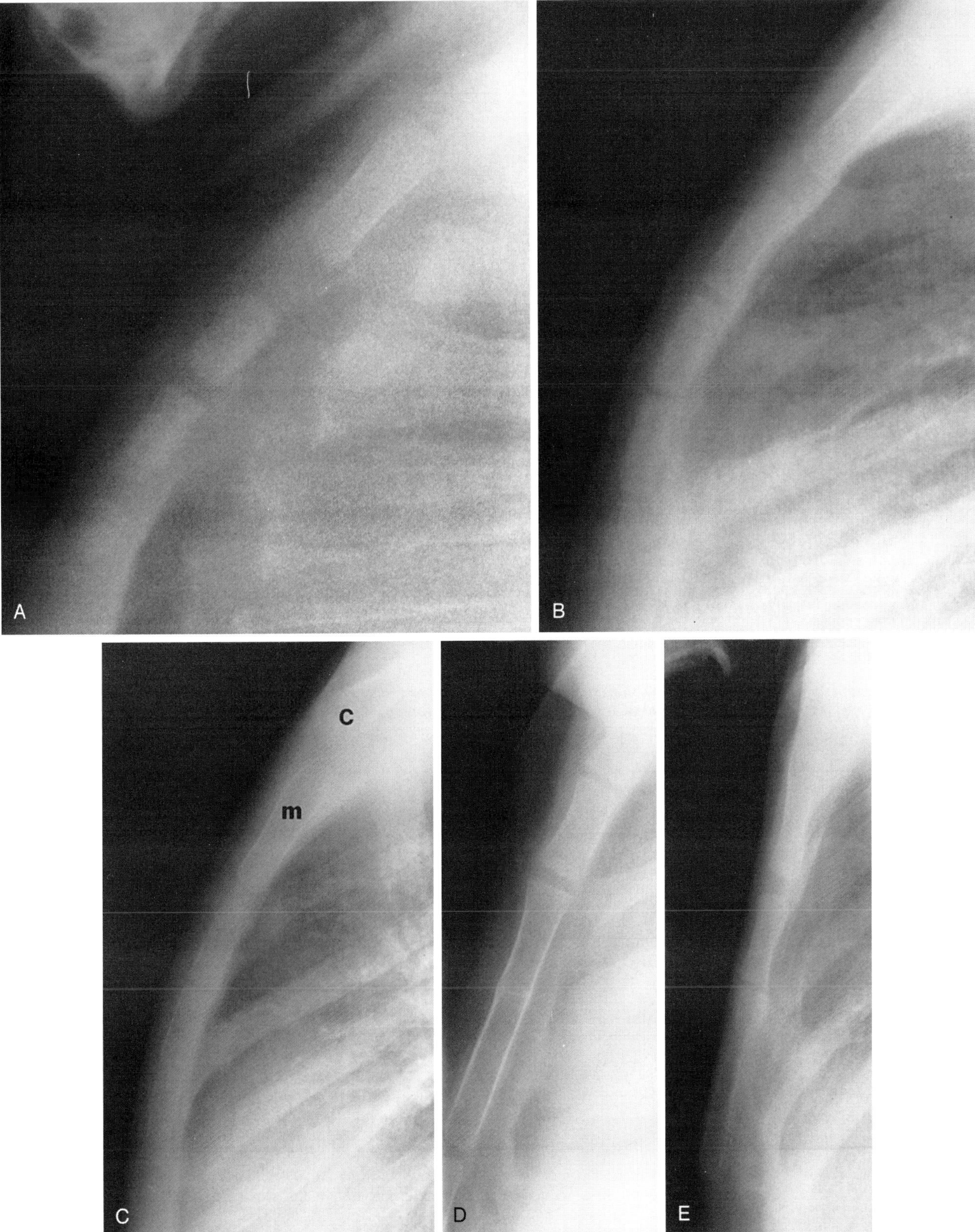

FIGURE 12–2. Skeletal maturation and normal development: Sternum.[1–3] A 2-month-old boy. At this age, the sternum is ossified but large gaps, filled with cartilage, remain between the individual segments. B 3-year-old girl. As ossification proceeds, the intersegmental gaps become narrower. C 7-year-old boy. The first, second, and third segments of the sternal body are beginning to fuse. The normal clavicle (c) should not be confused with a dislocation of the manubrium (m). D 12-year-old boy. The second and third segments have fused. E 14-year-old boy. The intersegmental centers have fused, but the manubriosternal junction remains open.

Illustration continued on following page

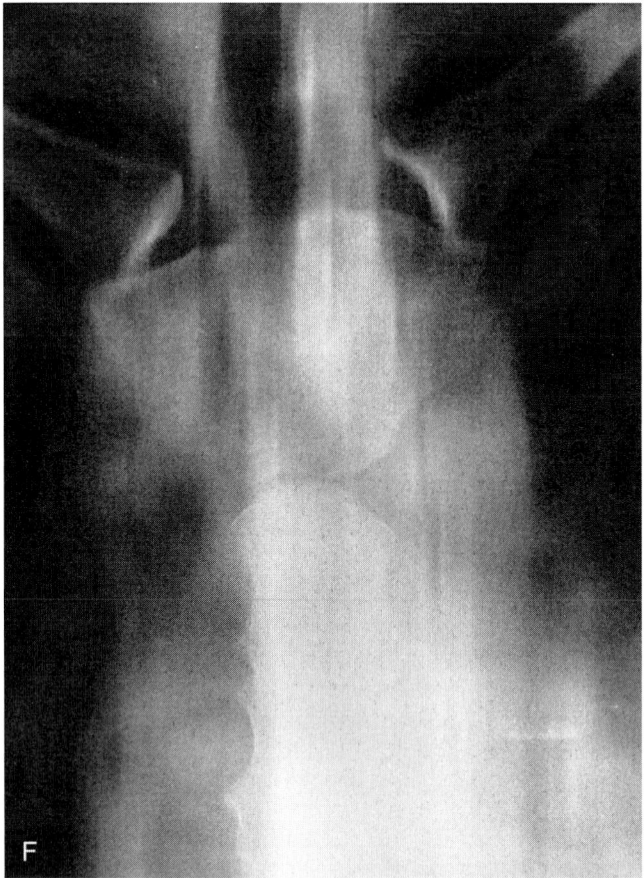

FIGURE 12–2 *Continued.* F Adult: 35-year-old woman. This coronal conventional tomogram reveals the sternoclavicular joints and manubriosternal junction. Observe that the manubrium has not fused to the sternal body.

The primary ossification centers of the manubrium and three or four segments of the sternal body typically are ossified at birth. The secondary ossification center of the xiphoid process first appears about the age of 15 years. The intersegmental centers of the sternal body fuse between the ages of 8 and 25 years. Fusion of the manubriosternal junction occurs only rarely. When it does, fusion occurs after the age of 30 years.

TABLE 12–2. Developmental Anomalies, Anatomic Variants, and Skeletal Dysplasias Affecting the Ribs and Sternum*

Entity	Figure(s)	Characteristics
Ribs		
Cervical rib[4–6]	2–34	Transverse processes of C7 typically are shorter than those of T1 Both elongated C7 transverse processes and cervical ribs may contribute to neurovascular compression at the thoracic outlet Cervical ribs are present in 10–15 per cent of patients with the Klippel-Feil syndrome (see also Table 2–4)
Transitional rib anomalies[3, 4]	4–7 12–3	Wide variation of hypoplastic, hyperplastic, and unusually shaped ribs may occur at the thoracolumbar transitional region; usually of no clinical significance Lumbar rib: anomalous supernumerary ribs articulating with the transverse processes of the first lumbar vertebra Other entities include horizontal ribs, asymmetric ribs, and ribs associated with vertebral anomalies
Intrathoracic rib[7–9]	12–4	Extremely rare anomaly in which a rib protrudes within the thoracic cavity Usually unilateral and generally asymptomatic Occasionally, the intrathoracic rib may have a fibrous diaphragmatic attachment, which can disrupt respiration

TABLE 12–2. Developmental Anomalies, Anatomic Variants, and Skeletal Dysplasias Affecting the Ribs and Sternum* *Continued*

Entity	Figure(s)	Characteristics
Rib foramen[5]		Rare anomaly; radiolucent foramen may involve any rib; no clinical significance; may simulate an osteolytic lesion
Bifurcated rib[3, 5]		Anomalous bifurcation in anterior aspect of rib near its costochondral junction; no clinical significance
Rib synostosis[3, 5]	12–5	Complete or incomplete anomalous fusion of two adjacent ribs, usually of no clinical significance Srb's anomaly: rare anomalous synostosis of the first and second ribs Osseous bridging of small segments of two adjacent ribs, with or without pseudarthrosis, also has been reported
Congenital pseudarthrosis[5]		Anomalous failure of ossification of the central portion of the first rib Margins are smooth and well-corticated but may have bulbous appearance Usually painless but may simulate fatigue fracture
Costochondral cartilage calcification or ossification[3, 10]	12–6	Calcification or ossification of the costochondral cartilage may begin as early as age 20 years; appears to be a physiologic reaction to muscular contraction related to the relative rigidity of chest wall On frontal radiographs, the ossification appears fork-like in men and tongue-like in women On lateral radiographs, large calcified masses may be seen overlying the sternum Especially prevalent in older individuals, and usually of no clinical significance Also found in children with hyperthyroidism
Achondroplasia[5]		Symmetric shortening of ribs; may not completely extend around the thorax
Osteopetrosis[5]		Diffuse sclerosis of ribs with predisposition to rib fracture
Sternum		
Sternal foramen[11]		Vascular channel within the lower sternal body; occurs in as many as 20 per cent of adults; asymptomatic variant of no clinical significance
Sternal fissure (bifid sternum)[3, 12]		Rare anomalous failure of fusion of the sternal ridges resulting in a midline vertical split in any segment of the sternum Complete fissure often associated with anomalies of diaphragm, heart, and other organs Incomplete fissure not usually associated with other anomalies
Asymmetry of developing ossification centers[3, 4]		Numerous anatomic variants and anomalies of development frequently result in asymmetric or unusual shape of the manubrium, body, and xiphoid process
Accessory ossicles[3]		Variant seen in as many as 4 per cent of adults Os episternalia (or suprasternalia) located above the manubrium; often paired Os parasternalia located lateral to the manubrium in the cartilage of the first ribs
Absent xiphoid process[3]		Normal finding in 47 per cent of women and in 9 per cent of men
Pectus excavatum[3, 13]	12–7	Funnel chest: common chest wall deformity; may be an isolated anomaly or it may accompany Marfan syndrome or Ehlers-Danlos syndrome Depression of sternum seen best on physical examination and on lateral radiographs; displacement of heart toward left hemithorax may obscure right heart border on frontal radiographs
Pectus carinatum[3, 5]		Pigeon breast: deformity characterized by anterior displacement of the sternum; may be an isolated anomaly or may be associated with Morquio's syndrome
Cleidocranial dysplasia[3, 5]		Hypoplasia or aplasia of the sternoclavicular joint found in combination with clavicular abnormalities

*See also Tables 1–1 and 1–2.

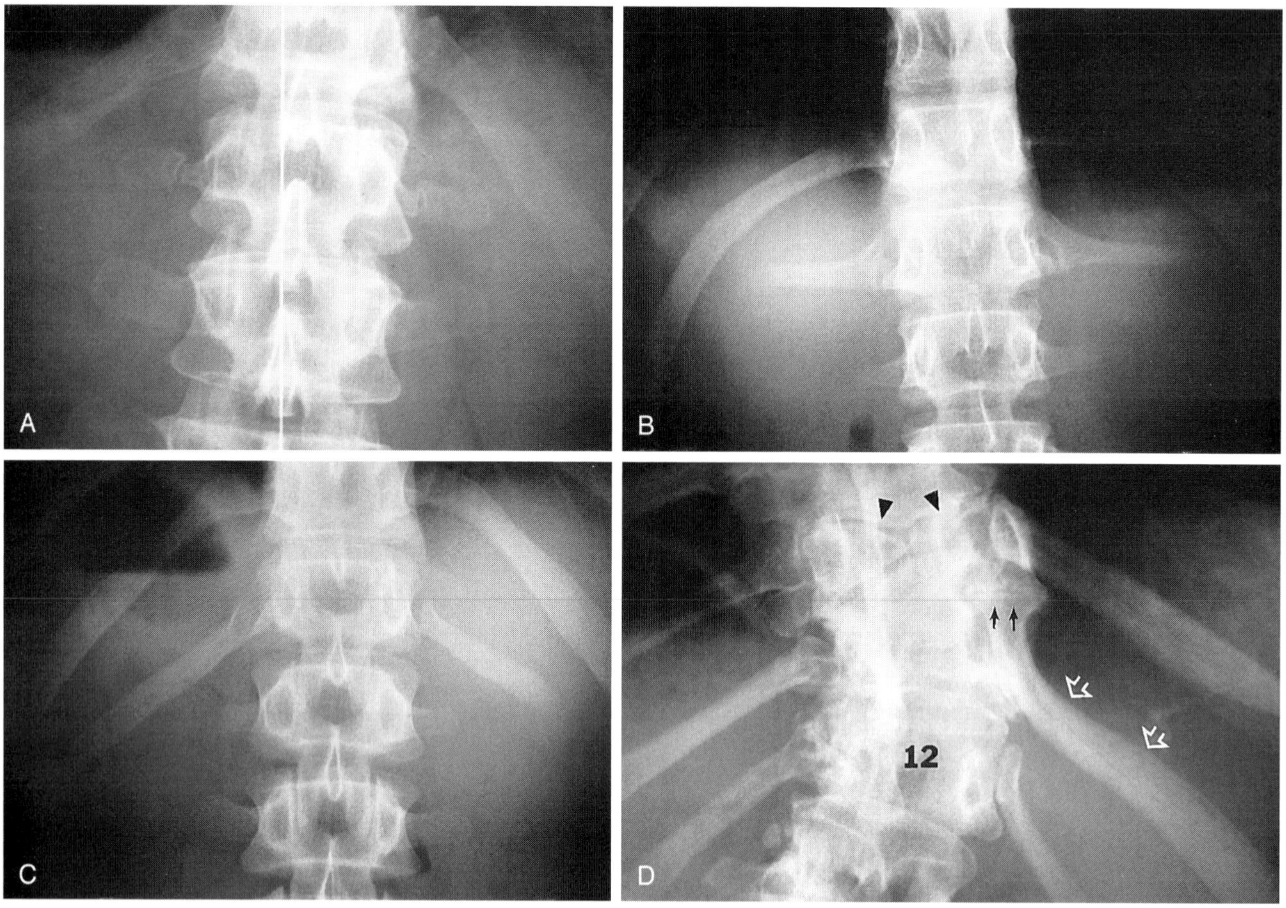

FIGURE 12–3. Transitional rib anomalies and anatomic variations.[3, 4] A Lumbar ribs. Observe the small articulating ribs arising from the L1 transverse processes. B Horizontal twelfth ribs. The twelfth ribs are short, straight, and oriented horizontally. C Asymmetric twelfth ribs. Observe the variation in the length of the two twelfth ribs. D Anomalous ribs associated with spinal anomalies. A short, angular kyphosis is associated with a T10 butterfly vertebra (arrowheads). The eleventh thoracic vertebra is wedge-shaped. The left eleventh rib has an abnormal costovertebral articulation (arrows) and exhibits stress-induced reactive sclerosis (open arrows).

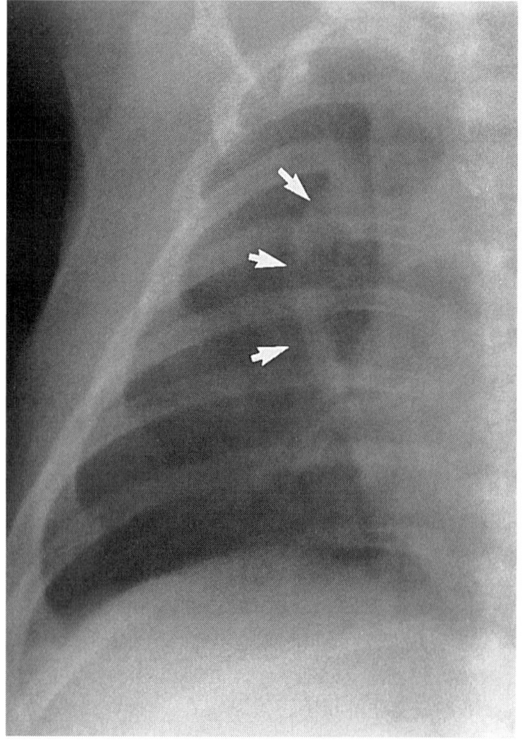

FIGURE 12–4. Intrathoracic rib.[7–9] An anomalous rib (arrows) arises from the posteroinferior margin of the right fourth rib and is projected over the inner portion of the lung field in this frontal projection. *(Courtesy of S. Hilton, M.D., San Diego, California)*

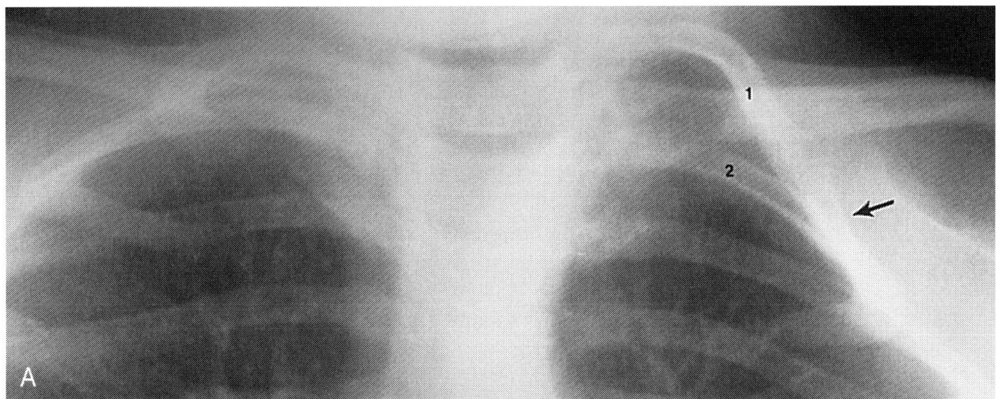

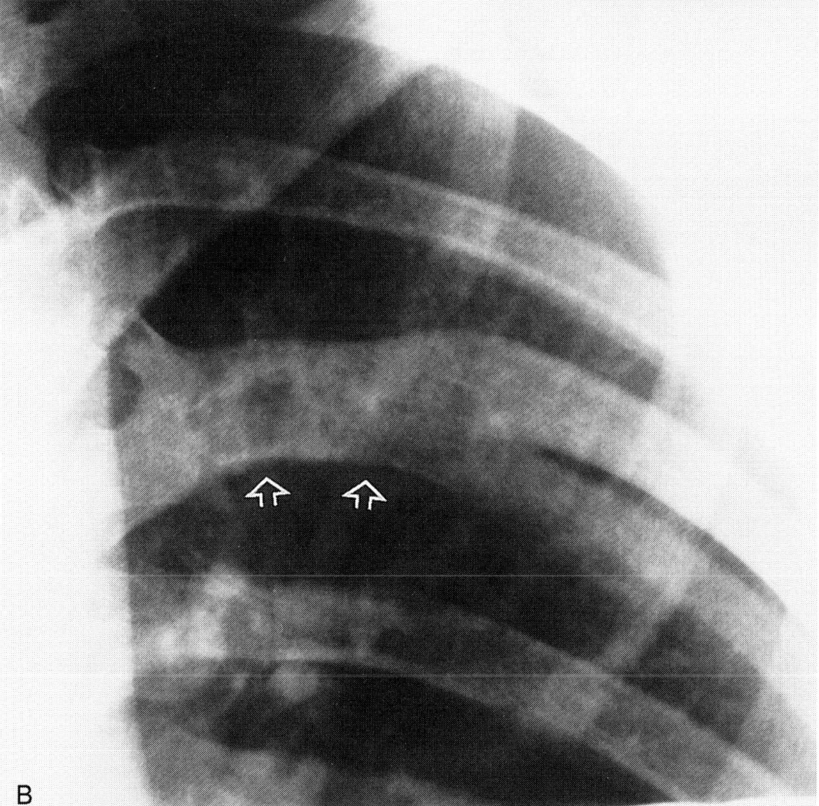

FIGURE 12–5. Rib synostosis.[3, 5] A Posteroanterior chest film in this 6-year-old child reveals anomalous fusion (arrow) of the left first (1) and second (2) ribs, resulting in an unusual depression of the left side of the thoracic cage. Such synostosis of the first and second ribs has been referred to as Srb's anomaly. B Observe the fusion of the proximal portion of the fourth and fifth ribs (open arrows) in this patient. The synostosis was asymptomatic and was discovered as an incidental finding on an earlier chest radiograph.

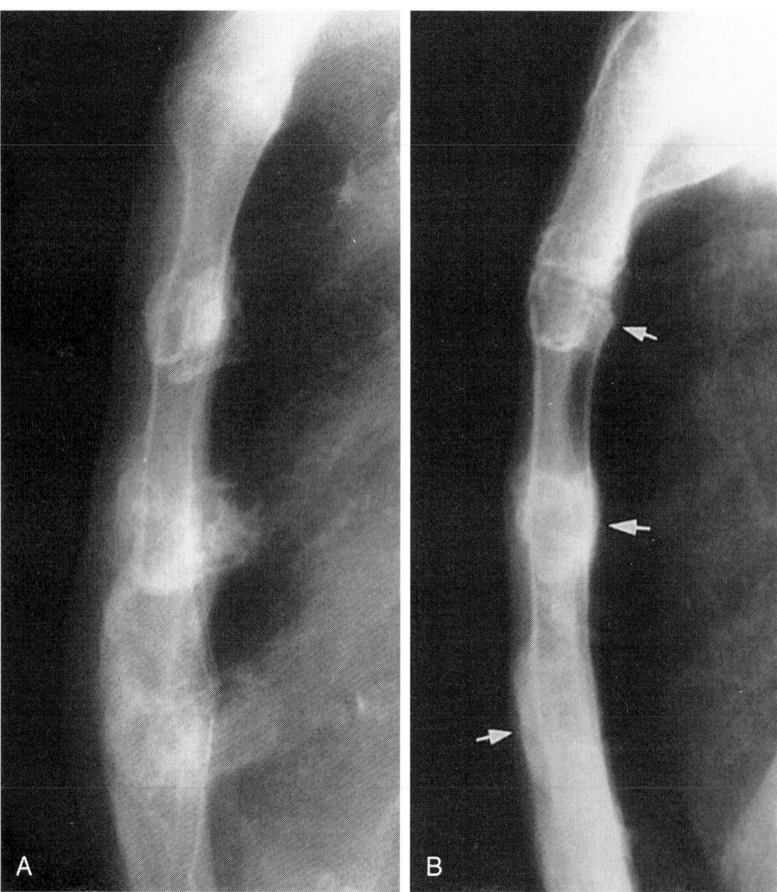

FIGURE 12–6. Costochondral calcification or ossification.[3, 10] A Lateral radiograph of the sternum reveals several bulbous zones of faintly calcified costal cartilage. B In another patient, observe the prominent, expansile appearance of calcified costal cartilages (arrows).

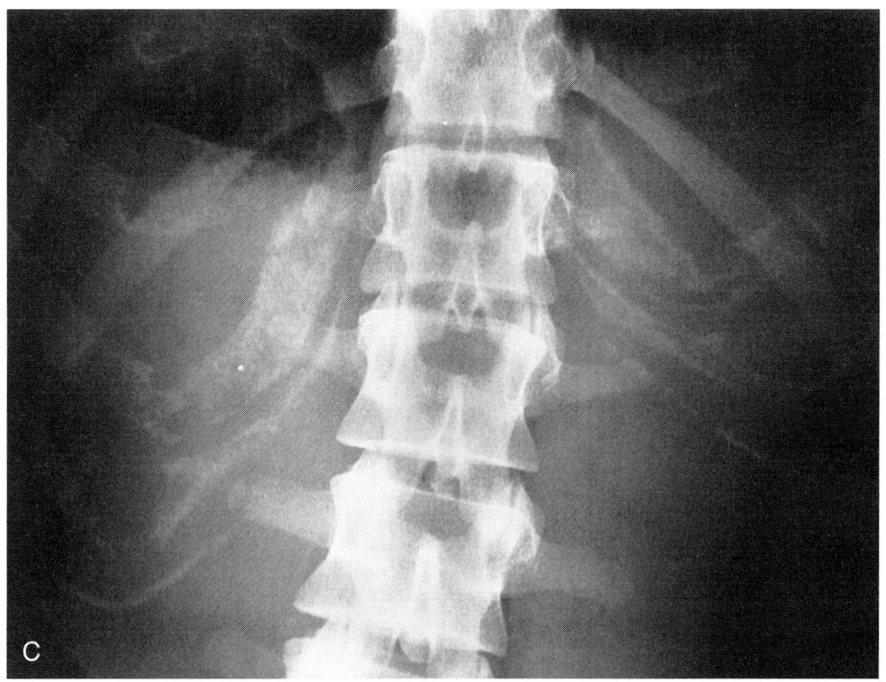

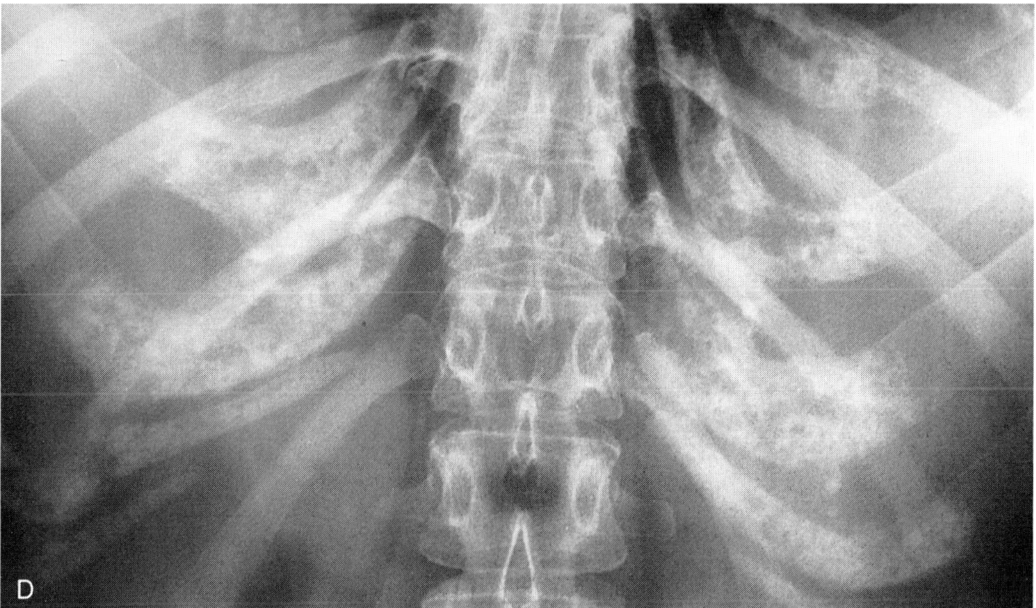

FIGURE 12–6 *Continued.* C, D In two additional patients, observe the diffuse calcification of the costochondral cartilages on frontal radiographs.

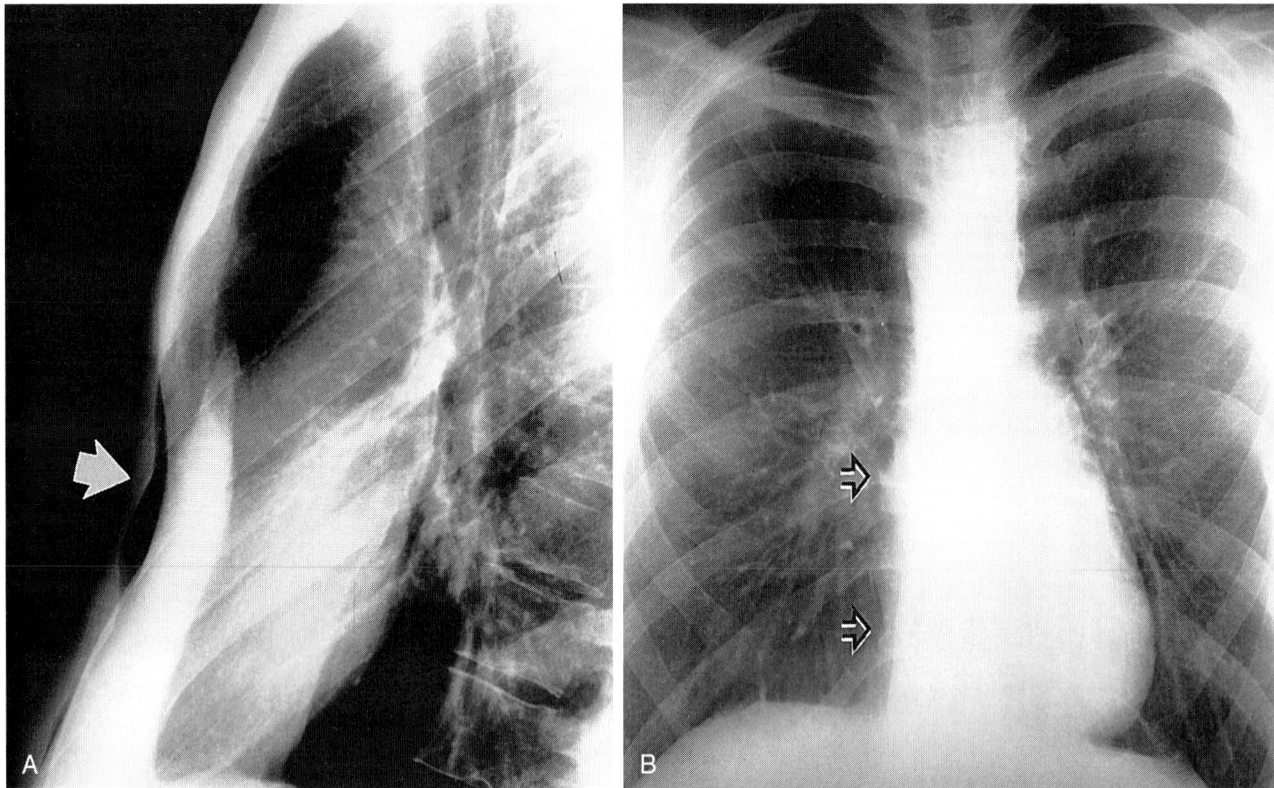

FIGURE 12–7. Pectus excavatum.[3, 13] Lateral (A) and posteroanterior (B) chest radiographs of a 27-year-old man reveal depression of the sternum (solid arrow) and displacement of the right heart border toward the left hemithorax (open arrows). This common chest wall deformity may be an isolated anomaly, or it may accompany Marfan syndrome or Ehlers-Danlos syndrome. *(Courtesy of I. Roug, D.C., Marietta, Georgia.)*

TABLE 12–3. Rib Notching[14]

Category	Specific Entities	Figure(s)	Characteristics
Normal variant	Normal persons		Prominent groove within the inferior aspect of the rib that may resemble pathologic destruction or erosion
Normal aging phenomenon	Osteoporosis in elderly patients		Postmenopausal or senile osteoporosis may result in indistinct cortical margins
Collagen vascular disease	Rheumatoid arthritis Systemic lupus erythematosus Sjögren syndrome Scleroderma		Symmetric groove-like indentations along the superior costal margins of the second to fifth ribs
Neurogenic tumors	Neurofibromatosis Thoracic neuroblastoma	See Fig. 12–37	Dysplastic bone formation contributes to twisted ribbon-like configuration of the ribs; superior and inferior erosions of adjacent ribs also may occur as a result of pressure from adjacent neurofibromas
Paralysis	Poliomyelitis Posttraumatic paralysis		Disuse osteoporosis may result in diminished mineralization of bone
Diminished muscle tone	Marfan syndrome		Thin ribs with superior and inferior defects
Subperiosteal resorption	Hyperparathyroidism Renal osteodystrophy		Subperiosteal resorption of cortical bone may resemble destructive osteolysis
Congenital heart disease and vascular disease	Coarctation of the aorta (Rösler sign) Venous dilatation Tetralogy of Fallot Surgery for congenital heart disease	12–8	Symmetric inferior (and occasionally superior) erosion, usually of the posterior margin of the fourth to eighth ribs Pressure erosion from prominent collateral circulation

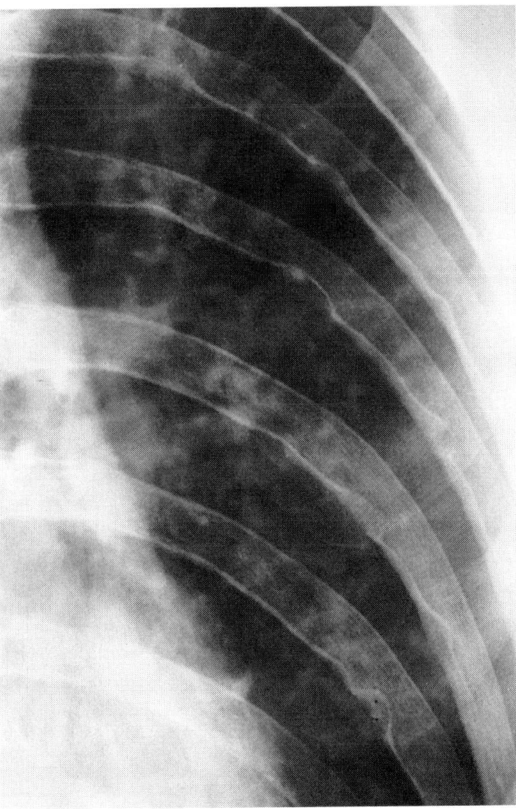

FIGURE 12–8. Coarctation of the aorta: rib notching.[14] Observe the undulating inferior rib margins in this patient. The fourth through eighth ribs were involved bilaterally. The rib notching seen in patients with coarctation of the aorta has been referred to as the Rösler sign. *(Courtesy of R. Arkless, M.D., Seabeck, Washington.)*

TABLE 12–4. Injuries of the Ribs and Sternum*

Entity	Figure(s)	Characteristics	Complications and Related Disorders
Ribs			
Acute rib fracture[15–17]	12–9 12–10	Direct injuries from falls or blows to the chest Multiple ribs commonly are fractured Crushing injuries may cause separation at the costochondral junctions or associated sternal fractures	Pneumothorax, hemothorax, lung contusion
		Fractures of first and second rib imply severe and unusual trauma	Vascular injury with fractures of upper two ribs
		Flail chest: two fractures in one rib, allowing that part of the thoracic cage to move independently of the remaining portion	Impaired ventilation, pendulum breathing, ineffective cough, hypoxia, and pulmonary edema may complicate flail chest
		Rib fractures and associated soft tissue hematoma, edema, and hemothorax also may be evaluated using diagnostic ultrasonography	

Table continued on following page

TABLE 12–4. Injuries of the Ribs and Sternum* *Continued*

Entity	Figure(s)	Characteristics	Complications and Related Disorders
Child abuse[18–20]	12–11	Any of the following findings should raise suspicion of child abuse: 1. Single or multiple rib fractures in children, especially between the ages of 1 and 4 2. Fractures at different phases of healing 3. Fractures of the rib heads adjacent to the costovertebral joints 4. Bilateral rib fractures	Multiple and unusual fractures and other signs elsewhere Child abuse may eventually result in repeated morbidity and even death if not detected and if abuse continues
Stress (fatigue) fracture of ribs[21–24]	12–12 12–13	Cough fracture: repeated coughing in bronchitis or other pulmonary disease Fatigue fractures also have been linked to carrying heavy packs and to activities associated with golf, rowing, and tennis Chronic stress from costovertebral osteoarthrosis or other articular disease may result in osteosclerotic reaction of rib	Difficulty breathing and impaired recuperation
Costovertebral joint dislocation[25]		Extremely rare, usually resulting from direct injury to the 1st, 11th, or 12th ribs Slipping rib syndrome: displacement of 10th rib at the costovertebral articulation caused by trauma; may result in upper abdominal or loin pain and may be accompanied by a snapping sensation and point tenderness	
Tietze's syndrome (costosternal syndrome)[26]		Benign, self-limited, painful enlargement of the upper costal cartilages occurring insidiously or after minor trauma Seen in as many as 10 per cent of patients with chest pain Radiographs usually normal but may reveal osteosclerosis of ribs and sternum	May simulate cardiogenic chest pain
Sternum			
Acute sternal fracture[27]	12–14	Direct trauma, such as chest-crushing injuries, result in fractures principally at the manubriosternal junction Direct blows to the upper region of the sternum may result in transverse fractures at the site of impact Indirect trauma rarely results in fracture of the sternum	Associated injury of ribs and costal cartilages Aortic, arterial, tracheal, cardiac, or pulmonary injuries may lead to death

TABLE 12–4. Injuries of the Ribs and Sternum* *Continued*

Entity	Figure(s)	Characteristics	Complications and Related Disorders
Stress (insufficiency) fracture of the sternum[28]	12–15	Severe osteoporosis and chronic progressive thoracic kyphosis infrequently result in insufficiency fractures of the sternum Osteomalacia, plasma cell myeloma, and renal osteodystrophy also may result in insufficiency fractures by the same mechanism	Progressive kyphosis
Sternoclavicular joint dislocation[29]	12–16	Sternoclavicular dislocations are rare Best evaluated by conventional tomography or computed tomography (CT) 1. Anterior dislocation: far more common than posterior dislocation; result from major, indirect trauma transmitted along the long axis of the clavicle from an injury to the shoulder region 2. Posterior dislocation: result from direct forces applied to the anteromedial aspect of the clavicle	Anterior dislocation may be associated with fractures of the ribs, sternum, and clavicle Posterior dislocations may impinge on the trachea, esophagus, great vessels, or other mediastinal structures, leading to vascular injury, cough, dysphagia, dyspnea, or even death
Manubriosternal junction dislocation[30]	12–17	Usually results from direct trauma or crushing injuries of the chest	May be associated with spinal, rib, and clavicle fractures May be complicated by injury to the aorta, other arteries, trachea, heart, and lung

*See also Tables 1–3 to 1–5.

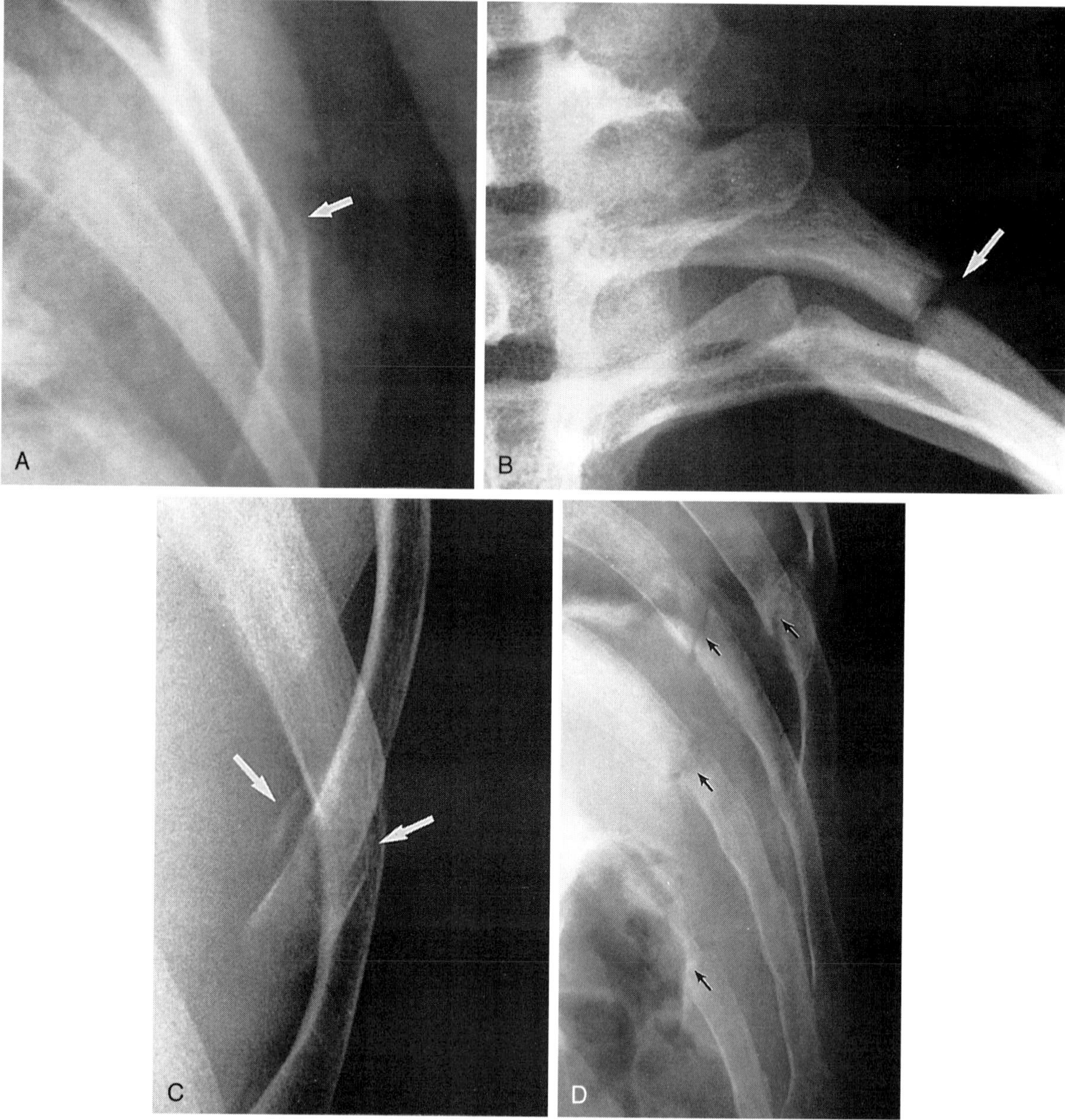

FIGURE 12–9. Acute rib fractures.[15–16] A Acute fracture in a 70-year-old man after a car accident. Observe the cortical offset of the sixth rib adjacent to the fracture site (arrow). B Acute first rib fracture. Frontal radiograph of the ribs in this 19-year-old man obtained after a body surfing injury at a rock concert shows a slightly displaced fracture of the first rib (arrow). Fractures of the first and second ribs generally occur with severe trauma and may be associated with vascular injury or other fractures of the shoulder girdle or spine. *(B, Courtesy of E.E. Bonic, D.C., Portland, Oregon.)* C Minimally displaced fracture of the eighth rib is seen 14 days after trauma. A faint zone of callus is evident (arrows). D Radiograph of the ribs, obtained 2 weeks after this rodeo bull-rider was thrown from a bull, shows multiple lower rib fractures (arrows).

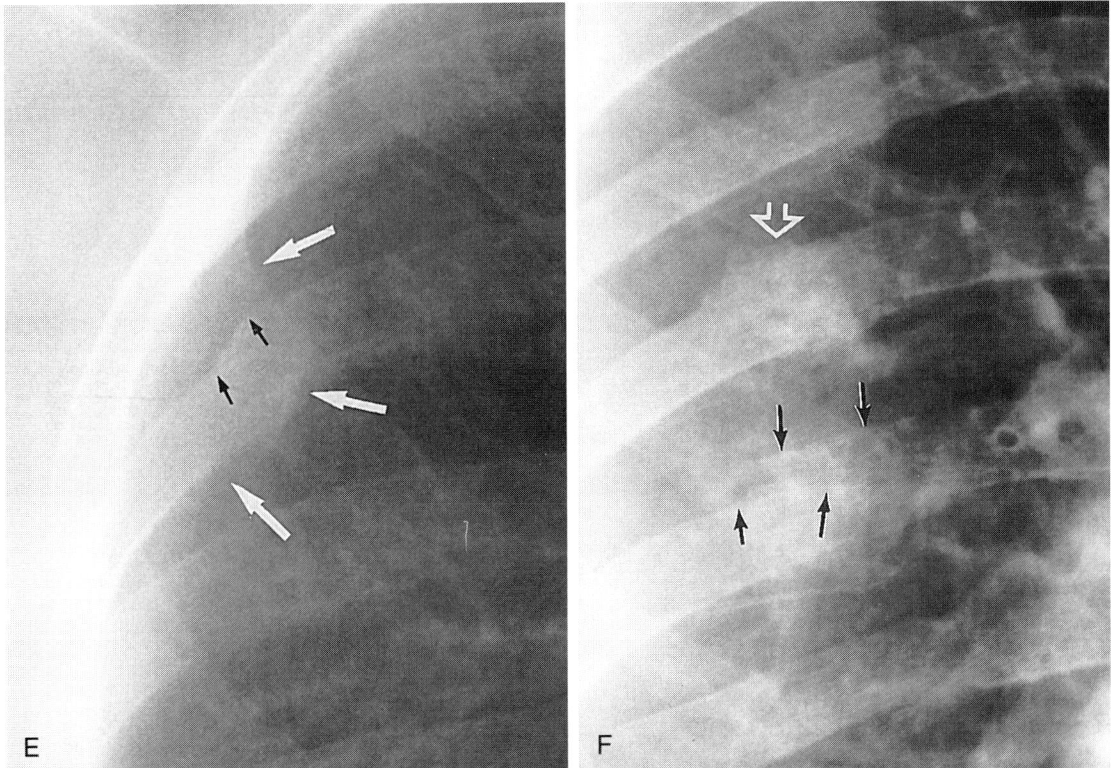

FIGURE 12–9 *Continued.* E Healing rib fracture seen in profile reveals bony offset (black arrows). A prominent extrapleural mass with tapering edges and a convex border protruding into the lung (white arrows) also is evident. F Rib displacement (arrows) and early callus formation (open arrow) are evident in another patient with rib fractures.

TABLE 12–5. Some Causes of an Extrapleural Mass[31, 32]*

	Figure(s)
Common Causes	
Rib fracture	See Fig. 12–9
Skeletal metastasis	See Fig. 12–26
Plasma cell myeloma	See Fig. 12–31
Fibrous dysplasia	See Fig. 12–38
Osteosarcoma	See Fig. 12–27
Ewing's sarcoma	See Fig. 12–30
Brown tumor	See Fig. 12–41
Chondrosarcoma	See Fig. 12–29
Mediastinal masses	
Rare Causes	
Hematoma	
Lipoma	
Neurofibroma	
Chest wall masses	
Postsurgical causes	
Chest wall infection	
Tuberculosis	
Subphrenic mass	

*An extrapleural mass is seen on chest radiographs as a radiodense area adjacent to the inner margin of the chest wall. The mass has a sharply convex margin that protrudes into and displaces the lung field. The upper and lower margins of the mass are tapered and may be concave toward the lung surface. This appearance has been termed the extrapleural sign.

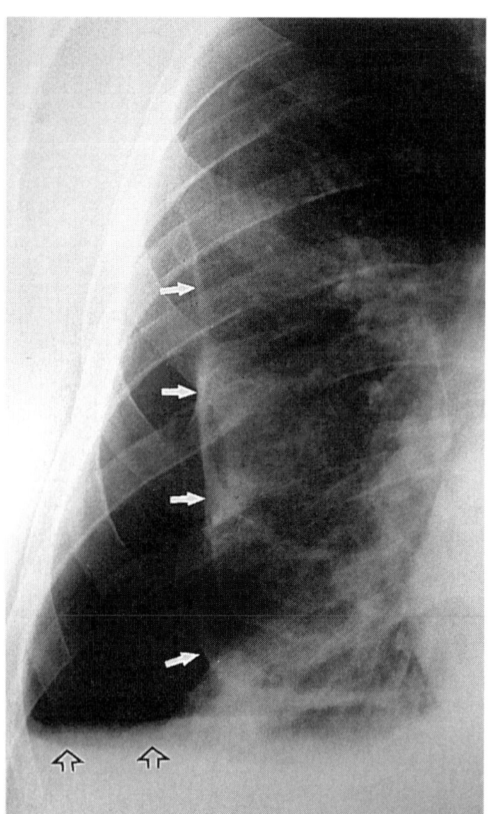

FIGURE 12–10. Posttraumatic pneumothorax.[17] This 61-year-old man sustained multiple rib fractures in a motor vehicle collision. He had severe pain and shortness of breath. Observe the medially displaced edge of the pleural margin (arrows), absence of lung markings peripherally, and excessive opacification of the lung tissue. Blunting of the costophrenic sulcus and a fluid level (open arrows) indicate the presence of a pleural effusion. Pneumothorax and hemothorax are important complications of rib fractures and other thoracic cage injuries.

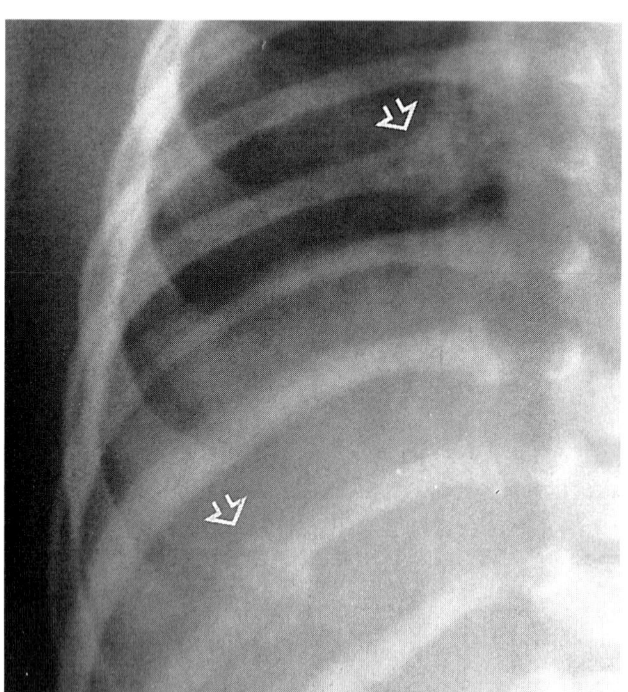

FIGURE 12–11. Child abuse.[18–20] Observe the multiple rib fractures (open arrows), a common finding in the abused child. Such fractures often are bilateral, are paravertebral, or involve the heads of the ribs. *(Courtesy of D. Edwards, M.D., San Diego, California.)*

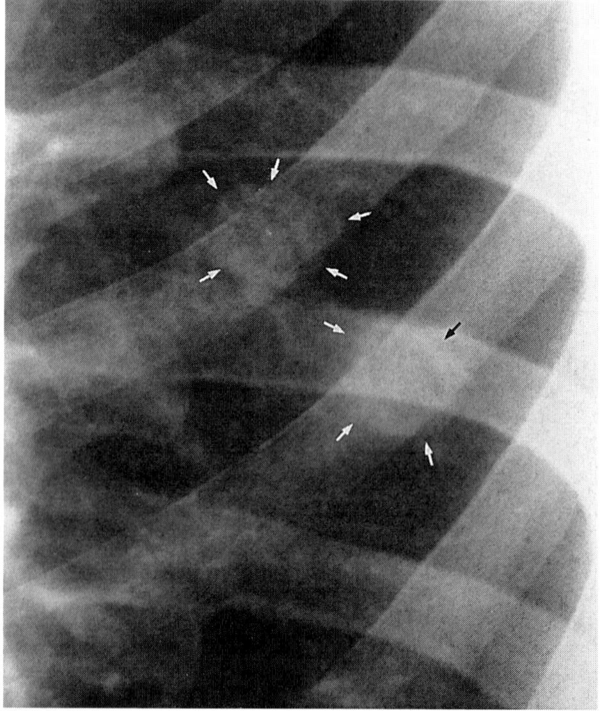

FIGURE 12–12. Stress (fatigue) fracture: Healing cough fracture.[21–24] This 39-year-old man with severe bronchitis sustained fatigue fractures of two of his ribs ("cough fractures"). Observe the callus formation surrounding the fracture sites (arrows) in these radiographs obtained 6 weeks after the initial fractures. *(Courtesy of G. Greenstein, D.C., Bridgeport, Connecticut.)*

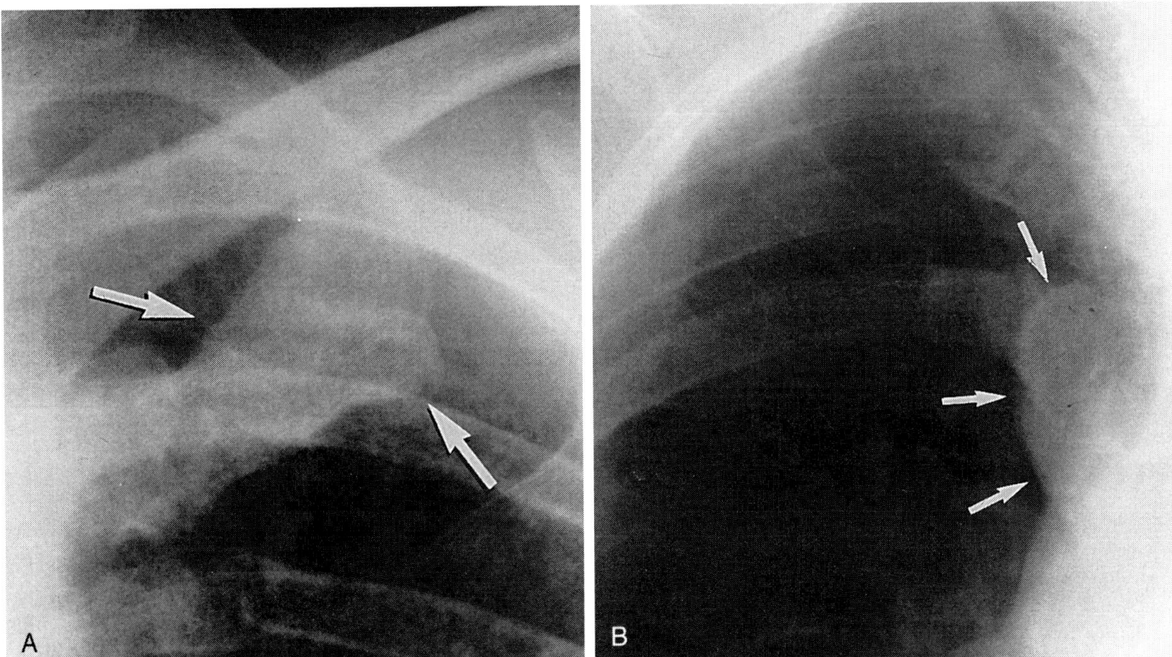

FIGURE 12–13. Stress (fatigue) fracture and reaction to stress.[21–24] A Fatigue fracture. Transverse radiolucent line with surrounding sclerosis (arrows) represents a healing fatigue fracture of the first rib secondary to repeated throwing activity. Other causes of stress fracture of this rib include golfing, carrying a back pack, coughing, or other physical activities. *(A, Courtesy of B. Groth, M.D., Mosinee, Wisconsin.)* B Reactive stress changes. Observe the diffuse sclerosis involving the posterior aspect of the rib and the costovertebral joint osteophytes in this patient with diffuse idiopathic skeletal hyperostosis (DISH) (arrows). This reactive sclerosis is seen in a variety of conditions, including costovertebral joint arthrosis, ankylosing spondylitis, and DISH.

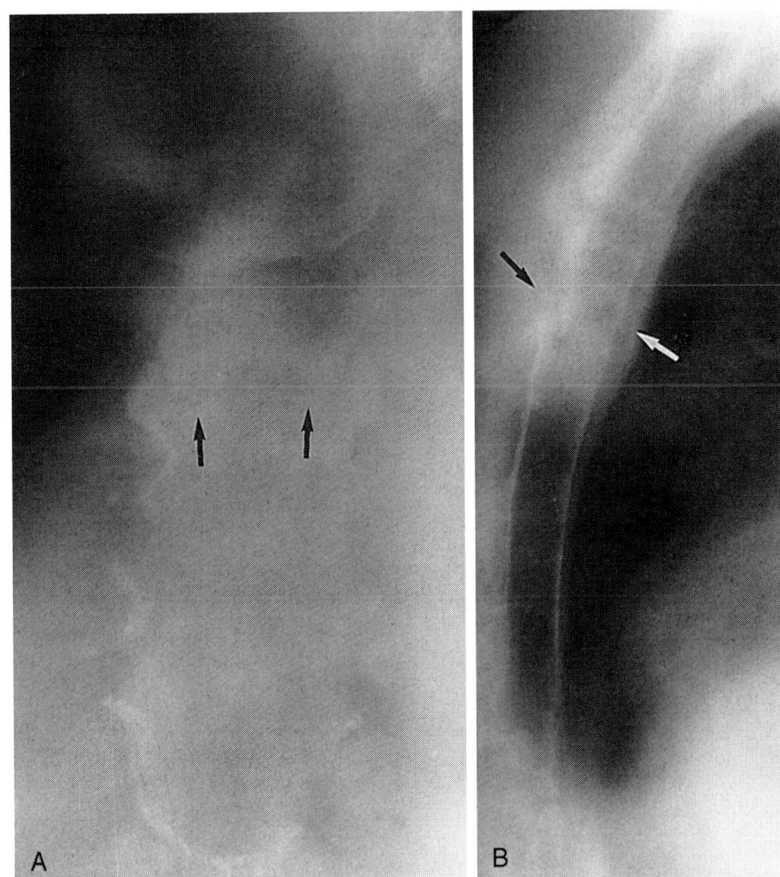

FIGURE 12–14. Acute sternal fracture.[27] Frontal (A) and lateral (B) radiographs show a transverse fracture of the sternal body, just below the manubrium (arrows). Biopsy revealed a nonpathologic fracture.

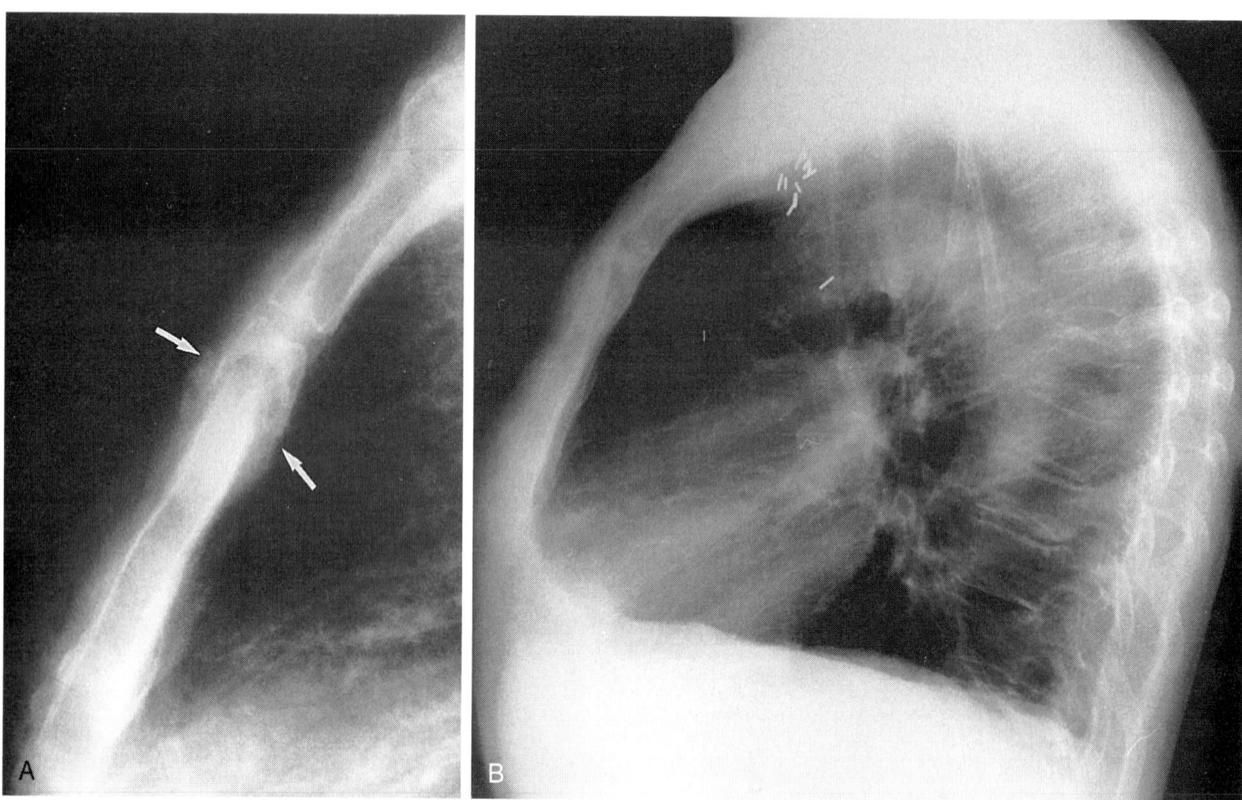

FIGURE 12–15. Stress (insufficiency) fracture of the sternum.[28] A Observe the fracture of the sternum (arrows) seen in association with progressive kyphosis in this 63-year-old woman. B Lateral chest radiograph in the same patient demonstrates osteoporosis, kyphosis, and multiple compression fractures. *(Courtesy of R. Kerr, M.D., Los Angeles, California.)*

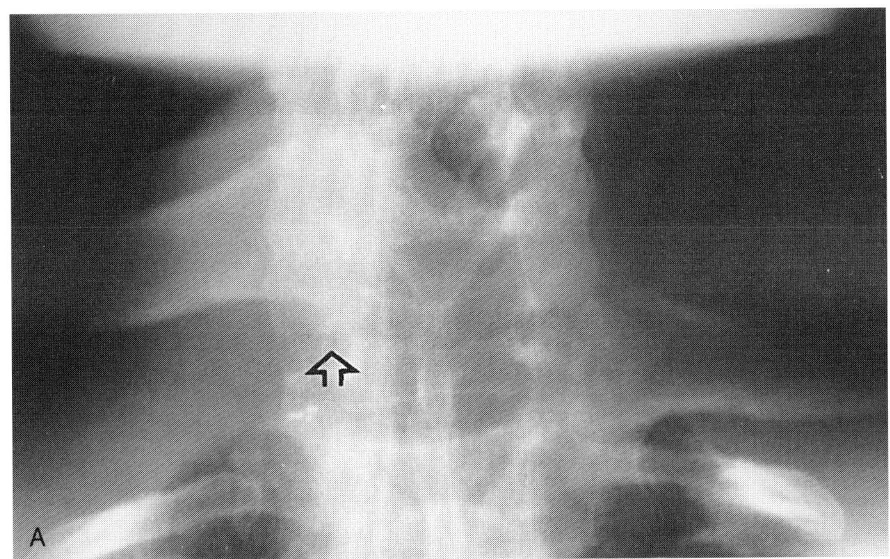

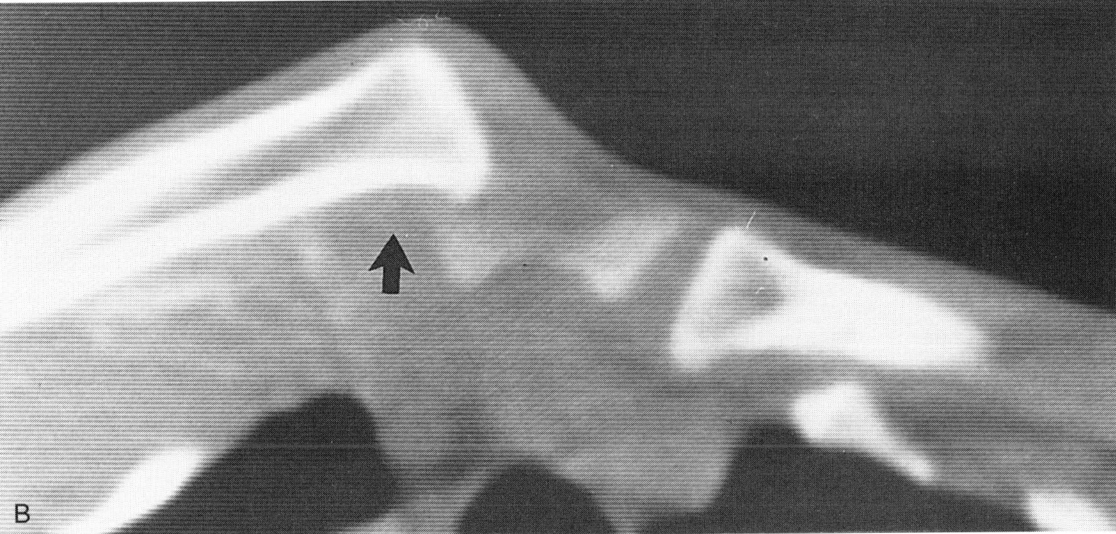

FIGURE 12–16. Sternoclavicular joint: Anterior dislocation.[29] A Frontal lordotic radiograph shows superior displacement of the right clavicle (open arrow) in relation to the opposite clavicle. B In another patient, a transaxial computed tomographic (CT) scan clearly displays the anterior dislocation of the sternoclavicular joint (arrow). Sternoclavicular joint dislocations are rare. Anterior dislocation, far more common than posterior dislocation, typically results from major, indirect trauma transmitted along the long axis of the clavicle from an injury to the shoulder region.

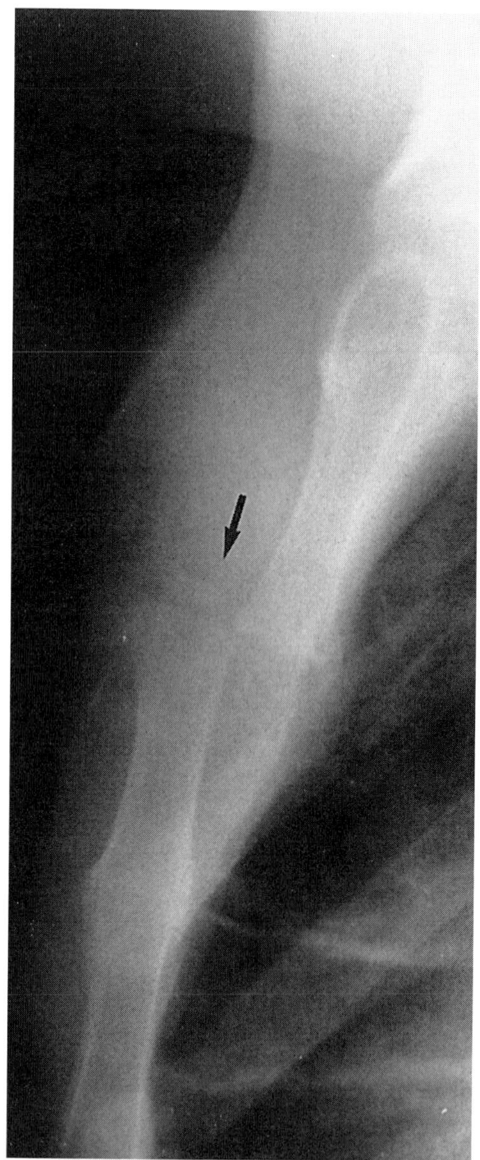

FIGURE 12–17. Manubriosternal junction dislocation.[30] Observe the anterior dislocation (arrow) of the body of the sternum at the manubriosternal junction.

Sternal dislocations may be associated with spine, rib, and clavicle fractures and may be complicated by injury to the major arteries, trachea, heart, and lung.

TABLE 12–6. Articular Disorders Affecting the Joints of the Thoracic Cage*

Entity	Figure(s)	Characteristic Sites of Involvement	Characteristics
Degenerative and related disorders			
Osteoarthrosis[3, 33, 34]	3–32 12–18	Costovertebral joint Sternoclavicular joint First sternocostal joint	Narrowed articular space Osteophytes (may simulate pulmonary lesions) Subchondral bone sclerosis
Inflammatory disorders			
Rheumatoid arthritis[34–37]	12–19	Manubriosternal junction (30–70 per cent of patients) Sternoclavicular joint (30 per cent of patients)	Unilateral or bilateral subchondral erosions and, rarely, extensive osteolysis Absence of osteophytes and other osseous outgrowths
Ankylosing spondylitis[38–40]	12–20	Sternoclavicular joint	Bilateral or unilateral involvement Erosion, sclerosis, and, occasionally, ankylosis
Psoriatic arthritis[38, 39]	12–21	Sternoclavicular joint Manubriosternal junction	Findings can be severe and may be associated with pain and soft tissue swelling Osteoporosis, subchondral erosion, hyperostosis, and synostosis May resemble rheumatoid arthritis or ankylosing spondylitis
SAPHO syndrome[41]		Sternum Anterior portions of ribs Clavicle Sternoclavicular joint Manubriosternal junction	SAPHO is an acronym for the findings of synovitis (S), acne (A), pustulosis (P), hyperostosis (H), and osteitis (O) Arthro-osteitis associated with acne or pustulosis palmaris et plantaris; closely related to sternocostoclavicular hyperostosis, psoriasis, and chronic recurrent multifocal osteomyelitis Prominent hyperostosis and painful osteitis of the anterior chest wall as well as synovitis of the nearby joints
Sternocostoclavicular hyperostosis[41]	12–22	Sternum Upper ribs Clavicle	Bilateral bone overgrowth and soft tissue ossification Associated with pustulosis palmaris et plantaris in 30–50 per cent of patients (see SAPHO syndrome earlier) Age 40 to 60 years; men > women Clinical findings: pain, swelling, tenderness, and local heat overlying the anterior upper chest wall
Reiter's syndrome[38, 42]		Manubriosternal junction	Osseus erosion and bony proliferation Findings identical to those of psoriatic and rheumatoid arthritis Associated with urethritis and conjunctivitis
Dermatomyositis and polymyositis[43]	12–23	Muscles and subcutaneous tissues of chest wall	Diffuse subcutaneous, intermuscular, and intramuscular calcification of chest wall
Infection			
Pyogenic septic arthritis[44]	12–24	Sternoclavicular joint Manubriosternal junction Costosternal joint	Intravenous drug abusers predisposed to sternoclavicular joint infections Unilateral joint space widening and destruction Soft tissue mass or abscess variable Osseous ankylosis rare

*See also Tables 1–6 to 1–9.

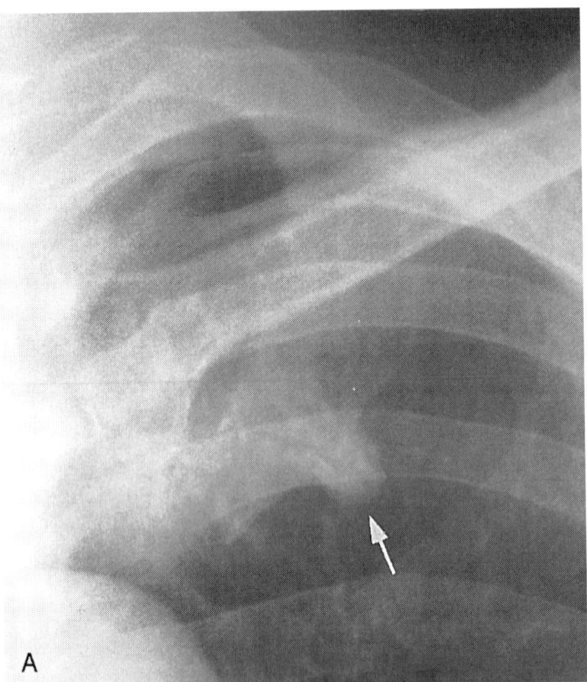

FIGURE 12–18. Osteoarthrosis.[3, 33, 34] A First sternocostal joint. Observe the prominent osteophytes arising from the first sternocostal articulation (arrow). Degenerative disease is a frequent finding at this site and may simulate a pulmonary mass. B, C Sternoclavicular joint. This 69-year-old woman had undergone mediastinal surgery 1 year before these radiographs were taken. In B, an oblique radiograph shows the nonspecific finding of an indistinct subchondral margin of the manubrial surface of the right sternoclavicular joint (arrows). In C, a coronal conventional tomogram more clearly shows the sclerosis, the poorly defined margin of the medial aspect of the clavicle, and subchondral cyst formation (arrows) within the manubrium adjacent to the joint.

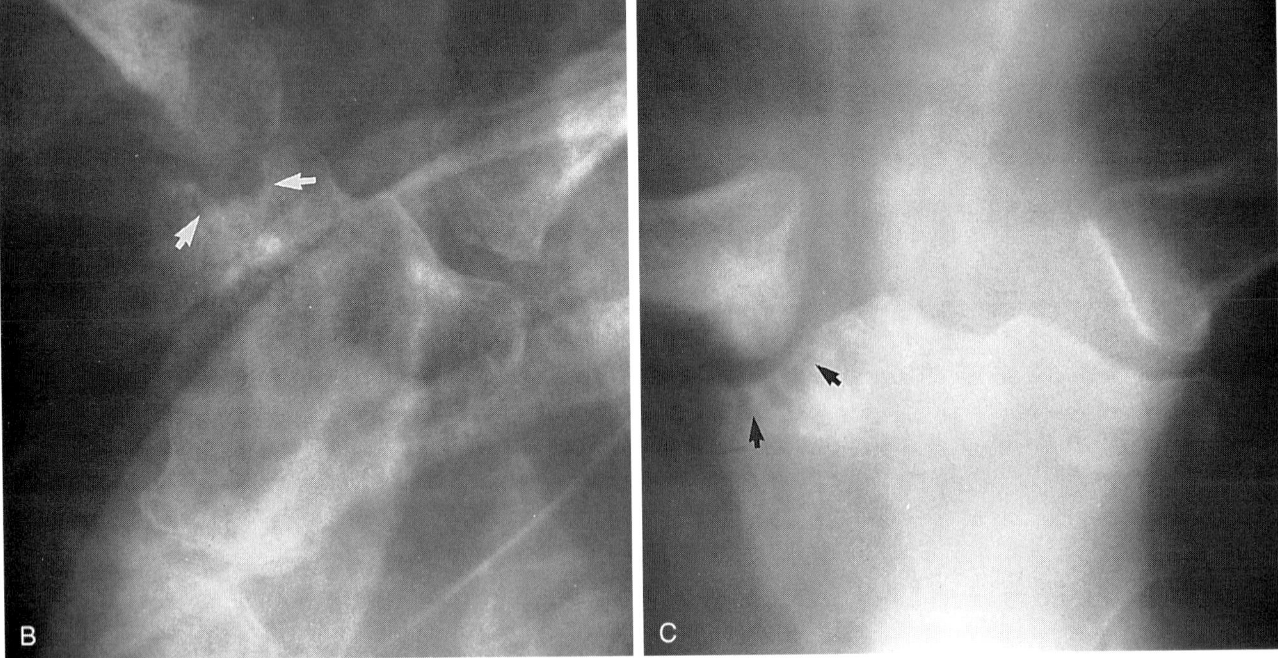

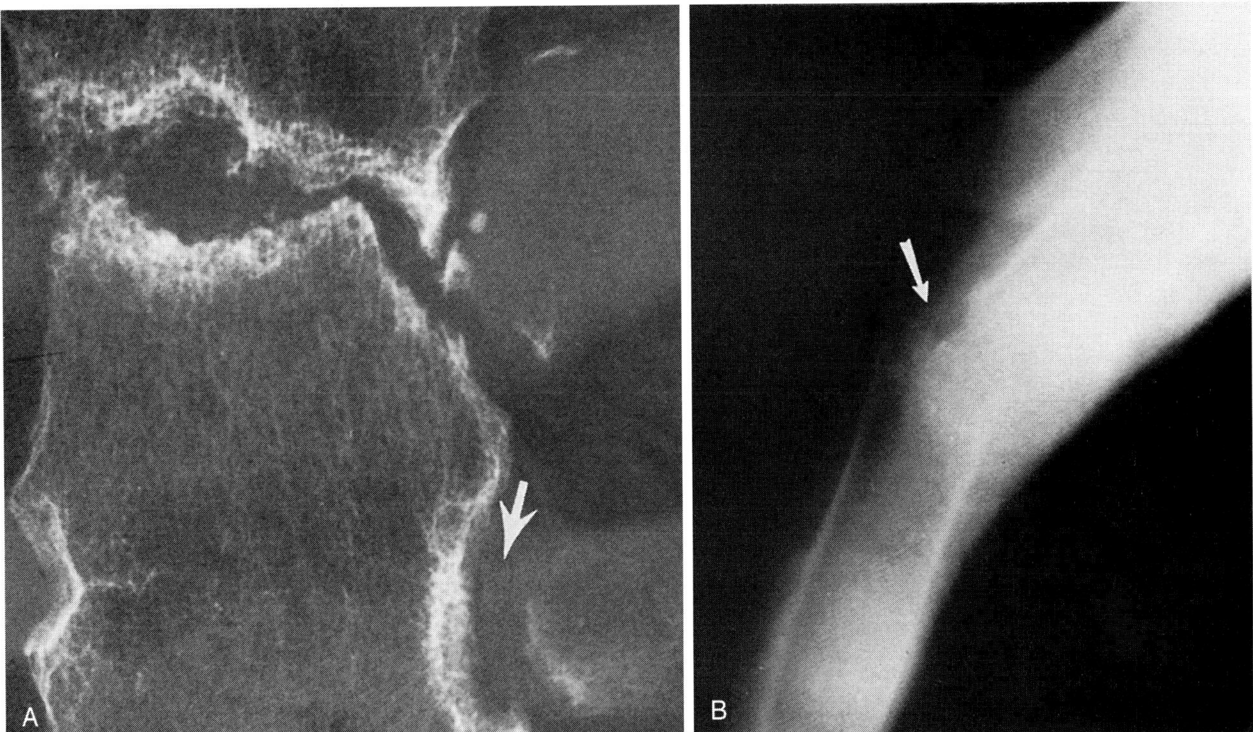

FIGURE 12–19. Rheumatoid arthritis: manubriosternal junction.[34–37] **A** Radiographic abnormalities of the manubriosternal junction are illustrated in this coronal section of the sternum. They include osseous erosions and sclerosis. Note also irregularity of the sternocostal joints (arrow). **B** Lateral radiograph from another rheumatoid arthritis patient reveals spontaneous subluxation of the manubriosternal junction (arrow). *(From Resnick D: Diagnosis of Bone and Joint Disorders. 3rd Ed. Philadelphia, WB Saunders, 1995, p 906.)*

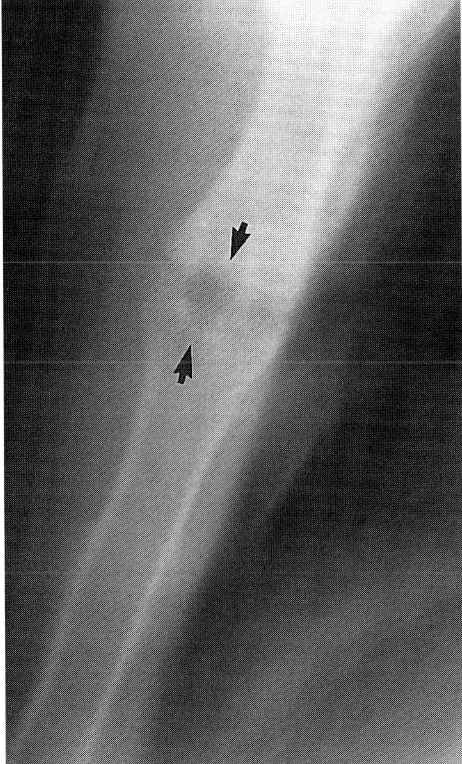

FIGURE 12–20. Ankylosing spondylitis.[38–40] The manubriosternal junction is narrowed and indistinct, and the subchondral bone is eroded (arrows) in this 49-year-old man with a 10-year history of ankylosing spondylitis.

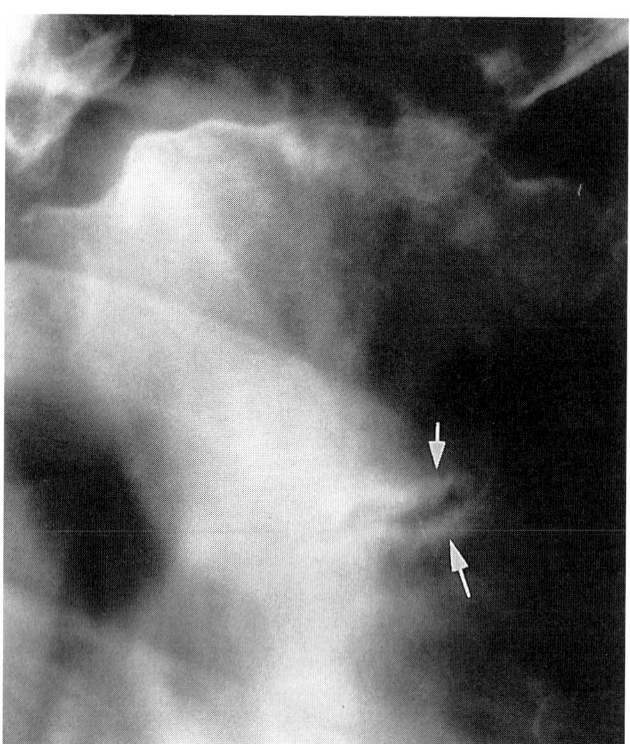

FIGURE 12–21. Psoriatic arthropathy: manubriosternal junction.[38, 39] Observe the joint space irregularity and sclerosis of the manubriosternal junction (arrows) in this 53-year-old man with psoriatic skin lesions and foot involvement.

Radiographic changes in psoriatic arthritis that affect the manubriosternal junction may resemble those seen in rheumatoid arthritis and ankylosing spondylitis and include osteoporosis, subchondral erosion, sclerosis, and synostosis.

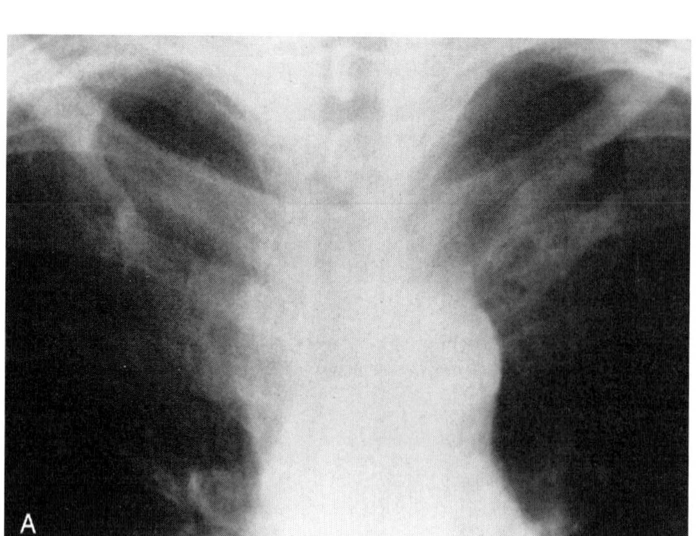

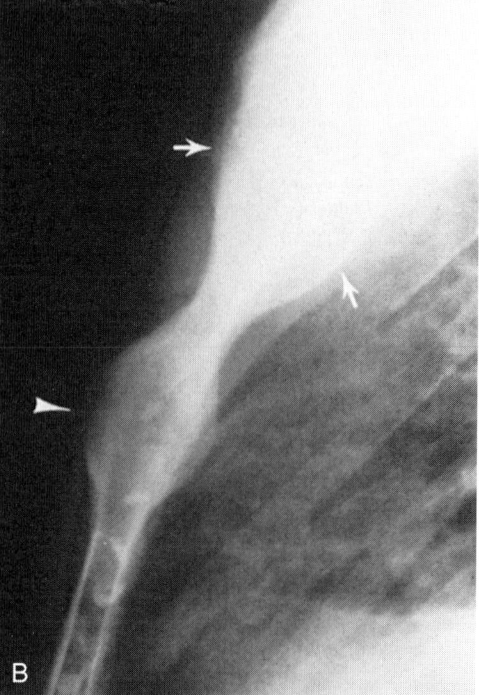

FIGURE 12–22. Sternocostoclavicular hyperostosis.[41] Progressive soft tissue prominence developed in the upper anterior chest wall in this 53-year-old woman. **A** Osseous mass is projected over the upper chest on both sides. Observe also the obliteration of the inferior aspects of the clavicles, the anterior margins of the first ribs, and the sternoclavicular joints. **B** Lateral radiograph reveals the ossified mass (arrows) as well as ossification of the manubriosternal junction (arrowhead). *(From Resnick D: Diagnosis of Bone and Joint Disorders. 3rd Ed. Philadelphia, WB Saunders, 1995, p 4454. Courtesy of R. Kerr, M.D., Los Angeles, California.)*

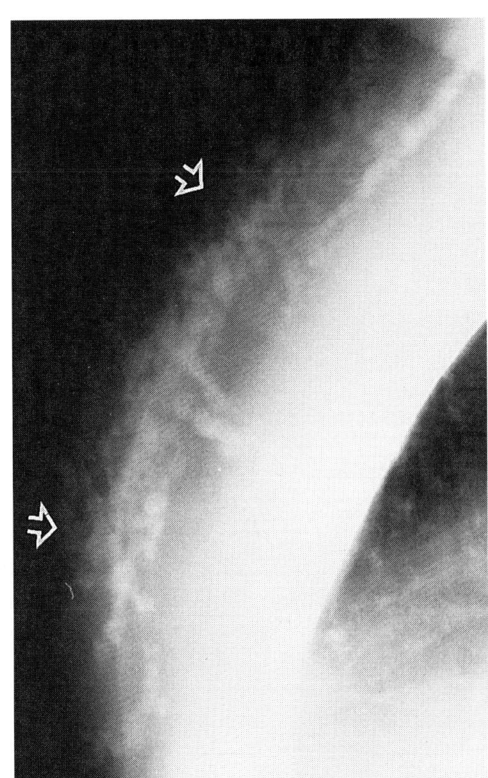

FIGURE 12–23. Dermatomyositis and polymyositis: Anterior chest wall.[43] Diffuse soft tissue calcification is seen in the pectoral region anterior to the sternum (open arrows) in this patient with diffuse dermatomyositis and polymyositis. *(Courtesy of C. Pineda, M.D., Mexico City, Mexico.)*

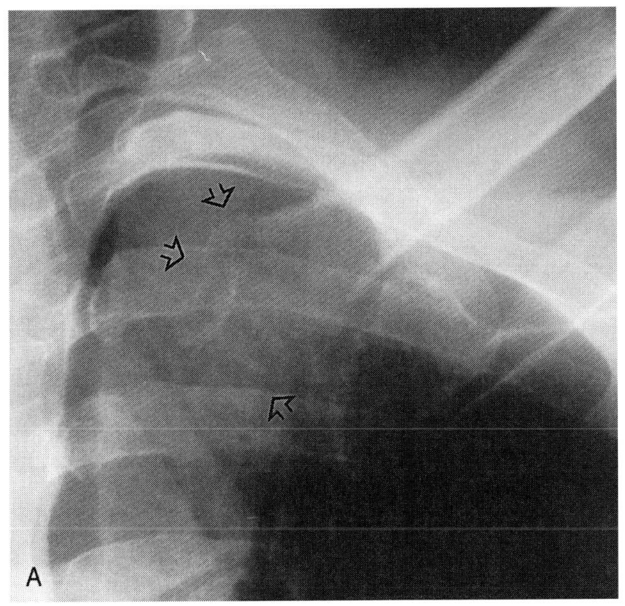

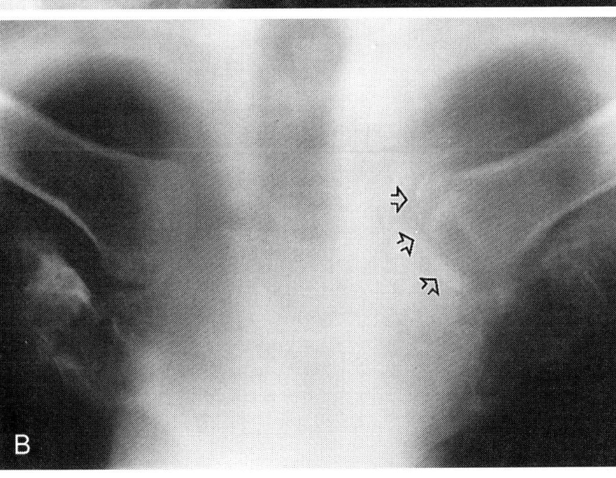

FIGURE 12–24. Pyogenic septic arthritis: Sternoclavicular joint.[44] In a 53-year-old female intravenous drug addict, a frontal radiograph (A) and conventional tomogram (B) of the sternoclavicular joint show joint space narrowing, osteopenia, and erosions of the subchondral bone (open arrows), typical of septic arthritis. *Staphylococcus aureus* was cultured from the joint.

TABLE 12–7. Neoplasms Affecting the Ribs and Sternum*

Entity	Figure(s)	Characteristics
Secondary malignant neoplasms of bone		
Skeletal metastasis[45–47]	12–25 12–26	Ribs are commonly involved in skeletal metastasis; sternum infrequently involved Pancoast tumor: Bronchogenic carcinoma of the superior sulcus frequently invades and destroys the upper ribs and cervicothoracic spine by direct extension or by hematogenous or lymphatic dissemination; associated with apical lung mass; clinical findings of ptosis, myosis, and anhydrosis (Horner's syndrome)
Primary malignant neoplasms of bone		
Osteosarcoma[48–50]	12–27 12–28	Fewer than 3 per cent of osteosarcomas affect the ribs Most rib osteosarcomas are secondary, arising from malignant transformation of Paget's disease or irradiated bone; primary osteosarcomas of ribs are extremely rare Osteolytic, osteoblastic, and mixed patterns of bone destruction Pulmonary metastases from osteosarcoma may be seen on radiographs of the chest or thoracic spine: multiple ossified masses within the lung field
Osteoblastoma (aggressive)[51]		Two per cent of aggressive osteoblastomas affect the ribs Expansile osteolytic lesion that may be partially ossified or contain calcium
Chondrosarcoma[52, 53]	12–29	Approximately 20 per cent of chondrosarcomas affect the ribs; 2 per cent affect the sternum Most rib lesions are conventional or mesenchymal forms Tend to be osteolytic lesions, sometimes containing a bulky cartilaginous cap and frequently containing calcifications Soft tissue masses common
Ewing's sarcoma[54]	12–30	Eight per cent of Ewing's sarcomas affect the ribs Aggressive permeative or moth-eaten pattern of bone destruction Central metadiaphyseal location and soft tissue mass are common
Myeloproliferative disorders		
Plasma cell (multiple) myeloma[55]	12–31	Seventy-five percent of all plasma cell myeloma is the multiple form Twenty-five per cent of myeloma patients with skeletal lesions have rib involvement; 15 per cent have sternal involvement Diffuse osteopenia or punctate osteolytic lesions
Hodgkin's disease[56]		Sixteen per cent of skeletal lesions in Hodgkin's disease occur in the ribs; 4 per cent occur in the sternum
Primary lymphoma (non-Hodgkin's)[57]	12–32	Approximately 2 per cent of patients with primary non-Hodgkin's lymphoma have rib involvement May result in multiple moth-eaten or permeative osteolytic lesions Diffuse or localized sclerotic lesions are rare
Primary benign neoplasms of bone		
Enostosis[58]		Twelve per cent of enostoses occur in the ribs
Osteoid osteoma[59–61]	12–33	Fewer than 1 per cent of osteoid osteomas occur in the ribs Central radiolucent nidus with surrounding reactive sclerosis
Osteoblastoma (conventional)[62]		Fewer than 5 per cent of osteoblastomas involve the ribs
Enchondroma (solitary)[53, 63]	12–34	Five per cent of solitary enchondromas affect the ribs Usually osteolytic and frequently are expansile and multiloculated Matrix may be calcified

TABLE 12–7. Neoplasms Affecting the Ribs and Sternum* *Continued*

Entity	Figure(s)	Characteristics
Maffucci's syndrome[53]		More than 30 per cent of patients with Maffucci's syndrome have rib involvement Soft tissue hemangiomas in addition to multiple enchondromas Higher risk of malignant transformation than with solitary enchondroma
Osteochondroma (solitary)[64]	12–35	Fewer than 5 per cent of solitary osteochondromas occur in the ribs Often bulky cartilaginous lesions arising from the anterior aspect of the ribs adjacent to costal cartilage
Intraosseous lipoma[65]		Approximately 8 per cent of lipomas occur in the ribs Radiolucent solitary lesion
Hemangioma[66]	12–36	Approximately 9 per cent of hemangiomas occur in the ribs Osseous expansion and trabecular striation within lesions
Aneurysmal bone cyst[67]		Almost 10 per cent of aneurysmal bone cysts involve the ribs Eccentric, thin-walled, expansile, multiloculated osteolytic lesion
Tumor-like lesions		
Paget's disease[68]		Rare involvement of ribs Usually polyostotic and may exhibit unilateral involvement
Neurofibromatosis 1 (von Recklinghausen's disease)[69]	12–37	Commonly affects ribs Mesodermal dysplasia (and occasionally pressure erosion) results in thin ribbon-like ribs with widened intercostal spaces Circumscribed osteolytic lesions occasionally appear
Monostotic fibrous dysplasia[70]	12–38 A	Approximately 28 per cent of all monostotic lesions affect the ribs Most common benign lesion of the rib cage, representing 30 per cent of primary benign chest wall lesions Thick rim of sclerosis surrounding a radiolucent lesion or radiodense lesion; ground-glass appearance of matrix; tends to affect entire rib; anterior end of rib may appear bulbous and expanded Most rib lesions, whether monostotic or polyostotic, are unilateral, assisting in the differentiation from lesions such as metastasis and hyperparathyroidism, diseases that typically are more widely disseminated
Polyostotic fibrous dysplasia[70]	12–38 B	Rib involvement is seen in over 50 per cent of cases of polyostotic fibrous dysplasia Unilateral (or infrequently, bilateral asymmetric) involvement of the ribs
Langerhans' cell histiocytosis[71]		Five per cent of lesions affect the ribs, most frequently eosinophilic granuloma Single or multiple osteolytic lesions frequently result in pathologic fracture

*See also Tables 1–10 to 1–12.

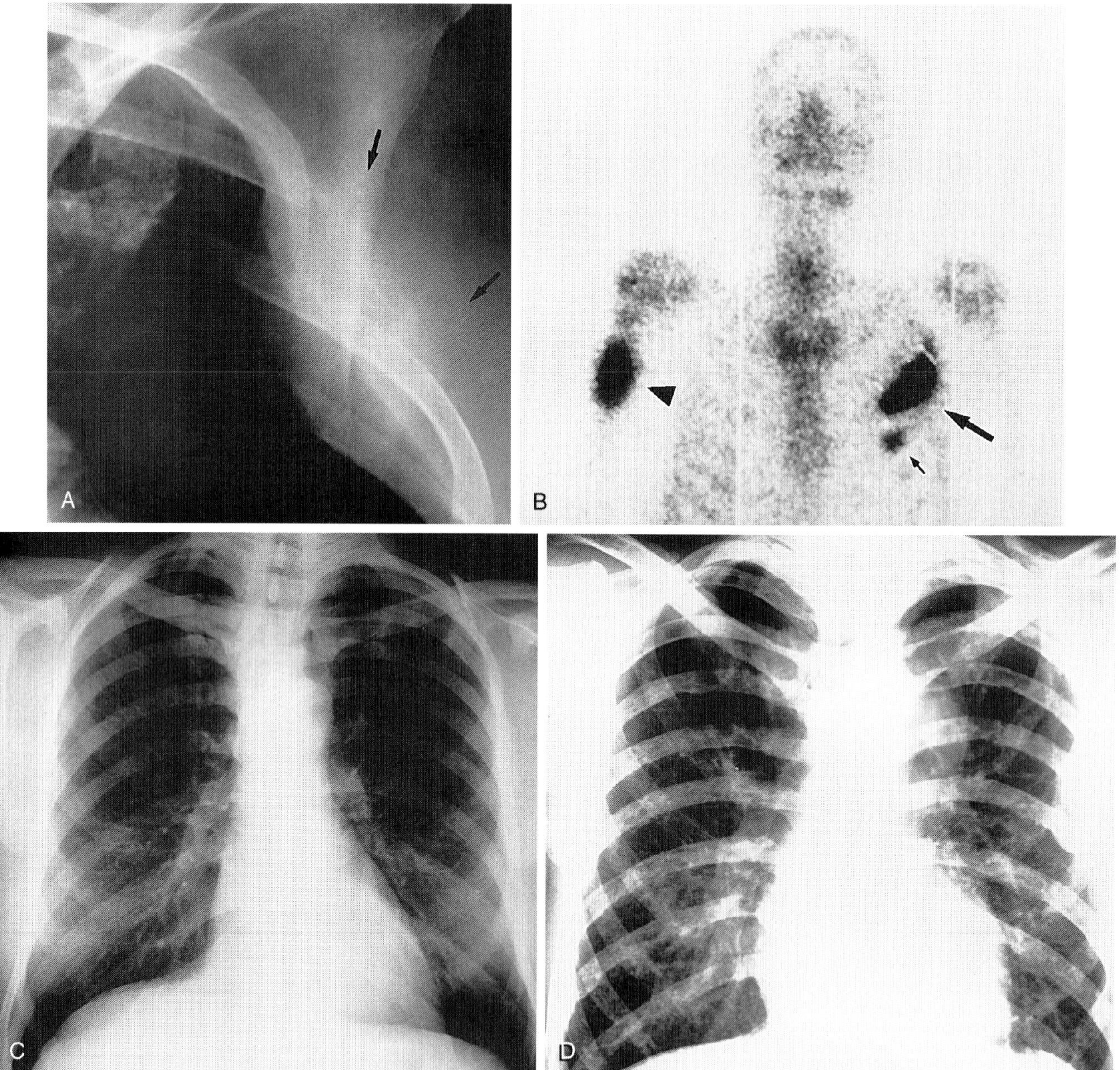

FIGURE 12–25. Skeletal metastasis: Ribs—various patterns.[45–47] A, B Osteolytic pattern. A 61-year-old man with known prostate carcinoma had rib pain. In A, an anteroposterior view of the rib shows widespread osteolytic destruction of the posterolateral aspect of the left third rib (arrows). In B, a bone scan reveals increased accumulation of the bone-seeking radionuclide in the affected ribs (arrows) and in the contralateral humerus (arrowhead). Several other sites (not shown), including the pelvis and spine, revealed widespread metastases. C Osteoblastic pattern. Radiograph of the chest and thoracic cage in this man with prostate carcinoma shows a diffuse osteoblastic pattern of metastatic disease. No evidence of bone enlargement, scalloping, or coarsened trabeculae is seen. D Mixed pattern. A 20-year-old man with a medulloblastoma metastatic to the skeleton complained of severe bone pain. His radiographs reveal a mixed pattern of metastasis with both osteolytic and osteoblastic lesions throughout the bones of the thoracic cage.

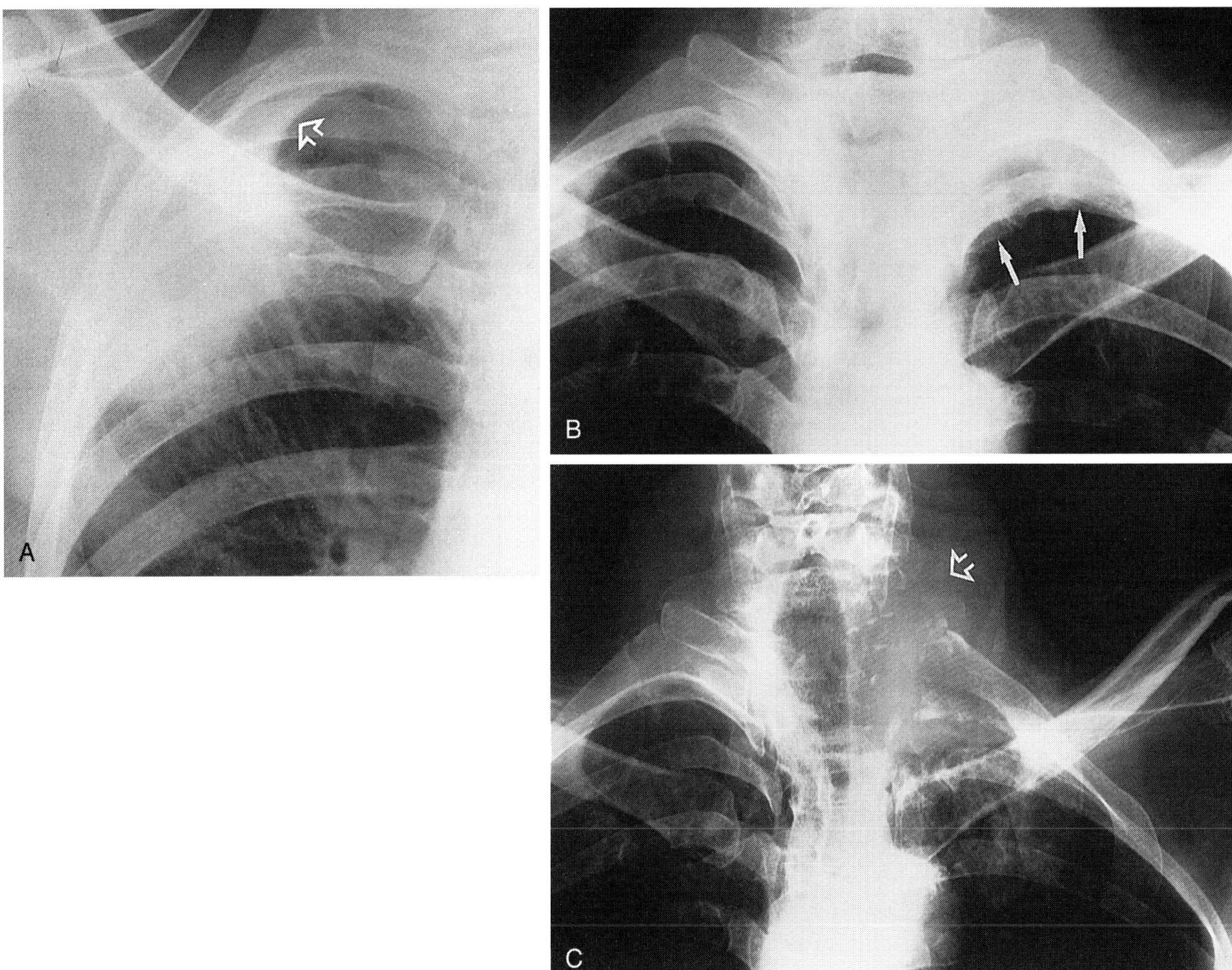

FIGURE 12–26. Skeletal metastasis: Pancoast tumor.[45–47] A Large radiopaque soft tissue mass is present in the right lung apex in this patient with carcinoma of the lung. Underlying rib destruction, not well seen on this chest radiograph, is suggested by the tapering extrapleural sign at the edge of the lesion (open arrow). B In another patient with a Pancoast tumor, a subtle radiopaque area is noted in the left lung apex (arrows). C In a third patient, extensive osteolytic destruction of the upper ribs and thoracic vertebrae is evident (open arrow).

In Pancoast tumors, carcinoma of the apex of the lung invades adjacent ribs or cervicothoracic vertebrae by direct extension. In other cases, contiguous spread of tumor into the adjacent bone may result from hematogenous or lymphatic dissemination. *(Courtesy of B.A. Howard, M.D., Charlotte, North Carolina.)*

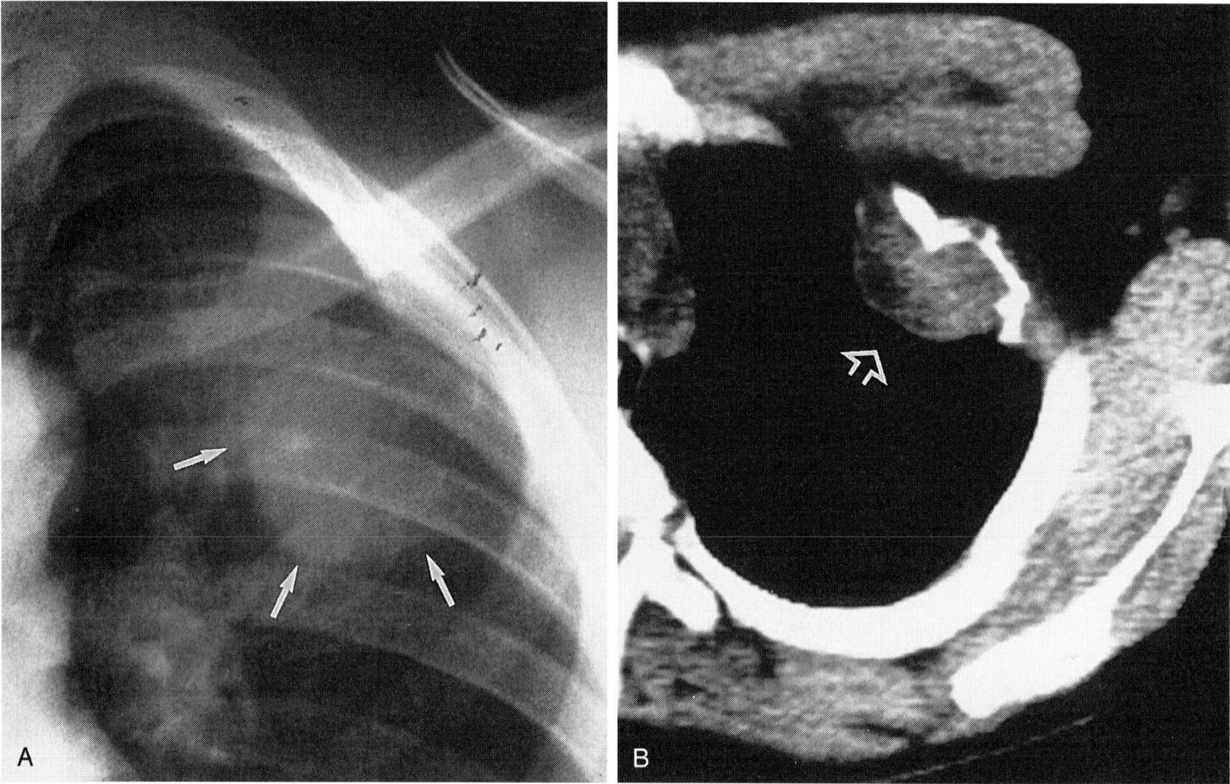

FIGURE 12–27. Primary osteosarcoma.[48–50] A 10 year-old boy had pain along the anterior aspect of the rib cage. **A** Posteroanterior chest radiograph shows a large, lobulated extrapleural soft tissue mass overlying the upper lung field (arrows). **B** Transaxial computed tomographic (CT) scan localizes the lesion to the anterior aspect of the rib, revealing osseous destruction and a large associated soft tissue mass (open arrow).

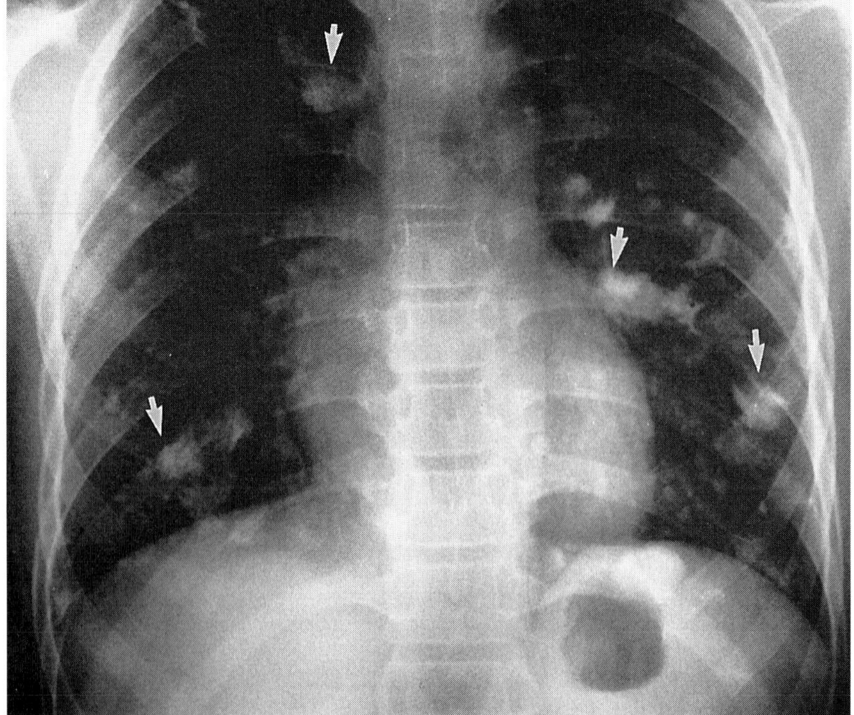

FIGURE 12–28. Osteosarcoma: pulmonary metastasis.[50] Posteroanterior chest radiograph of this 12-year-old boy with known osteosarcoma in the femur reveals multiple ossified masses throughout the lungs (arrows).

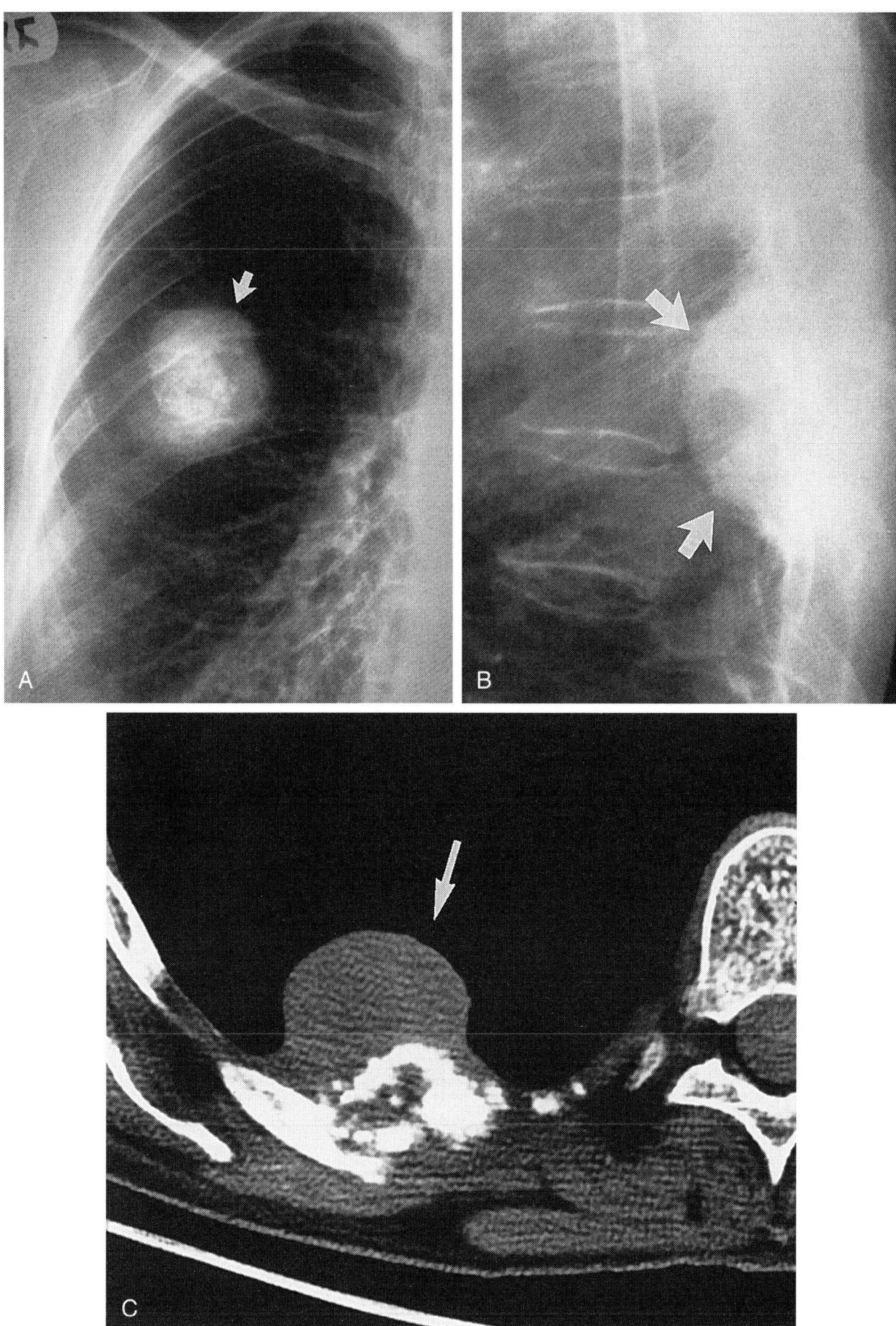

FIGURE 12–29. Mesenchymal chondrosarcoma.[52, 53] This 51-year-old woman had a 1-month history of right posterior chest wall pain. **A, B** The posteroanterior (**A**) and lateral (**B**) chest radiographs demonstrate a pleural-based mass in the periphery of the right hemithorax, adjacent to the eighth rib (arrows). **C** Transaxial computed tomographic (CT) scan shows a calcified mass arising from the anterior aspect of the posterolateral portion of the right eighth rib (arrow). The lesion was resected and examined, and the histologic diagnosis was mesenchymal chondrosarcoma.

Mesenchymal chondrosarcoma is a particularly aggressive form, characterized by a poor prognosis and a greater tendency to metastasize than conventional chondrosarcoma. *(Courtesy of G. Greenway, M.D., Dallas, Texas.)*

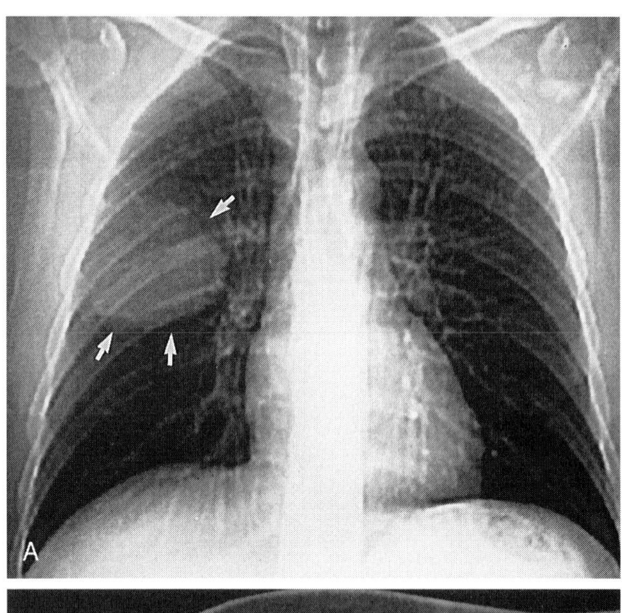

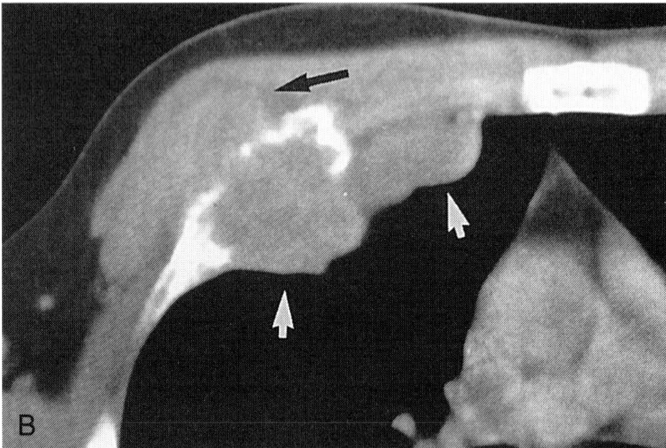

FIGURE 12–30. Ewing's sarcoma.[54] This 28-year-old male patient had a painless, enlarging right upper chest wall mass. A Frontal computed tomographic (CT) localizer scan shows a large extrapleural mass overlying the right lung field (arrows). B Transaxial CT scan delineates more clearly the extent and nature of this expansile lesion involving the anterior aspect of the third rib. The lesion, which destroys the bone, also is associated with a large soft tissue mass (arrows). *(Courtesy of G. Greenway, M.D., Dallas, Texas.)*

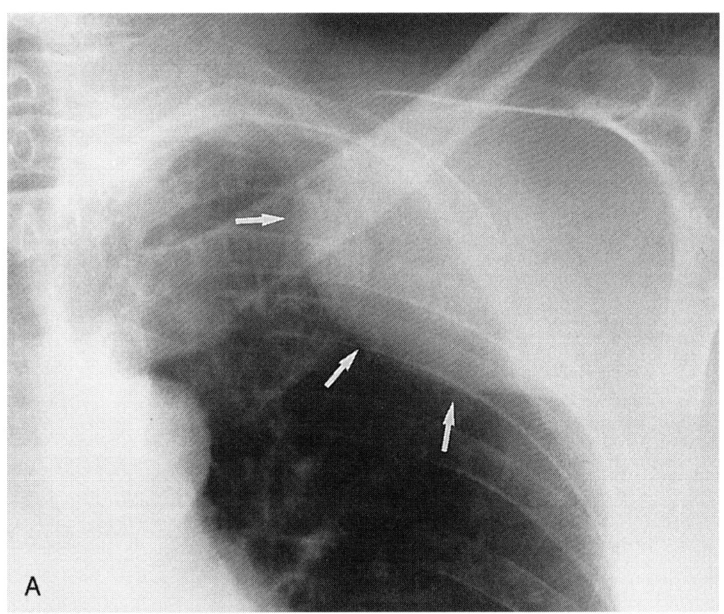

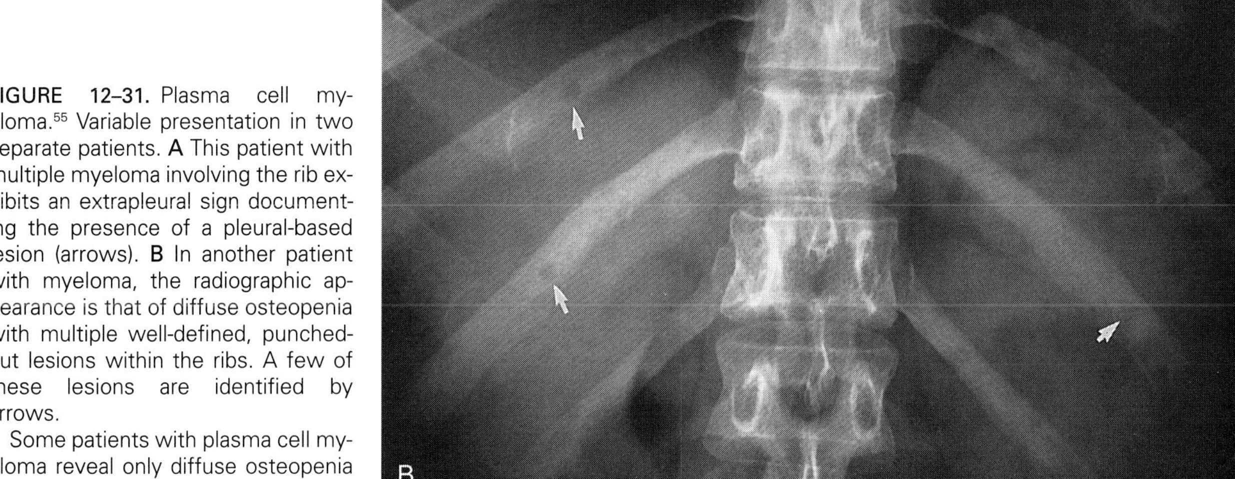

FIGURE 12–31. Plasma cell myeloma.[55] Variable presentation in two separate patients. A This patient with multiple myeloma involving the rib exhibits an extrapleural sign documenting the presence of a pleural-based lesion (arrows). B In another patient with myeloma, the radiographic appearance is that of diffuse osteopenia with multiple well-defined, punched-out lesions within the ribs. A few of these lesions are identified by arrows.

Some patients with plasma cell myeloma reveal only diffuse osteopenia on radiographs.

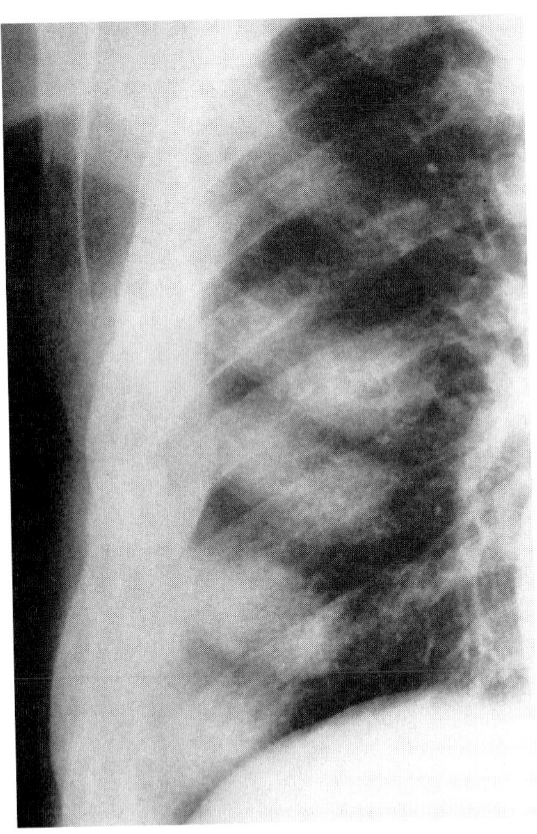

FIGURE 12–32. Primary non-Hodgkin's lymphoma.[57] Observe the diffuse osteosclerotic, expansile appearance of the ribs in this 58-year-old man with long-standing, untreated primary lymphoma. Similar changes were evident throughout most of the skeleton. *(Courtesy of R. Arkless, M.D., Seabeck, Washington.)*

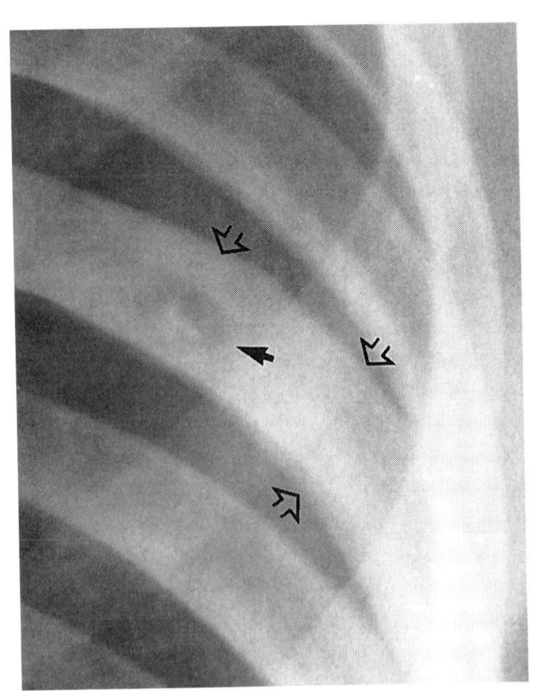

FIGURE 12–33. Osteoid osteoma.[59–61] An ovoid radiolucent area (arrow) containing a central opaque region is surrounded by bone sclerosis and hypertrophy (open arrows) within the rib of this young patient. The radiolucent area represents the nidus of the tumor, and the surrounding hyperostosis is a reactive phenomenon. *(Courtesy of A. Brower, M.D., Norfolk, Virginia.)*

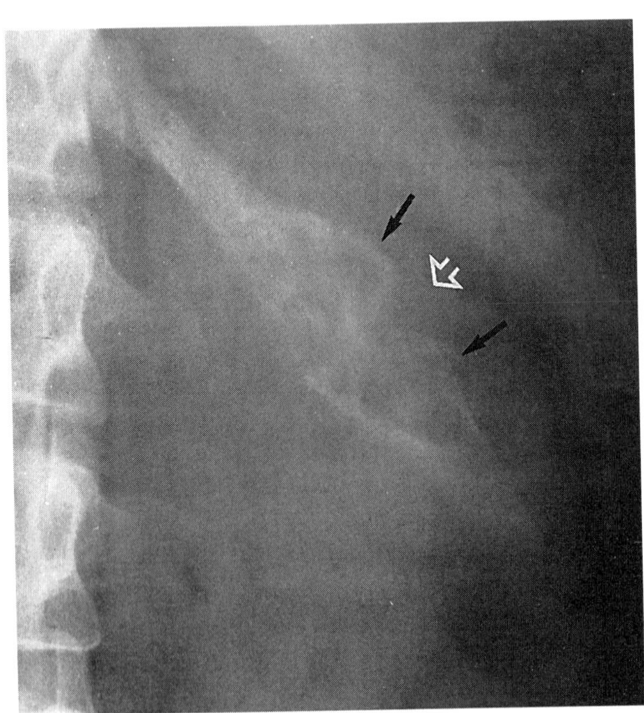

FIGURE 12–34. Enchondroma.[53, 63] This lesion appears multiloculated (black arrows), demonstrates osseous expansion, and possesses a questionable area in which the cortex is difficult to visualize (open arrow). Biopsy confirmed that the lesion was a benign enchondroma. More typically cartilage lesions develop at the costochondral junction.

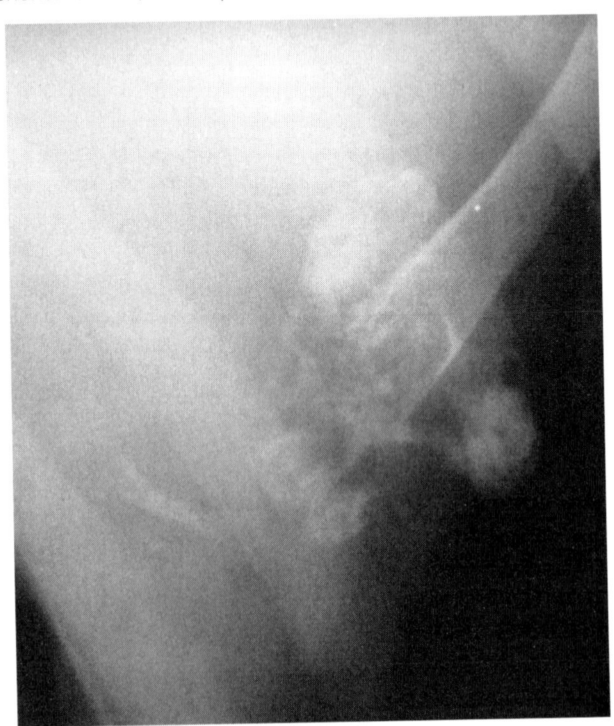

FIGURE 12–35. Osteochondroma.[64] A cauliflower-shaped ossified lesion arises from the costochondral junction of the seventh rib. The costochondral region is the most likely site for a rib osteochondroma owing to the presence in this area of normal cartilaginous tissue. *(Courtesy of B.L. Harger, D.C., Portland, Oregon.)*

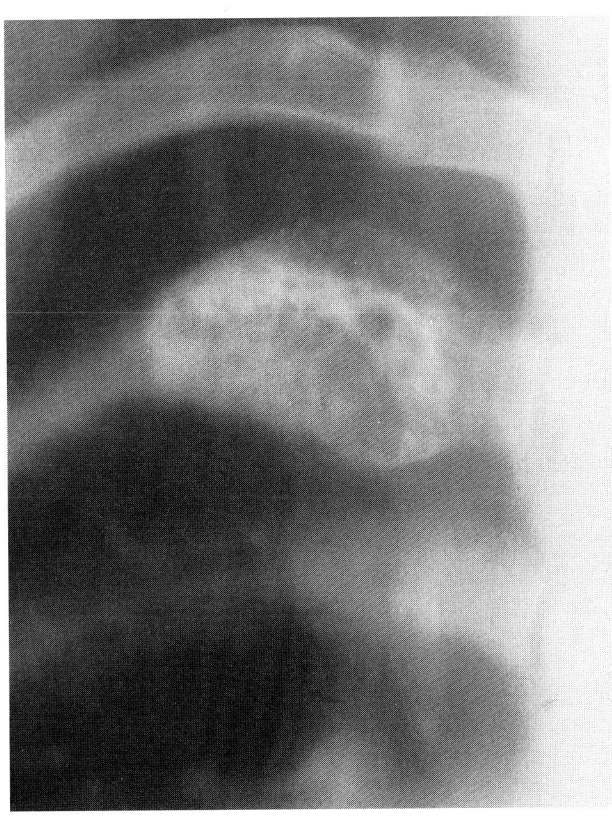

FIGURE 12–36. Hemangioma.[66] Conventional tomogram shows osseous expansion of this striated osteolytic rib lesion. About 9 per cent of all hemangiomas occur in the ribs. Most lesions are asymptomatic.

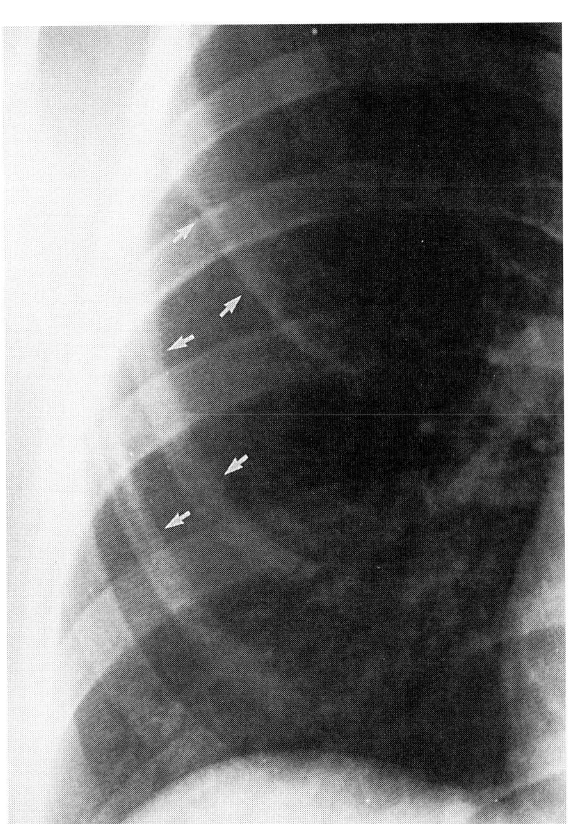

FIGURE 12–37. Neurofibromatosis: rib involvement.[69] In a 20-year-old woman, extensive narrowing and irregularity of the anterior portions of several ribs (arrows) are evident. This appearance reflects a generalized mesodermal dysplasia typical of neurofibromatosis. Pressure erosions of the ribs from neurofibromas (not evident in this patient) also may occur. *(Courtesy of R. Arkless. M.D., Seabeck, Washington.)*

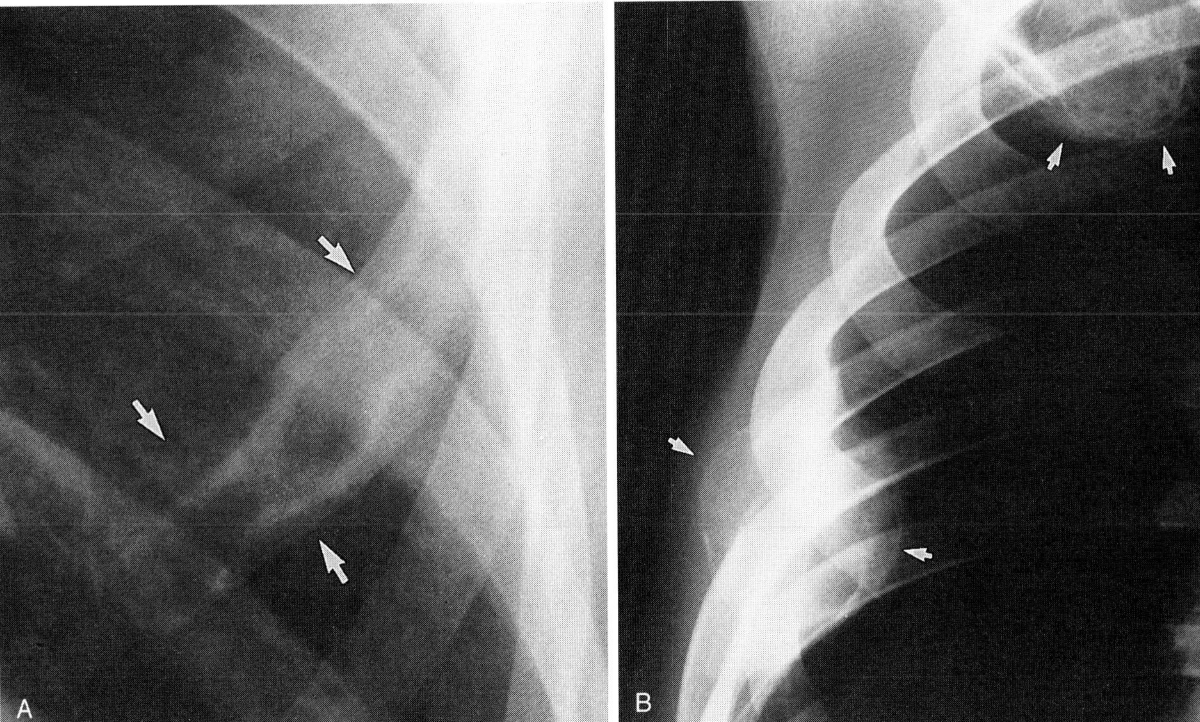

FIGURE 12–38. Fibrous dysplasia.[70] A Monostotic form. An undulating sclerotic margin is seen adjacent to this slightly expansile, radiolucent rib lesion (arrows). B Polyostotic form. In another patient, expansile lesions of the first and fifth ribs are seen (arrows). Observe the extrapleural sign associated with each lesion.

TABLE 12–8. Metabolic, Hematologic, and Infectious Disorders Affecting the Ribs and Sternum*

Entity	Figure(s)	Characteristics
Generalized osteoporosis[72]	12–9, 12–15	Uniform decrease in radiodensity, thinning of cortices Frequently results in insufficiency fractures of the ribs and, less frequently, the sternum Acute rib fractures may occur with minimal trauma in osteoporotic patients
Osteogenesis imperfecta[73]		Osteoporosis and bone fragility Thin, gracile appearance of ribs with pectus carinatum Severe rib deformities and multiple fractures common
Osteomalacia[74]	12–39	Diffuse osteopenia Liberty Bell chest: Bone softening results in a bell-shaped deformity of the thoracic cage Decreased trabeculae; remaining trabeculae appear prominent and coarsened Looser's zones (pseudofractures)—transverse fractures of ribs
Rickets[74]	12–40	Rachitic rosary: bulbous appearance of ribs adjacent to costochondral junction resulting from metaphyseal widening Osteopenia with rib fractures
Hyperparathyroidism and renal osteodystrophy[75]	12–41	Brown tumor (osteoclastoma): solitary or multiple expansile osteolytic lesions containing fibrous tissue and giant cells; may disappear after treatment for hyperparathyroidism Subperiosteal resorption may result in rib notching or erosion Osteosclerosis more common in renal osteodystrophy
Hemodialysis treatment[76, 77]	12–42	Diffuse osteopenia and spontaneous rib fractures Amyloidosis of sternoclavicular joints
Thalassemia[78]	12–43	Marrow hyperplasia within ribs produces an expansile appearance of the proximal ends of the ribs adjacent to the costovertebral joints
Acromegaly[3]		Elongation of the inferior body of the rib with marginal sclerosis Widening of anterior costal end of rib and dentate costocartilage interface
Myelofibrosis[79]		Diffuse osteosclerosis of bones of thoracic cage Occasional periosteal bone apposition or periostitis, osteolysis, or osteopenia
Infantile cortical hyperostosis (Caffey's disease)[80]		Uncommon disease of infancy Cortical hyperostosis of the ribs in a monostotic, unilateral, or diffuse pattern Predilection for the lateral arches of the ribs Osseous bridging of ribs may occur with healing Pleural effusions ipsilateral to the side of involvement are common
Osteomyelitis[81]		Acute pyogenic osteomyelitis frequently involves the bones about the sternoclavicular region in intravenous drug abusers Sternal infections may occur after median sternotomy for open chest surgery Typical organisms in chest wall infections include staphylococcus, pseudomonas, actinomyces, aspergillus, coccidioides, brucella, mycobacterium
Chronic recurrent multifocal osteomyelitis (CRMO)[82]		Occurs mainly in children and adolescents Involves the bones of the anterior chest wall and clavicle Initial lytic destruction of metaphysis adjacent to growth plate with no periosteal bone formation or sequestration Closely related to the SAPHO (synovitis, acne, pustulosis, hyperostosis, and osteitis) syndrome (Table 12–6)

*See also Tables 1–13 to 1–17.

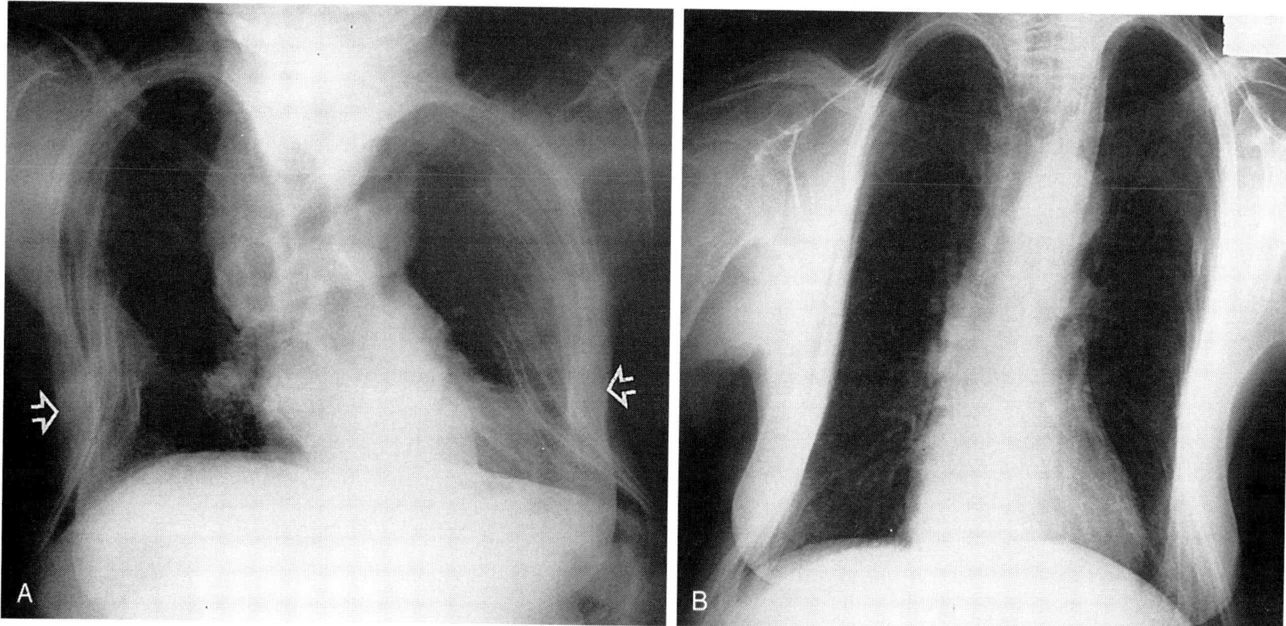

FIGURE 12–39. Osteomalacia.[74] A Bone softening in this patient with osteomalacia secondary to gluten enteropathy has resulted in multiple rib deformities. The bilateral central indentation of the thoracic cage (open arrows), has been termed the "Liberty Bell" chest. Note also the diffuse osteopenia throughout the skeleton. B In this 60-year-old woman with osteomalacia and hyperparathyroidism, similar findings are evident.

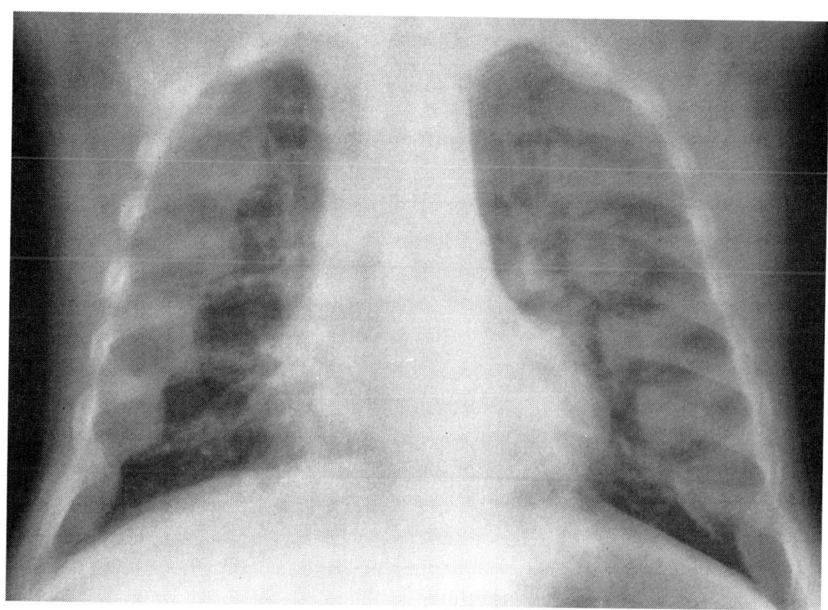

FIGURE 12–40. Rickets: rachitic rosary.[74] Bulbous expansion of the anterior aspect of the ribs at the costochondral junctions, the so-called rachitic rosary, is a classic finding in children with advanced rickets.

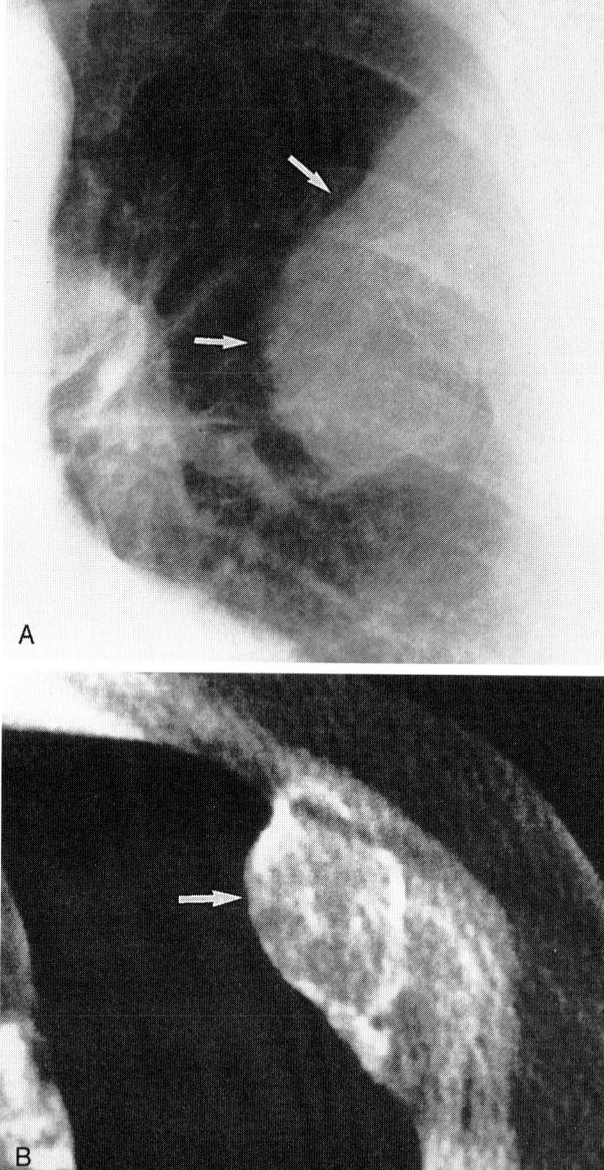

FIGURE 12–41. Hyperparathyroidism: Brown tumor.[75] Routine radiograph (A) and a transaxial computed tomographic (CT) scan (B) in a patient with primary hyperparathyroidism demonstrate a large expansile mass in the rib that causes an extrapleural sign (arrows). The computed tomographic (CT) scan displays the lesion to best advantage.

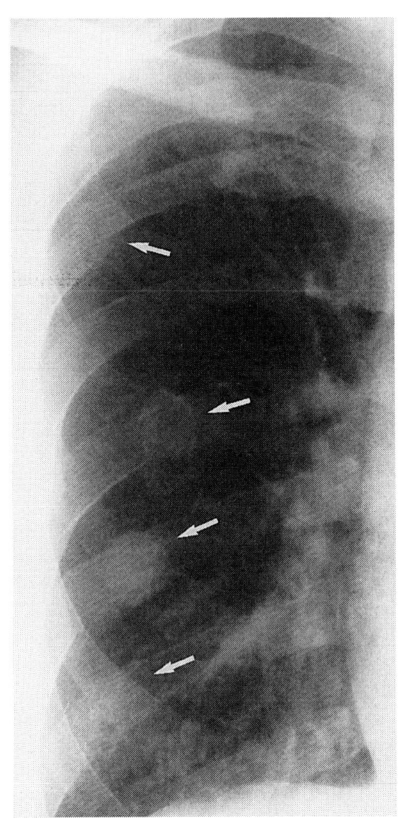

FIGURE 12–42. Hemodialysis treatment: Spontaneous fractures.[76, 77] Radiograph of this patient on long-term hemodialysis therapy for chronic renal failure demonstrates diffuse osteopenia and multiple healing rib fractures (arrows). The ribs are the most frequent site of spontaneous fractures in a hemodialysis patient whose condition is poorly managed.

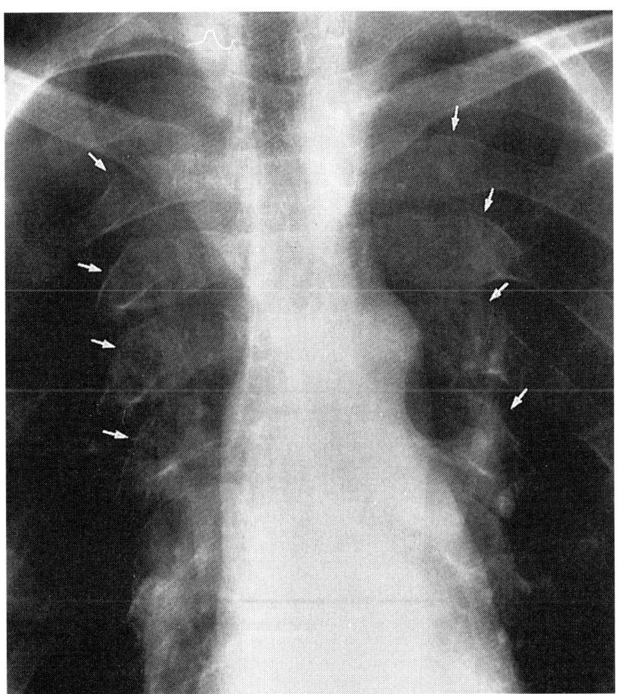

FIGURE 12–43. Thalassemia.[78] Extensive expansion of the posterior aspect of the ribs (arrows) is seen as a manifestation of marrow hyperplasia in this 27-year-old man with thalassemia major.

REFERENCES

1. Edeiken J, Dalinka M, Karasick D: Edeiken's Roentgen Diagnosis of Diseases of Bone. 4th Ed. Baltimore, Williams & Wilkins, 1990.
2. Keats TE, Smith TH: An Atlas of Normal Developmental Roentgen Anatomy. 2nd Ed. Chicago, Year Book, 1988.
3. Köhler A, Zimmer EA: Borderlands of Normal and Early Pathologic Findings in Skeletal Radiography. 4th Ed. New York, Thieme Medical Publishers, 1993.
4. Keats TE: Atlas of Normal Roentgen Variants That May Simulate Disease. 6th Ed. Chicago, Year Book Medical Publishers, 1996.
5. Yochum TR, Rowe LJ: Essentials of Skeletal Radiology. 2nd Ed. Baltimore, Williams & Wilkins, 1996.
6. Adson AW: Surgical treatment for symptoms produced by cervical ribs and the scalenus anticus syndrome. Clin Orthop 207:3, 1986.
7. Weinstein AS, Mueller CF: Intrathoracic rib. AJR 94:587, 1965.
8. Stark P, Lawrence DD: Intrathoracic rib—CT features of a rare chest wall anomaly. Comput Radiol 6:365, 1984.
9. Kelleher J, O'Connell DJ, MacMahon H: Intrathoracic rib: Radiographic features of two cases. Br J Radiol 52:181, 1979.
10. Senac MO, Lee FA, Gilsnaz V: Early costochondral calcification in adolescent hyperthyroidism. Radiology 156:375, 1985.
11. Resnik CS, Brower AC: Midline circular defect of the sternum. Radiology 130:657, 1979.
12. Larsen LL, Ibach HF: Complete congenital fissure of the sternum. AJR 87:1062, 1962.
13. Morse RP, Rockenmacher S, Pyeritz RE, et al: Diagnosis and management of infantile Marfan's syndrome. Pediatrics 86:888, 1990.
14. Eisenberg RL: Clinical Imaging: An Atlas of Differential Diagnosis. Rockville, MD, Aspen, 1988.
15. Mariacher-Gehler S, Michel BA: Sonography: A simple way to visualize rib fractures. AJR 163:1268, 1994.
16. Kattan KR: Trauma to the bony thorax. Semin Roentgenol 13:69, 1978.
17. Kinasewitz GT: Pneumothorax. Semin Respir Crit Care Med 16:293, 1995.
18. Kleinman PK, Marks SC, Nimkin K, et al: Rib fractures in 31 abused infants: Postmortem radiologic-histopathologic study. Radiology 200:807, 1996.
19. Leventhal JM, Thomas SA, Rosenfeld NS, et al: Fractures in young children: Distinguishing child abuse from unintentional injuries. Am J Dis Child 147:87, 1993.
20. Strouse PJ, Owings CL: Fractures of the first rib in child abuse. Radiology 197:763, 1995.
21. Roberge RJ, Morgenstern MJ, Osborn H: Cough fracture of the ribs. Am J Emerg Med 2:513, 1984.
22. Gurtler R, Pavlov H, Torg JS: Stress fracture of the ipsilateral first rib in a pitcher. Am J Sports Med 13:277, 1985.
23. Sacchetti AD, Beswick DR, Morse SK: Rebound rib: Stress-induced first rib fracture. Ann Emerg Med 12:177, 1983.
24. Huang G-S, Park Y-H, Taylor JAM, et al: Hyperostosis of ribs: Association with vertebral hyperostosis. J Rheumatol 20:2073, 1993.
25. Spence EK, Rosato EF: The slipping rib syndrome. Arch Surg 118:1330, 1983.
26. Jurik AG, Justesen T, Graudal H: Radiographic findings in patients with clinical Tietze's syndrome. Skeletal Radiol 16:517, 1987.
27. Brookes JG, Dunn RJ, Rogers LR: Sternal fractures: A retrospective analysis of 272 cases. J Trauma 35:46, 1993.
28. Chen C, Chandnani V, Kang HS, et al: Insufficiency fracture of the sternum caused by osteopenia: Plain film findings in seven patients. AJR 154:1025, 1990.
29. Levinsohn EM, Bunnell WP, Yuan HA: Computed tomography in the diagnosis of dislocations of the sternoclavicular joint. Clin Orthop 140:13, 1979.
30. Gopalakrishnan KC, El Masri WS: Fractures of the sternum associated with spinal injury. J Bone Joint Surg [Br] 68:178, 1986.
31. Felson B: Chest Roentgenology. Philadelphia, WB Saunders, 1973.
32. Greenfield GB: Radiology of Bone Diseases. 2nd Ed. Philadelphia, JB Lippincott, 1975.
33. Kier R, Wain SL, Apple J, et al: Osteoarthritis of the sternoclavicular joint. Invest Radiol 21:227, 1986.
34. Brossmann J, Stäbler A, Preidler KW, et al: Sternoclavicular joint: MR imaging–anatomic correlation. Radiology 198:193, 1996.
35. Kalliomaki JL, Viitanen S-M, Virtama P: Radiological findings of sternoclavicular joints in rheumatoid arthritis. Acta Rheumatol Scand 14:233, 1968.
36. Laitenen H, Saksanen S, Suoranta H: Involvement of the manubriosternal articulation in rheumatoid arthritis. Acta Rheumatol Scand 16:40, 1970.
37. Schils JP, Resnick D, Haghighi PN, et al: Pathogenesis of discovertebral and manubriosternal junction abnormalities in rheumatoid arthritis: A cadaveric study. J Rheumatol 16:291, 1989.
38. Jurik AG: Anterior chest wall involvement in seronegative arthritides: A study of the frequency of changes at radiography. Rheumatol Int 12:7, 1992.
39. Grosbois B, Paxlotsky Y, Chales G, et al: Clinical and radiological study of the manubrio-sternal joint. Rev Rhum Mal Osteoartic 49:232, 1982.
40. Reuler JB, Girard DE, Nardone DA: Sternoclavicular joint involvement in ankylosing spondylitis. South Med J 71:1480, 1978.
41. Boutin RD, Resnick D: The SAPHO syndrome: An evolving concept for unifying several idiopathic disorders of bone and skin. AJR 170:585, 1998.
42. Candardjis G, Saudan Y, DeBosset P: Etude radiologique de l'articulation manubrio-sternale dans la pelvispondylite rhumatismale et le syndrome de Reiter. J Radiol Electrol Med Nucl 59:93, 1978.
43. Hernandez RJ, Keim DR, Sullivan DB, et al: Magnetic resonance imaging appearance of the muscles in childhood dermatomyositis. J Pediatr 117:546, 1990.
44. Brancós MA, Peris P, Miró JM, et al: Septic arthritis in heroin addicts. Semin Arthritis Rheum 21:81, 1991.
45. Kleinman GM, Hochberg FH, Richardson EP Jr: Systemic metastases from medulloblastoma: Report of two cases and review of the literature. Cancer 48:2296, 1981.
46. Wong DA, Fornasier VL, MacNab I: Spinal metastases: The obvious, the occult, and the impostors. Spine 15:1, 1990.
47. Garrett IR: Bone destruction in cancer. Semin Oncol 20:4, 1993.
48. Dahlin DC, Unni KK: Osteosarcoma of bone and its important recognizable varieties. Am J Surg Pathol 1:61, 1977.
49. Abdulrahman RE, White CS, Templeton PA, et al: Primary osteosarcoma of the ribs: CT findings. Skeletal Radiol 24:127, 1995.
50. St James AT: Resection of multiple metastatic pulmonary lesions of osteogenic sarcoma. JAMA 169:943, 1959.
51. Mitchell M, Ackerman LV: Metastatic and pseudomalignant osteoblastoma: A report of two unusual cases. Skeletal Radiol 15:213, 1986.
52. Nakashima Y, Unni KK, Shives TC, et al: Mesenchymal

chondrosarcoma of bone and soft tissue: A review of 111 cases. Cancer 57:2444, 1986.
53. Brien EW, Mirra JM, Kerr R: Benign and malignant cartilage tumors of bone and joint: Their anatomic and theoretical basis with an emphasis on radiology, pathology and clinical biology. 1. The intramedullary cartilage tumors. Skeletal Radiol 26:325, 1997.
54. Levine E, Levine C: Ewing tumor of rib: Radiologic findings and computed tomography contribution. Skeletal Radiol 9:227, 1983.
55. Kyle RA: Multiple myeloma: Review of 869 cases. Mayo Clin Proc 50:29, 1975.
56. Franczyk J, Samuels T, Rubenstein J, et al: Skeletal lymphoma. J Can Assoc Radiol 40:75, 1989.
57. Hermann G, Klein MJ, Fikry Abedlewahab I, et al: MRI appearance of primary non-Hodgkin's lymphoma of bone. Skeletal Radiol 26:629, 1997.
58. Greenspan A: Bone island (enostosis): Current concept—a review. Skeletal Radiol 24:111, 1995.
59. McGuire MH, Mankin HJ: Osteoid osteoma: An unusual presentation as a rib lesion. Orthopedics 7:305, 1984.
60. Shankman S, Desai P, Beltran J: Subperiosteal osteoid osteoma: Radiographic and pathologic manifestations. Skeletal Radiol 26:457, 1997.
61. Kayser F, Resnick D, Haghighi P, et al: Evidence of the subperiosteal origin of osteoid osteomas in tubular bones: Analysis by CT and MR imaging. AJR 170:609, 1998.
62. Lichtenstein L, Sawyer WF: Benign osteoblastoma: Further observations and report of twenty additional cases. J Bone Joint Surg [Am] 46:755, 1964.
63. Keating RB, Wright PW, Staple TW: Enchondroma protuberans of the rib. Skeletal Radiol 13:55, 1985.
64. Geirnaerdt MJA, Bloem JL, Eulderink F, et al: Cartilaginous tumors: Correlation of gadolinium-enhanced MR imaging and histopathologic findings. Radiology 186:813, 1993.
65. Milgram JW: Intraosseous lipoma: A clinicopathologic study of 66 cases. Clin Orthop 231:277, 1988.
66. Sherman RS, Wilner D: The roentgen diagnosis of hemangioma of bone. AJR 86:1146, 1961.
67. De Dios AMV, Bond JR, Shives TC, et al: Aneurysmal bone cyst: A clinico-pathologic study of 238 cases. Cancer 69:2921, 1992.
68. Mirra JM, Brien EW, Tehranzadeh J: Paget's disease of bone: Review with emphasis on radiologic features. Part II. Skeletal Radiol 24:173, 1995.
69. Crawford AH Jr, Bogamery N: Osseous manifestations of neurofibromatosis in childhood. J Pediatr Orthop 6:72, 1986.
70. Gibson MJ, Middlemiss JH: Fibrous dysplasia of bone. Br J Radiol 44:1, 1971.
71. Kilpatrick SE, Wenger DE, Gilchrist GS, et al: Langerhans' cell histiocytosis (histiocytosis X) of bone: A clinicopathologic analysis of 263 pediatric and adult cases. Cancer 76:2471, 1995.
72. Taylor JAM, Resnick D, Sartoris DJ: Radiographic-pathologic correlation. *In* Sartoris DJ (ed): Osteoporosis: Diagnosis and Treatment. New York, Marcel Dekker, 1996, p 147.
73. Hanscom DA, Winter RB, Lutter L, et al: Osteogenesis imperfecta: Radiographic classification, natural history and treatment of spinal deformity. J Bone Joint Surg [Am] 74:598, 1992.
74. Mankin HJ: Rickets, osteomalacia, and renal osteodystrophy. Orthop Clin North Am 21:81, 1990.
75. Chew FS, Huang-Hellinger F: Brown tumor. AJR 160:752, 1993.
76. Simpson W, Kerr DNS, Hill AVL, et al: Skeletal changes in patients on regular hemodialysis. Radiology 107:313, 1971.
77. Cameron EW, Resnik CS, Light PD, et al: Hemodialysis-related amyloidosis of the sternoclavicular joint. Skeletal Radiol 26:428, 1997.
78. Resnick D: Hemoglobinopathies and other anemias. *In* Resnick D (ed): Diagnosis of Bone and Joint Disorders. 3rd Ed. Philadelphia, WB Saunders, 1995, p 2128.
79. Bouroncle BA, Doan CA: Myelofibrosis: clinical, hematologic and pathologic study of 110 patients. Am J Med Sci 243:697, 1962.
80. Gentry RR, Rust RS, Lohr JA, et al: Infantile cortical hyperostosis of the ribs (Caffey's disease) without mandibular involvement. Pediatr Radiol 13:236, 1983.
81. Tecce PM, Fishman EK: Spiral CT with multiplanar reconstruction in the diagnosis of sternoclavicular osteomyelitis. Skeletal Radiol 24:275, 1995.
82. Jurik AG, Egund N: MRI in chronic recurrent multifocal osteomyelitis. Skeletal Radiol 26:230, 1997.

CHAPTER 13

Clavicle, Scapula, and Shoulder

Normal Developmental Anatomy

Accurate interpretation of radiographs of the pediatric shoulder requires a thorough understanding of normal developmental anatomy. Table 13–1 outlines the age of appearance and fusion of the primary and secondary ossification centers. Figures 13–1 and 13–2 demonstrate the radiographic appearance of many important ossification centers and other developmental landmarks at selected ages from birth to skeletal maturity.

Developmental Anomalies, Anatomic Variants, and Sources of Diagnostic Error

The shoulder is a frequent site of anomalies, anatomic variations, and other sources of diagnostic error that may simulate disease and potentially result in misdiagnosis. Table 13–2 and Figures 13–3 to 13–12 represent selected examples of some of the more common processes affecting the clavicle, the scapula, and the proximal portion of the humerus.

Skeletal Dysplasias and Other Congenital Diseases

The bones and joints about the shoulder are frequent sites of skeletal dysplasias and other congenital diseases. Table 13–3 lists some of the more frequently occurring conditions, and Figures 13–13 and 13–14 illustrate two examples of dysplasia.

Physical Injury

Physical injury to the shoulder region results in a wide variety of fractures of the clavicle, the scapula, and the proximal portion of the humerus. Additionally, dislocations of the glenohumeral joint and the acromioclavicular joint frequently are encountered. Table 13–4 lists the most common types of fractures, and Table 13–5 outlines the various types of shoulder dislocation. Several examples of these injuries are illustrated in Figures 13–15 to 13–23. Injuries of the sternoclavicular joint are discussed in Chapter 12, and fractures of the humeral diaphysis are discussed and illustrated in Chapter 14.

Internal Joint Derangements and Other Soft Tissue Injuries

The shoulder is second only to the knee in frequency of internal joint derangements. Common abnormalities of tendons, ligaments, joint capsules, and labral structures are listed in Table 13–6. Table 13–6 also lists a number of other miscellaneous traumatic disorders. Figures 13–24 to 13–28 illustrate several examples of the conditions discussed in Table 13–6.

Articular Disorders

The glenohumeral, acromioclavicular, and coracoclavicular joints are frequent target sites of involvement for many degenerative, inflammatory, crystal-induced, and infectious articular disorders. Table 13–7 outlines these diseases and their characteristics. Figures 13–29 to 13–46 illustrate the typical radiographic manifestations of the most common articular disorders affecting the shoulder.

Neoplasms

The clavicle and the scapula are infrequent sites of involvement for benign, malignant, and tumor-like lesions of bone. Table 13–8 describes the range of such neoplasms, many of which are illustrated in Figures 13–47 to 13–54.

Metabolic, Hematologic, and Infectious Disorders

Several metabolic, hematologic, and infectious disorders affect the bones and soft tissue structures about the shoulder region. Table 13–9 lists some of the more common disorders and discusses their characteristics. Figures 13–55 to 13–59 illustrate the typical imaging findings of many of these disorders.

Miscellaneous Disorders Resulting in Clavicular Osteosclerosis, Periostitis, or Bone Enlargement

Table 13–10 describes a variety of conditions that result in osteosclerosis, periostitis, or bone enlargement of the clavicle. Figures 13–60 to 13–62 illustrate some of the more common examples.

TABLE 13–1. Shoulder: Approximate Age of Appearance and Fusion of Ossification Centers[1–4] (Figs. 13–1 and 13–2)

Ossification Center	Primary or Secondary	No. of Centers (Per Bone)	Age of Appearance* (Years)	Age of Fusion* (Years)	Comments
Clavicle					
Shaft	P	1	Birth		
Proximal epiphysis	S	1	16–20	22–25	Fuses with shaft
Scapula					
Body	P	1	Birth		
Coracoid process	S	1	Birth–1	16–19	Fuses with body
Coracoid tip epiphysis	S	2	15–19	20–24	Fuses with coracoid process
Subcoracoid epiphysis	S	1	10	20–24	Fuses with coracoid process
Margin of glenoid	S	1	14–19	20–24	Fuses with body
Border and angle epiphyses	S	2	15–17	20–24	Fuses with body
Acromion process	S	2	14–17	19–22	Fuses with body
Proximal portion of humerus			**(months)**		
Humeral head epiphysis	S	1	Birth–1 mo	4–6	Fuses with greater tuberosity
Greater tuberosity	S	1	3–27 mo	4–6	Fuses with humeral head
Lesser tuberosity	S	1	3–27 mo	20–23	Fuses with humeral head
Humeral metaphysis				20–23	Head and tuberosity fuse to metaphysis

*Ages of appearance and fusion of ossification centers in girls typically precede those of boys. Ethnic differences also exist.
P, Primary; S, secondary.

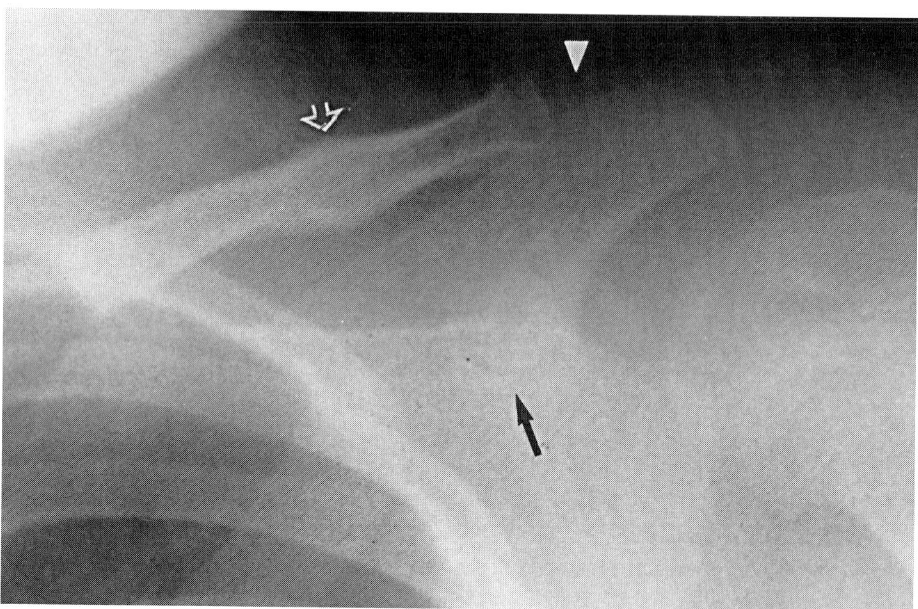

FIGURE 13–1. Skeletal maturation and normal development: Clavicle, young child. Frontal projection of the clavicle in this 2-year-old girl shows a normal expansion at the junction of the middle and distal thirds of the clavicle (open arrow) and is the result of its curved contour. Note the unfused ossification center of the coracoid process (arrow) and the wide acromioclavicular articulation (arrowhead). The clavicle is the first bone of the body to ossify during fetal life. It ossifies from membrane with cartilage growth at the ends. An epiphyseal ossification center appears at the medial end of the clavicle between the ages of 16 and 20 years. The appearance of the clavicle is dependent on its position and, as a result, may appear bowed or twisted.

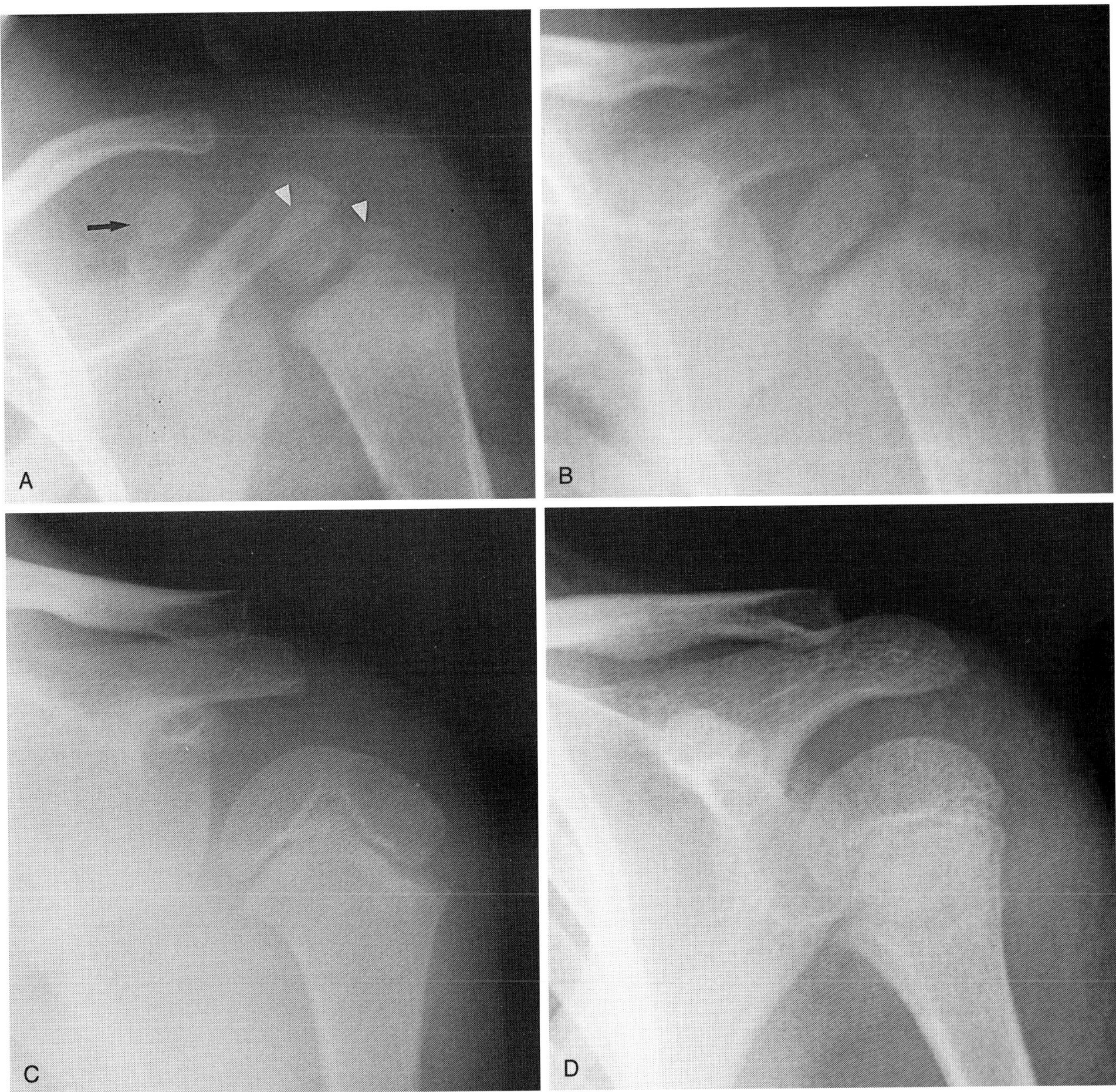

FIGURE 13–2. Skeletal maturation and normal development: Shoulder.[1–4] A 16-month-old girl. Observe the paired proximal humeral capital epiphyses (arrowheads) and the adjacent radiodense area of the zone of provisional calcification. The secondary ossification center of the coracoid process is evident (arrow) and has not yet fused to the scapula. The acromioclavicular joint is characteristically wide. B 2-year-old boy. The humeral capital epiphyses are larger, and the zone of provisional calcification in the humeral metaphysis remains radiodense. C 5-year-old girl. The paired humeral capital epiphyses have fused together and conform to the chevron-shaped humeral metaphysis. D 8-year-old girl. The humeral capital epiphysis is now the same width as the adjacent metaphysis. The acromioclavicular joint remains wide.

Illustration continued on following page

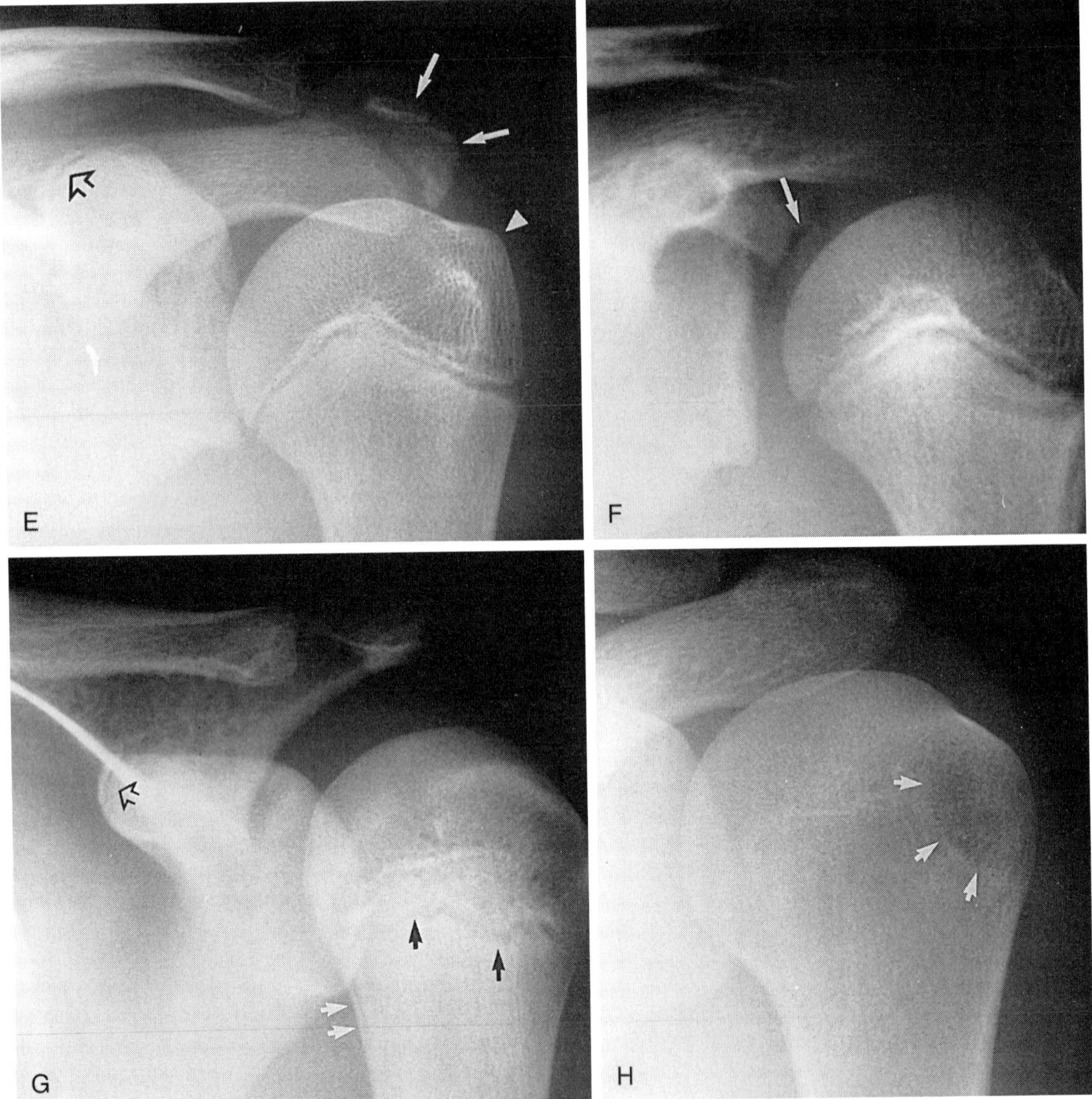

FIGURE 13–2 *Continued.* E 12-year-old girl. Secondary ossification centers for the acromion (arrows) and coracoid processes (open arrow) are apparent. The greater tuberosity is now distinctly visible (arrowhead). F 12-year-old boy. A normal physiologic intra-articular vacuum phenomenon (arrow) is present, outlining the articular cartilage of the humeral head. G 14-year-old boy. On this internal rotation radiograph, the physeal line of the humeral capital epiphysis is seen as an irregular transverse line (black arrows) just before closure. This should not be confused with a fracture. The greater tuberosity forms a superimposed arc of radiodensity overlying the humeral head. A secondary ossification center is present at the coracoid process (open arrow). Unusual projection of the cortex simulates periostitis of the humeral metaphysis (white arrows). H 16-year-old girl. This radiograph reveals normal adult proportions and closure of all ossification centers. A small, normal humeral pseudocyst is present within the greater tuberosity (arrows). The acromioclavicular joint is of normal adult width.

TABLE 13–2. Developmental Anomalies, Anatomic Variants, and Sources of Diagnostic Error Affecting the Shoulder

Entity	Figure(s)	Characteristics
Clavicle		
Fork deformity of the medial end of clavicle[5]	13–3	In young people, the medial articular surface of the clavicle appears fork-shaped before completion of development May persist into adulthood in otherwise normal persons and should not be mistaken for a disease process
Ununited ossification centers[5]	13–4	Ossification centers of the medial ends of the clavicles may persist into adulthood and simulate fractures
Rhomboid fossa[5, 6]	13–5	Scalloped undersurface of the medial aspect of the clavicles at the attachment of the rhomboid ligament between the clavicle and first rib Often bilateral but not always symmetric Normal anatomic variant that may simulate destructive lesion of the clavicle or a cavitating lesion of the lung apex
Congenital pseudarthrosis[7]	13–6	Congenital pseudarthrosis affects the right clavicle almost exclusively; bilateral in 10 per cent of cases; left side involvement frequently associated with dextrocardia Pseudarthrosis may occur as an isolated phenomenon or in association with neurofibromatosis and fibrous dysplasia
Clavicular companion shadow[8]	13–7	Normal radiodense area paralleling the superior aspect of the clavicle represents the normal soft tissue shadows, such as the platysma muscle, adjacent to the clavicle Should not be mistaken for an apical lung lesion, periostitis, or subperiosteal hemorrhage
Coracoclavicular joint[9]	13–8	Anomalous osseous flange arising from the undersurface of the clavicle that articulates with the coracoid process Normal variant in the region of the coracoclavicular ligament; usually of no clinical significance Infrequently painful after trauma; surgical resection may relieve the pain Heterotopic ossification of coracoclavicular ligaments after acromioclavicular dislocation may simulate a coracoclavicular joint
Scapula		
Sprengel's deformity[6, 10]	13–9	Developmental anomaly involving elevation of the scapula Present in approximately 25 per cent of patients with the Klippel-Feil syndrome Also may be seen as an isolated anomaly
Omovertebral bone[6, 10]	13–9	Anomalous bone, cartilage, or fibrous tissue extending from the superior angle of the scapula to the spinous process, lamina, or transverse process of the C5 or C6 vertebra Present in 30–40 per cent of patients with Sprengel's deformity
Hypoplasia of the glenoid neck[11]	13–10	Also termed scapular dysplasia and dentated glenoid anomaly Findings: scapular neck hypoplasia, notched articular surface of the glenoid cavity, and widening of the inferior aspect of the glenohumeral articular surface Usually bilateral and relatively symmetric Family history of similar abnormalities observed in some cases Many patients have pain and limited shoulder motion Approximately 25% have multidirectional glenohumeral instability
Ununited ossification centers[5]		Failure of ossification of several secondary ossification centers occurs about the acromion (os acromiale), coracoid process, glenoid, and inferior angle of the scapula (infrascapular bone)
Os acromiale[12, 13]		Ossification center of the tip of the acromion usually fuses with the acromion before the person reaches 25 years of age; persists into adulthood in as many as 15 per cent of persons Triangular shape; may simulate fracture May be associated with pain and an increased prevalence of shoulder impingement syndrome and rotator cuff tears
Prominent vascular channel[5]	13–11	Vascular channels within the wing of the scapula may be prominent and resemble fractures—often parallel the scapular spine
Proximal portion of humerus		
Humeral pseudocyst[14]	13–2 H, 13–12	Zone of diminished trabeculae within the spongiosa bone of the greater tubercle of the humerus May simulate destructive neoplasm such as chondroblastoma

See also Table 1–1.

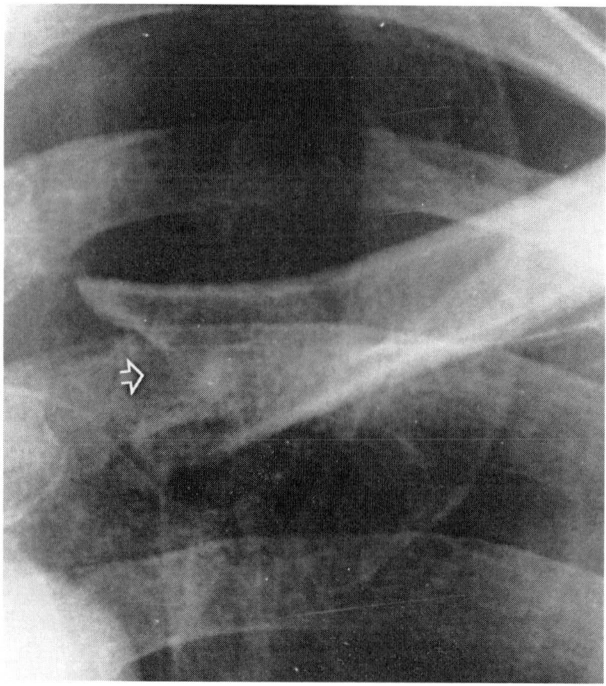

FIGURE 13–3. Fork deformity of the medial end of the clavicle.[5] In young people, the medial articular surface of the clavicle appears fork-shaped before completion of development. This appearance may persist into adulthood in otherwise normal persons and should not be mistaken for osseous destruction or other pathologic condition.

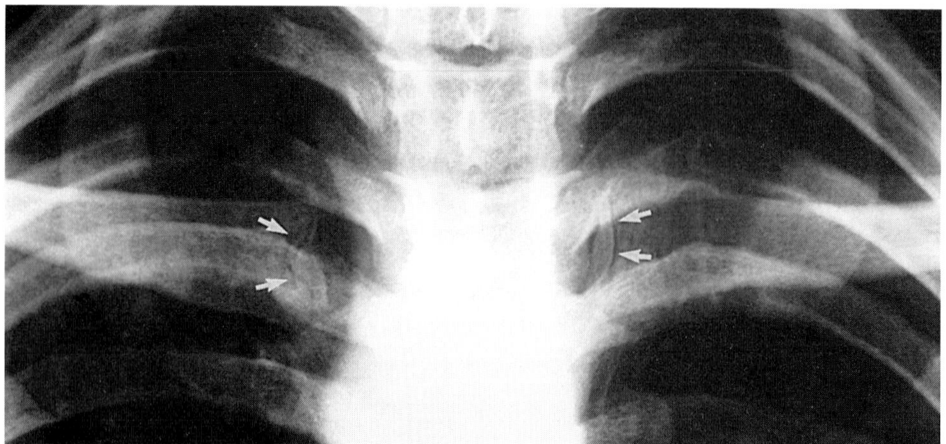

FIGURE 13–4. Ununited ossification centers.[5] Observe the failure of ossification of the secondary ossification centers of the medial ends of the clavicles (arrows) in this 30-year-old man. This ossification center typically begins to ossify between the ages of 16 and 20 years and fuses between the ages of 22 and 25 years.

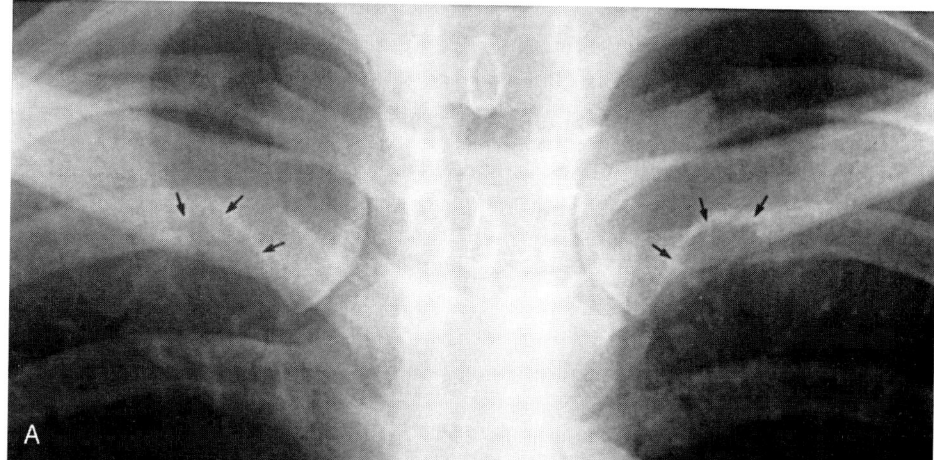

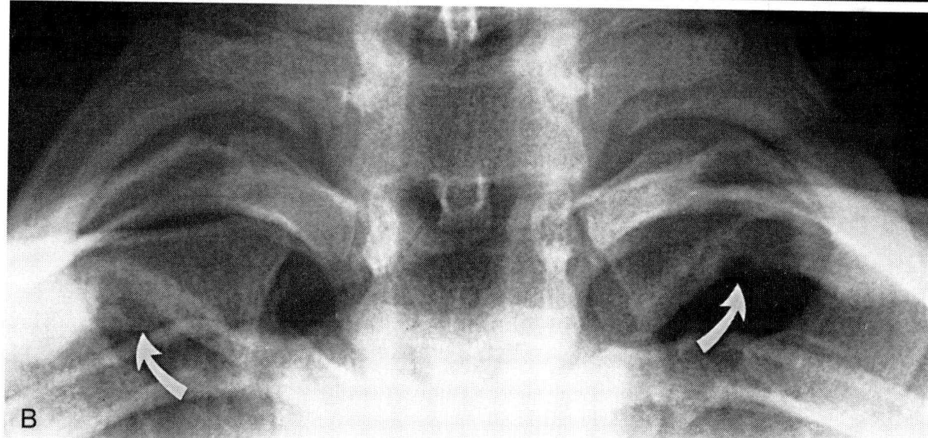

FIGURE 13–5. Rhomboid fossae.[5, 6] A Note the scalloped appearance of the undersurface of the medial aspect of both clavicles (arrows). B Another bilateral example in a 16-year-old boy (curved arrows). Rhomboid fossae are normal anatomic variants that may simulate destructive lesions of the clavicle or cavitating lesions of the lung apex.

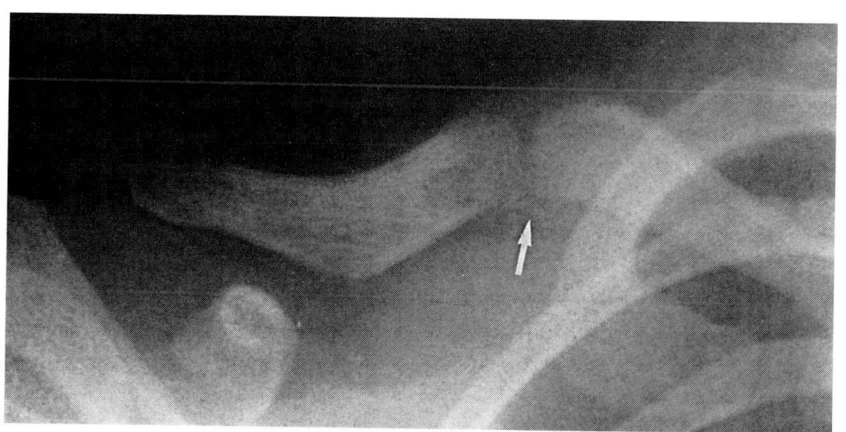

FIGURE 13–6. Congenital pseudarthrosis of the clavicle.[7] Observe the radiolucent defect in the mid-diaphysis of the clavicle in this infant (arrow). Callus formation is absent, and the bone edges adjacent to the pseudarthrosis are rounded. *(Courtesy of A. D' Abreu, M.D., Porto Alegre, Brazil.)*

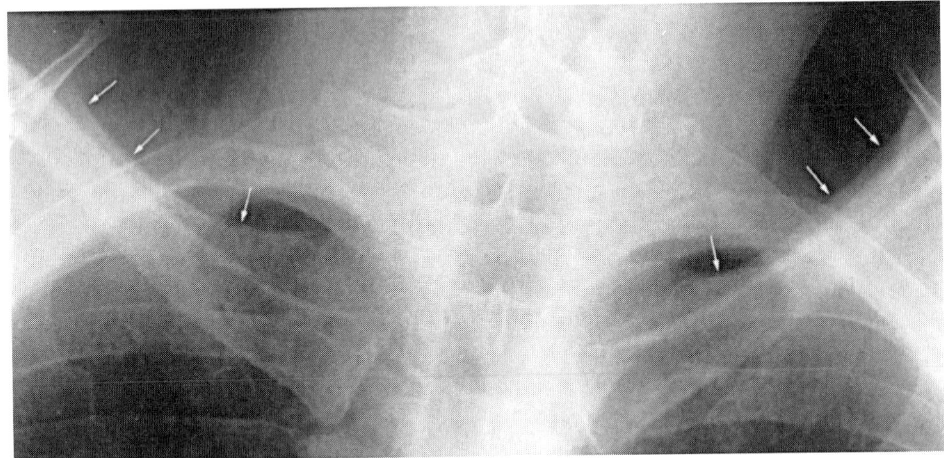

FIGURE 13–7. Clavicular companion shadow.[8] Observe the normal radiodense shadow paralleling the superior aspect of the clavicle (arrows). This finding represents the normal subcutaneous soft tissues adjacent to the clavicle and should not be mistaken for an apical lung lesion, periostitis, or subperiosteal hemorrhage.

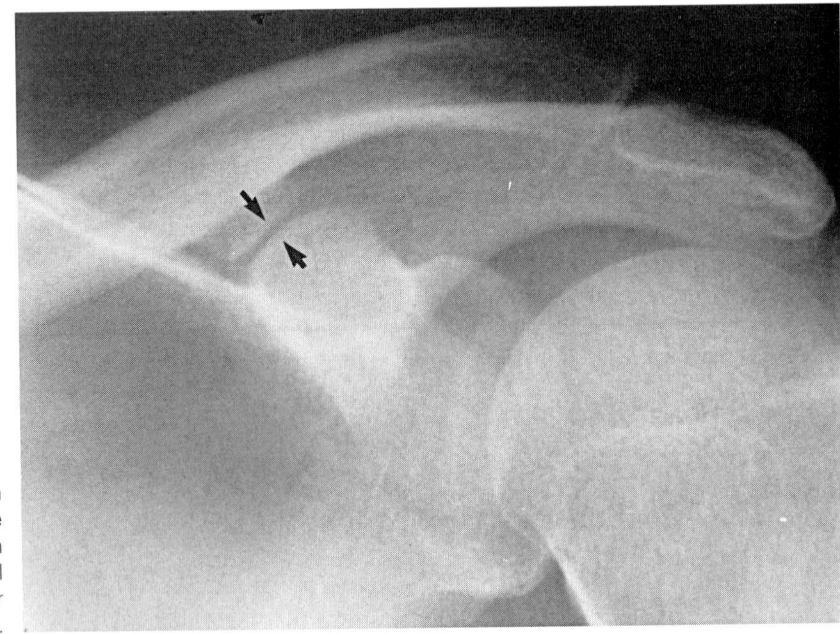

FIGURE 13–8. Coracoclavicular joint.[9] An anomalous osseous flange arising from the undersurface of the clavicle articulates with the coracoid process (arrows). This normal variant in the region of the coracoclavicular ligament usually is of no clinical significance.

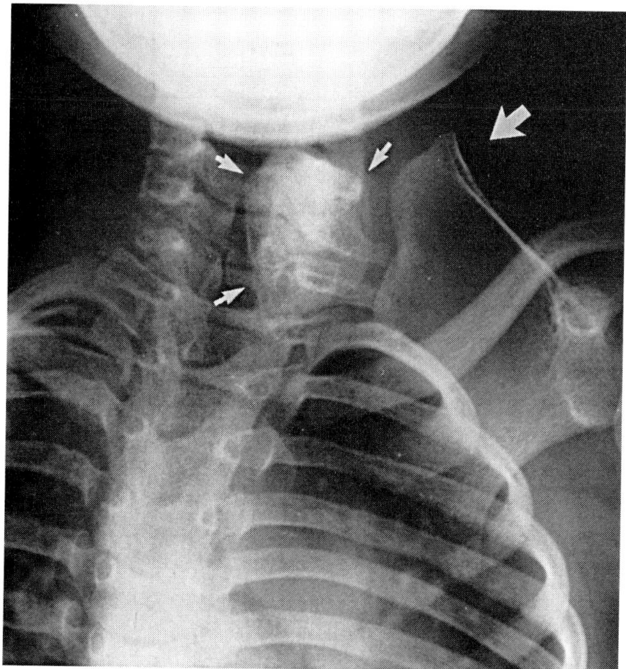

FIGURE 13–9. Sprengel's deformity and omovertebral bone: Klippel-Feil syndrome.[6, 10] Observe the elevation of the scapula (Sprengel's deformity) (large arrow), omovertebral bone (small arrows), and multiple other cervical spine anomalies in this patient with Klippel-Feil syndrome. Sprengel's deformity is present in about 25 per cent of patients with Klippel-Feil syndrome.

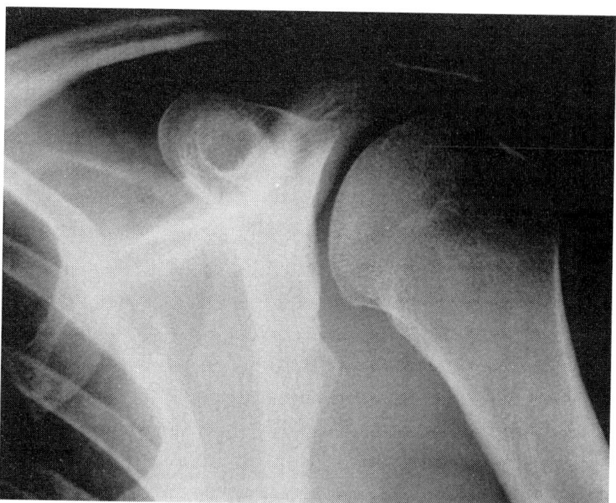

FIGURE 13–10. Glenoid hypoplasia (scapular dysplasia).[11] This patient exhibits typical findings, including scapular neck hypoplasia, notched articular surface of the glenoid, and widening of the inferior articular surface. *(Courtesy of A. Brower, M.D., Norfolk, Virginia.)*

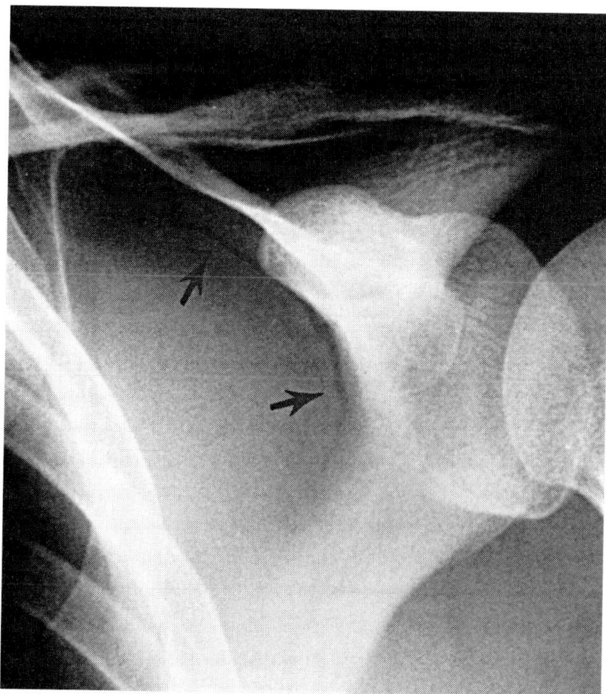

FIGURE 13–11. Prominent vascular channel.[5] A curvilinear radiolucent vascular groove in the wing of the scapula is seen (arrows). Such vascular grooves may simulate fractures. *(Courtesy of L. E. Hoffman, D.C., Portland, Oregon.)*

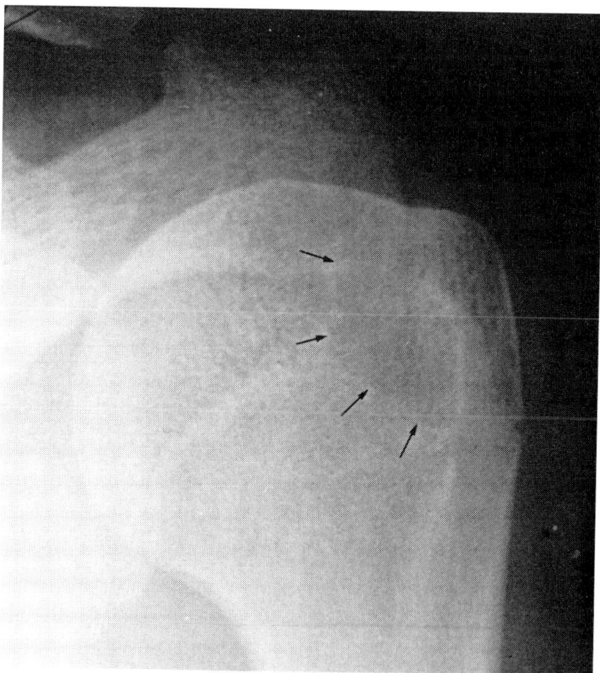

FIGURE 13–12. Humeral pseudocyst.[14] The circular area of radiolucency adjacent to and within the greater tuberosity (arrows) is a normal zone of trabecular diminution termed the humeral pseudocyst. The curvilinear inferior margin separates the relatively porous lateral region from the more densely compact spongiosa located medially.

TABLE 13–3. Skeletal Dysplasias and Other Congenital Diseases Affecting the Shoulder

Entity	Figure(s)	Characteristics
Achondroplasia[15]		Splaying of the proximal portion of the humerus Metaphyseal cupping
Infantile cortical hyperostosis (Caffey's disease)[16, 122]		Clinical triad: hyperirritability, palpable masses overlying affected bones, and soft tissue swelling Bilateral symmetric periosteal new bone formation along the clavicular shaft and, less commonly, the scapula May be associated with Erb-Duchenne palsy
Fibrodysplasia ossificans progressiva[17]		Extensive soft tissue ossification involving the shoulder girdle musculature, tendons, fascia, and ligaments
Osteopoikilosis[18]	13–13	Proximal portion of humerus and glenoid region frequently affected Multiple circular zones of osteosclerosis tend to accumulate in a periarticular distribution
Osteopetrosis[19]		Diffuse sclerosis of clavicle, scapula, and humerus Flared proximal humeral metaphysis May lead to pathologic fracture
Melorheostosis[20]		Hemimelic distribution of flowing hyperostosis along humeral shaft or scapula Occasional soft tissue ossification
Cleidocranial dysplasia[21]	13–14	Failure of ossification of the clavicular growth centers resulting in hypoplasia or complete absence (10 per cent of cases) of clavicles Scapulae may be hypoplastic or deformed Marked shoulder hypermobility often leads to glenohumeral joint dislocations

See also Table 1–2.

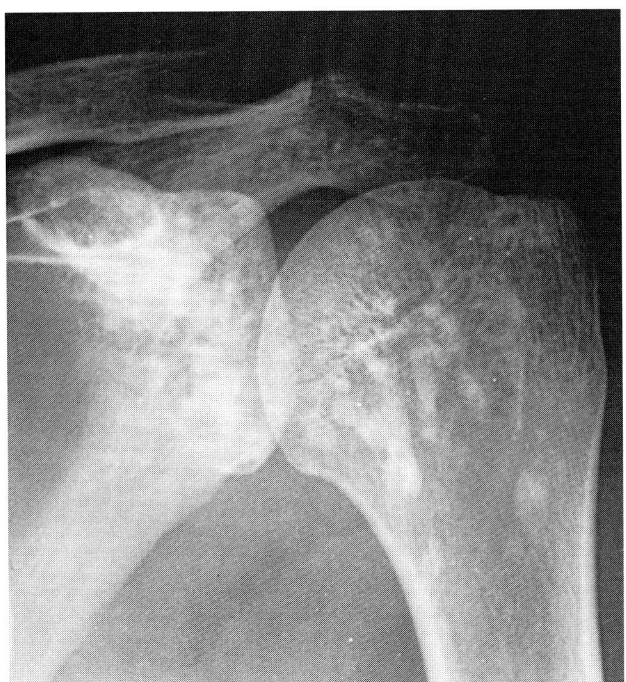

FIGURE 13–13. Osteopoikilosis.[18] Note the circular and ovoid osteosclerotic foci localized within the humerus and scapula. A symmetric periarticular distribution is characteristic of this fairly common sclerosing dysplasia. Although the epiphysis may be affected, most lesions occur predominantly in the metaphysis. Osteopoikilosis typically is a process that affects several bones about the major joints.

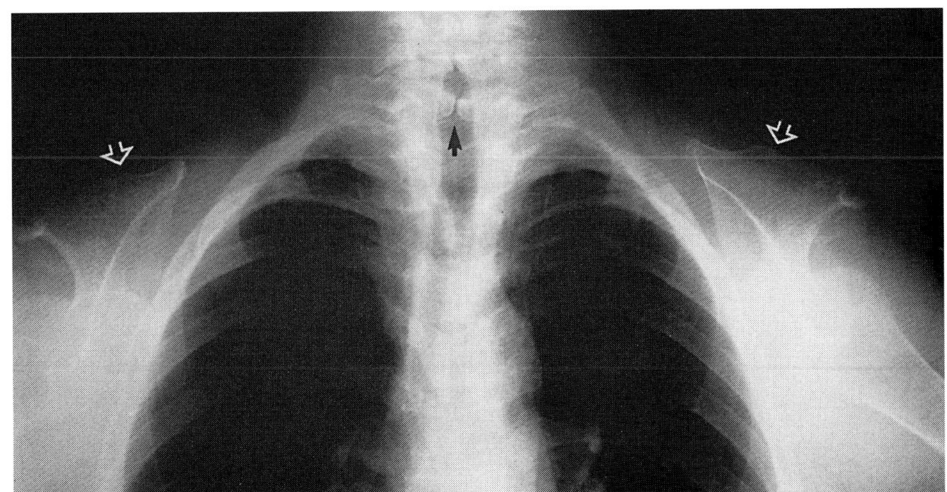

FIGURE 13–14. Cleidocranial dysplasia.[21] Complete absence of the clavicles, spina bifida occulta (arrow), and hypoplastic scapulae (open arrows) are evident. Involved patients have varying degrees of hypermobility and drooping of the shoulders. Any portion of the clavicle may be absent, but the middle and outer portions are affected most commonly. Total clavicular agenesis is evident in only 10 per cent of cases. The scapula may be underdeveloped with a small glenoid cavity.

TABLE 13–4. Fractures About the Shoulder

Injury	Figure(s), Table(s)	Characteristics	Complications and Related Injuries
Fractures of the proximal portion of the humerus			
Acute fractures in adults[22, 23]	13–15	Middle-aged and elderly adults Osteoporosis significant predisposing factor Classified as one-part to four-part fractures based on the degree and the location of displacement among: Surgical neck Anatomic neck Greater and lesser tuberosities	May be associated with lipohemarthrosis, drooping shoulder, intra-articular bodies, degenerative disease, delayed union, heterotopic bone formation, rotator cuff injury, injury of brachial plexus and axillary artery, marked humeral head rotation, and osteonecrosis
Growth plate injuries in children[24, 25]	13–16	Type I physeal injury: Slipped humeral epiphysis Boys aged 11 to 16 years Little League shoulder syndrome: epiphysiolysis of the humeral epiphysis	Limb shortening in 10 per cent of patients
Fractures of the clavicle[26, 27]	13–17	Most common bone fractured during childbirth Frequent accidental injury in children Infrequent injury in child abuse	All types: Nonunion uncommon (<1 per cent) Posttraumatic pseudarthrosis also rare First rib fracture *Children:* clavicle fractures heal rapidly without significant deformity *Adults:* resultant deformity secondary to excessive callus formation may be observed
Intermediate segment	13–17 A, E, F	Seventy-five to 80 per cent of clavicle fractures Fall on outstretched arm or fall on shoulder	Occasional cosmetic deformity Neurovascular compression by large callus (rare)
Distal (lateral) segment	13–17 B, C	Fifteen to 20 per cent of clavicle fractures Downward forces on humerus and scapula	Delayed union or nonunion rarely Posttraumatic osteolysis of the clavicle Acromioclavicular and coracoclavicular joint injuries
Proximal (medial) segment	13–17 D	Five per cent of clavicle fractures Direct trauma Intra-articular and transverse types	Degenerative joint disease with intra-articular type Sternoclavicular joint injuries
Fractures of the scapula[28–30]		Five to 7 per cent of all fractures about the shoulder	All types: 95 per cent associated with fractures of the clavicle, ribs, and skull or dislocation of the acromioclavicular joint
Scapular body	13–18 A, B	Most frequent site: 50–70 per cent of scapular fractures	
Scapular neck		Second most frequent site Direct blow Bankart lesion: occurs in 20 per cent of glenohumeral dislocations	Labral injuries
Glenoid fossa and articular surface	13–18 C	Stress fracture: inferior margin of the glenoid in baseball pitchers (rare)	Labral injuries
Scapular spine		Rare injury Direct trauma	
Acromion process	13–18 D	Direct trauma or muscular traction Most common injury of the scapula in child abuse; partial avulsion or complete fracture; usually unilateral and left-sided	Significant neurologic injury to brachial plexus
Coracoid process	13–18 E	*Mechanisms* 1. Direct injury from dislocating humeral head 2. Direct force on tip 3. Avulsion from traction of coracoclavicular ligament 4. Stress fracture in trapshooters	Significant neurologic injury to brachial plexus
Floating shoulder	13–18 F	Combined fractures of the scapular neck and ipsilateral clavicle Result in disruption of the stability of the suspensory structures of the shoulder	Muscle forces and the weight of the arm typically pull the glenoid fragment distally and anteromedially
Fractures of the first and second ribs[31]	12–9 B; Table 12–4	Major trauma to the thorax or shoulder Stress fracture from heavy backpacking and weightlifting	Rupture of the lung apex or subclavian artery, aneurysm of the aortic arch, tracheoesophageal fistula, pleurisy, hemothorax, cardiac alterations, neurologic injury, and other fractures, especially of cervicothoracic transverse processes

*See also Tables 1–3 and 1–4.

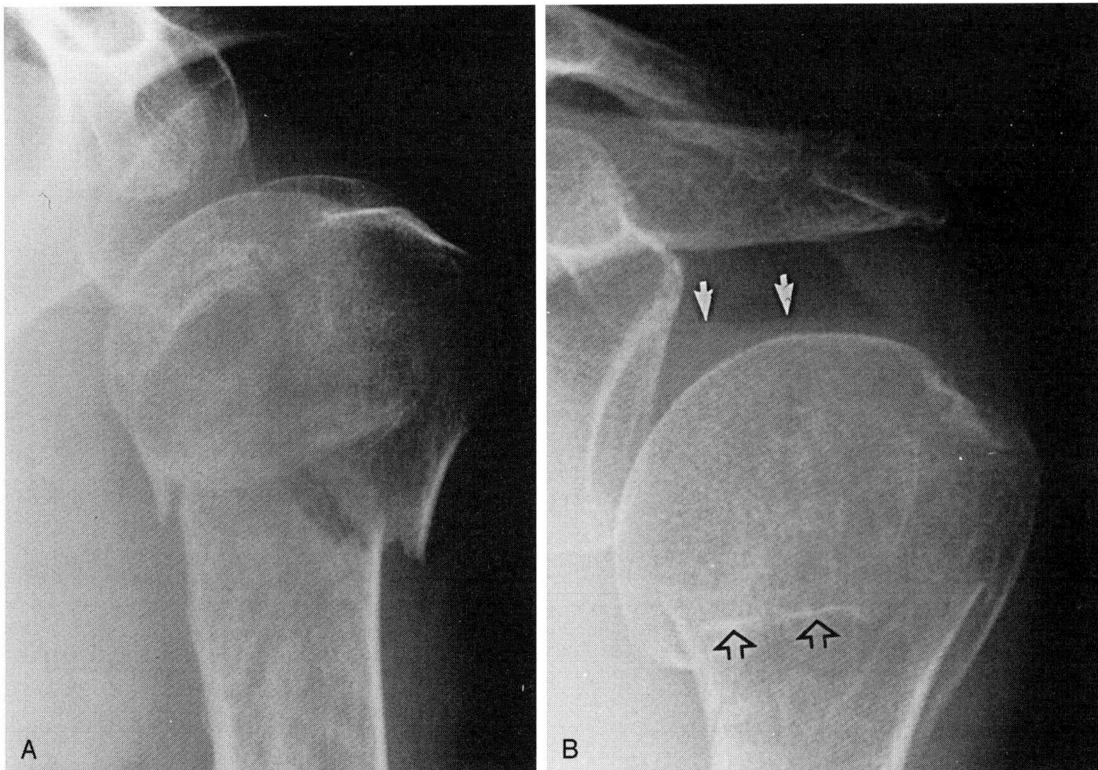

FIGURE 13–15. Fractures of the proximal portion of the humerus.[22, 23] A This 74-year-old osteoporotic man had fallen on his shoulder 3 weeks before this radiograph was obtained. The radiograph reveals a minimally displaced three-part fracture of the surgical neck and greater tuberosity of the humerus. A computed tomographic (CT) scan revealed that the lesser tuberosity was intact. B In another patient, fracture of the surgical neck of the humerus (open arrows) is accompanied by a lipohemarthrosis, which is seen as a fat-fluid level (arrows) and represents release of fat from the bone marrow into the joint fluid. Observe also the inferior subluxation of the humeral head relative to the glenoid fossa, a condition that may be caused by a large joint effusion and is termed a drooping shoulder. Fractures of the proximal portion of the humerus occur most frequently in patients older than 45 years of age, especially osteoporotic persons. They are classified as one-part to four-part on the basis of the degree and the location of displacement among four regions of the humerus: head, shaft, greater tuberosity, and lesser tuberosity.

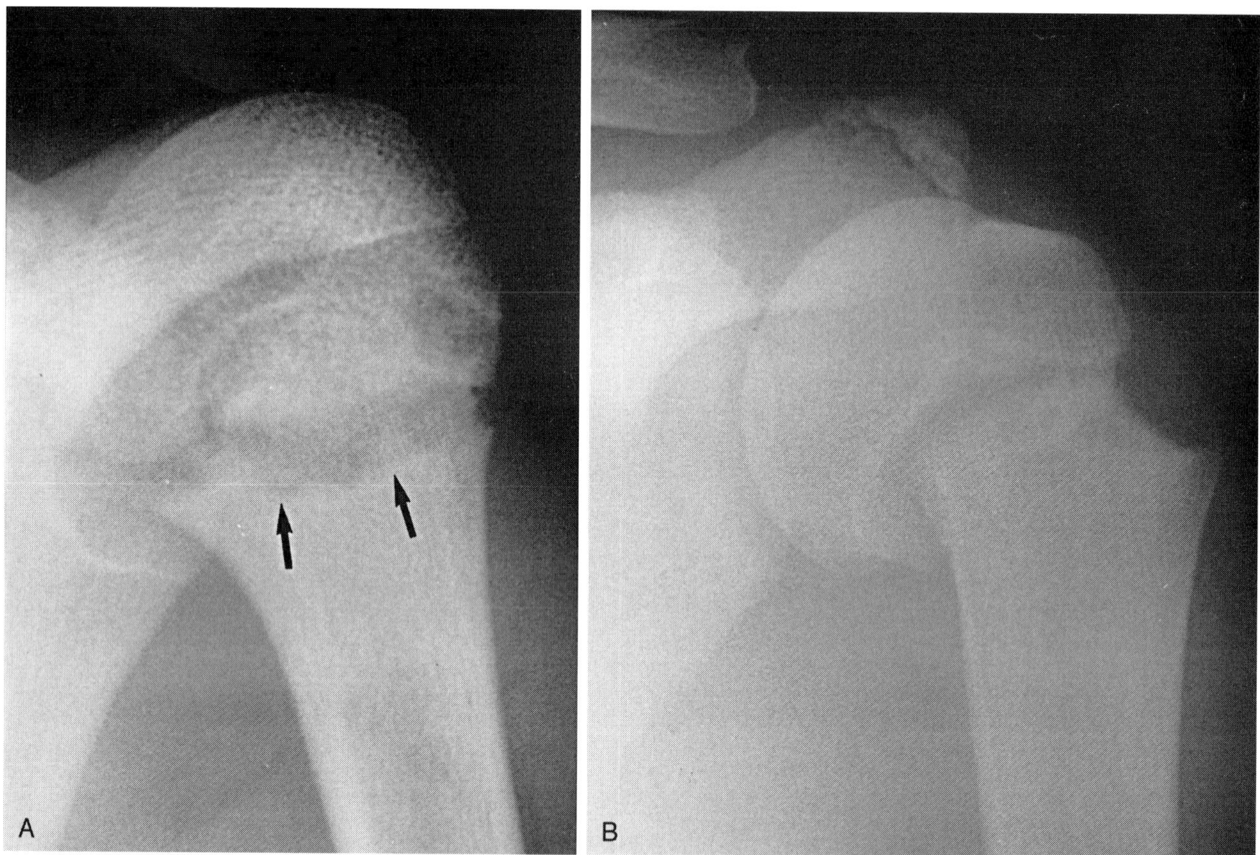

FIGURE 13–16. Growth plate injury: Little League shoulder syndrome.[24, 25] A This 13-year-old baseball pitcher developed progressive shoulder pain in his pitching arm. Observe the widening and irregularity of the humeral physis (arrows) and the sclerosis of the adjacent metaphyseal margin. (A, *Courtesy of G. Greenway, M.D., Dallas, Texas.*) B A more severe example shows a fracture through the growth plate of the proximal end of the humerus in a 14-year-old baseball pitcher. Note the obvious displacement of the humeral epiphysis. Little League shoulder syndrome represents epiphysiolysis of the proximal humeral epiphysis in adolescent baseball pitchers. It is a Salter-Harris type I growth plate injury that may result in shortening of the limb. Such injuries also may occur as a result of a fall on an outstretched arm with the wrist and elbow fully extended.

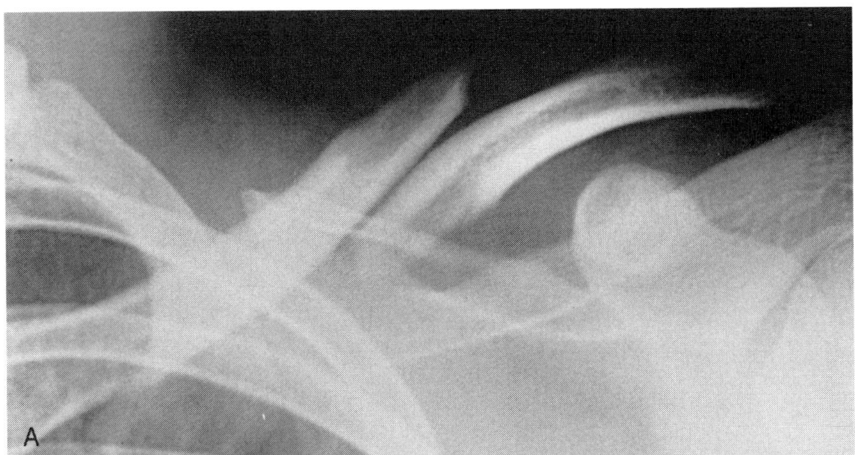

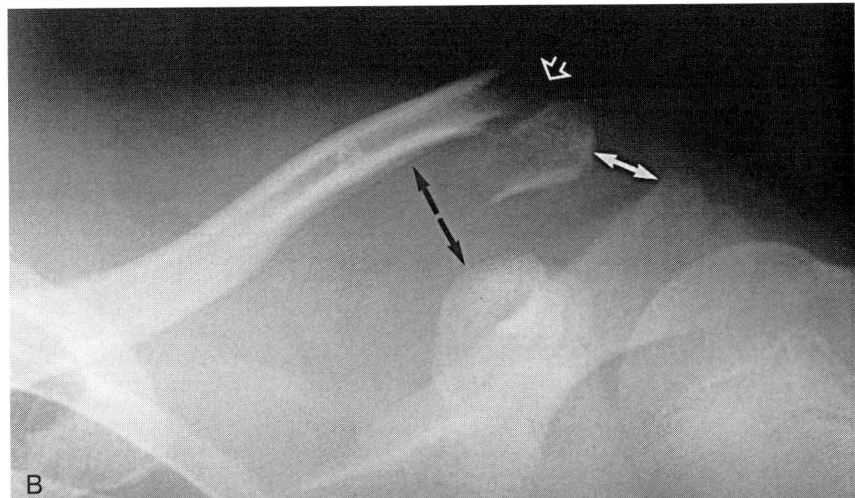

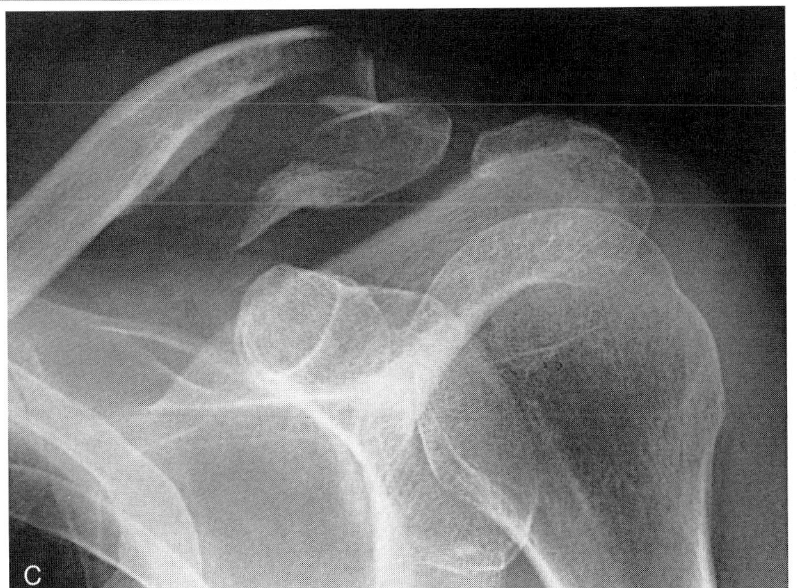

FIGURE 13–17. Clavicle fractures.[26, 27] **A** Intermediate segment. Note the fracture at the junction of the distal and intermediate thirds of the clavicle. The intermediate or middle segment of the clavicle is pulled upward by the sternocleidomastoid muscle, and the distal segment is pulled downward by the weight of the arm and inward by the pull of the pectoralis major and latissimus dorsi muscles on the scapula and the humerus. This parallel offset of the two fragments is termed bayonet apposition, a common finding in fractures of the intermediate segment. **B** Lateral segment. A fracture of the distal end of the clavicle (open arrow) is associated with complete rupture of the coracoclavicular ligaments (black arrows) and acromioclavicular ligaments (double-headed white arrow) in a 13-year-old boy. Observe the widened coracoclavicular distance and superior displacement of the proximal portion of the clavicle. **C** A similar fracture of the lateral segment is seen in an adult. Note the comminuted fragments and upward displacement of the medial portion of the clavicle.

Illustration continued on following page

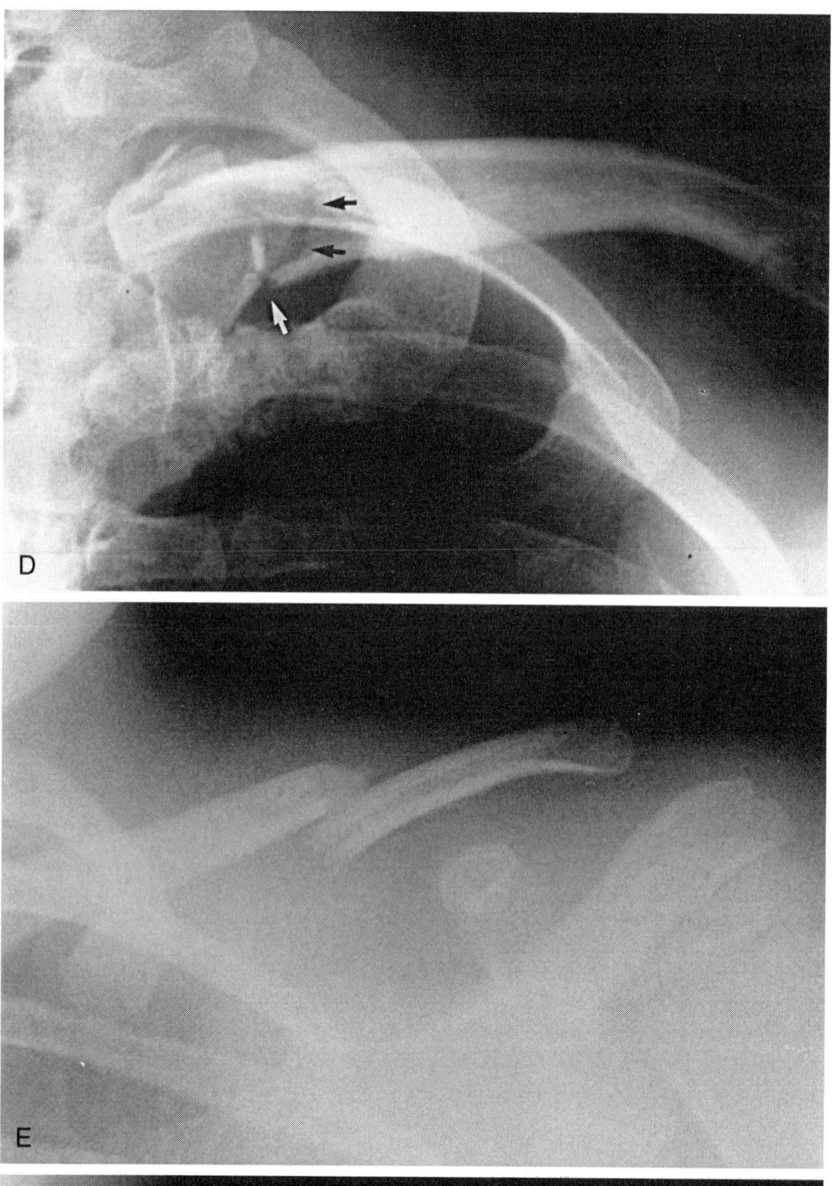

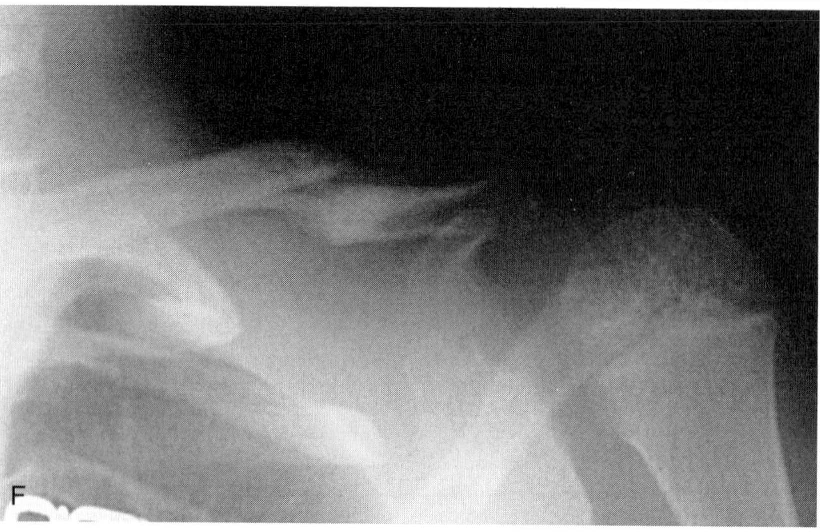

FIGURE 13–17 *Continued.* D Medial segment. Observe the comminuted fracture of the medial segment of the clavicle (arrows). E, F Normal healing in a child. In this 5-year-old child, the initial radiograph **(E)** shows a fracture of the intermediate segment with bayonet apposition. The medial portion of the clavicle is pulled upward, and the lateral segment is pulled downward and toward the midline. A subsequent radiograph **(F)**, obtained 65 days after injury, demonstrates solid bone fusion with abundant callus formation and remodeling despite poor apposition of fracture fragments.

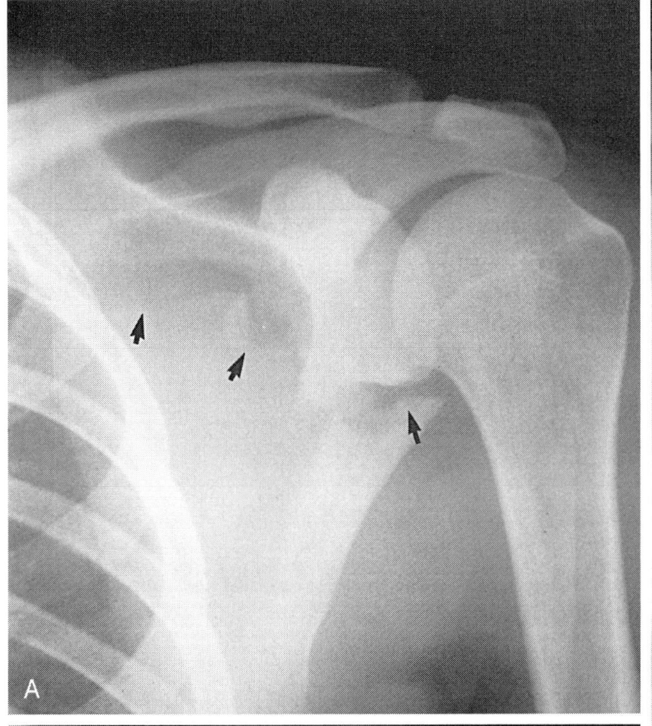

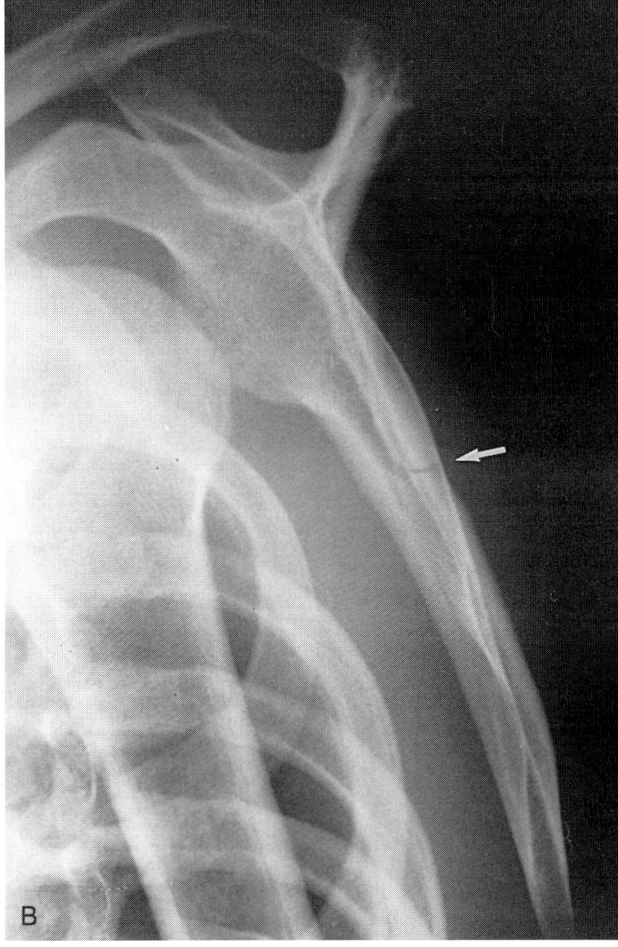

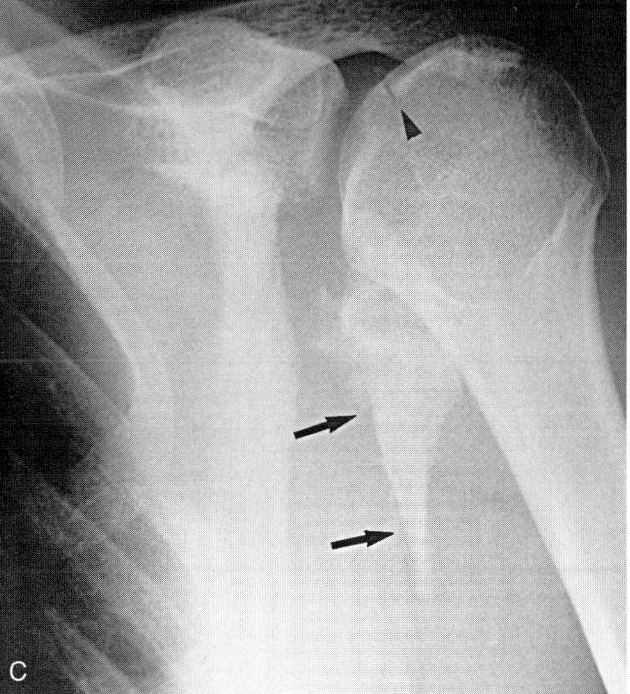

FIGURE 13–18. Scapular fractures.[28–30] A Body of scapula. Observe the jagged transverse fracture through the entire body of the scapula (arrows). About 50 to 70 per cent of scapular fractures involve the body and result from direct force. B Value of scapular Y projection. In another patient, the scapular Y view clearly demonstrates a fracture of the body of the scapula (arrow) associated with anterior subcoracoid glenohumeral dislocation. C Complex fracture of glenoid and body. In this patient, a comminuted intra-articular fracture of the glenoid and scapular body with severe inferior displacement of the fracture fragment is evident (arrows). The greater tuberosity of the humerus also is fractured (arrowhead). *(C, Courtesy of R. Crokin, D.C., Portland, Oregon.)*

Illustration continued on following page

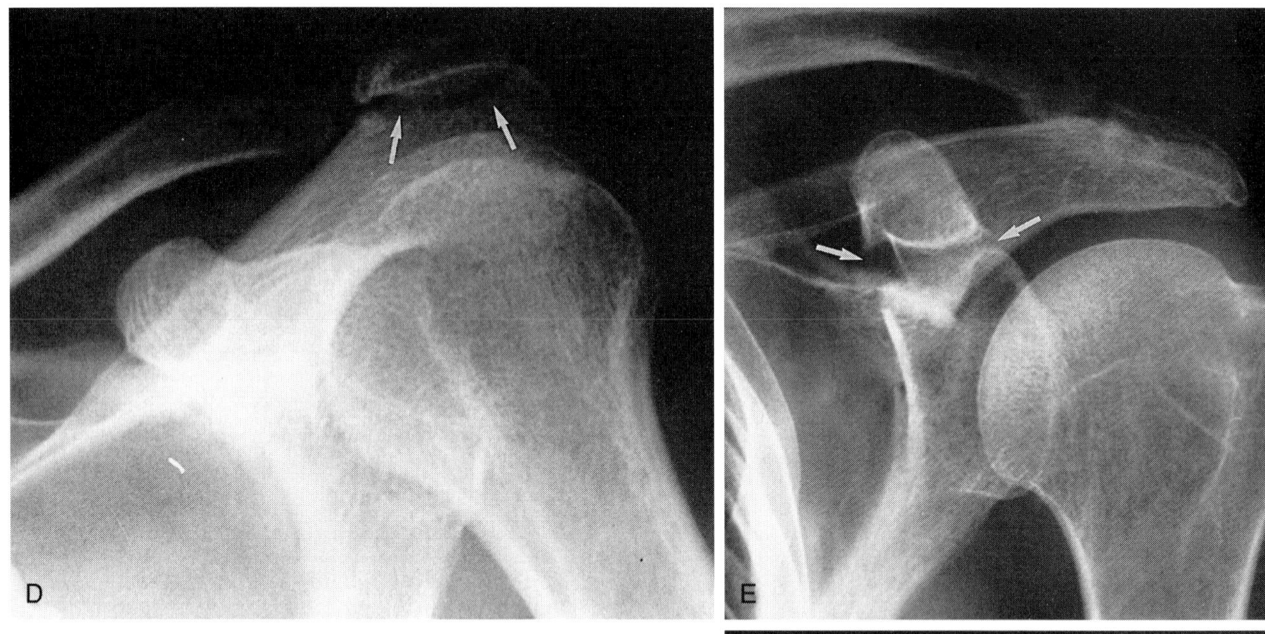

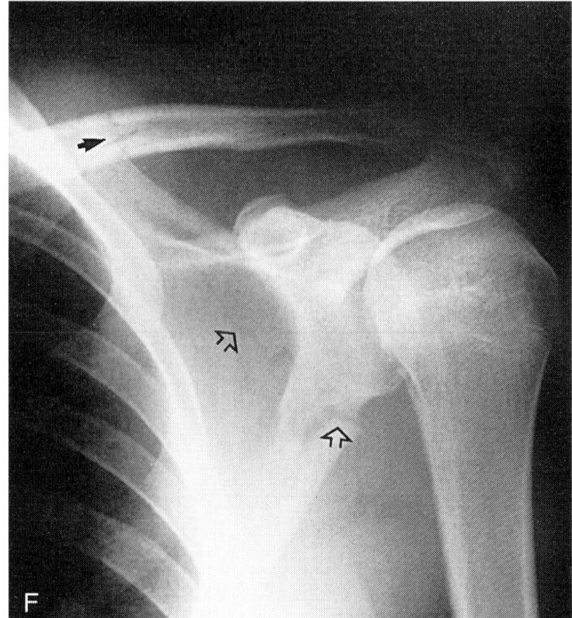

FIGURE 13–18 *Continued.* **D** Acromion fracture. A transverse fracture line through the base of the acromion (arrows) is evident. Brachial plexus injury is a rare but well-recognized complication of acromion fractures. **E** Coracoid process fracture. Observe the fracture through the coracoid process (arrows). Fractures of the coracoid process usually result from direct trauma or from an avulsion of the coracoclavicular ligament, the short head of the biceps, or the coracobrachialis muscle. Patients with this type of fracture should be observed carefully for associated fractures and neurologic injury. **F** Floating shoulder. Observe the transverse fractures through the body of the scapula (open arrows) and the intermediate segment of the clavicle (arrow). Combined fractures of the scapular neck and ipsilateral clavicle disrupt the stability of the suspensory structures of the shoulder, a condition termed floating shoulder. Scapular fractures often are associated with pneumothorax and fractures of the ribs, clavicle, and skull.

TABLE 13–5. Dislocations of the Shoulder*

Entity	Figure(s), Table(s)	Characteristics	Complications and Related Injuries
Glenohumeral joint dislocation		Eighty-eight per cent of all shoulder dislocations	
Anterior dislocation[32–35]	13–19	Ninety-five per cent of glenohumeral joint dislocations Four types: 1. Subcoracoid 2. Subglenoid 3. Subclavicular 4. Intrathoracic	Recurrence (40 per cent of cases), Hill-Sachs lesion, Bankart lesion, avulsion fracture of greater tuberosity, labral injury, brachial plexus injury, rotator cuff injury, rib fractures
Posterior dislocation[36]	13–20	Two to 4 per cent of glenohumeral joint dislocations Three major types: 1. Subacromial 2. Subglenoid 3. Subspinous More than 50 per cent initially unrecognized	Secondary degenerative disease, disruption of posterior capsule, fracture of posterior glenoid rim (reverse Bankart lesion), lesser tuberosity avulsion, subscapularis tendon injury
Superior dislocation[37]	13–21	Rare injury	Rotator cuff, capsule and biceps tendon injury, fractures of clavicle, acromion, coracoid process, and humeral tuberosities
Inferior dislocation (luxatio erecta)[38]		Rare injury	Fractures of greater tuberosity, acromion, coracoid process, clavicle, and inferior glenoid rim Axillary artery and brachial plexus injury, recurrent dislocations, and adhesive capsulitis
Drooping shoulder[39]	13–22	Rare occurrence: in patients with fractures of the surgical neck of the humerus Cause unknown but may relate to atony of deltoid muscle or hemarthrosis Results in self-limited displacement that corrects in weeks	Associated humeral fracture
Acromioclavicular (AC) joint dislocation[40, 41, 128]	13–23	Ten per cent of all shoulder dislocations Frequent injury between ages 16 and 40 years Old terminology: shoulder separation	Complications of all types: Premature degenerative disease CC ligament calcification or ossification Posttraumatic osteolysis of the clavicle Persistent instability if untreated
Type I injury		Mild sprain AC joint capsule partially disrupted Normal appearance on radiographs Surgery not indicated	
Type II injury		Moderate sprain AC joint capsule and CC ligaments partially disrupted AC joint space widened on radiographs Surgery not indicated	
Type III injury		Severe sprain AC joint capsule and CC ligaments completely disrupted Superior displacement of clavicle on radiographs Surgery optional	
Type IV injury		Type III with avulsion of CC ligament from clavicle Penetration of clavicle through periosteal sleeve or major soft tissue injury Surgery indicated	
Type V injury		Type III with a posterior dislocation of clavicle behind acromion Surgery indicated	
Type VI injury		Type III with inferolateral dislocation of lateral end of clavicle Surgery indicated	
Sternoclavicular joint dislocation[42]	12–16; Table 12–4	Rare: only 2–3 per cent of all shoulder dislocations Severe trauma	*Anterior dislocation:* avulsion of inferior margin of clavicle, growth plate injury *Posterior dislocation:* injury to trachea, esophagus, great vessels, or nerves in the superior mediastinum; may lead to cough, dyspnea, dysphagia, and even death

*See also Table 1–5.
AC = acromioclavicular; CC = coracoclavicular.

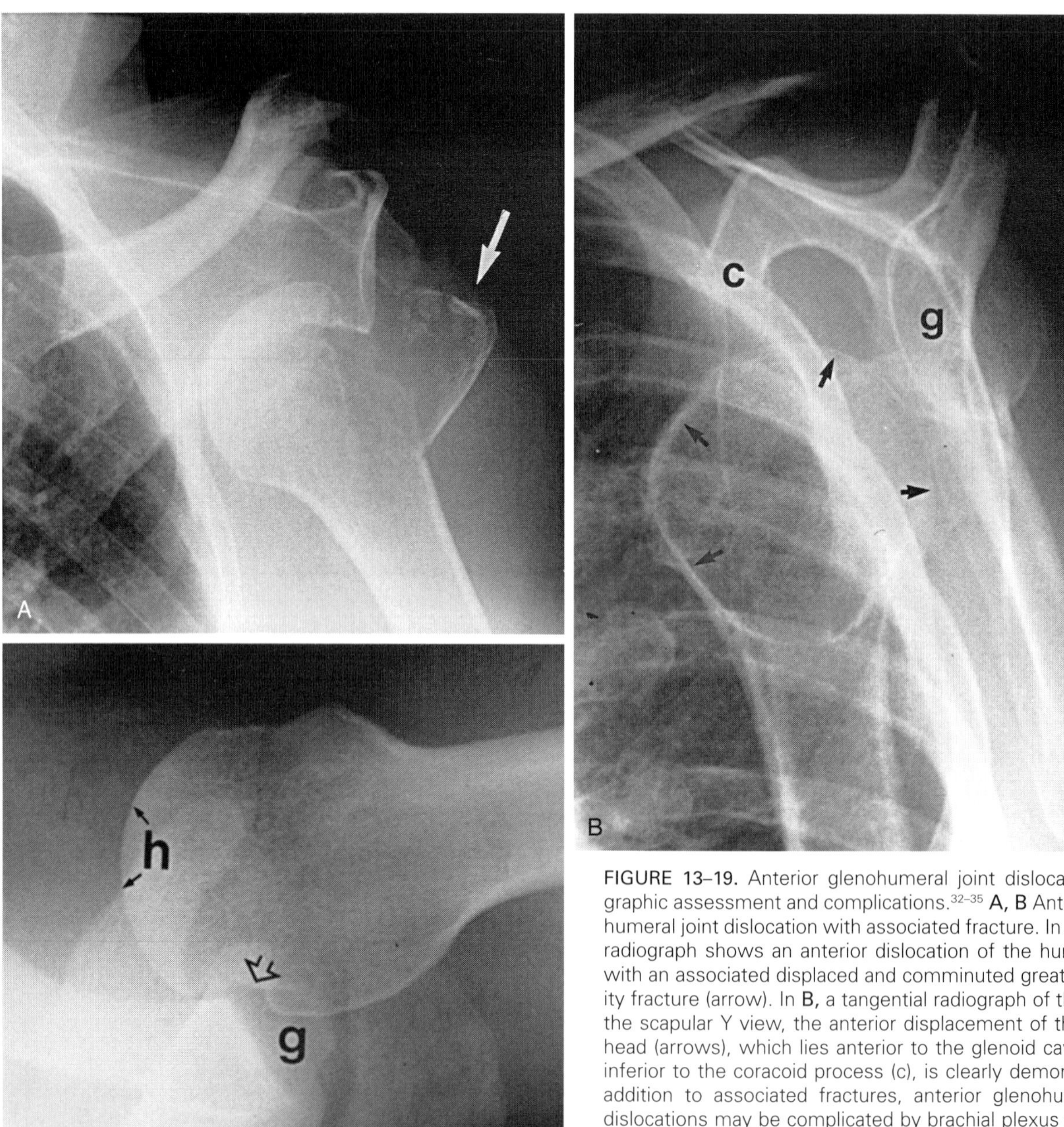

FIGURE 13–19. Anterior glenohumeral joint dislocation: radiographic assessment and complications.[32–35] A, B Anterior glenohumeral joint dislocation with associated fracture. In A, a frontal radiograph shows an anterior dislocation of the humeral head with an associated displaced and comminuted greater tuberosity fracture (arrow). In B, a tangential radiograph of the scapula, the scapular Y view, the anterior displacement of the humeral head (arrows), which lies anterior to the glenoid cavity (g) and inferior to the coracoid process (c), is clearly demonstrated. In addition to associated fractures, anterior glenohumeral joint dislocations may be complicated by brachial plexus and rotator cuff injuries. C Axillary radiograph. This view clearly demonstrates the anterior dislocation of the humeral head articular surface (h) (arrows) with respect to the glenoid cavity (g). This projection often is difficult to obtain while the humeral head remains displaced. A Hill-Sachs impaction fracture of the humeral head also is seen (open arrow).

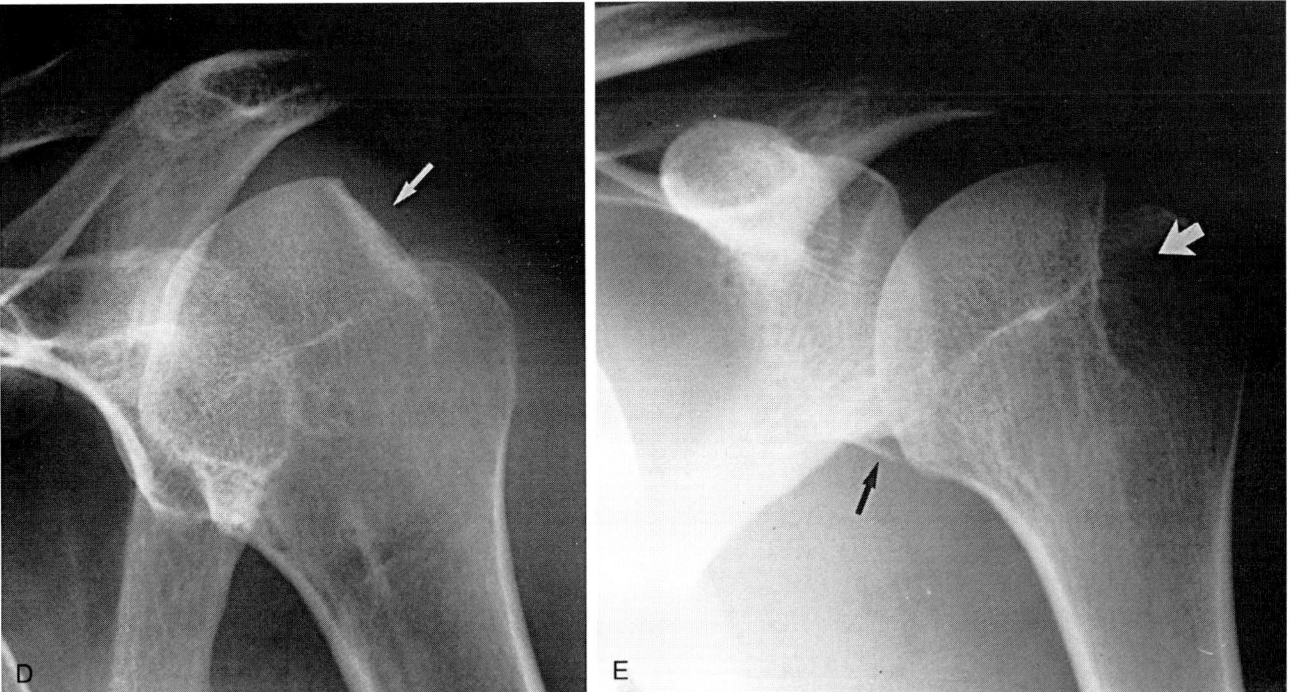

FIGURE 13–19 *Continued.* **D** Hill-Sachs lesion. In a patient with recurrent anterior dislocation, observe the compression fracture of the posterolateral aspect of the humeral head (arrow). **E** Bankart and Hill-Sachs lesions. In a patient with recurrent dislocations and a Hill-Sachs lesion (white arrow), observe the bone fragment adjacent to the glenoid rim (black arrow). The Hill-Sachs lesion is a compression fracture of the posterolateral aspect of the humeral head that is produced by impaction of the humerus against the anterior rim of the glenoid; it is reported to be present in 50 to 100 per cent of recurrent dislocations. Bankart lesions are fractures of the anterior glenoid rim caused by impaction of the humeral head as it dislocates. Osseous lesions may be seen via routine radiography, but purely cartilaginous labral injuries may require computed tomographic (CT) arthrography or magnetic resonance (MR) imaging.

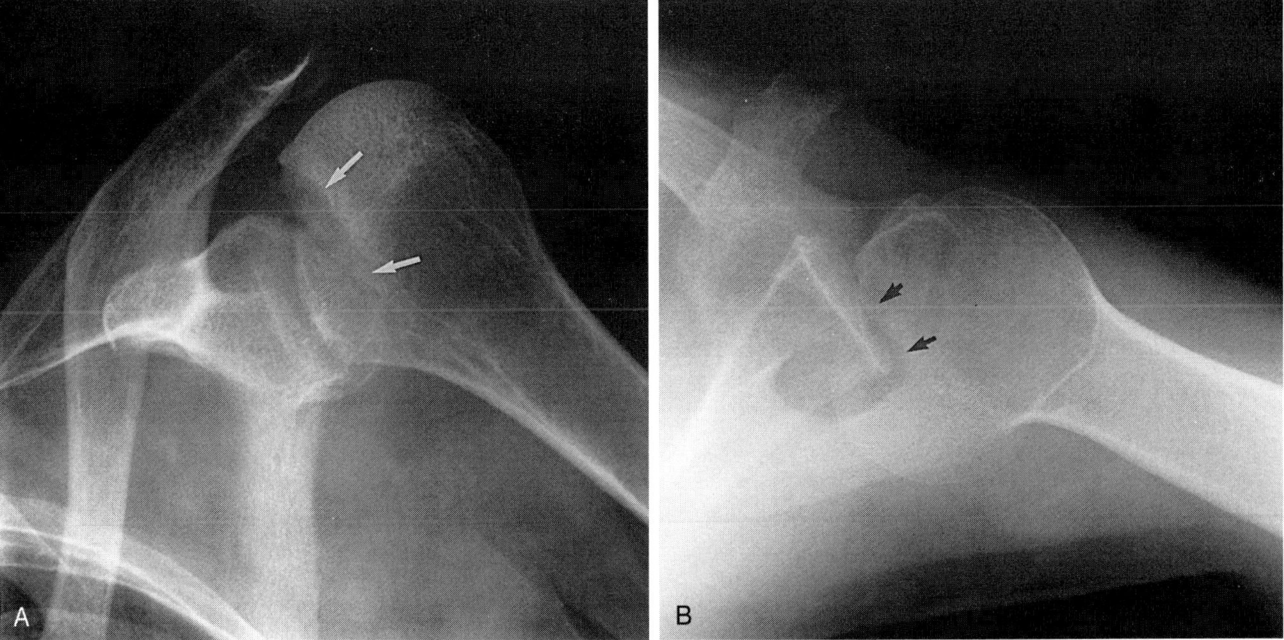

FIGURE 13–20. Posterior glenohumeral joint dislocation.[36] This patient with a chronic irreducible posterior dislocation is unable to externally rotate the arm at the glenohumeral joint. **A** Internal rotation radiograph shows the characteristic trough fracture (arrows) caused by impaction of the humeral head against the posterior rim of the glenoid. **B** Axillary radiograph clearly shows the posteriorly dislocated humeral head in relation to the glenoid and trough fracture (arrows). Posterior dislocations represent only 2 to 4 per cent of all shoulder dislocations. More than half of these dislocations are unrecognized on initial evaluation. Bilateral posterior dislocations may be seen in patients after seizures and electrical shocks.

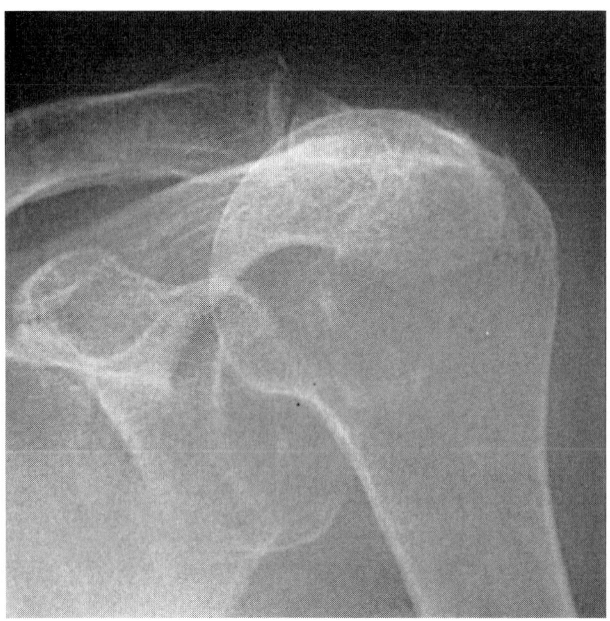

FIGURE 13–21. Superior glenohumeral joint dislocation.[37] Observe the elevation of the humeral head with respect to the glenoid cavity with acute superior dislocation of the humerus. Note that the inferior surface of the acromion is located inferiorly with respect to the superior aspect of the humeral head. This is a rare and unusual pattern of dislocation. Fractures of adjacent bones and injuries to the rotator cuff, joint capsule, biceps tendon, and surrounding muscles frequently complicate superior dislocations.

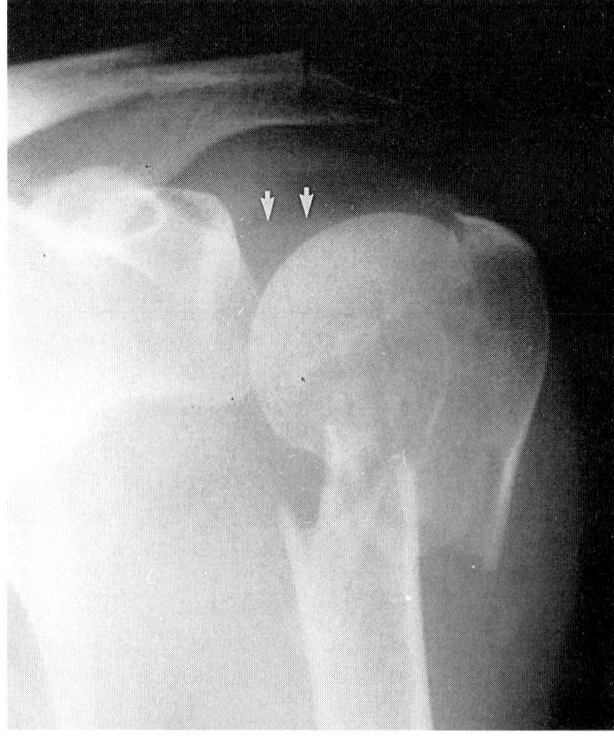

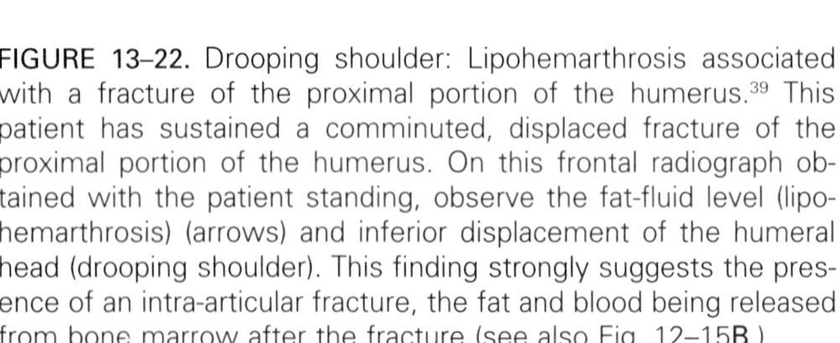

FIGURE 13–22. Drooping shoulder: Lipohemarthrosis associated with a fracture of the proximal portion of the humerus.[39] This patient has sustained a comminuted, displaced fracture of the proximal portion of the humerus. On this frontal radiograph obtained with the patient standing, observe the fat-fluid level (lipohemarthrosis) (arrows) and inferior displacement of the humeral head (drooping shoulder). This finding strongly suggests the presence of an intra-articular fracture, the fat and blood being released from bone marrow after the fracture (see also Fig. 12–15**B**.)

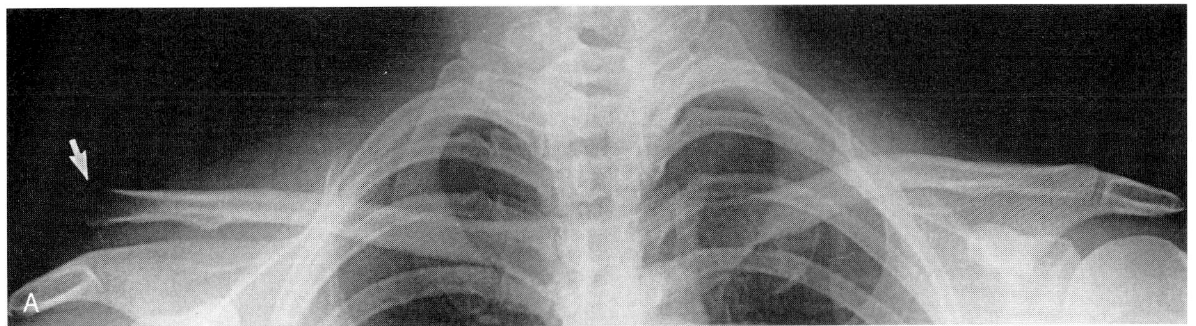

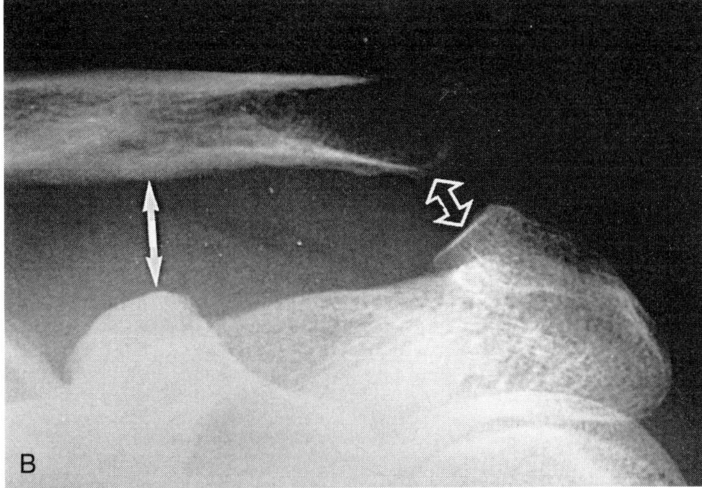

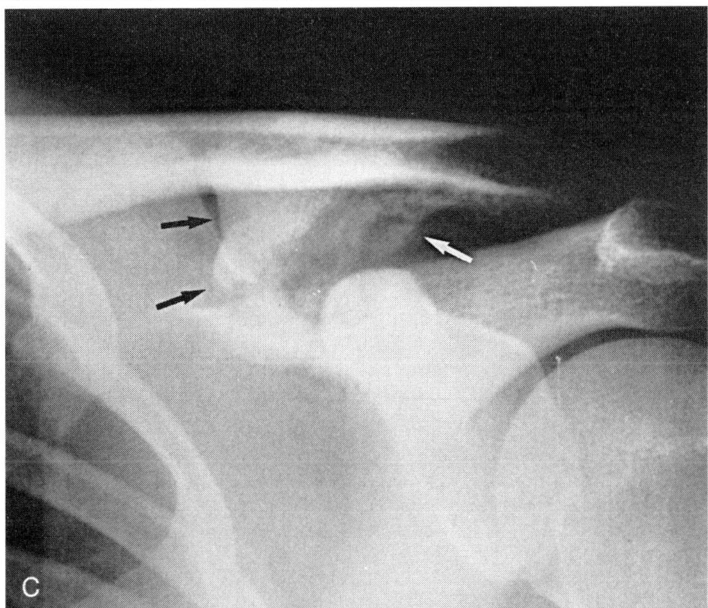

FIGURE 13–23. Acromioclavicular joint dislocation.[40, 41, 128] **A** Acute grade V injury. Frontal stress radiograph obtained while the patient held a weight in both hands reveals marked widening of the coracoclavicular and acromioclavicular joint spaces, resulting in superior displacement of the clavicle (arrow). The type V injury is a severe sprain characterized by disruption of both the acromioclavicular and coracoclavicular ligaments with acromioclavicular joint dislocation. The clavicle is elevated above the adjacent acromion. **B** In another patient, a grade III or V acromioclavicular joint sprain (dislocation) is seen as widening of the coracoclavicular space (double-headed white arrow) and the acromioclavicular joint space (double-headed open arrow). *(**B**, Courtesy T. Dobson, D.C., Portland, Oregon.)* **C** Chronic heterotopic ossification. Observe the extensive sheet-like ossification in the region of the coracoclavicular ligaments (arrows) in this man, who had sustained a severe acromioclavicular joint dislocation several years earlier. Posttraumatic heterotopic ossification is a well-known complication of such ligamentous injuries, but its presence does not appear to influence the eventual prognosis. In addition to radiographs taken with and without weights, anteroposterior shoulder radiographs obtained in internal rotation also may be used in diagnosing some grade III or V acromioclavicular joint dislocations.

TABLE 13–6. Internal Joint Derangements and Other Soft Tissue Injuries Affecting the Shoulder*

Entity	Figure(s), Table(s)	Characteristics
Shoulder impingement syndrome[43]		Repeated impingement and eventual tears of the tendons of the rotator cuff or the long head of the biceps brachii muscle between the humeral head and the coracohumeral arch Primary impingement occurs mainly in nonathletic persons; related to alterations of the coracoacromial arch, such as acromioclavicular joint osteoarthrosis, and developmental or posttraumatic abnormalities Secondary impingement occurs mainly in athletes involved in activities requiring overhead movement of the arm; related to glenohumeral or scapular instability Three stages: 1. Reversible edema and hemorrhage in patients younger than the age of 25 years 2. Fibrosis and tendinosis in patients between the ages of 25 and 40 years 3. Tendon rupture and subacromial enthesophytes, usually in patients older than 40 years of age
Rotator cuff tendon tear[44–46]	13–24, 13–25	Full-thickness or partial-thickness tear of the supraspinatus (most common), infraspinatus, subscapularis, or teres minor tendons predominate in patients older than 40 years of age *Acute tears:* occur suddenly or as a result of a definite injury; fewer than 10 per cent of all rotator cuff tears *Chronic tears:* present for months or years; most common type May complicate rheumatoid arthritis, ankylosing spondylitis, septic arthritis, and other articular disorders Depth of tear: 1. Full-thickness tear: extends from bursal surface to articular surface 2. Partial-thickness tear: involves only the bursal or articular surface 3. Intrasubstance tear: confined within the substance of the tendon and does not extend to the surface Causes: trauma, attrition, ischemia, impingement Radiographic findings (chronic tears only): 1. Elevation of the humeral head related to narrowing of the acromiohumeral space 2. Inferior acromial concavity 3. Cyst formation and sclerosis within the apposing surfaces of the acromion and humeral head Arthrography, ultrasonography, and magnetic resonance (MR) imaging are useful techniques for evaluation of acute and chronic tears; more accurate in assessing full-thickness tears than partial-thickness tears
Rotator cuff tendinitis[47]		Ischemic or degenerative pathologic conditions of the tendon; the terms tendinosis and tendinopathy are more appropriate than tendinitis Common in manual laborers involved in occupations requiring frequent arm elevation and the use of hand tools and in athletes participating in sports involving frequent shoulder movement Routine radiographs not useful in evaluation MR imaging findings: increased signal intensity within tendon on T1-weighted and proton density–weighted spin echo images and, to a lesser extent, on T2-weighted images
Calcific tendinitis and bursitis[64]	Table 13–7	See discussion on Calcium hydroxyapatite crystal deposition
Adhesive capsulitis[48]		Also termed capsulitis, periarthritis, and frozen shoulder Severe painful restriction of glenohumeral joint motion; usually self-limited, lasting about 12 to 18 months Most patients are between the ages of 40 and 70 years May be primary, with no apparent cause, or secondary, in patients with previous trauma Predisposing factors: trauma, hemiplegia, cerebral hemorrhage, diabetes mellitus, hyperthyroidism, cervical spondylosis, and immobilization Routine radiographs usually are not helpful; arthrography most useful

TABLE 13–6. Internal Joint Derangements and Other Soft Tissue Injuries Affecting the Shoulder*
Continued

Entity	Figure(s), Table(s)	Characteristics
Biceps tendinitis and tenosynovitis[49, 50]		Inflammation of the tendon of the long head of the biceps may occur as a result of two mechanisms: 1. Impingement: tendon becomes trapped between the humeral head, the acromion, and the coracoacromial ligament during elevation and rotation of the arm 2. Attrition: stenosis of the bicipital groove related to periostitis leads to tendon attrition, peritendinous synovitis, and, in some cases, tendon rupture Most common in fifth or sixth decade of life Associated with activities such as golf, swimming, and throwing sports Symptoms include anterior shoulder pain, referred pain to the humeral insertion of the deltoid, and tenderness over the bicipital groove Radiographs not helpful; computed tomography (CT), arthrography, and MR imaging more useful
Rupture of long head of biceps brachii tendon[50]		*Complete rupture:* usually occurs proximally within the extracapsular portion of the tendon of the long head of the biceps brachii muscle May result from impingement or tendon degeneration Clinical findings include audible pop, ecchymoses, and a change in contour of the soft tissues of the arm *Partial rupture:* clinical findings more subtle MR imaging and ultrasonography are useful in evaluating both complete and partial ruptures of the tendon; arthrography less reliable
Capsular, ligamentous, and labral abnormalities[51]		Glenohumeral joint instability and dislocation frequently are associated with injuries of the capsule, ligaments, and labrum Computed arthrotomography and MR arthrography appear to be most useful in evaluation
Erb-Duchenne paralysis[52]	13–26	Upper extremity palsy caused by brachial plexus injury at birth Hypoplasia of the glenoid neck, coracoid process, and humeral head, overhanging of the distal portion of the clavicle and acromion process
Posttraumatic osteolysis of the clavicle[53, 54]	13–27	Progressive resorption of the outer end of the clavicle Usually begins after single or repeated episodes of local trauma Traumatic insult may be minor or related to chronic stress as in weight-lifters Possible association also with spinal cord injury Symptoms include pain, local crepitation, and diminished strength and mobility Osteolysis begins as early as 2 weeks and as late as several years after injury 0.5 to 3 cm of the distal part of the clavicle may undergo osteolysis over a 12- to 18-month period Other findings include soft tissue swelling and dystrophic calcification Findings are self-limited, resulting in eventual reconstitution over a period of 4 to 6 months; the acromioclavicular joint may remain permanently widened
Heterotopic ossification[55]	13–28	Periarticular heterotopic ossification occurs in patients after brain and spinal cord injury Osseous deposits begin as poorly defined opaque areas appearing 2 to 6 months after injury and progress to large radiodense lesions possessing trabeculae Complete osseous ankylosis of the shoulder may result

*See also Table 1–5.

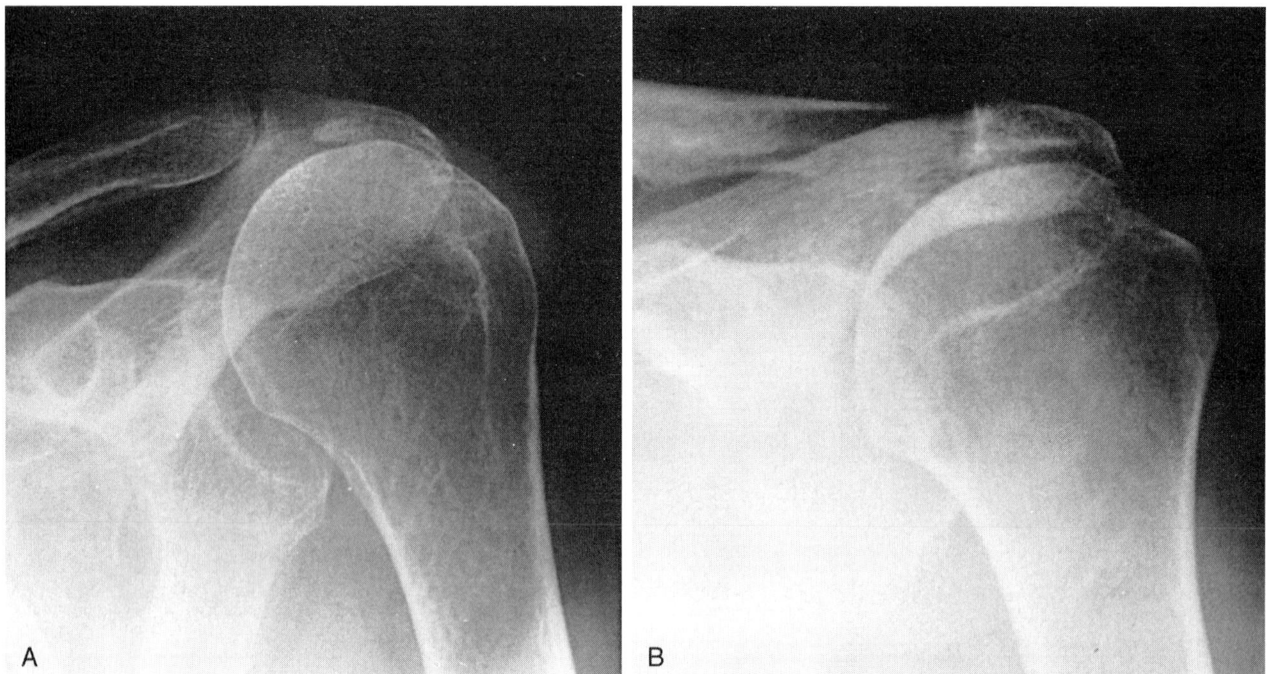

FIGURE 13–24. Chronic degenerative rotator cuff tear: routine radiographic abnormalities.[44, 45] A Radiograph of the shoulder in a patient with a chronic rotator cuff tear reveals elevation of the humeral head with respect to the glenoid, leading to obliteration of the acromiohumeral space, contact of the humeral head and the acromion, and scalloping of the inferior surface of the acromion. B This 83-year-old man had chronic shoulder pain. Observe the narrowing of the acromiohumeral space and the concavity of the undersurface of the acromion and clavicle resulting from degenerative remodeling.

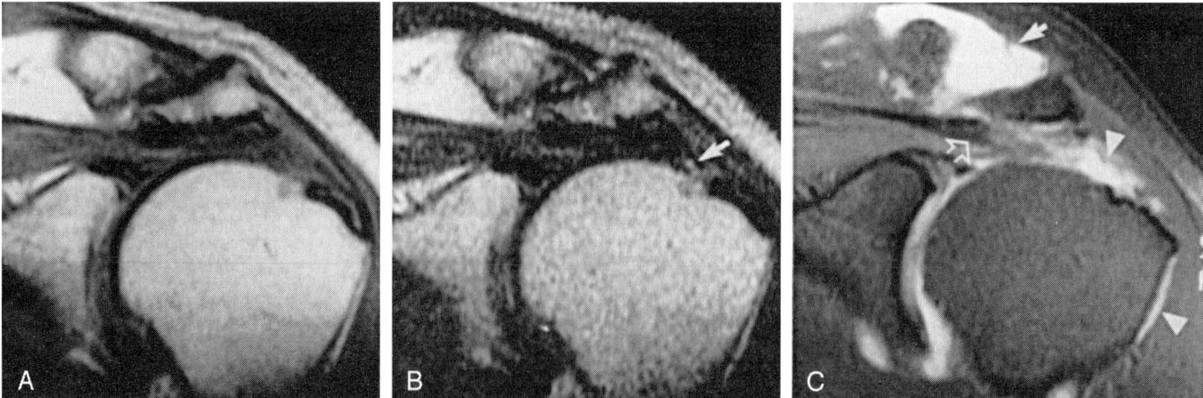

FIGURE 13–25. Full-thickness rotator cuff tear: magnetic resonance (MR) imaging and MR arthrography.[45–47] A, B Coronal oblique proton density–weighted (TR/TE, 2000/20) (A) and T2-weighted (TR/TE, 2000/80) (B) spin echo MR images show osteoarthrosis of the acromioclavicular joint and an enlarged and irregular distal portion of the supraspinatus tendon. Only one region of the tendon, however, reveals increased signal intensity in B (arrow). C A coronal oblique T1-weighted (TR/TE, 650/20) spin echo MR image obtained with chemical presaturation of fat (ChemSat) after the intra-articular administration of a gadolinium compound revealed the high signal intensity of the contrast agent in the glenohumeral joint, subacromial-subdeltoid bursa (arrowheads), and acromioclavicular joint (solid arrow). Note the completely torn and retracted supraspinatus tendon (open arrow). *(From Resnick D, Kang HS: Internal Derangements of Joints. Philadelphia, WB Saunders, 1997, p 205.)*

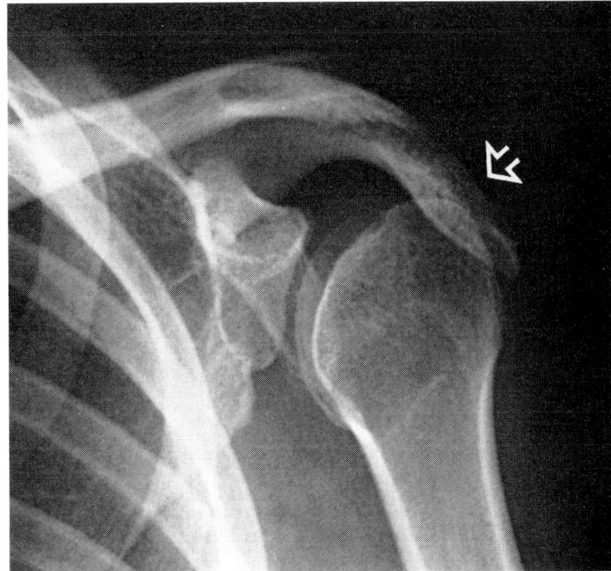

FIGURE 13–26. Erb-Duchenne paralysis.[52] Hypoplasia of the glenoid neck, coracoid process, and humeral head are associated with overhanging of the distal end of the clavicle and acromion process (open arrow). These findings are characteristic in patients with Erb-Duchenne paralysis, an upper extremity palsy caused by a brachial plexus injury at birth.

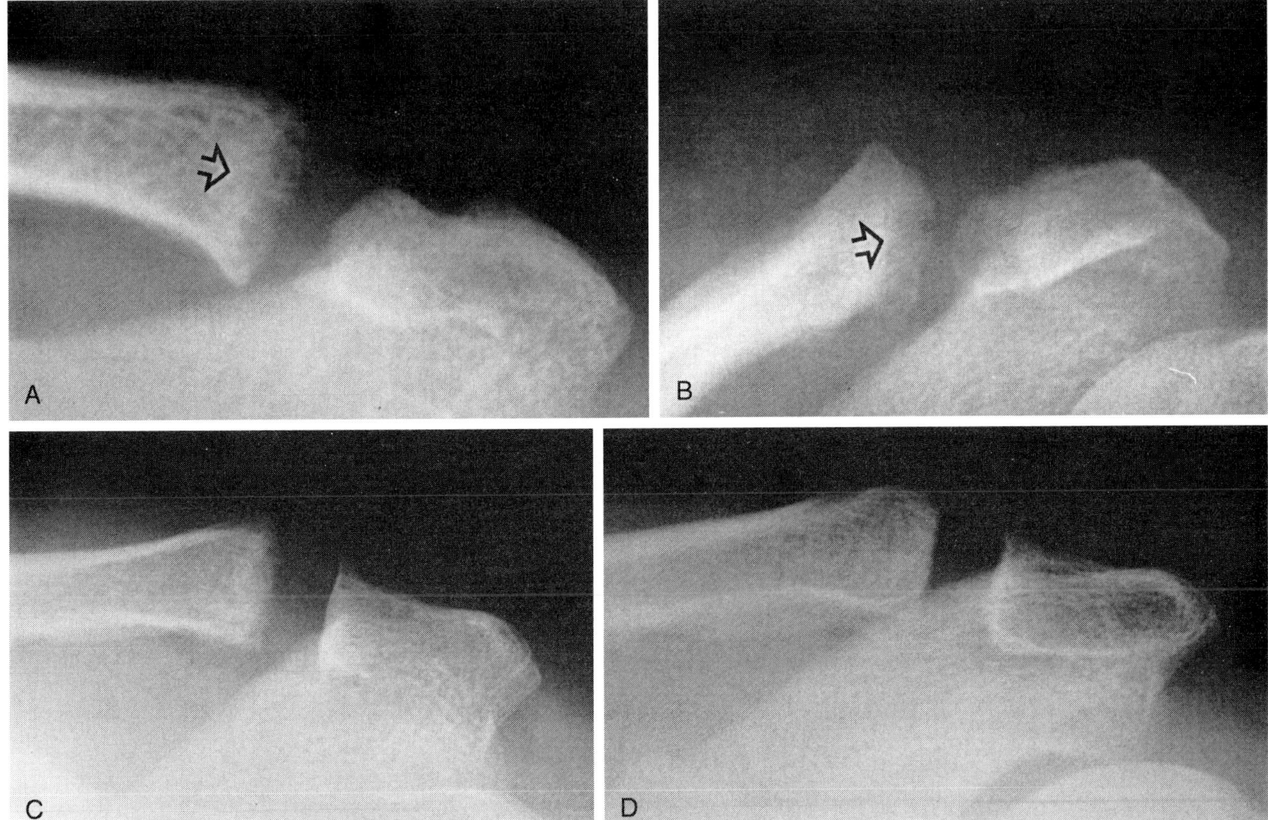

FIGURE 13–27. Posttraumatic osteolysis of the clavicle.[53, 54] A, B Two radiographs of the acromioclavicular joint in this competitive weightlifter show an indistinct articular surface of the distal end of the clavicle (open arrow) and minimal joint space widening. Stress radiographs failed to reveal acromioclavicular joint dislocation. C, D A similar appearance is evident in another patient with shoulder pain that developed gradually after heavy lifting and participation in volleyball. In C, observe the widening of the acromioclavicular joint space and indistinct subchondral bone surface of the clavicle. In D, a radiograph obtained 6 months later when the patient was asymptomatic, reconstitution of the clavicular articular surface is evident, but the joint space remains widened. The appearance in these two patients is typical of posttraumatic osteolysis of the clavicle. *(C, D, Courtesy of D. Lonquist, D.C., Delta, Colorado.)*

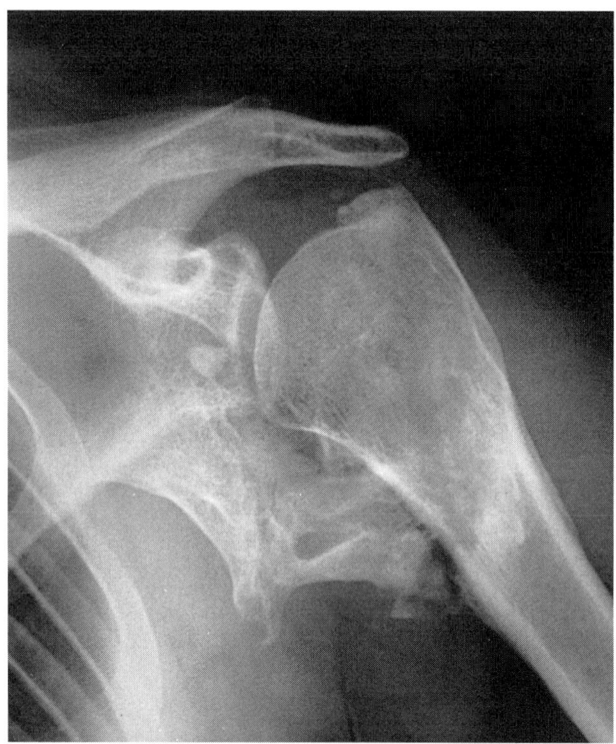

FIGURE 13–28 Heterotopic ossification.[55] This 43-year-old man sustained a head injury and was comatose for 3 days. Observe the extensive ossification surrounding the glenohumeral joint, resulting in almost complete osseous ankylosis. Brain and spinal cord injury may result in heterotopic ossification. This appearance may resemble the findings seen in fibrodysplasia ossificans progressiva.

TABLE 13–7. Articular Disorders Affecting the Shoulder

Entity	Figure(s)	Characteristics
Degenerative and related disorders		
Osteoarthrosis: glenohumeral joint[56]	13–29	Primary osteoarthrosis of the glenohumeral joint occurs only infrequently Usually secondary to local trauma or disease processes, such as alkaptonuria, acromegaly, epiphyseal dysplasia, crystal deposition diseases, and hemophilia *Radiographic findings* Osteophytes: glenoid, humeral head, and bicipital groove region Subchondral sclerosis Subchondral cysts Elevation of humeral head: secondary to rotator cuff degeneration and disruption
Osteoarthrosis: acromioclavicular joint[43, 57]	13–30	Almost universal in elderly persons Diffuse pain or discomfort in the shoulder region; may radiate to upper arm; worse when arm is elevated between 120 and 180 degrees *Radiographic findings* Joint space narrowing, osteophytes, and sclerosis Hypertrophy and superior subluxation of distal end of clavicle Osseous proliferation of superior surface of acromion Subacromial osteophytes may lead to impingement of the rotator cuff Osseous excrescences at site of coracoclavicular ligament may appear in elderly patients

TABLE 13–7. Articular Disorders Affecting the Shoulder *Continued*

Entity	Figure(s)	Characteristics
Inflammatory disorders		
Rheumatoid arthritis[58, 59]	13–31	1. Glenohumeral joint Disability, pain, tenderness, restriction of motion, and soft tissue swelling *Radiographic findings* Bilateral symmetric, concentric joint space narrowing Marginal subchondral erosions Cystic changes in superolateral region of humeral head adjacent to greater tuberosity Mild sclerosis of humeral head Elevation of humeral head secondary to rotatory cuff atrophy or tear Eventual deformity and flattening of humeral articular surface in severe disease Synovial cysts, rotator cuff tears, synovial abnormalities, and subacromial bursitis may be demonstrated by magnetic resonance (MR) imaging or arthrography 2. Acromioclavicular joint Bilateral or unilateral involvement Pain, tenderness, and local soft tissue swelling Soft tissue swelling, subchondral osteopenia, erosions, subluxation Erosions predominate on the clavicle; may eventually result in extensive tapered or irregular osteolysis of the outer one third of the clavicle with apparent joint space widening 3. Coracoclavicular joint Elongated shallow erosions on the undersurface of the clavicle adjacent to the coracoid process (also seen in ankylosing spondylitis and hyperparathyroidism) Similar erosions within the upper ribs also may be observed
Juvenile chronic arthritis[60]		Diffuse concentric joint space narrowing, periarticular osteoporosis, bone enlargement, and erosions of the humeral head, and subluxation
Ankylosing spondylitis[61]	13–32	1. Glenohumeral joint Thirty-two per cent of patients with long-standing ankylosing spondylitis have glenohumeral joint involvement Bilateral > unilateral Osteoporosis and diffuse joint space narrowing Erosive changes of the superolateral portion of the humerus may be extensive, resulting in destruction of the entire outer aspect of the humerus (the hatchet sign) Elevation of humeral head secondary to rotator cuff atrophy and tear Joint ankylosis occurs infrequently 2. Acromioclavicular joint Bilateral erosive changes of distal end of clavicle may result in extensive resorption and widening of the joint space 3. Coracoclavicular joint Scalloped clavicular erosion similar to that of rheumatoid arthritis Ossification of coracoclavicular ligaments may occur infrequently
Psoriatic arthropathy[62]	13–33	Shoulder involvement similar to, but less frequent than, ankylosing spondylitis Glenohumeral and acromioclavicular joints may be involved Findings range from minor erosions to severe osteolysis
Scleroderma (progressive systemic sclerosis)[63]	13–34	Globular accumulations of periarticular soft tissue calcinosis Bone resorption of the acromion and distal end of the clavicle Extensive osseous resorption may occur
Crystal deposition and metabolic disorders		
Calcium hydroxyapatite crystal deposition[64]	13–35	Calcium hydroxyapatite crystal deposition in tendons and bursae, as well as in capsules and ligaments about the shoulder, results in calcific tendinitis and bursitis May be asymptomatic or may be associated with painful episodes Acute symptoms: pain, tenderness on pressure, local edema or swelling, restricted active or passive motion and infrequently, mild fever Chronic symptoms: mild, nonincapacitating pain and tenderness Single or multiple cloud-like linear, triangular, or circular soft tissue calcifications within the rotator cuff tendons and subacromial and subdeltoid bursae Most frequently involved sites are the tendons of the supraspinatus, infraspinatus, teres minor, subscapularis, biceps, and pectoralis major muscles and the subacromial (subdeltoid) bursa Occasionally, large tumor-like accumulations of calcification also will be seen about the shoulder in patients with chronic renal disease or collagen vascular disorders

Table continued on following page

TABLE 13–7. Articular Disorders Affecting the Shoulder *Continued*

Entity	Figure(s)	Characteristics
Calcium pyrophosphate dihydrate (CPPD) crystal deposition[65, 66]	13–36	Joint space narrowing, subchondral sclerosis, cysts, osteophytes, chondrocalcinosis; capsular, tendinous, and bursal deposits and rotator cuff tears Advanced destruction and fragmentation of the glenohumeral and acromioclavicular joints occasionally may resemble neuropathic osteoarthropathy in severe cases
Milwaukee shoulder syndrome[67, 68]	13–37	Also termed rapid destructive arthritis of the shoulder, hemorrhagic shoulder of the elderly, apatite-associated destructive arthritis Cause is unclear; believed to be related to a generalized process such as osteonecrosis or intra-articular deposition of mixed calcium phosphate crystals Predominates in elderly women with a history of trauma Symptoms mild in comparison with severe radiographic manifestations Severe rapid atrophic destruction of humerus and rotator cuff tear Bilateral in as many as 65 per cent of patients Differential diagnosis: neuropathic osteoarthropathy, rheumatoid arthritis, secondary osteoarthrosis, CPPD crystal deposition disease, septic arthritis, or ochronotic arthropathy
Gouty arthropathy[69]	13–38	Involvement of glenohumeral and acromioclavicular joints is uncommon Soft tissue swelling, erosions, cysts, joint space narrowing, and proliferative changes of the glenohumeral joint; erosion of the distal end of the clavicle and irregular splaying of the acromioclavicular joint
Amyloid deposition[70]		Amyloid deposition within the soft tissues of the shoulder may occur as a primary process or in association with hemodialysis treatment, gout, inflammatory arthropathy, neoplasm, plasma cell myeloma, and collagen vascular disease Radiographic manifestations include osteoporosis, osteolytic lesions, pathologic fractures, osteonecrosis, soft tissue nodules and swelling, subchondral cysts and erosions, joint subluxations and contractures, and neuropathic osteoarthropathy Huge collections may result in hard rubbery masses about the shoulders, termed the shoulder pad sign
Hemochromatosis[71]	13–39	Rare disorder exhibiting findings identical to those of CPPD crystal deposition disease with chondrocalcinosis and secondary osteoarthrosis Prominent osteophytes, joint space narrowing, and irregularity of the humeral head may be seen
Infectious disorders		
Pyogenic septic arthritis[72]	13–40	Surgery, penetrating injury, immunosuppression, and debilitating illness, such as diabetes mellitus, all predispose to joint infection In intravenous drug abusers, the acromioclavicular joint frequently is involved, often with atypical organisms such as *Pseudomonas* *Radiographic findings* Rapid concentric loss of joint space Poorly defined or "fuzzy" subchondral bone margins Periarticular osteoporosis Loss of definition and destruction of subchondral bone Capsular distention Erosions Slipped capital humeral epiphysis Metaphyseal osteomyelitis
Tuberculous arthritis[73, 74]	13–41	Typically monoarticular disease in older patients Various degrees of soft tissue swelling Gradual joint space narrowing Juxta-articular osteoporosis Peripherally located erosions Subchondral erosions Periarticular abscess Periostitis Subacromial (subdeltoid) bursitis may occur
Miscellaneous disorders		
Pigmented villonodular synovitis[75, 76]	13–42	Cystic erosions on both sides of the joint Hemorrhagic joint effusion Eventual osteoporosis Well-preserved joint space until late in the disease Extra-articular form is termed giant cell tumor of the tendon sheath

TABLE 13–7. Articular Disorders Affecting the Shoulder *Continued*

Entity	Figure(s)	Characteristics
Idiopathic synovial osteochondromatosis[77, 78]	13–43	Multiple intra-articular or periarticular collections of calcification of variable size and density; monoarticular process Erosion of adjacent humerus and scapula may occur Secondary osteoarthrosis common Noncalcified bodies are best demonstrated with arthrography Secondary synovial osteochondromatosis may occur as a result of degenerative joint disease
Acromegalic arthropathy[79]	13–44	Abnormal cartilage proliferation results in secondary osteoarthrosis Joint space: widening in initial stages; narrowing in advanced stages Sclerosis, osseous fragmentation, and beak-like osteophytes on the inferior aspect of the humeral head
Hemophilic arthropathy[80]	13–45	Glenohumeral joint involvement includes secondary osteoarthrosis, osteoporosis, epiphyseal enlargement, joint space narrowing, subchondral erosion, sclerosis, and cyst formation Rotator cuff disruption is a frequent finding
Neuropathic osteoarthropathy[81]	13–46	As many as 25 per cent of patients with syringomyelia develop neuropathic osteoarthropathy, especially in the glenohumeral joint Fragmentation and sclerosis of the humeral head are common Cyst formation, dislocation, disorganization, and osseous debris Pathologic fractures of humerus, scapula, and clavicle

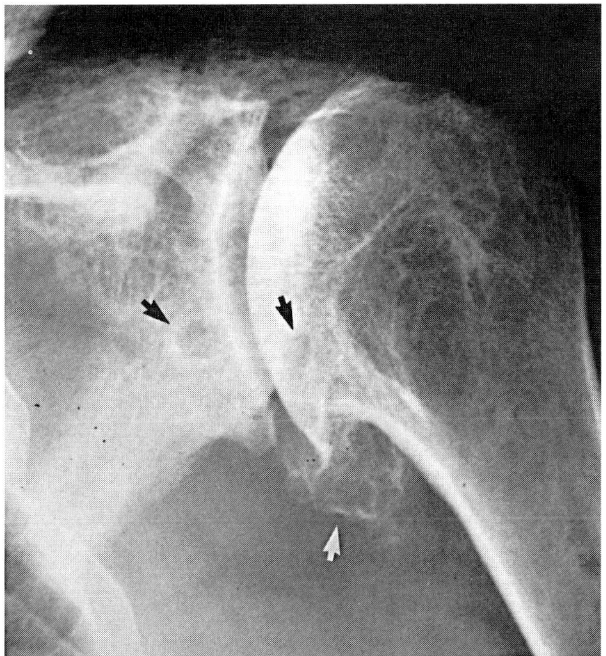

FIGURE 13–29. Osteoarthrosis (degenerative joint disease): Glenohumeral joint.[56] In this patient with generalized osteoarthrosis of several joints, dramatic changes of the glenohumeral joint are seen. A large osteophyte (white arrow), nonuniform loss of joint space, subchondral sclerosis, and cyst formation (black arrows) are apparent. Poor visualization of the superolateral aspect of the humeral head is a photographic artifact and is not related to erosion or destruction. Degenerative disease of the glenohumeral joint is rare in the absence of trauma or other predisposing factors. *(Courtesy of R. Shapiro, M.D., Sacramento, California.)*

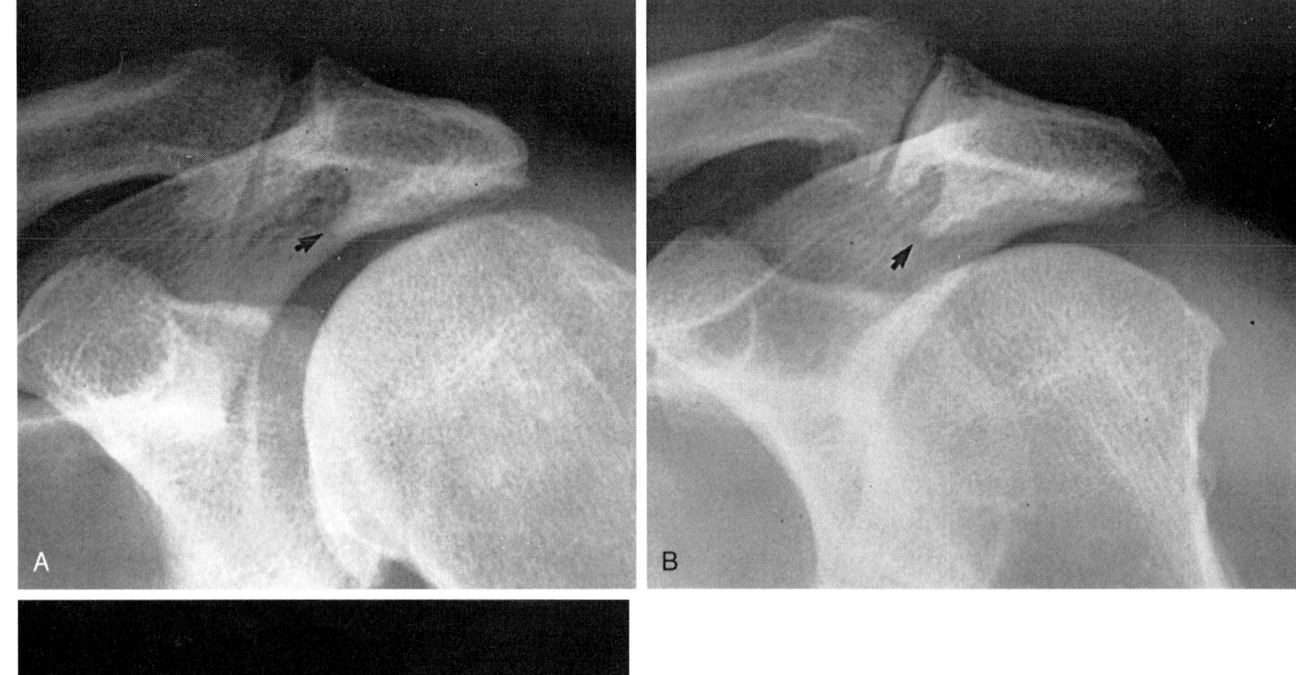

FIGURE 13–30. Osteoarthrosis (degenerative joint disease): acromioclavicular joint.[43, 56, 57] A, B External rotation (A) and internal rotation (B) views of the shoulder reveal nonuniform joint space narrowing, osteophytes, subchondral sclerosis, and a large subacromial enthesophyte (arrows). Enthesopathy at this site is implicated as an aggravating factor in the shoulder impingement syndrome and may contribute to rotator cuff tears. C In another patient with severe degenerative joint disease, extensive osteophyte formation and ossification of the intra-articular meniscus are present.

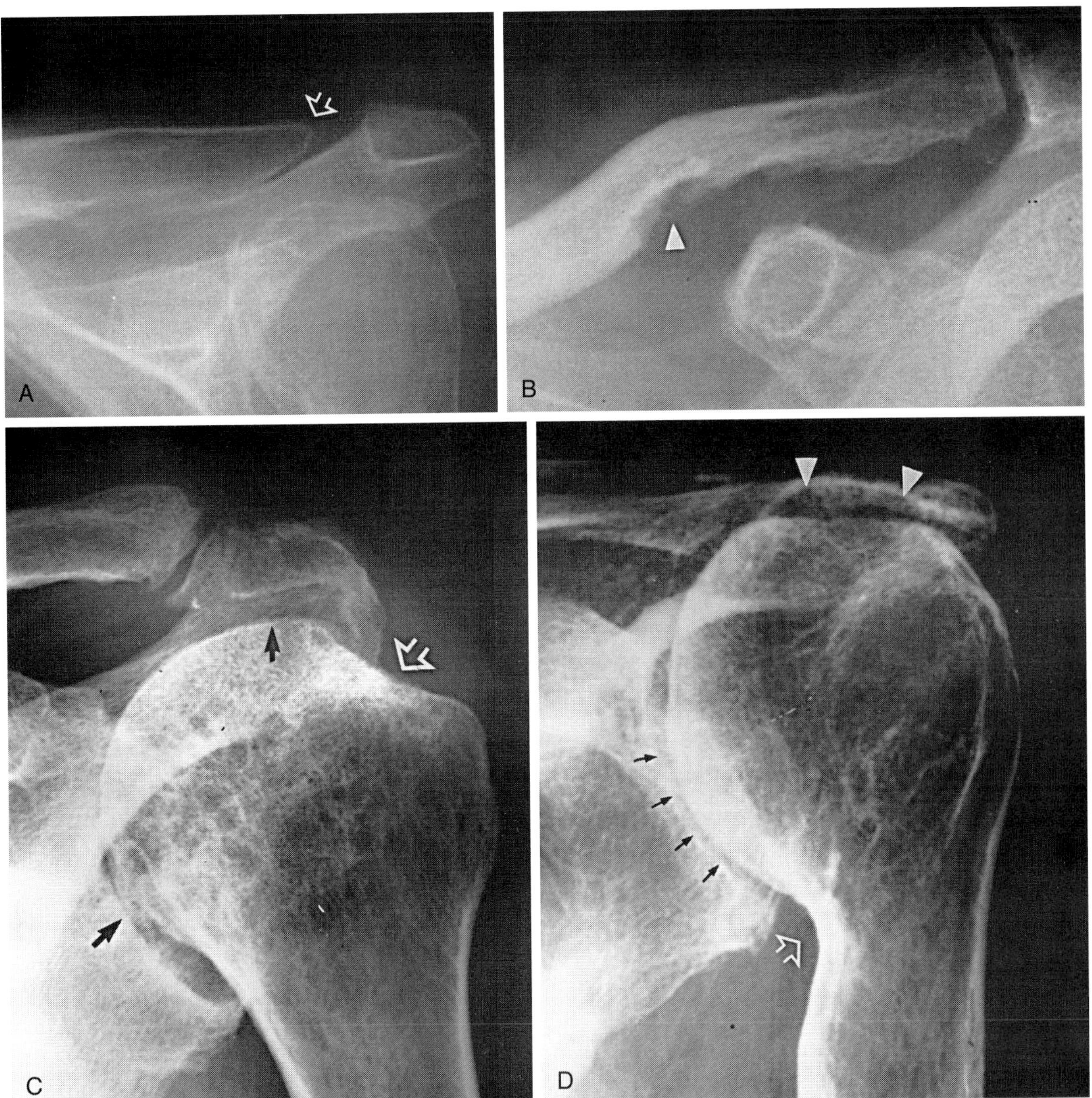

FIGURE 13–31. Rheumatoid arthritis.[58, 59] A, B Abnormalities of the acromioclavicular joint and clavicle. In A, resorption of the distal end of the clavicle results in tapering of the bone (open arrow) and widening of the acromioclavicular joint. In B, a prominent erosion is seen at the site of attachment of the coracoclavicular ligament (arrowhead), a frequent site of involvement in rheumatoid arthritis. A similar finding may be seen in hyperparathyroidism and ankylosing spondylitis. C, D Abnormalities of the glenohumeral joint and acromiohumeral space. In C, the radiographic findings include superior subluxation of the humerus, acromiohumeral space and glenohumeral joint space narrowing (arrows), intraosseous cystic erosions within the humeral head and glenoid, and a large superolateral erosion of the humeral head resembling a Hill-Sachs lesion (open arrow). In D, another patient with long-standing rheumatoid arthritis, observe the obliteration of the acromiohumeral space and glenohumeral joint space (arrows), diffuse osteopenia, erosion of the undersurface of the acromion (arrowheads), and a large erosion of the medial aspect of the humeral neck (open arrow). Rotator cuff tear is common in rheumatoid arthritis and accounts for the narrowing of the acromiohumeral space and subsequent erosion of the inferior aspect of the acromion and distal end of the clavicle.

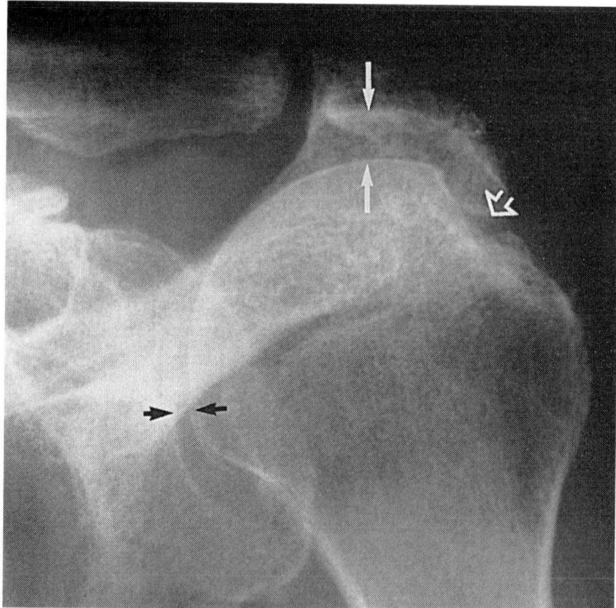

FIGURE 13–32. Ankylosing spondylitis.[61] Observe the elevation of the humerus and narrowing of the acromiohumeral space (white arrows) in this patient with ankylosing spondylitis and resultant rotator cuff tear. The glenohumeral joint space is narrowed (black arrows) and a large erosive defect is present along the lateral aspect of the humeral head (open arrow). The glenohumeral joint is involved in approximately 32 per cent of patients with long-standing ankylosing spondylitis.

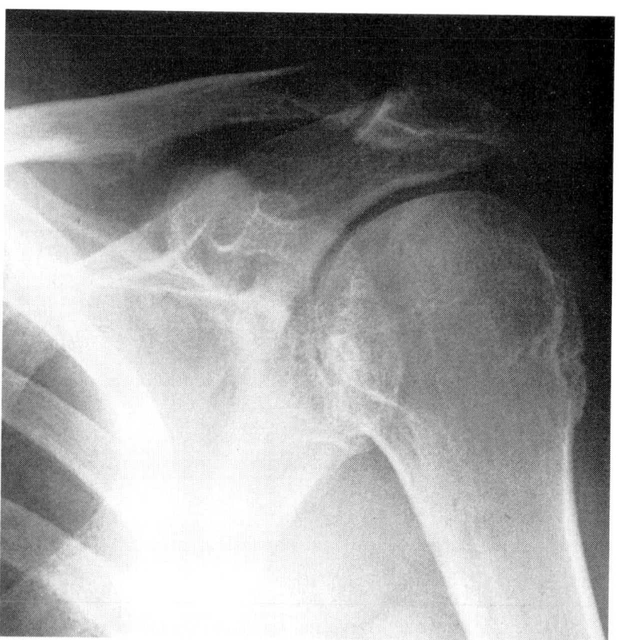

FIGURE 13–33. Psoriatic arthropathy.[62] Patient is a 49-year-old man with psoriasis and polyarticular joint disease. Frontal radiograph reveals fluffy bony excrescences arising from the humeral head, acromion, coracoid process, and site of attachment of the coracoclavicular ligament on the clavicle. The glenohumeral joint space also is narrowed. These findings are consistent with the appearance of a seronegative spondyloarthropathy.

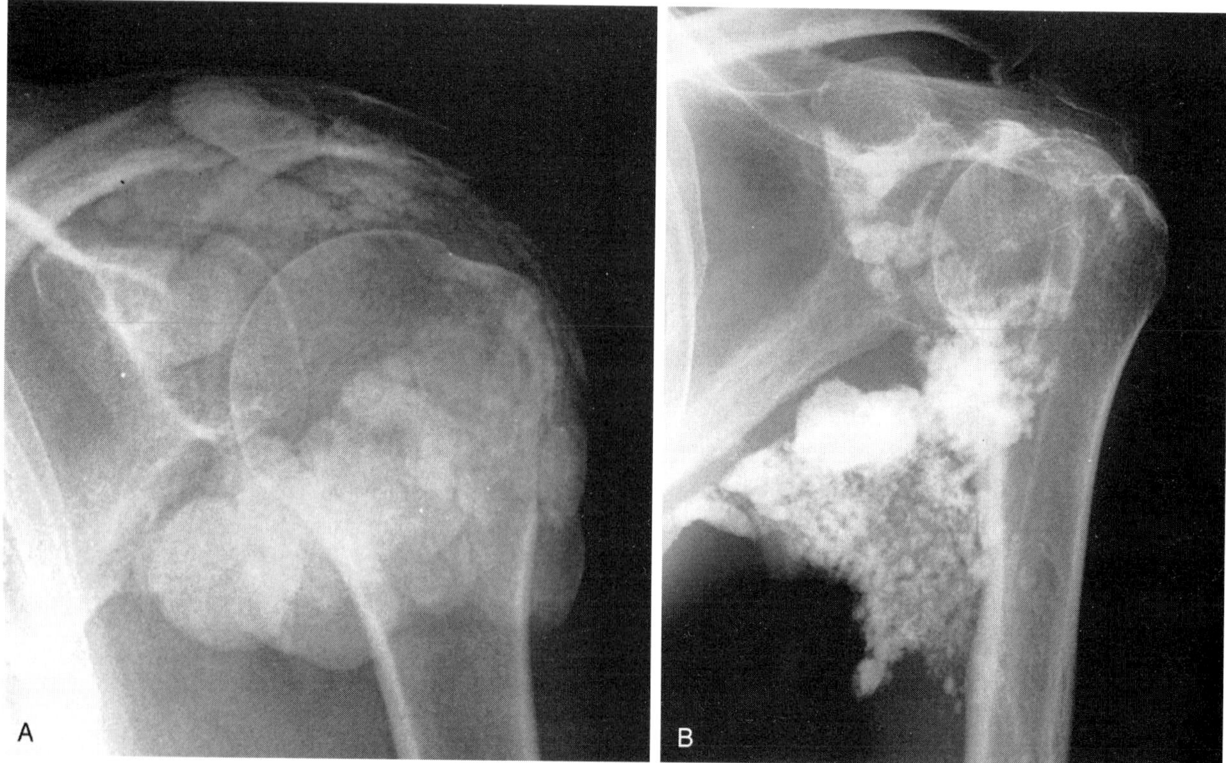

FIGURE 13–34. Scleroderma (progressive systemic sclerosis).[63] A Cloudy accumulations of soft tissue calcification are seen adjacent to the glenohumeral joint and axilla in this 54-year-old man with polyarticular joint disease and esophageal abnormalities. B In another patient, a sheet-like pattern of dense calcification predominates.

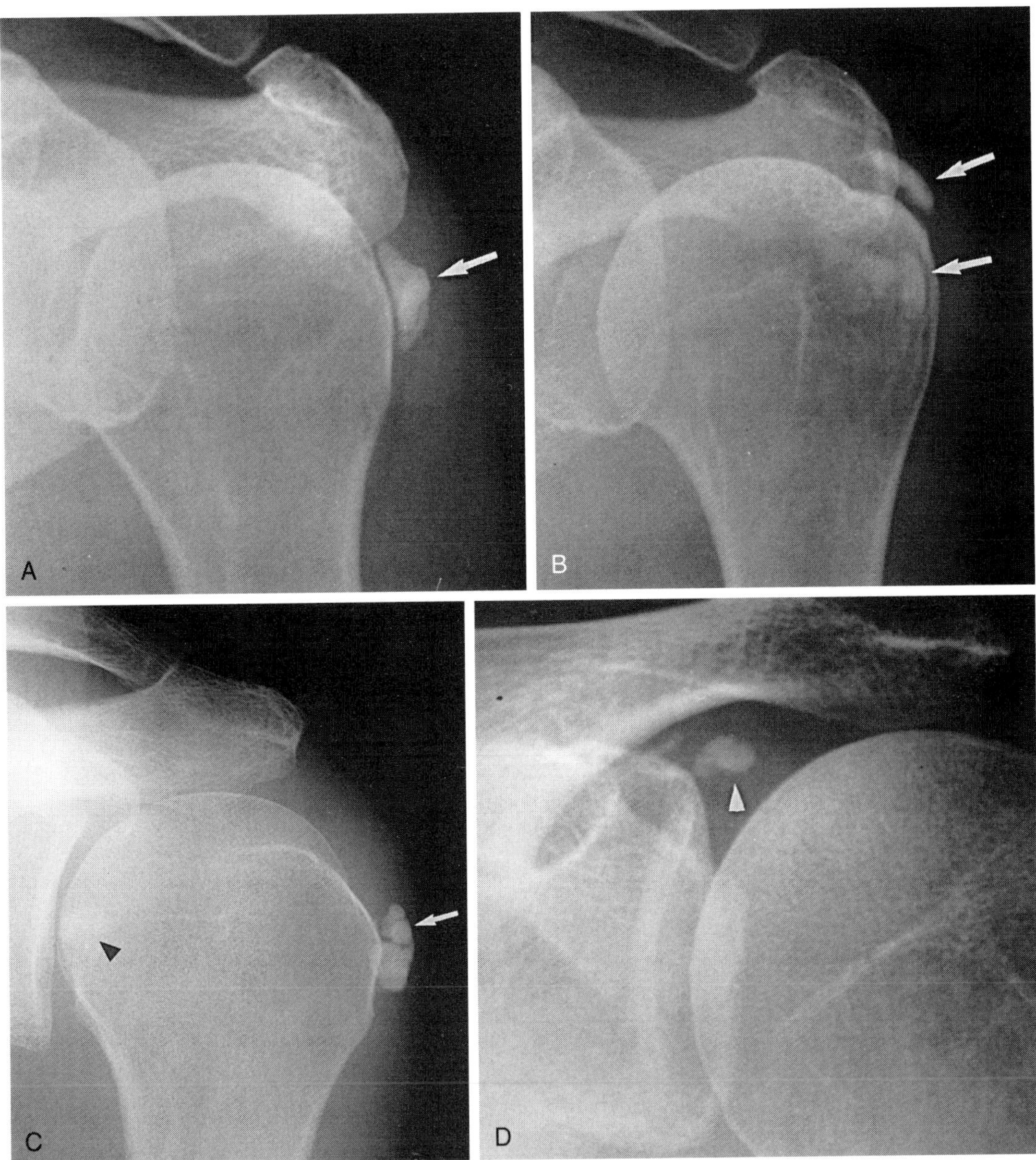

FIGURE 13–35. Calcium hydroxyapatite crystal deposition: calcific tendinitis.[64] A–C Rotator cuff tendons. A, B Internal rotation (A) and external rotation (B) radiographs reveal multiple accumulations of cloud-like calcification (arrows) within the tendons of the supraspinatus and infraspinatus muscles. In C, internal rotation radiograph shows globular calcification within the infraspinatus and teres minor tendons that appear lateral to the humeral head (arrow). Another accumulation of calcification is present overlying the medial aspect of the humeral head (arrowhead), within the subscapularis tendon. *(A, B, Courtesy of D. Jones, M.D., Southport, Australia.)* D Long head of the biceps brachii tendon. External rotation radiograph reveals calcification (arrowhead) in the vicinity of the biceps tendon near its attachment to the superior margin of the glenoid.

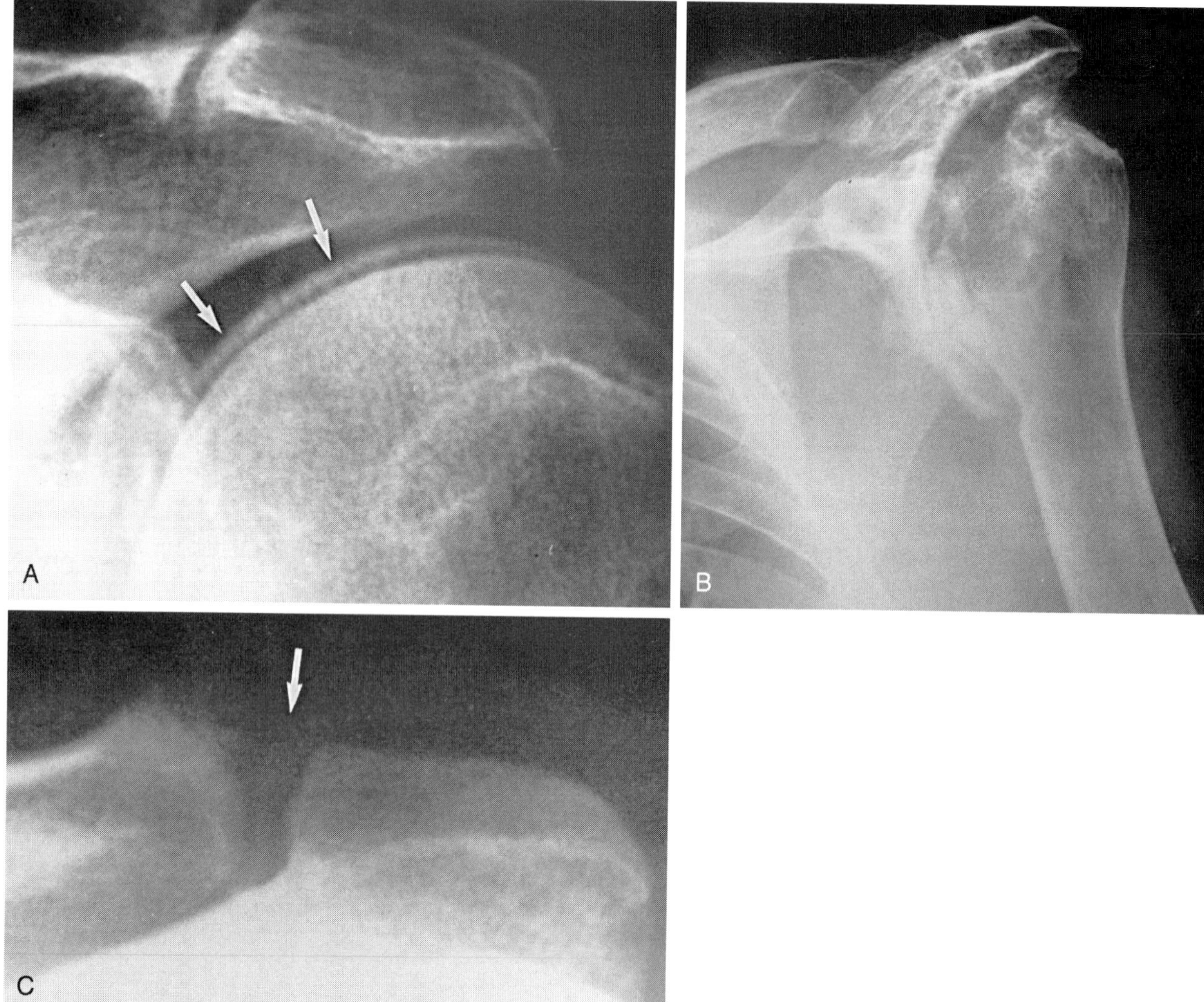

FIGURE 13–36. Calcium pyrophosphate dihydrate (CPPD) crystal deposition disease.[65, 66] A, B Glenohumeral joint. In A, chondrocalcinosis is present. Curvilinear calcification of the articular hyaline cartilage (arrows) within the glenohumeral joint parallels the humeral head. B, Pyrophosphate arthropathy. In another patient with CPPD crystal deposition disease, severe destructive osseous changes involving the proximal portion of the humerus, glenoid, and medial humeral metaphysis resemble the changes of neuropathic joint disease and Milwaukee shoulder syndrome. C Acromioclavicular joint. Chondrocalcinosis is seen within the intra-articular cartilaginous disc of the acromioclavicular joint (arrow). About 24 per cent of patients with CPPD crystal deposition disease have acromioclavicular joint involvement. Other changes at this site may include soft tissue swelling, osseous sclerosis, joint space narrowing, and even tumor-like masses.

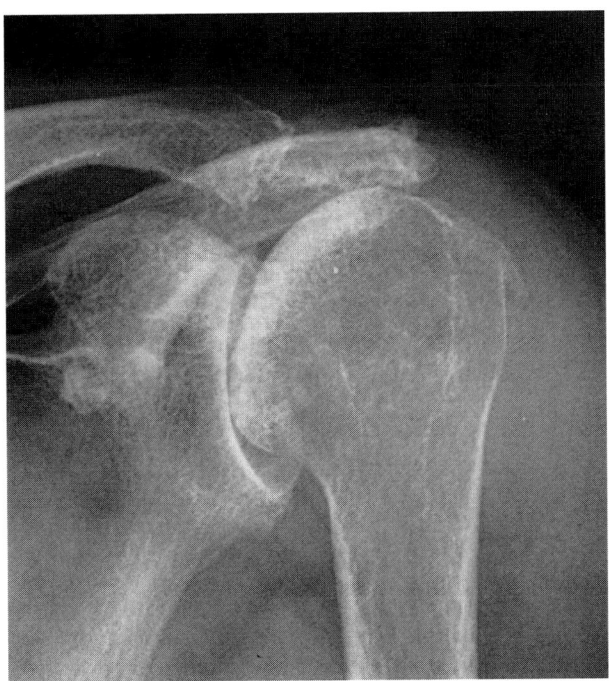

FIGURE 13–37. Milwaukee shoulder syndrome: intra-articular crystal deposition.[67, 68] In a 75-year-old man, radiographic findings include joint space narrowing, elevation of the humerus from a rotator cuff tear, subchondral bone sclerosis, and flattening of the humeral head. Other findings include glenoid deformity, osteopenia, and erosions of the undersurface of the acromion and medial aspect of the humeral metaphysis. The Milwaukee shoulder syndrome refers to structural joint damage in patients with intra-articular accumulation of calcium hydroxyapatite and, to a lesser extent, calcium pyrophosphate crystals.

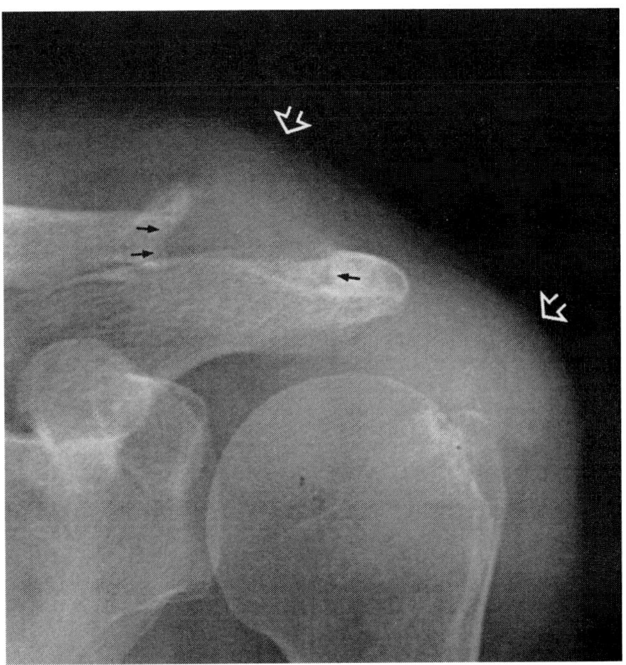

FIGURE 13–38. Gouty arthropathy.[69] This 53-year-old man has chronic tophaceous gout, gouty nephritis, and chronic renal insufficiency. Observe the extensive destruction of the subarticular bone about the acromioclavicular joint (arrows). Large accumulations of radiodense soft tissue nodules in the subacromial-subdeltoid bursa and adjacent to the acromioclavicular joint (open arrows) may represent deposition of tophaceous material, calcium hydroxyapatite crystals, or amyloid secondary to chronic renal disease. *(Courtesy of C. Chen, M.D., Taipei, Taiwan.)*

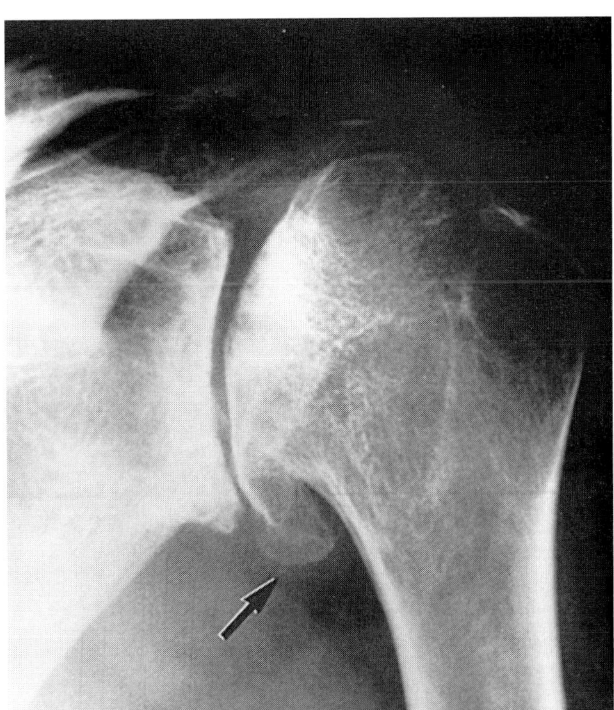

FIGURE 13–39. Hemochromatosis.[71] Radiographic findings in the shoulder include joint space narrowing, subchondral sclerosis, deformity of the humeral head, and a large osteophyte arising from the inferior aspect of the humeral head (arrow). *(Courtesy of V. Vint, M.D., San Diego, California.)*

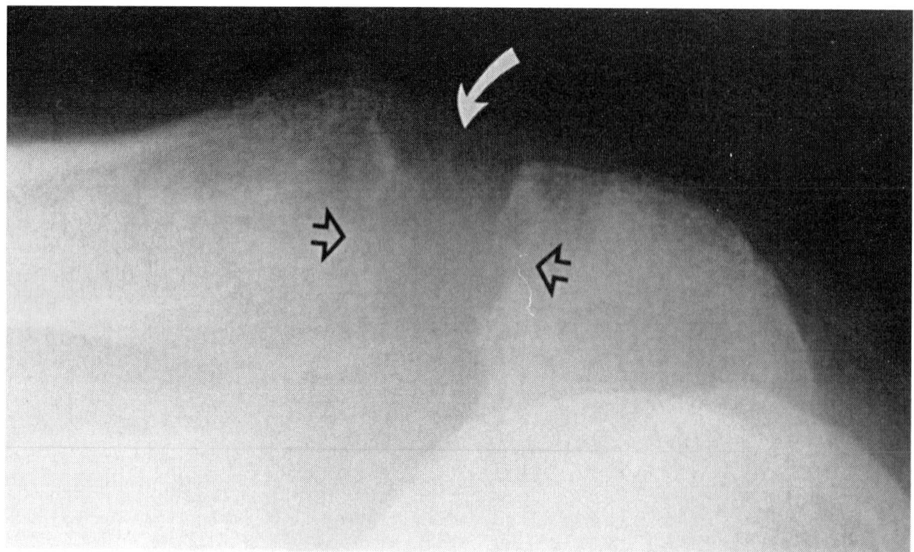

FIGURE 13–40. Pyogenic septic arthritis: acromioclavicular joint.[72] This intravenous heroin abuser developed gradual onset of shoulder pain. Frontal radiograph reveals widening of the joint space (curved arrow) and subchondral erosion of both the clavicle and the acromion (open arrows). Joint aspirate contained *Pseudomonas* organisms. Intravenous drug abusers are predisposed to *Staphylococcus* and *Pseudomonas* infections of the acromioclavicular, sternoclavicular, spinal, and sacroiliac joints, as well as of the symphysis pubis.

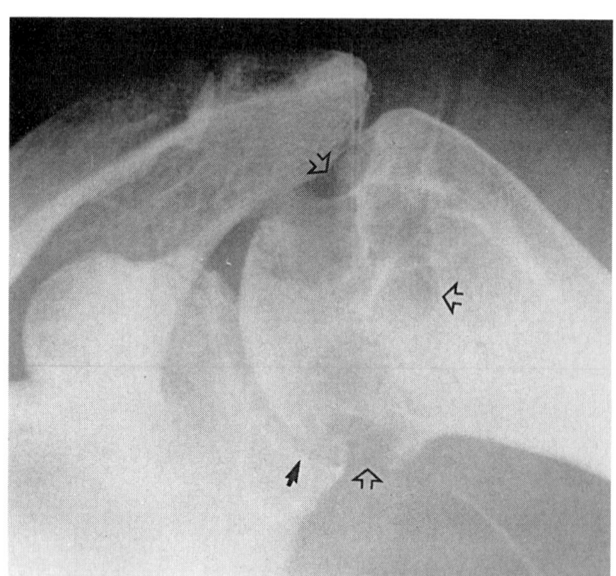

FIGURE 13–41. Tuberculous arthritis: glenohumeral joint.[73, 74] Epiphyseal osteomyelitis is seen as widespread osteolytic cyst-like erosions within the humeral head (open arrows). The infection has disseminated to the glenohumeral joint and is characterized by marked joint space narrowing (small black arrow). The acromioclavicular joint does not appear to be affected.

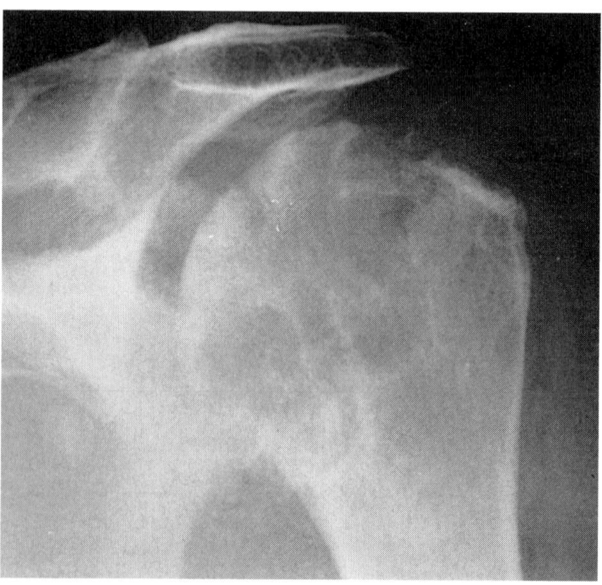

FIGURE 13–42. Pigmented villonodular synovitis.[75, 76] The radiographic findings in this patient with chronic shoulder pain include large erosions involving the entire humeral head, widening of the glenohumeral joint space, and erosion of the subarticular bone of the glenoid. This synovial proliferative disorder of unknown cause usually is monoarticular, and 50 per cent of patients report a history of previous trauma.

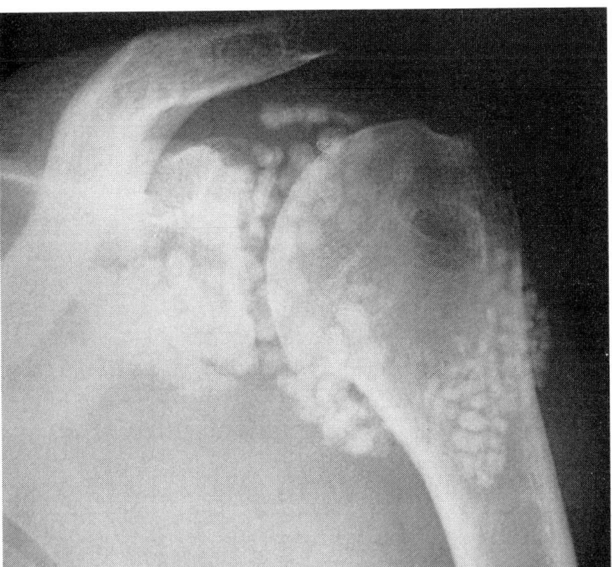

FIGURE 13–43. Idiopathic synovial osteochondromatosis.[77, 78] Numerous juxta-articular radiodense, osteocartilaginous bodies are present within the shoulder capsule. Idiopathic synovial osteochondromatosis represents metaplastic or neoplastic proliferation of cartilaginous bodies by the synovial membrane. It typically occurs in patients between the ages of 20 and 40 years and is twice as common in men. Secondary synovial osteochondromatosis also may occur as a result of degenerative joint disease. *(Courtesy of J. Slivka, M.D., San Diego, California.)*

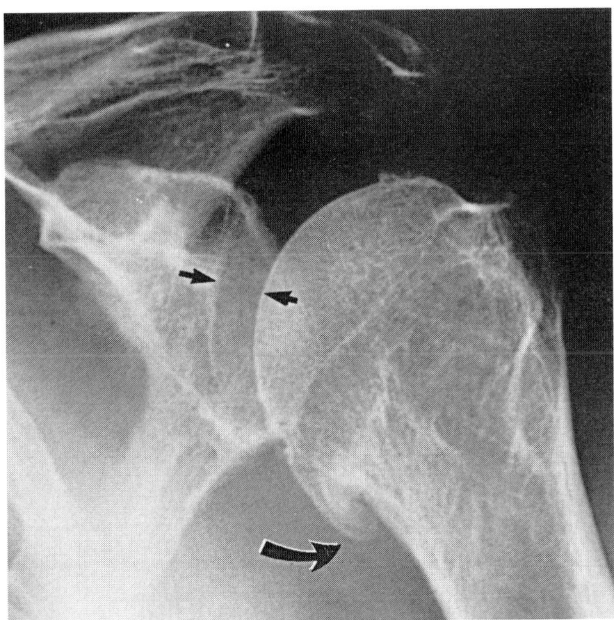

FIGURE 13–44. Acromegalic arthropathy.[79] Radiograph of the shoulder in this 53-year-old man reveals a large osteophyte (curved arrow), indicating accelerated degenerative joint disease of the glenohumeral joint. Cartilage proliferation has resulted in widening of the glenohumeral joint (arrows). Most radiographic changes in acromegalic arthropathy relate to overgrowth of bone and soft tissues.

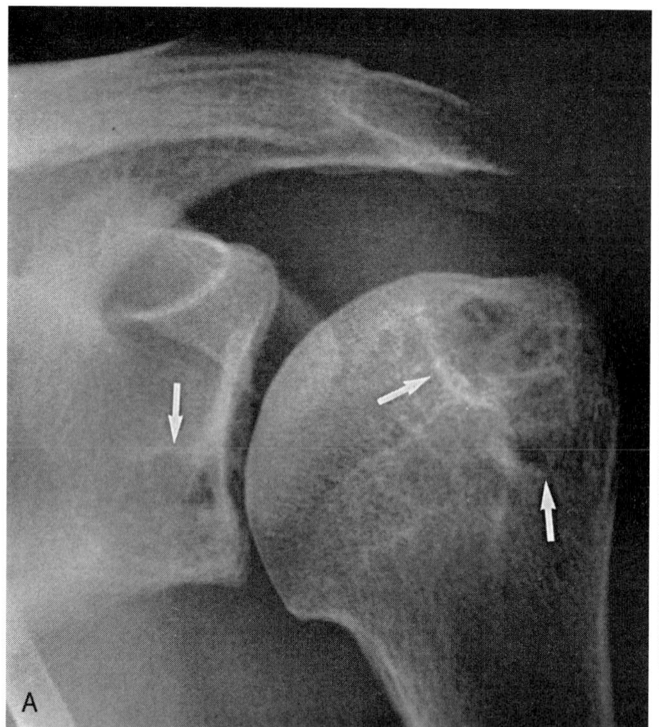

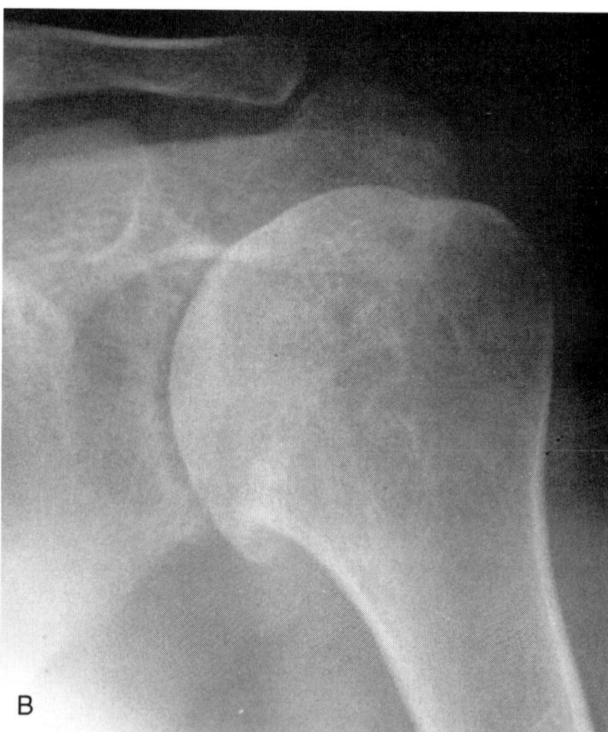

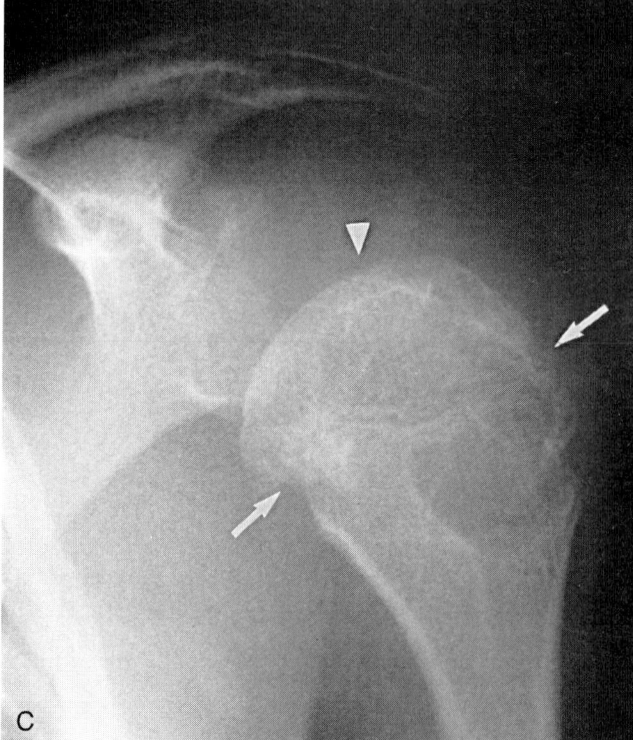

FIGURE 13–45. Hemophilic arthropathy.[80] A This 29-year-old hemophilic man had a history of severe episodes of hemarthrosis of the glenohumeral joint. Observe the subchondral cysts within the glenoid and humeral head (arrows). B In another 29-year-old man, uniform joint space narrowing, sclerosis, osteophytosis, and cyst formation are seen. C This 17-year-old boy has had long-standing hemophilia and has sustained several episodes of hemarthrosis. A frontal radiograph reveals a large joint effusion, probably a hemarthrosis, leading to inferior subluxation of the humeral head with respect to the glenoid cavity (arrowhead). Significant articular surface erosions of the humeral head are apparent (arrows). Both shoulders exhibited symmetric changes typical of hemophilic arthropathy. These changes closely resemble those of juvenile chronic (rheumatoid) arthritis.

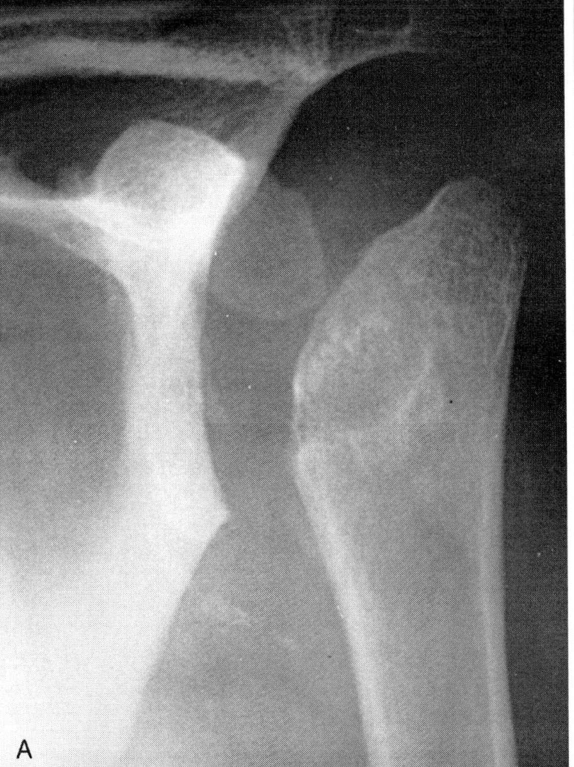

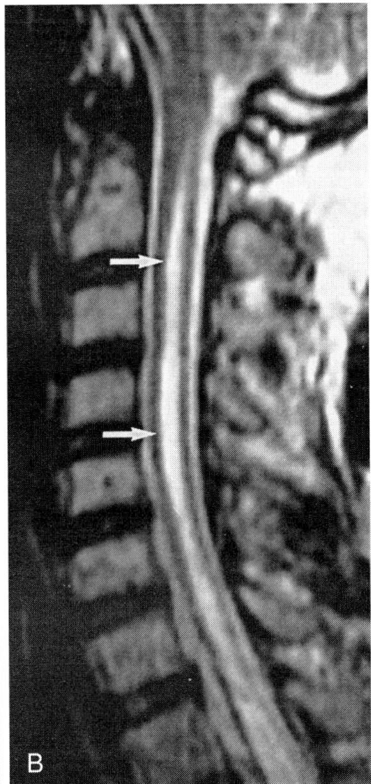

FIGURE 13–46. Neuropathic osteoarthropathy: syringomyelia.[81] **A** Extensive atrophic destruction of the humeral head and glenoid are seen in this patient with a C3-C7 syrinx. Faint osseous debris also is present within the joint. **B** In another patient, a sagittal T2-weighted (TR/TE, 3600/96) fast spin echo magnetic resonance (MR) image reveals an expanded high signal intensity cerebrospinal fluid–filled cavity within the cervical and upper thoracic cord (arrows). *(Courtesy of D. Forrester, M.D., and R. Kerr, M.D., Los Angeles, California.)*

TABLE 13–8. Neoplasms Affecting the Clavicle and Scapula

Entity	Figure(s)	Characteristics
Secondary malignant neoplasms of bone		
Skeletal metastasis[82]		Osteolytic, osteoblastic, or mixed lesions occasionally occur within the sternum and clavicle Irradiation of primary breast or lung carcinoma may result in radiation-induced sarcoma, osteoporosis, and osteonecrosis
Primary malignant neoplasms of bone		
Osteosarcoma[83, 84]	13–47	One per cent of osteosarcomas affect the scapula; fewer than 1 per cent affect the clavicle Most osteosarcomas of the clavicle and scapula are secondary, arising from malignant transformation of Paget's disease or irradiated bone
Osteoblastoma (aggressive)[85]		As many as 4 per cent of aggressive osteoblastomas affect the scapula; fewer than 1 per cent affect the clavicle Expansile osteolytic lesion that may be partially ossified or contain calcium
Chondrosarcoma[86]		Approximately 5 per cent of chondrosarcomas affect the scapula; 1 per cent affect the clavicle Tend to be osteolytic lesions sometimes containing a bulky cartilaginous cap and frequently containing calcifications Soft tissue masses common
Fibrosarcoma[87]		Approximately 2 per cent of fibrosarcomas affect the scapula; 1 per cent affect the clavicle
Ewing's sarcoma[88]	13–48	As many as 5 per cent of Ewing's sarcomas affect the scapula; 2 per cent affect the clavicle Aggressive permeative or moth-eaten pattern of bone destruction often associated with periostitis and soft tissue mass Most lesions central and metadiaphyseal in location

Table continued on following page

TABLE 13–8. Neoplasms Affecting the Clavicle and Scapula *Continued*

Entity	Figure(s)	Characteristics
Myeloproliferative disorders		
Plasma cell (multiple) myeloma[89]	13–49	Seventy-five percent of all plasma cell myeloma is the multiple form Approximately 5 per cent of myeloma patients with skeletal lesions have scapular involvement; 10 per cent have clavicular involvement Diffuse osteopenia or punctate osteolytic lesions
Solitary plasmacytoma[90]		Approximately 3 per cent of plasmacytomas affect the scapula; 5 per cent affect the clavicle
Hodgkin's disease[91]		Approximately 3 per cent of skeletal lesions in Hodgkin's disease occur in the scapula; 1 per cent occur in the clavicle
Primary lymphoma (non-Hodgkin's)[92]		Approximately 4 per cent of patients with primary non-Hodgkin's lymphoma of bone have scapular involvement; 2 per cent have clavicular involvement May result in multiple moth-eaten or permeative osteolytic rib lesions Diffuse or localized sclerotic lesions are rare
Primary benign neoplasms of bone		
Osteoid osteoma[93, 94]		Rare occurrence within scapula and clavicle Central radiolucent nidus with surrounding reactive sclerosis
Osteoblastoma (conventional)[94]		Approximately 1 per cent of conventional osteoblastomas affect the scapula; fewer than 1 per cent affect the clavicle
Enchondroma (solitary)[95]		Approximately 1 per cent of solitary enchondromas affect the scapula; fewer than 1 per cent affect the clavicle
Maffucci's syndrome[96]		Over 26 per cent of patients with Maffucci's syndrome have scapular lesions; fewer than 3 per cent have clavicular lesions Soft tissue hemangiomas in addition to multiple enchondromas Higher risk of malignant transformation than solitary enchondroma
Chondroblastoma[97]		Approximately 2 per cent of chondroblastomas involve the scapula; fewer than 1 per cent involve the clavicle Radiolucent lesion, typically in a subchondral, epiphyseal, or apophyseal location Proximal humeral epiphysis is one of the most common sites (see Chapter 14)
Osteochondroma (solitary)[98]	13–50	Approximately 4 per cent of solitary osteochondromas arise from the scapula; fewer than 1 per cent arise from the clavicle
Hemangioma[99]	13–51	Approximately 2 per cent of hemangiomas occur in the scapula; 1 per cent occur in the clavicle Osseous expansion and trabecular striation within lesions
Aneurysmal bone cyst[100]	13–52	Approximately 2 per cent of aneurysmal bone cysts involve the scapula and 3 per cent involve the clavicle; one of the most common benign tumors of the clavicle Eccentric, thin-walled, expansile, multiloculated osteolytic lesion
Tumor-like lesions		
Paget's disease[101, 102]	13–53	Paget's disease involves the scapula and clavicle infrequently Usually polyostotic and may exhibit unilateral involvement
Neurofibromatosis 1 (von Recklinghausen's disease)[103]		Involvement of scapula and clavicle is uncommon Clavicular pseudarthrosis may result from improper fracture healing
Monostotic fibrous dysplasia[104]		Approximately 2 per cent of all monostotic lesions affect the scapula; fewer than 1 per cent affect the clavicle Improper fracture healing may result in clavicular pseudarthrosis
Polyostotic fibrous dysplasia[104]		Scapula is involved in over 33 per cent of cases and clavicle is involved in 10 per cent of cases of polyostotic fibrous dysplasia Unilateral (or infrequently, bilateral asymmetric) involvement
Langerhans' cell histiocytosis[105, 106]	13–54	Five per cent of lesions affect the clavicle and scapula Histiocytic infiltration of bone Eosinophilic granuloma is the most frequently encountered form

*See also Tables 1–10 to 1–12.

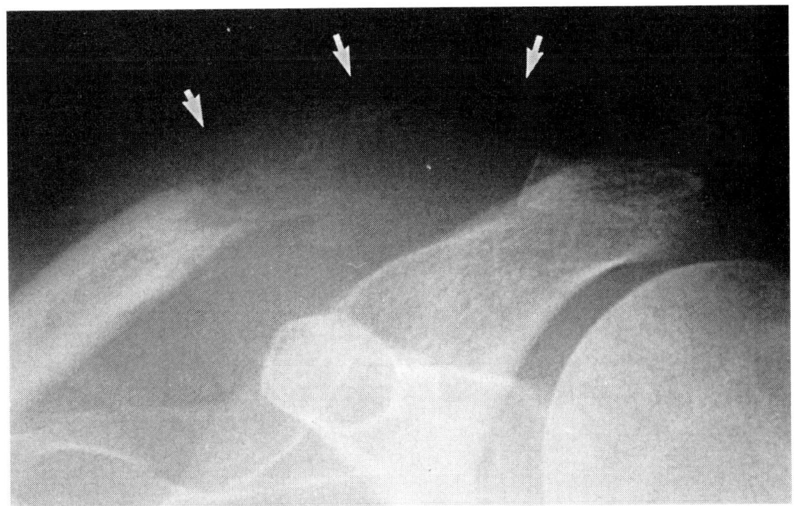

FIGURE 13–47. Osteosarcoma.[83, 84] This 50-year-old man had severe shoulder pain. Radiographs reveal extensive osteolytic destruction of the distal end of the clavicle (arrows). The histologic diagnosis was osteosarcoma.

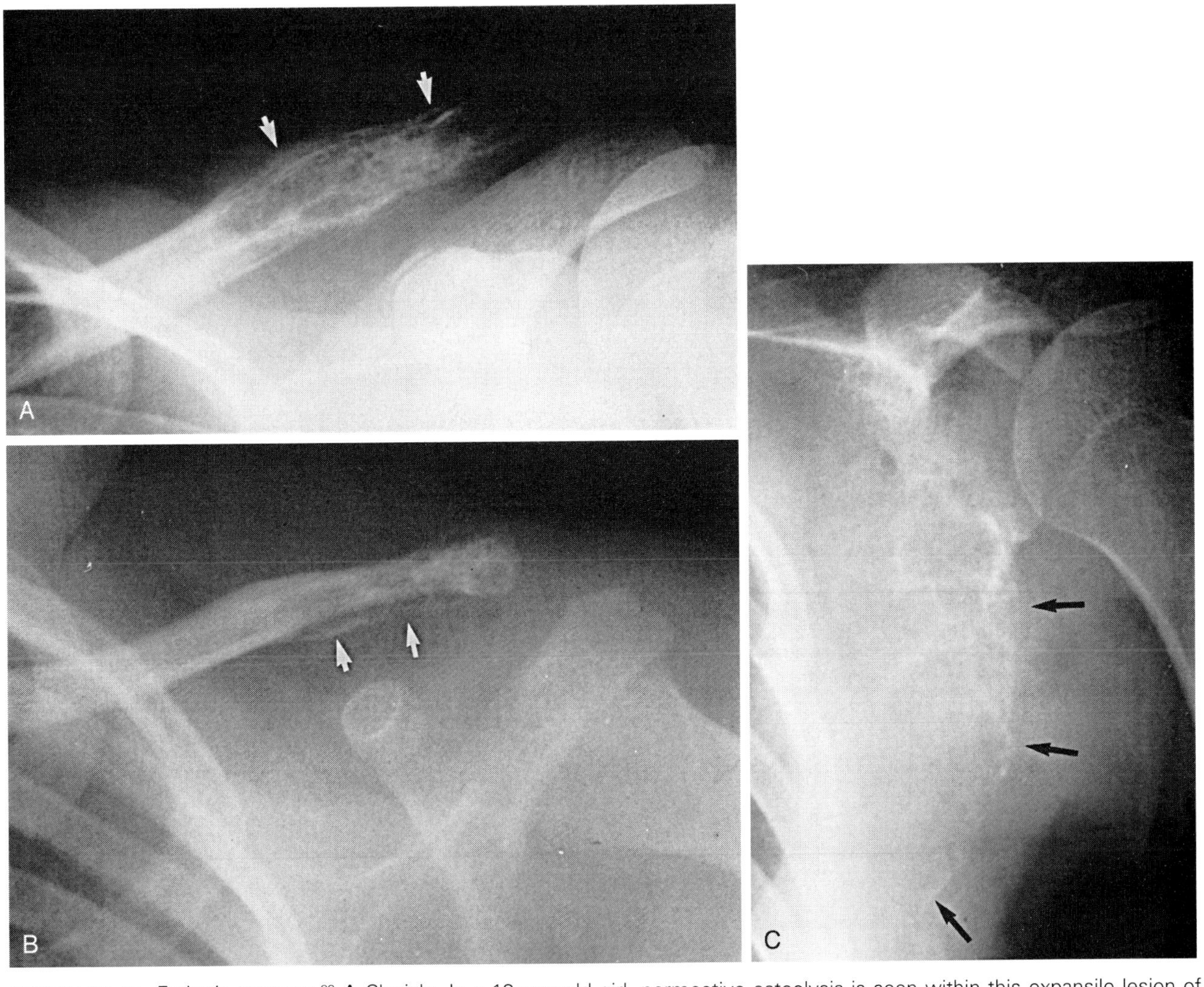

FIGURE 13–48. Ewing's sarcoma.[88] A Clavicle. In a 13-year-old girl, permeative osteolysis is seen within this expansile lesion of the clavicle (arrows). B Clavicle. A radiograph of the clavicle of this 3-year-old child with Ewing's sarcoma shows a permeative pattern of osteolysis with a laminated periosteal response (arrows). C Scapula. A radiograph of the shoulder in this 15-year-old girl shows an expansile, multiloculated osteolytic lesion involving the majority of the body of the scapula (arrows). *(C, Courtesy of R. Kerr, M.D., Los Angeles, California.)*

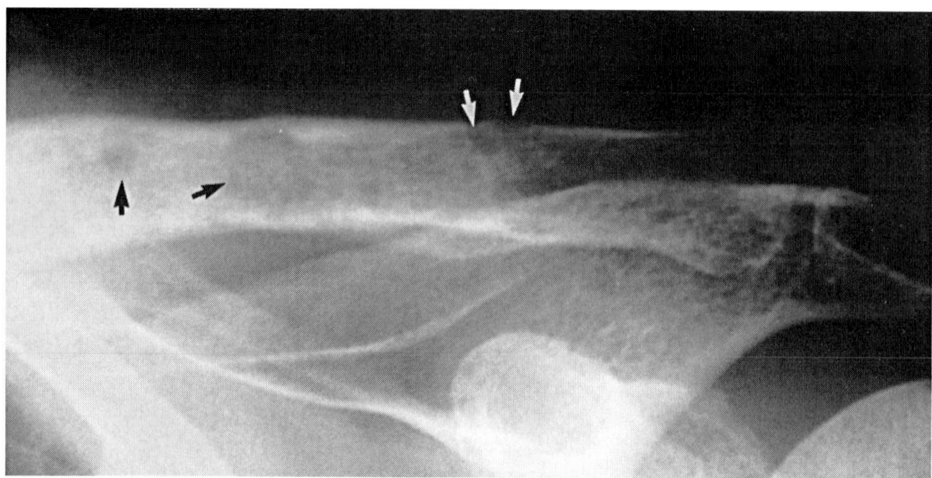

FIGURE 13–49. Plasma cell myeloma.[89] Several small and large punctate osteolytic lesions (arrows) are present throughout the clavicle.

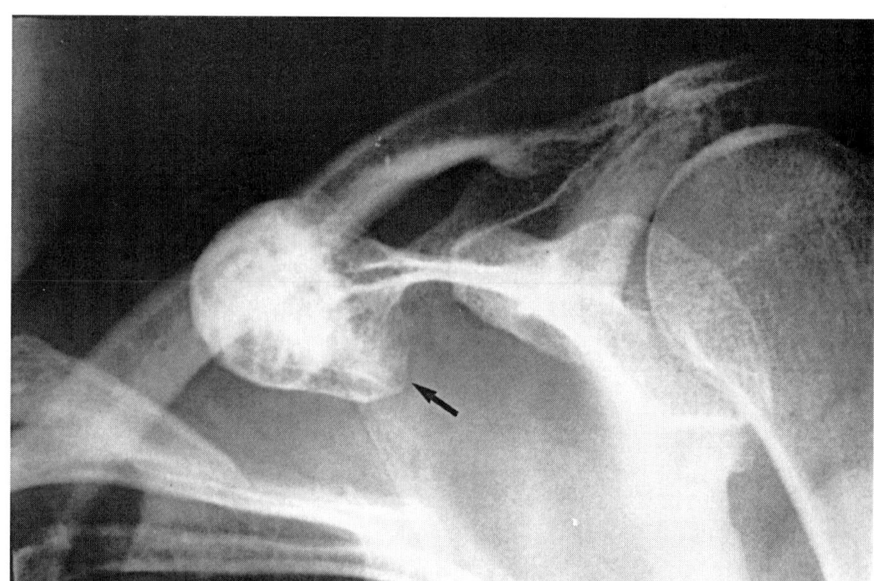

FIGURE 13–50. Osteochondroma.[98] Observe the bulbous osteochondroma arising from the medial border of the scapula (arrow) in this 34-year-old man with hereditary multiple exostoses.

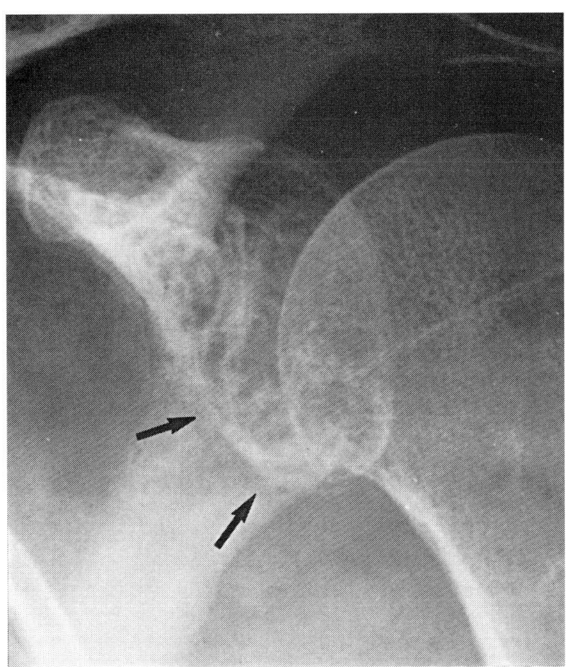

FIGURE 13–51. Hemangioma.[99] Note the trabeculated osteolytic lesion affecting the glenoid of the scapula (arrows), an incidental finding in this 55-year-old woman who was undergoing radiographic examination for evaluation of a shoulder injury.

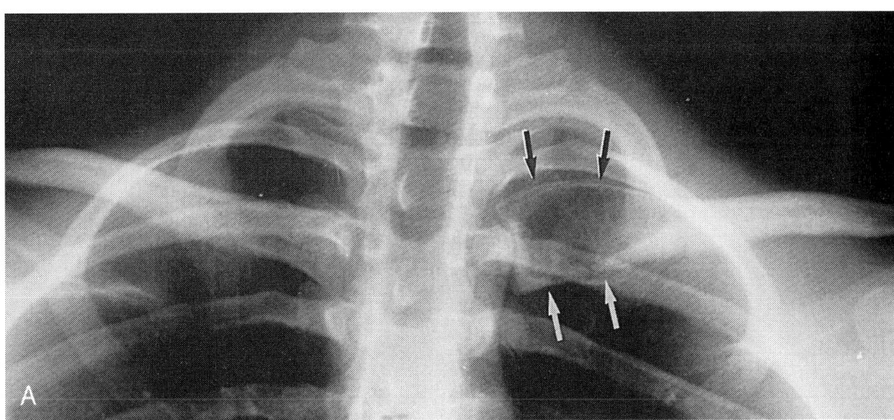

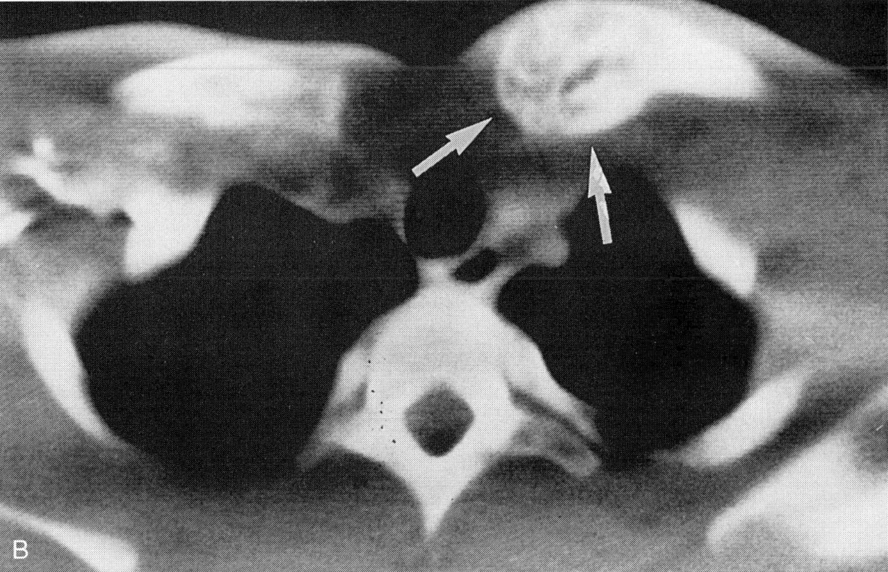

FIGURE 13–52. Aneurysmal bone cyst.[100] This 18-year-old man had sternoclavicular pain. A Frontal radiograph. Comparison of the clavicles reveals an expansile osteolytic lesion involving the proximal portion of the left clavicle (arrows). B Transaxial computed tomographic (CT) image confirms the expansile osteolytic nature of the tumor (arrows) and demonstrates that the cortex is intact; no adjacent soft tissue mass is present. *(Courtesy of M. Mitchell, M.D., Halifax, Nova Scotia, Canada.)*

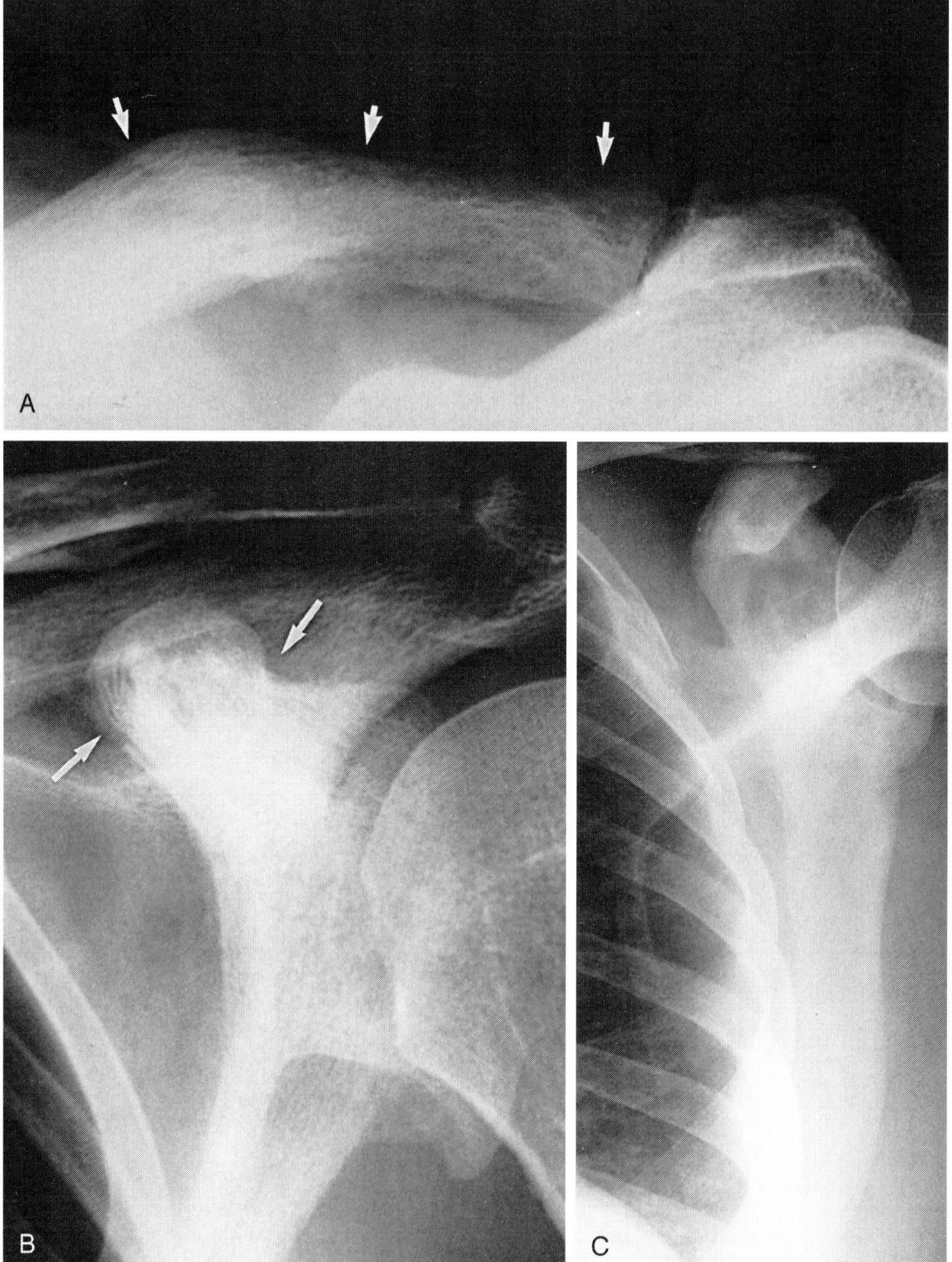

FIGURE 13–53. Paget's disease.[101, 102] A Clavicle. Bone enlargement and trabecular coarsening (arrows) predominate in the clavicle of this patient with Paget's disease. B Scapula. Observe the osteosclerotic appearance and enlargement of the coracoid process (arrows), scapular neck, and glenoid. C Body of the scapula. Note the osteosclerosis, cortical enlargement, and thickening and coalescence of the trabeculae throughout the scapula of this 65-year-old woman with Paget's disease. The adjacent ribs and humerus were not affected. *(C, Courtesy of E. Dal Mas, D.C., Portland, Oregon.)*

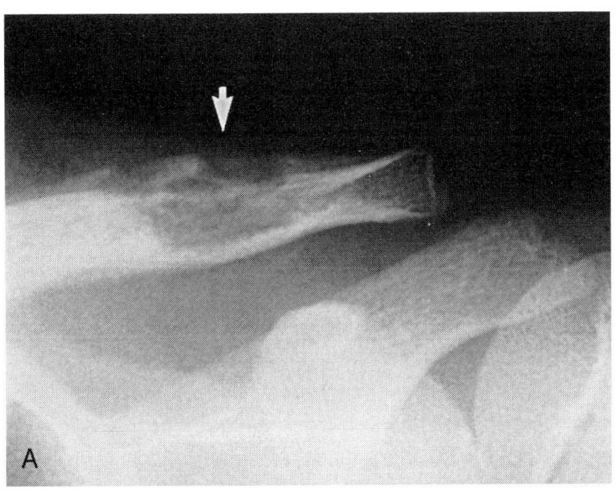

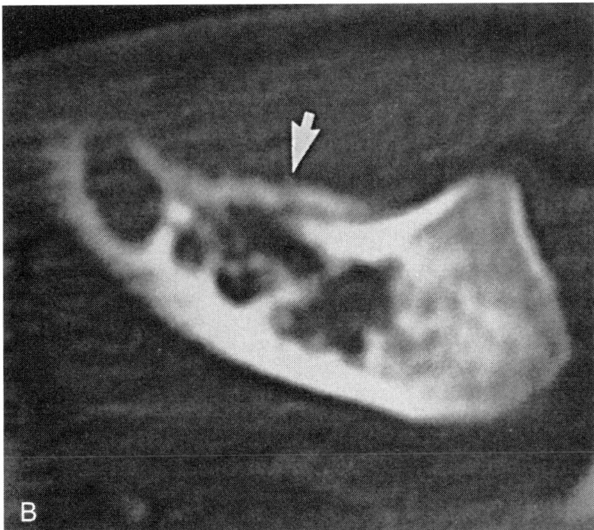

FIGURE 13–54. Langerhans' cell histiocytosis: eosinophilic granuloma.[105, 106] **A** Frontal radiograph of a 9-year-old boy shows an expansile lesion with periostitis and a permeative pattern of osteolytic destruction involving the distal clavicular diaphysis (arrow). **B** Transaxial computed tomographic (CT), image further documents the osteolytic, expansile, and septated appearance of the lesion (arrow). Biopsy revealed eosinophilic granuloma of bone, the most frequent and mildest form of Langerhans' cell histiocytosis. *(Courtesy of G. Greenway, M.D., Dallas, Texas.)*

TABLE 13–9. Metabolic, Hematologic and Infectious Disorders Affecting the Shoulder

Disorder	Figure(s)	Characteristics
Generalized osteoporosis[107]		Major complication: fractures of the proximal portion of the humerus (see Chapter 14)
Osteomalacia and rickets[108]		*Osteomalacia* Osteopenia Decreased trabeculae; remaining trabeculae appear prominent and coarsened Looser's zones or pseudofractures *Rickets* Findings most prominent in the proximal portion of the humerus Metaphyseal demineralization: frayed, widened, cupped metaphyses Bowing of bones Osteopenia
Hyperparathyroidism and renal osteodystrophy[109–111]	13–55	Bone resorption and erosion of the distal end of the clavicle and the undersurface of the clavicle at the attachment site of the coracoclavicular ligaments Occasional bone sclerosis (more common with renal osteodystrophy) Chondrocalcinosis (CPPD crystal deposition) Brown tumors Soft tissue calcification Slipped capital humeral epiphysis Pathologic fracture
Milk-alkali syndrome[112]	13–56	Metastatic periarticular soft tissue calcification in persons who ingest large quantities of milk and alkaline substances Patients with chronic peptic ulcer disease and renal insufficiency Osseous tissues are normal Widespread calcification also occurs in blood vessels, kidneys, falx cerebri, and ligaments
Osteonecrosis[113, 114]	13–57	Also termed ischemic necrosis or avascular necrosis of the humeral head Sclerosis, subchondral cysts, subchondral bone collapse, and eventual flattening of the humeral head; snowcap appearance may occur Predisposing factors include corticosteroid use, hemoglobinopathies, Gaucher's disease, trauma, and alcoholism
Radiation changes of bone[115]	13–58	Radiation therapy for carcinoma of the breast or lung apex may result in radiation osteitis, osteonecrosis, and sarcoma formation Radiographic findings of osteitis and osteonecrosis include subchondral bone destruction, osseous debris, and joint disorganization resembling neuropathic osteoarthropathy
Pyogenic osteomyelitis[116]	13–59	Clavicle and scapula infrequently involved Initial latent period in which no radiographic signs are present—days to weeks Early signs: soft tissue swelling with obliteration of soft tissue planes Late signs: osteoporosis, osteolysis, cortical lucency, periostitis, involucrum formation, sequestration, and sinus tracts May be associated with septic arthritis of adjacent joints

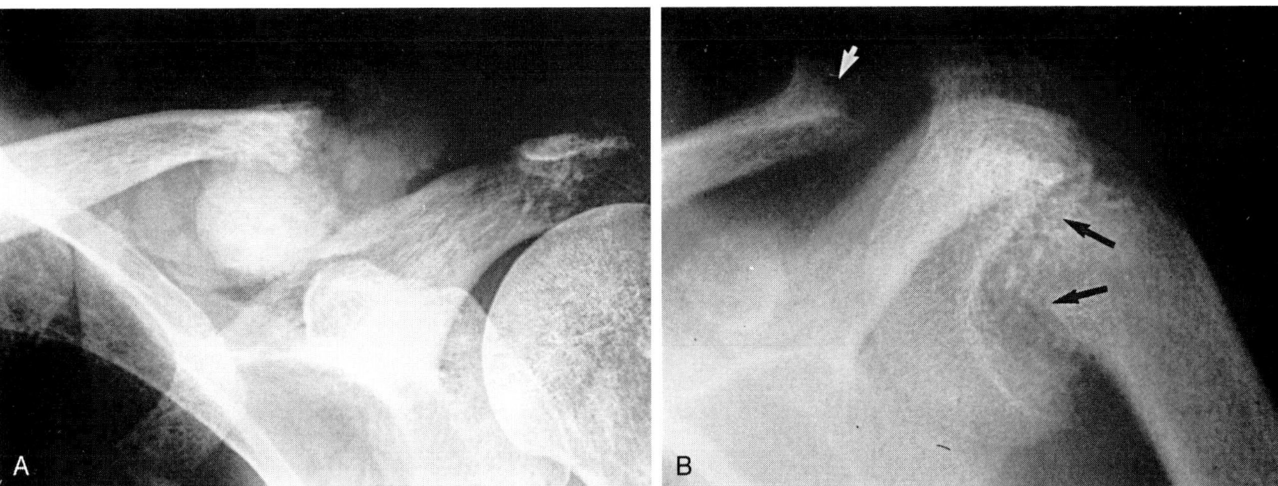

FIGURE 13–55. Renal osteodystrophy.[109–111] A Observe the extensive erosion of the distal end of the clavicle and widening of the acromioclavicular joint in this 65-year-old renal transplant patient. Prominent soft tissue calcification also is present. B Routine radiograph of this child's shoulder reveals osteopenia, widening of the physis, and a type I growth plate injury with displacement of the humeral epiphysis (black arrows). These findings of subchondral resorption and resultant epiphyseal slippage often are seen in the proximal humeral epiphysis in children with chronic renal disease and resemble the physeal changes seen in rickets. Extensive resorption of the distal portion of the clavicle (white arrow) results in widening of the acromioclavicular joint. *(B, Courtesy of M.N. Pathria, M.D., San Diego, California.)*

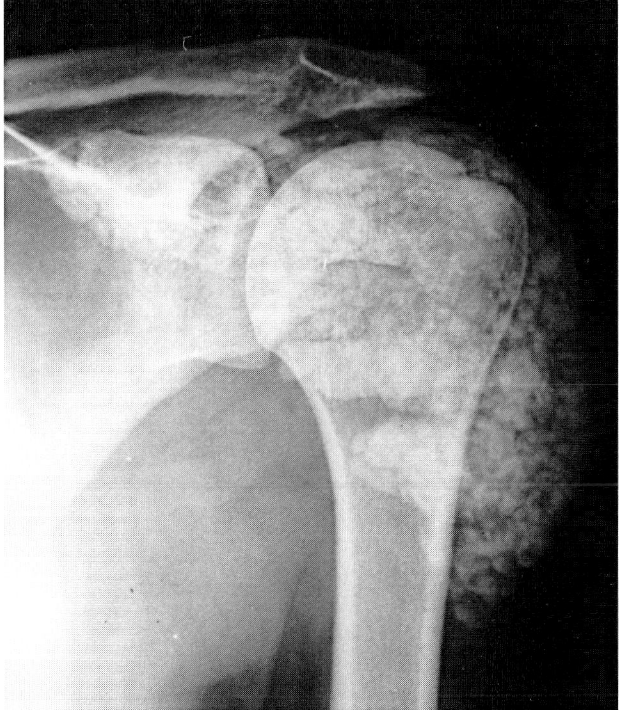

FIGURE 13–56. Milk-alkali syndrome.[112] Observe the extensive soft tissue calcinosis in this patient who was drinking excessive amounts of milk and calcium carbonate for his heartburn. Milk-alkali syndrome represents metastatic periarticular soft tissue calcification in persons who ingest large quantities of milk and alkaline substances simultaneously.

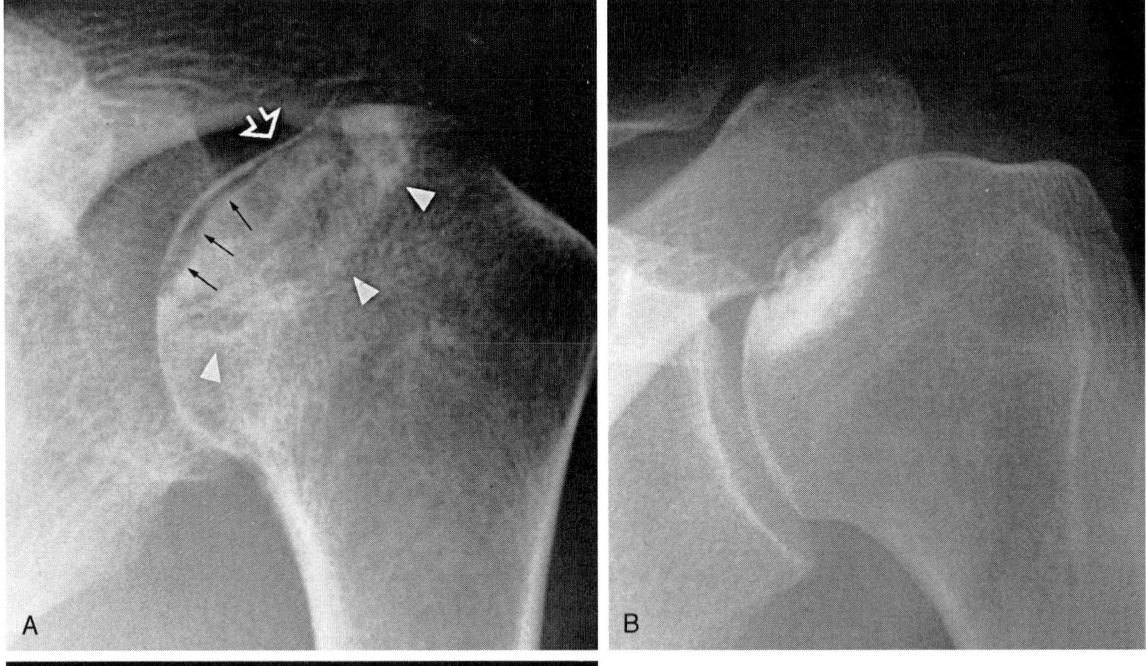

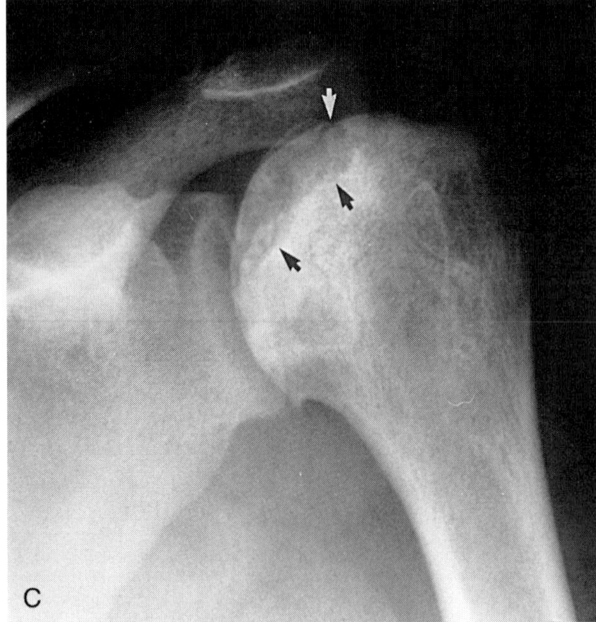

FIGURE 13–57. Osteonecrosis.[113, 114] A, B Corticosteroid-induced osteonecrosis. In A, a 47-year-old man with shoulder pain, the radiographic findings include collapse and fragmentation of the humeral head articular surface (open arrow), a curvilinear subarticular radiolucency (crescent sign) (arrows), and a combination of radiolucency and radiodensity in the humeral head (arrowheads). In B, a radiograph of a 39-year-old woman on long-term corticosteroid therapy demonstrates a zone of sclerosis (snowcap appearance) with a small zone of radiolucent destruction of the proximal humeral articular surface. The glenohumeral joint space is preserved. C Hemoglobinopathy. This 30-year-old woman with sickle cell anemia has an epiphyseal infarct, a common complication of vascular occlusion. Note the sclerotic zone adjacent to the subchondral radiolucent area (black arrows) and the articular collapse (white arrow).

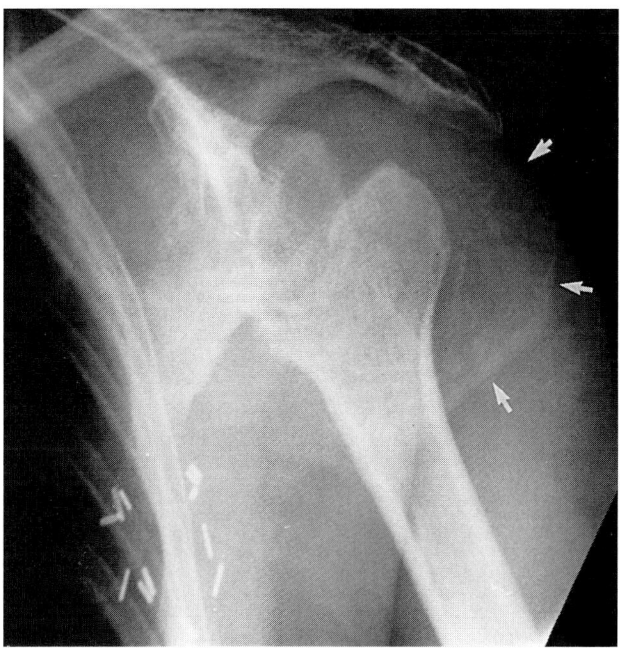

FIGURE 13–58. Radiation changes.[115] This patient underwent radiation therapy for carcinoma of the breast. Observe the destruction of subchondral bone in the humeral head, widening of the superior aspect of the glenohumeral joint space, and bursal distention with osseous debris (arrows). Radiation osteitis and osteonecrosis are believed to be responsible for these changes. This appearance resembles that of neuropathic joint disease associated with syringomyelia.

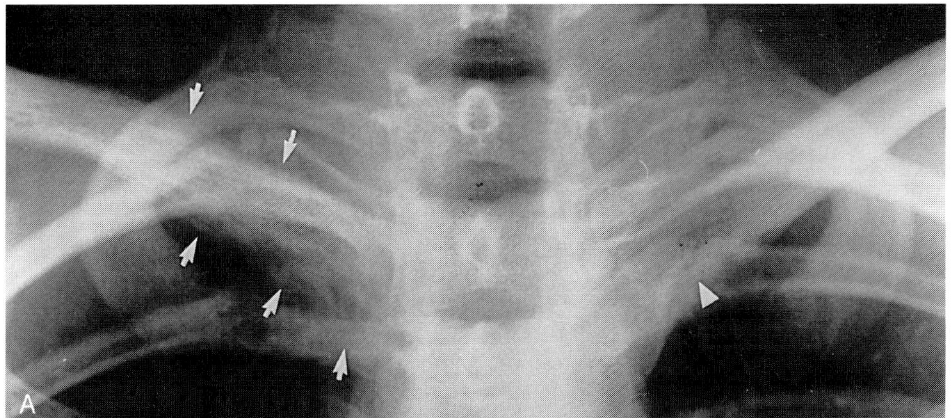

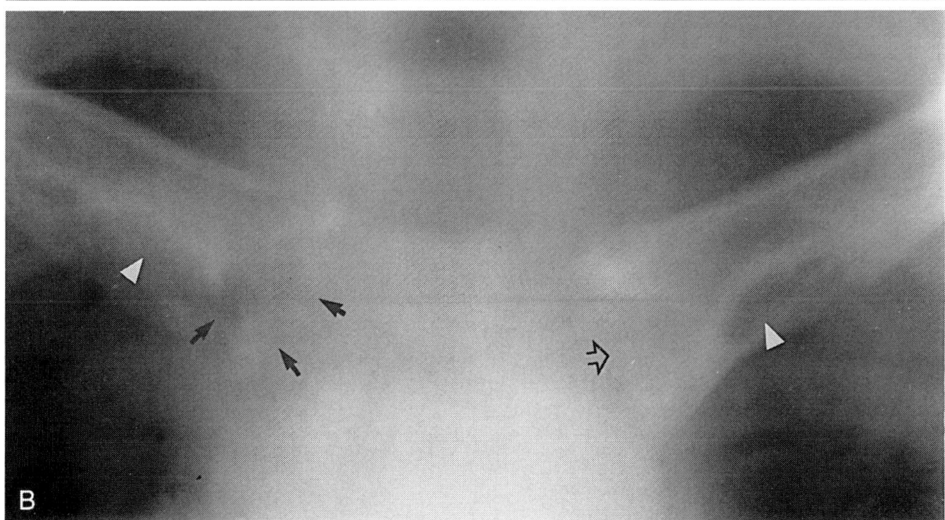

FIGURE 13–59. Pyogenic osteomyelitis: clavicle.[116] Frontal radiograph (A) and conventional tomogram (B) of the clavicles of this 18-year-old male patient show permeative destruction of the medial portion of the right clavicle with destruction of its articular end (arrows). Of incidental note are bilateral rhomboid fossae (arrowheads) and a fork-shaped medial end of the left clavicle (open arrow), both of which are normal variants.

TABLE 13–10. Miscellaneous Disorders Resulting in Clavicular Osteosclerosis, Periostitis, or Bone Enlargement

Entity	Figure(s)	Typical Age of Onset (Years)	Characteristics
SAPHO syndrome[117]		Variable	SAPHO is an acronym for the findings of synovitis (S), acne (A), pustulosis (P), hyperostosis (H), and osteitis (O) Arthro-osteitis associated with acne or pustulosis palmaris et plantaris; closely related to sternocostoclavicular hyperostosis, psoriasis, and chronic recurrent multifocal osteomyelitis Prominent hyperostosis and painful osteitis of the clavicles and anterior chest wall as well as synovitis of the nearby joints
Sternocostoclavicular hyperostosis[117, 118]		40–60	Bilateral clavicle overgrowth and soft tissue ossification Associated with pustulosis palmaris et plantaris in 30–50 per cent of patients (see SAPHO syndrome above) Men > women; cause unknown Clinical findings: pain, swelling, tenderness, and local heat overlying the anterior upper chest wall
Condensing osteitis of the clavicle[117, 119]	13–60	20–50	Also termed osteitis condensans clavicle Painful swelling and sclerosis of the medial ends of the clavicles Encountered in young women involved in heavy lifting or sports activities Cause unknown
Chronic recurrent multifocal osteomyelitis[117, 120]	13–61	5–10	Closely related to SAPHO syndrome Also termed plasma cell osteomyelitis, and primary chronic osteomyelitis Pain, tenderness, and swelling affecting the medial ends of the clavicles Radiographic findings: intense sclerosis, bone enlargement, osteolysis, and periostitis involving the clavicle
Friedrich's disease[4, 121]		5–20	Ischemic necrosis of the medial clavicular epiphysis Soft tissue swelling, tenderness to palpation over medial end of clavicle Osteosclerosis of entire clavicular head; often associated with notch-like defect of medial end of clavicle Benign, self-limited process
Infantile cortical hyperostosis (Caffey's disease)[16, 122]		Younger than 5 months	Diffuse periostitis and cortical hyperostosis of the clavicles and, less commonly, the scapulae May become extreme See also Table 13–3
Acromegaly[123]		Older than 20	Osseous proliferation at ligament attachments on the undersurface of the distal end of the clavicle
Primary hypertrophic osteoarthropathy (pachydermoperiostosis)[124]		15–20	Diaphyseal, metaphyseal, and epiphyseal periostitis Shaggy, irregular excrescences Diaphyseal expansion
Secondary hypertrophic osteoarthropathy[125]	13–62	Adults; rare in children	Bilateral diaphyseal and metaphyseal periostitis of the clavicle Single layer or laminated, regular or irregular proliferation Periarticular osteoporosis, soft tissue swelling Underlying primary visceral disease such as bronchogenic carcinoma and mesothelioma
Hypervitaminosis A[126]		Older than 1 year	Megadoses of vitamin A in children may result in undulating diaphyseal periostitis of the tubular bones including the clavicle Self-limited with cessation of vitamin A ingestion
Prostaglandin periostitis[127]		Neonates: within first 60 days of life	Prostaglandin E_1 and E_2 are medications used in the treatment of neonates with congenital heart disease Long-term infusion (40 days or more) or, rarely, short-term therapy (9 to 14 days) may result in bilateral periostitis and cortical thickening of tubular bones including the clavicle Self-limited; complete resolution usually occurs within 6 months to 1 year
Paget's disease[101, 102]	13–53A	Older than 55	Bilateral or unilateral trabecular coarsening, bone enlargement, osteosclerosis, osteolysis, or combined pattern of osteolysis and sclerosis See also Table 13–8

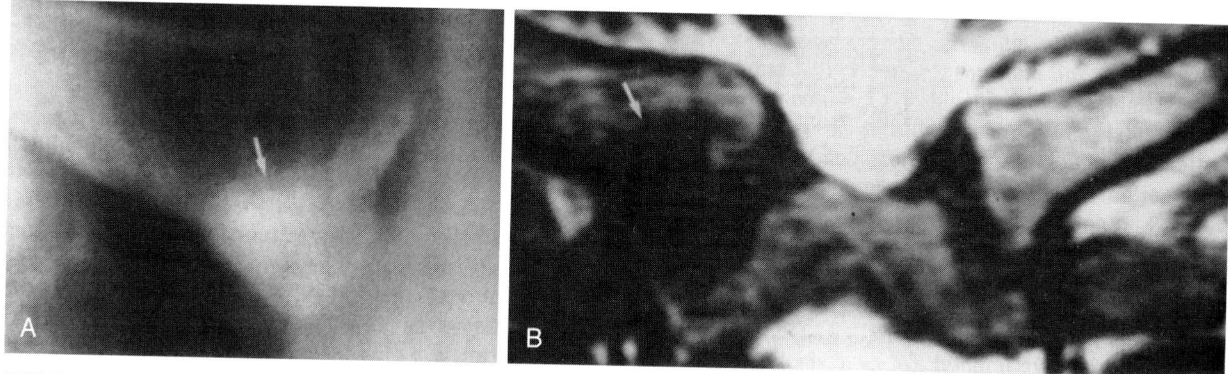

FIGURE 13–60. Condensing osteitis of the clavicle.[117, 118] A 40-year-old woman developed pain and tenderness over the medial end of the right clavicle. A Conventional tomography reveals bone sclerosis involving the inferomedial aspect of the bone (arrow). B Coronal T1-weighted (TR/TE, 300/11) spin echo magnetic resonance (MR) image shows low signal intensity in this area (arrow). The diminished signal intensity persisted on T2-weighted spin echo and gradient echo images (not shown). *(From Resnick D: Diagnosis of Bone and Joint Disorders. Philadelphia, WB Saunders, 1995, p 2100.)*

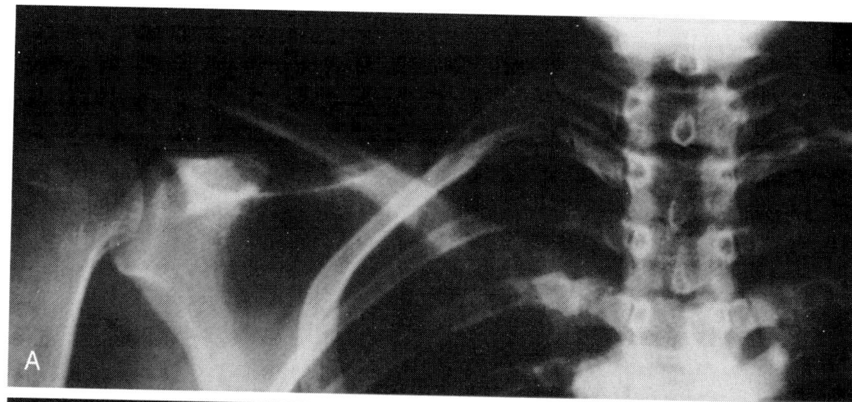

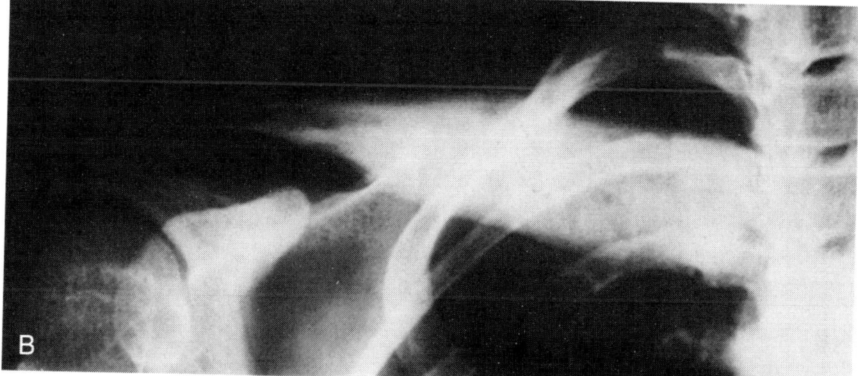

FIGURE 13–61. Chronic recurrent multifocal osteomyelitis.[117, 120] A 16-year-old girl developed pain and progressive enlargement of the medial portion of the right clavicle over a 6-month period. She had no fever or erythema. Radiographs obtained 8 months apart reveal a process that is associated initially (A) with permeative bone destruction and subsequently (B) with massive enlargement of the clavicle. Biopsy and histologic evaluation indicated only chronic osteitis. Cultures were negative. *(From Resnick D: Diagnosis of Bone and Joint Disorders. Philadelphia, WB Saunders, 1995, p 2389.)*

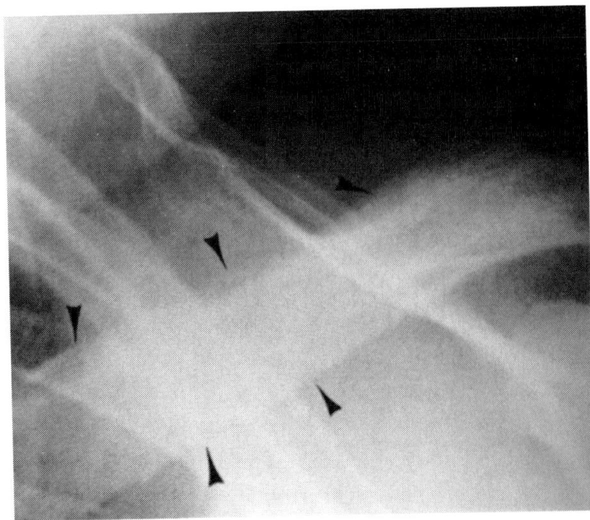

FIGURE 13–62. Secondary hypertrophic osteoarthropathy: periostitis.[125] Deposition of new bone (arrowheads) has resulted in diffuse enlargement of the clavicle. The process was bilateral and affected several tubular bones in this patient. *(From Resnick D: Diagnosis of Bone and Joint Disorders. Philadelphia, WB Saunders, 1995, p 4430.)*

REFERENCES

1. Edeiken J, Dalinka M, Karasick D: Edeiken's Roentgen Diagnosis of Diseases of Bone. 4th Ed. Baltimore, Williams & Wilkins, 1990.
2. Keats TE, Smith TH: An Atlas of Normal Developmental Roentgen Anatomy. 2nd Ed. Chicago, Year Book Medical Publishers, 1988.
3. Greenfield GB: Radiology of Bone Diseases. 2nd Ed. Philadelphia, JB Lippincott, 1975.
4. Köhler A, Zimmer EA: Borderlands of Normal and Early Pathologic Findings in Skeletal Radiography. 4th Ed. New York, Thieme Medical Publishers, 1993.
5. Keats TE: Atlas of Normal Roentgen Variants That May Simulate Disease. 6th Ed. Chicago, Year Book Medical Publishers, 1996.
6. Yochum TR, Rowe LJ: Essentials of Skeletal Radiology. 2nd Ed. Baltimore, Williams & Wilkins, 1996.
7. Schnall SB, King JD, Marrero G: Congenital pseudoarthrosis of the clavicle: A review of the literature and surgical results of six cases. J Pediatr Orthop 8:316, 1988.
8. Juhl JH, Kuhlman JE: Methods of examination, techniques, and anatomy of the chest. *In* Juhl JH, Crummy AB, Kuhlman JE (eds): Paul and Juhl's Essentials of Radiologic Imaging. 7th Ed. Philadelphia, Lippincott-Raven, 1998, p 800.
9. Haramati N, Cook RA, Raphael B, et al: Coraco-clavicular joint: Normal variant in humans. A radiographic demonstration in the human and non-human primate. Skeletal Radiol 23:117, 1994.
10. Ogden JA, Conlogue GJ, Phillips SB, et al: Sprengel's deformity: Radiology of the pathologic deformation. Skeletal Radiol 4:204, 1979.
11. Trout TE, Resnick D: Glenoid hypoplasia and its relationship to instability. Skeletal Radiol 25:37, 1996.
12. Edelson JG, Zuckerman J, Hershkovitz I: Os acromiale: Anatomy and surgical implications. J Bone Joint Surg [Br] 74:551, 1993.
13. Park JG, Lee JK, Phelps CT: Os acromiale associated with rotator cuff impingement: MR imaging of the shoulder. Radiology 193:255, 1994.
14. Resnick D, Cone RO: The nature of humeral pseudocysts. Radiology 150:27, 1984.
15. Langer LO, Baumann PA, Gorlin RJ: Achondroplasia. AJR 100:12, 1967.
16. Machlachlan AK, Gerrard JW, Houston CS, et al: Familial infantile cortical hyperostosis in a large Canadian family. Can Med Assoc J 130:1172, 1984.
17. Cramer SF, Ruehl A, Mandel MA: Fibrodysplasia ossificans progressiva: A distinctive bone-forming lesion of the soft tissue. Cancer 48:1016, 1981.
18. Benli IT, Akalin S, Boysan E, et al: Epidemiological, clinical, and radiological aspects of osteopoikilosis. J Bone Joint Surg [Br] 74:504, 1992.
19. Kovanlikaya A, Loro ML, Gilsanz V: Pathogenesis of osteosclerosis in autosomal dominant osteopetrosis. AJR 168:929, 1997.
20. Yu JS, Resnick D, Vaughan LM, et al: Melorheostosis with an ossified soft tissue mass. Skeletal Radiol 24:367, 1995.
21. Chitayat D, Hodgkinson KA, Azouz EM: Intrafamilial variability in cleidocranial dysplasia: A three generation family. Am J Med Genet 42:298, 1992.
22. Kilcoyne RF, Shuman WP, Matsen FA III, et al: The Neer classification of displaced proximal humeral fractures: Spectrum of findings on plain radiographs and CT scans. AJR 154:1029, 1990.
23. Ovesen J, Nielsen S: Experimental distal subluxation in the glenohumeral joint. Arch Orthop Trauma Surg 104:78, 1985.
24. Barnett LS: Little League shoulder syndrome: Proximal humeral epiphysiolysis in adolescent baseball pitchers. J Bone Joint Surg [Am] 67:495, 1985.
25. Rogers LF, Poznanski AK: Imaging of epiphyseal injuries. Radiology 191:297, 1994.
26. Weinberg B, Seife B, Alonso P: The apical oblique view of the clavicle: Its usefulness in neonatal and childhood trauma. Skeletal Radiol 20:201, 1991.

27. Robinson CM: Fractures of the clavicle in the adult: Epidemiology and classification. J Bone Joint Surg [Br] 80:476, 1998.
28. Ada JR, Miller ME: Scapular fractures: Analysis of 113 cases. Clin Orthop 269:174, 1991.
29. Froimson AI: Fracture of the coracoid process of the scapula. J Bone Joint Surg [Am] 60:710, 1978.
30. Herscovici D Jr, Fiennes AGTW, Allgöwer M, et al: The floating shoulder: Ipsilateral clavicle and scapular neck fractures. J Bone Joint Surg [Br] 74:362, 1992.
31. Strouse PJ, Owings CL: Fractures of the first rib in child abuse. Radiology 197:763, 1995.
32. Deutsch AL, Resnick D, Mink JH, et al: Computed tomography of the glenohumeral joint: Normal anatomy and clinical experience. Radiology 153:603, 1984.
33. Richards RD, Sartoris DJ, Pathria MN, et al: Hill-Sachs lesion and normal humeral groove: MR imaging features allowing their differentiation. Radiology 190:665, 1994.
34. Workman TL, Burkhard TK, Resnick D, et al: Hill-Sachs lesion: Comparison of detection with MR imaging, radiography, and arthroscopy. Radiology 185:847, 1992.
35. Gonzalez D, Lopez RA: Concurrent rotator-cuff tear and brachial plexus palsy associated with anterior dislocation of the shoulder: A report of two cases. J Bone Joint Surg [Am] 73:620, 1991.
36. Hawkins RJ, Neer CS II, Pianta RM, et al: Locked posterior dislocation of the shoulder. J Bone Joint Surg [Am] 69:9, 1987.
37. Downey EF Jr, Curtis DJ, Brower AC: Unusual dislocations of the shoulder. AJR 140:1207, 1983.
38. Davids JR, Talbott RD: Luxatio erecta humeri: A case report. Clin Orthop 252:144, 1990.
39. Arger PH, Oberkircher PE, Miller WT: Lipohemarthrosis. AJR 121:97, 1974.
40. Väätäinen U, Pirinen A, Mäkelä A: Radiologic evaluation of the acromioclavicular joint. Skeletal Radiol 20:115, 1991.
41. Vanarthos WJ, Ekman EF, Bohrer SP: Radiographic diagnosis of acromioclavicular joint separation without weight bearing: Importance of internal rotation of the arm. AJR 162:120, 1994.
42. Levinsohn EM, Bunnell WP, Yuan HA: Computed tomography in the diagnosis of dislocations of the sternoclavicular joint. Clin Orthop 140:13, 1979.
43. Jim YF, Chang CY, Wu JJ, et al: Shoulder impingement syndrome: Impingement view and arthrography based on 100 cases. Skeletal Radiol 21:449, 1992.
44. DeSmet AA, Ting YM: Diagnosis of rotator cuff tear on routine radiographs. J Can Assoc Radiol 28:54, 1977.
45. Patte D: Classification of rotator cuff lesions. Clin Orthop 254:81, 1990.
46. Patten RM, Spear RP, Richardson ML: Diagnostic performance of magnetic resonance imaging for the diagnosis of rotator cuff tears using supplementary images in the oblique and sagittal plane. Invest Radiol 29:87, 1994.
47. Rafii M, Firooznia H, Sherman O, et al: Rotator cuff lesions: Signal patterns at MR imaging. Radiology 177:817, 1990.
48. Resnick D: Frozen shoulder. Ann Rheum Dis 44:805, 1985.
49. Middleton WD, Remus WR, Totty WG, et al: Ultrasonographic evaluation of the rotator cuff and biceps tendon. J Bone Joint Surg [Am] 68:440, 1986.
50. van Leersum M, Schweitzer ME: Magnetic resonance imaging of the biceps complex. MRI Clin North Am 1:77, 1993.
51. Schweitzer ME: MR arthrography of the labral-ligamentous complex of the shoulder. Radiology 190:641, 1994.
52. Pollock AN, Reed MH: Shoulder deformities from obstetrical brachial plexus paralysis. Skeletal Radiol 18:295, 1989.
53. Kaplan PA, Resnick D: Stress-induced osteolysis of the clavicle. Radiology 158:139, 1986.
54. Roach NA, Schweitzer ME: Does osteolysis of the distal clavicle occur following spinal cord injury? Skeletal Radiol 26:16, 1997.
55. Garland DE, Blum CE, Waters RL: Periarticular heterotopic ossification in head-injured adults: Incidence and location. J Bone Joint Surg [Am] 62:1143, 1980.
56. Neer CS II: Replacement arthroplasty for glenohumeral osteoarthritis. J Bone Joint Surg [Am] 56:1, 1974.
57. Brossman J, Preidler KW, Pedowitz RA, et al: Shoulder impingement syndrome: Influence of shoulder position on rotator cuff impingement. AJR 167:1511, 1996.
58. Resnick D, Niwayama G: Resorption of the undersurface of the distal clavicle in rheumatoid arthritis. Radiology 120:75, 1976.
59. Babini JC, Gusis SE, Babini SM, et al: Superolateral erosions of the humeral head in chronic inflammatory arthropathies. Skeletal Radiol 21:515, 1992.
60. Reed MH, Wilmot DM: The radiology of juvenile rheumatoid arthritis: A review of the English language literature. J Rheumatol 18:2, 1991.
61. Resnick D: Patterns of peripheral joint disease in ankylosing spondylitis. Radiology 110:523, 1974.
62. Resnick D, Niwayama G: On the nature and significance of bony proliferation in "rheumatoid variant" disorders. AJR 129:275, 1977.
63. Czirjak L, Nagy Z, Szegedi G: Systemic sclerosis in the elderly. Clin Rheumatol 11:483, 1992.
64. Holt PD, Keats TE: Calcific tendinitis: A review of the usual and unusual. Skeletal Radiol 22:1, 1993.
65. Steinbach LS, Resnick D: Calcium pyrophosphate dihydrate crystal deposition disease revisited. Radiology 200:1, 1996.
66. Huang G-S, Bachmann D, Taylor JAM, et al: Calcium pyrophosphate dihydrate crystal deposition disease and pseudogout of the acromioclavicular joint: Radiographic and pathologic features. J Rheumatol 20:2077, 1993.
67. Halverson PB, Carrera GF, McCarthy DJ: Milwaukee shoulder syndrome: Fifteen additional cases and a description of contributing factors. Arch Intern Med 150:677, 1990.
68. Nguyen VD: Rapid destructive arthritis of the shoulder. Skeletal Radiol 25:107, 1996.
69. Miller-Blair D, White R, Greenspan A: Acute gout involving the acromioclavicular joint following treatment with gemfibrozil. J Rheumatol 19:166, 1992.
70. Katz GA, Peter JB, Pearson CM, et al: The shoulder pad sign—a diagnostic feature of amyloid arthropathy. N Engl J Med 288:354, 1973.
71. Faraawi R, Harth M, Kertesz A, et al: Arthritis in hemochromatosis. J Rheumatol 20:448, 1993.
72. Brancós MA, Peris P, Miró JM, et al: Septic arthritis in heroin addicts. Semin Arthritis Rheum 21:81, 1991.
73. Antti-Poika I, Vankka E, Santavirta S, et al: Two cases of shoulder joint tuberculosis. Acta Orthop Scand 62:81, 1991.
74. Haygood T, Williamson SL: Radiographic findings of extremity tuberculosis in childhood: Back to the future? RadioGraphics 14:561, 1994.
75. Schwartz HS, Unni KK, Pritchard DJ: Pigmented villo-

nodular synovitis: A retrospective review of affected larger joints. Clin Orthop 247:243, 1989.

76. Hughes TH, Sartoris DJ, Schweitzer ME, et al: Pigmented villonodular synovitis: MRI characteristics. Skeletal Radiol 24:7, 1995.
77. Varma BP, Ramakrishna YJ: Synovial chondromatosis of the shoulder. Aust NZ J Surg 46:44, 1976.
78. Kramer J, Recht M, Deely DM, et al: MR appearance of idiopathic synovial osteochondromatosis. J Comput Assist Tomogr 17:772, 1993.
79. Melo-Gomes J, Viana-Queiroz M: Acromegalic arthropathy: A reversible rheumatic disease. J Rheumatol 14:393, 1987.
80. MacDonald PB, Locht RC, Lindsay D, et al: Haemophilic arthropathy of the shoulder. J Bone Joint Surg [Br] 72:470, 1990.
81. Kolawole T, Banna M, Hawass N, et al: Neuropathic arthropathy as a complication of post-traumatic syringomyelia. Br J Radiol 60:702, 1987.
82. Garrett IR: Bone destruction in cancer. Semin Oncol 20:4, 1993.
83. Dahlin DC, Unni KK: Osteosarcoma of bone and its important recognizable varieties. Am J Surg Pathol 1:61, 1977.
84. Logan PM, Munk PL, O'Connell JX, et al: Post-radiation osteosarcoma of the scapula. Skeletal Radiol 25:596, 1996.
85. Mitchell ML, Ackerman LV: Metastatic and pseudomalignant osteoblastoma: A report of two unusual cases. Skeletal Radiol 15:213, 1986.
86. Smith J, McLachlan DL, Huvos AG, et al: Primary tumors of the clavicle and scapula. AJR 124:113, 1975.
87. Taconis WK, Mulder JD: Fibrosarcoma and malignant fibrous histiocytoma of long bones: Radiographic features and grading. Skeletal Radiol 11:237, 1984.
88. Dahlin DC, Coventry MB, Scanlon PW: Ewing's sarcoma: A critical analysis of 165 cases. J Bone Joint Surg [Am] 43:185, 1961.
89. Kyle RA: Multiple myeloma: Review of 869 cases. Mayo Clin Proc 50:29, 1975.
90. McLauchlan J: Solitary myeloma of the clavicle with long survival after total excision: Report of a case. J Bone Joint Surg [Br] 55:357, 1973.
91. Franczyk J, Samuels T, Rubenstein J, et al: Skeletal lymphoma. J Can Assoc Radiol 40:75, 1989.
92. Hermann G, Klein MJ, Fikry Abedlewahab I, et al: MRI appearance of primary non-Hodgkin's lymphoma of bone. Skeletal Radiol 26:629, 1997.
93. Mosheiff R, Liebergall M, Ziv I, et al: Osteoid osteoma of the scapula: A case report and review of the literature. Clin Orthop 262:129, 1991.
94. Loizaga JM, Calvo M, Barea FL, et al: Osteoblastoma and osteoid osteoma: Clinical and morphologic features of 162 cases. Pathol Res Pract 189:33, 1993.
95. Schiller AL: Diagnosis of borderline cartilage lesions of bone. Semin Diagn Pathol 2:42, 1985.
96. Ben-Itzhak I, Denolf FA, Versfeld GA, et al: The Maffucci syndrome. J Pediatr Orthop 8:345, 1988.
97. Kurt AM, Unni KK, Sim FH, et al: Chondroblastoma of bone. Hum Pathol 20:965, 1989.
98. Schmale GA, Conrad EV, Raskind WH: The natural history of hereditary multiple exostosis. J Bone Joint Surg [Am] 76:986, 1994.
99. Sherman RS, Wilner D: The roentgen diagnosis of hemangioma of bone. AJR 86:1146, 1961.
100. De Dios AMV, Bond JR, Shives TC, et al: Aneurysmal bone cyst: A clinico-pathologic study of 238 cases. Cancer 69:2921, 1992.
101. Matfin G, McPherson F: Paget's disease of bone: Recent advances. J Orthop Rheumatol 6:127, 1993.
102. Mirra JM, Brien EW, Tehranzadeh J: Paget's disease of bone: Review with emphasis on radiologic features. II. Skeletal Radiol 24:173, 1995.
103. Crawford AH Jr, Bogamery N: Osseous manifestations of neurofibromatosis in childhood. J Pediatr Orthop 6:72, 1986.
104. Gibson MJ, Middlemiss JH: Fibrous dysplasia of bone. Br J Radiol 44:1, 1971.
105. Stull MA, Kransdorf MJ, Devaney KO: Langerhans cell histiocytosis of bone. RadioGraphics 12:801, 1992.
106. Kilpatrick SE, Wenger DE, Gilchrist GS, et al: Langerhans' cell histiocytosis (histiocytosis X) of bone: A clinicopathologic analysis of 263 pediatric and adult cases. Cancer 76:2471, 1995.
107. Taylor JAM, Resnick D, Sartoris DJ: Radiographic-pathologic correlation. *In* Sartoris DJ (ed): Osteoporosis: Diagnosis and treatment. New York, Marcel Dekker, 1996, p 147.
108. Mankin HJ: Rickets, osteomalacia, and renal osteodystrophy. Orthop Clin North Am 21:81, 1990.
109. Wolfson BJ, Capitanio MA: The wide spectrum of renal osteodystrophy in children. CRC Crit Rev Diagn Imaging 27:297, 1987.
110. Resnick D, Niwayama G: Subchondral resorption of bone in renal osteodystrophy. Radiology 118:315, 1976.
111. Tigges S, Nance EP, Carpenter WA, et al: Renal osteodystrophy: Imaging findings that mimic those of other diseases. AJR 165:143, 1995.
112. Schuman CA, Jones HW III: The "milk-alkali" syndrome: Two case reports with discussion of pathogenesis. Q J Med 55:119, 1985.
113. Kofoed H: Revascularization of the humeral head: A report of two cases of fracture-dislocation of the shoulder. Clin Orthop 179:175, 1983.
114. Lee DK, Hansen HR: Post-traumatic avascular necrosis of the humeral head in displaced proximal humerus fractures. J Trauma 21:788, 1984.
115. Langlands AO, Souter WA, Samuel E, et al: Radiation osteitis following irradiation for breast cancer. Clin Radiol 28:93, 1977.
116. Gersovich EO, Greenspan A: Osteomyelitis of the clavicle: Clinical, radiologic, and bacteriologic findings in ten patients. Skeletal Radiol 23:205, 1994.
117. Boutin RD, Resnick D: The SAPHO syndrome: An evolving concept for unifying several idiopathic disorders of bone and skin. AJR 170:585, 1998.
118. Köhler H, Uehlinger E, Kutzner K, et al: Sternocostoclavicular hyperostosis: Painful swelling of the sternum, clavicles, and upper ribs: Report of two new cases. Ann Intern Med 87:192, 1977.
119. Greenspan A, Gerscovich E, Szabo RM, et al: Condensing osteitis of the clavicle: A rare but frequently misdiagnosed condition. AJR 156:1011, 1991.
120. Rosenberg ZS, Shankman S, Klein M, et al: Chronic recurrent multifocal osteomyelitis. AJR 151:142, 1988.
121. Levy M, Goldberg I, Fischel RE, et al: Friedrich's disease: Aseptic necrosis of the sternal end of the clavicle. J Bone Joint Surg [Br] 63:539, 1981.
122. Holzman D: Infantile cortical hyperostosis of the scapula presenting as an ipsilateral Erb's palsy. J Pediatr 81:785, 1972.
123. Melo-Gomes J, Viana-Queiroz M: Acromegalic arthropathy: A reversible rheumatic disease. J Rheumatol 14:393, 1987.

124. Herbert DA, Fessel WJ: Idiopathic hypertrophic osteoarthropathy (pachydermoperiostosis). West J Med 134:354, 1981.
125. Kroon HMJA, Pauwels EKJ: Bone scintigraphy for the detection and follow-up of hypertrophic osteoarthropathy. Diagn Imaging 51:47, 1982.
126. Gamble JG, Ip SC: Hypervitaminosis A in a child from megadosing. J Pediatr Orthop 5:219, 1985.
127. Høst A, Halken S, Andersen PE Jr: Reversibility of cortical hyperostosis following long-term prostaglandin E_1 therapy in infants with ductus-dependent congenital heart disease. Pediatr Radiol 18:149, 1988.
128. Miller ME, Ada JR: Injuries to the shoulder girdle. *In* Browner BD, Jupiter JB, Levine AM, et al (eds): Skeletal Trauma: Fractures, Dislocations, Ligamentous Injuries. Philadelphia, WB Saunders, 1992, p 1306.

CHAPTER 14

Humerus

- Developmental Anomalies, Anatomic Variants, and Sources of Diagnostic Error
- Physical Injury
- Bone Tumors
- Metabolic, Hematologic, and Infectious Disorders

Developmental Anomalies, Anatomic Variants, and Sources of Diagnostic Error

Few developmental anomalies and anatomic variants affect the humerus. Table 14–1 and Figures 14–1 and 14–2 represent selected examples.

Physical Injury

Acute fractures of the humeral diaphysis occur infrequently, and the muscles of the upper arm are a frequent site for posttraumatic heterotopic ossification. These conditions are described in Table 14–2 and are illustrated in Figures 14–3 and 14–4. Injuries of the proximal and distal portions of the humerus are covered in Chapters 13 and 15, respectively.

Bone Tumors

The humerus is a frequent site of malignant and benign tumors and tumor-like processes. Tables 14–3 to 14–5 list the major characteristics of these disorders. Their radiographic manifestations are illustrated in Figures 14–5 to 14–19.

Metabolic, Hematologic, and Infectious Disorders

A wide variety of metabolic, hematologic, and infectious disorders may involve the humerus. Table 14–6 lists some of the more common disorders and describes their characteristics. Their radiographic features are illustrated in Figures 14–20 to 14–23. Further manifestations of these disorders within the proximal and distal portions of the humerus are covered in Chapters 13 and 15, respectively.

TABLE 14–1. Developmental Anomalies, Anatomic Variants, and Sources of Diagnostic Error

Disorder	Figure(s)	Characteristics
Humeral pseudocyst[1]	13–2 H, 13–12	Zone of diminished trabeculae within the spongiosa bone of the greater tubercle of the humerus May simulate destructive neoplasm, such as chondroblastoma
Supracondylar process[2–4]	14–1	Rare anomaly affecting less than 1 per cent of population Anomalous elongated projection or flange of bone arising from the anteromedial cortical surface of the distal humeral metadiaphysis, projecting toward the elbow joint May be connected to the medial epicondyle of the humerus by a fibrous band termed the ligament of Struthers Median nerve and, occasionally, the brachial artery pass beneath this fibrous band Peripheral median nerve entrapment has been reported
Chevron sign[5]	14–2	Obliquely oriented trabeculae within the distal portion of the humerus may appear very prominent on frontal radiographs, simulating the appearance of osteoporosis or bone destruction This normal finding represents the typical herringbone or chevron pattern of trabecular bone and is of no clinical significance
Supratrochlear foramen[6]		Failure of complete ossification of the thin membranous bone separating the olecranon fossa from the coronoid fossa of the distal portion of the humerus results in an unossified circular hole that is of no clinical significance Present in 4 to 13 per cent of the population Left > right Women > men
Simulated periostitis[6]	13–2 G	Periostitis of the proximal metaphysis of the humerus may be simulated by the intertubercular groove in neonates or by overlying projection of the cortices in adults Bilateral "physiologic periostitis of newborn infants" may be visible in the humeral diaphyses beginning about the age of 1 month and persisting throughout the first year of life Periostitis of the lateral epicondyle may be simulated by normal flanges of bone along the cortex of the distal humeral metaphyses Simulated periostitis may be mistaken for a pathologic condition but is of no clinical significance
Upper humeral notches[3, 7]		Irregularity of the cortex of the medial aspect of the proximal humeral metaphysis in children between 10 and 16 years of age These notches may be bilateral and resemble cortical destruction Normal variant
Prominent deltoid tuberosity[3]		Insertion site of the deltoid muscle on the anterolateral aspect of the humeral diaphysis may appear as a prominent cortical outgrowth simulating a neoplasm

See also Table 1–1.

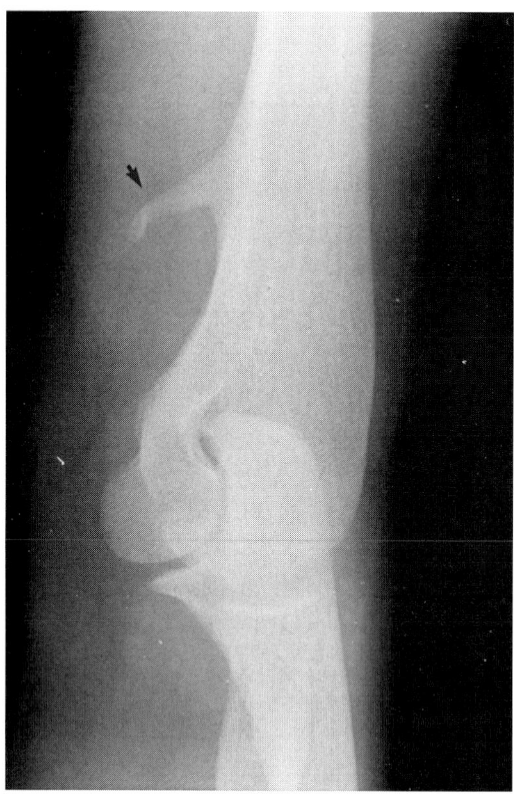

FIGURE 14–1. Supracondylar process.[2–4] An osseous outgrowth arises from the anteromedial surface of the distal portion of the humerus approximately 5 to 7 cm above the medial condyle (arrow). This anomaly, present in 1 to 3 per cent of the general population, usually is an incidental finding and does not cause signs or symptoms. The process may be joined to the medial epicondyle by the ligament of Struthers, a band of fibrous tissue that may occasionally lead to peripheral entrapment of the median nerve.

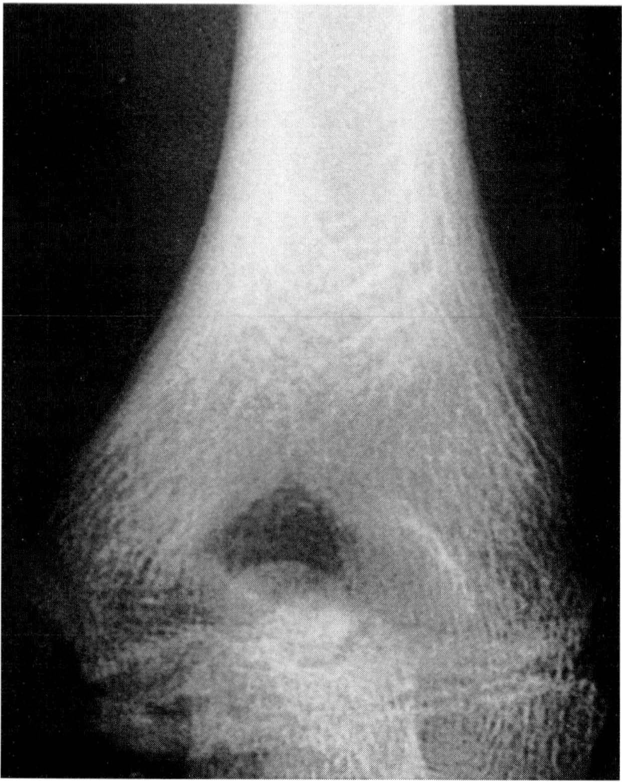

FIGURE 14–2. Chevron sign.[5] Observe the normal, obliquely oriented trabeculae within the cancellous bone of the distal portion of the humerus. This herringbone or chevron arrangement of trabeculae may simulate the appearance of osteoporosis or osteolytic destruction, but it is of no clinical significance.

TABLE 14–2. **Physical Injury: Humeral Diaphysis and Soft Tissues**

Fractures	Figure(s)	Characteristics	Complications and Related Injuries
Fractures of the humeral diaphysis			
Acute fractures[8–10]	14–3	Fractures of humeral diaphysis account for about 3 per cent of all fractures Adults > children Most common site: junction of distal and middle thirds Transverse orientation—50 to 70 per cent of all humeral diaphyseal fractures; oblique—20 per cent; spiral—20 per cent Direct trauma: automobile accidents, gunshot wounds, physical assault Indirect trauma: throwing a ball, shot putting, arm wrestling, childbirth injury	Delayed union or nonunion when fracture is transverse or distracted Radial nerve injury in 5 to 15 per cent of cases Brachial artery injury Characteristic displacements related to sites of muscular attachment: Fractures above insertion of pectoralis major result in rotator cuff displacing proximal fragment into abduction and external rotation; fractures between insertion of pectoralis major proximally and the deltoid distally result in adduction of the proximal fragment; fractures distal to deltoid insertion result in abduction of the proximal fragment and proximal displacement of the distal fragment
Child abuse[11]		Humerus is second only to the ribs as the most common site of fracture in child abuse Fractures may be single or multiple Spiral fractures of the humeral diaphysis are highly suggestive, but not invariably diagnostic, of abuse in children, especially the nonambulating infant; left-sided diaphyseal fractures most frequent; periosteal reaction suggests healing fracture Metaphyseal lesions of distal end of the humerus and epiphyseal displacement (Salter-Harris type I injury) of the distal humeral epiphysis suggestive of abuse (see Chapter 13)	Fractures or injuries in other locations Fractures in different phases of healing
Soft tissue injury			
Posttraumatic heterotopic ossification[12]	14–4	Also termed posttraumatic myositis ossificans Faint calcific intermuscular or intramuscular shadow may appear within 2 to 6 weeks of injury Well-defined region of ossification aligned parallel to the long axis of the humerus may be evident within 6 to 8 weeks Associated periostitis may relate to subperiosteal hemorrhage	Limitation of motion May result in abnormal shoulder or elbow biomechanics and lead to premature degeneration May resemble aggressive neoplasms, such as osteosarcoma or Ewing's sarcoma

See also Tables 1–3 and 1–4.
See Chapter 13 for injuries to the proximal portion of the humerus and Chapter 15 for injuries to the distal portion of the humerus.

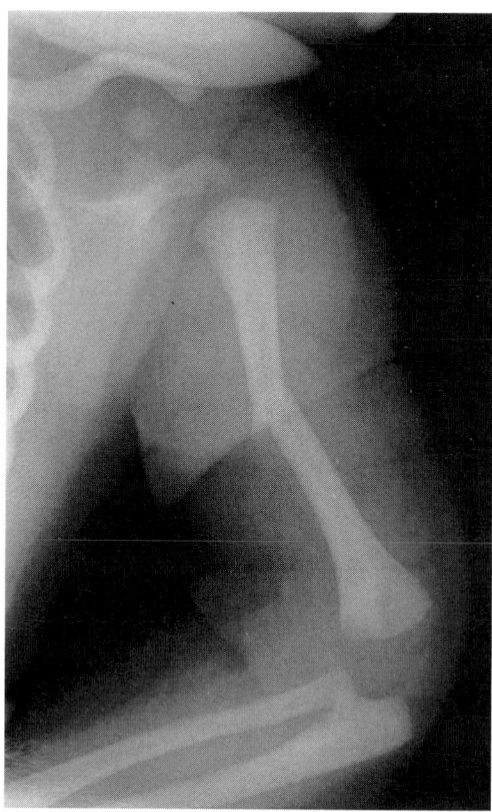

FIGURE 14–3. Humeral shaft fracture.[8–10] A difficult shoulder delivery resulted in a fracture of the humeral shaft in this newborn infant. Note the lateral displacement of the distal fragment. Radial nerve injury, and, less likely, vascular injury, malunion, and nonunion, may complicate humeral shaft fractures.

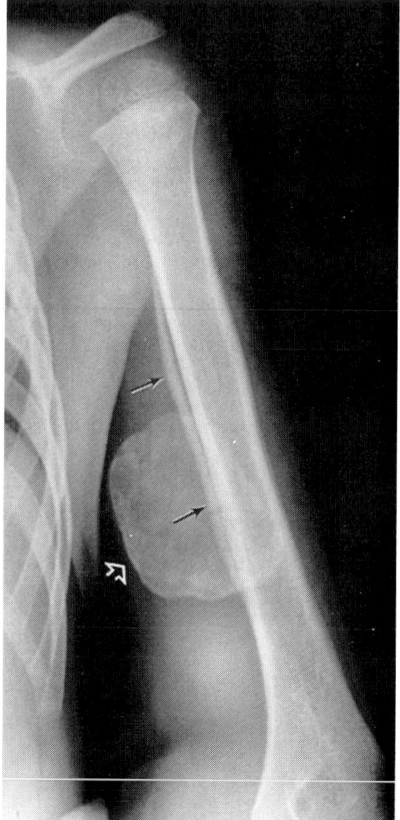

FIGURE 14–4. Heterotopic ossification: posttraumatic myositis ossificans.[12] This 4-year-old boy fell on his elbow. A radiograph taken 1 year later shows a well-organized hematoma (open arrow) with solid periosteal new bone formation (arrows) involving the medial humeral diaphysis. *(Courtesy of D. Witte, M.D., Memphis, Tennessee.)*

TABLE 14–3. Malignant Tumors Affecting the Humerus*

Tumor	Figure(s)	Characteristics
Secondary malignant neoplasms of bone		
Skeletal metastasis[13, 14]	14–5	Fewer than 10 per cent of skeletal metastatic lesions affect the humerus Seventy-five percent exhibit permeative or moth-eaten osteolysis Twenty-five percent exhibit diffuse or patchy osteosclerosis or a mixed pattern of lysis and sclerosis Usually multiple sites of involvement Pathologic fracture *Cortical metastasis* Prevalent in the long tubular bones of patients with metastasis, especially from bronchogenic carcinoma Small radiolucent, eccentric, saucer-shaped, scalloped erosions, which sometimes occur near the entrance of nutrient arteries into the bone, are referred to as "cookie bite" lesions
Malignant transformation of benign processes[15]	14–6	Several benign tumors and tumor-like lesions may undergo sarcomatous malignant transformation: Paget's disease, fibrous dysplasia, neurofibromatosis, hereditary multiple exostoses, Ollier's disease, Maffucci's syndrome, and infrequently solitary primary benign tumors
Primary malignant neoplasms of bone		
Osteosarcoma (conventional)[16]	14–6, 14–7	Ten to 15 per cent of osteosarcomas occur in the humerus Osteolytic, osteosclerotic, or mixed patterns of medullary and cortical destruction Prominent periosteal reaction common Preference for the proximal metaphyseal region
Osteosarcoma (parosteal)[17]		Fifteen per cent of parosteal osteosarcomas occur in the humerus Osteosclerotic surface lesion of bone Large radiodense, oval, sessile mass with smooth or irregular margins Peripheral portion of lesion may have cleavage plane separating it from the humerus Ossification begins centrally and progresses outward, opposite that of benign heterotopic bone formation (myositis ossification)
Chondrosarcoma (conventional)[18, 19]		Ten per cent of chondrosarcomas occur in the humerus Tend to be osteolytic lesions, sometimes containing a bulky cartilaginous cap and frequently containing calcifications May have soft tissue mass
Giant cell tumor (aggressive)[20]		More than 10 per cent of aggressive giant cell tumors occur in the humerus Eccentrically located, subarticular osteolytic lesion extending into the metaphysis Cortical destruction and soft tissue mass are variable findings Radiographic appearance is an inaccurate guide to determining malignancy of lesion—biopsy is necessary
Fibrosarcoma[21]		Eleven per cent of fibrosarcomas involve the humerus Purely osteolytic destruction with no associated sclerotic reaction or periostitis
Malignant fibrous histiocytoma[21]		Fewer than 10 per cent of malignant fibrous histiocytomas involve the humerus Pathologic fracture common Metaphyseal location with frequent spread to epiphysis and diaphysis Moth-eaten or permeative osteolysis, frequently resembling fibrosarcoma
Ewing's sarcoma[22]	14–8	Ten percent of Ewing's sarcomas occur in the humerus Permeative or moth-eaten osteolysis, aggressive cortical erosion or violation, laminated or spiculated periostitis, and soft tissue masses Most lesions central and diametaphyseal in location

Table continued on following page

TABLE 14–3. Malignant Tumors Affecting the Humerus* *Continued*

Tumor	Figure(s)	Characteristics
Myeloproliferative disorders		
Plasma cell (multiple) myeloma[23]	14–9	Fifteen per cent of multiple myeloma lesions occur in the humerus Early: Normal radiographs or diffuse osteopenia Later: Widespread well-circumscribed osteolytic lesions with discrete margins, which appear uniform in size Ninety-seven per cent osteolytic; 3 per cent osteoblastic False-negative bone scans common
Solitary plasmacytoma[23]		Fourteen per cent of solitary plasmacytomas occur in the humerus Solitary, geographic, expansile, osteolytic lesion that frequently results in pathologic fracture Seventy per cent eventually develop into multiple myeloma
Primary lymphoma (non-Hodgkin's)[24, 25]	14–10	Approximately 11 per cent of lesions in primary lymphoma occur in the humerus Multiple moth-eaten or permeative osteolytic lesions Diffuse or localized sclerotic lesions are rare Common cause of pathologic fracture
Leukemia[26]	14–11	Humerus frequently involved Diffuse osteopenia, radiolucent or radiodense transverse metaphyseal bands, osteolytic lesions, periostitis, and, infrequently, osteosclerosis Radiodense metaphyses more frequent in patients undergoing chemotherapy for leukemia; may resemble lead poisoning

* See also Table 1–10.

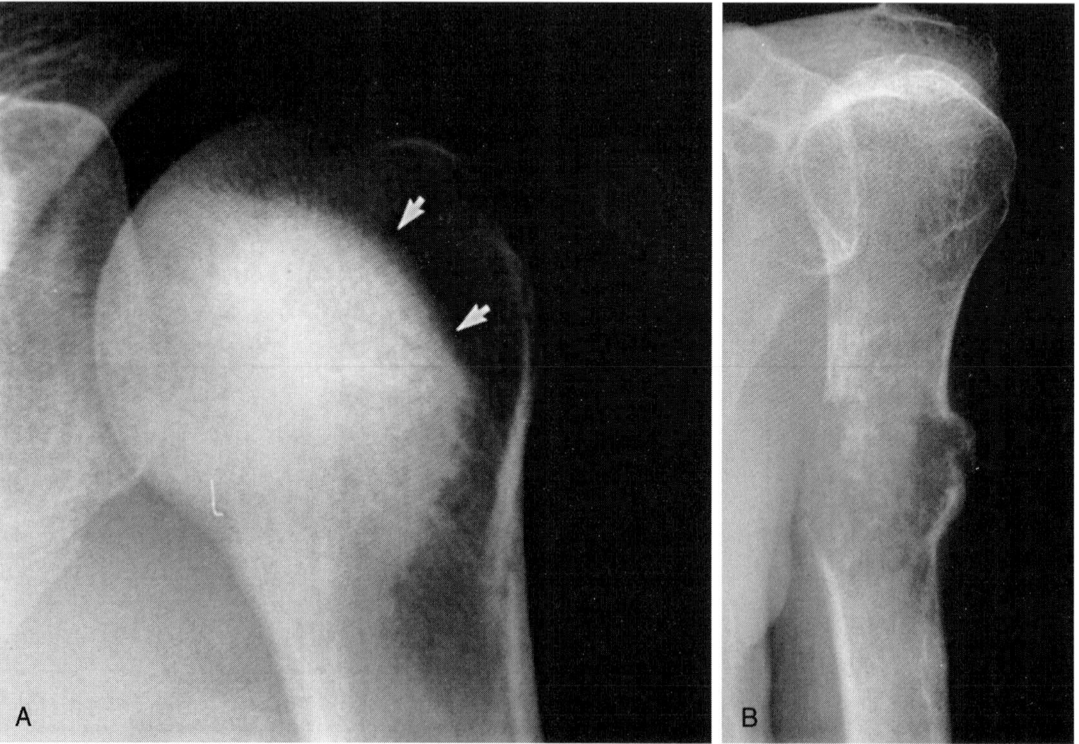

FIGURE 14–5. Skeletal metastasis: various patterns.[13, 14] A This 54-year-old man was diagnosed as having carcinoma of the prostate several years before this radiographic examination. The radiograph shows a zone of osteosclerosis within the head of the humerus (arrows). B In another patient, a 56-year-old man with carcinoma of the tonsils, a permeative pattern of osteolytic destruction involving the proximal portion of the humerus has resulted in a pathologic fracture.

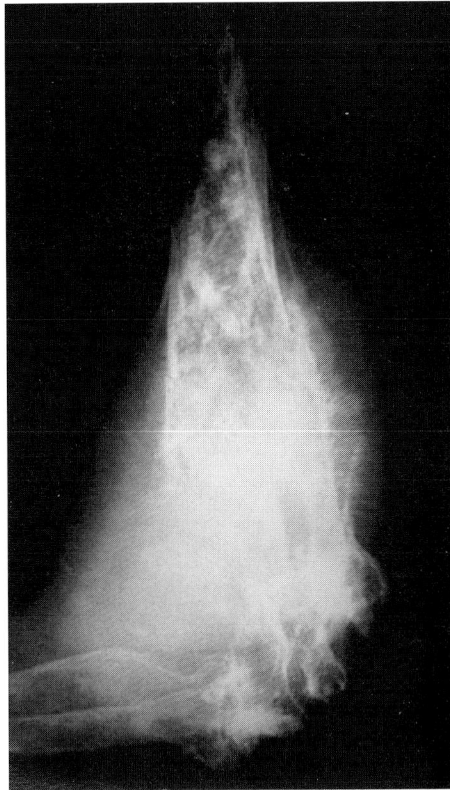

FIGURE 14–6. Osteosarcoma: Malignant transformation from fibrous dysplasia.[15] This patient with known fibrous dysplasia developed new onset of pain. Radiographs reveal a highly aggressive, destructive lesion involving the distal portion of the humerus. Bone expansion, cortical destruction, spiculated periostitis, and a soft tissue mass are evident. Biopsy revealed osteosarcoma developing in an area of fibrous dysplasia. Malignant transformation occurs in fewer than 1 per cent of reported cases of fibrous dysplasia. Osteosarcoma and fibrosarcoma are the most frequently encountered tumor types, occurring in both monostotic and polyostotic fibrous dysplasia. *(Courtesy of G. Greenway, M.D., Dallas, Texas.)*

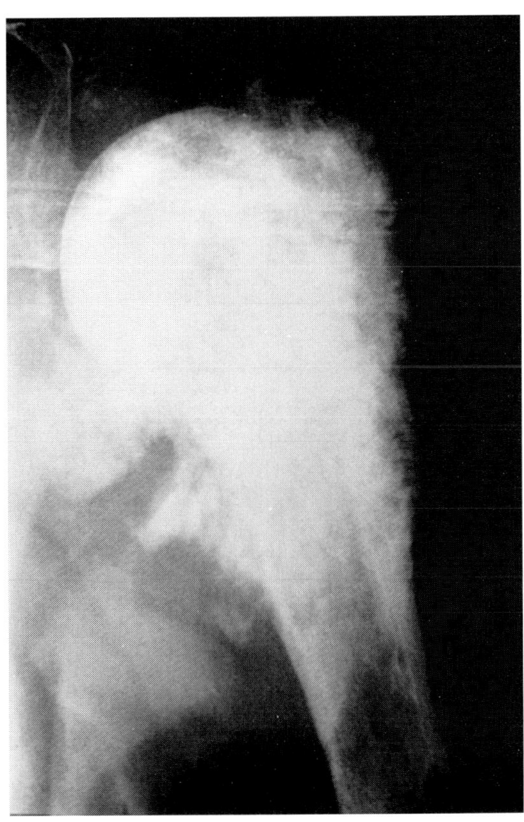

FIGURE 14–7. Conventional osteosarcoma.[16] An 80-year-old woman had shoulder pain. A frontal radiograph demonstrates extensive osteoblastic new bone deposition within the entire proximal portion of the humerus. The periosteal margins are spiculated, and the tumor appears very aggressive.

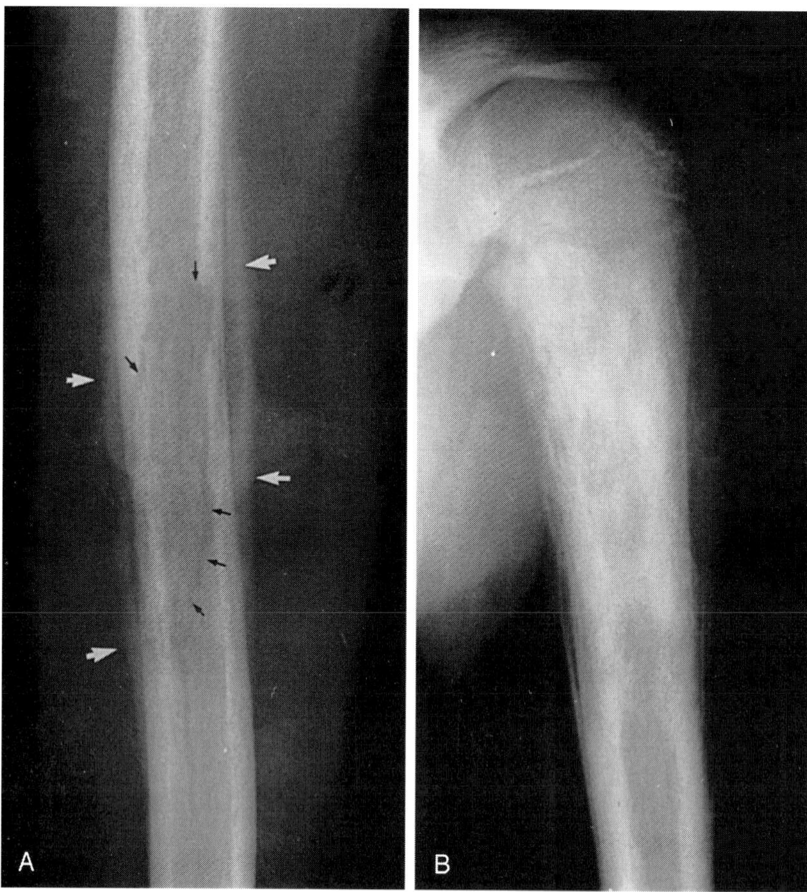

FIGURE 14–8. Ewing's sarcoma.[22] A Radiograph of the humerus shows a pathologic fracture (black arrows) through an area of extensive permeative destruction of the medullary and cortical bone. Observe also the thick periostitis throughout the diaphysis (white arrows). B Laminated periosteal response results in radiodensity of the humeral metadiaphysis in another patient with Ewing's sarcoma. (B, *Courtesy of P.H. VanderStoep, M.D., St. Cloud, Minnesota.*)

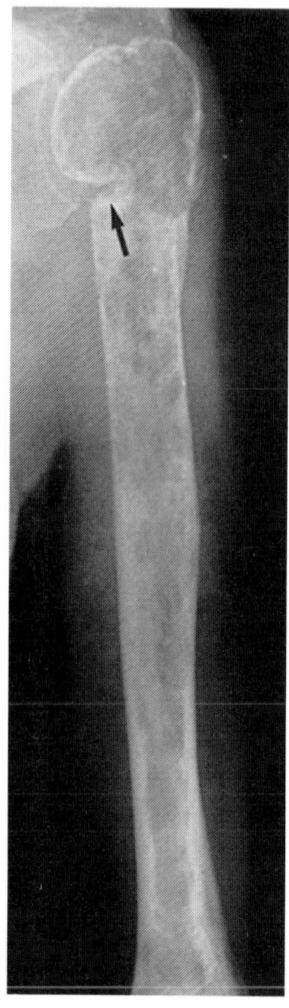

FIGURE 14–9. Plasma cell (multiple) myeloma.[23] Numerous osteolytic scalloped lesions are seen throughout the entire humerus. A pathologic fracture of the surgical neck has occurred (arrow).

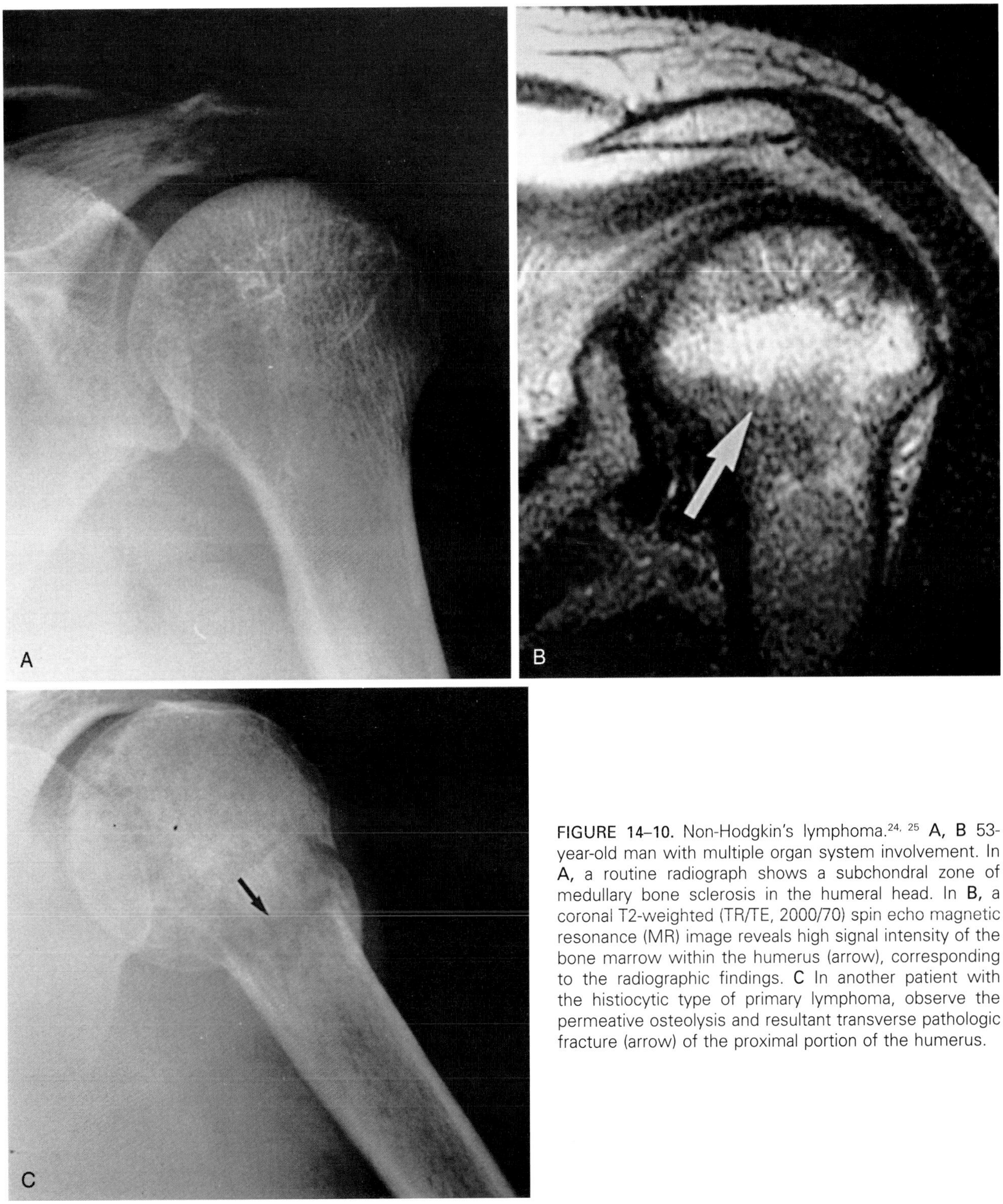

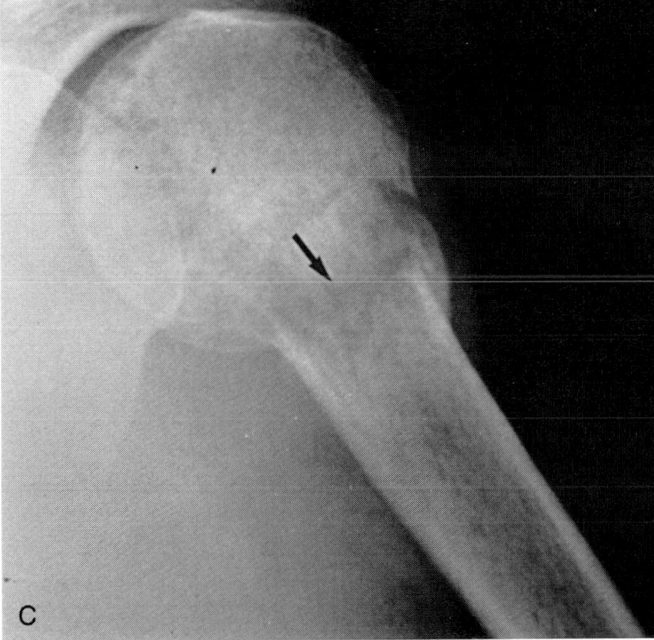

FIGURE 14–10. Non-Hodgkin's lymphoma.[24, 25] A, B 53-year-old man with multiple organ system involvement. In A, a routine radiograph shows a subchondral zone of medullary bone sclerosis in the humeral head. In B, a coronal T2-weighted (TR/TE, 2000/70) spin echo magnetic resonance (MR) image reveals high signal intensity of the bone marrow within the humerus (arrow), corresponding to the radiographic findings. C In another patient with the histiocytic type of primary lymphoma, observe the permeative osteolysis and resultant transverse pathologic fracture (arrow) of the proximal portion of the humerus.

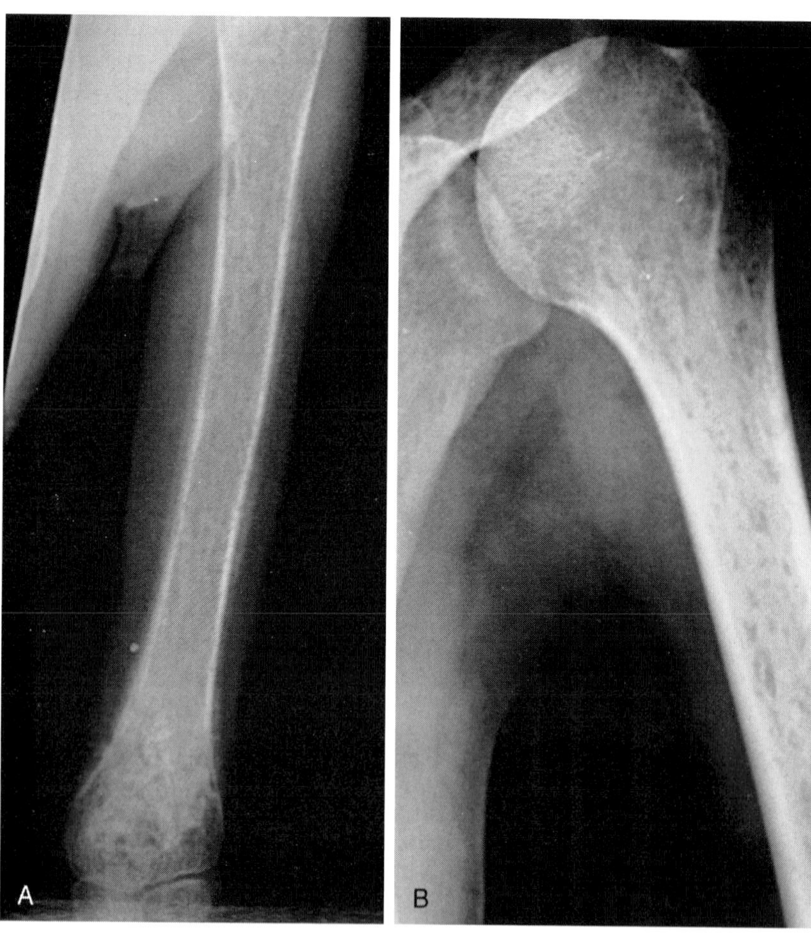

FIGURE 14–11. Acute childhood leukemia.[26] A Permeative osteolysis with periostitis is seen throughout the humerus of this child with leukemia. B In another patient with acute childhood leukemia, observe the moth-eaten osteolytic destructive lesions throughout the humeral diaphysis and metaphysis, resembling the punched-out lesions of plasma cell myeloma.

TABLE 14–4. Benign Tumors Affecting the Humerus*

Tumor	Figure(s)	Characteristics
Enostosis[27]		Fewer than 10 per cent of enostoses (bone islands) occur in the humerus Solitary, rarely multiple, painless, discrete foci of osteosclerosis within the spongiosa of bone Round, ovoid, or oblong with brush border composed of radiating osseous spicules that intermingle with the surrounding trabeculae of the spongiosa
Osteoid osteoma[28, 29]		Seven per cent of osteoid osteomas occur in the humerus Cortical or subperiosteal lesion with reactive sclerosis surrounding central radiolucent nidus Nidus less than 1 cm in diameter and usually not visible on routine radiographs
Osteoblastoma (conventional)[30]		Fewer than 3 per cent of conventional osteoblastomas involve the humerus Osteolytic, osteosclerotic, or both Expansile lesion that may be subperiosteal Partially calcified matrix in many cases Cortical thinning Often resembles large osteoid osteoma
Enchondroma (solitary)[31]	14–12	Approximately 7 per cent of solitary enchondromas involve the humerus Central or eccentric, medullary osteolytic lesion Lobulated endosteal scalloping Approximately 50 per cent have stippled calcification within the matrix
Enchondromatosis (Ollier's disease)[31]		Multiple enchondromas; frequently involve the humerus
Maffucci's syndrome[31]		Humerus is involved in over 40 per cent of cases of Maffucci's syndrome Multiple enchondromas and soft tissue hemangiomas Unilateral distribution in 50 per cent of cases
Chondroblastoma[32, 33]	14–13	Approximately 22 per cent of chondroblastomas affect the humerus Circular osteolytic lesion affecting predominantly the proximal humeral epiphyses May exhibit calcification in matrix Occasionally periosteal reaction and edema may be seen on magnetic resonance (MR) imaging

TABLE 14–4. Benign Tumors Affecting the Humerus* *Continued*

Tumor	Figure(s)	Characteristics
Osteochondroma (solitary)[34, 35]	14–14	As many as 20 per cent of solitary osteochondromas arise from the humerus Pedunculated or sessile, cartilage-covered osseous excrescence arising from the surface of the metaphysis of the proximal or distal portion of the humerus Cortex and medulla are continuous with the host bone May occur spontaneously or after accidental or iatrogenic injury Typically grow away from the adjacent joint Complications: pathologic fracture, neurovascular compression, and malignant transformation (fewer than 1 per cent of cases)
Hereditary multiple exostoses[36–38]		Multiple osteochondromas, sometimes numbering in the hundreds Proximal humeral metaphysis frequently involved May result in neurovascular compression or malignant transformation (fewer than 5 per cent of cases)
Nonossifying fibroma and fibrous cortical defect[39]	14–15	Five per cent of nonossifying fibromas and fibrous cortical defects involve the humerus Eccentric, multiloculated osteolytic lesion arising from the metaphyseal cortex Resembles a well-circumscribed, blister-like shell of bone arising from the cortex Cortical thinning often is present Eventually disappears, filling in with normal bone Nonossifying fibromas typically are larger than fibrous cortical defects
Giant cell tumor (benign)[20]		Approximately 6 per cent of benign giant cell tumors occur in the humerus Eccentric osteolytic neoplasm with a predilection for the subarticular region Often multiloculated and expansile Radiographs are inaccurate in distinguishing benign from aggressive giant cell tumors
Intraosseous lipoma[40]		Fewer than 10 per cent of intraosseous lipomas occur in the humerus Osteolytic lesion surrounded by a thin, well-defined sclerotic border Central calcified or ossified nidus is common Occasional osseous expansion Cortical destruction and periostitis absent
Simple bone cyst[41, 42]	14–16	Over half of all simple bone cysts occur in the humerus Mildly expansile, solitary osteolytic lesion within medullary cavity of proximal portion of humerus May be multiloculated Pathologic fracture with characteristic "fallen fragment" sign
Aneurysmal bone cyst[43]		Fewer than 10 per cent of aneurysmal bone cysts occur in the humerus Eccentric, thin-walled, expansile osteolytic lesion of the humeral metaphysis Thin trabeculation with multiloculated appearance Buttressing at edge of lesion

* See also Table 1–11.

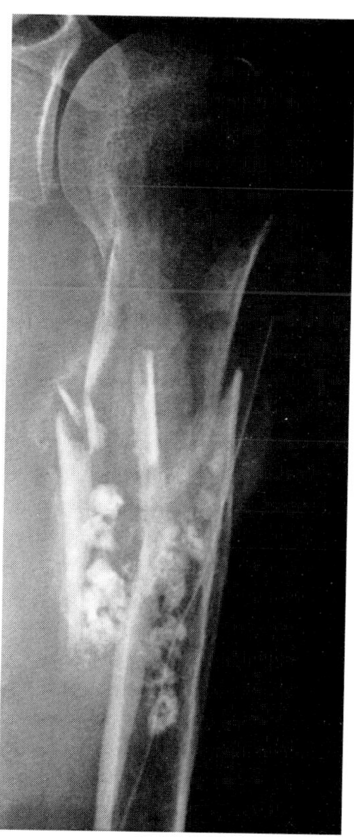

FIGURE 14–12. Enchondroma: pathologic fracture.[31] An 80-year-old male patient had fallen 1 month before these radiographs were obtained. He had decreased range of motion. An elongated, heavily calcified tumor with a healing, comminuted pathologic fracture is seen within the humeral diaphysis.

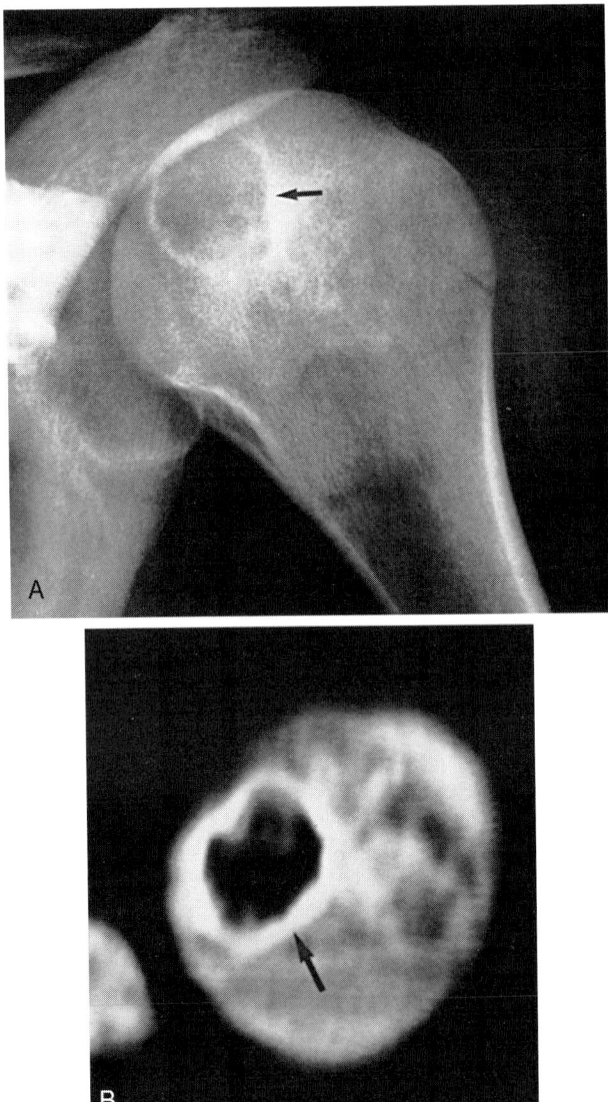

FIGURE 14–13. Chondroblastoma.[32, 33] A 17-year-old boy with shoulder pain. A Frontal radiograph of the humerus reveals a well-defined osteolytic epiphyseal lesion (arrow), that appears well defined. B Transaxial computed tomographic (CT) scan clearly defines the lesion (arrow) and shows the sclerotic margin to good advantage. *(Courtesy of R. Sweet, M.D., Pomona, California.)*

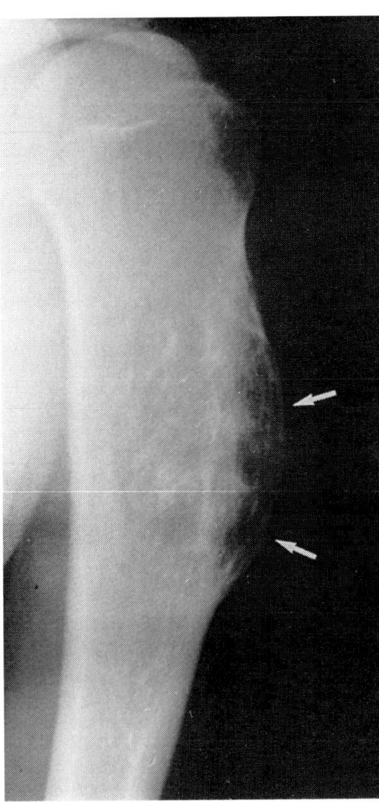

FIGURE 14–14. Solitary osteochondroma.[34, 35] An expansile, sessile osteochondroma arising from the proximal metadiaphysis of the humerus is seen on a routine radiograph (arrows).

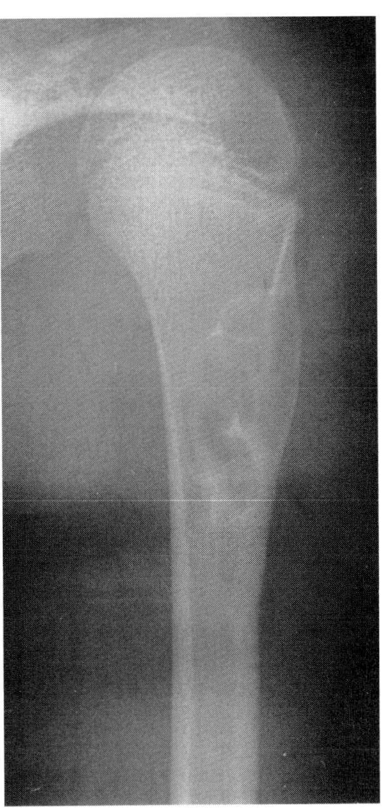

FIGURE 14–15. Nonossifying fibroma.[39] Routine radiograph of the proximal portion of the humerus in this 11-year-old girl reveals a large, eccentric, expansile, multiloculated, geographic osteolytic lesion. Cortical thinning and endosteal scalloping also are evident.

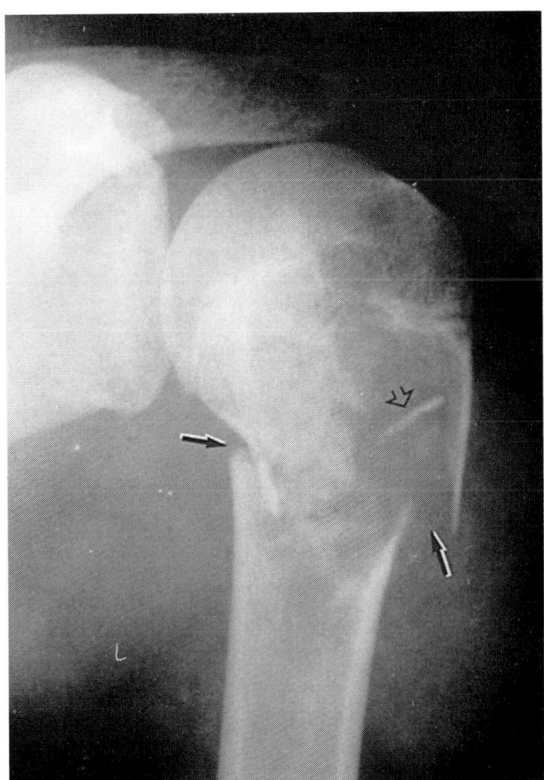

FIGURE 14–16. Simple bone cyst: Pathologic fracture.[41, 42] This young patient with a simple bone cyst in the proximal portion of the humerus sustained a transverse pathologic fracture through the weakened bone (arrows). Routine radiograph exhibits the classic "fallen fragment sign," in which a sliver of fractured cortical bone migrates to a dependent position within the fluid matrix of the lesion (open arrow). On serial radiographs of the humerus, simple bone cysts may appear to migrate away from the physis owing to normal longitudinal metaphyseal growth between the physis and the lesion. *(Courtesy of D. Pate, D.C., San Diego, California and Terry R. Yochum, D.C., Denver, Colorado.)*

TABLE 14–5. Tumor-Like Lesions Affecting the Humerus*

Tumor-Like Lesion	Figure(s)	Characteristics
Paget's disease[44, 45]	14–17	Humerus is a commonly affected site Usually polyostotic and may have unilateral involvement Coarsened trabeculae and bone enlargement Diaphyseal and metaphyseal involvement with extension into epiphysis Stages of involvement: osteolytic (50 per cent), osteosclerotic (25 per cent), and mixed (25 per cent), malignant transformation (less than 2 per cent) Pathologic fractures, deformities, pseudofractures
Monostotic fibrous dysplasia[46]	14–6, 14–18	Fewer than 4 per cent of monostotic lesions affect the humerus Thick rim of sclerosis surrounding a radiolucent lesion Ground-glass appearance of fibrous matrix
Polyostotic fibrous dysplasia[46]		Fifty per cent of patients have humeral lesions Unilateral or bilateral, asymmetric humeral involvement Lesions appear the same as monostotic form but frequently are larger, more expansile, and more multiloculated than monostotic lesions
Langerhans' cell histiocytosis[47, 48]	14–19	Humerus is involved in about 7 per cent of cases Osteolytic lesions may be multiloculated and expansile Eosinophilic granuloma is the most frequent and mildest form of this disorder characterized by histiocytic infiltration of tissues

* See also Table 1–10.

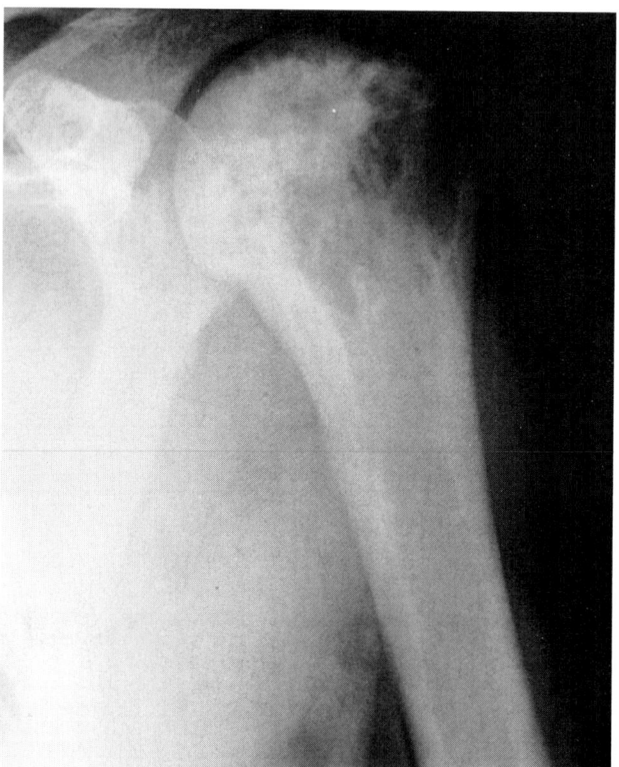

FIGURE 14–17. Paget's disease: humerus.[44, 45] Observe the areas of thickened, coarsely trabeculated bone with radiolucent regions of varying size extending into the subchondral region of the humerus. The combined stage of Paget's disease, as seen in this patient, involves both osteolytic and osteosclerotic osseous changes.

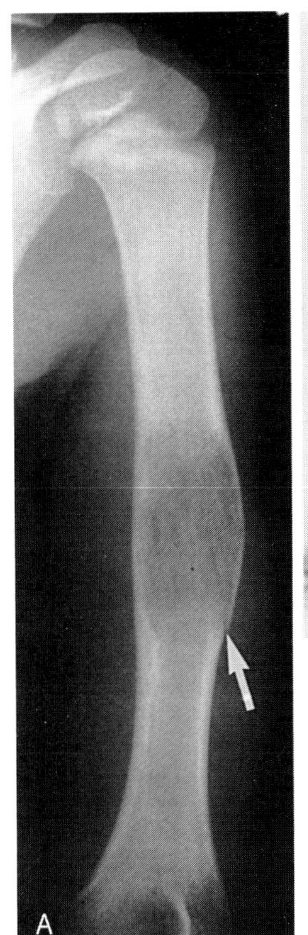

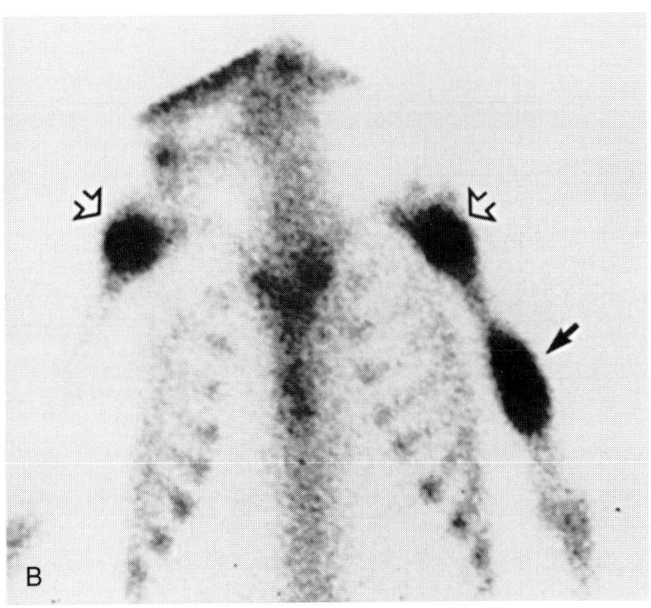

FIGURE 14–18. Monostotic fibrous dysplasia.[46] In a 4-year-old girl, a radiograph (A) shows an expansile diaphyseal lesion with endosteal scalloping, typical ground-glass hazy appearance of the matrix, and pathologic fracture (arrow). A ^{99m}Tc-methylene diphosphonate bone scan (B) shows focal concentration of radionuclide in the vicinity of the lesion (arrow) and normal increased uptake at the growing epiphyses (open arrows).

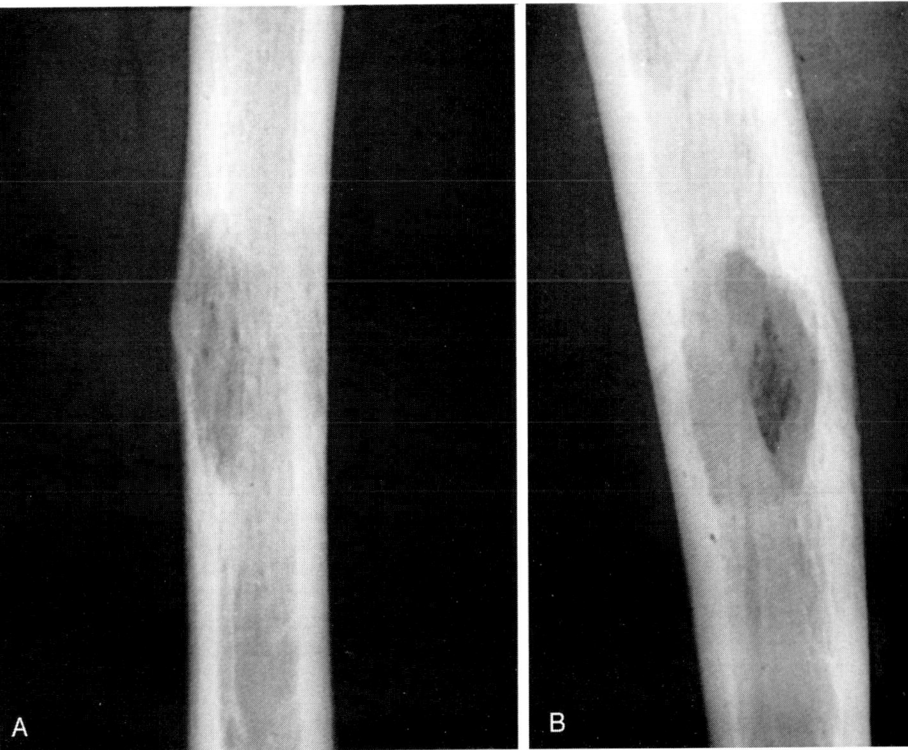

FIGURE 14–19. Langerhans' cell histiocytosis: eosinophilic granuloma.[47, 48] Anteroposterior (A) and lateral (B) radiographs of the humerus in this 23-year-old woman reveal a permeative pattern of osteolytic destruction. Biopsy analysis revealed eosinophilic granuloma. The lesion appears aggressive on the frontal radiograph (A) and shows geographic destruction on the lateral radiograph (B). Eosinophilic granuloma of bone is the most frequent and mildest form of Langerhans' cell histiocytosis, a disease characterized by histiocytic infiltration of tissues. *(Courtesy of R. Kerr, M.D., Los Angeles, California.)*

TABLE 14–6. Metabolic, Hematologic, and Infectious Disorders Affecting the Humerus*

Disorder	Figure(s)	Characteristics
Generalized osteoporosis[49]		Uniform decrease in radiodensity, thinning of cortices, accentuation of trabeculae May result in insufficiency fractures of the humerus
Osteogenesis imperfecta[50]		Osteoporosis and bone fragility Thin, gracile appearance of entire skeleton Severe deformities and fractures commonly affect the humerus
Osteomalacia and rickets[51]		*Osteomalacia* Diffuse osteopenia Decreased trabeculae; remaining trabeculae appear prominent and coarsened Looser's zones (pseudofractures) *Rickets* Metaphyseal demineralization resulting in frayed metaphyses Bowing deformities Osteopenia Looser's zones
Gaucher's disease[52]	14–20	Marrow infiltration results in osteopenia, osteolytic lesions, cortical diminution, and medullary widening of tubular bones Osseous weakening results in pathologic fractures Modeling deformities: Erlenmeyer flask deformity (widening of the distal diametaphysis of the humerus) Osteonecrosis of humeral metadiaphysis and humeral head
Secondary hypertrophic osteoarthropathy[53]		Syndrome characterized by digital clubbing, arthritis, and bilateral symmetric periostitis of humerus and other tubular bones Complication of many diseases, including bronchogenic carcinoma, mesothelioma, and other intrathoracic and intra-abdominal diseases
Acute osteomyelitis[54]	14–21	Acute pyogenic osteomyelitis frequently involves the metaphysis in children Poorly defined permeative bone destruction In infants and young children, streptococcal infection may be causative
Chronic osteomyelitis[55]	14–22	Humerus is a common site of this rare disease Osteosclerosis and cortical thickening Thick, single layer periosteal bone proliferation Poorly defined areas of osteolysis and osteosclerosis Sequestrum and involucrum Cloaca formation
Collagen vascular disease: soft tissue calcification[56]	14–23	Dermatomyositis, polymyositis, scleroderma, and other collagen vascular diseases may result in calcinosis in the soft tissues of the upper arm Differential diagnosis: hyperparathyroidism, neurologic injury, melorheostosis, posttraumatic heterotopic ossification, soft tissue neoplasms, fibrodysplasia ossificans progressiva

* See also Tables 1–13 to 1–17.

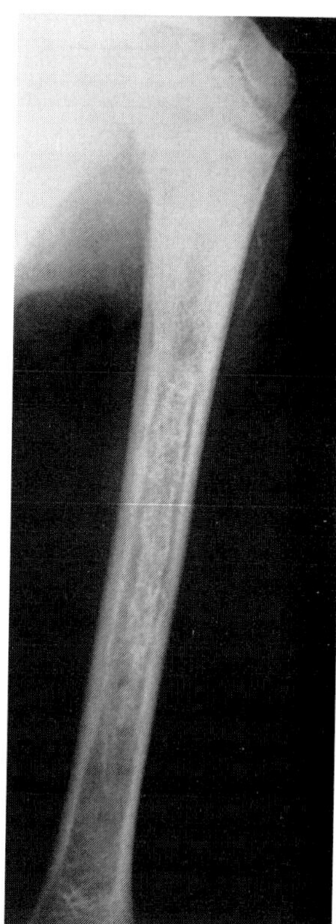

FIGURE 14–20. Gaucher's disease: medullary infarct.[52] Radiograph of the humerus in this 10-year-old boy with Gaucher's disease reveals diaphyseal medullary sclerosis characteristic of a medullary infarct. Gaucher's disease also may be manifested as osteopenia, cortical thinning, or erosion, coarsened trabecular pattern, osteolytic lesions, modeling deformity (such as Erlenmeyer flask deformity), and epiphyseal osteonecrosis.

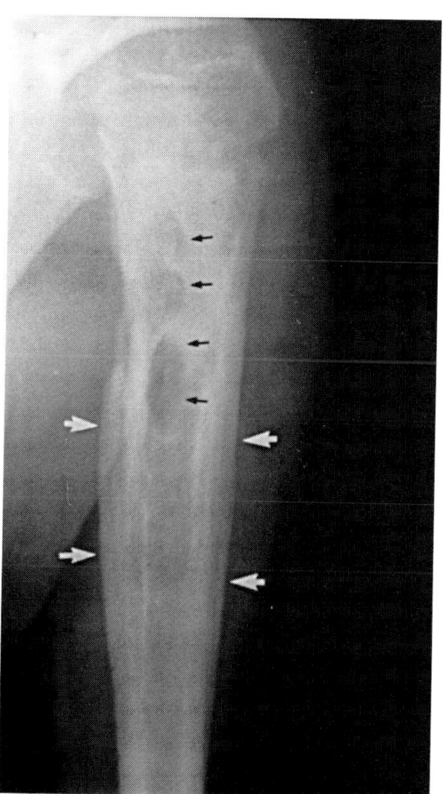

FIGURE 14–21. Acute pyogenic osteomyelitis.[54] In this 12-year-old patient, observe the diffuse solid layer of periosteal new bone formation (white arrows), the increased density, and the central, elongated osteolytic lesions (black arrows) within the proximal humeral metadiaphysis.

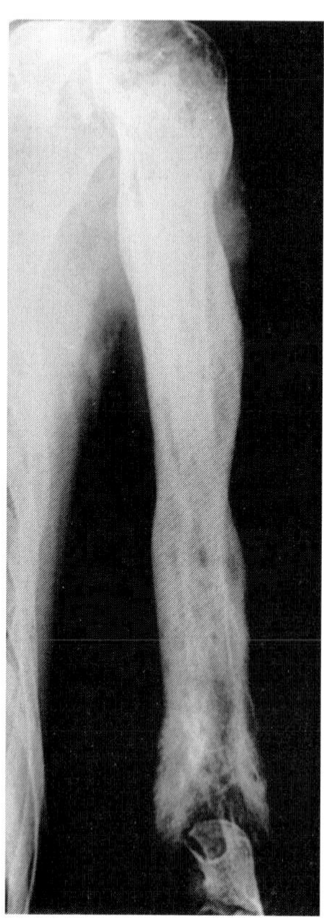

FIGURE 14–22. Chronic osteomyelitis: *Staphylococcus aureus*.[55] A bizarre cloak of ossification is seen surrounding the entire diaphysis and both metaphyses of the humerus. Circular osteolytic foci are present in the distal aspect of the shaft. This patient had long-standing chronic osteomyelitis that showed no change on serial radiographs. Radiographic signs of activity in chronic osteomyelitis include a change from previous radiographs, poorly defined areas of osteolysis, thin linear periostitis, and sequestration, none of which were present in this patient. *(Courtesy of C. Pineda, M.D., Mexico City, Mexico.)*

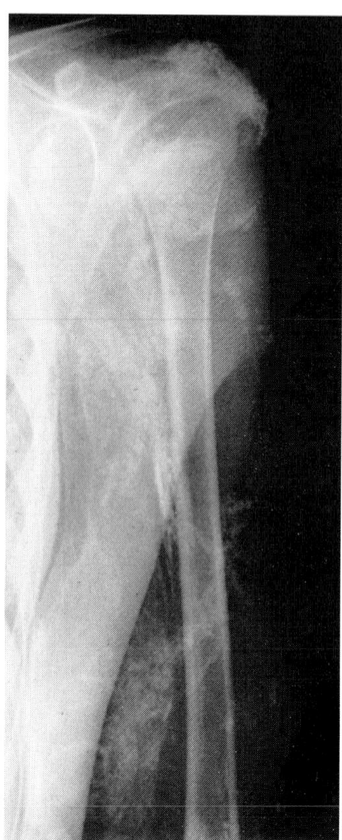

FIGURE 14–23. Collagen vascular disease: Dermatomyositis and polymyositis.[56] Observe the sheet-like periarticular, muscular, and subcutaneous calcification adjacent to the humerus in this 16-year-old girl with dermatomyositis-polymyositis. A number of collagen vascular diseases may result in localized or diffuse soft tissue calcification. *(Courtesy of C. Van Lom, M.D., San Diego, California.)*

REFERENCES

1. Resnick D, Cone RO: The nature of humeral pseudocysts. Radiology 150:27, 1984.
2. Wertsch JJ, Melvin J: Median nerve anatomy and entrapment syndromes: A review. Arch Phys Med Rehabil 63:623, 1982.
3. Keats TE: Atlas of Normal Roentgen Variants That May Simulate Disease. 6th Ed. Chicago, Year Book Medical Publishers, 1996.
4. Yochum TR, Rowe LJ: Essentials of Skeletal Radiology. 2nd Ed. Baltimore, Williams & Wilkins, 1996.
5. Resnick D, Niwayama G: Osteoporosis. *In* Resnick D: Diagnosis of Bone and Joint Disorders. 3rd Ed. Philadelphia, WB Saunders, 1995, p 1832.
6. Köhler A, Zimmer EA: Borderlands of Normal and Early Pathologic Findings in Skeletal Radiography. 4th Ed. New York, Thieme Medical Publishers, 1993.
7. Ozonoff MB, Zeiter FM Jr: The upper humeral notch: A normal variant in children. Radiology 113:699, 1974.
8. Ward EF, Savoie FH, Hughes JL: Fractures of the diaphyseal humerus. *In* Browner BD, Jupiter JB, Levine AM, et al (eds): Skeletal Trauma: Fractures, Dislocations, Ligamentous Injuries. Philadelphia, WB Saunders, 1992, p 1177.
9. Mast JW, Spiegel PG, Harvey JP Jr, et al: Fractures of the humeral shaft: A retrospective study of 240 adult fractures. Clin Orthop 112:254, 1975.
10. Rogers LF: Radiology of Skeletal Trauma. 2nd Ed. New York, Churchill Livingstone, 1992.
11. Thomas SA, Rosenfield NS, Leventhal JM, et al: Long-bone fractures in young children: Distinguishing accidental injuries from child abuse. Pediatrics 88:471, 1991.
12. Nuovo MA, Norman A, Chumas A, et al: Myositis ossificans with atypical clinical, radiographic, or pathologic findings: A review of 23 cases. Skeletal Radiol 21:87, 1992.
13. Greenspan A, Norman A: Osteolytic cortical destruction: An unusual pattern of skeletal metastasis. Skeletal Radiol 17:402, 1988.
14. Resnik C, Garver P, Resnick D: Bony expansion in skeletal metastasis from carcinoma of the prostate as seen by bone scintigraphy. South Med J 77:1331, 1984.
15. Huvos AG, Higinbotham NL, Miller TR: Bone sarcomas arising in fibrous dysplasia. J Bone Joint Surg [Am] 54:1047, 1972.
16. Dahlin DC, Unni KK: Osteosarcoma of bone and its important recognizable varieties. Am J Surg Pathol 1:61, 1977.
17. Ritschl P, Wurnig C, Lechner G, et al: Parosteal osteosarcoma: 2–23 year follow-up of 33 patients. Acta Orthop Scand 62:195, 1991.
18. Henderson ED, Dahlin DC: Chondrosarcoma of bone—a study of two hundred and eighty-eight cases. J Bone Joint Surg [Am] 45:1450, 1963.
19. Brien EW, Mirra JM, Kerr R: Benign and malignant cartilage tumors of bone and joint: Their anatomic and theoretical basis with an emphasis on radiology, pathology and clinical biology. 1. The intramedullary cartilage tumors. Skeletal Radiol 26:325, 1997.
20. Dahlin DC: Giant cell tumor of bone: Highlights of 407 cases. AJR 144:955, 1985.
21. Taconis WK, Mulder JD: Fibrosarcoma and malignant fibrous histiocytoma of long bones: Radiographic features and grading. Skeletal Radiol 11:237, 1984.
22. Dahlin DC, Coventry MB, Scanlon PW: Ewing's sarcoma: A critical analysis of 165 cases. J Bone Joint Surg [Am] 43:185, 1961.
23. Kyle RA: Multiple myeloma: Review of 869 cases. Mayo Clin Proc 50:29, 1975.
24. Hermann G, Klein MJ, Fikry Abedlewahab I, et al: MRI appearance of primary non-Hodgkin's lymphoma of bone. Skeletal Radiol 26:629, 1997.
25. Clayton F, Butler JJ, Ayala AG, et al: Non-Hodgkin's lymphoma in bone: Pathologic and radiologic features with clinical correlates. Cancer 60:2494, 1987.
26. Benz G, Brandeis WE, Willich E: Radiological aspects of leukemia in childhood: An analysis of 89 children. Pediatr Radiol 4:201, 1976.
27. Greenspan A: Bone island (enostosis): Current concept—a review. Skeletal Radiol 24:111, 1995.
28. Cronemeyer RL, Kirchmer NA, DeSmet AA, et al: Intra-articular osteoid osteoma of the humerus simulating synovitis of the elbow: A case report. J Bone Joint Surg [Am] 63:1172, 1981.
29. Kayser F, Resnick D, Haghighi P, et al: Evidence of the subperiosteal origin of osteoid osteomas in tubular bones: Analysis by CT and MR imaging. AJR 170:609, 1998.
30. Tonai M, Campbell CJ, Ahn GH, et al: Osteoblastoma: Classification and report of 16 cases. Clin Orthop 167:222, 1982.
31. Schiller AL: Diagnosis of borderline cartilage lesions of bone. Semin Diagn Pathol 2:42, 1985.
32. Bloem JL, Mulder JD: Chondroblastoma: A clinical and radiological study of 104 cases. Skeletal Radiol 14:1, 1985.
33. Weatherall PT, Maale GE, Mendelsohn DB, et al: Chondroblastoma: Classic and confusing appearance at MR imaging. Radiology 190:467, 1994.
34. Milgran JW: The origins of osteochondromas and enchondromas: A histopathologic study. Clin Orthop 174:264, 1983.
35. Karasick D, Schweitzer ME, Eschelman DJ: Symptomatic osteochondromas: Imaging features. AJR 168:1507, 1997.
36. Shapiro F, Simon S, Glimcher MJ: Hereditary multiple exostoses: Anthropometric, roentgenologic and clinical aspects. J Bone Joint Surg [Am] 61:815, 1979.
37. Solomon L: Chondrosarcoma in hereditary multiple exostosis. S Afr Med J 48:671, 1974.
38. Schmale GA, Conrad EV, Raskind WH: The natural history of hereditary multiple exostosis. J Bone Joint Surg [Am] 76:986, 1994.
39. Ritschl P, Karnel F, Hajek P: Fibrous metaphyseal defects—determination of their origin and natural history using a radiomorphological study. Skeletal Radiol 17:8, 1988.
40. Milgram JW: Intraosseous lipoma: A clinicopathologic study of 66 cases. Clin Orthop 231:277, 1988.
41. Chigira M, Maehara S, Arita S, et al: The aetiology and treatment of simple bone cysts. J Bone Joint Surg [Br] 65:633, 1983.
42. McGlynn FJ, Mickelson MR, El-Khoury GY: The fallen fragment sign in unicameral bone cysts. Clin Orthop 156:157, 1981.
43. De Dios AMV, Bond JR, Shives TC, et al: Aneurysmal bone cyst: A clinico-pathologic study of 238 cases. Cancer 69:2921, 1992.
44. Matfin G, McPherson F: Paget's disease of bone: Recent advances. J Orthop Rheumatol 6:127, 1993.
45. Mirra JM, Brien EW, Tehranzadeh J: Paget's disease of bone: Review with emphasis on radiologic features. Part II. Skeletal Radiol 24:173, 1995.

46. Gibson MJ, Middlemiss JH: Fibrous dysplasia of bone. Br J Radiol 44:1, 1971.
47. Stull MA, Kransdorf MJ, Devaney KO: Langerhans cell histiocytosis of bone. RadioGraphics 12:801, 1992.
48. Kilpatrick SE, Wenger DE, Gilchrist GS, et al: Langerhans' cell histiocytosis (histiocytosis X) of bone: A clinicopathologic analysis of 263 pediatric and adult cases. Cancer 76:2471, 1995.
49. Taylor JAM, Resnick D, Sartoris DJ: Radiographic-pathologic correlation. *In* Sartoris DJ: Osteoporosis: Diagnosis and Treatment. New York, Marcel Dekker, 1996, p 147.
50. Root L: The treatment of osteogenesis imperfecta. Orthop Clin North Am 15:775, 1984.
51. Mankin HJ: Rickets, osteomalacia, and renal osteodystrophy. Orthop Clin North Am 21:81, 1990.
52. Greenfield GB: Bone changes in chronic adult Gaucher's disease. AJR 110:800, 1970.
53. Pineda C: Diagnostic imaging in hypertrophic osteoarthropathy. Clin Exp Rheumatol 10:27, 1992.
54. Gold RH, Hawkins RA, Katz RD: Bacterial osteomyelitis: Findings on plain radiography, CT, MR, and scintigraphy. AJR 157:365, 1991.
55. Tumeh SS, Aliabadi P, Weissman BN, et al: Disease activity in osteomyelitis: Role of radiography. Radiology 165:781, 1987.
56. Pachman LN: Juvenile dermatomyositis. Pediatr Clin North Am 33:1097, 1986.

CHAPTER 15

Elbow

- Normal Developmental Anatomy
- Developmental Anomalies, Anatomic Variants, Sources of Diagnostic Error, and Skeletal Dysplasias
- Dislocations and Fractures
- Elbow Joint Effusion: Intracapsular Fat Pad Displacement
- Soft Tissue Injuries
- Articular Disorders
- Metabolic, Hematologic, and Infectious Disorders

Normal Developmental Anatomy

Accurate interpretation of radiographs of the pediatric elbow requires a complete understanding of normal developmental anatomy. Table 15–1 outlines the age of appearance and fusion of the primary and secondary ossification centers. Figures 15–1 and 15–2 demonstrate the radiographic appearance of many important ossification centers and other developmental landmarks at selected ages from birth to skeletal maturity. Figure 15–3 illustrates a special view for evaluating the radial head.

Developmental Anomalies, Anatomic Variants, Sources of Diagnostic Error, and Skeletal Dysplasias

Several anomalies, anatomic variants, skeletal dysplasias, and other sources of diagnostic error about the elbow may simulate disease and potentially result in misdiagnosis. Table 15–2 and Figures 15–4 to 15–6 represent selected examples of some of the more common processes affecting this region.

Dislocations and Fractures

Physical injury to the elbow region may result in a wide variety of dislocations and fractures. Table 15–3 lists the most common types of such injuries, and several examples of these are illustrated in Figures 15–8 to 15–18. Injuries to the humeral shaft are discussed in Chapter 14, and fractures of the diaphyses of the radius and ulna are discussed and illustrated in Chapter 16.

Elbow Joint Effusion: Intracapsular Fat Pad Displacement

Displacement (elevation) of both the posterior and anterior intracapsular fat pads of the elbow indicates the presence of joint effusion. Table 15–4 lists a number of causes of joint effusion, and Figure 15–7 illustrates two examples.

Soft Tissue Injuries

The elbow is a frequent site of injuries to tendons, ligaments, and joint capsules. The more common injuries are listed in Table 15–5. Figures 15–19 to 15–21 illustrate several examples of these posttraumatic conditions.

Articular Disorders

The joints of the elbow are frequent target sites of involvement for many degenerative, inflammatory, crystal-induced, and infectious articular disorders. Table 15–6 outlines these diseases and their characteristics. Figures 15–22 to 15–32 illustrate the typical radiographic manifestations of the most common articular disorders affecting the elbow.

Metabolic, Hematologic, and Infectious Disorders

Several metabolic, hematologic, and infectious disorders affect the bones and soft tissue structures about the elbow region. Table 15–7 lists some of the more common disorders and describes their characteristics. Figures 15–33 and 15–34 illustrate the characteristic imaging findings of many of these disorders. Additionally, osteonecrosis of the juvenile capitulum (Panner's disease) is illustrated in Figure 15–35.

TABLE 15–1. Elbow: Approximate Age of Appearance and Fusion of Ossification Centers[1–5] (Figs. 15–1 to 15–3)

Ossification Center	Primary or Secondary	No. of Centers (Per Bone)	Age of Appearance* (Years)	Age of Fusion* (Years)	Comments
Capitulum epiphysis	S	1	2	13	Fuses to trochlea
				12–13	Fuses to lateral epicondyle
				16	Fuses to humerus
Medial humeral epicondyle	S	1	4–6	16	Fuses to humerus
Radial head epiphysis	S	1	5	16	Fuses to radius
Trochlear epiphysis	S	1	8	13	Fuses to capitulum
				16	Fuses to humerus
Olecranon epiphysis	S	1 or 2	9	12–15	Fuses to ulna
Lateral humeral epicondyle	S	1	10	12–13	Fuses to capitulum
				15	Fuses to humerus

*Ages of appearance and fusion of ossification centers in girls typically precede those of boys. Ethnic differences also exist.
P, primary; S, secondary.

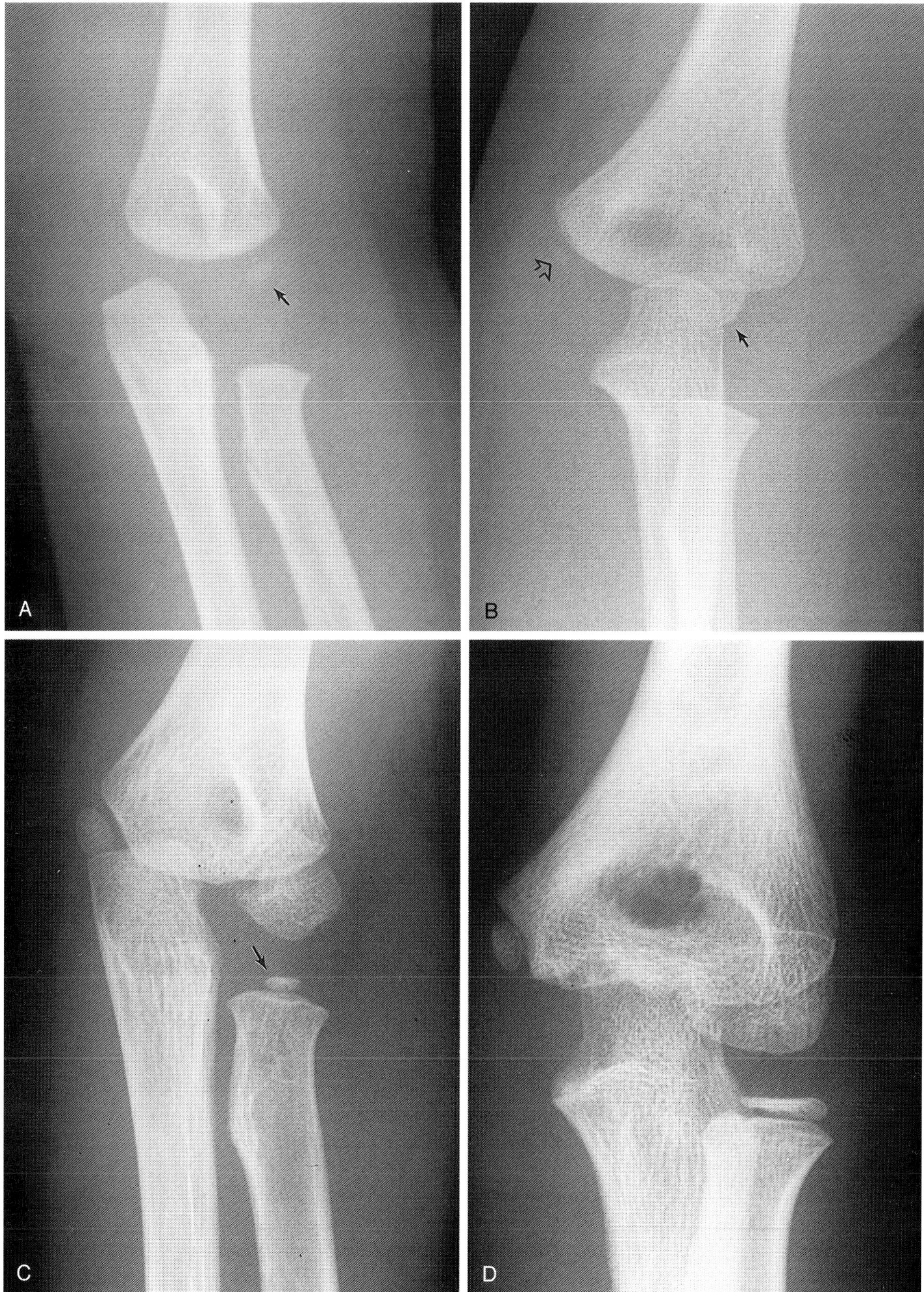

FIGURE 15–1. Skeletal maturation and normal development: anteroposterior elbow radiographs.[1–5] A 1-year-old girl. The secondary ossification center of the capitulum has begun to ossify (arrow). B 2-year-old girl. The secondary ossification center of the medial epicondyle is beginning to ossify (open arrow), and the capitulum is larger (arrow). C 5-year-old girl. The secondary ossification center of the radial head has begun to ossify (arrow). D 8-year-old boy. The normal radial head ossification center frequently is radiodense, as in this case. The distal humeral metaphysis has widened significantly.

Illustration continued on following page

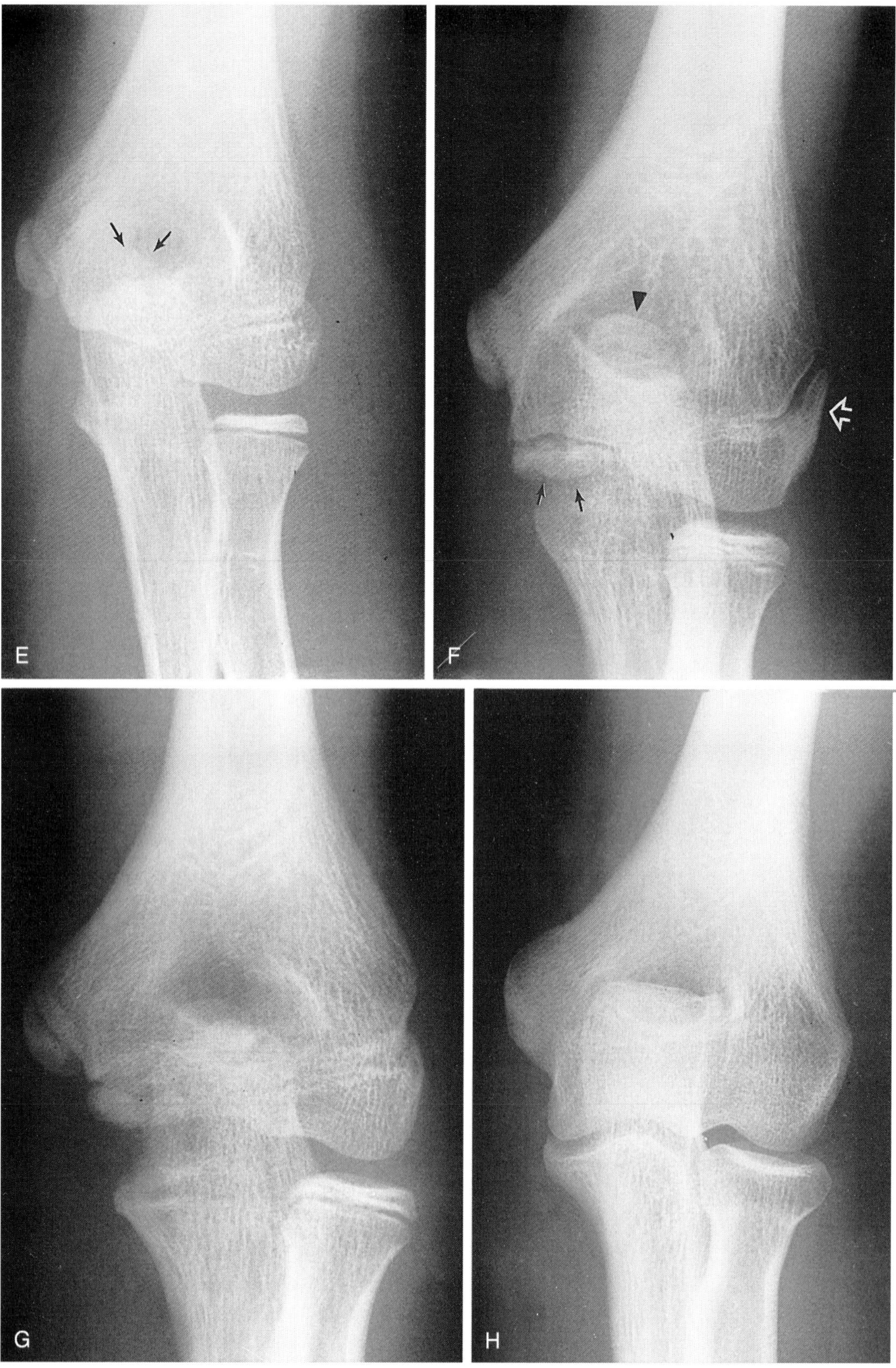

FIGURE 15–1 *Continued.* E 10-year-old girl. The existing ossification centers have enlarged and begun to conform to their adjacent metaphyses. The olecranon ossification center has begun to appear (arrows), a finding that is better seen on lateral radiographs. F 12-year-old girl. The secondary ossification center for the trochlea is beginning to ossify (arrows), and the center for the capitulum has a lateral projection that extends proximally along the humeral metaphysis (open arrow). The olecranon ossification center is enlarging (arrowhead). G 12-year-old boy. The ossification centers of the capitulum and trochlea have fused together, and the olecranon ossification center is large and prominent. H 16-year-old girl. Complete fusion of all ossification centers has occurred, and the elbow exhibits adult proportions.

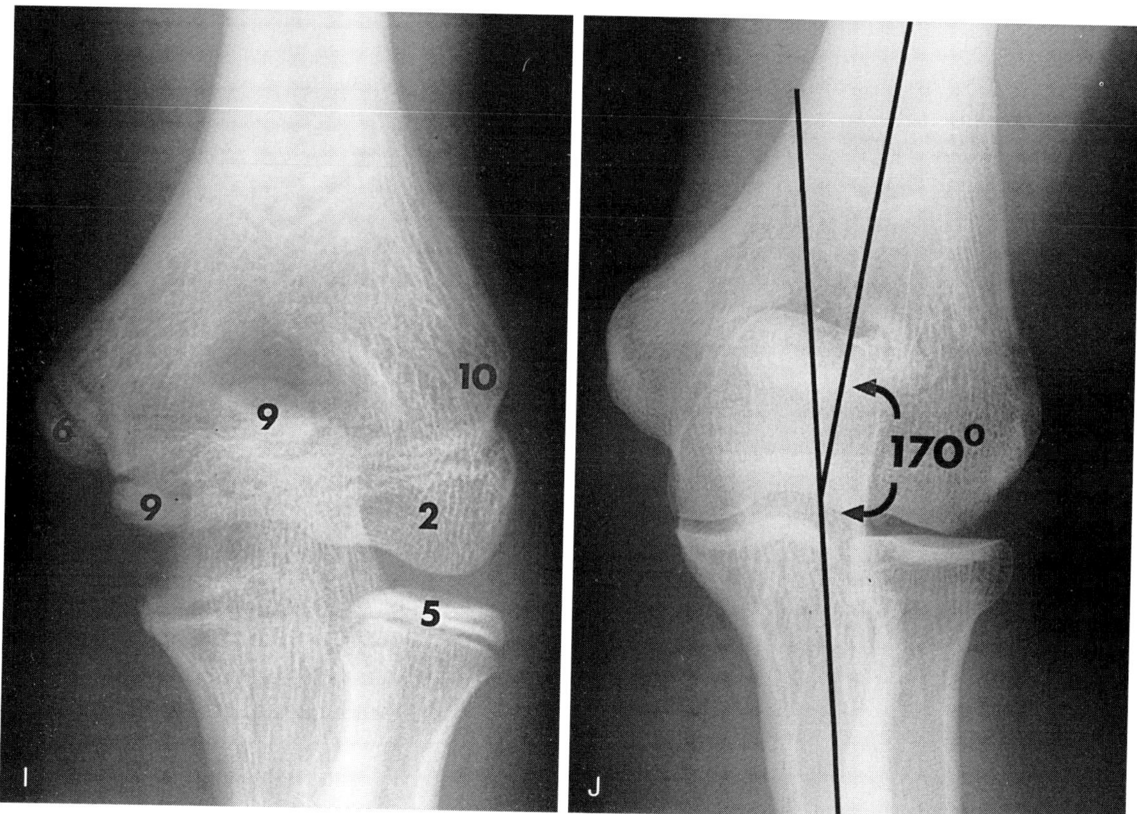

FIGURE 15–1 *Continued.* **I** Normal pattern of ossification about the elbow. Numbers indicate approximate age in years at which the center begins to ossify (Table 15–1). **J** Adult: 43-year-old man. The normal carrying angle of the elbow ranges from 154 to 178 degrees, averages 169 degrees, and may be altered as a result of fracture or other deformity.

Clinical Note: The normal appearances of the developing radial head and neck often are misinterpreted as evidence of trauma because (1) the radial neck of an infant is slightly angulated medially in the frontal projection, simulating a dislocation of the radial head; (2) the early physis of the proximal portion of the radius is wedge-shaped, mimicking an avulsion fracture of the head; and (3) notches and clefts in the metaphysis of the proximal portion of the radius may closely resemble posttraumatic abnormalities.[5]

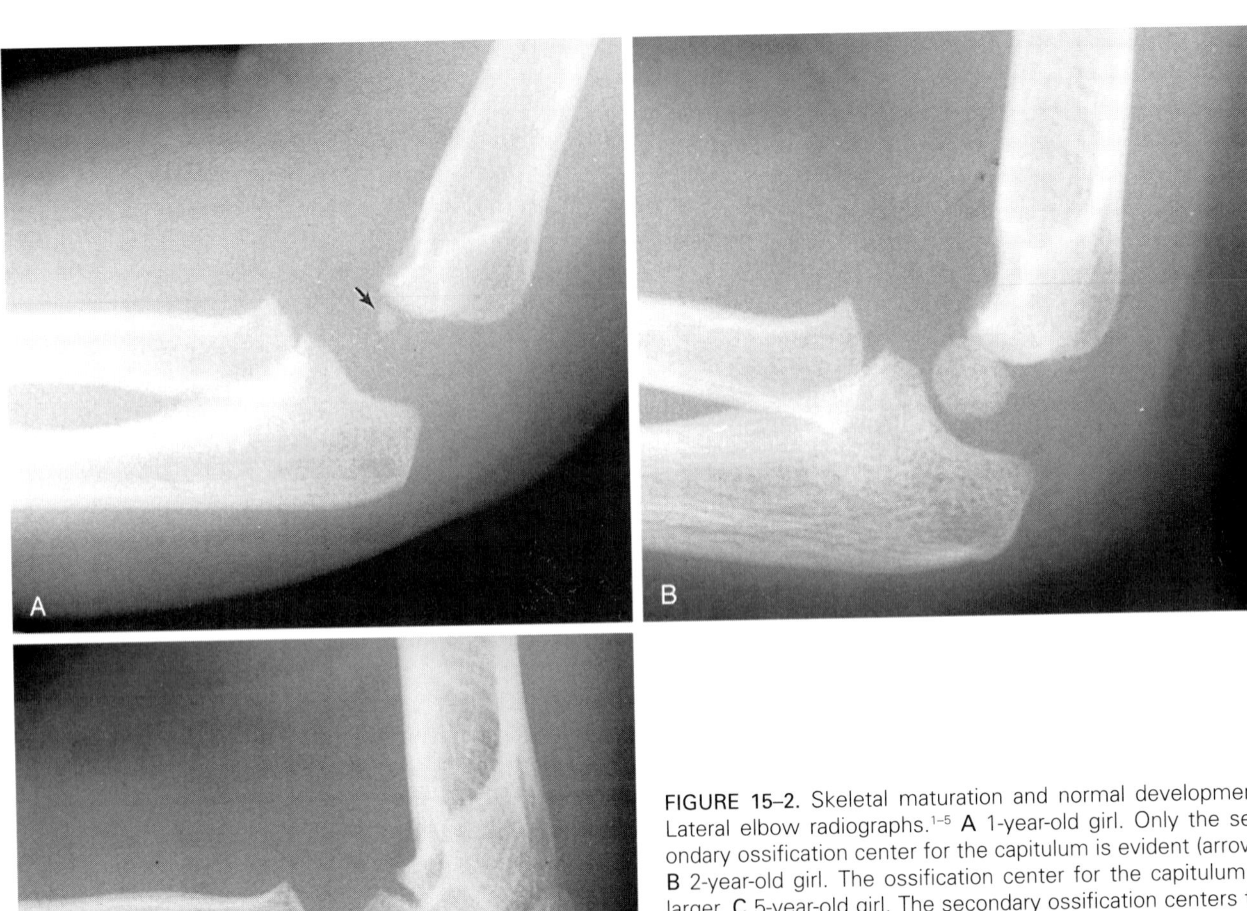

FIGURE 15–2. Skeletal maturation and normal development: Lateral elbow radiographs.[1–5] A 1-year-old girl. Only the secondary ossification center for the capitulum is evident (arrow). B 2-year-old girl. The ossification center for the capitulum is larger. C 5-year-old girl. The secondary ossification centers for the radial head (arrow) and medial epicondyle (open arrow) are present. These usually appear at the ages of 5 and 6 years, respectively.

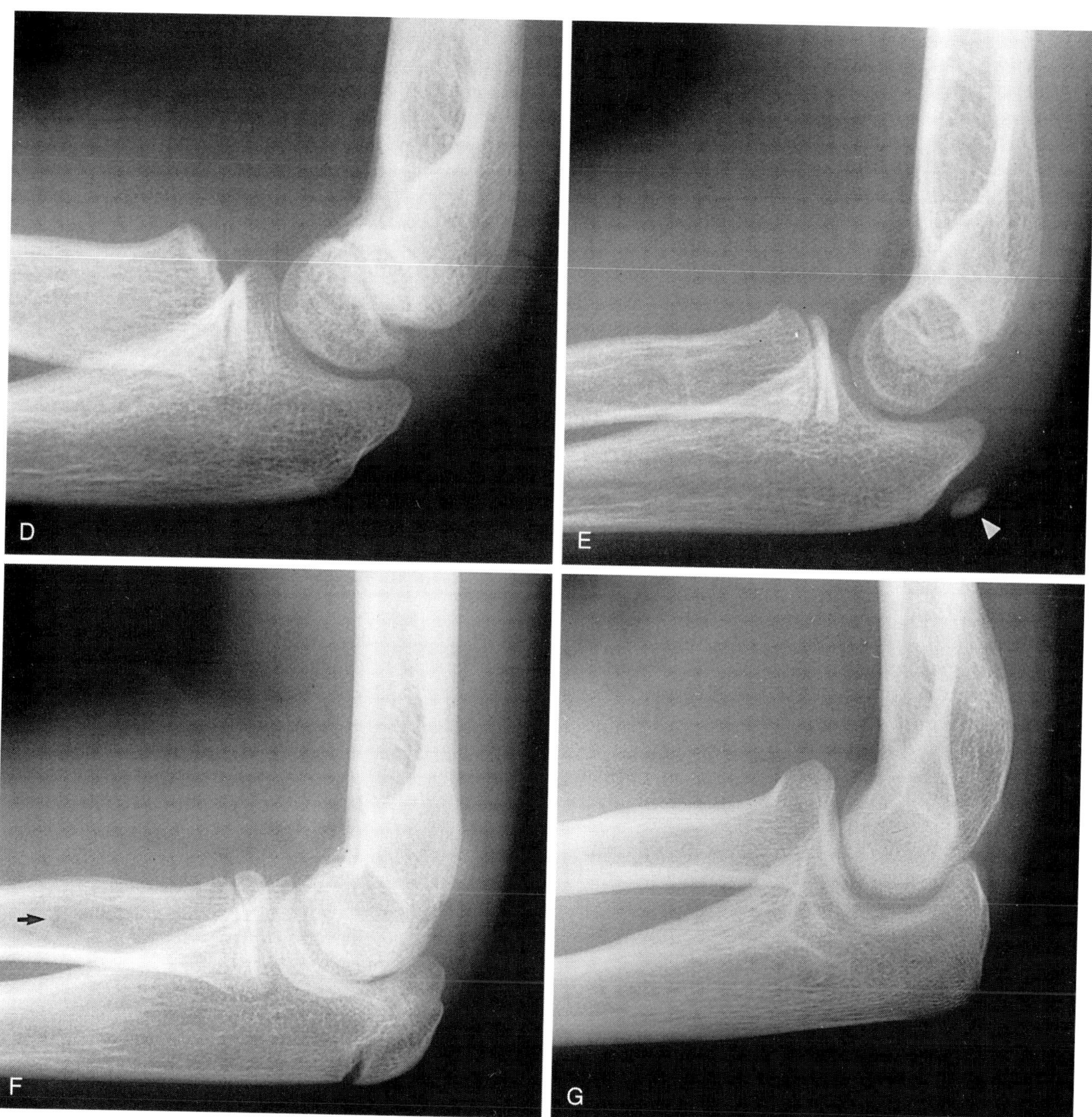

FIGURE 15–2 *Continued.* D 8-year-old boy. The radial head ossification center normally is radiodense, as in this case. The capitulum ossification center conforms to the shape of the humeral metaphysis. E 10-year-old girl. The secondary ossification center for the olecranon has begun to ossify (arrowhead). F 13-year-old boy. The secondary ossification center for the olecranon is beginning to fuse to the ulna. The radiolucent area in the radius represents the normal trabecular pattern in the cancellous bone of the radial tuberosity (arrow) and should not be mistaken for a destructive lesion. G 16-year-old girl. Complete fusion of all ossification centers has occurred, and the elbow exhibits adult proportions.

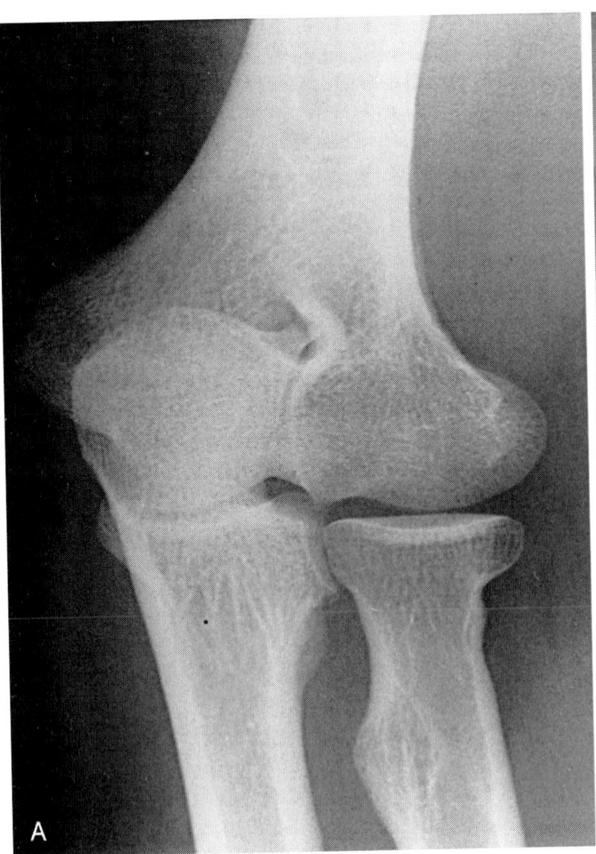

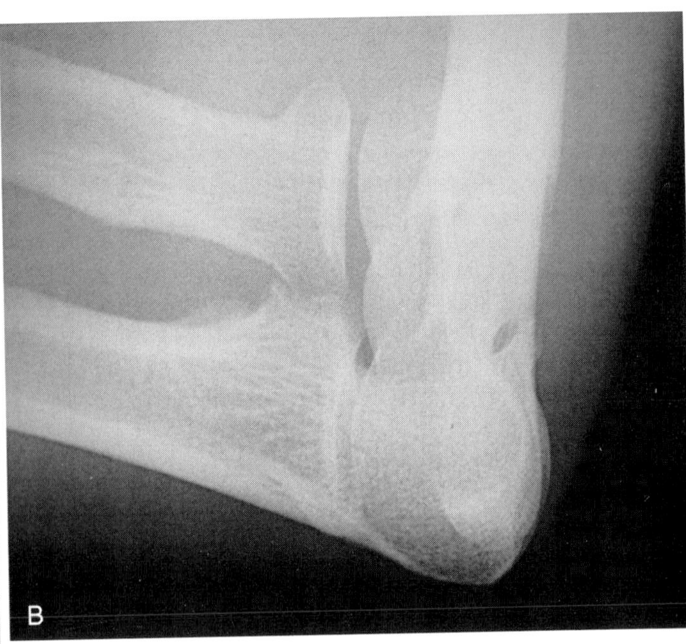

FIGURE 15–3. A, B Normal radial head projections.[6] Special angulated views of the radial head clearly depict the anatomy of the proximal radioulnar region and are particularly useful in analyzing fractures of the radial head and neck.

TABLE 15–2. Developmental Anomalies, Anatomic Variants, Sources of Diagnostic Error, and Skeletal Dysplasias

Disorder	Figure(s)	Characteristics
Simulated periostitis[7, 8]	13–2 G	See Table 14–1
Supracondylar process[7, 8]	14–1	See Table 14–1
Chevron sign[9]	14–2	See Table 14–1
Supratrochlear foramen[7, 8, 10]		See Table 14–1
Radiolucent radial tuberosity[8]	15–2 F, 16–1	Normal radiolucency of the cancellous bone within the radial tuberosity may simulate a destructive lesion or a cyst No clinical significance
Incomplete union of ossification centers[8]	15–4	In children, incompletely fused ossification centers may simulate fractures Common sites: olecranon, epicondyles, trochlea, capitulum, radial head Irregularities of the growing epiphyses about the elbow are common Olecranon ossification center may arise from two or more nuclei, simulating a fracture Nonunion of ossification centers may persist into adulthood
Patella cubiti[11]		Sesamoid bone within the triceps tendon just above the olecranon Rare anomaly that may simulate heterotopic ossification within the triceps tendon
Radioulnar synostosis[12]	15–5	Anomalous osseous fusion of the proximal portions of the radius and the ulna Bilateral in 60 per cent of patients Restricts normal forearm supination and pronation Additional anomalies may accompany radioulnar synostosis
Hereditary osteo-onychodysostosis (HOOD syndrome)[13]	15–6	Dislocation of the radial head due to asymmetric development of the humeral condyles and hypoplasia of the radial head and capitulum Also termed Fong's syndrome or nail-patella syndrome Associated abnormalities of the fingernails and toenails, absence or hypoplasia of the patella, and presence of iliac horns
Osteopoikilosis[14]	15–7	Multiple circular zones of osteosclerosis tend to accumulate in a periarticular distribution

See also Table 1–1.

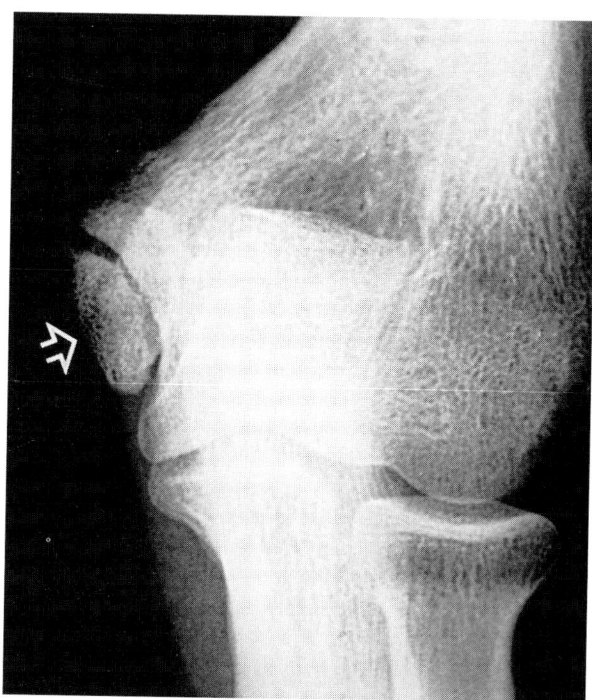

FIGURE 15–4. Unfused ossification center.[8] A well-corticated, circular osseous fragment is seen at the medial epicondyle of the humerus (open arrow) in this 35-year-old man. This ossicle represents failure of union of the ossification center. Ossification of the medial epicondyle usually begins to appear on radiographs between the ages of 2 and 7 years, and in most persons, fusion is complete by the age of 20 years.

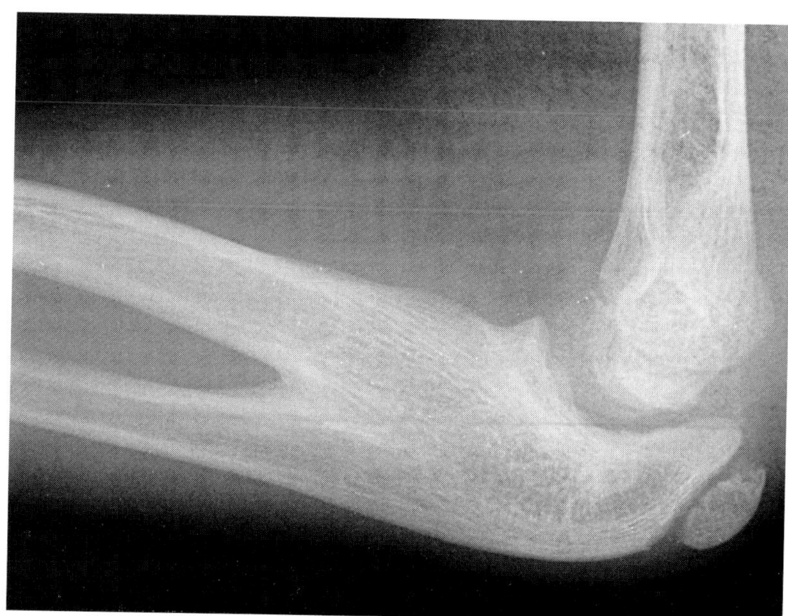

FIGURE 15–5. Radioulnar synostosis.[12] Complete osseous fusion of the proximal portions of the radius and ulna is seen. This anomaly, which is bilateral in 60 per cent of patients, interferes with normal forearm supination. Additional anomalies may accompany radioulnar synostosis. (The olecranon ossification center has not yet fused in this child.)

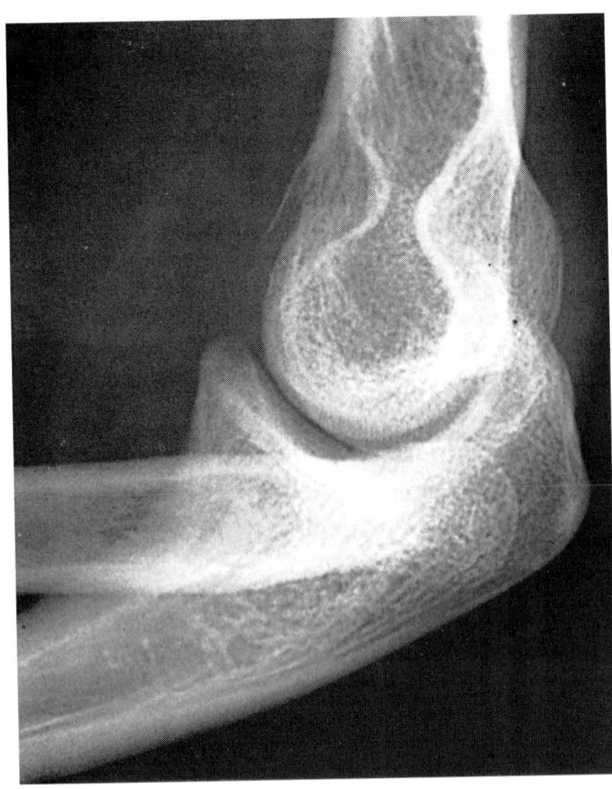

FIGURE 15–6. Hereditary osteo-onychodysostosis (HOOD syndrome).[13] Observe the dislocation of the radial head owing to asymmetric development of the humeral condyles and hypoplasia of the capitulum and radial head. This condition, also referred to as Fong's syndrome or nail-patella syndrome, is characterized by associated abnormalities of the fingernails and toenails, absence or hypoplasia of the patella, and presence of iliac horns. *(Courtesy of R. Sweet, M.D., Pomona, California.)*

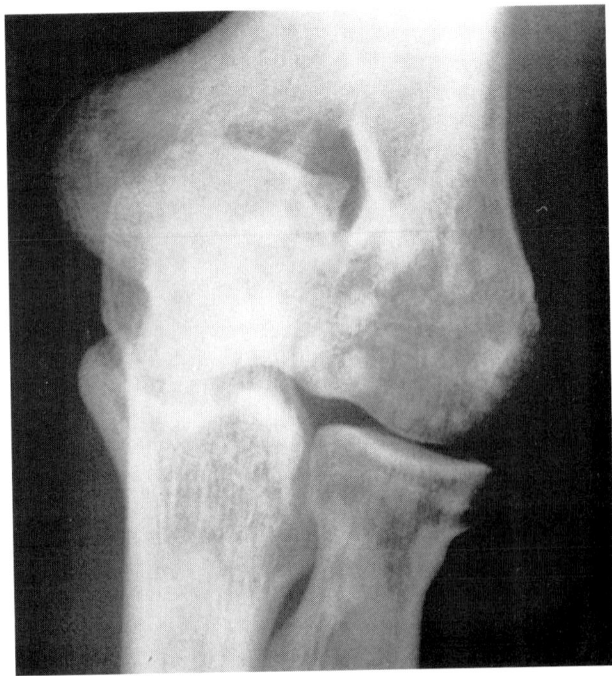

FIGURE 15–7. Osteopoikilosis.[14] Note the circular and ovoid osteosclerotic foci within the radius, ulna, and humerus. The symmetric, periarticular distribution is characteristic of this fairly common sclerosing dysplasia. Although the epiphysis may be affected, most lesions occur in the metaphysis. *(Courtesy of L. Danzig, M.D., Santa Ana, California.)*

TABLE 15–3. Dislocations and Fractures

Injury	Figure(s)	Characteristics	Complications and Related Disorders
Elbow dislocation		Most frequent site of dislocation in children	
Posterior dislocation of elbow[18]	15–9	Usual mechanism: hyperextension Eighty to 90 per cent are posterior dislocations of both ulna and radius in relation to the humerus	Children: Often associated with medial epicondyle avulsion Adults: Associated with fractures of radial head and coronoid process of ulna Median nerve entrapment
Radial head dislocation[19]	15–10	Children: "nursemaid's elbow" or "pulled elbow" Sudden pull on child's arm while in pronated position Very common	Annular ligament entrapment (rare)
		Adults: Isolated radial head dislocation is rare May become chronic	Associated ulnar fracture
Monteggia fracture-dislocation[20]	16–6	Common in adults; rare in children Radial head dislocation associated with ulnar fracture Four types have been described based on the location of the fracture and direction of dislocation See Table 16–2	All of the above plus heterotopic ossification Radial nerve injury (20 per cent of cases)
Extra-articular fractures of the distal portion of the humerus			
Supracondylar fracture[21]		60 per cent of all elbow fractures in children Rare in adults Extension (95 per cent) and flexion (5 per cent) types Paradoxic posterior fat pad sign Supracondylar process, if present, may fracture Disruption of anterior humeral line on lateral radiograph	Brachial artery injury Median, ulnar, or radial nerve injury Alignment abnormalities Heterotopic ossification Volkmann's ischemic contracture
Intra-articular fractures of the distal portion of the humerus			
Transcondylar fracture[21]		Intra-articular fracture resembling supracondylar fracture Horizontal through both condyles Extension and flexion varieties	Heterotopic ossification Coronoid process entrapment
Intercondylar fracture[21, 22]	15–11	Most common in persons over the age of 50 years; rare fracture Vertical and horizontal or oblique component Comminuted with Y or T configuration	Nerve and vessel injury Instability Loss of elbow function Delayed union or nonunion Ischemic necrosis
Condylar fracture[21]		Relatively uncommon fracture seen most frequently in children Lateral condyle > medial condyle	Instability Restriction of motion
Capitulum fracture[23]	15–12	Rare injuries caused by direct forces applied through the radial head Type I (Hahn-Steinthal type): Displacement of large segment of bone Type II (Kocher-Lorenz type): Mainly displacement of cartilage	Tear of medial collateral ligament
Epicondylar fracture[21]		More frequent in children than adults Rare injury See growth plate injuries below	Ulnar nerve injury

Table continued on following page

TABLE 15–3. Dislocations and Fractures About the Elbow *Continued*

Injury	Figure(s)	Characteristics	Complications and Related Disorders
Fractures of the proximal portion of the ulna			
Olecranon process fracture[24]	15–13	Fracture through semilunar notch Proximal displacement of fragment from pull of triceps muscle Often comminuted	Disruption of triceps mechanism Decreased range of motion Degenerative joint disease Nonunion (5 per cent of cases) Ulnar nerve damage (10 per cent of cases)
Coronoid process fracture[25]	15–14	Rare isolated injury Often associated with posterior elbow dislocation Avulsion from brachialis tendon or impaction against the trochlea	Decreased range of motion Degenerative joint disease
Fractures of the proximal portion of the radius		Radial head projections often helpful Joint effusion results in positive fat pad sign (Table 15–4)	
Radial head fractures[6, 26]	15–15	Most common elbow fracture in adults From indirect trauma Classification: Four types after Mason I: undisplaced fractures II: marginal fractures with displacement III: comminuted fractures IV: fractures associated with dislocation Radiographic findings may be subtle Offset in cortical continuity of radial head and neck Vertical split of radial head termed chisel fracture	Limited range of motion Degenerative joint disease Heterotopic ossification May be associated with fractures of wrist and forearm (Monteggia's fracture-dislocation) May be a component of an Essex-Lopresti injury: comminuted and displaced radial head fracture combined with diastasis of the distal radioulnar joint
Radial neck fractures[6]		Impaction fracture of radial neck without radial head fracture is encountered frequently Findings of cortical offset may be subtle	Limited range of motion Degenerative joint disease Heterotopic ossification
Child abuse[27]		Humerus is second most common site of fracture (ribs most common site) Subperiosteal hemorrhage with periostitis Metaphyseal corner fractures Physeal injuries Multiple fractures at different stages of healing	Continued morbidity and even death
Growth plate injuries			
Distal portion of the humerus[28]		Common: 16.7 per cent of all physeal injuries	Growth arrest, joint deformity and osteonecrosis
Medial epicondyle[29]	15–16	Type I injuries most common: epiphysiolysis	Entrapment of epiphysis within joint
Lateral condyle[28, 29]		Type IV injuries in children younger than age 10 years	
Distal humeral epiphysis[28]		Type I or II in children from birth to age 5 years	Cubitus varus deformity
Proximal portion of the radius[28]		Injury in children aged 8 to 13 years	
Stress injuries[30]		Stress fracture of the coronoid process of ulna from ball throwing	
Osteochondritis dissecans and osteochondral fractures[31, 32]	15–17, 15–18	Usually involves capitulum or trochlea History of acute injury or chronic stress Frequently affects gymnasts	Joint locking Limited range of motion Degenerative joint disease Osteonecrosis

See also Tables 1–3 and 1–4.

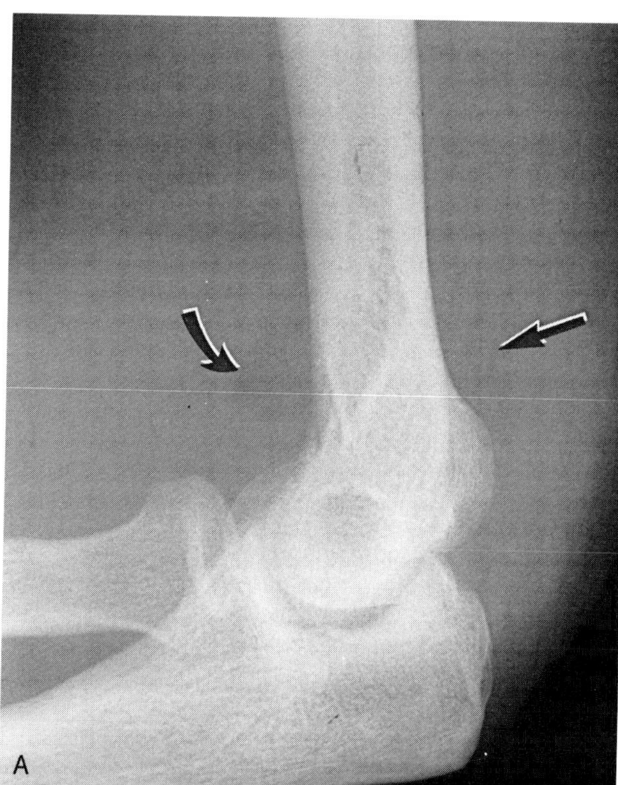

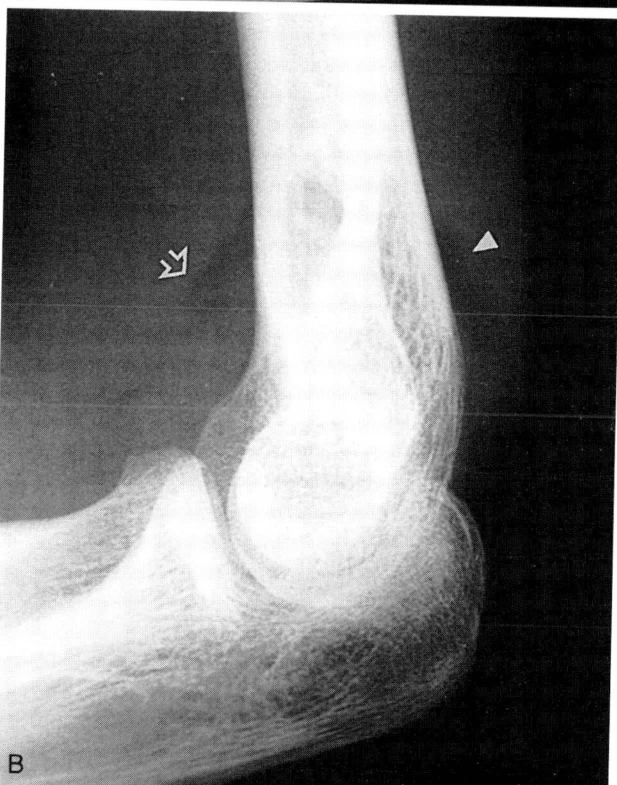

TABLE 15–4. Some Causes of Intracapsular Fat Pad Displacement in the Elbow*[15–17] (Fig. 15–8)

Blood
Intra-articular fracture
Hemophilia
Transudate
Rheumatoid arthritis
Other synovial arthropathies
Gout
Calcium pyrophosphate dihydrate (CPPD) crystal deposition
Osteoarthrosis
Neuropathic osteoarthropathy
Exudate
Infectious arthritis
Neoplasm
Leukemia
Metastasis
Synovial sarcoma
Osteoid osteoma
Other
Villonodular synovitis
Synovial osteochondromatosis
Osteochondritis dissecans

*Adapted from Murphy WA, Siegel MJ: Elbow fat pads with new signs and extended differential diagnosis. Radiology 124:659, 1977.

FIGURE 15–8. Elbow joint effusion: Intracapsular fat pad displacement.[15–17] A Elevation of both the anterior (curved arrow) and posterior (arrow) intracapsular fat pads of the elbow is evident in this patient with a radial head fracture (not seen). B In another patient with an intra-articular fracture of the radial head (fracture not seen), elevation of both anterior (open arrow) and posterior (arrowhead) fat pads indicates a joint effusion. This sign usually reflects the existence of intracapsular fluid or blood and has traditionally been synonymous with an occult intra-articular fracture. Recent evidence has shown that visualization of joint effusion without evidence of fracture on initial radiographs after trauma does not correlate with the presence of occult fracture in 83 per cent of pediatric cases. However, presence of persistent joint effusions on follow-up radiographs correlates with occult fractures.[17] Joint effusions also may be associated with a number of other pathologic processes (Table 15–4).

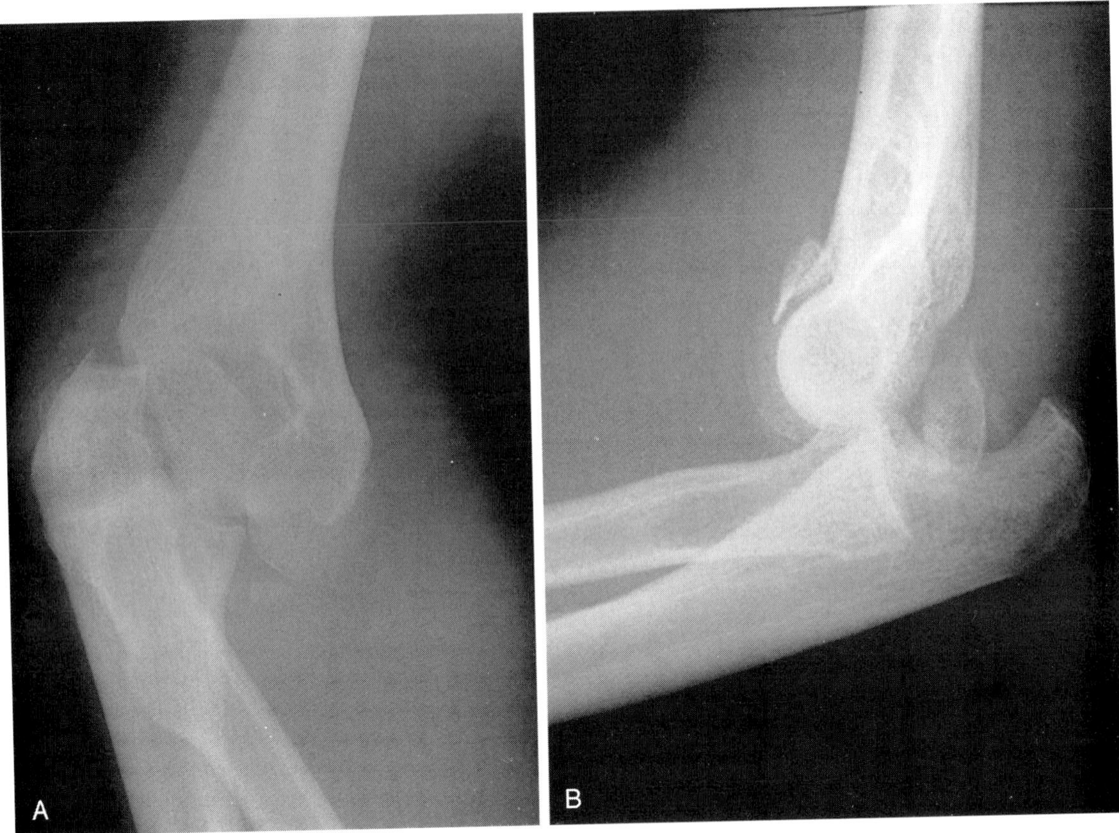

FIGURE 15–9. Posterior dislocation.[18] Frontal (A) and lateral (B) radiographs in this 28-year-old man reveal posterior dislocation of both the radius and the ulna with respect to the humerus. The lateral condyle of the humerus is fractured, and impingement of the radial head and capitulum is evident. This injury typically occurs from a fall on the outstretched hand while the elbow is hyperextended. The posterior type of dislocation represents about 80 to 90 per cent of all elbow dislocations. Complications include coronoid process fractures in adults and fracture (and possible entrapment) of the medial condylar ossification center in children and adolescents. Median nerve entrapment also may occur after reduction.

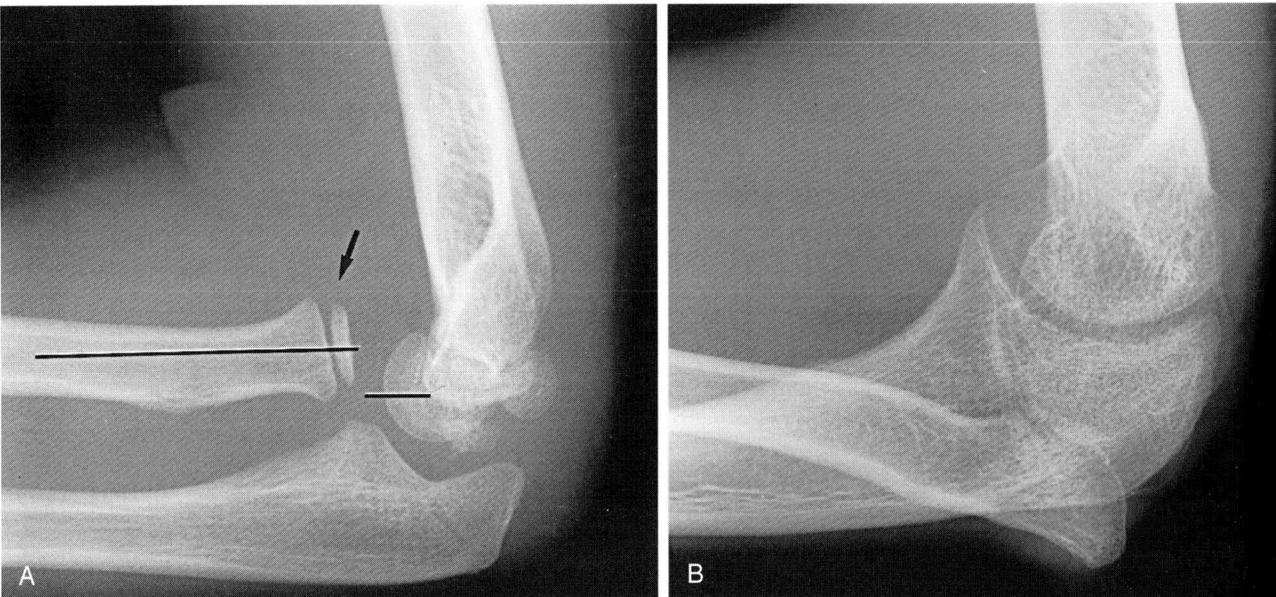

FIGURE 15–10. Traumatic radial head dislocation.[19] A Nursemaid's elbow. In this infant, observe the abnormal separation of the radius and ulna and the isolated anterior dislocation of the radial head (arrow) with respect to the capitulum. A line constructed through the center of, and parallel to, the long axis of the radius (radiocapitular line) should intersect the center of the capitulum in all ranges of flexion and extension of the elbow. Note the offset in this line. Isolated radial head dislocation occurs most frequently in children; it is also termed nursemaid's elbow or pulled elbow. This injury is caused by a sudden pull of the child's arm, resulting in sudden elbow hyperextension and slipping of the radial head beneath the annular ligament, which is torn from its attachment to the radial neck. The dislocation usually reduces spontaneously or on supination of the forearm by a physician, but surgical reduction occasionally is required. B Recurrent radial head dislocation. This 21-year-old man had recurrent traumatic radial head dislocations. Observe the posterior displacement of the radial head in relation to the ulna. The radial head appears small and dysplastic. Owing to the rarity of isolated radial head dislocations, all patients should undergo thorough investigation for associated ulnar fractures.

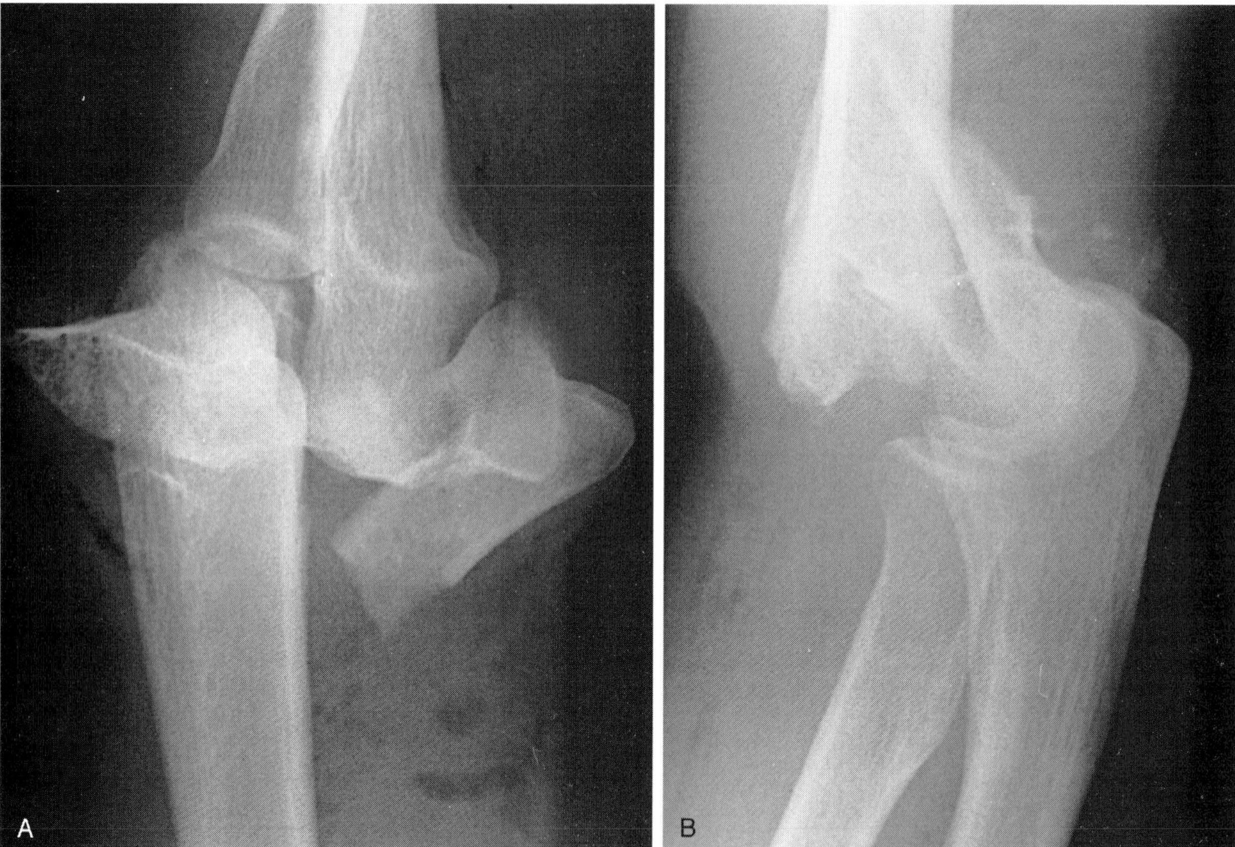

FIGURE 15–11. Intercondylar fracture.[21, 22] Frontal (A) and lateral (B) radiographs show an open comminuted fracture, which has led to separation of the trochlear and capitular fragments. The shaft of the humerus is displaced anteriorly, and extensive soft tissue emphysema is evident. Intercondylar fractures are relatively rare and occur primarily in patients older than 50 years of age. Rotation at the fracture site and incongruity of the articular surfaces are potential complications.

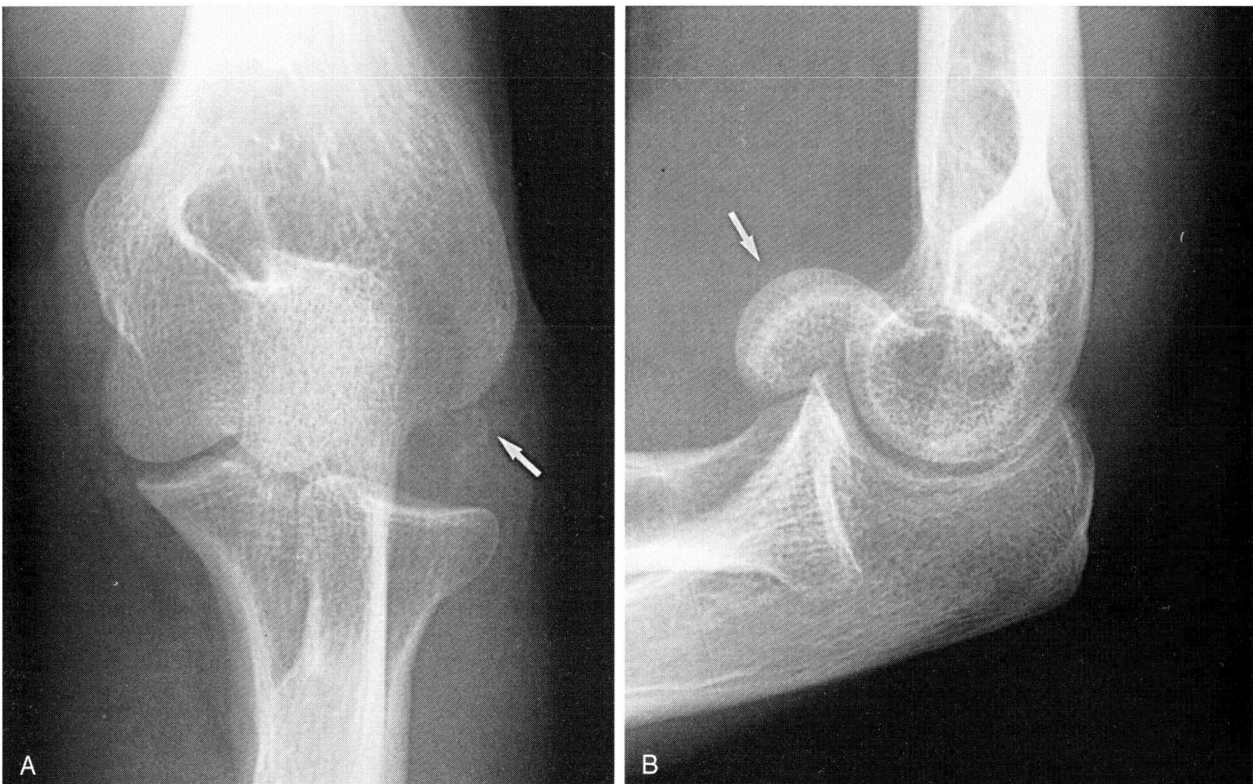

FIGURE 15–12. Fracture: Capitulum.[23] A Frontal radiograph shows absence of the capitulum adjacent to the lateral aspect of the distal end of the humerus. Small fragments of bone are evident (arrow). B Lateral radiograph shows displacement and rotation of the capitular fragment, which is lying within the radial fossa (arrow). The injury in this patient is the type I (Hahn-Steinthal type) fracture involving a coronally oriented fracture of a large segment of the capitulum with characteristic anterior and superior displacement of the fracture fragment. The injury is difficult to visualize on anteroposterior radiographs. The half-moon appearance of the capitular fragment on lateral films, however, is characteristic of this injury. Type II fractures (not shown) involve fracture of only the articular cartilage and uncapping of the capitulum, a condition difficult to observe on routine radiographs.

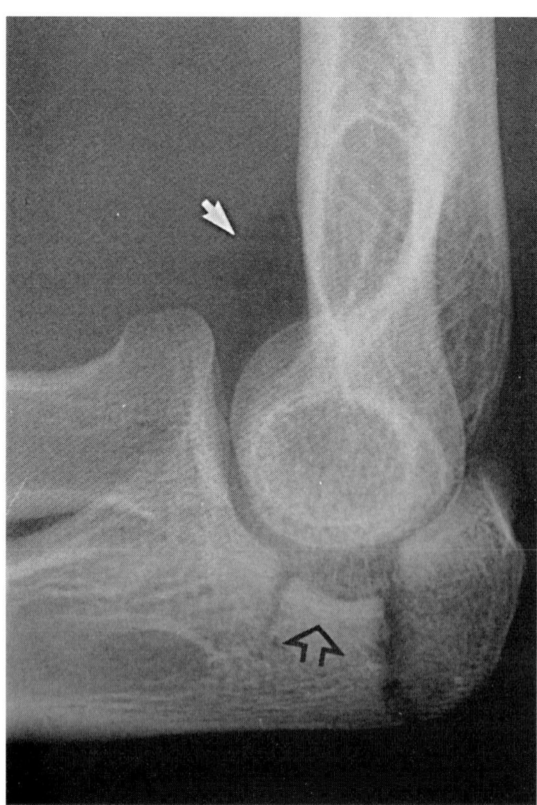

FIGURE 15–13. Olecranon process fracture.[24] Observe the comminuted intra-articular fracture with associated depression of the articular surface (open arrow), resulting in incongruity of the articular surface of the semilunar notch of the ulna. Also note elevation of the anterior intracapsular fat pad, indicating an associated joint effusion (arrow) that is not well seen on this view. The combination of posterior displacement of the olecranon fragment with anterior movement of the remaining portion of the ulna and radial head is a serious injury termed fracture-dislocation of the elbow. Complications of olecranon fractures include decreased range of motion, osteoarthrosis, nonunion, and ulnar nerve damage.

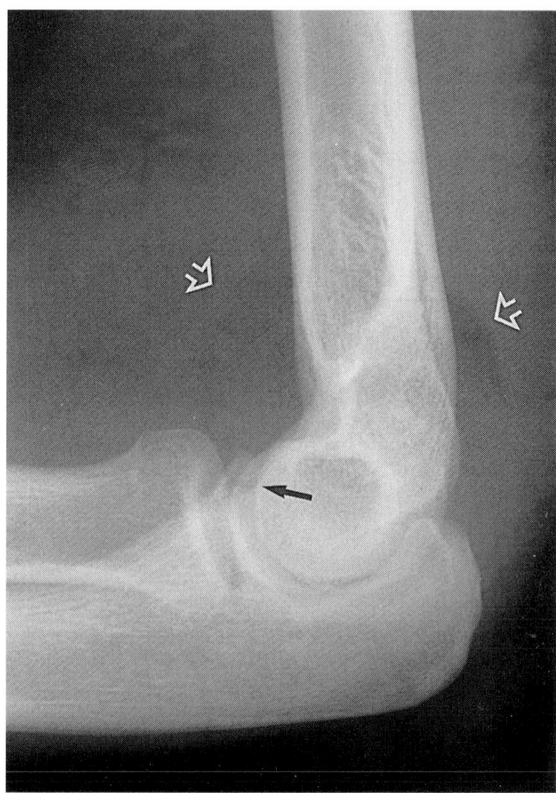

FIGURE 15–14. Coronoid process fracture.[25] A small, almost imperceptible fracture of the coronoid process is seen (arrow). Elevation of both the anterior and posterior intracapsular fat pads (open arrows) also is present. Isolated fractures of the ulnar coronoid process are rare and occur as a result of avulsion from the brachialis tendon or direct impaction against the trochlea. Coronoid process fractures more commonly are associated with posterior elbow dislocations.

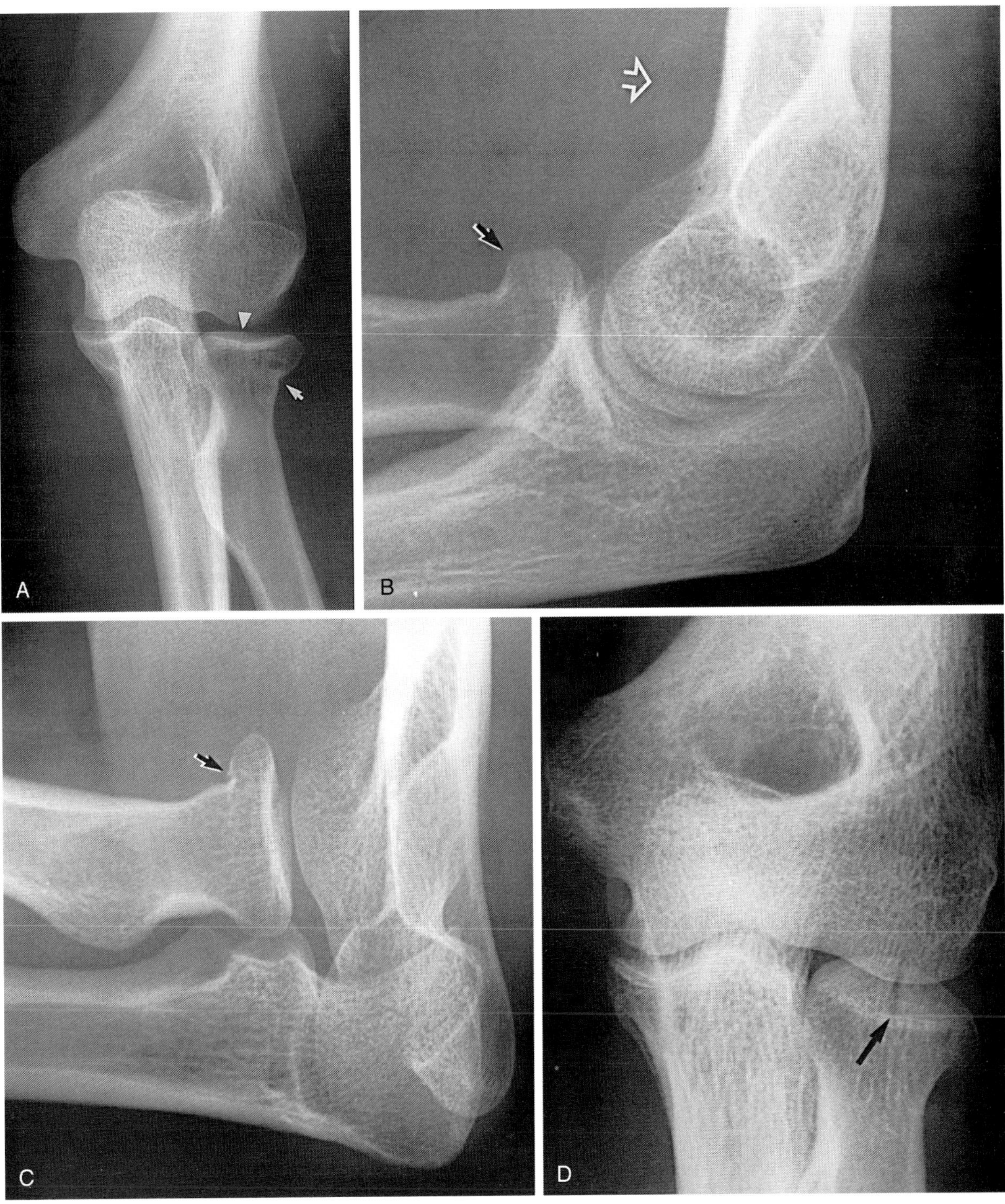

FIGURE 15–15. Radial head fracture.[6, 26] A–C This patient fell while skating. In A, a frontal radiograph shows a subtle longitudinal intra-articular fracture of the radial head (arrowhead) and an offset in the cortical margin of the head-neck junction (arrow). In B, the routine lateral radiograph reveals a subtle anterior fat pad sign (open arrow), suggesting a fracture, but the head-neck junction appears essentially normal (arrow). In C, a specialized radiographic projection, the radial head–capitulum view, projects the proximal portion of the radius away from the overlying ulna, allowing a clear depiction of the sharp, angular cortical defect characteristic of an impaction fracture (arrow). D In another patient, a longitudinal intra-articular fracture (chisel fracture) is seen (arrow).

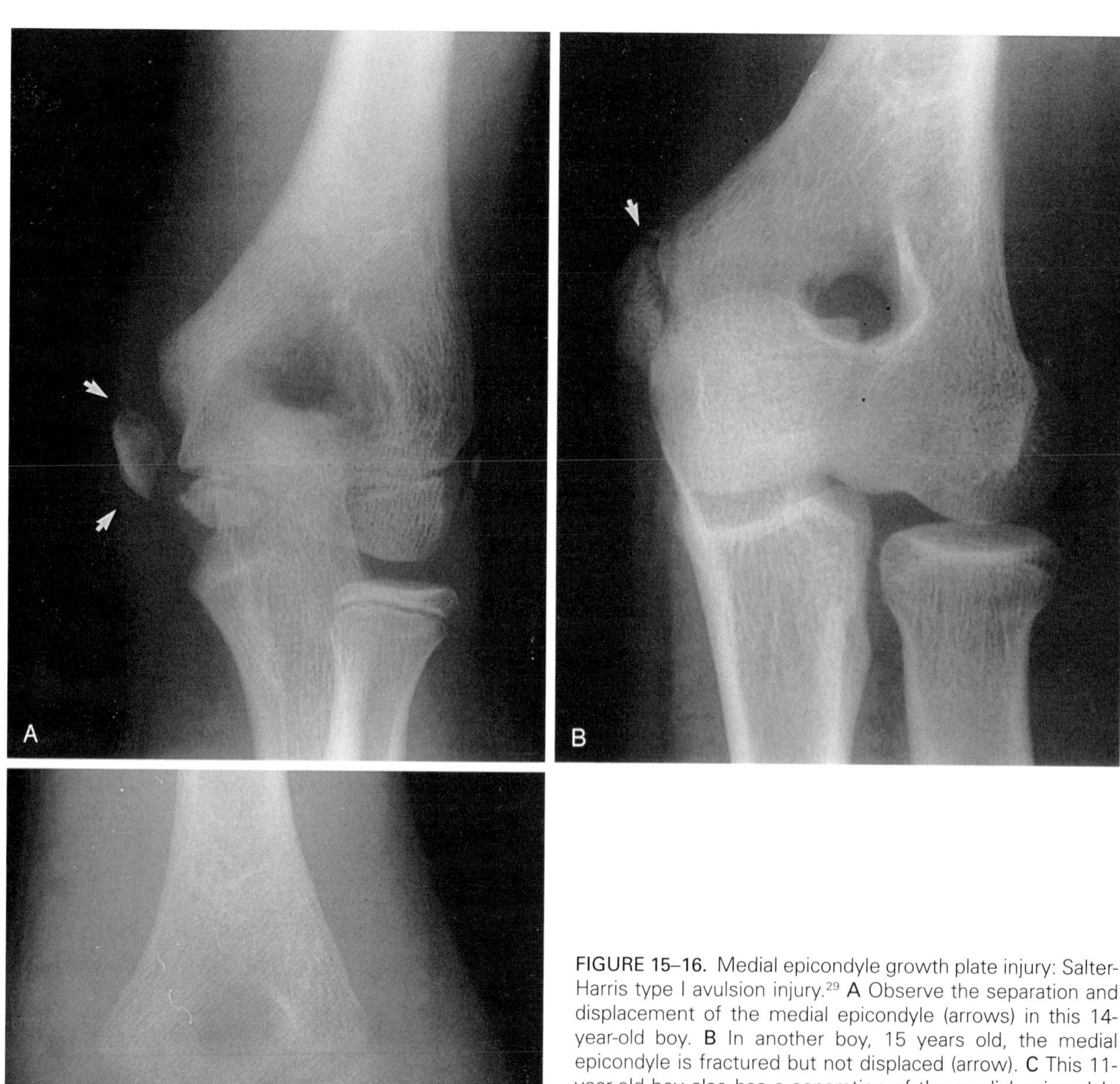

FIGURE 15–16. Medial epicondyle growth plate injury: Salter-Harris type I avulsion injury.[29] A Observe the separation and displacement of the medial epicondyle (arrows) in this 14-year-old boy. B In another boy, 15 years old, the medial epicondyle is fractured but not displaced (arrow). C This 11-year-old boy also has a separation of the medial epicondyle with extensive soft tissue swelling. This injury typically occurs as a result of valgus stress and consequent avulsion of the medial epicondyle ossification center by the attachment of the flexor pronator muscle group and the ulnar collateral ligament. The epicondyle may be drawn into the joint, becoming entrapped.

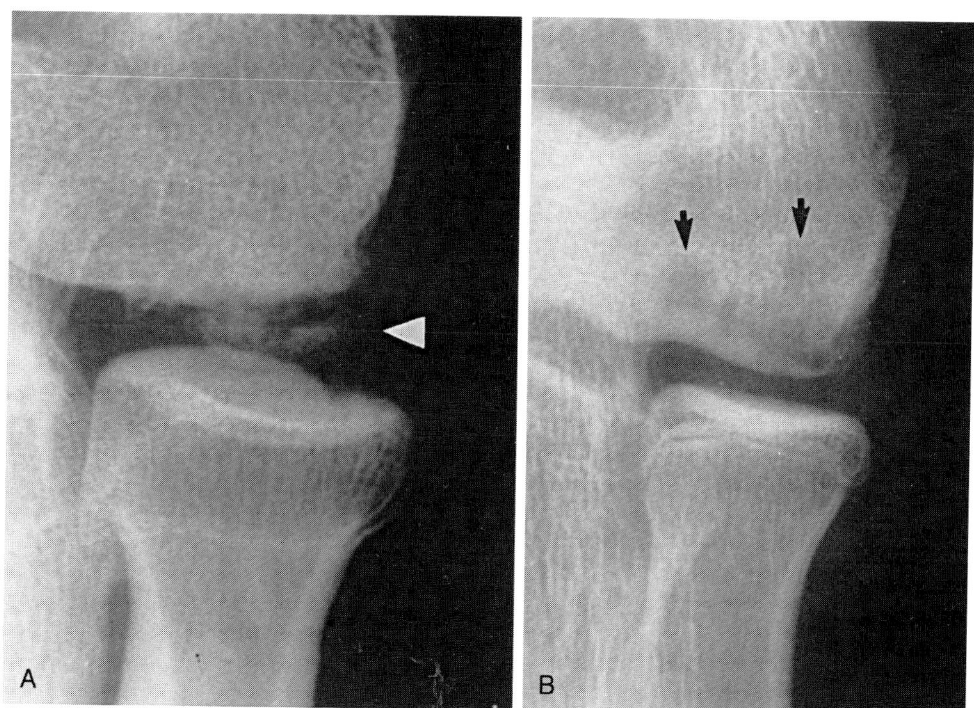

FIGURE 15–17. Osteochondritis dissecans: Capitulum.[31, 32] A This 29-year-old man had progressive elbow pain. Frontal radiograph shows an intra-articular fragment adjacent to the articular surface of the capitulum (arrowhead). *(A, Courtesy of V. Vint, M.D., San Diego, California.)* B In another patient, a 13-year-old high school football player, observe the radiolucent cyst-like lesions involving the subchondral surface of the capitulum (arrows). *(B, Courtesy of T. Mick, D.C., Bloomington, Minnesota.)* Although the radiographic appearance is similar, osteochondritis dissecans differs from Panner's disease in that Panner's disease occurs between the ages of 5 and 10 years, whereas osteochondritis dissecans occurs in adolescents and adults after ossification and fusion of the capitulum.

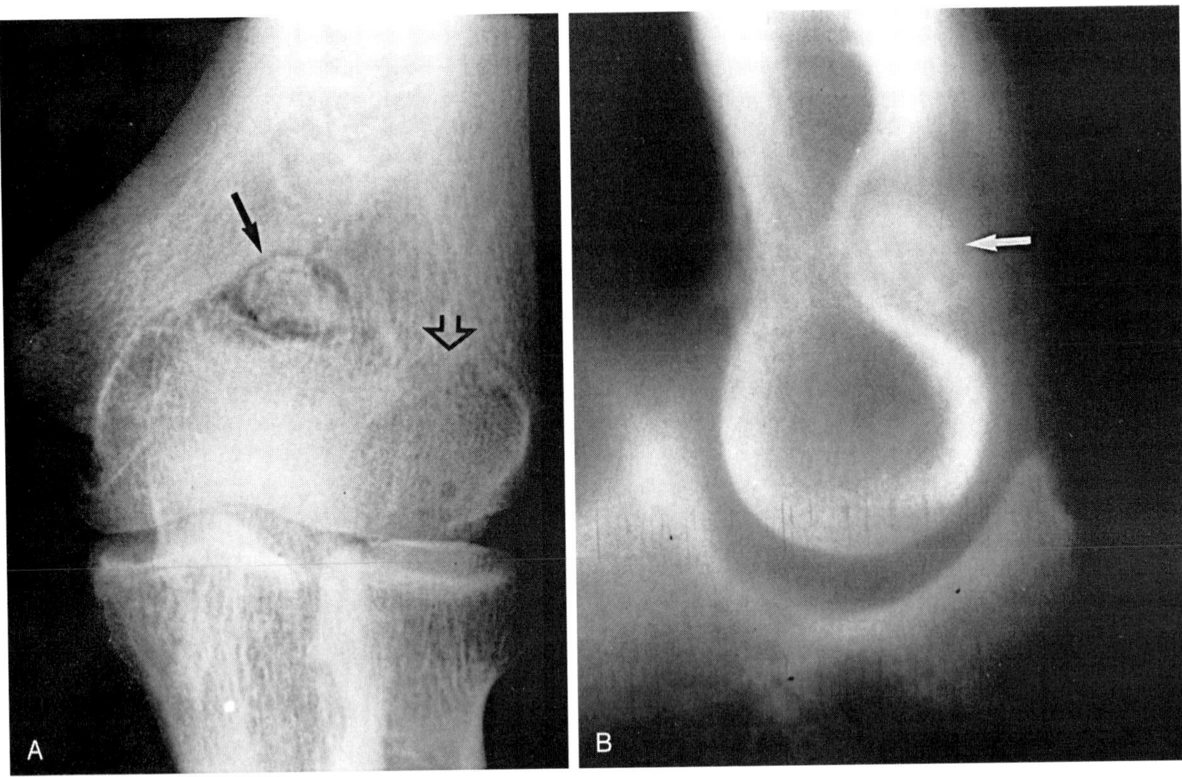

FIGURE 15–18. Osteochondral fracture: intra-articular osteochondral body.[31,32] This 20-year-old man with previous trauma noticed decreased range of motion in his elbow. A Routine frontal radiograph demonstrates an ovoid osseous body overlying the olecranon and coronoid fossae (arrow). The subchondral region of the capitulum appears somewhat radiolucent (open arrow). B Lateral conventional tomogram clearly reveals an osseous body deep within the olecranon fossa (arrow). Subsequent arthrotomy revealed loss of cartilage on the capitulum and radial head. Osteochondral bodies within the coronoid or olecranon fossa often are difficult to visualize on routine lateral radiographs owing to superimposed overlying structures. *(Courtesy of G. Greenway, M.D., Dallas, Texas.)*

TABLE 15–5. Soft Tissue Injuries About the Elbow*

Entity	Figure(s)	Characteristics
Ligamentous injuries		
Medial elbow instability[33]	15–19	Injury of the medial collateral ligament Single acute injury or repetitive injuries such as those encountered in baseball pitchers May also result in muscle tears, avulsion fractures, and ulnar nerve damage Valgus stress radiography useful in revealing ligament injury; arthrography and magnetic resonance (MR) imaging also useful Degenerative changes develop in chronic elbow instability
Lateral elbow instability[34]		Injury to the lateral collateral ligament complex Acute varus stress resulting in elbow dislocation is the most frequent cause of lateral elbow instability Repetitive injuries such as in throwing activities, not as frequent as acute injury Other causes: elbow subluxations, surgical injury MR imaging useful
Tendon injuries		Intratendinous tear: partial or complete Avulsion injuries may occur at the site of tendon attachment to bone Chronic injuries (overuse syndromes) usually result from sporting activities Acute injuries Spontaneous tendon ruptures may occur in patients with hyperparathyroidism, systemic lupus erythematosus, rheumatoid arthritis, and osteogenesis imperfecta MR imaging most useful in evaluating such injuries

TABLE 15–5. Soft Tissue Injuries About the Elbow* *Continued*

Entity	Figure(s)	Characteristics
Lateral tendons (lateral epicondylitis)[35]	15–20	Common extensor tendon injuries Lateral epicondylitis more common than acute injury—most common injury of the elbow in athletes Backhand stroke in tennis; wrist maintained in extension and radial deviation (tennis elbow) Radiographic changes: calcification in as many as 30 per cent of cases MR imaging may be helpful in diagnosis
Medial tendons (medial epicondylitis)[36]		Common flexor tendon injuries Medial epicondylitis more common than acute injury Medial epicondylitis also termed medial tennis elbow, golfer's elbow, or pitcher's elbow Also occurs in javelin throwers, racquetball and squash players, swimmers, and bowlers MR imaging useful in evaluation
Anterolateral tendons[37]	15–21	Injuries of the distal end of the biceps brachii tendon Fewer than 5 per cent of all biceps tendon injuries Single acute event may rupture biceps tendon or result in avulsion at the radial tuberosity Weightlifters: forceful hyperextension applied to a flexed and supinated forearm Partial tears more difficult to diagnose than complete tears
Posterior tendons[38]		Triceps brachii tendon injuries Uncommon injury Complete tears > partial tears Single acute event may rupture triceps tendon or result in avulsion of the olecranon process of the ulna *Mechanism:* Deceleration force applied to extended arm with contraction of triceps (as in a fall) Direct blow to attachment at olecranon process (infrequent injury)

*See also Table 1–5.

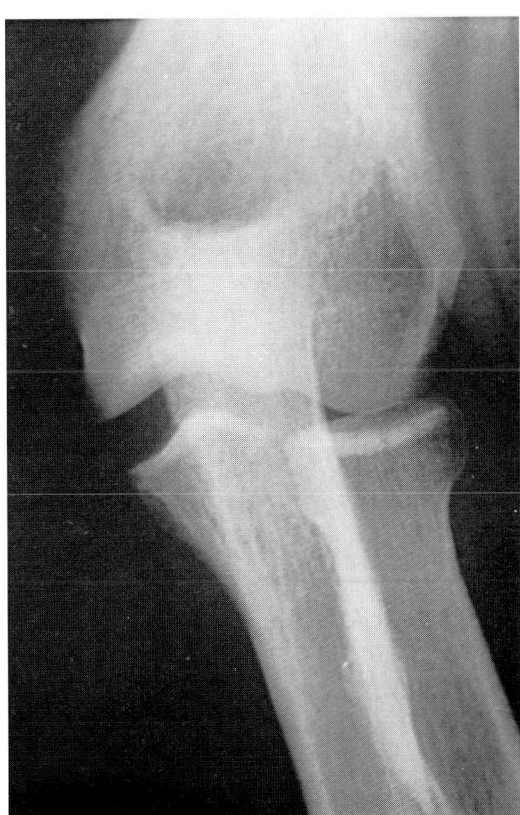

FIGURE 15–19. Medial elbow instability: Stress radiograph.[33] Radiograph obtained during the application of valgus stress to a partially flexed elbow reveals widening of the medial aspect of the joint, indicative of injury to the medial collateral ligament. *(From Resnick D, Kang HS: Internal Derangements of Joints. Philadelphia, WB Saunders, 1997, p 355.)*

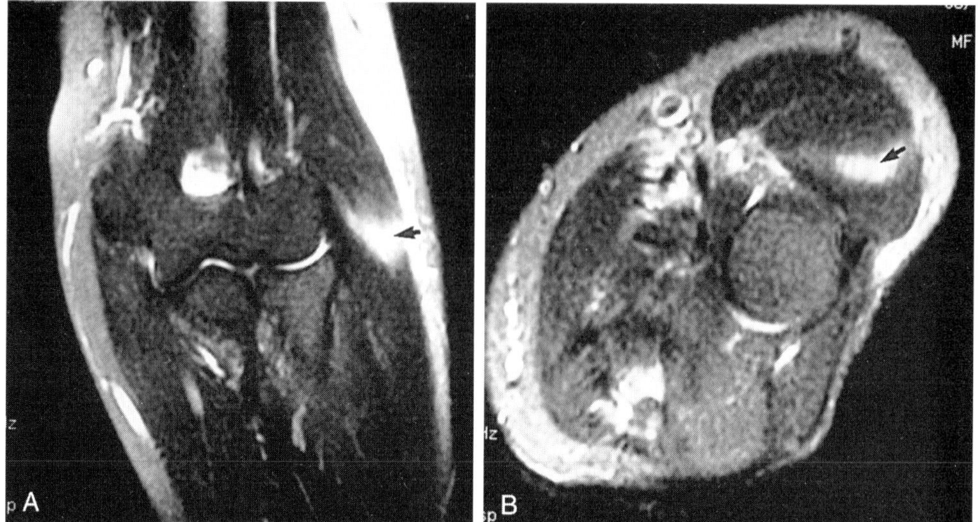

FIGURE 15–20. Lateral epicondylitis: Tears of the extensor carpi radialis brevis tendon and muscle.[35] These coronal (TR/TE, 3000/100) **(A)** and transaxial (TR/TE, 3000/90) **(B)** fat-suppressed fast spin echo magnetic resonance (MR) images in a patient with tennis elbow show the site of injury (arrows) as a region of high signal intensity. *(From Resnick D, Kang HS: Internal Derangements of Joints. Philadelphia, WB Saunders, 1997, p 366.)*

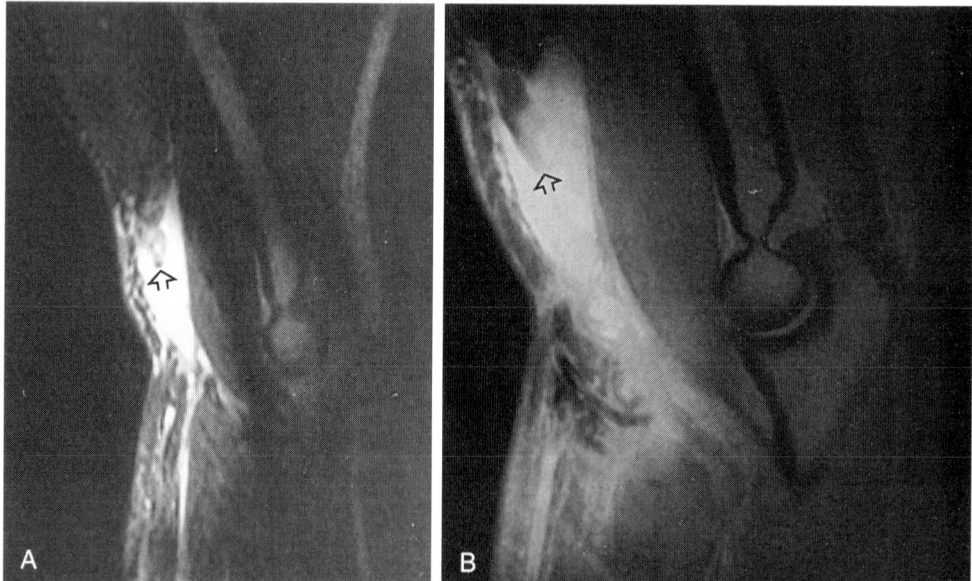

FIGURE 15–21. Biceps brachii tendon: Tear of the distal end.[37] Complete rupture at distal insertion site in a 44-year-old man is evident. Sagittal STIR (GR/TE, 3000/38; inversion time, 150 ms) **(A)** and fat-suppressed fast spin echo (TR/TE, 3300/17) **(B)** MR images reveal the retracted tendon (open arrows) and high signal intensity characteristic of soft tissue edema and hemorrhage. *(From Resnick D, Kang HS: Internal Derangements of Joints. Philadelphia, WB Saunders, 1997, p 362.)*

TABLE 15–6. Articular Disorders Affecting the Elbow

Entity	Figure(s)	Characteristics
Degenerative and related disorders		
Osteoarthrosis[39]	15–22	Primary osteoarthrosis of the elbow occurs only infrequently Usually secondary to local trauma or disease processes, such as alkaptonuria, acromegaly, epiphyseal dysplasia, crystal deposition diseases, and hemophilia *Radiographic findings:* Osteophytes Subchondral sclerosis Subchondral cysts Occasional intra-articular osteochondral bodies
Diffuse idiopathic skeletal hyperostosis (DISH)[40]	15–23	Olecranon enthesophytes present in 48 per cent of patients with DISH Hyperostosis along medial aspect of distal portion of the humerus
Inflammatory disorders		
Rheumatoid arthritis[41]	15–24	Bilateral symmetric, concentric joint space narrowing Marginal subchondral erosions Cystic changes Mild sclerosis of apposing joint surfaces
Juvenile chronic arthritis[42]		Diffuse concentric joint space narrowing Periarticular osteoporosis Erosions Subluxation
Ankylosing spondylitis[43, 44]	15–25	Twelve per cent of patients with long-standing ankylosing spondylitis have elbow joint involvement Bilateral or unilateral distribution Joint effusion Osteoporosis Diffuse joint space narrowing Osseous proliferation
Psoriatic arthropathy[44]		Elbow involvement rare Findings range from minor erosions to severe osteolysis
Scleroderma (progressive systemic sclerosis)[45]	15–26	Globular accumulations of periarticular soft tissue calcinosis Extensive osseous resorption may occur
Crystal deposition and metabolic disorders		
Gouty arthropathy[46]	15–27	Bilateral soft tissue swelling over the extensor surface of elbow—bursal inflammation Marginal and eccentric erosions and cyst-like lesions Osseous proliferation occasionally seen
Calcium pyrophosphate dihydrate (CPPD) crystal deposition[47, 48]	15–28	Chondrocalcinosis: capsular, tendinous, and triceps tendon deposits Joint space narrowing, subchondral sclerosis, cysts, and osteophytes Osseous resorption of proximal portions of radius and ulna Advanced destruction and fragmentation may resemble neuropathic osteoarthropathy in severe cases
Infectious disorders		
Pyogenic septic arthritis and bursitis[49]	15–29	Surgery, penetrating injury, immunosuppression, and debilitating illness, such as diabetes mellitus, all predispose to joint infection *Radiographic findings:* Rapid concentric loss of joint space Poorly defined or "fuzzy" subchondral bone margins Periarticular osteoporosis Loss of definition and destruction of subchondral bone Capsular distention Erosions Osteomyelitis of adjacent metaphyses
Tuberculous arthritis[50]		Typically monoarticular disease in older patients Various degrees of soft tissue swelling Gradual joint space narrowing Juxta-articular osteoporosis Peripherally located erosions Subchondral erosions Periarticular abscess Periostitis Olecranon bursitis may occur

Table continued on following page

TABLE 15–6. Articular Disorders Affecting the Elbow *Continued*

Entity	Figure(s)	Characteristics
Miscellaneous disorders		
Pigmented villonodular synovitis[51, 52]		Cystic erosions on both sides of the joint Hemorrhagic joint effusion Eventual osteoporosis Well-preserved joint space until late in the disease Extra-articular form is termed giant cell tumor of the tendon sheath
Idiopathic synovial osteochondromatosis[53, 54]	15–30	Multiple intra-articular or periarticular collections of calcification of variable size and density Monoarticular process Erosion of adjacent bones may occur Secondary osteoarthrosis common Noncalcified bodies within the coronoid and olecranon fossae are best demonstrated with arthrography Secondary synovial osteochondromatosis may occur as a result of degenerative joint disease
Acromegalic arthropathy[55]		Abnormal cartilage proliferation results in secondary osteoarthrosis Joint space: widening in initial stages, narrowing in advanced stages Sclerosis, osseous fragmentation, and osteophytes
Hemophilic arthropathy[56]	15–31	Elbow joint involvement is frequent in hemophilia Secondary osteoarthrosis, osteoporosis, epiphyseal enlargement, joint space narrowing, and subchondral erosion, sclerosis, and cyst formation Trochlear and radial notches may be widened from erosion, and the radial head may be enlarged as a result of epiphyseal overgrowth
Neuropathic osteoarthropathy[57]	15–32	As many as 25 per cent of patients with syringomyelia of the cervical cord develop neuropathic osteoarthropathy of the joints of the upper extremity Fragmentation, sclerosis, cyst formation, dislocation, disorganization, and osseous debris

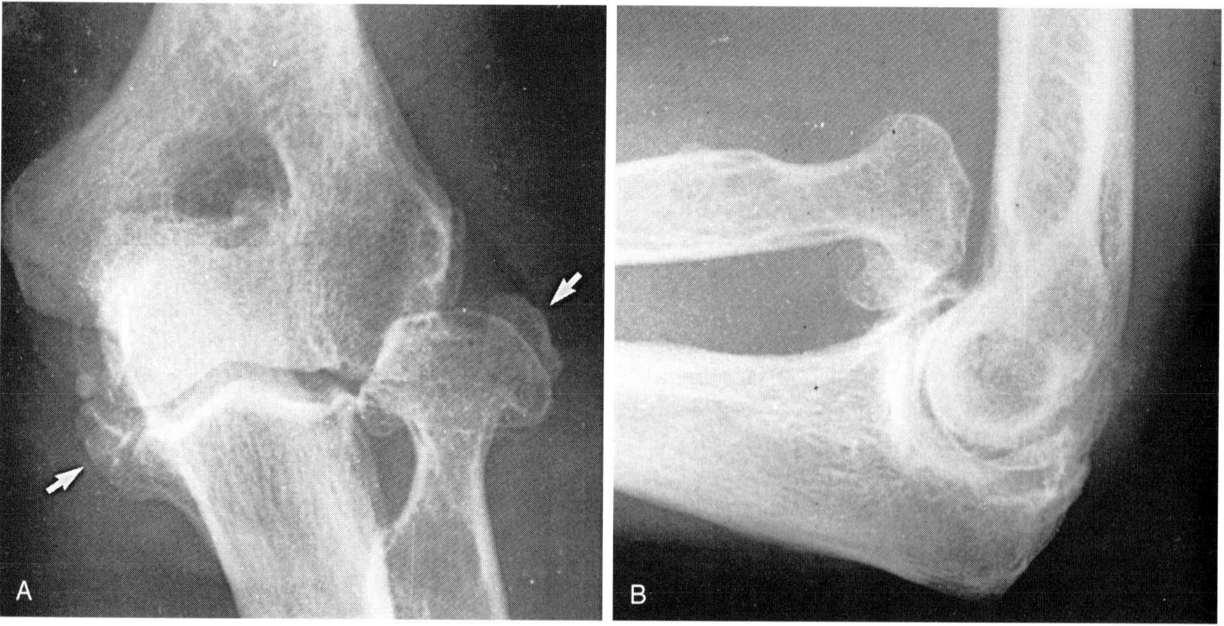

FIGURE 15–22. Osteoarthrosis.[39] This patient with a previous fracture and dislocation of the radial head had frontal (A) and lateral (B) radiographs of the elbow. They demonstrate nonuniform loss of joint space, radial head dislocation, and presence of osteophytes and intra-articular osseous bodies (arrows). Degenerative joint disease of the elbow is uncommon and usually is secondary to previous occupational or accidental trauma.

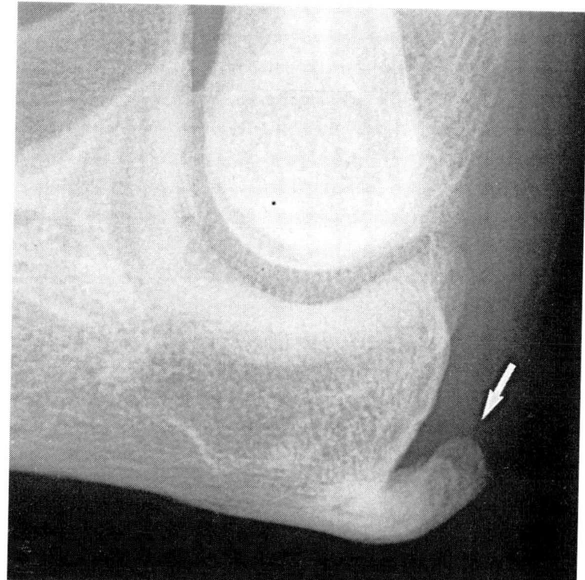

FIGURE 15–23. Diffuse idiopathic skeletal hyperostosis (DISH).[40] A prominent enthesophyte arises from the olecranon process (arrow) in this patient with DISH. The site of attachment of the triceps tendon is the characteristic location of enthesopathy in this disease, which occurs in about 48 per cent of persons with DISH.

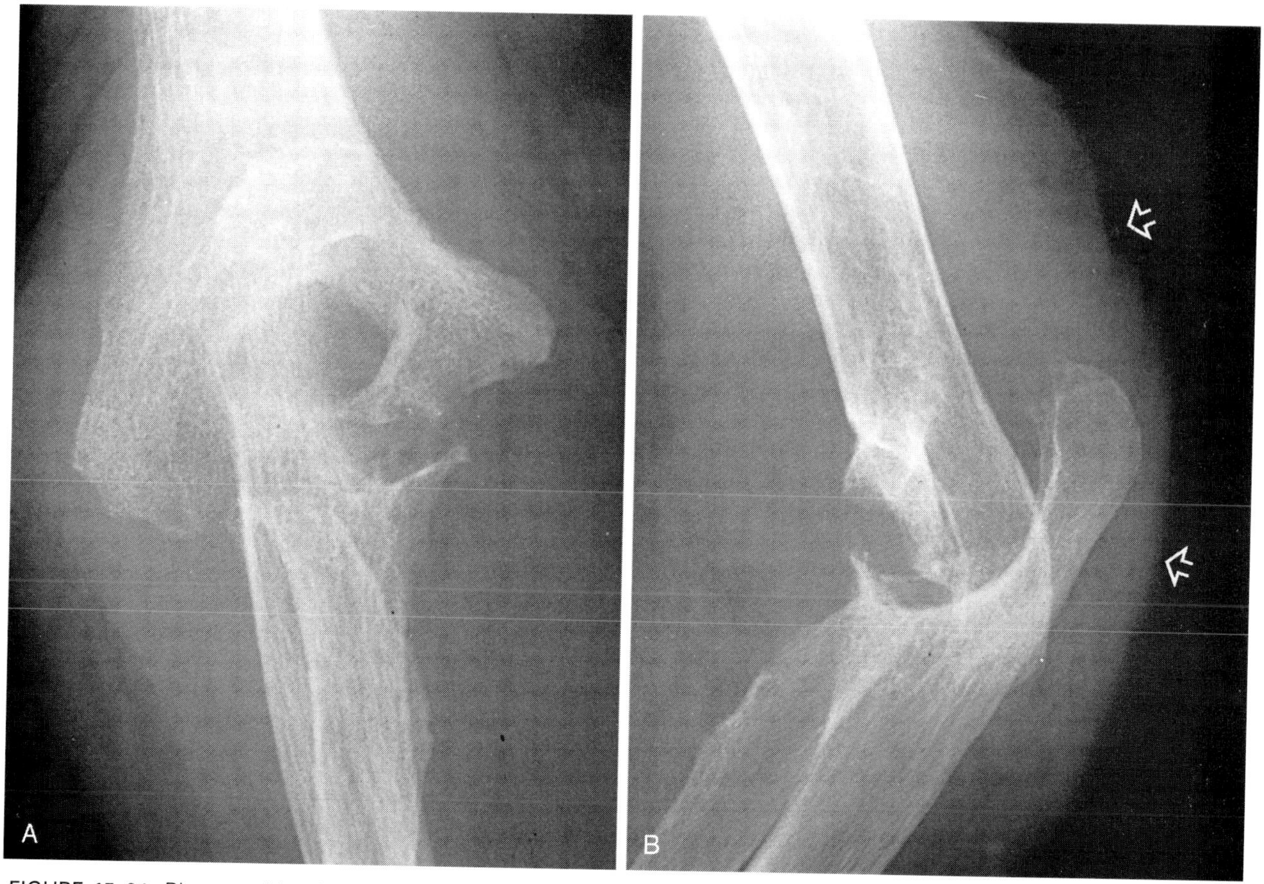

FIGURE 15–24. Rheumatoid arthritis.[41] A 55-year-old woman with a 20-year history of rheumatoid arthritis had severe elbow pain and swelling after twisting her arm. Frontal (A) and lateral (B) radiographs reveal marked erosive changes of the distal end of the humerus, olecranon, and radial head. Marked osteopenia is present, and there is no evidence of osteophyte formation. A large soft tissue prominence over the dorsal surface of the olecranon (open arrows) was proved by arthrography to be a synovial cyst. Culture of aspirated joint fluid yielded no evidence of infectious organisms. The elbow is involved in approximately 34 per cent of patients with long-standing rheumatoid arthritis. Involvement usually is bilateral, but the process may be more advanced in the dominant extremity.

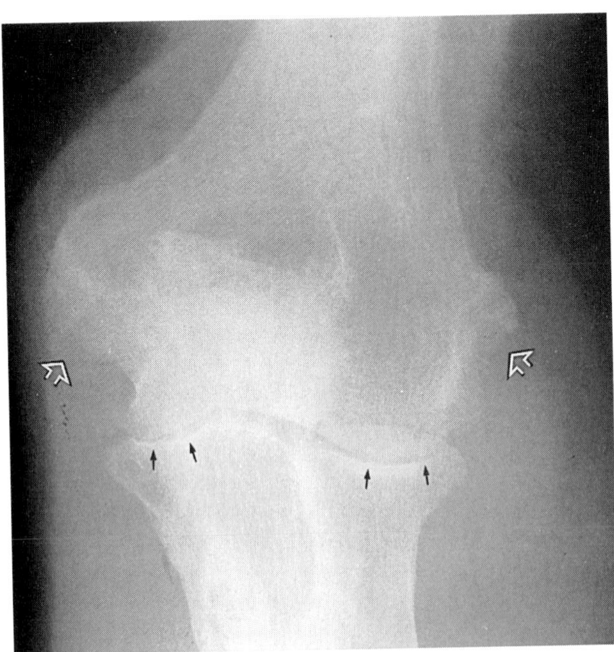

FIGURE 15–25. Ankylosing spondylitis.[43, 44] Anteroposterior radiograph of the elbow of this 55-year-old man with severe ankylosing spondylitis reveals diffuse joint space narrowing (arrows) and fluffy periarticular periostitis (open arrows). Elbow joint involvement occurs in only 12 per cent of persons with long-standing ankylosing spondylitis.

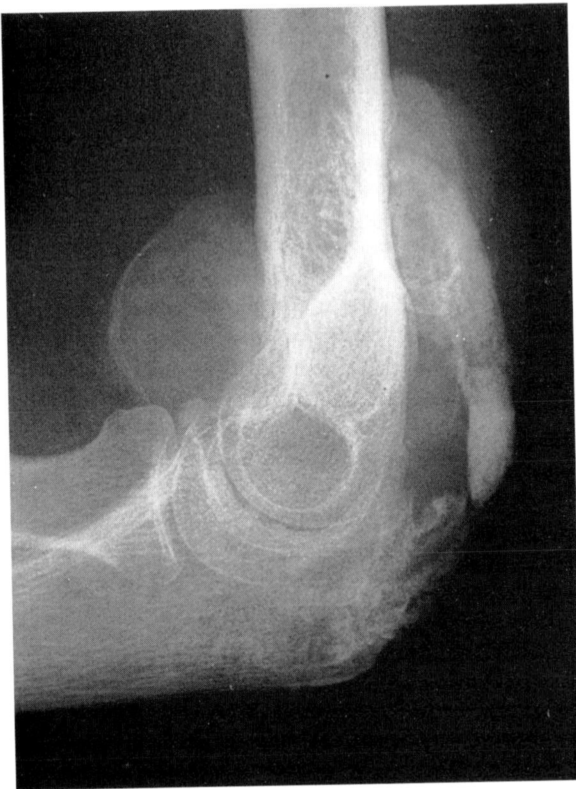

FIGURE 15–26. Scleroderma (progressive systemic sclerosis).[45] Prominent periarticular (and possibly intra-articular) calcinosis is seen in this patient with long-standing scleroderma. *(Courtesy of V. Vint, M.D., San Diego, California.)*

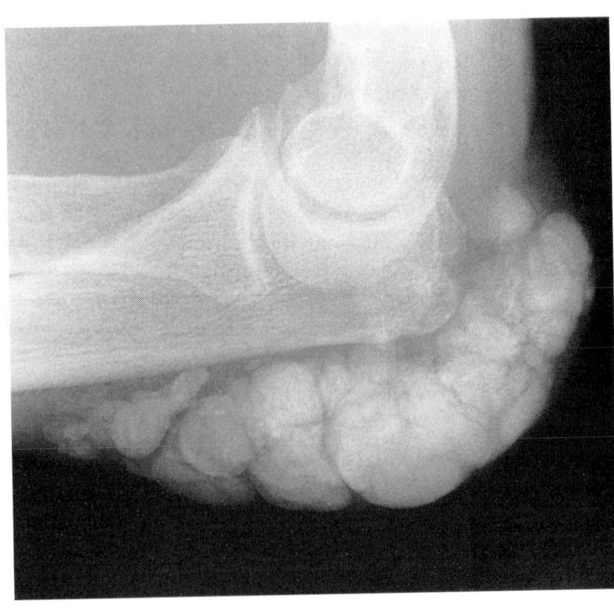

FIGURE 15–27. Gouty arthropathy.[46] Lateral radiograph of this 58-year-old man with long-standing gout and chronic renal disease reveals a large nodular collection of soft tissue calcification about the extensor surface of the olecranon. The calcification may represent tophi from gout or, alternatively, it may represent calcium hydroxyapatite deposition secondary to chronic renal disease.

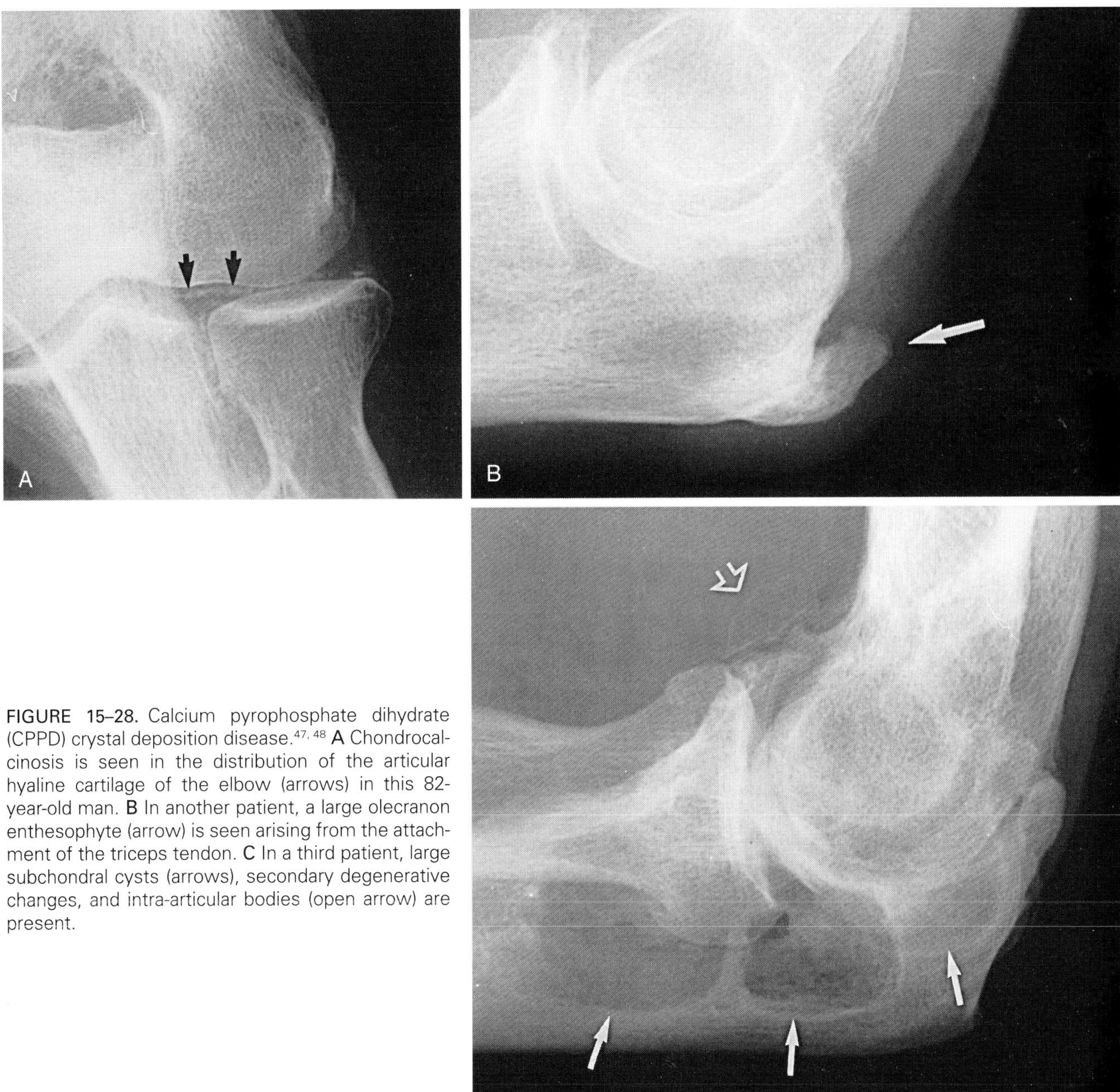

FIGURE 15–28. Calcium pyrophosphate dihydrate (CPPD) crystal deposition disease.[47, 48] A Chondrocalcinosis is seen in the distribution of the articular hyaline cartilage of the elbow (arrows) in this 82-year-old man. B In another patient, a large olecranon enthesophyte (arrow) is seen arising from the attachment of the triceps tendon. C In a third patient, large subchondral cysts (arrows), secondary degenerative changes, and intra-articular bodies (open arrow) are present.

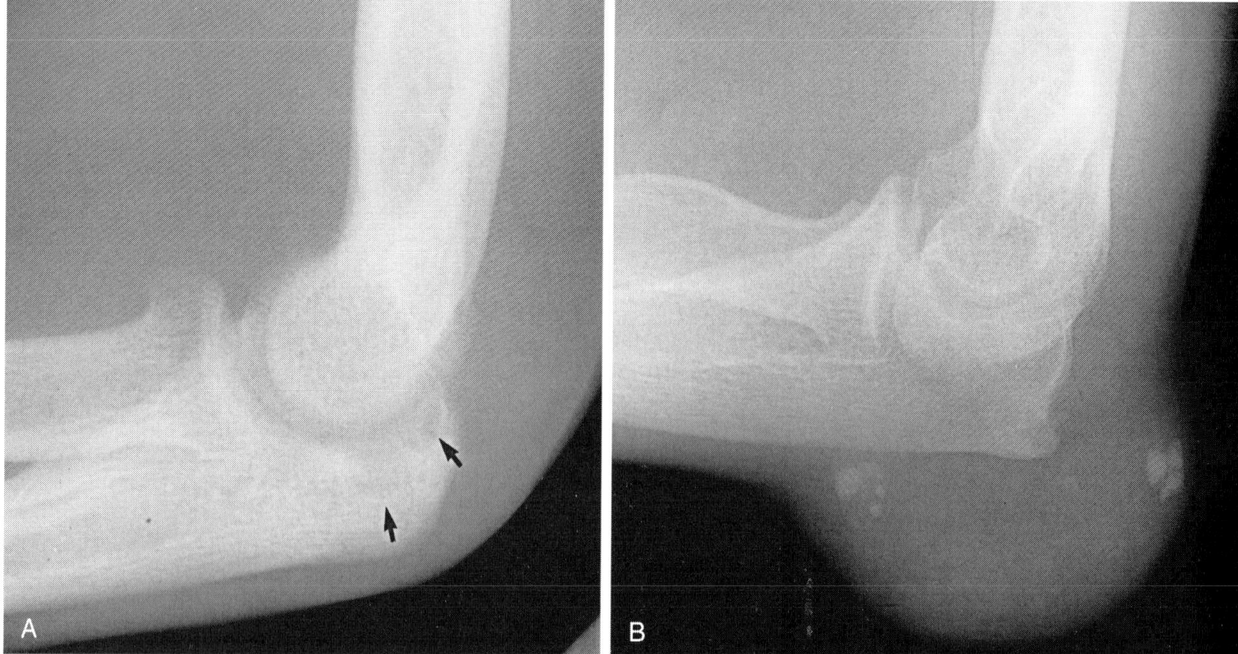

FIGURE 15–29. Pyogenic septic arthritis and bursitis.[49] A Septic arthritis: *Pseudomonas* infection. This 21-year-old man had pain and swelling over the elbow for 3 months. Routine radiograph reveals indistinct subchondral bone margins, joint space narrowing, and erosions (arrows). The joint was infected by *Pseudomonas,* presumably via hematogenous spread. B Septic bursitis. Observe the massive soft tissue swelling and soft tissue edema caused by *Staphylococcus aureus* infection of the subcutaneous olecranon bursa (olecranon bursitis). Areas of calcification are present within the bursa.

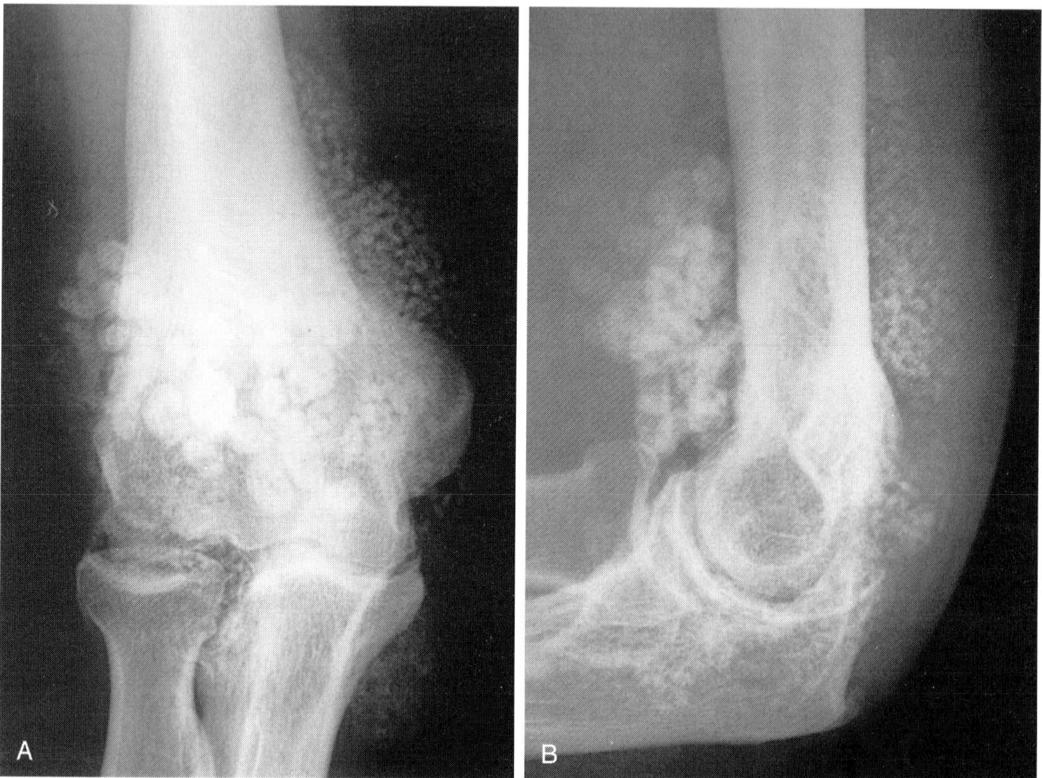

FIGURE 15–30. Idiopathic synovial osteochondromatosis.[53, 54] Frontal (A) and lateral (B) radiographs reveal multiple juxta-articular radiodense osteocartilaginous bodies within the synovial cavity of the elbow. Idiopathic synovial osteochondromatosis represents metaplastic or neoplastic proliferation of cartilaginous bodies by the synovial membrane. Secondary synovial osteochondromatosis also may occur as a result of degenerative joint disease. Noncalcified lesions are best evaluated with arthrography.

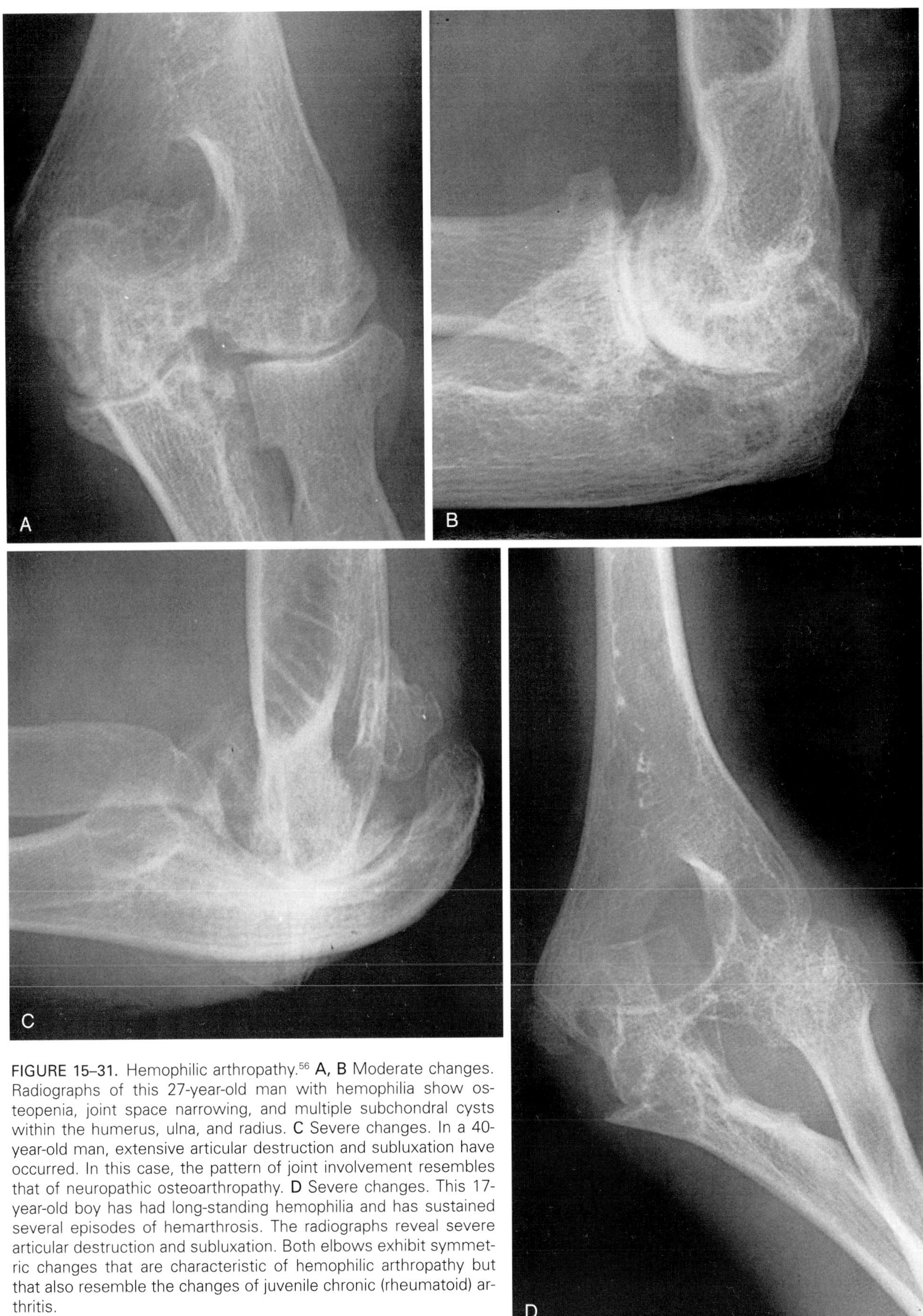

FIGURE 15–31. Hemophilic arthropathy.[56] A, B Moderate changes. Radiographs of this 27-year-old man with hemophilia show osteopenia, joint space narrowing, and multiple subchondral cysts within the humerus, ulna, and radius. C Severe changes. In a 40-year-old man, extensive articular destruction and subluxation have occurred. In this case, the pattern of joint involvement resembles that of neuropathic osteoarthropathy. D Severe changes. This 17-year-old boy has had long-standing hemophilia and has sustained several episodes of hemarthrosis. The radiographs reveal severe articular destruction and subluxation. Both elbows exhibit symmetric changes that are characteristic of hemophilic arthropathy but that also resemble the changes of juvenile chronic (rheumatoid) arthritis.

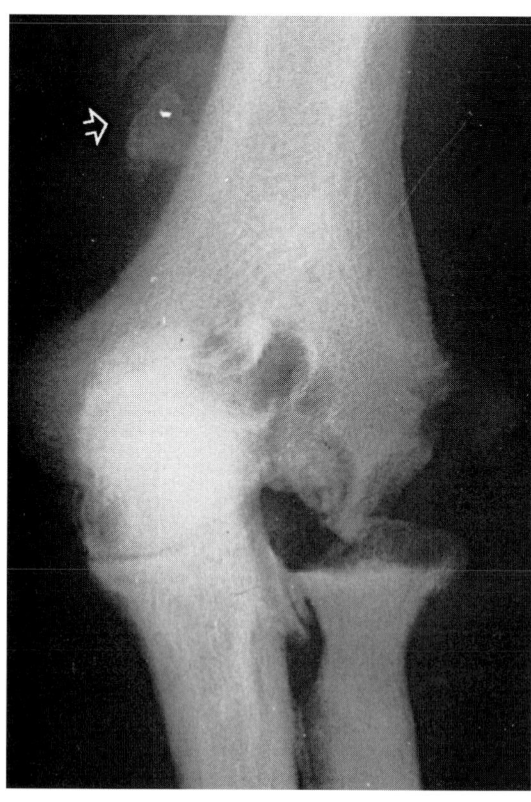

FIGURE 15–32. Neuropathic osteoarthropathy: syringomyelia.[57] Observe the extensive destruction of the capitulum, lateral epicondyle, and radial head in this patient with a cervical cord syrinx. Osseous debris also is evident (open arrow).

TABLE 15–7. Metabolic, Hematologic, and Infectious Disorders Affecting the Elbow

Disorder	Figure(s)	Characteristics
Rickets[58]		Prominent findings of the metaphyses about the elbow in patients with long-standing rickets Metaphyseal demineralization: frayed, widened, cupped metaphyses Bowing of bones Osteopenia
Hyperparathyroidism and renal osteodystrophy[59–62]	15–27	Occasional bone sclerosis (more common with renal osteodystrophy) Chondrocalcinosis (calcium pyrophosphate dihydrate [CPPD] crystal deposition) Brown tumors Soft tissue calcification Pathologic fracture
Heterotopic ossification: Brain injury[63]	15–33	Brain and spinal cord injury (as in burns, mechanical trauma, and venous stasis) may result in heterotopic ossification about the elbow and other major joints Osseous deposits typically begin as poorly defined opaque areas appearing 2 to 6 months after the injury and progress to large radiodense lesions possessing trabeculae May eventually result in complete ankylosis of the joint
Osteonecrosis: Panner's disease[64]	15–34	Osteonecrosis or altered sequence of ossification involving the capitulum of the humerus Occurs between the ages of 5 and 10 years, especially in gymnasts and baseball players Boys > girls Increased radiodensity, often with a peripheral zone of subchondral radiolucency Fragmentation and collapse of capitulum may result Complete regeneration and reconstitution of capitulum typically occurs without residual deformity or disability Radiographic appearance may resemble that of osteochondritis dissecans and osteochondral fracture

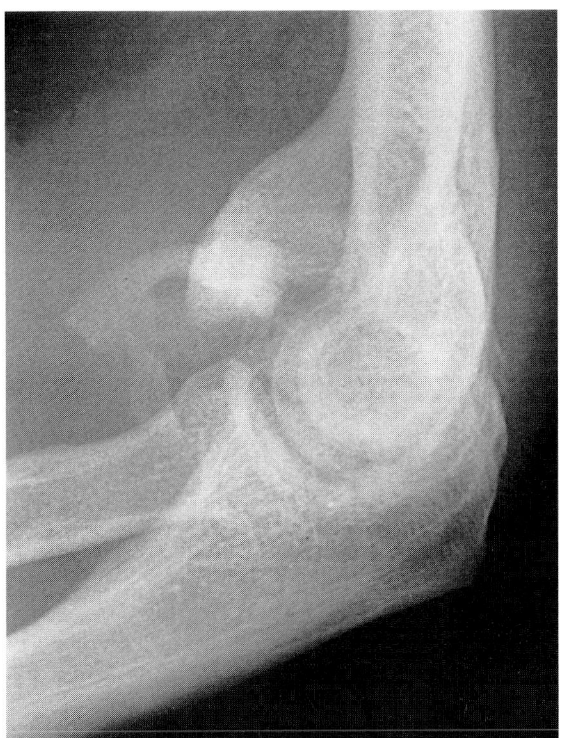

FIGURE 15–33. Heterotopic ossification.[63] This 43-year-old man sustained a head injury and was comatose for 3 days. Observe the extensive ossification surrounding the elbow joint. Such ossification may eventually result in complete osseous ankylosis. The ossification often involves several joints and may resemble the changes of fibrodysplasia ossificans progressiva.

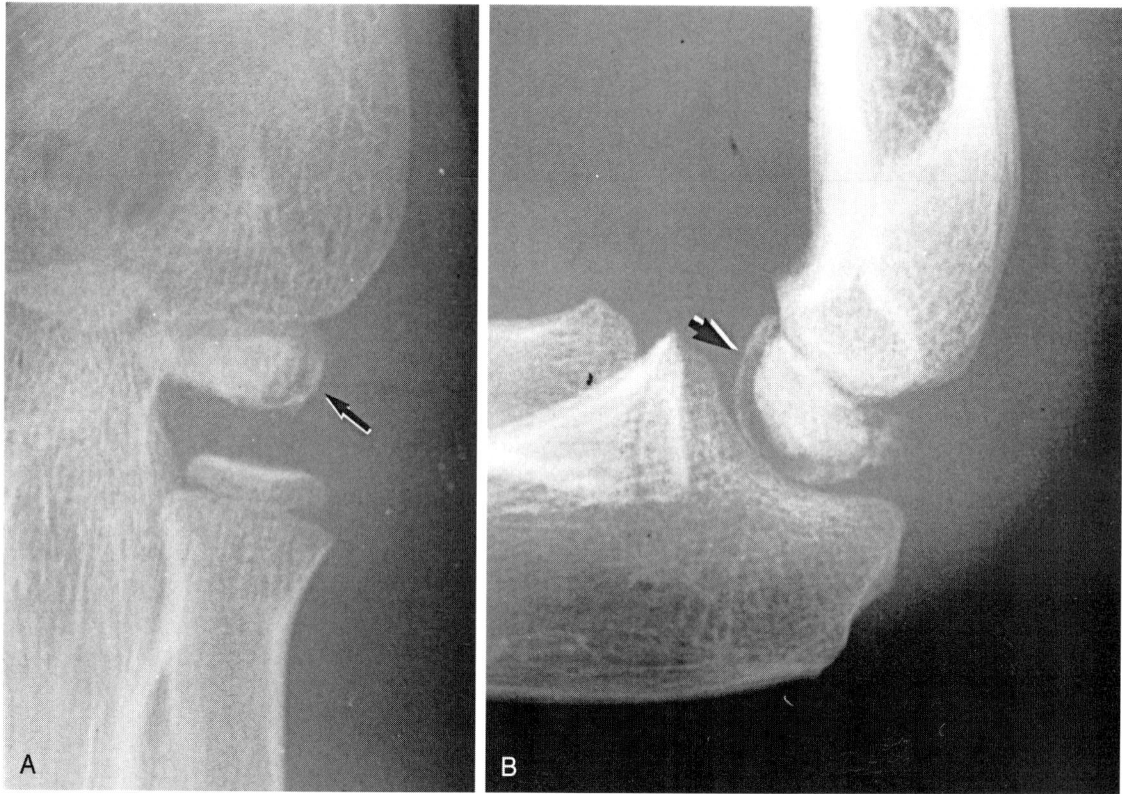

FIGURE 15–34. Panner's disease.[64] Frontal (A) and lateral (B) radiographs of this 7-year-old boy with elbow pain and stiffness reveal a linear region of subchondral radiolucency and diffuse increased radiodensity involving the capitulum (arrows). This osteonecrosis of the capitulum occurs in the juvenile epiphysis, typically between the ages of 5 and 10 years, and is more common in boys, especially baseball players and gymnasts. *(Courtesy of E. Bosch, M.D., Santiago, Chile.)* (B, *From Resnick D, Kang HS: Internal Derangements of Joints. Philadelphia, WB Saunders, 1997, p 372.)*

REFERENCES

1. Brodeur AE, Silberstein MJ, Graviss ER, et al: The basic tenets for appropriate evaluation of the elbow in pediatrics. Curr Probl Diagn Radiol 12:1, 1983.
2. Edeiken J, Dalinka M, Karasick D: Edeiken's Roentgen Diagnosis of Diseases of Bone. 4th Ed. Baltimore, Williams & Wilkins, 1990.
3. Keats TE, Smith TH: An Atlas of Normal Developmental Roentgen Anatomy. 2nd Ed. Chicago, Year Book, 1988.
4. Greenfield GB: Radiology of Bone Diseases. 2nd Ed. Philadelphia, JB Lippincott, 1975.
5. Silberstein MJ, Brodeur AE, Graviss ER: Some vagaries of the radial head and neck. J Bone Joint Surg [Am] 64:1153, 1982.
6. Greenspan A, Norman A: Radial head–capitellum view: An expanded imaging approach to elbow injury. Radiology 164:272, 1987.
7. Köhler A, Zimmer EA: Borderlands of Normal and Early Pathologic Findings in Skeletal Radiography. 4th Ed. New York, Thieme Medical Publishers, 1993.
8. Keats TE: Atlas of Normal Roentgen Variants That May Simulate Disease, 6th Ed. Chicago, Year Book, 1996.
9. Resnick D, Niwayama G: Osteoporosis. *In* Resnick D: Diagnosis of Bone and Joint Disorders. Philadelphia, WB Saunders, 1995, p 1837.
10. Yochum TR, Rowe LJ: Essentials of Skeletal Radiology. 2nd Ed. Baltimore, Williams & Wilkins, 1996.
11. Kattan KR, Babcock DS: Bilateral patella cubiti. Skeletal Radiol 4:249, 1979.
12. Mital MA: Congenital radioulnar synostosis and congenital dislocation of the radial head. Orthop Clin North Am 7:375, 1976.
13. Guidera KJ, Satterwhite Y, Ogden JA, et al: Nail patella syndrome: A review of 44 orthopaedic patients. J Pediatr Orthop 11:737, 1991.
14. Benli IT, Akalin S, Boysan E, et al: Epidemiological, clinical, and radiological aspects of osteopoikilosis. J Bone Joint Surg [Br] 74:504, 1992.
15. Bohrer SP: The fat pad sign following elbow trauma. Its usefulness and reliability in suspecting invisible fractures. Clin Radiol 21:90, 1970.
16. Murphy WA, Siegel MJ: Elbow fat pads with new signs and extended differential diagnosis. Radiology 124:659, 1977.
17. Donnelly LF, Klostermeier TT, Klosterman LA: Traumatic elbow effusions in pediatric patients: Are occult fractures the rule? AJR 171:243, 1998.
18. Floyd WE III, Gebhardt MC, Emans JB: Intra-articular entrapment of the median nerve after elbow dislocation in children. J Hand Surg [Am] 12:704, 1987.
19. Triantafyllou SJ, Wilson SC, Rychak JS: Irreducible pulled elbow in a child. A case report. Clin Orthop 284:153, 1992.
20. Ring D, Jupiter JB, Simpson NS: Monteggia fractures in adults. J Bone Joint Surg [Am] 80:1733, 1998.
21. Beltran J, Rosenberg ZS, Kawelblum M, et al: Pediatric elbow fractures: MRI evaluation. Skeletal Radiol 23:277, 1994.
22. Gabel GT, Hanson G, Bennett JB, et al: Intraarticular fractures of the distal humerus in the adult. Clin Orthop 216:99, 1987.
23. Schild H, Muller HA, Klose K: The halfmoon sign. Australas Radiol 26:273, 1982.
24. Horne JG, Tanzer TL: Olecranon fractures: A review of 100 cases. J Trauma 21:469, 1981.
25. Regan W, Morrey B: Fractures of the coronoid process of the ulna. J Bone Joint Surg [Am] 71:1348, 1989.
26. Bock GW, Cohen MS, Resnick D: Fracture-dislocation of the elbow with inferior radioulnar dissociation: A variant of the Essex-Lopresti injury. Skeletal Radiol 21:315, 1992.
27. Leventhal JM, Thomas SA, Rosenfield NS, et al: Fractures in young children: Distinguishing child abuse from unintentional injuries. Am J Dis Child 147:87, 1993.
28. Rogers LF, Poznanski AK: Imaging of epiphyseal injuries. Radiology 191:297, 1994.
29. De Jager LT, Hoffman EB: Fracture-separation of the distal humeral epiphysis. J Bone Joint Surg [Br] 73:143, 1991.
30. Daffner RH, Pavlov H: Stress fractures: Current concepts. AJR 159:245, 1992.
31. Bauer M, Jonsson K, Josefsson PO, et al: Osteochondritis dissecans of the elbow: A long term follow-up study. Clin Orthop 284:156, 1992.
32. Patten RM: Overuse syndromes and injuries involving the elbow: MR imaging findings. AJR 164:1205, 1995.
33. Mirowitz SA, London SL: Ulnar collateral ligament injury in baseball pitchers: MR imaging evaluation. Radiology 185:573, 1992.
34. Morrey BF, O'Driscoll SW: Lateral collateral ligament injury. *In* BF Morrey (ed): The Elbow and Its Disorders. 2nd Ed. Philadelphia, WB Saunders, 1993, p 573.
35. Caldwell GL Jr, Safran MR: Elbow problems in the athlete. Orthop Clin North Am 26:465, 1995.
36. Ho CP: Sports and occupational injuries of the elbow: MR imaging findings. AJR 164:1465, 1995.
37. Fitzgerald SW, Curry DR, Erickson SJ, et al: Distal biceps tendon injury: MR imaging diagnosis. Radiology 191:203, 1994.
38. Tiger E, Mayer DP, Glazer R: Complete avulsion of the triceps tendon: MRI diagnosis. Comput Med Imaging Graph 17:51, 1993.
39. Goodfellow JW, Bullough PG: The pattern of aging of the articular cartilage of the elbow joint. J Bone Joint Surg [Br] 49:175, 1967.
40. Beyeler CH, Schlapbach P, Gerber NJ, et al: Diffuse idiopathic skeletal hyperostosis (DISH) of the elbow: A cause of elbow pain? A controlled study. Br J Rheumatol 31:319, 1992.
41. Weston WJ: The synovial changes at the elbow in rheumatoid arthritis. Australas Radiol 15:170, 1971.
42. Reed MH, Wilmot DM: The radiology of juvenile rheumatoid arthritis: A review of the English language literature. J Rheumatol 18:2, 1991.
43. Resnick D: Patterns of peripheral joint disease in ankylosing spondylitis. Radiology 110:523, 1974.
44. Resnick D, Niwayama G: On the nature and significance of bony proliferation in "rheumatoid variant" disorders. AJR 129:275, 1977.
45. Czirjak L, Nagy Z, Szegedi G: Systemic sclerosis in the elderly. Clin Rheumatol 11:483, 1992.
46. Resnick D: Diagnosis of Bone and Joint Disorders. 3rd Ed. Philadelphia, WB Saunders, 1995, p 1511.
47. Resnick D, Niwayama G, Georgen TG, et al: Clinical, radiographic and pathologic abnormalities in calcium pyrophosphate dihydrate deposition disease (CPPD): Pseudogout. Radiology 122:1, 1977.
48. Steinbach LS, Resnick D: Calcium pyrophosphate dihydrate crystal deposition disease revisited. Radiology 200:1, 1996.
49. Ho G Jr, Mikolich DJ: Bacterial infection of superficial subcutaneous bursae. Clinics Rheum Dis 12:437, 1986.
50. Haygood TM, Williamson SL: Radiographic findings of extremity tuberculosis in childhood: Back to the future? RadioGraphics 14:561, 1994.

51. Schwartz HS, Unni KK, Pritchard DJ: Pigmented villonodular synovitis: A retrospective review of affected larger joints. Clin Orthop 247:243, 1989.
52. Hughes TH, Sartoris DJ, Schweitzer ME, et al: Pigmented villonodular synovitis: MRI characteristics. Skeletal Radiol 24:7, 1995.
53. Giustra PE, Furman RS, Roberts L, et al: Synovial chondromatosis involving the elbow. AJR 127:347, 1976.
54. Kramer J, Recht M, Deely DM, et al: MR appearance of idiopathic synovial osteochondromatosis. J Comput Assist Tomogr 17:772, 1993.
55. Melo-Gomes J, Viana-Queiroz M: Acromegalic arthropathy: A reversible rheumatic disease. J Rheumatol 14:393, 1987.
56. Hôgh J, Ludlam CA, Macnicol MF: Hemophilic arthropathy of the upper limb. Clin Orthop 218:225, 1987.
57. Resnik CS, Reed WW: Hand, wrist, and elbow arthropathy in syringomyelia. J Can Assoc Radiol 36:325, 1985.
58. Mankin HJ: Rickets, osteomalacia, and renal osteodystrophy. Orthop Clin North Am 21:81, 1990.
59. Wolfson BJ, Capitanio MA: The wide spectrum of renal osteodystrophy in children. CRC Crit Rev Diagn Imaging 27:297, 1987.
60. Resnick D, Niwayama G: Subchondral resorption of bone in renal osteodystrophy. Radiology 118:315, 1976.
61. Tigges S, Nance EP, Carpenter WA, et al: Renal osteodystrophy: Imaging findings that mimic those of other diseases. AJR 165:143, 1995.
62. Murphy MD, Sartoris DJ, Quale JL, et al: Musculoskeletal manifestations of chronic renal insufficiency. RadioGraphics 13:357, 1993.
63. Garland DE, Blum CE, Waters RL: Periarticular heterotopic ossification in head-injured adults: Incidence and location. J Bone Joint Surg [Am] 62:1143, 1980.
64. Bauer M, Jonsson K, Josefsson PO, et al: Osteochondritis dissecans of the elbow: A long term follow-up study. Clin Orthop 284:156, 1992.

CHAPTER 16

Radius and Ulna

- Developmental Anomalies, Anatomic Variants, Sources of Diagnostic Error, and Dysplasias
- Physical Injury
- Bone Tumors
- Metabolic, Hematologic, and Infectious Disorders

Developmental Anomalies, Anatomic Variants, Sources of Diagnostic Error, and Dysplasias

The most common developmental anomalies, anatomic variants, sources of diagnostic error, and skeletal dysplasias involving the radius and ulna are listed in Table 16–1. Figures 16–1 to 16–4 represent selected examples.

Physical Injury

Fractures and other physical injuries to the radius and ulna are described in Tables 16–2 and 16–3. These injuries are illustrated in Figures 16–5 to 16–15. Injuries to the proximal portions of the radius and ulna are discussed in Chapter 15, and injuries of the wrist are discussed in Chapter 17.

Bone Tumors

The radius and ulna are infrequent sites of malignant and benign neoplasms and tumor-like processes. Table 16–4 lists the major characteristics of these disorders. Their radiographic manifestations are illustrated in Figures 16–16 to 16–27.

Metabolic, Hematologic, and Infectious Disorders

A wide variety of metabolic, hematologic, and infectious disorders may involve the bones of the forearm. Table 16–5 lists some of the more common disorders and describes their characteristics. Their radiographic features are illustrated in Figures 16–28 to 16–36. Further manifestations of these disorders within the proximal and distal portions of the radius and ulna are discussed in Chapters 15 and 17, respectively.

TABLE 16–1. Developmental Anomalies, Anatomic Variants, and Skeletal Dysplasias Affecting the Radius and Ulna

Disorder	Figure(s)	Characteristics
Radioulnar synostosis[1]	15–5	Anomalous osseous fusion of the proximal portions of the radius and ulna Bilateral in 60 per cent of patients Restricts normal forearm supination and pronation Additional anomalies may accompany radioulnar synostosis
Radiolucent radial tuberosity[2]	15–2F 16–1	Normal radiolucency of the cancellous bone within the radial tuberosity may simulate a destructive lesion or a cyst No clinical significance
Madelung's deformity[3]	16–2	*Radiographic findings* Radius: Dorsal and ulnar curvature; decreased length; triangular distal epiphysis owing to premature fusion of medial half of epiphysis; ulnar and volar angulation of distal radial articular surface Ulna: Elongated ulna with dorsal subluxation; enlargement and distortion of ulnar head Carpal bones: Wedging of carpal bones between deformed radius and protruding ulna; triangular configuration of carpals with lunate at apex Inferior radioulnar joint: Increased width of inferior radioulnar joint Radiocarpal joint: V-shaped; decreased carpal angle Several forms of Madelung's deformity have been identified: 1. Isolated, idiopathic form: females > males; bilateral > unilateral; asymmetric in severity 2. Dysplastic form: seen in association with multiple hereditary exostosis and dyschondrosteosis 3. Genetic form: seen with Turner's syndrome 4. Posttraumatic form: from an extension injury to the radial epiphysis
Positive ulnar variance (ulnar abutment or impaction syndrome)[4–6]	16–3	Increased length of ulna in relation to the radius Results in limitation of rotation, subsequent ligamentous relaxation of the wrist, and a thinner triangular fibrocartilage complex (TFCC) Ulnar abutment (impaction) syndrome refers to the consequent degeneration, TFCC perforation, and lunotriquetral interosseous ligament disruption
Negative ulnar variance (ulna minus variant)[7–9]	16–4	Decreased length of ulna in relation to the radius measured at the distal end Present in about 20 per cent of normal patients Association between negative ulnar variance and Kienböck's disease has been proposed, but the significance of the correlation remains controversial May result in prominent fossa within the radial surface of the inferior radioulnar articulation that may simulate focal destruction

See also Tables 1–1 and 1–2.

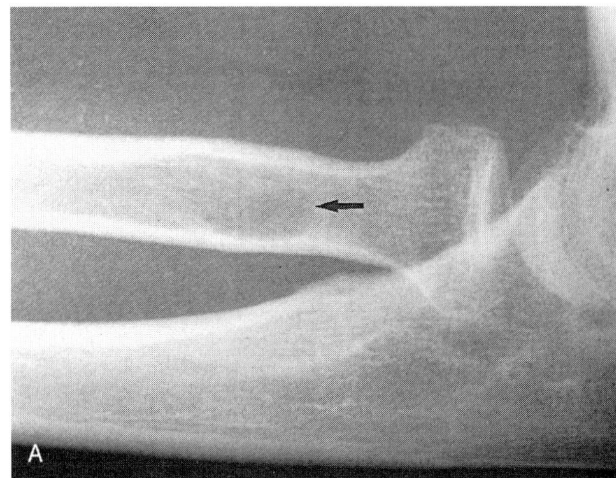

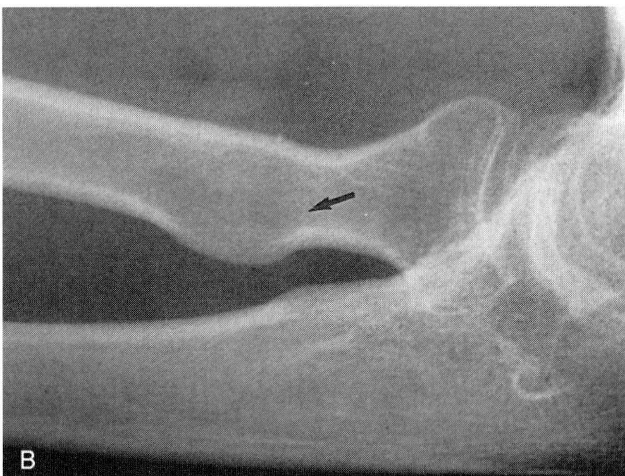

FIGURE 16–1. A, B Normal radiolucent radial tuberosity.[2] Two views of the proximal portion of the radius show an expansile radiolucent region representing the normal radial tuberosity (arrows). This appearance may mimic an osteolytic lesion, especially in the absence of a sclerotic margin.

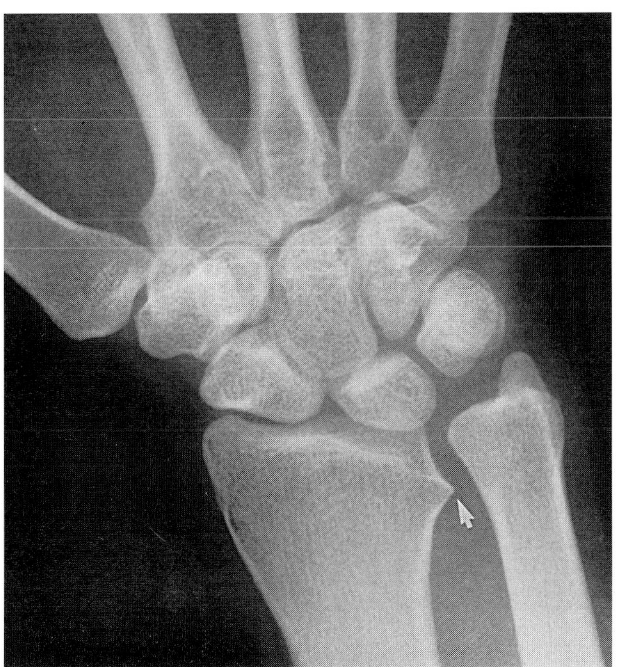

FIGURE 16–2. Madelung's deformity.[3] Findings include an increased width between the distal portions of the radius and ulna, a relatively long ulna in comparison with the radius, a decreased carpal angle, triangularization of the distal radial epiphysis, an osseous excrescence at the metaphyses of the radius (arrow), and wedging of the carpal bones between the deformed radius and protruding ulna. The lunate bone is at the apex of the wedge. The isolated idiopathic form of Madelung's deformity is more common in women and is more frequently bilateral than unilateral; the degree of severity is unequal on the two sides. *(Courtesy of G. Greenway, M.D., Dallas, Texas.)*

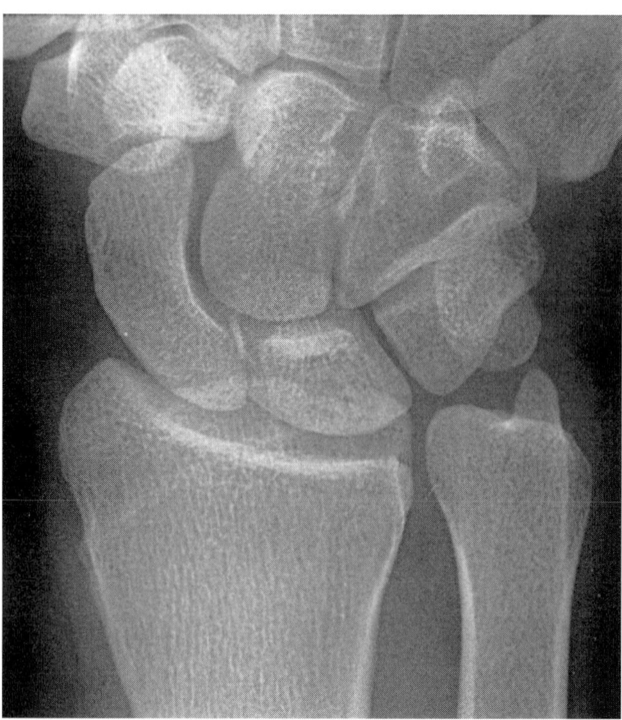

FIGURE 16–3. Positive ulnar variance: ulnar abutment (impaction) syndrome.[4–6] The ulna is relatively long in comparison with the radius, a finding termed positive ulnar variance. This form of variance results in limitation of rotation, subsequent ligamentous relaxation of the wrist, and a thinner triangular fibrocartilage complex (TFCC). The ulnar abutment (impaction) syndrome refers to the consequent degeneration, TFCC perforation, and lunotriquetral interosseous ligament disruption.

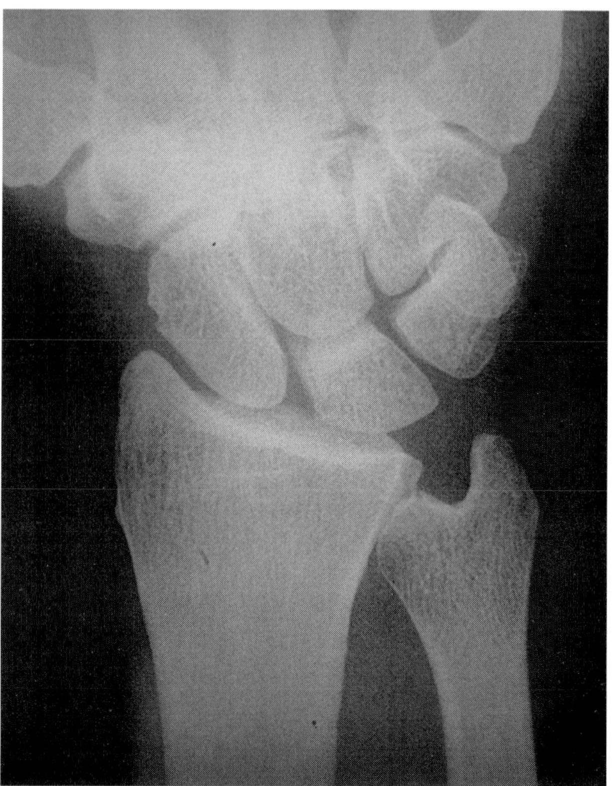

FIGURE 16–4. Negative ulnar variance (ulna minus).[7–9] On this posteroanterior radiograph of the wrist, the ulna is shorter than the radius, and mild osteoarthrosis of the distal radioulnar joint is evident. Note the discontinuity of the distal surfaces of the ulna and radius at the radiocarpal joint.

TABLE 16–2. Fractures and Dislocations of the Radial and Ulnar Diaphyses

Site	Figure(s)	Characteristics	Complications and Related Injuries
Ulna (alone)			
"Nightstick" fracture[10]	16–5	Direct blow to forearm Distal third ulna > middle third ulna > proximal third	Displacement at fracture site (uncommon)
Monteggia fracture-dislocation[11, 12]	16–6	Type I: fracture of middle or upper third of ulna with anterior dislocation of radial head (65 per cent of cases) Type II: fracture of middle or upper third of ulna with posterior dislocation of radial head (18 per cent of cases) Type III: fracture of ulna just distal to coronoid process with lateral dislocation of radial head (16 per cent of cases) Type IV: fracture of upper or middle third of ulna with anterior dislocation of radial head and fracture of proximal portion of radius (1 per cent of cases)	Injury to branches of radial nerve (20 per cent of cases)
Radius (alone)			
Proximal and middle segments[13]		Uncommon: usually associated with ulnar fracture	
Galeazzi's injury[14]	16–7	Fracture of the radial shaft with dislocation or subluxation of inferior radioulnar joint Caused by direct blow or fall on the outstretched hand with pronation of forearm Variable degree of displacement at fracture site	Angulation Entrapment of extensor carpi ulnaris tendon Delayed union or nonunion Limitation of supination and pronation of forearm Fractures of ulnar head and styloid process
Radius and ulna[15]		Closed or open Nondisplaced or displaced	Delayed union or nonunion (especially of ulna) Displacement more common in adults than in children Infection, especially in open fractures Nerve and vascular injuries, especially in open fractures and those with severe displacement Compartment syndromes Synostosis between radius and ulna (rare)
Stress injuries[16]	16–8	Stress fractures or stress reactions in the ulna of rodeo riders, tennis players, baseball pitchers, volleyball players, weightlifters, and patients using wheelchairs	

See also Tables 1–3 and 1–4; see Chapter 15 for injuries to the proximal portion of the radius and ulna and Chapter 17 for injuries to the wrist.

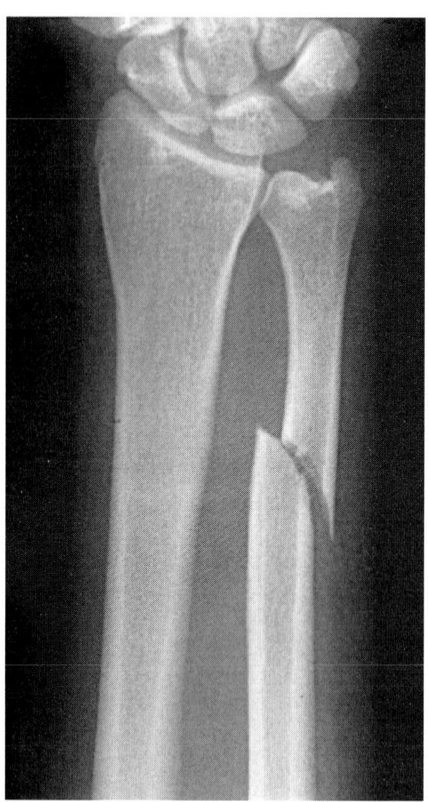

FIGURE 16–5. "Nightstick" fracture: Isolated fracture of the ulnar diaphysis.[10] Note the oblique, minimally displaced fracture of the distal portion of the ulna. The distal and proximal radioulnar joints and the radius were intact radiographically. These fractures occur as a result of a direct blow to the forearm during a violent assault by a hard object, such as a nightstick or club.

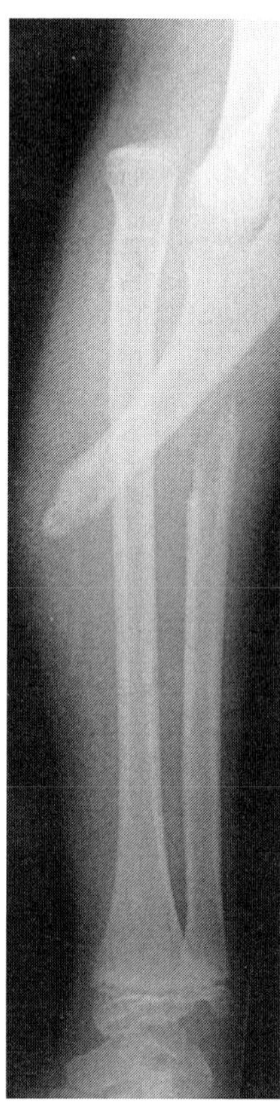

FIGURE 16–6. Monteggia's fracture-dislocation (type I).[11, 12] A displaced fracture of the proximal one third of the ulnar diaphysis and associated anterior dislocation of the radial head are evident in this 15-year-old boy. Monteggia injuries are common in adults but are rare and easily overlooked in children. Type I injuries represent 65 per cent of cases, but variations including types II, III, and IV also may occur.

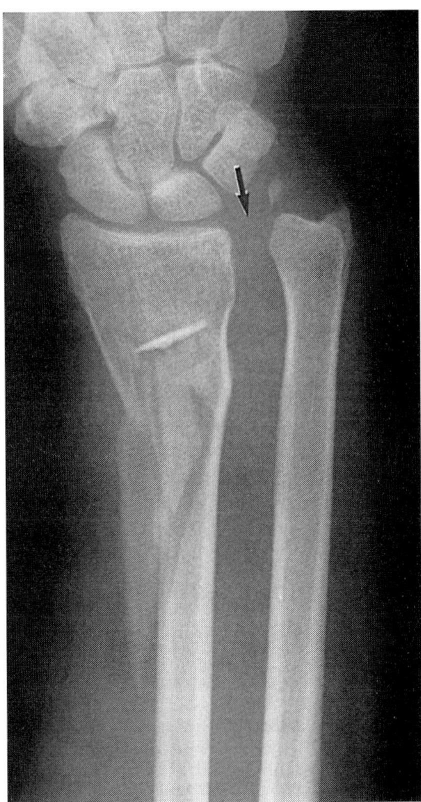

FIGURE 16–7. Galeazzi's fracture-dislocation.[14] This 21-year-old woman has a comminuted distal radius fracture, diastasis of the inferior radionulnar articulation (arrow), and a displaced fracture of the ulnar styloid process. The short oblique or transverse fracture usually occurs at the junction of the middle and distal thirds of the radial diaphysis, and the distal radial fragment is displaced in an ulnar direction. In addition to radioulnar diastasis, fractures of the ulnar head or styloid process often accompany the injury. Complications include nonunion, malunion, and limitation of supination and pronation ranges of motion.

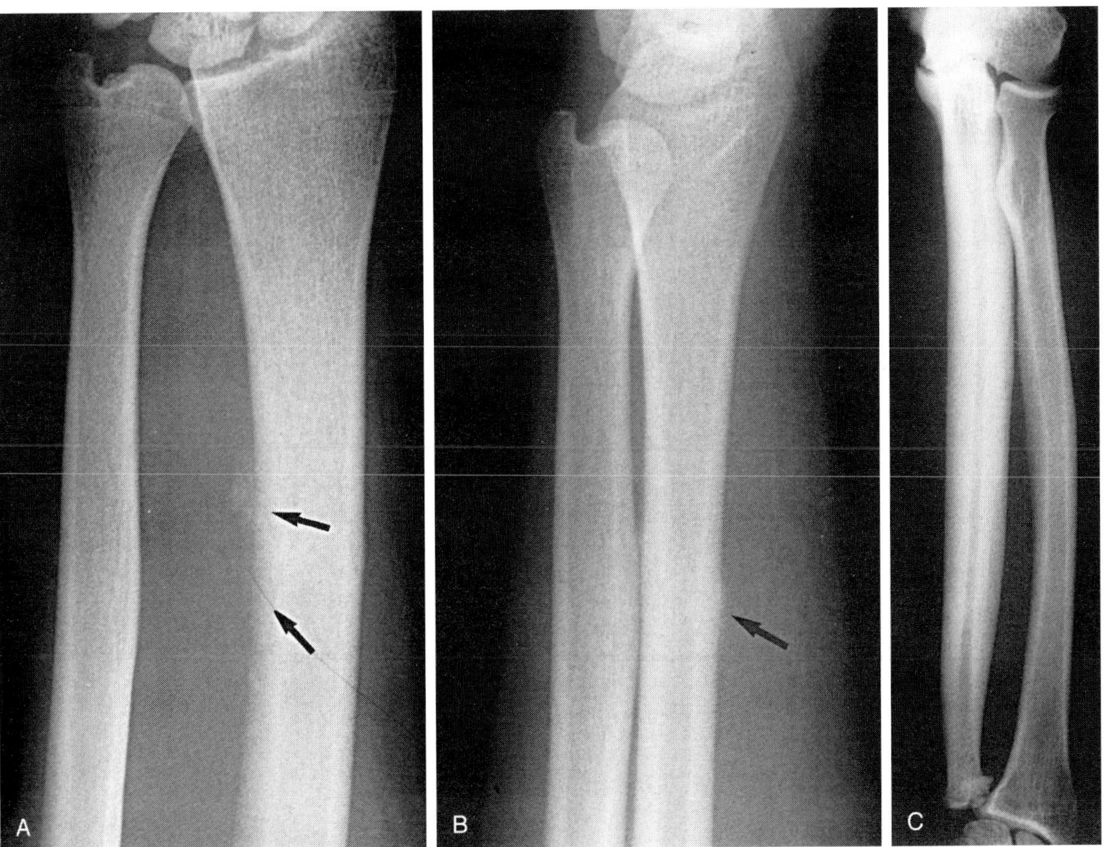

FIGURE 16–8. Reactions to stress.[16] A, B Stress (fatigue) fracture. Frontal (A) and lateral (B) radiographs of this 22-year-old professional pool player illustrate periosteal new bone formation (arrows). C Stress reaction. In another patient, a 27-year-old rodeo cowboy, a radiograph of the ulna exhibits diffuse cortical hyperostosis, a complication seen in members of this profession. *(C, Courtesy of G. Greenway, M.D., Dallas, Texas.)*

TABLE 16–3. Fractures and Dislocations About the Distal Portions of the Radius and Ulna

Fracture	Figure(s)	Characteristics	Complications and Related Injuries
Colles' (Pouteau's)[17] fracture	16–9	Mechanism: dorsiflexion Fracture of distal portion of radius with dorsal displacement Classification system based on extra-articular versus intra-articular location, presence or absence of ulnar fracture Varying amounts of radial displacement angulation, and shortening Ulnar styloid fracture in about 50 to 60 per cent of cases Associated injuries to carpus, elbow, humerus, and femur (in osteoporotic patients), inferior radioulnar joint	Deformity related to radial shortening and angulation Subluxation or dislocation of inferior radioulnar joint Reflex sympathetic dystrophy Injury to median or, less commonly, radial or ulnar nerve Osteoarthrosis Tendon rupture
Moore's fracture[17]		Combination of Colles' fracture, fracture of the ulnar styloid process, and disruption of the inferior radioulnar joint	
Incomplete pediatric fractures[18]	16–10	Mechanism: longitudinal forces insufficient to cause complete discontinuity of the bone Incomplete fractures of the distal portion of the radius and ulna in children are common Impaction fracture: subtle increased zone of radiodensity at site of impaction Torus fracture: buckling of the metaphyseal cortex of the radius and ulna Greenstick fracture: buckling or bending of one side of the cortex, with fracture of the opposite side; diaphysis or metaphysis	May initially be overlooked, especially without evidence of buckling
Barton's fracture[19]	16–11	Mechanism: dorsiflexion and pronation Fracture of dorsal rim of radius with intra-articular extension	Similar to those of Colles' fracture
Dislocation of the inferior radioulnar joint[14]		Isolated dislocation of the inferior radioulnar joint: rare injury Galeazzi injury: dislocation of the inferior radioulnar joint combined with fracture of the radial shaft Fracture may be comminuted and severely displaced Essex-Lopresti injury: dislocation of the inferior radioulnar joint combined with comminuted fracture of the radial head	Triangular fibrocartilage complex injury Fracture of ulnar head or styloid process Wrist and elbow instability
Radiocarpal fracture-dislocation[20]		Mechanism: dorsiflexion Uncommon and severe injury Associated fractures of dorsal rim and styloid process of radius, and the ulnar styloid process May be irreducible	Entrapment of tendons and ulnar nerve and artery
Hutchinson's (chauffeur's) fracture[21]	16–12	Mechanism: direct blow or avulsion by radial collateral ligament Fracture of styloid process of radius Usually nondisplaced	Scapholunate dissociation Degenerative joint disease Ligament damage
Smith's (reverse Colles') fracture[22]	16–13	Mechanism: variable Fracture of distal portion of radius with palmar displacement Less common than Colles' fracture Varying amounts of radial comminution, articular involvement	Complications similar to those of Colles' fracture Extensor tendon injury Associated fracture of ulnar styloid process
Ulnar styloid process[23]	16–14	Mechanism: dorsiflexion or avulsion by ulnar collateral or triangular ligament Usually associated with radial fractures, infrequently isolated Usually nondisplaced	Nonunion Triangular fibrocartilage injury
Child abuse[24]	16–15	Incomplete or complete fracture of the radius or ulna may occur Epiphyseal injuries Other fractures at different stages of healing	Other injuries

TABLE 16–3. Fractures and Dislocations About the Distal Portions of the Radius and Ulna *Continued*

Fracture	Figure(s)	Characteristics	Complications and Related Injuries
Growth plate injuries: distal portion of radius[25]		Mechanism: chronic stress in gymnastic athletes or compression and rotation from upper limb weight-bearing Fifty per cent of all growth plate injuries: distal portion of the radius is the most frequent site of physeal injuries Type I injury: usually occurs between ages 9 and 14 years May resemble metaphyseal changes of rickets and dysplasias	Retardation of limb growth Positive ulnar variance Inferior radioulnar joint abnormalities
Growth plate injuries: distal portion of ulna[25, 26]		Mechanism: acute injury 5.7 per cent of all growth plate injuries Ulna is not as common a site as radius Type I injury most common Stress injuries of the distal radial epiphysis occurs in young gymnasts: radiodense reactive sclerosis	Retardation of limb growth

See also Tables 1–3 and 1–4.

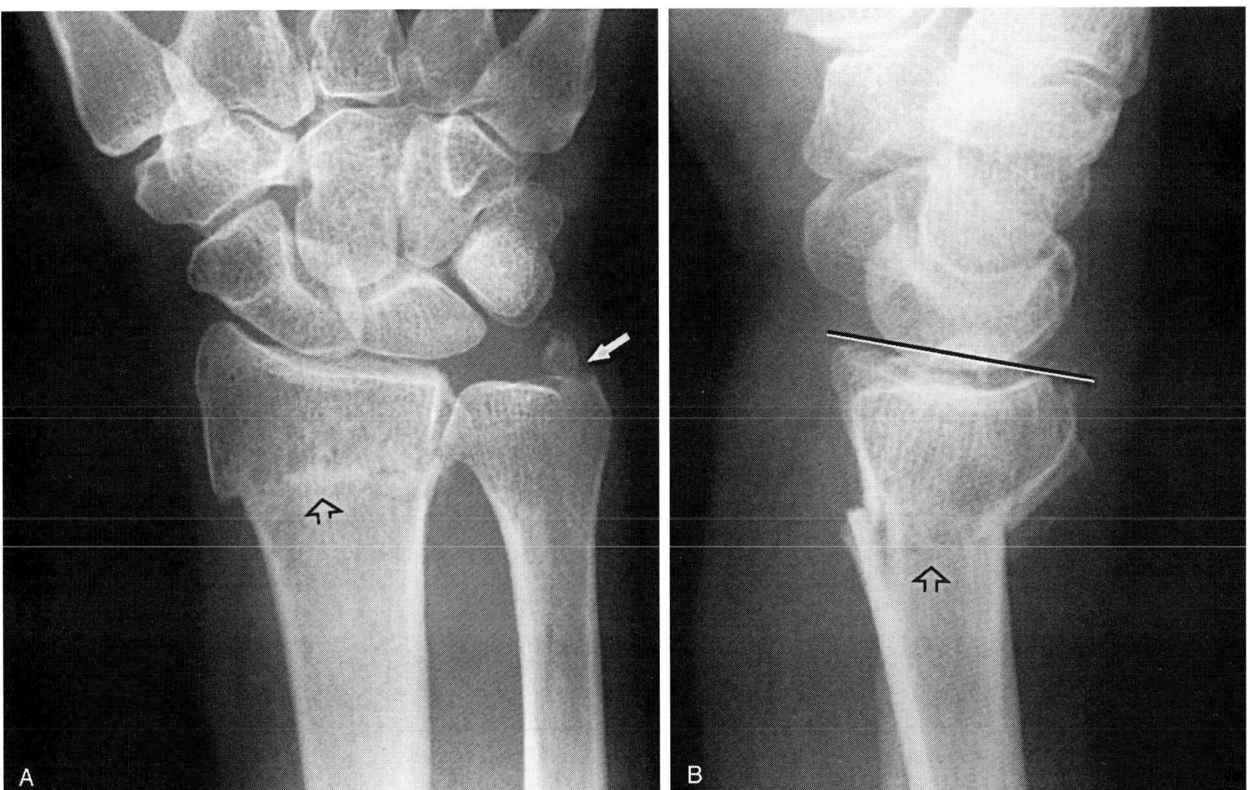

FIGURE 16–9. Colles' fracture.[17] Frontal **(A)** and lateral **(B)** radiographs of this 61-year-old woman reveal a transverse fracture of the distal radial metaphysis (open arrows) with dorsal angulation of the distal radial articular surface (line). The ulnar styloid also is fractured (arrow), and prominent soft tissue swelling is observed. *(Courtesy of A.L. Anderson, D.C., Portland, Oregon.)*

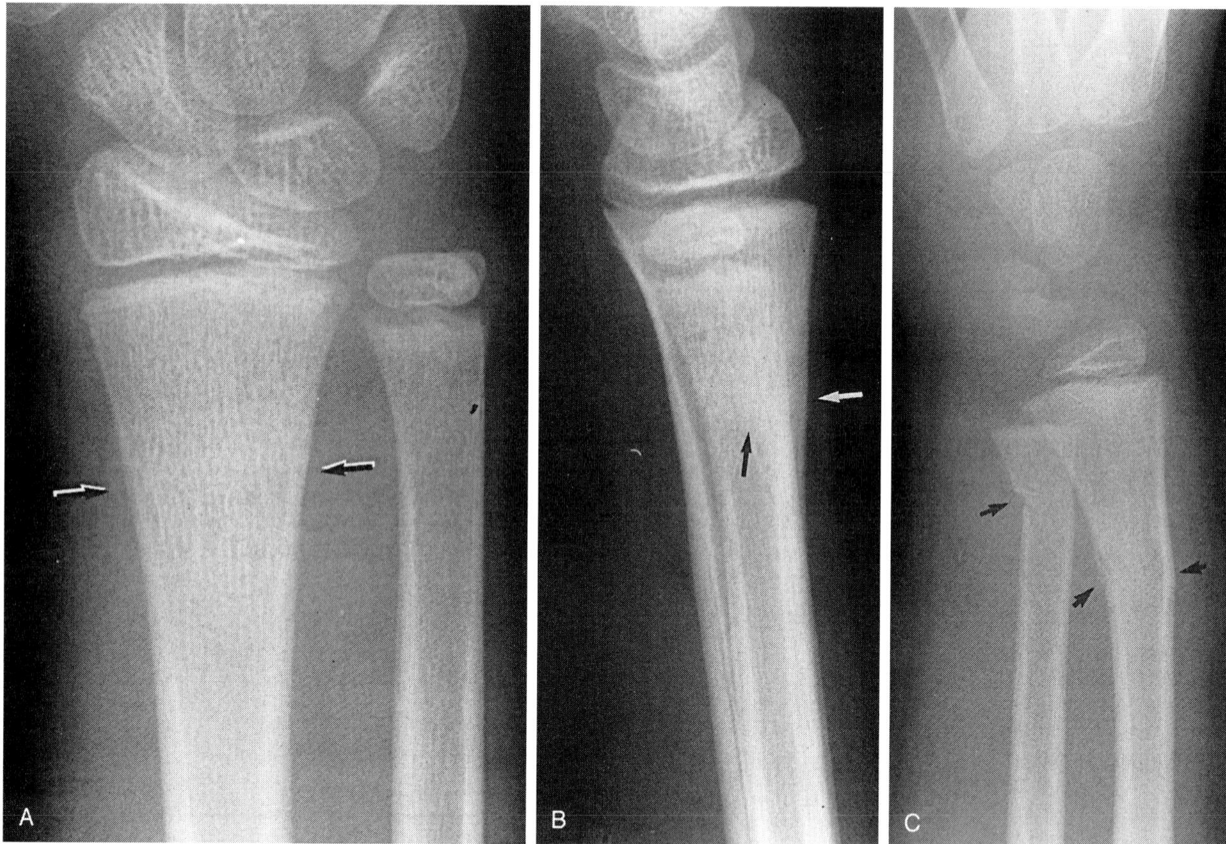

FIGURE 16–10. Pediatric fractures of the distal ends of the radius and ulna.[18] **A, B** Impaction fracture. Frontal **(A)** and lateral **(B)** radiographs of this 13-year-old patient show an impaction fracture of the distal radial metaphysis manifested only as a subtle increased zone of density at the site of impaction (arrows). **C** Torus fracture. Note the buckling of the metaphyseal cortices of the radius and ulna (arrows) in this 8-year-old child who fell on an outstretched arm.

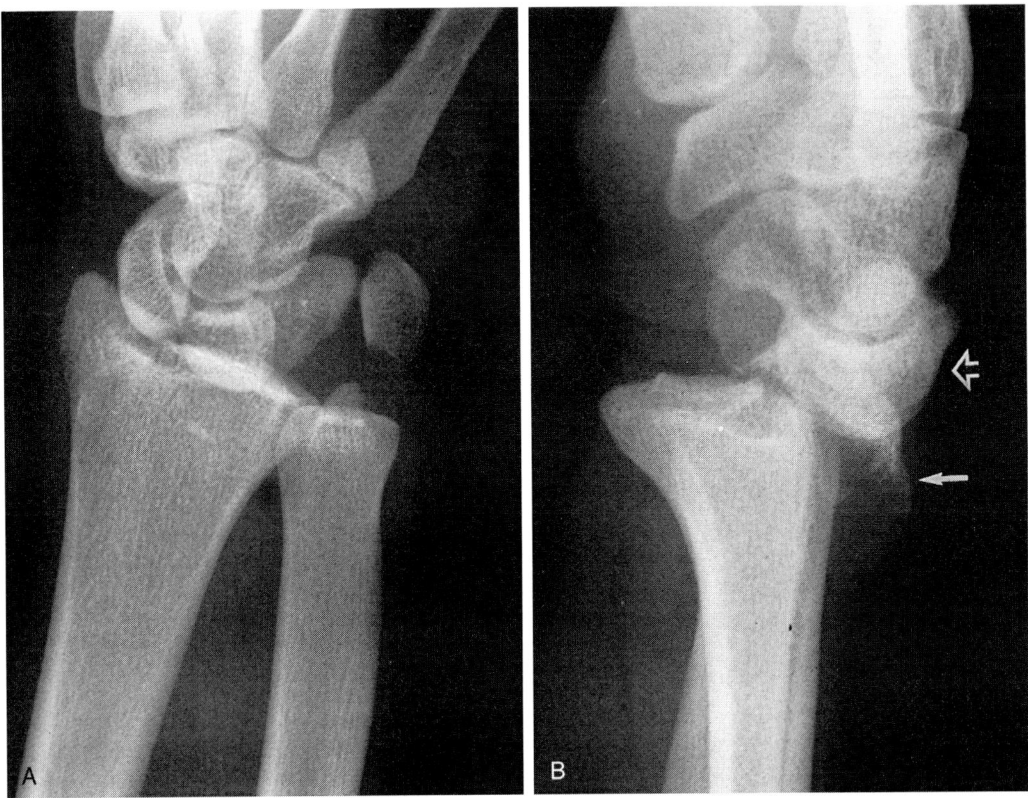

FIGURE 16–11. Barton's fracture.[19] This 24-year-old man injured his wrist in a fall. Frontal (A) and lateral (B) radiographs reveal fracture of the dorsal rim of the radius (arrow) with intra-articular extension into the radiocarpal joint and dorsal dislocation of the radiocarpal articulations (open arrow). These fractures generally are related to dorsiflexion and pronation of the forearm on the fixed wrist and occur frequently in young people involved in motorcycle accidents.

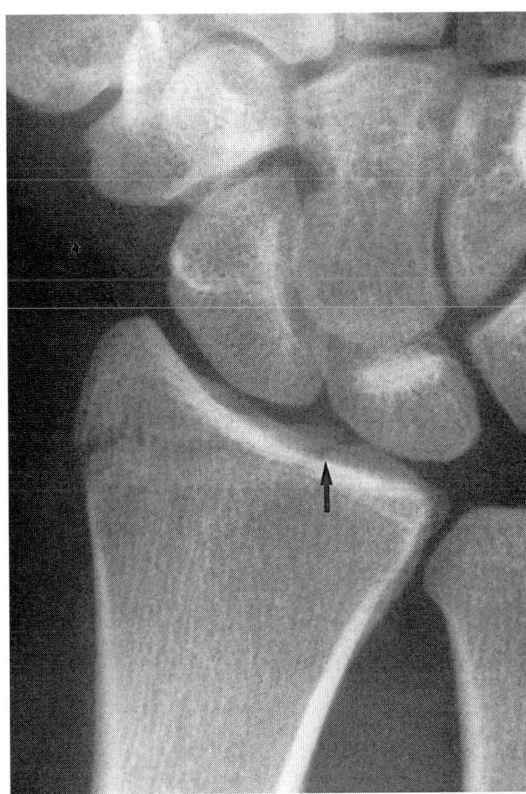

FIGURE 16–12. Hutchinson's (chauffeur's) fracture: Radial styloid process.[21] Observe the large triangular fragment in this nondisplaced fracture. Intra-articular extension (arrow) is an important component of this fracture. Hutchinson's fracture occurs as a result of a direct blow or as an avulsion of the radiocarpal or radial collateral ligament.

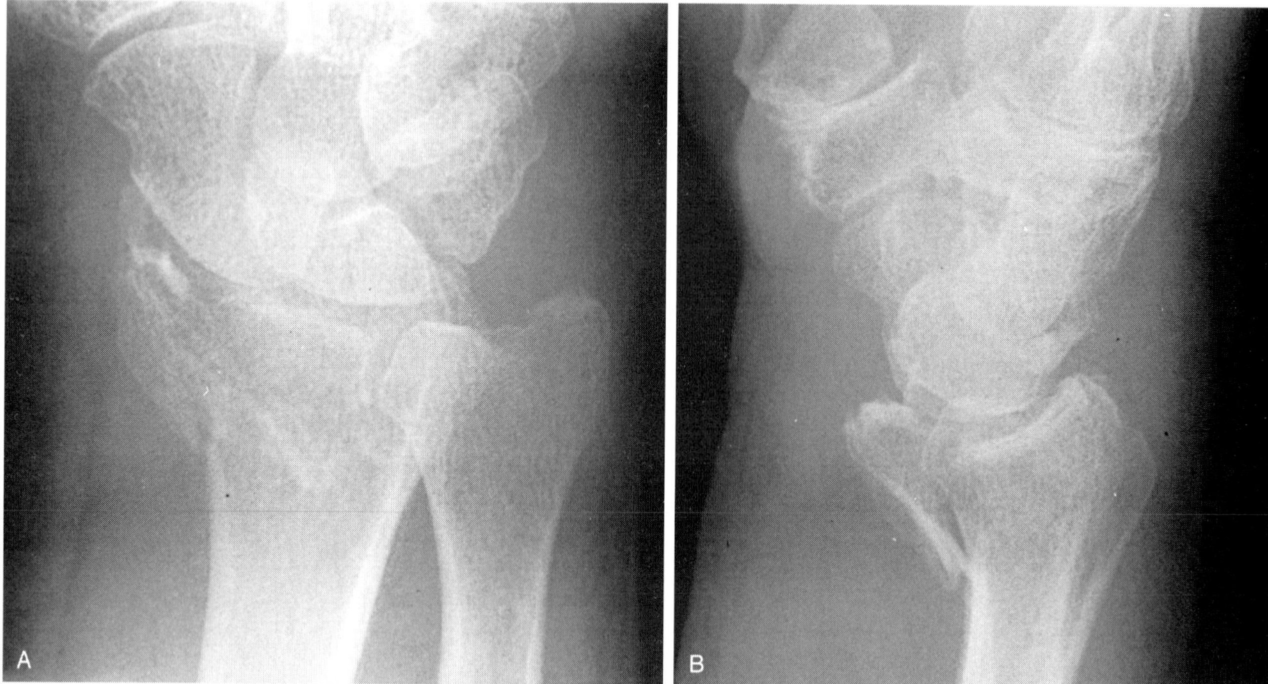

FIGURE 16–13. Smith's fracture: reverse Colles' fracture.[22] This 68-year-old woman had fallen, injuring her wrist. Frontal (A) and lateral (B) radiographs show a transverse fracture of the distal portion of the radius. The lateral radiograph (B) demonstrates mild volar and proximal displacement of the fracture fragment and the carpal bones as well as soft tissue swelling. This injury is less common than Colles' fracture and involves palmar angulation and anterior displacement of the distal radial surface. The fracture may be intra-articular or extra-articular, and it may be complicated by extensor tendon injury.

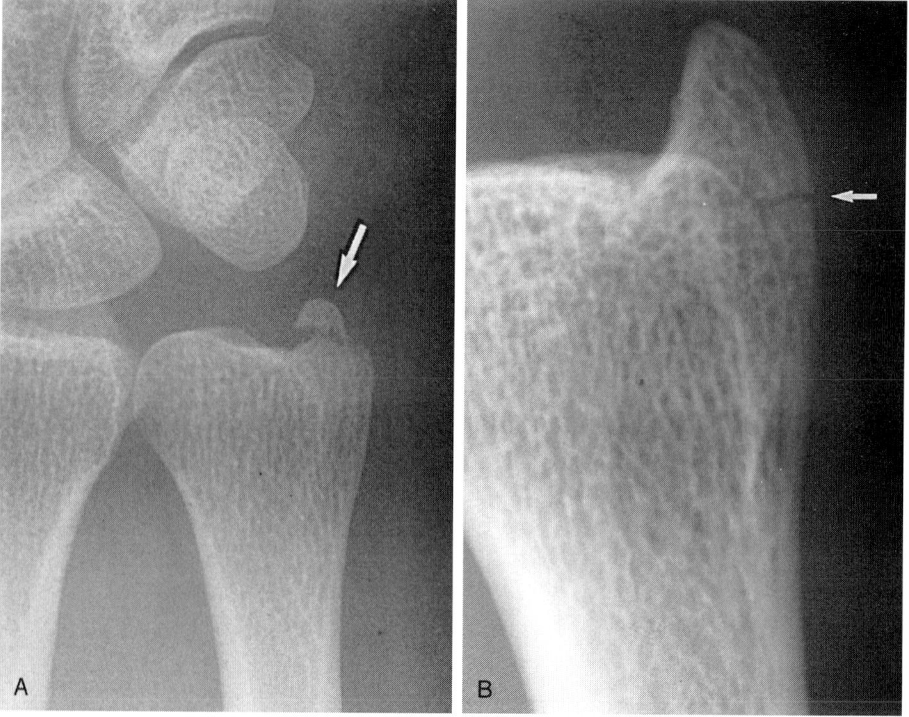

FIGURE 16–14. Isolated ulnar styloid process fracture.[23] A This isolated fracture of the ulnar styloid process has minimal displacement (arrow). B In another patient, magnification radiography shows a nondisplaced transverse fracture (arrow). Ulnar styloid process fractures often are a component of more complex wrist injuries, including Colles' fracture, but may occur as an isolated phenomenon related to avulsion by the ulnar collateral or triangular ligaments. Nonunion of such fractures may be a source of chronic wrist pain and may be difficult to differentiate from ununited ossification centers.

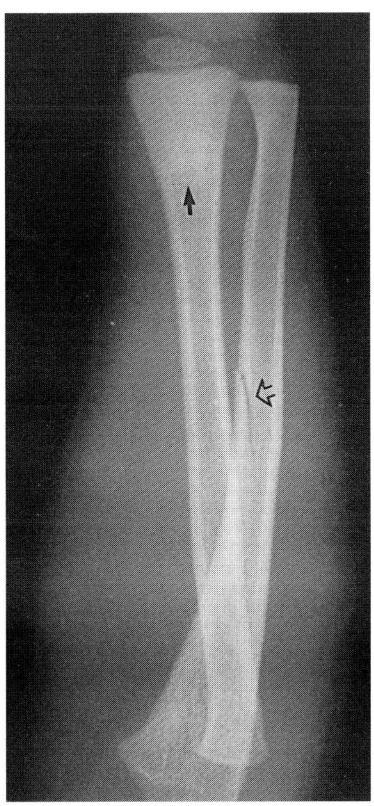

FIGURE 16–15. Child abuse.[24] An oblique ulnar fracture (open arrow) and an impacted radius fracture (arrow) are seen in this child who had been deliberately assaulted.

TABLE 16–4. **Tumors Affecting the Radius and Ulna**

Tumor	Figure(s)	Characteristics
Malignant neoplasms of bone		
Secondary malignant neoplasms of bone		
Skeletal metastasis[27, 28]	16–16	Acral metastasis rare: fewer than 10 per cent of skeletal metastatic lesions affect the radius and ulna Seventy-five per cent permeative or moth-eaten osteolysis Twenty-five diffuse or patchy osteosclerosis or mixed pattern of lysis and sclerosis Usually multiple sites of involvement Pathologic fracture Cortical metastasis ("cookie-bite" lesions), especially from bronchogenic carcinoma
Primary malignant neoplasms of bone		
Osteosarcoma (conventional)[29]		Fewer than 1 per cent of osteosarcomas occur in the radius and ulna Osteolytic, osteosclerotic, or mixed patterns of medullary and cortical destruction Prominent periosteal reaction common Preferential involvement of the metaphyseal region
Osteosarcoma (parosteal)[30]		Two per cent of parosteal osteosarcomas occur in the radius and 1 per cent occur in the ulna Osteosclerotic surface lesion of bone Large radiodense, oval, sessile mass with smooth or irregular margins Ossification begins centrally and progresses outward, opposite that of benign heterotopic bone formation (myositis ossification)
Giant cell tumor (aggressive)[31]		Approximately 4 per cent of aggressive giant cell tumors occur in the distal portion of the radius Eccentrically located, subarticular osteolytic lesion extending into the metaphysis Cortical destruction and soft tissue mass are variable findings Radiographic appearance is an inaccurate guide to determining malignancy of lesion; biopsy is necessary

Table continued on following page

TABLE 16–4. Tumors Affecting the Radius and Ulna *Continued*

Tumor	Figure(s)	Characteristics
Ewing's sarcoma[32]		Two per cent of Ewing's sarcomas occur in the radius and 1 per cent occur in the ulna Permeative or moth-eaten osteolysis, aggressive cortical erosion or violation, laminated or spiculated periostitis, and soft tissue masses Most lesions central and diametaphyseal in location
Myeloproliferative disorders		
Plasma cell (multiple) myeloma[33]	16–17	Approximately 4 per cent of multiple myeloma lesions occur in the radius and 1 per cent occur in the ulna Early: normal radiographs or diffuse osteopenia Later: widespread, well-circumscribed osteolytic lesions with discrete margins, which appear uniform in size Ninety-seven per cent osteolytic; 3 per cent osteoblastic False-negative bone scans common
Primary lymphoma (non-Hodgkin's)[34]	16–18	Approximately 2 per cent of lesions in cases of primary lymphoma occur in the ulna Multiple moth-eaten or permeative osteolytic lesions Diffuse or localized sclerotic lesions are rare Common cause of pathologic fracture
Leukemia[35]	16–19	Radius and ulna occasionally involved Diffuse osteopenia, radiolucent or radiodense transverse metaphyseal bands, osteolytic lesions, periostitis, and, infrequently, osteosclerosis Radiodense metaphyses more frequent in patients undergoing chemotherapy for leukemia: may resemble lead poisoning
Benign neoplasms of bone		
Osteoid osteoma[36]		Three per cent of osteoid osteomas occur in the ulna and 1 per cent occur in the radius Cortical or subperiosteal lesion with reactive sclerosis surrounding central radiolucent nidus Nidus less than 1 cm in diameter and usually not visible on routine radiographs Intracapsular lesions provoke less reactive sclerosis and are more likely to cause joint pain
Osteoblastoma (conventional)[37]		Two per cent of conventional osteoblastomas involve the ulna; 1 per cent involve the radius Osteolytic, osteosclerotic, or both Expansile lesion that may be subperiosteal Partially calcified matrix in many cases Cortical thinning Often resembles large osteoid osteoma
Enchondroma (solitary)[38]		Approximately 2 per cent of solitary enchondromas involve the radius; fewer than 1 per cent involve the ulna Solitary, central or eccentric, medullary osteolytic lesion Lobulated endosteal scalloping Approximately 50 per cent have stippled calcification within the matrix
Enchondromatosis (Ollier's disease)[38]		Multiple enchondromas Occasionally involves the radius and ulna
Maffucci's syndrome[38]		Radius and ulna are involved in over 40 per cent of cases of Maffucci's syndrome Multiple enchondromas and soft tissue hemangiomas Unilateral distribution in 50 per cent of cases
Osteochondroma (solitary)[39, 40]	16–20	One per cent of solitary osteochondromas arise from the radius and ulna Pedunculated or sessile cartilage-covered osseous excresence arising from the surface of the metaphysis Cortex and medulla are continuous with the host bone May occur spontaneously or after accidental or iatrogenic injury Typically grow away from the adjacent joint Complications: pathologic fracture, and malignant transformation (fewer than 1 per cent of cases)
Hereditary multiple exostosis[41, 42]	16–21	Occasional involvement of bones of forearm Proximal or distal metaphyses may be involved Frequently results in Madelung's deformity May result in malignant transformation (fewer than 5 per cent of cases)

TABLE 16–4. Tumors Affecting the Radius and Ulna *Continued*

Tumor	Figure(s)	Characteristics
Nonossifying fibroma and fibrous cortical defect[43]	16–22	Nonossifying fibromas favor the lower extremity and infrequently occur in the radius or ulna Eccentric, multiloculated osteolytic lesion arising from the metaphyseal cortex Resemble a well-circumscribed, blister-like shell of bone arising from the cortex Cortical thinning often is present Eventually disapppear, filling in with normal bone Nonossifying fibromas typically are larger than fibrous cortical defects
Giant cell tumor (benign)[31]	16–23	Approximately 10 per cent of benign giant cell tumors occur in the radius and 3 per cent occur in the ulna Eccentric osteolytic neoplasm with a predilection for the subarticular region of the distal end of the radius Often multiloculated and expansile Radiographs are inaccurate in distinguishing benign from aggressive giant cell tumors
Intraosseous lipoma[44]		Fewer than 2 per cent of intraosseous lipomas occur in the ulna; infrequently occur in the radius Osteolytic lesion surrounded by a thin, well-defined sclerotic border Central calcified or ossified nidus is common Occasional osseous expansion Cortical destruction and periostitis absent
Hemangioma (solitary)[45]	16–24	Rare in the radius and ulna Radiolucent, slightly expansile intraosseous lesion Radiating, lattice-like or web-like trabecular pattern Occasional cortical thinning Rarely periostitis, soft tissue mass, or osteosclerosis Intracortical and periosteal forms of hemangioma are extremely rare
Aneurysmal bone cyst[46]	16–25	Four per cent of aneurysmal bone cysts occur in the ulna and 3 per cent occur in the radius Eccentric, thin-walled, expansile osteolytic lesion of the humeral metaphysis Thin trabeculation with multiloculated appearance Buttressing at edge of lesion
Tumor-like lesions of bone		
Paget's disease[47, 48]	16–26	Radius and ulna are rarely involved in Paget's disease Usually polyostotic and may have unilateral involvement Coarsened trabeculae and bone enlargement Diaphyseal and metaphyseal involvement with extension into epiphysis Stages of involvement; osteolytic (50 per cent), osteosclerotic (25 per cent), and mixed (25 per cent), malignant transformation (less than 2 per cent) Bowing deformities frequently occur
Monostotic fibrous dysplasia[49]	16–27	Monostotic involvement of the radius or ulna is rare Thick rim of sclerosis surrounding a radiolucent lesion Ground-glass appearance of fibrous matrix
Polyostotic fibrous dysplasia[49]		Thirty to 40 per cent of patients have lesions in the radius or ulna Unilateral or bilateral, asymmetric humeral involvement Lesions appear the same as monostotic form but frequently are larger, more expansile, and more multiloculated than monostotic lesions
Langerhans' cell histiocytosis[50, 51]		Radius is involved in about 3 per cent of cases; ulna rarely involved Osteolytic lesions may be multiloculated and expansile Eosinophilic granuloma is the most frequent and mildest form of this disorder

See also Tables 1–10 to 1–12.

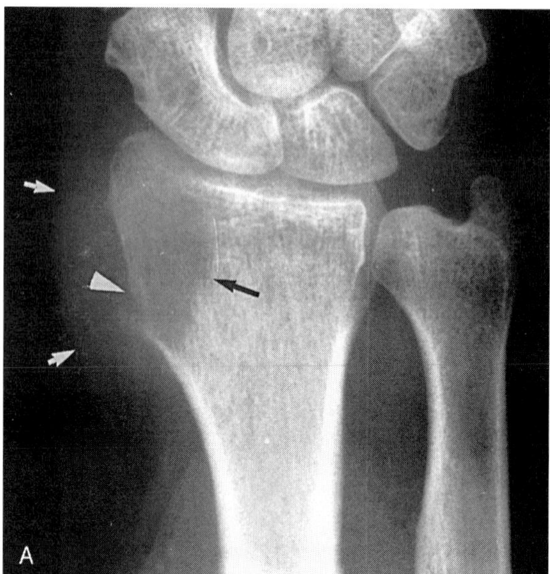

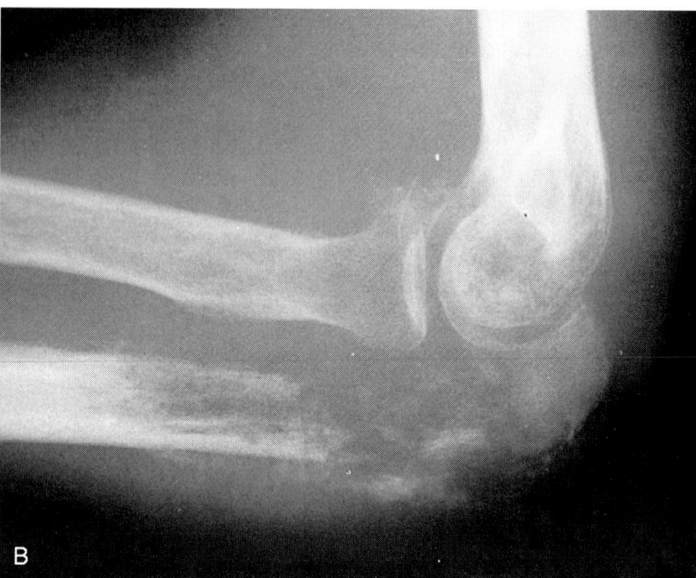

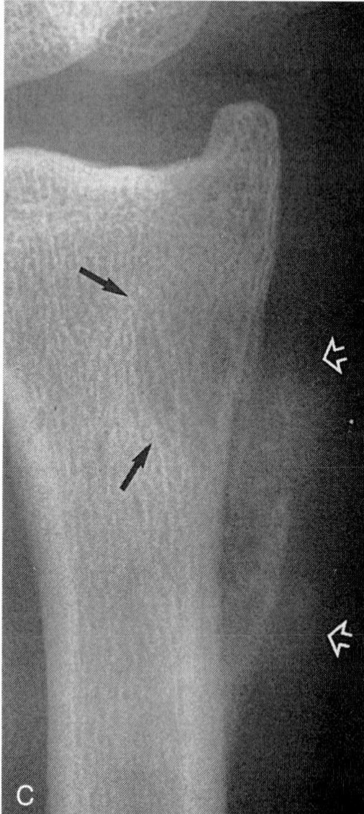

FIGURE 16–16. Skeletal metastasis.[27, 28] **A** Bronchogenic carcinoma. This 63-year-old man had bronchogenic carcinoma and wrist pain. A radiograph of the wrist reveals permeative osteolysis (black arrow), cortical perforation (white arrowhead), and a soft tissue mass (white arrows). **B** Bronchogenic carcinoma. In another patient, severe, permeative osteolytic destruction of bone is accompanied by prominent soft tissue swelling overlying the proximal portion of the ulna. **C** Malignant melanoma. This 23-year-old man had pain and swelling over the distal ulna. He reported having had a "skin cyst" removed several years previously. A radiograph of the ulna shows a moth-eaten or permeative destructive lesion with osteolysis of the distal portion of the ulna (arrows) and associated periosteal proliferation and soft tissue swelling (open arrows). At this time, no other osseous lesions were identified, and a preoperative diagnosis of a primary malignant tumor, probably Ewing's sarcoma, was made. The patient underwent surgery that revealed a lesion containing melanin. The histologic evaluation showed malignant melanoma. The patient developed widespread skeletal metastasis within months. Periosteal reaction and involvement of bone beyond the elbow or knee are seen more commonly with primary malignant tumors and are infrequent findings in cases of skeletal metastasis.

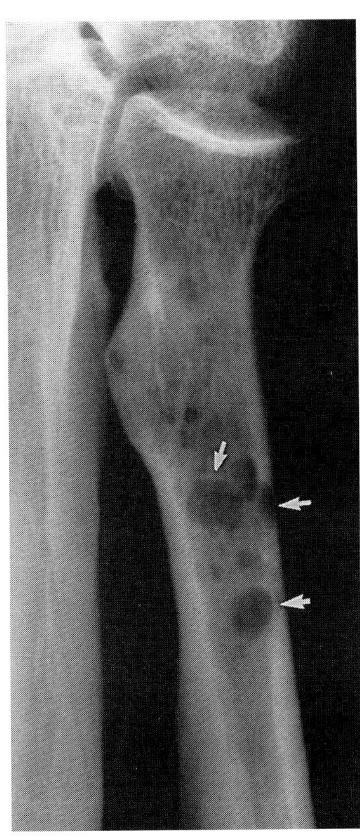

FIGURE 16–17. Plasma cell myeloma.[33] This patient is a 60-year-old man. Multiple, well-circumscribed osteolytic lesions are evident in the proximal portion of the radius (arrows). This patient had diffuse involvement of several sites throughout the skeleton.

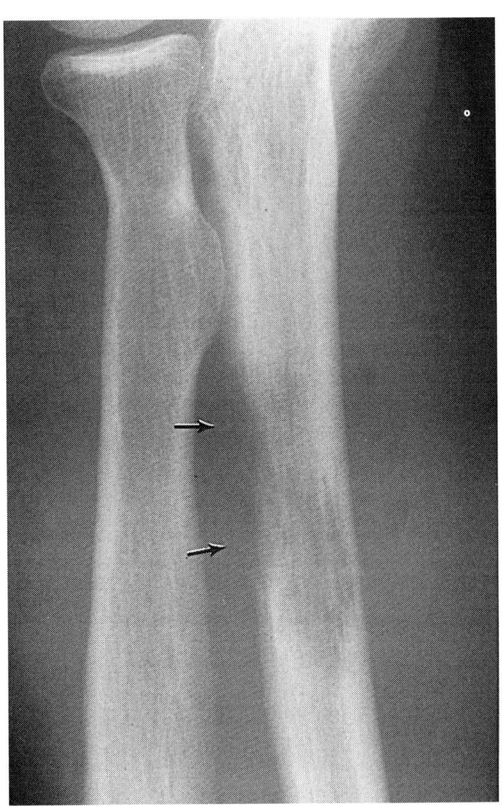

FIGURE 16–18. Lymphoma.[34] Observe the moth-eaten and permeative osteolysis with cortical perforation (arrows) involving the ulnar diaphysis of this 23-year-old man. Overall increased radiodensity of the ulna also is noted. The pathologic diagnosis was lymphoma, primary signet cell type. *(Courtesy of T. Broderick, M.D., Orange, California.)*

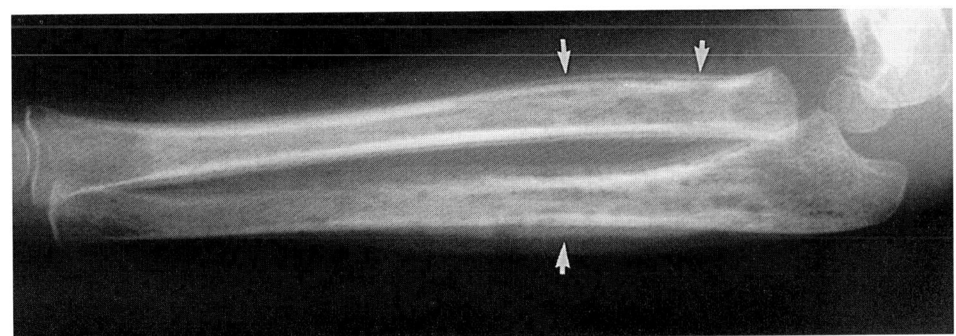

FIGURE 16–19. Acute childhood leukemia.[35] Permeative osteolysis with single layer periostitis (arrows) is seen throughout the radius and ulna of this child with leukemia. Radiographic changes in the skeleton occur in as many as 70 per cent of persons with acute childhood leukemia.

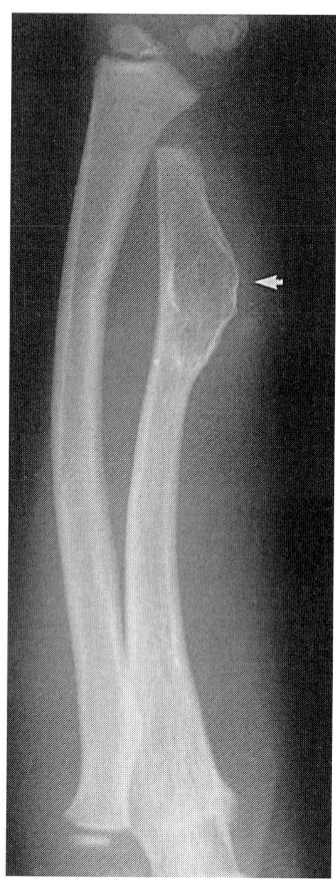

FIGURE 16–20. Solitary osteochondroma.[39, 40] A sessile, expansile osseous outgrowth involving the distal ulnar metadiaphysis (arrow) is present in this 4-year-old boy with a short ulna (reverse Madelung's deformity). The cortex overlying the lesion is intact, and no evidence of periosteal reaction or soft tissue mass is present. The ulna is an unusual location for a solitary osteochondroma. *(Courtesy of G. Greenway, M.D., Dallas, Texas.)*

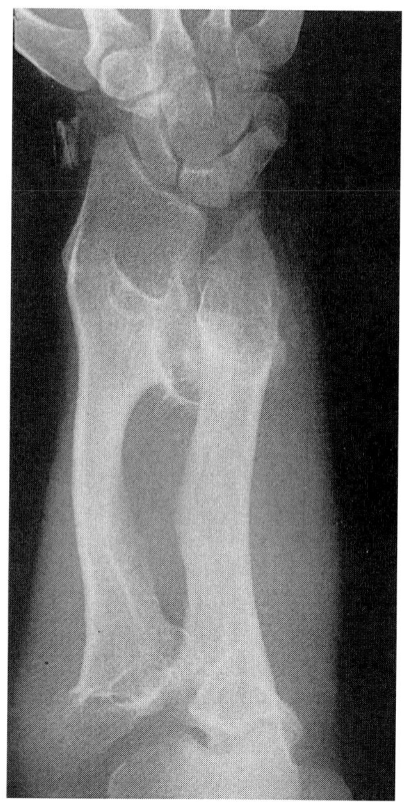

FIGURE 16–21. Hereditary multiple exostoses.[41, 42] Marked deformity of the radius and ulna is seen in this patient with hereditary multiple exostoses. The abnormalities include bowing of the radius, metaphyseal osteochondromas, shortening of the ulna, and an angulated articular surface of the radius. *(Courtesy of T. Broderick, M.D., Orange, California.)*

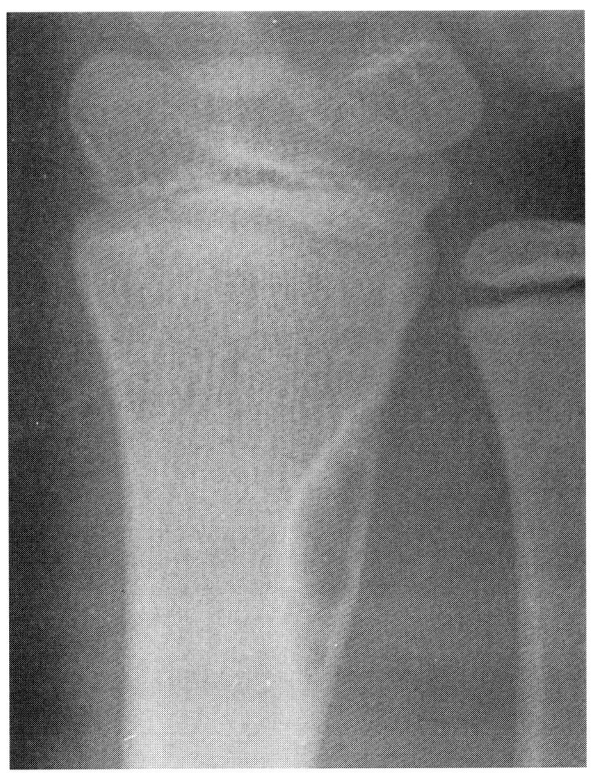

FIGURE 16–22. Nonossifying fibroma.[43] In this 11-year-old boy, an eccentric osteolytic lesion with a lobulated sclerotic margin is present in the metaphysis of the distal end of the radius.

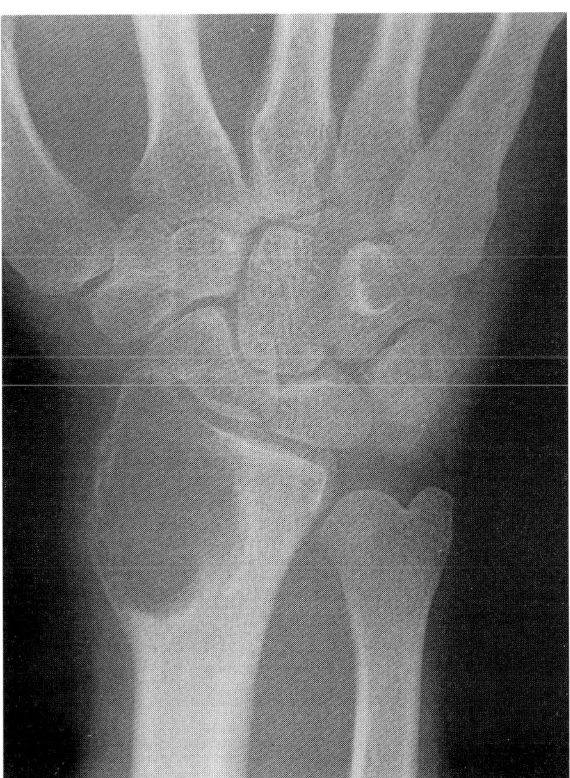

FIGURE 16–23. Giant cell tumor.[31] A radiograph of this 37-year-old man reveals an eccentric, osteolytic, geographic lesion extending into the subchondral region, producing cortical thinning and expansion and possessing a delicate trabecular pattern. Ten per cent of giant cell tumors affect the radius. The radiographic appearance of the giant cell tumor is an inaccurate guide to the histologic composition and clinical behavior of the lesion. Benign lesions may appear aggressive and aggressive lesions may appear benign. Giant cell tumors of the distal end of the radius have a higher likelihood of malignancy than giant cell tumors at any other skeletal site.

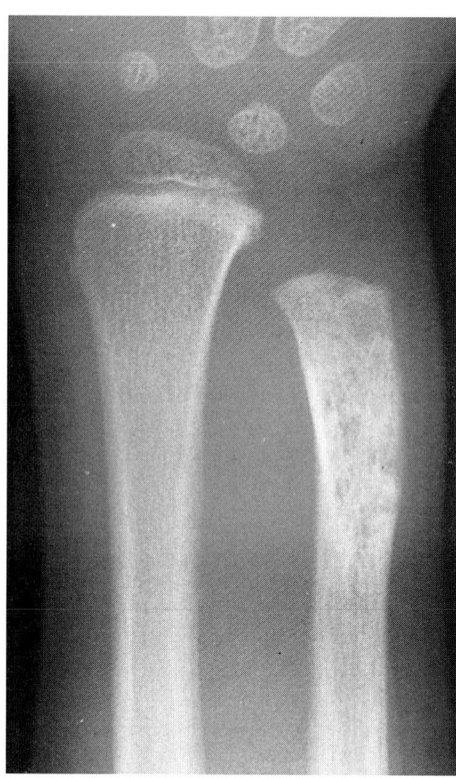

FIGURE 16–24. Hemangioma.[45] A radiograph of the forearm in this 5-year-old child shows a trabeculated lesion of the ulnar metadiaphysis. This benign hemangioma appears permeative and aggressive and should be considered possibly malignant until proved otherwise. The ulna is an extremely rare location for hemangioma.

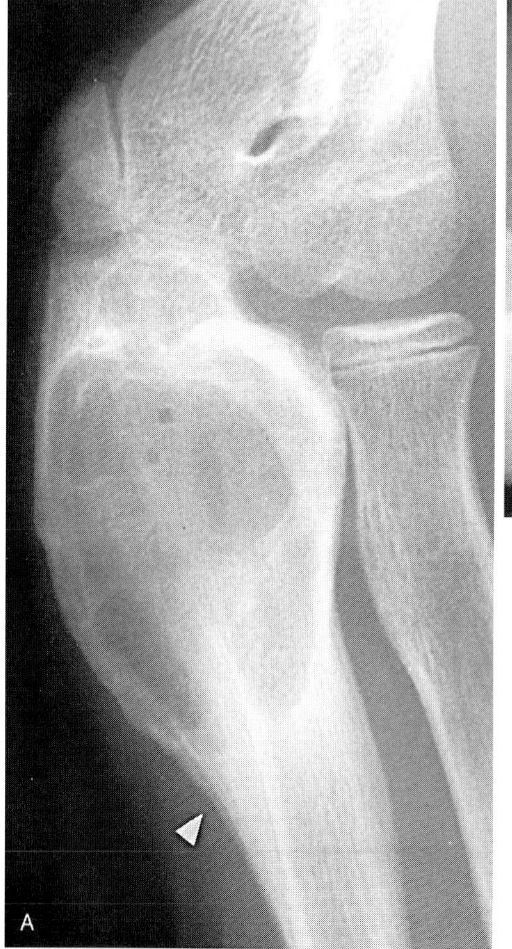

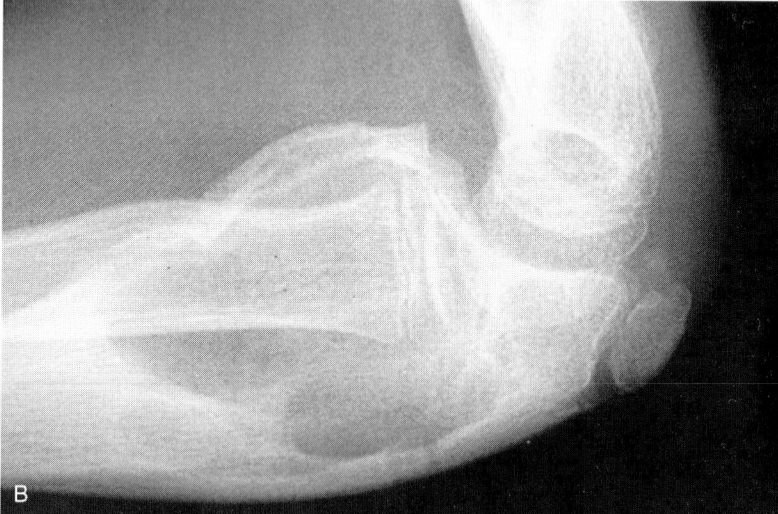

FIGURE 16–25. Aneurysmal bone cyst.[46] A 13-year-old boy had a painful mass on the elbow. Oblique (**A**) and lateral (**B**) radiographs show an expansile, multiloculated, geographic osteolytic lesion involving the proximal ulnar metaphysis and extending into the subarticular region. A triangular zone of cortical buttressing is present at the distal end of the lesion (arrowhead). No evidence of periostitis, soft tissue mass, or cortical disruption is present. The radius and humerus were normal.

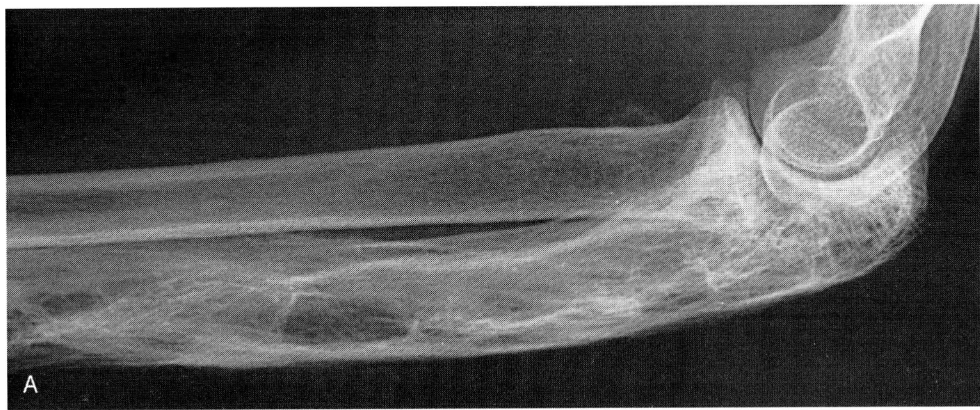

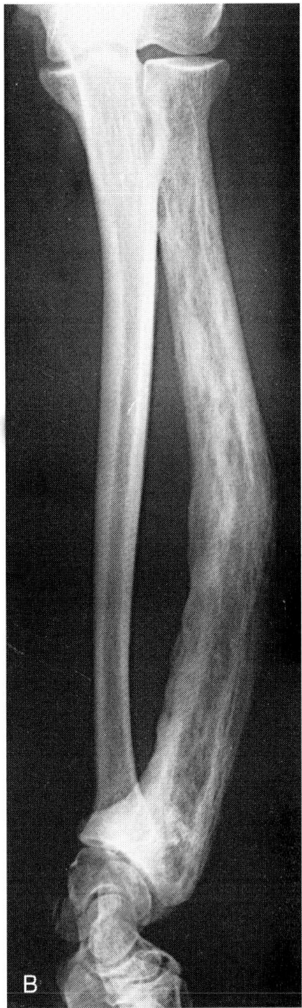

FIGURE 16–26. Paget's disease.[47, 48] A Ulna. A combined pattern of osteolysis and osteosclerosis is evident. Note the characteristically coarsened trabeculae with combined areas of osteosclerotic bone and vacuous radiolucent regions. Note also the typical subchondral distribution of the bone changes. B Radius. In another patient, observe the severe enlargement and bowing of the radius that often accompany this disease.

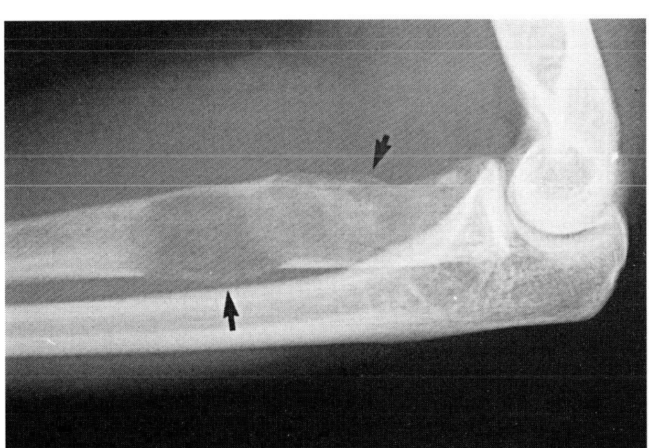

FIGURE 16–27. Monostotic fibrous dysplasia.[49] Endosteal thinning and a ground-glass appearance are noted in this slightly expansile metadiaphyseal lesion involving the proximal portion of the radius (arrows). *(Courtesy of G. Bock, M.D., Winnipeg, Manitoba, Canada.)*

TABLE 16–5. Metabolic, Hematologic, and Infectious Disorders Affecting the Radius and the Ulna

Disorder	Figure(s)	Characteristics
Generalized osteoporosis[52, 53]		Uniform decrease in radiodensity, thinning of cortices, accentuation of trabeculae Osteoporosis predisposes to fractures of the distal end of the radius in elderly patients: most common upper extremity fracture in patients with osteoporosis
Rickets and osteomalacia[54]	16–28	*Rickets* Findings are most prominent in patients with chronic disease Metaphyseal demineralization resulting in frayed metaphyses Bowing deformities Osteopenia Looser's zones *Osteomalacia* Diffuse osteopenia Decreased trabeculae; remaining trabeculae appear prominent and coarsened Looser's zones (pseudofractures) rare in radius and ulna
Renal osteodystrophy and hyperparathyroidism[55–57]	16–29	Brown tumor (osteoclastoma): solitary or multiple expansile osteolytic lesions containing fibrous tissue and giant cells; may disappear after treatment for hyperparathyroidism Osteosclerosis more common in renal osteodystrophy Rickets-like physeal changes in patients with chronic renal disease
Primary hypertrophic osteoarthropathy (pachydermoperiostosis)[58]	16–30	Primary form of hypertrophic osteoarthropathy (3 to 5 per cent of all cases of hypertrophic osteoarthropathy) Bilateral symmetric periostitis of the long tubular bones Clinical syndrome: enlargement of the hands and feet, digital clubbing, convexity of the nails, cutaneous abnormalities, and joint pains
Secondary hypertrophic osteoarthropathy[58]	16–31	Bilateral symmetric periostitis of radius and ulna as well as other tubular bones Syndrome characterized by digital clubbing, arthritis, and bilateral symmetric periostitis of humerus and other tubular bones Complication of many diseases including bronchogenic carcinoma, mesothelioma and other intrathoracic and intra-abdominal diseases
Lead poisoning[59, 60]	16–32	Prolonged ingestion, inhalation, or absorption of lead-containing materials Thick transverse radiodense metaphyseal lines in infants and children Similar radiodense lines also may be seen in the metaphyses, iliac crest, and vertebral bodies of adults Delayed skeletal development
Hemophilic pseudotumor[61, 62]	16–33	Massive periosteal or intraosseous hemorrhage results in an expanded radiolucent pseudotumor Well-defined osteolytic lesion within radius, ulna, or other bones
Acute pyogenic osteomyelitis[63]	16–34	Acute pyogenic osteomyelitis frequently involves the metaphysis in children Poorly defined permeative bone destruction and soft tissue swelling
Chronic recurrent multifocal osteomyelitis (CRMO)[64]	16–35	Unknown cause This unusual entity is controversial—not certain whether it is truly infectious in nature Occurs mainly in children and adolescents Radiographic findings suggest acute or subacute osteomyelitis Initial osteolytic destruction of metaphysis adjacent to growth plate with no periosteal bone formation or sequestration May be associated with pustular skin lesions (synovitis-acne-pustulosis-hyperostosis-osteomyelitis [SAPHO] syndrome) Typically causes significant symptoms but regresses without residual change
Collagen vascular disease: soft tissue calcification[65]	16–36	Dermatomyositis, polymyositis, scleroderma, and other collagen vascular diseases may result in calcinosis in the soft tissues of the upper arm Differential diagnosis: hyperparathyroidism, neurologic injury, melorheostosis, posttraumatic heterotopic ossification, soft tissue neoplasms, fibrodysplasia ossificans progressiva

See also Tables 1–13 to 1–17.

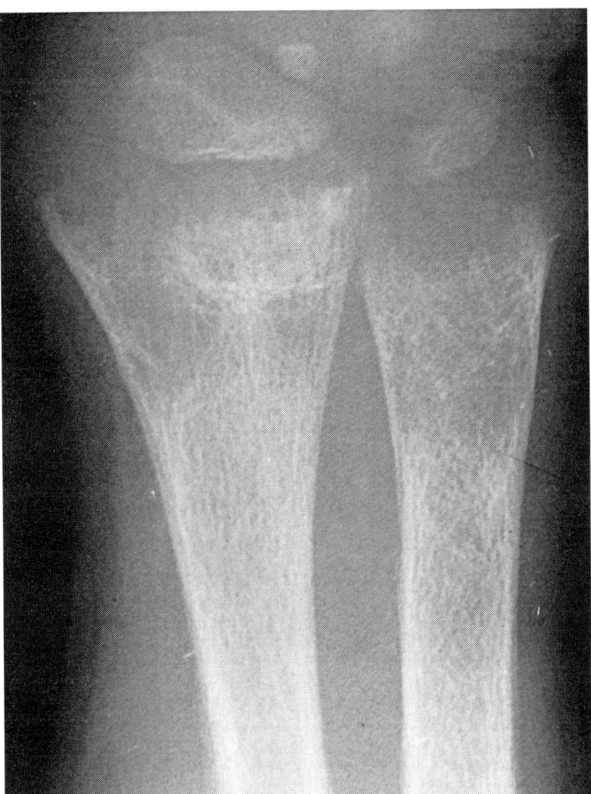

FIGURE 16–28. Rickets.[54] Physeal widening, metaphyseal disorganization, irregularity, and demineralization are characteristic findings in children with advanced rickets.

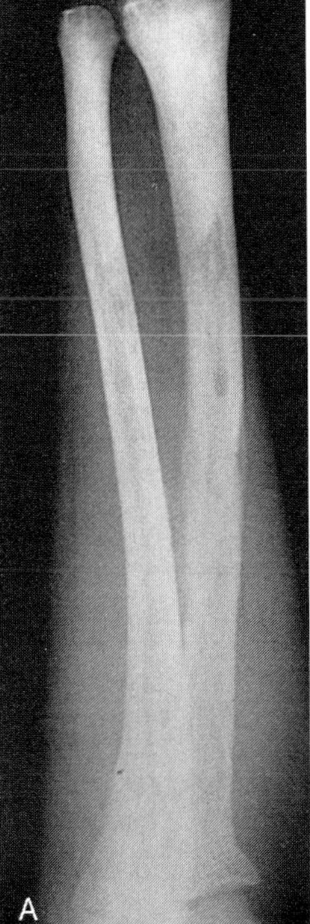

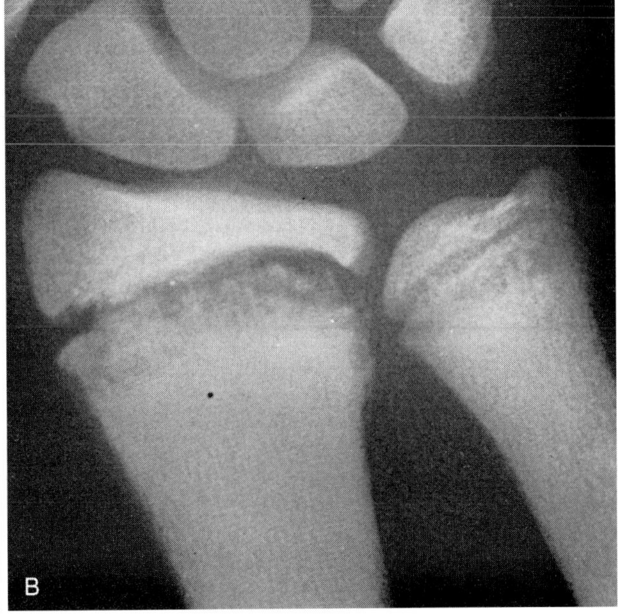

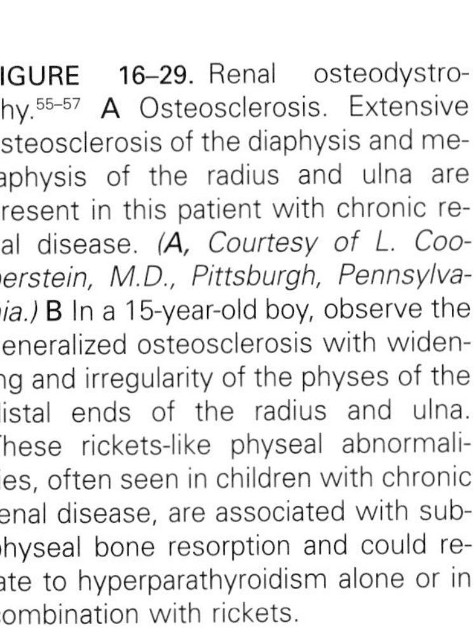

FIGURE 16–29. Renal osteodystrophy.[55–57] A Osteosclerosis. Extensive osteosclerosis of the diaphysis and metaphysis of the radius and ulna are present in this patient with chronic renal disease. *(A, Courtesy of L. Cooperstein, M.D., Pittsburgh, Pennsylvania.)* B In a 15-year-old boy, observe the generalized osteosclerosis with widening and irregularity of the physes of the distal ends of the radius and ulna. These rickets-like physeal abnormalities, often seen in children with chronic renal disease, are associated with subphyseal bone resorption and could relate to hyperparathyroidism alone or in combination with rickets.

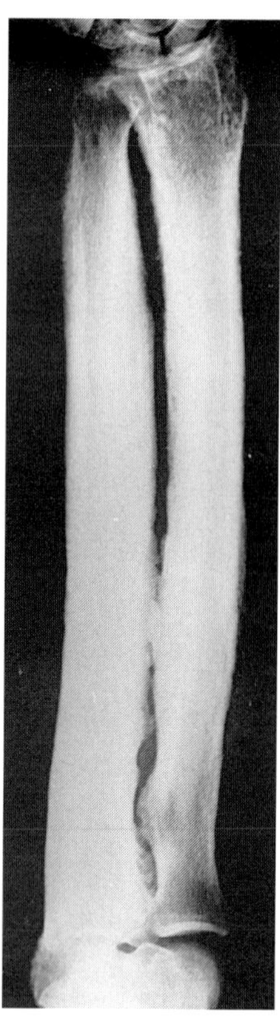

FIGURE 16–30. Primary hypertrophic osteoarthropathy: Pachydermoperiostosis.[58] Widespread, prominent periostitis affects the radius and ulna. The findings in this patient were bilateral and symmetric and involved several tubular bones throughout the skeleton. *(Courtesy of C. Chen, M.D., Kaohsiung, Taiwan, Republic of China.)*

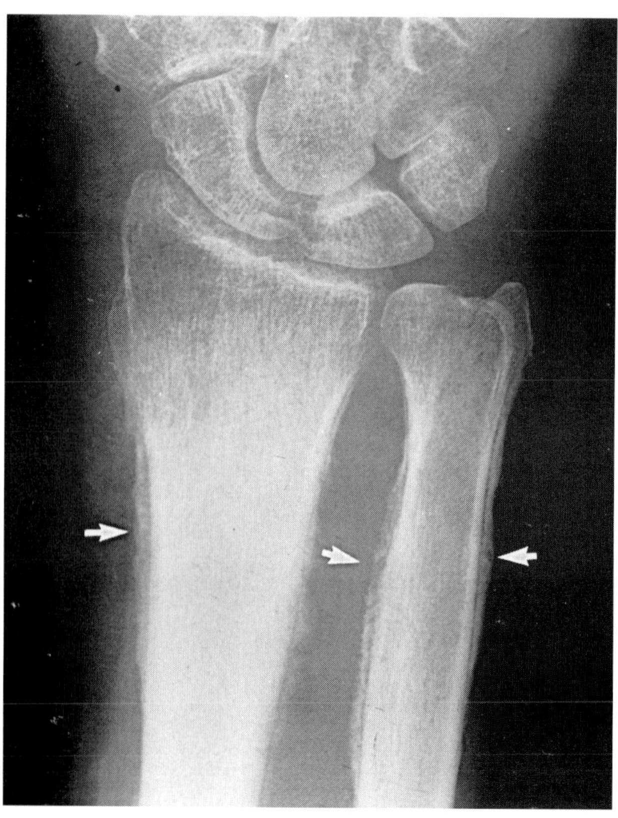

FIGURE 16–31. Secondary hypertrophic osteoarthropathy.[58] Radial and ulnar periostitis (arrows) is seen in this patient with bronchogenic carcinoma. The findings were bilateral and symmetric.

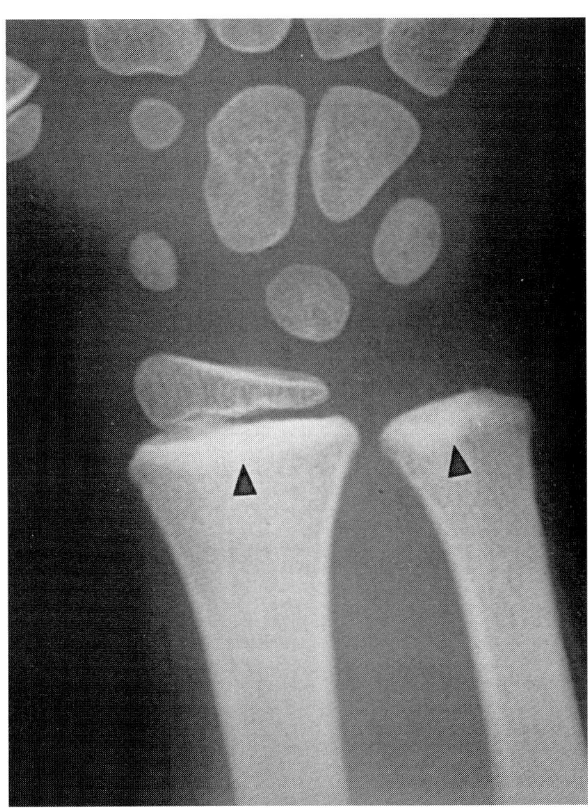

FIGURE 16–32. Lead poisoning.[59, 60] This 6-year-old boy had been eating paint for 1 year when this radiograph was obtained. Observe the transverse sclerotic bands within the metaphyses of the radius and ulna (arrowheads). These changes were present bilaterally. Other causes of metaphyseal density are treated rickets, scurvy, hypoparathyroidism, and hypervitaminosis A or D.

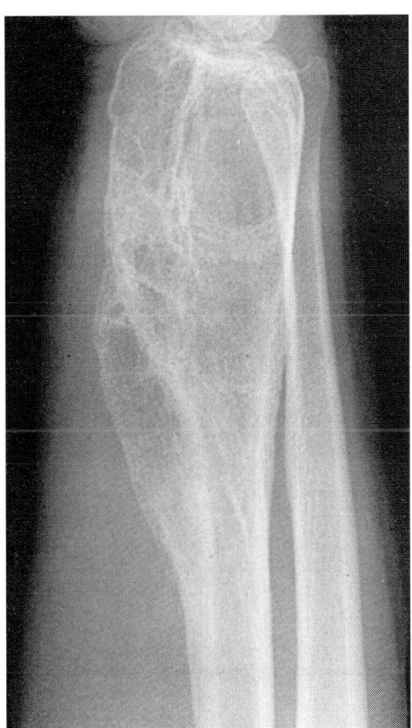

FIGURE 16–33. Hemophilia: pseudotumor.[61, 62] A large multiloculated, expansile osteolytic lesion extending from the mid-diaphysis to the epiphysis of the radius in this 19-year-old man represents a pseudotumor that accompanies intraosseous or periosteal bleeding in hemophilia. This lesion also resembles an aneurysmal bone cyst or giant cell tumor. *(Courtesy of A. Brower, M.D., Norfolk, Virginia.)*

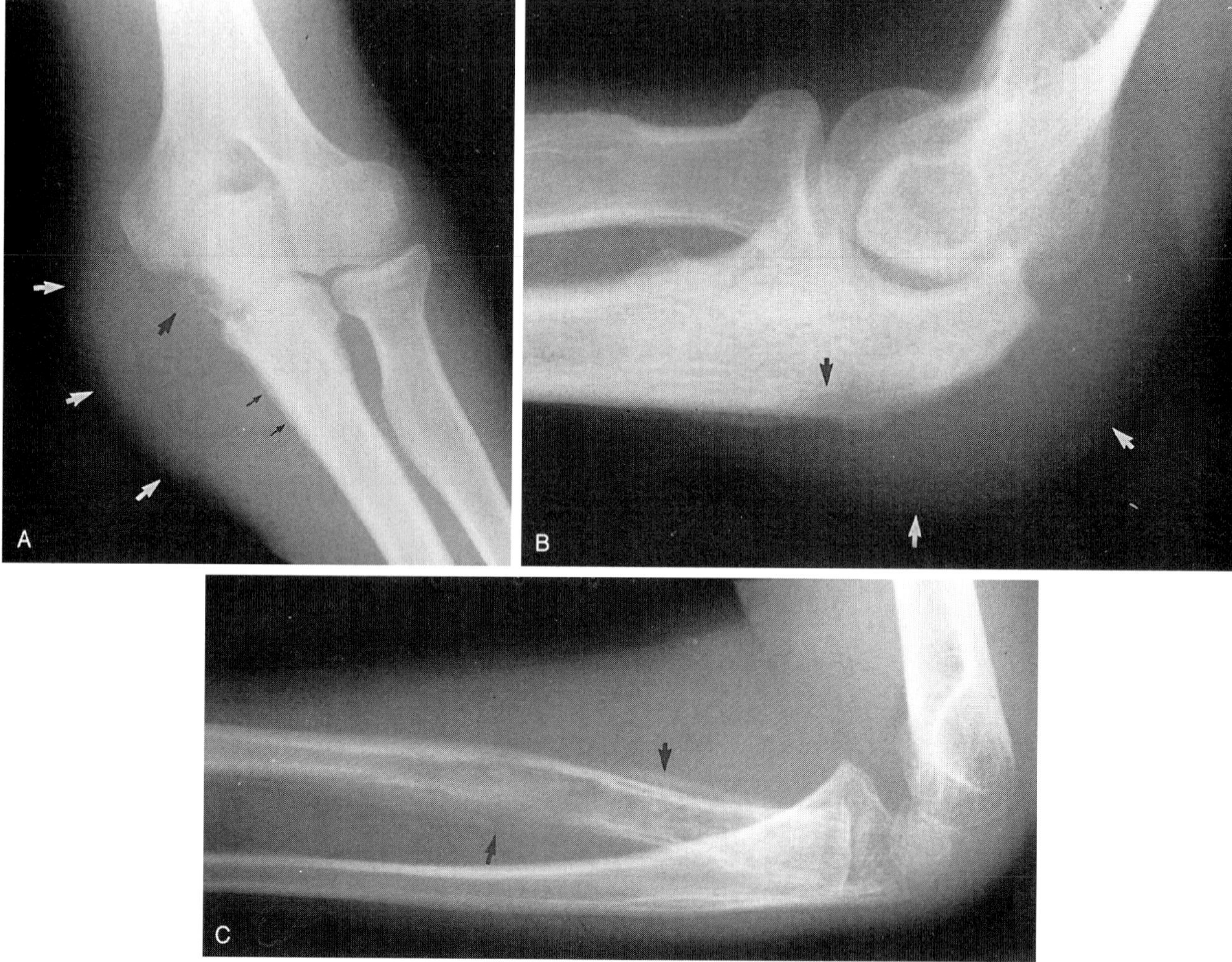

FIGURE 16–34. Acute pyogenic osteomyelitis.[63] A, B This 23-year-old man complained of pain and swelling about the elbow and forearm. Frontal (A) and lateral (B) radiographs of the elbow show marked soft tissue swelling (white arrows) as well as diffuse sclerosis of the proximal portion of the ulna, prominent osseous erosions of the medial olecranon (large black arrows), and periostitis (small black arrows). C In another patient, a child, a permeative pattern of osteolytic destruction and single-layer periostitis (arrows) is evident in the radius.

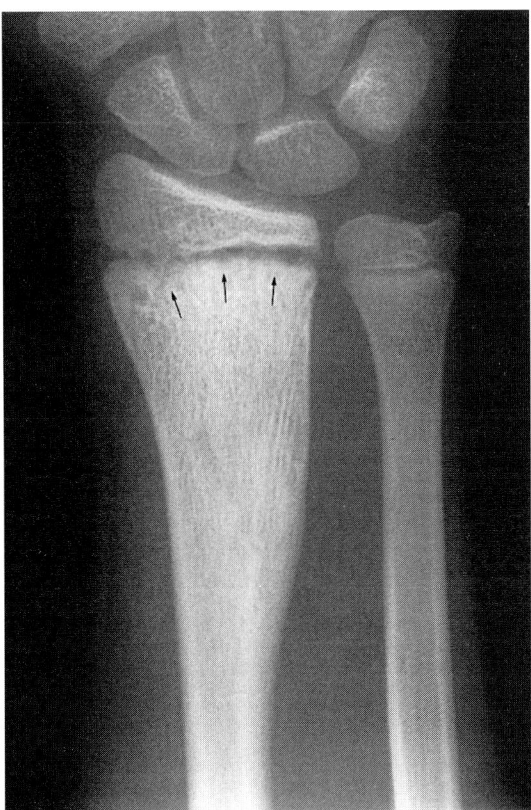

FIGURE 16–35. Chronic recurrent multifocal osteomyelitis.[64] This 12-year-old boy had had unilateral wrist pain and swelling of 12 months' duration. Eight months after the wrist pain subsided, he developed unilateral ankle pain and swelling. The erythrocyte sedimentation rate was slightly elevated, but all other serologic test results were normal. Radiographs revealed similar changes in both locations. The findings include striking metaphyseal sclerosis, periosteal bone expansion, and subchondral osteolysis of the metaphysis adjacent to the growth plate (arrows). *(Courtesy of S. Cassell, M.D., Eugene, Oregon.)*

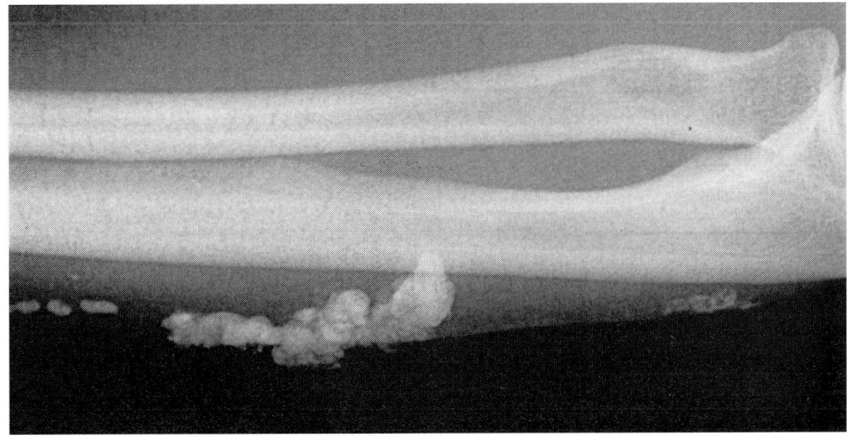

FIGURE 16–36. Scleroderma (progressive systemic sclerosis).[65] Globular masses of soft tissue calcification are seen adjacent to the dorsal surface of the ulna in this patient with long-standing scleroderma (progressive systemic sclerosis).

REFERENCES

1. Mital MA: Congenital radioulnar synostosis and congenital dislocation of the radial head. Orthop Clin North Am 7:375, 1976.
2. Köhler A, Zimmer EA: Borderlands of Normal and Early Pathologic Findings in Skeletal Radiography. 4th Ed. New York, Thieme Medical Publishers, 1993, p 163.
3. Fagg PS: Wrist pain in the Madelung's deformity of dyschondrosteosis. J Hand Surg [Br] 13:11, 1988.
4. Friedman SL, Palmer AK: The ulnar impaction syndrome. Hand Clin 7:295, 1991.
5. Imaeda T, Nakamura R, Shionoya K, Met al: Ulnar impaction syndrome: MR imaging findings. Radiology 201:495, 1996.
6. Escobedo EM, Bergman AG, Hunter JC: MR imaging of ulnar impaction. Skeletal Radiol 24:85, 1995.
7. Bonzar M, Firrell JC, Mah ET, et al: Kienböck disease and negative ulnar variance. J Bone Joint Surg [Am] 80:1154, 1998.
8. DeSmet L: Ulnar variance: Facts and fiction review article. Acta Orthop Belg 60:1, 1994.
9. Voorhees DR, Daffner RH, Nunley JA, et al: Carpal ligamentous disruptions and negative ulnar variance. Skeletal Radiol 13:257, 1985.
10. Goldberg HD, Young JWR, Reiner BI, et al: Double injuries of the forearm: A common occurrence. Radiology 185:223, 1992.
11. Olney BW, Menelaus MB: Monteggia and equivalent lesions in childhood. J Pediatr Orthop 9:219, 1989.
12. Ring D, Jupiter JB, Simpson NS: Monteggia fractures in adults. J Bone Joint Surg [Am] 80:1733, 1998.
13. Alpar EK, Thompson K, Owen R, et al: Midshaft fractures of the forearm bones in children. Injury 13:153, 1981.
14. Walsh HPJ, McLaren CAN, Owen R: Galeazzi fractures in children. J Bone Joint Surg [Br] 69:730, 1987.
15. Watson FM, Eaton RG: Post-traumatic radio-ulnar synostosis. J Trauma 18:467, 1978.
16. Anderson MW, Greenspan A: Stress fractures. Radiology 199:1, 1996.
17. Cautilli RA, Joyce MF, Gordon E, et al: Classifications of fractures of the distal radius. Clin Orthop 103:163, 1974.
18. Light TR, Ogden DA, Ogden JA: The anatomy of metaphyseal torus fractures. Clin Orthop 188:103, 1984.
19. DeOliveira JC: Barton's fractures. J Bone Joint Surg [Am] 55:586, 1973.
20. Bilos ZJ, Pankovich AM, Yelda S: Fracture-dislocation of the radiocarpal joint. J Bone Joint Surg [Am] 59:198, 1977.
21. Helm RH, Tonkin MA: The chauffeur's fracture: Simple or complex? J Hand Surg [Br] 17:156, 1992.
22. Thomas WG, Kershaw CJ: Entrapment of the extensor tendons in a Smith's fracture: Brief report. J Bone Joint Surg [Br] 70:491, 1988.
23. Burgess RC, Watson HK: Hypertrophic ulnar styloid nonunions. Clin Orthop 228:215, 1988.
24. Kleinman PK, Marks SC Jr, Richmond JM, et al: Inflicted skeletal injury: Post mortem radiologic-histopathologic study in 31 infants. AJR 165:647, 1995.
25. Manoli A II: Irreducible fracture-separation of the distal radial epiphysis: Report of a case. J Bone Joint Surg [Am] 64:1095, 1982.
26. Chang CY, Shih C, Penn IW, et al: Wrist injuries in adolescent gymnasts of a Chinese opera school: Radiography survey. Radiology 195:861, 1995.
27. Greenspan A, Norman A: Osteolytic cortical destruction: An unusual pattern of skeletal metastasis. Skeletal Radiol 17:402, 1988.
28. Resnik C, Garver P, Resnick D: Bony expansion in skeletal metastasis from carcinoma of the prostate as seen by bone scintigraphy. South Med J 77:1331, 1984.
29. Dahlin DC, Unni KK: Osteosarcoma of bone and its important recognizable varieties. Am J Surg Pathol 1:61, 1977.
30. Ritschl P, Wurnig C, Lechner G, et al: Parosteal osteosarcoma: 2-23-year follow-up of 33 patients. Acta Orthop Scand 62:195, 1991.
31. Dahlin DC: Giant cell tumor of bone: Highlights of 407 cases. AJR 144:955, 1985.
32. Dahlin DC, Coventry MB, Scanlon PW: Ewing's sarcoma: A critical analysis of 165 cases. J Bone Joint Surg [Am] 43:185, 1961.
33. Kyle RA: Multiple myeloma: Review of 869 cases. Mayo Clin Proc 50:29, 1975.
34. Clayton F, Butler JJ, Ayala AG, et al: Non-Hodgkin's lymphoma in bone: Pathologic and radiologic features with clinical correlates. Cancer 60:2494, 1987.
35. Benz G, Brandeis WE, Willich E: Radiological aspects of leukemia in childhood: An analysis of 89 children. Pediatr Radiol 4:201, 1976.
36. Kayser F, Resnick D, Haghighi P, et al: Evidence of the subperiosteal origin of osteoid osteomas in tubular bones: Analysis by CT and MR imaging. AJR 170:609, 1998.
37. Tonai M, Campbell CJ, Ahn GH, et al: Osteoblastoma: Classification and report of 16 cases. Clin Orthop 167:222, 1982.
38. Schiller AL: Diagnosis of borderline cartilage lesions of bone. Semin Diagn Pathol 2:42, 1985.
39. Milgran JW: The origins of osteochondromas and enchondromas: A histopathologic study. Clin Orthop 174:264, 1983.
40. Karasick D, Schweitzer ME, Eschelman DJ: Symptomatic osteochondromas: Imaging features. AJR 168:1507, 1997.
41. Burgess RC, Cates H: Deformities of the forearm in patients who have multiple cartilaginous exostosis. J Bone Joint Surg [Am] 75:13, 1993.
42. Schmale GA, Conrad EV, Raskind WH: The natural history of hereditary multiple exostosis. J Bone Joint Surg [Am] 76:986, 1994.
43. Ritschl P, Karnel F, Hajek P: Fibrous metaphyseal defects: Determination of their origin and natural history using a radiomorphological study. Skeletal Radiol 17:8, 1988.
44. Milgram JW: Intraosseous lipoma: A clinicopathologic study of 66 cases. Clin Orthop 231:277, 1988.
45. Sherman RS, Wilner D: The roentgen diagnosis of hemangioma of bone. AJR 86:1146, 1961.
46. De Dios AMV, Bond JR, Shives TC, et al: Aneurysmal bone cyst: A clinico-pathologic study of 238 cases. Cancer 69:2921, 1992.
47. Matfin G, McPherson F: Paget's disease of bone: Recent advances. J Orthop Rheumatol 6:127, 1993.
48. Mirra JM, Brien EW, Tehranzadeh J: Paget's disease of bone: Review with emphasis on radiologic features, part II. Skeletal Radiol 24:173, 1995.
49. Gibson MJ, Middlemiss JH: Fibrous dysplasia of bone. Br J Radiol 44:1, 1971.
50. Stull MA, Kransdorf MJ, Devaney KO: Langerhans cell histiocytosis of bone. RadioGraphics 12:801, 1992.
51. Kilpatrick SE, Wenger DE, Gilchrist GS, et al: Langerhans' cell histiocytosis (histiocytosis X) of bone: A clinicopathologic analysis of 263 pediatric and adult cases. Cancer 76:2471, 1995.
52. Taylor JAM, Resnick D, Sartoris DJ: Radiographic-pathologic correlation. *In* Sartoris DJ: Osteoporosis: Diagno-

sis and Treatment. New York, Marcel Dekker, 1996, p 147.
53. Brien E, Healey JH: *In* Sartoris DJ: Osteoporosis: Diagnosis and Treatment. New York, Marcel Dekker, 1996, p 116.
54. Mankin HJ: Rickets, osteomalacia, and renal osteodystrophy. Orthop Clin North Am 21:81, 1990.
55. Wolfson BJ, Capitanio MA: The wide spectrum of renal osteodystrophy in children. CRC Crit Rev Diagn Imaging 27:297, 1987.
56. Tigges S, Nance EP, Carpenter WA, et al: Renal osteodystrophy: Imaging findings that mimic those of other diseases. AJR 165:143, 1995.
57. Sundaram M: Renal osteodystrophy. Skeletal Radiol 18:415, 1989.
58. Pineda C: Diagnostic imaging in hypertrophic osteoarthropathy. Clin Exp Rheumatol 10:27, 1992.
59. Sachs HK: The evolution of the radiologic lead line. Radiology 19:81, 1981.
60. Raber SA: The dense metaphyseal band sign. Radiology 211:773, 1999.
61. Jaovisidha S, Nam Ryu K, Hodler J, et al: Hemophilic pseudotumor: Spectrum of MR findings. Skeletal Radiol 26:468, 1997.
62. Wilson DA, Prince JR: MR imaging of hemophilic pseudotumors. AJR 150:349, 1988.
63. Gold RH, Hawkins RA, Katz RD: Bacterial osteomyelitis: Findings on plain radiography, CT, MR, and scintigraphy. AJR 157:365, 1991.
64. Rosenberg ZS, Shankman S, Klein M, et al: Chronic recurrent multifocal osteomyelitis. AJR 151:142, 1988.
65. Czirjak L, Nagy Z, Szegedi G: Systemic sclerosis in the elderly. Clin Rheumatol 11:483, 1992.

CHAPTER 17

Wrist and Hand

Normal Developmental Anatomy

A thorough understanding of normal developmental anatomy is essential for accurate interpretation of radiographs of the pediatric wrist and hand. Table 17–1 outlines the age of appearance and fusion of the primary and secondary ossification centers. Figure 17–1 illustrates examples of radiographs of children from 13 months to 15 years of age. Both the chronological age and skeletal age are listed for each of these examples. These radiographs show the radiographic appearance of many important ossification centers and other developmental landmarks from infancy through adolescence. For precise assessment of skeletal age, the Gruehlich and Pyle atlas[1] or similar publications should be consulted.

Figure 17–2 shows the normal appearance of the phalangeal ungual tufts.

Developmental Anomalies, Anatomic Variants, and Sources of Diagnostic Error

The bones and soft tissues of the wrist and hand are frequent sites of anomalies, anatomic variations, and other sources of diagnostic error that may simulate disease and potentially result in misdiagnoses. Furthermore, many of these alterations may represent a component of a more complex developmental malformation syndrome or chromosomal abnormality. Table 17–2 and Figures 17–3 to 17–12 illustrate selected examples of some of the more common processes.

Skeletal Dysplasias and Other Congenital Diseases

Table 17–3 outlines a number of the skeletal dysplasias and congenital disorders that may affect the wrist and hand. Figures 17–13 to 17–17 show the radiographic manifestations of some of these disorders.

Physical Injury

Physical injury to the wrist and hand may result in a wide variety of fractures, dislocations, and soft tissue injuries. Table 17–4 and Figures 17–18 to 17–26 pertain to fractures and dislocations of the carpal bones.

Table 17–5 and Figures 17–27 to 17–30 describe and illustrate the most common patterns of ligamentous instability of the wrist. Table 17–6 and Figures 17–31 to 17–37 refer to fractures and dislocations of the metacarpal bones and phalanges.

Soft Tissue Disorders

Several disorders of the soft tissues are encountered about the wrist and hand. Table 17–7 represents a list of some of the more frequently occurring conditions, some of which are illustrated in Figures 17–38 to 17–40.

Articular Disorders

The articulations of the wrist and hand are frequent target sites for degenerative, inflammatory, crystal-induced, and infectious articular disorders. Table 17–8 outlines these diseases and their radiographic characteristics. Table 17–9 is a compartmental analysis emphasizing the target sites of joint involvement typical of some of the more common disorders. Figures 17–41 to 17–65 illustrate the typical radiographic manifestations of the most common articular disorders affecting this region.

Tumors and Tumor-like Lesions

Malignant tumors of bone involve the bones of the hand and wrist much less frequently than benign tumors. Table 17–10 lists and characterizes these malignant neoplasms, many of which are illustrated in Figures 17–66 to 17–71. Table 17–11 describes benign tumors and tumor-like lesions that characteristically involve the bones of the wrist and hand. These are illustrated in Figures 17– 72 to 17–80.

Metabolic, Hematologic, Vascular, and Infectious Disorders

Several metabolic, hematologic, vascular, and infectious disorders involve the bones of the wrist and hand and the surrounding soft tissue structures. Table 17–12 lists some of the more common disorders and describes their characteristics. Figures 17–81 to 17–92 illustrate the characteristic imaging findings of several of these disorders.

Osteonecrosis

Osteonecrosis of the bones about the wrist and hand may occur spontaneously or result from trauma or other predisposing factors. Table 17–13 discusses these disorders. An example of Kienböck's disease—osteonecrosis of the lunate bone—is shown in Figure 17–93. Posttraumatic osteonecrosis of the scaphoid bone is illustrated earlier in the chapter (Fig. 17–18*D*).

Acquired Deformities

Several well-recognized patterns of deformity occur about the wrist and hand. Most of these acquired deformities result from complications of inflammatory articular disorders or from physical injury. Table 17–14 describes a number of these deformities, many of which are illustrated throughout the chapter as they are manifested in several of the causative disorders.

Phalangeal Resorption

Table 17–15 lists several disorders that result in phalangeal resorption or acro-osteolysis and identifies the site of resorption characteristic of each disorder. Examples of phalangeal resorption are illustrated throughout the chapter as they characteristically appear in relation to many of the disorders. Figure 17–94 is a schematic diagram of the different sites of resorption.

Soft Tissue Calcification

Table 17–16 lists several disorders that result in soft tissue calcification about the terminal phalanges. Many examples of such calcification are illustrated throughout the chapter.

TABLE 17–1. Wrist and Hand: Approximate Age of Appearance and Fusion of Ossification Centers[1–5] (Figs. 17–1 and 17–2)

Ossification Center	Primary or Secondary	No. of Centers	Age of Appearance*	Age of Fusion* (Years)
Wrist				
Capitate	P	1	Birth–6 months	
Hamate	P	1	Birth–6 months	
Triquetrum	P	1	1–3.5 years	
Lunate	P	1	1.5–4.5 years	
Navicular	P	1	3–9 years	
Trapezium	P	1	3–9 years	
Trapezoid	P	1	3–9 years	
Pisiform	P	1	7–13 years	
Distal radial epiphysis	S	1	6 24 months	20–25
Distal ulnar epiphysis	S	1	5.5–9.5 years	19–25
Hand				
Metacarpal heads (second through fifth)	S	4	10–24 months	14–21
Metacarpal base (first)	S	1	1–3.5 years	14–21
Phalangeal bases (second through fifth)	S	4	1–2.5 years	14 21
Phalangeal bases (first)	S	1	1–2.5 years	14–21

*Ages of appearance and fusion of ossification centers in girls typically precede those of boys. Ethnic differences also exist.
P, Primary; S, secondary.

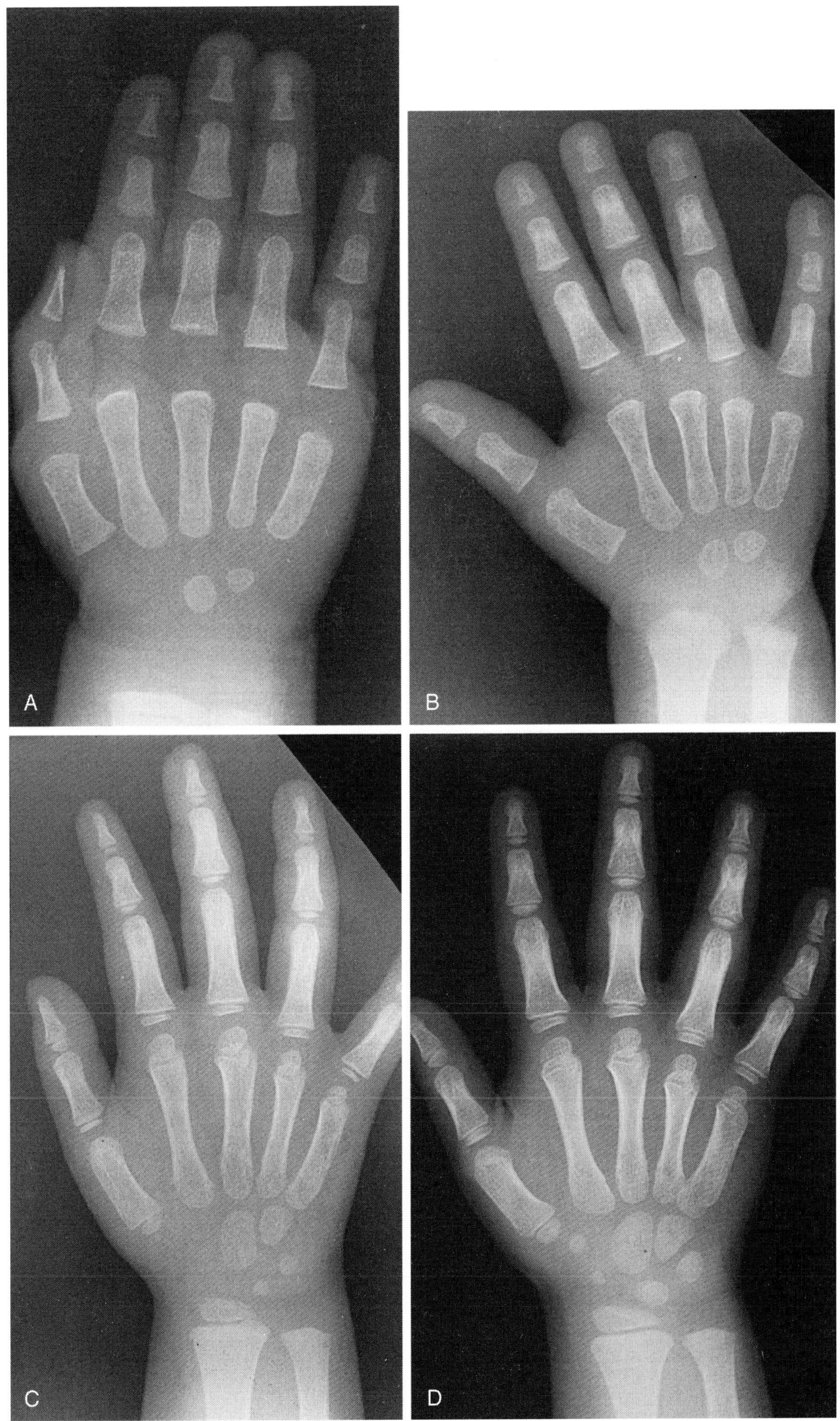

FIGURE 17–1. Skeletal maturation and normal development: Posteroanterior radiographs of the hand and wrist.[1–5] A Male; CA = 13 mo; SA = 15 mo; SD ± 2.1. B Male; CA = 20 mo; SA = 18 mo; SD ± 2.7. C Female; CA = 3 yr; SA = 3 yr; SD ± 6.0. D Female; CA = 4 yr 5 mo; SA = 4 yr; SD ± 7.0.

Illustration continued on following page

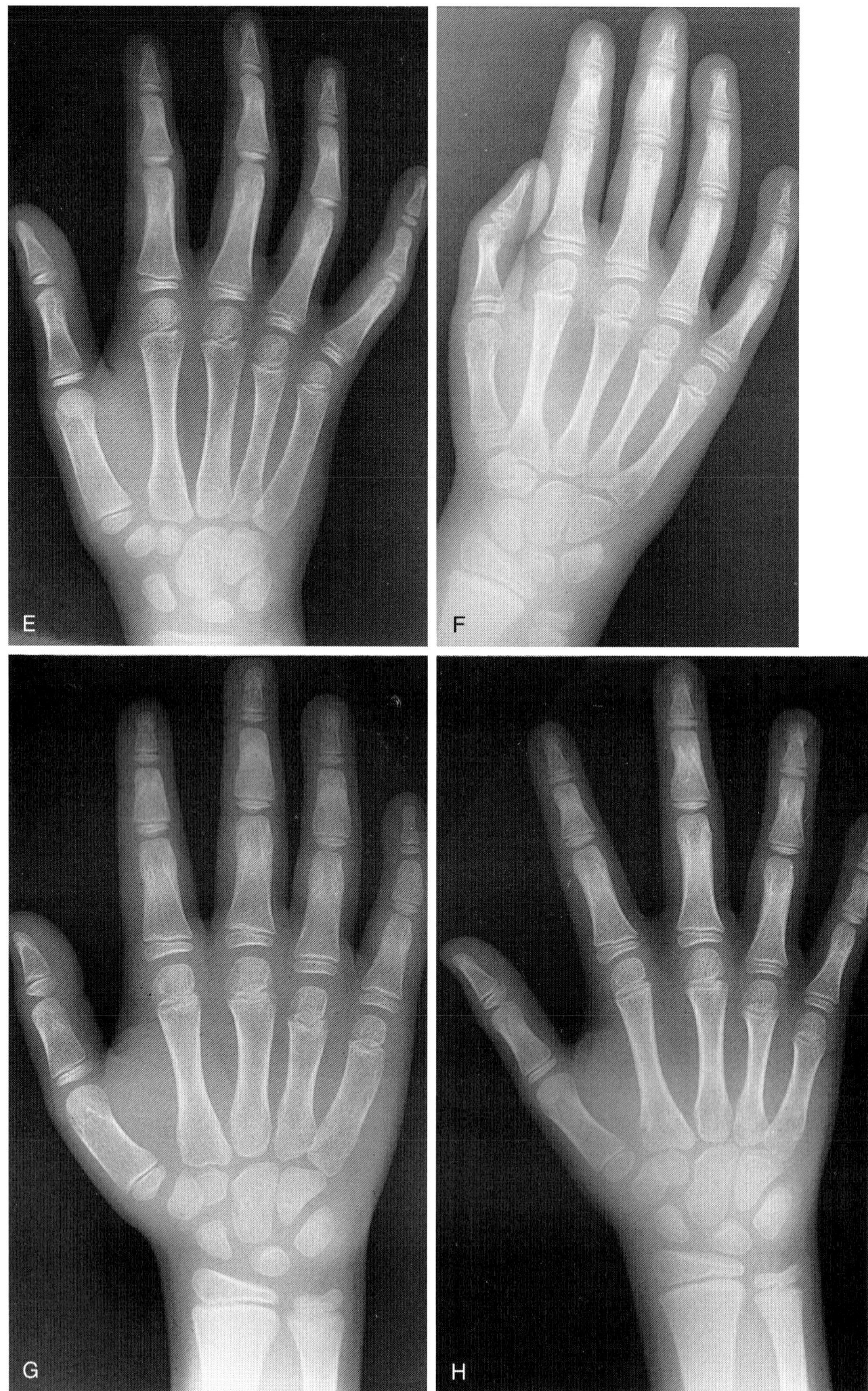

FIGURE 17–1 *Continued.* **E** Male; CA = 7 yr; SA = 7 yr; SD ± 10.0. **F** Female; CA = 8 yr; SA = 8 yr 6 mo; SD ± 10.9. **G** Male; CA = 8 yr 4 mo; SA = 9 yr; SD ± 11.0. **H** Male; CA = 10 yr; SA = 10 yr; SD ± 11.4.

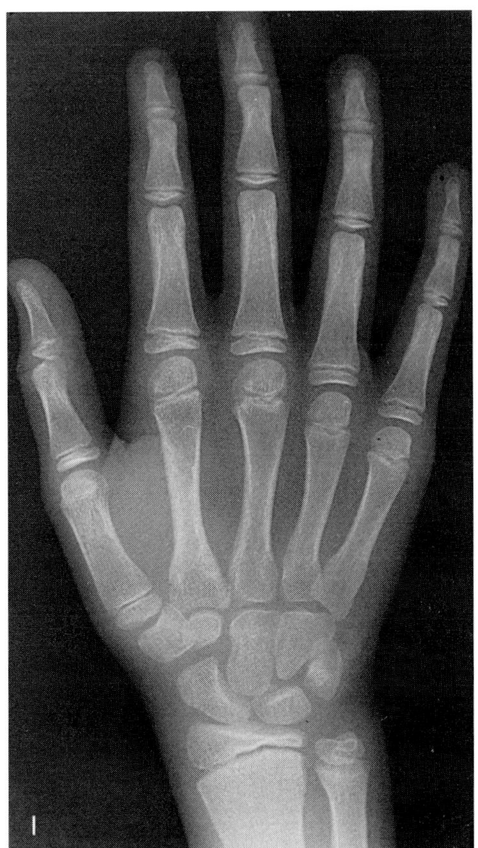

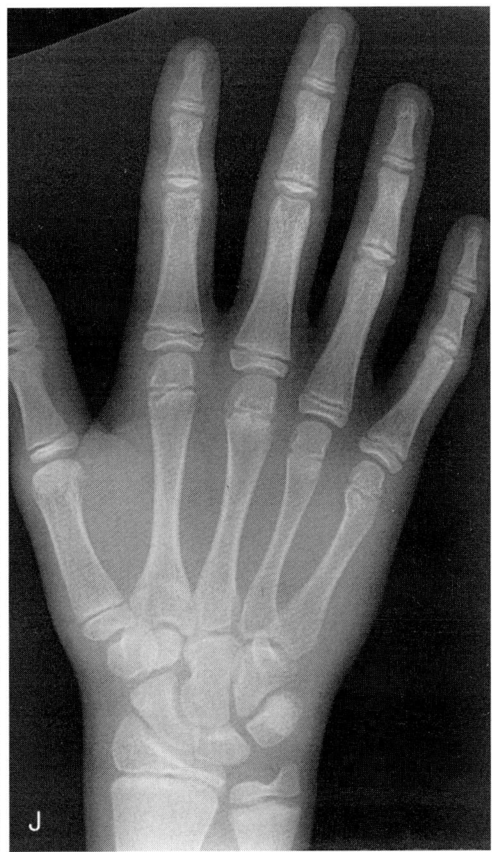

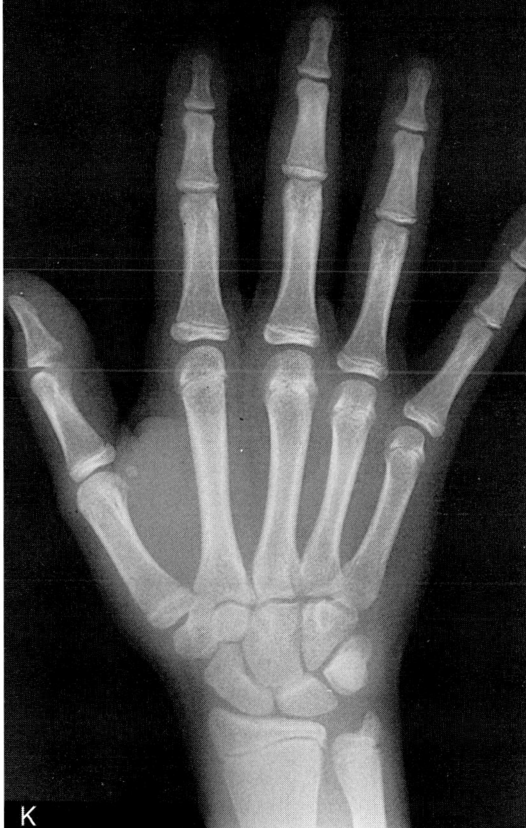

FIGURE 17–1 *Continued.* **I** Male; CA = 11 yr; SA = 11 yr; SD ± 10.5. **J** Male; CA = 14 yr; SA = 13 yr 6 mo; SD ± 11.5. **K** Female; CA = 15 yr; SA = 13 yr 6 mo; SD ± 13.6.

CA, Chronologic age in months (mo) or years (yr); SA, estimated skeletal age in months (mo) or years (yr); SD, standard deviation from the mean expressed in months.

Note: These radiographs were randomly selected from teaching files from a variety of sources to demonstrate only general trends in osseous development. For precise and accurate assessment of skeletal maturity of the hand and wrist, refer to Greulich WW, Pyle SI: *Radiographic Atlas of Skeletal Development of the Hand and Wrist.* 2nd Ed. Palo Alto, Stanford University Press, 1959.

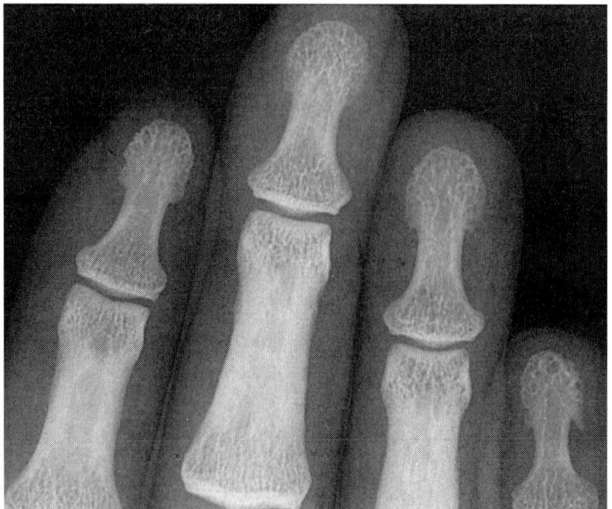

FIGURE 17–2. Normal ungual tufts: Terminal phalanges.[2–5] Note the normally bulbous end of the terminal tuft. The trabeculae may appear somewhat lace-like and should not be confused with a pathologic condition.

TABLE 17–2. Developmental Anomalies, Anatomic Variants, and Sources of Diagnostic Error*

Entity	Figure(s)	Characteristics	Associated Syndromes or Disorders
Madelung's deformity[6, 7]	16–2	*Radius* Dorsal and ulnar curvature; decreased length; triangular distal epiphysis owing to premature fusion of medial half of epiphysis; ulnar and volar angulation of distal radial articular surface *Ulna* Elongated ulna with dorsal subluxation; enlargement and distortion of ulnar head *Carpal bones* Wedging of carpal bones between deformed radius and protruding ulna; triangular configuration of carpals with lunate at apex *Inferior radioulnar joint* Increased width of inferior radioulnar joint *Radiocarpal joint* V-shaped; decreased carpal angle See also Table 16–1	Isolated idiopathic form Dysplastic form: multiple hereditary exostosis and dyschondrosteosis Genetic form: Turner's syndrome Posttraumatic form: extension injury to radial epiphysis

TABLE 17–2. Developmental Anomalies, Anatomic Variants, and Sources of Diagnostic Error*
Continued

Entity	Figure(s)	Characteristics	Associated Syndromes or Disorders
Carpal synostosis (coalition)[8, 9]	17–3	Lunate-triquetrum: most frequent site; often bilateral Capitate-hamate: second most frequent site Synostoses of carpal bones in the same row usually are isolated anomalies of no clinical significance Occasional painful osteoarthrosis may develop at site of partial fusion Scapholunate space may be widened with intact scapholunate ligament in lunotriquetral coalition Synostosis of more than two carpal bones or of carpal bones across both rows occurs infrequently and may be related to congenital malformation syndromes	Arthrogryposis Ellis–van Creveld syndrome Hand-foot-uterus syndrome Symphalangism Dyschondrosteosis Holt-Oram syndrome Cleft hand and foot Polydactyly Symphalangism Tarsal coalition Acquired: Inflammatory arthropathy may result in ankylosis
Scaphoid anomalies[10]		*Rare anomalies:* Bipartite scaphoid Hypoplastic scaphoid *Variants:* Irregular distal pole Normal scaphoid tubercle	Often mistaken for fractures or other pathologic condition
Accessory carpal bones[10]	17–4	Additional ossification centers result in extra carpal bones Unfused ossicles (accessory bones) represent normal anatomic variants that usually are of no clinical significance; infrequently result in symptoms; frequently simulate fractures Typical location and smooth, well-corticated margins help to distinguish ossicles from fractures	May be mistaken for fractures Occasionally syndrome-related
Bipartite carpal bones[10, 176, 177]		Any carpal bone may arise from more than one ossification center Bipartite scaphoid and hook of the hamate have been reported	May be mistaken for fractures
Os styloideum[11]	17–5	Also termed carpal boss, carpe bossu, or dorsal boss Accessory ossicle or dorsal bony prominence overlying the dorsal surface of the second and third carpometacarpal joints Often painful owing to bursitis, osteophyte, osseous proliferation, adjacent ganglion, or slippage of extensor tendon	Occasionally mistaken for a ganglion

Table continued on following page

TABLE 17–2. Developmental Anomalies, Anatomic Variants, and Sources of Diagnostic Error*
Continued

Entity	Figure(s)	Characteristics	Associated Syndromes or Disorders
Brachydactyly (brachymesophalangy)[10]	17–6	Developmental shortening of middle phalanx Fifth digit most common Normal variant: 20 per cent of Asian population; 1 per cent of white population Occasionally related to syndrome	Trisomy 21 (60 per cent of patients) Often accompanies clinodactyly
Short metacarpal bone[12]	17–7	Variant of brachydactyly Isolated or syndrome-related forms Usually affects fourth metacarpal bone Premature closure of metacarpal ossification centers Positive metacarpal sign	Isolated anomaly Turner's syndrome Pseudohypoparathyroidism Pseudospseudohypoparathyroidism Sickle cell anemia
Epiphyseal variations[5, 10]		Normal metacarpal and phalangeal epiphyses may be broad, irregular, asymmetric, divided by a cleft, or cone-shaped Additional metacarpal epiphyses occur infrequently Persistent unfused ossification center at the ulnar styloid is a common anomaly (os triangulare)	May mimic fracture or posttraumatic disorder Cleidocranial dysplasia
Syndactyly[10]		Developmental lack of differentiation between two or more digits Fusion of two digits may be partial or complete Osseous or soft tissue involvement Occurs as an isolated anomaly or in association with a generalized syndrome Syndactyly of the second and third digits is most likely an isolated anomaly	May be associated with polydactyly: polysyndactyly Poland syndrome: absent pectoral muscles Many associated chromosomal, craniofacial, and other syndromes
Phalangeal synostosis (symphalangism)[10]	17–8	Nonsegmentation of one phalanx to another within the same digit usually related to absence of ossification centers Usually involves several digits of the same hand May be bilateral	Should not be mistaken for acquired fusion of inflammatory arthropathies
Polydactyly[10]		Developmental duplication of a digit Postaxial: duplicated digits on ulnar side of hand Preaxial: duplicated digits on radial side of hand	Associated anomalies: polydactyly, duplications, absent bones Most frequently an isolated anomaly but may be related to a generalized syndrome
Bifid thumb[10, 14]	17–9	Form of polydactyly in which two terminal phalanges are present side by side or the terminal phalanx is bifurcated	Usually isolated anomaly Down syndrome Fanconi anemia Acrocephalosyndactyly syndromes
Triphalangeal thumb[10, 14]	17–10	Rare normal variant Extra phalanx between proximal and distal phalanges of the thumb	Associated anomalies: polydactyly, duplications, absent bones Associated syndromes: Holt-Oram, trisomy 13–15, and Blackfan-Diamond anemia

TABLE 17–2. Developmental Anomalies, Anatomic Variants, and Sources of Diagnostic Error* *Continued*

Entity	Figure(s)	Characteristics	Associated Syndromes or Disorders
Clinodactyly[10]		Medial or lateral curvature of a finger Most frequently an incidental finding associated with brachydactyly of the fifth digit	Infrequently associated with many different hand and foot syndromes, chromosomal disorders, and craniofacial syndromes Traumatic clinodactyly also may follow injury
Kirner deformity (dystelephalangy)[15]	17–11	Normal variation: palmar bending of the shafts of the fifth terminal phalanges Usually bilateral and painless	Usually isolated variant Epiphyseal separation may occur
Macrodactyly[16, 17]	17–12	Also termed localized or focal gigantism Localized overgrowth of both soft tissues and osseous elements of a digit Isolated congenital form: present at birth	Neurofibromatosis Soft tissue hemangioma Macrodystrophia lipomatosa Lymphangioma Proteus syndrome

See also Table 1–1.
*For a more extensive discussion of these disorders, see Poznanski AK: The Hand in Radiologic Diagnosis. 2nd Ed. Philadelphia, WB Saunders, 1984.

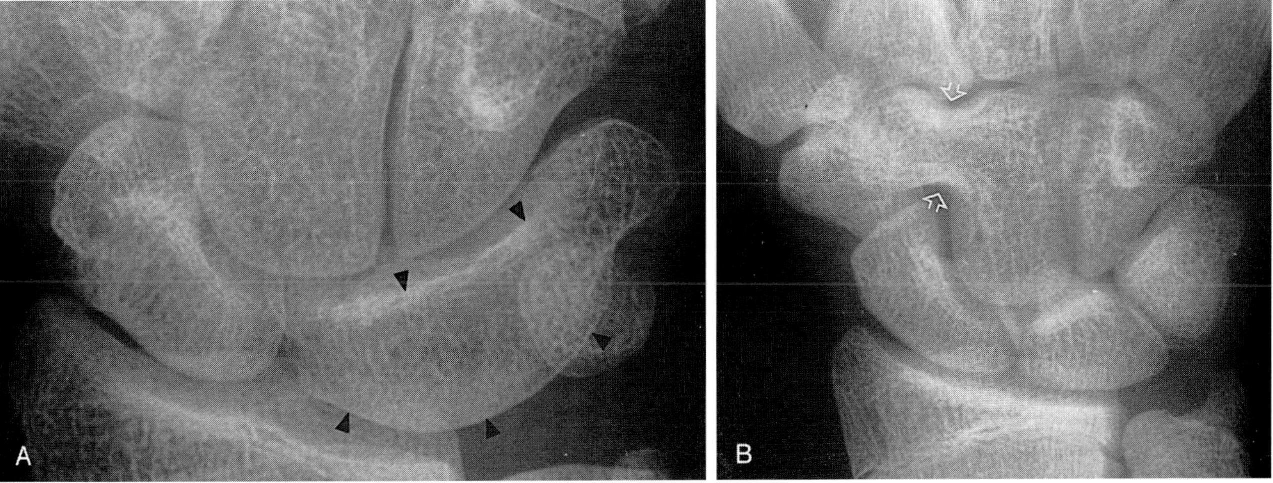

FIGURE 17–3. Carpal synostosis (coalition).[8, 9] **A** Lunotriquetral coalition. Osseous fusion of the lunate bone and the triquetrum is seen in this patient (arrowheads). The lunotriquetral articulation is the most common site of carpal coalition. **B** Capitellotrapezoidal coalition. Osseous ankylosis of the capitellum and trapezoid bones, as seen in this patient (open arrows), is infrequent. Isolated fusions involving bones in the same carpal row (proximal or distal) are common and of no clinical significance. Fusion of carpal bones across different rows may be related to congenital malformation syndromes and deserves further investigation.

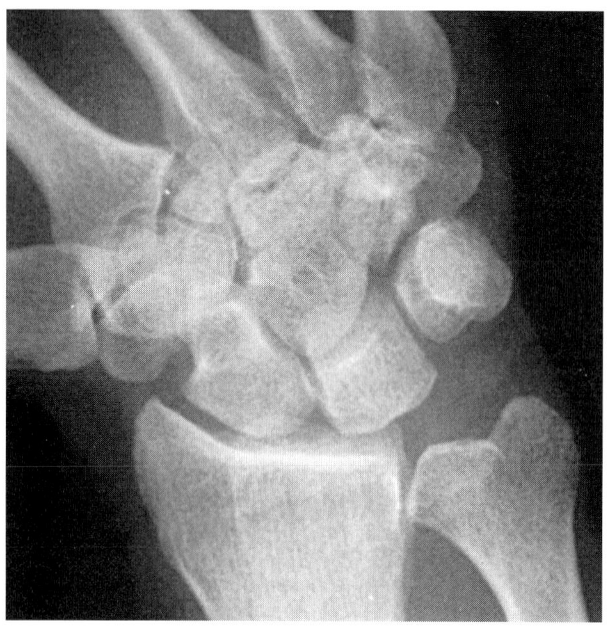

FIGURE 17–4. Accessory carpal bones.[10] Extra ossification centers may appear in the wrist, resulting in extra bones in addition to the eight normal carpal bones. These supernumerary carpal bones usually cause no symptoms or signs, but they must be differentiated from small fracture fragments. Accessory carpal bones may occasionally be found as a component of other heritable or congenital syndromes.

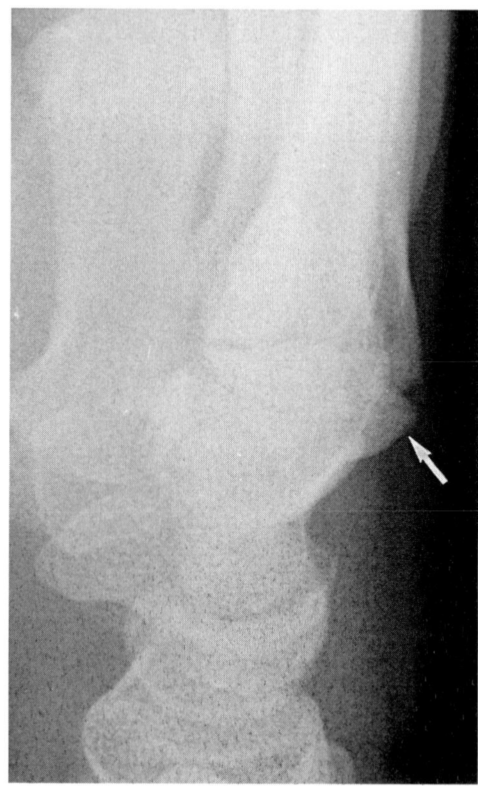

FIGURE 17–5. Os styloideum (carpal boss).[11] A typical os styloideum is seen as a triangular ossicle of bone on an angulated lateral radiograph (arrow). The carpal boss, or carpe bossu, is located overlying the dorsum of the wrist at the bases of the second and third metacarpal bones. It may be asymptomatic or painful, resulting in limitation of hand motion.

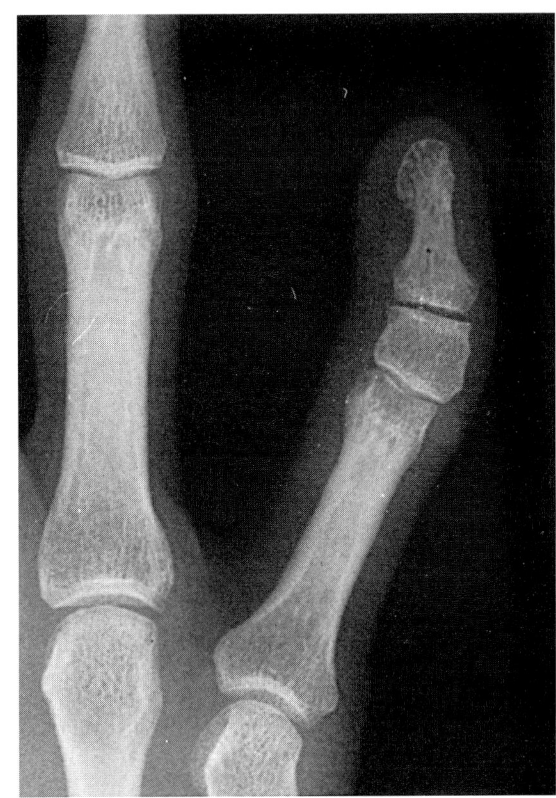

FIGURE 17–6. Brachydactyly.[10] The middle phalanx of the fifth digit is shorter on its radial side than on its ulnar side, resulting in slight radial clinodactyly. Shortening of the fifth middle phalanx is the most common form of phalangeal shortening and is also the most common hand anomaly. This anomaly usually is an isolated phenomenon, but it may be related to trisomy 21 and other syndromes. *(Courtesy of G. Greenway, M.D., Dallas, Texas.)*

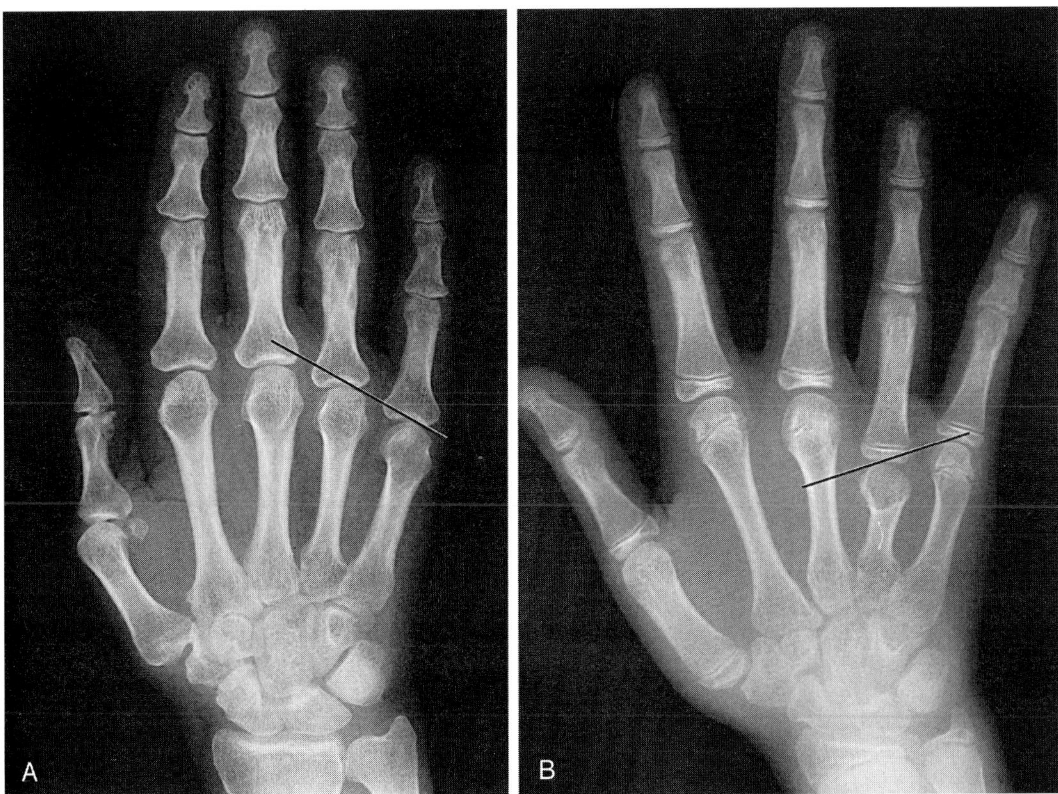

FIGURE 17–7. Short fourth metacarpal bone.[12] **A** Metacarpal sign. In normal persons, a line drawn tangent to the distal ends of the fourth and fifth metacarpals should not intersect the end of the third metacarpal or should just contact its articular surface. In patients with a shortened fourth metacarpal bone, the line intersects the third metacarpal bone, a finding termed positive metacarpal sign. **B** Isolated anomaly. Observe the shortened fourth metacarpal bone, resulting in a positive metacarpal sign (the line intersects the third metacarpal bone). This bilateral and symmetric anomaly was due to premature closure of the metacarpal ossification center in this 12-year-old girl. Metacarpal shortening, an anomalous variant often is seen as a familial trait in normal persons, but it also may be evident in persons with Turner's syndrome (Fig. 17–13).

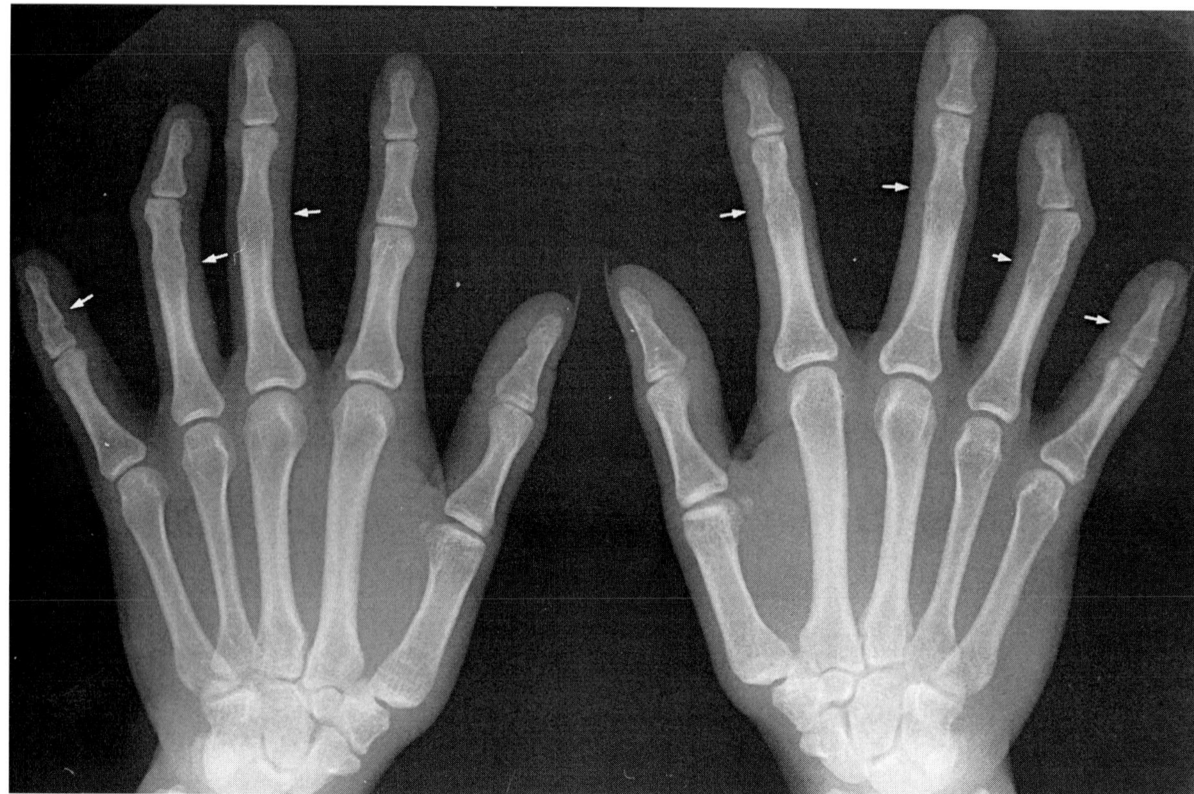

FIGURE 17–8. Phalangeal synostosis (symphalangism).[10] Observe the smooth bilateral osseous fusion of the proximal interphalangeal joints of the second to fourth fingers and the distal interphalangeal joints of the fifth fingers (arrows). Occasionally, a small rudimentary lucent cleft is seen at the site of the articulation. This condition, which represents fusion of one phalanx to another within the same digit, usually is inherited as a dominant trait, but it may also be syndrome related. Symphalangism likewise must be differentiated from acquired intra-articular fusion, such as that seen in juvenile chronic arthritis and psoriatic arthritis.

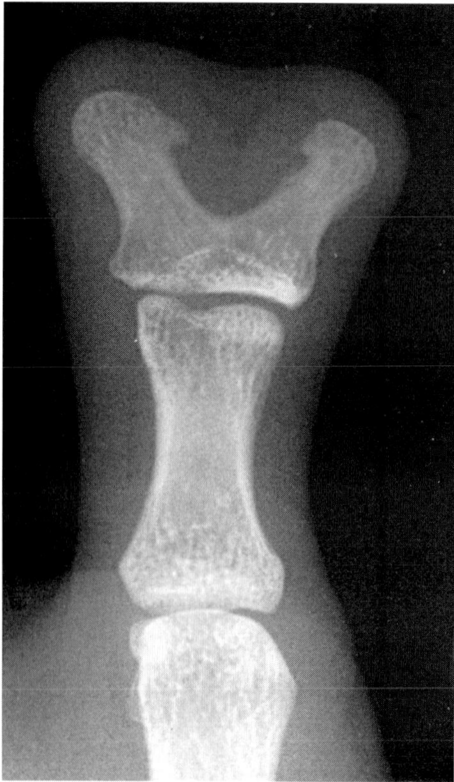

FIGURE 17–9. Bifid thumb.[10, 14] Note the fork-shaped partial duplication of the terminal phalanx in this patient. This is a form of polydactyly, which may occur as an isolated anomaly or as an associated finding in Down syndrome, Fanconi's anemia, and some other syndromes.

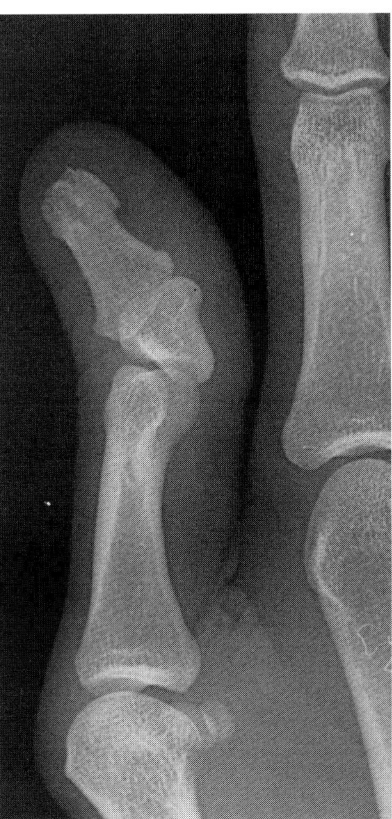

FIGURE 17–10. Triphalangeal thumb.[10, 14] An extra phalanx is located between the proximal and distal phalanges of the thumb. This anomaly is a rare familial disorder that can occur as an isolated finding or in association with other anomalies, such as polydactyly, duplications, absent bones, and some syndromes (Holt-Oram syndrome, trisomy 13–15, and Blackfan-Diamond anemia).

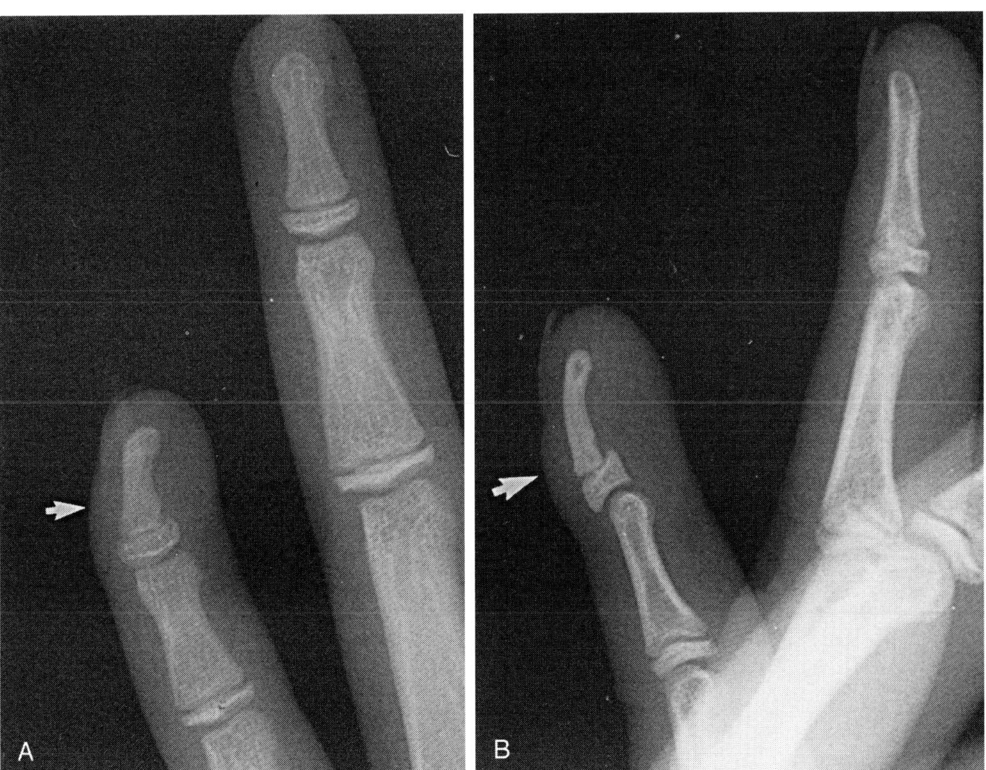

FIGURE 17–11. Kirner's deformity.[15] A Frontal radiograph. B Lateral radiograph. Palmar bending of the shaft of the terminal fifth phalanx (arrows) was found incidentally in this 11-year-old girl. This deformity usually is bilateral and may occur in association with epiphyseal separation, but usually it is painless and is considered a variation of normal.

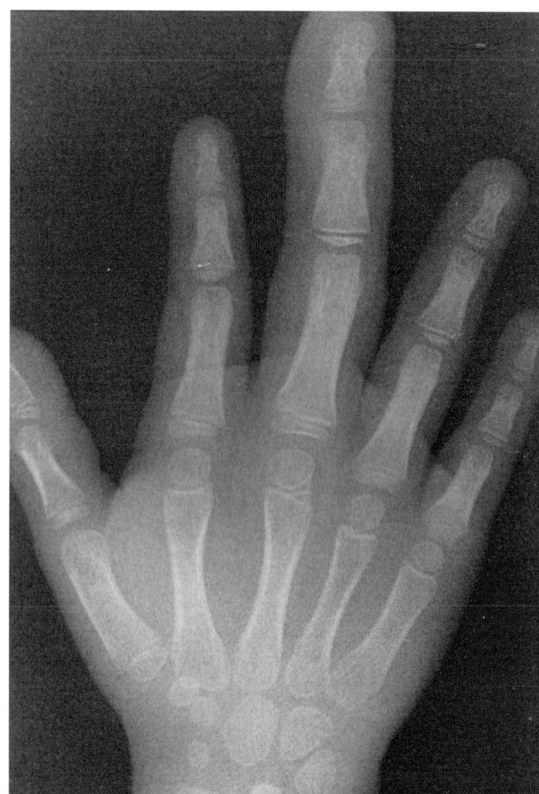

FIGURE 17–12. Macrodactyly (localized gigantism).[16, 17] In this 7-year-old girl, observe the characteristic overgrowth of both the bones and soft tissues of the third digit. Localized gigantism may be an isolated phenomenon or may be associated with vascular anomalies, neurofibromatosis, macrodystrophia lipomatosis, or the Proteus syndrome.

TABLE 17–3. Skeletal Dysplasias and Other Congenital Diseases Affecting the Wrist and Hand

Entity	Figure(s)	Characteristics
Turner's syndrome[12, 18]	17–13	Gonadal dysgenesis Short fourth metacarpal bone Delayed epiphyseal fusion Drumstick-shaped phalanges
Marfan sydrome[19–21]	17–14	Arachnodactyly: long slender fingers Hypermobility of wrist and finger joints Elongated thumb: when the hand is clenched, the thumb projects beyond the ulnar margin of the hand near the hypothenar eminence Metacarpal index: ratio of the length to midshaft width of the second to fifth metacarpal bones; ratio in normal men is less than 8.8; in normal women is less than 9.4; increased in patients with Marfan disease
Achondroplasia[22]		Short digits Divergent fingers: trident hand Metaphyseal cupping and irregularity Bones short but well formed in adults
Fibrodysplasia (myositis) ossificans progressiva[23]		Multiple congenital anomalies: hypoplasia of thumb, clinodactyly, polydactyly, and syndactyly
Osteogenesis imperfecta[24]		Bones of hand often are spared except in severe disease Osteoporosis with pencil-thin cortices Fractures seen occasionally Rare cystic form—ballooning of bone, metaphyseal flaring, and honeycombed appearance of thick trabeculae
Osteopoikilosis[25]	17–15	Multiple round or oval radiodense areas within spongiosa Periarticular location, especially in carpal bones

TABLE 17–3. Skeletal Dysplasias and Other Congenital Diseases Affecting the Wrist and Hand *Continued*

Entity	Figure(s)	Characteristics
Melorheostosis[26, 27]	17–16	Occasional involvement of hands Unilateral, hemimelic involvement is typical Cortical thickening and flowing hyperostosis resembling flowing candle wax extending from the forearm down the metacarpal bones and phalanges
Ehlers-Danlos syndrome[28]		Elongated ulnar styloid process Acro-osteolysis: rare Joint hypermobility
Hurler's syndrome (MPS 1-H)[29]	17–17	Major changes appear about 1 year of age Tapering of the proximal portion of the metacarpal bones Widening of the proximal and middle phalangeal shafts Late appearance of carpal bones Flexion contractures of fingers V-shaped deformity of the distal portions of the radius and ulna Osteoporosis Clinical findings: clouding of the cornea, mental retardation, normal or slightly reduced stature, stiff joints, hirsutism, flexion of the hands, atlantoaxial subluxation, and aortic regurgitation
Macrodystrophia lipomatosa[16, 17]		Rare condition of unknown cause Bizarre digital overgrowth of fatty tissue within the soft tissues of the hand

See also Table 1–2.

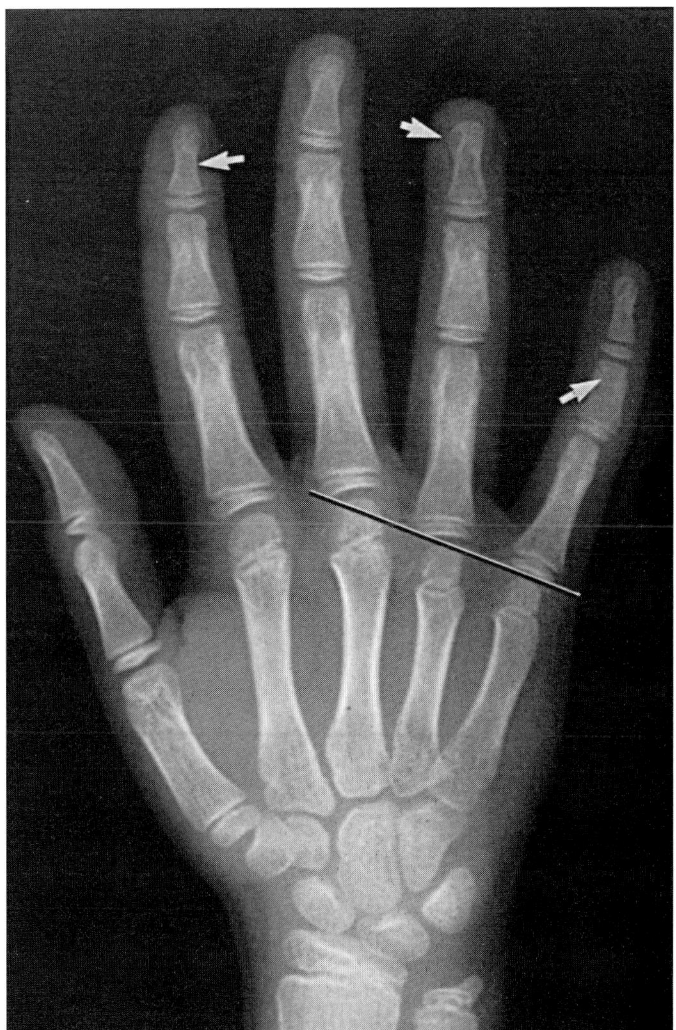

FIGURE 17–13. Turner's syndrome.[12, 18] The fourth metacarpal bone is short in relation to the adjacent metacarpal bones (positive metacarpal sign). Elongated phalanges, subtle cyst-like changes in the phalanges (arrows), and osteopenia throughout the bones of the hand are evident in this 12½-year-old girl with gonadal dysgenesis. Other findings in Turner's syndrome that may be observed are delayed epiphyseal fusion and drumstick-shaped phalanges.

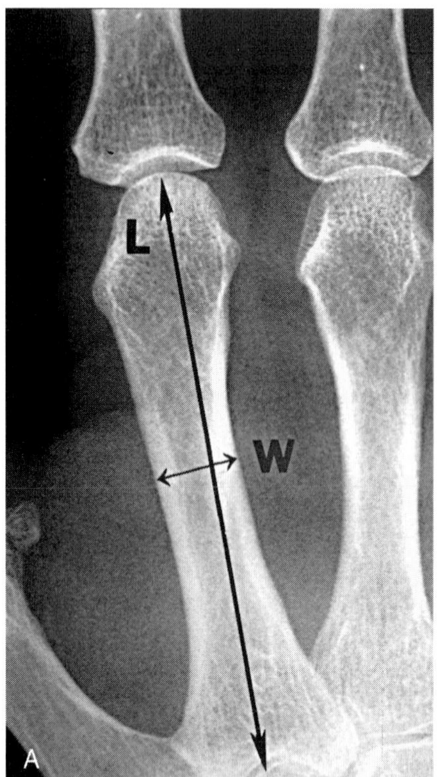

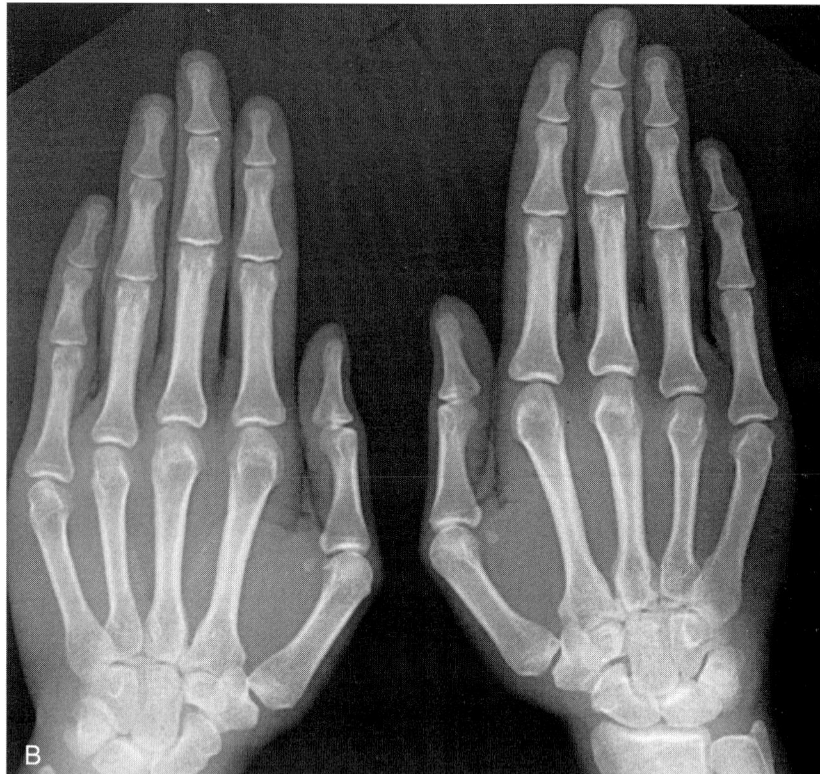

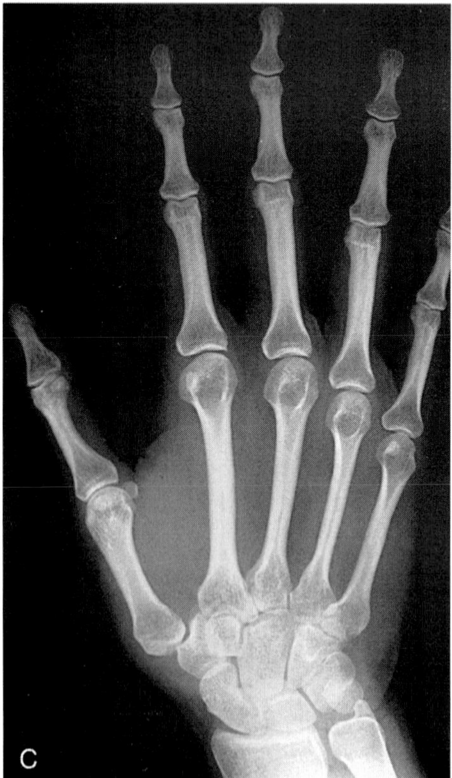

FIGURE 17–14. Marfan syndrome: Arachnodactyly.[19–21] **A** Metacarpal index: Normal situation. The metacarpal index is used to determine the relative slenderness of the metacarpal bones. It is defined as the average of ratios of the length (L) divided by the midpoint widths (W) of the second to fifth metacarpal bones. In normal men, the ratio is less than 8.8; in normal women, it is less than 9.4. The ratio typically is increased in patients with Marfan syndrome. **B** In this 27-year-old African-American woman, arachnodactyly is seen as elongation of the metacarpal bones and phalanges and normal bone density. **C** In another patient with Marfan syndrome, observe the long slender metacarpal bones and phalanges and the relative absence of subcutaneous fat. *(C, Courtesy of B.L. Harger, D.C., Portland, Oregon.)*

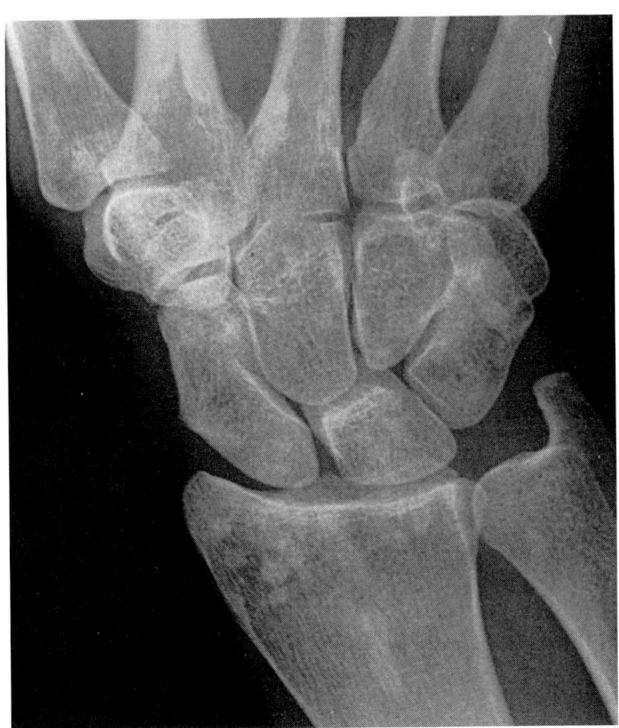

FIGURE 17–15. Osteopoikilosis.[25] Note the circular and ovoid osteosclerotic foci localized within the metacarpal and carpal bones, radius, and ulna. The symmetric periarticular distribution is characteristic of this fairly common sclerosing dysplasia. Although the epiphysis may be affected, most lesions usually predominate in the metaphysis.

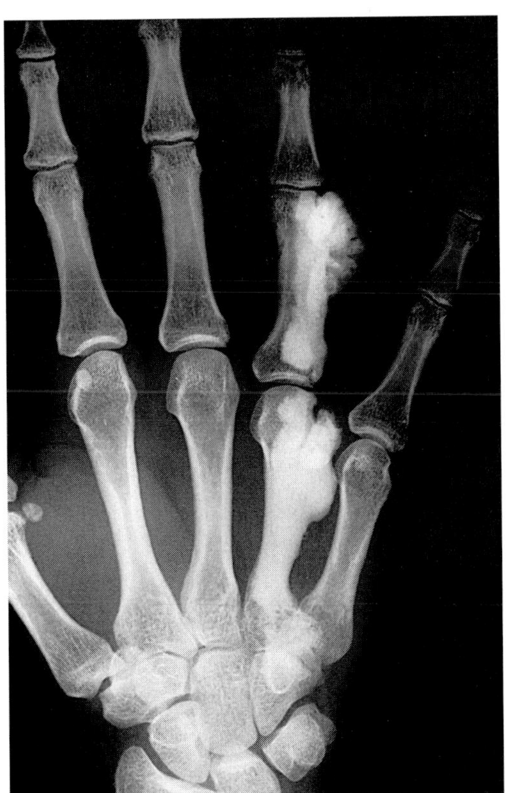

FIGURE 17–16. Melorheostosis.[26, 27] Dramatic asymmetric periosteal and endosteal hyperostosis simulating flowing candle wax involves the ulnar side of the fourth metacarpal bone and proximal phalanx. The asymmetric hemimelic distribution of one digit is characteristic of this disease. Melorheostosis is a sclerosing dysplasia of bone that can result in joint swelling and contracture, pain, restriction of motion, growth disturbances, muscle weakness and atrophy, and skin changes. It may be positive on a bone scan. *(Courtesy of A. Newberg, M.D., Boston, Massachusetts.)*

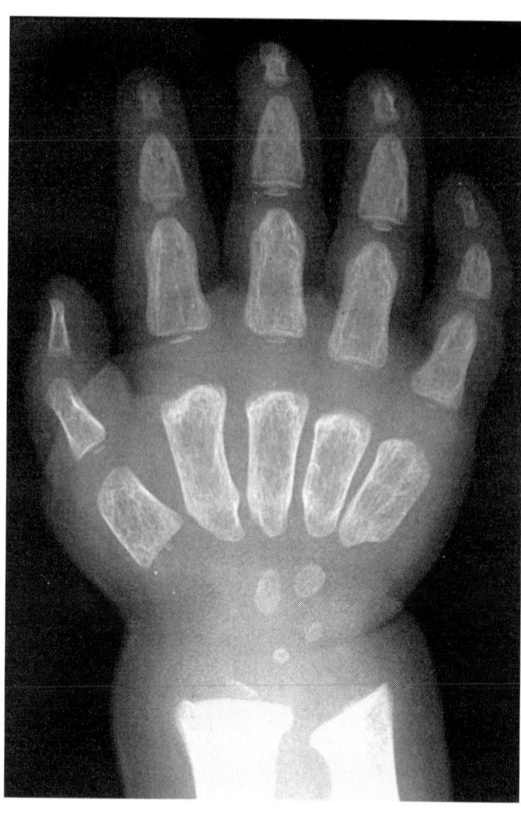

FIGURE 17–17. Hurler's syndrome (MPS 1-H).[29] Radiograph of the hand in this 3-year-old girl with Hurler's syndrome demonstrates osteopenia, pointing of the proximal portion of the metacarpal bones, widening of the proximal and middle phalangeal shafts, small carpal bones, flexion of the fingers, and a V-shaped deformity of the distal ends of the radius and ulna.

TABLE 17–4. Carpal Fractures and Dislocations

Entity	Figure(s)	Characteristics	Complications and Related Injuries
Isolated carpal fractures			
Scaphoid fracture[30–33]	17–18	Most common carpal fracture and most frequent site for occult fracture Usually occurs between ages 15 and 40 years *Mechanism* Fall on outstretched hand Proximal pole: (20 per cent) Waist: (70 per cent) Distal (10 per cent): distal body, tuberosity, distal articular surface Waist fractures typically take 6 to 8 weeks or more to heal Tuberosity fractures typically take 4 to 6 weeks to heal Magnetic resonance (MR) imaging can reveal occult wrist fractures when findings are normal or equivocal	Nonunion in 5 to 15 per cent of cases Ischemic necrosis in 10 to 15 per cent of cases; most common in proximal pole fractures; prevalence of ischemic necrosis increases by 30 to 40 per cent in cases of nonunion Degenerative joint disease Tendon ruptures as a result of nonunion Occasionally associated with other wrist fractures and ligament disruptions 16 per cent of scaphoid fractures are missed on initial radiographic evaluation
Triquetrum fracture[30, 34]	17–19	Three to 4 per cent of all carpal fractures Dorsal surface typically fractured *Mechanism* Contact with hamate or ulnar styloid process or avulsion by the dorsal radiotriquetral ligaments Best seen on lateral and steep oblique views	
Lunate fracture[30, 34]		Two to 7 per cent of all carpal fractures Dorsal or volar aspect or any portion of the body may fracture Usually avulsion fractures	Ischemic necrosis

TABLE 17–4. Carpal Fractures and Dislocations *Continued*

Entity	Figure(s)	Characteristics	Complications and Related Injuries
Hamate fracture[30, 34–36]	17–20	Two to 4 percent of all carpal fractures Hook is most common site of hamate fracture *Mechanism* Direct force from racquet, bat, or club; also from fall on a dorsiflexed wrist	Nonunion Ischemic necrosis Ulnar or median nerve injury Tendon rupture
Pisiform fracture[34, 36]	17–21	*Mechanism* Direct crushing injury from fall on outstretched hand	Ulnar nerve injury
Capitate fracture[30, 34]		Infrequent	May be combined with scaphoid fracture (scaphocapitate syndrome)
Trapezium fracture[30, 34]		Infrequent	
Trapezoid fracture[30, 34]		Infrequent	
Carpal dislocations and fracture-dislocations			
Lesser arc injuries (lunate and perilunate dislocation)[37–39]	17–22, 17–23	Lunate dislocation: most common isolated carpal dislocation Hyperextension of the wrist Lateral view shows volar displacement and rotation of lunate; the capitate remains aligned with the radius Lunate appears triangular on the frontal view with the apex pointing distally ("pie sign") Perilunate dislocation: on the lateral view, the lunate remains aligned with the radius while the other carpal bones dislocate, usually dorsally On the frontal view, the capitate overlaps the lunate Often accompanies transscaphoid fracture (see greater arc injuries)	Wrist instability Osteonecrosis Predictable sequence of events after traumatic loading and impaction upon the thenar eminence, initially injuring the radial side of the wrist Stage I: scapholunate dissociation Stage II: perilunate instability owing to failure of radiocapitate ligament or radial styloid process fracture; leads to perilunate dislocation Stage III: further ligament disruption resulting in triquetral malrotation, triquetrolunate diastasis, or triquetral fracture Stage IV: Disruption of dorsal radiocarpal ligaments leading to lunate dislocation
Greater arc injuries[37, 38, 40]	17–22, 17–24	Predictable fracture-dislocation patterns passing through the greater arc consisting of scaphoid, capitate, hamate, and triquetrum Examples: Transscaphoid perilunate fracture-dislocation (relatively common) Transscaphoid, transcapitate, perilunate fracture-dislocation (scaphocapitate syndrome) Transscaphoid, transcapitate, transhamate, transtriquetral perilunate fracture-dislocation (rare injury)	Complications similar to those of carpal dislocations and wrist instability
Scaphoid dislocation[41]		Infrequent injury Two types: Isolated scaphoid dislocation—requires closed reduction Dislocation in conjunction with axial carpal disruption—requires open reduction to stabilize carpals	Residual rotary subluxation of the scaphoid Median nerve compression
Common carpometacarpal joint dislocation[42]	17–25	Rare injury, typically involves ulnar aspect of wrist Dorsal dislocation, usually of 1 or 2 metacarpals in relation to the carpals CT useful in evaluation	Ulnar or median nerve injury Extensor tendon rupture Metacarpal fractures
First carpometacarpal joint dislocation[43]	17–26	Rare injury	Often associated with Bennett's fracture-subluxation of the base of the first metacarpal bone

See also Tables 1–3 to 1–5.

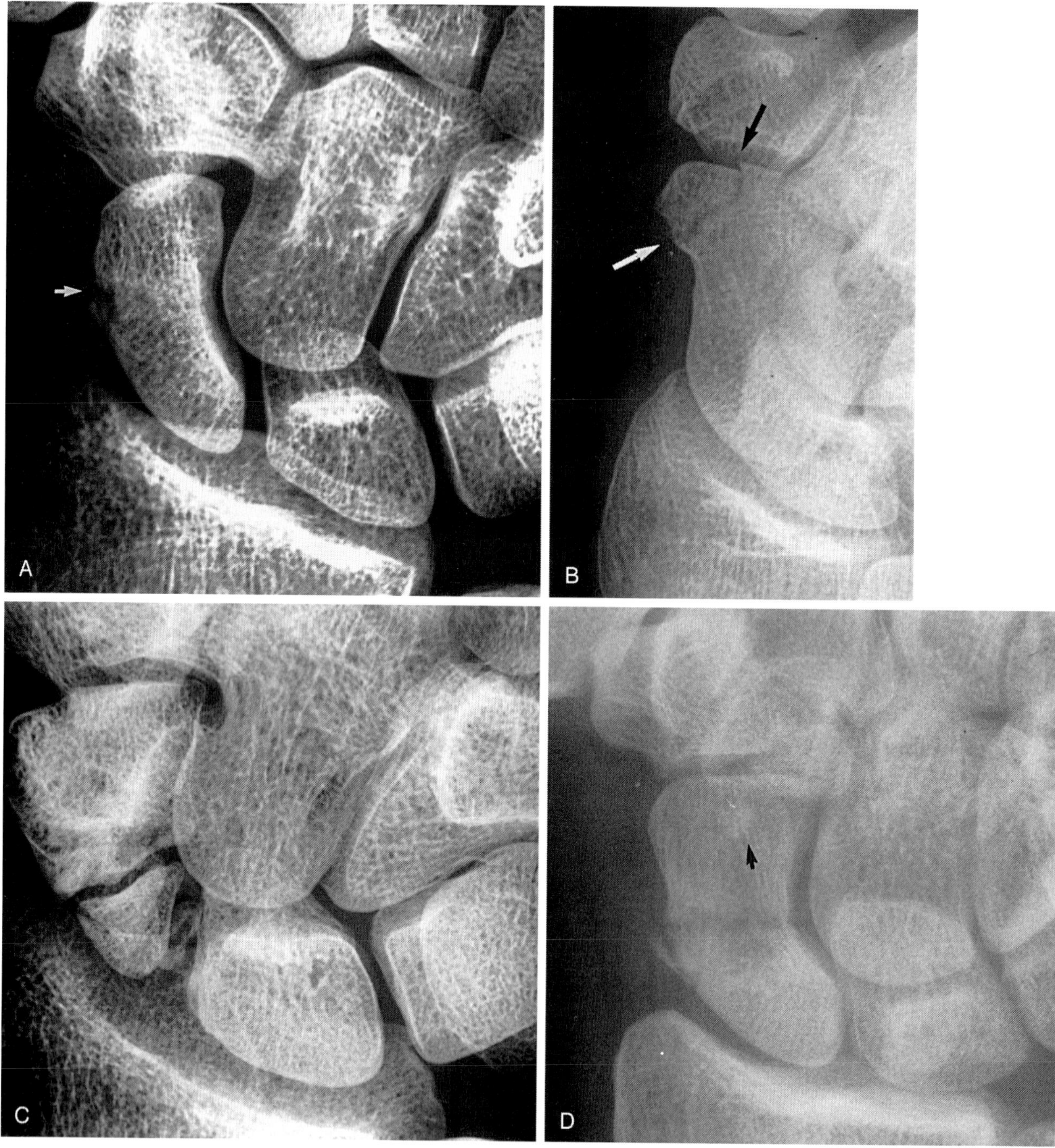

FIGURE 17–18. Carpal fractures: scaphoid bone.[30–33] A Scaphoid waist fracture: A fracture line is seen traversing the midwaist of the scaphoid bone (arrow). B Distal scaphoid fracture. Oblique view shows a fracture of the scaphoid tuberosity (arrows). C Complication: nonunion. In another patient, observe the widened fracture cleft and the rounded sclerotic margins at the fracture site. Subchondral cyst formation and widening of the scapholunate articulation also are evident. D Complication: osteonecrosis. A transverse radiolucent fracture line is evident through the waist of the scaphoid. The proximal fracture fragment is osteosclerotic, a sign of osteonecrosis. A small bone island (enostosis) is noted incidentally in the distal pole (arrow). *(A, C, Courtesy of U. Mayer, M.D., Klagenfurt, Austria.)*

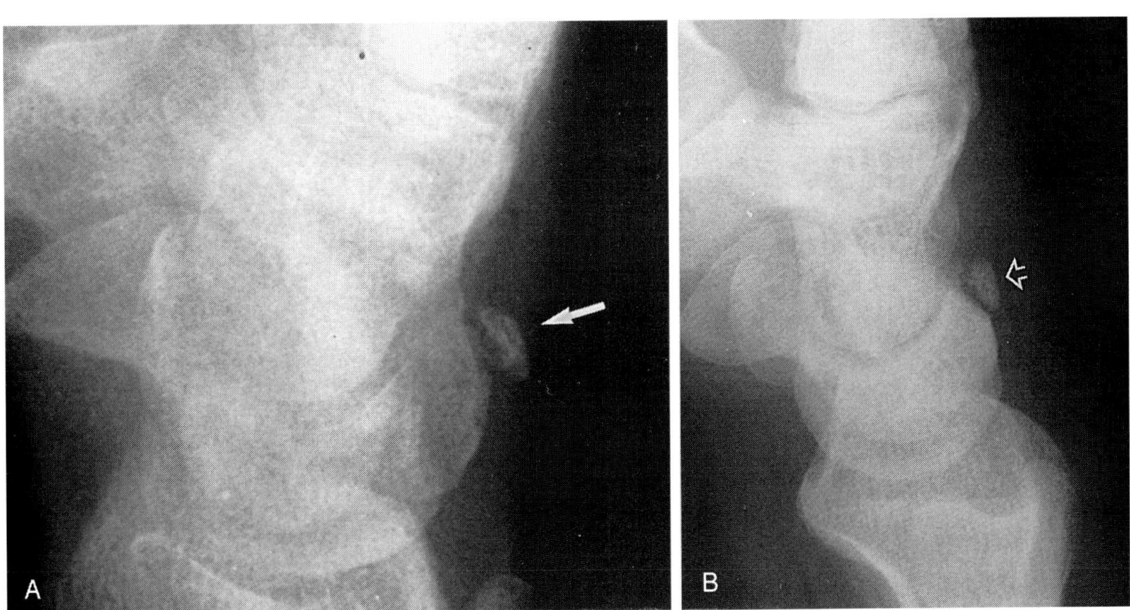

FIGURE 17–19. Carpal fractures: Dorsal surface of triquetrum.[30, 34] A Lateral radiograph reveals the fracture fragment adjacent to the dorsal surface of the triquetrum (arrow). B A similar fracture of the triquetrum is evident in another patient (open arrow).

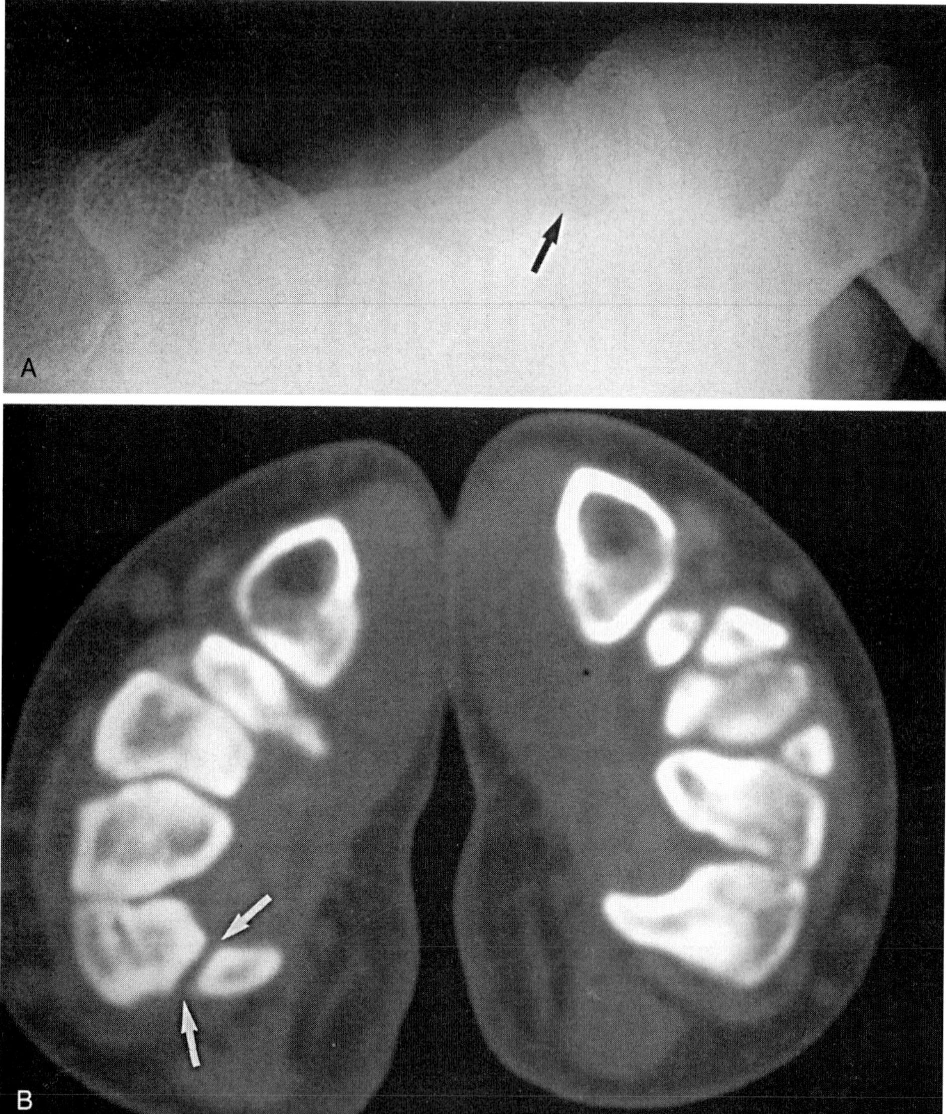

FIGURE 17–20. Carpal fractures: Hamate bone.[30, 34–36] This patient had had several months of pain after an injury sustained while swinging a golf club. Carpal tunnel radiograph **(A)** and transaxial computed tomographic (CT) scan **(B)** reveal the fracture through the hook of the hamate bone (arrows). Compare with the normal contralateral side in **B.** *(Courtesy of G. Greenway, M.D., Dallas, Texas.)*

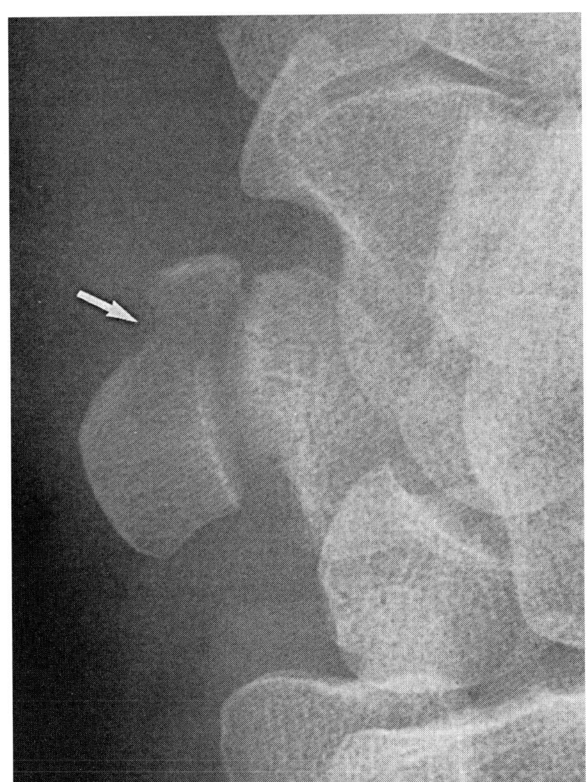

FIGURE 17–21. Carpal fractures: Pisiform bone.[34, 36] Semisupinated oblique radiograph reveals a minimally displaced fracture of the pisiform bone (arrow). Pisiform fractures result from a crushing mechanism, usually sustained by breaking a fall with an outstretched hyperextended wrist, and may be complicated by ulnar nerve damage.

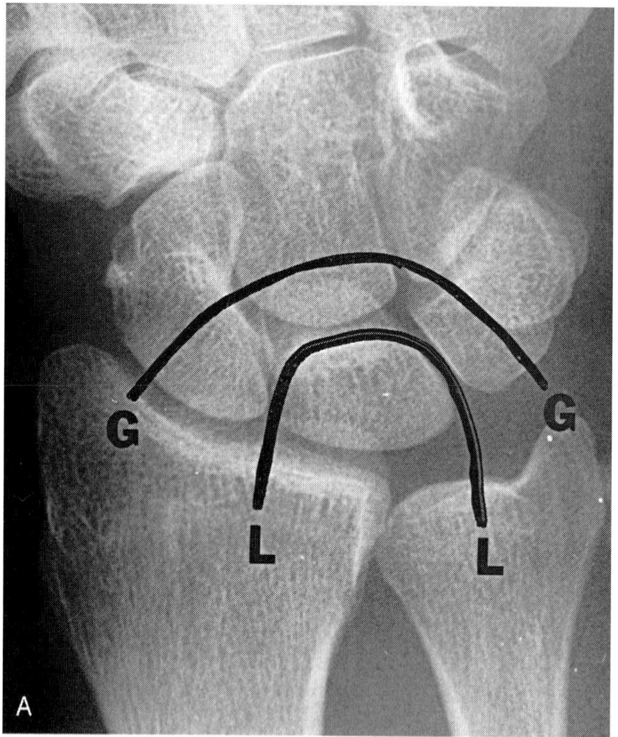

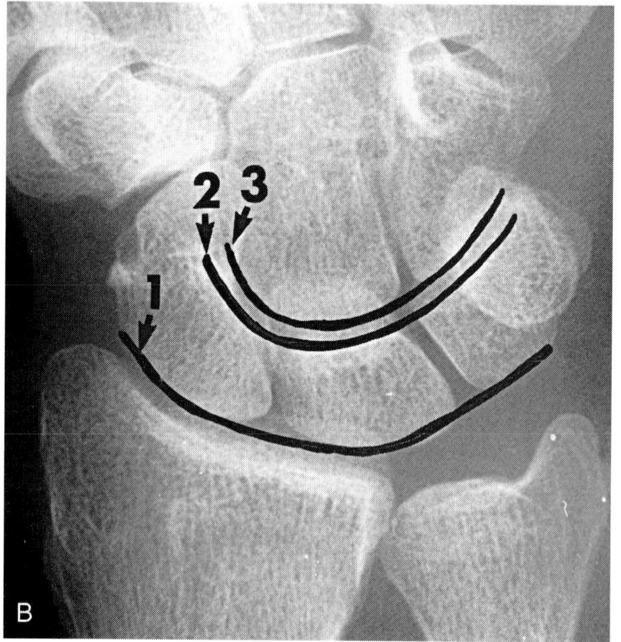

FIGURE 17–22. Wrist injuries: Carpal relationships—the normal arcs.[37–40] **A** Greater (G) and lesser (L) arc locations are shown. Fractures and dislocations along these arcs occur in predictable patterns. A pure greater arc injury consists of a trans-scaphoid, transcapitate, transhamate, transtriquetral fracture-dislocation. A pure lesser arc injury is a perilunate or lunate dislocation. Various combinations of these injury patterns are seen clinically. **B** Normal arcs of proximal and distal carpal rows. On routine posteroanterior radiographs of the wrist, three arcs are demonstrated. Arc 1 (proximal carpal articular surfaces of the proximal carpal row) joins the outer curvatures of the proximal articular surfaces of the scaphoid, lunate, and triquetrum (1). Arc II (distal carpal articular surfaces of the proximal carpal row) connects the distal smooth curves of these same three bones (2). Arc III (proximal carpal articular surfaces of the distal carpal row) connects the distal smooth surfaces of the capitate and hamate bones (3).

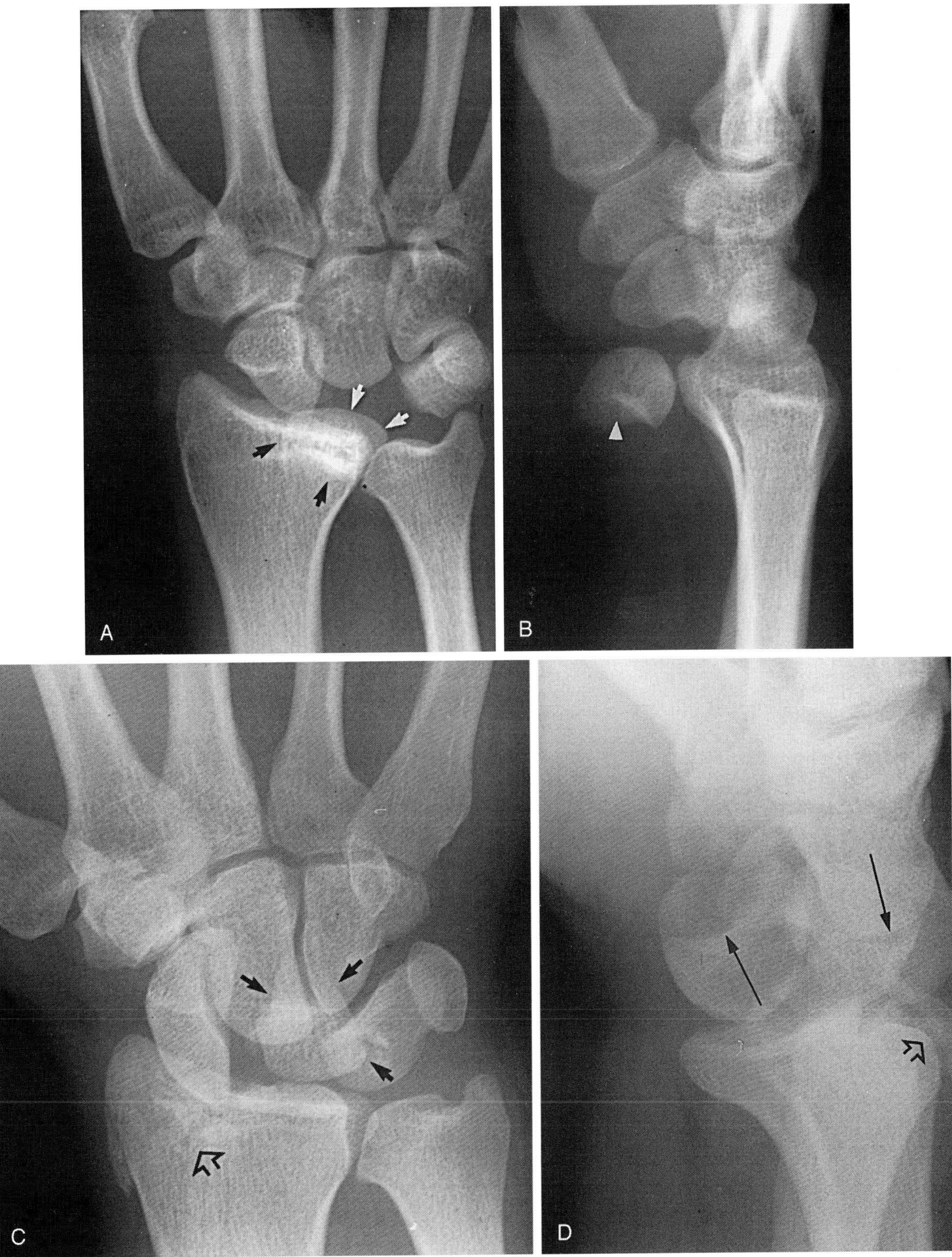

FIGURE 17–23. Lesser arc wrist injuries.[37–39] A, B Lunate dislocation. In A, a frontal radiograph demonstrates volar dislocation of the lunate bone. The lunate bone is displaced proximally and overlies the volar surface of the distal end of the radius (arrows). The space proximal to the capitate bone is vacant. In B, the lateral radiograph is most diagnostic, showing volar displacement. In addition, the lunate bone has rotated 180 degrees; therefore, the distal surface (arrowhead) is directed proximally. Neither the lunate nor the capitate bone is truly aligned with the distal surface of the radius, indicating the difficulty encountered in classifying such injuries as either lunate or perilunate dislocation. C, D Perilunate dislocation. In C, a posteroanterior radiograph shows overlap of the lunate bone with respect to the capitate and hamate bones and the triquetrum (arrows). A radial styloid fracture (open arrows) also is present. Observe the disruption of the lesser arc and the severe scapholunate dissociation. In D, the lateral radiograph clearly demonstrates the normal relationship between the lunate bone, the distal end of the radius, and the dorsal displacement of the capitate bone with respect to the lunate bone. (In the normal situation, the arrows within the capitate and lunate bones should be aligned.)

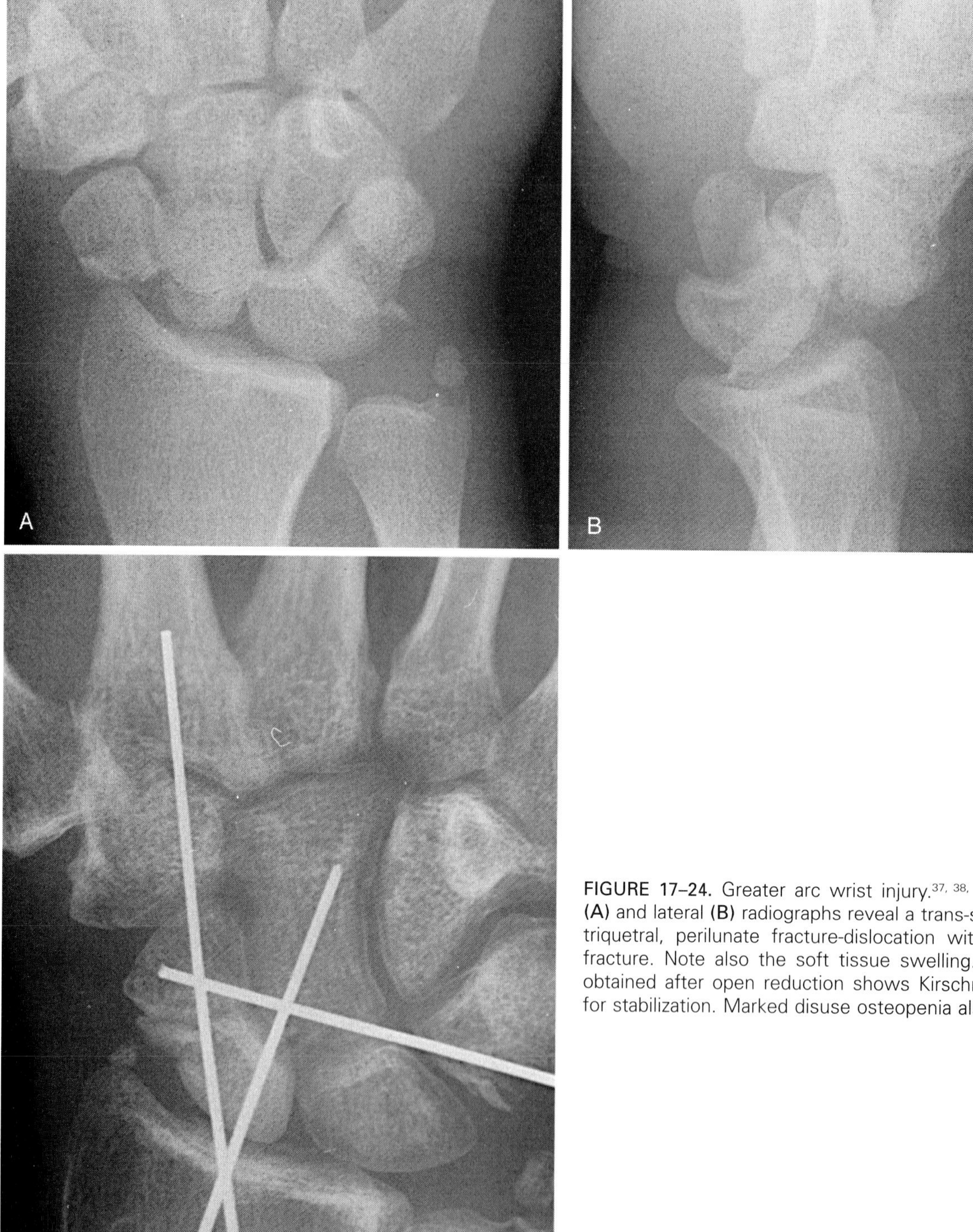

FIGURE 17–24. Greater arc wrist injury.[37, 38, 40] A, B Frontal (A) and lateral (B) radiographs reveal a trans-scaphoid, trans-triquetral, perilunate fracture-dislocation with ulnar styloid fracture. Note also the soft tissue swelling. C Radiograph obtained after open reduction shows Kirschner wires used for stabilization. Marked disuse osteopenia also is present.

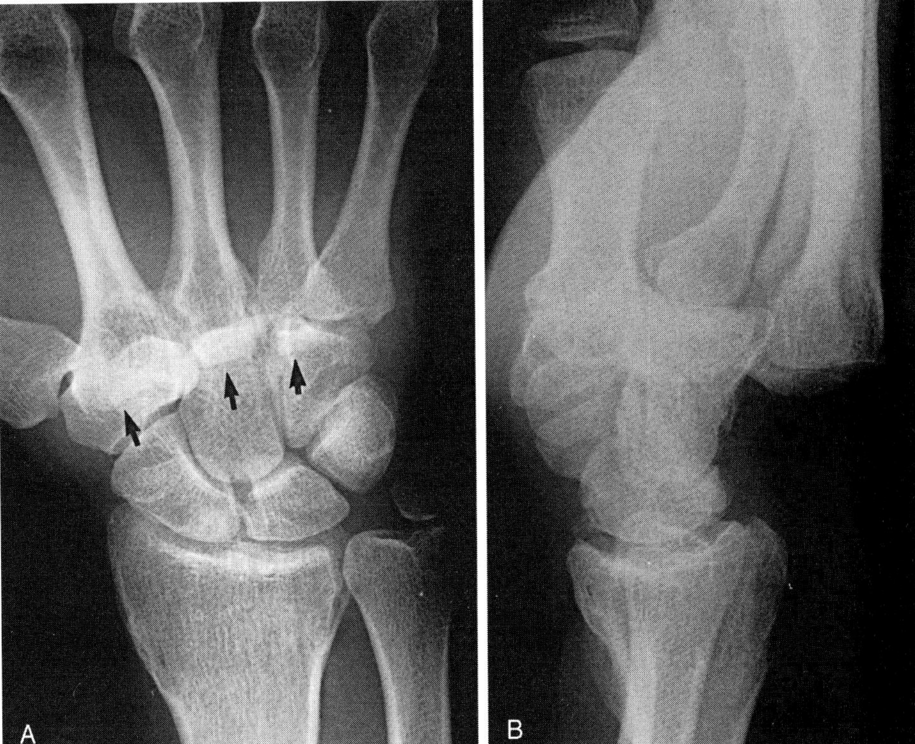

FIGURE 17–25. Dislocations of the common carpometacarpal joints.[42] Frontal (A) and lateral (B) radiographs show dorsal dislocation of the lateral four metacarpal bases with respect to the adjacent carpal bones. The metacarpal bases overlap the distal carpal row (arrows). No associated fractures are evident.

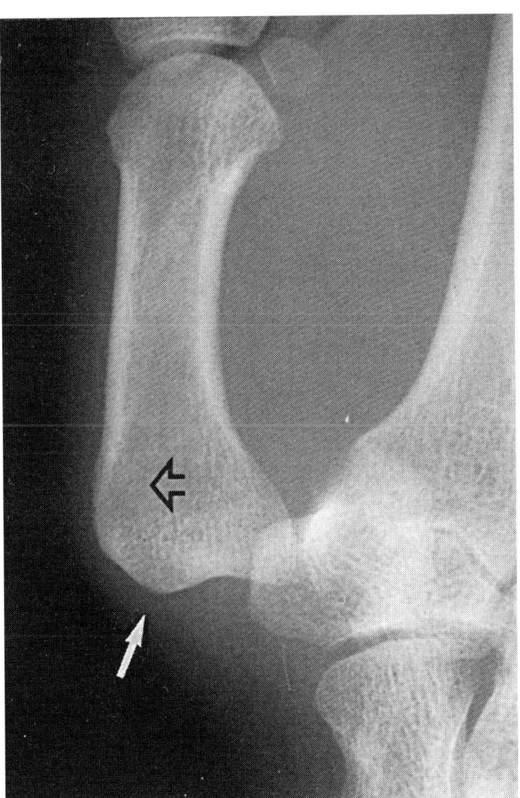

FIGURE 17–26. Dislocation of the first carpometacarpal joint.[43] Loss of continuity is seen between the trapezium and the base of the dorsally and medially dislocated first metacarpal bone (arrow). The open arrow indicates the direction of displacement of the first metacarpal bone.

TABLE 17–5. Ligamentous Instability of the Wrist*

Entity	Figure(s)	Characteristics	Complications and Related Injuries
Overview of wrist instability[44]		Several different patterns of instability have been identified Criteria that suggest carpal instability: abnormal carpal alignment on routine radiographs; scapholunate joint or ligament pain; reproducible painful clicking or popping; positive radiographic instability pattern in which abnormal motion is documented	Complications of all types of instability: Disabling wrist pain Osteoarthrosis Disability
Rotary subluxation of scaphoid and scapholunate dissociation[44–46]	17–27	Rotary subluxation of the scaphoid: most common type of wrist instability *Radiographic findings* "Ring" sign—shortened scaphoid and ring produced by the cortex of the distal pole of the scaphoid on frontal radiograph Wide scapholunate joint Overlapping of saphoid and capitate Increased scapholunate angle Scapholunate dissociation: frequent component of rotary subluxation of scaphoid and other patterns of instability Disruption of scapholunate interosseous ligament Scapholunate separation on frontal radiograph: 2 mm (suggested) or 4 mm (definite); "Terry Thomas" or "David Letterman" sign Occasionally, widened scapholunate joint may be normal variant	Predisposing disorders: Acute and chronic trauma Rheumatoid arthritis Calcium pyrophosphate dihydrate (CPPD) crystal deposition disease Other patterns of wrist instability
Dorsal intercalated segmental instability (DISI)[44, 47, 48]	17–28	Common midcarpal instability Often associated with scapholunate dissociation Dorsally tilted lunate, flexed scaphoid, scapholunate angle greater than 80 degrees, and capitolunate angle greater than 30 degrees May occur with or without scapholunate dissociation	
Ventral intercalated carpal instability (VISI)[44, 47, 48]	17–29	Less common than DISI Ventrally tilted lunate, scapholunate angle is less than 30 degrees, and capitolunate angle is greater than 30 degrees	
Scapholunate advanced collapse (SLAC wrist)[49]	17–30	Pattern of posttraumatic osteoarthrosis Narrowing of radioscaphoid and capitolunate spaces leading to scapholunate dissociation and eventual DISI	Associated with the following: Osteoarthrosis Calcium pyrophosphate dihydrate (CPPD) crystal deposition disease

*Only the most frequent patterns are discussed here. For a more detailed discussion of wrist instability, see Yin Y, Mann FA, Hodge JC, et al: Roentgenographic interpretation of ligamentous instabilities of the wrist: Static and dynamic instabilities. *In* Gilula L, Yin Y (Eds): Imaging of the Hand and Wrist. Philadelphia, WB Saunders, 1996, p 203.

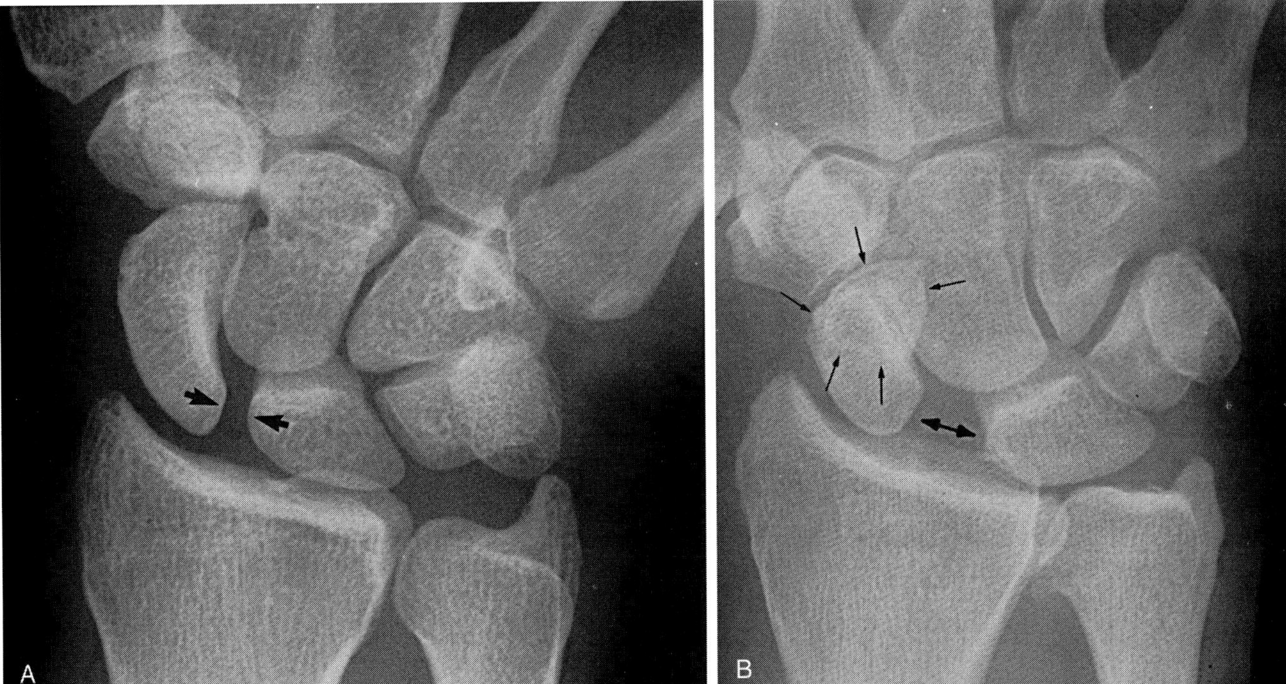

FIGURE 17–27. Scapholunate dissociation (rotary subluxation of the scaphoid).[44–46] A The scapholunate distance is widened (arrows). B Radiograph of this 58-year-old man with wrist pain demonstrates widening of the scapholunate interosseous space (double-headed arrow) and a markedly shortened appearance of the scaphoid bone. Additionally, the distal pole of the scaphoid appears as a characteristic ring-like structure owing to rotation of this bone (small arrows). Scapholunate dissociation is suggested when the space between the scaphoid and lunate bones is 2 mm or wider, and it can be diagnosed with certainty if the distance is 4 mm or greater. Scapholunate separation results from perforation or disruption of the scapholunate interosseous ligament, and in cases in which the scaphoid has rotated in a palmar direction, a tear of the volar radiocarpal ligament is also present. In addition to routine radiographic projections, frontal radiographs should be obtained with ulnar deviation and radial deviation and with the patient's fist tightly clenched.

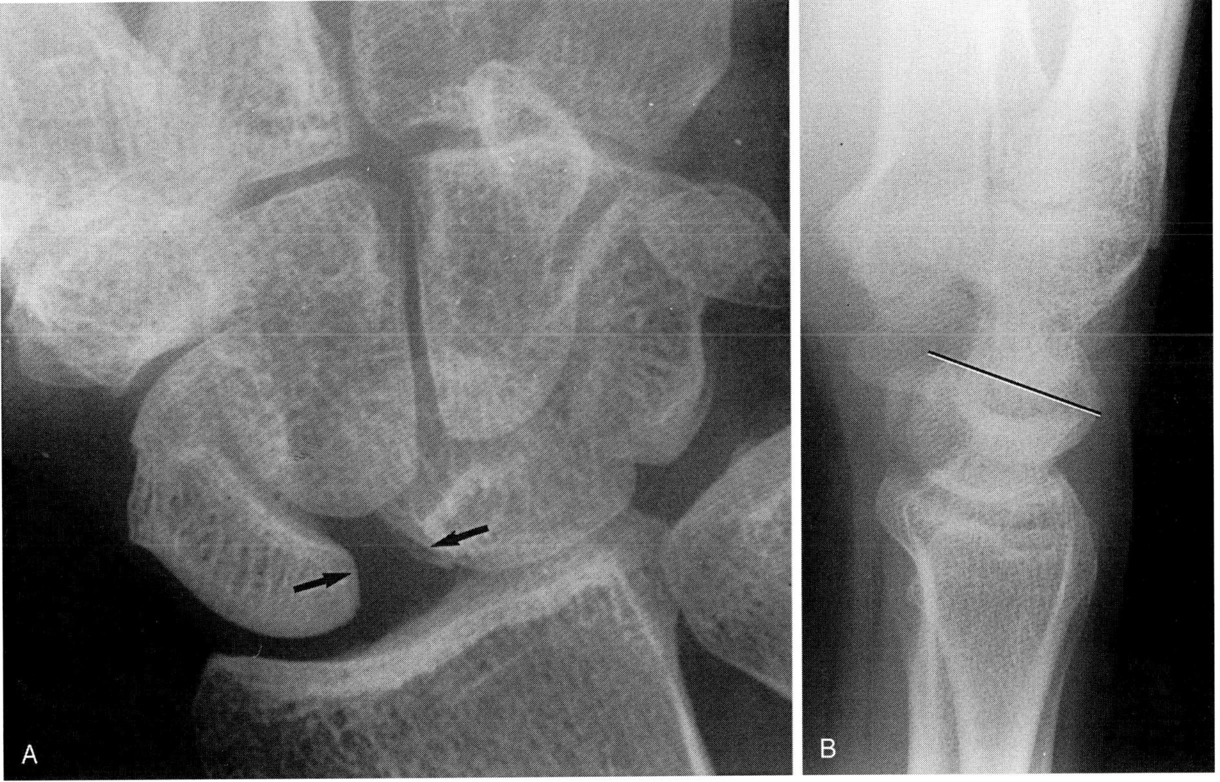

FIGURE 17–28. A, B Carpal instability: dorsal intercalated segmental instability (DISI).[44, 47, 48] Findings include scapholunate joint space widening (arrows) and dorsiflexion of the lunate bone (line). The radiocarpal and midcarpal joint spaces are narrowed.

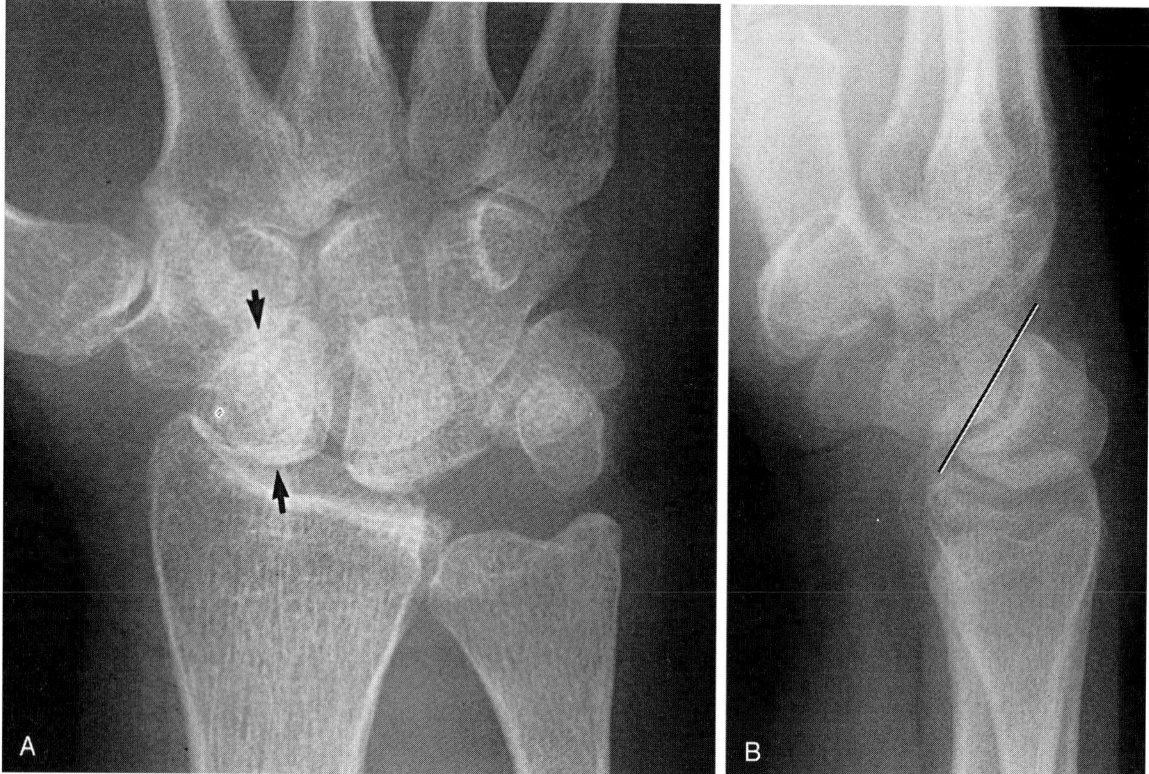

FIGURE 17–29. A, B Carpal instability: volar intercalated segmental instability (VISI).[44, 47, 48] In this 72-year-old woman, the distal pole of the scaphoid bone shows palmar displacement, resulting in a ring-like shadow (arrows) and volar tilting of the lunate bone (line).

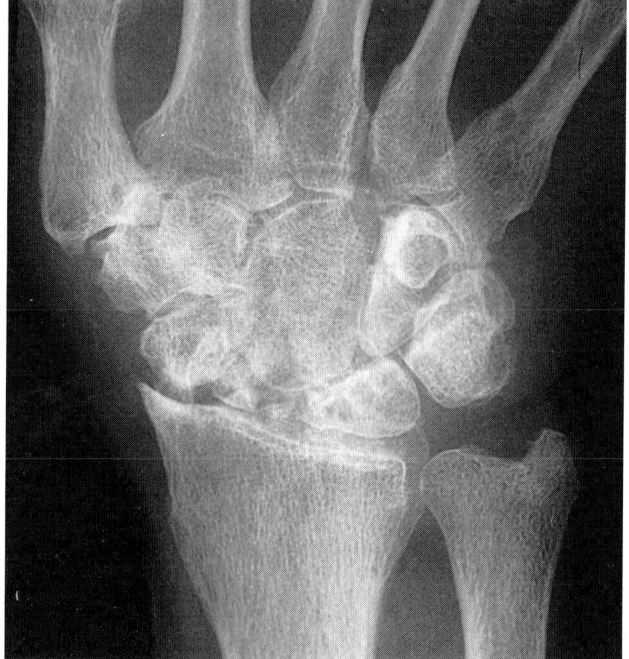

FIGURE 17–30. Carpal instability: scapholunate advanced collapse (SLAC) wrist.[49] In this patient with severe degenerative joint disease, observe the presence of scapholunate dissociation, narrowing of the radiocarpal and midcarpal articulations, and flattening of the scaphoid and lunate bones. These radiographic findings, seen in association with degenerative joint disease or calcium pyrophosphate dihydrate (CPPD) crystal deposition disease, are termed SLAC wrist.

TABLE 17–6. Fractures and Dislocations of the Hand

Entity	Figure(s)	Characteristics	Complications and Related Injuries
Metacarpophalangeal (MCP) joint dislocations[30, 50]		Second to fifth MCP joints *Mechanism* Forced hyperextension from fall on an outstretched hand Index finger most common site Classified as simple (reducible) or complex (potentially irreducible) Metacarpal head usually is displaced into the palm	Disruption of volar plate Interposition and entrapment of the volar plate or sesamoid bone
Interphalangeal joint dislocations[51]	17–31	Proximal interphalangeal joint dislocations very common Usually involve only one joint Posterior dislocation results from hyperextension injury Anterior dislocations less common	Associated phalangeal fracture Associated ligamentous and volar plate injuries common Intra-articular fracture-dislocation with joint instability Interposition of volar plate or flexor tendon Entrapment of sesamoid bone of thumb can prevent reduction
Bennett's fracture-dislocation[52]	17–32	Intra-articular fracture of the base of the first metacarpal bone Axial blow to a partially flexed first metacarpal bone Fracture of a small fragment of the volar lip Base of metacarpal bone is displaced dorsally and radially	Osteoarthrosis
Rolando's fracture[52, 53]	17–33	Y- or T-shaped comminuted fracture of the base of the first metacarpal bone	Osteoarthrosis
Gamekeeper's thumb[54–56]	17–34	Disruption of the ulnar collateral ligaments (UCL) of the first MCP joint A common mechanism is the ski pole injury–violent abduction-extension (valgus) force applied to the thumb; 6 per cent of all ski injuries Unstable condition involving rupture of the ulnar collateral ligaments *Clinical findings* Pain, swelling, tenderness, edema, and pinch instability Routine radiographs cannot help differentiate between displaced and nondisplaced tears; however, magnetic resonance (MR) imaging is effective in depicting such displacement Initial radiographs may appear normal, or they may show a small fragment of avulsed bone at the base of the proximal phalanx in some cases Stress radiography may be useful in revealing excessive motion and subluxation Multiple radiographic projections allow a more complete evaluation of alignment and apposition of phalangeal fractures	Pinch instability Avulsion of bone with rotation of fragments Stener lesion: abnormal folded position of the UCL in which the ligament becomes displaced and trapped superficially to the adductor pollicis aponeurosis; interferes with healing and necessitates surgery
Dorsal dislocation of the first MCP joint[57]		Results from forcible hyperextension of the thumb	Ligament injury with instability Interposition and entrapment of a sesamoid bone

Table continued on following page

TABLE 17–6. Fractures and Dislocations of the Hand *Continued*

Entity	Figure(s)	Characteristics	Complications and Related Injuries
Metacarpal fractures[30, 58]	17–35	Most commonly involve first and fifth metacarpal bones Typical sites: shaft and neck of fifth metacarpal (bar-room fracture) Shaft of third or fourth metacarpal bone (or both of these) (boxer's fracture)	Displacement, angulation, or rotation commonly encountered Rotation, if not corrected, may lead to serious disability
Phalangeal fractures[30, 59, 60]	17–36 A	More frequent than metacarpal fractures Distal phalanx most common, followed by proximal and middle phalanges	Associated tendon injuries and dislocations
	17–36 B, C	Fractures with intra-articular extension or rotational deformity Small intra-articular fractures may be subtle on routine radiographs and may require multiple projections	May result in marked disability or loss of functional capacity
	17–36 D	Mallet fracture: avulsion injury at the base of the dorsal surface of the terminal phalanx with disruption of the extensor mechanism	Damage to the extensor tendon mechanism: mallet finger with persistent flexion deformity
		Volar plate fracture: dorsal dislocation of a proximal interphalangeal joint is associated with an avulsion fracture in the middle phalanx at the site of attachment of the volar plate	Damage to the flexor tendon mechanism resulting in inability to flex the finger at proximal interphalangeal joint
	17–36 E	Nailbed injury: open skin surface may expose bone or joint	Secondary infection
	17–36 F	Growth plate fractures: involve the distal phalangeal physes in children	Growth plate injury in children Deformity and growth abnormalities
Phalangeal stress injuries[61, 62]	17–37	Extremely rare injuries Phalanges: bowlers Phalangeal tufts: guitar players	
Child abuse[63]		Torus fractures of the metacarpal bones and phalanges have been reported Most likely mechanism is forced hyperextension of fingers	Other fractures and injuries at different sites

See also Tables 1–3 and 1–4.

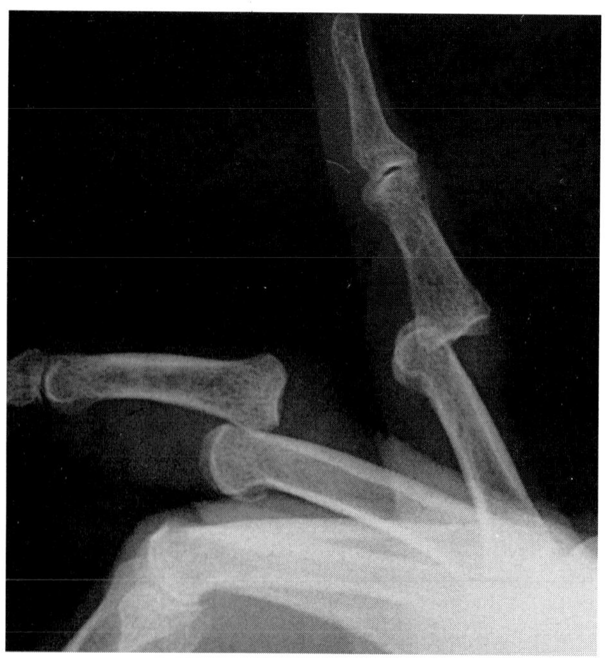

FIGURE 17–31. Interphalangeal joint dislocation.[51] Dorsal dislocations of the fourth and fifth proximal interphalangeal joints are evident. No associated fractures are observed. Such dislocations are common, occur as a result of hyperextension, and usually affect only one interphalangeal joint. Radiographs should be observed carefully for associated fractures.

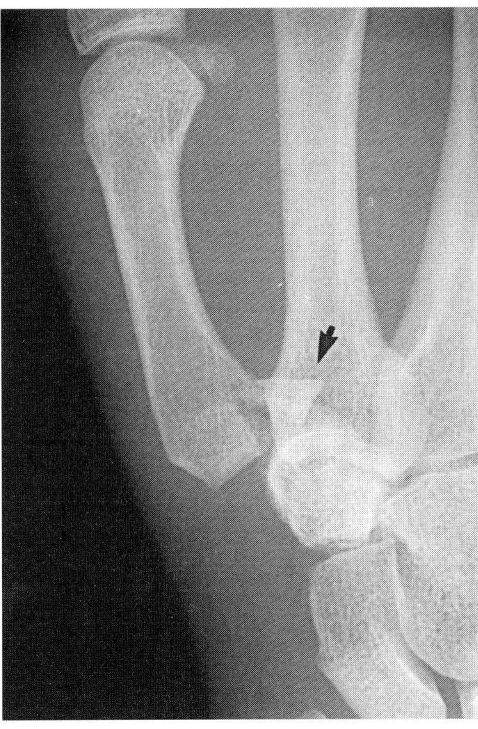

FIGURE 17–32. Intra-articular injuries of the first metacarpal base: Bennett's fracture-dislocation.[52] A typical oblique fracture of the volar lip of the first metacarpal base with a single displaced fragment (arrow) is evident on this radiograph. Bennett's fracture is a relatively common intra-articular injury that occurs at the base of the first metacarpal bone. It involves an axial force applied to a partially flexed metacarpal bone. The base of the metacarpal bone is pulled dorsally and radially and is separated by an oblique fracture line from a fragment of bone from the volar lip.

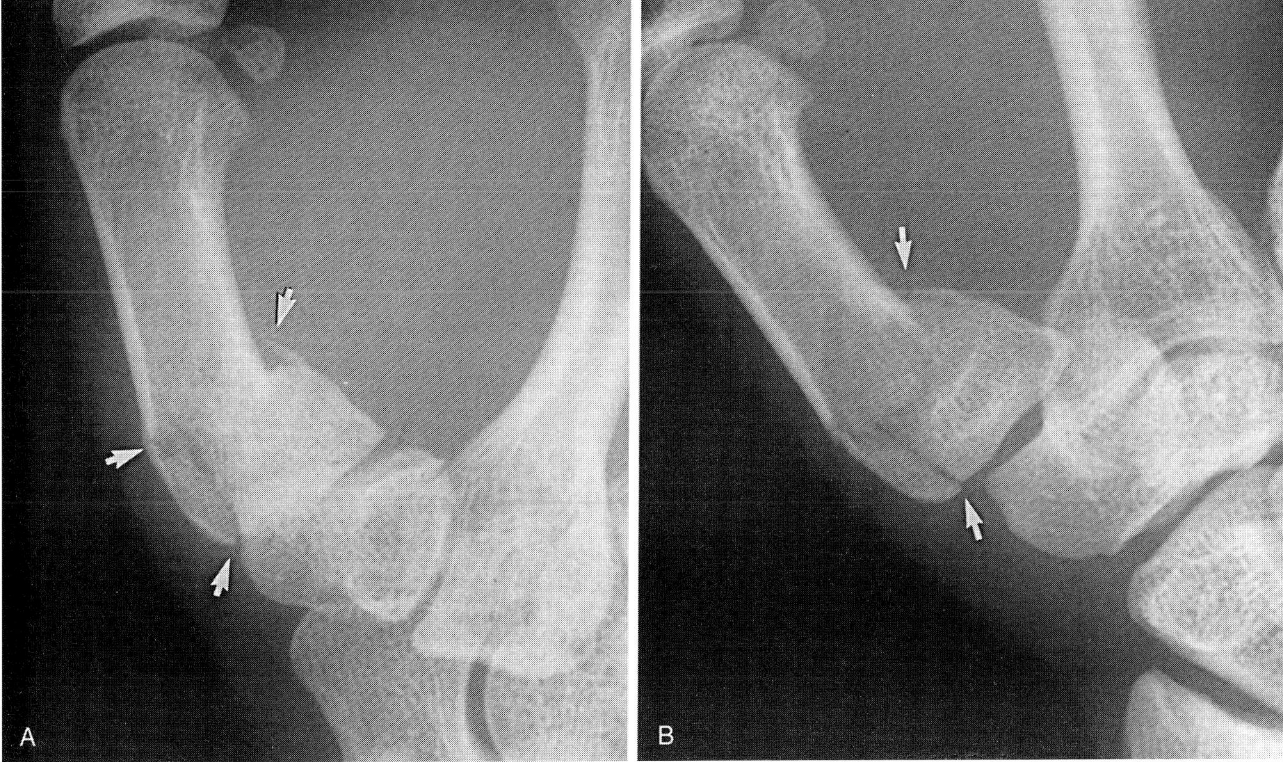

FIGURE 17–33. A, B Intra-articular injuries of the first metacarpal base: Rolando's fracture.[52, 53] Two projections of the thumb reveal a comminuted intra-articular fracture at the base of the first metacarpal bone (arrows).

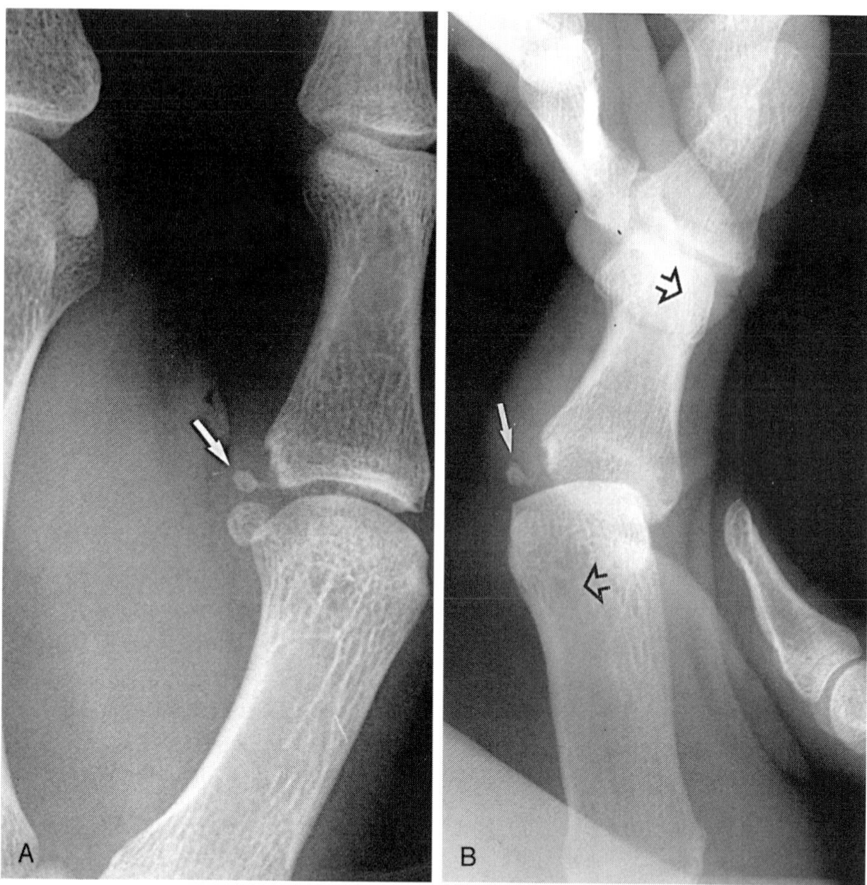

FIGURE 17–34. Gamekeeper's thumb.[54–56] A Routine posteroanterior radiograph shows a small osseous fragment (arrow) avulsed from the base of the first proximal phalanx. B Radiograph obtained with the application of radial stress reveals excessive motion at the metacarpophalangeal joint. The open arrows indicate the direction of stress applied by the examiner, and the white arrow indicates the osseous fragment.

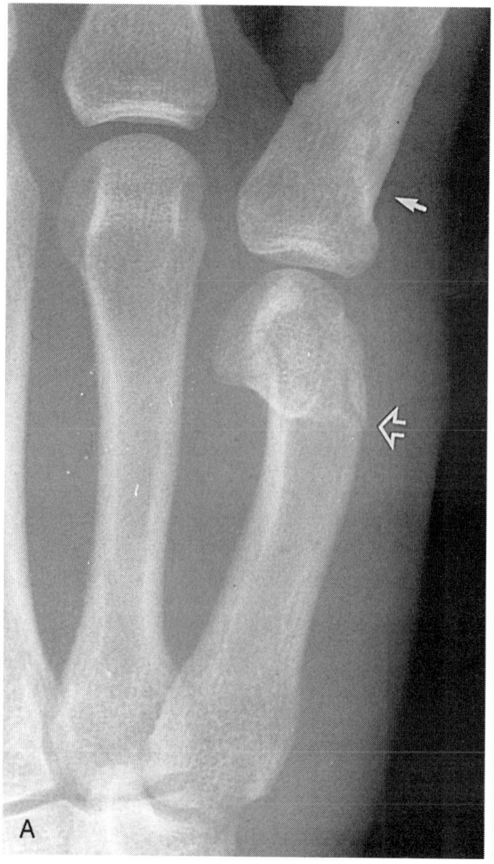

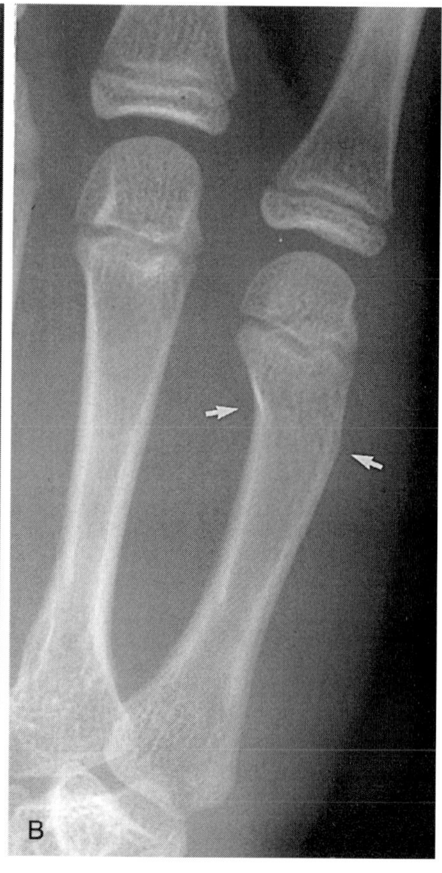

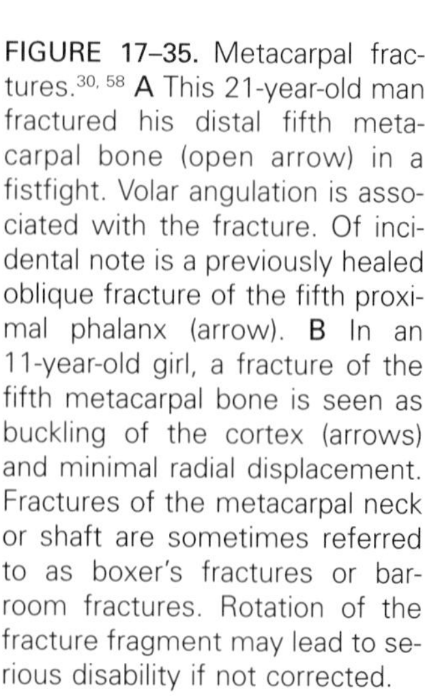

FIGURE 17–35. Metacarpal fractures.[30, 58] A This 21-year-old man fractured his distal fifth metacarpal bone (open arrow) in a fistfight. Volar angulation is associated with the fracture. Of incidental note is a previously healed oblique fracture of the fifth proximal phalanx (arrow). B In an 11-year-old girl, a fracture of the fifth metacarpal bone is seen as buckling of the cortex (arrows) and minimal radial displacement. Fractures of the metacarpal neck or shaft are sometimes referred to as boxer's fractures or barroom fractures. Rotation of the fracture fragment may lead to serious disability if not corrected.

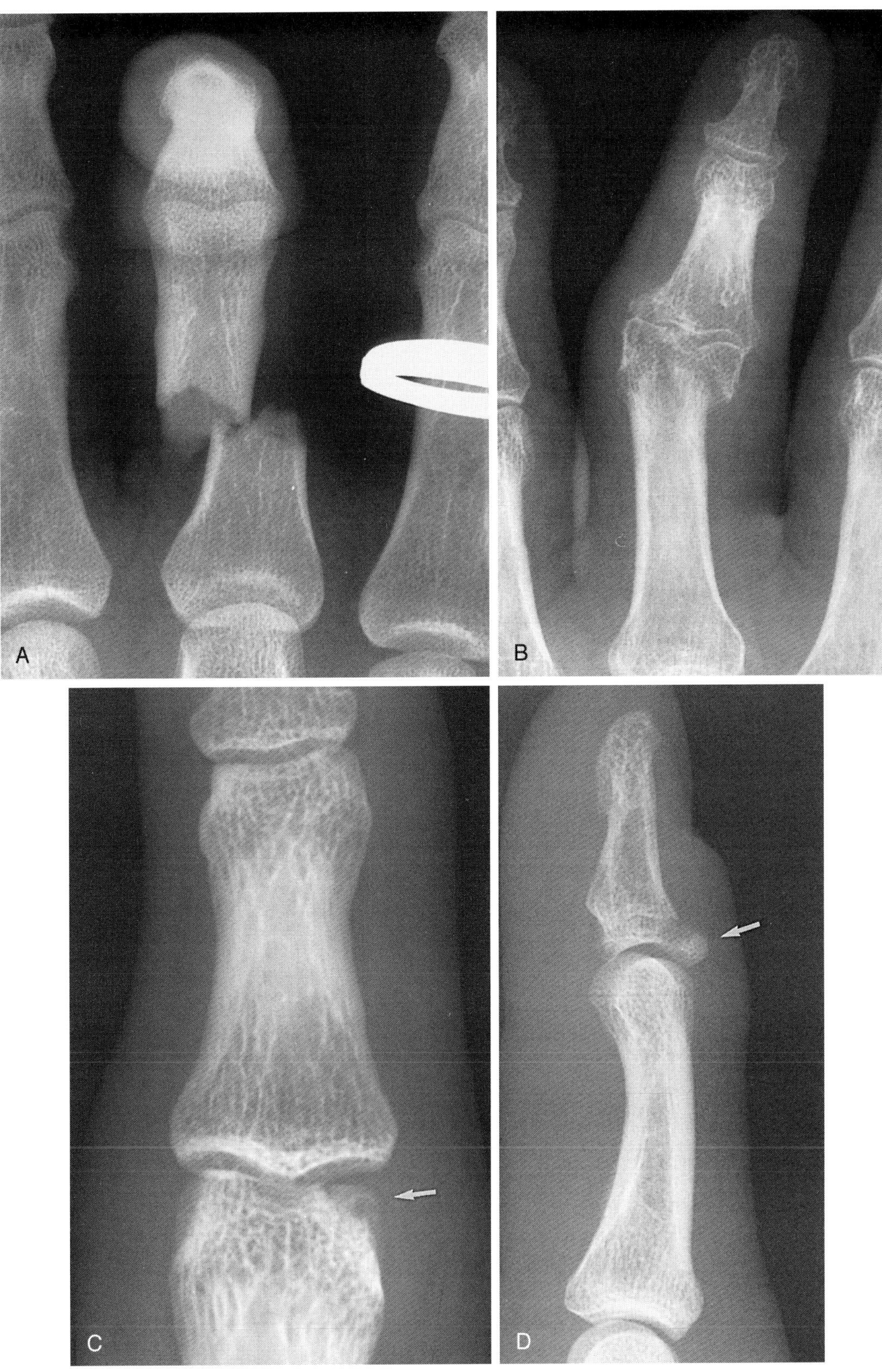

FIGURE 17–36. Phalangeal fractures.[30, 59, 60] A Displaced fracture of the midshaft of the phalanx shows poor alignment and apposition. B Radiograph of another patient shows a displaced intra-articular fracture of the distal end of the proximal phalanx with ulnar deviation of the distal fragment. C In yet another patient, an intra-articular fracture of the head of the proximal phalanx is demonstrated (arrow). D Mallet finger. Observe the small fragment of bone at the proximal portion of the extensor surface of the distal phalanx (arrow). This injury results from avulsion at the insertion of the extensor tendon mechanism. It is typically associated with a 40- to 45-degree flexion deformity, and the patient has loss of active extension at the distal interphalangeal joint.

Illustration continued on following page

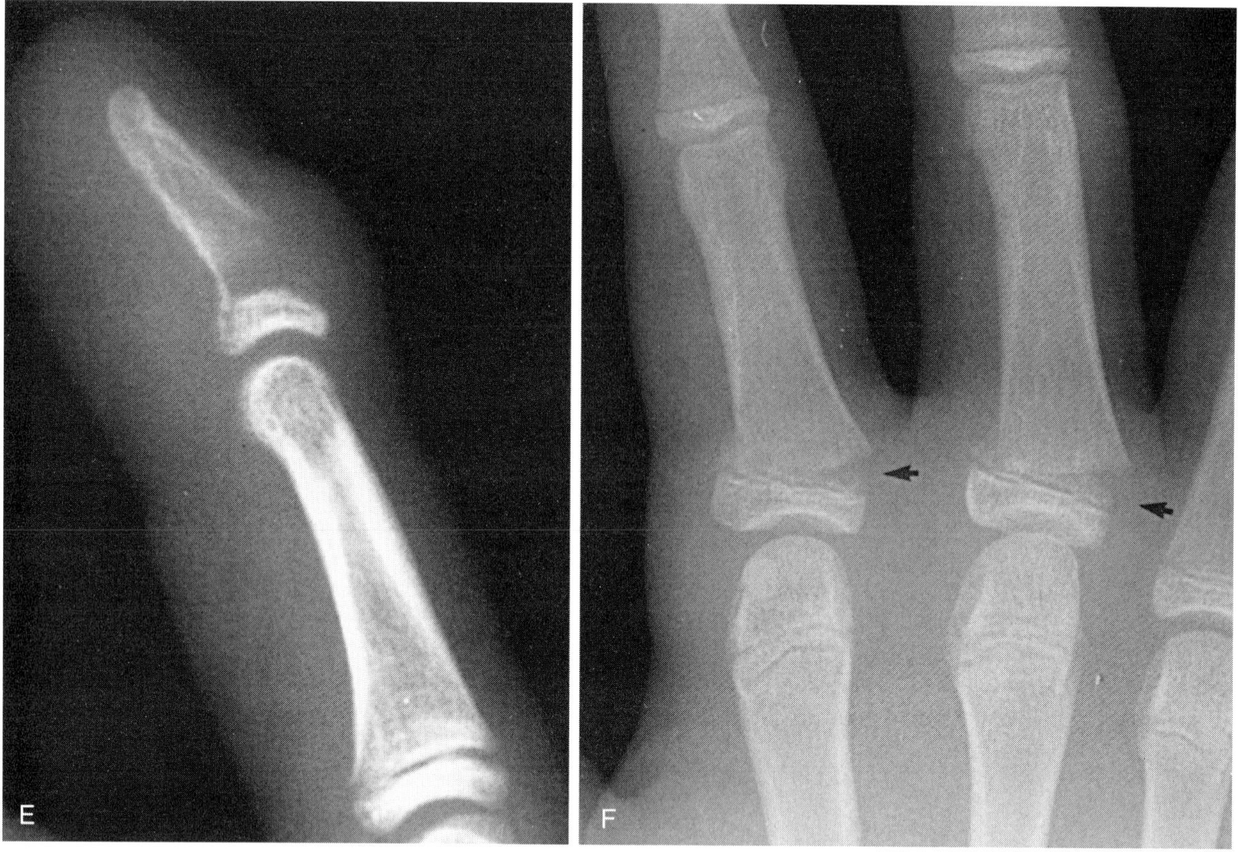

FIGURE 17–36 *Continued.* E Nail-bed injury. This 14-year-old boy sustained a hyperflexion injury of his finger. A Salter-Harris type I fracture of the terminal phalanx is present, with epiphyseal displacement, bone resorption, and soft tissue swelling. This type of injury usually disrupts the nail bed, exposing the underlying tissues to the environment and rendering them susceptible to infection. F Growth plate injuries. Salter-Harris type II fractures of the second and third proximal phalangeal bases are seen (arrows).

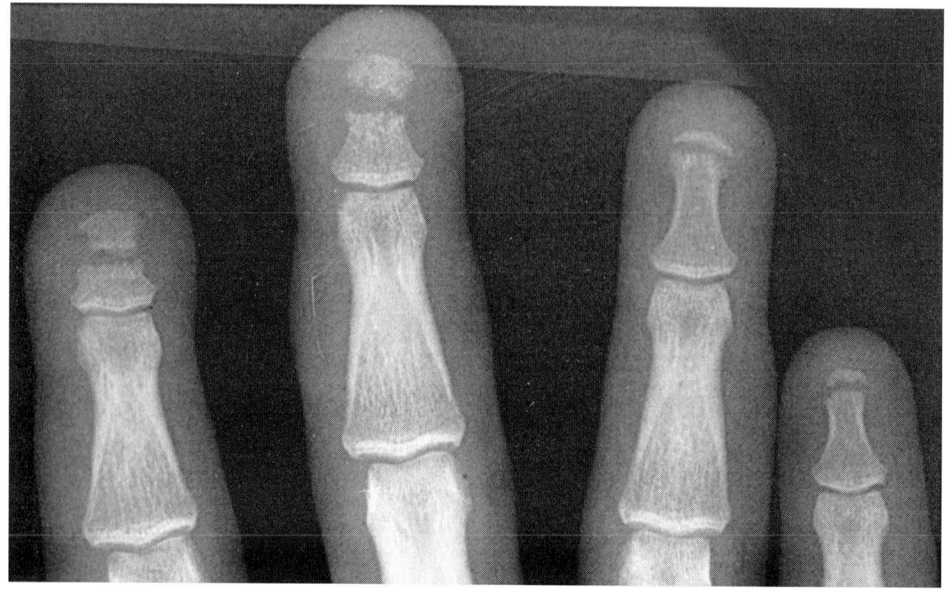

FIGURE 17–37. Phalangeal stress fractures: Guitar player acro-osteolysis.[61, 62] This enthusiastic guitar player sustained fatigue fractures of several terminal phalanges, a condition that has been termed guitar player acro-osteolysis. Observe the radiolucent bands traversing the terminal tufts.

TABLE 17–7. Soft Tissue Disorders Affecting the Wrist and Hand

Entity	Figure(s)	Characteristics
Ligament injuries[44]		See wrist instability (Table 17–5)
Lesions of the triangular fibrocartilage (TFC) complex[64, 65]	17–38	Full-thickness and partial-thickness defects occur as a result of degeneration or trauma Traumatic avulsion from ulnar or radial attachments also may occur Arthrography and magnetic resonance (MR) imaging have limited usefulness owing to the occurrence of communicating defects of the TFC complex in asymptomatic persons
Abnormalities of the extensor and flexor tendons and tendon sheaths[66]	17–39	Spectrum of abnormalities: Tendinitis and tenosynovitis: inflammation of tendons and tendon sheaths (i.e., De Quervain's syndrome: tenosynovitis of the abductor pollicis longus and extensor brevis tendons) Tendon rupture: partial or complete disruption with retraction of tendon or avulsion of tendon sheath; may result in inability to extend or flex the fingers (i.e., mallet finger with disruption of extensor tendon resulting in persistent flexion deformity at distal interphalangeal joint [Fig. 17–36D]) MR imaging is the most useful imaging study for most of these disorders
Carpal tunnel syndrome[67]	17–40	Entrapment of median nerve within the carpal tunnel Some causes: tenosynovitis of the flexor tendon sheaths, rheumatologic disorders, infiltrative diseases, trauma, neoplasms, anatomic factors, diabetes mellitus, pregnancy, osteoarthrosis; idiopathic Clinical history, physical examination, and electromyography, usually diagnostic Ultrasonography, computed tomography (CT), and MR imaging play a minor role in evaluation *MR imaging findings* Swelling of median nerve (at level of pisiform bone) Flattening of median nerve (at level of hamate bone) Palmar bowing of flexor retinaculum (at level of hamate bone) Increased signal intensity of median nerve on T2-weighted images
Ganglion cyst[68, 69]		Most commonly occurring soft tissue mass about the wrist Fibrous walled mass containing clear mucinous fluid Arises from joint capsules, tendons, or tendon sheaths, especially on extensor surface of wrist Ultrasonography and MR imaging often useful in evaluation
Glomus tumor[70]		Benign soft tissue lesion at base of nail that may involve the terminal phalanx Shallow well-marginated erosion of adjacent bone
Giant cell tumor of tendon sheath[71]		Benign giant cell tumors of soft tissues may arise from tendon sheaths about the wrist or, more frequently, in the fingers Closely resembles pigmented villonodular or nodular synovitis Soft tissue mass may result in erosion of adjacent bone

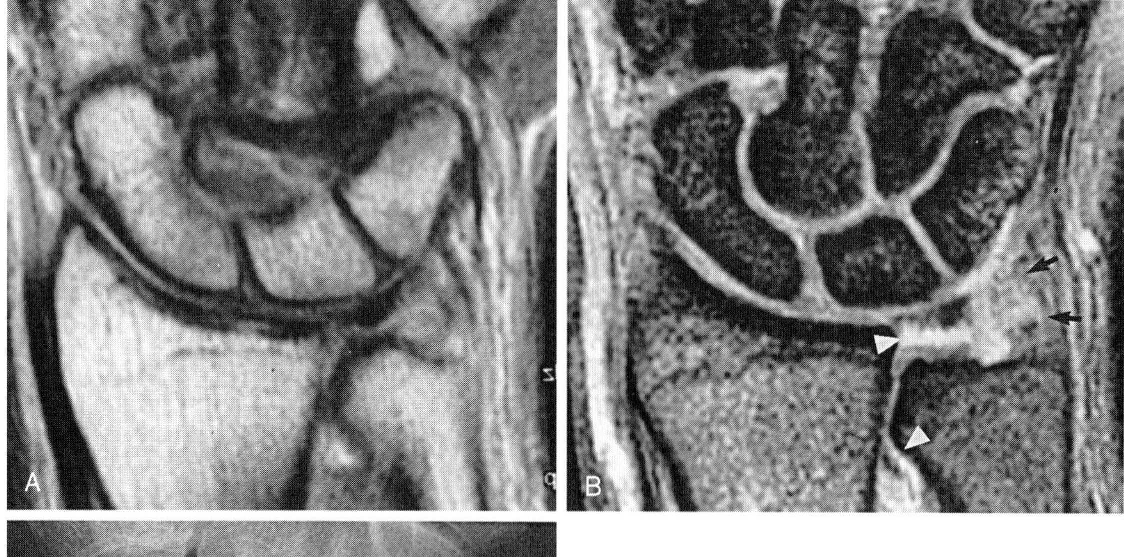

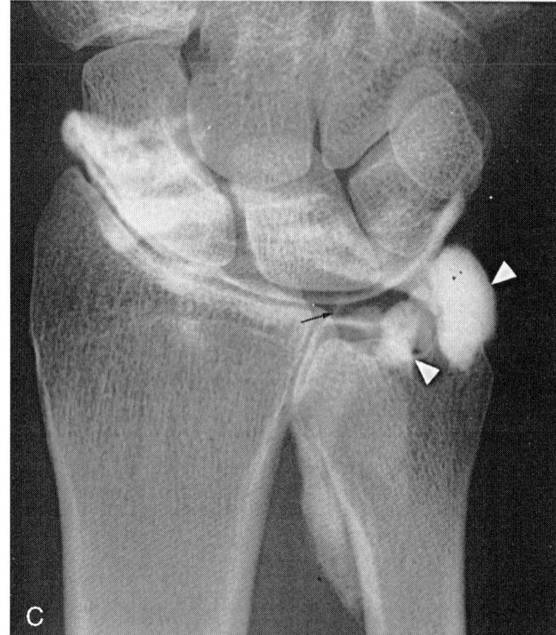

FIGURE 17–38. Triangular fibrocartilage complex: Ulnar detachment.[64, 65] A, B Coronal proton density–weighted (TR/TE, 2500/20) spin echo (A) and multiplanar gradient recalled (MPGR) (TR/TE, 549/15; flip angle, 35 degrees). (B) Magnetic resonance (MR) images show abnormal separation of the triangular fibrocartilage complex from the distal portion of the ulna and absence of visualization of the ulnar-sided attachments of the complex. In B, abnormal high signal intensity (arrows) is evident in this region, and fluid is present in the distal radioulnar joint (arrowheads). C Radiocarpal joint arthrogram shows a communicating defect in the triangular fibrocartilage complex (arrow), abnormal collections of contrast agent about the ulna (arrowheads), and proximal extravasation of contrast material from the distal radioulnar joint. *(From Resnick D, Kang HS: Internal Derangements of Joints. Philadelphia, WB Saunders, 1997, p 415.)*

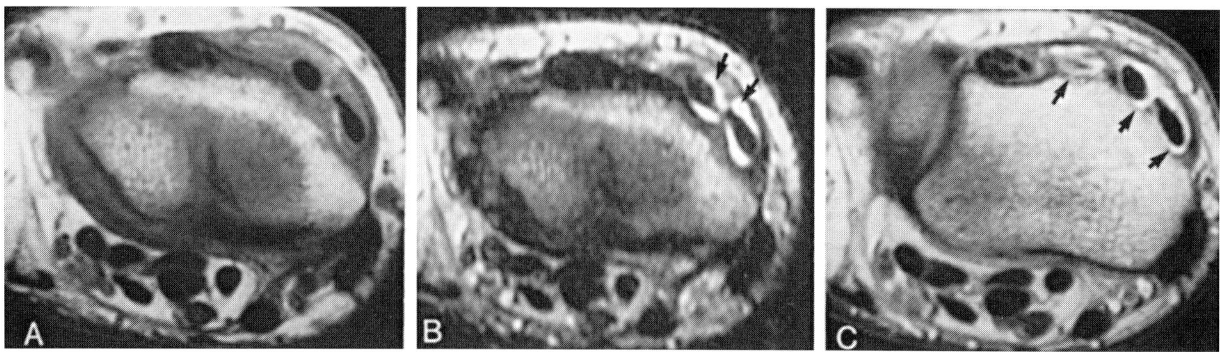

FIGURE 17–39. Tenosynovitis of the tendon sheaths of the extensor pollicis longus and the extensor carpi radialis brevis and longus tendons: magnetic resonance (MR) imaging.[66] Transaxial T1-weighted (TR/TE, 700/17) (A) and T2-weighted (TR/TE, 2000/80) (B) spin echo MR images and a transaxial T1-weighted (TR/TE, 650/20) spin echo MR image after intravenous administration of gadolinium compound (C) show the enlarged tendon sheaths. The high signal intensity (arrows) in B and C is consistent with the presence of synovial inflammatory tissue. *(From Resnick D, Kang HS: Internal Derangements of Joints. Philadelphia, WB Saunders, 1997, p 448.)*

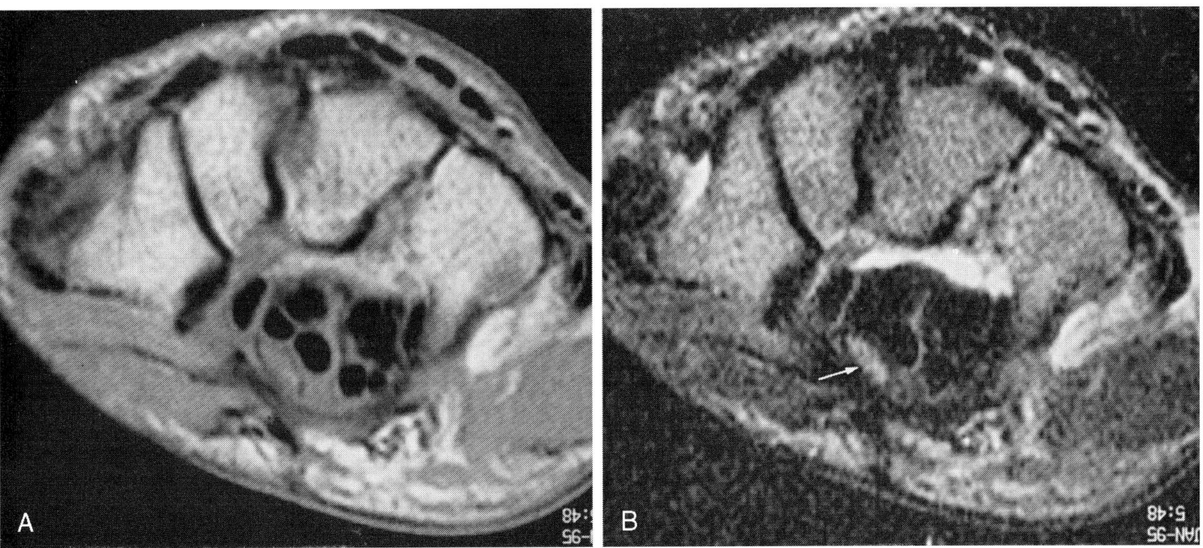

FIGURE 17–40. Carpal tunnel syndrome: magnetic resonance (MR) imaging.[67] Transverse proton density–weighted (TR/TE, 1800/20) (A) and T2-weighted (TR/TE, 1800/80) (B) spin echo MR images in a patient with clinical evidence of severe carpal tunnel syndrome show bowing of the flexor retinaculum, fluid dorsal to the flexor tendons and sheaths, and increased signal intensity of the median nerve (arrow) in B. *(From Resnick D, Kang HS: Internal Derangements of Joints. Philadelphia, WB Saunders, 1997, p 444.)*

TABLE 17–8. Articular Disorders of the Wrist and Hand

Entity	Figure(s)	Characteristics
Degenerative and related disorders		
Primary osteoarthrosis[72–75]	17–41	Primary osteoarthrosis involves predominantly the interphalangeal joints and first carpometacarpal joints May also be age-related
Secondary osteoarthrosis[76]	17–42	Secondary osteoarthrosis may involve any previously injured joint Repeated trauma to the metacarpophalangeal joints in boxers and manual laborers is referred to as boxer's arthropathy or Missouri metacarpal syndrome Nonuniform joint space narrowing Subchondral sclerosis Osteophytes Subluxation
Erosive (inflammatory) osteoarthritis[77–80]	17–43	Predilection for interphalangeal joints but also may involve the first carpometacarpal joint Acute painful inflammatory episodes in elderly patients Central erosions Nonuniform joint space narrowing Subchondral sclerosis Osteophytes Subluxation
Inflammatory disorders		
Rheumatoid arthritis[81, 82]	17–44	Bilateral symmetric, concentric joint space narrowing, erosion, periarticular osteopenia, deformities and subluxation
Juvenile chronic arthritis[83, 84]	17–45	Soft tissue swelling Diffuse, bilateral symmetric joint space loss and erosion, periarticular osteoporosis, ballooning of epiphyses, premature epiphyseal fusion, and joint ankylosis
Ankylosing spondylitis[85]	17–46	Erosions and periarticular enthesopathy (whiskering) predominates about the wrist Changes in fingers resemble those of psoriasis Infrequently, may result in partial or complete intra-articular osseous ankylosis

Table continued on following page

TABLE 17–8. Articular Disorders of the Wrist and Hand *Continued*

Entity	Figure(s)	Characteristics
Psoriatic arthropathy[78, 86–88]	17–47	Predilection for distal and proximal interphalangeal joints Central and peripheral erosions and fluffy, poorly defined periarticular periostitis Ray pattern: involvement of several joints within the same digit Diffuse soft tissue swelling: sausage digit Preservation of bone density
Reiter's syndrome[87–89]	17–48	Findings identical to those of psoriatic arthropathy but a greater predilection for lower extremity
Systemic lupus erythematosus[90]	17–49	Articular signs and symptoms present in as many as 90 per cent of patients Deforming nonerosive arthropathy Myositis, polyarthritis, subchondral cysts, tendon weakening and rupture, soft tissue calcification, acrosclerosis, tuft resorption
Jaccoud's arthropathy[91]	17–50	One form of nonerosive deforming arthropathy with reversible subluxations resulting from capsular inflammation and fibrosis; involves mainly the fourth and fifth metacarpophalangeal joints Seen in patients with rheumatic fever, systemic lupus erythematosus, scleroderma, and other collagen vascular disorders Nonerosive deforming arthropathy is seen less commonly in agammaglobulinemia, Ehlers-Danlos syndrome, sarcoidosis, and rheumatoid arthritis
Dermatomyositis and polymyositis[92]		Diffuse soft tissue calcification
Scleroderma (progressive systemic sclerosis)[93]	17–51	Tendon calcification Soft tissue, periarticular, and intra-articular calcification Acro-osteolysis of the ungual tufts Periarticular erosions
Crystal deposition and metabolic diseases		
Gouty arthropathy[94–96]	17–52	May involve any joint in wrist or hand Periarticular erosions often with overhanging margins Soft tissue tophi
Calcium pyrophosphate dihydrate (CPPD) crystal deposition disease[97–99]	17–53	Periarticular and intra-articular calcification (chondrocalcinosis) Pyrophosphate arthropathy involving radiocarpal and metacarpophalangeal joints Scapholunate advanced collapse (SLAC wrist)
Hemochromatosis[100, 101]	17–54	Rare involvement of wrist and hand Findings resemble those of CPPD crystal deposition disease Beak-like excrescences arising from radial aspect of metacarpal heads
Calcium hydroxyapatite crystal deposition disease[102, 103]	17–55	Periarticular calcification of ligaments and tendons about the wrist may be encountered Masses may diminish in size or disappear Most common site of calcification in the wrist is within the flexor carpi ulnaris tendon and in the hands about the interphalangeal and metacarpophalangeal joints
Miscellaneous disorders		
Multicentric reticulohistiocytosis[104]	17–56	Uncommon systemic disease of unknown cause that becomes apparent in adult life Characterized by proliferation of histiocytes in skin, mucosa, subcutaneous tissues, synovia, and, on occasion, bone and periosteum Bilateral symmetric central and marginal erosions of interphalangeal joints (75 per cent of patients), resulting in apparent separation of joint surfaces Soft tissue swelling and eventual arthritis mutilans
Sarcoidosis[105–107]	17–57	Chronic, multisystem disease of unknown cause characterized by the development of noncaseating granulomas Honeycomb or latticework trabecular pattern predominating in the phalanges and metacarpal bones Cystic defects, pathologic fracture, subcutaneous nodules, and osteosclerosis Acro-osteolysis and phalangeal sclerosis

TABLE 17–8. Articular Disorders of the Wrist and Hand *Continued*

Entity	Figure(s)	Characteristics
Idiopathic synovial osteochondromatosis[108, 109]	17–58	Multiple intra-articular or periarticular collections of intracapsular osteochondral or chondral bodies of variable size and density May result in erosion of adjacent bone Idiopathic form more common than secondary form in hand
Neuropathic osteoarthropathy[110]	17–59	Wrist and hand involvement: leprosy, congenital insensitivity to pain, syringomyelia *Radiographic findings* Prominent atrophic resorption of terminal tufts Joint space narrowing and obliteration, subluxation, disorganization, and destruction; bone fragmentation, destruction, and sclerosis
Frostbite[111, 112]	17–60	Local tissue damage from cellular injury as a result of the freezing process itself or from vascular insufficiency Soft tissue swelling, osteoporosis, periostitis, secondary infection, arthritis secondary to cartilage injury, terminal tuft resorption, epiphyseal abnormalities, and premature physeal fusion in children Thumb frequently is spared
Thermal and electrical injuries[113]	17–61	Soft tissue swelling, loss, or contracture; osteoporosis, acro-osteolysis, periostitis, epiphyseal injury and growth disturbance, articular abnormalities, osteolysis, osteosclerosis, and periarticular calcification and ossification
Silicone synovitis[114, 115]	17–62	Complication of silicone implant surgery for joint reconstruction Believed to be a reaction to shedded silicone particles embedded within the synovium, with resultant synovial hypertrophy and chronic inflammatory and giant cell infiltration of the synovial membrane Associated soft tissue swelling and preservation of cartilage spaces often is found Widespread joint destruction, cysts, and osseous fragmentation
Fracture blisters[116]	17–63	Infrequent complication of fractures Irregular blisters and nodules about the wrist and hand
Epidermolysis bullosa[117]	17–64	Rare chronic skin disorder resulting from insufficient adherence of the epidermis to the dermis, leading to formation of vesicles, bullae, and ulcerations that occur spontaneously or after minor trauma.
Osteolysis with detritic synovitis[118]	17–65	Rare disease characterized by pain, swelling, marked joint deformity, osseous resorption, osteolysis, erosion, and osseous debris

See also Tables 1–6 to 1–9.

TABLE 17–9. Compartmental Analysis of Wrist and Hand Disease*

		Articulations†								
Entity		**DIP**	**PIP**	**MCP**	**RC**	**DRU**	**MC**	**PT**	**CCMC**	**FIRST MCP**
Osteoarthrosis	17–41	+	+					+		+
Erosive (inflammatory) osteoarthritis	17–43	+	+				+			+
Rheumatoid arthritis	17–44		+	+	+	+	+	+	+	+
Scleroderma	17–51	+	+			+				+
Gouty arthropathy	17–52	+	+	+	+	+	+		+‡	+
CPPD crystal deposition disease	17–53			+	+		+			+

*Only the typical locations for each disease are indicated.
†DIP, Distal interphalangeal; PIP, proximal interphalangeal; MCP, metacarpophalangeal; RC, radiocarpal; DRU, distal radioulnar; MC, midcarpal; PT, pisiform-triquetral; CCMC, common carpometacarpal; MCP, metacarpophalangeal; CPPD, calcium pyrophosphate dihydrate.
‡Very severe abnormalities may be present in this compartment.

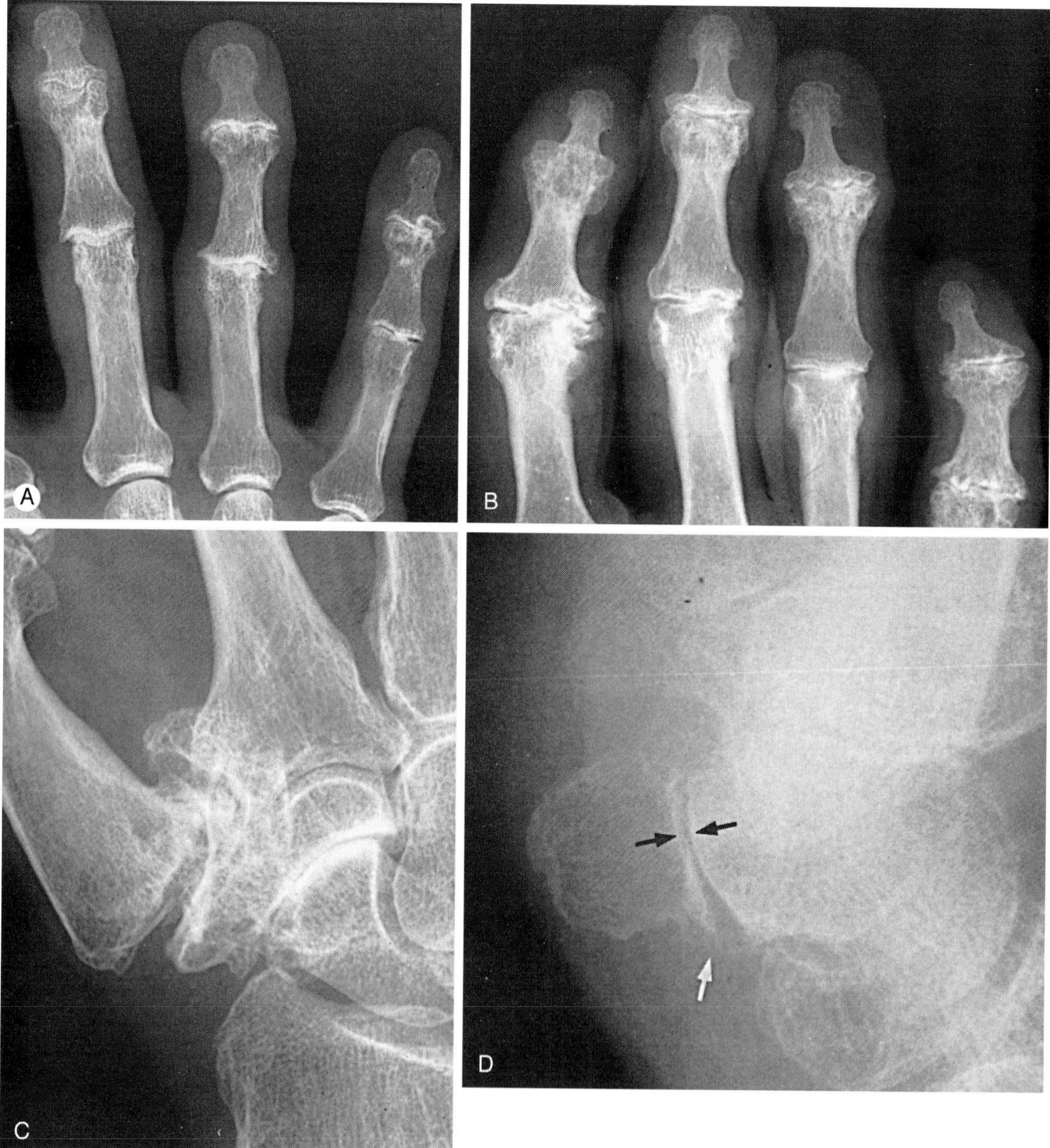

FIGURE 17–41. Primary osteoarthrosis: typical sites.[72–75] **A, B** Interphalangeal joints. In **A,** degenerative joint disease of the interphalangeal joints is characterized by osteophytes, nonuniform loss of joint space, subchondral sclerosis, and soft tissue prominence overlying the terminal interphalangeal joints (Heberden's nodes). The metacarpophalangeal joints are normal. In **B,** another patient, observe the prominent osteophytes, sclerosis, irregular joint space narrowing, and subluxations. **C** First carpometacarpal region. Degenerative changes are seen in the trapeziometacarpal, trapezioscaphoid, and trapeziotrapezoid articulations, common sites of involvement for osteoarthrosis. The changes are characterized by radial subluxation of the base of the first metacarpal bone, subchondral sclerosis, joint space narrowing, osteophyte formation, subchondral cysts, and intra-articular osseous bodies. **D** Pisiform-triquetral joint. Semisupinated oblique radiograph reveals joint space narrowing (black arrows), subchondral sclerosis, and osteophyte formation (white arrow) at the pisotriquetral articulation, a rare location for degenerative joint disease. *(D, Courtesy of R. Shapiro, M.D., Sacramento, California.)*

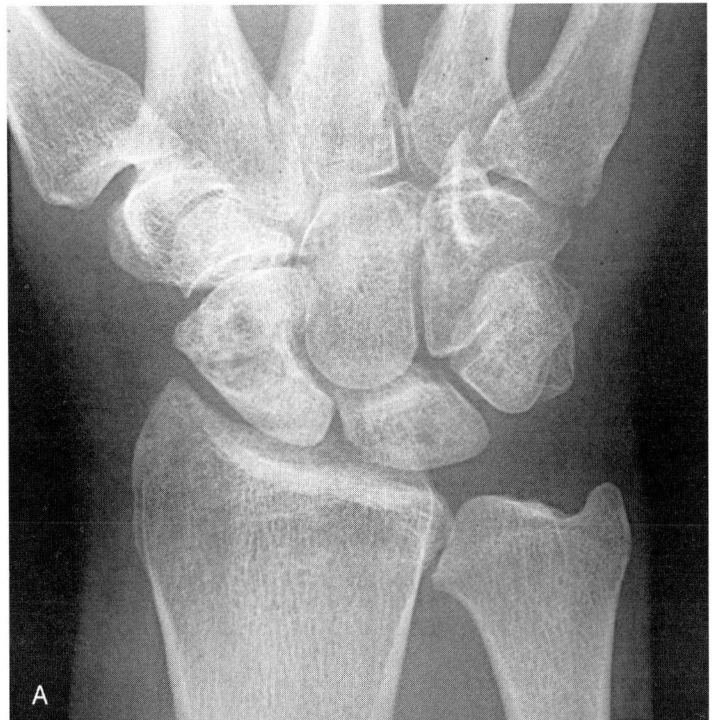

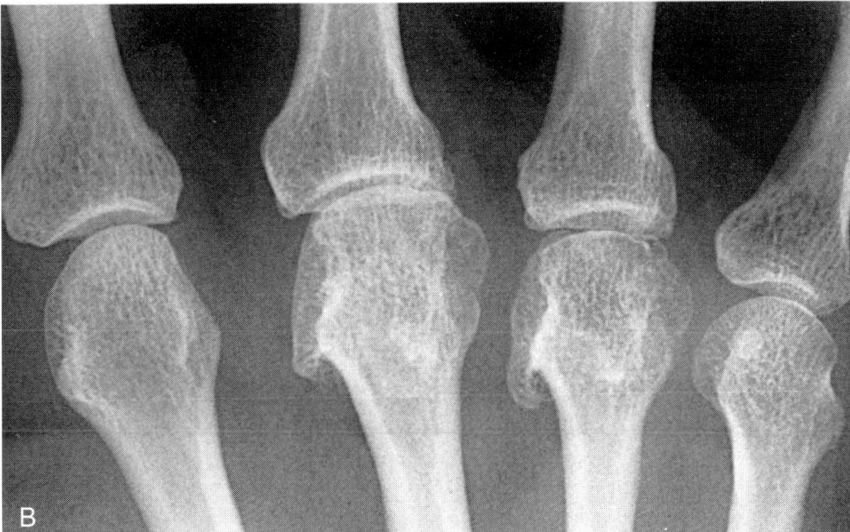

FIGURE 17–42. Secondary osteoarthrosis: posttraumatic.[76] A This 50-year-old retired boxer had persistent wrist pain. Large subchondral cysts are seen in the scaphoid and lunate bones. Joint space narrowing and osteophytes are not prominent in this patient. B Metacarpophalangeal joints. Degenerative joint disease is evident, characterized by nonuniform loss of joint space and osteophyte formation, with no evidence of erosion. Degenerative disease at this site is seen after repeated trauma, such as that sustained in boxers or manual laborers, and has been referred to as boxer's arthropathy or Missouri metacarpal syndrome. It may resemble pyrophosphate arthropathy seen in calcium pyrophosphate dihydrate (CPPD) crystal deposition disease and hemochromatosis. *(B, Courtesy of A. Brower, M.D., Norfolk, Virginia.)*

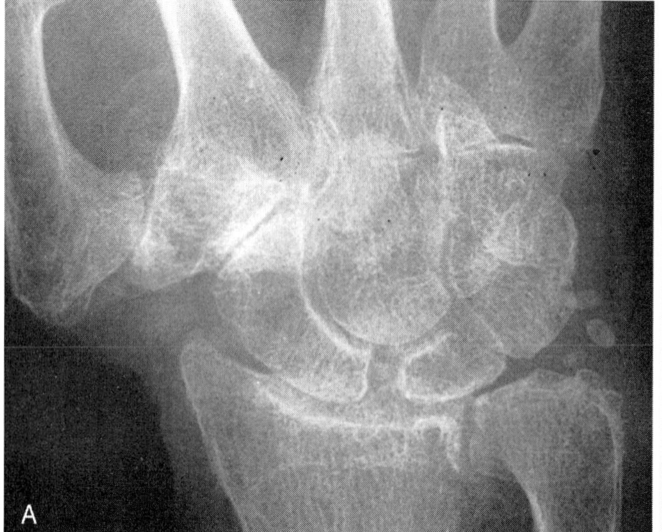

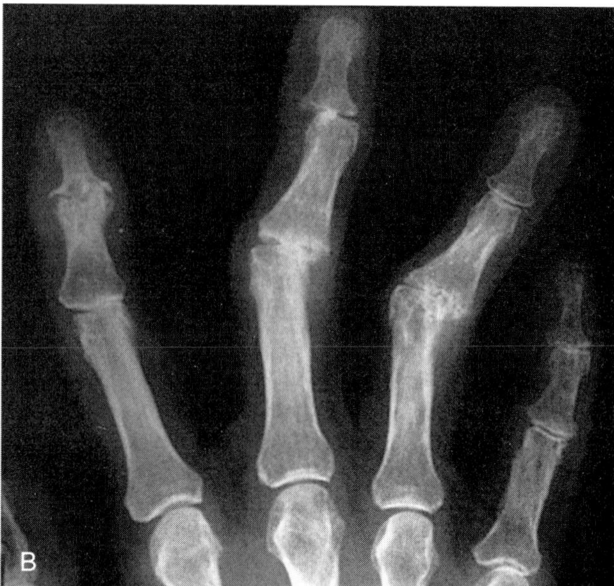

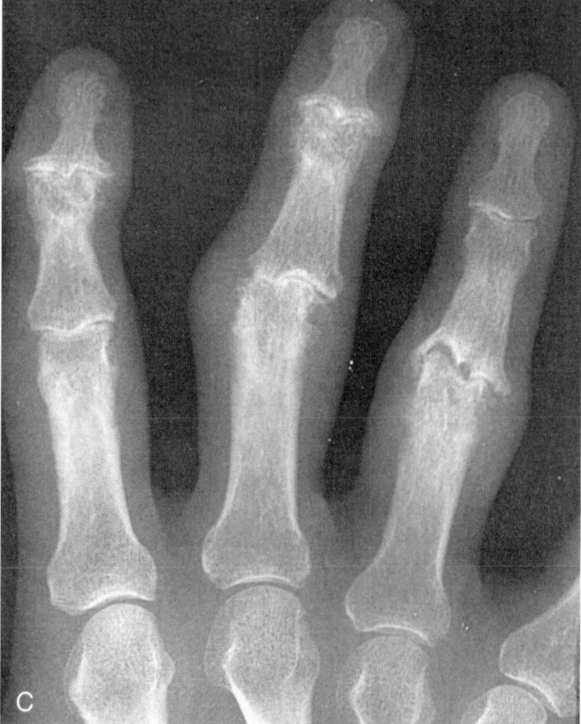

FIGURE 17–43. Erosive (inflammatory) osteoarthritis.[77–80] **A** Wrist involvement. Observe the severe subluxation and degenerative changes at the first carpometacarpal, trapezioscaphoid, and distal radioulnar joints. Scapholunate dissociation also is present, indicating probable disruption of the interosseous scapholunate ligament. **B, C** Interphalangeal joint involvement. In **B,** a 73-year-old woman, observe the central erosions of the subchondral bone, joint subluxations, soft tissue swelling, and preservation of the metacarpophalangeal joints. In **C,** another patient, similar changes are seen within the proximal and terminal interphalangeal joints. The metacarpophalangeal joints are not involved.

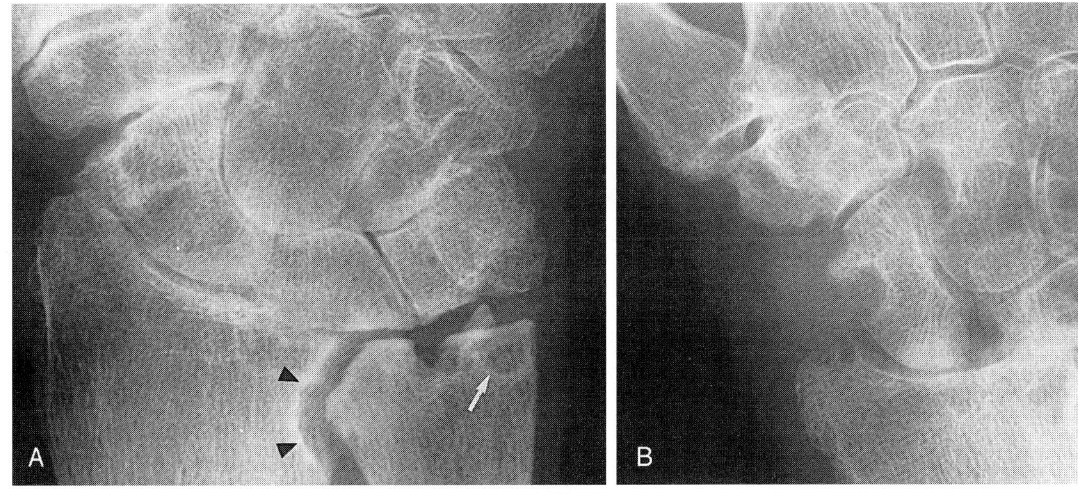

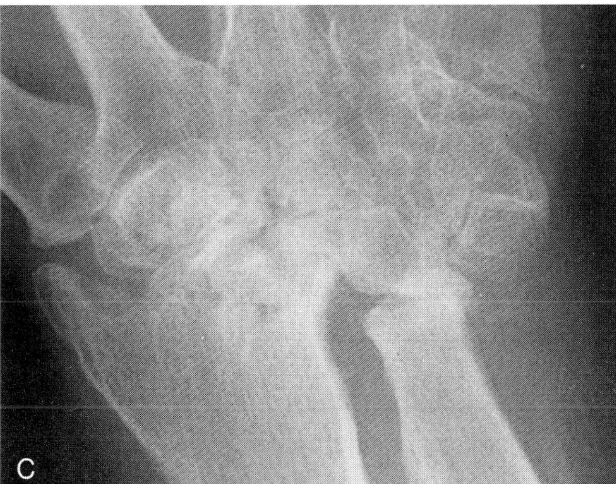

FIGURE 17–44. Rheumatoid arthritis.[81, 82] A–C Carpal abnormalities. In A, moderate changes of rheumatoid arthritis are seen. Widespread radiocarpal, midcarpal, and pericapitate joint space narrowing predominates in this patient. Observe the characteristic erosions of the ulnar styloid process (arrow) and distal radioulnar joint (arrowheads). In B, advanced changes (cystic form) are noted. The characteristic radiographic findings include soft tissue swelling, radiocarpal joint space narrowing, scapholunate widening, and multiple marginal erosions and subchondral cysts involving the carpal bones and the distal ends of the radius and ulna. In C, severe changes (pancarpal destruction) are evident in another patient. Observe the widespread erosive destruction of the joint spaces and the fragmentation and collapse of the carpal bones, radius, and ulna.

Illustration continued on following page

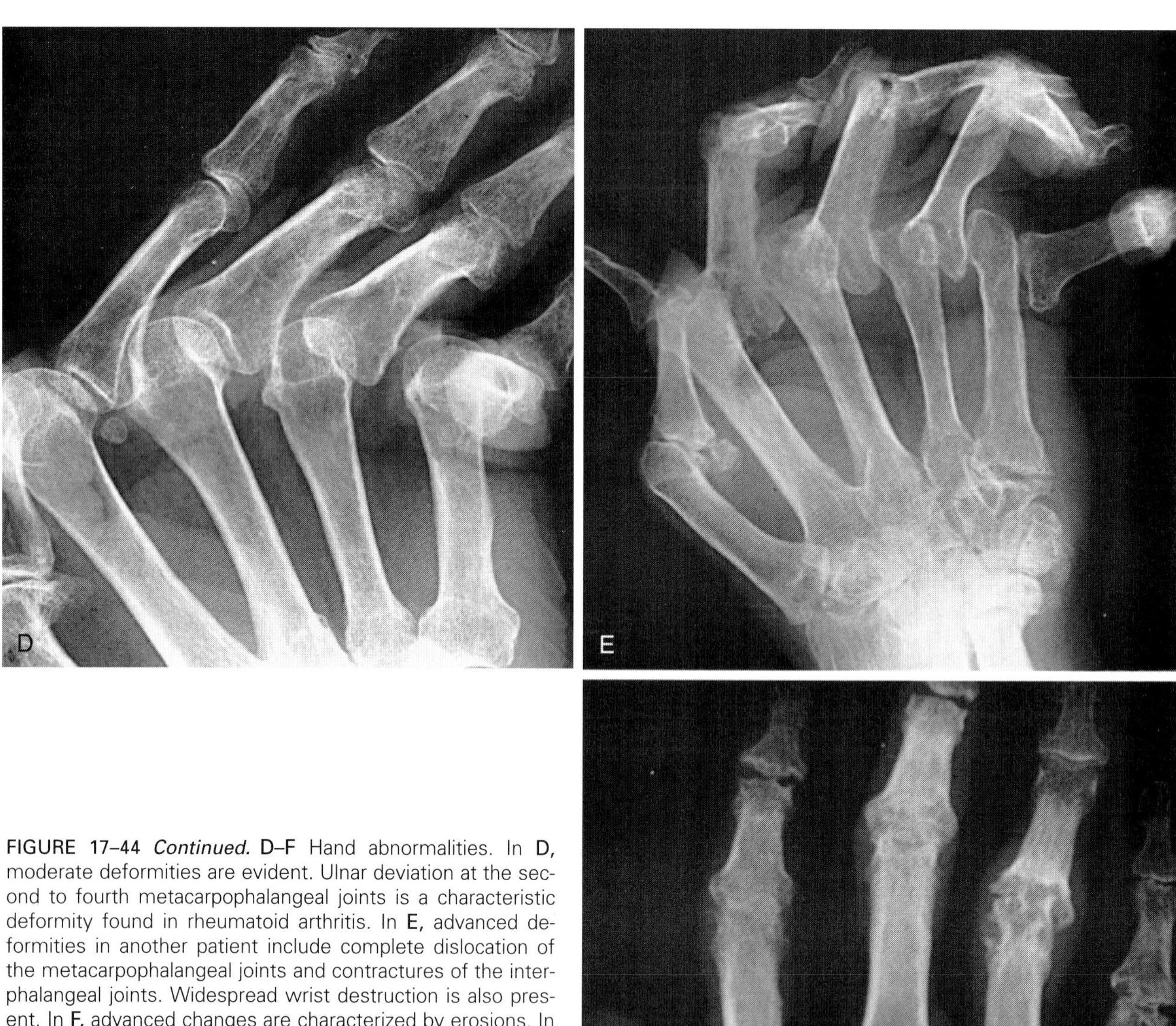

FIGURE 17–44 *Continued.* D–F Hand abnormalities. In **D,** moderate deformities are evident. Ulnar deviation at the second to fourth metacarpophalangeal joints is a characteristic deformity found in rheumatoid arthritis. In **E,** advanced deformities in another patient include complete dislocation of the metacarpophalangeal joints and contractures of the interphalangeal joints. Widespread wrist destruction is also present. In **F,** advanced changes are characterized by erosions. In a third patient, observe the numerous marginal and central erosions involving the metacarpophalangeal and proximal interphalangeal joints. Note also the uniform loss of joint space and periarticular osteopenia. Such changes in rheumatoid arthritis tend to spare the distal interphalangeal joints until late in the disease.

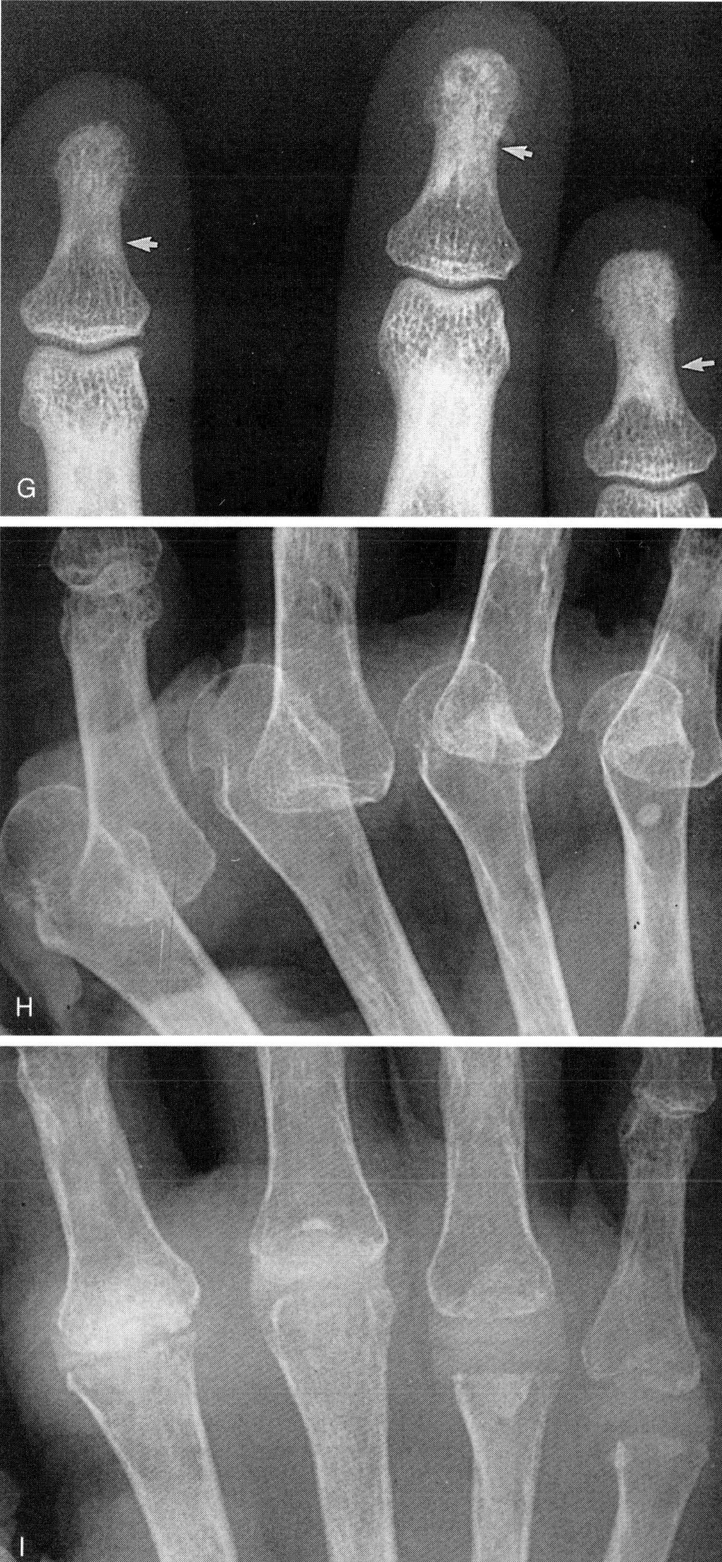

FIGURE 17–44 *Continued.* G Phalangeal sclerosis. The terminal phalanges are sclerotic (arrows), an infrequent complication of rheumatoid arthritis and other inflammatory arthropathies. H, I Surgical correction of deformities. In H, extensive volar dislocation of the second to fifth metacarpophalangeal joints is evident. In I, a postarthroplasty radiograph shows correction of the ulnar deviation and presence of joint prostheses.

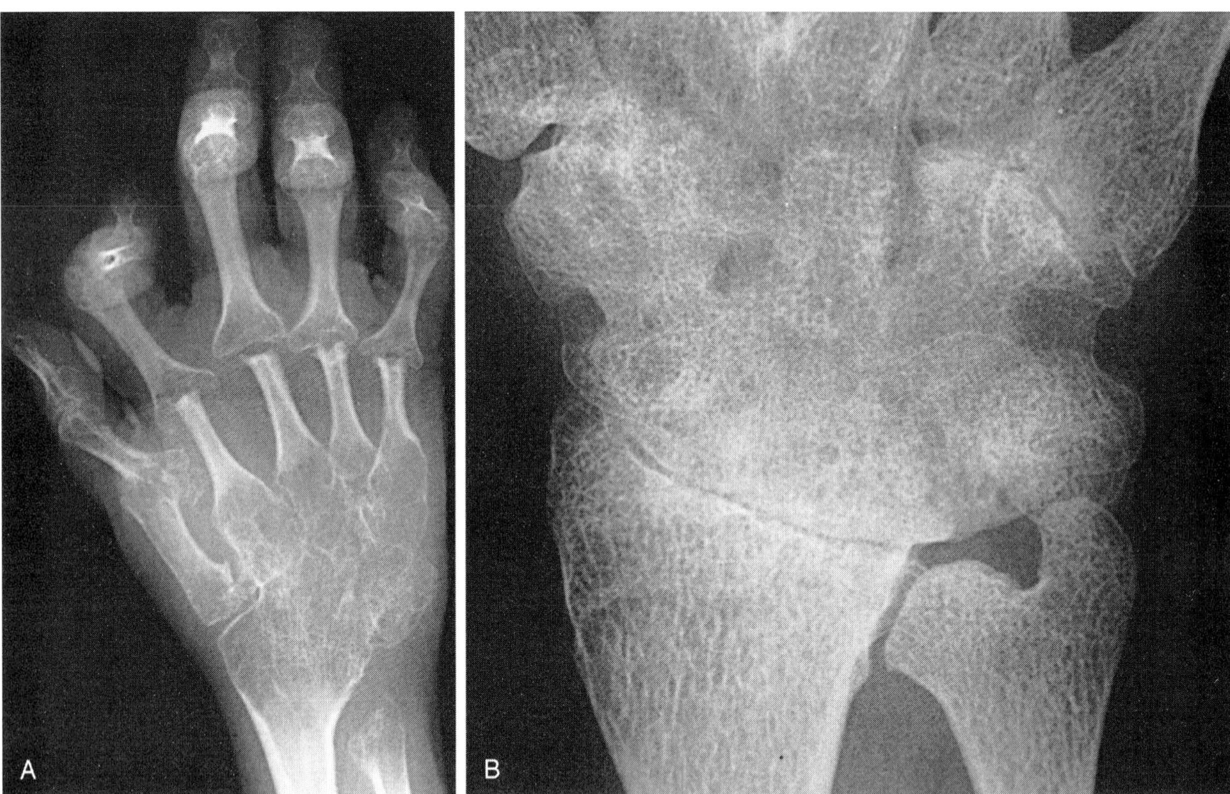

FIGURE 17–45. Juvenile chronic arthritis: Wrist and hand abnormalities.[83, 84] A This 23-year-old woman with a 10-year history of Still's disease has several characteristic radiographic findings, including periarticular osteopenia, wrist ankylosis, erosion and resorption of the distal end of the ulna, widespread joint space narrowing, and soft tissue atrophy. Flexion deformities of the proximal interphalangeal joints also are prominent. All the findings were bilateral and symmetric (other hand not shown). Interpretation of the changes about the metacarpophalangeal joints is complicated by previous surgery. B In this 27-year-old woman with juvenile rheumatoid arthritis, compete osseous ankylosis of the intercarpal and carpometacarpal articulations has occurred. The radiocarpal joint is severely narrowed. Some degree of carpal ankylosis has been reported in as many as 47 per cent of persons with juvenile chronic arthritis.

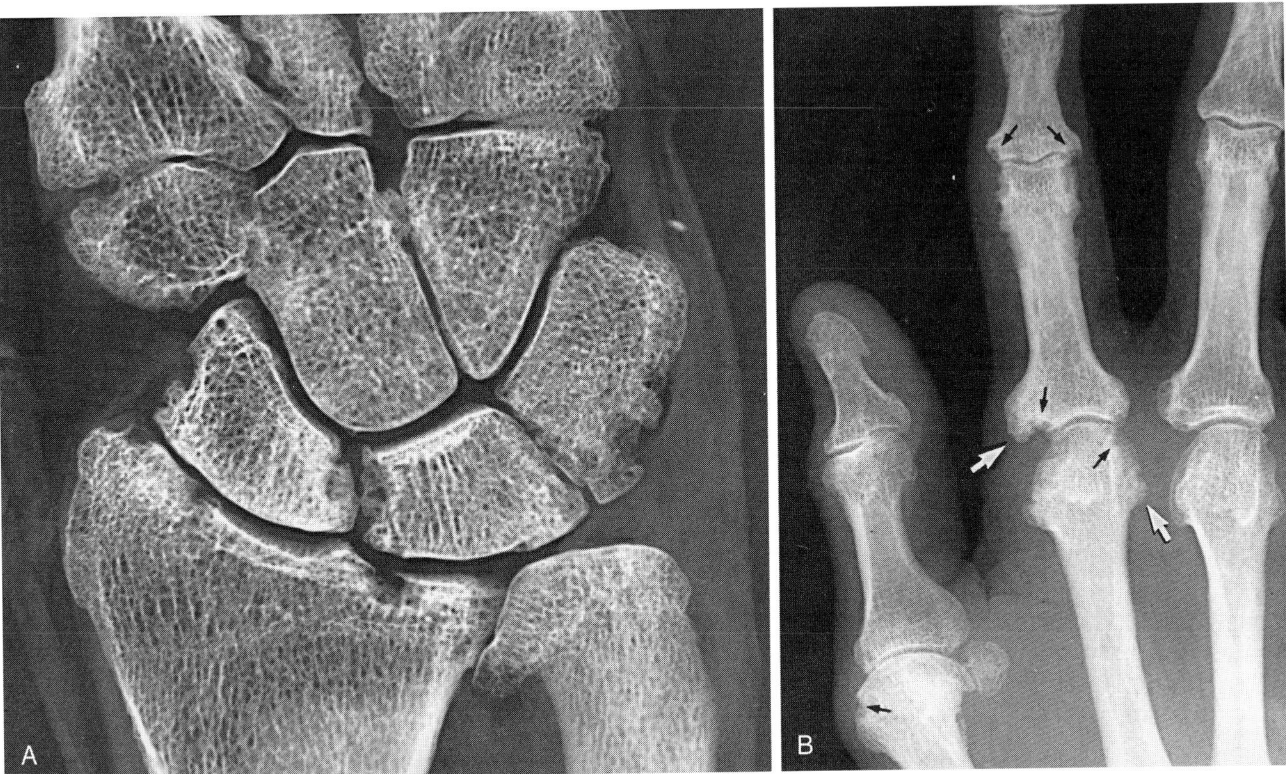

FIGURE 17–46. Ankylosing spondylitis.[85] A Wrist abnormalities. Observe the widespread erosions of the scaphoid and lunate bones and the triquetrum, as well as the distal end of the radius in this radiograph of a coronal cadaveric section from a person with ankylosing spondylitis. B Hand abnormalities. Prominent periarticular excrescences (enthesophytes) (large white arrows) are seen adjacent to the metacarpophalangeal and interphalangeal joints. Marginal erosions (small black arrows) and joint space narrowing also are evident. Note the absence of periarticular osteopenia. Asymmetric abnormalities of the hand and wrist occur in approximately 30 per cent of patients with severe ankylosing spondylitis.

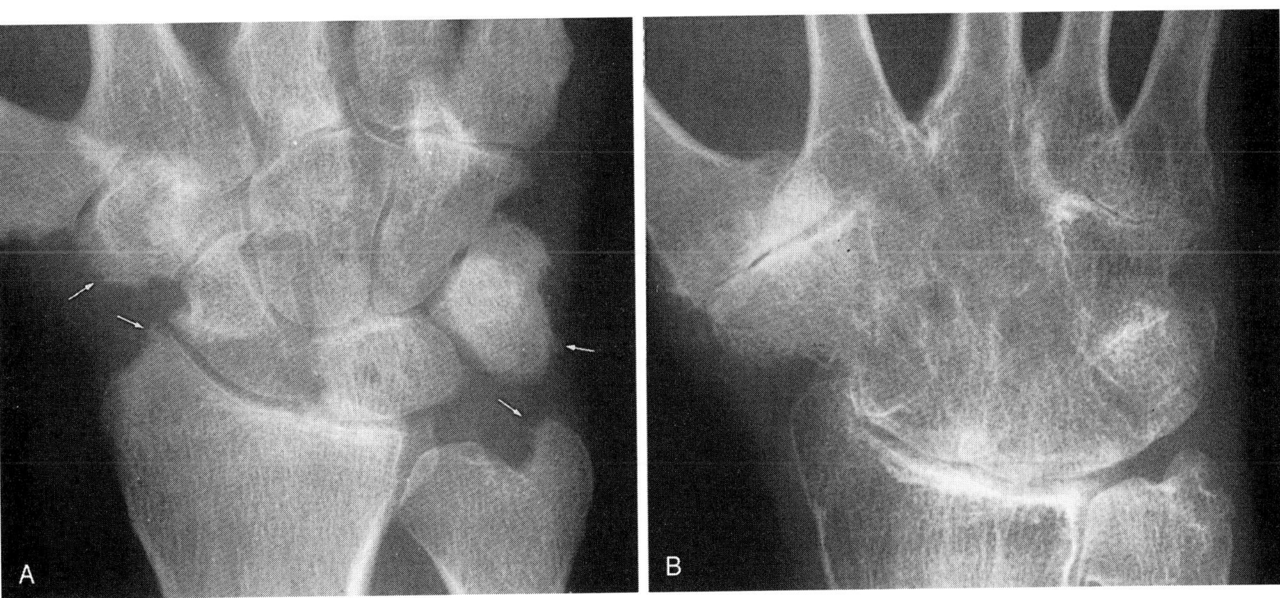

FIGURE 17–47. Psoriatic arthropathy.[78, 86–88] A, B Wrist abnormalities. In A, diffuse pancarpal joint space narrowing, cystic erosions, fluffy periostitis ("whiskering") (arrows), and absence of obvious osteopenia are typical features of the seronegative spondyloarthropathies. In B, diffuse osseous ankylosis of all intercarpal and carpometacarpal joints has occurred in a patient with advanced psoriatic arthritis. *(B, Courtesy of P. Kindynis, M.D., Geneva, Switzerland.)*

Illustration continued on following page

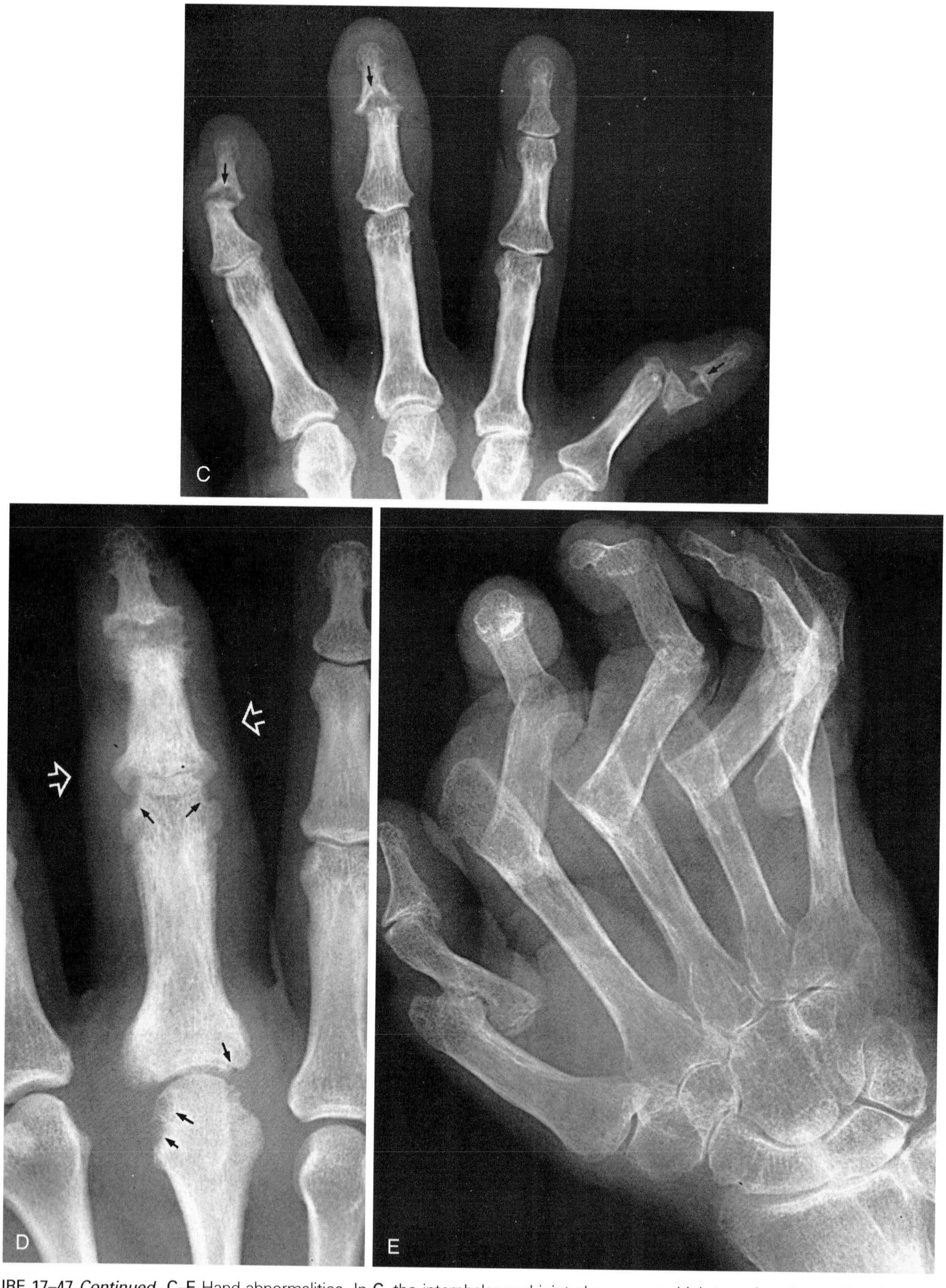

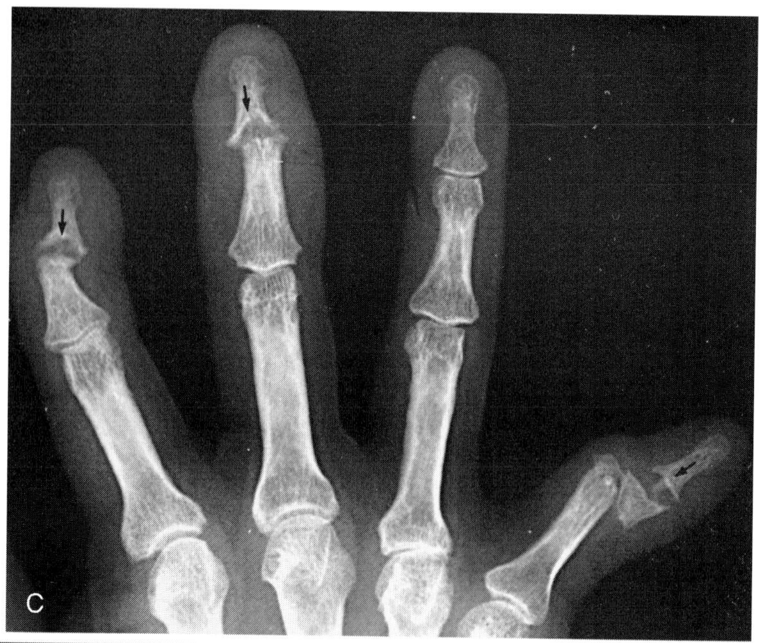

FIGURE 17–47 *Continued.* C–E Hand abnormalities. In **C,** the interphalangeal joint shows central joint erosions (arrows) and subluxation involving several distal interphalangeal joints and the fifth proximal interphalangeal joint. Prominent soft tissue swelling involving the second, third, and fifth digits is referred to as the "sausage digit" appearance. In **D,** the ray pattern is evident. Observe the prominent soft tissue swelling (sausage digit) (open arrows) and bone sclerosis rather than osteopenia. Marginal erosions (arrows) involving all the joints of the third digit with no evidence of involvement in the joints of the adjacent digits is referred to as the ray pattern and is typical of psoriasis and Reiter's syndrome. In **E,** a pattern of severely deforming resorptive arthropathy is evident in the hand of this 52-year-old woman with severe psoriasis. This pattern of deformity has been termed the *main en lorgnette* or opera glass appearance and involves a telescoping of the dislocated metacarpophalangeal joints and flexion contractures of the fingers. Diffuse osteopenia and tuft resorption also are present. Although this type of deformity may also occur in rheumatoid arthritis, absence of wrist involvement with such severe hand disease would be most unusual for rheumatoid arthritis. *(D, Courtesy of C. Pineda, M.D., Mexico City, Mexico.)*

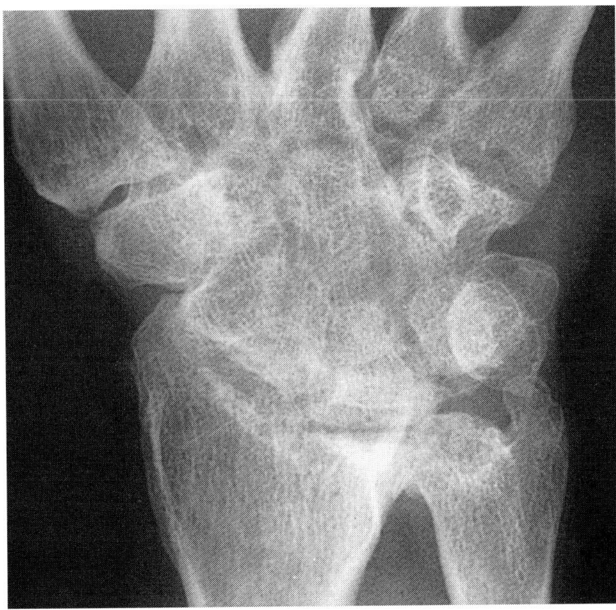

FIGURE 17–48. Reiter's syndrome: Wrist abnormalities.[87–89] In this 42-year-old man with a long history of Reiter's syndrome, pancarpal joint space narrowing, erosions, and ankylosis are seen. Observe also the undulating and indistinct cortical margins of the carpal bones. *(Courtesy of J. Schils, M.D., Cleveland, Ohio.)*

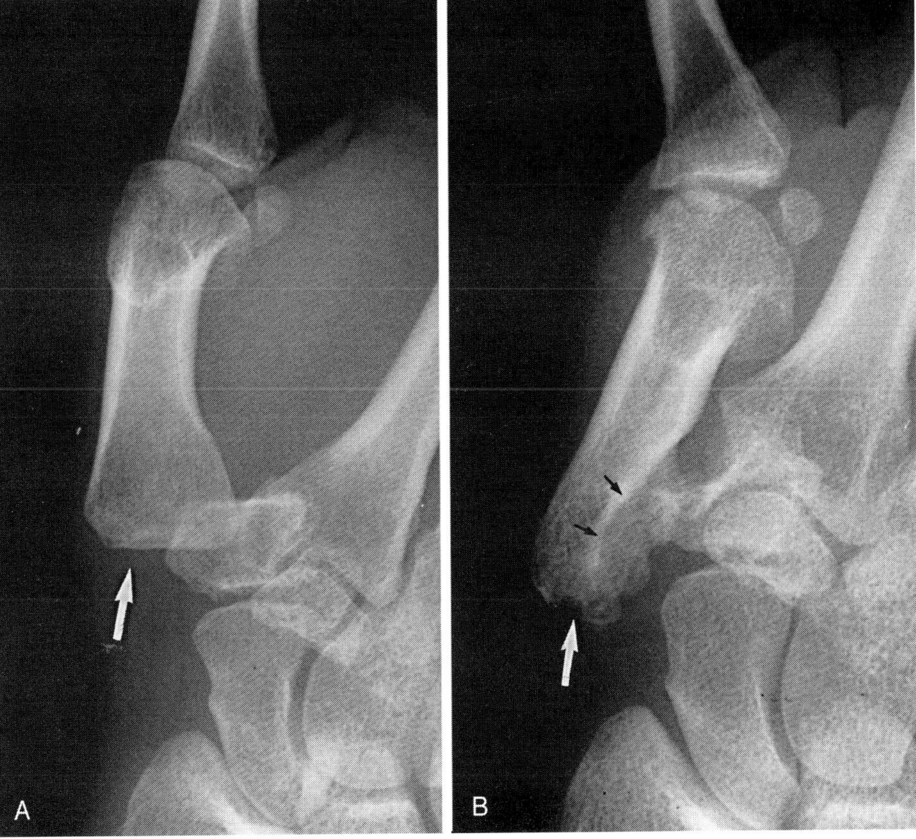

FIGURE 17–49. Systemic lupus erythematosus.[90] A, B First carpometacarpal joint abnormalities. In A, persistent ligament laxity has resulted in subluxation of the first trapeziometacarpal articulation (arrow). In B, a radiograph taken 5 years later reveals complete dislocation (white arrow) and mechanical erosion of the proximal portion of the first metacarpal bone (black arrows). The trapezium appears to have been dissolved and resorbed.

Illustration continued on following page

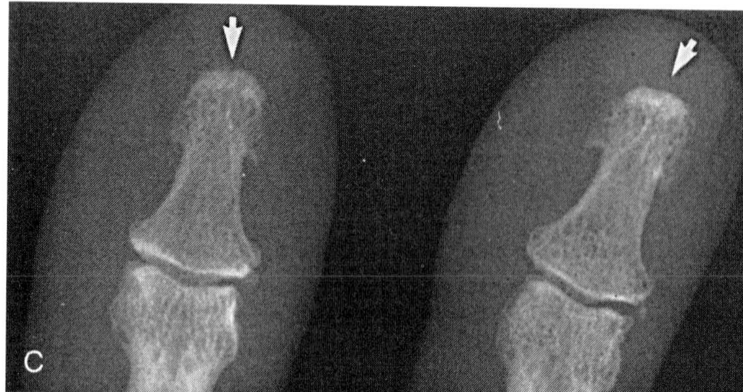

FIGURE 17–49 *Continued.* C Phalangeal sclerosis. In another patient, observe the sclerosis of the tips of the phalangeal tufts (arrows). D, E Reversible subluxations. In another patient with long-standing lupus erythematosus, marked ulnar deviation at the metacarpophalangeal joints and boutonnière deformity of the thumb are evident on the initial radiograph (D), and the reversible nature of the subluxations can be appreciated when the hand is pressed against the cassette (E). *(D, E Courtesy of C. Pineda, M.D., Mexico City, Mexico.)*

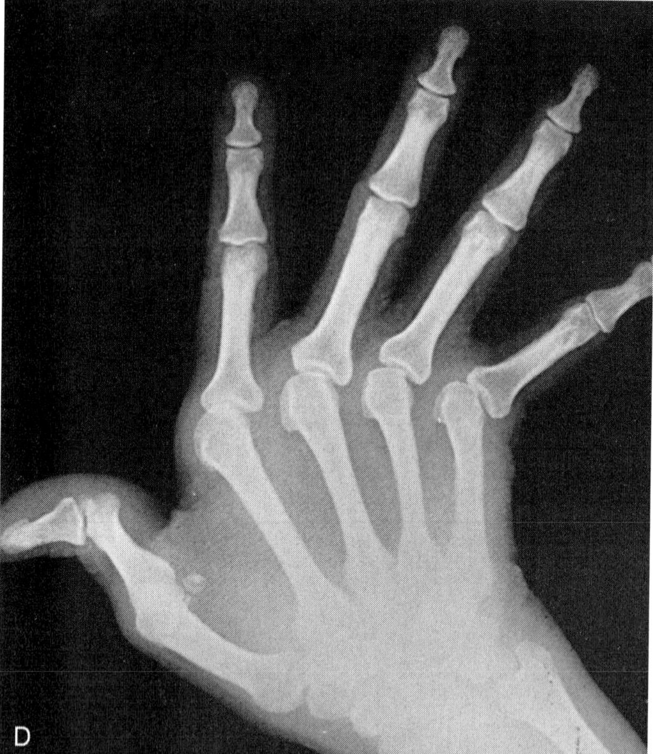

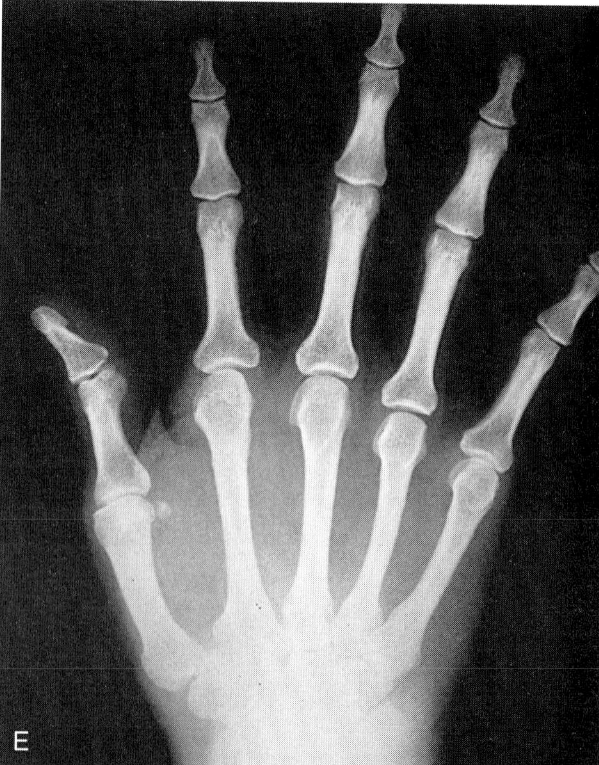

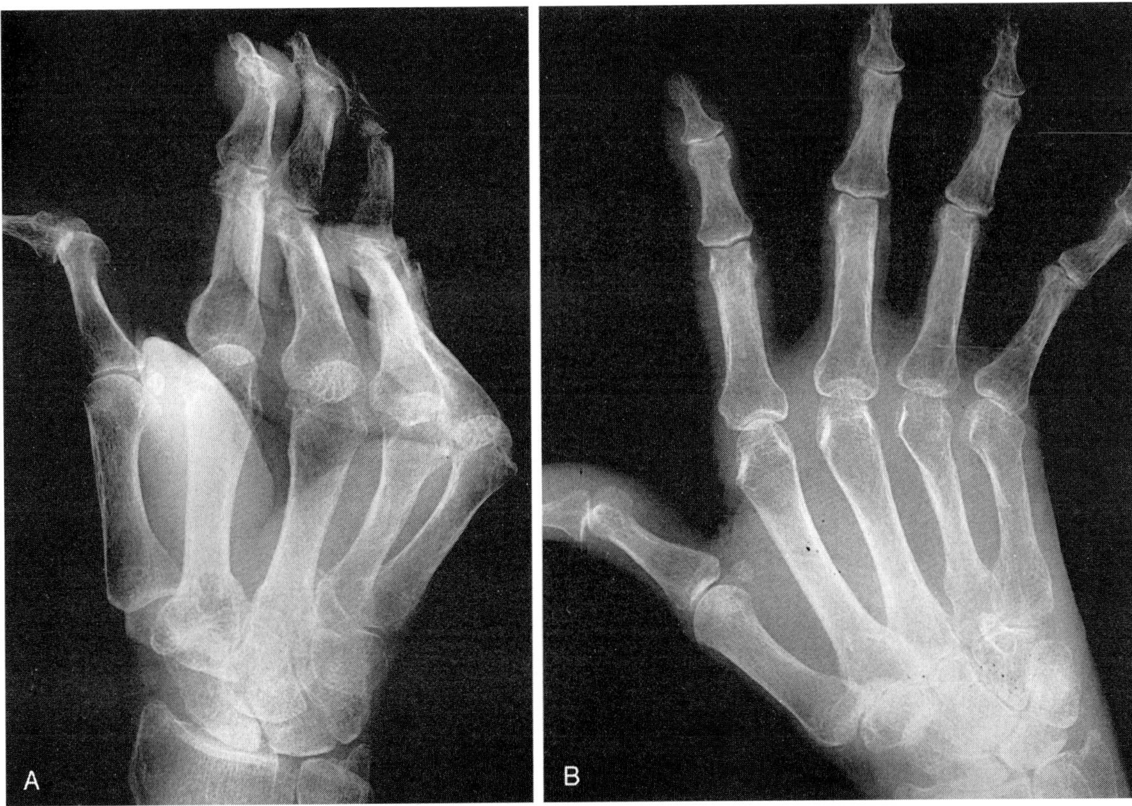

FIGURE 17–50. Jaccoud's arthropathy: nonerosive deforming arthropathy with reversible subluxations.[91] This 64-year-old woman had injured her hand. Marked swan-neck deformities of the hands were seen clinically. The patient could not remember ever having been diagnosed as having rheumatic fever or systemic lupus erythematosus. **A** Initial oblique radiograph shows osteoporosis and multiple swan-neck deformities with an absence of destructive or erosive lesions. **B** Another radiograph obtained the next day, with the hand pressed on the cassette, shows a reversal of most of the deformities. Ulnar deviation of the metacarpophalangeal joints, especially the fifth, persists. *(Courtesy of G. Greenway, M.D., Dallas, Texas.)*

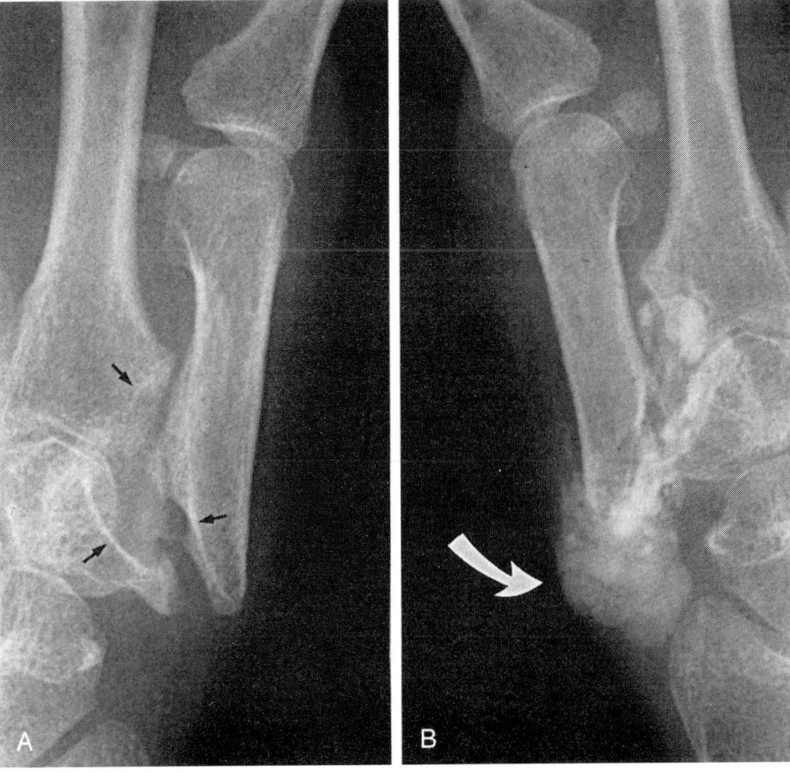

FIGURE 17–51. Scleroderma (progressive systemic sclerosis).[93] **A, B** Carpometacarpal abnormalities. This 53-year-old woman has had long-standing scleroderma. Radiographs of both wrists show characteristic changes at the first carpometacarpal joint. On the left **(A)**, scalloped erosions of the trapezium and the base of the metacarpal bones (arrows) are associated with dorsal and radial subluxation of the metacarpal base. Similar changes on the right **(B)** are accompanied by extensive intra-articular and periarticular globular calcification (curved arrow). *(***A, B,** *From Resnick D, Scavulli JF, Goergen TG, et al: Intra-articular calcification in scleroderma. Radiology 124:685, 1977.)*
Illustration continued on following page

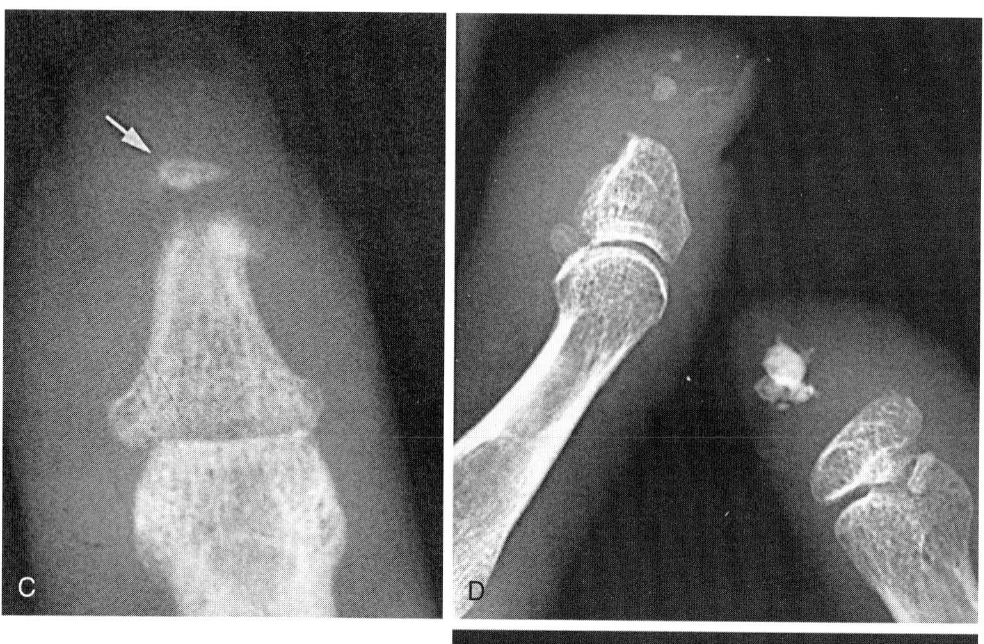

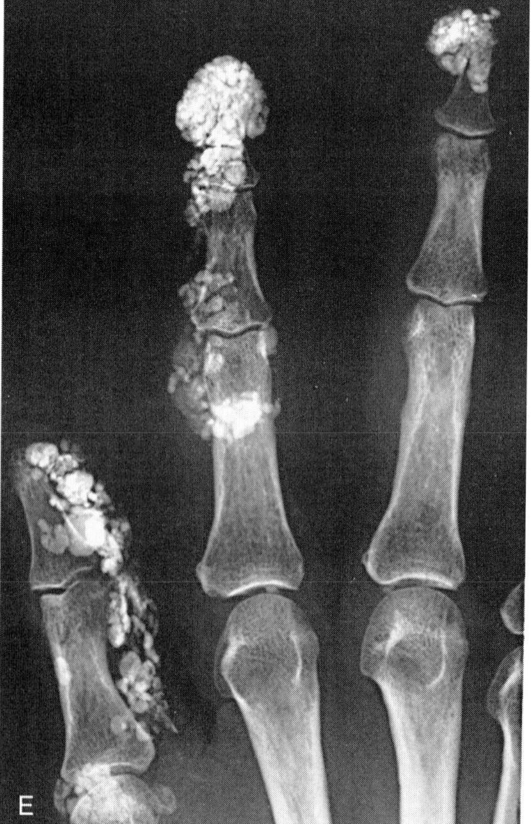

FIGURE 17–51 *Continued.* C–E Hand abnormalities. In **C,** band-like resorption of the terminal phalanx is seen (arrow). In **D,** acro-osteolysis of the terminal tufts of both thumbs is present in this patient with longstanding scleroderma. In **E,** extensive subcutaneous calcification is present in another patient with scleroderma. *(**D,** Courtesy of V. Vint, M.D., San Diego, California; **E,** courtesy of M. Alson, M.D., Stanford, California.)*

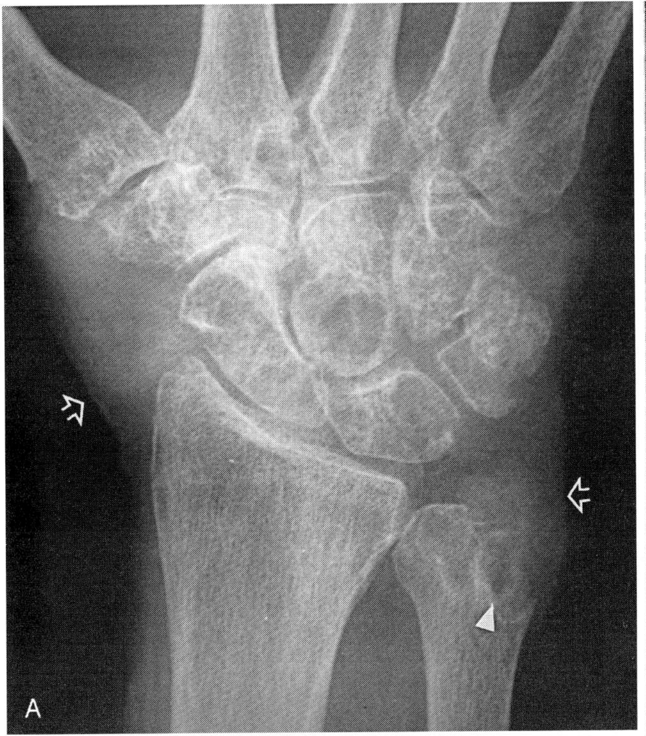

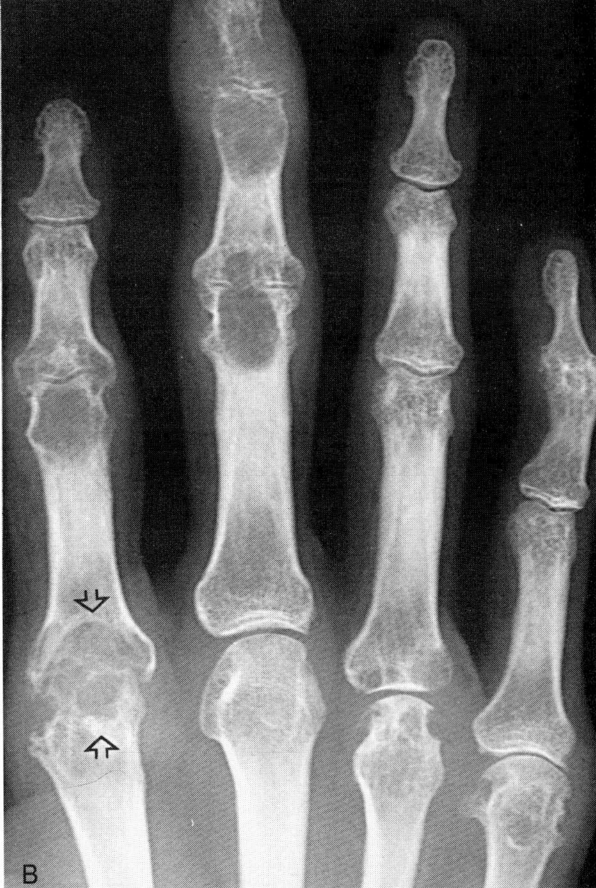

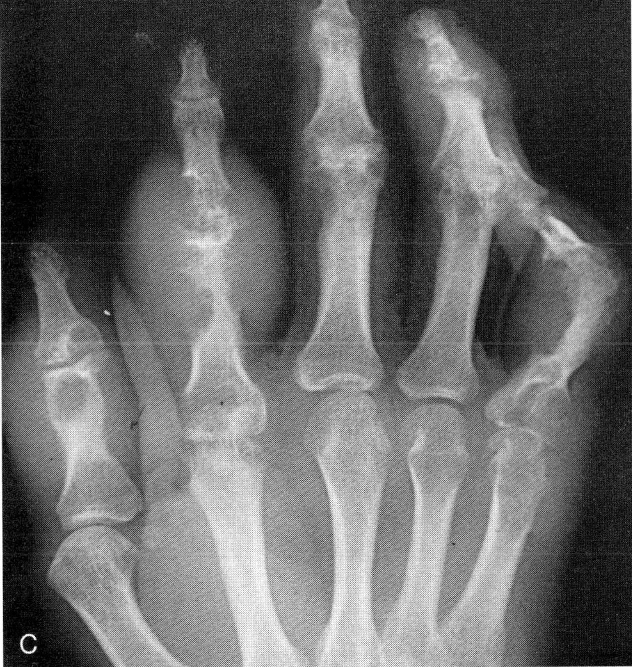

FIGURE 17–52. Gouty arthropathy.[94–96] **A** Wrist abnormalities. Extensive periarticular soft tissue swelling (open arrows) and cystic erosions of the carpal bones are seen in this 84-year-old man with long-standing gout. Observe the extensive erosion of the ulnar styloid process (arrowhead). *(A, Courtesy of T. Georgen, M.D., San Diego, California.)* **B, C** Hand abnormalities. In **B**, multiple periarticular marginal erosions and cystic changes can be seen involving several joints. Severe intra-articular erosions and joint destruction are evident at the second metacarpophalangeal joint (open arrows). Soft tissue swelling also is prominent, and the overall bone density is well preserved. In **C**, severe changes can be noted in another patient with chronic gout. Observe the extensive soft tissue swelling as well as marginal and nonmarginal erosions, some with overhanging margins.

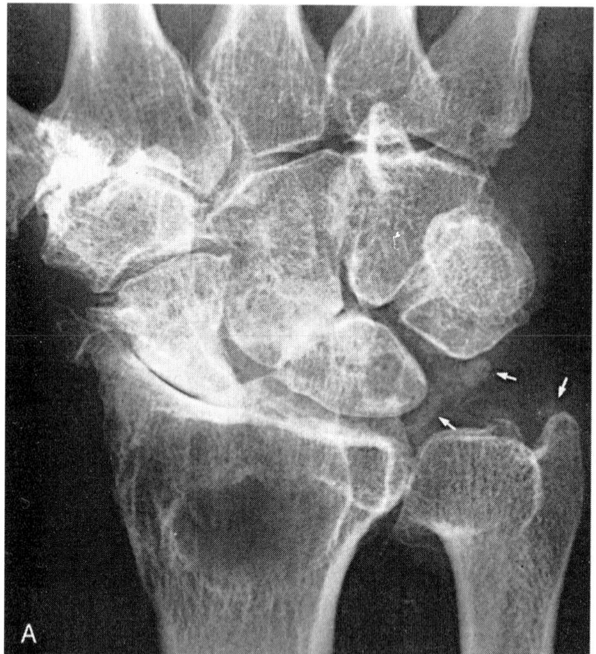

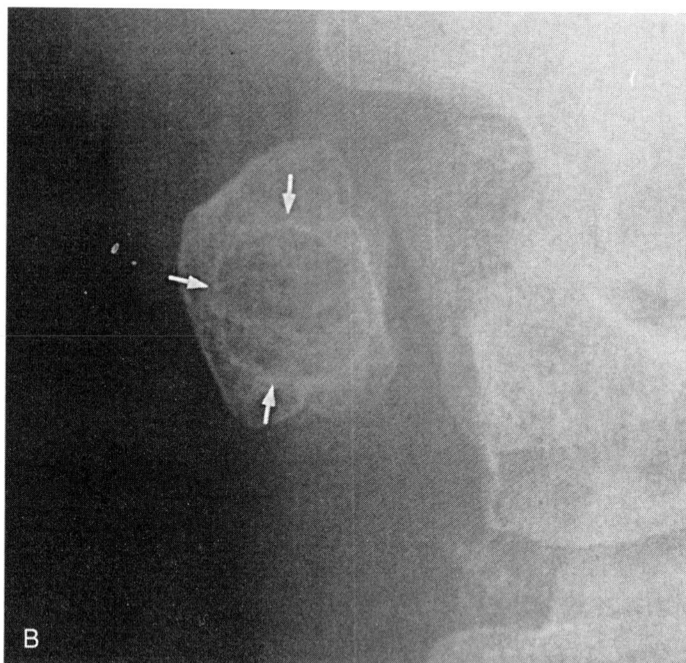

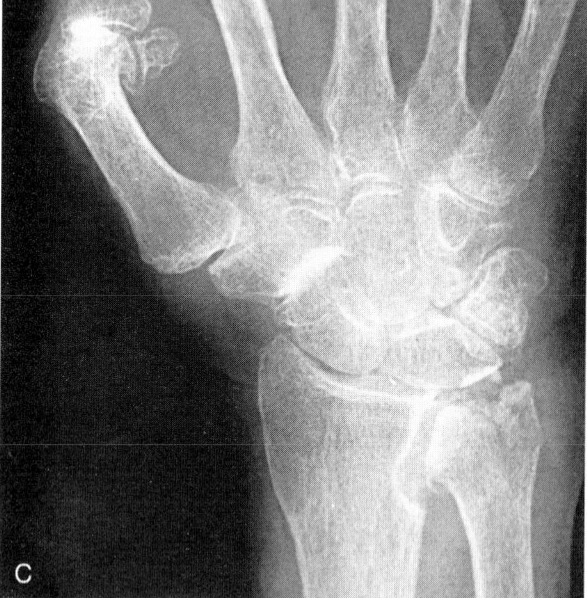

FIGURE 17–53. Calcium pyrophosphate dihydrate (CPPD) crystal deposition disease.[97–99] A Diffuse chondrocalcinosis (arrows), huge subchondral cysts, joint space narrowing, and scapholunate dissociation are evident in the wrist of this 67-year-old woman with CPPD crystal deposition disease. This pattern of carpal destruction and instability is termed scapholunate advanced collapse (SLAC) wrist. B In another patient, a prominent subchondral cyst is seen in the pisiform bone (arrows). C Pyrophosphate arthropathy affecting the first metacarpophalangeal and trapezioscaphoid joints in this 64-year-old woman is characterized by marked subchondral sclerosis, joint space narrowing, and osteophyte formation. Observe also the radiocarpal joint space narrowing and erosion of the radius at the distal radioulnar joint. Pyrophosphate arthropathy is found in more than 70 per cent of wrists in patients with CPPD crystal deposition disease.

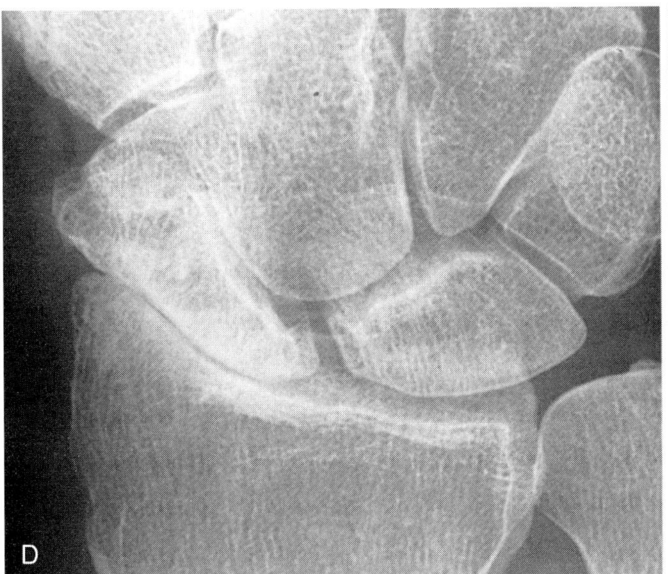

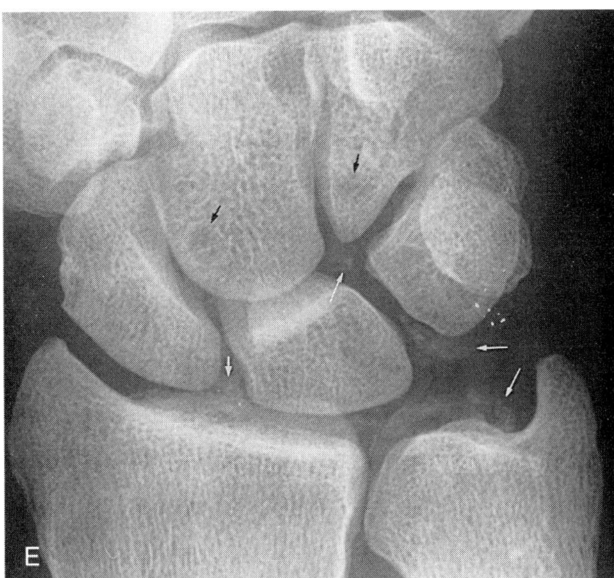

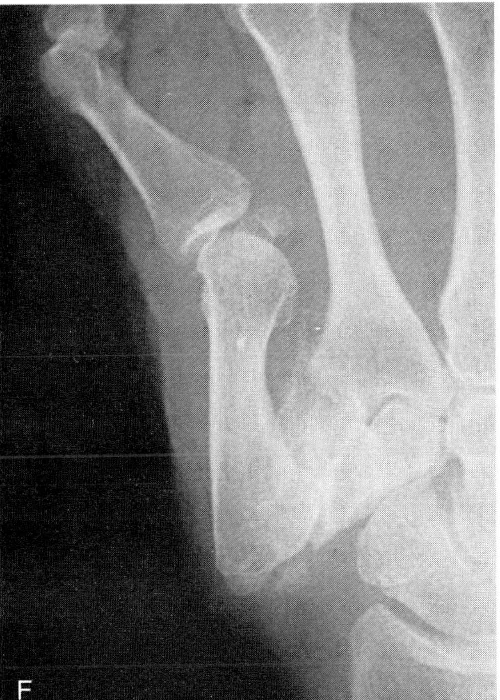

FIGURE 17–53 *Continued.* D Pyrophosphate arthropathy is manifested in this patient as narrowing of the radioscaphoid articulation, a common site of involvement in patients with CPPD crystal deposition disease. Dense sclerosis of the scaphoid bone is also characteristic of pyrophosphate arthropathy. E Chondrocalcinosis, seen as curvilinear articular cartilage calcification (white arrows), is found in more than 60 per cent of wrists of patients with CPPD crystal deposition disease. Note also the subchondral cysts (black arrows). F First carpometacarpal joint involvement. Observe the typical pyrophosphate arthropathy with nonuniform joint space narrowing, subchondral sclerosis, large osteophytes, and subluxation.

Illustration continued on following page

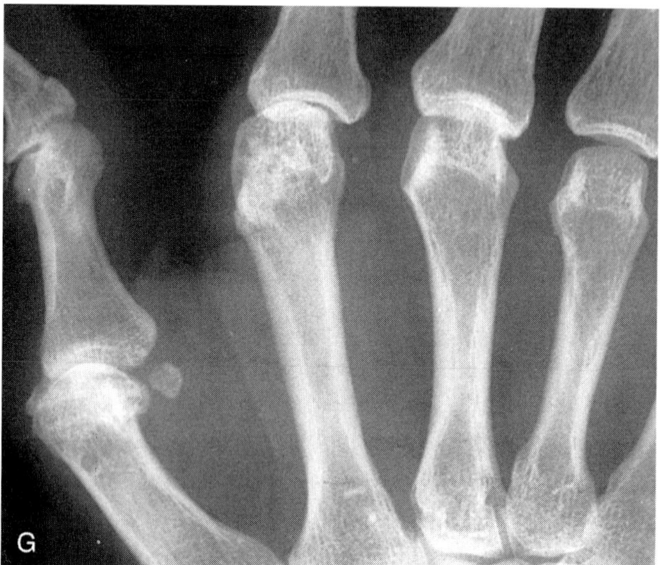

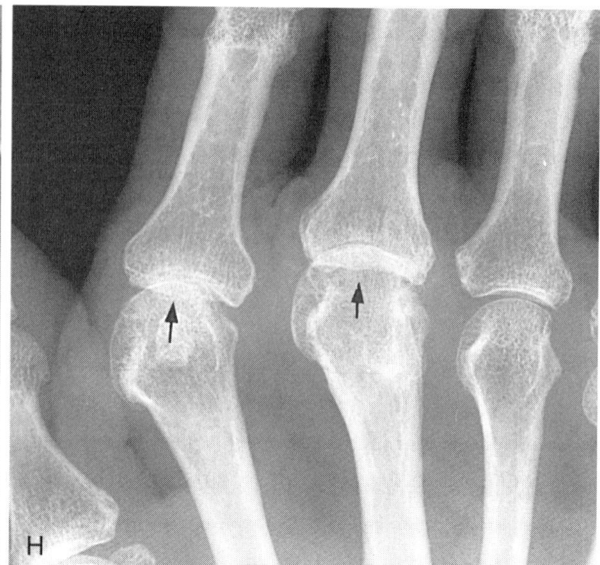

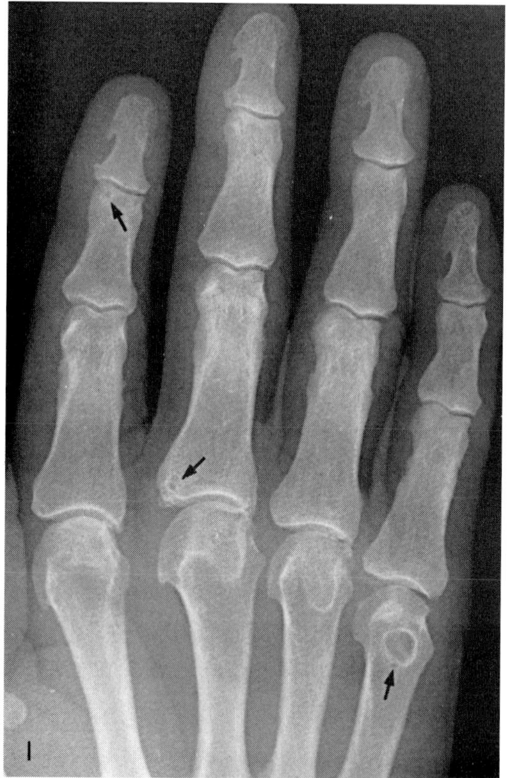

FIGURE 17–53 *Continued.* G Pyrophosphate arthropathy involving the first, second, and third metacarpophalangeal joints is seen as nonuniform loss of joint space, subchondral sclerosis, and osteophyte formation. H In another patient, an 80-year-old man, similar changes are identified in the second and third metacarpophalangeal joints (arrows). I In a 69-year-old man, cystic changes (arrows) predominate.

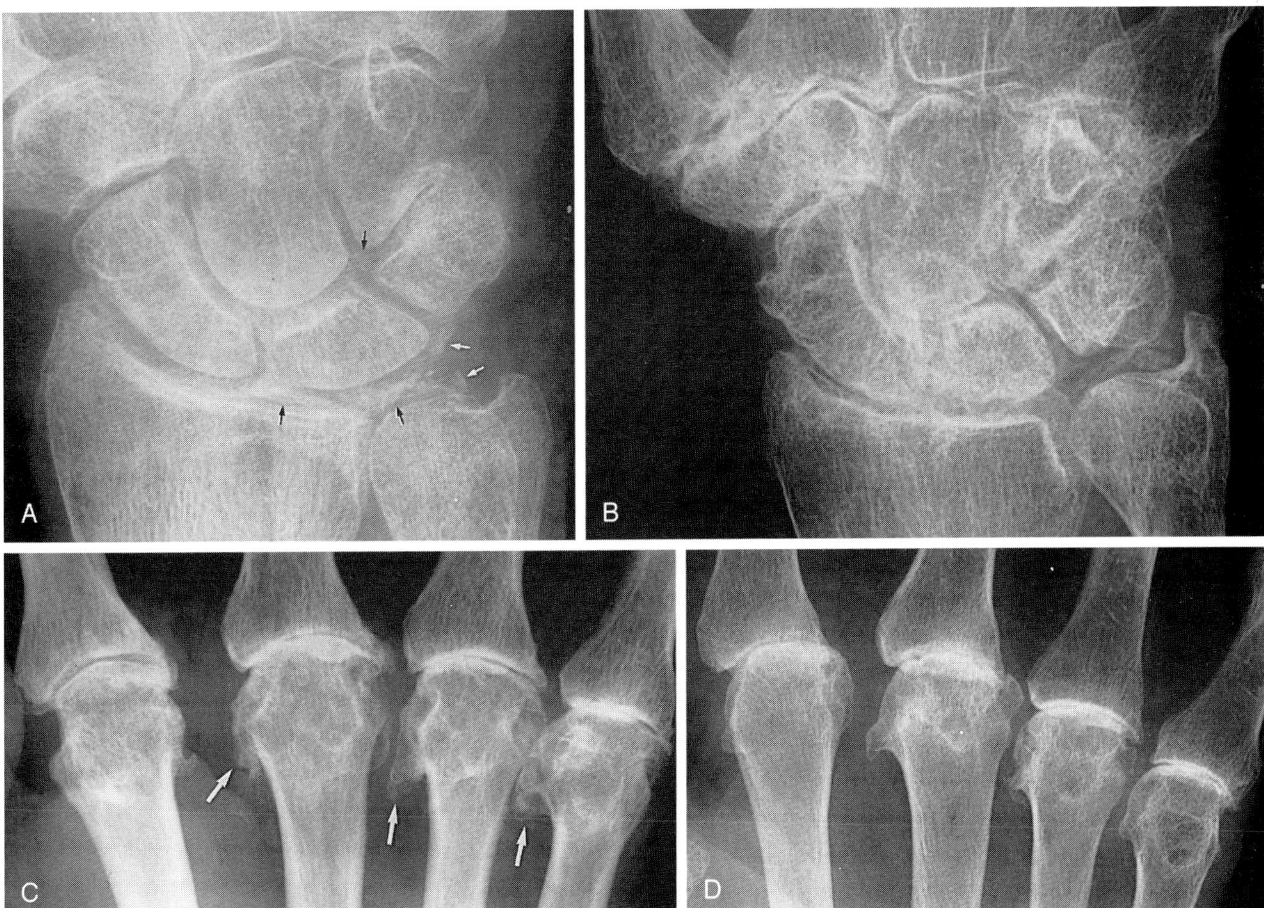

FIGURE 17–54. Hemochromatosis.[100, 101] A, B Wrist abnormalities. In A, chondrocalcinosis is manifested as linear calcification within the hyaline cartilage and fibrocartilage of the radiocarpal and midcarpal articulations and the triangular fibrocartilage complex (arrows). In B, arthropathy and chondrocalcinosis are present in another patient with long-standing hemochromatosis. Observe the prominent pancompartmental joint space narrowing, osteopenia, and chondrocalcinosis. C, D Metacarpophalangeal arthropathy. In C, nonuniform narrowing of the metacarpophalangeal joints is accompanied by subchondral sclerosis and prominent hook-shaped osteophytes (arrows). This arthropathy is characteristic of hemochromatosis. In D, another patient, similar findings are evident. *(C, Courtesy of V. Vint, M.D., San Diego, California.)*

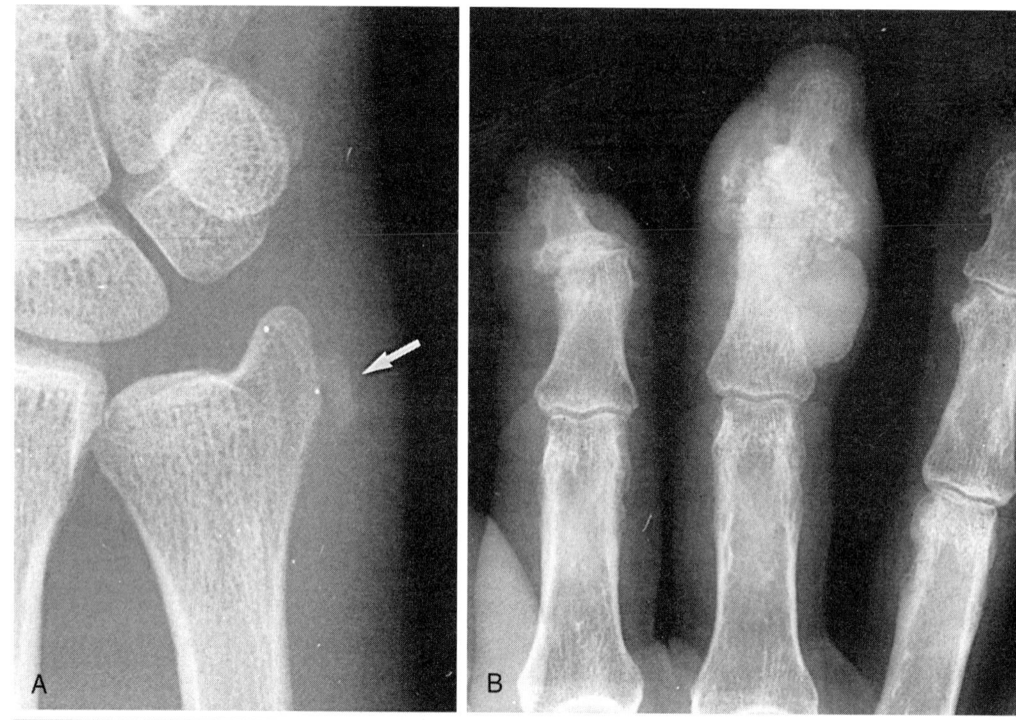

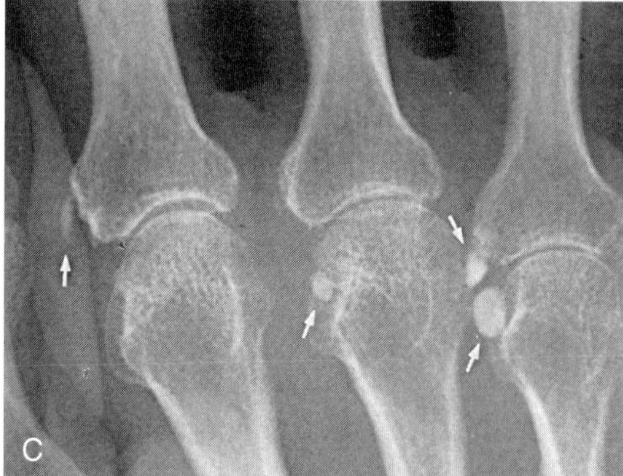

FIGURE 17–55. Calcium hydroxyapatite crystal deposition disease: calcific tendinitis.[102, 103] A Extensor carpi ulnaris tendon. Observe the globular accumulation of calcification adjacent to the ulnar aspect of the wrist (arrow) in this patient with persistent pain. B Periarticular hydroxyapatite crystal deposition. Globular periarticular accumulations of calcification are seen surrounding the terminal interphalangeal joint and distal tuft in this patient. *(B, Courtesy of V. Vint, M.D., San Diego, California.)* C In another patient, observe periarticular, globular collections of calcification (arrows). *(C, Courtesy of R. Shapiro, M.D., Sacramento, California.)*

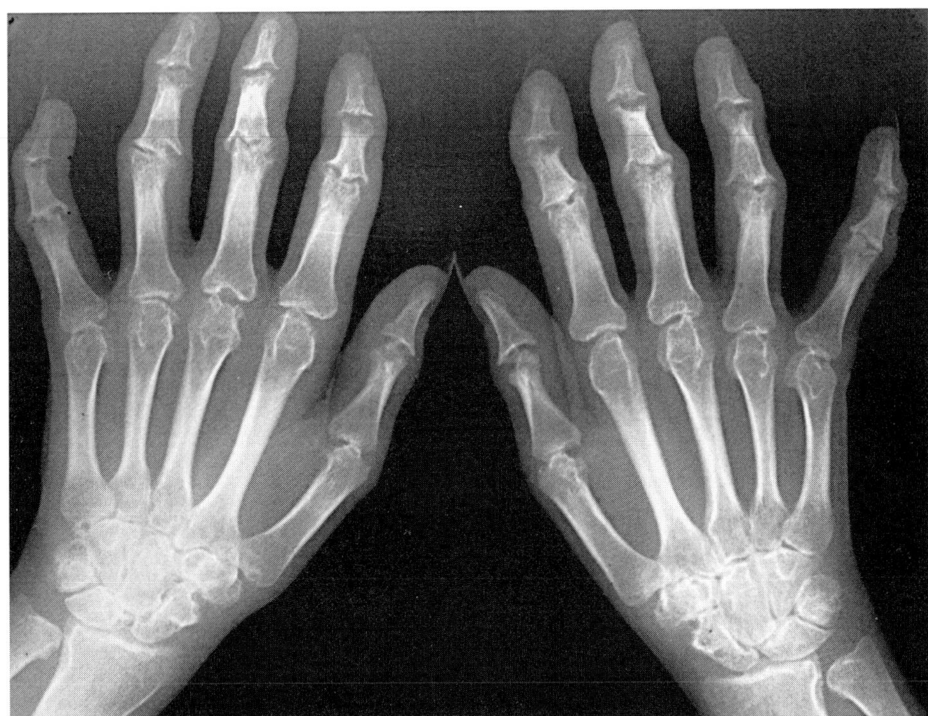

FIGURE 17–56. Multicentric reticulohistiocytosis.[104] Bilateral symmetric polyarticular joint disease is seen in this patient. Central articular erosions are present at all the interphalangeal joints as well as at many of the metacarpophalangeal joints. Similar erosions are seen in the carpal bones and the distal radioulnar joints. Periarticular osteopenia and minimal joint subluxations also are evident. *(Courtesy of A. Brower, M.D., Norfolk, Virginia.)*

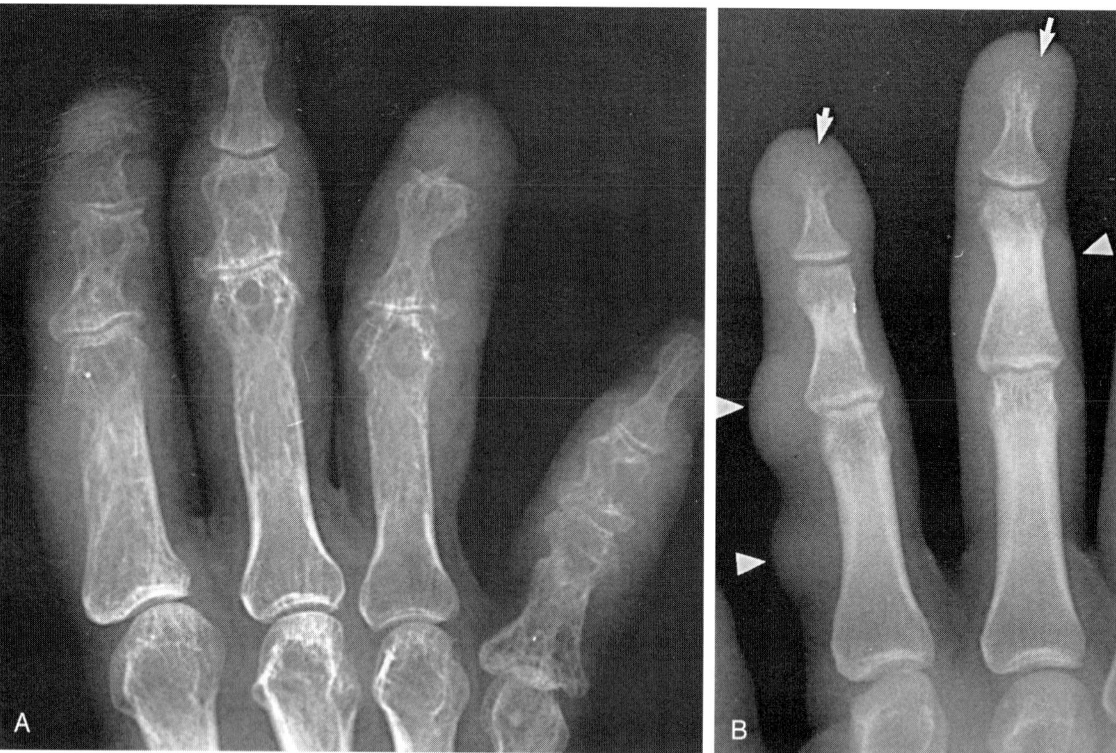

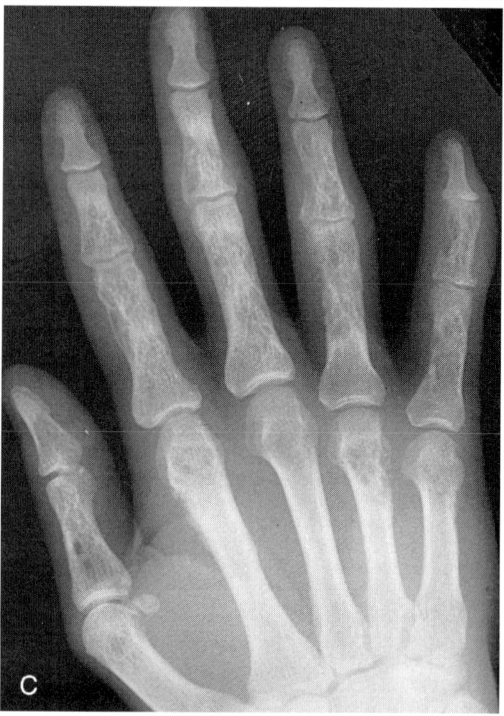

FIGURE 17–57. Sarcoidosis.[105–107] A An abnormal, coarsened, reticulated, or lace-like trabecular pattern is evident in the phalanges. Acro-osteolysis of the distal phalanges and subcutaneous nodules also are seen. *(A, Courtesy of M.N. Pathria, M.D., San Diego, California.)* B In another patient, observe the acro-osteolysis of the terminal tufts (arrows) and subcutaneous nodules (arrowheads). C In a third patient, lace-like trabeculae are present throughout the phalanges and metacarpal bones, frequent sites of involvement. *(C, Courtesy of B.N. Weissman, M.D., Boston, Massachusetts.)*

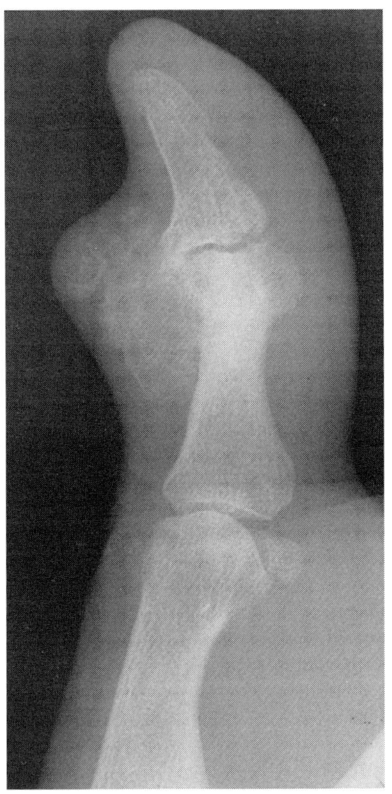

FIGURE 17–58. Extra-articular synovial osteochondromatosis.[108, 109] Observe the large collection of ossified osteocartilaginous bodies adjacent to the interphalangeal joint of the thumb, creating a bizarre soft tissue deformity. This metaplastic disorder of the synovium usually produces intra-articular bodies.

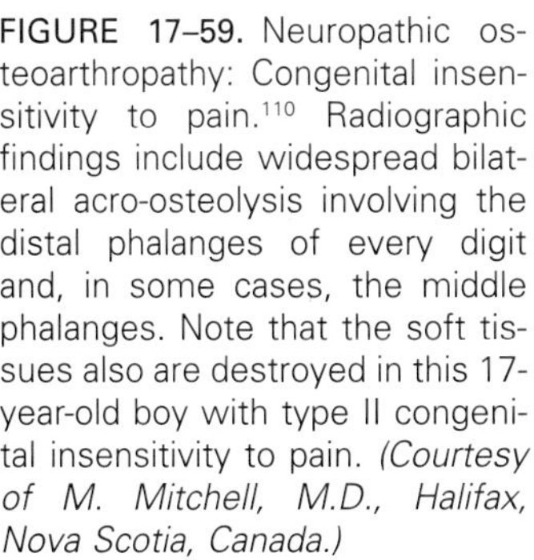

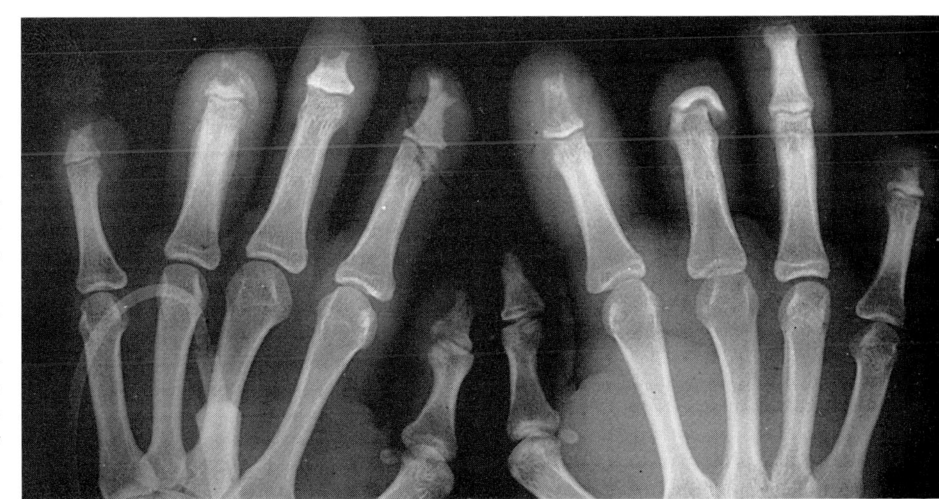

FIGURE 17–59. Neuropathic osteoarthropathy: Congenital insensitivity to pain.[110] Radiographic findings include widespread bilateral acro-osteolysis involving the distal phalanges of every digit and, in some cases, the middle phalanges. Note that the soft tissues also are destroyed in this 17-year-old boy with type II congenital insensitivity to pain. *(Courtesy of M. Mitchell, M.D., Halifax, Nova Scotia, Canada.)*

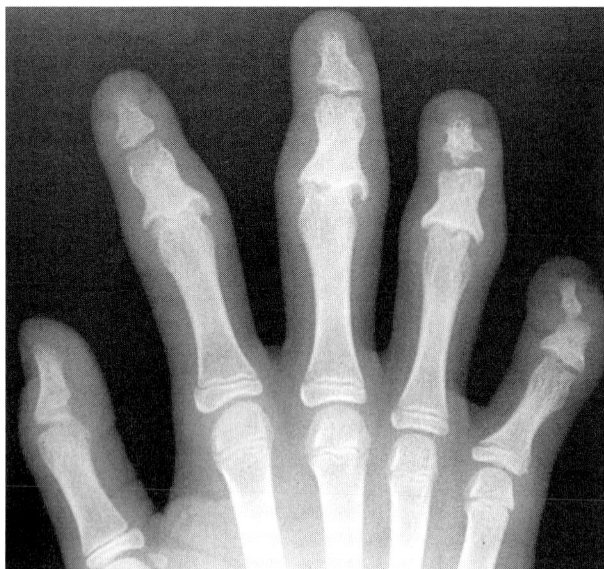

FIGURE 17–60. Frostbite.[111, 112] Osseous and cartilaginous destruction of the interphalangeal joints is evident. Subchondral erosion, collapse, and joint space narrowing simulate the findings of inflammatory (erosive) osteoarthritis. Soft tissue swelling is prominent, and deformity secondary to epiphyseal injury also is present. The thumb is spared because typically it is clenched in the fist and clasped within the palm during exposure to the cold. *(Courtesy of R. Stiles, M.D., Atlanta, Georgia.)*

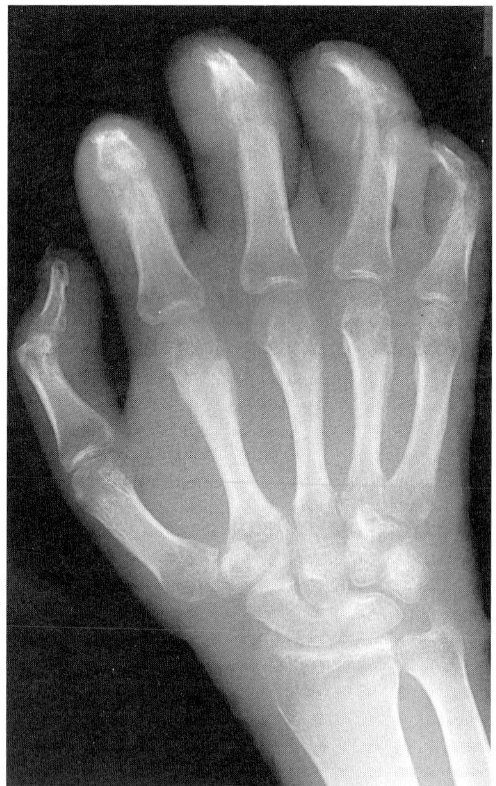

FIGURE 17–61. Thermal injury: Burns.[113] In a patient who recently burned his hand, early changes are present, including diffuse soft tissue swelling, severe periarticular osteoporosis, and osseous fusion of the interphalangeal joints. Osteolysis of the terminal phalanges and phalangeal periostitis also are seen.

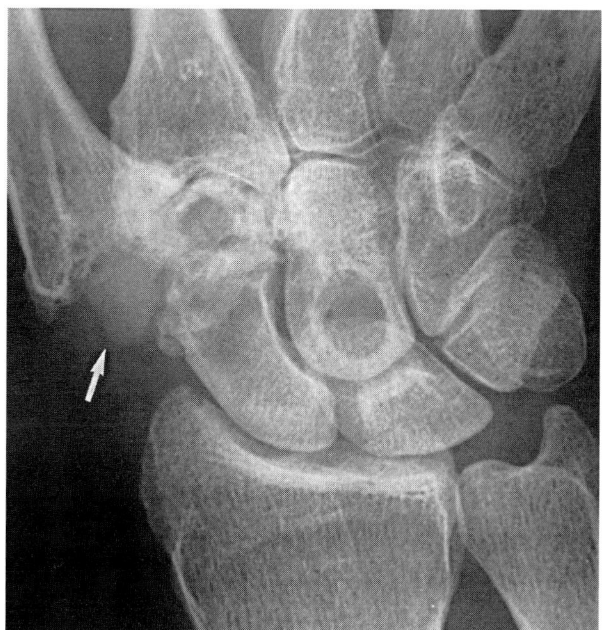

FIGURE 17–62. Silicone synovitis.[114, 115] This patient with severe erosive osteoarthritis had a silicone prosthetic implant to replace the trapezium (arrow). Observe the well-defined radiolucent defects and erosions in the adjacent carpal bones.

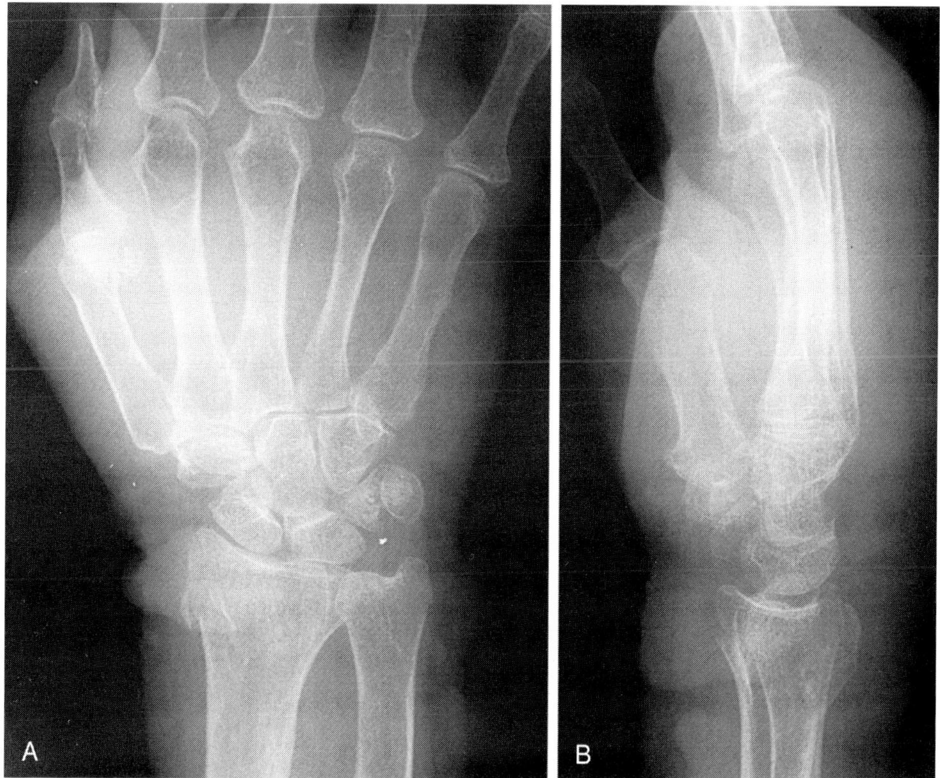

FIGURE 17–63. A, B Fracture blisters.[116] This 79-year-old woman sustained a Colles' fracture of the distal end of the radius and subsequently developed several irregular nodules about the wrist characteristic of fracture blisters. These blisters represent a rare complication of fractures.

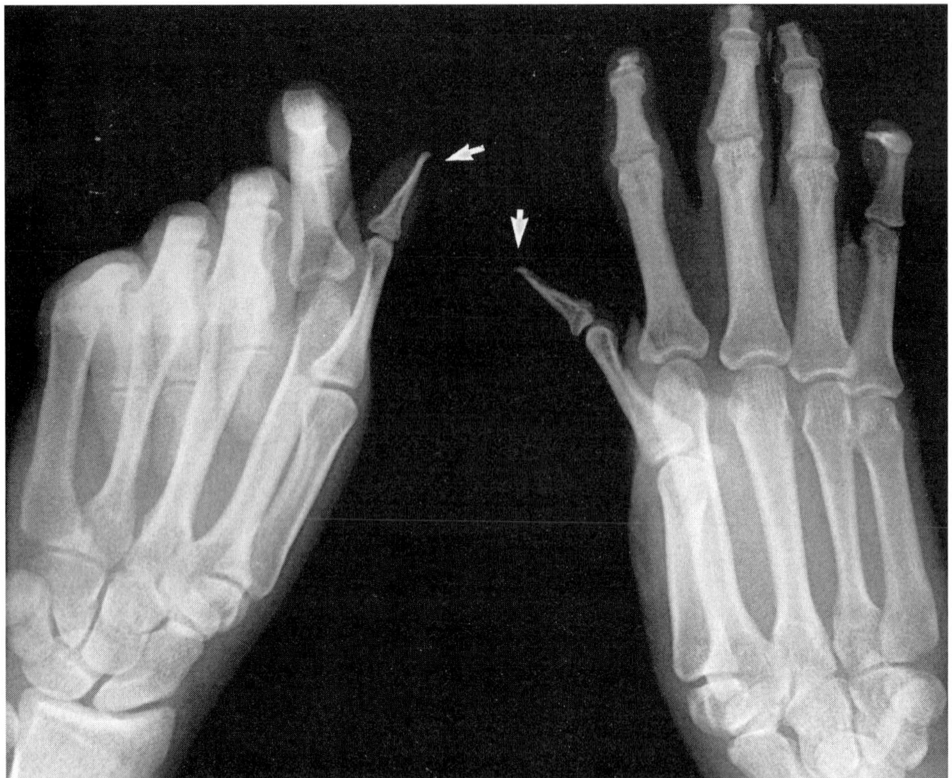

FIGURE 17–64. Epidermolysis bullosum.[117] Frontal view of both hands shows marked constriction around the metacarpal region with multiple flexion contractures. Close examination of the tufts reveals skin resorption, nonvisualization of the nails, and terminal phalangeal resorption, which is seen especially well on the thumbs (arrows). This radiographic appearance is virtually pathognomonic of epidermolysis bullosum.

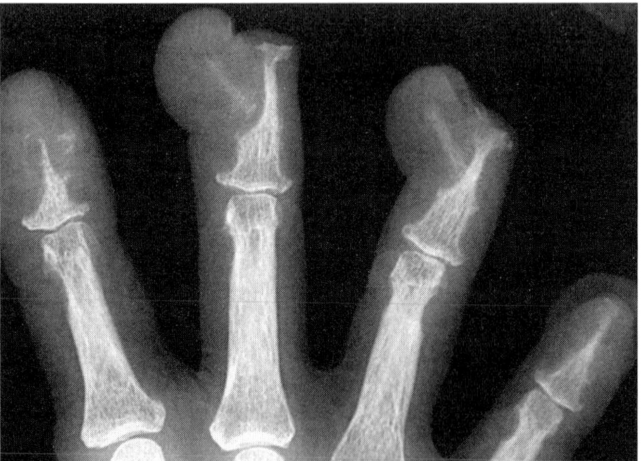

FIGURE 17–65. Osteolysis with detritic synovitis.[118] This 67-year-old woman developed pain and swelling of the interphalangeal joints of both hands. Radiographic findings were bilateral and symmetric and included severe resorption and osteolysis of the terminal tufts and, to a lesser extent, the middle and proximal phalanges of all fingers. Marked joint deformity is associated with osseous debris adjacent to the destructive lesions. Analysis of biopsy material revealed nonspecific inflammation. *(From Resnick D, Weisman M, Goergen TG, et al: Osteolysis with detritic synovitis. A new syndrome. Arch Intern Med 138:1003, 1978. Copyright 1978, American Medical Association.)*

TABLE 17–10. Malignant Tumors Affecting the Bones of the Wrist and Hand

Entity	Figure(s)	Characteristics
Malignant Neoplasms		
Secondary malignant tumors		
Skeletal metastasis[119, 120]	17–66	Fewer than 1 per cent of metastatic lesions affect the bones of the wrist and hand; predilection for the distal phalanges Acral metastases occur most frequently in patients with carcinoma of the lung and bronchus Irregular osteolysis and cortical destruction
Primary malignant tumors		
Osteosarcoma (conventional)[121]	17–67	Fewer than 1 per cent of osteosarcomas involve the bones of wrist and hand Osteolytic or osteosclerotic lesions or more frequently a mixed pattern Metaphyseal location preferred
Osteosarcoma (parosteal)[122]	17–68	Infrequently involves the bones of the wrist and hand Arises from surface of metaphyseal region Aggressive cortical destruction, periostitis, and soft tissue mass
Osteoblastoma (aggressive)[123]		Two per cent of aggressive osteoblastomas affect the bones of the wrist and hand Expansile osteolytic lesion that may be partially ossified or contain calcium
Fibrosarcoma[124]		Fewer than 1 per cent of fibrosarcomas affect the bones of the wrist and hand Purely osteolytic destruction with no associated sclerotic reaction or periostitis
Ewing's sarcoma[125]	17–69	One per cent of Ewing's sarcomas affect the bones of wrist and hand Central diaphyseal lesions of the tubular bones predominate Aggressive permeative or motheaten pattern of bone destruction with laminated or spiculated periostitis and soft tissue mass
Synovial sarcoma[126]	17–70	Uncommon malignant neoplasm frequently found in the soft tissues in extra-articular locations More common in lower extremity than in upper extremity Poor prognosis: frequent recurrence and metastases, especially to the lung Large soft tissue mass and aggressive osteolytic destruction of adjacent bone Approximately 20 to 30 per cent of synovial sarcomas contain calcification
Myeloproliferative disorders of bone		
Plasma cell (multiple) myeloma[127]	17–71	Only 1 per cent of multiple myeloma lesions occur in the bones of the wrist and hand Diffuse osteopenia or discrete osteolytic lesions

See also Table 1–10.

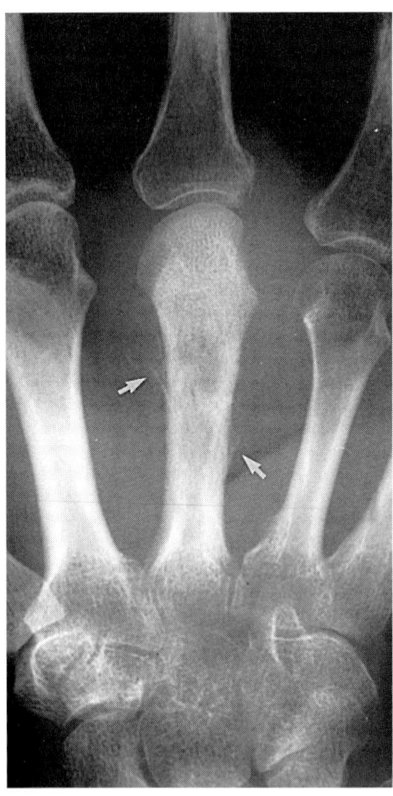

FIGURE 17–66. Skeletal metastasis: malignant melanoma.[119, 120] This 23-year-old man had pain and swelling over the distal end of the ulna. He reported having a "skin cyst" removed several years previously. An initial lesion was found in the ulna. The patient underwent surgery, which revealed a lesion containing melanin. The histologic evaluation revealed malignant melanoma. The patient developed widespread skeletal metastasis within months. This radiograph from a subsequent skeletal survey revealed a destructive mixed lytic-sclerotic lesion of the metacarpal bone and the proximal phalanx of the third finger, with periostitis and soft tissue swelling (arrows). Periosteal reaction and involvement of bone beyond the elbow or knee are seen more commonly in patients with primary malignant tumors and are infrequent findings in those with skeletal metastasis.

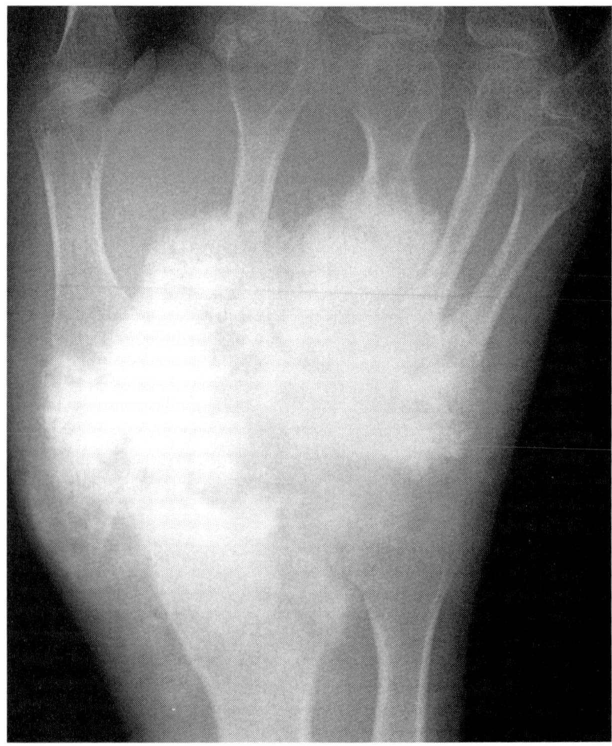

FIGURE 17–67. Conventional osteosarcoma.[121] Observe the widespread osteoblastic proliferation and destruction of the carpal bones with prominent soft tissue extension of osteosarcoma in this 19-year-old man. Osteosarcoma infrequently affects the carpal bones. *(Courtesy of L. White, M.D., Toronto, Ontario, Canada.)*

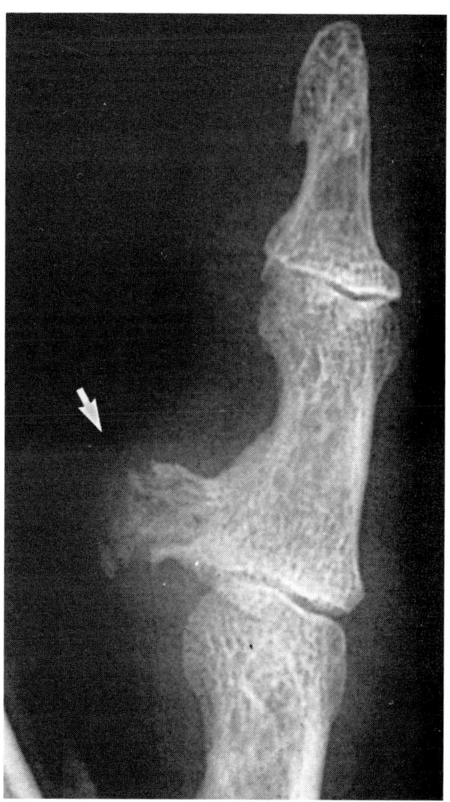

FIGURE 17–68. Parosteal osteosarcoma.[122] Routine radiograph of this 58-year-old man reveals a spiculated lesion growing horizontally from the cortex of the proximal portion of the middle phalanx (arrow). Parosteal osteosarcomas generally affect patients between 20 and 40 years of age. *(Courtesy of J. Slivka, M.D., San Diego, California.)*

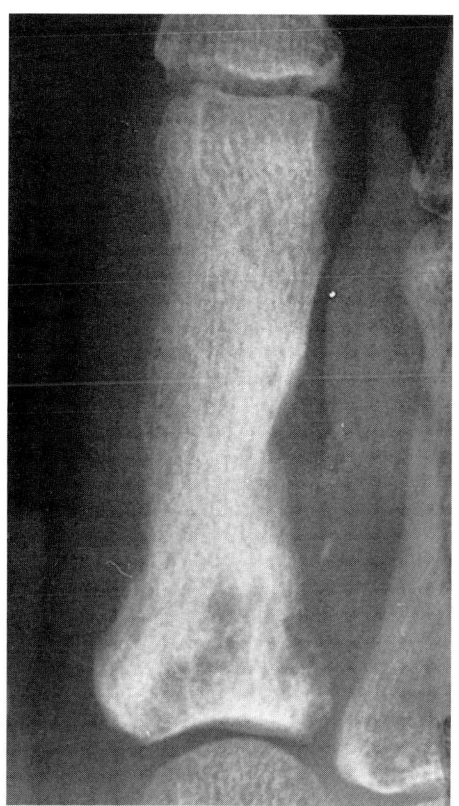

FIGURE 17–69. Ewing's sarcoma.[125] Radiographic abnormalities in the third proximal phalanx include considerable sclerosis, permeative cortical destruction, and minimal periostitis. A previous biopsy is responsible for the large cortical defect and radiodensity within the soft tissues. *(Courtesy of J. Rausch, M.D., Fort Wayne, Indiana.)*

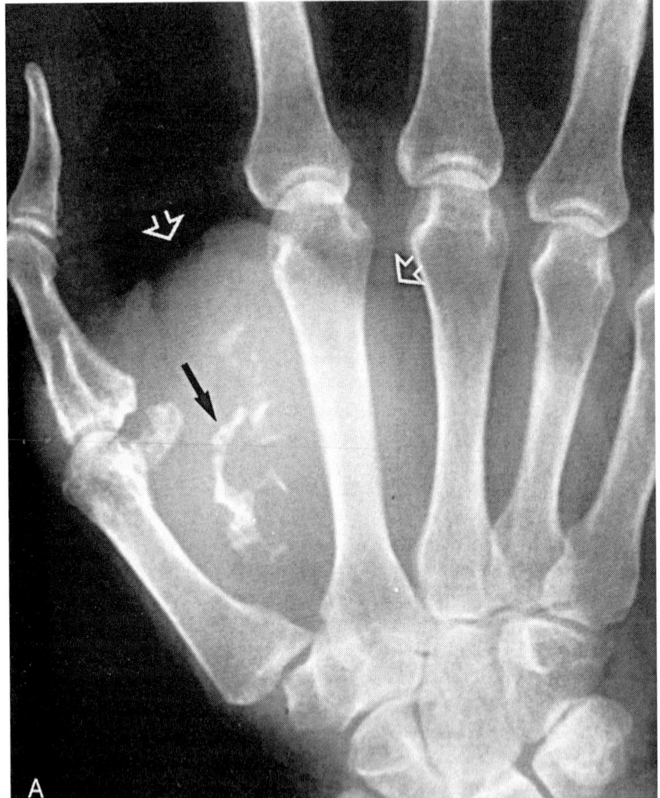

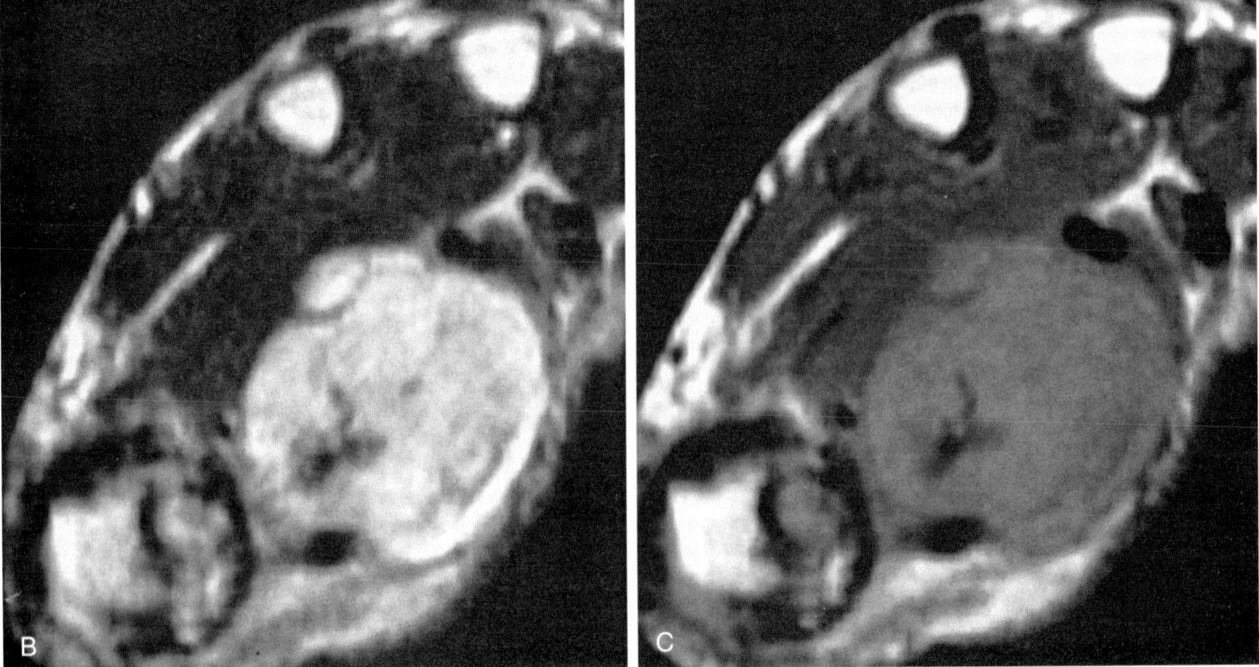

FIGURE 17–70. Synovial sarcoma.[126] A 75-year-old woman had an enlarging painful mass of the thenar eminence. **A** Frontal view of the hand shows a radiodense soft tissue mass (open arrows) with a central, irregular zone of soft tissue calcification (arrow). **B, C** A large soft tissue mass is of high signal intensity on the transaxial T2-weighted **(B)** (TR/TE, 1800/70) magnetic resonance (MR) image and of intermediate signal intensity on the proton density–weighted **(C)** (TR/TE, 1800/20) image. The magnetic resonance (MR) images help to delineate the nature and extent of this aggressive neoplasm.

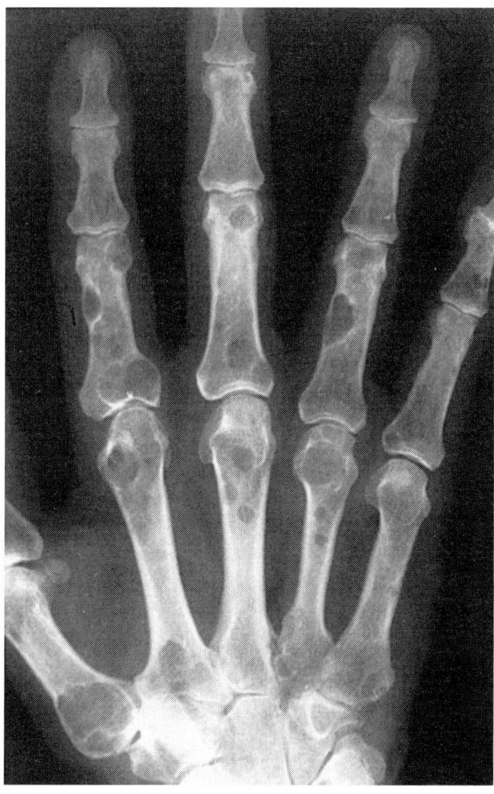

FIGURE 17–71. Plasma cell myeloma.[127] Well-circumscribed osteolytic lesions are disseminated throughout the bones of the hand. Some of the radiolucent foci possess sclerotic margins.

TABLE 17–11. Benign Tumors and Tumor-Like Lesions Affecting the Bones of the Wrist and Hand

Entity	Figure(s)	Characteristics
Primary benign tumors of bone		
Enostosis[128]	17–18D	Nine per cent of enostoses affect the bones of the wrist and hand Circular or ovoid osteosclerotic focus
Osteoid osteoma[129–132]	17–72	Nine per cent of osteoid osteomas occur in the bones of the wrist and hand Extremely painful lesion classically relieved by salicylates Central radiolucent area (nidus) less than 1 cm in diameter surrounded by reactive sclerosis Diaphyseal location, but may affect metaphysis, epiphysis, or carpal bones
Subungual exostosis[133]	17–73	Approximately 20 per cent of subungual exostoses involve the hand Solitary osteochondroma arising from the dorsal surface of the distal phalanx Pressure on the undersurface of the nail may cause severe pain Lesion possesses smooth continuation of cortical and medullary bone Most frequently affects thumb and index finger
Turret exostosis[134]		Infrequent osseous excrescence arising from the dorsal surface of a proximal or middle phalanx of a finger History of penetrating injury followed by pain and soft tissue swelling or lump *Radiographic findings* Initial soft tissue swelling leading to immature periostitis and broad-based osseous protuberance on surface of bone

Table continued on following page

TABLE 17–11. Benign Tumors and Tumor-Like Lesions Affecting the Bones of the Wrist and Hand *Continued*

Entity	Figure(s)	Characteristics
Enchondroma (solitary)[135, 136]	17–74	Fifty-seven per cent of solitary enchondromas affect the bones of the wrist and hand, especially the proximal phalanges, followed in decreasing frequency by the metacarpal bones, the middle phalanges, the terminal phalanges, and the carpal bones Solitary enchondroma is a benign neoplasm composed of hyaline cartilage that develops in the medullary cavity and usually is discovered in the third or fourth decade of life Most lesions are painless, and painful lesions should arouse the suspicion of malignant transformation, a complication that occurs only rarely in solitary lesions and as many as 20 to 30 per cent of cases of multiple lesions (Ollier's disease and Maffucci's syndrome) Osteolytic metadiaphyseal lesions, endosteal scalloping, matrix calcification (50 per cent of lesions)
Enchondromatosis (Ollier's disease)[136, 137]	17–75	More than 50 per cent of patients with Ollier's disease have lesions involving the wrist and hand Multiple enchondromas involving the metacarpal bones and phalanges Tubular radiolucent areas extending into the metaphysis from the physis Shortening and deformity of affected bones Frequent calcification of matrix
Maffucci's syndrome[136, 138]		Eighty-eight per cent of patients with Maffucci's syndrome have lesions involving the wrist and hand Multiple enchondromas with soft tissue hemangiomas—multiple phleboliths in the soft tissues Multiple central or eccentric radiolucent lesions containing variable amounts of calcification Shortening and deformity of affected bones
Giant cell tumor (benign)[139]		Four per cent of benign giant cell tumors are located in the bones of the wrist and hand, and an additional 4 per cent of lesions are located in the distal portion of the radius Osteolytic subarticular lesion that extends to the metaphyseal region
Simple bone cyst[140]		Only 1 per cent of simple bone cysts occur in the bones of the wrist and hand Multiloculated, eccentric lesion
Intraosseous lipoma[141]		Fewer than 1 per cent of intraosseous lipomas occur in the bones of the wrist and hand Geographic osteolytic lesion with sclerotic margins, often containing a central calcified or ossified nidus
Aneurysmal bone cyst[142]	17–76	Five per cent of aneurysmal bone cysts involve the bones of the wrist and hand Eccentric, thin-walled, expansile, multiloculated, osteolytic, metaphyseal lesion
Tumor-like lesions of bone		
Paget's disease[143, 144]	17–77	Infrequent involvement of the bones of the wrist and hand Usually polyostotic form
Fibrous dysplasia[145]	17–78	Involvement of the bones of the wrist and hand is rare in the monostotic form but present in about 55 per cent of patients with polyostotic disease
Intraosseous ganglion cyst[146, 147]	17–79	Intraosseous ganglia often are clinically silent; however, chronic pain, which sometimes increases with physical activity, may be evident Geographic cyst-like lesions of various sizes within the carpal bones, especially the lunate bone
Epidermoid (inclusion) cyst[148]	17–80	Well-defined osteolytic lesion of terminal phalanx Sclerotic margin and mild expansion Usually 2 cm or less in diameter History of blunt or penetrating trauma

See also Tables 1–11 and 1–12.

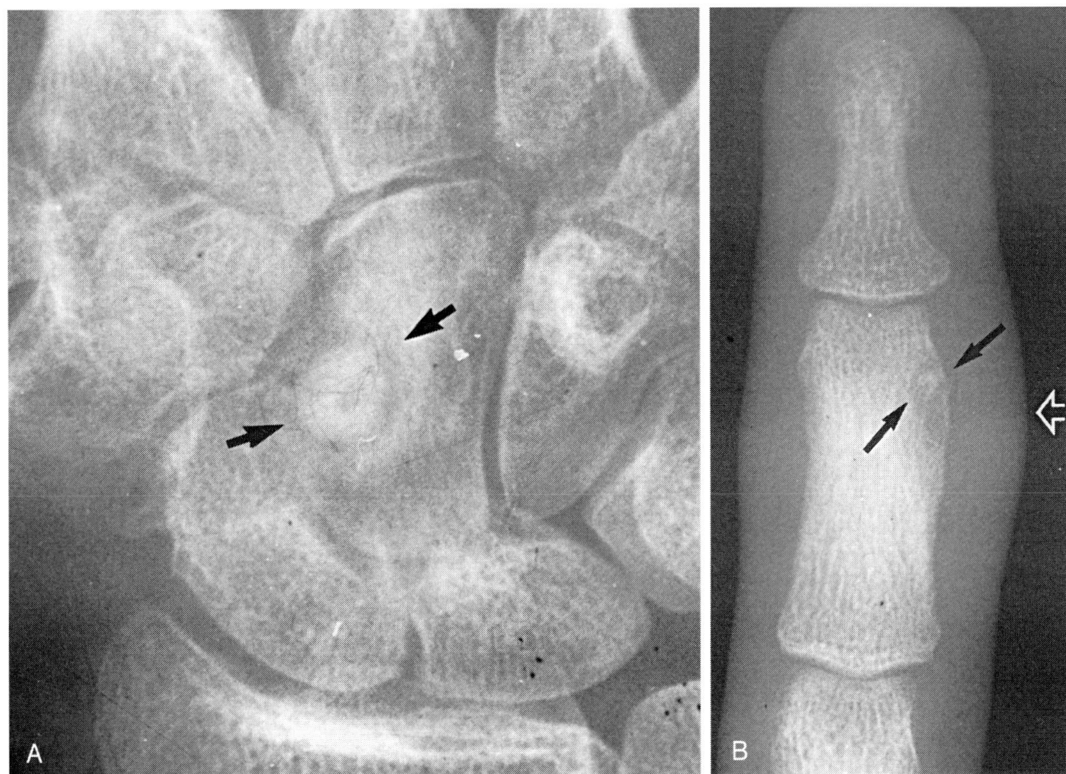

FIGURE 17–72. Osteoid osteoma.[129–132] A Carpal involvement. An eccentric circular radiolucent area with a central zone of calcification (arrows) surrounded by reactive sclerosis is evident in the capitate bone. Diffuse periarticular osteopenia throughout the carpus is the result of disuse and hyperemia. B Phalangeal involvement. A 23-year-old man had a painful swelling over the middle phalanx of the fourth finger. The radiograph reveals soft tissue swelling (open arrow) and an eccentric circular radiolucent area with a central zone of calcification (arrows) surrounded by reactive sclerosis. Approximately 9 per cent of osteoid osteomas occur in the bones of the wrist and hand, but the capitate bone is not frequently involved.

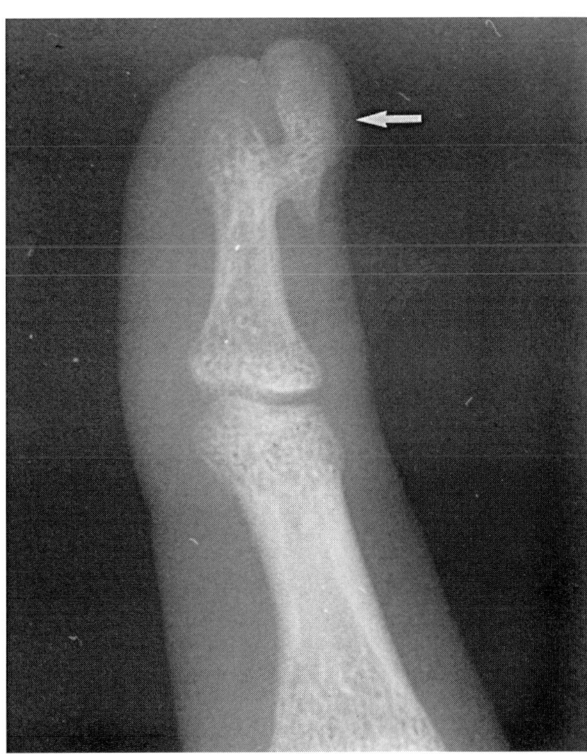

FIGURE 17–73. Subungual exostosis.[133] In this patient with a painful deformity of the fingernail, a pedunculated osseous excrescence arising from the dorsal surface of the terminal tuft is seen displacing the nail (arrow). The subungual exostosis is an uncommon, solitary, benign bone neoplasm arising from a distal phalanx at or adjacent to the nail bed. Histologically, it is identical to an osteochondroma. Rapid growth of an osteochondroma, although not diagnostic of malignant transformation, is an ominous sign requiring surgical removal of the lesion.

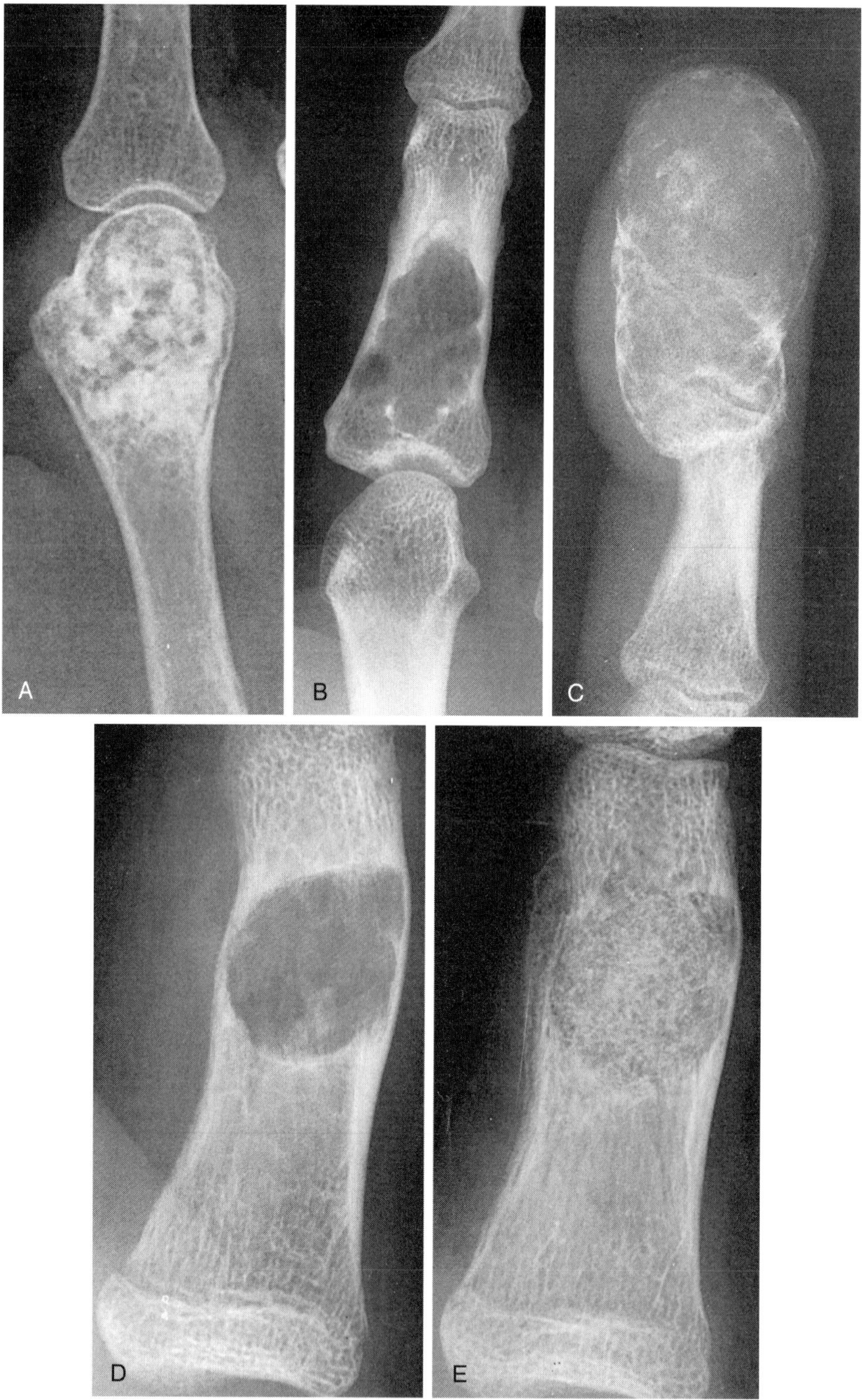

FIGURE 17–74. Solitary enchondroma: tubular bones of the hand.[135, 136] A Radiolucent lesion with endosteal scalloping involving the medullary cavity of the metaphysis and subchondral region of the metacarpal head is evident. Stippled calcification, present in about 50 per cent of cartilaginous tumors, is seen within the matrix. *(A, Courtesy of S.K. Brahme, M.D., San Diego, California.)* B Classic appearance of an enchondroma is seen. Radiographic findings include a radiolucent metadiaphyseal lesion with geographic margins, endosteal scalloping, and faint trabeculation. C Enchondromas in the terminal phalanx are rare. Observe the marked expansion within this atypical lesion. D, E In another patient, magnification radiographs of an enchondroma were taken before (D) and after (E) curettage and packing with bone chips. In D, this diaphyseal lesion is well circumscribed, with endosteal scalloping and faint trabeculation within the matrix. In E, the postsurgical radiograph reveals a mottled opacification of the matrix. This procedure is occasionally performed to strengthen the bone and to offset the likelihood of pathologic fracture. *(D, E, Courtesy of U. Mayer, M.D., Klagenfurt, Austria.)*

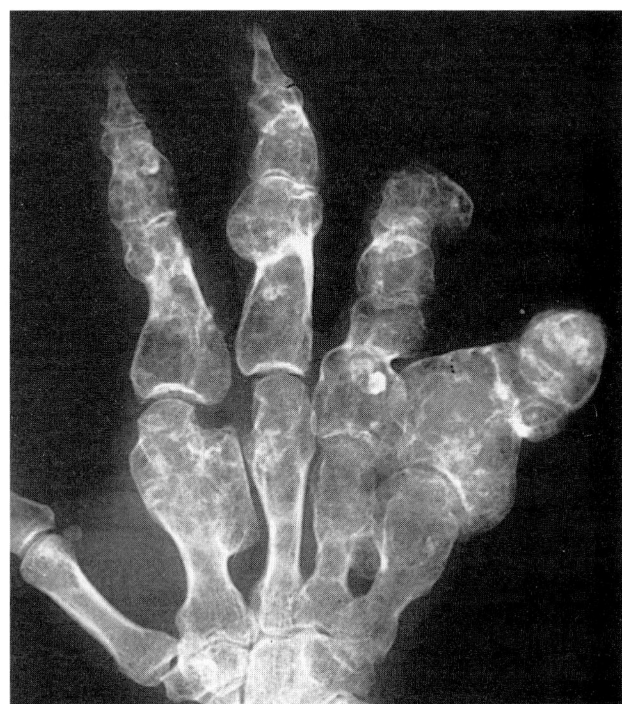

FIGURE 17–75. Enchondromatosis (Ollier's disease).[136, 137] Considerable deformity and multiple expansile, multiloculated radiolucent lesions are evident throughout most bones of the hand. Faint calcification is seen within the matrix. Malignant transformation to chondrosarcoma may occur in as many as 25 per cent of patients by the age of 40 years.

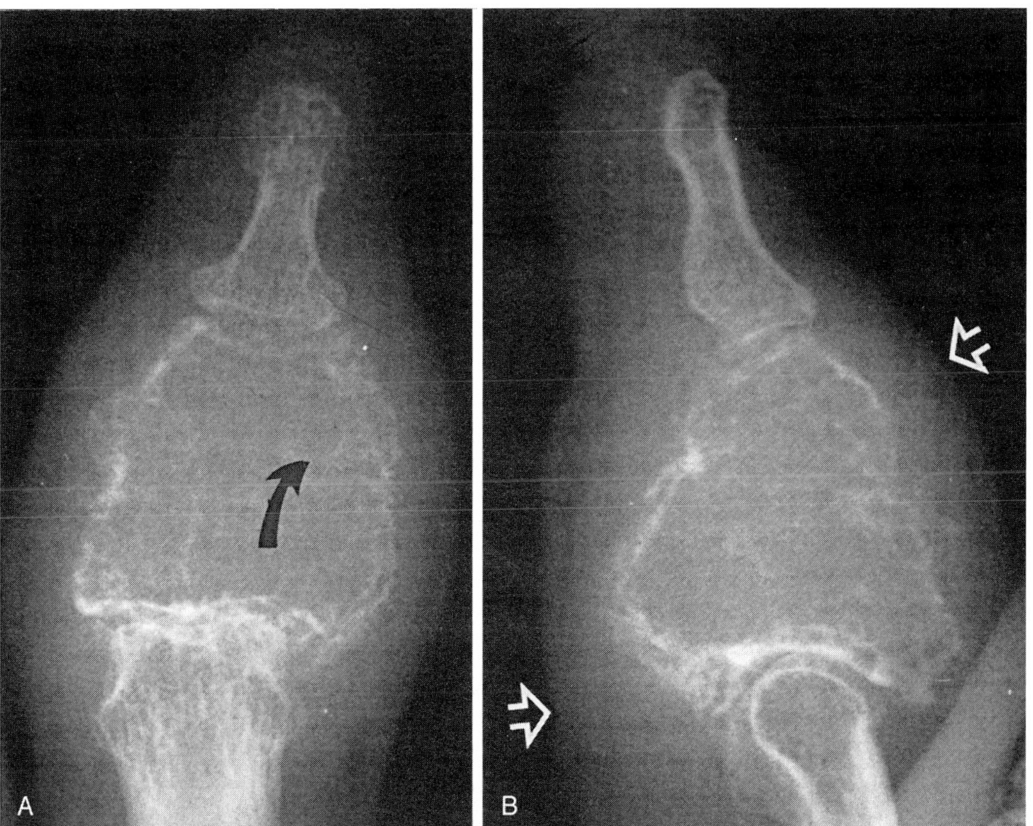

FIGURE 17–76. Aneurysmal bone cyst.[142] Frontal (A) and lateral (B) radiographs of the hand of this 57-year-old woman show an expansile, finely trabeculated (curved arrow) osteolytic lesion involving the entire middle phalanx of the third digit. Observe also the prominent soft tissue displacement and swelling (open arrows).

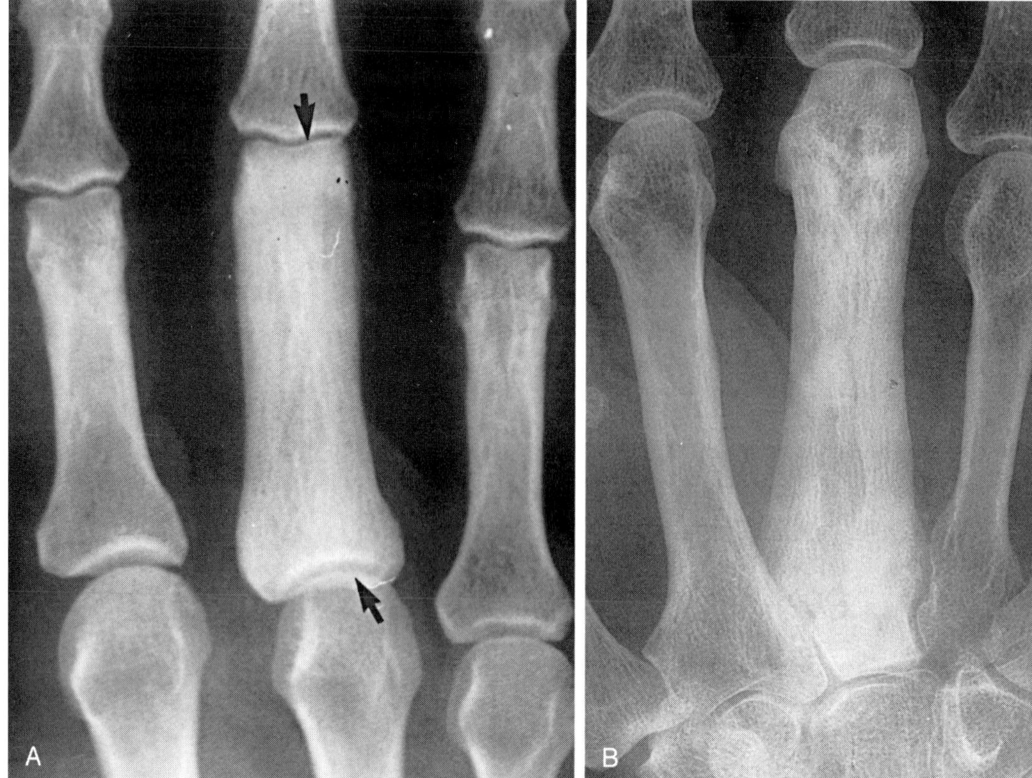

FIGURE 17–77. Paget's disease.[143, 144] A Typical alterations of Paget's disease in the proximal phalanx of this patient include diffuse increased sclerosis, bone enlargement, thickened and coarsened trabeculae, and subarticular distribution (arrows). B Posteroanterior radiograph of the metacarpal bone in this 86-year-old man reveals diffuse osseous enlargement, coarsened trabeculae, and increased radiodensity. When Paget's disease affects the hand, involvement of a single hand or single bone is not uncommon.

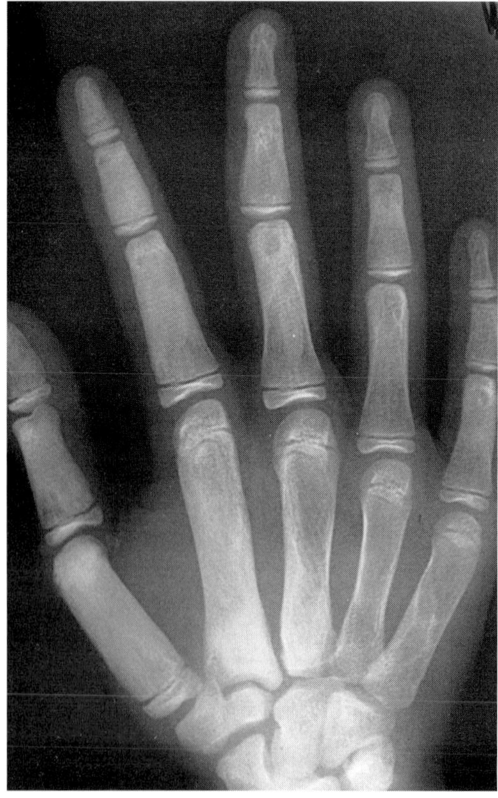

FIGURE 17–78. Polyostotic fibrous dysplasia.[145] Altered bone texture with osteosclerotic and osteolytic regions characterizes the bones of the hand in this child. The radiolucent lesions have the characteristic ground-glass appearance, and the more osteosclerotic lesions appear diffuse, with loss of definition between cortical and medullary bone.

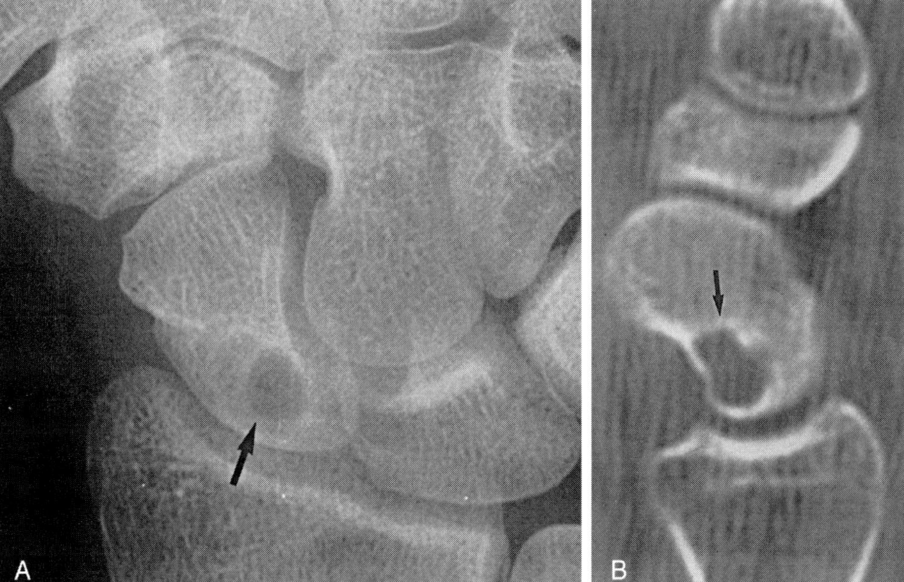

FIGURE 17–79. Intraosseous ganglion cyst.[146, 147] This 29-year-old man had chronic wrist pain. A Routine radiograph. A large, focal, well-marginated osteolytic lesion (arrow) is evident in the proximal pole of the scaphoid bone. B Sagittal computed tomographic (CT) image. The scan clearly demonstrates the extent of the lesion and its fluid-like density (arrow).

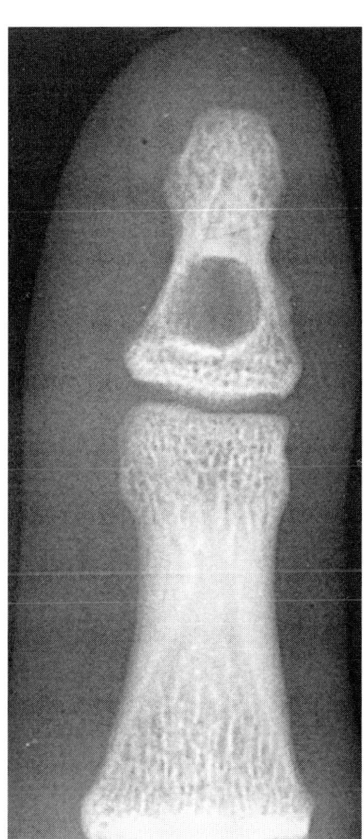

FIGURE 17–80. Epidermoid (inclusion) cyst.[148] A circular geographic osteolytic lesion with a sclerotic margin is seen in the terminal phalanx. It is believed that epidermoid cysts occur subsequent to implantation of ectodermal tissue after trauma to superficially located bone. They occur most frequently in the skull and the hand.

TABLE 17–12. Metabolic, Hematologic, Vascular, and Infectious Disorders Affecting the Wrist and Hand

Entity	Figure(s)	Characteristics
Generalized osteoporosis[149–151]	17–81	Uniform decrease in radiodensity, thinning of cortices Combined cortical thickness: at the midshaft of the second metacarpal, the transverse thickness of both cortices should be equal to or greater than the transverse thickness of the medullary cavity; in osteoporosis, however, the transverse cortical thickness is diminished Routine radiographs may suggest the presence of osteoporosis, but bone densitometry is necessary to assess bone mineral content accurately
Regional osteoporosis[151–153]	17–82	Osteopenia confined to a specific anatomic region may occur as a result of disuse and immobilization after a fracture or other injury; also seen in reflex sympathetic dystrophy, burns, frostbite, and paralysis Findings may be more widespread in paralyzed patients Band-like, patchy, spotty, or periarticular osteopenia Subperiosteal and intracortical bone resorption Subchondral and juxta-articular erosions
Hyperparathyroidism and renal osteodystrophy[154]	17–83	Brown tumors (osteoclastomas) Subperiosteal resorption, especially radial side of second and third middle phalanges Metastatic soft tissue calcification and vascular calcification Tuft resorption—acro-osteolysis
Amyloid deposition[155]	17–84	Patients on long-term hemodialysis develop amyloid deposition Deposits in carpal tunnel may lead to carpal tunnel syndrome and extensive carpal bone erosion
Hypothyroidism[156]	17–85	Delayed skeletal maturation, epiphyseal dysgenesis, carpal tunnel syndrome, soft tissue edema, neuropathy, myopathy, osteoporosis, erosive arthritis, and calcium pyrophosphate dihydrate (CPPD) crystal deposition
Pseudohypoparathyroidism (PHP) and pseudopseudohypoparathyroidism (PPHP)[157]		Premature physeal fusion: metacarpal shortening Soft tissue calcification and ossification
Acromegaly[158, 159]	17–86	Soft tissue overgrowth: prominent soft tissues of fingers, joint space widening, and clubbing of fingers Osseous overgrowth: enlargement of sesamoid bones and terminal tufts, periarticular excrescences Acromegalic arthropathy with eventual secondary osteoarthrosis
Primary hypertrophic osteoarthropathy[160]	17–87	Pachydermoperiostosis is the primary form of hypertrophic osteoarthropathy and represents only 3 to 5 per cent of all cases Clinical findings: enlargement of the hands and feet, digital clubbing, convexity of the nails, cutaneous abnormalities, and joint pains Radiographic findings: bilateral symmetric periostitis of the long tubular bones and digital clubbing
Secondary hypertrophic osteoarthropathy[161]	17–88	Most common form of hypertrophic osteoarthropathy Present in about 5 per cent of patients with bronchogenic carcinoma Predominant radiographic findings: bilateral symmetric periostitis and digital clubbing
Acute pyogenic osteomyelitis[162]	17–89	Pyogenic infection of bones and joints usually spreads from contiguous sources of infection, such as a felon or paronychia Especially prevalent in patients with diabetes mellitus and immunocompromised patients Soft tissue swelling, osteolytic destruction, and periostitis
Acute pyogenic septic arthritis[162, 163]	17–90	Septic arthritis: most joint infections begin as a monoarticular arthritis but frequently spread to adjacent bones and joints in the wrist or hand Rapid loss of joint space and destruction of subchondral bone Periarticular osteopenia, joint subluxation, and periostitis Human bite injury: direct implantation of organism into the metacarpophalangeal joint, usually resulting from a fistfight Most frequent organisms in this common type of infection are *Staphylococcus aureus*, *Streptococcus* species, and *Bacillus fusiformis*

TABLE 17–12. Metabolic, Hematologic, Vascular, and Infectious Disorders Affecting the Wrist and Hand *Continued*

Entity	Figure(s)	Characteristics
Tuberculous osteomyelitis and arthritis[164, 165]	17–91	Tuberculous infection is much less common than pyogenic infection in the wrist and hand; when it does occur, it has a predilection for the carpal region Mild symptoms and indolent course Most common organism: *Mycobacterium tuberculosis* Osteomyelitis: usually begins in epiphysis as an osteolytic lesion; may spread to metaphysis and diaphysis as moth-eaten or permeative pattern of destruction; may involve several bones of the hand Spina ventosa: tuberculous dactylitis; soft tissue swelling, bone destruction, periostitis, and bone expansion involving one or several digits; children > adults Arthritis: Juxta-articular osteoporosis, joint space narrowing, joint effusion, and periarticular erosions
Unusual and atypical infections[166]	17–92	Leprosy *(Mycobacterium leprae):* neuropathic osteoarthropathy—atrophic erosions of ungual tufts; osteomyelitis—periostitis and bone destruction; calcification of radial or ulnar nerves Leprosy is encountered infrequently in the United States but is more common in Africa, South America, and Asia *Coccidioidomycosis:* fungus found in Mexico and southwestern United States; results in osteolytic lesions; may be disseminated Congenital syphilis *(Treponema pallidum):* diametaphyseal gummas result in periostitis and aggressive bone destruction

See also Tables 1–13, 1–14, and 1–17.

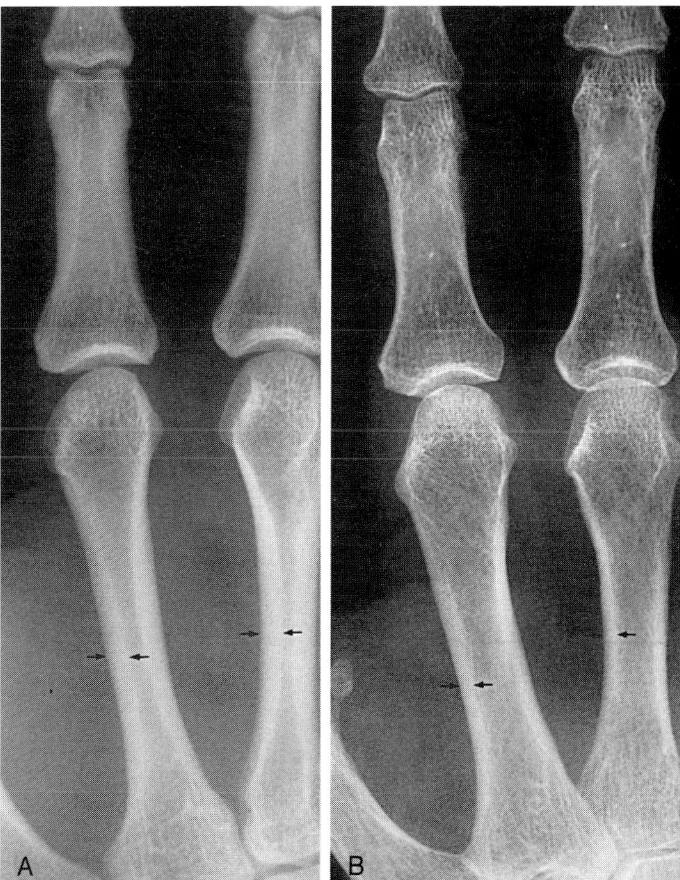

FIGURE 17–81. Generalized osteoporosis: routine radiography.[149–151] A Normal bone density: 26-year-old man. Note the normal mineralization of the metacarpal bones and phalanges. The cortices are thick (arrows), and there is no evidence of bone resorption. B Generalized osteoporosis: 71-year-old woman. Increased radiolucency and uniform thinning of all the cortices (arrows) are present.

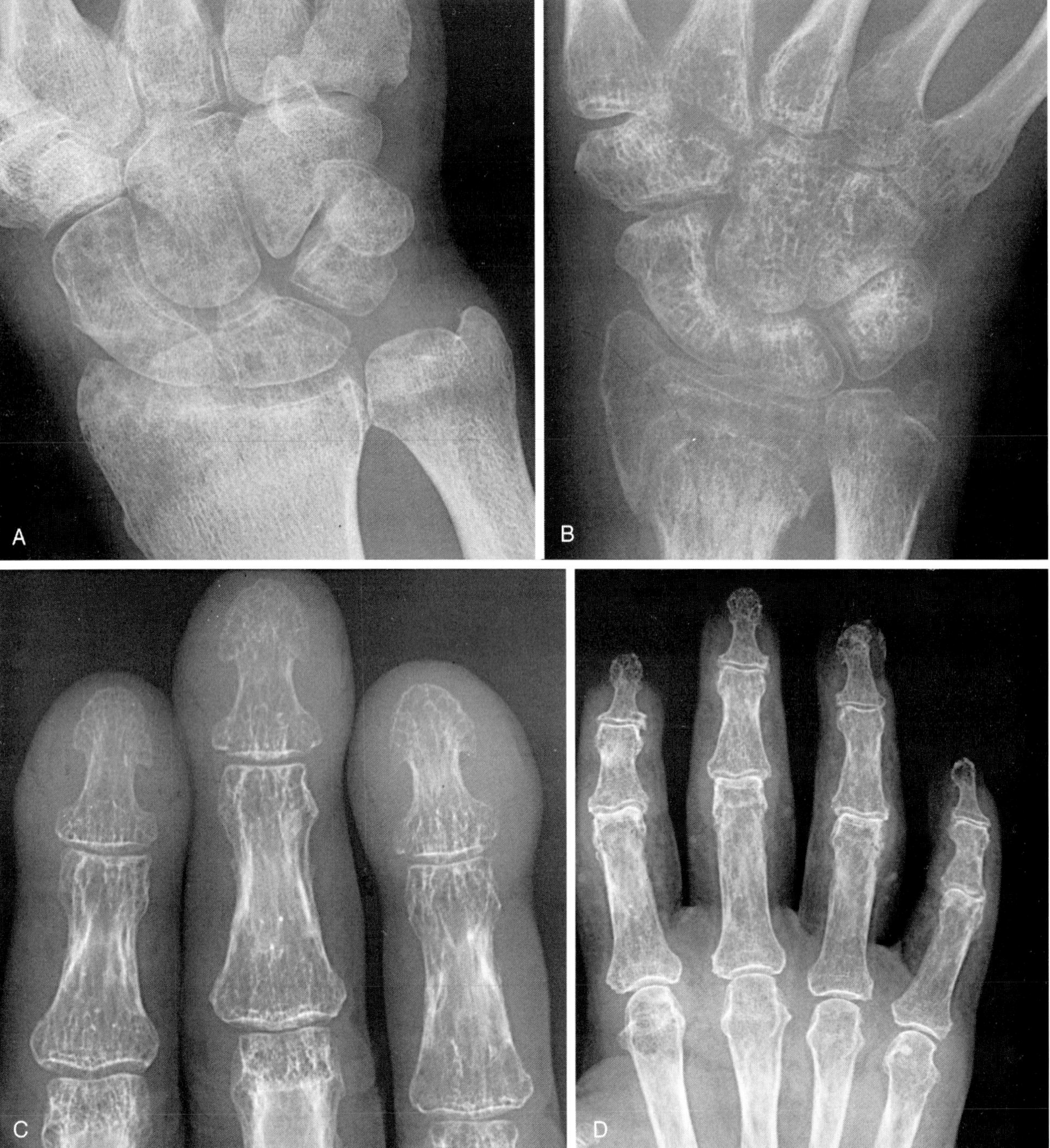

FIGURE 17–82. Regional osteoporosis.[151–153] A, B Immobilization (disuse) osteoporosis. In A, this patient's forearm and wrist were in a cast for 6 weeks. The radiograph exhibits a patchy pattern of periarticular osteopenia throughout the bones of the distal forearm and wrist. A band-like metaphyseal radiolucency is also recognized within the radius and ulna. In B, this 47-year-old woman with a Colles' fracture was immobilized for 6 weeks. Observe the spotty, patchy, and band-like osteopenia of the adjacent bones typical of disuse osteoporosis. This type of osteoporosis generally appears after 8 weeks of immobilization and may simulate the permeative appearance of malignancy. C, D Reflex sympathetic dystrophy. In C, findings include swelling of the soft tissues of the distal phalanges and osteoporosis characterized by subperiosteal, intracortical, and medullary resorption of bone. In D, a radiograph of another patient with reflex sympathetic dystrophy reveals diffuse soft tissue swelling and a patchy, permeative pattern of osteopenia. Spotty, patchy and band-like bone resorption is typical of rapid-onset osteoporosis such as that seen in disuse, burns, frostbite, paralysis, or reflex sympathetic dystrophy, an appearance that may simulate an aggressive neoplasm.

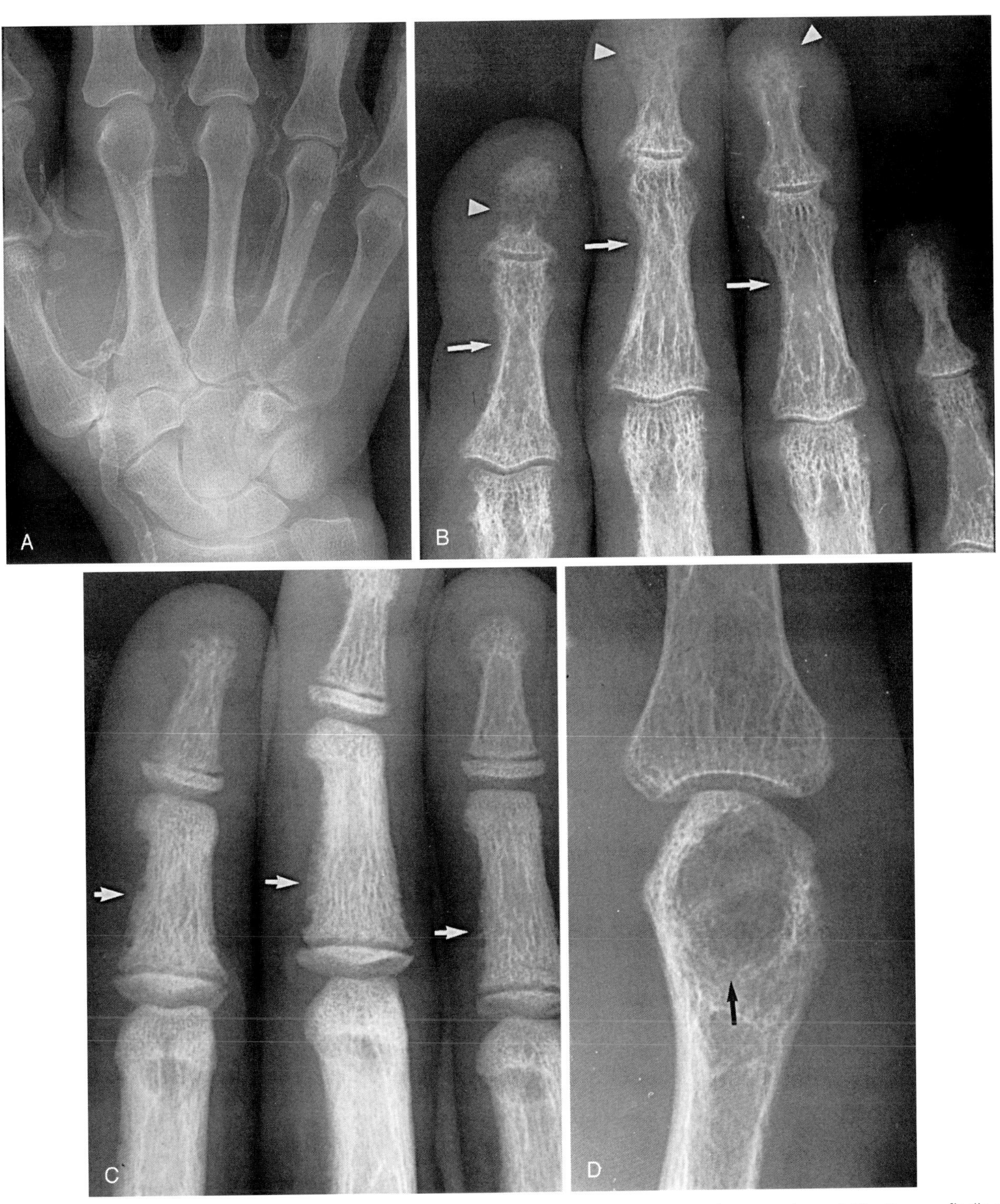

FIGURE 17–83. Hyperparathyroidism.[154] A Vascular calcification. Observe the extensive vascular calcification, a finding occurring more frequently in patients undergoing hemodialysis. B Subperiosteal resorption and acro-osteolysis. Subperiosteal resorption, predominantly on the radial aspect of the middle phalanges (arrows), and acro-osteolysis or tuft resorption (arrowheads) are frequent findings in hyperparathyroidism. C Subperiosteal resorption. Subperiosteal resorption (arrows) and osteosclerosis are seen in this renal transplant patient with secondary hyperparathyroidism. *(C, Courtesy of U. Mayer, M.D., Klagenfurt, Austria.)* D Brown tumor. An osteolytic lesion with well-defined sclerotic margins is seen in the metacarpal bone (arrow).

Illustration continued on following page

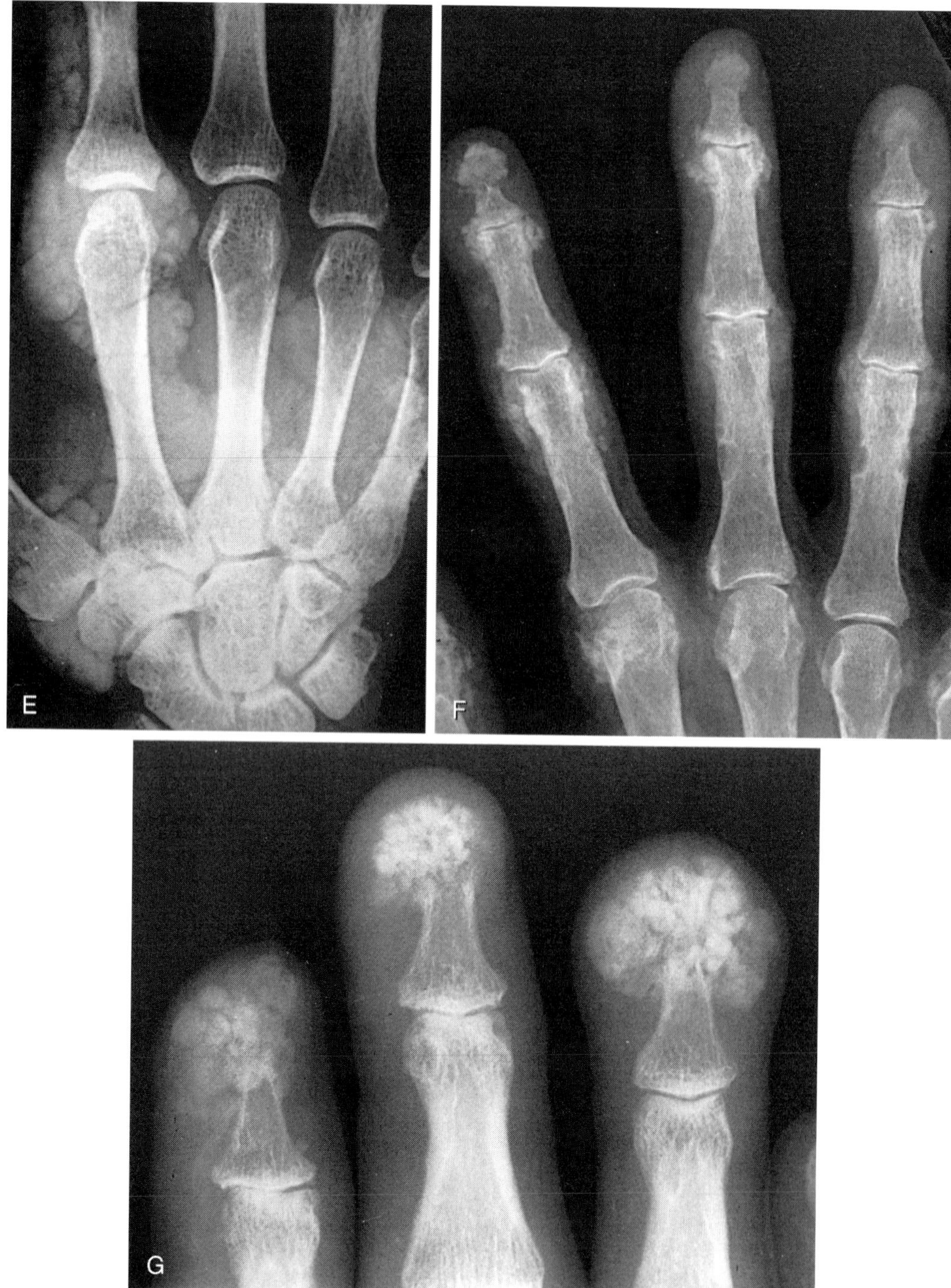

FIGURE 17–83 *Continued.* E–G Soft tissue calcification. In **E**, observe the extensive lobulated calcinosis of the subcutaneous tissues in a patient with secondary hyperparathyroidism. In **F**, a 64-year-old woman has evidence of extensive periarticular calcification and acro-osteolysis. In **G**, a radiograph of a 49-year-old man shows tumoral calcification surrounding the distal tuft, another manifestation of chronic renal failure. (*F, Courtesy of T. Broderick, M.D., Orange, California.*) These forms of metastatic soft tissue calcification are related to a disturbance in calcium or phosphorous metabolism and may accompany hyperparathyroidism and renal osteodystrophy.

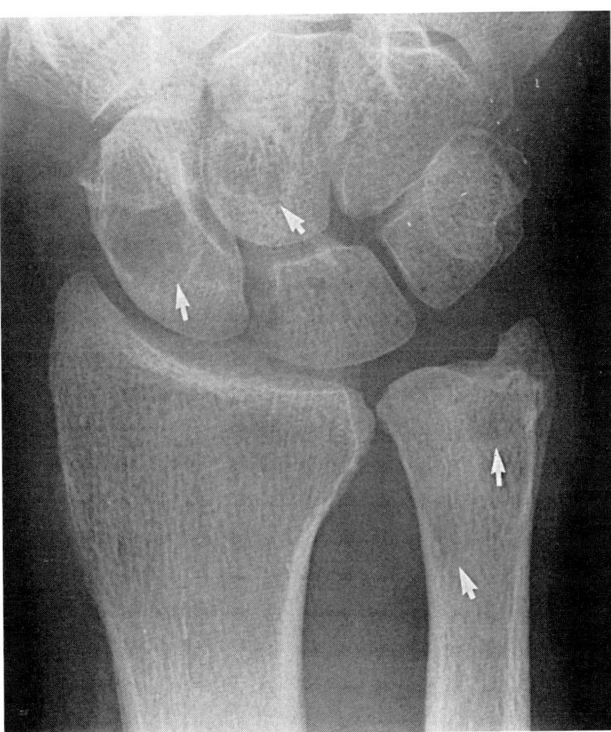

FIGURE 17–84. Amyloid deposition.[155] Long-term hemodialysis in a 55-year-old man with chronic renal failure. Multiple radiolucent cyst-like lesions are present in several carpal bones (arrows). Amyloid deposition is a well-established complication of hemodialysis. In the wrist, it may lead to multiple intraosseous osteolytic lesions, as in this patient, and carpal tunnel syndrome. *(Courtesy of G. Greenway, M.D., Dallas, Texas.)*

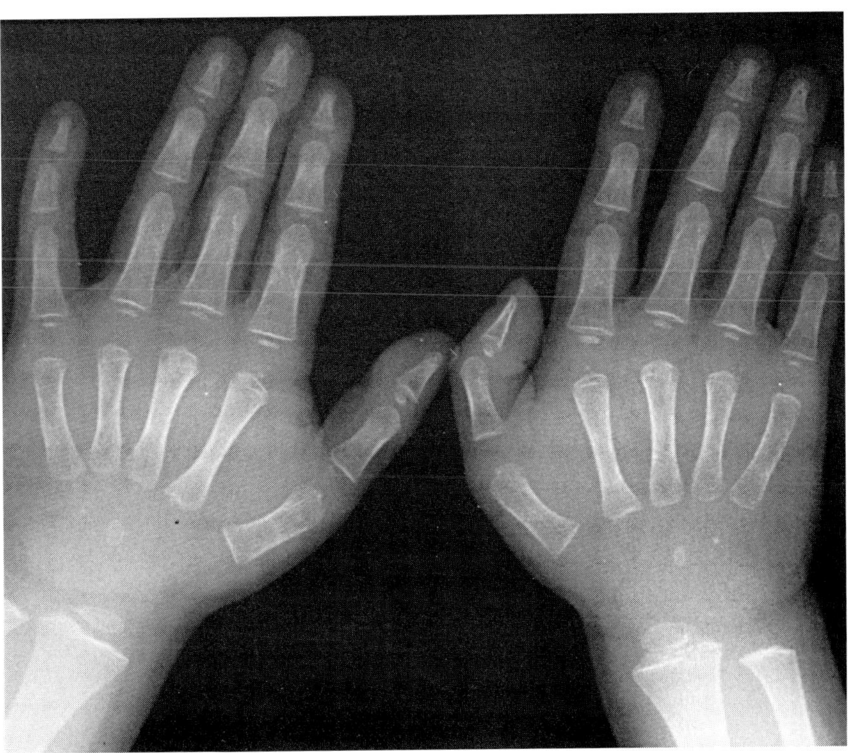

FIGURE 17–85. Hypothyroidism: Delayed skeletal maturation.[156] This boy with cretinism had a chronologic age of 9 years 9 months. Radiographs of both hands reveal a skeletal age of 2 years 8 months.

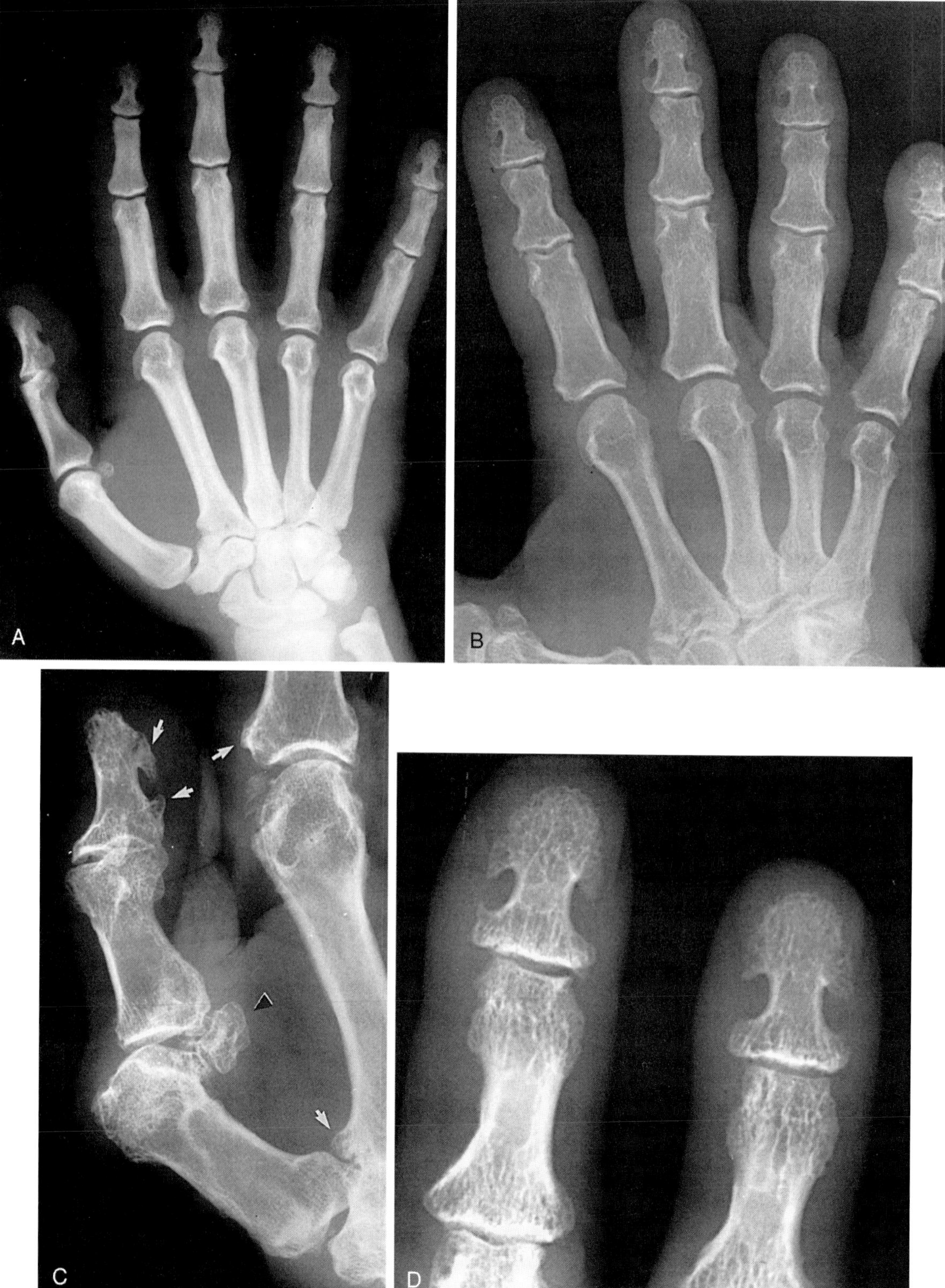

FIGURE 17–86. Acromegaly.[158, 159] A Diffuse soft tissue hypertrophy and widened metacarpophalangeal joint spaces are evident. B In another patient, soft tissue hypertrophy, widened joint spaces, spade-shaped terminal tufts, and thickening of the proximal phalangeal diaphyses are seen. C Hypertrophy of the sesamoid bones (arrowhead), as seen in this 62-year-old man, is a well-documented finding in acromegaly. Note also the periarticular and tuft bone proliferation (arrows). D Enlarged terminal tufts. The enlarged terminal phalanges are prominent and appear spade-shaped, a characteristic finding in acromegaly. Note also the prominent soft tissues.

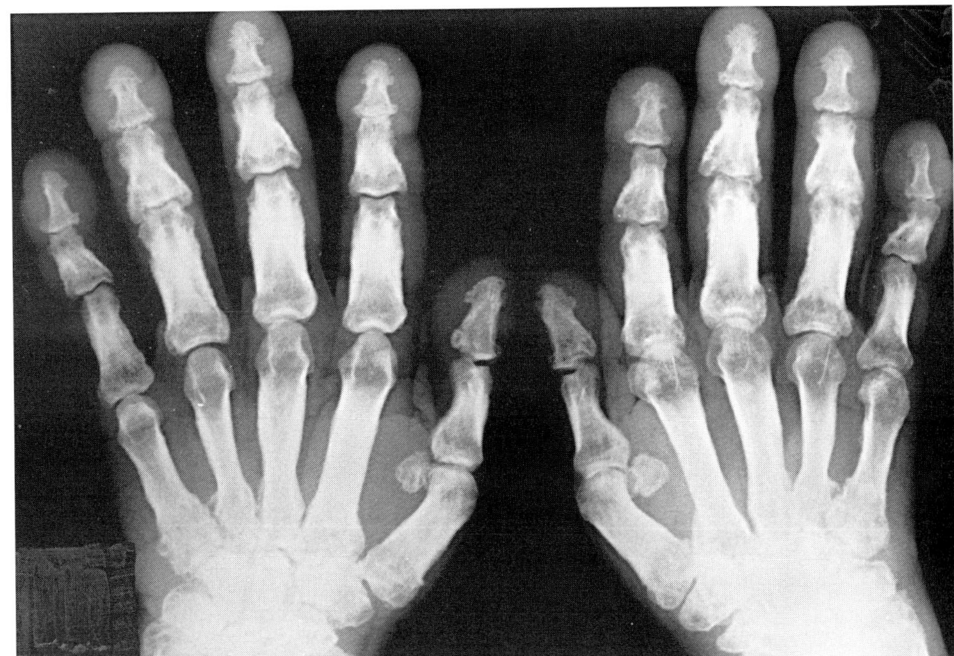

FIGURE 17–87. Primary hypertrophic osteoarthropathy: Pachydermoperiostosis.[160] Observe the bilaterally symmetric and widespread soft tissue clubbing and prominent periostitis affecting the tubular bones of the hands. The findings in this patient were present in several tubular bones throughout the skeleton. *(Courtesy of C. Chen, M.D., Kaohsiung, Taiwan.)*

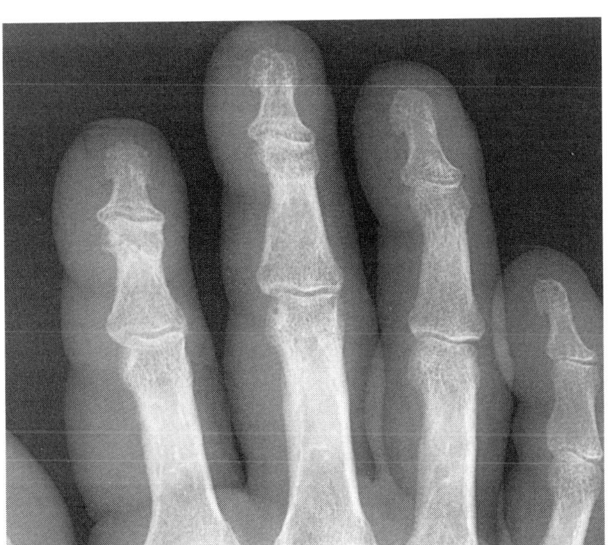

FIGURE 17–88. Digital clubbing: Secondary hypertrophic osteoarthropathy.[161] This 60-year-old man was diagnosed as having bronchogenic carcinoma. Characteristic bulbous hypertrophy of the soft tissues overlying the terminal phalanges is seen. This finding relates to thickening of the fibroelastic tissue at the base of the nail bed and consequent increased curvature of the nail itself. It may result in tuft resorption or hypertrophy. It often accompanies hypertrophic osteoarthropathy, a condition that occurs in approximately 5 per cent of patients with bronchogenic carcinoma and may also occur in many other diseases.

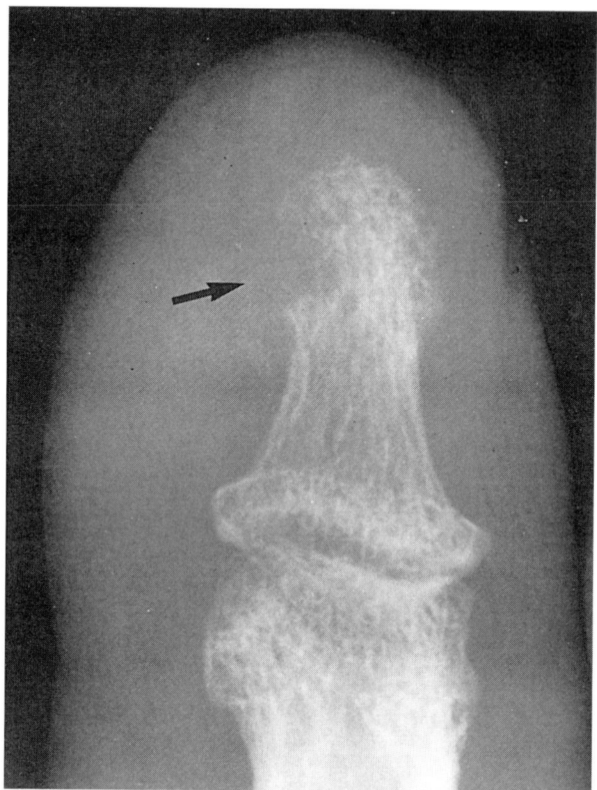

FIGURE 17–89. Acute pyogenic osteomyelitis: spread from a contiguous source.[162] Routine radiograph shows considerable soft tissue swelling. Infection from an adjacent felon has eroded into the tuft of the terminal phalanx (arrow). A felon is an infection in the terminal pulp space, and a paronychia is a subcuticular abscess of the nail fold. When these soft tissue infections are neglected, organisms may spread to the contiguous bone, joint, or tendon sheath.

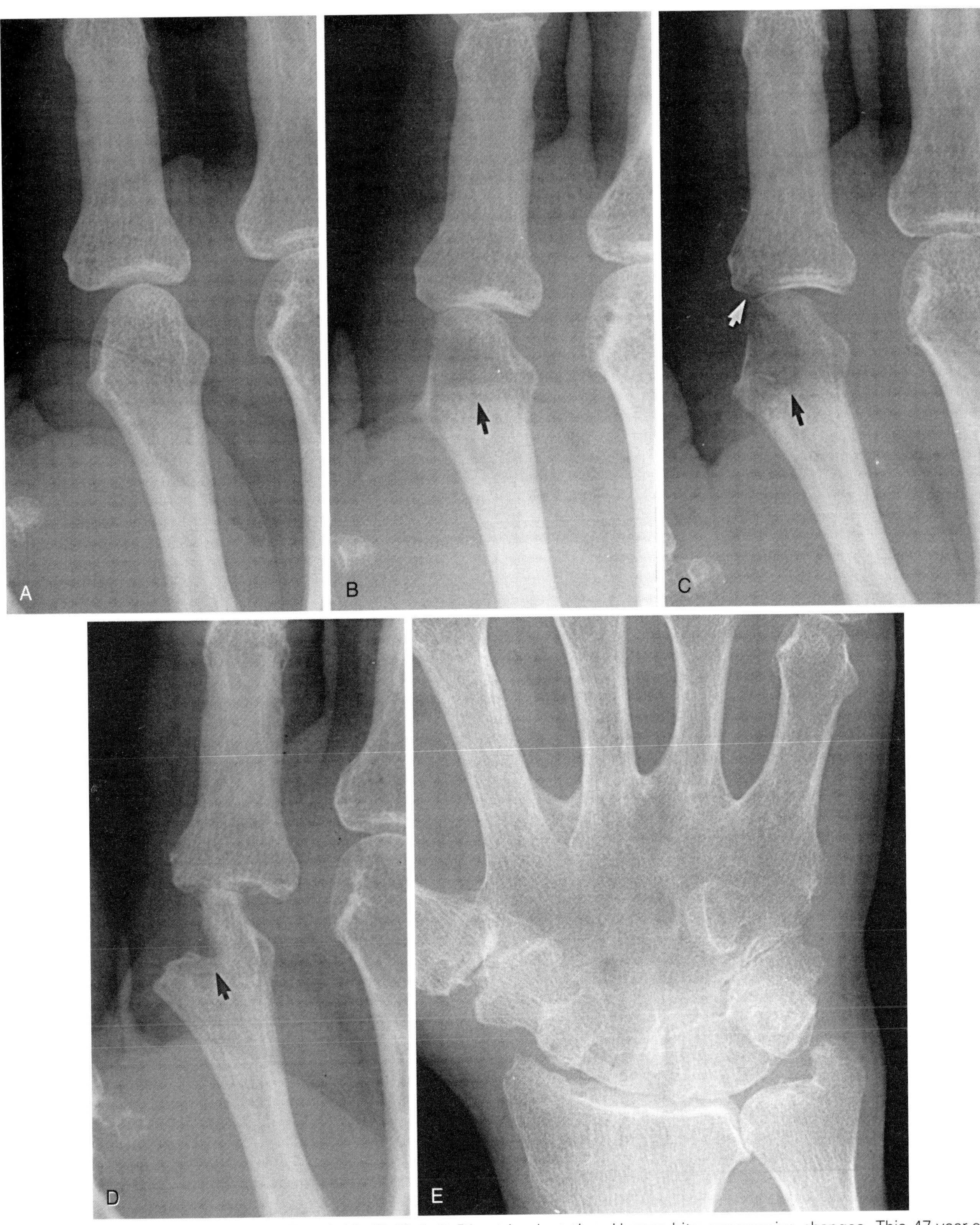

FIGURE 17–90. Acute pyogenic septic arthritis.[162, 163] A–D Direct implantation: Human bite, progressive changes. This 47-year-old man was involved in a fistfight in which his hand was lacerated and he developed severe swelling and erythema over the dorsum of his second metacarpophalangeal joint. Serial radiographs were obtained. A, January 15: one week after the altercation, the radiograph appears essentially normal. B, February 5: the joint space is narrowed and the metacarpal head appears osteopenic (black arrow). C, February 20: a large erosion is seen in the metacarpal head (black arrow), and an erosion of the subchondral bone of the proximal phalanx is becoming evident (white arrow). D, May 14: four months after the initial injury, widespread destruction of the metacarpal head (black arrow), joint space narrowing, and subluxation are apparent despite antibiotic treatment. E Wrist ankylosis. In another patient, complete osseous ankylosis of all the intercarpal and carpometacarpal articulations is consistent with the residual appearance of septic arthritis.

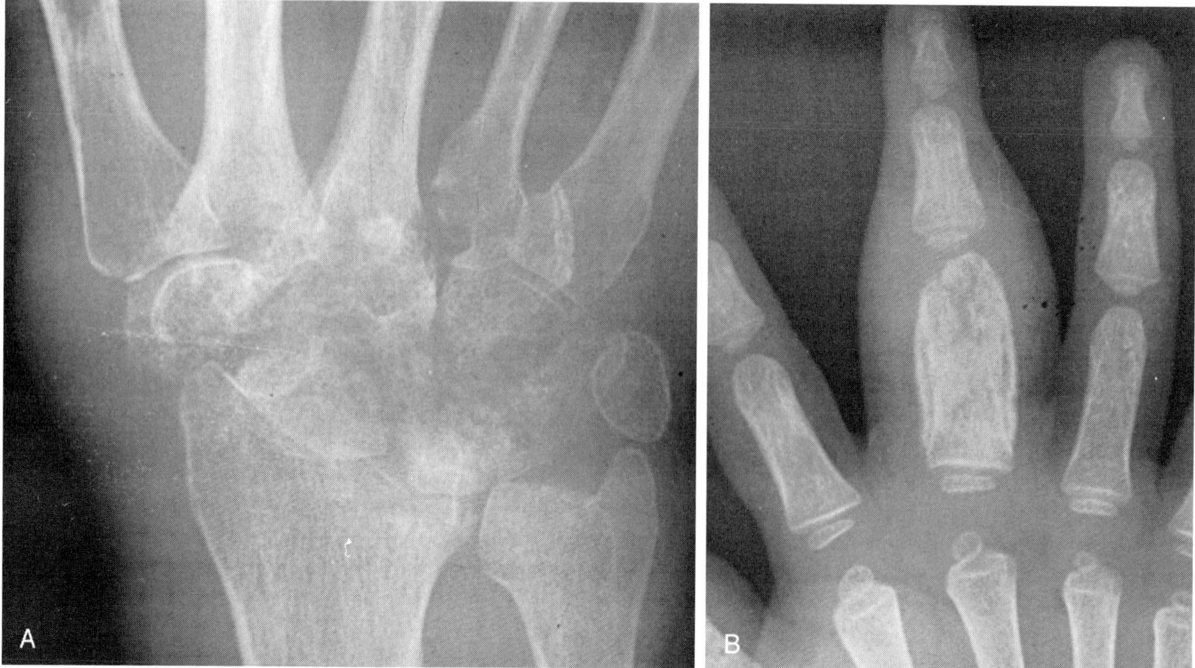

FIGURE 17–91. Tuberculous infection.[164, 165] A Tuberculous arthritis. In a 58-year-old man with long-standing pulmonary tuberculosis and wrist pain, abnormalities include soft tissue swelling, widespread joint space narrowing, periarticular osteopenia, osseous erosions, and collapse of the carpal bones and the distal articular surface of the radius. B Tuberculous osteomyelitis: dactylitis. Prominent soft tissue swelling and exuberant periostitis and enlargement of the proximal phalanx are characteristic of tuberculous dactylitis in this child. Lytic lesions may also predominate in tuberculosis involving the digits. Radiographic changes typically are much more gradual in tuberculous infections than they are in pyogenic infections.

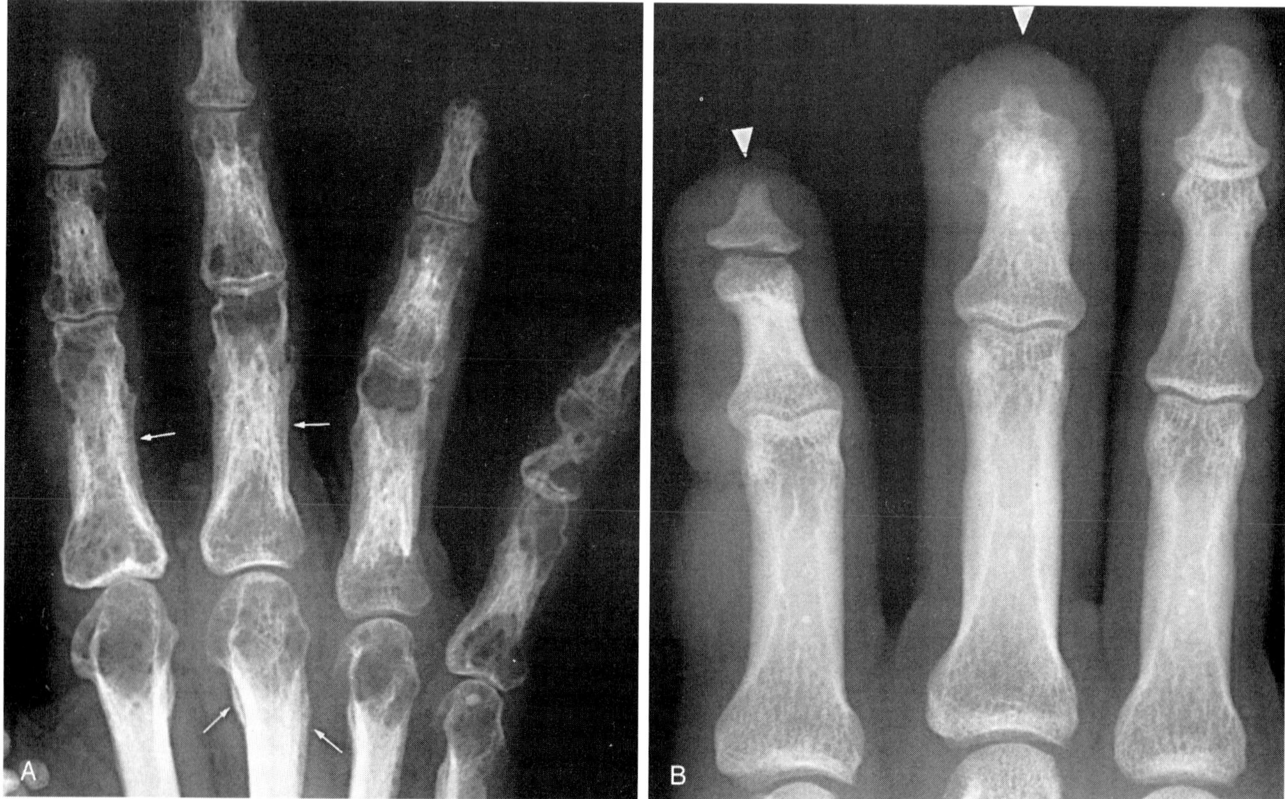

FIGURE 17–92. Leprosy.[166] A Osteomyelitis. Periostitis (arrows) and moth-eaten and permeative destruction of several metacarpal bones and phalanges are present. B Neuropathic lesions. In a second patient with long-standing leprosy, the tapered osseous surfaces of the second and third terminal phalanges represent phalangeal osteolysis. Note also the soft tissue swelling of these two digits. Involvement in both cases was bilateral and symmetric.

TABLE 17–13. Osteonecrosis

Entity	Figure(s)	Characteristics
Lunate bone (Kienböck's disease)[167]	17–93	Most frequent carpal bone to undergo osteonecrosis Magnetic resonance (MR) imaging most sensitive in comparison with radiography and scintigraphy Most common in patients with negative ulnar variance Occurs between the ages of 20 and 40 years
Scaphoid bone[168, 169]	17–18D	Idiopathic form (Preiser's disease) or posttraumatic form (most common) Proximal portion affected most frequently after fracture of the waist of the scaphoid
Capitate bone[170]		Idiopathic or after an injury
Hamate bone[171, 172]		Infrequent site of osteonecrosis Occurs after fractures of the body and hook of the hamate
Phalanges (Thiemann's disease)[173]		Osteonecrosis of the phalangeal epiphyses secondary to trauma Occurs between the ages of 11 and 19 years May result in pain and swelling about the interphalangeal joints

See also Table 1–16.

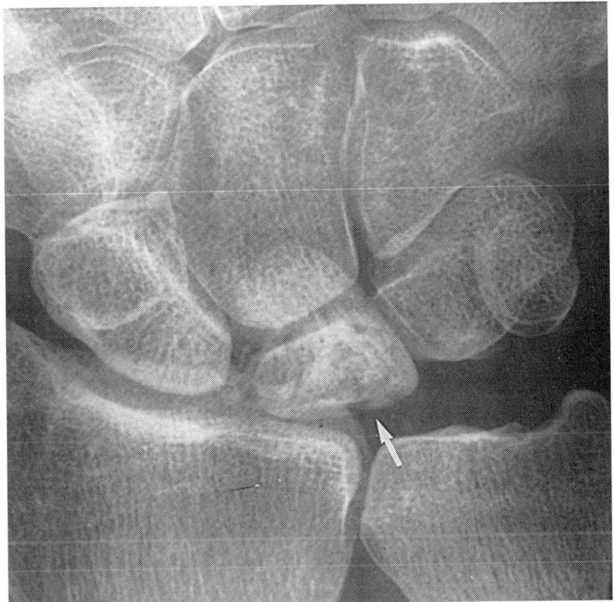

FIGURE 17–93. Kienböck's disease.[167] Observe the sclerosis and fragmentation of the carpal lunate bone (arrow). This form of osteonecrosis has a predilection for the right wrist and is especially prevalent in manual laborers. A history of trauma may be elicited, but this is not a constant feature. Progressive pain, swelling, and disability are the chief presenting clinical features. A short ulna (negative ulnar variance) is encountered in as many as 75 per cent of cases. Radiographs may appear normal early in the course of the disease, in which case scintigraphy and magnetic resonance (MR) imaging can be helpful.

TABLE 17–14. Acquired Deformities of the Wrist and Hand[174]

Entity	Characteristics	Causes
Wrist deformities		
Radial deviation of wrist	Carpal bones are displaced toward the radial side of the wrist in conjuction with ulnar deviation at the MCP joints See also zigzag deformity (below)	Rheumatoid arthritis
Ulnar deviation of wrist	Carpal bones are displaced toward the ulnar side of the wrist in conjunction with flexion deformity at the MCP joints	Juvenile chronic arthritis
Ulnar bayonet deformity	Ulnar migration of the carpal bones at the radiocarpal joint Ulna overrides the radius at the inferior radioulnar joint	Juvenile chronic arthritis
Finger deformities		
Boutonnière deformity	Hyperflexion at PIP joints and hyperextension at DIP joints	Rheumatoid arthritis Systemic lupus erythematosus
Flexion deformities	Hyperflexion at DIP and PIP joints	Rheumatoid arthritis Psoriatic arthritis Dupuytren's contracture
Swan-neck deformity	Hyperextension at PIP joints and hyperflexion at DIP joints	Rheumatoid arthritis Systemic lupus erythematosus
Mallet finger	Persistent flexion at the DIP joints Loosening or disruption of the distal attachment of the extensor tendon to the terminal phalanx Uncommon deformity	Rheumatoid arthritis Traumatic extensor tendon rupture
Ulnar deviation of MCP joints	Deviation of proximal phalanges toward ulnar side in relation to metacarpal bones	Rheumatoid arthritis Psoriatic arthropathy
Zigzag deformity	Combination of ulnar deviation at MCP joints and radial deviation of wrist	Rheumatoid arthritis
Z-shaped deformity of thumb	Also termed hitchhiker's thumb Boutonnière deformity of thumb—hyperextension at the interphalangeal joint and hyperflexion at the MCP joint	Systemic lupus erythematosus Rheumatoid arthritis
Main-en-lorgnette deformity	Arthritis mutilans or opera glass hand In cases of severe phalangeal and metacarpal erosions, the soft tissues of the fingers telescope on each other as the underlying struts of bone are resorbed, resembling a collapsed opera glass	Psoriatic arthropathy Juvenile chronic arthritis Rheumatoid arthritis Neuropathic osteoarthropathy
Nonerosive deforming arthropathy	Jaccoud's arthropathy Malalignment of joints in the absence of joint erosions Reversible subluxations: deformities may be present when the hand is gently placed on the cassette and disappear when the hand is pressed firmly against cassette	Systemic lupus erythematosus Rheumatic fever Scleroderma Rare: Agammaglobulinemia Ehlers-Danlos syndrome Sarcoidosis Rheumatoid arthritis
Pencil-in-cup deformity	Resorption of distal end of metacarpal bone or phalanx with associated cup-like erosion of proximal articulating surface of adjacent phalanx, resembling a pencil in a cup	Psoriatic arthropathy Rheumatoid arthritis

MCP, Metacarpophalangeal; PIP, proximal interphalangeal joint; DIP, distal interphalangeal joint.

TABLE 17–15. Characteristic Sites of Terminal Phalangeal Resorption in Various Disorders[175] (Fig. 17–94)

	Site*		
Entity	*Tuft*	*Midportion or Waist*	*Periarticular*
Scleroderma	+		+
Hyperparathyroidism	+	+	+
Thermal injury	+		+
Frostbite	+		+
Psoriasis	+		+
Epidermolysis bullosa	+		
Polyvinylchloride acro-osteolysis		+	
Neuropathic osteoarthropathy	+		
Multicentric reticulohistiocytosis	+		+
Inflammatory (erosive) osteoarthritis			+
Lesch-Nyhan syndrome	+		
Progeria	+		

*Only the characteristic sites of bone resorption are indicated, although in any single disease, considerable variability in these sites may exist.

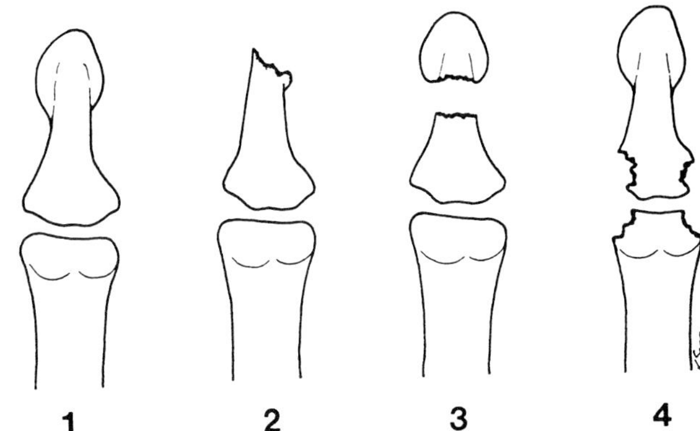

FIGURE 17–94. Phalangeal resorption: differential diagnosis.[175] The normal situation is depicted in diagram 1. Resorption of the tuft (2) can be seen in scleroderma, other collagen vascular disorders, thermal injuries, hyperparathyroidism, psoriasis, neuropathic osteoarthropathy, and epidermolysis bullosa. Band-like resorption of the terminal phalanx (3) is seen in familial and occupational acro-osteolysis, collagen vascular disorders, and hyperparathyroidism. Erosions about the distal interphalangeal joint (4) can occur in psoriatic arthropathy, multicentric reticulohistiocytosis, gout, thermal injuries, scleroderma, and hyperparathyroidism. *(From Resnick D [ed]: Diagnosis of Bone and Joint Disorders. 3rd Ed. Philadelphia, WB Saunders, 1995, p 1213.)*

TABLE 17–16. Some Causes of Soft Tissue Calcification About the Terminal Phalanges[174]

Scleroderma
Dermatomyositis
Systemic lupus erythematosus
Hyperparathyroidism
Epidermolysis bullosa
Raynaud's disease
Synovial osteochondromatosis
Calcium hydroxyapatite crystal deposition

REFERENCES

1. Greulich WW, Pyle SI: Radiographic Atlas of Skeletal Development of the Hand and Wrist. 2nd Ed. Palo Alto, Stanford University Press, 1959.
2. Edeiken J, Dalinka M, Karasick D: Edeiken's Roentgen Diagnosis of Diseases of Bone. 4th Ed. Baltimore, Williams & Wilkins, 1990.
3. Keats TE, Smith TH: An Atlas of Normal Developmental Roentgen Anatomy. 2nd Ed. Chicago, Year Book Medical Publishers, 1988.
4. Greenfield GB: Radiology of Bone Diseases. 2nd Ed. Philadelphia, JB Lippincott, 1975.
5. Köhler A, Zimmer EA: Borderlands of Normal and Early Pathologic Findings in Skeletal Radiography. 4th Ed. New York, Thieme Medical Publishers, 1993.
6. Keats TE: Atlas of Normal Roentgen Variants That May Simulate Disease. 6th Ed. Chicago, Year Book Medical Publishers, 1996.
7. Fagg PS: Wrist pain in the Madelung's deformity of dyschondrosteosis. J Hand Surg [Br] 13:11, 1988.
8. Metz VM, Schimmerl SM, Gilula LA, et al: Wide scapholunate joint space in lunotriquetral coalition: A normal variant? Radiology 188:557, 1993.
9. Simmons BP, McKenzie WD: Symptomatic carpal coalition. J Hand Surg [Am] 10:190, 1985.
10. Poznanski AK: The Hand in Radiologic Diagnosis: With Gamuts and Pattern Profiles. 2nd Ed. Philadelphia, WB Saunders, 1984.
11. Conway, WF, Destouet JM, Gilula LA, et al: The carpal boss: An overview of radiographic evaluation. Radiology 156:29, 1985.
12. Bloom R: The metacarpal sign. Br J Radiol 43:133, 1970.
13. Elkington SG, Hunstman RG: The Talbot fingers: A study in symphalangism. Br Med J 1:407, 1967.
14. Wood VE: Congenital thumb deformities. Clin Orthop 195:7, 1985.

15. Blank E, Girdany BR: Symmetric bowing of the terminal phalanges of the fifth fingers in a family (Kirner's deformity). AJR 93:367, 1965.
16. Pear J, Viljoen D, Beighton P: Limb overgrowth—clinical observations and nosological considerations. S Afr J Med 64:905, 1983.
17. Wang YC, Jeng CM, Marcantonio DR, et al: Macrodystrophia lipomatosa: MR imaging in three patients. Clin Imaging 21:323, 1997.
18. Kosowicz J: The roentgen appearance of the hand and wrist in gonadal dysgenesis. AJR 93:354, 1965.
19. Rand TC, Edwards DK, Bay CA, et al: The metacarpal index in normal children. Pediatr Radiol 9:31, 1980.
20. Joseph KN, Kane HA, Milner RS, et al: Orthopedic aspects of the Marfan phenotype. Clin Orthop 277:251, 1992.
21. Morse RP, Rockenmacher S, Pyeritz RE, et al: Diagnosis and management of infantile Marfan's syndrome. Pediatrics 86:888, 1990.
22. Bailey JA: Orthopaedic aspects of achondroplasia. J Bone Joint Surg [Am] 52:1285, 1970.
23. Bridges AL, Kou-Ching H, Singh A, et al: Fibrodysplasia (myositis) ossificans progressiva. Semin Arthritis Rheum 24:155, 1994.
24. Root L: The treatment of osteogenesis imperfecta. Orthop Clin North Am 15:775, 1984.
25. Benli IT, Akalin S, Boysan E, et al: Epidemiological, clinical, and radiological aspects of osteopoikilosis. J Bone Joint Surg [Br] 74:504, 1992.
26. Campbell CJ, Papademetriou T, Bonfiglio M: Melorheostosis: A report of the clinical, roentgenographic, and pathological findings in fourteen cases. J Bone Joint Surg [Am] 50:1281, 1968.
27. Caudle RJ, Stern PJ: Melorheostosis of the hand: A case report with long-term follow-up. J Bone Joint Surg [Am] 69:1229, 1987.
28. Ainsworth SR, Aulicino PL: A survey of patients with Ehlers-Danlos syndrome. Clin Orthop 286:250, 1993.
29. Watts RWE, Spellacy E, Kendall BE, et al: Computed tomography studies on patients with mucopolysaccharidosis. Neuroradiology 21:9, 1981.
30. Rogers LF: Radiology of Skeletal Trauma. 2nd. Ed. New York, Churchill Livingstone, 1992.
31. Duppe H, Johnell O, Lundborg G, et al: Long-term results of fracture of the scaphoid: A follow-up study of more than thirty years. J Bone Joint Surg [Am] 76:249, 1994.
32. Calandra JJ, Goldner RD, Hardaker WT: Scaphoid fractures: Assessment and treatment. Orthopedics 15:931, 1992.
33. Hunter JC, Escobedo EM, Wilson AJ, et al: MR imaging of clinically suspected scaphoid fractures. AJR 168:1287, 1997.
34. Cohen MS: Fractures of the carpal bones. Hand Clin 13:547, 1997.
35. Norman A, Nelson J, Green S: Fractures of the hook of the hamate: Radiographic signs. Radiology 154:49, 1985.
36. Lacey JD, Hodge JC: Pisiform and hamulus fractures: Easily missed fractures diagnosed on a reverse oblique radiograph. J Emerg Med 16:445, 1998.
37. Yin Y, Mann FA, Gilula LA, et al: Roentgenographic approach to complex bone abnormalities. *In* Gilula LA, Yin Y (eds): Imaging of the Hand and Wrist. Philadelphia, WB Saunders, 1996.
38. Johnson RP: The acutely injured wrist and its residuals. Clin Orthop 149:33, 1980.
39. Pai C-H, Wei D-C, Hu S-T: Carpal bone dislocation: An analysis of twenty cases with relative emphasis on the role of crushing mechanisms. J Trauma 35:28, 1993.
40. Yeager BA, Dalinka MK: Radiology of trauma to the wrist: Dislocations, fracture dislocations, and instability patterns. Skeletal Radiol 13:120, 1985.
41. Sides D, Laorr A, Greenspan A: Carpal scaphoid: Radiographic pattern of dislocation. Radiology 195:215, 1995.
42. Lawlis JF III, Gunther SF: Carpometacarpal dislocations: Long-term follow-up. J Bone Joint Surg [Am] 73:52, 1991.
43. Strauch RJ, Behrman MJ, Rosenwasser MP: Acute dislocation of the carpometacarpal joint of the thumb: An anatomic and cadaver study. J Hand Surg [Am] 19:93, 1994.
44. Yin Y, Mann FA, Hodge JC, et al: Roentgenographic interpretation of ligamentous instabilities of the wrist: Static and dynamic instabilities. *In* Gilula LA, Yin Y (eds): Imaging of the Hand and Wrist. Philadelphia, WB Saunders, 1996, p 203.
45. Cautilli GP, Wehbé MA: Scapho-lunate distance and cortical ring sign. J Hand Surg [Am] 16:501, 1991.
46. Watson H, Ottoni L, Pitts EC, et al: Rotary subluxation of the scaphoid: A spectrum of instability. J Hand Surg [Br] 18:62, 1993.
47. Zanetti M, Hodler J, Gilula LA: Assessment of dorsal or ventral intercalated segmental instability configurations of the wrist: Reliability of sagittal MR images. Radiology 206:339, 1998.
48. Truong NP, Mann FA, Gilula LA, et al: Wrist instability series: Increasing yield with clinical-radiologic screening criteria. Radiology 192:481, 1994.
49. Watson HK, Ballet FL: The SLAC wrist: Scapholunate advanced collapse pattern of degenerative arthritis. J Hand Surg [Am] 9:358, 1984.
50. Hubbard LF: Metacarpophalangeal dislocations. Hand Clin 4:39, 1988.
51. Lubahn JD: Dorsal fracture dislocations of the proximal interphalangeal joint. Hand Clin 4:15, 1988.
52. Pellegrini VD Jr: Fractures at the base of the thumb. Hand Clin 4:87, 1988.
53. Kontakis GM, Katonis PG, Steriopoulos KA: Rolando's fracture treated by closed reduction and external fixation. Arch Orthop Trauma Surg 117:84, 1998.
54. Spaeth HJ, Abrams RA, Bock GW, et al: Gamekeeper thumb: Differentiation of nondisplaced and displaced tears of the ulnar collateral ligament with MR imaging. Work in progress. Radiology 188:553, 1993.
55. Hinke DH, Erickson SJ, Chamoy L, et al: Ulnar collateral ligament of the thumb: MR findings in cadavers, volunteers, and patients with ligamentous injury (Gamekeeper's thumb). AJR 163:1431, 1994.
56. Haramati N, Hiller N, Dowdle J, et al: MRI of the Stener lesion. Skeletal Radiol 24:515, 1995.
57. Miller RJ: Dislocations and fracture dislocations of the metacarpophalangeal joint of the thumb. Hand Clin 4:45, 1988.
58. McKerrell J, Bowen V, Johnston G, et al: Boxer's fractures—conservative or operative management. J Trauma 27:486, 1987.
59. Street JM: Radiographs of phalangeal fractures: Importance of the internally rotated oblique projection for diagnosis. AJR 160:575, 1993.
60. Rogers LF, Poznanski AK: Imaging of epiphyseal injuries. Radiology 191:297, 1994.
61. Destouet JM, Murphy WA: Guitar player acro-osteolysis. Skeletal Radiol 6:275, 1981.
62. Baran R, Tosti A: Occupational acroosteolysis in a guitar player. Acta Derm Venereol 73:64, 1993.

63. Nimkin K, Spevak MR, Kleinman PK: Fractures of the feet and hands in child abuse: Imaging and pathologic features. Radiology 203:233, 1997.
64. Skahen JR III, Palmer AK, Levinsohn EM, et al: Magnetic resonance imaging of the triangular fibrocartilage complex. J Hand Surg [Am] 15:552, 1990.
65. Miller RJ, Totterman SMS: Triangular fibrocartilage in asymptomatic subjects: Investigation of abnormal MR signal intensity. Radiology 196:22, 1995.
66. Glajchen N, Schweitzer M: MRI features in de Quervain's tenosynovitis of the wrist. Skeletal Radiol 25:63, 1996.
67. Mesgarzadeh M, Schneck CD, Boakdarpour A, et al: Carpal tunnel: MR imaging. II. Carpal tunnel syndrome. Radiology 171:749, 1989.
68. Miller TT, Potter HG, McCormack RR Jr: Benign soft tissue masses of the wrist and hand: MRI appearances. Skeletal Radiol 23:327, 1994.
69. Vo P, Wright T, Hayden F, et al: Evaluating dorsal wrist pain: MRI diagnosis of occult dorsal wrist ganglion. J Hand Surg [Am] 20:667, 1995.
70. Drapé JL, Idy-Peretti I, Goettmann S, et al: Subungual glomus tumors: Evaluation with MR imaging. Radiology 195:507, 1995.
71. Jelinek JS, Kransdorf MJ, Shmookler BM, et al: Giant cell tumor of the tendon sheath: MR findings in nine cases. AJR 162:919, 1994.
72. Buckland-Wright JC, MacFarlane DG, Lynch JA: Relationship between joint space width and subchondral sclerosis in the osteoarthritic hand: A quantitative microfocal radiographic study. J Rheumatol 19:788, 1992.
73. Menon J: The problem of trapeziometacarpal degenerative arthritis. Clin Orthop 175:155, 1983.
74. Cooke KS, Singson RD, Glickel SZ, et al: Degenerative changes of the trapeziometacarpal joint: Radiologic assessment. Skeletal Radiol 24:523, 1995.
75. Paley D, McMurtry RY, Cruickshank B: Pathologic conditions of the pisiform and pisotriquetral joint. J Hand Surg [Am] 12:110, 1987.
76. Williams WV, Cope R, Gaunt WD, et al: Metacarpophalangeal arthropathy associated with manual labor: Missouri metacarpal syndrome. Arthritis Rheum 30:1362, 1987.
77. Cobby M, Cushnaghan J, Creamer P, et al: Erosive osteoarthritis: Is it a separate disease entity? Clin Radiol 42:258, 1990.
78. Martel W, Stuck KJ, Dworin AM, et al: Erosive osteoarthritis and psoriatic arthritis: A radiologic comparison in the hand, wrist, and foot. AJR 134:125, 1980.
79. Greenway G, Resnick D, Weisman M, et al: Carpal involvement in inflammatory (erosive) osteoarthritis. J Can Assoc Radiol 30:95, 1979.
80. Smith D, Braunstein EM, Brandt KD, et al: A radiographic comparison of erosive osteoarthritis and idiopathic nodal osteoarthritis. J Rheumatol 19:896, 1992.
81. Buckland-Wright JC, Clarke GS, Walker SR: Erosion number and area progression in the wrists and hands of rheumatoid patients: A quantitative microfocal radiographic study. Ann Rheum Dis 48:25, 1989.
82. Sugimoto H, Takeda A, Masuyama J, et al: Early-stage rheumatoid arthritis: Diagnostic accuracy of MR imaging. Radiology 198:185, 1996.
83. Evans DM, Ansell BM, Hall MA: The wrist in juvenile arthritis. J Hand Surg [Br] 16:293, 1991.
84. Azouz EM, Duffy CM: Juvenile spondyloarthropathies: Clinical manifestations and medical imaging. Skeletal Radiol 24:399, 1995.
85. Resnick D: Patterns of peripheral joint disease in ankylosing spondylitis. Radiology 110:523, 1974.
86. Resnick D, Broderick RW: Bony proliferation of terminal phalanges in psoriasis: The "ivory" phalanx. J Can Assoc Radiol 28:187, 1977.
87. Resnick D, Niwayama G: On the nature and significance of bony proliferation in "rheumatoid variant" disorders. AJR 129:275, 1977.
88. Forrester DM, Kirkpatrick J: Periostitis and pseudoperiostitis. Radiology 118:597, 1976.
89. Martel W, Braunstein EM, Borlaza G, et al: Radiologic features of Reiter's syndrome. Radiology 132:1, 1979.
90. Reilly PA, Evison G, McHugh NJ, et al: Arthropathy of the hands and feet in systemic lupus erythematosus. J Rheumatol 17:777, 1990.
91. Selby CL: Review and differential diagnosis of Jaccoud's arthropathy. IM 6:55, 1985.
92. Pachman LN: Juvenile dermatomyositis. Pediatr Clin North Am 33:1097, 1986.
93. Czirjak L, Nagy Z, Szegedi G: Systemic sclerosis in the elderly. Clin Rheumatol 11:483, 1992.
94. Garcia-Porrua C, Gonzalez-Gay MA, Vazquez-Caruncho M: Tophaceous gout mimicking tumoral growth. J Rheumatol 26:508, 1999.
95. Yu JS, Chung C, Recht M, et al: MR imaging of tophaceous gout. AJR 168:523, 1997.
96. Holland NW, Jost D, Beutler A, et al: Finger pad tophi in gout. J Rheumatol 23:690, 1996.
97. Resnick D, Niwayama G, Georgen TG, et al: Clinical, radiographic and pathologic abnormalities in calcium pyrophosphate dihydrate deposition disease (CPPD): Pseudogout. Radiology 122:1, 1977.
98. Steinbach LS, Resnick D: Calcium pyrophosphate dihydrate crystal deposition disease revisited. Radiology 200:1, 1996.
99. Bourqui M, Vischer TL, Stasse P, et al: Pyrophosphate arthropathy in the carpal and metacarpophalangeal joints. Ann Rheum Dis 42:626, 1983.
100. Faraawi R, Harth M, Kertesz A, et al: Arthritis in hemochromatosis. J Rheumatol 20:448, 1993.
101. Jonge-Bok JMD, Macfarlane JD: The articular diversity of early haemochromatosis. J Bone Joint Surg [Br] 69:41, 1987.
102. Holt PD, Keats TE: Calcific tendinitis: A review of the usual and unusual. Skeletal Radiol 22:1, 1993.
103. McCarthy GM, Carrera GF, Ryan LM: Acute calcific periarthritis of the finger joints: A syndrome of women. J Rheumatol 20:1077, 1993.
104. Nakajima Y, Sato K, Morita H, et al: Severe progressive erosive arthritis in multicentric reticulohistiocytosis: Possible involvement of cytokines in synovial proliferation. Arthritis Rheum 19:1643, 1992.
105. Kalb RE, Epstein W, Grossman ME: Sarcoidosis with subcutaneous nodules. Am J Med 85:731, 1988.
106. Rivera-Sanfeliz G, Resnick D, Haghighi P: Sarcoidosis of hands. Skeletal Radiol 25:786, 1996.
107. Adelaar RS: Sarcoidosis of the upper extremity: Case presentation and literature review. J Hand Surg [Am] 8:492, 1983.
108. Ishizuki M, Isobe Y, Arai T, et al: Osteochondromatosis of the finger joints. Hand 9:198, 1977.
109. Kramer J, Recht M, Deely DM, et al: MR appearance of idiopathic synovial osteochondromatosis. J Comput Assist Tomogr 17:772, 1993.
110. Hasegawa Y, Ninomiya M, Yamada Y, et al: Osteoarthropathy in congenital sensory neuropathy with anhidrosis. Clin Orthop 258:232, 1990.
111. Brown FE, Spiegel PK, Boyle WE Jr: Digital deformity:

An effect of frostbite in children. Pediatrics 71:955, 1983.
112. Reed MH: Growth disturbances in the hands following thermal injuries in children. 2. Frostbite. J Can Assoc Radiol 39:95, 1988.
113. Schiele HP, Hubbard RB, Bruck HM: Radiographic changes in burns of the upper extremity. Radiology 104:13, 1972.
114. Atkinson RE, Smith RJ: Silicone synovitis following silicone implant arthroplasty. Hand Clin 2:291, 1986.
115. Chan M, Chowchuen P, Workman T, et al: Silicone synovitis: MR imaging in five patients. Skeletal Radiol 27:13, 1998.
116. Resnick D, Niwayama G: Soft tissues. *In* Resnick D [ed]: Diagnosis of Bone and Joint Disorders. 3rd Ed. Philadelphia, WB Saunders, 1995, p 4603.
117. Wong WL, Pemberton J: The musculoskeletal manifestations of epidermolysis bullosa: An analysis of 19 cases with review of the literature. Br J Radiol 65:480, 1992.
118. Resnick D, Weisman M, Goergen TG, et al: Osteolysis with detritic synovitis, a new syndrome. Arch Int Med 138:1003, 1978.
119. Galmarini CM, Kertesz A, Oliva R, et al: Metastasis of bronchogenic carcinoma to the thumb. Med Oncol 15:282, 1998.
120. Gelberman RH, Stewart WR, Harrelson JM: Hand metastasis from melanoma: A case study. Clin Orthop 136:264, 1978.
121. Okada K, Wold LE, Beabout JW, et al: Osteosarcoma of the hand: A clinicopathologic study of 12 cases. Cancer 72:719, 1993.
122. Ritschl P, Wurnig C, Lechner G, et al: Parosteal osteosarcoma: 2-23-year follow-up of 33 patients. Acta Orthop Scand 62:195, 1991.
123. Lucas DR, Unni KK, McLeod RA, et al: Osteoblastoma: Clinicopathologic study of 306 cases. Hum Pathol 25:117, 1994.
124. Taconis WK, Mulder JD: Fibrosarcoma and malignant fibrous histiocytoma of long bones: Radiographic features and grading. Skeletal Radiol 11:237, 1984.
125. Reinus WR, Gilula LA, Shirley SK, et al: Radiographic appearance of Ewing sarcoma of the hands and feet: Report from the Intergroup Ewing Sarcoma Study. AJR 144:331, 1985.
126. Buck P, Mickelson MR, Bonfiglio M: Synovial sarcoma: A review of 33 cases. Clin Orthop 156:211, 1981.
127. Kyle RA: Multiple myeloma: Review of 869 cases. Mayo Clin Proc 50:29, 1975.
128. Greenspan A: Bone island (enostosis): Current concept—a review. Skeletal Radiol 24:111, 1995.
129. Riester J, Mosher JF: Osteoid osteoma of the capitate: A case report. J Hand Surg [Am] 9:278, 1984.
130. Shankman S, Desai P, Beltran J: Subperiosteal osteoid osteoma: Radiographic and pathologic manifestations. Skeletal Radiol 26:457, 1997.
131. Lamb DW, Del Castillo F: Phalangeal osteoid osteoma in the hand. Hand 13:291, 1981.
132. Kayser F, Resnick D, Haghighi P, et al: Evidence of the subperiosteal origin of osteoid osteomas in tubular bones: Analysis by CT and MR imaging. AJR 170:609, 1998.
133. Carroll RE, Chance JT, Inan Y: Subungual exostosis in the hand. J Hand Surg [Br] 17:569, 1992.
134. Rubin JA, Steinberg DR: Turret exostosis of the metacarpal: A case report. J Hand Surg [Am] 21:296, 1996.
135. Jewusiak EM, Spence KF, Sell KW: Solitary benign enchondroma of the long bones of the hand: Results of curettage and packing with freeze-dried cancellous-bone allograft. J Bone Joint Surg [Am] 53:1587, 1971.
136. Brien EW, Mirra JM, Kerr R: Benign and malignant cartilage tumors of bone and joint: Their anatomic and theoretical basis with an emphasis on radiology, pathology and clinical biology. 1. The intramedullary cartilage tumors. Skeletal Radiol 26:325, 1997.
137. Meinzer F, Minagi H, Steinbach HL: The variable manifestation of multiple enchondromatosis. Radiology 99:377, 1971.
138. Collins PS, Han W, Williams LR, et al: Maffucci's syndrome (hemangiomatosis osteolytica): A report of four cases. J Vasc Surg 16:364, 1992.
139. Dahlin DC: Giant cell tumor of bone: Highlights of 407 cases. AJR 144:955, 1985.
140. Lokiec F, Wientroub S: Simple bone cyst: Etiology, classification, pathology, and treatment. J Pediatr Orthop [Br] 7:262, 1998.
141. Blacksin MF, Ende N, Benevenia J: Magnetic resonance imaging of intraosseous lipomas: A radiologic-pathologic correlation. Skeletal Radiol 24:37, 1995.
142. De Dios AMV, Bond JR, Shives TC, et al: Aneurysmal bone cyst. A clinico-pathologic study of 238 cases. Cancer 69:2921, 1992.
143. Friedman AC, Orcutt H, Madewell JE: Paget disease of the hand: Radiographic spectrum. AJR 138:691, 1982.
144. Mirra JM, Brien EW, Tehranzadeh J: Paget's disease of bone: Review with emphasis on radiologic features, part II. Skeletal Radiol 24:173, 1995.
145. Gibson MJ, Middlemiss JH: Fibrous dysplasia of bone. Br J Radiol 44:1, 1971.
146. Iwahara T, Hirayama T, Takemitu Y: Intraosseous ganglion of the lunate. J Hand Surg [Br] 15:297, 1983.
147. Magee TH, Rowedder AM, Degnan GG: Intraosseous ganglia of the wrist. Radiology 195:517, 1995.
148. Trias A, Beauregard G: Epidermoid cyst of bone. Can J Surg 17:1, 1974.
149. Bloom RA, Pogrund H, Libson E: Radiogrammetry of the metacarpal: A critical reappraisal. Skeletal Radiol 10:5, 1983.
150. Genant HK, Engelke K, Fuerst T, et al: Noninvasive assessment of bone mineral and structure: State of the art. J Bone Miner Res 11:707, 1996.
151. Taylor JAM, Resnick D, Sartoris DJ: Radiographic-pathologic correlation. *In* Sartoris DJ: Osteoporosis: Diagnosis and Treatment. New York, Marcel Dekker, 1996, p 147.
152. Clouston WM, Lloyd HM: Immobilization-induced hypercalcemia and regional osteoporosis. Clin Orthop 216:247, 1987.
153. Schwarzman RJ, McLellan TL: Reflex sympathetic dystrophy: A review. Arch Neurol 44:555, 1987.
154. Mankin HJ: Metabolic bone disease. J Bone Joint Surg [Am] 76:760, 1994.
155. Kurer MHJ, Baillod RA, Madgwick JCA: Musculoskeletal manifestations of amyloidosis: A review of 83 patients on haemodialysis for at least 10 years. J Bone Joint Surg [Br] 73:271, 1991.
156. Hernandez RJ, Poznanski AW, Hopwood NJ: Size and skeletal maturation of the hand in children with hypothyroidism and hypopituitarism. AJR 133:405, 1979.
157. Cherninkov Z, Cherninkova S: Two cases of pseudohypoparathyroidism in a family with type E brachydactylia. Radiol Diagn [Berlin] 30:57, 1989.
158. Lang EK, Bessler WT: The roentgenologic features of acromegaly. AJR 86:321, 1961.

159. Bluestone R, Bywaters EGL, Hartog M, et al: Acromegalic arthropathy. Ann Rheum Dis 30:243, 1971.
160. Pineda C: Diagnostic imaging in hypertrophic osteoarthropathy. Clin Exp Rheumatol 10:27, 1992.
161. Vázquez-Abad D, Pineda C, Martinez-Lavin M: Digital clubbing: A numerical assessment of the deformity. J Rheumatol 16:518, 1989.
162. Resnick D: Osteomyelitis and septic arthritis complicating hand injuries and infections: Pathogenesis of roentgenographic abnormalities. J Can Assoc Radiol 27:21, 1976.
163. Gonzalez MH, Papierski P, Hall RF Jr: Osteomyelitis of the hand after a human bite. J Hand Surg [Am] 18:520, 1993.
164. Robins RH: Tuberculosis of the wrist and hand. Br J Surg 54:211, 1967.
165. Feldman F, Auerbach R, Johnston A: Tuberculous dactylitis in the adult. AJR 112:460, 1971.
166. MacMoran JW, Brand PW: Bone loss in limbs with decreased or absent sensation: Ten year follow-up of the hands in leprosy. Skeletal Radiol 16:452, 1987.
167. Mirabello SC, Rosenthal DI, Smith RJ: Correlation of clinical and radiographic findings in Kienböck's disease. J Hand Surg [Am] 12:1049, 1987.
168. Gelberman RH, Menon J: The vascularity of the scaphoid bone. J Hand Surg [Am] 5:508, 1980.
169. Sherman SB, Greenspan A, Norman A: Osteonecrosis of the distal pole of the carpal scaphoid following fracture—a rare complication. Skeletal Radiol 9:189, 1983.
170. Arcalis AA, Pedemonte JJP, Massons AJM: Idiopathic necrosis of the capitate. Acta Orthop Belg 62:46, 1996.
171. Telfer JR, Evans DM, Bingham JB: Avascular necrosis of the hamate. J Hand Surg [Br] 19:389, 1994.
172. Failla JM: Osteonecrosis associated with nonunion of the hook of the hamate. Orthopedics 16:217, 1993.
173. Gewanter H, Baum J: Thiemann's disease. J Rheumatol 12:150, 1985.
174. Resnick D [Ed]: Diagnosis of Bone and Joint Disorders. 3rd Ed. Philadelphia, WB Saunders, 1995.
175. Resnick D: Scleroderma (progressive systemic sclerosis). *In* Resnick D [ed]: Diagnosis of Bone and Joint Disorders. 3rd Ed. Philadelphia, WB Saunders, 1995, p 1213.
176. Doman AN, Marcus NW: Congenital bipartite scaphoid. J Hand Surg [Am] 15:869, 1990.
177. Pierre-Jerome C, Roug IK: MRI of bilateral bipartite hamulus. Surg Radiol Anat 20:299, 1998.

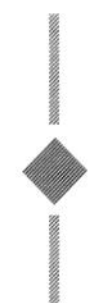

Index

Note: Page numbers in *italics* refer to illustrations; page numbers followed by t refer to tables.

A

B

C

E

I

J

K

N

O

R

S

ISBN 0-7216-7510-7